Student Resources for Abrams' Clinical Drug Therapy, Eighth Edition

These reliable resources accompany the text and provide additional tools to help you succeed!

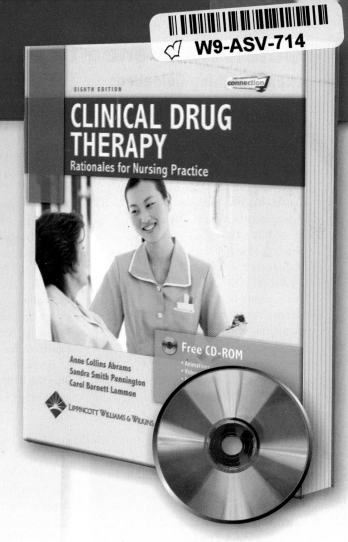

A FREE CD-ROM in the back of the book includes:

- **A Medication Administration video**.
- **NCLEX-style review questions** with rationales.
- **Drug Monographs** for the top 100 most commonly prescribed drugs!.
- **Animations** help you understand concepts including:
  - Absorption
  - Nerve Synapse
  - Distribution
  - Muscle Contraction
  - Drug Binding
  - Immune Response
  - Excretion
  - Cell Cycle
  - Hypertension
  - Intramuscular Injection
  - Intravenous Injection
  - Gas Exchange in Alveoli
  - Heart Failure
  - Stroke
  - Hemostasis

Plus, A FREE Photo Atlas of Medication Administration, shrink-wrapped with the book, illustrates techniques for safe drug administration. Rationales to help you understand every nursing action are included.

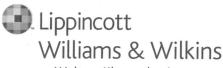

Lippincott
Williams & Wilkins
a Wolters Kluwer business

Quick Reference to Features

Client Teaching Guidelines

Safe and Effective Use of Prescription Medications   55
Safe and Effective Use of Over-the-Counter (OTC) Medications   57
General Information About Herbal and Dietary Supplements   61
Opioid (Narcotic) Analgesics   93
Acetaminophen, Aspirin, and Other NSAIDs   120
Drugs Used in Migraines   121
Antianxiety and Sedative-Hypnotic Drugs   143
Antipsychotic Drugs   163
Antidepressants and Lithium   183
Antiseizure Medications   204
Antiparkinson Drugs   220
Skeletal Muscle Relaxants   231
Methylphenidate and Dexmethyl-phenidate   258
Adrenergic Drugs   280
Alpha$_2$ Agonists and Alpha-Blocking Drugs   298
Beta-Blocking Drugs   299
Cholinergic Drugs   313
Anticholinergic Drugs   326
Growth Hormone   347
Fertility Drugs   347
Long-Term Corticosteroid Therapy   362
Levothyroxine   379
Propylthiouracil or Methimazole   380
Drugs for Osteoporosis   396
Antidiabetic Drugs   420
Hormone Replacement Therapy   447
Oral Contraceptives   448
Androgens   460
Antimicrobial Drugs   477
Oral Penicillins   495
Oral Cephalosporins   496
Oral Fluoroquinolones   509
Oral Tetracyclines   522
Oral Sulfonamides   523
Macrolides and Ketolides   534
Isoniazid, Rifampin, and Pyrazinamide   552
Miscellaneous Antiviral Drugs   572
Antiretroviral Drugs   573
Oral and Topical Antifungal Drugs   594
Antiparasitic Drugs   614
Vaccinations   644
Blood Cell and Immune System Stimulants   658
Immunosuppressant Drugs   677
Managing Chemotherapy   710
Antiasthmatic Drugs   740
Antihistamines   756
Nasal Decongestants, Anticough Medications, and Multi-Ingredient Cold Remedies   766

Digoxin   786
Antidysrhythmic Drugs   807
Antianginal Drugs   824
Antihypertensive Drugs   852
Diuretics   869
Drugs to Prevent or Treat Blood Clots   889
Dyslipidemic Drugs   905
Nutritional Support Products, Vitamins, and Minerals   935
Weight Management and Drugs That Aid Weight Loss   961
Antiulcer and Anti-Heartburn Drugs   979
Laxatives   992
Antidiarrheals   1005
Antiemetic Drugs   1016
Topical Eye Medications   1032
Topical Medications for Skin Disorders   1050
Drug Use During Pregnancy and Lactation   1074

Nursing Actions

Drug Administration   44
Monitoring Drug Therapy   70
Opioid Analgesics   99
Analgesic–Antipyretic–Anti-Inflammatory, and Related Drugs   126
Antianxiety and Sedative-Hypnotic Drugs   149
Antipsychotic Drugs   168
Antidepressants   188
Antiseizure Drugs   209
Antiparkinson Drugs   222
Skeletal Muscle Relaxants   232
Central Nervous System Stimulants   260
Adrenergic Drugs   284
Antiadrenergic Drugs   302
Cholinergic Drugs   315
Anticholinergic Drugs   329
Hypothalamic and Pituitary Hormones   348
Corticosteroids   369
Thyroid and Antithyroid Drugs   383
Drugs Used in Calcium and Bone Disorders   400
Antidiabetic Drugs   428
Estrogens, Progestins, and Hormonal Contraceptives   451
Androgens and Anabolic Steroids   461
Antimicrobial Drugs   481
Beta-Lactam Antibacterials   499
Aminoglycosides and Fluoroquinolones   512
Tetracyclines, Sulfonamides, and Urinary Agents   524

Macrolides, Ketolides, and Miscellaneous Antibacterials   536
Antitubercular Drugs   556
Antiviral Drugs   576
Antifungal Drugs   598
Antiparasitics   615
Immunizing Agents   647
Hematopoietic and Immunostimulant Agents   661
Immunosuppressants   684
Antineoplastic Drugs   715
Drugs for Asthma and Other Bronchoconstrictive Disorders   744
Antihistamines   758
Nasal Decongestants, Antitussives, and Cold Remedies   768
Cardiotonic-Inotropic Drugs   789
Antidysrhythmic Drugs   810
Antianginal Drugs   826
Drugs Used in Hypotension and Shock   835
Antihypertensive Drugs   858
Diuretics   872
Drugs That Affect Blood Coagulation   892
Drugs for Dyslipidemia   907
Nutritional Products, Vitamins, and Mineral–Electrolytes   945
Drugs for Weight Loss and Maintenance   967
Antiulcer Drugs   983
Laxatives and Cathartics   994
Antidiarrheals   1006
Antiemetics   1018
Ophthalmic Drugs   1034
Dermatologic Drugs   1054
Abortifacients, Prostaglandins, Tocolytics, and Oxytocics   1075

Research Briefs

Patient-Controlled Analgesia Using a Skin Patch   95
Rebound Headaches Associated With Overuse of Analgesics   130
Rasagiline (Agilect), A New Antiparkinson Drug   221
Smoking Cessation   249
Epinephrine vs. Vasopressin: A Look at Selected Current Research   281
Use of Cardioselective Beta Blockers in Clients With Chronic Obstructive Pulmonary Disease   296
Use of Alternative Medicines in Diabetes Mellitus   416
Adjuvant Chemotherapy in Treatment of Breast Cancer   713
Use of Digoxin in Men and Women   783
Effects of Vitamin E Supplementation   939
Commercial Weight-Loss Programs   965

CLINICAL DRUG THERAPY

Rationales for Nursing Practice

EIGHTH EDITION

CLINICAL DRUG THERAPY
Rationales for Nursing Practice

Anne Collins Abrams, RN, MSN *Associate Professor, Emeritus*
Department of Baccalaureate and Graduate Nursing
College of Health Sciences
Eastern Kentucky University
Richmond, Kentucky
Chapters 1–6, 12–15, 34–42, 57, 58, 63–65

Carol Barnett Lammon, RN, PhD *Associate Professor*
University of Alabama School of Nursing
University of Alabama at Birmingham
Birmingham, Alabama
Chapters 7–10, 16–20, 26, 29–33, 56, 59–62

Sandra Smith Pennington, RN, PhD *Professor of Nursing*
Berea College
Berea, Kentucky
Professor and Graduate Program Director, DSc in Nursing Program
Rocky Mountain University of Health Professions
Provo, Utah
Chapters 11, 21–25, 27, 28, 43–55

CONSULTANT
Tracey L. Goldsmith, PharmD *Independent Legal and Healthcare Consultant*
Magnolia, Texas

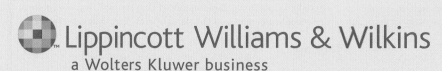
. Lippincott Williams & Wilkins
a Wolters Kluwer business

Philadelphia · Baltimore · New York · London
Buenos Aires · Hong Kong · Sydney · Tokyo

Senior Acquisitions Editor: Margaret Zuccarini
Developmental Editor: Megan Klim
Editorial Assistant: Delema Caldwell-Jordan
Production Editors: Audrey Lickwar, Sandra Cherrey Scheinin
Director of Nursing Production: Helen Ewan
Senior Managing Editor/Production: Erika Kors
Creative Director: Doug Smock
Manufacturing Coordinator: Karin Duffield
Indexer: Michael Ferreira
Compositor: Circle Graphics
Printer: RR Donnelley/Willard

8th Edition

9 8 7 6 5 4 3 2 1

Library of Congress Cataloging-in-Publication Data

Abrams, Anne Collins.
  Clinical drug therapy : rationales for nursing practice / Anne Collins Abrams, Carol Barnett Lammon, Sandra Smith Pennington ; consultant, Tracey L. Goldsmith.—8th ed.
    p. ; cm.
  Includes bibliographical references and index.
  ISBN 0-7817-6263-4
  1. Chemotherapy. 2. Drugs. 3. Nursing.
  [DNLM: 1. Pharmaceutical Preparations—Nurses' Instruction. 2. Drug Therapy—Nurses' Instruction.   QV 55 A161c 2007] I. Lammon, Carol Barnett.   II. Pennington, Sandra Smith.
III. Title.
RM262.A27 2007
615.5'8—dc22
                                                        2005029110

Care has been taken to confirm the accuracy of the information presented and to describe generally accepted practices. However, the author, editors, and publisher are not responsible for errors or omissions or for any consequences from application of the information in this book and make no warranty, express or implied, with respect to the content of the publication.

The authors, editors, and publisher have exerted every effort to ensure that drug selection and dosage set forth in this text are in accordance with the current recommendations and practice at the time of publication. However, in view of ongoing research, changes in government regulations, and the constant flow of information relating to drug therapy and drug reactions, the reader is urged to check the package insert for each drug for any change in indications and dosage and for added warnings and precautions. This is particularly important when the recommended agent is a new or infrequently employed drug.

Some drugs and medical devices presented in this publication have Food and Drug Administration (FDA) clearance for limited use in restricted research settings. It is the responsibility of the health care provider to ascertain the FDA status of each drug or device planned for use in his or her clinical practice.

CONTRIBUTORS

Sondra G. Ferguson, RN, MSN, ANP, APRN, BC
Assistant Professor of Nursing
Berea College
Berea, Kentucky
Chapters 47, 48, 52, 54, 55

Tracey Goldsmith, PharmD
Independent Legal and Healthcare Consultant
Magnolia, Texas
Chapters 29–33

Kathleen E. Jenks, BSN, MSEd, RN
Associate Professor
Mercy College of Northwest Ohio
Toledo, Ohio
Applying Your Knowledge Features

REVIEWERS

Mary C. Bielski
Clinical Education Coordinator,
Nursing Faculty
Triton College
River Grove, Illinois

Karen Damron, RN, BSN, MSN
Assistant Professor of Nursing
Pikeville College
Pikeville, Kentucky

Karen M. Fite, RN, MSN
Level I Coordinator, Professor
Calhoun Community College
Decatur, Alabama

Charlene Beach Gagliardi, RN, BSN, MSN
Professor of Nursing
Mount Saint Mary's College
Los Angeles, California

Susan Holmes, RN, MSN, CRNP
Instructor
Auburn University of Nursing
Auburn, Alabama

Elsie Klish, MEd, MS, RN, ARNP-FNP
Associate Professor of Nursing
Newman University
Wichita, Kansas

Andrea Knesek, MSN, RN, BC
Nursing Faculty
Macomb Community College
Clinton Township, Michigan

Elizabeth M. Long, RN, MSN, CGNP, CNS
Nursing Instructor
Lamar University
Beaumont, Texas

Karen Malloy, RN, MSN
Department Chair, ADN Mobility
Program
San Jacinto College—South
Houston, Texas

Karen S. March, RN, MSN, CCRN, APRN-BC
Assistant Professor of Nursing
York College of Pennsylvania
York, Pennsylvania

Darlene Mathis, RN, MSN, APRN, BC, NP-C, CRNP
Assistant Professor, Family Nurse
Practitioner
Samford University
Birmingham, Alabama

Carol L. Moore, PhD, ARNP, BC
Chairperson & Associate Professor of
Nursing
Bethel College
North Newton, Kansas

Julie Nauser, RN, MSN
Research College of Nursing
Kansas City, Missouri

Winnie Pickering, RN, MSN
Associate Professor in
Nursing/Nursing Faculty
James A. Rhodes State College
Lima, Ohio

Kathleen Pickrell
Associate Professor and Chair
Indiana State University
Terre Haute, Indiana

Donna Roberson, MSN, APRN, BC
Clinical Instructor/Faculty
East Carolina University School of
Nursing
Greenville, North Carolina

Patricia A. Roper, RN, MS
Professor of Nursing
Columbus State Community College
Columbus, Ohio

Sally P. Scavone, RN, BS, MS
Professor of Nursing
Erie Community College
Buffalo, New York

Carol Smith, MSN, RN, PhD Student
Assistant Professor
Bellarmine University
Louisville, Kentucky

Teryl M. Ward, RN, MSN
Nursing Instructor
Modesto Junior College
Modesto, California

Laurel A. Danes-Webb, RN, MS, CS, FNP, CDE
Professor of Nursing
Hocking College
Nelsonville, Ohio

Deborah White, MSN, RN
Professor
Jefferson Community College
Louisville, Kentucky

Linda S. Williams, MSN, RNBC
Professor of Nursing
Jackson Community College
Jackson, Mississippi

Thomas Worms, RN, MSN
Professor of Nursing
Truman College
Chicago, Illinois

PREFACE

PURPOSE

The basic precepts underlying previous editions of *Clinical Drug Therapy* also guided the writing of this eighth edition. The overall purpose is to promote safe, effective, and rational drug therapy by

- Providing information that accurately reflects current practices in drug therapy
- Facilitating the acquisition, comprehension, and application of knowledge related to drug therapy. Application requires knowledge about the drug and the client receiving it.
- Identifying knowledge and skills the nurse can use to smooth the interface between a drug and the client receiving it

GOALS AND RESPONSIBILITIES OF NURSING CARE RELATED TO DRUG THERAPY

- Preventing the need for drug therapy, when possible, by promoting health and preventing conditions that require drug therapy
- Using appropriate and effective nonpharmacologic interventions instead of, or in conjunction with, drug therapy when indicated. When used with drug therapy, such interventions may promote lower drug dosage, less frequent administration, and fewer adverse effects.
- Enhancing therapeutic effects by administering drugs accurately and considering clients' individual characteristics that influence responses to drug therapy
- Preventing or minimizing adverse drug effects by knowing the major adverse effects associated with particular drugs, identifying clients with characteristics that may increase their risks of experiencing adverse effects, and actively monitoring for the occurrence of adverse effects. When adverse effects occur, early recognition allows interventions to minimize their severity. Because all drugs may cause adverse effects, nurses must maintain a high index of suspicion that signs and symptoms, especially new ones, may be drug induced.
- Teaching clients and caregivers about accurate administration of medications, nonpharmacologic treatments to use with or instead of pharmacologic treatments, and when to contact a health care provider

ORGANIZATIONAL FRAMEWORK

The content of *Clinical Drug Therapy* is organized into ten sections, primarily by therapeutic drug groups and their effects on particular body systems. This approach helps students make logical connections between major drug groups and the conditions for which they are used. It also provides a foundation for learning about new drugs, most of which fit into known groups.

The first section contains the basic information required to learn, understand, and apply drug knowledge. The chapters in this section include information about drug names, classifications, prototypes, costs, laws and standards, schedules of controlled substances, drug approval processes, and learning strategies (Chapter 1); cellular physiology, drug transport, pharmacokinetic processes, the receptor theory of drug action, types of drug interactions, and factors that influence drug effects on body tissues (Chapter 2); dosage forms and routes and methods of accurate drug administration (Chapter 3); and guidelines for using the nursing process in drug therapy and general principles of drug therapy (Chapter 4).

Most drug sections include an initial chapter that reviews the physiology of a body system, followed by several chapters that discuss drug groups used to treat disorders of that body system. The seven physiology review chapters are designed to facilitate understanding of drug effects on a body system. These include the central nervous system; the autonomic nervous system; and the endocrine, hematopoietic and immune, respiratory, cardiovascular, and digestive systems. Other chapters within each section emphasize therapeutic classes of drugs and prototypical or commonly used individual drugs, those used to treat common disorders, and those likely to be encountered in clinical nursing practice. Drug chapter content is presented in a consistent format and includes a description of a condition (or conditions) for which a drug group is used; a general description of a drug group, including mechanism(s) of action, indications for use, and contraindications; and descriptions and tables of individual drugs, with recommended dosages and routes of administration.

Additional clinically relevant information is presented under the headings of **Nursing Process, Principles of Therapy,** and **Nursing Actions.**

Nursing Process sections emphasize the importance of the nursing process in drug therapy, including assessment of the client's condition in relation to the drug group, nursing diagnoses, expected outcomes, needed interventions, and evaluation of the client's progress toward expected outcomes. **Client Teaching Guidelines** are displayed separately from other interventions to emphasize their importance and for easy student reference.

Principles of Therapy sections present guidelines for maximizing benefits and minimizing adverse effects of drug therapy in various circumstances and populations, including middle-aged and older adults, children and adolescents, and clients with impaired kidney or liver function. General principles are included in Chapter 4; specific principles related to drug groups are included in the chapters where those drug groups are discussed. This approach, rather than separate chapters on pediatric and geriatric pharmacology, for example, was chosen because knowledge about a drug is required before that knowledge can be applied to a specific population with distinctive characteristics and needs in relation to drug therapy.

Each drug chapter includes a **Nursing Actions** display that provides specific nursing responsibilities related to drug administration and client observation.

Other drug sections include products used to treat infectious, ophthalmic, and dermatologic disorders plus drugs used during pregnancy, labor and delivery, and lactation.

NEW TO THIS EDITION

This thoroughly updated edition includes new content and features:

- **Updated Drug Information.** Many new drugs have been added: some are additions to well-known drug groups, such as antidiabetic drugs (Chapter 26) and anti-retroviral drugs (Chapter 35); others represent advances in the drug therapy of some disease processes, such as newer anticancer agents (Chapter 42).

  In addition, continuing trends in drug dosage formulations are reflected in the increased numbers of fixed-dose combination drug products, long-acting preparations, and nasal or oral inhalation products.
- **Major Revision of Many Chapters.** Chapter revisions reflect current practices in drug therapy, integrate new drugs, and explain the major characteristics of new drug groups.
- **Applying Your Knowledge.** These threaded case studies provide real-world examples and lend significance to conceptual content. Each drug chapter opens with a client scenario, which builds throughout the chapter. Case-based questions test students' critical thinking, and special "How Do You Avoid This Medication Error?" questions promote safe and accurate drug administration.
- **Research Briefs.** The briefs summarize important research related to drug therapy and provide nursing implications.
- **New Illustrations.** Several new illustrations have been developed to enhance understanding of drug actions.

SPECIAL FEATURES

- **Four-Color Design.** The striking design enhances the liveliness of the text and promotes student interest and interactivity.
- **Readability.** Since the first edition of *Clinical Drug Therapy* was published in 1983, many students and faculty have commented about the book's clear presentation style.
- **Organizational Framework.** The book's organizational framework allows it to be used effectively as both a textbook and as a reference. Used as a textbook, students can read chapters in their entirety to learn the characteristics of major drug classes, their prototypical drugs or commonly used representatives, their uses and effects in prevention or treatment of disease processes, and their implications for nursing practice. Used as a reference book, students can readily review selected topics for classroom use or clinical application. Facilitating such uses are a consistent format and frequent headings that allow readers to identify topics at a glance.
- **Chapter Objectives.** Learning objectives at the beginning of each chapter focus students' attention on important chapter content.
- **Drugs at a Glance Tables.** These tables highlight and summarize pertinent drug information, including drug names, dosages, and other related facts.
- **Boxed Displays.** These include information to promote understanding of drug therapy for selected conditions.
- **Herbal and Dietary Supplements.** Commonly used products are introduced in Chapter 4 and included in selected later chapters. Safety aspects are emphasized.
- **Client Teaching Guidelines.** This feature is designed to meet several goals. One is to highlight the importance of teaching clients and caregivers how to manage drug therapy at home, where most medications are taken. This is done by separating teaching from other nursing interventions. Another goal is to promote active and knowledgeable client participation in drug therapy regimens, which helps to maximize therapeutic effects and minimize adverse effects. In addition, written guidelines allow clients and caregivers to have a source of reference when questions arise in the home setting. A third goal is to make client teaching easier and less time consuming. Using the guidelines as a foundation, the nurse can simply add or delete information according to a client's individual needs. To assist both the nurse and client further, the guidelines contain minimal medical jargon.
- **Principles of Therapy.** This unique section describes important drug- and client-related characteristics that need to be considered in drug therapy regimens. Such considerations can greatly increase safety and therapeutic effects, and all health care providers associated with drug therapy should be aware of them. Most chap-

ters contain principles with the headings of **Use in Children, Use in Older Adults, Use in Clients with Renal Impairment, Use in Clients with Hepatic Impairment,** and **Use in Home Care** to denote differences related to age, developmental level, pathophysiology, and setting. Some chapters include principles related to these headings as well: **Genetic and Ethnic Considerations, Use in Critical Illness,** and **Management of Drug Toxicity or Drug Withdrawal.**

- **Nursing Actions Displays.** These displays emphasize nursing interventions during drug therapy within the following categories: Administer accurately, Observe for therapeutic effects, Observe for adverse effects, and Observe for drug interactions. The inclusion of rationales for interventions provides a strong knowledge base and scientific foundation for clinical practice and critical thinking.

- **Review and Application Exercises.** Located at the end of each chapter, these exercises include two types of questions. **Short Answer** questions encourage students to rehearse clinical application strategies in a nonclinical, nonstressful, nondistracting environment. They also promote self-testing in chapter content and can be used to promote classroom discussion. To help students prepare for the licensing examination, this edition adds **NCLEX-style** questions to each drug chapter. Answers and rationales for these exercises can be found on the **Instructor's Resource CD-ROM.**

- **Appendices.** These include recently approved and miscellaneous drugs, the International System of Units, therapeutic serum drug concentrations for selected drugs, Canadian drug laws and standards, Canadian drug names, and anesthetics.

- **Extensive Index.** Listings of generic and trade names of drugs, nursing process, and other topics provide rapid access to desired information.

TEACHING–LEARNING PACKAGE

Nursing students must develop skills in critical thinking, information processing, decision making, collaboration, and problem solving. How can a teacher assist students to develop these skills in relation to drug therapy? The ancillary package assists both students and teachers in this development.

The **Study Guide** engages students' interest and active participation by providing a variety of learning exercises and opportunities to practice cognitive skills. Worksheets promote the learning of concepts, principles, and characteristics and uses of major drug groups and can be completed independently or by small groups as in-class learning activities. Applying Your Knowledge scenarios promote appropriate data collection, critical analysis of both drug- and client-related data, and application of the data in client care.

The **Connection** companion Web site, http://connection. lww.com/go/abrams8e, provides online updates for faculty and students, links to newly approved drugs, and more.

The free **Student Resource CD-ROM** is an invaluable learning tool that provides 3-D animated demonstrations of pharmacology concepts, medication administration video, NCLEX-style review questions, and monographs of the most commonly prescribed drugs.

The **Instructor's Resource CD-ROM** facilitates use of the text in designing and implementing courses of study. To fulfill this purpose, the CD-ROM contains

- General observations and comments about teaching and learning pharmacology in relation to nursing
- A sample syllabus for a separate 3-credit-hour, 1-semester pharmacology course that may be taught in a traditional classroom or a nontraditional, online setting
- General teaching strategies for pharmacology and specific teaching strategies for each chapter
- Answers to the review exercises from the book
- Brownstone test bank that includes approximately 1,000 multiple-choice test items in NCLEX format, a test generator, and a grade book. These materials can assist the instructor in evaluating students' knowledge of drug information and their ability to apply that information in client care.
- PowerPoint slides that include text and art from *Clinical Drug Therapy* to provide significant classroom or online teaching support.

These varied materials allow each instructor to choose or adapt them relevant to his or her circumstances. The authors and publisher hope these resources are truly helpful in easing the day-to-day rigors of teaching pharmacology and invite comments from instructors regarding the materials.

Anne Collins Abrams, RN, MSN
Carol Barnett Lammon, RN, PhD
Sandra Smith Pennington, RN, PhD

HOW TO USE Clinical Drug Therapy

Drugs at a Glance tables give students characteristics as well as routes and dosage ranges in an easy-to-read format. **Prototype drugs** are highlighted in the tables and in the text.

Table 6-1 Drugs at a Glance: Opioid Analgesics

GENERIC/TRADE NAME	ROUTES AND DOSAGE RANGES	
	Adults	Children
Agonists **Codeine**	*Pain:* PO, Sub-Q, IM 15–60 mg q4–6h PRN; usual dose 30 mg; maximum, 360 mg/24 h *Cough:* PO 10–20 mg q4h PRN; maximum, 120 mg/24 h	*1 y or older, Pain:* PO, Sub-Q, IM 0.5 mg/kg q4–6h PRN *2–6 y, Cough:* PO 2.5–5 mg q4–6h; maximum, 30 mg/24 h *6–12 y, Cough:* PO 5–10 mg q4–6h; maximum, 60 mg/24 h
Fentanyl (Sublimaze)	Preanesthetic sedation, IM 0.05–0.1 mg 30–60 min before surgery Analgesic adjunct to general anesthesia, IV total dose of 0.002–0.05 mg/kg, depending on the surgical procedure Adjunct to regional anesthesia, IM or slow IV (over 1–2 min) 0.05–0.1 mg PRN Postoperative analgesia, IM 0.05–0.1 mg, repeat in 1–2 h if needed General anesthesia, IV 0.05–0.1 mg/kg with oxygen and a muscle relaxant (maximum dose 0.15 mg/kg with open-heart surgery, other major surgeries, and complicated neurologic or orthopedic procedures) Chronic pain, transdermal system 2.5–10 mg every 72 h	*Weight at least 10 kg:* Conscious sedation or preanesthetic sedation, 5–15 mcg/kg of body weight (100–400 mcg), depending on weight, type of procedure, and other factors. Maximum dose, 400 mcg, regardless of age and weight. *2–12 y:* General anesthesia induction and maintenance, IV 2–3 mcg/kg

---

OBJECTIVES

After studying this chapter, you will be able to:

1. Identify types and potential causes of seizures.
2. Discuss major factors that influence choice of an antiseizure drug for a client with a seizure disorder.
3. Give characteristics and effects of commonly used antiseizure drugs.
4. Differentiate between older and more recent antiseizure drugs.
5. Compare advantages and disadvantages between monotherapy and combination drug therapy for seizure disorders.
6. Apply the nursing process with clients receiving antiseizure drugs.
7. Describe strategies for prevention and treatment of status epilepticus.
8. Discuss the use of antiseizure drugs in special populations.

Chapter Objectives let students know what they're going to learn in each and every chapter.

APPLYING YOUR KNOWLEDGE 10-1:
HOW CAN YOU AVOID THIS MEDICATION ERROR?
Mr. Mehring is talking with his pastor when you arrive to administer his medication. He asks you to just leave the medication and he will take it when he finishes his visit. You leave the medication with Mr. Mehring and chart it as given.

APPLYING YOUR KNOWLEDGE

While in the hospital, Carl Mehring, age 70, is diagnosed with chronic depression secondary to his chronic heart failure, hypertension, diabetes mellitus, and renal insufficiency. As Mr. Mehring's health has declined, so has his interest in his family, friends, and hobbies. His physician prescribes sertraline 50 mg PO twice a day.

APPLYING YOUR KNOWLEDGE: ANSWERS

10-1 The nurse should never leave an antidepressant at the bedside. Charting the medication as given when it has not yet been taken by the client is not truthful, and the client may forget to take the medication or may hold the medication for a later time and save up multiple doses. This is especially problematic with a client suffering from depression because he or she may have suicidal ideations.

10-2 Some antidepressant medications, such as sertraline, are in the class of selective serotonin reuptake inhibitors (SSRIs), which may not reach a therapeutic effect for up to 2 to 4 weeks. Provide appropriate teaching for both the client and his wife regarding therapeutic effect. Check to make sure that Mr. Mehring is taking the right dosage. Encourage him to continue taking the medication.

10-3 Check with the physician to see if Mr. Mehring's dose can be taken once a day in the morning. If this is not possible, then check to see if a different SSRI can be given that has once-a-day dosing. Taking the dose in the morning may solve Mr. Mehring's sleeping difficulty if the problem is due to the drug and not due to the depression.

Applying Your Knowledge features help students apply concepts to client care. Most chapters open with a client scenario, which is then carried through the chapter. Applying Your Knowledge questions require students to take the content they have learned and apply it to the client in the case study, and special "How Do You Avoid This Medication Error?" questions reinforce safe drug administration. Answers are provided at the end of each chapter, allowing students to monitor their progress.

Nursing Process material helps students think about drug therapy in terms of the nursing process.

400 mg three times a day) and deciding for themselves whether their symptoms improve (eg, less pain, improved ability to walk) and whether they want to continue.

NURSING PROCESS

Assessment

- Assess for signs and symptoms of pain, such as location, severity, duration, and factors that cause or relieve the pain (see Chap. 6).
- Assess for fever (thermometer readings above 99.6°F [37.3°C] are usually considered fever). Hot, dry skin; flushed face; reduced urine output; and concentrated urine may accompany fever if the person also is dehydrated.
- Assess for inflammation. Local signs are redness, heat, edema, and pain or tenderness; systemic signs include fever, elevated white blood cell count (leukocytosis), and weakness.
- With arthritis or other musculoskeletal disorders, assess for pain and limitations in activity and mobility.
- Ask about use of OTC analgesic, antipyretic, or anti-inflammatory drugs and herbal or dietary supplements.
- Ask about allergic reactions to aspirin or NSAIDs.
- Assess for history of peptic ulcer disease, GI bleeding, or kidney disorders.
- With migraine, assess severity and patterns of occurrences.

Nursing Diagnoses

- Acute Pain
- Chronic Pain
- Activity Intolerance related to pain
- Risk for Poisoning: Acetaminophen overdose
- Risk for Injury related to adverse drug effects (GI bleeding, renal insufficiency)
- Deficient Knowledge: Therapeutic and adverse effects of commonly used drugs
- Deficient Knowledge: Correct use of OTC drugs for pain, fever, and inflammation

Planning/Goals

The client will

- Experience relief of discomfort with minimal adverse drug effects
- Experience increased mobility and activity tolerance
- Inform health care providers if taking aspirin, an NSAID or acetaminophen regularly.
- Self-administer the drugs safely
- Avoid overuse of the drugs
- Use measures to prevent accidental ingestion or overdose, especially in children
- Experience fewer and less severe attacks of migraine

Interventions

Implement measures to prevent or minimize pain, fever, and inflammation.

- Treat the disease processes (eg, infection, arthritis) or circumstances (eg, impaired blood supply, lack of physical activity, poor positioning or body alignment) thought to be causing pain, fever, or inflammation.
- Treat pain as soon as possible; early treatment may prevent severe pain and anxiety and allow the use of milder analgesic drugs. Use distraction, relaxation techniques, or other nonpharmacologic techniques along with drug therapy, when appropriate.
- With acute musculoskeletal injuries (eg, sprains), cold applications can decrease pain, swelling, and inflammation. Apply for approximately 20 minutes, then remove.
- Assist clients with migraine to identify and avoid "triggers." Assist clients to drink 2 to 3 liters of fluid daily when taking an NSAID regularly. This strategy decreases gastric irritation and helps to maintain good kidney function. With long-term use of aspirin, fluids help to prevent precipitation of salicylate crystals in the urinary tract. With antigout drugs, fluids help to prevent precipitation of urate crystals and formation of urate kidney stones. Fluid intake is especially important initially when serum uric acid levels are high and large amounts of uric acid are being excreted.

Provide appropriate teaching for any drug therapy (see accompanying displays).

Evaluation

- Interview and observe regarding relief of symptoms.
- Interview and observe regarding mobility and activity levels.
- Interview and observe regarding safe, effective use of the drugs.
- Select drugs appropriately.

APPLYING YOUR KNOWLEDGE 7–3
Given Julie's medication regimen, what nursing measures should be implemented to decrease the probability of GI bleeding?

PRINCIPLES OF THERAPY

Use of Aspirin

When pain, fever, or inflammation is present, aspirin is effective across a wide range of clinical conditions. Like any other drug, aspirin must be used appropriately to maximize therapeutic benefits and minimize adverse reactions.

Client Teaching Guidelines give students specific information they may need to educate patients.

Herbal and Dietary Supplement content is highlighted so students become aware of how these alternative therapies can affect traditional medications.

 Herbal Supplement

St. John's wort (*Hypericum perforatum*) is an herb that is widely self-prescribed for depression. Several studies, most of which used about 900 milligrams daily of a standardized extract, indicate its usefulness in mild to moderate depression, with fewer adverse effects than antidepressant drugs. A 3-year, multicenter study by the National Institutes of Health concluded that the herb is not effective in major depression.

Antidepressant effects are attributed mainly to hypericin, although several other active components have also been identified. The mechanism of action is unknown, but the herb is thought to act similarly to antidepressant drugs. Some herbalists refer to St. John's wort as "natural Prozac."

Adverse effects, which are usually infrequent and mild, include constipation, dizziness, dry mouth, fatigue, GI distress, nausea, photosensitivity, restlessness, skin rash, and sleep disturbances. These symptoms are relieved by stopping the herb.

Drug interactions may be extensive. St. John's wort should not be combined with alcohol, antidepressant drugs (eg, MAO inhibitors, SSRIs, TCAs), nasal decongestants or other over-the-counter cold and flu medications, bronchodilators, opioid analgesics, or amino acid supplements containing phenylalanine and tyrosine. All of these interactions may result in hypertension, possibly severe.

NURSING ACTIONS

Antiseizure Drugs

Nursing Actions give students specific instructions on administration of drugs and observations of client responses, with rationales for each step.

NURSING ACTIONS	RATIONALE/EXPLANATION
1. Administer accurately	
a. Give on a regular schedule about the same time each day.	To maintain therapeutic blood levels of drugs
b. Give most oral antiseizure drugs after meals or with a full glass of water or other fluid; levetiracetam, oxcarbazepine, topiramate, and zonisamide may be taken with or without food.	Most antiseizure drugs cause some gastric irritation, nausea, or vomiting. Taking the drugs with food or fluid helps decrease gastrointestinal side effects.
c. To give phenytoin:	
(1) Shake oral suspensions of the drug vigorously before pouring and always use the same measuring equipment.	In suspensions, particles of drug are suspended in water or other liquid. On standing, drug particles settle to the bottom of the container. Shaking the container is necessary to distribute drug particles in the liquid vehicle. If the contents are not mixed well every time a dose is given, the liquid vehicle will be given initially, and the concentrated drug will be given later. That is, underdosage will occur at first, and little if any therapeutic benefit will result. Overdosage will follow, and the risks of serious toxicity are greatly increased. Using the same measuring container ensures consistent dosage. Calibrated medication cups or measuring teaspoons or tablespoons are acceptable. Regular household teaspoons and tablespoons used for eating and serving are not acceptable because sizes vary widely.
(2) Do not mix parenteral phenytoin in the same syringe with any other drug.	Phenytoin solution is highly alkaline (pH approximately 12) and physically incompatible with other drugs. A precipitate occurs if mixing is attempted.
(3) Give phenytoin as an undiluted intravenous (IV) bolus injection at a rate not exceeding 50 mg/min, then flush the IV line with normal saline or dilute in 50–100 mL of normal saline (0.9% NaCl) and administer over approximately 30–60 minutes. If piggybacked into a primary IV line, the primary IV solution must be normal saline or the line must be flushed with normal saline before and after administration of phenytoin. An in-line filter is recommended.	Phenytoin cannot be diluted or given in IV fluids other than normal saline because it precipitates within minutes. Slow administration and dilution decrease local venous irritation from the highly alkaline drug solution. Rapid administration must be avoided because it may produce myocardial depression, hypotension, cardiac dysrhythmias, and even cardiac arrest.
d. To give IV fosphenytoin:	
(1) Check the physician's order and the drug concentration carefully.	The dose is expressed in phenytoin equivalents (PE; fosphenytoin 50 mg PE = phenytoin 50 mg).
(2) Dilute the dose in 5% dextrose or 0.9% sodium chloride solution to a concentration of 1.5 mg PE/mL to 25 mg PE/mL and infuse no faster than 150 mg PE/min.	The drug is preferably diluted in the pharmacy and labeled with the concentration and duration of the infusion. For a 100-mg PE dose, diluting with 4 mL yields the maximum concentration of 25 mg PE/mL; this amount could be infused in about 1 min at the maximal recommended rate. A 1-g loading dose could be added to 50 mL of 0.9% sodium chloride and infused in approximately 10 min at the maximal recommended rate.
(3) Consult a pharmacist or the manufacturer's literature if any aspect of the dose or instructions for administration are unclear.	To avoid error
e. To give carbamazepine and phenytoin suspensions by nasogastric (NG) feeding tube, dilute with an equal amount of	Absorption is slow and decreased, possibly because of drug adherence to the NG tube. Dilution and tube irrigation decrease such adherence.

Review and Application Exercises provide students with the opportunity to review what they just learned. These include both short-answer exercises and NCLEX-style questions.

11-1 Monitor the phenytoin level. The normal free phenytoin level is 0.8 to 2 mcg/mL. Adequate serum levels are needed for seizure control.

11-2 Ask if Frank is taking a monoamine oxidase (MAO) inhibitor, which may be used to treat depression. Carbamazepine should not be taken within 14 days of an MAO inhibitor.

11-3 The client must always taper the dosage of an AED gradually, or the seizures may exacerbate.

Review and Application Exercises

Short Answer Exercises

1. For a client with a newly developed seizure disorder, why is it important to verify the type of seizure by electroencephalogram before starting AEDs?

2. What are the indications for use of the major AEDs?

3. What are the major adverse effects of commonly used AEDs, and how can they be minimized?

4. What are the advantages and disadvantages of treatment with a single drug and of treatment with multiple drugs?

5. Which of the benzodiazepines are used as AEDs?

6. What are the advantages of carbamazepine and valproic acid compared with the benzodiazepines, phenytoin, and phenobarbital?

7. How are the newer drugs similar to or different from phenytoin?

8. What is the treatment of choice for an acute convulsion or status epilepticus?

9. Why is it important when teaching clients to emphasize that none of the AEDs should be stopped abruptly?

10. How can a home care nurse monitor AED therapy during a home visit?

NCLEX-Style Questions

11. An 18-year-old client presents to the clinic with complaints of breast tenderness, nausea, vomiting, and absence of menses for 2 months. She has a history of a seizure disorder that is well controlled with oxcarbazepine (Trileptal). She believes that she has been taking her oral contraceptives as directed but asks if she could be pregnant. The nurse recognizes that the best response to the client's question is which of the following?
    a. "Oxcarbazepine can decreases the effectiveness of oral contraceptive drugs, so we need to do a pregnancy test."
    b. "You can't be pregnant if you have been taking your pills correctly."
    c. "Don't worry; birth control pills are very effective."
    d. "Taking antiseizure drugs with oral contraceptives significantly decreases your risk of pregnancy."

12. A client scheduled for her next dose of phenytoin (Dilantin) has a serum plasma phenytoin level of 16 mcg/mL. Based on this information, the nurse should do which of the following?
    a. Administer the drug.

ACKNOWLEDGMENTS

Anne Abrams is extremely pleased to welcome Carol Lammon and Sandra Pennington as coauthors. As contributors to the sixth and seventh editions and as coauthors of the eighth edition, they exhibited high levels of nursing scholarship and clinical expertise. As experienced nurse educators, they have well-developed skills in assessing and meeting the learning needs of nursing students. Their talents add greatly to the quality of this text and are much appreciated.

Sincere appreciation is also expressed to the following people who assisted in the preparation of this book:

Margaret Zuccarini, Senior Acquisitions Editor at Lippincott Williams & Wilkins, who has continued to guide the development of this text with grace and vision.

Tracey Goldsmith, PharmD, who reviewed all chapters and revised Chapters 29–33 as a contributor.

Mary Jo Kirkpatrick, RN, MSN, who authored the Study Guide.

Joanne Carlson, MSN, APRN, who prepared the test bank and PowerPoint slides.

Diane Schweisguth, RN, BSN, who revised the material on the Instructor's Resource CD-ROM.

CONTENTS

SECTION 1
Foundations of Drug Therapy 1

CHAPTER 1 Introduction to Pharmacology 3

A Message to Students 3
Pharmacology and Drug Therapy 3
Understanding Grouping and Naming of Drugs 4
Prescription and Nonprescription Drugs 4
Sources of Drugs 6
Drug Development and Approval 6
Pharmacoeconomics 8
Sources of Drug Information 8
Strategies for Studying Pharmacology 8

CHAPTER 2 Basic Concepts and Processes 10

Introduction 10
Cellular Physiology 10
Drug Transport Through Cell Membranes 12
Pharmacokinetics 12
Pharmacodynamics 17
Variables That Affect Drug Actions 18
Adverse Effects of Drugs 25
Toxicology: Drug Overdose 26

CHAPTER 3 Administering Medications 31

Introduction 31
General Principles of Accurate Drug Administration 31
Legal Responsibilities 32
Medication Errors 32
Medication Systems 33
Medication Orders 33
Drug Preparations and Dosage Forms 34
Calculating Drug Dosages 36
Routes of Administration 38

CHAPTER 4 Nursing Process in Drug Therapy 50

Introduction 50
Nursing Process in Drug Therapy 51
Integrating Nursing Process, Critical Paths, and Drug Therapy 56
General Principles of Drug Therapy 62

SECTION 2
Drugs Affecting the Central Nervous System 73

CHAPTER 5 Physiology of the Central Nervous System 75

Introduction 75
Basic Unit of the Central Nervous System: The Neuron 75
Neurotransmission 75
Major Components of the Central Nervous System 78
Drugs That Affect the Central Nervous System 80

CHAPTER 6 Opioid Analgesics and Opioid Antagonists 82

Introduction 82
General Characteristics of Opioid Analgesics 83
Individual Drugs 85
Principles of Therapy 92

CHAPTER 7 Analgesic–Antipyretic– Anti-Inflammatory and Related Drugs 103

Introduction 103
General Characteristics of Analgesic–Antipyretic– Anti-Inflammatory and Related Drugs 104
Classifications and Individual Drugs 109
Principles of Therapy 119

CHAPTER 8 Antianxiety and Sedative-Hypnotic Drugs 132

Introduction 132
General Characteristics of Benzodiazepines 135
Individual Drugs 138
Principles of Therapy 142

CHAPTER 9 Antipsychotic Drugs 153

Introduction 153
General Characteristics of Antipsychotic Drugs 154
Individual Drugs 155
Principles of Therapy 163

CHAPTER 10 Antidepressants and Mood Stabilizers 174

Introduction 174
General Characteristics of Antidepressant Drugs 176
Types of Antidepressants and Individual Drugs 177
Principles of Therapy 182

CHAPTER 11 Antiseizure Drugs 193

Introduction 193
General Characteristics of Antiseizure Drugs 194
Individual Drugs 195
Principles of Therapy 203

CHAPTER 12 Antiparkinson Drugs 214

Introduction 214
General Characteristics of Antiparkinson Drugs 214
Individual Antiparkinson Drugs 216
Principles of Therapy 220

CHAPTER 13 Skeletal Muscle Relaxants 227

Introduction 227
General Characteristics of
Skeletal Muscle Relaxants 228
Individual Drugs 228
Principles of Therapy 231

CHAPTER 14 Substance Abuse Disorders 235

Introduction 235
Central Nervous System Depressants 237
Central Nervous System Stimulants 242
Principles of Therapy 250

CHAPTER 15 Central Nervous System Stimulants 253

Introduction 253
General Characteristics of Stimulants 254
Individual Drugs 254
Principles of Therapy 258

SECTION 3

Drugs Affecting the Autonomic Nervous System 263

CHAPTER 16 Physiology of the Autonomic Nervous System 265

Introduction 265
Structure and Function of the
Autonomic Nervous System 265
Characteristics of Autonomic Drugs 271

CHAPTER 17 Adrenergic Drugs 272

Introduction 272
General Characteristics of Adrenergic Drugs 272
Individual Drugs 275
Principles of Therapy 279

CHAPTER 18 Antiadrenergic Drugs 289

Introduction 289
General Characteristics of Antiadrenergic Drugs 289
Individual Drugs 291
Principles of Therapy 298

CHAPTER 19 Cholinergic Drugs 307

Introduction 307
General Characteristics of Cholinergic Drugs 308
Individual Drugs 309
Principles of Therapy 312

CHAPTER 20 Anticholinergic Drugs 319

Introduction 319
General Characteristics of Anticholinergic Drugs 319
Individual Drugs 321
Principles of Therapy 326

SECTION 4

Drugs Affecting the Endocrine System 333

CHAPTER 21 Physiology of the Endocrine System 335

Introduction 335
Endocrine System–Nervous System Interactions 336
General Characteristics of Hormones 336
Use of Hormonal Drugs 338

CHAPTER 22 Hypothalamic and Pituitary Hormones 339

Introduction 339
Types of Hormones 339
Individual Drugs 341
Principles of Therapy 347

CHAPTER 23 Corticosteroids 352

Introduction 352
General Characteristics of
Exogenous Corticosteroids 355
Principles of Therapy 363

CHAPTER 24 Thyroid and Antithyroid Drugs 373

Introduction 373
General Characteristics of Thyroid
and Antithyroid Drugs 374
Individual Drugs 376
Principles of Therapy 379

CHAPTER 25 Hormones That Regulate Calcium
and Bone Metabolism 387

Introduction 387
Individual Drugs 390
Principles of Therapy 396

CHAPTER 26 Antidiabetic Drugs 404

Introduction 404
Hypoglycemic Drugs 407
Principles of Therapy 419

CHAPTER 27 Estrogens, Progestins, and
Hormonal Contraceptives 436

Introduction 436
General Characteristics of Estrogens, Progestins,
and Hormonal Contraceptives 438
Individual Drugs 440
Principles of Therapy 447

CHAPTER 28 Androgens and
Anabolic Steroids 455

Introduction 455
General Characteristics of Androgens and Anabolic
Steroids Used As Drugs 457
Individual Drugs 458
Principles of Therapy 460

SECTION 5

Drugs Used to Treat Infections 465

CHAPTER 29 General Characteristics
of Antimicrobial Drugs 467

Introduction 467
Microorganisms and Infections 467
Characteristics of Antimicrobial Drugs 474
Principles of Therapy 476

CHAPTER 30 Beta-Lactam Antibacterials:
Penicillins, Cephalosporins,
and Other Drugs 485

Introduction 485
Penicillins 485
Cephalosporins 489
Carbapenems 491
Monobactam 494
Principles of Therapy 495

CHAPTER 31 Aminoglycosides
and Fluoroquinolones 504

Introduction 504
Aminoglycosides 504
Fluoroquinolones 507
Principles of Therapy 509

CHAPTER 32 Tetracyclines, Sulfonamides,
and Urinary Agents 515

Introduction 515
Principles of Therapy 522

CHAPTER 33 Macrolides, Ketolides, and
Miscellaneous Antibacterials 528

Introduction 528
Macrolides and Ketolides 528
Miscellaneous Antibacterial Drugs 530
Principles of Therapy 533

CHAPTER 34 Drugs for Tuberculosis and
Mycobacterium avium Complex
(MAC) Disease 542

Introduction 542
Antitubercular Drugs 544
Treatment of Active Tuberculosis 550
Mycobacterium avium Complex Disease 550
Principles of Therapy 552

CHAPTER 35 Antiviral Drugs 560

Introduction 560
Antiviral Drugs 562
Principles of Therapy 571

CHAPTER 36 Antifungal Drugs 582

Introduction 582
Antifungal Drugs 583
Principles of Therapy 595

CHAPTER 37 Antiparasitics 603

Introduction 603
Antiparasitic Drugs 606
Principles of Therapy 614

SECTION 6

Drugs Affecting Hematopoiesis and the Immune System 619

CHAPTER 38 Physiology of the Hematopoietic and Immune Systems 621

Introduction 621
Hematopoietic Cytokines 621
Overview of Body Defense Mechanisms 624
Immunity 624
Immune Cells 626
Immune System Cytokines 629
Client-Related Factors That Influence
Immune Function 629
Immune Disorders 631
Drugs That Alter Hematopoietic and
Immune Responses 632

CHAPTER 39 Immunizing Agents 633

Introduction 633
General Characteristics of Immunizing Agents 634
Individual Immunizing Agents 634
Principles of Therapy 644

CHAPTER 40 Hematopoietic and Immunostimulant Drugs 651

Introduction 651
General Characteristics of Hematopoietic and
Immunostimulant Drugs 651
Classifications and Individual Drugs 655
Principles of Therapy 658

CHAPTER 41 Immunosuppressants 665

Introduction 665
Classifications and Individual Drugs 668
Principles of Therapy 676

CHAPTER 42 Drugs Used in Oncologic Disorders 691

Introduction 691
Traditional Cytotoxic Antineoplastic Drugs 694
Biologic Targeted Antineoplastic Drugs 699
Antineoplastic Hormone Inhibitor Drugs 702
Cytoprotectant Drugs 705
Principles of Therapy 709

SECTION 7

Drugs Affecting the Respiratory System 723

CHAPTER 43 Physiology of the Respiratory System 725

Overview of the Respiratory System 725
Disorders of the Respiratory System 727
Drug Therapy 727

CHAPTER 44 Drugs for Asthma and Other Bronchoconstrictive Disorders 729

Introduction 729
Bronchodilators 732
Anti-Inflammatory Agents 735
Principles of Therapy 739

CHAPTER 45 Antihistamines and Allergic Disorders 747

Introduction 747
General Characteristics of Antihistamines 750
Classifications and Individual Drugs 753
Principles of Therapy 755

CHAPTER 46 Nasal Decongestants, Antitussives, and Cold Remedies 760

Introduction 760
General Characteristics of Drugs Used in/for
Respiratory Disorders 761
Individual Drugs 762
Principles of Therapy 766

SECTION 8

Drugs Affecting the Cardiovascular System 771

CHAPTER 47 Physiology of the Cardiovascular System 773

Introduction 773
Heart 773
Blood Vessels 774
Blood 775
Cardiovascular Disorders 776
Drug Therapy Used for Cardiovascular Disorders 776

CHAPTER 48 Drug Therapy for
Heart Failure 777

Introduction 777
Inotropes 778
Human B-Type Natriuretic Peptide (Nesiritide) 783
Endothelin Receptor Antagonists (Bosentan) 784
Principles of Therapy 785

CHAPTER 49 Antidysrhythmic Drugs 794

Introduction 794
General Characteristics of
Antidysrhythmic Drugs 796
Classifications and Individual Drugs 796
Principles of Therapy 807

CHAPTER 50 Antianginal Drugs 814

Introduction 814
Antianginal Drugs: Classifications and
Individual Drugs 817
Principles of Therapy 823

CHAPTER 51 Drugs Used in Hypotension
and Shock 829

Introduction 829
General Characteristics of Antishock Drugs 830
Individual Drugs 830
Principles of Therapy 833

CHAPTER 52 Antihypertensive Drugs 838

Introduction 838
Antihypertensives: Classifications and
Individual Drugs 842
Principles of Therapy 851

CHAPTER 53 Diuretics 861

Introduction 861
General Characteristics of Diuretic Drugs 863
Types of Diuretics and Individual Drugs 865
Principles of Therapy 868

CHAPTER 54 Drugs That Affect Blood
Coagulation 876

Introduction 876
Drugs Used in Thrombotic and Thromboembolic
Disorders: Classifications and Individual Drugs 879
Principles of Therapy 888

CHAPTER 55 Drugs for Dyslipidemia 897

Introduction 897
General Characteristics of Drugs Used for
Management of Dyslipidemia 900
Dyslipidemic Drugs: Classifications and
Individual Drugs 901
Principles of Therapy 905

SECTION 9
Drugs Affecting the Digestive System 911

CHAPTER 56 Physiology of the
Digestive System 913

Introduction 913
Structures of the Digestive System 913
Secretions of the Digestive System 915
Effects of Drugs on the Digestive System 916

CHAPTER 57 Nutritional Support Products,
Vitamins, and
Mineral–Electrolytes 917

Introduction 917
Nutritional Deficiency States 917
Nutritional Products 918
Agents Used in Mineral–Electrolyte Imbalances 925
Principles of Therapy 935

CHAPTER 58 Drugs to Aid Weight
Management 952

Introduction 952
General Characteristics of Drugs for Obesity 957
Individual Drugs 957
Principles of Therapy 960

CHAPTER 59 Drugs Used for Peptic Ulcer and
Acid Reflux Disorders 970

Introduction 970
Classifications and Individual Drugs 972
Principles of Therapy 980

CHAPTER 60 Laxatives and Cathartics 987

Introduction 987
General Characteristics of Laxatives and Cathartics 988
Classifications and Individual Drugs 988
Principles of Therapy 992

CHAPTER 61 Antidiarrheals 997

Introduction 997
Characteristics, Classifications, and
Individual Antidiarrheal Drugs 998
Principles of Therapy 1004

CHAPTER 62 Antiemetics 1010

Introduction 1010
General Characteristics of Antiemetic Drugs 1011
Classifications and Individual Drugs 1011
Principles of Therapy 1015

SECTION 10
Drugs Used in Special Conditions 1021

CHAPTER 63 Drugs Used in
Ophthalmic Conditions 1023

Introduction 1023
Ophthalmic Drug Therapy 1024
Principles of Therapy 1032

CHAPTER 64 Drugs Used in
Dermatologic Conditions 1039

Introduction 1039
Dermatologic Drug Therapy 1042
Principles of Therapy 1049

CHAPTER 65 Drug Use During Pregnancy
and Lactation 1057

Introduction 1057
Pregnancy 1057
Fetal Therapeutics 1059
Maternal Therapeutics 1059
Drugs That Alter Uterine Motility 1069
Drugs Used During Labor and Delivery at Term 1071
Neonatal Therapeutics 1072
Principles of Therapy 1073

APPENDIX A Recently Approved and Miscellaneous Drugs 1079

APPENDIX B The International System of Units 1082

APPENDIX C Serum Drug Concentrations 1083

APPENDIX D Canadian Drug Laws and Standards 1084

APPENDIX E Canadian Drug Names 1087

APPENDIX F Anesthetics, Adjunctive Drugs,
and Nursing Considerations 1095

INDEX 1101

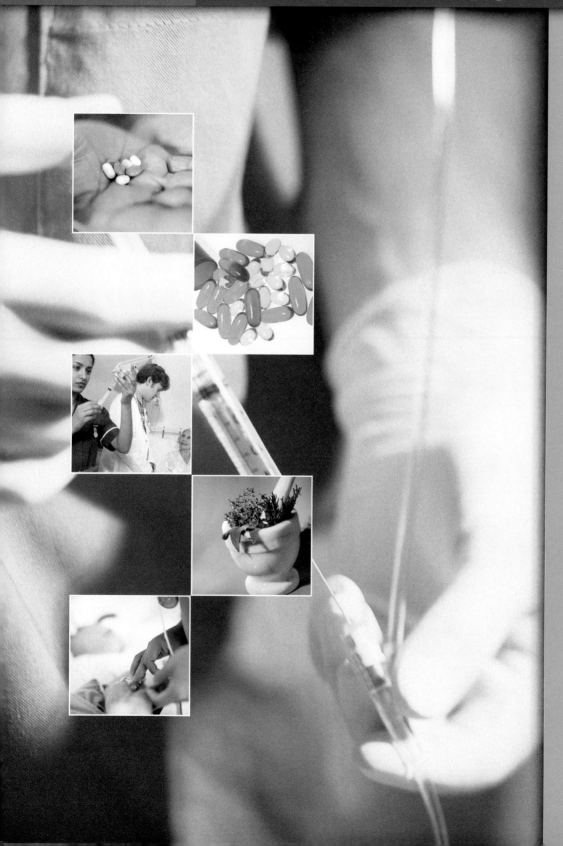

SECTION

1

Foundations of Drug Therapy

CHAPTER OUTLINE

1 Introduction to Pharmacology

2 Basic Concepts and Processes

3 Administering Medications

4 Nursing Process in Drug Therapy

Introduction to Pharmacology

OBJECTIVES

After studying this chapter, you will be able to:

1. Differentiate between pharmacology and drug therapy.
2. Distinguish between generic and trade names of drugs.
3. Define a prototypical drug.
4. Select authoritative sources of drug information.
5. Discuss major drug laws and standards.
6. Describe the main categories of controlled substances in relation to therapeutic use and potential for abuse.
7. Identify nursing responsibilities in handling controlled substances correctly.
8. Discuss the role of the Food and Drug Administration.
9. Analyze the potential impact of drug costs on drug therapy regimens.
10. Develop personal techniques for learning about drugs and using drug knowledge in client care.

A MESSAGE TO STUDENTS

You have probably been taking medicines and seeing other people take medicines most of your life. Perhaps you have given medicines to your children, parents, grandparents, or others. Have you ever wondered why it's usually okay to give children Tylenol but not aspirin? Why do a lot of middle-aged and older people take an aspirin a day? Why do people with high blood pressure, heart failure, or diabetes take ACE inhibitors, and what are ACE inhibitors? When should an antibiotic NOT be prescribed for an infection?

You are embarking on an exciting journey of discovery as you begin or continue your study of pharmacology. Much of what you learn will apply to your personal and family life as well as your professional life as a nurse. The purpose of this book is to help you learn about medications and why, how, when, and where they are used in daily life. Bon voyage!!

PHARMACOLOGY AND DRUG THERAPY

Pharmacology is the study of drugs (chemicals) that alter functions of living organisms. Drug therapy, also called *pharmacotherapy,* is the use of drugs to prevent, diagnose, or treat signs, symptoms, and disease processes. When prevention or cure is not a reasonable goal, relief of symptoms can greatly improve a client's quality of life and ability to function in activities of daily living. Drugs given for therapeutic purposes are called *medications.*

Medications may be given for various reasons. In many instances, drug therapy aims to lessen disease processes rather than to cure them. To meet this goal, drugs may be given for local or systemic effects. Drugs with local effects, such as sunscreen lotions and local anesthetics, act mainly at the site of application. Those with systemic effects are taken into the body, circulated through the bloodstream to their sites of action in various body tissues, and eventually eliminated from the body. *Most drugs are given for their systemic effects.* Drugs may also be given for relatively immediate effects (ie, for acute problems such as pain or infection) or long-term effects (eg, to relieve signs and symptoms of chronic disorders). Many drugs are given for their long-term effects.

UNDERSTANDING GROUPING AND NAMING OF DRUGS

Drug Classifications

Drugs are classified, or *grouped,* according to their effects on particular body systems, their therapeutic uses, and their chemical characteristics. For example, morphine can be classified as a central nervous system depressant, a narcotic or opioid analgesic, and as an opiate (derived from opium). The names of therapeutic classifications usually reflect the conditions for which the drugs are used (eg, antidepressants, antihypertensives, antidiabetic drugs). The names of many drug groups reflect their chemical characteristics rather than their therapeutic uses (eg, adrenergics, antiadrenergics, benzodiazepines). Many commonly used drugs fit into multiple groups because they have wide-ranging effects on the human body and because they can be grouped according to various characteristics.

Prototype Drugs

Individual drugs that represent groups of drugs are called *prototypes.* Prototypes, which are often the first drug of a particular group to be developed, are usually the standard with which newer, similar drugs are compared. For example, morphine is the prototype of opioid analgesics; penicillin is the prototype of antibacterial drugs.

Drug classifications and prototypes are quite stable, and most new drugs can be assigned to a group and compared with an established prototype. However, some groups lack a universally accepted prototype and some prototypes are replaced over time by newer, more commonly used drugs.

Drug Names

Individual drugs may have several different names, but the two that are most commonly used are the generic name and the trade name (also called the brand name). The *generic name* (eg, amoxicillin) is related to the chemical or official name and is independent of the manufacturer. The generic name often indicates the drug group (eg, drugs with generic names ending in "cillin" are penicillins). The *trade name* is designated and patented by the manufacturer. For example, amoxicillin is manufactured by several pharmaceutical companies, some of which assign a specific trade name (eg, Amoxil, Trimox) and several of which use only the generic name. In drug literature, trade names are capitalized and generic names are presented in lowercase unless used in a list or at the beginning of a sentence. Drugs may be prescribed and dispensed by generic or trade name.

PRESCRIPTION AND NONPRESCRIPTION DRUGS

Legally, American consumers have two routes of access to therapeutic drugs. One route is by prescription or order from a licensed health care provider, such as a physician, dentist, or nurse practitioner. The other route is the over-the-counter (OTC) purchase of drugs that do not require a prescription.

Various drug laws regulate both of these routes. Acquiring and using prescription drugs for nontherapeutic purposes, by persons who are not authorized to have the drugs or for whom they are not prescribed, is illegal.

American Drug Laws and Standards

Current drug laws and standards have evolved over many years. Their main goal is to protect the public by ensuring that drugs marketed for therapeutic purposes, whether prescription or OTC, are safe and effective. Their main provisions are summarized in Table 1-1.

The Food, Drug, and Cosmetic Act of 1938 has been especially important because this law and its amendments regulate the manufacture, distribution, advertising, and labeling of drugs. It also confers official status on drugs listed in the *United States Pharmacopeia.* The names of these drugs may be followed by the letters *USP.* Official drugs must meet standards of purity and strength as determined by chemical analysis or by animal response to specified doses (bioassay). The Durham-Humphrey Amendment has designated drugs that must be prescribed by a physician and dispensed by a pharmacist. The Food and Drug Administration (FDA) is charged with enforcing the law. In addition, the Public Health Service regulates vaccines and other biologic products, and the Federal Trade Commission can suppress misleading advertisements of nonprescription drugs.

Another important law is the Comprehensive Drug Abuse Prevention and Control Act, passed in 1970. Title II of this law, called the Controlled Substances Act, regulates the manufacture and distribution of narcotics, stimulants, depressants, hallucinogens, and anabolic steroids. These drugs are categorized according to therapeutic usefulness and potential for abuse (Box 1-1) and are labeled as controlled substances (eg, morphine, a Schedule II drug, is labeled C–II [C = Controlled Substance]).

The Drug Enforcement Administration (DEA) is charged with enforcing the Controlled Substances Act. Individuals and companies legally empowered to handle controlled substances must be registered with the DEA, keep accurate records of all transactions, and provide for secure storage. Physicians are assigned a number by the DEA and must

TABLE 1-1 American Drug Laws and Amendments

YEAR	NAME	MAIN PROVISION(S)
1906	Pure Food and Drug Act	Established official standards and requirements for accurate labeling of drug products
1912	Sherley Amendment	Prohibited fraudulent claims of drug effectiveness
1914	Harrison Narcotic Act	Restricted the importation, manufacture, sale, and use of opium, cocaine, marijuana, and other drugs that the act defined as narcotics
1938	Food, Drug, and Cosmetic Act	• Required proof of safety from the manufacturer before a new drug could be marketed • Authorized factory inspections • Established penalties for fraudulent claims and misleading labels
1945	Amendment	Required governmental certification of biologic products, such as insulin and antibiotics
1952	Durham-Humphrey Amendment	Designated drugs that must be prescribed by a physician and dispensed by a pharmacist (eg, controlled substances, drugs considered unsafe for use except under supervision by a health care provider, and drugs limited to prescription use under a manufacturer's new drug application)
1962	Kefauver-Harris Amendment	• Required a manufacturer to provide evidence (from well-controlled research studies) that a drug was effective for claims and conditions identified in the product's labeling • Gave the federal government the authority to standardize drug names
1970	Comprehensive Drug Abuse Prevention and Control Act; Title II, Controlled Substances Act	• Regulated distribution of narcotics and other drugs of abuse • Categorized these drugs according to therapeutic usefulness and potential for abuse
1978	Drug Regulation Reform Act	• Established guidelines for research studies and data to be submitted to the FDA by manufacturers • Shortened the time required to develop and market new drugs
1983	Orphan Drug Act	• Decreased taxes and competition for manufacturers who would produce drugs to treat selected serious disorders affecting relatively few people
1987		• Established new regulations designed to speed up the approval process for high-priority medications
1992	Prescription Drug User Fee Act	• Allowed the FDA to collect user fees from pharmaceutical companies, with each new drug application, to shorten the review time (eg, by hiring more staff) • Specified a review time of 12 months for standard drugs and 6 months for priority drugs
1997	FDA Modernization Act	• Updated regulation of biologic products • Increased client access to experimental drugs and medical devices • Accelerated review of important new drugs • Allowed drug companies to disseminate information about off-label (non–FDA-approved) uses and costs of drugs • Extended user fees

FDA, Food and Drug Administration.

include the number on all prescriptions they write for a controlled substance. Prescriptions for Schedule II drugs cannot be refilled; a new prescription is required. Nurses are responsible for storing controlled substances in locked containers, administering them only to people for whom they are prescribed, recording each dose given on agency narcotic sheets and on the client's medication administration record, maintaining an accurate inventory, and reporting discrepancies to the proper authorities.

In addition to federal laws, state laws also regulate the sale and distribution of controlled drugs. These laws may be more stringent than federal laws; if so, the stricter laws usually apply.

Box 1-1 Categories of Controlled Substances

Schedule I

Drugs that are not approved for medical use and have high abuse potentials: flunitrazepam (Rohypnol) gamma hydroxybutyric acid (GHB), heroin, lysergic acid diethylamide (LSD), marijuana, 3,4-methylenedioxy-methamphetamine (MDMA or ecstasy), mescaline, peyote, tetrahydrocannabinol.

Schedule II

Drugs that are used medically and have high abuse potentials: opioid analgesics (eg, codeine, hydromorphone, methadone, meperidine, morphine, oxycodone, oxymorphone), central nervous system (CNS) stimulants (eg, cocaine, methamphetamine, methylphenidate), and barbiturate sedative-hypnotics (amobarbital, pentobarbital, secobarbital).

Schedule III

Drugs with less potential for abuse than those in Schedules I and II, but abuse may lead to psychological or physical dependence:

androgens and anabolic steroids, ketamine, some CNS stimulants (eg, benzphetamine), and mixtures containing small amounts of controlled substances (eg, codeine, barbiturates not listed in other schedules).

Schedule IV

Drugs with some potential for abuse: benzodiazepines (eg, diazepam, lorazepam, temazepam), other sedative-hypnotics (eg, phenobarbital, chloral hydrate), and some prescription appetite suppressants (eg, mazindol, phentermine).

Schedule V

Products containing moderate amounts of controlled substances. They may be dispensed by the pharmacist without a physician's prescription but with some restrictions regarding amount, record keeping, and other safeguards. Included are antidiarrheal drugs, such as diphenoxylate and atropine (Lomotil).

Canadian Drug Laws and Standards

Canada and its provinces have laws and standards that parallel those of the United States, particularly as related to controlled substances (see Appendix D).

SOURCES OF DRUGS

Where do medications come from? Historically, drugs were mainly derived from plants (eg, morphine), animals (eg, insulin), and minerals (eg, iron). Now, most drugs are synthetic chemical compounds manufactured in laboratories. Chemists, for example, often create a useful new drug by altering the chemical structure of an existing drug. Such techniques and other technologic advances have enabled the production of new drugs as well as synthetic versions of many drugs originally derived from plants and animals. Synthetic drugs are more standardized in their chemical characteristics, more consistent in their effects, and less likely to produce allergic reactions. Semisynthetic drugs (eg, many antibiotics) are naturally occurring substances that have been chemically modified.

Biotechnology is also an important source of drugs. This process involves manipulating deoxyribonucleic acid (DNA) and ribonucleic acid (RNA) and recombining genes into hybrid molecules that can be inserted into living organisms (*Escherichia coli* bacteria are often used) and repeatedly reproduced. Each hybrid molecule produces a genetically identical molecule, called a *clone*. Cloning makes it possible to identify the DNA sequence in a gene and produce the protein product encoded by a gene, such as insulin. Cloning also allows production of adequate amounts of the drug for therapeutic or research purposes.

DRUG DEVELOPMENT AND APPROVAL

The FDA is responsible for assuring that new drugs are safe and effective before approving the drugs and allowing them to be marketed. The FDA reviews research studies (usually conducted or sponsored by a pharmaceutical company) about proposed new drugs; the organization does not test the drugs.

Before passage of the Food, Drug, and Cosmetic Act, many drugs were marketed without confirmation of safety or efficacy. Since 1962, however, newly developed drugs are extensively tested before being marketed for general use. The drugs are carefully evaluated at each step. Testing usually proceeds if there is evidence of safety and effectiveness, but it may be stopped at any time due to inadequate effectiveness or excessive toxicity. Many potential drugs are discarded and never marketed; some drugs are marketed but later withdrawn, usually because of adverse effects that become evident only when the drug is used in a large, diverse population.

Testing and Clinical Trials

The testing process begins with animal studies to determine potential uses and effects. The next step involves FDA review of the data obtained in the animal studies. The drug then undergoes clinical trials in humans. Most clinical trials use a randomized, controlled experimental design that involves selection of subjects according to established criteria, random assignment of subjects to experimental groups, and administration of the test drug to one group and a control substance to another group.

In Phase I, a few doses are given to a few healthy volunteers to determine safe dosages, routes of administration, absorption, metabolism, excretion, and toxicity. In Phase II, a few doses are given to a few subjects with the disease or symptom for which the drug is being studied, and responses are compared with those of healthy subjects. In Phase III, the drug is given to a larger and more representative group of subjects. In double-blind, placebo-controlled designs, half of the subjects receive the new drug and half receive a placebo, with neither subjects nor researchers knowing who receives which formulation. In crossover studies, subjects serve as their own control; each subject receives the experimental drug during half the study and a placebo during the other half. Other research methods include control studies in which some clients receive a known drug rather than a placebo; in subject matching, clients are paired with others of similar characteristics. Phase III studies help to determine whether the potential benefits of the drug outweigh the risks.

In Phase IV, the FDA evaluates the data from the first three phases for drug safety and effectiveness, allows the drug to be marketed for general use, and requires manufacturers to continue monitoring the drug's effects. Some adverse drug effects may become evident during the postmarketing phase as the drug is more widely used. Several drugs have been withdrawn in recent years, partly or mainly because of increased post-marketing surveillance. Critics contend that changes enacted to streamline the approval process have allowed unsafe drugs to be marketed; proponents claim that the faster review process helps clients with serious diseases to gain effective treatment more quickly.

The FDA has increased efforts to monitor marketed drugs in recent years, especially for their adverse effects. One such effort involves contracts with some commercial companies that provide access to databases containing information on the actual use of prescription drugs in adults and children. Examples of information include how long nonhospitalized patients stay on prescribed medications, which combinations of medications are being prescribed to patients, and the use of prescription drugs in hospitalized children. Individual patients are not identified in these databases.

Food and Drug Administration Approval

The FDA approves many new drugs annually. In 1992, procedures were changed to accelerate the approval process, especially for drugs used to treat acquired immunodeficiency syndrome. Since then, new drugs are categorized according to their review priority and therapeutic potential. A status of "1P" indicates a new drug reviewed on a priority basis and with some therapeutic advantages over similar drugs already available; a status of "1S" indicates standard review and drugs with few, if any, therapeutic advantages (ie, the new drug is similar to one already available). Most newly approved drugs are "1S" prescription drugs.

The FDA also approves drugs for OTC availability, including the transfer of drugs from prescription to OTC status, and may require additional clinical trials to determine the safety and effectiveness of OTC use. Numerous drugs have been transferred from prescription to OTC status in recent years, and the trend continues. For drugs taken orally, indications for use may be different, and recommended doses are usually lower for the OTC formulation. For example, for OTC ibuprofen, which is available under its generic name as well as under several trade names (eg, Advil) in 200-mg tablets and used for pain, fever, and dysmenorrhea, the recommended dose is usually 200 to 400 milligrams three or four times daily. With prescription ibuprofen, Motrin is the common trade name and dosage may be 400, 600, or 800 milligrams three or four times daily.

Food and Drug Administration approval of a drug for OTC availability involves evaluation of evidence that the consumer can use the drug safely, using information on the product label, and shifts primary responsibility for safe and effective drug therapy from health care professionals to consumers. With prescription drugs, a health care professional diagnoses the condition, often with the help of laboratory and other diagnostic tests, and determines a need for the drug. With OTC drugs, the client must make these decisions, with or without consultation with a health care provider. Questions to be answered include the following:

- Can consumers accurately self-diagnose the condition for which a drug is indicated?
- Can consumers read and understand the label well enough to determine the dosage, interpret warnings and contraindications and determine whether they apply, and recognize drugs already being taken that might interact adversely with the drug being considered?
- Is the drug effective when used as recommended?
- Is the drug safe when used as instructed?

Having drugs available OTC has potential advantages and disadvantages for consumers. Advantages include greater autonomy, faster and more convenient access to effective treatment, possibly earlier resumption of usual activities of daily living, fewer visits to a health care provider, and possibly increased efforts by consumers to learn about their symptoms/conditions and recommended treatments. Disadvantages include inaccurate self-diagnoses and potential risks of choosing a wrong or contraindicated drug, delaying treatment by a health care professional, and developing adverse drug reactions and interactions.

When a drug is switched from prescription to OTC status, pharmaceutical companies' sales and profits increase and insurance companies' costs decrease. Costs to consumers increase because health insurance policies do not cover OTC drugs.

Drug Marketing

A new drug is protected by patent for 14 years, during which time only the pharmaceutical manufacturer that developed it can market it. This is seen as a return on the company's investment in developing a drug, which may require years of work and millions of dollars, and as an incentive for developing other drugs. Other pharmaceutical companies cannot manufacture and market the drug until the patent expires. However, for new drugs that are popular and widely used, other companies often produce similar drugs, with different generic and trade names. For example, the marketing of fluoxetine (Prozac) led to the introduction of similar drugs from different companies, such as paroxetine (Paxil) and sertraline (Zoloft). Prozac was approved in 1987 and its patent expired in 2001, meaning that any pharmaceutical company could then manufacture and market the generic formulation of fluoxetine. Generic drugs are required to be therapeutically equivalent and are much less expensive than trade-name drugs.

PHARMACOECONOMICS

Pharmacoeconomics involves the costs of drug therapy, including costs of purchasing; dispensing (ie, salaries of pharmacists, pharmacy technicians); storage; administration (ie, salaries of nurses, costs of supplies); laboratory and other tests used to monitor client responses; and losses due to expiration. Length of illness or hospitalization is also considered.

Because costs are a major factor in choosing medications, the number of research projects that study and compare cost has increased. The goal of most studies is to define drug therapy regimens that provide the desired benefits at the least cost. For drugs or regimens of similar efficacy and toxicity, there is considerable pressure on prescribers to prescribe less costly drugs.

SOURCES OF DRUG INFORMATION

There are many sources of drug data, including pharmacology textbooks, drug reference books, journal articles, and Internet sites. For the beginning student of pharmacology, a textbook is usually the best source of information because it describes groups of drugs in relation to therapeutic uses. Drug reference books are most helpful in relation to individual drugs. Two authoritative sources are the *American Hospital Formulary Service* and *Drug Facts and Comparisons.* The former is published by the American Society of Health-System Pharmacists and updated periodically. The latter is published by the Facts and Comparisons division of Lippincott Williams & Wilkins and is updated monthly (looseleaf edition) or annually (hardbound edition). A widely available but less authoritative source is the *Physicians' Desk Reference (PDR).* The *PDR,* published yearly, compiles manufacturers' package inserts for selected drugs.

Numerous drug handbooks (eg, *Lippincott's Nursing Drug Guide,* published annually) and pharmacologic, medical, and nursing journals also contain information about drugs. Journal articles often present information about drug therapy for clients with specific disease processes and may thereby facilitate application of drug knowledge in clinical practice.

STRATEGIES FOR STUDYING PHARMACOLOGY

Several approaches or strategies facilitate the learning of pharmacology. Some guidelines for effective study include the following:

- Concentrate on therapeutic classifications and their prototypes. For example, morphine is the prototype of opioid analgesics (see Chap. 6). Understanding morphine makes learning about other opioid analgesics easier because they are compared with morphine.
- Compare a newly encountered drug with a prototype or similar drug when possible. Relating the unknown to the known aids learning and retention of knowledge.
- Try to understand how the drug acts in the body. This understanding allows you to predict therapeutic effects and to predict, prevent, or minimize adverse effects by early detection and treatment.
- Concentrate study efforts on major characteristics. Such characteristics include the main indications for use, common and potentially serious adverse effects, conditions in which the drug is contraindicated or must be used cautiously, and related nursing care needs.
- Keep an authoritative, up-to-date drug reference readily available. A drug reference is a more reliable source of drug information than memory, especially for dosage ranges. Use the reference freely whenever you encounter an unfamiliar drug or when a question arises about a familiar one.
- Use your own words when taking notes or writing drug information cards. Also, write notes, answers to review questions, definitions of new terms, and trade names of drugs encountered in clinical practice settings directly into your pharmacology textbook. The mental processing required for these activities helps in both initial learning and later retention and application of knowledge.
- Rehearse applying drug knowledge in nursing care by asking yourself, "What if I have a client who is receiving this drug? What must I do to safely administer the drug? For what must I assess the client before giving the drug and for what must I observe the client after drug administration? What if my client is an elderly person or a child?"

Review and Application Exercises

Short Answer Exercises

1. What is the difference between local and systemic effects of drugs?

2. Can a client experience systemic effects of local drugs and local effects of systemic drugs? Why or why not?

3. Why is it helpful for nurses to know the generic names of commonly used medications?

4. Why is it helpful to study prototypes of drug groups?

5. List at least three strategies for studying pharmacology.

6. List at least three authoritative sources of drug information.

NCLEX-Style Questions

7. Most modern medications are
   a. natural products derived from plants
   b. natural products derived from minerals
   c. synthetic products manufactured in laboratories
   d. synthetic modifications of natural products

8. Which of the following statements is true?
   a. A drug can belong to only one group or classification.
   b. A prototype drug is the standard by which similar drugs are compared.
   c. Drug groups and prototypes change frequently.
   d. The generic name of a drug changes among manufacturers.

9. Controlled drugs are
   a. categorized according to prescription or non-prescription status
   b. regulated by state and local laws more than federal laws
   c. those that must demonstrate high standards of safety
   d. scheduled according to medical use and potential for abuse

10. Over-the-counter drugs
    a. are considered safe for any consumers to use
    b. are not available for treatment of most commonly occurring symptoms
    c. often differ in indications for use and recommended dosages from their prescription versions
    d. are paid for by most insurance policies

11. With a new drug, the Food and Drug Administration is responsible for
    a. testing the drug with animals
    b. testing the drug with healthy people
    c. marketing the drug to health care providers
    d. evaluating the drug for safety and effectiveness

Selected References

Brass, E. P. (2001). Changing the status of drugs from prescription to over-the-counter availability. *New England Journal of Medicine, 345*(11), 810–816.

Lipsky, M. S., & Sharp, L. K. (2001). From idea to market: The drug approval process. *Journal of the American Board of Family Practice, 14*(5), 362–367.

U.S. Food and Drug Administration. *Frequently asked questions.* Retrieved June 6, 2005, from http://www.fda.gov/opacom/faqs/faqs.html

Basic Concepts and Processes

APPLYING YOUR KNOWLEDGE

Mrs. Green, an 89-year-old widow, has recently switched to a new antihypertension medication. She prides herself on being independent and able to manage on her own, despite failing memory and failing health. When you visit as a home health nurse, you assess therapeutic and adverse effects of her medications.

INTRODUCTION

All body functions and disease processes and most drug actions occur at the cellular level. Drugs are chemicals that alter basic processes in body cells. They can stimulate or inhibit normal cellular functions and activities; however, they cannot add functions and activities. To act on body cells, drugs given for systemic effects must reach adequate concentrations in the blood and in the other tissue fluids surrounding the cells. Thus, they must enter the body and be circulated to their sites of action (target cells). After they act on cells, they must be eliminated from the body.

How do systemic drugs reach, interact with, and leave body cells? How do people respond to drug actions? The answers to these questions are derived from cellular physiology, pathways and mechanisms of drug transport, pharmacokinetics, pharmacodynamics, and other basic concepts and processes. These

concepts and processes form the foundation of rational drug therapy and the content of this chapter.

CELLULAR PHYSIOLOGY

Cells are dynamic, busy "factories" (Box 2-1). That is, they take in raw materials, manufacture various products required to maintain cellular and bodily functions, and deliver those products to their appropriate destinations in the body. Although cells differ from one tissue to another, their common characteristics include the ability to

- Exchange materials with their immediate environment
- Obtain energy from nutrients
- Synthesize hormones, neurotransmitters, enzymes, structural proteins, and other complex molecules
- Duplicate themselves (reproduce)

Box 2-1 Cell Structures and Functions

Protoplasm comprises the internal environment of body cells. Protoplasm is composed of water, electrolytes (potassium, magnesium, phosphate, sulfate, and bicarbonate), proteins, lipids, and carbohydrates.

- **Water** makes up 70%–85% of most cells; cellular enzymes, electrolytes, and other chemicals are dissolved or suspended in the water.
- **Electrolytes** provide chemicals for cellular reactions and are required for some processes (eg, transmission of electrochemical impulses in nerve and muscle cells).
- **Proteins** comprise 10%–20% of the cell mass. They consist of "physical" proteins that form the structure of cells and "chemical" proteins that function mainly as enzymes within the cell. These enzymatic proteins come into direct contact with other substances in the cell fluid and catalyze chemical reactions within the cell.
- **Lipids,** mainly phospholipids and cholesterol, form the membranes that separate structures inside the cell and the cell itself from surrounding cells and body fluids.
- **Carbohydrates** play a minor role in cell structure, but a major role in cell nutrition. Glucose is present in extracellular fluid and is readily available to supply the cell's need for energy. In addition, a small amount of carbohydrate is stored within the cell as glycogen, a storage form of glucose that can be rapidly converted when needed.

The **nucleus** might be called the "manager" of cellular activities because it regulates the types and amounts of proteins, enzymes, and other substances to be produced.

The **cytoplasm** surrounds the nucleus and contains the working units of the cell.

The **endoplasmic reticulum** (ER) contains ribosomes, which synthesize enzymes and other proteins. These enzymes include those that synthesize glycogen, triglycerides, and steroids and those that detoxify drugs and other chemicals. The ER is important in the production of hormones by glandular cells and the production of plasma proteins and drug-metabolizing enzymes by liver cells.

The **Golgi complex** stores hormones and other substances produced by the ER. It also packages these substances into secretory granules, which then move out of the Golgi complex into the cytoplasm and, after an appropriate stimulus, are released from the cell through the process of exocytosis.

Mitochondria generate energy for cellular activities and require oxygen.

Lysosomes are membrane-enclosed vesicles that contain enzymes capable of digesting nutrients (proteins, carbohydrates, fats), damaged cellular structures, foreign substances (eg, bacteria), and the cell itself. When a cell becomes worn out or damaged, the membrane around the lysosome breaks and the enzymes (hydrolases) are released. However, lysosomal contents also are released into extracellular spaces, destroying surrounding cells. Normally, the enzymes are inactivated by enzyme inhibitors and excessive tissue destruction is prevented.

The **cell membrane,** a complex structure composed of phospholipids, proteins, cholesterol, and carbohydrates, separates intracellular contents from the extracellular environment; provides receptors for hormones and other biologically active substances; participates in electrical events that occur in nerve and muscle cells; and helps regulate growth and proliferation.

The cell membrane, which covers the entire surface of the cell, consists of a thin, double layer of lipids interspersed with proteins. The lipid layer is composed of phospholipid (fatty acid and phosphate) molecules. The phosphate end of each phospholipid molecule, located on the external surface and in contact with the tissue fluids surrounding the cell, is soluble in water. The fatty-acid end of the phospholipid molecule, located in the middle of the membrane, is soluble only in fat. Thus, this portion of the membrane allows easy penetration of fat-soluble substances such as oxygen and alcohol, but is impermeable to water-soluble substances such as ions and glucose.

Cell membrane proteins, most of which are combined with a carbohydrate as glycoproteins, include integral and peripheral proteins. *Integral proteins* penetrate through the entire membrane so that each end is available to interact with other substances. The protein portion protrudes on the intracellular side of the cell membrane; the glyco portion protrudes to the outside of the cell, dangling outward from the cell surface. Some of these proteins provide structural channels or pores through which water and water-soluble substances (eg, sodium, potassium, and calcium ions) can diffuse between extracellular and intracellular fluids. Other proteins act as carriers to transport substances that otherwise could not penetrate the lipid layer of the membrane. Still others act as enzymes to catalyze chemical reactions within the cell. *Peripheral proteins* do not penetrate the cell membrane. They are usually attached to the intracellular side of the membrane and to integral proteins. These proteins function as enzymes and other substances that regulate intracellular function.

Cell membrane carbohydrates occur mainly in combination with proteins (glycoproteins) or lipids (glycolipids). Glycoproteins composed of carbohydrate around a small, inner core of protein (called proteoglycans) often are attached to and cover the entire outside surface of the cell. As a result, the carbohydrate molecules are free to interact with extracellular substances and perform several important functions. First, many have a negative electrical charge, which gives most cells an overall negative surface charge that repels other negatively charged substances.

(continued)

Box 2-1 Cell Structures and Functions (continued)

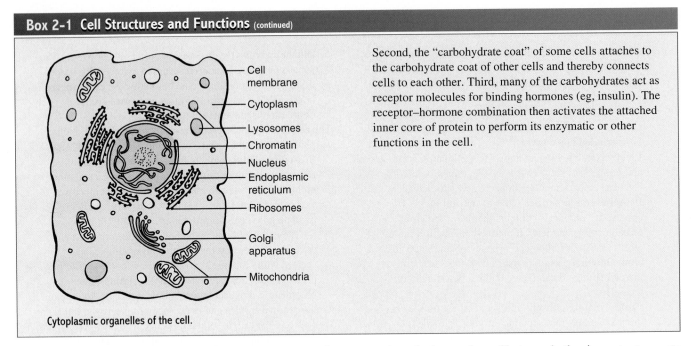

Cytoplasmic organelles of the cell.

Second, the "carbohydrate coat" of some cells attaches to the carbohydrate coat of other cells and thereby connects cells to each other. Third, many of the carbohydrates act as receptor molecules for binding hormones (eg, insulin). The receptor–hormone combination then activates the attached inner core of protein to perform its enzymatic or other functions in the cell.

● Communicate with one another via various biologic chemicals, such as neurotransmitters and hormones

DRUG TRANSPORT THROUGH CELL MEMBRANES

Drugs, as well as physiologic substances such as hormones and neurotransmitters, must reach and interact with or cross the cell membrane to stimulate or inhibit cellular function. Most drugs are given for effects on body cells that are distant from the sites of administration (ie, systemic effects). To move through the body and reach their sites of action, metabolism, and excretion (Fig. 2-1), drug molecules must cross numerous cell membranes. For example, molecules of most oral drugs must cross the membranes of cells in the gastrointestinal tract, liver, and capillaries to reach the bloodstream, circulate to their target cells, leave the bloodstream and attach to receptors on cells, perform their action, return to the bloodstream, circulate to the liver, reach drug-metabolizing enzymes in liver cells, re-enter the bloodstream (usually as metabolites), circulate to the kidneys, and be excreted in urine. Several transport pathways and mechanisms are used to move drug molecules through the body. Box 2-2 describes these pathways and mechanisms.

PHARMACOKINETICS

Pharmacokinetics involves drug movement through the body (ie, "what the body does to the drug") to reach sites of action, metabolism, and excretion. Specific processes are absorption, distribution, metabolism (biotransformation), and excretion. Overall, these processes largely determine serum drug levels; onset, peak, and duration of drug actions; drug half-life; ther-

apeutic and adverse drug effects; and other important aspects of drug therapy.

Absorption

Absorption is the process that occurs from the time a drug enters the body to the time it enters the bloodstream to be circulated. Onset of drug action is largely determined by the rate of absorption; intensity is determined by the extent of

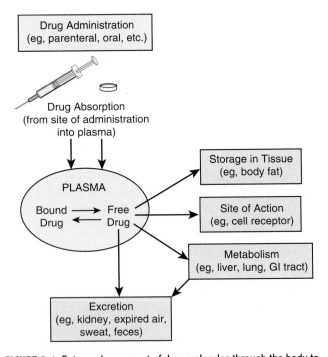

FIGURE 2-1 Entry and movement of drug molecules through the body to sites of action, metabolism, and excretion.

Box 2-2 Drug Transport Pathways and Mechanisms

Pathways

There are three main pathways of drug movement across cell membranes. The most common pathway is *direct penetration* of the membrane by lipid-soluble drugs, which are able to dissolve in the lipid layer of the cell membrane. Most systemic drugs are formulated to be lipid soluble so they can move through cell membranes, even oral tablets and capsules that must be sufficiently water soluble to dissolve in the aqueous fluids of the stomach and small intestine.

A second pathway involves passage through *protein channels* that go all the way through the cell membrane. Only a few drugs are able to use this pathway because most drug molecules are too large to pass through the small channels. Small ions (eg, sodium and potassium) use this pathway, but their movement is regulated by specific channels with a gating mechanism. The gate is a flap of protein that opens for a few milliseconds to allow ion movement across the cell membrane, then closes (ie, blocks the channel opening) to prevent additional ion movement. On sodium channels, the gates are located on the outside of the cell membrane; when the gates open, sodium ions (Na^+) move from extracellular fluid into the cell. On potassium channels, the gates are located on the inside of the cell membrane; when the gates open, potassium ions (K^+) move from the cell into extracellular fluid.

The stimulus for opening and closing the gates may be voltage gating or chemical (also called ligand) gating. With voltage gating, the electrical potential across the cell membrane determines whether the gate is open or closed. With chemical gating, a chemical substance (a ligand) binds with the protein forming the channel and changes the shape of the protein to open or close the gate. Chemical gating (eg, by neurotransmitters such as acetylcholine) is very important in the transmission of signals from one nerve cell to another and from nerve cells to muscle cells to cause muscle contraction.

The third pathway involves *carrier proteins* that transport molecules from one side of the cell membrane to the other. All of the carrier proteins are selective in the substances they transport; a drug's structure determines which carrier will transport it. These transport systems are an important means of moving drug molecules through the body. They are used, for example, to carry oral drugs from the intestine to the bloodstream, to carry hormones to their sites of action inside body cells, and to carry drug molecules from the blood into renal tubules.

Mechanisms

After they are absorbed into the body, drugs are transported to and from target cells by such mechanisms as passive diffusion, facilitated diffusion, and active transport.

Passive diffusion, the most common mechanism, involves movement of a drug from an area of higher concentration to one of lower concentration. For example, after oral administration, the initial concentration of a drug is higher in the gastrointestinal tract than in the blood. This promotes movement of the drug into the bloodstream. When the drug is circulated, the concentration is higher in the blood than in body cells, so that the drug moves (from capillaries) into the fluids surrounding the cells or into the cells themselves. Passive diffusion continues until a state of equilibrium is reached between the amount of drug in the tissues and the amount in the blood.

Facilitated diffusion is a similar process, except that drug molecules combine with a carrier substance, such as an enzyme or other protein.

In *active transport*, drug molecules are moved from an area of lower concentration to one of higher concentration. This process requires a carrier substance and the release of cellular energy.

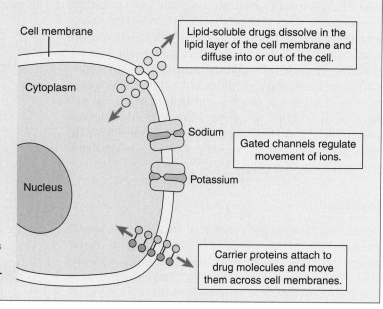

Drug transport pathways. Drug molecules cross cell membranes to move into and out of body cells by directly penetrating the lipid layer, diffusing through open or gated channels, or attaching to carrier proteins.

Cell membrane

Lipid-soluble drugs dissolve in the lipid layer of the cell membrane and diffuse into or out of the cell.

Cytoplasm

Sodium

Gated channels regulate movement of ions.

Potassium

Nucleus

Carrier proteins attach to drug molecules and move them across cell membranes.

absorption. Numerous factors affect the rate and extent of drug absorption, including dosage form, route of administration, blood flow to the site of administration, gastrointestinal function, the presence of food or other drugs, and other variables. Dosage form is a major determinant of a drug's *bioavailability* (the portion of a dose that reaches the systemic circulation and is available to act on body cells). An intravenous drug is virtually 100% bioavailable; an oral drug is virtually always less than 100% bioavailable because some of it is not absorbed from the gastrointestinal tract and some goes to the liver and is partially metabolized before reaching the systemic circulation.

Most oral drugs must be swallowed, dissolved in gastric fluid, and delivered to the small intestine (which has a large surface area for absorption of nutrients and drugs) before they are absorbed. Liquid medications are absorbed faster than tablets or capsules because they need not be dissolved. Rapid movement through the stomach and small intestine may increase drug absorption by promoting contact with absorptive mucous membrane; it also may decrease absorption because some drugs may move through the small intestine too rapidly to be absorbed. For many drugs, the presence of food in the stomach slows the rate of absorption and may decrease the amount of drug absorbed.

Drugs injected into subcutaneous (Sub-Q) or intramuscular (IM) tissues are usually absorbed more rapidly than oral drugs because they move directly from the injection site to the bloodstream. Absorption is rapid from IM sites because muscle tissue has an abundant blood supply. Drugs injected intravenously (IV) do not need to be absorbed because they are placed directly into the bloodstream.

Other absorptive sites include the skin, mucous membranes, and lungs. Most drugs applied to the skin are given for local effects (eg, sunscreens). Systemic absorption is minimal from intact skin but may be considerable when the skin is inflamed or damaged. Also, a number of drugs are formulated in adhesive skin patches for absorption through the skin (eg, clonidine, fentanyl, nitroglycerin). Some drugs applied to mucous membranes also are given for local effects. However, systemic absorption occurs from the mucosa of the oral cavity, nose, eye, vagina, and rectum. Drugs absorbed through mucous membranes pass directly into the bloodstream. The lungs have a large surface area for absorption of anesthetic gases and a few other drugs.

Distribution

Distribution involves the transport of drug molecules within the body. After a drug is injected or absorbed into the bloodstream, it is carried by the blood and tissue fluids to its sites of pharmacologic action, metabolism, and excretion. Most drug molecules enter and leave the bloodstream at the capillary level, through gaps between the cells that form capillary walls. Distribution depends largely on the adequacy of blood circulation. Drugs are distributed rapidly to organs receiving

a large blood supply, such as the heart, liver, and kidneys. Distribution to other internal organs, muscle, fat, and skin is usually slower.

Protein binding is an important factor in drug distribution (Fig. 2-2). Most drugs form a compound with plasma proteins, mainly albumin, which act as carriers. Drug molecules bound to plasma proteins are pharmacologically inactive because the large size of the complex prevents their leaving the bloodstream through the small openings in capillary walls and reaching their sites of action, metabolism, and excretion. *Only the free or unbound portion of a drug acts on body cells.* As the free drug acts on cells, the decrease in plasma drug levels causes some of the bound drug to be released.

Protein binding allows part of a drug dose to be stored and released as needed. Some drugs also are stored in muscle, fat, or other body tissues and released gradually when plasma drug levels fall. These storage mechanisms maintain lower, more even blood levels and reduce the risk of toxicity. Drugs that are highly bound to plasma proteins or stored extensively in other tissues have a long duration of action.

Drug distribution into the central nervous system (CNS) is limited because the blood–brain barrier, which is composed of capillaries with tight walls, limits movement of drug molecules into brain tissue. This barrier usually acts as a selectively permeable membrane to protect the CNS. However, it also can make drug therapy for CNS disorders more difficult because drugs must pass *through* cells of the capillary wall rather than *between* cells. As a result, only drugs that are lipid soluble or have a transport system can cross the blood–brain barrier and reach therapeutic concentrations in brain tissue.

Drug distribution during pregnancy and lactation is also unique (see Chap. 65). During pregnancy, most drugs cross the placenta and may affect the fetus. During lactation, many drugs enter breast milk and may affect the nursing infant.

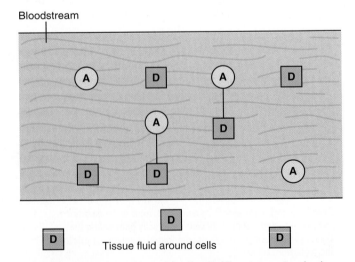

FIGURE 2-2 Plasma proteins, mainly albumin (A), act as carriers for drug molecules (D). Bound drug (A–D) stays in the bloodstream and is pharmacologically inactive. Free drug (D) can leave the bloodstream and act on body cells.

Metabolism

Metabolism is the method by which drugs are inactivated or biotransformed by the body. Most often, an active drug is changed into one or more inactive metabolites, which are then excreted. Some active drugs yield metabolites that are also active and that continue to exert their effects on body cells until they are metabolized further or excreted. Other drugs (called *prodrugs*) are initially inactive and exert no pharmacologic effects until they are metabolized.

Most drugs are lipid soluble, a characteristic that aids their movement across cell membranes. However, the kidneys, which are the primary excretory organs, can excrete only water-soluble substances. Therefore, one function of metabolism is to convert fat-soluble drugs into water-soluble metabolites. Hepatic drug metabolism or clearance is a major mechanism for terminating drug action and eliminating drug molecules from the body.

Most drugs are metabolized by cytochrome P450 (CYP) enzymes in the liver; red blood cells, plasma, kidneys, lungs, and gastrointestinal mucosa also contain drug-metabolizing enzymes. The CYP system consists of 12 groups, 9 of which metabolize endogenous substances and 3 of which metabolize drugs. The drug-metabolizing groups are labeled CYP1, CYP2, and CYP3. Of the many drugs metabolized by the liver, the CYP3 group of enzymes is thought to metabolize about 50%, the CYP2 group about 45%, and the CYP1 group about 5%. Individual members of the groups, each of which metabolizes specific drugs, are further categorized. For example, many drugs are metabolized by CYP3A4 enzymes.

CYP enzymes, located within hepatocytes, are complex proteins with binding sites for drug molecules (and endogenous substances). They catalyze the chemical reactions of oxidation, reduction, hydrolysis, and conjugation with endogenous substances, such as glucuronic acid or sulfate. With chronic administration, some drugs stimulate liver cells to produce larger amounts of drug-metabolizing enzymes (called *enzyme induction*). Enzyme induction accelerates drug metabolism because larger amounts of the enzymes (and more binding sites) allow larger amounts of a drug to be metabolized during a given time. As a result, larger doses of the rapidly metabolized drug may be required to produce or maintain therapeutic effects. Rapid metabolism may also increase the production of toxic metabolites with some drugs (eg, acetaminophen). Drugs that induce enzyme production also may increase the rate of metabolism for endogenous steroidal hormones (eg, cortisol, estrogens, testosterone, vitamin D). However, enzyme induction does not occur for 1 to 3 weeks after an inducing agent is started, because new enzyme proteins must be synthesized.

Metabolism also can be decreased or delayed in a process called *enzyme inhibition,* which most often occurs with concurrent administration of two or more drugs that compete for the same metabolizing enzymes. In this case, smaller doses of the slowly metabolized drug may be needed to avoid adverse reactions and toxicity from drug accumulation. Enzyme inhibition occurs within hours or days of starting an inhibiting agent. Cimetidine, a gastric acid suppressor, inhibits several CYP enzymes (eg, 1A2, 2C, 3A) and can greatly decrease drug metabolism. The rate of drug metabolism also is reduced in infants (their hepatic enzyme system is immature), in people with impaired blood flow to the liver or severe hepatic or cardiovascular disease, and in people who are malnourished or on low-protein diets.

When drugs are given orally, they are absorbed from the gastrointestinal tract and carried to the liver through the portal circulation. Some drugs are extensively metabolized in the liver, with only part of a drug dose reaching the systemic circulation for distribution to sites of action. This is called the *first-pass effect* or *presystemic metabolism.*

Excretion

Excretion refers to elimination of a drug from the body. Effective excretion requires adequate functioning of the circulatory system and of the organs of excretion (kidneys, bowel, lungs, and skin). Most drugs are excreted by the kidneys and eliminated (unchanged or as metabolites) in the urine. Some drugs or metabolites are excreted in bile and then eliminated in feces; others are excreted in bile, reabsorbed from the small intestine, returned to the liver (called *enterohepatic recirculation*), metabolized, and eventually excreted in urine. Some oral drugs are not absorbed and are excreted in the feces. The lungs mainly remove volatile substances, such as anesthetic gases. The skin has minimal excretory function. Factors impairing excretion, especially severe renal disease, lead to accumulation of numerous drugs, which may cause severe adverse effects if dosage is not reduced.

Serum Drug Levels

A *serum drug level* is a laboratory measurement of the amount of a drug in the blood at a particular time (Fig. 2-3). It reflects dosage, absorption, bioavailability, half-life, and the rates of metabolism and excretion. A *minimum effective concentration* (MEC) must be present before a drug exerts its pharmacologic action on body cells; this is largely determined by the drug dose and how well it is absorbed into the bloodstream. A *toxic concentration* is an excessive level at which toxicity occurs. Toxic concentrations may stem from a single large dose, repeated small doses, or slow metabolism that allows the drug to accumulate in the body. Between these low and high concentrations is the therapeutic range, which is the goal of drug therapy—that is, enough drug to be beneficial, but not enough to be toxic.

For most drugs, serum levels indicate the onset, peak, and duration of drug action. When a single dose of a drug is given,

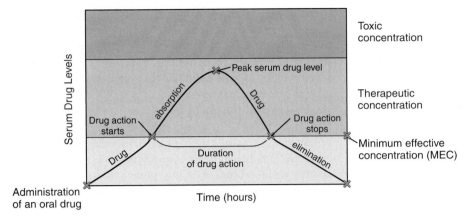

Drug action in relation to serum drug levels and time after a single dose.

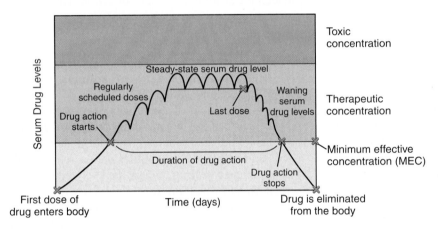

Drug action in relation to serum drug levels with repeated doses.

FIGURE 2-3 Serum drug levels with single and multiple oral drug doses. Drug action starts when enough drug is absorbed to reach the minimum effective concentration (MEC), continues as long as the serum level is above the MEC, wanes as drug molecules are metabolized and excreted (if no more doses are given), and stops when the serum level drops below the MEC. The goal of drug therapy is to maintain serum drug levels in the therapeutic range.

onset of action occurs when the drug level reaches the MEC. The drug level continues to climb as more of the drug is absorbed, until it reaches its highest concentration and peak drug action occurs. Then, drug levels decline as the drug is eliminated (ie, metabolized and excreted) from the body. Although there may still be numerous drug molecules in the body, drug action stops when drug levels fall below the MEC. The *duration of action* is the time during which serum drug levels are at or above the MEC. When multiple doses of a drug are given (eg, for chronic, long-lasting conditions), the goal is usually to give sufficient doses often enough to maintain serum drug levels in the therapeutic range and avoid the toxic range.

In clinical practice, measuring serum drug levels is useful in several circumstances:

● When drugs with a low therapeutic index are given. These are drugs with a narrow margin of safety because their therapeutic doses are close to their toxic doses (eg, digoxin, aminoglycoside antibiotics, lithium).
● To document the serum drug levels associated with particular drug dosages, therapeutic effects, or possible adverse effects

● To monitor unexpected responses to a drug dose such as decreased therapeutic effects or increased adverse effects
● When a drug overdose is suspected

Serum Half-Life

Serum half-life, also called *elimination half-life,* is the time required for the serum concentration of a drug to decrease by 50%. It is determined primarily by the drug's rates of metabolism and excretion. A drug with a short half-life requires more frequent administration than one with a long half-life.

When a drug is given at a stable dose, four or five half-lives are required to achieve steady-state concentrations and develop equilibrium between tissue and serum concentrations. Because maximal therapeutic effects do not occur until equilibrium is established, some drugs are not fully effective for days or weeks. To maintain steady-state conditions, the amount of drug given must equal the amount eliminated from the body. When a drug dose is changed, an additional four to five half-lives are required to re-establish equilibrium; when a drug is discontinued, it is eliminated gradually over several half-lives.

PHARMACODYNAMICS

Pharmacodynamics involves drug actions on target cells and the resulting alterations in cellular biochemical reactions and functions (ie, "what the drug does to the body"). As previously stated, all drug actions occur at the cellular level.

Receptor Theory of Drug Action

Like the physiologic substances (eg, hormones, neurotransmitters) that normally regulate cell functions, most drugs exert their effects by chemically binding with receptors at the cellular level (Fig. 2-4). Most receptors are proteins located on the surfaces of cell membranes or within cells. Specific receptors include *enzymes* involved in essential metabolic or regulatory processes (eg, dihydrofolate reductase, acetylcholinesterase); *proteins* involved in transport (eg, sodium–potassium adenosine triphosphatase) or structural processes (eg, tubulin); and *nucleic acids* (eg, DNA) involved in cellular protein synthesis, reproduction, and other metabolic activities.

When drug molecules bind with receptor molecules, the resulting drug–receptor complex initiates physiochemical reactions that stimulate or inhibit normal cellular functions. One type of reaction involves activation, inactivation, or other alterations of intracellular enzymes. Because enzymes catalyze almost all cellular functions, drug-induced changes can markedly increase or decrease the rate of cellular metabolism. For example, an epinephrine–receptor complex increases the activity of the intracellular enzyme adenyl cyclase, which then causes the formation of cyclic adenosine monophosphate (cAMP). cAMP, in turn, can initiate any one of many different intracellular actions, the exact effect depending on the type of cell.

A second type of reaction involves changes in the permeability of cell membranes to one or more ions. The receptor protein is a structural component of the cell membrane, and its binding to a drug molecule may open or close ion channels. In nerve cells, for example, sodium or calcium ion channels may open and allow movement of ions into the cell. This movement usually causes the cell membrane to depolarize and excite the cell. At other times, potassium channels may open and allow movement of potassium ions out of the cell. This action inhibits neuronal excitability and function. In muscle cells, movement of the ions into the cells may alter intracellular functions, such as the direct effect of calcium ions in stimulating muscle contraction.

A third reaction may modify the synthesis, release, or inactivation of the neurohormones (eg, acetylcholine, norepinephrine, serotonin) that regulate many physiologic processes.

Additional elements and characteristics of the receptor theory include the following:

● The site and extent of drug action on body cells are determined primarily by specific characteristics of receptors and drugs. Receptors vary in type, location, number, and functional capacity. For example, many different types of receptors have been identified. Most types occur in most body tissues, such as receptors for epinephrine and norepinephrine (whether received from stimulation of the sympathetic nervous system or administration of drug formulations) and receptors for hormones, including growth hormone, thyroid hormone, and insulin. Some occur in fewer body tissues, such as receptors for opiates and benzodiazepines in the brain and subgroups of receptors for epinephrine in the heart (beta$_1$-adrenergic receptors) and lungs (beta$_2$-adrenergic receptors). Receptor type and location influence drug action. The receptor is often described as a lock into which the drug molecule fits as a key, and only those drugs able to bond chemically to the receptors in a particular body tissue can exert pharmacologic effects on that tissue. Thus, all body cells do not respond to all drugs, even though virtually all cell receptors are exposed to any drug molecules circulating in the bloodstream.

The number of receptor sites available to interact with drug molecules also affects the extent of drug action. Presumably, drug molecules must occupy a minimal number of receptors to produce pharmacologic effects. Thus, if many receptors are available but only a few are occupied by drug molecules, few drug effects occur. In this instance, increasing the drug dosage increases the pharmacologic effects. Conversely, if only a few receptors are available for many drug molecules, receptors may be saturated. In this instance, if most receptor sites are occupied, increasing the drug dosage produces no additional pharmacologic effect.

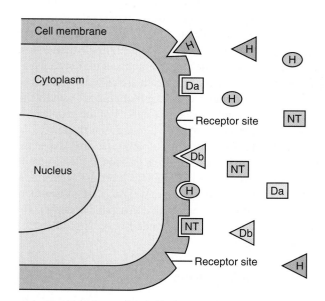

FIGURE 2-4 Cell membrane contains receptors for physiologic substances such as hormones (H) and neurotransmitters (NT). These substances stimulate or inhibit cellular function. Drug molecules (Da and Db) also interact with receptors to stimulate or inhibit cellular function.

Drugs vary even more widely than receptors. Because all drugs are chemical substances, chemical characteristics determine drug actions and pharmacologic effects. For example, a drug's chemical structure affects its ability to reach tissue fluids around a cell and bind with its cell receptors. Minor changes in drug structure may produce major changes in pharmacologic effects. Another major factor is the concentration of drug molecules that reach receptor sites in body tissues. Drug- and client-related variables that affect drug actions are further described later in this chapter.

● When drug molecules chemically bind with cell receptors, pharmacologic effects result from agonism or antagonism. *Agonists* are drugs that produce effects similar to those produced by naturally occurring hormones, neurotransmitters, and other substances. Agonists may accelerate or slow normal cellular processes, depending on the type of receptor activated. For example, epinephrine-like drugs act on the heart to increase the heart rate, and acetylcholine-like drugs act on the heart to slow the heart rate; both are agonists. *Antagonists* are drugs that inhibit cell function by occupying receptor sites. This strategy prevents natural body substances or other drugs from occupying the receptor sites and activating cell functions. After drug action occurs, drug molecules may detach from receptor molecules (ie, the chemical binding is reversible), return to the bloodstream, and circulate to the liver for metabolism and the kidneys for excretion.

● Receptors are dynamic cellular components that can be synthesized by body cells and altered by endogenous substances and exogenous drugs. For example, prolonged stimulation of body cells with an excitatory agonist usually reduces the number or sensitivity of receptors. As a result, the cell becomes less responsive to the agonist (a process called receptor desensitization or *down-regulation*). Prolonged inhibition of normal cellular functions with an antagonist may increase receptor number or sensitivity. If the antagonist is suddenly reduced or stopped, the cell becomes excessively responsive to an agonist (a process called receptor *up-regulation*). These changes in receptors may explain why some drugs must be tapered in dosage and discontinued gradually if withdrawal symptoms are to be avoided.

Nonreceptor Drug Actions

Relatively few drugs act by mechanisms other than combination with receptor sites on cells. Drugs that do not act on receptor sites include the following:

● Antacids, which act chemically to neutralize the hydrochloric acid produced by gastric parietal cells and thereby raise the pH of gastric fluid
● Osmotic diuretics (eg, mannitol), which increase the osmolarity of plasma and pull water out of tissues into the bloodstream

● Drugs that are structurally similar to nutrients required by body cells (eg, purines, pyrimidines) and that can be incorporated into cellular constituents, such as nucleic acids. This interferes with normal cell functioning. Several anticancer drugs act by this mechanism.
● Metal chelating agents combine with toxic metals (eg, lead) to form a complex that can be more readily excreted.

VARIABLES THAT AFFECT DRUG ACTIONS

Historically, expected responses to drugs were based on those occurring when a particular drug was given to healthy adult men (18 to 65 years of age) of average weight (150 lb [70 kg]). However, other groups (eg, women, children, older adults, different ethnic or racial groups, clients with diseases or symptoms that the drugs are designed to treat) receive drugs and respond differently than healthy adult men. As a result, newer clinical trials include more representatives of these groups. In any client, however, responses may be altered by both drug- and client-related variables, some of which are described in the following sections.

Drug-Related Variables

Dosage

Dosage refers to the frequency, size, and number of doses; it is a major determinant of drug actions and responses, both therapeutic and adverse. If the amount is too small or administered infrequently, no pharmacologic action occurs because the drug does not reach an adequate concentration at target cells. If the amount is too large or administered too often, toxicity (poisoning) may occur. *Overdosage* may occur with a single large dose or with chronic ingestion of smaller doses. Doses that produce signs and symptoms of toxicity are called *toxic doses*. Doses that cause death are called *lethal doses*.

Dosages recommended in drug literature are usually those that produce particular responses in 50% of the people tested. These dosages usually produce a mixture of therapeutic and adverse effects. The dosage of a particular drug depends on many characteristics of the drug (reason for use, potency, pharmacokinetics, route of administration, dosage form, and others) and of the recipient (age, weight, state of health, and function of cardiovascular, renal, and hepatic systems). Thus, recommended dosages are intended only as guidelines for individualizing dosages.

Route of Administration

Routes of administration affect drug actions and client responses largely by influencing absorption and distribution. For rapid drug action and response, the IV route is most effective because the drug is injected directly into the bloodstream.

For some drugs, the IM route also produces drug action within a few minutes because muscles have a large blood supply. The oral route usually produces slower drug action than parenteral routes. Absorption and action of topical drugs vary according to the drug formulation, whether the drug is applied to skin or mucous membranes, and other factors.

Drug–Diet Interactions

Food often slows absorption of oral drugs by slowing gastric emptying time and altering gastrointestinal secretions and motility. When tablets or capsules are taken with or soon after food, they dissolve more slowly and drug molecules are delivered to absorptive sites in the small intestine more slowly. Food also may decrease absorption by combining with a drug to form an insoluble drug–food complex. Interactions that alter drug absorption can be minimized by spacing food and medications.

In addition, some foods contain substances that react with certain drugs. One such interaction occurs between tyramine-containing foods and monoamine oxidase (MAO) inhibitor drugs. Tyramine causes the release of norepinephrine, a strong vasoconstrictive agent, from the adrenal medulla and sympathetic neurons. Normally, norepinephrine is active for only a few milliseconds before it is inactivated by MAO. However, because MAO inhibitor drugs prevent inactivation of norepinephrine, ingesting tyramine-containing foods with an MAO inhibitor may produce severe hypertension or intracranial hemorrhage. MAO inhibitors include the antidepressants isocarboxazid and phenelzine and the antineoplastic procarbazine. These drugs are rarely used now, partly because of this serious interaction and partly because other effective drugs are available. Tyramine-rich foods to be avoided by clients taking MAO inhibitors include beer, wine, aged cheeses, yeast products, chicken livers, and pickled herring.

An interaction may occur between warfarin (Coumadin), an oral anticoagulant, and foods containing vitamin K. Because vitamin K antagonizes the action of warfarin, large amounts of spinach and other green leafy vegetables may offset the anticoagulant effects and predispose the person to thromboembolic disorders.

A third interaction occurs between tetracycline, an antibiotic, and dairy products, such as milk and cheese. The drug combines with the calcium in milk products to form a nonabsorbable compound that is excreted in the feces.

Drug–Drug Interactions

The action of a drug may be increased or decreased by its interaction with another drug in the body. Most interactions occur whenever the interacting drugs are present in the body; some, especially those affecting the absorption of oral drugs, occur when the interacting drugs are given at or near the same time. The basic cause of many drug–drug interactions is altered drug metabolism. For example, drugs metabolized by the same enzymes compete for enzyme binding sites and there may not be enough binding sites for two or more drugs. Also, some drugs induce or inhibit the metabolism of other drugs. Protein binding is also the basis for some important drug–drug interactions. A drug with a strong attraction to protein-binding sites may displace a less tightly bound drug. The displaced drug then becomes pharmacologically active, and the overall effect is the same as taking a larger dose of the displaced drug.

Increased Drug Effects

Interactions that can increase the therapeutic or adverse effects of drugs include the following:

- *Additive effects* occur when two drugs with similar pharmacologic actions are taken.

  Example: ethanol + sedative drug → increased sedation
- *Synergism* or *potentiation* occurs when two drugs with different sites or mechanisms of action produce greater effects when taken together.

  Example: acetaminophen (nonopioid analgesic) + codeine (opioid analgesic) → increased analgesia
- *Interference* by one drug with the metabolism or elimination of a second drug may result in intensified effects of the second drug.

  Example: cimetidine inhibits CYP1A, 2C, and 3A drug-metabolizing enzymes in the liver and therefore interferes with the metabolism of many drugs (eg, benzodiazepine antianxiety and hypnotic drugs; calcium channel blockers; some antidysrhythmics, beta-blockers, and antiseizure drugs; warfarin). When these drugs are given concurrently with cimetidine, they are likely to cause adverse and toxic effects.
- *Displacement* of one drug from plasma protein-binding sites by a second drug increases the effects of the displaced drug. This increase occurs because the displaced drug, freed from its bound form, becomes pharmacologically active.

  Example: aspirin (an anti-inflammatory/analgesic/antipyretic agent) + warfarin (an anticoagulant) → increased anticoagulant effect

Decreased Drug Effects

Interactions in which drug effects are decreased are grouped under the term *antagonism*. Examples of such interactions are as follows:

- An *antidote* drug can be given to antagonize the toxic effects of another drug.

  Example: naloxone (a narcotic antagonist) + morphine (a narcotic or opioid analgesic) → relief of opioid-induced respiratory depression. Naloxone molecules displace morphine molecules from their receptor sites on nerve cells in the brain so that the morphine molecules cannot continue to exert their depressant effects.

- Decreased intestinal absorption of oral drugs occurs when drugs combine to produce nonabsorbable compounds.

  Example: aluminum or magnesium hydroxide (antacids) + oral tetracycline (an antibiotic) → binding of tetracycline to aluminum or magnesium, causing decreased absorption and decreased antibiotic effect of tetracycline

- Activation of drug-metabolizing enzymes in the liver increases the metabolism rate of any drug metabolized mainly by that group of enzymes. Several drugs (eg, phenytoin, rifampin) and cigarette smoking are known *enzyme inducers.*

  Example: phenobarbital (a barbiturate) + warfarin (an anticoagulant) → decreased effects of warfarin

- Increased excretion occurs when urinary pH is changed and renal reabsorption is blocked.

  Example: sodium bicarbonate + phenobarbital → increased excretion of phenobarbital. The sodium bicarbonate alkalinizes the urine and increases drug elimination by the kidneys. This interaction has been used to treat phenobarbital overdoses.

APPLYING YOUR KNOWLEDGE 2-1:
HOW CAN YOU AVOID THIS MEDICATION ERROR?

Mrs. Green has recently switched to felodipine 10 mg qd (a calcium channel blocker) to treat her hypertension. During your most recent visit (3 days ago), you instructed Mrs. Green to take her medication with a large glass of juice and cautioned her to swallow the tablet whole. You also checked her vital signs; her blood pressure was 148/70.

Today, you recheck her vital signs and her blood pressure is 96/60. You ask Mrs. Green about her medication and she tells you that she has been taking it with a large glass of grapefruit juice.

Client-Related Variables

Age

The effects of age on drug action are especially important in neonates, infants, and older adults. In children, drug action depends largely on age and developmental stage.

During pregnancy, drugs cross the placenta and may harm the fetus. Fetuses have no effective mechanisms for metabolizing or eliminating drugs because their liver and kidney functions are immature. Newborn infants (birth to 1 month) also handle drugs inefficiently. Drug distribution, metabolism, and excretion differ markedly in neonates, especially premature infants, because their organ systems are not fully developed. Older infants (1 month to 1 year) reach approximately adult levels of protein binding and kidney function, but liver function and the blood–brain barrier are still immature.

Children (1 to 12 years) have a period of increased activity of drug-metabolizing enzymes so that some drugs are rapidly metabolized and eliminated. Although the onset and duration of this period are unclear, a few studies have been done with particular drugs. Theophylline, for example, is cleared much faster in a 7-year-old child than in a neonate or adult (18–65 years). After approximately 12 years of age, healthy children handle drugs similarly to healthy adults.

In older adults (65 years and older), physiologic changes may alter all pharmacokinetic processes. Changes in the gastrointestinal tract include decreased gastric acidity, decreased blood flow, and decreased motility. Despite these changes, however, there is little difference in drug absorption. Changes in the cardiovascular system include decreased cardiac output and therefore slower distribution of drug molecules to their sites of action, metabolism, and excretion. In the liver, blood flow and metabolizing enzymes are decreased. Thus, many drugs are metabolized more slowly, have a longer action, and are more likely to accumulate with chronic administration. In the kidneys, there is decreased blood flow, decreased glomerular filtration rate, and decreased tubular secretion of drugs. All of these changes tend to slow excretion and promote accumulation of drugs in the body. *Impaired kidney and liver function greatly increase the risks of adverse drug effects.* In addition, older adults are more likely to have acute and chronic illnesses that require the use of multiple drugs or long-term drug therapy. Thus, possibilities for interactions among drugs and between drugs and diseased organs are greatly multiplied.

Body Weight

Body weight affects drug action mainly in relation to dose. The ratio between the amount of drug given and body weight influences drug distribution and concentration at sites of action. In general, people heavier than average may need larger doses, provided that their renal, hepatic, and cardiovascular functions are adequate. Recommended doses for many drugs are listed in terms of grams or milligrams per kilogram of body weight.

Genetic and Ethnic Characteristics

Drugs are given to elicit certain responses that are relatively predictable for most drug recipients. When given the same drug in the same dose, however, some people experience inadequate therapeutic effects, and others experience unusual or exaggerated effects, including increased toxicity. These interindividual variations in drug response are often attributed to genetic or ethnic differences in drug pharmacokinetics or pharmacodynamics. As a result, there is increased awareness that genetic and ethnic characteristics are important factors and that diverse groups must be included in clinical trials.

Genetics

A person's genetic characteristics may influence drug action in several ways. For example, genes determine the types and amounts of proteins produced in the body. When most drugs enter the body, they interact with proteins (eg, in plasma, tissues, cell membranes, drug receptor sites) to reach their sites of action, and they interact with other proteins (eg, drug-metabolizing enzymes in the liver and other organs) to be biotransformed and eliminated from the body. Genetic characteristics that alter any of these proteins can alter drug pharmacokinetics or pharmacodynamics.

One of the earliest genetic variations to be identified derived from the observation that some people taking usual doses of isoniazid (an antitubercular drug), hydralazine (an antihypertensive agent), or procainamide (an antidysrhythmic) showed no therapeutic effects, whereas toxicity developed in other people. Research established that these drugs are normally metabolized by acetylation, a chemical conjugation process in which the drug molecule combines with an acetyl group of acetyl coenzyme A. The reaction is catalyzed by a hepatic drug-metabolizing enzyme called *acetyltransferase*. It was further established that humans may acetylate the drug rapidly or slowly, depending largely on genetically controlled differences in acetyltransferase activity. Clinically, rapid acetylators may need larger-than-usual doses to achieve therapeutic effects, and slow acetylators may need smaller-than-usual doses to avoid toxic effects. In addition, several genetic variations of the cytochrome P450 drug-metabolizing system have been identified. Specific variations may influence any of the chemical processes by which drugs are metabolized.

As another example of genetic variation in drug metabolism, some people are deficient in glucose-6-phosphate dehydrogenase, an enzyme normally found in red blood cells and other body tissues. These people may have hemolytic anemia when given antimalarial drugs, sulfonamides, analgesics, antipyretics, and other drugs.

Ethnicity

Most drug information has been derived from clinical drug trials using white men. Interethnic variations became evident when drugs and dosages developed for Caucasian people produced unexpected responses, including toxicity, when given to individuals from other ethnic groups.

One common variation is that African Americans are less responsive to some antihypertensive drugs than are Caucasians. For example, angiotensin-converting enzyme (ACE) inhibitors and beta-adrenergic blocking drugs are less effective as single-drug therapy. In general, African-American hypertensive clients respond better to diuretics or calcium channel blockers than to ACE inhibitors and beta-blockers. Another variation is that Asians usually require much smaller doses of some commonly used drugs, including beta-blockers and several psychotropic drugs (eg, alprazolam, an antianxiety agent; and haloperidol, an antipsychotic). Some documented interethnic variations are included in later chapters.

Gender

Except during pregnancy and lactation, gender has been considered a minor influence on drug action. Most research studies related to drugs have involved men, and clinicians have extrapolated the findings to women. Several reasons have been advanced for excluding women from clinical drug trials, including the risks to a fetus if a woman becomes pregnant and the greater complexity in sample size and data analysis. However, because differences between men and women in responses to drug therapy are being identified, the need to include women in drug studies is evident.

Some gender-related differences in responses to drugs may stem from hormonal fluctuations in women during the menstrual cycle. Altered responses have been demonstrated in some women taking clonidine, an antihypertensive; lithium, a mood-stabilizing agent; phenytoin, an anticonvulsant; propranolol, a beta-adrenergic blocking drug used in the management of hypertension, angina pectoris, and migraine; and antidepressants. In addition, a significant percentage of women with arthritis, asthma, depression, diabetes mellitus, epilepsy, and migraine experience increased symptoms premenstrually. The increased symptoms may indicate a need for adjustments in their drug therapy regimens. Women with clinical depression, for example, may need higher doses of antidepressant medications premenstrually, if symptoms exacerbate, and lower doses during the rest of the menstrual cycle.

Another example is that women with schizophrenia require lower dosages of antipsychotic medications than men. If given the higher doses required by men, women are likely to have adverse drug reactions.

Pathologic Conditions

Pathologic conditions may alter pharmacokinetic processes (Table 2-1). In general, all pharmacokinetic processes are decreased in cardiovascular disorders characterized by decreased blood flow to tissues, such as heart failure. In addition, the absorption of oral drugs is decreased with various gastrointestinal disorders. Distribution is altered in liver or kidney disease and other conditions that alter plasma proteins. Metabolism is decreased in malnutrition (eg, inadequate protein to synthesize drug-metabolizing enzymes) and severe liver disease; it may be increased in conditions that increase body metabolism, such as hyperthyroidism and fever. Excretion is decreased in kidney disease.

(text continues on page 25)

TABLE 2-1 Effects of Pathologic Conditions on Drug Pharmacokinetics

PATHOLOGIC CONDITION	PHARMACOKINETIC CONSEQUENCES
Cardiovascular disorders that impair the pumping ability of the heart, decrease cardiac output, or impair blood flow to body tissues (eg, acute myocardial infarction, heart failure, hypotension, shock)	*Absorption, distribution, metabolism,* and *excretion* are impaired because of decreased blood flow to sites of drug administration, sites of drug action, the liver, and the kidneys (respectively).
Central nervous system (CNS) disorders that alter respiration or circulation (eg, brain trauma or injury, brain ischemia caused by inadequate cerebral blood flow, drugs that depress or stimulate brain function)	CNS impairment may alter pharmacokinetics by causing hypo- or hyperventilation and acid–base imbalances. Also, cerebral irritation due to head injuries may lead to stimulation of the sympathetic nervous system and increased cardiac output. Increased blood flow may accelerate all pharmacokinetic processes. With faster *absorption* and *distribution,* drug action may be more rapid, but faster *metabolism* and *excretion* may shorten duration of action.
Gastrointestinal (GI) disorders that interfere with GI function or blood flow (eg, trauma or surgery of the GI tract, abdominal infection, paralytic ileus, pancreatitis)	Impaired GI function often occurs with both GI and non-GI disorders, and many patients cannot take oral medications. Those who can take oral drugs may have impaired *absorption* because of vomiting, diarrhea, concurrent use of drugs that raise the pH of gastric fluids (eg, antacids, proton pump inhibitors), or concurrent ingestion of foods or tube feedings that decrease drug absorption. Conversely, crushing tablets or opening capsules to give a drug through a GI tube accelerates absorption.
Inflammatory bowel disorders (eg, Crohn's disease, ulcerative colitis)	*Absorption* of oral drugs is variable. It may be increased because GI hypermotility rapidly delivers drug molecules to sites of absorption in the small intestine and drugs tend to be absorbed more rapidly by inflamed tissue. It may be decreased because hypermotility and diarrhea may move the drug through the GI tract too rapidly to be adequately absorbed.
Endocrine disorders that impair function or change hormonal balance	
Diabetes-induced cardiovascular disorders	Impaired circulation may decrease all pharmacokinetic processes.
Thyroid disorders	The main effect is on *metabolism.* Hypothyroidism slows metabolism, which prolongs drug action and slows elimination. Hyperthyroidism accelerates metabolism, producing a shorter duration of action and a faster elimination rate. Effective treatment of a thyroid disorder returns thyroid function and drug metabolism to normal.
Adrenal disorders resulting from the underlying illness or the stress response that accompanies illness	Increased adrenal function (ie, increased amounts of circulating catecholamines and cortisol) affects drug action by increasing cardiac output, redistributing cardiac output (more blood flow to the heart and brain, less to kidneys, liver, and GI tract), causing fluid retention, and increasing blood volume. Stress also changes plasma protein levels, which can affect the unbound portion of a drug dose. Decreased adrenal function causes hypotension and shock, which impairs all pharmacokinetic processes.
Hepatic disorders that impair hepatic function and blood flow (eg, hepatitis, cirrhosis)	Hepatic *metabolism* depends on hepatic blood flow, hepatic enzyme activity, and plasma protein binding. Increased blood flow increases delivery of drug molecules to hepatocytes, where metabolism occurs, and thereby accelerates drug metabolism. Decreased hepatic blood flow slows metabolism. Severe liver disease or cirrhosis may impair all pharmacokinetic processes. *Absorption* of oral drugs may be decreased in clients with cirrhosis due to edema in the GI tract. *Distribution* may be impaired if the liver is unable

TABLE 2-1 Effects of Pathologic Conditions on Drug Pharmacokinetics (continued)

PATHOLOGIC CONDITION	PHARMACOKINETIC CONSEQUENCES
	to synthesize adequate amounts of plasma proteins, especially albumin. Also, liver impairment leads to inadequate *metabolism* and accumulation of substances (eg, serum bilirubin) that can displace drugs from protein-binding sites. With decreased protein binding, the serum concentration of active drug is increased and the drug is distributed to sites of action and elimination more rapidly. Thus, onset of drug action may be faster, peak blood levels may be higher and cause adverse effects, and the duration of action may be shorter because the drug is metabolized and excreted more quickly. In clients with cirrhosis, oral drugs are distributed directly into the systemic circulation rather than going through the portal circulation and the liver first. This shunting of blood around the liver means that oral drugs that are normally extensively metabolized during their first pass through the liver (eg, propranolol) must be given in reduced doses to prevent high blood levels and toxicity. *Metabolism* may be impaired by disorders that reduce hepatic blood flow. In addition, an impaired liver may not be able to synthesize adequate amounts of drug-metabolizing enzymes. *Excretion* may be increased when protein binding is impaired because larger amounts of free drug are circulating in the bloodstream and being delivered more rapidly to sites of metabolism and excretion. The result is a shorter half-life and duration of action. Excretion is decreased when the liver is unable to metabolize lipid-soluble drugs into water-soluble metabolites that can be excreted by the kidneys.
Renal impairments (eg, acute renal failure [ARF] and chronic renal failure [CRF]) that interfere with GI function (eg, delayed gastric emptying, changes in gastric pH, symptoms such as vomiting and diarrhea); cardiovascular function (eg, changes in extracellular fluid volume [ECF], plasma protein binding, and tissue binding); acid–base balance, or liver function	*Absorption* of oral drugs may be decreased due to GI changes. In CRF, gastric pH may be increased by the use of antacids to bind phosphate. This may decrease the absorption of oral drugs that dissolve in an acidic environment and increase absorption of drugs that dissolve in an alkaline environment. *Distribution* of many drugs may be altered. Water-soluble drugs are distributed throughout the ECF, including edema fluid, which is usually increased because the kidney is less able to eliminate water and sodium. Binding of acidic drugs with albumin is usually decreased because of less albumin or decreased binding capacity of albumin for a drug. Causes of decreased albumin include hypermetabolic states (eg, trauma, sepsis) in which protein breakdown exceeds protein synthesis, nephrotic states in which albumin is lost in the urine, and liver disease that decreases hepatic synthesis of albumin. Causes of reduced binding capacity include structural changes in the albumin molecule and uremic toxins that compete with drugs for binding sites. When less of a drug is bound to albumin, the higher serum drug levels of unbound or active drug can result in drug toxicity. In addition, more unbound drug is available for distribution into tissues and sites of metabolism and excretion so that faster elimination can decrease drug half-life and therapeutic effects. For basic drugs (eg, clindamycin, propafenone), alpha$_1$-acid glycoprotein (AAG) is the main binding protein. The amount of AAG increases in some patients,

(continued)

TABLE 2-1 Effects of Pathologic Conditions on Drug Pharmacokinetics (continued)

PATHOLOGIC CONDITION	PHARMACOKINETIC CONSEQUENCES
	including those who have received renal transplants and those receiving hemodialysis. If these patients are given a basic drug, a larger amount is bound, and a smaller amount is free to exert a pharmacologic effect. Finally, some conditions that often occur in renal impairment (eg, metabolic acidosis, respiratory alkalosis) may alter tissue distribution of some drugs. For example, digoxin can be displaced from tissue-binding sites by metabolic products that cannot be adequately excreted by impaired kidneys. *Metabolism* can be increased, decreased, or unaffected. One factor is alteration of drug metabolism in the liver. In uremia, reduction and hydrolysis reactions may be slower, but oxidation by cytochrome P450 enzymes and conjugation with glucuronide or sulfate usually proceed at normal rates. Another factor is the inability of impaired kidneys to eliminate drugs and pharmacologically active metabolites, which may lead to accumulation and adverse drug reactions with long-term drug therapy. Metabolites may have pharmacologic activity similar to or different from that of the parent drug. A third factor may be impaired renal metabolism of drugs. Although the role of the kidneys in excretion of drugs is well known, their role in drug metabolism has received little attention. The kidney itself contains many of the same metabolizing enzymes found in the liver, including renal cytochrome P450 enzymes, which metabolize a variety of chemicals and drugs. *Excretion* of many drugs and metabolites is reduced. The kidneys normally excrete both the parent drug and metabolites produced by the liver and other tissues. Processes of renal excretion include glomerular filtration, tubular secretion, and tubular reabsorption, all of which may be affected by renal impairment. If the kidneys are unable to excrete drugs and metabolites, some of which may be pharmacologically active, these substances may accumulate and cause adverse or toxic effects.
Respiratory impairment	Respiratory impairment may indirectly affect drug *metabolism.* For example, hypoxemia leads to decreased enzyme production in the liver, decreased efficiency of the enzymes that are produced, and decreased oxygen available for drug biotransformation. Mechanical ventilation leads to decreased blood flow to the liver.
Sepsis-induced alterations in cardiovascular function and hepatic blood flow	Sepsis may affect all pharmacokinetic processes. Early sepsis is characterized by hyperdynamic circulation, with increased cardiac output and shunting of blood to vital organs. As a result, *absorption, distribution, metabolism,* and *excretion* may be accelerated. Late sepsis is characterized by hypodynamic circulation, with diminished cardiac output and reduced blood flow to major organs. Thus, *absorption, distribution, metabolism,* and *excretion* may be impaired.
Shock-induced alterations in cardiovascular function and blood flow	Shock may inhibit all pharmacokinetic processes. *Absorption* is impaired by decreased blood flow to sites of administration; *distribution* is impaired by decreased blood flow to all body tissues; *metabolism* is impaired by decreased blood flow to the liver; and *excretion* is impaired by decreased blood flow to the kidneys.

Psychological Considerations

Psychological considerations influence individual responses to drug administration, although specific mechanisms are unknown. An example is the *placebo response.* A placebo is a pharmacologically inactive substance. Placebos are used in clinical drug trials to compare the medication being tested with a "dummy" medication. Interestingly, recipients often report both therapeutic and adverse effects from placebos.

Attitudes and expectations related to drugs in general, a particular drug, or a placebo influence client response. They also influence compliance or the willingness to carry out the prescribed drug regimen, especially with long-term drug therapy.

Tolerance and Cross-Tolerance

Drug *tolerance* occurs when the body becomes accustomed to a particular drug over time so that larger doses must be given to produce the same effects. Tolerance may be acquired to the pharmacologic action of many drugs, especially opioid analgesics, alcohol, and other CNS depressants. Tolerance to pharmacologically related drugs is called *cross-tolerance.* For example, a person who regularly drinks large amounts of alcohol becomes able to ingest even larger amounts before becoming intoxicated—this is tolerance to alcohol. If the person is then given sedative-type drugs or a general anesthetic, larger-than-usual doses are required to produce a pharmacologic effect—this is cross-tolerance.

Tolerance and cross-tolerance are usually attributed to activation of drug-metabolizing enzymes in the liver, which accelerates drug metabolism and excretion. They also are attributed to decreased sensitivity or numbers of receptor sites.

ADVERSE EFFECTS OF DRUGS

As used in this book, the term *adverse effects* refers to any undesired responses to drug administration, as opposed to *therapeutic effects,* which are desired responses. Most drugs produce a mixture of therapeutic and adverse effects; all drugs can produce adverse effects. Adverse effects may produce essentially any sign, symptom, or disease process and may involve any body system or tissue. They may be common or rare, mild or severe, localized or widespread—depending on the drug and the recipient.

Some adverse effects occur with usual therapeutic doses of drugs (often called *side effects*); others are more likely to occur and to be more severe with high doses. Common or serious adverse effects include the following:

- *CNS effects* may result from CNS stimulation (eg, agitation, confusion, delirium, disorientation, hallucinations, psychosis, seizures) or CNS depression (eg, dizziness, drowsiness, impaired level of consciousness, sedation, coma, impaired respiration and circulation). CNS effects may occur with many drugs, including most therapeutic groups, substances of abuse, and over-the-counter preparations.
- *Gastrointestinal effects* (anorexia, nausea, vomiting, constipation, diarrhea) are common adverse reactions. Nausea and vomiting occur with many drugs as a result of local irritation of the gastrointestinal tract or stimulation of the vomiting center in the brain. Diarrhea occurs with drugs that cause local irritation or increase peristalsis. More serious effects include bleeding or ulceration (most often with aspirin and nonsteroidal anti-inflammatory agents) and severe diarrhea/colitis (most often with antibiotics).
- *Hematologic effects* (blood coagulation disorders, bleeding disorders, bone marrow depression, anemias, leukopenia, agranulocytosis, thrombocytopenia) are relatively common and potentially life threatening. Excessive bleeding is most often associated with anticoagulants and thrombolytics; bone marrow depression is usually associated with antineoplastic drugs.
- *Hepatic effects* (hepatitis, liver dysfunction or failure, biliary tract inflammation or obstruction) are potentially life threatening. Because most drugs are metabolized by the liver, the liver is especially susceptible to drug-induced injury. Drugs that are hepatotoxic include acetaminophen (Tylenol), isoniazid (INH), methotrexate (Trexall), phenytoin (Dilantin), and aspirin and other salicylates. In the presence of drug- or disease-induced liver damage, the metabolism of many drugs is impaired. Consequently, drugs metabolized by the liver tend to accumulate in the body and cause adverse effects. Besides hepatotoxicity, many drugs produce abnormal values in liver function tests without producing clinical signs of liver dysfunction.
- *Nephrotoxicity* (nephritis, renal insufficiency or failure) occurs with several antimicrobial agents (eg, gentamicin and other aminoglycosides), nonsteroidal anti-inflammatory agents (eg, ibuprofen and related drugs), and others. It is potentially serious because it may interfere with drug excretion, thereby causing drug accumulation and increased adverse effects.
- *Hypersensitivity* or *allergy* may occur with almost any drug in susceptible clients. It is largely unpredictable and unrelated to dose. It occurs in those who have previously been exposed to the drug or a similar substance (antigen) and who have developed antibodies. When readministered, the drug reacts with the antibodies to cause cell damage and the release of histamine and other intracellular substances. These substances produce reactions ranging from mild skin rashes to anaphylactic shock. Anaphylactic shock is a life-threatening hypersensitivity reaction characterized by respiratory distress and cardiovascular collapse. It occurs within a few minutes after drug administration and requires emergency treatment with epinephrine. Some allergic reactions (eg, serum sickness) occur 1 to 2 weeks after the drug is given.

- *Drug fever* is a fever associated with administration of a medication. Drugs can cause fever by several mechanisms, including allergic reactions, damaging body tissues, increasing body heat or interfering with its dissipation, or acting on the temperature-regulating center in the brain. The most common mechanism is an allergic reaction. Fever may occur alone or with other allergic manifestations (eg, skin rash, hives, joint and muscle pain, enlarged lymph glands, eosinophilia), and its pattern may be low grade and continuous or spiking and intermittent. It may begin within hours after the first dose if the client has taken the drug before, or within approximately 10 days of continued administration if the drug is new to the client. If the causative drug is discontinued, fever usually subsides within 48 to 72 hours unless drug excretion is delayed or significant tissue damage has occurred (eg, hepatitis).

  Many drugs have been implicated as causes of drug fever, including most antimicrobials, several cardiovascular agents (eg, beta-blockers, hydralazine, procainamide, quinidine), drugs with anticholinergic properties (eg, atropine, some antihistamines, phenothiazine antipsychotic agents, tricyclic antidepressants), and some anticonvulsants.

- *Idiosyncrasy* refers to an unexpected reaction to a drug that occurs the first time it is given. These reactions are usually attributed to genetic characteristics that alter the person's drug-metabolizing enzymes.

- *Drug dependence* (see Chap. 14) may occur with mind-altering drugs, such as opioid analgesics, sedative-hypnotic agents, antianxiety agents, and CNS stimulants. Dependence may be physiologic or psychological. Physiologic dependence produces unpleasant physical symptoms when the dose is reduced or the drug is withdrawn. Psychological dependence leads to excessive preoccupation with drugs and drug-seeking behavior.

- *Carcinogenicity* is the ability of a substance to cause cancer. Several drugs are carcinogens, including some hormones and anticancer drugs. Carcinogenicity apparently results from drug-induced alterations in cellular DNA.

- *Teratogenicity* is the ability of a substance to cause abnormal fetal development when taken by pregnant women. Drug groups considered teratogenic include analgesics, diuretics, antiepileptic drugs, antihistamines, antibiotics, antiemetics, and others.

TOXICOLOGY: DRUG OVERDOSE

Drug toxicity (also called poisoning, overdose, or intoxication) results from excessive amounts of a drug and may cause reversible or irreversible damage to body tissues. It is a common problem in both adult and pediatric populations. It may result from a single large dose or prolonged ingestion of smaller doses and may involve alcohol or prescription, over-the-counter, or illicit drugs. Poisoned clients may be seen in essentially any setting but are especially likely to be encountered in hospital emergency departments.

In some cases, the client or someone accompanying the client may know the toxic agent (eg, accidental overdose of a therapeutic drug, use of an illicit drug, a suicide attempt). Often, however, multiple drugs have been ingested, the causative drugs are unknown, and the circumstances may involve traumatic injury or impaired mental status that make the client unable to provide useful information. Clinical manifestations are often nonspecific for drug overdoses and may indicate other disease processes. Because of the variable presentation of drug intoxication, health care providers must have a high index of suspicion so that toxicity can be rapidly recognized and treated.

Most poisoned or overdosed clients are treated in emergency rooms and discharged to their homes. A few are admitted to intensive care units (ICUs), often because of unconsciousness and the need for endotracheal intubation and mechanical ventilation. Unconsciousness is a major toxic effect of several commonly ingested substances such as benzodiazepine antianxiety and sedative agents, tricyclic antidepressants, ethanol, and opiates. Serious cardiovascular effects (eg, cardiac arrest, dysrhythmias, circulatory impairment) are also common and warrant admission to an ICU.

The main goals of treatment for a poisoned client are starting treatment as soon as possible after drug ingestion, supporting and stabilizing vital functions, preventing further damage from the toxic agent by reducing absorption or increasing elimination, and administering specific antidotes when available and indicated. General aspects of care are described in Box 2-3; selected antidotes are listed in Table 2-2; and specific aspects of care are described in relevant chapters.

Box 2-3 General Management of Toxicity

- The first priority is support of vital functions, as indicated by rapid assessment of vital signs and level of consciousness. In serious poisonings, an electrocardiogram is indicated and findings of severe toxicity (eg, dysrhythmias, ischemia) justify aggressive care. Standard cardiopulmonary resuscitation (CPR) measures may be needed to maintain breathing and circulation. An intravenous (IV) line is usually needed to administer fluids and drugs, and invasive treatment or monitoring devices may be inserted.

  Endotracheal intubation and mechanical ventilation are often required to maintain breathing (in unconscious patients), correct hypoxemia, and protect the airway. Hypoxemia must be corrected quickly to avoid brain injury, myocardial ischemia, and cardiac dysrhythmias. Ventilation with positive end expiratory pressure (PEEP) should be used cautiously in hypotensive patients because it decreases venous return to the heart and worsens hypotension.

  Serious cardiovascular manifestations often require drug therapy. Hypotension and hypoperfusion may be treated with inotropic and vasopressor drugs to increase cardiac output and raise blood pressure. Dysrhythmias are treated according to Advanced Cardiac Life Support (ACLS) protocols.

  Recurring seizures or status epilepticus requires treatment with anticonvulsant drugs.

- For unconscious patients, as soon as an IV line is established, some authorities recommend a dose of naloxone (2 mg IV) for possible narcotic overdose and thiamine (100 mg IV) for possible brain dysfunction due to thiamine deficiency. In addition, a fingerstick blood glucose test should be done and, if hypoglycemia is indicated, a 50% dextrose solution (50 mL IV) should be given.

- After the patient is out of immediate danger, a thorough physical examination and efforts to determine the drug(s), the amounts, and the time lapse since exposure are needed. If the patient is unable to supply needed information, interview anyone else who may be able to do so. Ask about the use of prescription and over-the-counter drugs, alcohol, and illicit substances.

- There are no standard laboratory tests for poisoned patients, but baseline tests of liver and kidney function are usually indicated. Screening tests for toxic substances are not very helpful because test results may be delayed, many substances are not detected, and the results rarely affect initial treatment. Specimens of blood, urine, or gastric fluids may be obtained for laboratory analysis. Serum drug levels are needed when acetaminophen, alcohol, digoxin, lithium, aspirin, or theophylline is known to be an ingested drug, to assist with treatment.

- For most orally ingested drugs, the initial and major treatment is a single dose of activated charcoal. Sometimes called the "universal antidote," it is useful in many poisonings because it adsorbs many toxins and rarely causes complications. When given within 30 minutes of drug ingestion, it decreases absorption of the toxic drug by about 90%; when given an hour after ingestion, it decreases absorption by about 37%. Activated charcoal (1 g/kg of body weight or 50–100 g) is usually mixed with 240 mL of water (25–50 g in 120 mL of water for children) to make a slurry, which is gritty and unpleasant to swallow. It is often given by nasogastric tube. The charcoal blackens subsequent bowel movements. If used with whole bowel irrigation (WBI; see below), activated charcoal should be given before the WBI solution is started. If given during WBI, the binding capacity of the charcoal is decreased. Activated charcoal does not significantly decrease absorption of some drugs (eg, ethanol, iron, lithium, metals).

  Multiple doses of activated charcoal may be given in some instances (eg, ingestion of sustained-release drugs). One regimen is an initial dose of 50 to 100 grams, then 12.5 grams every 1, 2, or 4–6 hours for a few doses.

  Adverse effects of both single and multiple doses of activated charcoal include pulmonary aspiration and bowel obstruction from impaction of the charcoal–drug complex. To prevent these effects, unconscious patients should not receive the drug until the airway is secure against aspiration, and many patients are given a laxative (eg, sorbitol) to aid removal of the charcoal–drug complex.

  Other procedures for gastrointestinal decontamination are no longer routinely used because of minimal effectiveness and potential complications (eg, ipecac-induced vomiting, gastric lavage). Ipecac is rarely used in hospital settings and is no longer recommended to treat poisonings in children in home settings. Parents should call a poison control center or a health care provider. Gastric lavage may be beneficial in serious overdoses if performed within an hour of drug ingestion. If the ingested agent delays gastric emptying (eg, drugs with anticholinergic effects), the time limit may be extended. When used after ingestion of pills or capsules, the tube lumen should be large enough to allow removal of pill fragments.

- Whole bowel irrigation (WBI) with a polyethylene glycol solution (eg, Colyte) is a newer technique for removing toxic ingestions of long-acting, sustained-release drugs (eg, many beta-blockers, calcium channel blockers, and theophylline preparations); enteric-coated drugs; and toxins that do not bind well with activated charcoal (eg, iron, lithium). It may also be helpful in removing packets of illicit drugs, such as cocaine or heroin. When used, 500–2000 mL per hour are given orally or by nasogastric tube until bowel contents are clear. Vomiting is the most common adverse effect. WBI is contraindicated in patients with serious bowel disorders (eg, obstruction, perforation, ileus), hemodynamic instability, or respiratory impairment (unless intubated).

- Urinary elimination of some drugs and toxic metabolites can be accelerated by changing the pH of urine (eg, alkalinizing with IV sodium bicarbonate for salicylate overdose); diuresis; or hemodialysis. Hemodialysis is the treatment of choice in severe lithium and aspirin (salicylate) poisoning.

- Specific antidotes can be administered when available and as indicated by the client's clinical condition. Available antidotes vary widely in effectiveness. Some are very effective and rapidly reverse toxic manifestations (eg, naloxone for opiates, flumazenil for benzodiazepines, specific Fab fragments for digoxin).

  When an antidote is used, its half-life relative to the toxin's half-life must be considered. For example, the half-life of naloxone, a narcotic antagonist, is relatively short compared with the half-life of the longer-acting opiates such as methadone. Similarly, flumazenil has a shorter half-life than most benzodiazepines. Thus, repeated doses of these agents may be needed to prevent recurrence of the toxic state.

TABLE 2-2 Antidotes for Overdoses of Selected Therapeutic Drugs

OVERDOSED DRUG (POISON)	ANTIDOTE	ROUTE AND DOSAGE RANGES	COMMENTS
Acetaminophen (see Chap. 7)	Acetylcysteine (Mucomyst)	PO 140 mg/kg initially, then 70 mg/kg q4h for 17 doses	Dilute 20% solution to a 5% solution with a cola or other soft drink for oral administration
Anticholinergics (atropine; see Chap. 20)	Physostigmine	IV, IM 2 mg; give IV slowly, over at least 2 min	Infrequently used because of its toxicity.
Benzodiazepines (see Chap. 8)	Flumazenil	IV 0.2 mg over 30 sec; if no response, may give additional 0.3 mg over 30 sec. Additional doses of 0.5 mg may be given at 1-min intervals up to a total amount of 3 mg	Should not be given to patients with overdose of unknown drugs or drugs known to cause seizures in overdose (eg, cocaine, lithium)
Beta blockers (see Chap. 18)	Glucagon	IV 50–150 mcg/kg (5–10 mg for adults) over 1 min initially, then 2–5 mg/h by continuous infusion as needed	Glucagon increases myocardial contractility; not FDA-approved for this indication
Calcium channel blockers (see Chaps. 50, 52)	Calcium gluconate 10%	IV 1 g over 5 min; may be repeated	Increases myocardial contractility
Cholinergics (see Chap. 19)	Atropine	Adults: IV 2 mg, repeated as needed Children: IV 0.05 mg/kg, up to 2 mg	If poisoning is due to organophosphates (eg, insecticides), pralidoxime may be given with the atropine.
Digoxin (see Chap. 48)	Digoxin immune Fab (Digibind)	IV 40 mg (1 vial) for each 0.6 mg of digoxin ingested Reconstitute each vial with 4 mL Water for Injection, then dilute with sterile isotonic saline to a convenient volume and give over 30 min, through a 0.22-micron filter. If cardiac arrest seems imminent, may give the dose as a bolus injection.	Recommended for severe toxicity; reverses cardiac and extracardiac symptoms in a few minutes *Note:* Serum digoxin levels increase after antidote administration, but the drug is bound and therefore inactive.
Heparin (see Chap. 54)	Protamine sulfate	IV 1 mg/100 units of heparin, slowly, over at least 10 min; a single dose should not exceed 50 mg	
Iron (see Chap. 57)	Deferoxamine	IM 1 g q8h PRN IV 15 mg/kg/h if hypotensive	Indicated for serum iron levels >500 mg/dL or serum levels >350 mg/dL with GI or cardiovascular symptoms Can bind and remove a portion of an ingested dose; urine becomes red as iron is excreted
Isoniazid (INH)	Pyridoxine	IV 1 g per gram of INH ingested, at rate of 1 g q2–3 min. If	Indicated for management of seizures and correction of acidosis

TABLE 2-2 Antidotes for Overdoses of Selected Therapeutic Drugs (continued)

OVERDOSED DRUG (POISON)	ANTIDOTE	ROUTE AND DOSAGE RANGES	COMMENTS
		amount of INH unknown, give 5 g; may be repeated.	
Lead	Succimer (Chemet)	Children: PO 10 mg/kg q8h for 5 days	
Opioid analgesics (Chap. 6)	Naloxone (Narcan)	Adults: IV 0.4–2 mg PRN Children: IV 0.1 mg/kg per dose	Can also be given IM, Sub-Q, or by endo-tracheal tube
Phenothiazine anti-psychotic agents (see Chap. 9)	Diphenhydramine (Benadryl)	Adults: IV 50 mg Children: IV 1–2 mg/kg, up to a total of 50 mg	Given to relieve extrapyra-midal symptoms (move-ment disorders)
Thrombolytics (see Chap. 54)	Aminocaproic acid (Amicar)	PO, IV infusion, 5 g ini-tially, then 1–1.25 g/h for 8 h or until bleed-ing is controlled; max-imum dose, 30 g/24h	
Tricyclic antidepressants (see Chap. 10)	Sodium bicarbonate	IV 1–2 mEq/kg initially, then continuous IV drip to maintain serum pH of 7.5	To treat cardiac dysrhyth-mias, conduction distur-bances, and hypotension
Warfarin (see Chap. 54)	Vitamin K₁	PO 5–10 mg daily IV (severe overdose) continuous infusion at rate no faster than 1 mg/min	

APPLYING YOUR KNOWLEDGE: ANSWER

2-1 Grapefruit juice interacts with many medications, including felodipine. The serum drug level of felodip-ine increases because the grapefruit juice inhibits the isozyme of cytochrome P450 that is important in the metabolism of felodipine. As the blood level of the drug increases, serious toxic effects can occur. Other juices do not impact cytochrome P450, so it would be safe to have Mrs. Green take her medication with another type of juice or with water. Notify the physi-cian regarding Mrs. Green's hypotension and the drug–food interaction. If Mrs. Green remains on felodipine, she must be cautioned to eliminate grape-fruit juice from her diet.

Review and Application Exercises

Short Answer Exercises

1. Why do nurses need to understand cellular physi-ology in relation to drug therapy?

2. What are some factors that decrease absorption of an oral drug?

3. Drug dosage is a major determinant of both thera-peutic and adverse drug effects. How can you use this knowledge in monitoring a client's response to drug therapy?

4. Does protein binding speed or slow drug distribu-tion to sites of action? Why?

5. Are drugs equally distributed throughout the body? Why or why not?

6. What are the implications of hepatic enzyme induction and inhibition in terms of drug metabo-lism and elimination from the body?

7. For a drug in which biotransformation produces active metabolites, is drug action shortened or lengthened? What difference does this make in client care?

8. Which pharmacokinetic processes are likely to be impaired with severe cardiovascular disease and with severe renal disease?

9. What are the main elements of the receptor theory of drug action?

10. When drug–drug interactions occur, are drug actions increased or decreased?

11. What are some reasons for individual differences in responses to drugs?

NCLEX-Style Questions

12. Pharmacokinetics involve
   a. drug effects on human cells
   b. drug binding with receptors
   c. drug absorption, distribution, metabolism, and elimination
   d. drug stimulation of normal cell functions

13. What is meant by the "first-pass effect"?
   a. drugs initially bind to plasma proteins
   b. initial renal function in drug excretion
   c. the way drugs reach their target cells
   d. initial metabolism of an oral drug before it reaches the systemic circulation

14. A client with liver disease may have impaired
   a. absorption
   b. distribution
   c. metabolism
   d. excretion

15. A client with an overdose of an oral drug usually receives
   a. a specific antidote
   b. activated charcoal
   c. syrup of ipecac
   d. a strong laxative

16. Characteristics of receptors include which of the following?
   a. They are carbohydrates located in cell membranes or inside cells.
   b. They are constantly synthesized and degraded in the body.
   c. They bind with molecules of any drug circulating in the bloodstream.
   d. They regulate the actions of all drugs.

Selected References

Aschenbrenner, D. S., & Chu, J. J. (2004). The treatment of poisoning in children. *American Journal of Nursing, 104*(2), 75–77.

Bauer, L. A. (2002). Clinical pharmacokinetics and pharmacodynamics. In J. T. DiPiro, R. L. Talbert, G. C. Yee, G. R. Matzke, B. G. Wells, & L. M. Posey (Eds.), *Pharmacotherapy: A pathophysiologic approach* (5th ed., pp. 33–54). New York: McGraw-Hill.

Chyka, P. A. (2002). Clinical toxicology. In J. T. DiPiro, R. L. Talbert, G. C. Yee, G. R. Matzke, B. G. Wells, & L. M. Posey (Eds.), *Pharmacotherapy: A pathophysiologic approach* (5th ed., pp. 99–121). New York: McGraw-Hill.

Diasio, R. B. (2004). Principles of drug therapy. In L. Goldman & D. Ausiello (Eds.), *Cecil textbook of medicine* (22nd ed., pp. 124–134). Philadelphia: W. B. Saunders.

Drug facts and comparisons. (Updated monthly). St. Louis: Facts and Comparisons.

Ford, M. D. (2004). Acute poisoning. In L. Goldman & D. Ausiello (Eds.), *Cecil textbook of medicine* (22nd ed., pp. 628–640). Philadelphia: W. B. Saunders.

Green, G. B., Harris, I. S., Lin, G. A., et al. (Eds.). (2004). *The Washington manual of medical therapeutics* (31st ed.). Philadelphia: Lippincott Williams & Wilkins.

Smeltzer, S. C., & Bare, B. G. (2004). *Brunner & Suddarth's textbook of medical-surgical nursing* (10th ed.). Philadelphia: Lippincott Williams & Wilkins.

Administering Medications

OBJECTIVES

After studying this chapter, you will be able to:

1. List the "rights" of drug administration.
2. Discuss knowledge and skills needed to implement the "rights" of drug administration.
3. List requirements of a complete drug order or prescription.
4. Accurately interpret drug orders containing common abbreviations.
5. Differentiate drug dosage forms for various routes and purposes of administration.
6. Discuss advantages and disadvantages of oral, parenteral, and topical routes of drug administration.
7. Identify supplies, techniques, and observations needed for safe and accurate administration of drugs by different routes.

APPLYING YOUR KNOWLEDGE

Juan Sanchez is transferred to your rehabilitation facility after a cerebral vascular accident (stroke) 2 weeks ago. When you review his chart, it indicates he has right-sided hemiparesis and memory deficits.

INTRODUCTION

Drugs given for therapeutic purposes are called *medications.* Giving medications to clients is an important nursing responsibility in many health care settings, including ambulatory care, hospitals, long-term care facilities, and clients' homes. The basic requirements for accurate drug administration are often called the "five rights":

1. Right *drug*
2. Right *dose*
3. Right *client*
4. Right *route*
5. Right *time*

Some people add a sixth "right:" *documentation.* These "rights" require knowledge of the drugs to be given and the clients who are to receive them as well as specific nursing skills and interventions. When one of these "rights" is violated, medication errors can occur. Nurses need to recognize circumstances in which errors are likely to occur and intervene to prevent errors and protect clients. This chapter is concerned with safe and accurate medication administration.

GENERAL PRINCIPLES OF ACCURATE DRUG ADMINISTRATION

The following principles should be followed:

- Follow the "rights" consistently.
- Learn essential information about each drug to be given (eg, indications for use, contraindications, therapeutic effects, adverse effects, any specific instructions about administration).
- Interpret the prescriber's order accurately (ie, drug name, dose, frequency of administration). Question the prescriber if any information is unclear or if the drug seems inappropriate for the client's condition.
- Read labels of drug containers for the drug name and concentration (usually in milligrams per tablet, capsule, or milliliter of solution). Many medications are available in different dosage forms and concentrations, and it is extremely important that the correct ones be used.
- Minimize the use of abbreviations for drug names, doses, routes of administration, and times of administration.

This promotes safer administration and reduces errors. When abbreviations are used by prescribers or others, interpret them accurately or question the writers about intended meanings.

- Calculate doses accurately. Current nursing practice requires few dosage calculations (most are done by pharmacists). However, when they are needed, accuracy is essential. For medications with a narrow safety margin or potentially serious adverse effects, ask a pharmacist or a colleague to do the calculation also and compare the results. This is especially important when calculating children's dosages.

- Measure doses accurately. Ask a colleague to double-check measurements of insulin and heparin, unusual doses (ie, large or small), and any drugs to be given intravenously.

- Use the correct procedures and techniques for all routes of administration. For example, use appropriate anatomic landmarks to identify sites for intramuscular (IM) injections, follow the manufacturers' instructions for preparation and administration of intravenous (IV) medications, and use sterile materials and techniques for injectable and eye medications.

- Seek information about the client's medical diagnoses and condition in relation to drug administration (eg, ability to swallow oral medications; allergies or contraindications to ordered drugs; new signs or symptoms that may indicate adverse effects of administered drugs; heart, liver, or kidney disorders that may interfere with the client's ability to eliminate drugs).

- Verify the identity of all clients before administering medications; check identification bands on clients who have them (eg, in hospitals or long-term care facilities).

- Omit or delay doses as indicated by the client's condition, and report or record omissions appropriately.

- Be especially vigilant when giving medications to children, because there is a high risk of medication errors for several reasons (Box 3-1).

Box 3-1 Factors Contributing to Medication Errors in Children

- Children vary greatly: in age, from birth to 18 years; and in weight, from 2–3 kilograms (kg) to 100 kg or more.
- Most drugs have not been tested in children.
- Many drugs are marketed in dosage forms and concentrations suitable for adults, often requiring dilution, calculation, preparation, and administration of very small doses.
- Children have limited sites for administration of intravenous (IV) drugs, and several drugs may be given through the same site. In many cases, the need for small volumes of fluid limits flushing between drugs (which may produce undesirable interactions with other drugs and IV solutions).

In 1998, the Food and Drug Administration (FDA) published a requirement that new drugs likely to be important or frequently used in the treatment of children should be labeled with instructions for safe pediatric use.

LEGAL RESPONSIBILITIES

Registered and licensed practical nurses are legally empowered, under state nurse practice acts, to give medications ordered by licensed physicians and dentists. In some states, nurse practitioners may prescribe medications.

When giving medications, the nurse is legally responsible for safe and accurate administration. This means that the nurse may be held liable for not giving a drug or for giving a wrong drug or a wrong dose. In addition, *the nurse is expected to have sufficient drug knowledge to recognize and question erroneous orders.* If, after questioning the prescriber and seeking information from other authoritative sources, the nurse considers that giving a drug is unsafe, the nurse must refuse to give the drug. The fact that a physician wrote an erroneous order does not excuse the nurse from legal liability if he or she carries out that order.

The nurse also is legally responsible for actions delegated to people who are inadequately prepared for or legally barred from administering medications (eg, nursing assistants). However, certified medical assistants (CMAs) may administer medications in physicians' offices, and certified medication aides (nursing assistants with a short course of training, also called CMAs) often administer medications in long-term care facilities.

The nurse who consistently follows safe practices in giving medications does not need to be excessively concerned about legal liability. The basic techniques and guidelines described in this chapter are aimed at safe and accurate preparation and administration. Most errors result when these practices are not followed.

Legal responsibilities in other aspects of drug therapy are less clear-cut. However, in general, nurses are expected to monitor clients' responses to drug therapy (eg, therapeutic and adverse effects) and to teach clients safe and effective self-administration of drugs when indicated. These aspects are described more fully in Chapter 4.

MEDICATION ERRORS

Increasing attention is being paid to medication errors. Much of this interest stems from a 1999 report of the Institute of Medicine, which estimated that 44,000 to 98,000 deaths occur each year in the United States because of medical errors, including medication errors. The report cited studies indicating that in 1993, 7,000 deaths resulted from medication errors. In a later study of 1,116 hospitals, 430,586 medication errors occurred in approximately 5% of admitted patients. In 913 of these hospitals, more than 17,000 errors

(0.25% of admitted patients) reportedly caused adverse client outcomes (usually described as serious illness, conditions that prolong hospitalization or require additional treatment, or death). Other studies have reported that common errors include giving an incorrect dose, not giving an ordered drug, and giving an unordered drug. Specific drugs often associated with errors include insulin, heparin, and warfarin.

Because many errors are associated with medication orders and administration in hospitals, two systems may be used to reduce errors.

- Computerized ordering, in which a health care provider types a medication order directly into a computer. This decreases errors associated with illegible handwriting and erroneous transcription or dispensing.
- Bar coding of medications and patients' identification bands, which is being implemented. In 2004, the FDA passed a regulation requiring drug manufacturers to put bar codes on current prescription medications and non-prescription medications that are commonly used in hospitals by early 2006. New drugs must have bar codes within 60 days of their approval.

Several steps and numerous people are involved in giving the proper dose of a medication to the intended client. Each step or person has a potential for contributing to a medication error or preventing a medication error. All health care providers involved in drug therapy must be extremely vigilant in all phases of drug administration.

MEDICATION SYSTEMS

Each health care facility has a system for distributing drugs. The unit-dose system, in which most drugs are dispensed in single-dose containers for individual clients, is widely used. In this system, drug orders are checked by a pharmacist or pharmacy technician, who then places the indicated number of doses in the client's medication drawer at scheduled intervals. When a dose is due to be taken, the nurse removes the medication and gives it to the client. *Unit-dose wrappings of oral drugs should be left in place until the nurse is in the presence of the client and ready to give the medication.* Each dose of a drug must be recorded on the client's medication administration record (MAR) as soon as possible after administration. With bar-code scanning systems, doses are recorded automatically.

Increasingly, institutions are using automated, computerized, locked cabinets for which each nurse on a unit has a password or code for accessing the cabinet and obtaining a drug dose. An inventory is maintained, and drugs are restocked as needed.

Controlled drugs, such as opioid analgesics, are usually kept as a stock supply in a locked drawer or automated cabinet and replaced as needed. Each dose is signed for and recorded on the client's MAR. Each nurse must comply with legal regulations and institutional policies for dispensing and recording controlled drugs.

Bar-coding technology also may be implemented. Bar codes operate with other hospital computer systems and databases that contain a patient's medication orders and MAR. The bar code on the drug label contains the identification number, strength, and dosage form of the drug, and the bar code on the patient's wristband contains the MAR, which can be displayed when a nurse uses a handheld scanning device.

When administering medications, the nurse scans the bar code on the drug label, on the patient's identification band, and on the nurse's personal identification badge. A wireless computer network processes the scanned information; gives an error message on the scanner if the drug, dose, or time is incorrect for the patient; and updates the MAR. The FDA estimates that it will take about 20 years for all U.S. hospitals to implement this system of bar codes for medication administration.

For nurses, implementing the bar-coding technology increases the time requirements and interferes with their ability to individualize client care in relation to medications. Since 1995, the Veterans Health Administration (VHA) has used bar coding. In 2000, the VHA mandated that all its medical centers label medications with bar codes that could be scanned using handheld devices, and it required the use of bar codes on IV medications by November 30, 2002.

The VHA system, which continues to be updated, works well with routine medications, but nonroutine situations (eg, variable doses or times of administration) may pose problems. In addition, in long-term care facilities, it may be difficult to maintain legible bar codes on patient identification bands. Despite some drawbacks, bar coding increases patient safety and therefore should be supported by nurses as it continues to develop.

MEDICATION ORDERS

Medication orders should include the full name of the client; the generic or trade name of the drug; the dose, route, and frequency of administration; ~~and the~~ date, time, and signature of the prescriber.

Orders in a health care facility may be handwritten on an order sheet in the client's medical record or typed into a computer (the preferred method). Occasionally, verbal or telephone orders are acceptable. They are written on the client's order sheet, signed by the person taking the order, and later countersigned by the prescriber. After the order is written, a copy is sent to the pharmacy, where the order is recorded and the drug is dispensed to the appropriate client care unit. In many facilities, pharmacy staff prepare a computer-generated MAR for each 24-hour period.

For clients in ambulatory care settings, the procedure is essentially the same for drugs to be given immediately. For drugs to be taken at home, written prescriptions are given. In addition to the previous information, a prescription should include instructions for taking the drug (eg, dose, frequency) and whether the prescription can be refilled. Prescriptions for Schedule II controlled drugs cannot be refilled.

To interpret medication orders accurately, the nurse must know commonly used abbreviations for routes, dosages, and times of drug administration (Table 3-1). If the nurse cannot read the physician's order or if the order seems erroneous, he or she must question the order before giving the drug.

APPLYING YOUR KNOWLEDGE 3-1:
HOW CAN YOU AVOID THIS MEDICATION ERROR?

You are administering 6 A.M. medications to a client on a busy medical unit. You enter Mr. Gonzales's room, gently shake him awake, and call him by name. He slowly awakens and appears groggy. You explain that you have his medications, which he takes and then quickly falls back to sleep. On exiting the room, you look at the room number and realize that you just gave medications to Mr. Sanchez.

TABLE 3-1 Common Abbreviations

ROUTES OF DRUG ADMINISTRATION

IM	intramuscular
IV	intravenous
OD	right eye*
OS	left eye*
OU	both eyes*
PO	by mouth, oral
SL	sublingual
Sub-Q	subcutaneous

DRUG DOSAGES

cc	cubic centimeter
g	gram
gr	grain
gt	drop†
mg	milligram
mL	milliliter
oz	ounce
tbsp	tablespoon
tsp	teaspoon

TIMES OF DRUG ADMINISTRATION

ac	before meals
ad lib	as desired
bid	twice daily
hs	bedtime
pc	after meals
PRN	as needed
qd	every day, daily
q4h	every four hours
qid	four times daily
qod	every other day
stat	immediately
tid	three times daily

---

*Because of errors made with the abbreviations, some authorities recommend spelling out the site (eg, right eye).

†drops, gtt.

DRUG PREPARATIONS AND DOSAGE FORMS

Drug preparations and dosage forms vary according to the drug's chemical characteristics, reason for use, and route of administration. Some drugs are available in only one dosage form, and others are available in several forms. Characteristics of various dosage forms are described as follows and in Table 3-2.

Dosage forms of systemic drugs include liquids, tablets, capsules, suppositories, and transdermal and pump delivery systems. Systemic liquids are given orally, or PO (Latin *per os,* "by mouth"), or by injection. Those given by injection must be sterile.

Tablets and capsules are given PO. Tablets contain active drug plus binders, colorants, preservatives, and other substances. Capsules contain active drug enclosed in a gelatin capsule. Most tablets and capsules dissolve in the acidic fluids of the stomach and are absorbed in the alkaline fluids of the upper small intestine. Enteric-coated tablets and capsules are coated with a substance that is insoluble in stomach acid. This delays dissolution until the medication reaches the intestine, usually to avoid gastric irritation or to keep the drug from being destroyed by gastric acid. Tablets for sublingual (under the tongue) or buccal (held in cheek) administration must be specifically formulated for such use.

Several controlled-release dosage forms and drug delivery systems are available, and more continue to be developed. These formulations maintain more consistent serum drug levels and allow less frequent administration, which is more convenient for clients. Oral tablets and capsules are called by a variety of names (eg, timed release, sustained release, extended release) and their names usually include SR, XL, or other indications that they are long-acting formulations. Most of these formulations are given once or twice daily. Some drugs (eg, alendronate for osteoporosis, fluoxetine for major depression) are available in formulations that deliver a full week's dosage in one oral tablet. *Because controlled-release tablets and capsules contain high amounts of drug intended to be absorbed slowly and act over a prolonged period of time, they should never be broken, opened, crushed, or chewed. Such an action allows the full dose to be absorbed immediately and constitutes an overdose, with potential organ damage or death.* Transdermal (skin patch) formulations include systemically absorbed clonidine, estrogen, fentanyl, and nitroglycerin. These medications are slowly absorbed from the skin patches over varying periods of time (eg, 1 week for clonidine and estrogen). Pump delivery systems may be external or implanted under the skin and refillable or long acting without refills. Pumps are used to administer insulin, opioid analgesics, antineoplastics, and other drugs.

TABLE 3-2 Drug Dosage Forms

DOSAGE FORMS AND THEIR ROUTES OF ADMINISTRATION	CHARACTERISTICS	CONSIDERATIONS/PRECAUTIONS
Tablets		
Regular: PO, GI tube (crushed and mixed with water)	• Contain active drug plus binders, dyes, preservatives • Dissolve in gastric fluids	8 oz of water recommended when taken orally, to promote dissolution and absorption
Chewable: PO	Colorful and flavored, mainly for young children who are unable to swallow or who refuse regular tablets	Colors and flavors appeal to children; keep out of reach to avoid accidental overdose.
Enteric coated: PO	Dissolve in small intestine rather than stomach; mainly used for medications that cause gastric irritation	*Do not crush;* instruct clients not to chew or crush.
Extended release (XL): PO	• Also called sustained release (SR), long acting (LA), and others • Formulated for slow absorption and prolonged action • Effects of most last 12–24 hours • Contain relatively large doses of active drug	**Warning:** Crushing to give orally or through a GI tube administers an overdose, with potentially serious adverse effects or death!! *Never crush;* instruct clients not to chew or crush.
Sublingual: Under the tongue *Buccal:* Held in cheek	• Dissolve quickly • Medication absorbed directly into the bloodstream and exerts rapid systemic effects	Few medications formulated for administration by these routes
Capsules		
Regular: PO	• Contain active drug, fillers, and preservatives in a gelatin capsule • Gelatin capsules dissolve in gastric fluid and release medication	As with oral tablets, 8 oz of fluid recommended to promote dissolution of capsule and absorption of medication
Extended release (XL): PO	• Also called sustained release (SR), long acting (LA), and others • Formulated for slow absorption and prolonged action • Effects of most last 12–24 hours • Contain relatively large doses of active drug	**Warning:** Emptying a capsule to give the medication orally or through a GI tube administers an overdose, with potentially serious adverse effects or death!! Instruct clients not to bite, chew, or empty these capsules.
Solutions		
Oral: PO, GI tube	• Absorbed rapidly because they do not need to be dissolved	Use of appropriate measuring devices and accurate measurement are extremely important.
Parenteral: IV, IM, Sub-Q, intradermal	• Medications and all administration devices must be sterile • IV produces rapid effects; Sub-Q is used mainly for insulin and heparin; IM is used for only a few drugs; intradermal is used mainly to inject skin-test material rather than therapeutic drugs.	Use of appropriate equipment (eg, needles, syringes, IV administration sets) and accurate measurement are extremely important. Insulin syringes should always be used for insulin, and tuberculin syringes are recommended for measuring small amounts of other drugs.

(continued)

TABLE 3-2 Drug Dosage Forms (continued)

DOSAGE FORMS AND THEIR ROUTES OF ADMINISTRATION	CHARACTERISTICS	CONSIDERATIONS/PRECAUTIONS
Suspensions PO, Sub-Q (eg, NPH, Lente insulins)	• These are particles of active drug suspended in a liquid; the liquid must be rotated or shaken before measuring a dose.	Drug particles settle to the bottom on standing. If not remixed, the liquid vehicle is given rather than the drug dose.
Dermatologic Creams, Lotions, Ointments Topically to skin	• Most are formulated for minimal absorption through skin and for local effects at the site of application; medications in skin patch formulations are absorbed and exert systemic effects.	Formulations vary with intended uses and are not interchangeable. When removed from the client, skin patches must be disposed of properly to prevent someone else from being exposed to the active drug remaining in the patch.
Solutions and Powders for Oral or Nasal Inhalation, Including Metered Dose Inhalers (MDIs)	• Oral inhalations are used mainly for asthma; nasal sprays for nasal allergies (allergic rhinitis) • Effective with less systemic effect than oral drugs • Deliver a specified dose per inhalation	Several research studies indicate that patients often do not use MDIs correctly and sometimes are incorrectly taught by health care providers. Correct use is essential to obtaining therapeutic effects and avoiding adverse effects.
Eye Solutions and Ointments	• Should be sterile • Most are packaged in small amounts, to be used by a single patient	Can be systemically absorbed and cause systemic adverse effects
Throat Lozenges	• Used for cough and sore throat	
Ear Solutions	• Used mainly for ear infections	
Vaginal Creams and Suppositories	• Formulated for insertion into the vagina • Commonly used to treat vaginal infections	
Rectal Suppositories and Enemas	• Formulated for insertion into the rectum • Suppositories may be used to administer sedatives, analgesics, laxatives • Medicated enemas are used to treat inflammatory bowel diseases (eg, ulcerative colitis)	Effects somewhat unpredictable because absorption is erratic

GI, gastrointestinal; IM, intramuscular; IV, intravenous; PO, oral; Sub-Q, subcutaneous.

Solutions, ointments, creams, and suppositories are applied topically to skin or mucous membranes. They are formulated for the intended route of administration. For example, several drugs are available in solutions for nasal or oral inhalation; they are usually self-administered as a spray into the nose or mouth.

Many combination products containing fixed doses of two or more drugs are also available. Commonly used combinations include analgesics, antihypertensive drugs, and cold remedies. Most are oral tablets, capsules, or solutions.

CALCULATING DRUG DOSAGES

When calculating drug dosages, the importance of accuracy cannot be overemphasized. Accuracy requires basic skills in mathematics, knowledge of common units of measurement, and methods of using data in performing calculations.

Systems of Measurement

The most commonly used system of measurement is the *metric system,* in which the meter is used for linear measure, the gram for weight, and the liter for volume. One milliliter (mL) equals 1 cubic centimeter (cc), and both equal 1 gram (g) of water. The *apothecary system,* now obsolete and rarely used, has units called grains, minims, drams, ounces, pounds, pints, and quarts. The *household system,* with units of drops, teaspoons, tablespoons, and cups, is infrequently used in health care agencies but may be used at home. Table 3-3 lists equivalent measurements within and among these systems. Equivalents are approximate.

A few drugs are ordered and measured in terms of units or milliequivalents (mEq). *Units* express biologic activity in animal tests (ie, the amount of drug required to produce a particular response). Units are unique for each drug. For example, concentrations of insulin and heparin are both expressed in units, but there is no relation between a unit of insulin and a unit of heparin. These drugs are usually ordered in the number of units per dose (eg, NPH insulin 30 units subcutaneously [Sub-Q] every morning, or heparin 5000 units Sub-Q q12h) and labeled in number of units per milliliter (U 100 insulin contains 100 units/mL; heparin may have 1000, 5000, or 10,000 units/mL). *Milliequivalents* express the ionic activity of a drug. Drugs such as potassium chloride are ordered and labeled in the number of milliequivalents per dose, tablet, or milliliter.

Mathematical Calculations

Most drug orders and labels are expressed in metric units of measurement. If the amount specified in the order is the same as that on the drug label, no calculations are required, and preparing the right dose is a simple matter. For example, if the order reads "ibuprofen 400 mg PO" and the drug label reads "ibuprofen 400 mg per tablet," it is clear that one tablet is to be given.

What happens if the order calls for a 400-mg dose and 200-mg tablets are available? The question is, "How many 200-mg tablets are needed to give a dose of 400 mg?" In this case, the answer can be readily calculated mentally to indicate two tablets. This is a simple example that also can be used to illustrate mathematical calculations. This problem can be solved by several acceptable methods; the following formula is presented because of its relative simplicity for students lacking a more familiar method.

$$\frac{D}{H} = \frac{X}{V}$$

D = desired dose (dose ordered, often in milligrams)
H = on-hand or available dose (dose on the drug label; often in mg per tablet, capsule, or milliliter)
X = unknown (number of tablets, in this example)
V = unit (one tablet, in this example)

$$\frac{400 \text{ mg}}{200 \text{ mg}} = \frac{X \text{ tablet}}{1 \text{ tablet}}$$

Cross multiply:

$$200X = 400$$

$$X = \frac{400}{200} = 2 \text{ tablets}$$

What happens if the order and the label are written in different units? For example, the order may read "amoxicillin 0.5 g" and the label may read "amoxicillin 500 mg/capsule." To calculate the number of capsules needed for the dose, the first step is to convert 0.5 g to the equivalent number of milligrams, or convert 500 mg to the equivalent number of grams. The desired or ordered dose and the available or label dose *must* be in the same units of measurement. Using the equivalents (ie, 1 g = 1000 mg) listed in Table 3-3, an equation can be set up as follows:

$$\frac{1 \text{ g}}{1000 \text{ mg}} = \frac{0.5 \text{ g}}{X \text{ mg}}$$

$$X = 0.5 \times 1000 = 500 \text{ mg}$$

The next step is to use the new information in the formula, which then becomes:

$$\frac{D}{H} = \frac{X}{V}$$

$$\frac{500 \text{ mg}}{500 \text{ mg}} = \frac{X \text{ capsules}}{1 \text{ capsule}}$$

TABLE 3-3 Equivalents

METRIC	APOTHECARY	HOUSEHOLD
1 mL = 1 cc	= 15 or 16 minims	= 15 or 16 drops
4 or 5 mL	= 1 fluid dram	= 1 tsp
60 or 65 mg	= 1 gr	
30 or 32 mg	= ½ gr	
30 g = 30 mL	= 1 oz	= 2 tbsp
250 mL	= 8 oz	= 1 cup
454 g	= 1 lb	
500 mL = 500 cc	= 16 oz	= 1 pint
1 L = 1000 mL	= 32 oz	= 1 quart
1000 mcg	= 1 mg	
1000 mg	= 1 g	
1000 g = 1 kg	= 2.2 lb	= 2.2 lb
0.6 g = 600 mg or 650 mg	= 10 gr	

gr, grain; mcg, microgram.

$$500X = 500$$

$$X = \frac{500}{500} = 1 \text{ capsule}$$

The same procedure and formula can be used to calculate portions of tablets or doses of liquids. These are illustrated in the following problems:

1. Order: 25 mg PO
   Label: 50-mg tablet

   $$\frac{25 \text{ mg}}{50 \text{ mg}} = \frac{X \text{ tablet}}{1 \text{ tablet}}$$

   $$50X = 25$$

   $$X = \frac{25}{50} = 0.5 \text{ tablet}$$

2. Order: 25 mg IM
   Label: 50 mg in 1 cc

   $$\frac{25 \text{ mg}}{50 \text{ mg}} = \frac{X \text{ cc}}{1 \text{ cc}}$$

   $$50X = 25$$

   $$X = \frac{25}{50} = 0.5 \text{ cc}$$

3. Order: 4 mg IV
   Label: 10 mg/mL

   $$\frac{4 \text{ mg}}{10 \text{ mg}} = \frac{X \text{ mL}}{1 \text{ mL}}$$

   $$10X = 4$$

   $$X = \frac{4}{10} = 0.4 \text{ mL}$$

4. Order: Heparin 5000 units
   Label: Heparin 10,000 units/mL

   $$\frac{5000 \text{ units}}{10,000 \text{ units}} = \frac{X \text{ mL}}{1 \text{ mL}}$$

   $$10,000X = 5000$$

   $$X = \frac{5000}{10,000} = 0.5 \text{ mL}$$

5. Order: KCl 20 mEq
   Label: KCl 10 mEq/5 mL

   $$\frac{20 \text{ mEq}}{10 \text{ mEq}} = \frac{X \text{ mL}}{5 \text{ mL}}$$

   $$10X = 100$$

   $$X = \frac{100}{10} = 10 \text{ mL}$$

ROUTES OF ADMINISTRATION

Routes of administration depend on drug characteristics, client characteristics, and desired responses. The major routes are oral, parenteral, and topical. Each has advantages, disadvantages, indications for use, and specific techniques of administration (Table 3-4).

Oral and Topical Medications

Both oral and topical drugs are known for their ease of administration (see Table 3-4).

Parenteral Medications

The term *parenteral* refers to any route other than gastrointestinal (enteral) but is commonly used to indicate Sub-Q, IM, and IV injections. Injections require special drug preparations, equipment, and techniques. General characteristics are described below; specific considerations for the IV route are described in Box 3-2.

Parenteral drugs must be prepared, packaged, and administered in ways to maintain sterility. Vials are closed glass or plastic containers with rubber stoppers through which a sterile needle can be inserted for withdrawing medication. Single-dose vials usually do not contain a preservative and must be discarded after a dose is withdrawn. Multiple-dose vials contain a preservative and may be reused if aseptic technique is maintained.

Ampules are sealed glass containers, the tops of which must be broken off to allow insertion of a needle and withdrawal of the medication. Broken ampules and any remaining medication are discarded; they are no longer sterile and cannot be reused. When vials or ampules contain a powder form of the drug, a sterile solution of water or 0.9% sodium chloride must be added and the drug dissolved before withdrawal. Use a filter needle to withdraw the medication from an ampule or vial because broken glass or rubber fragments may need to be removed from the drug solution. Replace the filter needle with a regular needle before injecting the client.

Many injectable drugs (eg, morphine, heparin) are available in prefilled syringes with attached needles. These units are inserted into specially designed holders and used like other needle/syringe units.

Equipment for Injections

Sterile needles and syringes are used to measure and administer parenteral medications; they may be packaged together or separately. Needles are available in various gauges and lengths. The term *gauge* refers to lumen size, with larger numbers indicating smaller lumen sizes. For example, a 25-gauge needle is smaller than an 18-gauge needle. Choice of needle gauge and length depends on the route of administration, the viscosity (thickness) of the solution to be given, and the size of

TABLE 3-4 Routes of Drug Administration

ROUTE AND DESCRIPTION	ADVANTAGES	DISADVANTAGES	COMMENTS
Oral	• Simple and can be used by most people • Convenient; does not require complex equipment • Relatively inexpensive	• Amount of drug acting on body cells is unknown because varying portions of a dose are absorbed and some drug is metabolized in the liver before reaching the bloodstream for circulation • Slow drug action • Irritation of gastrointestinal mucosa by some drugs	The oral route should generally be used when possible, considering the client's condition and ability to take or tolerate oral drugs.
Gastrointestinal (GI) tubes (eg, nasogastric, gastrostomy)	• Allows use of GI tract in clients who cannot take oral drugs • Can be used over long periods of time, if necessary • May avoid or decrease injections	• With nasogastric tubes, medications may be aspirated into the lungs • Small-bore tubes often become clogged • Requires special precautions to give correctly and avoid complications	• Liquid preparations are preferred over crushed tablets and emptied capsules, when available. • Tube should be rinsed before and after instilling medication.
Subcutaneous (Sub-Q) injection—injection of drugs under the skin, into the underlying fatty tissue	• Relatively painless • Very small needles can be used • Insulin and heparin, commonly used medications that often require multiple daily injections, can be given Sub-Q	• Only a small amount of drug (up to 1 mL) can be given • Drug absorption is relatively slow • Only a few drugs can be given Sub-Q	The Sub-Q route is commonly used for only a few drugs because many drugs are irritating to Sub-Q tissues. Such drugs may cause pain, necrosis, and abscess formation if injected Sub-Q.
Intramuscular (IM) injection—injection of drugs into selected muscles	• May be used for several drugs • Drug absorption is rapid because muscle tissue has an abundant blood supply	• A relatively small amount of drug (up to 3 mL) can be given • Risks of damage to blood vessels or nerves if needle is not positioned correctly	It is very important to use anatomic landmarks when selecting IM injection sites.
Intravenous (IV) injection—injection of a drug into the bloodstream	• Allows medications to be given to a patient who cannot take fluids or drugs by GI tract • Bypasses barriers to drug absorption that occur with other routes • Rapid drug action • Larger amounts can be given than by Sub-Q and IM routes • Allows slow administration when indicated	• Time and skill required for venipuncture and maintaining an IV line • After it is injected, drug cannot be retrieved if adverse effects or overdoses occur • High potential for adverse reactions due to rapid drug action and possible complications of IV therapy (ie, bleeding, infection, fluid overload, extravasation) • Phlebitis commonly occurs and increases risks of thrombosis • Phlebitis and thrombosis cause discomfort or pain, may take days or weeks to subside, and limit the veins available for future therapy	• The nurse should wear latex gloves to start IV infusions, for protection against exposure to bloodborne pathogens. • Phlebitis and thrombosis result from injury to the endothelial cells that form the inner lining (intima) of veins and may be caused by repeated venipunctures, the IV catheter, hypertonic IV fluid, or irritating drugs.

(continued)

TABLE 3-4 Routes of Drug Administration (continued)

ROUTE AND DESCRIPTION	ADVANTAGES	DISADVANTAGES	COMMENTS
Topical administration—application to skin or mucous membranes. Application to mucous membranes includes drugs given by nasal or oral inhalation; by instillation into the lungs, eyes, or nose; and by insertion under the tongue (sublingual), into the cheek (buccal), and into the vagina or rectum.	• With application to intact skin, most medications act at the site of application, with little systemic absorption or systemic adverse effects. • Some drugs are given topically for systemic effects (eg, medicated skin patches). Effects may last several days, and the patches are usually convenient for clients. • With application to mucous membranes, most drugs are well and rapidly absorbed	• Some drugs irritate skin or mucous membranes and cause itching, rash, or discomfort • With inflamed, abraded, or damaged skin, drug absorption is increased and systemic adverse effects may occur • Application to mucous membranes may cause systemic adverse effects (eg, beta blocker eye drops, used to treat glaucoma, can cause bradycardia just as oral beta blockers can) • Specific drug preparations must be used for the various routes (ie, dermatologics for skin; ophthalmics for eyes; sublingual, buccal, vaginal, and rectal preparations for those sites).	When available and effective, topical drugs are often preferred over oral or injected drugs, because of fewer and/or less severe systemic adverse effects.

the client. Usually, a 25-gauge, ⅝-inch needle is used for Sub-Q injections, and a 22- or 20-gauge, 1½-inch needle is used for IM injections. Other needle sizes are available for special uses, such as for insulin or intradermal injections. When needles are used, avoid recapping them and dispose of them in appropriate containers. Such containers are designed to prevent accidental needle-stick injuries to health care and housekeeping personnel.

In many settings, needleless systems are being used. These systems involve a plastic tip on the syringe that can be used to enter vials and injection sites on IV tubing. Openings created by the tip reseal themselves. Needleless systems were developed because of the risk of injury and spread of blood-borne pathogens, such as the viruses that cause acquired immunodeficiency syndrome and hepatitis B.

Syringes also are available in various sizes. The 3-milliliter size is probably used most often. It is usually plastic and is available with or without an attached needle. Syringes are calibrated so that drug doses can be measured accurately. However, the calibrations vary according to the size and type of syringe.

Insulin and tuberculin syringes are used for specific purposes. Insulin syringes are calibrated to measure up to 100 units

of insulin. Safe practice requires that *only* insulin syringes be used to measure insulin and that they be used for no other drugs. Tuberculin syringes have a capacity of 1 milliliter. They should be used for small doses of any drug because measurements are more accurate than with larger syringes.

Sites for Injections

Common sites for subcutaneous injections are the upper arms, abdomen, back, and thighs (Fig. 3-1). Sites for intramuscular injections are the deltoid, dorsogluteal, ventrogluteal, and vastus lateralis muscles. These sites must be selected by first identifying anatomic landmarks (Fig. 3-2). Common sites for intravenous injections are the veins on the back of the hands and on the forearms (Fig. 3-3). Other sites (eg, subclavian and jugular veins) are also used, mainly in critically ill clients. Additional parenteral routes include injection into layers of the skin (intradermal), arteries (intra-arterial), joints (intra-articular), and cerebrospinal fluid (intrathecal). Nurses may administer drugs intradermally or intra-arterially (if an established arterial line is present), and physicians administer intra-articular and intrathecal medications.

Box 3-2 Principles and Techniques With Intravenous Drug Therapy

Methods

Intravenous (IV) injection or **IV** push is the direct injection of a medication into the vein. The drug may be injected through an injection site on IV tubing or an intermittent infusion device. Most IV push medications should be injected slowly. The time depends on the particular drug, but is often 2 minutes or longer for a dose. Rapid injection should generally be avoided because the drug produces high blood levels and is quickly circulated to the heart and brain, where it may cause adverse or toxic effects. Although IV push may be useful with a few drugs or in emergency situations, slower infusion of more dilute drugs is usually preferred.

Intermittent infusion is administration of intermittent doses, often diluted in 50–100 mL of fluid and infused over 30–60 minutes. The drug dose is usually prepared in a pharmacy and connected to an IV administration set that controls the amount and flow rate. Intermittent infusions are often connected to an injection port on a primary IV line, through which IV fluids are infusing continuously. The purpose of the primary IV line may be to provide fluids to the client or to keep the vein open for periodic administration of medications. The IV fluids are usually stopped for the medication infusion, then restarted. Drug doses may also be infused through an intermittent infusion device (eg, a heparin lock) to conserve veins and allow freedom of motion between drug doses. The devices decrease the amount of IV fluids given to patients who do not need them (ie, those who are able to ingest adequate amounts of oral fluids) and those who are at risk of fluid overload, especially children and older adults.

An intermittent infusion device may be part of an initial IV line or used to adapt a continuous IV for intermittent use. The devices include a heparin lock or a resealable adapter added to a peripheral or central IV catheter. These devices must be flushed routinely to maintain patency. If the IV catheter has more than one lumen, all must be flushed, whether being used or not. Saline is probably the most commonly used flushing solution; heparin may also be used if recommended by the device's manufacturer or required by institutional policy. For example, heparin (3–5 mL of 100 units/mL, after each use or monthly if not in use) is recommended for implanted catheters.

Continuous infusion indicates medications mixed in a large volume of IV fluid and infused continuously, over several hours. For example, vitamins and minerals (eg, potassium chloride) are usually added to liters of IV fluids. Greater dilution of the drug and administration over a longer time decreases risks of accumulation and toxicity, as well as venous irritation and thrombophlebitis.

Equipment

Equipment varies considerably from one health care agency to another. Nurses must become familiar with the equipment available in their work setting, including IV catheters, types of IV tubing, needles and needleless systems, types of volume control devices, and electronic infusion devices (IV pumps).

Catheters vary in size (both gauge and length), design, and composition (eg, polyvinyl chloride, polyurethane, silicone).

The most common design type is over the needle; the needle is used to start the IV, then it is removed. When choosing a catheter to start an IV, one that is much smaller than the lumen of the vein is recommended. This allows good blood flow and rapidly dilutes drug solutions as they enter the vein. This, in turn, prevents high drug concentrations and risks of toxicity. Also, after a catheter is inserted, it is very important to tape it securely so that it does not move around. Movement of the catheter increases venous irritation and risks of thrombophlebitis and infection. If signs of venous irritation and inflammation develop, the catheter should be removed and a new one inserted at another site. Additional recommendations include application of a topical antibiotic or antiseptic ointment at the IV site after catheter insertion, a sterile occlusive dressing over the site, and limiting the duration of placement to a few days.

Many medications are administered through peripherally inserted central catheters (PICC lines) or central venous catheters, in which the catheter tips are inserted into the superior vena cava, next to the right atrium of the heart. Central venous catheters may have single, double, or triple lumens. Other products, which are especially useful for long-term IV drug therapy, include a variety of implanted ports, pumps, and reservoirs.

If a catheter becomes clogged, do not irrigate it. Doing so may push a clot into the circulation and result in a pulmonary embolus, myocardial infarction, or stroke. It may also cause septicemia, if the clot is infected.

Needleless systems are one of the most important advances in IV therapy. Most products have a blunt-tipped plastic insertion device and an injection port that opens. These systems greatly decrease needle-stick injuries and exposure to bloodborne pathogens.

Electronic infusion devices allow amounts and flow rates of IV drug solutions to be set and controlled by a computer. Although the devices save nursing time because the nurse does not need to continually adjust flow rates, the biggest advantage is the steady rate of drug administration. The devices are used in most settings where IV drugs and IV fluids are administered, but they are especially valuable in pediatrics, where very small amounts of medication and IV fluid are needed, and in intensive care units, where strong drugs and varying amounts of IV fluid are usually required. Several types of pumps are available, even within the same health care agency. It is extremely important that nurses become familiar with the devices used in their work setting, so that they can program them accurately and determine whether or not they are functioning properly (ie, delivering medications as ordered).

Site Selection

IV needles are usually inserted into a vein on the hand or forearm; IV catheters may be inserted in a peripheral site or centrally (the catheter tip ends in the superior vena cava, near the right atrium of the heart, and medications and fluids are rapidly diluted and flow directly into the heart). In general, recommendations are:

- Start at the most distal location. This conserves more proximal veins for later use, if needed. Veins on the back of the hand and

(continued)

Box 3-2 Principles and Techniques With Intravenous Drug Therapy (continued)

on the forearm are often used. These sites usually provide more comfort and freedom of movement for clients than other sites.

- Use veins with a large blood volume flowing through them when possible. Many drugs cause irritation and phlebitis in small veins.
- When possible, avoid the antecubital vein on the inner surface of the elbow, veins over or close to joints, and veins on the inner aspect of the wrists. Reasons include the difficulty of stabilizing and maintaining an IV line at these sites. In addition, the antecubital vein is often used to draw blood samples for laboratory analysis and inner wrist venipunctures are very painful. *Do not perform venipuncture in foot or leg veins.* The risks of serious or fatal complications are too high.
- Rotate sites when long-term use (more than a few days) of IV fluid or drug therapy is required. Venous irritation occurs with longer duration of site use and with the administration of irritating drugs or fluids. When it is necessary to change an IV site, use the opposite arm if possible.

Drug Preparation

Most IV drugs are prepared for administration in pharmacies and this is the safest practice. When a nurse must prepare a medication, considerations include the following.

- Only drug formulations manufactured for IV use should be given IV. Other formulations contain various substances that are not sterile, pure enough, or soluble enough to be injected into the bloodstream. *In recent years, there have been numerous reports of medication errors resulting from IV administration of drug preparations intended for oral use!!* Such errors can and should be prevented. For example, when liquid medications intended for oral use are measured or dispensed in a syringe (as they often are for children, adults with difficulty in swallowing tablets and capsules, or for administration through a gastrointestinal [GI] tube), the syringe should have a blunt tip that will not connect to or penetrate IV tubing injection sites.
- Use sterile technique during all phases of IV drug preparation.
- Follow the manufacturer's instructions for mixing and diluting IV medications. Some liquid IV medications need to be diluted prior to IV administration, and powdered medications must be reconstituted appropriately (eg, the correct amount of the recommended diluent added). The diluent recommended by the drug's manufacturer should be used because different drugs require different diluents. In addition, be sure any reconstituted drug is completely dissolved to avoid particles that may be injected into the systemic circulation and lead to thrombus formation or embolism. A filtered aspiration needle should be used when withdrawing medication from a vial or ampule, to remove any particles in the solution. The filter needle should then be discarded, to prevent filtered particles from being injected when the medication is added to the IV fluid. Filters added to IV tubing also help to remove particles.
- Check the expiration date on all IV medications. Many drugs have a limited period of stability after they are reconstituted or diluted for IV administration.
- IV medications should be compatible with the infusing IV fluids. Most are compatible with 5% dextrose in water or saline solutions.

- If adding a medication to a container of IV fluid, invert the container to be sure the additive is well mixed with the solution.
- For any IV medication that is prepared or added to an IV bag, label the medication vial or IV bag with the name of the patient, drug, dosage, date, time of mixing, expiration date, and the preparer's signature.

Drug Administration

- Most IV medications are injected into a self-sealing site in any of several IV set-ups, including a scalp–vein needle and tubing; a plastic catheter connected to a heparin lock or other intermittent infusion device; or IV tubing and a plastic bag containing IV fluid.
- Before injecting any IV medication, be sure the IV line is open and functioning properly (eg, catheter not clotted, IV fluid not leaking into surrounding tissues, phlebitis not present). If leakage occurs, some drugs are very irritating to subcutaneous tissues and may cause tissue necrosis.
- Maintain sterility of all IV fluids, tubings, injection sites, drug solutions, and equipment coming into contact with the IV system. Because medications and fluids are injected directly into the bloodstream, breaks in sterile technique can lead to serious systemic infection (septicemia) and death.
- When two or more medications are to be given one after the other, flush the IV tubing and catheter (with the infusing IV fluid or with sterile 0.9% sodium chloride injection) so that the drugs do not come into contact with each other.
- If a medication is to be injected or infused through an intermittent infusion device containing heparin, the drug should be compatible with heparin or the device should be irrigated with sterile saline before and after medication administration. After irrigation, heparin then needs to be reinstilled. This is not a common event, because most heparin locks and other intermittent infusion devices are filled with saline rather than heparin.
- In general, administer slowly to allow greater dilution of the drug in the bloodstream. Most drugs given by IV push (direct injection) can be given over 2–5 minutes and most drugs diluted in 50–100 mL of IV fluid can be infused in 30–60 minutes.
- When injecting or infusing medications into IV solutions that contain other additives (eg, vitamins, insulin, minerals such as potassium or magnesium), be sure the medications are compatible with the other substances. Consult compatibility charts (usually available on nursing units) or pharmacists when indicated.
- IV flow rates are usually calculated in mL/hour and drops per minute. Required information includes the amount of solution or medication to be infused, the time or duration of the infusion, and the drop factor of the IV administration set to be used. The drop factor of macrodrip sets may be 10, 15, or 20 drops per mL, depending on the manufacturer. Most agencies use mainly one manufacturer's product. The drop factor of all microdrip sets is 60 drops per mL. Following is a sample calculation:

    Order: Cefazolin 1 g IV q8h

    Label: Cefazolin 1 g in 100 mL of 0.9% sodium chloride injection; infuse over 60 minutes

    Solution: Divide 100 by 60 to determine mL/min (1.66). Multiply 1.66 by the drop factor to determine drops/min (eg, with a drop factor of 20 drops/mL, 33 drops/min would deliver the dose). Count drops and regulate the flow rate manually or program an IV pump to deliver the dose.

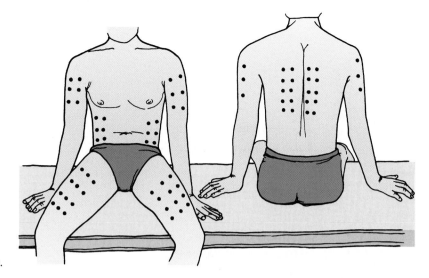

FIGURE 3-1 Subcutaneous injection sites.

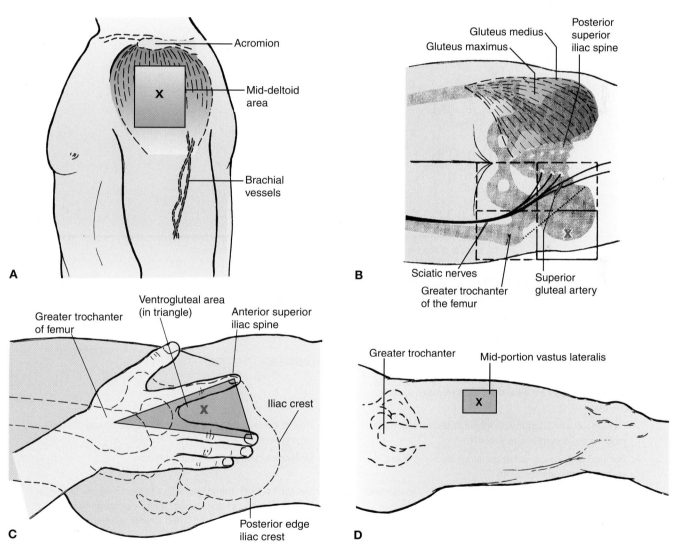

FIGURE 3-2 IM injection sites. **(A)** Placement of the needle for insertion into the deltoid muscle. The area of injection is bounded by the lower edge of the acromion on the top to a point on the side of the arm opposite the axilla on the bottom. The side boundaries of the rectangular site are parallel to the arm and one third and two thirds of the way around the side of the arm. **(B)** Proper placement of the needle for an intramuscular injection into the dorsogluteal site. It is above and outside a diagonal line drawn from the greater trochanter of the femur to the posterior superior iliac spine. Notice how this site allows the nurse to avoid entering an area near the sciatic nerves and the superior gluteal artery. **(C)** Placement of the needle for insertion into the ventrogluteal area. Notice how the nurse's palm is placed on the greater trochanter and the index finger is placed on the anterior superior iliac spine. The middle finger is spread posteriorly as far as possible along the iliac crest. The injection is made in the middle of the triangle formed by the nurse's fingers and the iliac crest. **(D)** Placement of the needle for insertion into the vastus lateralis. It is usually easier to have the client lying on his or her back. However, the client may be sitting when using this site for intramuscular injections. It is a suitable site for children when the nurse grasps the muscle in her hand to concentrate the muscle mass for injection.

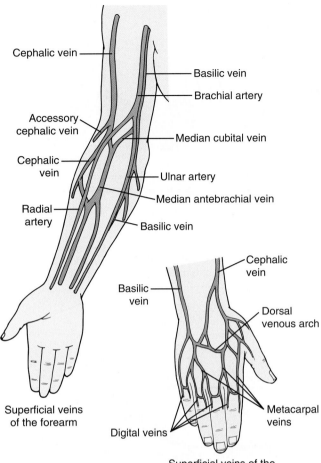

Superficial veins
of the forearm

Superficial veins of the
dorsal aspect of the hand

FIGURE 3-3 Veins of the hand and forearm that may be used to administer intravenous fluids and medications.

N U R S I N G   A C T I O N S

Drug Administration

NURSING ACTIONS	RATIONALE/EXPLANATION
1. Follow general rules for administering medications safely and effectively.	
a. Prepare and give drugs in well-lighted areas, as free of interruptions and distractions as possible.	To prevent errors in selecting ordered drugs, calculating dosages, and identifying clients
b. Perform hand hygiene before preparing medications and, if needed, during administration.	To prevent infection and cross-contamination
c. Use sterile technique in preparing and administering injections.	To prevent infection. Sterile technique involves using sterile needles and syringes, using sterile drug solutions, not touching sterile objects to any unsterile objects, and cleansing injection sites with an antiseptic.
d. Read the medication administration record (MAR) carefully. Read the label on the drug container, and compare with the MAR in terms of drug, dosage or concentration, and route of administration. Scan bar codes, if available.	For accurate drug administration. Most nursing texts instruct the nurse to read a drug label three times: when removing the container, while measuring the dose, and before returning the container.
e. Do not leave medications unattended.	To prevent accidental or deliberate ingestion by anyone other than the intended person and to prevent contamination or spilling of medications.

NURSING ACTIONS	RATIONALE/EXPLANATION
f. Identify the client, preferably by comparing the identification wristband to the medication sheet. Scan barcodes if available.	This is the best way to verify identity. Calling by name, relying on the name on a door or bed, and asking someone else are unreliable methods, although they must be used occasionally when the client lacks a name band.
g. Identify yourself, if indicated, and state your reason for approaching the client. For example, "I'm . . . I have your medication for you."	Explaining actions helps to decrease client anxiety and increase cooperation in taking prescribed medication.
h. Position the client appropriately for the intended route of administration.	To prevent complications, such as aspiration of oral drugs into the lungs
i. Provide water or other supplies as needed.	To promote comfort of the client and to ensure drug administration
j. Do not leave medications at the bedside as a general rule. Common exceptions are antacids, nitroglycerin, and eye medications.	To prevent omitting or losing the drug or hoarding of the drug by the client
k. Do not give a drug when signs and symptoms of toxicity are present. Notify the physician, and record that the drug was omitted and why.	Additional doses of a drug increase toxicity. However, drugs are not omitted without a careful assessment of the client's condition and a valid reason.
l. Record drug administration (or omission) as soon as possible and according to agency policies.	To maintain an accurate record of drugs received by the client
m. Evaluate whether missed scheduled doses should be given at a later time or omitted. Generally, give drugs ordered once or twice daily at a later time. For others, omit the one dose, and give the drug at the next scheduled time.	Clients may be unable to take the drug at the scheduled time because of diagnostic tests or many other reasons. A temporary change in the time of administration—usually for one dose only—may be necessary to maintain therapeutic effects.
n. For medications ordered as needed (PRN), assess the client's condition; check the physician's orders or MAR for the name, dose, and frequency of administration; and determine the time of the most recently administered dose.	Administration of PRN medications requires nursing assessment and decision making. Analgesics, antiemetics, and antipyretics are often ordered PRN.
o. For narcotics and other controlled substances, sign drugs out on separate narcotic records according to agency policies.	To meet legal requirements for dispensing controlled substances
p. If, at any time during drug preparation or administration, any question arises regarding the drug, the dose, or whether the client is supposed to receive it, check the original physician's order. If the order is not clear, call the physician for clarification before giving the drug.	To promote safety and prevent errors. The same procedure applies when the client questions drug orders at the bedside. For example, the client may state he has been receiving different drugs or different doses.
2. For oral medications:	
a. With adults	
(1) To give tablets or capsules, open the unit-dose wrapper, place medication in a medicine cup, and give the cup to the client. For solutions, hold the cup at eye level, and measure the dosage at the bottom of the meniscus. For suspensions, shake or invert containers to mix the medication before measuring the dose.	To maintain clean technique and measure doses accurately. Suspensions settle on standing, and if not mixed, diluent may be given rather than the active drug.
(2) Have the client in a sitting position when not contraindicated.	To decrease risks of aspirating medication into lungs. Aspiration may lead to difficulty in breathing and aspiration pneumonia.
(3) Give before, with, or after meals as indicated by the specific drug.	Food in the stomach usually delays drug absorption and action. It also decreases gastric irritation, a common side effect of oral drugs. Giving drugs at appropriate times in relation to food intake can increase therapeutic effects and decrease adverse effects.
(4) Give most oral drugs with a full glass (8 oz) of water or other fluid.	To promote dissolution and absorption of tablets and capsules. Also, to decrease gastric irritation by diluting drug concentration.

(continued)

NURSING ACTIONS	RATIONALE/EXPLANATION
b. With children, liquids or chewable tablets are usually given.	Children under 5 years of age are often unable to swallow tablets or capsules.
(1) Measure and give liquids to infants with a dropper or syringe, placing medication on the tongue or buccal mucosa and giving slowly.	For accurate measurement and administration. Giving slowly decreases risks of aspiration.
(2) Medications are often mixed with juice, applesauce, or other vehicle.	To increase the child's ability and willingness to take the medication. If this is done, use a small amount, and be sure the child takes all of it; otherwise, less than the ordered dose is given.
c. Do not give oral drugs if the client is:	
(1) NPO (receiving nothing by mouth)	Oral drugs and fluids may interfere with diagnostic tests or be otherwise contraindicated. Most drugs can be given after diagnostic tests are completed. If the client is having surgery, preoperative drug orders are cancelled. New orders are written postoperatively.
(2) Vomiting	Oral drugs and fluids increase vomiting. Thus, no benefit results from the drug. Also, fluid and electrolyte problems may result from loss of gastric acid.
(3) Excessively sedated or unconscious	To avoid aspiration of drugs into the lungs owing to impaired ability to swallow
3. For medications given by nasogastric tube:	
a. Use a liquid preparation when possible. If necessary, crush a tablet or empty a capsule into about 30 mL of water and mix well. **Do not crush enteric-coated or sustained-release products, and do not empty sustained-release capsules.**	Particles of tablets or powders from capsules may obstruct the tube lumen. Altering sustained-release products increases risks of overdosage and adverse effects.
b. Use a clean bulb syringe or other catheter-tipped syringe.	The syringe allows aspiration and serves as a funnel for instillation of medication and fluids into the stomach.
c. Before instilling medication, aspirate gastric fluid and check pH or use another method to check tube placement.	To be sure the tube is in the stomach
d. Rinse the tube, instill medication by gravity flow, and rinse the tube again with at least 50 mL of water. Do not allow the syringe to empty completely between additions.	Gravity flow is safer than applying pressure. Water "pushes" the drug into the stomach and rinses the tube, thereby maintaining tube patency. Additional water or other fluids may be given according to fluid needs of the client. Add fluids to avoid instilling air into the stomach unnecessarily, with possible client discomfort.
e. Clamp off the tube from suction or drainage for at least 30 minutes.	To avoid removing the medication from the stomach
4. For subcutaneous (Sub-Q) injections:	
a. Use only sterile drug preparations labeled or commonly used for Sub-Q injections.	Many parenteral drugs are too irritating to subcutaneous tissue for use by this route.
b. Use a 25-gauge, ⅝-inch needle for most Sub-Q injections.	This size needle is effective for most clients and drugs.
c. Select an appropriate injection site, based on client preferences, drug characteristics, and visual inspection of possible sites. In long-term therapy, such as with insulin, rotate injection sites. Avoid areas with lumps, bruises, or other lesions.	These techniques allow the client to participate in his or her care; avoid tissue damage and unpredictable absorption, which occur with repeated injections in the same location; and increase client comfort and cooperation
d. Cleanse the site with an alcohol sponge.	To prevent infection
e. Tighten the skin or pinch a fold of skin and tissue between thumb and fingers.	Either is acceptable for most clients. If the client is obese, tightening the skin may be easier. If the client is very thin, the tissue fold may keep the needle from hitting bone.
f. Hold the syringe like a pencil, and insert the needle quickly at a 45- or 90-degree angle. Use enough force to penetrate the skin and subcutaneous tissue in one smooth movement.	To give the drug correctly with minimal client discomfort.

NURSING ACTIONS	RATIONALE/EXPLANATION
g. Release the skin so that both hands are free to manipulate the syringe. Pull back gently on the plunger (aspirate). If no blood enters the syringe, inject the drug. If blood is aspirated into the syringe, remove the needle, and reprepare the medication.	To prevent accidental injection into the bloodstream. Blood return in the syringe is an uncommon occurrence. Aspiration is not recommended with heparin injections and possibly not needed with insulin injections.
h. Remove the needle quickly and apply gentle pressure for a few seconds.	To prevent bleeding
5. For intramuscular (IM) injections:	
a. Use only drug preparations labeled or commonly used for IM injections. Check label instructions for mixing drugs in powder form.	Some parenteral drug preparations cannot be given safely by the IM route.
b. Use a 1½-inch needle for most adults and a ⅝- to 1½-inch needle for children, depending on the size of the client.	A long needle is necessary to reach muscle tissue, which underlies subcutaneous fat.
c. Use the smallest-gauge needle that will accommodate the medication. A 22-gauge is satisfactory for most drugs; a 20-gauge may be used for viscous medications.	To decrease tissue damage and client discomfort
d. Select an appropriate injection site, based on client preferences, drug characteristics, anatomic landmarks, and visual inspection of possible sites. Rotate sites if frequent injections are being given, and avoid areas with lumps, bruises, or other lesions.	To increase client comfort and participation and to avoid tissue damage. Identification of anatomic landmarks is mandatory for safe administration of IM drugs.
e. Cleanse the site with an alcohol sponge.	To prevent infection
f. Tighten the skin, hold the syringe like a pencil, and insert the needle quickly at a 90-degree angle. Use enough force to penetrate the skin and subcutaneous tissue into the muscle in one smooth motion.	To give the drug correctly with minimal client discomfort
g. Aspirate (see 4g, Sub-Q injections).	
h. Remove the needle quickly and apply pressure for several seconds.	To prevent bleeding
6. For intravenous (IV) injections:	
a. Use only drug preparations that are labeled for IV use.	Others are not pure enough for safe injection into the bloodstream or are not compatible with the blood pH (7.35–7.45).
b. Check label instructions for the type and amount of fluid to use for dissolving or diluting the drug.	Some drugs require special preparation techniques to maintain solubility or pharmacologic activity. Most drugs in powder form can be dissolved in sterile water or sodium chloride for injection. Most drug solutions can be given with dextrose or dextrose and sodium chloride IV solutions.
c. Prepare drugs just before use, as a general rule. Also, add drugs to IV fluids just before use.	Some drugs are unstable in solution. In most agencies, drugs are mixed and added to IV fluids in the pharmacy. This is the preferred method because sterility can be better maintained.
d. For venipuncture and direct injection into a vein, apply a tourniquet, select a site in the arm, cleanse the skin with an antiseptic (eg, povidone-iodine or alcohol), insert the needle, and aspirate a small amount of blood into the syringe to be sure that the needle is in the vein. Remove the tourniquet, and inject the drug slowly. Remove the needle and apply pressure until there is no evidence of bleeding.	For safe and accurate drug administration with minimal risk to the client. The length of time required to give the drug depends on the specific drug and the amount. Slow administration, over several minutes, allows immediate discontinuation if adverse effects occur.
e. For administration by an established IV line:	
(1) Check the infusion for patency and flow rate. Check the venipuncture site for signs of infiltration and phlebitis before each drug dose.	The solution must be flowing freely for accurate drug administration. If infiltration or phlebitis is present, do not give the drug until a new IV line is begun.
(2) For direct injection, cleanse an injection site on the IV tubing, insert the needle, and inject the drug slowly.	Most tubings have injection sites to facilitate drug administration.

(continued)

NURSING ACTIONS	RATIONALE/EXPLANATION
(3) To use a volume-control set, fill it with 50–100 mL of IV fluid, and clamp it so that no further fluid enters the chamber and dilutes the drug. Inject the drug into an injection site after cleansing the site with an alcohol sponge and infuse, usually in 1 hour or less. After the drug is infused, add solution to maintain the infusion.	This method is used for administration of antibiotics on an intermittent schedule. Dilution of the drug decreases adverse effects.
(4) To use a "piggyback" method, add the drug to 50–100 mL of IV solution in a separate container. Attach the IV tubing and a needle. Insert the needle in an injection site on the main IV tubing after cleansing the site. Infuse the drug over 15–60 minutes, depending on the drug.	This method is also used for intermittent administration of antibiotics and other drugs. Whether a volume-control or piggyback apparatus is used depends on agency policy and equipment available.
f. When more than one drug is to be given, flush the line between drugs. Do not mix drugs in syringes or in IV fluids unless the drug literature states that the drugs are compatible.	Physical and chemical interactions between the drugs may occur and cause precipitation, inactivation, or increased toxicity. Most nursing units have charts depicting drug compatibility, or information may be obtained from the pharmacy.
7. For application to skin:	
a. Use drug preparations labeled for dermatologic use. Cleanse the skin, remove any previously applied medication, and apply the drug in a thin layer. For broken skin or open lesions, use sterile gloves, tongue blade, or cotton-tipped applicator to apply the drug.	To promote therapeutic effects and minimize adverse effects
8. For instillation of eye drops:	
a. Use drug preparations labeled for ophthalmic use. Wash your hands, open the eye to expose the conjunctival sac, and drop the medication into the sac, not on the eyeball, without touching the dropper tip to anything. Provide a tissue for blotting any excess drug. If two or more eye drops are scheduled at the same time, wait 1–5 minutes between instillations.	Ophthalmic preparations must be sterile to avoid infection. Blot any excess drug from the inner canthus near the nose to decrease systemic absorption of the drug.
With children, prepare the medication, place the child in a head-lowered position, steady the hand holding the medication on the child's head, gently retract the lower lid, and instill the medication into the conjunctival sac.	Careful positioning and restraint to avoid sudden movements are necessary to decrease risks of injury to the eye.
9. For instillation of nose drops and nasal sprays:	
a. Have the client hold his or her head back, and drop the medication into the nostrils. Give only as ordered	When nose drops are used for rhinitis and nasal congestion accompanying the common cold, overuse results in a rebound congestion that may be worse than the original symptom.
With children, place in a supine position with the head lowered, instill the medication, and maintain the position for 2–3 minutes. Then, place the child in a prone position.	
10. For instillation of ear medications:	
a. Open the ear canal by pulling the ear up and back for adults, down and back for children, and drop the medication on the side of the canal.	To straighten the canal and promote maximal contact between medication and tissue
11. For rectal suppositories:	
a. Lubricate the end with a water-soluble lubricant, wear a glove or finger cot, and insert into the rectum the length of the finger. Place the suppository next to the mucosal wall.	To promote absorption.
b. If the client prefers and is able, provide supplies for self-administration.	Allowing self-administration may prevent embarrassment to the client. Be sure the client knows the correct procedure.
12. For vaginal medications:	
a. Use gloves or an applicator for insertion. If an applicator is used, wash thoroughly with soap and water after each use.	
b. If the client prefers and is able, provide supplies for self-administration.	Some women may be embarrassed and prefer self-administration. Be sure the client knows the correct procedure.

APPLYING YOUR KNOWLEDGE: ANSWER

3-1 This medication error occurred because the medication was given to the wrong client. You did not check the client's name band and relied on the client to respond to your calling his name. In this situation, the client had been asleep and may have been responding simply to being awakened. Also, Mr. Sanchez's memory deficits and altered mental status may have contributed. Accurate identification of the client is imperative, especially when the client may be confused or unable to respond appropriately.

Review and Application Exercises

Short Answer Exercises

1. When giving an oral medication, what are some interventions to aid absorption and hasten therapeutic effects?

2. What are the advantages and disadvantages of the PO route and the IV route of drug administration?

3. For a client who receives all medications through a nasogastric feeding tube, which dosage forms are acceptable? Which are unacceptable, and why?

4. What are some legal factors that influence a nurse's administration of medications?

5. When administering medications, what safety precautions are needed with various routes?

6. What safety precautions must the nurse practice consistently to avoid self-injury and exposure to bloodborne pathogens?

7. With a client who refuses an important medication, what approaches or interventions might persuade the client to take the medication? Would the same approach be indicated if the medication were a vitamin supplement or a laxative?

NCLEX-Style Questions

8. An important safety measure in drug administration is
   a. calling the client by name
   b. using appropriate techniques for the ordered route of administration
   c. asking a coworker about an ordered drug
   d. leaving medications at the bedside

9. Drinking 8 oz of water with a tablet or capsule aids which of the following pharmacokinetic processes?
   a. absorption
   b. distribution
   c. biotransformation
   d. excretion

10. When administering medications by nasogastric tube, which of the following nursing actions is indicated?
    a. Verify the position of the tube before giving the drugs.
    b. Aspirate and discard stomach contents.
    c. Mix medications with tube-feeding formulas.
    d. Have the client sit in a chair.

11. Maintaining sterile technique is necessary while administering which of the following types of medication?
    a. oral suspensions
    b. vaginal suppositories
    c. nasal inhalation products
    d. injections

12. Anatomic landmarks are very important in which of the following routes of drug administration?
    a. oral
    b. inhalation
    c. intramuscular
    d. topical (to skin)

Selected References

Beckwith, M. C., Feddema, S. S., Barton, R. G., et al. (2004). A guide to drug therapy in patients with enteral feeding tubes: Dosage form selection and administration methods. *Hospital Pharmacy, 39*(3), 225–237.

Cohen, H., Robinson, E. S., & Mandrack, M. (2003). Getting to the root of medication errors: Survey results. *Nursing 2003, 33*(9), 36–45.

Dickerson, R. N. (2004). Medication administration considerations for patients receiving enteral tube feedings. *Hospital Pharmacy, 39*(1), 84, 89, 96.

Drug facts and comparisons. (Updated monthly). St. Louis: Facts and Comparisons.

Huffman, S., Jarczyk, K. S., O'Brien, E., et al. (2004). Methods to confirm feeding tube placement: Application of research in practice. *Pediatric Nursing, 30*(1), 10–13.

Togger, D. A., & Brenner, P. S. (2001). Metered dose inhalers. *American Journal of Nursing, 101*(10), 26–32.

Weinstein, S. M. (2001). *Plumer's principles and practice of intravenous therapy* (7th ed.). Philadelphia: Lippincott Williams & Wilkins.

Nursing Process in Drug Therapy

OBJECTIVES

After studying this chapter, you will be able to:

1. Assess clients for conditions and factors that are likely to influence drug effects, including age, weight, health status, and lifestyle.
2. Obtain a medication history about the client's use of prescription, over-the-counter (OTC), and social drugs as well as herbal and dietary supplements.
3. Identify nondrug interventions to prevent or decrease the need for drug therapy.
4. Discuss interventions to increase therapeutic effects and decrease adverse effects of drug therapy.
5. Discuss guidelines for rational choices of drugs, dosages, routes, and times of administration.
6. Observe clients for therapeutic and adverse responses to drug therapy.
7. Teach clients and family members how to use prescription and OTC drugs safely and effectively.
8. When indicated, teach clients about the potential effects of herbal and dietary supplements.
9. For clients who use herbal and dietary supplements, provide—or assist them in obtaining—reliable information.
10. Describe major considerations in drug therapy for clients with impaired renal or hepatic function or critical illness.
11. Discuss application of the nursing process in home care settings.

APPLYING YOUR KNOWLEDGE

You are making the first home visit for Robert Walker, an 80-year-old client with arthritis and hypertension. Upon reading his file, you learn that Mr. Walker lives alone but has a daughter who lives in the area. She visits him once a week and runs his errands. You note he is taking the following medications:

Ibuprofen 400 mg every 4 hours
Furosemide 20 mg once daily
Captopril 25 mg twice a day
Famotidine 20 mg at bedtime

INTRODUCTION

Drug therapy involves the use of drugs to prevent or treat disease processes and manifestations. It may save lives, improve the quality of life, and otherwise benefit recipients. It also may cause adverse effects. Adverse effects and failure to achieve therapeutic effects may occur with correct use, but they are more likely to occur with incorrect use. Physicians, pharmacists, clients, and nurses all have important roles to play in the safe and effective use of drugs.

For the nurse, drug therapy is one of many responsibilities in client care. To fulfill this responsibility, the nurse must be knowledgeable about pharmacology (drugs and their effects on the body), physiology (normal body functions), and pathophysiology (alterations in mental and physical functions due to disease processes) and must be adept at using all steps of the nursing process.

Chapter 1 included general information about drugs and suggested strategies for studying pharmacology. Chapter 2 described cellular physiology and concepts and processes essential to understanding drug effects in humans. Chapter 3 emphasized drug preparation and administration. Although the importance of safe and accurate administration cannot be overemphasized, this is only one aspect of the nursing process in drug therapy. The nurse also must monitor responses to drug therapy, both therapeutic and adverse, and teach clients about drugs, both prescribed and OTC. To help the nurse continue to acquire knowledge and skills related to drug therapy, this chapter includes nursing process guidelines, general principles of drug therapy, and general nursing actions. Guidelines, principles, and actions related to specific drug groups and individual drugs are included in appropriate chapters throughout this text.

NURSING PROCESS IN DRUG THERAPY

The nursing process is a systematic way of gathering and using information to plan and provide individualized client care and to evaluate the outcomes of care. It involves both cognitive and psychomotor skills. Knowledge of, and skill in, the nursing process are required for drug therapy as in other aspects of client care. The five steps of the nursing process are assessment, nursing diagnosis, planning and establishing goals for nursing care, interventions, and evaluation. One might say that assessment and interventions are the "action" phases, whereas analysis of assessment data, establishing nursing diagnoses and goals, and evaluation are "thinking" phases. However, knowledge and informed, rational thinking should underlie all data collection, decision making, and interventions.

Assessment

Assessment involves collecting data about client characteristics known to affect drug therapy. This includes observing and interviewing the client, interviewing family members or others involved in client care, completing a physical assessment, reviewing medical records for pertinent laboratory and diagnostic test reports, and other methods. Although listed as the first step in the nursing process, assessment is a component of all steps and occurs with every contact with the client.

The initial assessment needs to be thorough and should use all available sources of data to provide a sound basis for planning care. Later assessments of a client's response to treatment are ongoing; they provide a basis for rational decisions about continuing or revising nursing care. Guidelines for obtaining needed assessment data follow.

- On initial contact, assess age, weight, vital signs, health status, pathologic conditions, and ability to function in usual activities of daily living. The effects of these client-related factors on drug therapy are discussed in Chapter 2.
- Assess for previous and current use of prescription, nonprescription, and nontherapeutic (eg, alcohol, caf-

feine, nicotine, cocaine, marijuana) drugs. A medication history (Box 4-1) is useful, or the information can be incorporated into any data collection tool.

Specific questions and areas of assessment include the following:

- What are current drug orders?
- What does the client know about current drugs? Is teaching needed?
- What drugs has the client taken before? Include any drugs taken regularly, such as those taken for chronic illnesses (eg, hypertension, diabetes mellitus, arthritis). It also may be helpful to ask about nonprescription drugs for headaches, colds, indigestion, or constipation, because some people do not think of these preparations as drugs.
- Has the client ever had an allergic reaction to a drug? If so, what signs and symptoms occurred and how were they managed?
- What are the client's attitudes about drugs? Try to assess whether the client is likely to comply with a prescribed drug regimen or is likely to abuse drugs.
- If long-term drug therapy is likely, is the client able to buy or obtain medications and see a health care provider for monitoring and follow-up care?
- Is the client able to communicate verbally; can he or she swallow oral medications?
- Does the client have pathologic conditions that influence drug therapy? For example, all seriously ill clients should be assessed for impaired function of vital organs. Early recognition and treatment may prevent or decrease organ impairment.
- Assess for previous or current use of herbal or dietary supplements (eg, echinacea, gingko, glucosamine/chondroitin). If so, ask for names, how much is taken and how often, for how long, their reason for use, and perceived benefits or adverse effects.
- In addition to nursing assessment data, use progress notes, laboratory reports, and other sources as available to obtain baseline data for monitoring therapeutic or adverse drug effects. Laboratory tests of liver, kidney, and bone marrow function are often helpful because some drugs may damage these organs. Also, if liver or kidney damage exists, drug metabolism or excretion may be altered. Some specific laboratory tests include serum potassium levels before diuretic therapy, culture and susceptibility studies before antimicrobial therapy, and blood clotting tests before anticoagulant therapy.
- Seek information about ordered drugs, if needed.

After assessment data are obtained, they need to be analyzed for their relevance to the client's current condition and nursing care needs. In general, nurses must provide care based on available information while knowing that assessment data are always relatively incomplete. As a result, continued

Box 4-1 Medication History

Name_____ Age_____

Health problems, acute and chronic

Are you allergic to any medications?

If yes, describe specific effects or symptoms.

Part 1: Prescription Medications

1. Do you take any prescription medications on a regular basis?
2. If yes, ask the following about each medication.

Name	Dose
Frequency	Specific times
How long taken	Reason for use

3. Do you have any difficulty in taking your medicines? If yes, ask to specify problem areas.
4. Have you had any symptoms or problems that you think are caused by your medicines? If yes, ask to specify.
5. Do you need help from another person to take your medicines?
6. Do you take any prescription medications on an irregular basis? If yes, ask the following about each medication.

Name	Dose
Frequency	Reason
How long taken	

Part 2: Nonprescription Medications

Do you take over-the-counter medications?

		Medication		
Problem	*Yes/No*	*Name*	*Amount*	*Frequency*
Pain				
Headache				
Sleep				
Cold				
Indigestion				
Heartburn				
Diarrhea				
Constipation				
Other				

Part 3: Social Drugs

	Yes/No	*Amount/day*
Coffee		
Tea		
Cola drinks		
Alcohol		
Tobacco		

Part 4: Herbal or Dietary Supplements

Do you take any herbal or dietary supplements (eg, gingko, glucosamine/chondroitin, kava)? If so, ask for names, how much and how often taken, reason for use, perceived effectiveness, any adverse effects.

---

assessment is needed in relation to therapeutic and adverse drug effects as well as in regard to other aspects of safe and effective drug therapy.

APPLYING YOUR KNOWLEDGE 4-1

Review Mr. Walker's current medication regimen. Look up the medications, and note the drug class for each. Why do you think this client is taking them? Are the dosages appropriate for an 80-year-old?

Nursing Diagnoses

These statements, as developed by the North American Nursing Diagnosis Association, describe client problems or needs and are based on assessment data. They should be individualized according to the client's condition and the drugs prescribed. Thus, the nursing diagnoses needed to adequately reflect the client's condition vary considerably. Because almost any nursing diagnosis may apply in specific circumstances, this text emphasizes those diagnoses that generally apply to drug therapy.

- Deficient Knowledge: Drug therapy regimen (eg, drug ordered; reason for use; expected effects; monitoring of response by health care providers, including diagnostic tests and office visits)
- Deficient Knowledge: Safe and effective self-administration (when appropriate)
- Risk for Injury related to adverse drug effects
- Noncompliance: Overuse
- Noncompliance: Underuse

Planning/Goals

This step involves the expected outcomes of prescribed drug therapy. As a general rule, *goals should be stated in terms of client behavior, not nurse behavior.* For example, the client will

- Receive or take drugs as prescribed
- Experience relief of signs and symptoms
- Avoid preventable adverse drug effects
- Self-administer drugs safely and accurately
- Verbalize essential drug information
- Keep appointments for monitoring and follow-up
- Use any herbal and dietary supplements with caution and report such use to health care providers

Interventions

This step involves implementing planned activities and includes any task performed on a client's behalf. Areas of intervention may include assessment, drug administration, teaching about medications, solving problems related to drug therapy, promoting compliance with prescribed drug therapy, identifying barriers to compliance, and identifying resources (eg, financial assistance for obtaining medications).

General interventions include promoting health, preventing or decreasing the need for drug therapy, and using nondrug measures to enhance therapeutic effects or decrease adverse effects. Some examples include

- Promoting healthful lifestyles in terms of nutrition, fluids, exercise, rest, and sleep
- Handwashing and other measures to prevent infection
- Ambulating, positioning, exercising
- Assisting to cough and deep breathe
- Applying heat or cold
- Increasing or decreasing sensory stimulation
- Scheduling activities to allow periods of rest or sleep
- Recording vital signs, fluid intake, urine output, and other assessment data
- Implementing interventions indicated by a particular drug or the client's condition. For example, weighing clients helps in calculating dosages of several drugs and in assessing changes in fluid balance or nutritional status; ensuring that blood samples for serum drug levels are drawn at correct times in relation to drug admin-

istration helps to increase the accuracy of these tests in monitoring the client's condition; and, in clients at risk for developing acute renal failure (ARF), ensuring adequate fluid intake and blood pressure and avoiding or following safety precautions with nephrotoxic drugs (eg, aminoglycoside antibiotics) helps to prevent ARF.

- Client teaching (discussed in the following paragraphs, because it is of great importance)

Teaching about drug therapy is essential because most medications are self-administered and clients need information and assistance to use therapeutic drugs safely and effectively. When medications are given by another caregiver, rather than self-administered, the caregiver needs to understand information about the medications. Adequate knowledge and preparation are required to fulfill teaching responsibilities. Teaching aids to assist the nurse in this endeavor include *Box 4-2: Preparing to Teach a Client or Caregiver; Client Teaching Guidelines: Safe and Effective Use of Prescription Medications;* and *Client Teaching Guidelines: Safe and Effective Use of Over-the-Counter (OTC) Medications.* Later drug-related chapters contain client teaching guidelines for the drugs discussed in those particular chapters.

Most chapters also present specific interventions that are needed when a drug is ordered, as a separate feature entitled *Nursing Actions.* These actions relate to administering accurately, assessing for therapeutic and adverse effects, and observing for drug interactions. Rationales for the interventions are included.

In addition, interventions are often integrated with background information and client characteristics to assist in individualizing care. These interventions are presented under the heading of "Principles of Therapy." This chapter includes general principles or guidelines; later drug chapters include those related to particular drug groups.

Evaluation

This step involves evaluating the client's status in relation to stated goals and expected outcomes. Some outcomes can be evaluated within a few minutes of drug administration (eg, relief of acute pain after administration of an analgesic). Most, however, require much longer periods of time, often extending from hospitalization and direct observation by the nurse to self-care at home and occasional contact with a health care provider.

With the current emphasis on outpatient treatment and short hospitalizations, the client is likely to experience brief contacts with many health care providers. Minimal contact, plus a client's usual reluctance to admit noncompliance, contributes to difficulties in evaluating outcomes of drug therapy. These difficulties can be managed by using appropriate techniques and criteria of evaluation. General techniques include

- Directly observing the client's status
- Interviewing the client or others about the client's response to drug therapy

Box 4-2 Preparing to Teach a Client or Caregiver

- Assess learning needs, especially when new drugs are added or new conditions are being treated. This includes finding out what the person already knows about a particular drug. If the client has been taking a drug for a while, verify by questions and observations that he or she already knows essential drug information and takes the drug correctly. Do not assume that teaching is unneeded.

- Assess ability to manage a drug therapy regimen (ie, read printed instructions and drug labels, remember dosage schedules, self-administer medications by ordered routes). A medication history (see Box 4-1) helps to assess the client's knowledge and attitudes about drug therapy.

- From assessment data, develop an individualized teaching plan. This saves time for both nurse and client by avoiding repetition of known material. It also promotes compliance with prescribed drug therapy.

- Try to decrease client's and caregiver's anxiety and provide positive reinforcement for effort. They may feel overwhelmed by complicated medication regimens and are more likely to make errors with large numbers of medications or changes in the medication regimen.

- Choose an appropriate time (eg, when the client is mentally alert and not in acute distress [eg, due to pain, difficulty in breathing, or other symptoms]) and a place with minimal noise and distractions.

- Proceed slowly, in small steps; emphasize essential information; and provide ample opportunities to express concerns or ask questions.

- Try to provide a combination of verbal and written instructions, which is more effective than either alone. Minimize medical jargon and be aware that clients may have difficulty understanding and retaining the material being taught because of the stress of the illness.

- When explaining a drug therapy regimen to a hospitalized client, describe the name, purpose, expected effects, and so on. In many instances, the drug is familiar and can be described from personal knowledge. If the drug is unfamiliar, use available resources (eg, drug reference books, pharmacists) to learn about the drug and provide accurate information to the client.

  The client should know the name, preferably both the generic and a trade name, of any drugs being taken. Such knowledge is

a safety measure, especially if an allergic or other potentially serious adverse reaction or overdose occurs. It also decreases the risk of mistaking one drug for another and promotes a greater sense of control and responsibility regarding drug therapy. The client should also know the purpose of prescribed drugs. Although people vary in the amount of drug information they want and need, the purpose can usually be simply stated in terms of symptoms to be relieved or other expected benefits.

- When teaching a client about medications to be taken at home, provide specific instructions about taking the medications. Also teach the client and caregiver to observe for beneficial and adverse effects. If adverse effects occur, teach them how to manage minor ones and which ones to report to a health care provider. In addition, discuss specific ways to take medications so that usual activities of daily living are minimally disrupted. Planning with a client to develop a convenient routine, within the limitations imposed by individual drugs, may help increase compliance with the prescribed regimen. Allow time for questions and try to ensure that the client understands how, when, and why to take the medications.

- When teaching a client about potential adverse drug effects, the goal is to provide needed information without causing unnecessary anxiety. Most drugs produce undesirable effects; some are minor, some are potentially serious. Many people stop taking a drug rather than report adverse reactions. If reactions are reported, it may be possible to continue drug therapy by reducing dosage, changing the time of administration, or other measures. The occurrence of severe reactions indicates that the drug should be stopped and the prescribing physician should be notified.

- Throughout the teaching session and perhaps at times of other contacts, emphasize the importance of taking medications as prescribed. Common client errors include taking incorrect doses, taking doses at the wrong times, forgetting to take doses, and stopping a medication too soon. Treatment failure can often be directly traced to these errors. For example, missed doses of glaucoma medication can lead to optic nerve damage and blindness.

- Reassess learning needs when medication orders are changed (eg, when medications are added because of a new illness or stopped).

- Checking appropriate medical records, including medication records and diagnostic test reports
- With outpatients, performing "pill counts" to compare doses remaining with the number prescribed during a designated time

General criteria include

- Progress toward stated outcomes, such as relief of symptoms
- Accurate administration

- Avoidance of preventable adverse effects
- Compliance with instructions

Specific criteria indicate the parameters that must be measured to evaluate responses to particular drugs (eg, blood sugar with antidiabetic drugs, blood pressure with antihypertensive drugs).

APPLYING YOUR KNOWLEDGE 4-2

Think back to the case of Mr. Walker. Identify possible nursing diagnoses.

CLIENT TEACHING GUIDELINES

Safe and Effective Use of Prescription Medications

General Considerations

✔ Use drugs cautiously and only when necessary because all drugs affect body functions and may cause adverse effects.

✔ Use nondrug measures, when possible, to prevent the need for drug therapy or to enhance beneficial effects and decrease adverse effects of drugs.

✔ Do not take drugs left over from a previous illness or prescribed for someone else, and do not share prescription drugs with anyone else. The likelihood of having the right drug in the right dose is remote, and the risk of adverse effects is high in such circumstances.

✔ Keep all health care providers informed about all the drugs being taken, including over-the-counter (OTC) products and herbal or dietary supplements. One way to do this is to keep a written record of all current medicines, including their names and dosages and how they are taken. It is a good idea to carry a copy of this list at all times. This information can help avoid new prescriptions or OTC drugs that have similar effects or cancel each other's effects.

✔ Take drugs as prescribed and for the length of time prescribed; notify a health care provider if unable to obtain or take a medication. Therapeutic effects greatly depend on taking medications correctly. Altering the dose or time may cause underdosage or overdosage. Stopping a medication may cause a recurrence of the problem for which it was given or withdrawal symptoms. Some medications need to be tapered in dosage and gradually discontinued. If problems occur with taking the drug, report them to the prescribing physician rather than stopping the drug. Often, an adjustment in dosage or other aspect of administration may solve the problem.

✔ Follow instructions for follow-up care (eg, office visits, laboratory or other diagnostic tests that monitor therapeutic or adverse effects of drugs). Some drugs require more frequent monitoring than others. However, safety requires periodic checks with essentially all medications. With long-term use of a medication, responses may change over time with aging, changes in kidney function, and so on.

✔ Take drugs in current use when seeing a physician for any health-related problem. It may be helpful to remind the physician periodically of the medications being taken and ask if any can be discontinued or reduced in dosage.

✔ Get all prescriptions filled at the same pharmacy, when possible. This is an important safety factor in helping to avoid several prescriptions of the same or similar drugs and to minimize undesirable interactions of newly prescribed drugs with those already in use.

✔ Report any drug allergies to all health care providers, and wear a medical identification emblem that lists allergens.

✔ Ask questions (and write down the answers) about newly prescribed medications, such as:

What is the medicine's name?

What is it supposed to do (ie, what symptoms or problems will it relieve)?

How and when do I take it, and for how long?

Should it be taken with food or on an empty stomach?

While taking this medicine, should I avoid certain foods, beverages, other medications, certain activities? (For example, alcoholic beverages and driving a car should be avoided with medications that cause drowsiness or decrease alertness.)

Will this medication work safely with the others I'm already taking?

What side effects are likely and what do I do if they occur?

Will the medication affect my ability to sleep or work?

What should I do if I miss a dose?

Is there a drug information sheet I can have?

✔ Store medications out of reach of children and never refer to medications as "candy," to prevent accidental ingestion.

✔ Develop a plan for renewing or refilling prescriptions so that the medication supply does not run out when the prescribing physician is unavailable or the pharmacy is closed.

✔ When taking prescription medications, talk to a doctor, pharmacist, or nurse before starting an OTC medication or herbal or dietary supplement. This is a safety factor to avoid undesirable drug interactions.

✔ Inform health care providers if you have diabetes or kidney or liver disease. These conditions require special precautions with drug therapy.

✔ If pregnant, consult your obstetrician before taking any medications prescribed by another physician.

✔ If breast-feeding, consult your obstetrician or pediatrician before taking any medications prescribed by another physician.

Self-Administration

✔ Develop a routine for taking medications (eg, at the same time and place each day). A schedule that minimally disrupts usual household activities is more convenient and more likely to be followed accurately.

✔ Take medications in a well-lighted area and read labels of containers to ensure taking the intended drug. Do not take medications if you are not alert or cannot see clearly.

✔ Most tablets and capsules should be taken whole. If unable to take them whole, ask a health care provider before splitting, chewing, or crushing tablets or taking the medication out of capsules. Some long-acting preparations are dangerous if altered so that the entire dose is absorbed at the same time.

✔ As a general rule, take oral medications with 6–8 oz of water, in a sitting or standing position. The water helps tablets and capsules dissolve in the stomach, "dilutes" the drug so that it is less likely to upset the stomach, and promotes absorption of the drug into the bloodstream. The upright position helps the drug reach the stomach rather than getting stuck in the throat or esophagus.

✔ Take most oral drugs at evenly spaced intervals around the clock. For example, if ordered once daily, take about the same time every day. If ordered twice daily or morning and evening, take about 12 hours apart.

(continued)

CLIENT TEACHING GUIDELINES

CLIENT TEACHING GUIDELINES
Safe and Effective Use of Prescription Medications (Continued)

✔ Follow instructions about taking a medication with food or on an empty stomach; taking with other medications; or taking with fluids other than water. Prescription medications often include instructions to take on an empty stomach or with food. If taking several medications, ask a health care provider whether they may be taken together or at different times. For example, an antacid usually should not be taken at the same time as other oral medications because the antacid decreases absorption of many other drugs.

✔ If a dose is missed, most authorities recommend taking the dose if remembered soon after the scheduled time and omitting the dose if it is not remembered for several hours. If a dose is omitted, the next dose should be taken at the next scheduled time. Do not double the dose.

✔ If taking a liquid medication (or giving one to a child), measure with a calibrated medication cup or measuring spoon. A dose cannot be measured accurately with household teaspoons or tablespoons because they are different sizes and deliver varying amounts of medication. If the liquid medication is packaged with a measuring cup that shows teaspoons or tablespoons, that should be used to measure doses, for adults or children. This is especially important

for young children because most of their medications are given in liquid form.

✔ Use other types of medications according to instructions. If not clear how a medication is to be used, be sure to ask a health care provider. Correct use of oral or nasal inhalers, eye drops, and skin medications is essential for therapeutic effects.

✔ Report problems or new symptoms to a health care provider.

✔ Store medications safely, in a cool, dry place. Do not store them in a bathroom; heat, light, and moisture may cause them to decompose. Do not store them near a dangerous substance, which could be taken by mistake. Keep medications in the container in which they were dispensed by the pharmacy, where the label identifies it and gives directions. Do not put several different tablets or capsules in one container. Although this may be more convenient, especially when away from home for work or travel, it is never a safe practice because it increases the likelihood of taking the wrong drug.

✔ Discard outdated medications; do not keep drugs for long periods. Drugs are chemicals that may deteriorate over time, especially if exposed to heat and moisture. In addition, having many containers increases the risks of medication errors and adverse drug interactions.

INTEGRATING NURSING PROCESS, CRITICAL PATHS, AND DRUG THERAPY

In many agencies, nursing responsibilities related to drug therapy are designated in critical paths (also called *clinical pathways* or *care maps*). Critical paths are guidelines for the care of clients with particular conditions. Major components include a medical diagnosis, aspects of care related to the medical diagnosis, desired client outcomes, and time frames (usually days) for achieving the desired outcomes during the expected length of stay.

Medical diagnoses for which critical paths are developed are those often encountered in an agency and those that often result in complications or prolonged lengths of stay (eg, clients having coronary artery bypass grafts, myocardial infarction, hip or knee replacement). Development and implementation of the critical paths should be an interdisciplinary, collaborative effort. Thus, all health care professionals involved in the care of a client should be represented. Critical paths may be used in most health care settings. For clients, a comprehensive pathway extending from illness onset through treatment and recovery could promote continuity of care among agencies and health care providers. In hospital settings, case managers, who may be non-nurses, usually assess clients' conditions daily to evaluate progress toward the desired outcomes.

Depending on the medical diagnoses, many clinical pathways have specific guidelines related to drug therapy. These guidelines may affect any step of the nursing process. With assessment, for example, the critical path may state, "Assess for bleeding if on anticoagulant."

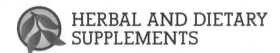 ## HERBAL AND DIETARY SUPPLEMENTS

In recent years, a nursing concern has emerged in the form of herbal and dietary supplements. These supplements are increasingly being used, and clients who take them are likely to be encountered in any clinical practice setting. Herbal medicines, also called *botanicals, phytochemicals,* and *nutraceuticals,* are derived from plants; other dietary supplements may be derived from a variety of sources. The 1994 Dietary Supplement Health and Education Act (DSHEA) defined a dietary supplement as "a vitamin, a mineral, an herb or other botanical used to supplement the diet." Under this law, herbs can be labeled according to their possible effects on the human body, but the products cannot claim to diagnose, prevent, relieve, or cure specific human diseases unless approved by the FDA. Most products have not been studied sufficiently to evaluate their safety or effectiveness; most available information involves self-reports of a few people. Overall, the effects of these products on particular con-

CLIENT TEACHING GUIDELINES

Safe and Effective Use of Over-the-Counter (OTC) Medications

☑ Read product labels carefully. The labels contain essential information about the name, ingredients, indications for use, usual dosage, when to stop using the medication or when to see a doctor, possible adverse effects, and expiration dates.

☑ Use a magnifying glass, if necessary, to read the fine print. If you do not understand the information on labels, ask a physician, pharmacist, or nurse.

☑ Do not take OTC medications longer or in higher doses than recommended.

☑ Note that all OTC medications are not safe for everyone. Many OTC medications warn against use with certain illnesses (eg, hypertension, thyroid disorders). Consult a health care provider before taking the product if you have one of the contraindicated conditions. If taking any prescription medications, consult a health care provider before taking any nonprescription drugs to avoid undesirable drug interactions and adverse effects. Some specific precautions include the following:

Avoid alcohol if taking antihistamines, cough or cold remedies containing dextromethorphan, or sleeping pills. Because all these drugs cause drowsiness, combining any of them with alcohol may result in excessive—potentially dangerous—sedation.

Avoid OTC sleeping aids if you are taking a prescription sedative-type drug (eg, for nervousness or depression).

Ask a health care provider before taking products containing aspirin if you are taking an anticoagulant (eg, Coumadin).

Ask a health care provider before taking other products containing aspirin if you are already taking a regular dose of aspirin to prevent blood clots, heart attack, or stroke. Aspirin is commonly used for this purpose, often in doses of 81 mg (a child's dose) or 325 mg.

Do not take a laxative if you have stomach pain, nausea, or vomiting, to avoid worsening the problem.

☑ Do not take a nasal decongestant (eg, Sudafed), a multi-symptom cold remedy containing pseudoephedrine (eg, Actifed, Sinutab), or an antihistamine-decongestant combination (eg, Claritin D), if you are taking a prescription medication for high blood pressure. Such products can raise blood pressure and decrease or cancel the blood pressure–lowering effect of the prescription drug. This could lead to severe hypertension and stroke.

☑ Store OTC drugs in a cool, dry place, in their original containers; check expiration dates periodically and discard those that have expired.

☑ If pregnant, consult your obstetrician before taking any OTC medications.

☑ If breast-feeding, consult your pediatrician or family doctor before taking any OTC medications.

☑ For children, follow any age limits on the label.

☑ Measure liquid OTC medications with the measuring device that comes with the product (some have a dropper or plastic cup calibrated in milliliters, teaspoons, or tablespoons). If such a device is not available, use a measuring spoon. It is not safe to use household teaspoons or tablespoons because they are different sizes and deliver varying amounts of medication. Accurate measurement of doses is especially important for young children because most of their medications are given in liquid form.

☑ Do not assume continued safety of an OTC medication you have taken for years. Older people are more likely to have adverse drug reactions and interactions because of changes in the heart, kidneys, and other organs that occur with aging and various disease processes.

☑ Note tamper-resistant features and do not buy products with damaged packages.

sumers, in combination with other herbal and dietary supplements, and in combination with pharmaceutical drugs, are essentially unknown.

What is the nursing role in relation to these products and drug therapy? Two major concerns are that use of supplements may keep the client from seeking treatment from a health care provider when indicated and that the products may interact with prescription drugs to decrease therapeutic effects or increase adverse effects. In general, nurses need to have an adequate knowledge base and to incorporate their knowledge in all steps of the nursing process. Some suggestions include the following:

● Seek information from authoritative, objective sources rather than product labels, advertisements, or personal testimonials from family members, friends, or celebrities. With the continued caution that little reliable information is known about most of these products, several resources are provided in this text:

● Table 4-1 describes some commonly used supplements. In later chapters, when information is available and deemed clinically relevant, selected supplements with some scientific support for their use are described in more detail. For example, in Chapter 7, some products reported to be useful in relieving pain, fever, inflammation, or migraine are described.

● *Client Teaching Guidelines.* In this chapter, general information is provided (see *Client Teaching Guidelines: General Information About Herbal and Dietary Supplements*). In later chapters, guidelines may emphasize avoidance or caution in using supplements thought to interact adversely with prescribed drugs or particular client conditions.

● Assessment guidelines. In this chapter, general information about the use or nonuse of supplements is assessed. In later chapters, specific supplements that may interact with particular drug group(s) are

(text continues on page 61)

TABLE 4-1 Herbal and Dietary Supplements

NAME/USES	CHARACTERISTICS	REMARKS
Black Cohosh • Most often used to relieve symptoms of menopause (eg, flushes, vaginal dryness, irritability) • May also relieve premenstrual syndrome (PMS) and dysmenorrhea	• May relieve menopausal symptoms by suppressing the release of luteinizing hormone (LH) from the pituitary gland and dysmenorrhea by relaxing uterine muscle • Well tolerated; in overdose may cause nausea, vomiting, dizziness, visual disturbances, and reduced pulse rate • Most clinical trials done with Remefemin, in small numbers of women; other trade names include Estroven and Femtrol	• No apparent advantage over traditional estrogen replacement therapy (ERT) • May be useful when ERT is contraindicated for a client or the client refuses ERT • Recommended dose is 1 tablet standardized to contain 20 mg of herbal drug, twice daily. • Not recommended for use longer than 6 months • Apparently has no effect on endometrium
Capsaicin (Chap. 6) • Used to treat pain associated with neuralgia, neuropathy, and osteoarthritis • Self-defense as the active ingredient in "pepper spray"	• A topical analgesic that may inhibit the synthesis, transport, and release of substance P, a pain transmitter • Derived from cayenne pepper • Adverse effects include skin irritation, itching, redness, and stinging	Applied topically
Chamomile Used mainly for antispasmodic effects in the gastrointestinal (GI) tract; may relieve abdominal cramping	• Usually ingested as a tea; may delay absorption of oral medications • May cause contact dermatitis and severe hypersensitivity reactions, including anaphylaxis, in people allergic to ragweed, asters, and chrysanthemums • May increase risks of bleeding	Few studies and little data to support use and effectiveness in GI disorders
Chondroitin (Chap. 7) Arthritis	• Derived from the trachea cartilage of slaughtered cattle • Usually taken with glucosamine • Adverse effects minor, may include GI upset, nausea, and headache	Several studies support use.
Creatine Athletes take creatine supplements to gain extra energy, to train longer and harder, and to improve performance	• An amino acid produced in the liver and kidneys and stored in muscles • Causes weight gain, usually within 2 weeks of starting use • Legal and available in health food stores as a powder to be mixed with water or juice, as a liquid, and as tablets and capsules	• Not recommended for use by children because studies have not been done and effects are unknown • Nurses and parents need to actively discourage children and adolescents from using creatine supplements.
Echinacea Most often used for the common cold, but also advertised for many other uses (immune system stimulant, anti-infective)	• Many species, but *E. purpurea* most often used medicinally • Effects on immune system include stimulation of phagocytes and monocytes • Contraindicated in persons with immune system disorders • Hepatotoxic with long-term use	• Hard to interpret validity of medicinal claims because various combinations of species and preparations used in reported studies • A few studies support use in clients with the common cold, with possibly shorter durations and less severe symptoms.

TABLE 4-1 Herbal and Dietary Supplements (continued)

NAME/USES	CHARACTERISTICS	REMARKS
Feverfew (Chap. 7) Migraines, menstrual irregularities, arthritis	• May increase risk of bleeding • May cause hypersensitivity reactions in people allergic to ragweed, asters, daisies, or chrysanthemums • May cause a withdrawal syndrome if use is stopped abruptly	Some studies support use in clients with migraine.
Garlic Used to lower serum cholesterol and for antihypertensive and antibiotic effects, but there is little reliable evidence for such uses	• Active ingredient thought to be allicin • Has antiplatelet activity and may increase risk of bleeding • Adverse effects include allergic reactions (asthma, dermatitis), dizziness, irritation of GI tract, nausea, vomiting	Medicinal effects probably exaggerated, especially those of deodorized supplements
Ginger Used mainly to treat nausea, including motion sickness and postoperative nausea	• Inhibits platelet aggregation; may increase clotting time • Gastroprotective effects in animal studies	Should not be used for morning sickness associated with pregnancy—may increase risk of miscarriage
Ginkgo Biloba Used mainly to improve memory and cognitive function in people with Alzheimer's disease; may be useful in treating peripheral arterial disease	• May increase blood flow to the brain and legs, improve memory, and decrease intermittent claudication • Inhibits platelet aggregation; may increase risks of bleeding with any drug that has antiplatelet effects (eg, aspirin) • Adverse effects include GI upset, headache, bleeding, allergic skin reaction	• Some studies indicate slight improvement in Alzheimer's disease. • A disadvantage is a delayed response, up to 6–8 weeks, and a recommendation to use no longer than 3 months.
Ginseng Used to increase stamina, strength, endurance, and mental acuity; also to promote sleep and relieve depression	• Has a variety of pharmacologic effects that vary with dose and duration of use (eg, inhibits platelet aggregation, may depress or stimulate central nervous system [CNS]) • Adverse effects include hypertension, nervousness, depression, insomnia, skin rashes, epistaxis, palpitations, vomiting • May increase risks of bleeding with any drug that has antiplatelet effects (eg, aspirin) • Increases risk of hypoglycemic reactions if taken with antidiabetic agents • Should not be taken with other herbs or drugs that inhibit monoamine oxidase (eg, St. John's wort, selegiline); headache, mania, and tremors may occur	• A few small studies in humans support benefits in improving psychomotor and cognitive functioning and sleep. • A ginseng abuse syndrome, with insomnia, hypotonia, and edema, has been reported. Caution clients to avoid ingesting excessive amounts. • Instruct clients with cardiovascular disease, diabetes mellitus, or hypertension to check with their primary physician before taking ginseng. • Instruct any client taking ginseng to avoid long-term use. Siberian ginseng should not be used longer than 3 weeks.

(continued)

TABLE 4-1 Herbal and Dietary Supplements (continued)

NAME/USES	CHARACTERISTICS	REMARKS
Glucosamine (Chap. 7) Arthritis	• Usually used with chondroitin • Has beneficial effects on cartilage • Adverse effects mild, may include GI upset, drowsiness	Several studies support use.
Kava (Chap. 8) Used to treat anxiety, stress, emotional excitability, and restlessness; additional claims include treatment of depression, insomnia, asthma, pain, rheumatism, and muscle spasms, and promotion of wound healing	• Produces mild euphoria and sedation; may have antiseizure effects • Adverse effects include impaired coordination, gait, and judgment; pupil dilation • Chronic heavy use may cause hematologic abnormalities (eg, decreased platelets, lymphocytes, plasma proteins), weight loss, and hepatotoxicity • May increase effects of alcohol and other CNS depressants	• Use as a calming agent is supported by limited evidence from a few small clinical trials; other therapeutic claims are poorly documented. • Should be used cautiously by people with renal disease, thrombocytopenia, or neutropenia • Should be avoided by people with hepatic disease, during pregnancy and lactation, and in children under 12 years old
Melatonin (Chap. 8) Used mainly for treatment of insomnia and prevention and treatment of jet lag	• Several studies of effects on sleep, energy level, fatigue, mental alertness, and mood indicate some improvement, compared with placebo • Contraindicated in persons with hepatic insufficiency or a history of cerebrovascular disease, depression, or neurologic disorders • Adverse effects include altered sleep patterns, confusion, headache, sedation, tachycardia	Patients with renal impairment should use cautiously.
Saint John's Wort (Chap. 10) Used for treatment of depression	• Active component may be hypericin or hyperforin • May act similarly to fluoxetine (Prozac), which increases serotonin in the brain • Studies (most lasting 6 months or less) indicate improvement in mild to moderate depression; *not* effective in major or serious depression • Adverse effects include confusion, dizziness, GI upset, photosensitivity • May interact with numerous drugs	• Should not be combined with monoamine oxidase inhibitor (MAOI) or selective serotonin reuptake inhibitor (SSRI) antidepressants • Can decrease effectiveness of birth control pills, antineoplastic drugs, antivirals used to treat acquired immunodeficiency syndrome (AIDS), and organ transplant drugs (eg, cyclosporine)
Saw Palmetto Used to relieve urinary symptoms in men with benign prostatic hyperplasia (BPH)	• Action unknown; may have anti-androgenic effects • Generally well tolerated; adverse effects usually minor but may include GI upset, headache. Diarrhea may occur with high doses.	• Reportedly effective in doses of 320 mg/d for 1–3 months • Men should have a prostate-specific antigen (PSA) test before starting saw palmetto, because the herb can reduce levels of PSA and produce a false-negative result.

TABLE 4-1 Herbal and Dietary Supplements (continued)

NAME/USES	CHARACTERISTICS	REMARKS
Valerian (Chap. 8) Used mainly to promote sleep and allay anxiety and nervousness; also has muscle relaxant effects	• Adverse effects with acute overdose or chronic use include blurred vision, drowsiness, dizziness, excitability, hypersensitivity reactions, insomnia; also, risk of liver damage from combination products containing valerian and from overdoses averaging 2.5 g • Additive sedation if taken with other CNS depressants	• Should not be combined with sedative drugs and should not be used regularly • Many extract products contain 40%–60% alcohol. • Most studies flawed—experts do not believe there is sufficient evidence to support the use of valerian for treatment of insomnia.

discussed. For example, some supplements are known to increase blood pressure (see Chap. 52) or risk of excessive bleeding (see Chap. 54).

● End-of-chapter references.

● A good source of information is the National Center for Complementary and Alternative Medicine (NCCAM) at the National Institutes of Health: NCCAM Clearinghouse
PO Box 8218

Silver Spring, MD 20907-8218
Tel: 1-888-644-6226
Web site: http://nccam.nih.gov

● Ask clients whether they use herbal medicines or other dietary supplements. If so, try to determine the name, dose, and frequency and duration of use.

● Teach clients about these products and their possible interactions with one another and with prescription drugs (when such information is available).

CLIENT TEACHING GUIDELINES

General Information About Herbal and Dietary Supplements

✔ Herbal and dietary products are chemicals that have druglike effects in people. Unfortunately, their effects are largely unknown and may be dangerous for some people because there is little reliable information about them. For most products, little research has been done to determine either their benefits or their adverse effects.

✔ The safety and effectiveness of these products are not documented or regulated by laws designed to protect consumers, as are pharmaceutical drugs. As a result, the types and amounts of ingredients may not be standardized or even identified on the product label. In fact, most products contain several active ingredients and it is often not known which ingredient has the desired pharmacologic effect. In addition, components and active ingredients of plants can vary considerably, depending on the soil, water, and climate where the plants are grown.

✔ These products can be used more safely if they are manufactured by a reputable company that states the ingredients are standardized (meaning that the dose of medicine in each tablet or capsule is the same).

✔ The product label should also state specific percentages, amounts, and strengths of active ingredients. With herbal medicines especially, different brands of the same herb vary in the amounts of active ingredients per recommended dose. Dosing is also difficult because a particular herb may be available in sev-

eral different dosage forms (eg, tablet, capsule, tea, extract) with different amounts of active ingredients.

✔ These products are often advertised as "natural." Many people interpret this to mean the products are safe and better than synthetic or man-made products. This is not true; "natural" does not mean safe, especially when taken concurrently with other herbals, dietary supplements, or drugs.

✔ When taking herbal or dietary supplements, follow the instructions on the product label. Inappropriate use or taking excessive amounts may cause dangerous side effects.

✔ Inform health care providers when taking any kind of herbal or dietary supplement, to reduce risks of severe adverse effects or drug–supplement interactions.

✔ Most herbal and dietary supplements should be avoided during pregnancy or lactation and in young children.

✔ The American Society of Anesthesiologists recommends that all herbal products be discontinued 2–3 weeks before any surgical procedure. Some products (eg, echinacea, feverfew, garlic, gingko, ginseng, kava, valerian, and St. John's wort) can interfere with or increase the effects of some drugs, affect blood pressure or heart rhythm, or increase risks of bleeding; some have unknown effects when combined with anesthetics, other perioperative medications, and surgical procedures.

✔ Store herbal and dietary supplements out of the reach of children.

GENERAL PRINCIPLES OF DRUG THERAPY

Goals and Guidelines

The goals of drug therapy are to maximize beneficial effects and minimize adverse effects. To help meet this goal, general guidelines include the following:

- Expected benefits should outweigh potential adverse effects. Thus, drugs usually should not be prescribed for trivial problems or problems for which nondrug measures are effective.
- Drug therapy should be individualized. Many variables influence a drug's effects on the human body. Failure to consider these variables may decrease therapeutic effects or increase risks of adverse effects to an unacceptable level.
- Drug effects on quality of life should be considered in designing a drug therapy regimen. Quality-of-life issues are also being emphasized in research studies, with expectations of measurable improvement as a result of drug therapy.

Drug Selection and Dosage

Numerous factors must be considered when choosing a drug and dosage range for a particular client, including the following:

- For the most part, use as few drugs in as few doses as possible. Minimizing the number of drugs and the frequency of administration increases client compliance with the prescribed drug regimen and decreases risks of serious adverse effects, including hazardous drug–drug interactions. There are notable exceptions to this basic rule. For example, multiple drugs are commonly used to treat hypertension and serious infections.
- Although individual drugs allow greater flexibility of dosage than fixed-dose combinations, fixed-dose combinations are increasingly available and commonly used, mainly because clients are more likely to take them. Also, many of the combination products are formulated to be long acting, which also promotes compliance.
- The least amount of the least potent drug that yields therapeutic benefit should be given to decrease adverse reactions. For example, if a mild nonopioid and a strong opioid analgesic are both ordered, give the nonopioid drug *if it is effective in relieving pain.*
- In drug literature, recommended dosages are listed in amounts likely to be effective for most people. However, they are only guidelines to be interpreted according to the client's condition. For example, clients with serious illnesses may require larger doses of some drugs than clients with milder illnesses; clients with severe kidney disease often need much smaller doses of renally excreted drugs.

- A drug can be started rapidly or slowly. If it has a long half-life and optimal therapeutic effects do not usually occur for several days or weeks, the prescriber may order a limited number of relatively large (loading) doses followed by a regular schedule of smaller (maintenance) doses. When drug actions are not urgent, therapy may be initiated with a maintenance dose.

Drug Therapy in Special Populations

Drug Therapy in Children

Drug therapy in neonates (birth to 1 month), infants (1 month to 1 year), and children (1 to 12 years) requires special consideration because of the child's changing size, developmental level, and organ function. Physiologic differences alter drug pharmacokinetics (Table 4-2), and drug therapy is less predictable than in adults. Neonates are especially vulnerable to adverse drug effects because of their immature liver and kidney function; neonatal therapeutics are discussed further in Chapter 65.

Most drug use in children is empiric because few studies have been done in that population. For many drugs, manufacturers' literature states "safety and effectiveness for use in children have not been established." Most drugs given to adults also are given to children, and general principles, techniques of drug administration, and nursing process guidelines apply.

All aspects of pediatric drug therapy must be guided by the child's age, weight, and level of growth and development. For safety, keep all medications in childproof containers, out of reach of children, and do not refer to medications as "candy." Additional principles and guidelines are discussed in the following sections.

Drug Selection and Dosage
- Choice of drug is often restricted because many drugs commonly used in adult drug therapy have not been sufficiently investigated to ensure safety and effectiveness in children.
- Safe therapeutic dosage ranges are less well defined for children than for adults. Some drugs are not recommended for use in children, and therefore dosages have not been established. For many drugs, doses for children are extrapolated from those established for adults. When pediatric dosage ranges are listed in drug literature, these should be used. Often, however, dosages are expressed as the amount of drug to be given per kilogram of body weight or square meter of body surface area, and the amount needed for a specific dose must be calculated as a fraction of the adult dose. Body surface area (BSA) is based on height and weight and can be estimated using a nomogram (Fig. 4-1). Use the estimated BSA in the following formula to calculate the child's dose:

$$\frac{\text{Body surface area (in square meters)}}{1.73 \text{ square meters } (m^2)} \times \text{adult dose} = \text{child's dose}$$

TABLE 4-2 Neonates, Infants, and Children: Physiologic Characteristics and Pharmacokinetic Consequences

PHYSIOLOGIC CHARACTERISTICS	PHARMACOKINETIC CONSEQUENCES
Increased thinness and permeability of skin in neonates and infants	Increased absorption of topical drugs (eg, corticosteroids may be absorbed sufficiently to suppress adrenocortical function)
Immature blood–brain barrier in neonates and infants	Increased distribution of drugs into the central nervous system because myelinization (which creates the blood–brain barrier to the passage of drugs) is not mature until approximately 2 years of age
Increased percentage of body water (70%–80% in neonates and infants, compared with 50%–60% in children older than 2 years of age and adults)	Usually increased volume of distribution in infants and young children, compared with adults. This would seem to indicate a need for larger doses. However, prolonged drug half-life and decreased rate of drug clearance may offset. The net effect is often a need for decreased dosage.
Altered protein binding until approximately 1 year of age, when it reaches adult levels	The amount and binding capacity of plasma proteins may be reduced. This may result in a greater proportion of unbound or pharmacologically active drug and greater risks of adverse drug effects. Dosage requirements may be decreased or modified by other factors. Drugs with decreased protein binding in neonates, compared with older children and adults, include ampicillin (Principen, others), diazepam (Valium), digoxin (Lanoxin), lidocaine (Xylocaine), nafcillin, phenobarbital, phenytoin (Dilantin), salicylates (eg, aspirin), and theophylline (Theolair).
Decreased glomerular filtration rate in neonates and infants, compared with older children and adults. Kidney function develops progressively during the first few months of life and is fairly mature by 1 year of age.	In neonates and infants, slowed excretion of drugs eliminated by the kidneys. Dosage of these drugs may need to be decreased, depending on the infant's age and level of growth and development.
Decreased activity of liver drug-metabolizing enzyme systems in neonates and infants	Decreased capacity for biotransformation of drugs. This results in slowed metabolism and elimination, with increased risks of drug accumulation and adverse effects.
Increased activity of liver drug-metabolizing enzyme systems in children	Increased capacity for biotransformation of some drugs. This results in a rapid rate of metabolism and elimination. For example, theophylline is cleared about 30% faster in a 7-year-old child than in an adult and approximately four times faster than in a neonate.

● Dosages obtained from calculations are approximate and must be individualized. These doses can be used initially and then increased or decreased according to the child's response.

Drug Administration
● Use the oral route of drug administration when possible. Try to obtain the child's cooperation; never force oral medications because forcing may lead to aspiration.
● Site selection for intramuscular injections depends on age and size. In infants, use thigh muscles because the deltoid muscles are quite small and the gluteal muscles do not develop until the child is walking. In children older than 18 months of age, use deltoid muscles; injections are considered less painful than in thigh muscles. In children older than 3 years of age, ventrogluteal injections are considered less painful than those in anterior thigh or dorsogluteal areas.

● Children are fearful of injections. With an immunization schedule that calls for 20 or more injections during childhood plus procedures required by illnesses, measures are needed to decrease the pain and fear associated with injections, venipunctures, and other "shots." One technique is the application of EMLA (eutectic mixture of lidocaine and prilocaine local anesthetics). A disadvantage is that EMLA must be applied an hour before the painful injection. Having parents present and using distraction techniques may also be helpful.

Drug Therapy in Older Adults

Aging is a continuum; precisely when a person becomes an "older adult" is not clearly established, but in this book, the term *older adult* refers to people 65 years of age and older. In this population, general nursing process guidelines and principles of drug therapy apply.

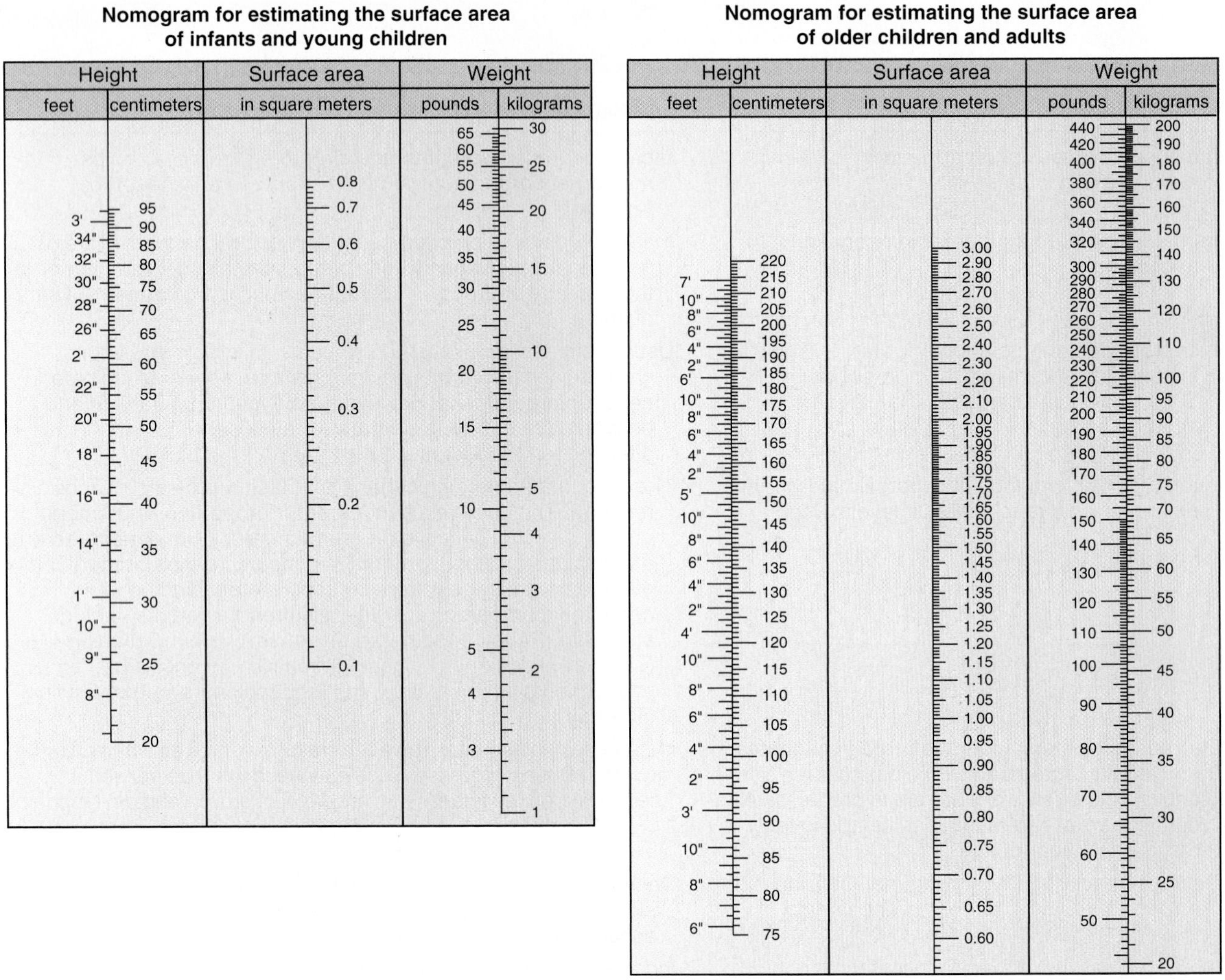

**Nomogram for estimating the surface area
of infants and young children**

Height		Surface area	Weight	
feet	centimeters	in square meters	pounds	kilograms

**Nomogram for estimating the surface area
of older children and adults**

Height		Surface area	Weight	
feet	centimeters	in square meters	pounds	kilograms

FIGURE 4-1 Body surface nomograms. To determine the surface area of the client, draw a straight line between the point representing his or her height on the left vertical scale to the point representing weight on the right vertical scale. The point at which this line intersects the middle vertical scale represents the client's surface area in square meters (courtesy of Abbott Laboratories).

Adverse effects are more likely because of physiologic changes associated with aging (Table 4-3), pathologic changes due to disease processes, multiple drug therapy for acute and chronic disorders, impaired memory and cognition, and difficulty in complying with drug orders. Overall, the goal of drug therapy may be "care" rather than "cure," with efforts to prevent or control symptoms and to maintain the client's ability to function in usual activities of daily living. Additional principles include the following:

● Although age in years is important, older adults are quite heterogeneous in their responses to drug therapy and responses differ widely within the same age group. Responses also differ in the same person over time. Physiologic age (ie, organ function) is more important than chronologic age.

● It may be difficult to separate the effects of aging from the effects of disease processes or drug therapy, particularly long-term drug therapy. Symptoms attributed to aging or disease may be caused by medications. This occurs because older adults are usually less able to metabolize and excrete drugs efficiently. As a result, drugs are more likely to accumulate. *When a client develops new symptoms or becomes less capable of functioning in usual activities of daily living, consider the possibility of adverse drug effects.* Because new signs and symptoms are often attributed to aging or disease, they may be ignored or treated by prescribing a new drug, when stopping or reducing the dose of an old drug is the indicated intervention.

● Use nondrug measures to decrease the need for drugs and to increase their effectiveness or decrease their

TABLE 4-3 Older Adults: Physiologic Characteristics and Pharmacokinetic Consequences

PHYSIOLOGIC CHARACTERISTICS	PHARMACOKINETIC CONSEQUENCES
Decreased gastrointestinal secretions and motility	Minimal effects on absorption of most oral drugs; effects on extended-release formulations are unknown
Decreased cardiac output	• Slower absorption from some sites of administration (eg, gastrointestinal tract, subcutaneous or muscle tissue); effects on absorption from skin and mucous membranes are unknown • Decreased distribution to sites of action in tissues, with potential for delaying the onset and reducing the extent of therapeutic effects
Decreased blood flow to the liver and kidneys	Delayed metabolism and excretion, which may lead to drug accumulation and increased risks of adverse or toxic effects
Decreased total body water and lean body mass per kg of weight; increased body fat	Water-soluble drugs (eg, ethanol, lithium) are distributed into a smaller area, with resultant higher plasma concentrations and higher risks of toxicity with a given dose. Fat-soluble drugs (eg, diazepam) are distributed to a larger area, accumulate in fat, and have a longer duration of action in the body.
Decreased serum albumin	Decreased availability of protein for binding and transporting drug molecules. This increases serum concentration of free, pharmacologically active drug, especially for those that are normally highly protein bound (eg, aspirin, warfarin). This may increase risks of adverse effects. However, the drug also may be metabolized and excreted more rapidly, thereby offsetting at least some of the risks. In addition, drug interactions occur with co-administration of multiple drugs that are highly protein bound. The drugs compete for protein-binding sites and are more likely to cause adverse effects with decreased levels of serum albumin. As above, the result is larger concentrations of free drug.
Decreased blood flow to the liver; decreased size of the liver; decreased number and activity of the cytochrome P450 (CYP) oxidative drug-metabolizing enzymes	Slowed metabolism and detoxification of many drugs, with increased risks of drug accumulation and toxic effects. (Numerous drugs metabolized by the CYP enzymes are often prescribed for older adults, including beta blockers, calcium channel blockers, antimicrobials, the statin cholesterol-lowering drugs, and anti-ulcer drugs. Metabolism of drugs metabolized by conjugative reactions [eg, acetaminophen, diazepam, morphine, steroids] does not change significantly with aging).
Decreased blood flow to the kidneys; decreased number of functioning nephrons; decreased glomerular filtration rate; and decreased tubular secretion	• Impaired drug excretion, prolonged half-life, and increased risks of toxicity • Age-related alterations in renal function are consistent and well described. When renal blood flow is decreased, less drug is delivered to the kidney for elimination. Renal mass is also decreased and older adults may be more sensitive to drugs that further impair renal function (eg, nonsteroidal anti-inflammatory drugs such as ibuprofen, which older adults often take for pain or arthritis).

adverse effects. For example, insomnia is a common complaint among older adults. Preventing it (eg, by avoiding excessive caffeine and napping) is much safer than taking sedative-hypnotic drugs.

Drug Selection and Dosage

● Any prescriber should review current medications, including nonprescription drugs, before prescribing new drugs. A regimen of several drugs increases the risks of adverse drug reactions and interactions.

● Medications—both prescription and nonprescription drugs—should be taken only when necessary. When drug therapy is required, the choice of drug should be based on available drug information regarding effects in older adults.

● The basic principle of giving the smallest effective number of drugs applies especially to older adults. In addition, all drugs should be given for the shortest effective time. This interval is not established for most drugs, and many drugs are continued for years.

Some drugs, especially with long-term use, need to be tapered in dosage and discontinued gradually to avoid withdrawal symptoms.

- Health care providers must reassess drug regimens periodically to see whether drugs, dosages, or other aspects need to be revised. This is especially important when a serious illness or significant changes in health status have occurred.

- The smallest number of effective doses should be prescribed. This strategy allows less disruption of usual activities and promotes compliance with the prescribed regimen. When any drug is started, the dosage should usually be smaller than for younger adults. The dosage can then be increased or decreased according to response. If increased dosage is indicated, increments should be smaller and made at longer intervals in older adults. This conservative, safe approach is sometimes called "start low, go slow."

Drug Administration

Older adults often take multiple medications, and many older adults are unable to self-administer more than three or four drugs correctly. For people receiving long-term drug therapy at home, use measures to help them take drugs safely and effectively:

- If vision is impaired, label drug containers with large lettering for easier readability. A magnifying glass also may be useful.

- Be sure the client can open drug containers. For example, avoid childproof containers for an older adult with arthritic hands.

- Several devices may be used to schedule drug doses and decrease risks of omitting or repeating doses. These devices include written schedules, calendars, and charts. Also available are drug containers with each dose prepared and clearly labeled as to the day and time it is to be taken. With the latter system, the client can tell at a glance whether a dose has been taken.

- Enlist family members or friends when necessary.

APPLYING YOUR KNOWLEDGE 4-3
Given Mr. Walker's age and his drug regimen, what factors related to medication administration should you consider?

Drug Therapy in Clients With Renal Impairment

Many clients have or are at risk for impaired renal function. Clients with disease processes such as diabetes, hypertension, or heart failure may have renal insufficiency on first contact, and this may be worsened by illness, major surgery or trauma, or administration of nephrotoxic drugs. In clients with normal renal function, renal failure may develop from depletion of intravascular fluid volume, shock due to sepsis or blood loss, seriously impaired cardiovascular function, major surgery, nephrotoxic drugs, or other conditions. Acute renal failure (ARF) may occur in any illness in which renal blood flow or function is impaired. Chronic renal failure (CRF) usually results from disease processes that destroy renal tissue.

With ARF, renal function may recover if the impairment is recognized promptly, contributing factors are eliminated or treated effectively, and medication dosages are adjusted according to the extent of renal impairment. With CRF, effective treatment can help to conserve functioning nephrons and delay progression to end-stage renal disease (ESRD). If ESRD develops, dialysis or transplantation is required.

In relation to drug therapy, the major concern is that the kidneys are unable or less able to excrete drugs and drug metabolites. Guidelines have been established for the use of many drugs; health care providers need to use these recommendations to maximize the safety and effectiveness of drug therapy. Some general guidelines are discussed here; specific guidelines for particular drug groups are included in the appropriate chapters.

- Drug therapy must be approached with special caution because of the high risks of drug accumulation and adverse effects. When possible, nephrologists should design drug therapy regimens. However, all health care providers need to be knowledgeable about risk factors for development of renal impairment; illnesses and their physiologic changes (eg, hemodynamic, renal, hepatic, and metabolic alterations) that affect renal function; and the effects of commonly used drugs on renal function.

- Renal status should be monitored in any client with renal insufficiency or risk factors for developing renal insufficiency. Signs and symptoms of ARF include decreased urine output (<600 mL/24 hours), increased blood urea nitrogen or increased serum creatinine (>2 mg/dL or an increase of ≥0.5 mg/dL over a baseline value of <3.0 mg/dL). In addition, an adequate fluid intake is required to excrete drugs by the kidneys. Any factors that deplete extracellular fluid volume (eg, inadequate fluid intake; diuretic drugs; loss of body fluids with blood loss, vomiting, or diarrhea) increase the risk of worsening renal impairment in clients with impairment or of causing impairment in those with previously normal function.

- Clients with renal impairment may respond to a drug dose or serum concentration differently than clients with normal renal function because of physiologic and biochemical changes. Thus, drug therapy must be individualized according to the extent of renal impairment. This individualization is usually determined by measuring serum creatinine, which is then used to calculate creatinine clearance. Estimations of creatinine clearance are more accurate for clients with stable renal function and average muscle mass (for their age, weight, and height). Estimations are less accurate for emaciated and obese clients and for those with changing renal function, as often occurs in acute illness. If a client is oliguric (<400 mL urine/24 hours), for example, the creatinine clearance should be estimated to be less than 10 milliliters per minute, regardless of the serum creatinine concentration. Also, in elderly clients, serum creatinine is an unreliable indicator of renal function because these clients usually have diminished muscle mass. As a result, they may have a normal serum level of creatinine even if their renal function is markedly reduced.

● Some medications can increase serum creatinine levels and create a false impression of renal failure. These drugs, which include cimetidine and trimethoprim, interfere with secretion of creatinine into kidney tubules. As a result, serum creatinine levels are increased without an associated decrease in renal function.

Drug Selection and Dosage

● Drug selection should be guided by baseline renal function and the known effects of drugs on renal function, when possible. Many commonly used drugs may adversely affect renal function, including nonsteroidal anti-inflammatory drugs such as ibuprofen (eg, Motrin, Advil). Some drugs are excreted exclusively (eg, aminoglycoside antibiotics, lithium), and most are excreted, to some extent, by the kidneys. Some drugs are contraindicated in renal impairment (eg, tetracyclines except doxycycline); others can be used if safety guidelines are followed (eg, reducing dosage, monitoring serum drug levels and renal function tests, avoiding dehydration). Drugs known to be nephrotoxic should be avoided when possible. In some instances, however, there are no effective substitutes and nephrotoxic drugs must be given. Some commonly used nephrotoxic drugs include aminoglycoside antibiotics, amphotericin B, and cisplatin.

● Dosage of many drugs needs to be decreased in clients with renal failure, including dosage of aminoglycoside antibiotics, most cephalosporin antibiotics, fluoroquinolones, and digoxin. In general, the most effective dosage adjustments are based on the client's clinical responses and serum drug levels.

● For clients receiving renal replacement therapy (eg, hemodialysis or some type of filtration), the treatment removes variable amounts of drugs that are usually excreted through the kidneys. With some drugs, such as many antimicrobials, a supplemental dose may be needed to maintain therapeutic blood levels of drug.

Drug Therapy in Clients With Hepatic Impairment

Most drugs are eliminated from the body by hepatic metabolism, renal excretion, or both. Hepatic metabolism depends mainly on blood flow and enzyme activity in the liver and protein binding in the plasma. Clients at risk for impaired liver function include those with primary liver disease (eg, hepatitis, cirrhosis) and those with disease processes that impair blood flow to the liver (eg, heart failure, shock, major surgery, trauma) or hepatic enzyme production. An additional factor is hepatotoxic drugs. Fortunately, although the liver is often damaged, it has a great capacity for cell repair and may be able to function with as little as 10% of undamaged hepatic cells.

In relation to drug therapy, acute liver impairment may interfere with drug metabolism and elimination, whereas chronic cirrhosis or severe liver impairment may affect all pharmacokinetic processes. It is difficult to predict the effects of drug therapy because of wide variations in liver function and few helpful diagnostic tests. In addition, with severe hepatic impairment, extrahepatic sites of drug metabolism (eg, intestine, kidneys, lungs) may become more important in eliminating drugs from the body. Thus, guidelines for drug selection, dosage, and duration of use are not well established. Some general guidelines for increasing drug safety and effectiveness are discussed here; known guidelines for particular drug groups are included in the appropriate chapters.

During drug therapy, clients with impaired liver function require close monitoring for signs and symptoms (eg, nausea, vomiting, jaundice, liver enlargement) and abnormal results of laboratory tests of liver function. Liver function tests should be monitored in clients with or at risk for liver impairment, especially when clients are receiving potentially hepatotoxic drugs. Indicators of hepatic impairment include serum bilirubin levels above 4 to 5 milligrams per deciliter, a prothrombin time greater than 1.5 times control, a serum albumin below 2.0 grams per deciliter, and elevated serum alanine (ALT) and aspartate (AST) aminotransferases. In some clients, abnormal liver function test results may occur without indicating severe liver damage and are often reversible.

Drug Selection and Dosage

● Drug selection should be based on knowledge of drug effects on hepatic function. Hepatotoxic drugs should be avoided when possible. If they cannot be avoided, they should be used in the smallest effective doses, for the shortest effective time. Commonly used hepatotoxic drugs include acetaminophen, isoniazid, and cholesterol-lowering statins. Alcohol is toxic to the liver by itself and increases the risks of hepatotoxicity with other drugs.

● In addition to hepatotoxic drugs, many other drugs can cause or aggravate liver impairment by decreasing hepatic blood flow and drug-metabolizing capacity. For example, epinephrine and related drugs may cause vasoconstriction in the hepatic artery and portal vein, the two main sources of the liver's blood supply. Beta-adrenergic blocking agents (eg, propranolol) decrease hepatic blood flow by decreasing cardiac output. Several drugs (eg, cimetidine, fluoxetine) inhibit hepatic metabolism of many co-administered drugs. The consequence may be toxicity from the inhibited drugs if the dose is not decreased.

● Dosage should be reduced for drugs that are extensively metabolized in the liver because, if doses are not reduced, serum drug levels are higher, elimination is slower, and toxicity is more likely to occur in a client with hepatic disease. For example, parenteral lidocaine is normally rapidly deactivated by hepatic metabolism. If blood flow is impaired so that lidocaine molecules in the blood are unable to reach drug-metabolizing liver cells, more drug stays in the bloodstream longer. Also, some oral drugs are normally extensively metabolized during their "first pass" through the liver, so that a relatively small portion of an oral dose reaches the systemic circulation. In clients with cirrhosis, the blood carrying the drug molecules is shunted around the liver so that oral drugs go directly into the systemic circulation. Some drugs whose dosages should be decreased in clients with hepatic failure include cefoperazone, cimetidine, clindamycin, diazepam, labetalol, lorazepam, morphine, phenytoin, propranolol, quinidine, ranitidine, theophylline, and verapamil.

Drug Therapy in Clients With Critical Illness

The term *critical illness,* as used here, denotes clients who are experiencing acute, serious, or life-threatening illness. Critically ill clients are at risk for multiple organ dysfunction, including cardiovascular, renal, and hepatic impairments that influence all aspects of drug therapy. In general, these clients exhibit varying degrees of organ impairment and their conditions tend to change rapidly, so that drug pharmacokinetics and pharmacodynamics vary widely. Although blood volume is often decreased, drug distribution is usually increased because of less protein binding and increased extracellular fluid. Drug elimination is usually impaired because of decreased blood flow and decreased function of the liver and kidneys.

Although critical care nursing is a specialty area and much of critical care is performed in an intensive care unit (ICU), nurses in numerous other settings also care for these clients. For example, nurses in emergency departments often initiate and maintain treatment for several hours; nurses on other hospital units care for clients who are transferred to or from ICUs; and, increasingly, clients formerly cared for in an ICU are on medical-surgical hospital units, in long-term care facilities, or even at home. Moreover, increasing numbers of nursing students are introduced to critical care during their educational programs, many new graduates seek employment in critical care settings, and experienced nurses may transfer to an ICU. Thus, all nurses need to know about drug therapy in critically ill clients. Some general guidelines are discussed here; more specific guidelines related to particular drugs are included in the appropriate chapters.

● Drug therapy in critically ill clients is often more complex, more problematic, and less predictable than in most other populations. One reason is that clients often have multiple organ impairments that alter drug effects and increase the risks of adverse drug reactions. Another reason is that critically ill clients often require aggressive treatment with large numbers, large doses, and combinations of highly potent medications. Overall, therapeutic effects may be decreased and adverse effects may be increased because the client's body may be unable to process or respond to drugs effectively.

In this at-risk population, safe and effective drug therapy requires that all involved health care providers be knowledgeable about common critical illnesses, the physiologic changes (eg, hemodynamic, renal, hepatic, and metabolic alterations) that can be caused by the illnesses, and the drugs used to treat the illnesses. Nurses need to be especially diligent in administering drugs and vigilant in observing client responses.

● Drugs used in clients with critical illness represent most drug classifications and are also discussed in other chapters. Commonly used drugs include analgesics, antimicrobials, cardiovascular agents, gastric acid suppressants, neuromuscular blocking agents, and sedatives. In many instances, the goal of drug therapy is to support vital functions and relieve life-threatening symptoms until healing can occur or definitive treatment can be instituted.

● Laboratory tests are often needed before and during drug therapy for critical illnesses to assess the client's condition (eg, cardiovascular, renal, and hepatic functions; fluid and electrolyte balance) and response to treatment. Other tests may include measurement of serum drug levels. The results of these tests may indicate that changes are needed in drug therapy.

● Serum protein levels should be monitored in critically ill clients because drug binding may be significantly altered. Serum albumin, which binds acidic drugs such as phenytoin and diazepam, is usually decreased during critical illness for a variety of reasons, including inadequate production by the liver. If there is not enough albumin to bind a drug, blood levels of the drug are higher and may cause adverse effects. Also, unbound molecules are metabolized and excreted more readily so that therapeutic effects may be decreased.

Alpha$_1$-acid glycoprotein binds basic drugs, and its synthesis may increase during critical illness. As a result, the bound portion of a dose increases for some drugs (eg, propranolol, imipramine) and therapeutic blood levels may not be achieved unless higher doses are given. In addition, these drugs are eliminated more slowly than usual.

Drug Selection and Dosage

Drug selection should be guided by the client's clinical status (eg, symptoms, severity of illness) and organ function, especially cardiovascular, renal, and hepatic functions.

- Dosage requirements may vary considerably among clients and within the same client at different times during an illness. A standard dose may be effective, sub-therapeutic, or toxic. Thus, it is especially important that initial dosages are individualized according to the severity of the condition being treated and the client's characteristics, such as age and organ function, and that maintenance dosages are titrated according to client responses and changes in organ function (eg, as indicated by symptoms or laboratory tests).
- Weigh clients when possible, initially and periodically, because dosage of many drugs is based on weight. In addition, periodic weights help to assess clients for loss of body mass or gain in body water, both of which affect the pharmacokinetics of the drugs administered.

Drug Administration

Route of administration should also be guided by the client's clinical status. Most drugs are given intravenously (IV) because critically ill clients are often unable to take oral medications and require many drugs, rapid drug action, and relatively large doses. In addition, the IV route achieves more reliable and measurable blood levels.

- When a drug is given IV, it reaches the heart and brain quickly because the sympathetic nervous system and other homeostatic mechanisms attempt to maintain blood flow to the heart and brain at the expense of blood flow to other organs such as the kidneys, gastrointestinal tract, liver, and skin. As a result, cardiovascular and central nervous system (CNS) effects may be faster, more pronounced, and longer lasting than usual. If the drug is a sedative, effects may include excessive sedation and cardiac depression.
- If the client is able to take oral medications, this is usually the preferred route. However, many factors may interfere with drug effects (eg, impaired function of the gastrointestinal tract, heart, kidneys, or liver) and drug–drug and drug–diet interactions may occur if precautions are not taken. For example, antiulcer drugs, which are often given to prevent stress ulcers and gastrointestinal bleeding, may decrease absorption of other drugs.
- For clients who receive oral medications or nutritional solutions through a nasogastric, gastrostomy, or jejunostomy tube, there may be drug–food interactions that impair drug absorption. In addition, crushing tablets or opening capsules to give a drug by a gastrointestinal (GI) tube may alter the absorption and chemical stability of the drug.
- Sublingual, oral inhalation, and transdermal medications may be used effectively in some critically ill clients. However, few drugs are available in these formulations.
- For clients with hypotension and shock, drugs usually should not be given orally, subcutaneously, intramuscularly, or by skin patch because shock impairs absorp-

tion from their sites of administration; distribution to body cells is unpredictable; the liver cannot metabolize drugs effectively; and the kidneys cannot excrete drugs effectively.
- With many drugs, the timing of administration may be important in increasing therapeutic effects and decreasing adverse effects. Once-daily drug doses should be given at approximately the same time each day; multiple daily doses should be given at approximately even intervals around the clock.

Drug Therapy in Home Care

The continuing trend toward outpatient care and brief hospitalizations has greatly expanded home care as clients are often discharged to their homes for follow-up care and recovery. Skilled nursing care, such as managing medication regimens, is often required during follow-up. Most general principles and nursing responsibilities related to drug therapy apply in home care as in other health care settings. Clients may require short- or long-term drug therapy. In most instances, the role of the nurse is to teach the client or caregiver to administer medications and monitor their effects. However, there are some general considerations:

- Remember that the nurse is a guest in the client's home and must work within the environment to establish rapport, elicit cooperation, and provide nursing care.
- When making initial contact (usually by telephone), schedule a home visit, preferably at a convenient time for the client and caregiver. In addition, state the main purpose of the visit and approximately how long the visit will be. Establish a method for contact in case the appointment must be canceled by either party.
- Assess the client's attitude toward the prescribed medication regimen and his or her ability to provide self-care. If the client is unable to provide self-care, determine who will be the primary caregiver for medication administration and will be observing for medication effects. Determine the learning needs of the client or caregiver in relation to the medication regimen.
- Ask to see all prescribed and OTC medications that the client takes, and ask how and when the client takes each one. With this information, you may be able to reinforce the client's compliance or identify potential problem areas (eg, differences between instructions and client usage of medications, drugs with opposing or duplicate effects, continued use of medications that were supposed to be discontinued, drugs discontinued because of adverse effects).
- Ask if the client takes any herbal medicines or dietary supplements. If so, try to determine the amount, frequency, duration of use, reasons for use, and perceived beneficial or adverse effects. Explain that you need this information because some herbal and

dietary supplements may cause various health problems or react adversely with prescription or OTC medications.

- Assess the environment for potential safety hazards (eg, risk of infection with corticosteroids and other immunosuppressants, risk of falls and other injuries with opioid analgesics and other drugs with sedating effects). In addition, assess the client's ability to obtain medications and keep appointments for follow-up visits to health care providers.

- Provide whatever information and assistance is needed for home management of the drug therapy regimen. Most people are accustomed to taking oral drugs, but they may need information about timing in relation to food intake, whether a tablet can be crushed, when to omit the drug, and other aspects. With other routes, you may initially need to demonstrate administration or coach the client or caregiver through each step. Demonstrating and having the client or caregiver do a return demonstration is a good way to teach psychomotor skills such as giving a medication through a GI tube, preparing and administering an injection, or manipulating an IV infusion pump.

- In addition to safe and accurate administration, teach the client and caregiver to observe for beneficial and adverse effects. If adverse effects occur, teach them how to manage minor ones and which ones to report to a health care provider.

- Between home visits, maintain contact with clients and caregivers to monitor progress, answer questions, identify problems, and provide reassurance. Clients and caregivers should be given a telephone number to call with questions about medications, adverse effects, and so forth. You may wish to schedule a daily time for receiving and making nonemergency calls. For clients and nurses with computers and Internet access, e-mail may be a convenient and efficient method of communication.

N U R S I N G   A C T I O N S

Monitoring Drug Therapy

NURSING ACTIONS	RATIONALE/EXPLANATION
1. Prepare medications for administration.	If giving medications to a group of patients, start preparing about 30 minutes before the scheduled administration time when possible, to avoid rushing and increasing the risk of errors.
a. Assemble appropriate supplies and equipment.	Medications and supplies are usually kept on a medication cart in a hospital or long-term care facility.
b. Calculate doses when indicated.	Except for very simple calculations, use pencil and paper to decrease the risk of errors. If unsure about the results, ask a colleague or a pharmacist to do the calculation. Compare results. Accuracy is vital.
c. Check vital signs when indicated.	Check blood pressure (recent recordings) before giving antihypertensive drugs. Check temperature before giving an antipyretic.
d. Check laboratory reports when indicated.	Commonly needed reports include serum potassium levels before giving diuretics; prothrombin time or international normalized ratio (INR) before giving Coumadin; culture and susceptibility reports before giving an antibiotic.
e. Check drug references when indicated.	This is often needed to look up new or unfamiliar drugs; other uses include assessing a drug in relation to a particular client (eg, Is it contraindicated? Is it likely to interact with other drugs the client is taking? Does the client's ordered dose fit within the dosage range listed in the drug reference? Can a tablet be crushed or a capsule opened without decreasing therapeutic effects or increasing adverse effects?)
2. Administer drugs accurately (see Chap. 3).	
a. Practice the five rights of drug administration (right drug, right client, right dose, right route, and right time).	These rights are ensured if the techniques described in Chapter 3 are consistently followed. The time may vary by approximately 30 minutes. For example, a drug ordered for 9 A.M. can be usually given between 8:30 A.M. and 9:30 A.M. No variation is allowed in the other rights.
b. Use correct techniques for different routes of administration.	For example, sterile equipment and techniques are required for injection of any drug.

NURSING ACTIONS	RATIONALE/EXPLANATION
c. Follow label instructions regarding mixing or other aspects of giving specific drugs.	Some drugs require specific techniques of preparation and administration.
d. In general, do not give antacids with any other oral drugs. When both are ordered, administer at least 2 hours apart.	Antacids decrease absorption of many oral drugs.
2. Observe for therapeutic effects.	
a. Look for improvement in signs and symptoms, laboratory or other diagnostic test reports, or ability to function.	In general, the nurse should know the expected effects and when they are likely to occur.
b. Ask questions to determine whether the client is feeling better.	Specific observations depend on the specific drug or drugs being given.
3. Observe for adverse effects.	
a. Look for signs and symptoms of new problems or worsening of previous disorders. If noted, compare the client's symptoms with your knowledge base about adverse effects associated with the drugs or consult a drug reference.	All drugs are potentially harmful, although the incidence and severity of adverse reactions vary among drugs and clients. People most likely to have adverse reactions are those with severe liver or kidney disease, those who are very young or very old, those taking several drugs, and those receiving large doses of any drug. Specific adverse effects for which to observe depend on the drugs being given.
b. Check laboratory (eg, complete blood count [CBC], electrolytes, blood urea nitrogen and serum creatinine, liver function tests) and other diagnostic test reports for abnormal values.	
c. Assess for decreasing ability to function at previous levels.	
d. Ask questions to determine how the client is feeling and whether he or she is having difficulties that may be associated with drug therapy.	
4. Observe for drug interactions.	Interactions may occur whenever the client is receiving two or more drugs concurrently and the number of possible interactions is very large. Although no one can be expected to know or recognize all potential or actual interactions, it is helpful to build a knowledge base about important interactions with commonly used drugs (eg, warfarin, sedatives, cardiovascular drugs).
a. Consider a possible interaction when a client does not experience expected therapeutic effects or develops adverse effects.	
b. Look for signs and symptoms of new problems or worsening of previous ones. If noted, compare the client's symptoms with your knowledge base about interactions associated with the drugs or consult a drug reference to validate your observations.	

APPLYING YOUR KNOWLEDGE: ANSWERS

4-1 Ibuprofen is used to manage Mr. Walker's arthritis. Hypertension is an indication for both furosemide and captopril. Most likely, Mr. Walker takes famotidine to treat heartburn.

4-2 Sample nursing diagnoses include Noncompliance, Risk for Injury related to Adverse Drug Effects, Risk for Injury related to Overdose, Risk for Loneliness, and Deficient Knowledge related to Drug Administration.

4-3 Mr. Walker takes several medications in various amounts at several times during the day. Older adults often have trouble administering more than three or four drugs. Mr. Walker is currently taking four different medications. Implement strategies to make sure Mr. Walker is taking the right drug, in the right dose, at the right time. Make sure that Mr. Walker's drugs are clearly labeled. Create a chart clearly depicting his medication regimen, or use/prepare a special drug con- tainer with prepared doses labeled with the correct time. Enlist his daughter's help.

Review and Application Exercises

Short Answer Exercises

1. Why do nurses need to know the therapeutic and adverse effects of the drugs they give?

2. Given a newly assigned client, what information is needed about present and previous medications or herbal and dietary supplements?

3. With children, what are some potential difficulties with drug administration, and how can they be prevented or minimized?

4. With older adults, what are some potential difficulties with drug administration, and how can they be prevented or minimized?

5. For older adults, explain what is meant by "start low, go slow" and why it is a good approach to drug therapy.

6. Why is client teaching about drug therapy needed, and what information should usually be included?

7. Describe at least three important nursing considerations for clients who have renal or hepatic impairment or critical illness.

8. For the home care nurse assisting with a medication regimen, what are some likely differences between the nursing care needed by a child and an adult?

9. For a client who reports using particular herbal or dietary supplements, how can the nurse evaluate whether they are safe or unsafe in view of the client's condition and drug therapy regimen?

NCLEX-Style Questions

10. During an initial nursing assessment, the client reports that he is allergic to a particular medicine. The nurse should
    a. Ask what symptoms occurred with the allergic reaction.
    b. Conduct a detailed medical history and physical examination.
    c. Disregard the information as unimportant.
    d. Suspect that the client overdosed on the drug.

11. Interventions to increase safety and effectiveness of drug therapy include
    a. avoiding the use of nondrug measures during drug therapy
    b. using multiple drugs to relieve most symptoms or problems
    c. teaching clients about their drug therapy regimens
    d. avoiding instructions to alter usual activities of daily living

12. When evaluating a client's response to drug therapy, the nurse should keep in mind that
    a. Few drugs cause adverse effects.
    b. Drugs may cause virtually any symptom or problem.

    c. Patients usually report adverse drug effects without being asked.
    d. Therapeutic effects are more important than adverse effects.

13. Considerations in individualizing drug therapy for a child include
    a. age and development
    b. equivalent drug selection and dosage for adults
    c. length of illness
    d. the child's usual diet

14. In teaching a client about adverse effects of a newly ordered drug, which of the following should be included?
    a. a detailed list of all potential adverse effects
    b. percentages of particular adverse effects that occurred during clinical trials of the drug
    c. adverse effects that the client is likely to see or feel
    d. research data about rare adverse effects

Selected References

DerMarderosian, A. (Ed.). (2001). *The review of natural products*. St. Louis: Facts and Comparisons.

DeSmet, P. (2002). Herbal remedies. *New England Journal of Medicine, 347*(25), 2046–2056.

Diasio, R. B. (2004). Principles of drug therapy. In L. Goldman & D. Ausiello (Eds.), *Cecil textbook of medicine* (22nd ed., pp. 124–134). Philadelphia: W. B. Saunders.

Hanlon, J. T., Ruby, C. M., Guay, D., et al. (2002). Geriatrics. In J. T. DiPiro, R. L. Talbert, G. C. Yee, G. R. Matzke, B. G. Wells, & L. M. Posey (Eds.), *Pharmacotherapy: A pathophysiologic approach* (5th ed., pp. 79–89). New York: McGraw-Hill.

Hatcher, T. (2001). The proverbial herb. *American Journal of Nursing, 101*(2), 36–43.

Metzl, J., Small, E., & Levine, S. R. (2001). Creatine use among young athletes. *Pediatrics, 108*(2), 421–425.

Minaker, K. L. (2004). Common clinical sequelae of aging. In L. Goldman & D. Ausiello (Eds.), *Cecil textbook of medicine* (22nd ed., pp. 105–111). Philadelphia: W. B. Saunders.

Nahata, M. C., & Taketomo, C. (2002). Pediatrics. In J. T. DiPiro, R. L. Talbert, G. C. Yee, G. R. Matzke, B. G. Wells, & L. M. Posey (Eds.), *Pharmacotherapy: A pathophysiologic approach* (5th ed., pp. 69–77). New York: McGraw-Hill.

Straus, S. E. (2004). Complementary and alternative medicine. In L. Goldman & D. Ausiello (Eds.), *Cecil textbook of medicine* (22nd ed., pp. 170–174). Philadelphia: W. B. Saunders.

Waddell, D. L., Hummel, M. E., & Sumners, A. D. (2001). Three herbs you should get to know. *American Journal of Nursing, 101*(4), 48–53.

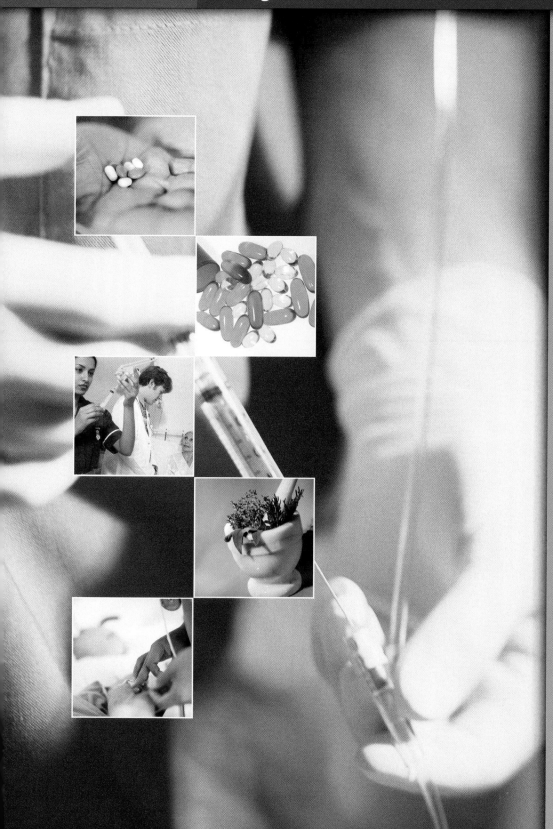

SECTION 2

Drugs Affecting the Central Nervous System

CHAPTER OUTLINE

5 Physiology of the Central Nervous System

6 Opioid Analgesics and Opioid Antagonists

7 Analgesic-Antipyretic-Anti-Inflammatory and Related Drugs

8 Antianxiety and Sedative-Hypnotic Drugs

9 Antipsychotic Drugs

10 Antidepressants and Mood Stabilizers

11 Antiseizure Drugs

12 Antiparkinson Drugs

13 Skeletal Muscle Relaxants

14 Substance Abuse Disorders

15 Central Nervous System Stimulants

Physiology of the Central Nervous System

OBJECTIVES

After studying this chapter, you will be able to:

1. Describe the process of neurotransmission.
2. Describe major neurotransmitters and their roles in central nervous system (CNS) functioning.
3. Discuss signs and symptoms of CNS depression.
4. Discuss general types and characteristics of CNS depressant drugs.

INTRODUCTION

The central nervous system (CNS), which is composed of the brain and spinal cord, acts as the control center for regulating physical and mental body processes. Afferent or sensory neurons carry messages to the CNS, and efferent or motor neurons carry messages away from the CNS. More specifically, the CNS constantly receives information about blood levels of oxygen and carbon dioxide, body temperature, and sensory stimuli and sends messages to effector organs to adjust the environment toward homeostasis. It is also concerned with higher intellectual functions (eg, thought, learning, reasoning, problem solving, memory) and with muscle function, both skeletal and smooth.

Complex interactions occur between the CNS and other parts of the body as well as among components of the CNS. Individual components of brain function are often studied separately, but it is the overall coordination of the mind–body connections that produces mental and physical health. A lack of coordination or imbalance in the CNS may lead to mental or physical disorders. Thus, emotions can strongly influence neural control of body function, and alterations in neural functions can strongly influence mood and behavior. More specific characteristics are reviewed to aid understanding of drugs that act by altering CNS functions.

BASIC UNIT OF THE CENTRAL NERVOUS SYSTEM: THE NEURON

Neurons are the basic functional units of the CNS. The *glia,* the other main cell type found in the CNS, protect, support, and nourish the neurons. Most neurons are composed of a cell body, a dendrite, and an axon. A *dendrite* has a branching structure with many synapses or sites for receiving stimuli or messages, which are then conducted toward the cell body. An *axon* is a finger-like projection that carries impulses away from the cell body. The end of the axon branches into presynaptic fibers that end with small, knob-like structures called *vesicles,* which project into the synapse and contain the granules where neurotransmitters are stored. Many axons are covered by a fatty substance called *myelin.* The myelin cover or sheath protects and insulates the axon. An axon together with its myelin sheath is called a *nerve fiber.* Nerve fibers that transmit the same type of impulses (eg, pain signals) are found together in a common pathway or tract.

NEUROTRANSMISSION

Neurons must be able to communicate with other neurons and body tissues. This communication involves a complex network of electrical and chemical signals that receive, interpret, modify, and send messages. Characteristics that allow neurons to communicate with other cells include excitability (the ability to produce an action potential or to be stimulated) and conductivity (the ability to convey electrical impulses). More specific components of the communication network include neurotransmitters, synapses, and receptors; descriptions of each of these follow.

Neurotransmitters

Neurotransmitters are chemical substances that carry messages from one neuron to another or from a neuron to other body tissues, such as cardiac or skeletal muscle. They are synthesized and stored in presynaptic nerve terminals and released in response to an electrical impulse (action potential), arriving at the end of the first neuron (presynaptic fiber). The basis for the action potential is the transient opening of ion channels. The entry of calcium ions is required for neurotransmitter release from storage sites in small sacs called *synaptic vesicles.*

When molecules of neurotransmitter are released from the synaptic vesicles, they cross the synapse, bind to receptors in the cell membrane of the postsynaptic neuron (Fig. 5-1), and excite or inhibit postsynaptic neurons. Free neurotransmitter molecules (ie, those not bound to receptors) are rapidly removed from the synapse by three mechanisms: transportation back into the presynaptic nerve terminal (reuptake) for reuse, diffusion into surrounding body fluids, or destruction by enzymes (eg, acetylcholine is degraded by cholinesterase; norepinephrine is metabolized by monoamine oxidase and catechol-O-methyltransferase).

Three main types of neurotransmitters are amines, amino acids, and peptides, all of which are derived from body proteins. Most acute CNS responses are caused by fast-acting neurotransmitters such as acetylcholine, the amines (dopamine, norepinephrine, serotonin), and amino acids (aspartate, gamma-aminobutyric acid [GABA], glutamate, and glycine). Most prolonged CNS responses are caused by slow-acting neurotransmitters, such as the neuropeptide hormones (eg, adrenocorticotropic hormone [ACTH or corticotropin] and antidiuretic hormone [ADH]), substance P, and others. Prolonged effects are thought to involve closure of calcium channels, changes in cellular metabolism, changes in activation or deactivation of specific genes in the cell nucleus, and alterations in the numbers of excitatory or inhibitory postsynaptic membrane receptors. Some peptides (eg, ADH) serve as chemical messengers in both the nervous system and the endocrine system. Substance P plays a role in transmitting pain signals from peripheral tissues to the CNS and the stress response to noxious stimuli.

Several factors affect the availability and function of neurotransmitters. These factors include the following:

- The availability of precursor proteins and enzymes required to synthesize particular neurotransmitters
- The number and binding capacity of receptors in the cell membranes of presynaptic and postsynaptic nerve endings
- Acid–base imbalances (acidosis decreases and alkalosis increases synaptic transmission)
- Hypoxia, which causes CNS depression (coma occurs within seconds without oxygen)
- Drugs, which may alter neurotransmitter synthesis, release, degradation, or binding to receptors to cause either CNS stimulation or depression

Synapses

Neurons in a chain are separated by a microscopic gap called a *synapse* or *synaptic cleft.* Synapses may be electrical, in which sodium and potassium ions can rapidly conduct an electrical impulse from one neuron to another, or chemical, in which a neurotransmitter conducts the message to the next neuron. The chemical synapse is more commonly used to communicate with other neurons or target cells. Neurotransmitter release and removal occur in the synapses.

Receptors

Receptors are proteins embedded in the cell membranes of neurons. In the CNS, most receptors are on postsynaptic neurons, but some are on presynaptic nerve terminals. A neurotransmitter must bind to receptors to exert an effect on the next neuron in the chain. Some receptors act rapidly to open ion channels, and others interact with a variety of intracellular proteins to initiate a second messenger system. For example, when norepinephrine binds with adrenergic receptors, intracellular events include activation of the enzyme adenyl cyclase and the production of cyclic adenosine monophosphate (cAMP). In this case, the cAMP is a second messenger that activates cellular functions and the physiologic responses controlled by the adrenergic receptors. A neurotransmitter–receptor complex may have an excitatory or inhibitory effect on the postsynaptic neuron.

Receptors are constantly being synthesized and degraded. They increase in number and activity (up-regulation) when there is underactivity at the synapse. They decrease in number and activity (down-regulation) when there is overactivity. Overall, receptors work with other control mechanisms of the nervous system to readjust abnormally stimulated or depressed nerve function toward normal.

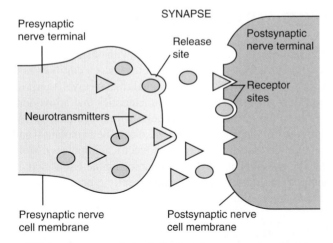

FIGURE 5-1 Neurotransmission in the central nervous system. Neurotransmitter molecules (eg, norepinephrine, acetylcholine), released by the presynaptic nerve, cross the synapse and bind with receptor proteins in the cell membrane of the postsynaptic nerve.

Neurotransmission Systems

Neurons function through communication networks that may be called *neurotransmission systems,* the major elements of which are neurotransmitters, synapses, and receptors. Although these elements are discussed separately here, it is the inter-action among these elements that promotes order or disorder in the body's physical and mental processes. Major neurotransmission systems are the cholinergic, dopaminergic, GABA-ergic, noradrenergic, and serotonergic networks.

The **cholinergic system** uses acetylcholine as its neurotransmitter. Acetylcholine is located in many areas of the brain, with especially high concentrations in the motor cortex and basal ganglia. It is also a neurotransmitter in the autonomic nervous system and at peripheral neuromuscular junctions. Acetylcholine exerts excitatory effects at synapses and nerve–muscle junctions and inhibitory effects at some peripheral sites, such as organs supplied by the vagus nerve. In the CNS, acetylcholine is associated with level of arousal, memory, motor conditioning, and speech.

The **dopaminergic system** uses dopamine as its neurotransmitter. Dopamine is found in the substantia nigra, the midbrain, and the hypothalamus. Much of the information about dopamine is derived from studies of antipsychotic drugs (see Chap. 9) and Parkinson's disease, a disorder caused by destruction of dopamine-producing neurons in the substantia nigra. Dopamine also is found outside the brain, in renal and mesenteric blood vessels.

In the CNS, dopamine is thought to be inhibitory in the basal ganglia but may be excitatory in other areas. Repeated stimulation of dopamine receptors decreases their numbers (down-regulation) and their sensitivity to dopamine (desensitization). Prolonged blockade of dopamine receptors increases their numbers and sensitivity to dopamine. Some receptors (called *autoreceptors*) occur on the presynaptic nerve terminal. When released, dopamine stimulates these receptors and a negative feedback system is initiated that inhibits further dopamine synthesis and release.

Two groups of dopamine receptors have been identified. They are differentiated by the intracellular events that follow dopamine–receptor binding. One group includes D1 and D5 receptors, which activate adenyl cyclase to produce cAMP. The other group includes D2, D3, and D4 receptors. D2 receptors have been described most thoroughly; they are thought to inhibit activation of adenyl cyclase and subsequent production of cAMP, suppress calcium ion currents, and activate potassium ion currents. The functions of D3 and D4 receptors have not been delineated. Overall, dopamine actions at the cellular level depend on the subtype of receptor to which it binds and the simultaneous effects of other neurotransmitters at the same target neurons.

The **GABA-ergic system** uses GABA as its neurotransmitter. GABA is found in the brain and spinal cord in abundant amounts. It is the major inhibitory neurotransmitter in the CNS, with a role in many neuronal circuits (estimated at nearly one third of CNS synapses). GABA receptors have been divided into two main types, A and B. The $GABA_A$ receptor is a chloride ion channel that opens when GABA is released from presynaptic neurons. The $GABA_B$ receptor is associated with potassium conductance. There is evidence of multiple subtypes of GABA receptors and important functional differences among them.

The **noradrenergic system** uses norepinephrine as its neurotransmitter. Norepinephrine is a catecholamine that is found in relatively large amounts in the hypothalamus and the limbic system and in smaller amounts in most areas of the brain, including the reticular formation. Norepinephrine is mainly an excitatory neurotransmitter that stimulates the brain to generalized increased activity. However, it is inhibitory in a few areas because of inhibitory receptors at some nerve synapses.

Norepinephrine receptors in the CNS are divided into alpha- and beta-adrenergic receptors and their subtypes. Activation of alpha$_1$, beta$_1$, and beta$_2$ receptors is thought to stimulate activity of intracellular adenyl cyclase and the production of cAMP. Activation of alpha$_2$ receptors is associated with inhibition of adenyl cyclase activity and decreased production of cAMP. In addition, alpha$_2$ receptors on the presynaptic nerve ending are believed to regulate norepinephrine release. In other words, when high levels of extracellular norepinephrine act on presynaptic alpha$_2$ receptors, the effect is similar to that of a negative feedback system that inhibits the release of norepinephrine. Overall, the noradrenergic system is associated with mood, motor activity, regulation of arousal, and reward. It is thought to play an important role in producing rapid eye movement (REM) sleep, during which dreaming occurs.

The **serotonergic system** uses serotonin (also called 5-hydroxytryptamine, or 5-HT) as its neurotransmitter. Serotonin-synthesizing neurons are widely distributed in the CNS. Because serotonin is synthesized from the amino acid tryptophan, the amount of tryptophan intake in the diet and the enzyme tryptophan hydroxylase control the rate of serotonin production. CNS serotonin is usually an inhibitory neurotransmitter and is associated with mood, the sleep–wake cycle, habituation, and sensory perceptions, including inhibition of pain pathways in the spinal cord. Serotonin is thought to produce sleep by inhibiting CNS activity and arousal.

Serotonin receptors are found in regions of the CNS that are associated with mood and anxiety and are also thought to be involved in temperature regulation. Activation of some receptors leads to hyperpolarization and neuronal inhibition. Several subtypes of serotonin receptors have been identified, some of which are linked to inhibition of adenyl cyclase activity or to regulation of potassium or calcium ion channels.

Serotonin is also found outside the CNS, mainly in mast cells of the lungs and platelets. It plays a major role in the blood coagulation process, during which it is released from platelets and causes vasoconstriction. It may also be involved in the vascular spasm associated with some pulmonary allergic reactions (during which it is released from mast cells) and migraine headaches. However, peripheral serotonin cannot cross the blood–brain barrier.

The **amino acid system** includes several amino acids that may serve as both structural components for protein synthesis and neurotransmitters. Amino acids were recognized as neurotransmitters relatively recently, and their roles and functions in this regard have not been completely elucidated. A summary of their characteristics follows.

Aspartate is an excitatory neurotransmitter found in high concentrations in the brain.

Glycine is an inhibitory neurotransmitter found in the brain stem and spinal cord. Glycine receptors have many of the features described for GABA$_A$ receptors; subtypes have been identified but their functions are unknown.

Glutamate is the most important excitatory neurotransmitter in the CNS; it occurs in high concentrations in virtually every area. Several subtypes of glutamate receptors have been identified, each with a unique distribution in the CNS. The functions of these receptor subtypes have not been established, but research suggests that the *N*-methyl D-aspartate (NMDA) glutamate receptor subtype plays a role in memory.

Although some glutamate is needed for normal neurotransmission, exposure of neurons to high concentrations can lead to neuronal cell death. Events leading to neuronal death are triggered by excessive activation of NMDA receptors and movement of calcium ions into the neurons. This process may be similar to the neurotoxicity associated with brain injury (eg, from ischemia, hypoglycemia, or hypoxia), where increased release and impaired reuptake of glutamate lead to excessive stimulation of glutamate receptors and subsequent cell death. Altered glutamate metabolism may also lead to the formation of free radicals, which are implicated in neuronal cell death associated with some neurodegenerative diseases and toxic chemicals, including some drugs of abuse.

Neurotransmission Systems in Selected Central Nervous System Disorders

Abnormalities in neurotransmission systems (eg, dysfunction or destruction of the neurons that normally produce neurotransmitters; altered receptor response to neurotransmitters) are implicated in many CNS disorders. For example, decreased acetylcholine is a characteristic of Alzheimer's disease; dopamine abnormalities occur in psychosis and Parkinson's disease; GABA abnormalities occur in anxiety, hyperarousal states, and seizure disorders; glutamate has been implicated in the pathogenesis of epilepsy, schizophrenia, stroke, and Huntington's disease; and serotonin abnormalities are thought to be involved in mental depression and sleep disorders.

Although most research has focused on single neurotransmitters and their respective receptors, CNS function in both health and disease probably results from interactions among neurotransmission systems. In health, for example, complex mechanisms regulate the amounts and binding capacities of neurotransmitters and receptors, as well as the balance between excitatory and inhibitory forces. When abnormalities occur in any of these elements, the resulting dysregulation and imbalances lead to signs and symptoms of CNS disorders. Overall, then, neurotransmission systems function interdependently; one system may increase, decrease, or otherwise modify the effects of another system.

Except for mental depression, most psychiatric symptoms result from CNS stimulation and usually involve physical and mental hyperactivity. Such hyperactivity reflects a wide range of observable behaviors and nonobservable thoughts and feelings. In most people, manifestations may include pleasant feelings of mild euphoria and high levels of enthusiasm, energy, and productivity. In people with psychiatric illnesses, such as severe anxiety or psychosis, manifestations include unpleasant feelings of tension, psychomotor agitation, nervousness, and decreased ability to rest and sleep, even when very tired. Many psychiatric disorders, therapeutic drugs, and drugs of abuse may cause varying degrees of CNS stimulation. In general, the pathogenesis of excessive CNS stimulation may involve one or more of the following mechanisms:

- Excessive amounts of excitatory neurotransmitters (eg, norepinephrine, glutamate)
- Increased numbers or sensitivity of excitatory receptors
- Insufficient amounts of inhibitory neurotransmitters (eg, GABA)
- Decreased numbers or sensitivity of inhibitory receptors

MAJOR COMPONENTS OF THE CENTRAL NERVOUS SYSTEM

Cerebral Cortex

The *cerebral cortex* is involved in all conscious processes, such as learning, memory, reasoning, verbalization, and voluntary body movements. Some parts receive incoming nerve impulses and are called *sensory areas*. Other parts send impulses to peripheral structures and are called *motor areas*. Around the sensory and motor areas are the "association" areas, which occupy the greater portion of the cortex. These areas analyze the information received by the sensory areas and decide on the appropriate response. In some instances, the response may be to store the perception in memory; in others, it may involve stimulation of motor centers to produce movement or speech.

Thalamus

The *thalamus* receives impulses carrying sensations such as heat, cold, pain, and muscle position sense. These sensations produce only a crude awareness at the thalamic level. They are relayed to the cerebral cortex, where they are interpreted regarding location, quality, intensity, and significance. The thalamus also relays motor impulses from the cortex to the spinal cord.

Hypothalamus

The *hypothalamus* has extensive neurologic and endocrine functions. In the CNS, it is connected with the thalamus, medulla oblongata, spinal cord, reticular activating system, and limbic system. In the autonomic nervous system, it is the center for motor control. In the endocrine system, it controls the secretion of all pituitary hormones, is anatomically connected to the posterior pituitary gland, and regulates the activity of the anterior pituitary. The hypothalamus constantly collects information about the internal environment of the body and helps maintain homeostasis by making continuous adjustments in water balance, body temperature, hormone levels, arterial blood pressure, heart rate, gastrointestinal motility, and other body functions. It is stimulated or inhibited by nerve impulses from different portions of the nervous system and by concentrations of nutrients, electrolytes, water, and hormones in the blood.

Specific neuroendocrine functions of the hypothalamus are

- Producing oxytocin and antidiuretic hormone (ADH), which are stored in the posterior pituitary gland and released in response to nerve impulses from the hypothalamus. Oxytocin initiates uterine contractions to begin labor and delivery and helps release milk from breast glands during breastfeeding. ADH helps maintain fluid balance by controlling water excretion.
- Regulating body temperature. When body temperature is elevated, sweating and dilation of blood vessels in the skin lower the temperature. When body temperature is low, sweating ceases, and vasoconstriction occurs. When heat loss is decreased, the temperature is raised.
- Assisting in regulation of arterial blood pressure by its effects on the vasomotor center. The vasomotor center in the medulla oblongata and pons maintains a state of partial contraction in blood vessels (vasomotor tone). The hypothalamus can exert excitatory or inhibitory effects on the vasomotor center. When nerve impulses from the hypothalamus excite the vasomotor center, vasomotor tone or vasoconstriction is increased, and blood pressure is raised. When the impulses from the hypothalamus inhibit the vasomotor center, vasomotor tone or vasoconstriction is decreased, with the overall effect of relative vasodilation and lowering of arterial blood pressure.
- Regulating anterior pituitary hormones, including thyroid-stimulating hormone, ACTH, and growth hormone. The hypothalamus secretes "releasing factors," which cause the anterior pituitary to secrete these hormones. There is a hypothalamic releasing factor for each hormone. The hypothalamic factor called *prolactin-inhibiting factor* inhibits secretion of prolactin, another anterior pituitary hormone.
- Regulating food and water intake by the hypothalamic thirst, appetite, hunger, and satiety centers.
- Regulating the physical changes associated with emotions (eg, increased blood pressure and heart rate). The hypothalamus, thalamus, and cerebral cortex interact to produce the feelings associated with emotions.

Medulla Oblongata

The *medulla oblongata* contains groups of neurons that form the vital cardiac, respiratory, and vasomotor centers. For example, if the respiratory center is stimulated, respiratory rate and depth are increased. If the respiratory center is depressed, respiratory rate and depth are decreased. The medulla also contains reflex centers for coughing, vomiting, sneezing, swallowing, and salivating. The medulla and pons varolii also contain groups of neurons from which cranial nerves 5 through 12 originate.

Reticular Activating System

The *reticular activating system* is a network of neurons that extends from the spinal cord through the medulla and pons to the thalamus and hypothalamus. It receives impulses from all parts of the body, evaluates the significance of the impulses, and decides which impulses to transmit to the cerebral cortex. It also excites or inhibits motor nerves that control both reflex and voluntary movement. Stimulation of these neurons produces wakefulness and mental alertness, and depression causes sedation and loss of consciousness.

Limbic System

The *limbic system* borders and interconnects with the thalamus, hypothalamus, basal ganglia, hippocampus, amygdala, and septum. It participates in regulation of feeding behavior, the sleep–wake cycle, emotions (eg, pleasure, fear, anger, sadness), and behavior (eg, aggression, laughing, crying). Many nerve impulses from the limbic system are transmitted through the hypothalamus; thus, physiologic changes in blood pressure, heart rate, respiration, and hormone secretion occur in response to the emotions.

Cerebellum

The *cerebellum,* which is connected with motor centers in the cerebral cortex and basal ganglia, coordinates muscular activity. For example, when several skeletal muscles are involved, some are contracted and some are relaxed for smooth, purposeful movements. It also helps maintain balance and posture by receiving nerve impulses from the inner ear that produce appropriate reflex responses.

Basal Ganglia

The *basal ganglia* are concerned with skeletal muscle tone and orderly activity. Normal function is influenced by dopamine. Degenerative changes in one of these areas, the substantia nigra, cause dopamine to be released in decreased amounts. This process is a factor in the development of Parkinson's disease, which is characterized by rigidity and increased muscle tone.

Pyramidal and Extrapyramidal Systems

The pyramidal and extrapyramidal systems are pathways out of the cerebral cortex that intermingle in the spinal cord. Disease processes affecting higher levels of the CNS involve both tracts.

In the *pyramidal* or *corticospinal tract,* nerve fibers originate in the cerebral cortex, go down the brain stem to the medulla, where the fibers cross, and continue down the spinal cord, where they end at various levels. Impulses are then carried from the spinal cord to skeletal muscle. Because the fibers cross in the medulla, impulses from the right side of the cerebral cortex control skeletal muscle movements of the left side of the body, and impulses from the left control muscle movements of the right side.

In the *extrapyramidal system,* fibers originate mainly in the premotor area of the cerebral cortex and travel to the basal ganglia and brain stem. The fibers are called *extrapyramidal* because they do not enter the medullary pyramids and cross over.

Brain Metabolism

To function properly, the brain must have an adequate and continuous supply of oxygen, glucose, and thiamine.

Oxygen is carried to the brain by the carotid and vertebral arteries. The brain requires more oxygen than any other organ. Cerebral cortex cells are very sensitive to lack of oxygen (hypoxia), and interruption of blood supply causes immediate loss of consciousness. Brain stem cells are less sensitive to hypoxia. People in whom hypoxia is relatively prolonged may survive, although they may have irreversible brain damage.

Glucose is required as an energy source for brain cell metabolism. Hypoglycemia (low blood sugar) may cause mental confusion, dizziness, convulsions, loss of consciousness, and permanent damage to the cerebral cortex.

Thiamine is required for production and use of glucose. Thiamine deficiency can reduce glucose use by approximately half and can cause degeneration of the myelin sheaths of nerve cells. Such degeneration in central neurons leads to a form of encephalopathy known as Wernicke-Korsakoff syndrome. Degeneration in peripheral nerves leads to polyneuritis and muscle atrophy, weakness, and paralysis.

Spinal Cord

The *spinal cord* is continuous with the medulla oblongata and extends down through the vertebral column to the sacral area. It consists of 31 segments, each of which is the point of origin for a pair of spinal nerves. The cord is a pathway between the brain and the peripheral nervous system. It carries impulses to and from the brain, along sensory and motor nerve fibers, and is a center for reflex actions. *Reflexes* are involuntary responses to certain nerve impulses received by the spinal cord (eg, the knee-jerk and pupillary reflexes).

DRUGS THAT AFFECT THE CENTRAL NERVOUS SYSTEM

Drugs that affect the CNS, sometimes called *centrally active drugs,* are broadly classified as depressants or stimulants.

CNS depressants (eg, antipsychotics, opioid analgesics, sedative-hypnotics) produce a general depression of the CNS when given in sufficient dosages. Mild CNS depression is characterized by lack of interest in surroundings and inability to focus on a topic (short attention span). Moderate CNS depression is characterized by drowsiness or sleep; decreased muscle tone; decreased ability to move; and decreased perception of sensations such as pain, heat, and cold. Severe CNS depression is characterized by unconsciousness or coma, loss of reflexes, respiratory failure, and death.

Central nervous system stimulants produce a variety of effects. Mild stimulation is characterized by wakefulness, mental alertness, and decreased fatigue. Increasing stimulation produces hyperactivity, excessive talking, nervousness, and insomnia. Excessive stimulation can cause convulsive seizures, cardiac dysrhythmias, and death. Because it is difficult to avoid excessive, harmful CNS stimulation by these drugs, CNS stimulants are less useful for therapeutic purposes than are CNS depressants.

Review and Application Exercises

Short Answer Exercises

1. Where are neurotransmitters synthesized and stored?

2. What events occur at the synapse between two neurons?

3. After a neurotransmitter is released and acts on receptors, how are the remaining molecules inactivated?

4. What are the main functions of acetylcholine, dopamine, GABA, norepinephrine, and serotonin?

5. What part of the brain is concerned mainly with thoughts, reasoning, and learning?

6. What part of the brain contains vital respiratory and cardiovascular centers?

7. How would you expect a person with CNS depression to look and behave?

8. How would you expect a person with excessive CNS stimulation to look and behave?

Selected References

Carroll, E. W., & Curtis, R. L. (2005). Organization and control of neural function. In C. M. Porth, *Pathophysiology: Concepts of altered health states* (7th ed., pp. 1113–1157). Philadelphia: Lippincott Williams & Wilkins.

Rhoades, R. A., & Tanner, G. A. (2003). *Medical physiology* (2nd ed.). Philadelphia: Lippincott Williams & Wilkins.

Opioid Analgesics and Opioid Antagonists

OBJECTIVES

After studying this chapter, you will be able to:

1. Discuss major types and characteristics of pain.
2. Discuss the nurse's role in assessing and managing clients' pain.
3. List characteristics of opioid analgesics in terms of mechanism of action, indications for use, and major adverse effects.
4. Describe morphine as the prototype of opioid analgesics.
5. Discuss morphine dosage forms and dosage ranges for various clinical uses.
6. Explain why higher doses of opioid analgesics are needed when the drugs are given orally.
7. Contrast the use of opioid analgesics in opiate-naive and opiate-tolerant clients.
8. Assess level of consciousness and respiratory status before and after administering opioids.
9. Teach clients about safe, effective use of opioid analgesics.
10. Describe characteristics and treatment of opioid toxicity.
11. Discuss principles of therapy for using opioid analgesics in special populations.

APPLYING YOUR KNOWLEDGE

Moe Harris is a 53-year-old male who had a lumbar laminectomy with spinal fusion today. Mr. Harris has experienced chronic low back pain for more than 10 years. During this time, he has been treated with a number of over-the-counter (OTC) and prescription medications for his pain. These drugs have included ibuprofen and hydrocodone with acetaminophen. He is a construction worker, married with three children, a nonsmoker, and drinks beer regularly.

Mr. Harris returns from the postanesthesia recovery room to your care at 10:00 A.M. His vital signs are stable on initial assessment. To treat his pain, the physician has ordered the following:

Morphine 4–8 mg IV, every 2–4 hours as needed, to be given over 5 minutes

After 24 hours, oxycodone 5 mg with acetaminophen 500 mg PO every 4–6 hours, PRN, not to exceed 6 doses in 24 hours

INTRODUCTION

Pain is the most common symptom prompting people to seek health care. This unpleasant, uncomfortable sensation usually indicates tissue damage and impels a person to remove the cause of the damage or seek relief from the pain. When not managed effectively, pain may greatly impair quality of life and ability to perform activities of daily living. In 2003, the Joint Commission on the Accreditation of Healthcare Organizations emphasized the importance of pain by incorporating effective assessment and management of pain for all patients in the standards by which it evaluates health care organizations. Opioid (narcotic) analgesics are drugs that relieve moderate to severe pain. To aid understanding of drug actions, selected characteristics of pain and endogenous pain-relieving substances are described.

Physiology of Pain

Pain occurs when tissue damage activates the free nerve endings (pain receptors or nociceptors) of peripheral nerves. Nociceptors are abundant in the skin and underlying soft tissue, muscle fascia, joint surfaces, arterial walls, and periosteum. Nociceptors are scarce in most internal organs, such as lung and uterine tissue. Causes of tissue damage may be physical, such as heat, cold, pressure, stretch, spasm, or ischemia, or they may be chemical, such as pain related to substances released from damaged cells and products of inflammation (eg, bradykinin, prostaglandins). Bradykinin, one of the strongest pain-producing substances, is quickly metabolized and therefore may be involved mainly in acute pain. Prostaglandins increase the pain-provoking effects of bradykinin by increasing the sensitivity of pain receptors. Several other substances are also thought to produce pain, including acetylcholine, adenosine triphosphate, histamine, leukotrienes, potassium, serotonin, and substance P. In general, these chemical mediators produce pain by activating and sensitizing peripheral nociceptors or stimulating the release of pain-producing substances.

For a person to feel pain, the signal from the nociceptors in peripheral tissues must be transmitted to the spinal cord, then to the hypothalamus and cerebral cortex in the brain. The signal is carried to the spinal cord by two types of peripheral nerve cells, A-delta fibers and C fibers. A-delta fibers, which are myelinated and found mainly in skin and muscle, transmit fast, sharp, well-localized pain signals. These fibers release glutamate and aspartate (excitatory amino acid neurotransmitters) at synapses in the spinal cord. C fibers, which are unmyelinated and found in muscle, mesentery, abdominal viscera, and periosteum, conduct the pain signal slowly and produce a poorly localized, dull or burning type of pain. Tissue damage resulting from an acute injury often produces an initial sharp pain transmitted by A-delta fibers followed by a dull ache or burning sensation transmitted by C fibers. C fibers release somatostatin and substance P at synapses in the spinal cord. Glutamate, aspartate, substance P, and perhaps other chemical mediators are thought to enhance transmission of the pain signal.

The dorsal horn of the spinal cord is the control center or relay station for information from the A-delta and C nerve fibers, for local modulation of the pain impulse, and for descending influences from higher centers in the central nervous system (CNS; eg, attention, emotion, memory). Here, nociceptive nerve fibers synapse with non-nociceptive nerve fibers (neurons that carry information other than pain signals). The brain also contains powerful descending pathways that modify nociceptive input. Some brain nuclei are serotonergic and project to the dorsal horn of the spinal cord, where they suppress nociceptive transmission. Another major inhibitory pathway is noradrenergic and originates in the pons. Thus, increasing the concentration of norepinephrine and serotonin in the synapse interrupts or inhibits transmission of nerve impulses that carry pain signals to the brain and spinal cord. (This is thought to account for the pain-relieving effects of the tricyclic antidepressants [TCAs], drugs that increase the amounts of serotonin and norepinephrine in the synapse by inhibiting their reuptake by presynaptic nerve endings.)

In the brain, the thalamus is a relay station for incoming sensory stimuli, including pain. Perception of pain is a primitive awareness in the thalamus, and sensation is not well localized or specific. From the thalamus, pain messages are relayed to the cerebral cortex, where they are perceived more specifically and analyzed to determine actions needed.

Pain may be classified according to point of origin in body structures (eg, somatic, visceral, neuropathic), duration (eg, acute, chronic), or cause (eg, cancer). These types of pain are described in Box 6-1.

Endogenous Analgesia System

The CNS has its own system for suppressing the transmission of pain signals from peripheral nerves. The system can be activated by nerve signals entering the periaqueductal gray area of the brain or by morphine-like drugs. Important elements include opiate receptors and endogenous peptides with actions similar to those of morphine. Opiate receptors are highly concentrated in some regions of the CNS, including the ascending and descending pain pathways and portions of the brain essential to the endogenous analgesia system. The opioid peptides (ie, the enkephalins, dynorphins, and beta-endorphins) interact with opiate receptors to inhibit pain transmission. All are important in the endogenous opiate system, but the three types of peptides differ in precursors and anatomic locations. Enkephalins are believed to interrupt the transmission of pain signals at the spinal cord level by inhibiting the release of substance P from C nerve fibers. The endogenous analgesia system may also inhibit pain signals at other points in the pain pathway.

GENERAL CHARACTERISTICS OF OPIOID ANALGESICS

Opioid analgesics are drugs that relieve moderate to severe pain by inhibiting the release of substance P in both central and peripheral nerves (which inhibits transmission of pain signals from peripheral tissues to the brain), reducing the perception of pain sensation in the brain, producing sedation, and decreasing the emotional upsets often associated with pain. They also inhibit the production of pain and inflammation by prostaglandins in peripheral tissues. Most of these analgesics are Schedule II drugs under federal narcotic laws and may lead to drug abuse and dependence. These drugs are called *opioids* because they act like morphine in the body.

Opioid analgesics are well absorbed with oral (PO), intramuscular (IM), or subcutaneous (Sub-Q) administration. Oral drugs undergo significant first-pass metabolism in the liver, which means that oral doses must be larger than parenteral doses to have equivalent therapeutic effects. The drugs are extensively metabolized in the liver, and metabolites are excreted in urine. Morphine and meperidine form pharmacologically active metabolites. Thus, liver impairment can interfere with metabolism, and kidney impairment can interfere with excretion. Drug accumulation and increased adverse effects may occur if dosage is not reduced.

Opioids exert widespread pharmacologic effects, especially in the CNS and the gastrointestinal (GI) system. These effects occur with usual doses and may be therapeutic or adverse, depending on the reason for use. CNS effects include analgesia; CNS depression, ranging from drowsiness to sleep to unconsciousness; decreased mental and physical activity;

Box 6-1 Types and Characteristics of Pain

Acute pain may be caused by injury, trauma, spasm, disease processes, and treatment or diagnostic procedures that damage skin, somatic structures, or visceral tissues. It is often described as sharp, lancing, or cutting. The intensity of the pain is usually proportional to the degree of tissue damage and the pain serves as a protective or warning system by demanding the sufferer's attention and compelling behavior to seek relief (ie, withdrawal from or avoidance of the pain-producing stimulus).

Acute pain is sometimes called *fast pain* because it is felt within about 0.1 second after a pain stimulus is applied. It is elicited by mechanical and thermal types of stimuli and conducted by A-delta fibers in the peripheral nerves to the spinal cord. Glutamate is the neurotransmitter secreted in the spinal cord at the type A-delta nerve fiber endings. Glutamate is an excitatory neurotransmitter in the CNS whose action lasts for only a few milliseconds.

Acute pain is often accompanied by anxiety and objective signs of discomfort (eg, facial expressions of distress; moaning or crying; positioning to protect the affected part; tenderness, edema, and skin color or temperature changes in the affected part; and either restlessness and excessive movement or limited movement, if movement increases pain). It usually responds to treatment and resolves within a few days to several weeks as tissue repair mechanisms heal the damaged area.

Chronic pain, usually defined as pain lasting 3 months or longer (some sources say 6 months), demands attention less urgently than acute pain, may not be characterized by visible signs, and is often accompanied by emotional stress, increased irritability, depression, social withdrawal, financial distress, loss of libido, disturbed sleep patterns, diminished appetite, weight loss, and decreased ability to perform usual activities of daily living. It may occur with or without evidence of tissue damage and may include acute pain that persists beyond the typical recovery time for the precipitating tissue injury; pain related to a chronic disease; pain without an identifiable cause; and pain associated with cancer. It may arise from viscera, muscle and connective tissue, and nerves (eg, neurologic disorders such as herpes zoster infection or diabetic neuropathy). It may be continuous or episodic or a combination of both.

Chronic pain may also be called *slow pain*, which begins after at least 1 second of exposure to a painful stimulus and increases slowly over several seconds or minutes. It can be elicited by mechanical, thermal, and chemical stimuli and is often described as burning, aching, or throbbing. Slow, chronic pain is transmitted by type C nerve fibers to the spinal cord and brain. Substance P is the neurotransmitter of type C nerve endings; it is released slowly and accumulates over seconds or minutes.

Cancer pain has characteristics of both acute and chronic pain and it may be constant or intermittent. Chronic cancer pain is caused mainly by tumor spread into pain-sensitive tissues (eg, bone, nerves, soft tissues, viscera) and the resulting tissue destruction. It usually progresses as the disease advances and can be severe and debilitating. Acute pain is usually associated with diagnostic procedures or treatment measures (eg, surgery, chemotherapy, radiation therapy).

Somatic pain results from stimulation of nociceptors in structural tissues (eg, skin, bone, muscle and soft tissue). It is usually well localized and described as sharp, burning, aching, gnawing, throbbing, or cramping. It may be intermittent or constant and acute or chronic. Sprains and other traumatic injuries are examples of acute somatic pain; the bone and joint pain of arthritis is an example of chronic somatic pain, although acute exacerbations may also occur. Somatic pain of low to moderate intensity may stimulate the sympathetic nervous system and produce increased blood pressure, pulse, and respiration; dilated pupils; and increased skeletal muscle tension, such as rigid posture or clenched fists.

Visceral pain results when many nociceptors are stimulated at the same time in abdominal or thoracic organs and their surrounding structural tissues. This type of pain, which can be severe, includes pain associated with cholecystitis, pancreatitis, uterine and ovarian disorders, and liver disease. Patients often describe visceral pain as deep, dull, aching, boring, or cramping. The cramping type of pain results from intermittent, rhythmical contractions or spasms of smooth muscle and often occurs with gastroenteritis, constipation, menstruation, gallbladder disease, and ureteral obstruction. Severe visceral pain stimulates the parasympathetic nervous system and produces decreased blood pressure and pulse; nausea and vomiting; weakness; syncope; and possibly loss of consciousness.

Visceral pain is diffuse and not well localized because it is transmitted through type C nerve fibers and can therefore only transmit the chronic, aching type of pain. It may be referred to a different part of the body (eg, pain from the liver can be referred to the right shoulder area; ischemic pain from the heart can be referred to the left arm or neck area).

Neuropathic pain results from direct injury of peripheral pain receptors, nerves, or the CNS. It is a relatively common cause of chronic pain and is usually described as severe, shooting, burning, or stabbing pain. It occurs with peripheral neuropathies associated with diabetes mellitus (diabetic neuropathy), herpes zoster infections (postherpetic neuralgia), traumatic nerve injuries, and some types of cancer or cancer treatments. It is very difficult to treat because standard analgesics (eg, nonsteroidal anti-inflammatory drugs and opioids) are less effective in neuropathic pain than in other types of pain. Tricyclic antidepressants (see Chap. 10), anticonvulsants (see Chap. 11), and corticosteroids (see Chap. 23) are often used along with analgesics.

respiratory depression; nausea and vomiting; and pupil constriction. Sedation and respiratory depression are major adverse effects and are potentially life threatening. Newer opioid analgesics were developed in an effort to find drugs as effective as morphine in relieving pain while causing less sedation, respiratory depression, and dependence. However, this effort has not been successful: **equianalgesic doses of these drugs produce sedative and respiratory depressant effects comparable with those of morphine.** In the GI tract, opioid analgesics slow motility and may cause constipation and smooth muscle spasms in the bowel and biliary tract.

Mechanism of Action

Opioids relieve pain mainly by binding to opioid receptors in the brain and spinal cord, and some receptors are found in peripheral tissues as well. When bound to an opioid drug, opioid receptors function like gates that close and thereby block or decrease transmission of pain impulses from one nerve cell to the next. Opioid receptors also activate the endogenous analgesia system. The major types of receptors are mu, kappa, and delta. Most opioid effects (analgesia; CNS depression, with respiratory depression and sedation; euphoria; decreased GI motility; and physical dependence) are attributed to activation of the mu receptors. Analgesia, sedation, and decreased GI motility also occur with activation of kappa receptors. Delta receptors are important in the endogenous analgesia system, but it is not clear whether they bind with opioid drugs. Opioid analgesics and opioid antagonists bind to different receptors to varying degrees, and their pharmacologic actions can be differentiated and classified on this basis.

Indications for Use

The main indication for the use of opioids is to prevent or relieve acute or chronic pain. Specific conditions in which opioids are used for analgesic effects include acute myocardial infarction, biliary colic, renal colic, burns and other traumatic injuries, postoperative states, and cancer. These drugs are usually given for chronic pain only when other measures and milder drugs are ineffective, as in terminal malignancy. Other clinical uses include

- Before and during surgery to promote sedation, decrease anxiety, facilitate induction of anesthesia, and decrease the amount of anesthesia required
- Before and during invasive diagnostic procedures, such as angiograms and endoscopic examinations
- During labor and delivery (obstetric analgesia)
- Treatment of GI disorders, such as abdominal cramping and diarrhea
- Treatment of acute pulmonary edema (morphine is used)
- Treatment of severe, unproductive cough (codeine is often used)

Contraindications to Use

Opioid analgesics are contraindicated or must be used very cautiously in people with respiratory depression, chronic lung disease, liver or kidney disease, prostatic hypertrophy, increased intracranial pressure, or hypersensitivity reactions to opioids and related drugs.

INDIVIDUAL DRUGS

The two main subgroups of opioid analgesics are agonists and agonists/antagonists. Agonists include morphine and morphine-like drugs. These agents have activity at mu and kappa opioid receptors and thus produce prototypical opioid effects. As their name indicates, the agonists/antagonists have both agonist and antagonist activity. In addition, numerous combinations of an opioid and acetaminophen, a nonopioid analgesic (see Chap. 7), are available and commonly used in both inpatient and outpatient health care settings. Opioid antagonists are antidote drugs that reverse the effects of opioid agonists. Individual drugs are described in the following sections. Trade names and dosages are listed in Table 6-1.

Opioid Agonists

[P] **Morphine**, the prototype, is a naturally occurring opium alkaloid used mainly to relieve severe acute or chronic pain. However, many physicians do not use morphine in clients with pain from pancreatic or biliary tract disease because of its spasm-producing effects. It is a Schedule II narcotic that is mainly given orally and parenterally. Client response depends on route of administration and dosage. After intravenous (IV) injection, maximal analgesia and respiratory depression usually occur within 10 to 20 minutes. After IM injection, these effects occur in about 30 minutes. With Sub-Q injection, effects may be delayed up to 60 to 90 minutes. With oral administration, peak activity occurs in about 60 minutes. The duration of action is 5 to 7 hours.

Morphine is about 30% bound to plasma proteins, and its half-life is 2 to 4 hours. It is metabolized in the liver and conjugated to an active metabolite that is excreted by the kidneys. Morphine and its metabolite accumulate in clients with impaired liver or kidney function and may cause prolonged sedation if dosage is not reduced. Older adults also may need small doses.

Oral administration of morphine is common for chronic pain associated with cancer. When given orally, relatively high doses are required, because part of each dose is metabolized in the liver and never reaches the systemic circulation. Concentrated solutions (eg, Roxanol, which contains 20 mg morphine/mL) and controlled-release tablets (eg, MS Contin, which contains 15–100 mg/tablet) have been developed for oral administration of these high doses.

In some cases of severe pain that cannot be controlled by other methods, morphine is administered as a continuous IV

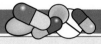 **Table 6-1 Drugs at a Glance: Opioid Analgesics**

	ROUTES AND DOSAGE RANGES	
GENERIC/TRADE NAME	**Adults**	**Children**
Agonists **Codeine**	*Pain*: PO, Sub-Q, IM 15–60 mg q4–6h PRN; usual dose 30 mg; maximum, 360 mg/24 h *Cough*: PO 10–20 mg q4h PRN; maximum, 120 mg/24 h	*1 y or older, Pain*: PO, Sub-Q, IM 0.5 mg/kg q4–6h PRN *2–6 y, Cough*: PO 2.5–5 mg q4–6h; maximum, 30 mg/24 h *6–12 y, Cough*: PO 5–10 mg q4–6h; maximum, 60 mg/24 h
Fentanyl (Sublimaze)	Preanesthetic sedation, IM 0.05–0.1 mg 30–60 min before surgery Analgesic adjunct to general anesthesia, IV total dose of 0.002–0.05 mg/kg, depending on the surgical procedure Adjunct to regional anesthesia, IM or slow IV (over 1–2 min) 0.05–0.1 mg PRN Postoperative analgesia, IM 0.05–0.1 mg, repeat in 1–2 h if needed General anesthesia, IV 0.05–0.1 mg/kg with oxygen and a muscle relaxant (maximum dose 0.15 mg/kg with open-heart surgery, other major surgeries, and complicated neurologic or orthopedic procedures) Chronic pain, transdermal system 2.5–10 mg every 72 h	*Weight at least 10 kg*: Conscious sedation or preanesthetic sedation, 5–15 mcg/kg of body weight (100–400 mcg), depending on weight, type of procedure, and other factors. Maximum dose, 400 mcg, regardless of age and weight. *2–12 y*: General anesthesia induction and maintenance, IV 2–3 mcg/kg
Hydromorphone (Dilaudid)	PO 2–4 mg q4–6h PRN IM, Sub-Q, IV 1–2 mg q4–6h PRN (may be increased to 4 mg for severe pain) Rectal suppository 3 mg q6–8h	Dosage not established
Levorphanol (Levo-Dromoran)	PO 2–3 mg q4–6h PRN	Dosage not established
Meperidine (Demerol)	IM, IV, Sub-Q, PO 50–100 mg q2–4h Obstetric analgesia, IM, Sub-Q 50–100 mg q2–4h for three or four doses	IM, Sub-Q, PO 1.1–1.75 mg/kg, up to adult dose, q3–4h
Methadone (Dolophine)	IM, Sub-Q, PO 2.5–10 mg q3–4h PRN	Not recommended; lack of data
Morphine (prototype) (MSIR, MS Contin, Roxanol, others)	PO immediate-release, 5–30 mg q4h PRN PO controlled-release, 30 mg or more q8–12h IM, Sub-Q 5–20 mg/70 kg q4h PRN IV injection, 2–10 mg/70 kg, diluted in 5 mL water for injection and injected slowly, over 5 min, PRN IV continuous infusion, 0.1–1 mg/mL in 5% dextrose in water solution, by controlled infusion pump Epidurally, 2–5 mg/24 h; intrathecally, 0.2–1 mg/24 h Rectal, 10–20 mg q4h	IM, Sub-Q 0.05–0.2 mg/kg (up to 15 mg) q4h
Oxycodone (OxyContin, Roxicodone, others)	PO, immediate release, 5 mg q6h PRN (OxyIR, Oxydose, OxyFAST); 10–30 mg q4h PRN for other formulations PO, controlled release, 10 mg q12h, increased if necessary	Not recommended for children <12 y
Oxymorphone (Numorphan)	IM, Sub-Q 1–1.5 mg q4–6h PRN IV 0.5 mg q4–6h PRN Rectal, 5 mg q4–6h PRN Obstetric analgesia, IM 0.5–1 mg	Dosage not established
Propoxyphene (Darvon)	Propoxyphene hydrochloride PO 65 mg q4h PRN (maximal daily dose, 390 mg) Propoxyphene napsylate PO 100 mg q4h PRN (maximal daily dose, 600 mg)	Not recommended Not recommended
Tramadol (Ultram)	PO 50–100 mg q4–6h PRN (maximum, 400 mg/d) Renal impairment (Crcl <30 mL/min): PO 50–100 mg q12h (maximum dose, 200 mg/d)	Dosage not established

	ROUTES AND DOSAGE RANGES	
GENERIC/TRADE NAME	Adults	Children
	Hepatic impairment (cirrhosis): PO 50 mg q12h Older adults (65–75 y): Same as adults, unless they also have renal or hepatic impairment Older adults (>75 y): <300 mg daily, in divided doses	
Agonists/Antagonists **Buprenorphine** (Buprenex)	IM or slow IV (over 2 min) 0.3 mg q6h PRN	Dosage not established
Butorphanol (Stadol)	IM, IV 1–4 mg q3–4h PRN Nasal spray 1 mg (one spray in one nostril) q3–4h PRN Older adults IM 1–2 mg q6–8h PRN Renal or hepatic impairment IM 1–2 mg q6–8h	Not recommended for children <18 y
Nalbuphine (Nubain)	IM, IV, Sub-Q 10 mg/70 kg q3–6h PRN	Not recommended

Crcl, creatinine clearance; GI, gastrointestinal; IM, intramuscular; IV, intravenous; PO, oral; PRN, as needed; Sub-Q, subcutaneous.

(Table 6-1 Drugs at a Glance: Opioid Analgesics (continued))

infusion. Other routes of administration include epidural, in which the drug is instilled through a catheter placed in the epidural space and slowly diffuses into the spinal cord, and intrathecal, in which the drug is injected directly into the spinal cord. Epidural and intrathecal morphine provide pain relief with very small doses, once or twice daily. When clients cannot take oral medications and injections are undesirable, rectal suppositories are often given.

Alfentanil (Alfenta), **fentanyl** (Sublimaze), **remifentanil** (Ultiva), and **sufentanil** (Sufenta) are potent opioid agonists with a short duration of action. They are most often used in anesthesia (see Appendix D) as analgesic adjuncts or primary anesthetic agents in open heart surgery or complicated neurologic and orthopedic procedures.

Fentanyl also is used for preanesthetic medication, postoperative analgesia, and chronic pain that requires an opioid analgesic. Because of a high risk of respiratory depression, recommended dosages must not be exceeded and the drug should be given only in an area with staff and equipment for emergency care (eg, intensive care unit, operating room, emergency department). As with other routes of administration, dosage of the oral lozenge should be individualized according to age, weight, illness, other medications, type of procedure and anesthesia, and other factors. A transdermal formulation (Duragesic) is used in the treatment of chronic pain. The active drug is deposited in the skin and slowly absorbed systemically. Thus, the skin patches have a slow onset of action (12 to 24 hours), but they last 3 days. When a patch is removed, the drug continues to be absorbed from the skin deposits for 24 hours or longer.

Codeine is a naturally occurring opium alkaloid, Schedule II drug used for analgesic and antitussive effects. Codeine produces weaker analgesic and antitussive effects and milder adverse effects than morphine. Compared with other opioid analgesics, codeine is more effective when given orally and is less likely to lead to abuse and dependence. The injected drug is more effective than the oral drug in relieving pain, but onset (15 to 30 minutes), peak (30 to 60 minutes), and duration of action (4 to 6 hours) are about the same. Half-life is about 3 hours. Larger doses are required for analgesic than for antitussive effects. Codeine is often given with acetaminophen for additive analgesic effects.

Codeine is metabolized to morphine, which is responsible for its analgesic effects, by the cytochrome P450 2D6 family of enzymes. As many as 10% of whites, Asians, and African Americans have inadequate amounts or activity of the 2D6 enzymes and may therefore receive less pain relief with usual therapeutic doses.

Hydrocodone, which is similar to codeine in its analgesic and antitussive effects, is a Schedule III drug. It is available in oral combination products for cough and with acetaminophen or ibuprofen for pain. Its half-life is about 4 hours and its duration of action is 4 to 6 hours. Hydrocodone is metabolized to hydromorphone by the cytochrome P450 2D6 enzymes.

Hydromorphone (Dilaudid) is a semisynthetic derivative of morphine that has the same actions, uses, contraindications, and adverse effects as morphine. It is more potent on a milligram basis and relatively more effective orally than morphine. Effects occur in 15 to 30 minutes, peak in 30 to

90 minutes, and last 4 to 5 hours. Hydromorphone produces less euphoria, nausea, and itching than morphine when given epidurally. It is metabolized in the liver to inactive metabolites that are excreted through the kidneys.

Levorphanol (Levo-Dromoran) is a synthetic drug with the same uses and adverse effects as morphine, although some reports indicate less nausea and vomiting. The average dose is probably equianalgesic with 10 milligrams of morphine. Maximal analgesia occurs 60 to 90 minutes after Sub-Q injection. Effects last 4 to 8 hours.

Meperidine (Demerol) is a synthetic drug that has a pharmacologic action similar to morphine. An injection of 80 to 100 milligrams is equivalent to 10 milligrams of morphine. After injection, analgesia occurs in 10 to 20 minutes, peaks in 1 hour, and lasts 2 to 4 hours. The oral form is only half as effective as the parenteral form because approximately half is metabolized in the liver and never reaches the systemic circulation. Compared with morphine, meperidine produces similar sedation and respiratory depression, but it has a shorter duration of action, requires more frequent administration, has little antitussive effect, causes less respiratory depression in newborns when used for obstetric analgesia, causes less smooth muscle spasm, and is preferred for clients with renal and biliary colic.

A unique feature of meperidine is that a neurotoxic metabolite (normeperidine) accumulates with chronic use, large doses, or renal failure. Normeperidine also accumulates more rapidly in patients who have taken drugs that induce hepatic drug-metabolizing enzymes (eg, phenytoin, isoniazid, rifampin) because faster metabolism of meperidine produces more normeperidine. Accumulation produces CNS stimulation characterized by agitation, convulsions, hallucinations, seizures, and tremors. The half-life of normeperidine is 15 to 30 hours, depending on renal function, and the effects of normeperidine are not reversible with opioid antagonist drugs.

As a result of these factors, the use of meperidine has greatly declined. Now, meperidine is recommended for short-term use in healthy individuals and is contraindicated for treatment of cancer pain, which often requires progressively higher doses over a long period of time. It is also contraindicated in patients who have taken amphetamines or monoamine oxidase inhibitor drugs (eg, phenelzine) within the past 21 days because this can precipitate a syndrome (called serotonin syndrome) of excitation, high fever, seizures, and death.

Methadone (Dolophine) is a synthetic drug similar to morphine, but with a longer duration of action. It is usually given orally, with which onset and peak of action occur in 30 to 60 minutes. Effects last 4 to 6 hours initially and longer with repeated use. Half-life is 15 to 30 hours, which also lengthens with repeated use. Methadone is used for severe pain and in the detoxification and maintenance treatment of opiate addicts.

Oxycodone (Roxicodone, others) is a semisynthetic derivative of codeine used to relieve moderate pain. It is less potent and less likely to produce dependence than morphine but is more potent and more likely to produce dependence than codeine. It is a Schedule II drug of abuse. Pharmacologic actions are similar to those of other opioid analgesics. Action starts in 15 to 30 minutes, peaks in 60 minutes, and lasts 4 to 6 hours. Its half-life is unknown. It is metabolized by the cytochrome P450 2D6 enzymes and excreted through the kidneys.

Oxycodone has been widely used for many years, often in combination with acetaminophen. It is also available alone in oral, immediate-release tablets and solutions. A few years ago, controlled-release tablets (OxyContin) in 10-, 20-, 40-, 80-, and 160-milligram sizes were marketed for extended treatment of moderate to severe pain (the 80- and 160-mg tablets should be used only by clients who have developed drug tolerance through long-term use of lesser doses). When given every 12 hours, the tablets could relieve pain around-the-clock. These effects are very advantageous to clients with terminal cancer or other chronically painful conditions. However, OxyContin soon became a popular drug of abuse, leading to dozens of deaths and much criminal activity. Most deaths have resulted from inappropriate use (ie, not legally prescribed for the user) and by chewing; crushing and snorting through the nose; or crushing and injecting the drug. Chewing or crushing destroys the long-acting feature and constitutes an overdose. Subsequently, the manufacturer and the Food and Drug Administration have issued precautions for prescribing OxyContin and warnings not to crush the product.

Oxymorphone (Numorphan) is a semisynthetic derivative of morphine. Its actions, uses, and adverse effects are similar to those of morphine, except that it has little antitussive effect. It is available as a solution for injection and as a rectal suppository. With injection, action starts in 5 to 10 minutes, peaks in 30 to 60 minutes, and lasts 3 to 6 hours.

Propoxyphene (Darvon) is a synthetic, Schedule IV drug that is chemically related to methadone. It is used for mild to moderate pain but is considered no more effective than 650 milligrams of aspirin or acetaminophen, with which it is usually given. Propoxyphene is abused (alone and with alcohol or other CNS depressant drugs), and deaths have occurred from overdoses. In addition, its metabolism produces an active metabolite, norpropoxyphene, which is eliminated in urine. Norpropoxyphene is not an opioid, but it has a long half-life and accumulates with repeated administration of propoxyphene. Accumulation is associated with dysrhythmias and pulmonary edema; there have also been reports of apnea, cardiac arrest, and death. Norpropoxyphene cannot be effectively removed by hemodialysis, and naloxone, an opioid antagonist, does not reverse its effects.

As a result of these characteristics, propoxyphene is not recommended for use in children, in clients at risk for suicide or addiction, older adults, or for long-term use. Despite these characteristics, dangers, and warnings from authoritative clinicians, the drug continues to be prescribed.

Tramadol (Ultram) is an oral, synthetic, centrally active analgesic for moderate to severe pain. It is effective and well tolerated in older adults and in people with acute or chronic pain, back pain, fibromyalgia, osteoarthritis, and neuropathic pain. Because it has a low potential for producing tolerance and abuse, it may be used long term for the management of chronic pain. It is not chemically related to opioids and is not a controlled drug. Its mechanism of action includes binding to mu opioid receptors and inhibiting reuptake of norepinephrine and serotonin in the brain, actions that interfere with transmission of pain signals. Analgesia occurs within 1 hour of administration and peaks in 2 to 3 hours. Tramadol causes significantly less respiratory depression than morphine but may cause other morphine-like adverse effects (eg, drowsiness, nausea, constipation, itching, orthostatic hypotension).

Tramadol is well absorbed after oral administration, even if taken with food. It is minimally bound (20%) to plasma proteins and its half-life is 6 to 7 hours. It is metabolized by the cytochrome P450 3A4 and 2D6 enzymes and forms an active metabolite. About 30% of a dose is excreted unchanged in the urine, and 60% is excreted as metabolites. Dosage should be reduced in people with renal or hepatic impairment. Tramadol is available in oral tablets alone and in combination with acetaminophen (Ultracet).

APPLYING YOUR KNOWLEDGE 6-1

At 12:00 P.M., you check on Mr. Harris. He complains of postoperative pain. He rates his pain as an 8 on a 10-point scale. Which pain medication will you give, and how much will you administer?

Opioid Agonists/Antagonists

These agents have agonist activity at some receptors and antagonist activity at others. Because of their agonist activity, they are potent analgesics with a lower abuse potential than pure agonists. Because of their antagonist activity, they may produce withdrawal symptoms in people with opiate dependence.

Buprenorphine (Buprenex) is a semisynthetic, Schedule V opioid with a long duration of action and a low incidence of causing physical dependence. These characteristics are attributed to its high affinity for and slow dissociation from mu receptors. With IM administration, analgesia occurs in 15 minutes, peaks in 60 minutes, and lasts approximately 6 hours. Buprenorphine may also be given IV. It is highly protein bound (96%) and has an elimination half-life of 2 to 3 hours. It is metabolized in the liver, and clearance is related to hepatic blood flow. It is excreted mainly in feces. Adverse effects include dizziness, sedation, hypoventilation, hypotension, and nausea and vomiting. Symptoms of opioid withdrawal rarely occur with co-administered opioids.

Butorphanol (Stadol) is a synthetic, Schedule IV agonist similar to morphine and meperidine in analgesic effects and ability to cause respiratory depression. It is used for moderate to severe pain and is given parenterally or topically to nasal mucosa by a metered spray (Stadol NS). After IM or IV administration, analgesia peaks in 30 to 60 minutes. After nasal application, analgesia peaks within 1 to 2 hours. Butorphanol also has antagonist activity and therefore should not be given to people who have been receiving opioid analgesics or who have opioid dependence. Other adverse effects include drowsiness and nausea and vomiting. Butorphanol is not recommended for use in children younger than 18 years of age.

Nalbuphine (Nubain) is a synthetic analgesic used for moderate to severe pain. It is not a controlled drug. It is given IV, IM, or Sub-Q. After IV injection, action starts in 2 to 3 minutes, peaks in 15 to 20 minutes, and lasts for 3 to 6 hours. After IM or Sub-Q injection, action begins in less than 15 minutes, peaks in 30 to 60 minutes, and lasts for 3 to 6 hours. Half-life is 5 hours. The most common adverse effect is sedation. Others include dizziness, sweating, headache, and psychotic symptoms, but these are reportedly minimal at doses of 10 milligrams or less.

Opioid Antagonists

Opioid antagonists reverse or block analgesia, CNS and respiratory depression, and other physiologic effects of opioid agonists. They compete with opioids for opioid receptor sites in the brain and thereby prevent opioid binding with receptors or displace opioids already occupying receptor sites. When an opioid cannot bind to receptor sites, it is "neutralized" and cannot exert its effects on body cells. Opioid antagonists do not relieve the depressant effects of other drugs, such as sedative-hypnotic, antianxiety, and antipsychotic agents. The chief clinical use of opioid antagonists is to relieve CNS and respiratory depression induced by therapeutic doses or overdoses of opioids. The drugs are also used to reverse postoperative opioid depression, and naltrexone is approved for the treatment of opioid and alcohol dependence. These drugs produce withdrawal symptoms when given to opioid-dependent people. Individual drugs are described in Table 6-2.

Naloxone (Narcan), **nalmefene** (Revex), and **naltrexone** (ReVia) are structurally and pharmacologically similar. Naloxone is the oldest and has long been the drug of choice to treat respiratory depression caused by an opioid drug. Therapeutic effects occur within minutes after IV, IM, or Sub-Q injection and last 1 to 2 hours. Naloxone has a shorter duration of action than opioids, and repeated injections are usually needed. For a long-acting drug such as methadone, injections may be needed for 2 to 3 days. Naloxone produces few adverse effects, and repeated injections can be given safely. This drug should be readily available in all health care settings in which opioids are given. Nalmefene is a newer agent whose main difference from naloxone is a longer duration of action. It may be preferred when opioid depression results from the use of long-acting drugs such as methadone. Nalmefene is

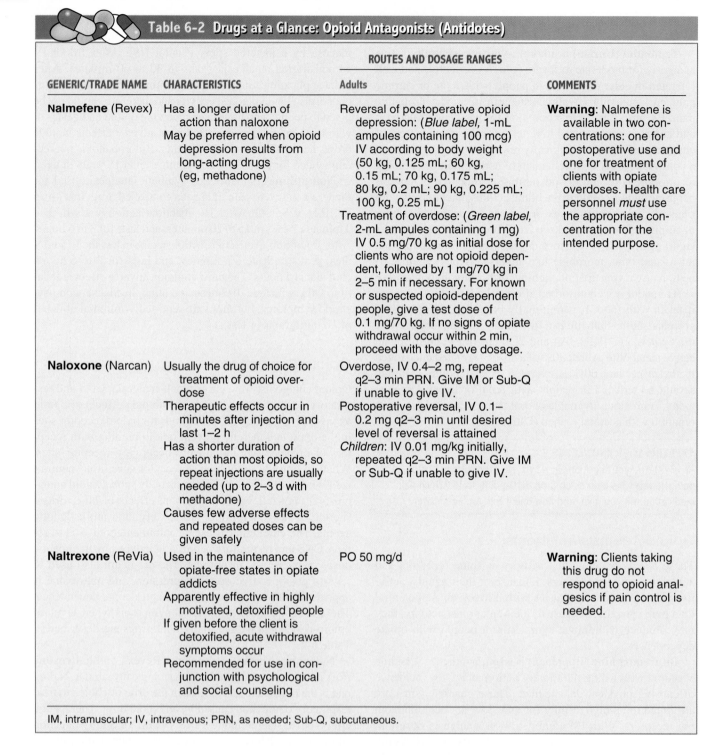

Table 6-2 Drugs at a Glance: Opioid Antagonists (Antidotes)

GENERIC/TRADE NAME	CHARACTERISTICS	ROUTES AND DOSAGE RANGES Adults	COMMENTS
Nalmefene (Revex)	Has a longer duration of action than naloxone May be preferred when opioid depression results from long-acting drugs (eg, methadone)	Reversal of postoperative opioid depression: (*Blue label,* 1-mL ampules containing 100 mcg) IV according to body weight (50 kg, 0.125 mL; 60 kg, 0.15 mL; 70 kg, 0.175 mL; 80 kg, 0.2 mL; 90 kg, 0.225 mL; 100 kg, 0.25 mL) Treatment of overdose: (*Green label,* 2-mL ampules containing 1 mg) IV 0.5 mg/70 kg as initial dose for clients who are not opioid dependent, followed by 1 mg/70 kg in 2–5 min if necessary. For known or suspected opioid-dependent people, give a test dose of 0.1 mg/70 kg. If no signs of opiate withdrawal occur within 2 min, proceed with the above dosage.	**Warning**: Nalmefene is available in two concentrations: one for postoperative use and one for treatment of clients with opiate overdoses. Health care personnel *must* use the appropriate concentration for the intended purpose.
Naloxone (Narcan)	Usually the drug of choice for treatment of opioid overdose Therapeutic effects occur in minutes after injection and last 1–2 h Has a shorter duration of action than most opioids, so repeat injections are usually needed (up to 2–3 d with methadone) Causes few adverse effects and repeated doses can be given safely	Overdose, IV 0.4–2 mg, repeat q2–3 min PRN. Give IM or Sub-Q if unable to give IV. Postoperative reversal, IV 0.1–0.2 mg q2–3 min until desired level of reversal is attained *Children*: IV 0.01 mg/kg initially, repeated q2–3 min PRN. Give IM or Sub-Q if unable to give IV.	
Naltrexone (ReVia)	Used in the maintenance of opiate-free states in opiate addicts Apparently effective in highly motivated, detoxified people If given before the client is detoxified, acute withdrawal symptoms occur Recommended for use in conjunction with psychological and social counseling	PO 50 mg/d	**Warning**: Clients taking this drug do not respond to opioid analgesics if pain control is needed.

IM, intramuscular; IV, intravenous; PRN, as needed; Sub-Q, subcutaneous.

available in two concentrations: one for postoperative use and one for treatment of clients with opioid overdoses. *Health care personnel must use the appropriate concentration.* Naltrexone is used in the maintenance of opiate-free states in opiate addicts. It is apparently effective in highly motivated, detoxified people. If given before clients are detoxified, acute withdrawal symptoms occur. Clients receiving naltrexone do not respond to analgesics if pain control is needed. The drug is rec-

ommended for use in conjunction with psychological and social counseling.

APPLYING YOUR KNOWLEDGE 6-2

At 1:00 P.M., you visit Mr. Harris's room. You note he is difficult to arouse and has a respiratory rate of 10 breaths per minute. What should be your nursing response?

Herbal and Dietary Supplement

Capsaicin (Zostrix), a product derived from cayenne chili peppers, is applied topically to the skin to relieve pain associated with osteoarthritis, rheumatoid arthritis, postherpetic neuralgia after a herpes zoster infection (shingles), diabetic neuropathy, postsurgical pain (including pain after mastectomy and amputation), and other neuropathic pain and complex pain syndromes. It may be most effective in relieving arthritic pain in joints close to skin surfaces (eg, fingers, elbows, knees). Its analgesic effects are attributed to depletion of substance P in nerve cells. Substance P is a mediator in the transmission of painful stimuli from peripheral tissues to the spinal cord. An additional analgesic effect may result from interference with production of prostaglandins and leukotrienes.

Capsaicin is available in a gel, creams, and lotions, in concentrations ranging from 0.025% to 0.25%, for topical application to the skin. It is most effective when applied 3 or 4 times daily; effects last about 4 to 5 hours. Less frequent application produces less effective analgesia. The main adverse effects are itching and stinging, which decrease with continued use.

Capsaicin also is the active ingredient in a popular non-lethal self-defense spray (pepper spray).

APPLYING YOUR KNOWLEDGE 6-3:
HOW CAN YOU AVOID THIS MEDICATION ERROR?
On the night after his surgery, Mr. Harris requests medication for pain. You note on his chart that the physician has ordered oral pain medication 24 hours after surgery. When Mr. Harris requests medication for pain, you administer Lortab 5/500.

NURSING PROCESS

Assessment

Pain is a subjective experience (whatever the person says it is), and humans display a wide variety of responses. Although pain thresholds (the point at which a tissue-damaging stimulus produces a sensation of pain) are similar, people differ in their perceptions, behaviors, and tolerance of pain. Differences in pain perception may result from psychological components. Stressors such as anxiety, depression, fatigue, anger, and fear tend to increase pain; rest, mood elevation, and diversionary activities tend to decrease pain. Differences in behaviors may or may not indicate pain to observers, and overt signs and symptoms are not reliable indicators of the presence or extent of pain. Especially with chronic pain, overt signs and symptoms may be absent. Differences in tolerance of pain (the amount or duration of pain a person is willing to suffer before seeking relief) often reflect the person's concern about the meaning of the pain and the type or intensity of the painful stimulus. Thus, pain is a complex physiologic, psychological, and sociocultural phenomenon that must be thoroughly assessed if it is to be managed effectively.

The nurse must assess every client in relation to pain, initially to determine appropriate interventions and later to determine whether the interventions were effective in preventing or relieving pain. Although the client is usually the best source of data, other people may be questioned about the client's words and behaviors that indicate pain. This is especially important with young children. During assessment, keep in mind that acute pain may coexist with or be superimposed on chronic pain. Specific assessment data usually include

- **Location.** Determining the location may assist in relieving the pain or identifying its underlying cause. Ask the client to show you where it hurts, if possible, and whether the pain stays in one place or radiates to other parts of the body. The term *referred pain* is used when pain arising from tissue damage in one area of the body is felt in another area. Patterns of referred pain may be helpful in diagnosis. For example, pain of cardiac origin may radiate to the neck, shoulders, chest muscles, and down the arms, often on the left side. This form of pain usually results from myocardial ischemia due to atherosclerosis of coronary arteries. Stomach pain is usually referred to the epigastrium and may indicate gastritis or peptic ulcer. Gallbladder and bile duct pain is often localized in the right upper quadrant of the abdomen. Uterine pain is usually felt as abdominal cramping or low back pain. Deep or chronic pain is usually more difficult to localize than superficial or acute pain.
- **Intensity or severity.** Because pain is a subjective experience and cannot be objectively measured, assessment of severity is based on the client's description and the nurse's observations. Various scales have been developed to measure and quantify pain. These include verbal descriptor scales in which the client is asked to rate pain as mild, moderate, or severe; numeric scales, with 0 representing no pain and 10 representing severe, intense pain; and visual analog scales, in which the client chooses the location indicating the level of pain on a continuum.
- **Relation to time, activities, and other signs and symptoms.** Specific questions include
  - When did the pain start?
  - What activities were occurring when the pain started?
  - Does the pain occur with exercise or when at rest?
  - Do other signs and symptoms occur before, during, or after the pain?
  - Is this the first episode or a recurrent pain?

● How long does the pain last?
● What, if anything, decreases or relieves the pain?
● What, if anything, aggravates the pain?

● **Other data.** For example, do not assume that postoperative pain is incisional and requires narcotic analgesics for relief. A person who has had abdominal surgery may have headache, musculoskeletal discomfort, or "gas pains." Also, restlessness may be caused by hypoxia or anxiety rather than pain.

Nursing Diagnoses

● Acute Pain
● Chronic Pain
● Impaired Gas Exchange related to sedation and decreased mobility
● Risk for Injury related to sedation and decreased mobility
● Constipation related to slowed peristalsis
● Deficient Knowledge: Effects and appropriate use of opioid analgesics
● Noncompliance: Drug dependence related to overuse

Planning/Goals

The client will
● Avoid or be relieved of pain.
● Use opioid analgesics appropriately.
● Avoid preventable adverse effects.
● Be closely monitored for excessive sedation and respiratory depression.
● Be able to communicate and perform other activities of daily living when feasible.

Interventions

Use measures to prevent, relieve, or decrease pain when possible. General measures include those that promote optimal body functioning and those that prevent trauma, inflammation, infection, and other sources of painful stimuli. Specific measures include the following:

● Encourage pulmonary hygiene techniques (eg, coughing, deep breathing, ambulation) to promote respiration and prevent pulmonary complications, such as pneumonia and atelectasis.
● Use sterile technique when caring for wounds, urinary catheters, or IV lines.
● Use exercises, ambulation, and position changes to promote circulation and musculoskeletal function.
● Handle any injured tissue very gently to avoid further trauma.
● Prevent bowel or bladder distention.
● Apply heat or cold.
● Use relaxation or distraction techniques.

● If a client is in pain on initial contact, try to relieve the pain as soon as possible. After pain is controlled, plan with the client to avoid or manage future episodes.
● If a client is not in pain initially but anticipates surgery or an uncomfortable diagnostic procedure, plan with the client ways to minimize and manage discomfort.

Client teaching guidelines for drug therapy with opioid analgesics are given in the accompanying display.

Evaluation

● Ask clients about their levels of comfort or relief from pain.
● Observe behaviors that indicate the presence or absence of pain.
● Observe participation and ability to function in usual activities of daily living.
● Observe for presence or absence of sedation and respiratory depression.
● Observe for drug-seeking behavior (possibly indicating dependence).

PRINCIPLES OF THERAPY

Goals of Therapy

The primary goal of therapy is to relieve pain and discomfort, thus promoting rest and relaxation. A secondary goal is to allow performance of the usual activities of daily living, as conditions permit. Studies often indicate that health care providers do not always meet these goals effectively, especially in cases of moderate to severe pain associated with surgery or cancer. Much of the difficulty has been attributed to inadequate or improper use of opioid analgesics, including administering the wrong drug, prescribing inadequate dosage, or leaving long intervals between doses. Even when opioid analgesics are ordered appropriately, nurses or clients and family members may not administer the drugs effectively. Traditionally, concerns about respiratory depression, excessive sedation, drug dependence, and other adverse effects have contributed to reluctance and delay in administering narcotic analgesics. Inadequate management of pain often leads to anxiety, depression, and other emotional upsets due to anticipation of pain.

A more humane approach to pain management has now evolved. Basic tenets of this approach are that no person should suffer pain needlessly; that pain occurs when the client says it does, and that pain should be relieved by whatever means are required, including pharmacologic and nonpharmacologic treatments; that doses of opioids should be titrated to achieve maximal effectiveness and minimal toxicity; and that dependence rarely results from drugs taken for physical pain. Proponents of this view emphasize the need to assess and monitor all clients receiving opioid analgesics.

CLIENT TEACHING GUIDELINES

Opioid (Narcotic) Analgesics

General Considerations

✔ Use nonpharmacologic treatments of pain (eg, exercise, heat and cold applications) instead of or along with analgesics, when effective.

✔ For pain that is not relieved by nondrug treatments, a non-narcotic analgesic (eg, acetaminophen or ibuprofen) may be taken.

✔ For pain that is not relieved by a non-narcotic analgesic, a narcotic may be alternated with a non-narcotic analgesic or a combination product containing a narcotic and non-narcotic may be effective. Use of a narcotic analgesic for acute pain is acceptable and unlikely to lead to addiction.

✔ Most combination products (eg, Lorcet, Lortab, Percocet, Vicodin, Tylenol No. 3) contain acetaminophen and there is a risk of liver failure from high doses of acetaminophen, or from lower doses in people who already have liver damage (eg, alcohol abusers). The maximum recommended daily dose, whether taken alone or in a combination product, is 4000 milligrams (eg, 8 tablets or capsules containing 500 mg each or 12 tablets containing 325 mg each). If unsure whether a combination product contains acetaminophen, ask a health care provider.

✔ For acute episodes of pain, most opioids may be taken as needed; for chronic pain, the drugs should be taken on a regular schedule, around the clock.

✔ When a choice of analgesics is available, use the least amount of the mildest drug that is likely to be effective in a particular situation.

✔ Take only as prescribed. If desired effects are not achieved, report to the physician. Do not increase the dose and do not take medication more often than prescribed. Although these principles apply to all medications, they are especially important with opioid analgesics because of potentially serious adverse reactions—including drug dependence—and because analgesics may mask pain for which medical attention is needed.

✔ Do not drink alcohol or take other drugs that cause drowsiness (eg, some antihistamines, sedative-type drugs for nervousness or anxiety, sleeping pills) while taking opioid analgesics. Combining drugs with similar effects may lead to excessive sedation, even coma, and difficulty in breathing.

✔ Do not smoke, cook, drive a car, or operate machinery when drowsy or dizzy or when vision is blurred from medication. Stay in bed at least 30–60 minutes after receiving an opioid analgesic by injection. Injected drugs may cause dizziness, drowsiness, and falls when walking around. If it is necessary to get out of bed, ask someone for assistance.

✔ When hospitalized, ask the physician or nurse about potential methods of pain management. For example, if anticipating surgery, ask how postoperative pain will be managed, how you need to report pain and request pain medication, and so on. It is better to take adequate medication and be able to cough, deep breathe, and ambulate than to avoid or minimize pain medication and be unable to perform activities that promote recovery and healing. Do not object to having bedrails up and asking for assistance to ambulate when receiving a strong narcotic analgesic. These are safety measures to prevent falls or other injuries because these analgesics may cause drowsiness, weakness, unsteady gait, and blurred vision.

✔ Constipation is a common adverse effect of opioid analgesics. It may be prevented or managed by eating high-fiber foods, such as whole-grain cereals, fruits, and vegetables; drinking 2–3 quarts of fluid daily; and being as active as tolerated. For someone unable to take these preventive measures, Metamucil daily or a mild laxative every other day may be needed.

Self-Administration

✔ Take oral narcotics with 6–8 oz of water, with or after food to reduce nausea.

✔ Do not crush or chew long-acting tablets (eg, MS Contin, OxyContin). The tablets are formulated to release the active drug slowly, over several hours. Crushing or chewing causes immediate release of the drug, with a high risk of overdose and adverse effects, and shortens the duration of action.

✔ Omit one or more doses if severe adverse effects occur (eg, excessive drowsiness, difficulty in breathing, severe nausea, vomiting, or constipation), and report to a health care provider.

Drug Selection

Morphine is often the drug of first choice for severe pain. It is effective, available in various dosage strengths and forms, and useful on a short- or long-term basis, and its adverse effects are well known. In addition, it is a "nonceiling" drug because there is no upper limit to the dosage that can be given to clients who have developed tolerance to previous dosages. This characteristic is especially valuable in clients with severe cancer-related pain, because the drug dosage can be increased and titrated to relieve pain when pain increases or tolerance develops. Thus, some clients have safely received extremely large doses. Other nonceiling drugs are hydromorphone, levorphanol, and methadone.

When more than one analgesic drug is ordered, the least potent drug that is effective in relieving pain should be used. For example, a nonopioid analgesic, such as acetaminophen, rather than an opioid analgesic, should be given when feasible.

Nonopioid analgesics may be alternated or given concurrently with opioid analgesics, especially in chronic pain. This strategy increases client comfort, reduces the likelihood of drug abuse and dependence, and decreases tolerance to the pain-relieving effects of the opioid analgesics. The drug preparation of choice may be one that combines an opioid and a nonopioid such as acetaminophen (Table 6-3). The nonopioids act by different mechanisms and therefore produce greater analgesic effects.

TABLE 6-3 Selected Combination Opioid–Acetaminophen Products

TRADE NAME/DOSAGE FORMS	SCHEDULE	OPIOID COMPONENT	AMOUNT OF ACETAMINOPHEN	AVERAGE ADULT DOSAGE RANGES
Hydrocet capsules	III	Hydrocodone 5 mg	500 mg	1–2 tabs q4–6h, up to 8 tabs/d
Lorcet-HD tablets	III	Hydrocodone 5 mg	500 mg	1–2 tabs q4–6h, up to 8 tabs/d
Lorcet Plus tablets	III	Hydrocodone 7.5 mg	650 mg	1 tab q4–6h
Lorcet 10/650 tablets	III	Hydrocodone 10 mg	650 mg	1 tab q4–6h
Lortab 2.5/500 tablets	III	Hydrocodone 2.5 mg	500 mg	1–2 tabs q4–6h, up to 8 tabs/d
Lortab 5/500 tablets	III	Hydrocodone 5 mg	500 mg	1–2 tabs q4–6h, up to 8 tabs/d
Lortab 7.5/500 tablets	III	Hydrocodone 7.5 mg	500 mg	1 tab q4–6h
Lortab 10/500 tablets	III	Hydrocodone 10 mg	500 mg	1 tab q4–6h up to 6/d
Percocet	II	Oxycodone 5 mg	325 mg	1 tab q6h
Roxicet tablets	II	Oxycodone 5 mg	325 mg	1 tab q6h
Roxicet oral solution	II	Oxycodone 5 mg	325 mg	5 mL q6h
Roxicet 5/500 caplets	II	Oxycodone 5 mg	500 mg	1 cap q6h
Tylenol with codeine elixir	V	Codeine 12 mg	120 mg	15 mL q4h
Tylenol with codeine No. 2 tablets	III	Codeine 15 mg	300 mg	1–4 tabs q4h
Tylenol with codeine No. 3 tablets	III	Codeine 30 mg	300 mg	0.5–2 tabs q4h
Tylenol with codeine No. 4 tablets	III	Codeine 60 mg	300 mg	1 tab q4h
Tylox capsules	II	Oxycodone 5 mg	500 mg	1 cap q6h
Ultracet tablets		Tramadol 37.5 mg	325 mg	2 tabs q4–6h
Vicodin tablets	III	Hydrocodone 5 mg	500 mg	1–2 tabs q4–6h, up to 8 tabs/d
Vicodin ES tablets	III	Hydrocodone 7.5 mg	750 mg	1 tab q4–6h, up to 5 tabs/d

Drug Dosage

Dosages of opioid analgesics should be sufficient to relieve pain without causing unacceptable adverse effects. Thus, dosages should be individualized according to the type and severity of pain; the client's age, size, and health status; whether the client is opiate naive (has not received sufficient opioids for development of tolerance) or opiate tolerant (has previously taken opioids and drug tolerance has developed, so that larger-than-usual doses are needed to relieve pain); whether the client has progressive or worsening disease; and other characteristics that influence responses to pain. Guidelines include the following:

- Small to moderate doses relieve constant, dull pain, and moderate to large doses relieve intermittent, sharp pain caused by trauma or conditions affecting the viscera.
- When an opioid analgesic is ordered in variable amounts (eg, 8–10 mg of morphine), the smaller amount should be given as long as it is effective in relieving pain.
- Dosages of opioid analgesics should be reduced for clients who also are receiving other CNS depressants, such as sedating, antianxiety, antidepressant, antihistaminic, antipsychotic, or other sedative-type drugs.

- Dosages often differ according to the route of administration, as discussed in the following section. Oral doses undergo extensive metabolism on their first pass through the liver, so oral doses are usually much larger than injected doses.

Drug Administration

Route of Administration

Opioid analgesics can be given by several routes, either noninvasively (orally, rectally, or transdermally) or invasively (Sub-Q, IV, or by spinal infusion). Oral drugs are preferred when feasible, and most clients achieve relief with short-acting or sustained-release oral preparations. *When the route is changed (eg, from oral to injection or vice versa), the dose must also be changed to prevent overdosage or underdosage.*

Intravenous injection is usually preferred for rapid relief of acute, severe pain. Small, frequent IV doses are often effective in relieving pain with minimal risk of serious adverse effects. This is especially advantageous during a serious illness or after surgery. Continuous IV infusion may be used to treat severe pain.

A technique called *patient-controlled analgesia* (PCA) allows self-administration. Devices may consist of a syringe of diluted drug connected to an IV line and infusion pump or a specially designed IV bag and special tubing. These devices deliver a dose when the client pushes a button. Some PCA pumps can also deliver a basic amount of analgesic by continuous infusion, with the client injecting additional doses when needed. The amount of drug delivered with each dose and the intervals between doses are preset and limited. PCA requires an alert, cooperative patient who can press a button when pain occurs. Studies indicate that analgesia is more effective, client satisfaction is high, and smaller amounts of drug are used than with conventional PRN administration. PCA is especially useful for patients with postoperative pain or high opioid requirements.

Two other routes of administration are used to manage acute pain. One route involves injection of opioid analgesics directly into the CNS through a catheter placed into the epidural or intrathecal space by an anesthesiologist or other physician. This method provides effective analgesia while minimizing depressant effects. This type of pain control was developed after opioid receptors were found on neurons in the spinal cord. The other route involves the injection of local anesthetics to provide local or regional analgesia. Both of these methods interrupt the transmission of pain signals and are effective in relieving pain, but they also require special techniques and monitoring procedures for safe use.

The epidural route can be used to administer PCA, and less opioid analgesic is required for pain relief than with the IV route. Morphine or fentanyl may be used alone or combined with the local anesthetic bupivacaine.

For clients with chronic pain and contraindications to oral or injected medications, some opioids are available in rectal suppositories or skin patches. Morphine, oxymorphone, and hydromorphone can be given rectally with similar potencies and half-lives as when given orally. For clients who cannot take oral medications and whose opioid requirement is too large for rectal administration, the transdermal route is preferred over IV or Sub-Q routes. A fentanyl skin patch (Duragesic) is effective and commonly used (see *Research Brief*). When first applied, pain relief is delayed approximately 12 hours (as the drug is gradually absorbed). Because of the delayed effects, doses of a short-acting opioid should be ordered and given as needed during the first 48 hours after the patch is applied. With continued use, the old patch is removed and a new one applied approximately every 72 hours. Opioid overdose can occur with fentanyl patches if the client has fever (hastens drug absorption) or liver impairment (slows drug metabolism).

Frequency of Administration

Opioid analgesics may be given as needed, within designated time limits, or on a regular schedule. Traditionally, the drugs have often been scheduled every 4 to 6 hours as needed (PRN). Numerous studies indicate that such a sched-

---

RESEARCH BRIEF

Patient-Controlled Analgesia Using a Skin Patch

PAINKILLING PATCH WORKS LIKE NEEDLE DELIVERY

Viscusi, E. R., Reynolds, L., Chung, F., et al. (2004). Patient-controlled transdermal fentanyl hydrochloride vs intravenous morphine pump for postoperative pain: A randomized controlled trial. *Journal of the American Medical Association, 291*(11), 1333–1341.

SUMMARY: In a study of 636 patients who had had major surgery, some received an adhesive skin patch that uses a minute electric current to deliver fentanyl and some received intravenous (IV) morphine. Both systems allowed patients to self-medicate. The skin patch, which resembles a credit card, is placed on the patient's upper arm or chest after surgery and patients can activate medication release as with IV patient-controlled analgesia systems. With the patch, 74% rated pain relief as good to excellent for the first 24 hours after surgery; 77% rated IV morphine highly. The system is being reviewed by the Food and Drug Administration.

NURSING IMPLICATIONS: The patch would be more comfortable for patients and allow them to move about more freely. It would also take less nursing time than maintaining an IV.

---

ule is often ineffective in managing clients' pain. Because these analgesics are used for moderate to severe pain, they should in general be scheduled to provide effective and consistent pain relief.

When analgesics are ordered PRN, have a clear-cut system by which the client reports pain or requests medication. The client should know that analgesic drugs are ordered and that they will be given promptly when needed. If a drug cannot be given or if administration must be delayed, explain this to the client. In addition, offer or give the drug when indicated by the client's condition rather than waiting for the client to request medication. When analgesics are needed, give them before conducting coughing and deep-breathing exercises or performing dressing changes and other therapeutic and diagnostic procedures.

For acute pain, opioid analgesics are most effective when given parenterally and at the onset of pain. In chronic, severe pain, opioid analgesics are most effective when given on a regular schedule, around the clock.

Opioids are not recommended for prolonged periods except for advanced malignant disease. Health care facilities usually have an automatic "stop order" for opioids after 48 to

72 hours; this means that the drug is discontinued when the time limit expires if it is not reordered by the prescriber.

Opioid Toxicity: Recognition and Management

Acute toxicity or opioid overdose can occur from therapeutic use or from abuse by drug-dependent people. Overdose may produce severe respiratory depression and coma. The main goal of treatment is to restore and maintain adequate respiratory function. This can be accomplished by inserting an endotracheal tube and starting mechanical ventilation, or by giving an opioid antagonist, such as naloxone or nalmefene. Thus, emergency supplies should be readily available in any setting where opioid analgesics are used, including ambulatory settings and clients' homes.

Opioid Withdrawal: Prevention and Management

Abstinence from opiates after chronic use produces a withdrawal syndrome characterized by anxiety; aggressiveness; restlessness; generalized body aches; insomnia; lacrimation; rhinorrhea; perspiration; pupil dilation; piloerection (goose flesh); anorexia, nausea, and vomiting; diarrhea; elevation of body temperature, respiratory rate, and systolic blood pressure; abdominal and other muscle cramps; dehydration; and weight loss. Although all opioids produce similar withdrawal syndromes, the onset, severity, and duration vary. With morphine, symptoms begin within a few hours of the last dose, reach peak intensity in 36 to 72 hours, and subside over approximately 10 days. With methadone, symptoms begin in 1 to 2 days, peak in approximately 3 days, and subside over several weeks. Heroin, meperidine, methadone, morphine, oxycodone, and oxymorphone are associated with more severe withdrawal symptoms than other opioids. If an opioid antagonist such as naloxone (Narcan) is given, withdrawal symptoms occur rapidly and are more intense but of shorter duration. Despite the discomfort that occurs, withdrawal from opioids is rarely life threatening unless other problems are present. An exception is opioid withdrawal in neonates, which has a high mortality rate if not treated effectively. Signs and symptoms in neonates include tremor, jitteriness, increased muscle tone, screaming, fever, sweating, tachycardia, vomiting, diarrhea, respiratory distress, and possibly seizures.

Recognition and treatment of early, mild symptoms of withdrawal can prevent progression to severe symptoms. Both opioids and nonopioids are used for treatment. Opioids may be used in two ways to provide a safe, comfortable, and therapeutic withdrawal. One technique is to give the opioid from which the person is withdrawing, which immediately reverses the signs and symptoms of withdrawal. Then, dosage is gradually reduced over several days. Another technique is to substitute a long-acting opioid (eg, methadone) for a short-acting

opioid of abuse. Methadone is usually given in an adequate dose to control symptoms, once or twice daily, and then is gradually tapered over 5 to 10 days. In neonates undergoing opioid withdrawal, methadone or paregoric may be used.

Clonidine, an antihypertensive drug, is a nonopioid that may be used to treat opioid withdrawal. Clonidine reduces the release of norepinephrine in the brain and thus reduces symptoms associated with excessive stimulation of the sympathetic nervous system (eg, anxiety, restlessness, insomnia). Blood pressure must be closely monitored during clonidine therapy. Other medications (nonopioid analgesics, antiemetics, antidiarrheals) are often required to treat other symptoms.

Treatment of Specific Disorders

Cancer

When opioid analgesics are required in clients with chronic pain associated with malignancy, the main consideration is client comfort, not preventing drug addiction. Effective treatment requires that pain be relieved and prevented from recurring. With disease progression and the development of drug tolerance, extremely large doses and frequent administration may be required. Additional guidelines include the following:

- Analgesics should be given on a regular schedule, around-the-clock. Clients should be awakened, if necessary, to prevent pain recurrence.
- Oral, rectal, and transdermal routes of administration are generally preferred over injections.
- A nonopioid analgesic (see Chap. 7) may be used alone for mild pain.
- Oxycodone or codeine can be used for moderate pain, often with a non-narcotic analgesic. A combination of the two types of drugs produces additive analgesic effects and may allow smaller doses of the opioid.
- Morphine or another strong opioid is given for severe pain. Although the dose of morphine can be titrated upward for adequate analgesia, unacceptable adverse effects (eg, excessive sedation, respiratory depression, nausea and vomiting) may limit the dose. Oral administration is preferred; the initial oral dosage of morphine is usually 10 to 20 milligrams every 3 to 4 hours.
- When long-acting forms of opioid analgesics are given on a regular schedule (eg, sustained-release forms of morphine, fentanyl skin patches), fast-acting forms also need to be ordered and available for "breakthrough" pain. If additional doses are needed frequently, the baseline dose of long-acting medication may need to be increased.
- In addition to opioid analgesics, other drugs may be used to increase client comfort. For example, tricyclic antidepressants (TCAs) have analgesic effects, especially in neuropathic pain. Lower doses of TCAs are required for analgesia than for depression, but anal-

gesic effects may not occur for 2 to 3 weeks. Antiemetics may be given for nausea and vomiting; laxatives or stool softeners are usually needed to prevent or relieve constipation because tolerance does not develop to the constipating effects of opioids.

Biliary, Renal, or Ureteral Colic

When opioid analgesics are used to relieve the acute, severe pain associated with various types of colic, an antispasmodic drug such as atropine may be needed as well. Opioid analgesics may increase smooth muscle tone and cause spasm. Atropine does not have strong antispasmodic properties of its own in usual doses, but it reduces the spasm-producing effects of opioid analgesics.

Postoperative Use

When analgesics are used postoperatively, the goal is to relieve pain without excessive sedation so that clients can do deep-breathing exercises, cough, ambulate, and implement other measures to promote recovery.

Burns

In severely burned clients, opioid analgesics should be used cautiously. A common cause of respiratory arrest in burned clients is excessive administration of analgesics. Agitation in a burned person usually should be interpreted as hypoxia or hypovolemia rather than pain, until proved otherwise. When opioid analgesics are necessary, they are usually given IV in small doses. Drugs given by other routes are absorbed erratically in the presence of shock and hypovolemia and may not relieve pain. In addition, unabsorbed drugs may be rapidly absorbed when circulation improves, with the potential for excessive dosage and toxic effects.

Use in Special Populations

Use in Opiate-Tolerant Clients

Whether opiate tolerance results from the use of prescribed, therapeutic drugs or the abuse of street drugs, there are two main considerations in using opioid analgesics in this population. First, larger-than-usual doses are required to treat pain. Second, signs and symptoms of withdrawal occur if adequate dosage is not maintained or if opioid antagonists are given.

Use in Children

In general, there is little understanding of the physiology, pathology, assessment, and management of pain in children. Many authorities indicate that children's pain is often ignored or undertreated, including children having surgical and other painful procedures for which adults routinely receive an anesthetic, a strong analgesic, or both. This is especially true

in preterm and full-term neonates. One reason for inadequate prevention and management of pain in newborns has been a common belief that they did not experience pain because of immature nervous systems. However, research indicates that neonates have abundant C fibers and that A-delta fibers are developing during the first few months of life. These are the nerve fibers that carry pain signals from peripheral tissues to the spinal cord. In addition, brain pain centers and the endogenous analgesia system seem to be developed and functional. Endogenous opioids are released at birth and in response to fetal and neonatal distress such as asphyxia or other difficulty associated with the birth process.

Older infants and children may experience pain even when analgesics have been ordered and are readily available. For example, children may fear injections or may be unable to communicate their discomfort. Health care providers or parents may fear adverse effects of opioid analgesics, including excessive sedation, respiratory depression, and addiction.

Other than reduced dosage, there have been few guidelines about the use of opioid analgesics in children. With increased knowledge about pain mechanisms and the recommendations prepared by the Acute Pain Management Guideline Panel in 1992, every nurse who works with children should be able to manage pain effectively. Specific considerations include the following:

- Opioid analgesics administered during labor and delivery may depress fetal and neonatal respiration. The drugs cross the blood–brain barrier of the infant more readily than that of the mother. Therefore, doses that do not depress maternal respiration may profoundly depress the infant's respiration. Respiration should be monitored closely in neonates, and the opioid antagonist naloxone should be readily available.
- Expressions of pain may differ according to age and developmental level. Infants may cry and have muscular rigidity and thrashing behavior. Preschoolers may behave aggressively or complain verbally of discomfort. Young school-aged children may express pain verbally or behaviorally, often with regression to behaviors used at younger ages. Adolescents may be reluctant to admit they are uncomfortable or need help. With chronic pain, children of all ages tend to withdraw and regress to an earlier stage of development.
- It is recommended that opioid analgesics be given by routes (eg, PO, IV, epidurally) other than IM injections, because IM injections are painful and frightening for children. For any child receiving parenteral opioids, vital signs and level of consciousness must be assessed regularly.
- Opioid formulations specifically for children are not generally available. When children's doses are calculated based on adult doses, the fractions and decimals that often result greatly increase the risk of a dosage error.

- Opioid rectal suppositories are used more often in children than in adults. Although useful when oral or parenteral routes are not indicated, the dose of medication actually received by the child is unknown because drug absorption is erratic and because adult suppositories are sometimes cut in half or otherwise altered.
- Opioid effects in children may differ from those expected in adults because of physiologic and pharmacokinetic differences. Assess regularly and be alert for unusual signs and symptoms.
- Hydromorphone, methadone, oxycodone, and oxymorphone are not recommended for use in children because safety, efficacy, and dosages have not been established.
- Like adults, children seem more able to cope with pain when they are informed about what is happening to them and are assisted in developing coping strategies. Age-appropriate doll play, a favorite videotape/DVD, diversionary activities, and other techniques can be used effectively. However, such techniques should be used in conjunction with adequate analgesia, not as a substitute for pain medication.

Use in Older Adults

Opioid analgesics should be used cautiously in older adults, especially if they are debilitated; have hepatic, renal, or respiratory impairment; or are receiving other drugs that depress the CNS. Older adults are especially sensitive to respiratory depression, excessive sedation, confusion, and other adverse effects. However, they should receive adequate analgesia, along with vigilant monitoring. Specific recommendations include the following:

- Use nondrug measures (eg, heat or cold applications, exercise) and nonopioid analgesics to relieve pain, when effective.
- When opioid analgesics are needed, use those with short half-lives (eg, oxycodone, hydromorphone) because they are less likely to accumulate.
- Start with low doses and increase doses gradually, if necessary.
- Give the drugs less often than for younger adults because the duration of action may be longer.
- Monitor carefully for sedation or confusion. Also, monitor voiding and urine output because acute urinary retention is more likely to occur in older adults.
- Assess older adults for ability to self-administer opioid analgesics safely. Those with short-term memory loss (common in this population) may require assistance and supervision.

Use in Clients With Renal Impairment

Most opioid analgesics and related drugs are extensively metabolized in the liver to metabolites that are then excreted in urine. In clients with renal impairment, the drugs should be given in minimal doses, for the shortest effective time, because usual doses may produce profound sedation and a prolonged duration of action. Morphine, for example, produces an active metabolite that may accumulate in clients with renal impairment. Meperidine should not be used because a toxic metabolite, normeperidine, may accumulate. Normeperidine is pharmacologically active and a CNS stimulant that may cause muscle spasms, seizures, and psychosis. These effects are not reversed by opioid antagonists such as naloxone.

Use in Clients With Hepatic Impairment

Because opioid analgesics and related drugs are extensively metabolized by the liver, they may accumulate and cause increased adverse effects in the presence of hepatic impairment. Dosages may need to be reduced, especially with chronic use.

Use in Clients With Critical Illness

Opioid analgesics are commonly used to manage pain associated with disease processes and invasive diagnostic and therapeutic procedures. In intensive care units, they are also used for synergistic effects with sedatives and neuromuscular blocking agents, which increases the risks of adverse drug reactions and interactions. In clients with critical illness, opioid analgesics are usually given by IV bolus or continuous infusion. Guidelines include the following:

- Assume that all critically ill clients are in pain or at high risk for development of pain.
- When pain is thought to be present, identify and treat the underlying cause when possible, rather than just treating the symptom.
- Assess for pain on a regular schedule around the clock (eg, every 1 to 2 hours in critical care units). Use a consistent method for assessing severity, such as a visual analog or numeric scale. If the client is able to communicate, ask about the location, severity, and so forth. If the client is unable to communicate needs for pain relief, as is often the case during critical illnesses, the nurse must evaluate posture, body language, risk factors, and other possible indicators of pain.
- Prevent pain when possible. Interventions include being very gentle when performing nursing care to avoid tissue trauma and positioning clients to prevent ischemia, edema, and misalignment. In addition, give analgesics before painful procedures, when indicated.
- When pain occurs, manage it appropriately to provide relief and prevent its recurrence. In general, opioid analgesics should be given continuously or on a regular schedule of intermittent doses, with supplemental or bolus doses when needed for breakthrough pain. When starting a continuous IV infusion of pain medication, a

loading dose should be given to attain therapeutic blood levels quickly.

- Opioid analgesics are often given by IV infusion over a prolonged period in clients with trauma and other critical illnesses. They may also be given orally, by transdermal patch, or by epidural infusion, depending on the client's condition.
- Opioid agonist drugs are preferred; morphine and fentanyl are commonly used. Partial agonists and mixed agonist–antagonist opioids are not recommended for use in critically ill clients. They may cause opioid withdrawal in those who have been receiving chronic opioid therapy and may also cause psychotomimetic effects.
- Consult specialists in pain management (eg, anesthesiologists, clinical pharmacists, nurses) when pain is inadequately controlled with the usual measures.

Use in Home Care

Opioid analgesics are widely used in the home for both acute and chronic pain. With acute pain, such as in postoperative recovery, the use of an opioid analgesic is often limited to a short period and clients self-administer their medications. The need for strong pain medication recedes as healing occurs. The home care nurse may teach clients and caregivers

safe usage of the drugs (eg, that the drugs decrease mental alertness and physical agility, so potentially hazardous activities should be avoided), nonpharmacologic methods of managing pain, and ways to prevent adverse effects of opioids (eg, excessive sedation, constipation). Physical dependence is uncommon with short-term use of opioid analgesics for acute pain.

With some types of chronic pain, such as those occurring with low back pain or osteoarthritis, opioid analgesics are not indicated for long-term use. Treatment involves nonopioid medications, physical therapy, and other measures. The home care nurse may need to explain the reasons for not using opioids on a long-term basis and to help clients and caregivers learn alternative methods of relieving discomfort.

With cancer pain, as previously discussed, the goal of treatment is to prevent or relieve pain and keep clients comfortable, without concern about addiction. Consequently, the home care nurse must assist clients and caregivers in understanding the appropriate use of opioid analgesics in cancer care, including administration on a regular schedule. The nurse also must be proficient in using and teaching various routes of drug administration and in arranging regimens with potentially very large doses and various combinations of drugs. In addition, an active effort is needed to prevent or manage adverse effects, such as a bowel program to prevent constipation.

NURSING ACTIONS

Opioid Analgesics

NURSING ACTIONS	RATIONALE/EXPLANATION
1. Administer accurately	
a. Check the rate, depth, and rhythm of respirations before each dose. If the rate is fewer than 12 per minute, delay or omit the dose and report to the physician.	Respiratory depression is a major adverse effect of strong analgesics. Assessing respirations before each dose can help prevent or minimize potentially life-threatening respiratory depression.
b. Have the client lie down to receive injections of opioid analgesics and for at least a few minutes afterward.	To prevent or minimize hypotension, nausea, and vomiting. These effects are more likely to occur in ambulatory clients. Also, clients may be sedated enough to increase risk of falls or other injuries if they try to ambulate.
c. When injecting opioid analgesics intravenously, give small doses; inject slowly over several minutes; and have opioid antagonist drugs, artificial airways, and equipment for artificial ventilation readily available.	Large doses or rapid intravenous injection may cause severe respiratory depression and hypotension.
d. Put siderails up; instruct the client not to smoke or try to ambulate without help. Keep the call light within reach.	To prevent falls or other injuries
e. When giving controlled-release tablets, do NOT crush them, and instruct the client not to chew them.	Crushing or chewing causes immediate release of the drug, with a high risk of overdose and toxicity.
f. To apply transdermal fentanyl:	Correct preparation of the site and application of the medicated adhesive patch are necessary for drug absorption and effectiveness.
(1) Clip (do not shave) hair, if needed, on a flat surface of the upper trunk.	

(continued)

NURSING ACTIONS	RATIONALE/EXPLANATION
(2) If it is necessary to cleanse the site, use plain water; do not use soaps, oils, lotions, alcohol, or other substances. Let the skin dry.	
(3) Apply the skin patch and press it in place for a few seconds.	
(4) Leave in place for 72 hours.	
(5) When a new patch is to be applied, *remove the old one,* fold it so that the medication is on the inside, and flush the patch down the toilet. Apply the new patch to a different skin site.	
2. Observe for therapeutic effects	Therapeutic effects depend on the reason for use, usually for analgesic effects, sometimes for antitussive or antidiarrheal effects.
a. A verbal statement of pain relief	
b. Decreased behavioral manifestations of pain or discomfort	
c. Sleeping	
d. Increased participation in usual activities of daily living, including interactions with other people in the environment	
e. Fewer and shorter episodes of nonproductive coughing when used for antitussive effects	Opioid analgesics relieve cough by depressing the cough center in the medulla oblongata.
f. Lowered blood pressure, decreased pulse rate, slower and deeper respirations, and less dyspnea when morphine is given for pulmonary edema	Morphine may relieve pulmonary edema by causing vasodilation, which in turn decreases venous return to the heart and decreases cardiac work.
g. Decreased diarrhea when given for constipating effects	These drugs slow secretions and motility of the gastrointestinal tract. Constipation is usually an adverse effect. However, in severe diarrhea or with ileostomy, the drugs decrease the number of bowel movements and make the consistency more paste-like than liquid.
3. Observe for adverse effects	
a. Respiratory depression—hypoxemia, restlessness, dyspnea, slow, shallow breathing, changes in blood pressure and pulse, decreased ability to cough	Respiratory depression is a major adverse effect of opioid analgesics and results from depression of the respiratory center in the medulla oblongata. Respiratory depression occurs with usual therapeutic doses and increases in incidence and severity with large doses or frequent administration.
b. Hypotension	Hypotension stems from drug effects on the vasomotor center in the medulla oblongata that cause peripheral vasodilation and lowering of blood pressure. This is a therapeutic effect with pulmonary edema.
c. Excessive sedation—drowsiness, slurred speech, impaired mobility and coordination, stupor, coma	This is caused by depression of the central nervous system (CNS) and is potentially life threatening.
d. Nausea and vomiting	Opioid analgesics stimulate the chemoreceptor trigger zone in the brain. Consequently, nausea and vomiting may occur with oral or parenteral routes of administration. They are more likely to occur with ambulation than with recumbency.
e. Constipation	This is caused by the drug's slowing effects on the gastrointestinal tract. Constipation may be alleviated by activity, adequate food and fluid intake, and regular administration of mild laxatives.
4. Observe for drug interactions	
a. Drugs that *increase* effects of opioid analgesics:	
(1) CNS depressants—alcohol, general anesthetics, benzodiazepine antianxiety and hypnotic agents, tricyclic antidepressants, sedating antihistamines, antipsychotic agents, barbiturates, and other drugs that cause sedation	All these drugs alone, as well as the opioid analgesics, produce CNS depression. When combined, additive CNS depression results. If dosage of one or more interacting drugs is high, severe respiratory depression, coma, and death may ensue.

NURSING ACTIONS	RATIONALE/EXPLANATION
(2) Anticholinergics—atropine and other drugs with anti-cholinergic effects (eg, antihistamines, tricyclic anti-depressants, phenothiazine antipsychotic drugs)	Increased constipation and urinary retention
(3) Antihypertensive drugs	Orthostatic hypotension, an adverse effect of both strong analgesics and antihypertensive drugs, may be increased if the two drug groups are given concurrently.
(4) Monoamine oxidase (MAO) inhibitors	These drugs interfere with detoxification of some opioid analgesics, especially meperidine. They may cause additive CNS depression with hypotension and respiratory depression or CNS stimulation with hyperexcitability and convulsions. If an MAO inhibitor is necessary, dosage should be reduced because the combination is potentially life threatening.
(5) Protease inhibitors—ritonavir, saquinavir, others	May increase CNS and respiratory depression
(6) Cimetidine	May increase CNS and respiratory depression, probably by inhibiting the cytochrome P450 enzymes that normally metabolize opioids
b. Drugs that *decrease* effects of opioid analgesics:	
(1) Opioid antagonists	These drugs reverse respiratory depression produced by opioid analgesics. This is their only clinical use, and they should not be given unless severe respiratory depression is present. They do not reverse respiratory depression caused by other CNS depressants.
(2) Butorphanol, nalbuphine	These analgesics are weak antagonists of opioid analgesics, and they may cause withdrawal symptoms in people who have been receiving opiates or who are physically dependent on opioid analgesics.

APPLYING YOUR KNOWLEDGE: ANSWERS

6-1 4 mg of morphine. Because this is the initial 24 hours after surgery and the pain is severe, morphine is the drug of choice. Start with the lowest effective dose and increase as needed. Larger doses have an increased risk of causing adverse effects. Also recognize that Mr. Harris has used pain medication for a long time and may require a higher dose of medication to control his pain.

6-2 Prepare to administer naloxone and assist with ventilation as needed. Naloxone is the drug of choice for opioid overdose.

6-3 Lortab is 5 mg of hydrocodone and 500 mg of acetaminophen. What is ordered is oxycodone. Roxicet 5/500 is 5 mg of oxycodone and 500 mg of acetaminophen. You must recognize the difference between oral pain medications and these two different opioids.

Review and Application Exercises

Short Answer Exercises

1. When assessing a client for pain, what are the major considerations?

2. What are some nonpharmacologic interventions for pain, and why should they be used instead of or along with analgesics?

3. What are the major adverse effects of opioid analgesics? How do opioid antagonists counteract adverse effects?

4. For a client who has had major surgery during the previous 24 to 72 hours, what type of analgesic is indicated? Why?

5. What are the potential differences in dosage between short-term (a few days) and long-term (weeks or months) administration of morphine?

6. Explain the rationale for using both opioid analgesics and nonopioid analgesics in the treatment of pain.

7. For a client with chronic cancer pain, what are the advantages and disadvantages of using opioid analgesics?

8. For a client with chronic cancer pain, should opioid analgesics be given as needed or on a regular schedule? Why?

9. For a client who is receiving large doses of an opioid analgesic, what signs and symptoms may indicate drug toxicity or overdose? What interventions are needed for suspected toxicity?

10. For a client who has been taking an opioid analgesic for a long time, what signs and symptoms would make you suspect opioid withdrawal? What interventions are needed for suspected withdrawal?

NCLEX-Style Questions

11. Opioid analgesics act mainly by
   a. causing sleep
   b. binding with opioid receptors in the brain and spinal cord
   c. increasing transmission of pain impulses between nerve cells
   d. decreasing the amount of norepinephrine and serotonin in synapses in the brain

12. A client receiving morphine should be assessed regularly for which of the following?
   a. respiratory depression
   b. hyperactive bowel sounds
   c. frequent urination
   d. insomnia

13. Long-term administration of an opioid results in which of the following?
   a. tolerance
   b. overdose
   c. withdrawal
   d. hepatotoxicity

14. The main advantage of patient-controlled analgesia systems is that they
   a. require less nursing time
   b. cause fewer adverse effects
   c. relieve pain more effectively
   d. can be used long term

15. For a client with severe cancer pain, an analgesic should be given
   a. when the client asks for it
   b. if a family member or friend asks that it be given
   c. when a client is restless
   d. on a regular schedule, around-the-clock

Selected References

Acute Pain Management Guideline Panel. (1992). Acute pain management: Operative or medical procedures and trauma. Clinical practice guideline. AHCRP Pub. No. 92-0032. Rockville, MD: Agency for Health Care Policy and Research, Public Health Service, U.S. Department of Health and Human Services for Health Care Policy and Research.

Ballantyne, J. C., & Mao, J. (2003). Opioid therapy for chronic pain. *New England Journal of Medicine, 349*(20), 1943–1953.

Barkin, R. L., & Barkin, D. (2001). Pharmacologic management of acute and chronic pain. *Southern Medical Journal, 94*(8), 756–812.

Baumann, T. J. (2002). Pain management. In J. T. DiPiro, R. L. Talbert, G. C. Yee, G. R. Matzke, B. G. Wells, & L. M. Posey (Eds.), *Pharmacotherapy: A pathophysiologic approach* (5th ed., pp. 1103–1117). New York: McGraw-Hill.

Devine, E. C. (2002). Somatosensory function and pain. In C. M. Porth, *Pathophysiology: Concepts of altered health states* (6th ed., pp. 1091–1122). Philadelphia: Lippincott Williams & Wilkins.

Drug facts and comparisons. (Updated monthly). St. Louis: Facts and Comparisons.

Green, G. B., Harris, I. S., Lin, G. A., et al. (Eds.). (2004). *The Washington manual of medical therapeutics* (31st ed.). Philadelphia: Lippincott Williams & Wilkins.

Howard, R. F. (2003). Current status of pain management in children. *Journal of the American Medical Association, 290*(18), 2464–2469.

Max, M. B. (2004). Pain. In L. Goldman & D. Ausiello (Eds.), *Cecil textbook of medicine* (22nd ed., pp. 138–145). Philadelphia: W. B. Saunders.

Spagrud, L. J., Piira, T., & von Baeyer, C. L. (2003). Children's self-report of pain intensity. *American Journal of Nursing, 103*(12), 62–64.

Viscusi, E. R., Reynolds, L., Chung, F., et al. (2004). Patient-controlled transdermal fentanyl hydrochloride vs intravenous morphine pump for postoperative pain: A randomized controlled trial. *Journal of the American Medical Association, 291*(11), 1333–1341.

Willens, J. S. (2004). Pain management. In S. C. Smeltzer & B. G. Bare, *Brunner & Suddarth's textbook of medical-surgical nursing* (10th ed., pp. 216–248). Philadelphia: Lippincott Williams & Wilkins.

Analgesic–Antipyretic–Anti-Inflammatory and Related Drugs

OBJECTIVES

After studying this chapter, you will be able to:

1. Discuss the role of prostaglandins in the etiology of pain, fever, and inflammation.
2. Discuss aspirin and other nonsteroidal anti-inflammatory drugs (NSAIDs) in terms of mechanism of action, indications for use, contraindications to use, nursing process, and principles of therapy.
3. Compare and contrast aspirin, other NSAIDs, and acetaminophen in terms of indications for use and adverse effects.
4. Differentiate among antiplatelet, analgesic, and anti-inflammatory doses of aspirin.
5. Differentiate between traditional NSAIDs and the cyclooxygenase-2 inhibitor, celecoxib.
6. Teach clients interventions to prevent or decrease adverse effects of aspirin, other NSAIDs, and acetaminophen.
7. Identify factors influencing the use of aspirin, NSAIDs, and acetaminophen in special populations.
8. Discuss recognition and management of acetaminophen toxicity.
9. Discuss the use of NSAIDs and antigout drugs.
10. Discuss the use of NSAIDs, triptans, and ergot antimigraine drugs.

APPLYING YOUR KNOWLEDGE

Julie McKay is a 32-year-old female who has chronic headache pain. Her first headaches began at age 18 as a combination of migraine type and tension headaches. For acute pain, she uses a combination of Excedrin Migraine (acetaminophen 250 mg, ASA 250 mg, and caffeine 65 mg per tablet), extra-strength acetaminophen (500 mg per tablet) and naproxen sodium (550 mg per tablet). For a typical headache, Julie takes two naproxen sodium tablets at the onset of her pain, followed by two tablets of the acetaminophen every 4 hours and two Excedrin Migraine tablets every 4 hours, starting 2 hours after the acetaminophen. If the pain is not relieved, she takes one naproxen sodium tablet in 12 hours and continues with the Excedrin Migraine and acetaminophen. The headache may last from 3 to 5 days.

INTRODUCTION

The analgesic–antipyretic–anti-inflammatory drug group includes chemically and pharmacologically diverse drugs that share the ability to relieve pain, fever, and/or inflammation, symptoms associated with many injuries and illnesses. Drugs discussed in this chapter include:

- **P** **Aspirin** (acetylsalicylic acid [ASA]), the prototype
- Aspirin-related drugs that are often called nonsteroidal anti-inflammatory drugs (NSAIDs), such as ibuprofen
- Acetaminophen
- Drugs used to prevent or treat gout and migraine

Aspirin, NSAIDs, and acetaminophen can also be called *antiprostaglandin drugs,* because they inhibit the synthesis of prostaglandins. Prostaglandins are chemical mediators found in most body tissues; they help regulate many cell functions and participate in the inflammatory response. They are formed when cellular injury occurs and phospholipids in cell membranes release arachidonic acid. Arachidonic acid is then metabolized by cyclooxygenase (COX) enzymes to produce prostaglandins, which act briefly in the area where they are produced and are then inactivated. Prostaglandins exert various and opposing effects in different body tissues (Table 7-1). To aid understanding of prostaglandins, their roles in pain, fever, and inflammation are described in the following sections.

Pain

Pain is the sensation of discomfort, hurt, or distress. It is a common human ailment and may occur with tissue injury and inflammation. Prostaglandins sensitize pain receptors and increase the pain associated with other chemical mediators of inflammation and immunity, such as bradykinin and histamine (Box 7-1).

Fever

Fever is an elevation of body temperature above the normal range. Body temperature is controlled by a regulating center

TABLE 7-1 Prostaglandins

PROSTAGLANDIN	LOCATIONS	EFFECTS
D_2	Airways, brain, mast cells	• Bronchoconstriction
E_2	Brain, kidneys, vascular smooth muscle, platelets	• Bronchodilation • Gastroprotection • Increased activity of GI smooth muscle • Increased sensitivity to pain • Increased body temperature • Vasodilation
F_2	Airways, eyes, uterus, vascular smooth muscle	• Bronchoconstriction • Increased activity of GI smooth muscle • Increased uterine contraction (eg, menstrual cramps)
I_2 (Prostacyclin)	Brain, endothelium, kidneys, platelets	• Decreased platelet aggregation • Gastroprotection • Vasodilation
Thromboxane A_2	Kidneys, macrophages, platelets, vascular smooth muscle	• Increased platelet aggregation • Vasoconstriction

GI, gastrointestinal.

in the hypothalamus. Normally, there is a balance between heat production and heat loss so that a constant body temperature is maintained. When there is excessive heat production, mechanisms to increase heat loss are activated. As a result, blood vessels dilate, more blood flows through the skin, sweating occurs, and body temperature usually stays within normal range. When fever occurs, the heat-regulating center in the hypothalamus is reset so that it tolerates a higher body temperature. Fever may be produced by dehydration, inflammation, infectious processes, some drugs, brain injury, or diseases involving the hypothalamus. Prostaglandin formation is stimulated by such circumstances and, along with bacterial toxins and other substances, prostaglandins act as pyrogens (fever-producing agents).

Inflammation

Inflammation is the normal body response to tissue damage from any source, and it may occur in any tissue or organ. It is an attempt by the body to remove the damaging agent and repair the damaged tissue. Local manifestations are redness, heat, edema, and pain. Redness and heat result from vasodilation and increased blood supply. Edema results from leakage of blood plasma into the area. Pain occurs when pain receptors on nerve endings are stimulated by heat, edema, pressure, chemicals released by the damaged cells, and prostaglandins. Systemic manifestations include leukocytosis, increased erythrocyte sedimentation rate, fever, headache, loss of appetite, lethargy or malaise, and weakness. Both local and systemic manifestations vary according to the cause and extent of tissue damage. In addition, inflammation may be acute or chronic.

Because inflammation may be a component of virtually any illness, anti-inflammatory drugs are needed when the inflammatory response is inappropriate, abnormal, or persistent, or destroys tissue. Common conditions that are characterized by pain, fever, and inflammation, and for which the drugs discussed in this chapter are used, are described in Box 7-2.

GENERAL CHARACTERISTICS OF ANALGESIC–ANTIPYRETIC– ANTI-INFLAMMATORY AND RELATED DRUGS

Mechanism of Action

Aspirin and other NSAIDs inhibit prostaglandin synthesis in the central nervous system (CNS) as well as the periphery, whereas the action of acetaminophen on prostaglandin inhibition is limited to the CNS. This selective action may explain the inability of acetaminophen to reduce inflammation, and the absence of adverse effects in the gastrointestinal (GI) tract, kidneys, and platelets. Aspirin, NSAIDs, and acetaminophen inactivate the COX enzymes, which are required for prostaglandin formation (Fig. 7-1). Two forms of COX, COX-1 and COX-2, have been identified. Aspirin and traditional nonselective NSAIDs inhibit both COX-1 and COX-2.

COX-1 is normally synthesized continuously and present in all tissues and cell types, especially platelets, endothelial cells, the GI tract, and the kidneys. Prostaglandins produced by COX-1 are important in numerous homeostatic functions and are associated with protective effects on the stomach and

Box 7-1 Chemical Mediators of Inflammation and Immunity

Bradykinin is a kinin in body fluids that becomes physiologically active with tissue injury. When tissue cells are damaged, white blood cells (WBCs) increase in the area and ingest damaged cells to remove them from the area. When the WBCs die, they release enzymes that activate kinins. The activated kinins increase and prolong the vasodilation and increased vascular permeability caused by histamine. They also cause pain by stimulating nerve endings for pain in the area. Thus, bradykinin may aggravate and prolong the erythema, heat, and pain of local inflammatory reactions. It also increases mucous gland secretion.

Complement is a group of plasma proteins essential to normal inflammatory and immunologic processes. More specifically, complement destroys cell membranes of body cells (eg, red blood cells, lymphocytes, platelets) and pathogenic microorganisms (eg, bacteria, viruses). The system is initiated by an antigen–antibody reaction or by tissue injury. Components of the system (called *C1* through *C9*) are activated in a cascade type of reaction in which each component becomes a proteolytic enzyme that splits the next component in the series. Activation yields products with profound inflammatory effects. C3a and C5a, also called *anaphylatoxins,* act mainly by liberating histamine from mast cells and platelets, and their effects are therefore similar to those of histamine. C3a causes or increases smooth muscle contraction, vasodilation, vascular permeability, degranulation of mast cells and basophils, and secretion of lysosomal enzymes by leukocytes. C5a performs the same functions as C3a and also promotes movement of WBCs into the injured area (chemotaxis). In addition, it activates the lipoxygenase pathway of arachidonic acid metabolism in neutrophils and macrophages, thereby inducing formation of leukotrienes and other substances that increase vascular permeability and chemotaxis.

In the immune response, the complement system breaks down antigen–antibody complexes, especially those in which the antigen is a microbial agent. It enables the body to produce inflammation and localize an infective agent. More specific reactions include increased vascular permeability, chemotaxis, and opsonization (coating a microbe or other antigen so it can be more readily phagocytized).

Cytokines may act on the cells that produce them, on surrounding cells, or on distant cells if sufficient amounts reach the bloodstream. Thus, cytokines act locally and systemically to produce inflammatory and immune responses, including increased vascular permeability and chemotaxis of macrophages, neutrophils, and basophils. Two major types of cytokines are interleukins (produced by leukocytes) and interferons (produced by T lymphocytes or fibroblasts). Interleukin-1 (IL-1) mediates several inflammatory responses, including fever; and IL-2 (also called T-cell growth factor) is required for the growth and function of T lymphocytes. Interferons are cytokines that protect nearby cells from invasion by intracellular microorganisms, such as viruses and rickettsiae. They also limit the growth of some cancer cells.

Histamine is formed (from the amino acid histidine) and stored in most body tissue, with high concentrations in mast cells, basophils, and platelets. Mast cells, which are abundant in skin and connective tissue, release histamine into the vascular system in response to stimuli (eg, antigen–antibody reaction, tissue injury, and some drugs). After it is released, histamine is highly vasoactive, causing vasodilation (increasing blood flow to the area and producing hypotension) and increasing permeability of capillaries and venules (producing edema). Other effects include contracting smooth muscles in the bronchi (producing bronchoconstriction and respiratory distress), gastrointestinal (GI) tract, and uterus; stimulating salivary, gastric, bronchial, and intestinal secretions; stimulating sensory nerve endings to cause pain and itching; and stimulating movement of eosinophils into injured tissue. Histamine is the first chemical mediator released in the inflammatory response and immediate hypersensitivity reactions (anaphylaxis).

When histamine is released from mast cells and basophils, it diffuses rapidly into other tissues. It then acts on target tissues through both histamine-1 (H_1) and histamine-2 (H_2) receptors. H_1 receptors are located mainly on smooth muscle cells in blood vessels and the respiratory and GI tracts. When histamine binds with these receptors, resulting events include contraction of smooth muscle, increased vascular permeability, production of nasal mucus, stimulation of sensory nerves, pruritus, and dilation of capillaries in the skin. H_2 receptors are also located in the airways, GI tract, and other tissues. When histamine binds to these receptors, there is increased secretion of gastric acid by parietal cells in the stomach mucosal lining, increased mucus secretion and bronchodilation in the airways, contraction of esophageal muscles, tachycardia, inhibition of lymphocyte function, and degranulation of basophils (with additional release of histamine and other mediators) in the bloodstream. In allergic reactions, both types of receptors mediate hypotension (in anaphylaxis), skin flushing, and headache. The peak effects of histamine occur within 1 to 2 minutes of its release and may last as long as 10 minutes, after which it is inactivated by histaminase (produced by eosinophils) or *N*-methyltransferase.

Leukotrienes, like prostaglandins, are derived from arachidonic acid metabolism. Leukotrienes, identified as LTB_4, LTC_4, LTD_4, and LTE_4, mediate inflammation and immune responses. LTB_4 plays a role in chemotaxis, mediating the aggregation of leukocytes at sites of injury. LTC_4, LTD_4, and LTE_4 produce smooth muscle contractility, bronchospasm, and increased vascular permeability.

Platelet-activating factor (PAF), like prostaglandins and leukotrienes, is derived from arachidonic acid metabolism and has multiple inflammatory activities. It is produced by mast cells, neutrophils, monocytes, and platelets. Because these cells are widely distributed, PAF effects can occur in virtually every organ and tissue. Besides causing platelet aggregation, PAF activates neutrophils, attracts eosinophils, increases vascular permeability, causes vasodilation, and causes IL-1 and tumor necrosis factor–alpha (TNF-alpha) to be released. PAF, IL-1, and TNF-alpha can induce each other's release.

Box 7-2 Selected Conditions for which Aspirin, Other NSAIDs, and Acetaminophen are Commonly Used

Bursitis—inflammation of a bursa (a cavity in connective tissue that contains synovial fluid; the fluid reduces friction between tendons and bones or ligaments). Common forms include acute painful shoulder, "tennis elbow," "housemaid's knee," and bunions.

Dysmenorrhea—pain associated with menstruation; thought to be caused by prostaglandins that increase contractility of the uterine muscle.

Gout—a disorder characterized by an inability to metabolize uric acid, a waste product of protein metabolism. The resulting hyperuricemia may be asymptomatic or may lead to urate deposits in various tissues. In the musculoskeletal system, often in the feet, urate deposits produce periodic episodes of severe pain, edema, and inflammation (gouty arthritis). In the kidneys, urate deposits may form renal calculi or cause other damage.

Migraine—a type of headache characterized by periodic attacks of pain, nausea, and increased sensitivity to light and sound. The pain is often worse on one side of the head; throbbing or pulsating in nature; moderate or severe in intensity; and disruptive of usual activities of daily living. The etiology is unknown, but one theory is that certain circumstances cause an imbalance of chemicals (eg, serotonin, prostaglandins) in the brain. This imbalance results in vasodilation, release of inflammatory mediators, and irritation of nerve endings. Numerous circumstances have been implicated as "triggers"

for the chemical imbalance and migraine, including alcohol (especially red wine), some foods (eg, chocolate, aged cheeses), some medications (eg, antihypertensives, oral contraceptives), irregular patterns of eating and sleeping, and physical and emotional stress. Migraine occurs more often in women than men and may be associated with menses.

Osteoarthritis (OA)—a disease that affects the cartilage of weight-bearing joints and produces pain, usually aggravated by movement, decreased range of motion, and progressive loss of mobility. As joint cartilage deteriorates over time, there is less padding and lubricating fluid; underlying bone is exposed; and friction and abrasion lead to inflammation of the synovial membrane lining of the joint. The joint becomes unstable, more susceptible to injury, and less efficient in repairing itself. Knee OA, a common type, often develops from repeated joint injury or repetitive motion. Pain in and around the knee occurs early in the disease process; joint stiffness, edema, and deformity occur as the disease advances.

Rheumatoid arthritis (RA)—a chronic, painful, inflammatory disorder that affects hingelike joints, tissues around these joints, and eventually other body organs (systemic effects). It is considered an autoimmune disorder in which the body attacks its own tissues. **Juvenile rheumatoid arthritis** is a chronic, inflammatory, systemic disease that may cause joint or connective tissue damage and visceral lesions throughout the body. Onset may occur before 16 years of age.

---

kidneys. In the stomach, the prostaglandins decrease gastric acid secretion, increase mucus secretion, and regulate blood circulation. In the kidneys, they help maintain adequate blood flow and function. In the cardiovascular system, they help regulate vascular tone (ie, vasoconstriction and vasodilation) and platelet function. Drug-induced inhibition of these prostaglandins results in the adverse effects associated with aspirin and related drugs, especially gastric irritation, ulceration, and bleeding. Inhibition of COX-1 activity in platelets may be more responsible for GI bleeding than inhibition in gastric mucosa.

COX-2 is also normally present in several tissues (eg, brain, bone, kidneys, GI tract, female reproductive system). However, it is thought to occur in small amounts or to be inactive until stimulated by pain and inflammation. In inflamed tissues, COX-2 is induced by inflammatory chemical mediators such as interleukin-1 and tumor necrosis factor–alpha. In the GI tract, COX-2 is also induced by trauma and *Helicobacter pylori* infection, a common cause of peptic ulcer disease. Overall, prostaglandins produced by COX-2 are associated with pain and other signs of inflammation. Inhibition of COX-2 results in the therapeutic effects of analgesia and anti-inflammatory activity. The COX-2 inhibitor drugs are NSAIDs designed to selectively inhibit COX-2 and relieve pain and inflammation with fewer adverse effects, especially stomach damage; however, with long-term use,

adverse effects still occur in the GI, renal, and cardiovascular systems.

To relieve pain, aspirin acts both centrally and peripherally to block the transmission of pain impulses. Related drugs act peripherally to prevent sensitization of pain receptors to various chemical substances released by damaged cells. To relieve fever, the drugs act on the hypothalamus to decrease its response to pyrogens and reset the "thermostat" at a lower level. For inflammation, the drugs prevent prostaglandins from increasing the pain and edema produced by other substances released by damaged cells. Although these drugs relieve symptoms and contribute greatly to the client's comfort and quality of life, they do not cure the underlying disorders that cause the symptoms.

Aspirin and traditional nonselective NSAIDs also have antiplatelet effects that differ in mechanism and extent. When aspirin is absorbed into the bloodstream, the acetyl portion dissociates, then binds irreversibly to platelet COX-1. This action prevents synthesis of thromboxane A_2, a prostaglandin derivative, thereby inhibiting platelet aggregation. A small single dose (325 mg) irreversibly acetylates circulating platelets within a few minutes, and effects last for the lifespan of the platelets (7 to 10 days). Most other NSAIDs bind reversibly with platelet COX-1 so that antiplatelet effects occur only while the drug is present in the blood. Thus, aspirin has greater effects, but all the drugs except acetaminophen and the

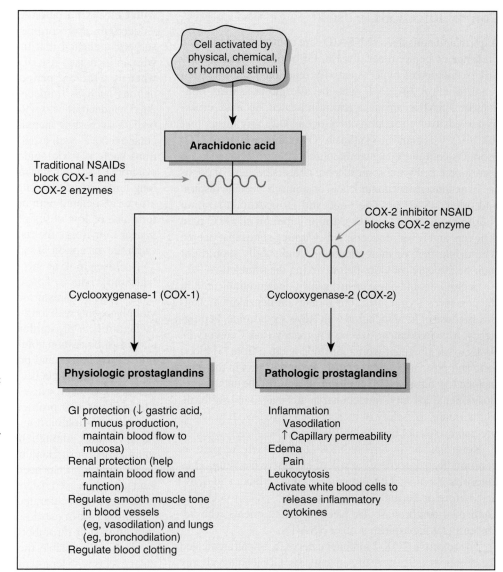

FIGURE 7-1 Physiologic and pathologic (ie, inflammatory) prostaglandins: actions of anti-prostaglandin drugs. Prostaglandins play important roles in normal body functions as well as inflammatory processes. Inhibition of both COX-1 and COX-2 by traditional nonsteroidal anti-inflammatory drugs (NSAIDs) produces adverse effects on the stomach (eg, irritation, ulceration, bleeding) as well as anti-inflammatory effects. Selective inhibition of COX-2 produces anti-inflammatory effects while maintaining protective effects on the stomach.

COX-2 inhibitors inhibit platelet aggregation, interfere with blood coagulation, and increase the risk of bleeding.

Indications for Use

Aspirin, NSAIDs, and acetaminophen are widely used to prevent and treat mild to moderate pain and/or inflammation associated with musculoskeletal disorders (eg, osteoarthritis [OA], tendinitis, gout), headache, dysmenorrhea, minor trauma (eg, athletic injuries such as sprains), minor surgery (eg, dental extraction, episiotomy), and other acute and chronic conditions. However, despite many similarities, aspirin and other NSAIDs differ in their approved uses. Although aspirin is effective in many disorders, its usage has declined for most indications, largely because of adverse effects on the GI tract and the advent of newer drugs. At the same time, low-dose aspirin is increasingly prescribed for clients at risk of myocardial infarction or stroke from thrombosis. This indication stems

from its antiplatelet activity and resultant effects on blood coagulation (ie, decreased clot formation). Some NSAIDs, such as ibuprofen (eg, Motrin) and related drugs, are widely used as anti-inflammatory agents and analgesics; ketorolac (eg, Toradol), which can be given orally and parenterally, is used only as an analgesic. Most of the other NSAIDs are too toxic to use as analgesics and antipyretics. They are used primarily to treat rheumatoid arthritis (RA) and other musculoskeletal disorders that do not respond to safer drugs. Celecoxib (Celebrex) is also used to treat familial adenomatous polyposis, in which the drug reduces the number of polyps and may decrease risks of colon cancer. Several NSAIDs are formulated as eye drops for use in treating eye disorders (see Chap. 63).

Acetaminophen, which differs chemically from aspirin and other NSAIDs, is commonly used as an aspirin substitute for pain and fever, but it lacks anti-inflammatory and antiplatelet effects.

Contraindications to Use

Aspirin and nonselective NSAIDs are contraindicated in the presence of peptic ulcer disease, GI or other bleeding disorders, history of hypersensitivity reactions, and impaired renal function. In people who are allergic to aspirin, non-aspirin NSAIDs are also contraindicated because cross-hypersensitivity reactions may occur with any drugs that inhibit prostaglandin synthesis. Over-the-counter (OTC) products containing acetaminophen or aspirin/NSAIDs are contraindicated for chronic alcohol abusers because of possible liver damage (acetaminophen) or stomach bleeding (aspirin and other NSAIDs). The Food and Drug Administration (FDA) requires an alcohol warning label on all OTC pain relievers and fever reducers. This warning states that people who drink three or more alcoholic drinks daily should ask their health care provider before taking the products.

In children and adolescents, aspirin is contraindicated in the presence of viral infections such as influenza or chickenpox because of its association with Reye's syndrome. In pregnancy, aspirin is categorized as Pregnancy Risk Category D. Risks to the pregnant woman include anemia from GI blood loss, and postpartum hemorrhage. Potential risks to the fetus include low birth weight, premature closure of the ductus arteriosus, renal toxicity, intracranial hemorrhage, and stillbirth. Furthermore, the safety of most nonselective NSAIDs during pregnancy has not been established.

Ketorolac, an injectable NSAID often used for pain, is contraindicated in clients at risk of excessive bleeding. Thus ketorolac should not be administered during labor and delivery; before or during any major surgery; with suspected or confirmed cerebrovascular bleeding; or to clients who are currently taking aspirin or other NSAIDs.

The selective COX-2 inhibitor celecoxib is contraindicated for clients with a history of peptic ulcers, GI bleeding, allergy to other NSAIDs, or severe renal impairment. Although celecoxib was formulated to have fewer adverse effects in the GI tract and renal system, long-term use and/or high dosages can result in GI bleeding and renal impairment. In addition, celecoxib is contraindicated in clients who are allergic to sulfonamides.

Long-term use of selective and nonselective NSAIDs is also associated with increased risk of serious adverse cardiovascular events such as myocardial infarction and stroke. Three COX-2 inhibitors have been marketed in the United States: celecoxib (Celebrex), rofecoxib (Vioxx), and valdecoxib (Bextra). Of these three drugs, only celecoxib remains available for prescription at this time. In September 2004, rofecoxib was voluntarily withdrawn from the market amid concerns resulting from evidence gathered in the Adenomatous Polyp Prevention on Vioxx (APPROVe) study, which showed a significant increase in myocardial infarctions and strokes in subjects receiving rofecoxib versus a placebo. Subsequent review of data from prevention studies involving celecoxib (National Cancer Institute's Adenoma Prevention

with Celecoxib trial or APC trial) and short-term studies of valdecoxib after coronary artery bypass grafting (CABG) surgery indicated that these drugs may also be associated with an increased risk of myocardial infarctions and strokes when used for long periods of time or in high-risk clinical situations such as immediately after heart surgery. In April 2005, valdecoxib was withdrawn from the U.S. market based on data suggesting increased potential for adverse cardiovascular events as well as an increased risk of serious skin reactions such as toxic epidermal necrolysis, Stevens-Johnson syndrome, and erythema multiforme. Although initial data from long-term clinical trials suggest that nonselective NSAIDs may also be associated with increased cardiovascular risk, short-term use of low doses of NSAIDs for pain relief does not appear to increase the risk of adverse cardiovascular events (with the exception of valdecoxib in post-CABG clients).

A closer look at the function of two contrasting prostaglandin products of the COX enzymes (in vitro) may suggest a possible mechanism for the occurrence of adverse cardiovascular events with long-term use of COX-2 inhibitors. Prostaglandin I_2, a prostaglandin product of COX-2, has been shown to be responsible for inhibition of platelet aggregation; vasodilation; and prevention of proliferation of vascular smooth muscle cells. Thromboxane A_2, a prostaglandin product of COX-1, causes platelet aggregation, vasoconstriction, and vascular proliferation. Aspirin and older nonselective NSAIDs inhibit both prostaglandin I_2 and thromboxane A_2 formation, though the COX-2 inhibitor medications inhibit only prostaglandin I_2 formation, leaving thromboxane A_2 unopposed. It has been proposed that this imbalance may lead to an increased risk of thrombotic events, elevated blood pressure, and accelerated atherogenesis, and ultimately an increased risk of cardiovascular events such as myocardial infarction and thrombotic stroke. Although this proposed mechanism is possible, the increased risk of adverse cardiovascular events with long-term use of some nonselective NSAIDs, which inhibit both COX-1 and COX-2 enzymes, cannot be fully explained by this mechanism. More research is needed to explain the increased cardiovascular risks attributed to the NSAID class of drugs.

The FDA has recommended that professional labeling for all prescription NSAIDs (both nonselective and COX-2 inhibitors) carry a black-box warning highlighting the increased risk of adverse cardiovascular events as well as the risk of severe and potentially life-threatening GI bleeding associated with the NSAID class of drugs. Nonprescription NSAID labels should include information regarding cardiovascular and GI risks as well as information regarding potential skin reactions associated with NSAIDs. COX-2 inhibitors may be appropriate for clients at high risk of GI bleeding or for those individuals with intolerance to the nonselective NSAIDs; however, prescribers should carefully evaluate the client's risk for cardiovascular events before prescribing these drugs.

Further FDA review of studies involving NSAIDs and cardiovascular risk is ongoing and may result in additional recommendations in the future. It is unclear at this time if rofecoxib and valdecoxib will return to the market in the United States.

CLASSIFICATIONS AND INDIVIDUAL DRUGS

Subgroups and selected individual drugs are described below. Indications for use, trade names, and dosage ranges of individual drugs are listed in Table 7-2.

Aspirin and Other Salicylates

P Aspirin is the prototype of the analgesic–antipyretic–anti-inflammatory drugs and the most commonly used salicylate. Because it is a nonprescription drug and is widely available, people tend to underestimate its usefulness. It is effective in pain of low to moderate intensity, especially that involving the skin, muscles, joints, and other connective tissue. It is useful in inflammatory disorders, such as arthritis, but many people prefer drugs that cause less gastric irritation.

Regular aspirin tablets are well absorbed after oral administration; their action starts within 15 to 30 minutes, peaks in 1 to 2 hours, and lasts 4 to 6 hours. Taking aspirin with food slows absorption but also decreases gastric irritation. Absorption of enteric-coated aspirin and rectal suppositories is slower and less complete.

Aspirin is distributed to all body tissues and fluids, including fetal tissues, breast milk, and the CNS. The highest concentrations are found in the plasma, liver, heart, and lungs. In plasma, aspirin binds to albumin (75% to 90%). Aspirin has a short half-life of 15 to 20 minutes because it is rapidly converted to salicylic acid, an active metabolite. Salicylic acid has a half-life of 2 to 3 hours at low doses and 6 to 12 hours at therapeutic anti-inflammatory doses. It undergoes oxidation and conjugation in the liver, and its metabolites are excreted through the kidneys. In alkaline urine (eg, pH of 8), renal excretion of salicylate is greatly increased.

Aspirin is a home remedy for headaches, colds, influenza and other respiratory infections, muscular aches, and fever. It can be purchased in plain, chewable, enteric-coated, and effervescent tablets and rectal suppositories. It is not marketed in liquid form because it is unstable in solution.

Diflunisal (Dolobid) is a salicylic acid derivative that differs chemically from aspirin. It is reportedly equal or superior to aspirin in mild to moderate pain, RA, and OA. Compared with aspirin, it has less antipyretic effect, causes less gastric irritation, and has a longer duration of action.

Choline salicylate (Arthropan) is also a salicylate with analgesic and antipyretic actions. Compared with aspirin, choline salicylate has a more rapid onset of action and peak action time and a shorter duration of action. It is indicated for reduction of fever, relief of moderate pain, and treatment of OA and RA. The drug is metabolized in the liver and excreted in the urine.

Salsalate (Disalcid) is a salicylate with antipyretic, analgesic, antirheumatic, and anti-inflammatory properties. It is indicated for relief of pain and fever as well as treatment of rheumatic fever, RA, and OA. It is absorbed in the small intestine rather than in the stomach and is reported to cause fewer GI adverse effects than aspirin. Onset, peak, and duration of action are similar to aspirin. The drug is metabolized in the liver and excreted in the urine.

NSAIDs

Propionic acid derivatives include fenoprofen (Nalfon), flurbiprofen (Ansaid), ibuprofen (Motrin, Advil), ketoprofen (Oruvail), naproxen (Naprosyn), and oxaprozin (Daypro). In addition to their use as anti-inflammatory agents, some are used as analgesics and antipyretics. Ibuprofen, ketoprofen, and naproxen are available OTC, with recommended doses smaller and durations of use shorter than those for prescription formulations. Although these drugs are usually better tolerated than aspirin, they are much more expensive and may cause all the adverse effects associated with aspirin and other prostaglandin inhibitors.

Ibuprofen, a commonly used drug, is well absorbed with oral administration. Its action starts in about 30 minutes, peaks in 1 to 2 hours, and lasts 4 to 6 hours. The drug is highly bound (about 99%) to plasma proteins and has a half-life of about 2 hours. It is metabolized in the liver and excreted by the kidneys. It is available by prescription and OTC, in tablets, chewable tablets, capsules, oral suspension, and oral drops, for use by adults and children.

Acetic acid derivatives include indomethacin (Indocin), sulindac (Clinoril), and tolmetin (Tolectin). These drugs have strong anti-inflammatory effects and more severe adverse effects than the propionic acid derivatives. Potentially serious adverse effects include GI ulceration, bone marrow depression, hemolytic anemia, mental confusion, depression, and psychosis. These effects are especially associated with indomethacin; sulindac and tolmetin were developed in an effort to find equally effective but less toxic derivatives. Adverse reactions occur less often with sulindac and tolmetin but are still common.

In addition to other uses, intravenous (IV) indomethacin is approved for treatment of patent ductus arteriosus in premature infants. (The ductus arteriosus joins the pulmonary artery to the aorta in the fetal circulation. When it fails to close, blood is shunted from the aorta to the pulmonary artery, causing severe cardiopulmonary problems.)

Related drugs are **etodolac** (Lodine), **ketorolac** (Toradol), and **nabumetone** (Relafen). Etodolac reportedly causes less gastric irritation, especially in older adults at high risk of GI bleeding. Ketorolac is used only for pain, and although it can be given orally, its unique characteristic is that it can be given by injection. Parenteral ketorolac reportedly compares with morphine and other opioids in analgesic effectiveness for moderate or severe pain. However, its use is

(text continues on page 114)

Table 7-2 Drugs at a Glance: Analgesic, Antipyretic, Anti-Inflammatory Drugs

GENERIC/TRADE NAME	INDICATIONS FOR USE	ROUTES AND DOSAGE RANGES		Comments
		Adults	**Children**	
Acetaminophen (Tylenol, others)	Pain Fever	PO 325–650 mg q4–6h, or 1000 mg three or four times per day; maximum 4 g/d	PO 10 mg/kg or according to age as follows: 0–3 mo, 40 mg; 4–11 mo, 80 mg; 1–2 y, 120 mg; 2–3 y, 160 mg; 4–5 y, 240 mg; 6–8 y, 320 mg; 9–10 y, 400 mg; 11 y, 480 mg. Doses may be given q4–6h to a maximum of 5 doses in 24 h.	**Warning:** Overdoses may cause fatal liver damage. Maximum recommended dose for adults is 4 g/d, from all sources. Parents and caregivers should ask pediatricians about the amounts of acetaminophen children may take safely.
		Rectal suppository 650 mg q4–6h, maximum of 6 in 24 h	Rectal suppository: age under 3 y, consult physician; age 3–6 y, 120 mg q4–6h, maximum, 720 mg in 24 h; age 6–12 y, 325 mg q4–6h, maximum 2.6 g in 24 h	
Aspirin	Pain, fever Osteoarthritis (OA), Rheumatoid Arthritis (RA) Prophylaxis of myocardial infarction (MI), transient ischemic attacks (TIAs), and stroke in men Rheumatic fever	*Pain, fever:* PO 325–650 mg q4h PRN; usual single dose, 650 mg *OA, RA:* PO 2–6 g/d in divided doses *Prophylaxis of MI, TIA, and stroke:* PO 81–325 mg/d *Acute rheumatic fever:* PO 5–8 g/d, in divided doses *TIAs;* PO 1300 mg/d in divided doses (650 mg twice a day or 325 mg four times a day)	*Pain, fever:* PO 10–15 mg/kg q4h, up to 60–80 mg/kg/d *Recommended doses for weight:* 24–35 lb (10.6–15.9 kg), 162 mg; 36–47 lb (16–21.4 kg), 243 mg; 48–59 lb (21.5–26.8 kg), 324 mg; 60–71 lb (26.9–32.3 kg), 405 mg; 72–95 lb (32.4–43.2 kg), 486 mg; 96 lb or above (43.3 kg or above), 648 mg *Juvenile RA:* PO 60–110 mg/kg/d in divided doses q6–8h *Acute rheumatic fever;* PO 100 mg/kg/d, in divided doses, for 2 wk, then 75 mg/kg/d for 4–6 wk	Therapeutic serum level of salicylate is 100–300 mcg/mL for treatment of arthritis and rheumatic fever; toxicity occurs at levels above 300 mcg/mL.

Table 7-2 Drugs at a Glance: Analgesic, Antipyretic, Anti-Inflammatory Drugs (continued)

GENERIC/TRADE NAME	INDICATIONS FOR USE	ROUTES AND DOSAGE RANGES		Comments
		Adults	Children	
Celecoxib (Celebrex)	OA RA Familial adenomatous polyposis (FAP)	*OA:* PO 100 mg twice daily or 200 mg once daily *RA:* PO 100–200 mg twice daily *FAP:* PO 200 mg twice daily	Dosage not established	200-mg doses should be taken with food.
Choline salicylate (Arthropan)	OA RA Pain, fever	Liquid PO: 870 mg (5 mL) q3–4h; maximum of 6 doses per day	Dosage not established for children <12 y	Should be taken with food
Diclofenac potassium (Cataflam) **Diclofenac sodium** (Voltaren, Voltaren XR)	OA RA Ankylosing spondylitis (AS) Pain, dysmenorrhea	*OA:* PO 100–150 mg/d in divided doses (eg, 50 mg two or three times or 75 mg twice or 100 mg once daily) *RA:* PO 150–200 mg/d in two, three, or four divided doses *AS:* PO 100–125 mg/d in four or five divided doses (eg, 25 mg four or five times daily) *Pain, dysmenorrhea:* (diclofenac potassium only) PO 50 mg three times daily	Dosage not established	Diclofenac potassium is available only in 50-mg, *immediate-release* tablets. It may be used for all indications. Diclofenac sodium is available in 25-, 50-, and 75-mg *delayed-release* tablets and a 100-mg *extended-release* (XR) tablet. It is not recommended for acute pain or dysmenorrhea.
Diflunisal (Dolobid)	OA RA Pain	*OA, RA:* PO 500–1000 mg/d, in two divided doses, increased to a maximum of 1500 mg/d if necessary *Pain:* PO 500–1000 mg initially, then 250–500 mg q8–12h	Not recommended for use in children <12 years of age	
Etodolac (Lodine, Lodine XL)	OA RA Pain	*OA, RA:* PO 600–1200 mg/d in two to four divided doses *Pain:* PO 200–400 mg q6–8h *Maximum according to weight:* 1200 mg/d for 60 kg (132 lbs) or more; 20 mg/kg/d for <60 kg	Dosage not established	Available in *immediate-release* and *extended-release* (XL) tablets of various strengths. The immediate-release forms should be used to treat acute pain.

(continued)

Table 7-2 Drugs at a Glance: Analgesic, Antipyretic, Anti-Inflammatory Drugs (continued)

GENERIC/TRADE NAME	INDICATIONS FOR USE	ROUTES AND DOSAGE RANGES		Comments
		Adults	**Children**	
Fenoprofen (Nalfon)	OA RA Pain	*OA, RA:* PO 300–600 mg three or four times per day *Pain:* PO 200 mg q4–6h PRN Maximum, 3200 mg/d	Dosage not established	
Flurbiprofen (Ansaid)	OA RA	*OA, RA:* PO 200–300 mg/d in two, three, or four divided doses	Dosage not established	
Ibuprofen (Advil, Motrin, PediaCare)	OA RA Pain, dysmenorrhea Fever	*OA, RA:* PO 300–600 mg 3 or 4 times per day; maximum, 2400 mg/d *Pain, dysmenorrhea:* PO 400 mg q4–6h PRN; maximum, 3200 mg/d	*1–12 y:* Fever, initial temperature 39.2°C (102.5°F) or less, PO 5 mg/kg q6–8h; initial temperature above 39.2°C (102.5°F), PO 10 mg/kg q6–8h; maximum dose, 40 mg/kg/d *Juvenile arthritis;* PO 20–40 mg/kg/d, in three or four divided doses	Available in numerous dosage forms and concentrations, including regular tablets; chewable tablets; capsules; oral suspensions (of 100 mg/5 mL); and oral drops (of 40 mg/mL, for infants)
Indomethacin (Indocin, Indocin SR)	OA RA AS Tendinitis Bursitis Acute painful shoulder Acute gout Closure of patent ductus arteriosus (IV only)	PO, rectal suppository; 75 mg/d initially, increased by 25 mg/d at weekly intervals to a maximum of 150–200 mg/d, if necessary *Acute gouty arthritis, acute painful shoulder;* PO 75–150 mg/d in three or four divided doses until pain and inflammation are controlled (eg, 3–5 d for gout; 7–14 d for painful shoulder), then discontinued	*Premature infants with patent ductus arteriosus;* IV 0.2–0.3 mg/kg q12h for a total of three doses	The sustained-release form is not recommended for acute gouty arthritis.
Ketoprofen (Oruvail)	Pain Dysmenorrhea OA RA	*Pain, dysmenorrhea:* PO 25–50 mg q6–8h PRN *OA, RA:* PO 150–300 mg/d in three or four divided doses Extended-release; 200 mg once daily Maximum; 300 mg/d for regular formulation; 200 mg/d for extended release; 100–150 mg/d for clients with impaired renal function	Do not give to children <16 years unless directed by a physician.	Extended-release capsules are available as generic ketoprofen and Oruvail. Note that the names do not contain any letters (eg, SR, XL) that indicate long-acting dosage forms.

Table 7-2 Drugs at a Glance: Analgesic, Antipyretic, Anti-Inflammatory Drugs (continued)

| GENERIC/TRADE NAME | INDICATIONS FOR USE | ROUTES AND DOSAGE RANGES | | Comments |
		Adults	Children	
Ketorolac (Toradol)	Moderately severe, acute pain, for short-term (up to 5 days) treatment	IV, IM 30 mg q6h PRN to a maximum of 120 mg/d PO 10 mg q4–6h to a maximum of 40 mg/d Older adults (>65 y), those with renal impairment, those with weight < 50 kg (110 lbs); IV, IM 15 mg q6h to a maximum of 60 mg/d	Dosage not established	Treatment is started with one or more injected doses, followed by oral doses when the client is able to take them. Maximum duration of both injected and oral doses, 5 days
Mefenamic acid (Ponstel, others)	Moderate pain (up to 1 wk) Dysmenorrhea	*Pain:* PO 500 mg initially followed by 250 mg q6h *Dysmenorrhea:* PO 500 mg initially then 250 mg q6h starting with onset of bleeding	Dosage not established for children <14 y	Should be taken with meals. Drug should not be needed more than 2–3 days; maximum duration not to exceed 1 wk.
Meloxicam (Mobic)	OA	PO 7.5 mg once daily; increased to 15 mg once daily if necessary	Dosage not established	May be taken without regard to meals
Nabumetone (Relafen)	OA RA	PO 1000–2000 mg/day in one or two doses	Dosage not established	Available in 500-mg and 750-mg tablets
Naproxen (Naprosyn) **Naproxen sodium** (Aleve, Anaprox, Naprelan)	OA RA Juvenile arthritis AS Pain Dysmenorrhea Bursitis Tendinitis Acute gout	*Naproxen:* PO 250–500 mg twice daily *Gout:* PO 750 mg initially, then 250 mg q8h until symptoms subside Maximum, 1250 mg/d *Naproxen sodium:* Pain, dysmenorrhea, acute tendinitis, bursitis: PO 550 mg q12h or 275 mg q6–8h Maximum, 1375 mg/d *OA, RA, AS:* PO 275–550 mg twice a day *Acute gout:* PO 825 mg initially, then 275 mg q8h until symptoms subside Controlled-release (Naprelan); 750–1000 mg once daily	*Juvenile arthritis (naproxen only):* PO 10 mg/kg/d in two divided doses. Oral suspension (125 mg/5 mL) twice daily according to weight: 13 kg (29 lb), 2.5 mL; 25 kg (55 lb), 5 mL; 39 kg (84 lb), 7.5 mL OTC preparation not recommended for children < 12 y	Available in several dosage strength tablets, in a suspension, and in immediate- and delayed-release formulations

(continued)

Table 7-2 Drugs at a Glance: Analgesic, Antipyretic, Anti-Inflammatory Drugs (continued)

| GENERIC/TRADE NAME | INDICATIONS FOR USE | ROUTES AND DOSAGE RANGES | | Comments |
		Adults	Children	
Oxaprozin (Daypro)	OA RA	PO 600–1200 mg once daily Maximum; 1800 mg/d or 26 mg/kg/d, whichever is lower, in divided doses	Dosage not established	Lower doses recommended for patients with low body weight or milder disease
Piroxicam (Feldene)	OA RA	PO 20 mg/d or 10 mg twice daily	Dosage not established	
Salsalate (Disalcid, others)	Pain, fever Rheumatic fever OA RA	PO 3000 mg/d in divided doses	Dosage not established	May be taken with food to decrease GI effects. Administer with full glass of water to prevent tablet or capsule from lodging in esophagus
Sulindac (Clinoril)	OA RA Ankylosing spondylitis Bursitis Tendinitis Acute painful shoulder Acute gout	PO 150–200 mg twice a day; maximum, 400 mg/d *Acute gout, acute painful shoulder:* PO 200 mg twice a day until pain and inflammation subside (eg, 7–14 d), then reduce dosage or discontinue	Dosage not established	
Tolmetin (Tolectin)	OA RA Juvenile rheumatoid arthritis	PO 400 mg three times daily initially, increased to 1800 mg/d if necessary	*Juvenile RA:* PO 20 mg/kg/d in three or four divided doses	

GI, gastrointestinal; IM, intramuscular; IV, intravenous; PO, oral; PRN, as needed.

limited to 5 days because it increases the risk of bleeding. Hematomas and wound bleeding have been reported with postoperative use.

Mefenamic acid (Ponstel) belongs to a family of NSAIDs called *fenamates*. The fenamates have anti-inflammatory, antipyretic, and analgesic properties. Mefenamic acid is used primarily for relief of moderate pain due to primary dysmenorrhea. Peak plasma concentrations of mefenamic acid are reached 2 to 4 hours after a single oral dose. About 50% of the drug is excreted in the urine and 20% is eliminated in the feces. The most common side effects occur in the GI tract, including dyspepsia and diarrhea accompanied by steatorrhea and inflammation of the bowel. A rare serious side effect is hemolytic anemia.

Oxicam drugs include meloxicam (Mobic) and piroxicam (Feldene). Meloxicam has a serum half-life of 15 to 20 hours and is excreted about equally in urine and feces. Piroxicam

has a half-life of about 50 hours. The long half-lives allow the drugs to be given once daily, but optimal efficacy may not occur for 1 to 2 weeks.

Diclofenac sodium (Voltaren) is chemically different from but pharmacologically similar to other NSAIDs. Formulations are delayed or extended-release, and onset of action is therefore delayed. Peak action occurs in about 2 hours and effects last 12 to 15 hours. The formulation of diclofenac potassium (Cataflam) is immediate-release; action starts quickly, peaks in about 20 minutes to 2 hours, and also lasts 12 to 15 hours. As a result, the potassium salt may be given for rapid relief of pain and primary dysmenorrhea. Diclofenac has a serum half-life of about 2 hours and is excreted mainly in the urine.

COX-2 inhibitors include celecoxib, rofecoxib, and valdecoxib. However, as previously discussed, only celecoxib is currently marketed in the United States due to concerns with increased risk of adverse cardiovascular events such as myocardial infarction and stroke. COX-2 inhibitors were designed to selectively block production of prostaglandins associated with pain and inflammation without blocking those associated with protective effects on gastric mucosa, renal function, and platelet aggregation. Thus, they produce less gastric irritation and renal impairment than aspirin and other NSAIDs. However, with prolonged use or high dosages, GI bleeding, renal impairment, and associated hypertension and edema are still risks. COX-2 inhibitors are not associated with increased risk of bleeding because they do not have the antiplatelet effects of aspirin and other NSAIDs.

Celecoxib (Celebrex) is well absorbed with oral administration; peak plasma levels and peak action occur approximately 3 hours after an oral dose. It is highly protein bound (97%) and its serum half-life is about 11 hours. It is metabolized by the cytochrome P450 enzymes in the liver to inactive metabolites that are then excreted in the urine. A small amount is excreted unchanged in the urine.

APPLYING YOUR KNOWLEDGE 7-1
Review Julie's medications. What would be the most likely adverse reaction to this medication regimen, considering the total amount of medication that Julie may take for her headaches?

Acetaminophen

Acetaminophen (also called APAP, an abbreviation of *N*-acetyl-*p*-aminophenol) is a nonprescription drug commonly used as an aspirin substitute because it does not cause nausea, vomiting, or GI bleeding, and it does not interfere with blood clotting. It is equal to aspirin in analgesic and antipyretic effects, but it lacks anti-inflammatory activity.

Acetaminophen is well absorbed with oral administration, and peak plasma concentrations are reached within 30 to 120 minutes. Duration of action is 3 to 4 hours.

Acetaminophen is metabolized in the liver; approximately 94% is excreted in the urine as inactive glucuronate and sulfate conjugates. Approximately 4% is metabolized to a toxic metabolite, which is normally inactivated by conjugation with glutathione and excreted in urine. With usual therapeutic doses, a sufficient amount of glutathione is available in the liver to detoxify acetaminophen. However, in acute or chronic overdose situations, the supply of glutathione may become depleted. In the absence of glutathione, the toxic metabolite combines with liver cells and causes damage or fatal liver necrosis. In people who abuse alcohol, usual therapeutic doses may cause or increase liver damage. The probable mechanism for increased risk of hepatotoxicity in this population is that ethanol induces drug-metabolizing enzymes in the liver. The resulting rapid metabolism of acetaminophen produces enough toxic metabolite to exceed the available glutathione.

Acetaminophen is available in tablet, liquid, and rectal suppository forms and is found in numerous combination products marketed as analgesics and cold remedies. It is often prescribed with codeine, hydrocodone, or oxycodone for added analgesic effects.

Drugs Used to Treat Gout and Hyperuricemia

Individual drugs are described below; dosages are listed in Table 7-3.

Allopurinol (Zyloprim) is used to prevent or treat hyperuricemia, which occurs with gout and with antineoplastic drug therapy. Uric acid is formed by purine metabolism and an enzyme called *xanthine oxidase*. Allopurinol prevents formation of uric acid by inhibiting xanthine oxidase. It is especially useful in treating chronic gout characterized by tophi (deposits of uric acid crystals in the joints, kidneys, and soft tissues) and impaired renal function. The drug promotes resorption of urate deposits and prevents their further development. Acute attacks of gout may result when urate deposits are mobilized. These may be prevented by concomitant administration of colchicine until serum uric acid levels are lowered.

Colchicine is an anti-inflammatory drug used to prevent or treat acute attacks of gout. In acute attacks, it is the drug of choice for relieving joint pain and edema. Colchicine decreases inflammation by decreasing the movement of leukocytes into body tissues containing urate crystals. It has no analgesic or antipyretic effects.

Probenecid (Benemid) increases the urinary excretion of uric acid. This uricosuric action is used therapeutically to treat hyperuricemia and gout. It is not effective in acute attacks of gouty arthritis but prevents hyperuricemia and tophi associated with chronic gout. Probenecid may cause acute gout until serum uric acid levels are within the normal range; concomitant administration of colchicine prevents this effect. (Probenecid also is used with penicillin, most often in treating sexually transmitted diseases. It increases blood levels and prolongs the action of penicillin by decreasing the rate of urinary excretion.)

Sulfinpyrazone (Anturane) is a uricosuric agent similar to probenecid. It is not effective in acute gout but prevents or decreases tissue changes of chronic gout. Colchicine is usually given during initial sulfinpyrazone therapy to prevent acute gout.

Drugs Used to Treat Migraine

Drugs used to treat migraine headaches can be divided into two categories: medications used to treat acute pain, and medications used to prevent migraine headaches from occurring. Drugs used for migraine prophylaxis are different in their classification and mechanism of action from medications useful in

Table 7-3 Drugs at a Glance: Drugs Used in Gout

GENERIC TRADE NAME	ROUTES AND DOSAGE RANGES	
	Adults	**Children**
Allopurinol (Zyloprim)	Mild gout, PO 200–400 mg/d Severe gout, PO 400–600 mg/d Hyperuricemia in clients with renal insufficiency, PO 100–200 mg/d Secondary hyperuricemia from anticancer drugs, PO 100–200 mg/d; maximum 800 mg/d	Secondary hyperuricemia from anticancer drugs: <6 y, PO 150 mg/d; 6–10 y, PO 300 mg/d
Colchicine	Acute attacks, PO 0.5 mg q1h until pain is relieved or toxicity (nausea, vomiting, diarrhea) occurs; 3-d interval between courses of therapy IV 1–2 mg initially, then 0.5 mg q3–6h until response is obtained; maximum total dose 4 mg Prophylaxis, PO 0.5–1 mg/d	Dosage not established
Probenecid (Benemid)	PO 250 mg twice a day for 1 wk, then 500 mg twice a day	>2 y, PO 40 mg/kg/d in divided doses
Sulfinpyrazone (Anturane)	PO 100–200 mg twice a day, gradually increased over 1 wk to a maximum of 400–800 mg/d	Dosage not established

IV, intravenous; PO, oral.

treating the acute pain of a migraine headache. Prophylactic drugs include beta blockers such as propranolol (see Chap. 18), calcium channel blockers such as nifedipine (see Chap. 50), tricyclic antidepressants such as imipramine (see Chap. 10), and anticonvulsants such as valproic acid (see Chap. 11). Drugs used for relieving the acute pain of migraine headaches are discussed in this section. Individual drugs are described below. Dosages are given in Table 7-4.

Almotriptan (Axert), **eletriptan** (Relpax), **frovatriptan** (Frova), **naratriptan** (Amerge), **rizatriptan** (Maxalt), **sumatriptan** (Imitrex), and **zolmitriptan** (Zomig), called "triptans," were developed specifically for the treatment of moderate or severe migraines. They are called *selective serotonin 5-HT₁ receptor agonists* because they act on a specific subtype of serotonin receptor to increase serotonin (5-hydroxytryptamine or 5-HT) in the brain. They relieve migraine by constricting blood vessels. Because of their vasoconstrictive properties, the drugs are contraindicated in clients with a history of angina pectoris, myocardial infarction, or uncontrolled hypertension. The drugs vary in onset of action, with subcutaneous sumatriptan acting the most rapidly and starting to relieve migraine headache within 10 minutes. Most clients obtain relief within

1 to 2 hours with all of the oral drugs. The drugs are metabolized in the liver by monoamine oxidase or cytochrome P450 enzymes; metabolism of eletriptan, rizatriptan, and zolmitriptan produces active metabolites. Subcutaneous sumatriptan produces more adverse effects than the oral drugs, which have similar adverse effects (eg, pain, paresthesias, nausea, dizziness, drowsiness). These are considered safer than ergot alkaloids.

Ergotamine tartrate (Ergomar) is an ergot alkaloid used only in the treatment of migraine. Ergot preparations relieve migraine by constricting blood vessels. Ergotamine is most effective when given sublingually or by inhalation at the onset of headache. When given orally, ergotamine is erratically absorbed, and therapeutic effects may be delayed for 20 to 30 minutes. Ergotamine is contraindicated during pregnancy and in the presence of severe hypertension, peripheral vascular disease, coronary artery disease, renal or hepatic disease, and severe infections.

Ergotamine tartrate and caffeine (Cafergot) is a commonly used antimigraine preparation. Caffeine reportedly increases the absorption and vasoconstrictive effects of ergotamine. **Dihydroergotamine mesylate** (DHE 45) is a semi-

Table 7-4 Drugs at a Glance: Drugs Used in Migraine

GENERIC/TRADE NAME	ROUTES AND DOSAGE RANGES
Serotonin Agonists (Triptans)	
Almotriptan (Axert)	PO 6.25 mg, repeat after 2 h if necessary. Maximum, 12.5 mg/24h
Eletriptan (Relpax)	PO 20–40 mg as a single dose, repeat after 2 h if necessary. Maximum dose, 80 mg/d
Frovatriptan (Frova)	PO 2.5 mg; repeat after 2 h if necessary. Maximum dose, 7.5 mg
Naratriptan (Amerge)	PO 1–2.5 mg as a single dose; repeat in 4 h if necessary. Maximum, 5 mg/d
Rizatriptan (Maxalt)	PO 5–10 mg as a single dose; repeat after 2 h if necessary. Maximum dose, 30 mg/d
Sumatriptan (Imitrex)	PO 25–100 mg as a single dose. Maximum dose, 300 mg/d Sub-Q 6 mg as a single dose. Maximum, 12 mg/d Nasal spray 5, 10, or 20 mg by unit-dose spray device. Maximum, 40 mg/d
Zolmitriptan (Zomig)	PO 1.25–2.5 mg as a single dose; may repeat after 2 h if necessary. Maximum dose, 10 mg/d Nasal spray 0.5, 1, 2.5, or 5 mg by unit-dose spray device. Maximum, 10 mg/d Orally disintegrating tablets (Zomig-ZMT) 2.5–5 mg as a single dose; may repeat after 2 h if necessary. Maximum dose, 10 mg/d
Ergot Preparations	
Dihydroergotamine mesylate (DHE 45)	IM 1 mg at onset of migraine, may be repeated hourly, if necessary, to a total of 3 mg IV 1 mg, repeated, if necessary, after 1 h; maximum dose 2 mg. Do not exceed 6 mg/wk.
Ergotamine tartrate (Ergomar)	PO, sublingually, 1–2 mg at onset of migraine, then 2 mg q30 min, if necessary, to a maximum of 6 mg/24 h or 10 mg/wk Inhalation, 0.36 mg (one inhalation) at onset of migraine, repeat in 5 min, if necessary, to a maximum of 6 inhalations/24 h
Ergotamine tartrate and caffeine (Cafergot)	*Adults:* PO 2 tablets at onset of migraine, then 1 tablet q30 min, if necessary, up to 6 tablets per attack or 10 tablets/wk Rectal suppository 0.5–1 suppository at onset of migraine, repeat in 1 h, if necessary, up to two suppositories per attack or five suppositories/wk *Children:* PO 0.5–1 tablet initially, then 0.5 tablet q30 min, if necessary, to a maximum of three tablets

IM, intramuscular; IV, intravenous; PO, oral; Sub-Q, subcutaneous.

synthetic derivative of ergotamine that is less toxic and less effective than the parent drug.

Herbal and Dietary Supplements

In addition to the drugs described above, many herbal medicines are used to relieve pain and/or inflammation. For most of these (eg, comfrey, marigold, pep-permint, primrose), such usage is anecdotal and unsupported by clinical studies. For a few supplements, there is some evidence of effectiveness with few adverse effects.

Chondroitin sulfate (CS), a supplement extracted from animal cartilage or manufactured synthetically and used to treat arthritis, is thought to delay the breakdown of joint cartilage (by inhibiting elastase, a proteolytic enzyme found in synovial membranes); to stimulate synthesis of new cartilage (by stimulating chondrocytes to produce collagen and proteoglycan); and to promote the "shock-absorbing" quality of cartilage (by retaining water).

Chondroitin is a normal component of joint cartilage, which also contains water (65% to 80%), collagen, proteoglycans, and chondrocytes that produce new collagen and proteoglycans. CS was first used as a dietary supplement because studies suggested that it would promote healing of cartilage damaged by inflammation or injury. The daily dose of CS is based on weight: less than 120 pounds, 800 milligrams; 120 to 200 pounds, 1200 milligrams; more than 200 pounds, 1600 milligrams. CS is usually taken with food, in two to four divided doses.

Proponents of CS cite clinical trials that indicate beneficial effects and low incidence of adverse effects. In 2003, a meta-analysis of 15 high-quality, randomized, double-blind controlled trials comparing chondroitin and glucosamine to placebo or active control concluded that oral CS significantly improved symptoms, including joint mobility, in clients with OA. Adverse effects were found to be statistically similar to placebo in all studies. The main adverse effect of CS is reportedly minor stomach upset. In addition, there is a theoretical risk of bleeding because of the drug's structural similarity to heparin, but there have been no reports of bleeding from the use of CS.

Opponents question whether CS is absorbed systemically, because of its large molecular size, and whether it is able to reach cartilage cells. They also state that little is known about long-term toxicity of the compound.

Feverfew is an herbal medicine with some evidence of effectiveness in migraine, especially in reducing incidence and severity. Its main active ingredient is thought to be parthenolide. Feverfew is thought to inhibit platelet aggregation, prostaglandin synthesis, and the release of inflammatory mediators such as histamine, but its exact mechanism in migraine prophylaxis is unknown. It is contraindicated in pregnant and lactating women.

In general, clients should be encouraged to try standard methods of preventing and treating migraine before taking products with uncertain benefits and risks. For example, commercial preparations of feverfew are not standardized and may contain different amounts of parthenolide. The usual recommended dose is 25 to 50 milligrams daily with food, but more studies are needed.

Adverse effects include hypersensitivity reactions in people who are allergic to ragweed, asters, chrysanthemums, or daisies, and stopping the preparation abruptly can result in withdrawal symptoms of pain and stiffness. No interactions with OTC or prescription drugs have been reported, but there is a potential for increasing risks of bleeding in clients taking an antiplatelet drug (eg, aspirin) or an anticoagulant (eg, warfarin).

Glucosamine, a synthetic supplement, is also taken for arthritis. Glucosamine is an essential structural component of joint connective tissue. With OA, glucosamine production is decreased, synovial fluid becomes thin and less effective in lubricating the joint, and joint cartilage deteriorates. The rationale for taking supplementary glucosamine is to reduce cartilage breakdown and improve cartilage production and repair.

Some studies indicate that glucosamine may decrease mild to moderate pain caused by OA in some clients, possibly as well as NSAIDs, Other studies indicate little or no benefit when glucosamine is compared with placebo. There is controversy about the ability of glucosamine to affect cartilage structure and delay joint deterioration. Most studies are criticized as being too small, of too short a duration, and of having flawed designs. A study of 212 clients with knee OA indicated that long-term use of glucosamine improves symptoms and prevents changes in joint structure. These clients took 1500 milligrams of glucosamine sulfate or placebo once a day for 3 years. Radiographs of the knees were taken before starting glucosamine and after 1 and 3 years of treatment. The researchers concluded that significant improvement of symptoms and less joint deterioration occurred in clients receiving glucosamine. Some reviewers of this study said the pain relief was minor and the radiographic changes were insignificant and did not indicate improvement in disease progression.

The previously mentioned 2003 meta-analysis, which compared chondroitin and glucosamine to placebo or controls, concluded that structural improvement as measured by joint-space narrowing was significantly demonstrated in clients receiving glucosamine. Glucosamine significantly improved joint structure and symptoms in clients with OA of the knee.

Glucosamine is available as a hydrochloride salt and as a sulfate salt. Most studies have been performed with glucosamine sulfate (GS), which is the preferred form. Dosage of GS is based on weight: less than 120 pounds, 1000 milligrams; 120 to 200 pounds, 1500 milligrams; more than 200 pounds, 2000 milligrams. GS is usually taken with food, in two to four divided doses.

There are no known contraindications to the use of glucosamine, but it should be avoided during pregnancy and lactation and in children, because effects are unknown. Adverse effects include GI upset (eg, epigastric pain, heartburn, nausea, constipation, diarrhea), drowsiness, headache, and skin rash. No interactions with OTC or prescription drugs have been reported.

Glucosamine and chondroitin can each be used alone, but are more often taken in combination, with the same dosages as listed above. Use of this combination greatly increased after it was highly praised in *The Arthritis Cure* by J. Theodosakis.

As with studies of the individual components, many of the studies involving glucosamine and chondroitin are flawed. The American College of Rheumatology and the Arthritis Foundation do not recommend the use of these supplements because they do not believe reported research studies adequately demonstrate significant relief of symptoms or slowing of the disease process. These organizations state that longer clinical trials with larger groups of people are needed. When questioned by clients, some physicians suggest taking the supplement for 3 months (glucosamine 500 mg and chondroitin

400 mg three times a day) and deciding for themselves whether their symptoms improve (eg, less pain, improved ability to walk) and whether they want to continue.

NURSING PROCESS

Assessment

- Assess for signs and symptoms of pain, such as location, severity, duration, and factors that cause or relieve the pain (see Chap. 6).
- Assess for fever (thermometer readings above 99.6°F [37.3°C] are usually considered fever). Hot, dry skin; flushed face; reduced urine output; and concentrated urine may accompany fever if the person also is dehydrated.
- Assess for inflammation. Local signs are redness, heat, edema, and pain or tenderness; systemic signs include fever, elevated white blood cell count (leukocytosis), and weakness.
- With arthritis or other musculoskeletal disorders, assess for pain and limitations in activity and mobility.
- Ask about use of OTC analgesic, antipyretic, or anti-inflammatory drugs and herbal or dietary supplements.
- Ask about allergic reactions to aspirin or NSAIDs.
- Assess for history of peptic ulcer disease, GI bleeding, or kidney disorders.
- With migraine, assess severity and patterns of occurrences.

Nursing Diagnoses

- Acute Pain
- Chronic Pain
- Activity Intolerance related to pain
- Risk for Poisoning: Acetaminophen overdose
- Risk for Injury related to adverse drug effects (GI bleeding, renal insufficiency)
- Deficient Knowledge: Therapeutic and adverse effects of commonly used drugs
- Deficient Knowledge: Correct use of OTC drugs for pain, fever, and inflammation

Planning/Goals

The Client Will
- Experience relief of discomfort with minimal adverse drug effects
- Experience increased mobility and activity tolerance
- Inform health care providers if taking aspirin, an NSAID or acetaminophen regularly.
- Self-administer the drugs safely
- Avoid overuse of the drugs
- Use measures to prevent accidental ingestion or overdose, especially in children
- Experience fewer and less severe attacks of migraine

Interventions

Implement measures to prevent or minimize pain, fever, and inflammation.
- Treat the disease processes (eg, infection, arthritis) or circumstances (eg, impaired blood supply, lack of physical activity, poor positioning or body alignment) thought to be causing pain, fever, or inflammation.
- Treat pain as soon as possible; early treatment may prevent severe pain and anxiety and allow the use of milder analgesic drugs. Use distraction, relaxation techniques, or other nonpharmacologic techniques along with drug therapy, when appropriate.
- With acute musculoskeletal injuries (eg, sprains), cold applications can decrease pain, swelling, and inflammation. Apply for approximately 20 minutes, then remove.
- Assist clients with migraine to identify and avoid "triggers." Assist clients to drink 2 to 3 liters of fluid daily when taking an NSAID regularly. This strategy decreases gastric irritation and helps to maintain good kidney function. With long-term use of aspirin, fluids help to prevent precipitation of salicylate crystals in the urinary tract. With antigout drugs, fluids help to prevent precipitation of urate crystals and formation of urate kidney stones. Fluid intake is especially important initially when serum uric acid levels are high and large amounts of uric acid are being excreted.

Provide appropriate teaching for any drug therapy (see accompanying displays).

Evaluation

- Interview and observe regarding relief of symptoms.
- Interview and observe regarding mobility and activity levels.
- Interview and observe regarding safe, effective use of the drugs.
- Select drugs appropriately.

APPLYING YOUR KNOWLEDGE 7-3
Given Julie's medication regimen, what nursing measures should be implemented to decrease the probability of GI bleeding?

PRINCIPLES OF THERAPY

Use of Aspirin

When pain, fever, or inflammation is present, aspirin is effective across a wide range of clinical conditions. Like any other drug, aspirin must be used appropriately to maximize therapeutic benefits and minimize adverse reactions.

(text continues on page 122)

CLIENT TEACHING GUIDELINES

Acetaminophen, Aspirin, and Other NSAIDs

General Considerations

✔ Aspirin and other nonsteroidal anti-inflammatory drugs (NSAIDs) such as ibuprofen (Advil, Motrin) are used to relieve pain, fever, and inflammation. Aspirin is as effective as the more costly NSAIDs, but is more likely to cause stomach irritation and bleeding problems. This advantage of NSAIDs may be minimal if high doses are taken.

Because these drugs are so widely used and available, there is a high risk of overdosing on different products containing the same drug or products containing similar drugs. Knowing drug names, reading product labels, and using the following precautions can increase safety in using these drugs:

1. If you are taking aspirin or an NSAID regularly for pain or inflammation, generally avoid taking additional aspirin in over-the-counter (OTC) aspirin or products containing aspirin (eg, Alka-Seltzer, Anacin, Arthritis Pain Formula, Ascriptin, Bufferin, Doan's Pills/Caplets, Ecotrin, Excedrin, Midol, Vanquish). There are two exceptions if you are taking a small dose of aspirin daily (usually 81–325 mg), to prevent heart attack and stroke. First, you should continue taking the aspirin if Celebrex is prescribed. Second, it is generally safe to take occasional doses of aspirin or an NSAID for pain or fever.

2. If you are taking any prescription NSAID regularly, avoid OTC products containing ibuprofen (eg, Advil, Dristan Sinus, Midol IB, Motrin IB, Sine-Aid IB), or naproxen (Aleve). Also, do not combine the OTC products with each other or with aspirin. These drugs are available as both prescription and OTC products. OTC ibuprofen is the same medication as prescription Motrin; OTC naproxen is the same as prescription Naprosyn; OTC ketoprofen is the same as prescription Orudis. Recommended doses are smaller for OTC products than for prescription drugs. However, any combination of these drugs could constitute an overdose.

✔ With NSAIDs, if one is not effective, another one may work because people vary in responses to the drugs. Improvement of symptoms depends on the reason for use. When taken for pain, the drugs usually act within 30 to 60 minutes; when taken for inflammatory disorders, such as arthritis, improvement may occur within 24 to 48 hours with aspirin and 1 to 2 weeks with other NSAIDs.

✔ Taking a medication for fever is not usually recommended unless the fever is high or is accompanied by other symptoms. Fever is one way the body fights infection.

✔ Do not take OTC ibuprofen more than 3 days for fever or 10 days for pain. If these symptoms persist or worsen, or if new symptoms develop, contact a health care provider.

✔ Avoid aspirin for approximately 2 weeks before and after major surgery or dental work to decrease the risk of excessive bleeding. If pregnant, do not take aspirin for approximately 2 weeks before the estimated delivery date.

✔ Inform any health care provider if taking acetaminophen aspirin, ibuprofen, or any other NSAID regularly.

✔ Inform health care providers if you have ever had an allergic reaction (eg, asthma, difficulty in breathing, hives), severe GI symptoms (eg, ulcer, bleeding), or a rash or other skin disorder after taking aspirin, ibuprofen, or similar drugs.

✔ Avoid or minimize alcoholic beverages because alcohol increases gastric irritation and risks of bleeding. The Food and Drug Administration requires an alcohol warning on the labels of OTC pain and fever relievers and urges people who drink three or more alcoholic drinks every day to ask their doctors before using the products.

✔ To avoid accidental ingestion and aspirin poisoning, store aspirin in a closed childproof container and keep out of children's reach.

Self-Administration

✔ Take aspirin, ibuprofen, and other NSAIDs with a full glass of liquid and food to decrease stomach irritation. Meloxicam (Mobic) may be taken without regard to food.

✔ Swallow enteric-coated aspirin (eg, Ecotrin) whole; do not chew or crush. The coating is applied to decrease stomach irritation by making the tablet dissolve in the intestine. Also, do not take with an antacid, which can cause the tablet to dissolve in the stomach.

✔ Swallow any long-acting pills or capsules whole; do not chew or crush. These include diclofenac *sodium* (Voltaren or Voltaren XR); diflunisal (Dolobid); etodolac (Lodine XL); ketoprofen or Oruvail extended-release capsules; naproxen delayed-release (EC-Naprosyn) or controlled-release (Naprelan) tablets.
Note: These are prescription drugs and most are also available in short acting products; if unsure whether the medicine you are taking is long acting, ask a health care provider.

✔ Drink 2–3 quarts of fluid daily when taking an NSAID regularly. This decreases gastric irritation and helps to maintain good kidney function.

✔ Report signs of bleeding (eg, nose bleed, vomiting blood, bruising, blood in urine or stools), difficulty breathing, skin rash or hives, ringing in ears, dizziness, severe stomach upset, or swelling and weight gain.

Acetaminophen

✔ Acetaminophen is often the initial drug of choice for relieving mild to moderate pain and fever because it is effective and does not cause gastric irritation or bleeding. It may be taken on an empty stomach.

✔ Acetaminophen is an effective aspirin substitute for pain or fever but not for inflammation or preventing heart attack or stroke.

✔ Acetaminophen is available in its generic form and with many OTC brand names (eg, Tylenol). Most preparations contain 500 mg of drug per tablet or capsule. In addition, almost all OTC pain relievers (often labeled "nonaspirin") and cold, flu, and sinus remedies contain acetaminophen. Thus, all consumers should read product labels carefully to avoid taking the drug in several products, with potential overdoses.

CLIENT TEACHING GUIDELINES

Acetaminophen, Aspirin, and Other NSAIDs (continued)

✔ Do not exceed recommended doses. For occasional pain or fever, 650–1000 mg may be taken three or four times daily. For daily, long-term use (eg, in osteoarthritis), do not take more than 4000 mg (eg, eight 500-mg or extra-strength tablets or capsules) daily. Larger doses may cause life-threatening liver damage. People who have hepatitis or other liver disorders and those who ingest alcoholic beverages frequently should take no more than 2000 mg daily.

✔ Do not exceed recommended duration of use (longer than 5 days in children, 10 days in adults, or 3 days for fever in adults and children) without consulting a physician.

✔ Avoid or minimize alcoholic beverages because alcohol increases risk of liver damage. The Food and Drug Administration requires an alcohol warning on the labels of OTC pain and fever relievers and urges people who drink three or more alcoholic drinks every day to ask their doctors before taking products containing acetaminophen.

Antigout Drugs

✔ When colchicine is taken for acute gout, pain is usually relieved in 4–12 hours with IV administration and 24–48 hours with oral administration. Inflammation and edema may not decrease for several days.

✔ With colchicine for chronic gout, carry the drug and start taking it as directed (usually one pill every hour for several hours until relief is obtained or nausea, vomiting, and diarrhea occur) when joint pain starts. This prevents or minimizes acute attacks of gout.

✔ Drink 2–3 quarts of fluid daily with antigout drugs. An adequate fluid intake helps prevent formation of uric acid kidney stones. Fluid intake is especially important initially, when uric acid levels in the blood are high and large amounts of uric acid are being excreted in the urine.

✔ When allopurinol is taken, blood levels of uric acid usually decrease to normal range within 1–3 weeks.

CLIENT TEACHING GUIDELINES

Drugs Used in Migraine

General Considerations

✔ Try to identify and avoid situations known to precipitate acute attacks of migraine.

✔ For mild or infrequent migraine attacks, acetaminophen, aspirin, or another nonsteroidal anti-inflammatory drug may be effective.

✔ For moderate-to-severe migraine attacks, the drug of first choice is probably sumatriptan (Imitrex) or a related drug, if not contraindicated (eg, by heart disease or hypertension). However, one of these drugs should not be taken if an ergot preparation has been taken within the previous 24 hours.

✔ If you have frequent or severe migraine attacks, consult a physician about medications to prevent or reduce the frequency of acute attacks.

✔ Never take an antimigraine medication prescribed for someone else or allow someone else to take yours. The medications used to relieve acute migraine can constrict blood vessels, raise blood pressure, and cause serious adverse effects.

✔ Chronic overuse of analgesics, preparations containing sedatives or caffeine, triptans, opioids, or ergotamine may play a role in causing rebound headaches.

Self-Administration

✔ Take medication at onset of pain, when possible, to prevent development of more severe symptoms.

✔ With triptans, take oral drugs (except for rizatriptan and zolmitriptan orally disintegrating tablets) with fluids. If symptoms recur, a second dose may be taken. However, do not take a second dose of almotriptan, eletriptan, frovatriptan, rizatriptan, or zolmitriptan sooner than 2 hours after the first dose, or a second dose of naratriptan sooner than 4 hours after the first dose. Do not take more than 12.5 mg of almotriptan, 80 mg of eletriptan, 7.5 mg of frovatriptan, 5 mg of naratriptan, 30 mg of rizatriptan, or 10 mg of zolmitriptan in any 24-hour period.

✔ Rizatriptan and zolmitriptan are available in a regular tablet, which can be taken with fluids, and in an orally disintegrating tablet, which can be dissolved on the tongue and swallowed without fluids. The tablet should be removed from its package with dry hands and placed on the tongue immediately. Zolmitriptan is also available as a nasal spray. The usual dose is one spray into one nostril, not to exceed 10 mg/d (2 doses).

✔ Sumatriptan can be taken by mouth, injection, or nasal spray. Instructions should be strictly followed for the prescribed method of administration. For the nasal spray, the usual dose is one spray into one nostril. If symptoms return, a second spray may be taken 2 hours or longer after the first spray. Do not take more than 40 mg of nasal spray or 200 mg orally or by injection in any 24-hour period. If self-administering injectable sumatriptan, be sure to give in fatty tissue under the skin. This drug must not be taken intravenously; serious, potentially fatal reactions may occur.

✔ If symptoms of an allergic reaction (eg, shortness of breath, wheezing, heart pounding, swelling of eyelids, face or lips, skin rash, or hives) occur after taking a triptan drug, tell your prescribing physician immediately and do not take any additional doses without specific instructions to do so.

✔ With ergot preparations, report signs of poor blood circulation, such as tingling sensations or coldness, numbness, or weakness of the arms and legs. These are symptoms of ergot toxicity. To avoid potentially serious adverse effects, do not exceed recommended doses.

For *pain,* aspirin is useful alone when the discomfort is of low to moderate intensity. For more severe pain, aspirin may be combined with an oral opioid (eg, codeine) or given between opioid doses. Aspirin and opioid analgesics act by different mechanisms, so such use is rational. For acute pain, aspirin is taken when the pain occurs and is often effective within a few minutes. For chronic pain, a regular schedule of administration, such as every 4 to 6 hours, is more effective.

For *fever,* aspirin is effective if drug therapy is indicated. However, aspirin is contraindicated in children because of its association with Reye's syndrome.

For *inflammation,* aspirin is useful in both short- and long-term therapy of conditions characterized by pain and inflammation, such as RA or OA. Although effective, the high doses and frequent administration required for anti-inflammatory effects increase the risks of GI upset, ulceration, and bleeding.

For acute pain or fever, plain aspirin tablets are preferred. For chronic pain, long-term use in arthritis, and daily use for antiplatelet effects, enteric-coated tablets may be better tolerated. Rectal suppositories are sometimes used when oral administration is contraindicated.

Drug Dosage

The dose of aspirin given depends mainly on the condition being treated. Low doses are used for antiplatelet effects in preventing arterial thrombotic disorders such as myocardial infarction or stroke. Lower-than-average doses are needed for clients with low serum albumin levels, because a larger proportion of each dose is free to exert pharmacologic activity. Larger doses are needed for anti-inflammatory effects than for analgesic and antipyretic effects. In general, clients taking low-dose aspirin to prevent myocardial infarction or stroke should continue to take the aspirin if prescribed a COX-2 inhibitor NSAID. The COX-2 inhibitors have little effect on platelet function.

Toxicity: Recognition and Management

Salicylate intoxication (salicylism) may occur with an acute overdose or with chronic use of therapeutic doses, especially the higher doses taken for anti-inflammatory effects. Chronic ingestion of large doses saturates a major metabolic pathway, thereby slowing drug elimination, prolonging the serum half-life, and causing drug accumulation.

Prevention

To decrease risks of toxicity, plasma salicylate levels should be measured when an acute overdose is suspected and periodically when large doses of aspirin are taken long term. Therapeutic levels are 150 to 300 micrograms per milliliter. Signs of salicylate toxicity occur at serum levels greater than 200; severe toxic effects may occur at levels greater than 400.

Signs and Symptoms

Manifestations of salicylism include nausea, vomiting, fever, fluid and electrolyte deficiencies, tinnitus, decreased hearing, visual changes, drowsiness, confusion, hyperventilation, and others. Severe CNS dysfunction (eg, delirium, stupor, coma, seizures) indicates life-threatening toxicity.

Treatment

In mild salicylism, stopping the drug or reducing the dose is usually sufficient. In severe salicylate overdose, treatment is symptomatic and aimed at preventing further absorption from the GI tract; increasing urinary excretion; and correcting fluid, electrolyte, and acid–base imbalances. When the drug may still be in the GI tract, gastric lavage and activated charcoal help reduce absorption. IV sodium bicarbonate produces an alkaline urine in which salicylates are more rapidly excreted, and hemodialysis effectively removes salicylates from the blood. IV fluids are indicated when high fever or dehydration is present. The specific content of IV fluids depends on the serum electrolyte and acid–base status.

Use of NSAIDs

Nonaspirin NSAIDs are widely used and preferred by many people because of less gastric irritation and GI upset, compared with aspirin. Many NSAIDs are prescription drugs used primarily for analgesia and anti-inflammatory effects in arthritis and other musculoskeletal disorders. However, several are approved for more general use as an analgesic or antipyretic. Ibuprofen, ketoprofen, and naproxen are available by prescription and OTC. Clients must be instructed to avoid combined use of prescription and nonprescription NSAIDs because of the high risk of adverse effects. NSAIDs commonly cause gastric mucosal damage, and prolonged use may lead to gastric ulceration and bleeding. Because NSAIDs lead to renal impairment in some clients, blood urea nitrogen and serum creatinine should be checked approximately 2 weeks after starting any of the agents.

NSAIDs inhibit platelet activity only while drug molecules are in the bloodstream, not for the life of the platelet (approximately 1 week) as aspirin does. Thus, they are not prescribed therapeutically for antiplatelet effects.

Effects of NSAIDs on Other Drugs

NSAIDs decrease effects of certain drugs. With **angiotensin-converting enzyme (ACE) inhibitors,** decreased antihypertensive effects are probably caused by sodium and water retention. With **beta blockers,** decreased antihypertensive effects are attributed to NSAID inhibition of renal prostaglandin synthesis, which allows unopposed pressor systems to produce hypertension. With **diuretics,** decreased effects on hypertension and edema are attributed to retention of sodium and water.

NSAIDs increase effects of other drugs. With **anticoagulants,** prothrombin time may be prolonged, and risks of bleeding are increased by NSAID-induced gastric irritation and antiplatelet effects. With **cyclosporine,** nephrotoxicity associated with both drugs may be increased. With **digoxin,** ibuprofen and indomethacin may increase serum levels. With **phenytoin,** serum drug levels and pharmacologic effects, including adverse or toxic effects, may be increased. With **lithium,** serum drug levels and risk of toxicity may be increased (except with sulindac, which has no effect or may decrease serum lithium levels). With **methotrexate** (MTX), risks of toxicity (eg, stomatitis, bone marrow suppression, nephrotoxicity) may be increased. Celecoxib and meloxicam apparently do *not* increase MTX toxicity.

Use of Acetaminophen

Acetaminophen is effective and widely used for the treatment of pain and fever. It has two major advantages over aspirin: acetaminophen does not cause gastric irritation or increase the risk of bleeding. It is the drug of choice for children with febrile illness (because of the association of aspirin with Reye's syndrome); elderly adults with impaired renal function (because aspirin and NSAIDs may cause further impairment); and pregnant women (because aspirin is associated with several maternal and fetal disorders, including bleeding).

Despite the high degree of safety of acetaminophen when used appropriately, it is probably not the drug of choice for people with hepatitis or other liver disorders or for those who drink substantial amounts of alcoholic beverages. The major drawback to acetaminophen use is potentially fatal liver damage with overdose. The kidneys and myocardium may also be damaged.

Toxicity: Recognition and Management

Acetaminophen poisoning may occur with a single large dose (possibly as little as 6 g, but usually 10–15 g) or with chronic ingestion of excessive doses (5–8 g/day for several weeks or 3–4 g/day for 1 year). Potentially fatal hepatotoxicity is the main concern and is most likely to occur with doses of 20 grams or more. Metabolism of acetaminophen produces a toxic metabolite that is normally inactivated by combining with glutathione. In overdose situations, the supply of glutathione is depleted and the toxic metabolite accumulates and directly damages liver cells. Acute renal failure may also occur.

Prevention

The recommended maximum daily dose is 4 grams for adults; additional amounts constitute an overdose. Ingestion of an overdose may be accidental or intentional. One contributing factor may be that some people think the drug is so safe that they can take any amount without harm. Another may be that people take the drug in several formulations without calculating or realizing that they are taking potentially harmful amounts. For example, numerous brand names of acetaminophen are available OTC, and acetaminophen is an ingredient in many prescription and OTC combination products (eg, Percocet; OTC cold, flu, headache, and sinus remedies). For chronic alcohol abusers, short-term ingestion of usual therapeutic doses may cause hepatotoxicity and it is recommended that these persons ingest no more than 2 grams daily.

If they ingest three or more alcoholic drinks daily, they should avoid acetaminophen or ask a physician before using even small doses. Another recommendation is to limit duration of use (5 days or less in children, 10 days or less in adults, and 3 days in both adults and children when used to reduce fever) unless directed by a physician.

Because of multiple reports of liver damage from acetaminophen poisoning, the FDA has strengthened the warning on products containing acetaminophen and emphasized that the maximum dose of 4 grams daily, from all sources, should not be exceeded.

Signs and Symptoms

Early symptoms (12–24 hours after ingestion) are nonspecific (eg, anorexia, nausea, vomiting, diaphoresis) and may not be considered serious or important enough to report or seek treatment. At 24 to 48 hours, symptoms may subside but tests of liver function (eg, aspartate aminotransferase, alanine aminotransferase, bilirubin, prothrombin time) begin to show increased levels. Later manifestations may include jaundice, vomiting, and CNS stimulation with excitement and delirium, followed by vascular collapse, coma, and death. Peak hepatotoxicity occurs in 3 to 4 days; recovery in nonfatal overdoses occurs in 7 to 8 days.

Plasma acetaminophen levels should be obtained when an overdose is known or suspected, preferably within 4 hours after ingestion and every 24 hours for several days. Minimal hepatotoxicity is associated with plasma levels of less than 120 micrograms per milliliter at 4 hours after ingestion, or less than 30 micrograms per milliliter at 12 hours after ingestion. With blood levels greater than 300 micrograms per milliliter at 4 hours after ingestion, about 90% of clients develop liver damage.

Treatment

Gastric lavage is recommended if overdose is detected within 4 hours after ingestion and activated charcoal can be given to inhibit absorption. In addition, the specific antidote is acetylcysteine (Mucomyst), a mucolytic agent given by inhalation in respiratory disorders. For acetaminophen poisoning, it is usually given orally (dosage is listed with other antidotes in Chap. 2). The drug provides cysteine, a precursor substance required for the synthesis of glutathione. Glutathione combines with a toxic metabolite and decreases hepatotoxicity if acetylcysteine is given. Acetylcysteine is most beneficial if given within 8 to 10 hours of acetaminophen ingestion, but may be helpful within 36 hours. It does not reverse damage that has already occurred.

APPLYING YOUR KNOWLEDGE 7-4
How much acetaminophen is Julie possibly consuming in a 24-hour time period, and what danger does this present?

Treatment of Specific Disorders

Arthritis

The primary goals of treatment are to control pain and inflammation and to minimize immobilization and disability. Rest, exercise, physical therapy, and drugs are used to attain these goals. Few of these measures prevent or slow joint destruction.

Osteoarthritis (OA)

The main goal of drug therapy is relief of pain. Acetaminophen is probably the initial drug of choice. For clients whose pain is inadequately relieved by acetaminophen, an NSAID is usually given. Ibuprofen and other propionic acid derivatives are often used, although available NSAIDs have comparable effectiveness. A drug may be given for 2 or 3 weeks on a trial basis. If therapeutic benefits occur, the drug may be continued; if no benefits seem evident or toxicity occurs, another drug may be tried. A COX-2 inhibitor may be preferred for clients at high risk of GI ulceration and bleeding. NSAIDs are usually given in analgesic doses for OA, rather than the larger anti-inflammatory doses given for RA.

Additional treatments for knee OA include topical capsaicin; oral chondroitin and glucosamine; and intra-articular injections of corticosteroids (see Chap. 23) or hyaluronic acid (eg, Synvisc, a product that helps restore the "shock-absorbing" ability of joint structures). Clients who continue to have severe pain and functional impairment despite medical treatment may need knee replacement surgery.

Rheumatoid Arthritis (RA)

Acetaminophen may relieve pain; aspirin or another NSAID may relieve pain and inflammation. Aspirin is effective, but many people are unable to tolerate the adverse effects associated with anti-inflammatory doses. When aspirin is used, dosage usually ranges between 2 and 6 grams daily but should be individualized to relieve symptoms, maintain therapeutic salicylate blood levels, and minimize adverse effects. For people who cannot take aspirin, another NSAID may be given. For those who cannot take aspirin or a nonselective NSAID because of GI irritation, peptic ulcer disease, bleeding disorders, or other contraindications, the selective COX-2 inhibitor NSAID, celecoxib, may be preferred. NSAIDs are usually given in larger, anti-inflammatory doses for RA, rather than the smaller, analgesic doses given for OA.

Second-line drugs for moderate or severe RA include corticosteroids and immunosuppressants. The goal of treatment with corticosteroids is to relieve symptoms. The treatment goal with immunosuppressants is to relieve symptoms and also slow tissue damage (so-called *disease-modifying effects*). Both groups of drugs may cause serious adverse effects, including greatly increased susceptibility to infection. MTX, which is also used in cancer chemotherapy, is given in smaller doses for RA. It is unknown whether MTX has disease-modifying effects or just improves symptoms and quality of life. About 75% of clients have a beneficial response, with improvement usually evident within 4 to 8 weeks (ie, less morning stiffness, pain, joint edema, and fatigue).

Three newer immunosuppressants used to treat RA are etanercept (Enbrel), infliximab (Remicade), and leflunomide (Arava) (see Chap. 41). Clinical improvement usually occurs within a few weeks. One of these drugs may be used alone or given along with MTX in clients whose symptoms are inadequately controlled by MTX alone.

Hyperuricemia and Gout

Opinions differ regarding treatment of asymptomatic hyperuricemia. Some authorities do not believe that drug therapy is indicated, and others believe that lowering serum uric acid levels may prevent joint inflammation and renal calculi. Allopurinol, probenecid, or sulfinpyrazone may be given for this purpose. Colchicine also should be given for several weeks to prevent acute attacks of gout while serum uric acid levels are being lowered. During initial administration of these drugs, a high fluid intake (to produce approximately 2000 mL of urine per day) and alkaline urine are recommended to prevent renal calculi. Urate crystals are more likely to precipitate in acid urine.

Acute Migraine

For infrequent or mild migraine attacks, acetaminophen, aspirin, or other NSAIDs may be effective. For example, NSAIDs are often effective to treat migraines associated with menstruation. For moderate to severe migraine attacks, sumatriptan and related drugs are effective and they cause fewer adverse effects than ergot preparations. They are usually well tolerated; adverse effects are relatively minor and usually brief. However, because they are strong vasoconstrictors, they should not be taken by people with coronary artery disease or hypertension. They are also expensive compared with other antimigraine drugs. If an ergot preparation is used, it should be given at the onset of headache, and the client should lie down in a quiet, darkened room.

Perioperative Use

Aspirin should generally be avoided for 1 to 2 weeks before and after surgery because it increases the risk of bleeding. Most other NSAIDs should be discontinued approximately 3 days before surgery; nabumetone and piroxicam have long half-lives and must be discontinued approximately 1 week before surgery. After surgery, especially after relatively minor procedures, such as dental extractions and episiotomies, an NSAID may be used to relieve pain. Caution is needed because of increased risk of bleeding, and the drug should not be given if there are other risk factors for bleeding. In addition, ketorolac, the only injectable NSAID, has been used to relieve postoperative pain. This drug has several advantages over opioid analgesics, but bleeding and hematomas may occur.

Cancer

Cancer often produces chronic pain from tumor invasion of tissues or complications of treatment (chemotherapy, surgery, or radiation). As with acute pain, acetaminophen, aspirin, or other NSAIDs prevent sensitization of peripheral pain receptors by inhibiting prostaglandin formation. They are especially effective for pain associated with bone metastases. For mild pain, acetaminophen or an NSAID may be used alone; for moderate to severe pain, these drugs may be continued and an opioid analgesic added. Nonopioid and opioid analgesics may be given together or alternated; a combination of analgesics is often needed to provide optimal pain relief. Aspirin is contraindicated for the client receiving chemotherapy that depresses the bone marrow because of the high risk of thrombocytopenia and bleeding.

Use in Special Populations

Use in Children

Acetaminophen is usually the drug of choice for pain or fever in children. Children seem less susceptible to liver toxicity than adults, apparently because they form less of the toxic metabolite during metabolism of acetaminophen. However, there is a risk of overdose and hepatotoxicity because acetaminophen is a very common ingredient in OTC cold, flu, fever, and pain remedies. An overdose can occur with large doses of one product or smaller amounts of several different products. In addition, toxicity has occurred when parents or caregivers have given the liquid concentration intended for children to infants. The concentrations are different and cannot be given interchangeably. Infants' doses are measured with a dropper, and children's doses are measured by teaspoon. Caution parents and caregivers to ask pediatricians for written instructions on giving acetaminophen to their children, to read the labels of all drug products very carefully, and to avoid giving children acetaminophen from multiple sources.

Ibuprofen also may be given for fever. Aspirin is not recommended because of its association with Reye's syndrome, a life-threatening illness characterized by encephalopathy, hepatic damage, and other serious problems. Reye's syndrome usually occurs after a viral infection, such as influenza or chickenpox, during which aspirin was given for fever. A rare, but serious, adverse effect of ibuprofen and NSAIDs in children is the occurrence of severe skin reactions, such as Stevens-Johnson syndrome or toxic epidermal necrolysis. For children with juvenile RA, aspirin, ibuprofen, naproxen, or tolmetin may be given. Pediatric indications for use and dosages have not been established for most of the other drugs.

When an NSAID is given during late pregnancy to prevent premature labor, it may adversely affect the kidneys of the fetus. When an NSAID is given shortly after birth to close a patent ductus arteriosus, it may adversely affect the kidneys of the neonate.

Use in Older Adults

Acetaminophen is usually safe in recommended doses unless liver damage is present or the person is a chronic alcohol abuser. Aspirin is usually safe in the small doses prescribed for prevention of myocardial infarction and stroke (antiplatelet effects). Aspirin and other NSAIDs are probably safe in therapeutic doses for occasional use as an analgesic or antipyretic. However, the incidence of musculoskeletal disorders (eg, OA) is higher in older adults, and an NSAID is often prescribed. Long-term use increases the risk of serious GI bleeding. Small doses, gradual increments, and taking the drug with food or a full glass of water may decrease GI effects. COX-2 inhibitor NSAIDs may be especially beneficial in older adults because they are less likely to cause gastric ulceration and bleeding. Older adults also are more likely than younger adults to acquire nephrotoxicity with NSAIDs, especially with high doses or long-term use, because the drugs may reduce blood flow to the kidneys.

Use in Clients With Renal Impairment

Acetaminophen, aspirin, and other NSAIDs can cause or aggravate renal impairment even though they are eliminated mainly by hepatic metabolism. Acetaminophen is normally metabolized in the liver to metabolites that are excreted through the kidneys; these metabolites may accumulate in clients with renal failure. In addition, acetaminophen is nephrotoxic in overdose because it forms a metabolite that attacks kidney cells and may cause necrosis. Aspirin is nephrotoxic in high doses, and protein binding of aspirin is reduced in clients with renal failure so that blood levels of active drug are higher. In addition, aspirin and other NSAIDs can decrease blood flow in the kidneys by inhibiting synthesis of prostaglandins that dilate renal blood vessels. When renal blood flow is normal, these prostaglandins have limited activity. However, when renal blood flow is decreased, synthesis of these prostaglandins is increased, and they protect the kidneys from ischemia and hypoxia by antagonizing the vasoconstrictive effects of angiotensin II, norepinephrine, and other substances. Thus, in clients who depend on prostaglandins to maintain an adequate renal blood flow, the prostaglandin-blocking effects of aspirin and NSAIDs result in constriction of renal arteries and arterioles; decreased renal blood flow; decreased glomerular filtration rate; and retention of salt and water. NSAIDs can also cause kidney damage by other mechanisms, including a hypersensitivity reaction that leads to acute renal failure, manifested by proteinuria, hematuria, or pyuria. Biopsy reports usually indicate inflammatory reactions such as glomerulonephritis or interstitial nephritis.

People at highest risk from the use of these drugs are those with pre-existing renal impairment; those older than 50 years of age; those taking diuretics; and those with hypertension, diabetes, or heart failure. Measures to prevent or minimize renal damage include avoiding nephrotoxic drugs when possible; treating the disorders that increase risk of renal damage; stopping the NSAID if renal impairment occurs; monitoring renal function; reducing dosage; and maintaining hydration.

The role of COX-2 inhibitor NSAIDs in renal impairment is not clear. Although it was hoped that these drugs would have protective effects on the kidneys as they do on the stomach, studies indicate that their effects on the kidneys are similar to those of the older NSAIDs.

Use in Clients With Hepatic Impairment

Except for acetaminophen, the effects of NSAIDs on liver function and the effects of hepatic impairment on most NSAIDs are largely unknown. Because the drugs are metabolized in the liver, they should be used with caution and in lower doses in people with impaired hepatic function or a history of liver disease. For example, some authorities recommend a maximum daily dose of 2 grams for people with hepatitis (compared with a maximum daily dose of 4 grams for people who do not have impaired liver function).

Acetaminophen can cause fatal liver necrosis in overdose because it forms a metabolite that can destroy liver cells. The hepatotoxic metabolite is formed more rapidly when drug-metabolizing enzymes in the liver have been stimulated by ingestion of alcohol; cigarette smoking; and drugs such as anticonvulsants and others. Thus, alcoholics are at high risk of hepatotoxicity with usual therapeutic doses.

In cirrhotic liver disease, naproxen and sulindac may be metabolized more slowly and aggravate hepatic impairment if dosage is not reduced. In liver impairment, blood levels of oral sumatriptan and related antimigraine drugs may be high because less drug is metabolized on its first pass through the liver and a higher proportion of a dose reaches the systemic circulation. Thus, the drugs should be used cautiously, possibly in reduced dosage.

Use in Clients With Critical Illness

Acetaminophen, aspirin, and other NSAIDs are infrequently used during critical illness, partly because they are usually given orally and many clients are unable to take oral medications. Pain is more likely to be treated with injectable opioid analgesics in this population. Acetaminophen may be given by rectal suppository for pain or fever in clients who are unable to take oral drugs.

These drugs may be risk factors for renal or hepatic impairment or bleeding disorders. For example, if a client has a history of taking aspirin, including the low doses prescribed for antithrombotic effects, there is a risk of bleeding from common therapeutic (eg, intramuscular injections, venipuncture, inserting urinary catheters or GI tubes) or diagnostic (eg, drawing blood, angiography) procedures. If a client has been taking an NSAID regularly, he or she may be more likely to experience renal failure if the critical illness causes dehydration or requires treatment with one or more nephrotoxic drugs. If a client presents with acute renal failure, NSAID ingestion must be considered as a possible cause. If a client is known to drink alcoholic beverages and take acetaminophen, he or she may be more likely to experience impaired liver function.

Use in Home Care

Home use of acetaminophen, NSAIDs, and other analgesic drugs is extremely widespread. Many people are aware of the beneficial effects of these drugs in relieving pain, but they may not be adequately informed about potential problems associated with use of the drugs. Thus, the home care nurse may need to assist clients in perceiving a need for additional information and provide that information. Specific suggestions include reading and following instructions on labels of OTC analgesics, not exceeding recommended dosages without consulting a health care provider, and avoiding multiple sources of acetaminophen or NSAIDs (eg, multiple OTC NSAIDs or an OTC and a prescription NSAID). In addition, adverse drug effects should be reviewed with clients, and clients should be assessed for characteristics (eg, older age group, renal impairment, overuse of the drugs) that increase the risks of adverse effects. The accompanying Research Brief illustrates the importance of educating individuals about the hazards of excessive, chronic use of analgesic medications.

NURSING ACTIONS

Analgesic–Antipyretic–Anti-Inflammatory, and Related Drugs

NURSING ACTIONS	RATIONALE/EXPLANATION
1. Administer accurately	
a. Give aspirin and other nonsteroidal anti-inflammatory drugs (NSAIDs) with a full glass of water or other fluid and with or just after food.	To decrease gastric irritation. Even though food delays absorption and decreases peak plasma levels of some of the drugs, it is probably safer to give them with food. Meloxicam may be given without regard to food.

NURSING ACTIONS	RATIONALE/EXPLANATION
b. Do not crush tablets or open capsules of long-acting dosage forms and instruct patients not to crush or chew the products. Examples include:	Breaking the tablets or capsules allows faster absorption, destroys the long-acting feature, and increases risks of adverse effects and toxicity from overdose.

    (1) Enteric-coated aspirin (eg, Ecotrin)

    (2) Diclofenac sodium (Voltaren or Voltaren XR)

    (3) Diflunisal (Dolobid)

    (4) Etodolac (Lodine XL)

    (5) Indomethacin or Indocin SR

    (6) Ketoprofen or Oruvail extended-release capsules

    (7) Naproxen delayed-release (EC-Naprosyn) or naproxen sodium controlled-release (Naprelan)

c. Give antimigraine preparations at the onset of headache.	To prevent development of more severe symptoms
d. Give rapidly disintegrating tablets for migraine relief by placing tablet on the tongue. Do not give with water.	Allows drug to dissolve and be absorbed

2. Observe for therapeutic effects

a. When drugs are given for pain, observe for decreased or absent manifestations of pain.	Pain relief is usually evident within 30–60 minutes.
b. When drugs are given for fever, record temperature every 2–4 hours, and observe for a decrease.	
c. When drugs are given for arthritis and other inflammatory disorders, observe for decreased pain, edema, redness, heat, and stiffness of joints. Also observe for increased joint mobility and exercise tolerance.	With aspirin, improvement is usually noted within 24–48 hours. With most of the NSAIDs, 1–2 weeks may be required before beneficial effects become evident.
d. When colchicine is given for acute gouty arthritis, observe for decreased pain and inflammation in involved joints.	Therapeutic effects occur within 4–12 hours after intravenous colchicine administration and 24–48 hours after oral administration. Edema may not decrease for several days.
e. When allopurinol, probenecid, or sulfinpyrazone is given for hyperuricemia, observe for normal serum uric acid level (approximately 2–8 mg/100 mL).	Serum uric acid levels usually decrease to normal range within 1–3 weeks.
f. When allopurinol, probenecid, or sulfinpyrazone is given for chronic gout, observe for decreased size of tophi, absence of new tophi, decreased joint pain and increased joint mobility, and normal serum uric acid levels.	
g. When triptans or ergot preparations are given to treat migraine headache, observe for relief of symptoms.	Therapeutic effects are usually evident within 15–30 minutes.

3. Observe for adverse effects

    a. With analgesic–antipyretic–anti-inflammatory and antigout agents, observe for:

(1) Gastrointestinal problems—anorexia, nausea, vomiting, diarrhea, bleeding, ulceration	These are common reactions, more likely with aspirin, indomethacin, piroxicam, sulindac, tolmetin, colchicine, and sulfinpyrazone and less likely with acetaminophen, celecoxib, diflunisal, etodolac, fenoprofen, ibuprofen, and naproxen.
(2) Hematologic problems—petechiae, bruises, hematuria, melena, epistaxis, and bone marrow depression (leukopenia, thrombocytopenia, anemia)	Bone marrow depression is more likely to occur with colchicine.
(3) Central nervous system effects—headache, dizziness, fainting, ataxia, insomnia, confusion, drowsiness	These effects are relatively common with indomethacin and may occur with most of the other drugs, especially with high dosages.

(continued)

NURSING ACTIONS	RATIONALE/EXPLANATION
(4) Skin rashes, dermatitis	Rare but serious skin reactions, such as Stevens-Johnson syndrome or toxic epidermal necrolysis, are possible.
(5) Hypersensitivity reactions with dyspnea, bronchospasm, skin rashes	These effects may simulate asthma in people who are allergic to aspirin and aspirin-like drugs; most likely to occur in patients with a history of nasal polyps.
(6) Tinnitus, blurred vision	Tinnitus (ringing or roaring in the ears) is a classic sign of aspirin overdose (salicylate intoxication). It occurs with NSAIDs as well.
(7) Nephrotoxicity—decreased urine output; increased blood urea nitrogen (BUN); increased serum creatinine; hyperkalemia; retention of sodium and water with resultant edema	More likely to occur in people with pre-existing renal impairment
(8) Cardiovascular effects—increased hypertension, edema. With long-term use, increased risk of myocardial infarction or stroke.	NSAIDs can cause sodium and water retention. Mechanism of adverse cardiovascular events is not fully understood; however, they may be partially explained by inhibition of prostaglandin I_2 formation, which increases risk of thromboembolic events.
(9) Hepatotoxicity—liver damage or failure	Occurs mainly with acetaminophen, in overdose or in people with underlying liver disease

b. With triptan antimigraine drugs, observe for:

NURSING ACTIONS	RATIONALE/EXPLANATION
(1) Chest tightness or pain, hypertension, drowsiness, dizziness, nausea, fatigue, paresthesias	Most adverse effects are mild and transient. However, because of their vasoconstrictive effects, they may cause or aggravate angina pectoris and hypertension.

c. With ergot antimigraine drugs, observe for:

NURSING ACTIONS	RATIONALE/EXPLANATION
(1) Nausea, vomiting, diarrhea	These drugs have a direct effect on the vomiting center of the brain and stimulate contraction of gastrointestinal smooth muscle.
(2) Symptoms of ergot poisoning (ergotism)—coolness, numbness, and tingling of the extremities; headache; vomiting; dizziness; thirst; convulsions; weak pulse; confusion; angina-like chest pain; transient tachycardia or bradycardia; muscle weakness and pain; cyanosis; gangrene of the extremities	The ergot alkaloids are highly toxic; poisoning may be acute or chronic. Acute poisoning is rare; chronic poisoning is usually a result of overdosage. Circulatory impairments may result from vasoconstriction and vascular insufficiency. Large doses also damage capillary endothelium and may cause thrombosis and occlusion. Gangrene of extremities rarely occurs with usual doses unless peripheral vascular disease or other contraindications are also present.
(3) Hypertension	Blood pressure may rise as a result of generalized vasoconstriction induced by the ergot preparation.
(4) Hypersensitivity reactions—local edema and pruritus, anaphylactic shock	Allergic reactions are relatively uncommon.

4. **Observe for drug interactions**

a. Drugs that *increase* effects of aspirin and other NSAIDs:

NURSING ACTIONS	RATIONALE/EXPLANATION
(1) Acidifying agents (eg, ascorbic acid)	Acidify urine and thereby decrease the urinary excretion rate of salicylates
(2) Alcohol	Increases gastric irritation and occult blood loss
(3) Anticoagulants, oral	Increase risk of bleeding substantially. People taking anticoagulants should avoid aspirin and aspirin-containing products.
(4) Codeine, hydrocodone, oxycodone	Additive analgesic effects because of different mechanisms of action. Aspirin or an NSAID can often be used with these drugs to provide adequate pain relief without excessive doses and sedation.
(5) Corticosteroids (eg, prednisone)	Additive gastric irritation and possible ulcerogenic effects

b. Drug that *increases* effects of celecoxib:

NURSING ACTIONS	RATIONALE/EXPLANATION
(1) Fluconazole (and possibly other azole antifungal drugs)	Inhibits liver enzymes that normally metabolize celecoxib; increases serum celecoxib levels

NURSING ACTIONS	RATIONALE/EXPLANATION
c. Drugs that *decrease* effects of aspirin and other NSAIDs:	
(1) Alkalinizing agents (eg, sodium bicarbonate)	Increase rate of renal excretion
(2) Misoprostol (Cytotec)	This drug, a prostaglandin, was developed specifically to prevent aspirin and NSAID-induced gastric ulcers.
d. Drug that *decreases* effects of fenoprofen:	
(1) Phenobarbital	Induces drug-metabolizing enzymes in the liver and decreases blood levels of fenoprofen. Dosage of fenoprofen may need to be increased if phenobarbital is started, or decreased if phenobarbital is discontinued.
e. Drugs that *increase* effects of indomethacin:	
(1) Anticoagulants, oral	Increase risk of gastrointestinal bleeding. Indomethacin causes gastric irritation and is considered an ulcerogenic drug.
(2) Corticosteroids	Increase ulcerogenic effect
(3) Salicylates	Increase ulcerogenic effect
(4) Heparin	Increases risk of bleeding. These drugs should not be used concurrently.
f. Drugs that *decrease* effects of indomethacin:	
(1) Antacids	Delay absorption from the gastrointestinal tract
g. Drugs that *decrease* effects of allopurinol, probenecid, and sulfinpyrazone:	
(1) Alkalinizing agents (eg, sodium bicarbonate)	Decrease risks of renal calculi from precipitation of uric acid crystals. Alkalinizing agents are recommended until serum uric acid levels return to normal.
(2) Colchicine	Decreases attacks of acute gout. Recommended for concurrent use until serum uric acid levels return to normal.
(3) Diuretics	Decrease uricosuric effects
(4) Salicylates	Mainly at salicylate doses of less than 2 grams per day, decrease uricosuric effects of probenecid and sulfinpyrazone but do not interfere with the action of allopurinol. Salicylates are uricosuric at doses greater than 5 grams per day.
h. Drugs that *increase* effects of ergot preparations:	
(1) Vasoconstrictors (eg, ephedrine, epinephrine, phenylephrine)	Additive vasoconstriction with risks of severe, persistent hypertension and intracranial hemorrhage
i. Drugs that *increase* effects of triptan antimigraine drugs:	
(1) Monoamine oxidase inhibitors (MAOIs)	Increase serum levels of triptans and may cause serious adverse effects, including cardiac dysrhythmias and myocardial infarction. **Triptans and MAOIs must not be taken concurrently; a triptan should not be taken for at least 2 weeks after an MAOI is discontinued.**
(2) Ergot preparations	**Triptans and ergot preparations should not be taken concurrently or within 24 hours of each other, because severe hypertension and stroke may occur.**
j. Drugs that *increase* effects of eletriptan (Relpax):	
(1) Any drug that inhibits CYP3A4 enzyme metabolism. Examples include ketoconazole (Nizoral), itraconazole (Sporanox), clarithromycin (Biaxin), ritonavir (Norvir), and nelfinavir (Viracept).	Inhibition of CYP3A4 enzymes increases the amount of eletriptan that remains in the body, resulting in toxicity.

RESEARCH BRIEF

Rebound Headaches Associated With Overuse of Analgesics

SOURCE:
Grassi, L., Andrasid, F., D'Amico, D., Usai, S., Rigamonti, A., Leone, M., & Bussone, G. (2003). Treatment of chronic daily headache with medication overuse. *Neurological Sciences, 24*(2), S125–S127.

SUMMARY:
Excessive use of simple analgesics and analgesics containing sedatives or caffeine, triptans, opioids, or ergotamine are believed to play a role in triggering overuse headaches, also called "rebound headaches." The most common clinical approach to management of overuse headaches involves cessation of the overused medication accompanied by temporary treatment of the rebound headache. Clients must be educated about the risks of chronic use of analgesics and encouraged to limit use of abortive and prophylactic migraine drugs appropriately. Use of nonpharmacologic therapies such as psychotherapy, biofeedback, and relaxation training may also be useful.

NURSING IMPLICATIONS:
The nurse should include the risks of rebound headache with chronic use of analgesic medications in the teaching plan for clients with headaches. Nonpharmacologic measures to relieve or prevent headache pain should be encouraged as part of the overall treatment plan.

APPLYING YOUR KNOWLEDGE: ANSWERS

7-1 GI bleeding. Taking ASA, caffeine, and naproxen sodium may lead to GI irritation and bleeding.

7-2 It is necessary to recognize that cold and flu medication frequently has acetaminophen added for analgesic effect. The cumulative effects of multiple medications with acetaminophen may lead to hepatic failure.

7-3 The client needs to increase fluid intake to 2 to 3 liters of fluid a day and take drugs with food. This will decrease gastric irritation and help maintain kidney function.

7-4 The total amount of acetaminophen may approach or exceed 9000 milligrams (9 g) in a 24-hour period, and this may lead to hepatic damage. The maximum recommended daily dose of acetaminophen should not exceed 4 grams in 24 hours.

Review and Application Exercises

Short Answer Exercises

1. How do aspirin and other NSAIDs produce analgesic, antipyretic, anti-inflammatory, and antiplatelet effects?

2. What adverse effects occur with aspirin and other NSAIDs, especially with daily ingestion?

3. Compare and contrast the uses and effects of aspirin, ibuprofen, and acetaminophen.

4. For a 6-year-old child with fever, would aspirin or acetaminophen be preferred? Why?

5. For a 50-year-old adult with RA, would aspirin, another NSAID, or acetaminophen be preferred? Why?

6. For a 75-year-old adult with OA and a long history of "stomach trouble," would aspirin, another NSAID, or acetaminophen be preferred? Why?

7. What are some nursing interventions to decrease the adverse effects of aspirin, other NSAIDs, and acetaminophen?

8. When teaching a client about home use of aspirin, other NSAIDs, and acetaminophen, what information must be included?

9. What is the rationale for using acetylcysteine in the treatment of acetaminophen toxicity?

10. What is the rationale for combining opioid and nonopioid analgesics in the treatment of moderate pain?

11. If you were a client, what information do you think would be most helpful in home management of migraine?

NCLEX-Style Questions

12. The nurse would question the pain medication order for which of the following clients?
    a. acetaminophen for OA in a 60-year-old man with peptic ulcer disease
    b. celecoxib for RA in a 48-year-old woman taking warfarin
    c. acetaminophen for a headache in a 55-year-old man scheduled for surgery in the morning
    d. aspirin for a feverish 12-year-old child with influenza

13. The most important laboratory tests the nurse should evaluate for a client who takes an overdose of acetaminophen are

a. plasma salicylate

b. aspartate aminotransferase and alanine amino-transferase, bilirubin, and prothrombin time

c. blood urea nitrogen and creatinine

d. hemoglobin, hematocrit, and complete blood count

14. Which of the following nursing interventions is most important when allopurinol is prescribed for the treatment of gout?

a. Monitor stools for occult blood.

b. Encourage an acid ash diet to acidify the urine.

c. Encourage fluid intake of at least 3000 mL of fluid per day.

d. Encourage the use of aspirin when an OTC analgesic is necessary.

15. Prior to administering sumatriptan for migraine headaches, the nurse should assess for

a. bradycardia

b. elevated blood glucose level

c. adequate urine output

d. use of ergot preparations in past 24 hours

Selected References

Ashkenazi, A., & Silberstein, S. D. (2003) The evolving management of migraine. *Current Opinion in Neurology, 16*(3), 341–345.

Barkin, R. L. & Barkin, D. (2001). Pharmacologic management of acute and chronic pain. *Southern Medical Journal, 94*(8), 756–812.

Bush, E. S., & Mayer, S. E. (2001). 5-Hydroxytryptamine (serotonin): Receptor agonists and antagonists. In J. G. Hardman & L. E. Limbird (Eds.), *Goodman & Gilman's The pharmacological basis of therapeutics* (10th ed., pp. 269–289). New York: McGraw-Hill.

Drug facts and comparisons. (Updated monthly). St. Louis: Facts and Comparisons.

Fetrow, C. W., Avila, J. R., & Margolis, S. (2003). *Professional's handbook of complementary & alternative medicines.* Springhouse, PA: Springhouse.

Fitzgerald, G. A. (2004). Coxibs and cardiovascular disease. *New England Journal of Medicine, 351*(17), 1709–1711.

Grassi, L., Andrasid, F., D'Amico, D., Usai, S., Rigamonti, A., Leone, M., & Bussone, G. (2003). Treatment of chronic daily headache with medication overuse. *Neurological Sciences, 24*(2), S125–S127.

Henderson, C. J. (2003–2004). Dietary outcomes in osteoarthritis disease management. *Bulletin on the Rheumatic Diseases: Evidence-Based Management of Rheumatic Diseases.* Retrieved March 22, 2004, from http://www.arthritis.org/research/Bulletin/Vol52No12/Introduction.asp

Hutchison, R. (2004). Cox-2 selective NSAIDS. *American Journal of Nursing, 104*(3), 52–56.

Richy, F., Bruyere, O., Cucherat, M., Henrotin, Y., & Reginster, J. Y. (2003). Structural and symptomatic efficacy of glucosamine and chondroitin in knee osteoarthritis, a comprehensive meta-analysis. *Archives of Internal Medicine, 163*, 1514–1522.

Roberts, L. J., & Morrow, J. D. (2001). Analgesic-antipyretic and anti-inflammatory agents and drugs employed in the treatment of gout. In J. G. Hardman & L. E. Limbird (Eds.), *Goodman & Gilman's The pharmacological basis of therapeutics* (10th ed., pp. 687–727). New York: McGraw-Hill.

Theodosakis, J. (1997). *The arthritis cure.* New York: St Martin's.

U.S. Food and Drug Administration. (2005). *FDA news: FDA announces series of changes to the class of marketed non-steroidal anti-inflammatory drugs (NSAIDs).* Retrieved July 25, 2005, from http://www.fda.gov/bbs/topics/news/2005/NEW01171.html

U.S. Food and Drug Administration. (2004). *FDA talk paper: FDA issues public advisory recommending limited use of cox-2 inhibitors.* Retrieved July 25, 2005, from http://www.fda.gov/bbs/topics/ANSWERS/2004/ans01336.html

Antianxiety and Sedative-Hypnotic Drugs

OBJECTIVES

After studying this chapter, you will be able to:

1. Discuss characteristics, sources, and signs and symptoms of anxiety.
2. Discuss functions of sleep and consequences of sleep deprivation.
3. Describe nondrug interventions to decrease anxiety and insomnia.
4. List characteristics of benzodiazepine antianxiety and hypnotic drugs in terms of mechanism of action, indications for use, nursing process implications, and potential for abuse and dependence.
5. Describe strategies for preventing, recognizing, or treating benzodiazepine withdrawal reactions.
6. Contrast characteristics of selected nonbenzodiazepines and benzodiazepines.
7. Teach clients guidelines for rational, safe use of antianxiety and sedative-hypnotic drugs.
8. Discuss the use of flumazenil and other treatment measures for overdose of benzodiazepines.

APPLYING YOUR KNOWLEDGE

Gertrude Portman is an 88-year-old woman who has been admitted for observation due to a syncopal episode. She is in the early stages of Alzheimer's disease and appears very anxious and agitated. Mrs. Portman has the following medical orders for sedation:

Alprazolam (Xanax) 0.25–0.5 mg 2–4 times daily for anxiety

Venlafaxine (Effexor XR) 75 mg daily

Zolpidem (Ambien) 5 mg PO at half strength (HS) for sleep

INTRODUCTION

Antianxiety and sedative-hypnotic agents are central nervous system (CNS) depressants that have similar effects. Antianxiety drugs and sedatives promote relaxation, and hypnotics produce sleep. The difference between the effects depends largely on dosage. Large doses of antianxiety and sedative agents produce sleep, and small doses of hypnotics produce antianxiety or sedative effects. In addition, therapeutic doses of hypnotics taken at bedtime may have residual sedative effects ("morning hangover") the following day. Because these drugs produce varying degrees of CNS depression, some are also used as anticonvulsants and anesthetics.

The main drugs used to treat anxiety and insomnia are the *benzodiazepines.* In addition, antidepressants (ie, tricyclics, selective serotonin reuptake inhibitors [SSRIs], and newer miscellaneous drugs) are increasingly being used to treat some types of anxiety. These medications are discussed in more detail in Chapter 10. The barbiturates, a historically important group of CNS depressants, are obsolete for most uses, including treatment of anxiety and insomnia. A few may be used as intravenous general anesthetics (see Appendix F), phenobarbital may be used to treat seizure disorders (see Chap. 11), and some are abused (see Chap. 14).

To promote understanding of the uses and effects of both benzodiazepines and nonbenzodiazepines, anxiety and insomnia are described in the following sections. The clinical manifestations of these disorders are similar and overlapping; that is, daytime anxiety may be manifested as nighttime difficulty in sleeping because the person cannot "turn off" worries, and difficulty in sleeping may be manifested as anxiety, fatigue, and decreased ability to function during usual waking hours.

Anxiety

Anxiety is a common disorder that may be referred to as *nervousness, tension, worry,* or other terms that denote an unpleasant feeling. It occurs when a person perceives a situation as threatening to physical, emotional, social, or economic well-being. Anxiety may occur in association with everyday events related to home, work, school, social activities, and chronic illness, or it may occur episodically, in association with acute illness, death, divorce, losing a job, starting a new job, or taking a test. *Situational anxiety* is a normal response to a stressful situation. It may be beneficial when it motivates the person toward constructive, problem-solving, coping activities. Symptoms may be quite severe, but they usually last only 2 to 3 weeks.

Although there is no clear boundary between normal and abnormal anxiety, when anxiety is severe or prolonged and impairs the ability to function in usual activities of daily living, it is called an *anxiety disorder*. The American Psychiatric Association delineates anxiety disorders as medical diagnoses in the *Diagnostic and Statistical Manual of Mental Disorders, 4th edition, Text Revision* (*DSM-IV-TR*). This classification includes several types of anxiety disorders (Box 8-1). Generalized anxiety disorder (GAD) is emphasized in this chapter.

The pathophysiology of anxiety disorders is unknown, but there is evidence of a biologic basis and possible imbalances among several neurotransmission systems. A simplistic view involves an excess of excitatory neurotransmitters (eg, norepinephrine) or a deficiency of inhibitory neurotransmitters (eg, gamma-aminobutyric acid [GABA]).

The noradrenergic system is associated with the hyperarousal state experienced by clients with anxiety (ie, feelings of panic, restlessness, tremulousness, palpitations, hyperventilation), which is attributed to excessive norepinephrine. Norepinephrine is released from the locus ceruleus (LC) in response to an actual or a perceived threat. The LC is a brain stem nucleus that contains many noradrenergic neurons and has extensive projections to the limbic system, cerebral cortex, and cerebellum. The involvement of the noradrenergic system in anxiety is supported by the observations that drugs that stimulate activity in the LC (eg, caffeine) may cause symptoms of anxiety, and drugs used to treat anxiety (eg, benzodiazepines) decrease neuronal firing and norepinephrine release in the LC.

Neuroendocrine factors also play a role in anxiety disorders. Perceived threat or stress activates the hypothalamic–pituitary–adrenal axis and corticotropin-releasing factor (CRF), one of its components. CRF activates the LC, which then releases norepinephrine and generates anxiety. Overall, CRF is considered important in integrating the endocrine, autonomic, and behavioral responses to stress.

GABA is the major inhibitory neurotransmitter in the brain and spinal cord. GABA$_A$ receptors are attached to chloride channels in nerve cell membranes. When GABA interacts with GABA$_A$ receptors, chloride channels open, chloride ions move into the neuron, and the nerve cell is less able to be excited (ie, generate an electrical impulse).

The serotonin system, although not as well understood, is also thought to play a role in anxiety. Both serotonin reuptake inhibitors and serotonin receptor agonists are now used to treat anxiety disorders. Research has suggested two possible roles for the serotonin receptor HT$_{1A}$. During embryonic development, stimulation of HT$_{1A}$ receptors by serotonin is thought to play a role in development of normal brain circuitry necessary for normal anxiety responses. However, during adulthood, SSRIs act through HT$_{1A}$ receptors to reduce anxiety responses. Additional causes of anxiety disorders include medical conditions (anxiety disorder due to a general medical condition according to the *DSM-IV*), psychiatric disorders, and substance abuse. Almost all major psychiatric illnesses may be associated with symptoms of anxiety (eg, dementia, major depression, mania, schizophrenia). Anxiety related to substance abuse is categorized in the *DSM-IV* as substance-induced anxiety disorder.

Sleep and Insomnia

Sleep is a recurrent period of decreased mental and physical activity during which a person is relatively unresponsive to sensory and environmental stimuli. Normal sleep allows rest, renewal of energy for performing activities of daily living, and alertness on awakening.

When a person retires for sleep, there is an initial period of drowsiness or sleep latency, which lasts about 30 minutes. After the person is asleep, cycles occur approximately every 90 minutes during the sleep period. During each cycle, the sleeper progresses from drowsiness (stage I) to deep sleep (stages III and IV). These stages are characterized by depressed body functions, non–rapid eye movement (non-REM), and nondreaming, and they are thought to be physically restorative. Activities that occur during these stages include *increased* tissue repair, synthesis of skeletal muscle protein, and secretion of growth hormone. At the same time, there is *decreased* body temperature, metabolic rate, glucose consumption, and production of catabolic hormones. Stage IV is followed by a period of 5 to 20 minutes of REM, dreaming, and increased physiologic activity.

REM sleep is thought to be mentally and emotionally restorative; REM deprivation can lead to serious psychological problems, including psychosis. It is estimated that a person spends about 75% of sleeping hours in non-REM sleep and about 25% in REM sleep. However, older adults often have a different pattern, with less deep sleep, more light sleep, more frequent awakenings, and generally more disruptions.

Insomnia, prolonged difficulty in going to sleep or staying asleep long enough to feel rested, is the most common sleep disorder. Insomnia has many causes, including such stressors as pain, anxiety, illness, changes in lifestyle or environment, and various drugs. Occasional sleeplessness is a normal response to many stimuli and is not usually harmful. As in anxiety, several neurotransmission systems are apparently involved in regulating sleep-wake cycles and producing insomnia.

Box 8-1 Anxiety Disorders

Generalized Anxiety Disorder (GAD)

Major diagnostic criteria for GAD include worry about two or more circumstances and multiple symptoms for 6 months or longer, and elimination of disease processes or drugs as possible causes. The frequency, duration, or intensity of the worry is exaggerated or out of proportion to the actual situation. Symptoms are related to motor tension (eg, muscle tension, restlessness, trembling, fatigue), overactivity of the autonomic nervous system (eg, dyspnea, palpitations, tachycardia, sweating, dry mouth, dizziness, nausea, diarrhea), and increased vigilance (feeling fearful, nervous, or keyed up; difficulty concentrating; irritability; insomnia).

Symptoms of anxiety occur with numerous disease processes, including medical disorders (eg, hyperthyroidism, cardiovascular disease, cancer) and psychiatric disorders (eg, mood disorders, schizophrenia, substance use disorders). They also frequently occur with drugs that affect the central nervous system (CNS). With CNS stimulants (eg, nasal decongestants, antiasthma drugs, nicotine, caffeine), symptoms occur with drug administration; with CNS depressants (eg, alcohol, benzodiazepines), symptoms are more likely to occur when the drug is stopped, especially if stopped abruptly.

When the symptoms are secondary to medical illness, they may decrease as the illness improves. However, most persons with GAD experience little relief when one stressful situation or problem is resolved. Instead, they quickly move on to another worry. Additional characteristics of GAD include its chronicity, although the severity of symptoms fluctuates over time; its frequent association with somatic symptoms (eg, headache, gastrointestinal complaints, including irritable bowel syndrome); and its frequent coexistence with depression, other anxiety disorders, and substance abuse or dependence.

Obsessive-Compulsive Disorder (OCD)

An obsession involves an uncontrollable desire to dwell on a thought or a feeling; a compulsion involves repeated performance of some act to relieve the fear and anxiety associated with an obsession. OCD is characterized by obsessions or compulsions that are severe enough to be time consuming (eg, take more than an hour per day), cause marked distress, or impair the person's ability to function in usual activities or relationships. The compulsive behavior provides some relief from anxiety but is not pleasurable. The person recognizes that the obsessions or compulsions are excessive or unreasonable and attempts to resist them. When patients resist or are prevented from performing the compulsive behavior, they experience increasing anxiety and often abuse alcohol or antianxiety, sedative-type drugs in the attempt to relieve anxiety.

Panic Disorder

Panic disorder involves acute, sudden, recurrent attacks of anxiety, with feelings of intense fear, terror, or impending doom. It may be accompanied by such symptoms as palpitations, sweat-ing, trembling, shortness of breath or a feeling of smothering, chest pain, nausea, or dizziness. Symptoms usually build to a peak over about 10 minutes and may require medication to be relieved. Afterward, the person is usually preoccupied and worried about future attacks.

A significant number (50–65%) of patients with panic disorder are thought to also have major depression. In addition, some patients with panic disorder also develop agoraphobia, a fear of having a panic attack in a place or situation where one cannot escape or get help. Combined panic disorder and agoraphobia often involves a chronic, relapsing pattern of significant functional impairment and may require lifetime treatment.

Post-Traumatic Stress Disorder (PTSD)

PTSD develops after seeing or being involved in highly stressful events that involve actual or threatened death or serious injury (eg, natural disasters, military combat, violent acts such as rape or murder, explosions or bombings, serious automobile accidents). The person responds to such an event with thoughts and feelings of intense fear, helplessness, or horror and develops symptoms such as hyperarousal, irritability, outbursts of anger, difficulty sleeping, difficulty concentrating, and an exaggerated startle response. These thoughts, feelings, and symptoms persist as the traumatic event is relived through recurring thoughts, images, nightmares, or flashbacks in which the actual event seems to be occurring. The intense psychic discomfort leads people to avoid situations that remind them of the event; become detached from other people; have less interest in activities they formerly enjoyed; and develop other disorders (eg, anxiety disorders, major depression, alcohol or other substance abuse).

The response to stress is highly individualized and the same event or type of event might precipitate PTSD in one person and have little effect in another. Thus, most people experience major stresses and traumatic events during their lifetimes, but many do not develop PTSD. This point needs emphasis because many people seem to assume that PTSD is the normal response to a tragic event and that intensive counseling is needed. For example, counselors converge upon schools in response to events that are perceived to be tragic or stressful. Some authorities take the opposing view, however, that talking about and reliving a traumatic event may increase anxiety in some people and thereby increase the likelihood that PTSD will occur.

Social Phobia

This disorder involves excessive concern about scrutiny by others, which may start in childhood and be lifelong. Affected persons are afraid they will say or do something that will embarrass or humiliate them. As a result, they try to avoid certain situations (eg, public speaking) or experience considerable distress if they cannot avoid them. They are often uncomfortable around other people or experience anxiety in many social situations.

GENERAL CHARACTERISTICS OF BENZODIAZEPINES

Benzodiazepines are widely used for anxiety and insomnia and are also used for several other indications. They have a wide margin of safety between therapeutic and toxic doses and are rarely fatal, even in overdose, unless combined with other CNS depressant drugs, such as alcohol. They are Schedule IV drugs under the Controlled Substances Act. They are drugs of abuse and may cause physiologic dependence; therefore, withdrawal symptoms occur if the drugs are stopped abruptly. To avoid withdrawal symptoms, benzodiazepines should be gradually tapered and discontinued. They do not induce drug-metabolizing enzymes or suppress REM sleep. They may cause characteristic effects of CNS depression, including excessive sedation, impairment of physical and mental activities, and respiratory depression. They are not recommended for long-term use.

Benzodiazepines differ mainly in their plasma half-lives, production of active metabolites, and clinical uses. Drugs with half-lives longer than 24 hours (eg, chlordiazepoxide, diazepam, clorazepate, flurazepam, quazepam) form active metabolites that also have long half-lives and tend to accumulate, especially in older adults and people with impaired liver function. These drugs require 5 to 7 days to reach steady-state serum levels. Therapeutic effects (eg, decreased anxiety or insomnia) and adverse effects (eg, sedation, ataxia) are more likely to occur after 2 or 3 days of therapy than initially. Such effects accumulate with chronic usage and persist for several days after the drugs are discontinued. Drugs with half-lives shorter than 24 hours (eg, alprazolam, lorazepam, midazolam, oxazepam, temazepam, triazolam) do not have active metabolites and do not accumulate. Although the drugs produce similar effects, they differ in clinical uses mainly because their manufacturers developed and promoted them for particular purposes.

Mechanism of Action

Benzodiazepines bind with benzodiazepine receptors in nerve cells of the brain; this receptor complex also has binding sites for GABA, an inhibitory neurotransmitter. This GABA–benzodiazepine receptor complex regulates the entry of chloride ions into the cell. When GABA binds to the receptor complex, chloride ions enter the cell and stabilize (hyperpolarize) the cell membrane so that it is less responsive to excitatory neurotransmitters, such as norepinephrine. Benzodiazepines bind at a different site on the receptor complex and enhance the inhibitory effect of GABA to relieve anxiety, tension, and nervousness and to produce sleep. The decreased neuronal excitability also accounts for the usefulness of benzodiazepines as muscle relaxants, hypnotics, and anticonvulsants.

At least two benzodiazepine receptors, called BZ1 and BZ2, have been identified in the brain. BZ1 is thought to be concerned with sleep mechanisms. BZ2 is associated with memory, motor, sensory, and cognitive functions.

Pharmacokinetics

Benzodiazepines are well absorbed with oral administration, and most are given orally. A few (eg, diazepam, lorazepam) are given both orally and parenterally. They are highly lipid soluble, widely distributed in body tissues, and highly bound to plasma proteins (85% to 98%). The high lipid solubility allows the drugs to easily enter the CNS and perform their actions. Then, the drugs are redistributed to peripheral tissues, from which they are slowly eliminated. Diazepam, for example, is an extremely lipid-soluble drug that enters the CNS and acts within 1 to 5 minutes after intravenous (IV) injection. However, the duration of action of a single IV dose is short (30 to 100 minutes) because the drug rapidly leaves the CNS and distributes peripherally. Thus, the pharmacodynamic effects (eg, sedation) do not correlate with plasma drug levels because the drugs move in and out of the CNS rapidly. This redistribution allows a client to awaken even though the drug may remain in the blood and other peripheral tissues for days or weeks before it is completely eliminated. The pharmacokinetic profile of some benzodiazepines is given in Table 8-1.

Benzodiazepines are mainly metabolized in the liver by the cytochrome P450 enzymes (3A4 subgroup) and glucuronide conjugation. Some (eg, midazolam) are also metabolized by CYP3A4 enzymes in the intestine. Most benzodiazepines are oxidized by the enzymes to metabolites that are then conjugated. For example, diazepam is converted to *N*-desmethyl-diazepam (N-DMDZ), an active metabolite with a long elimination half-life (up to 200 hours). N-DMDZ is further oxidized to oxazepam and then conjugated and excreted. With repeated drug doses, N-DMDZ accumulates and may contribute to both long-lasting antianxiety effects and to adverse effects. If oxidation is impaired (eg, in older adults; in individuals with liver disease; with concurrent use of drugs that inhibit oxidation), higher blood levels of both the parent drugs and metabolites increase the risks of adverse drug effects. In contrast, lorazepam, oxazepam, and temazepam are conjugated only, so their elimination is not impaired by the above factors. Drug metabolites are excreted through the kidneys.

Indications for Use

Major clinical uses of the benzodiazepines are as antianxiety, hypnotic, and anticonvulsant agents. They also are given for preoperative sedation, prevention of agitation and delirium tremens in acute alcohol withdrawal, and treatment of anxiety symptoms associated with depression, acute psychosis, or mania. Thus, they are often given concurrently with antidepressants, antipsychotics, and mood stabilizers.

Not all benzodiazepines are approved for all uses; Table 8-2 lists indications for the individual benzodiazepines.
(text continues on page 138)

TABLE 8-1 Pharmacokinetics of Benzodiazepines

GENERIC NAME	PROTEIN BINDING (%)	HALF-LIFE (H)	METABOLITE(S)	ACTION		
				Onset	Peak	Duration
Alprazolam	80	7–15	Active	30 min	1–2 h	4–6 h
Chlordiazepoxide	96	5–30	Active	10–15 min	1–4 h	2–3 d
Clonazepam	97	20–50	Inactive	varies	1–4 h	weeks
Clorazepate	97	40–50	Active	rapid	1–2 h	days
Diazepam	98	20–80	Active	PO 30–60 min	1–2 h	3 h
				IV 1–5 min	30 min	15–60 min
Estazolam	93	8–28	Inactive	30–60 min	2 h	24 h
Flurazepam	97	2–3	Active	15–45 min	30–60 min	6–8 h
Lorazepam	85	10–20	Inactive	PO 1–30 min	2–4 h	12–24 h
				IM 15–30 min	60–90 min	12–24 h
				IV 5–20 min	30 min	4 h
Midazolam		1–2	Active	15 min		30–60 min
Oxazepam	87	5–20	Inactive	slow	2–4 h	2–4 h
Quazepam	>95	41	Active	30 min	2 h	12–24 h
Temazepam	96	9–12	Inactive	30–60 min	2–3 h	6–8 h
Triazolam	78–89	2–5	Inactive	15–30 min	1–2 h	4–6 h

Table 8-2 Drugs at a Glance: Benzodiazepines

GENERIC/TRADE NAME	CLINICAL INDICATIONS	ROUTES AND DOSAGE RANGES	
		Adults	Children
Alprazolam (Xanax, Xanax XR)	Anxiety Panic disorder	*Anxiety:* PO 0.25–0.5 mg 3 times daily; maximum, 4 mg daily in divided doses *Older or debilitated adults:* PO 0.25 mg 2–3 times daily, increased gradually if necessary *Panic disorder:* PO 0.5 mg 3 times daily initially, gradually increase to 4–10 mg daily Xanax XR: PO 0.5–1 mg daily; gradually increase PRN to maximum dose of 3–6 mg daily	Dosage not established
Chlordiazepoxide (Librium)	Anxiety Acute alcohol withdrawal	PO 15–100 mg daily, once at bedtime or in 3–4 divided doses IM, IV 50–100 mg; maximum, 300 mg daily *Older or debilitated adults:* PO 5 mg 2–4 times daily; IM, IV 25–50 mg	*>6 y:* PO 5–10 mg 2–4 times daily *<6 y:* Not recommended
Clonazepam (Klonopin, Klonopin wafers)	Seizure disorders Panic disorder	*Seizure disorders:* PO 0.5 mg 3 times daily, increased by 0.5–1 mg every 3 days until seizures are controlled or adverse effects occur; maximum, 20 mg daily *Panic disorder:* PO 0.25 mg 2 times daily, increasing to 1 mg daily after 3 days	*Up to 10 y or 30 kg:* 0.01–0.03 mg/kg/d initially; not to exceed 0.05 mg/kg/d, in 2 or 3 divided doses; increase by 0.25–0.5 mg every third day until a daily dose of 0.1–0.2 mg/kg is reached

(continued)

Table 8-2 Drugs at a Glance: Benzodiazepines (continued)

GENERIC/TRADE NAME	CLINICAL INDICATIONS	ROUTES AND DOSAGE RANGES	
		Adults	Children
Clorazepate (Tranxene)	Anxiety Seizure disorders	PO 7.5 mg 3 times daily, increased by no more than 7.5 mg/wk; maximum, 90 mg daily	*9–12 y:* PO 7.5 mg 2 times daily, increased by no more than 7.5 mg/wk; maximum, 60 mg daily *<9 y:* Not recommended
ⓟ **Diazepam** (Valium)	Anxiety Seizure disorders Acute alcohol withdrawal Muscle spasm Preoperative sedation	PO 2–10 mg 2–4 times daily IM, IV 5–10 mg, repeated in 3–4 hours if necessary; give IV slowly, no faster than 5 mg (1 mL) per minute Older or debilitated adults: PO 2–5 mg once or twice daily, increased gradually if needed and tolerated	PO 1–2.5 mg 3–4 times daily, increased gradually if needed and tolerated *>30 d and < 5 y of age:* Seizures, IM, IV 0.2–0.5 mg/2–5 min to a maximum of 5 mg *5 y or older:* Seizures, IM, IV 1 mg/2–5 min to a maximum of 10 mg
Estazolam (ProSom)	Insomnia	PO 1–2 mg	Not for use in children < 18 years of age
Flurazepam (Dalmane)	Insomnia	PO 15–30 mg	Not for use in children < 15 years of age
Lorazepam (Ativan)	Anxiety Preoperative sedation	PO 2–6 mg/d in 2–3 divided doses IM 0.05 mg/kg to a maximum of 4 mg IV 2 mg, diluted with 2 mL of sterile water, sodium chloride, or 5% dextrose injection; do not exceed 2 mg/min *Older or debilitated adults:* PO 1–2 mg/d in divided doses	
Midazolam (Versed)	Preoperative sedation Sedation before short diagnostic tests and endoscopic examinations Induction of general anesthesia Supplementation of nitrous oxide/oxygen anesthesia for short surgical procedures	*Preoperative sedation:* IM 0.05–0.08 mg/kg approximately 1 h before surgery *Prediagnostic test sedation:* IV 0.1–0.15 mg/kg or up to 0.2 mg/kg initially; maintenance dose, approximately 25% of initial dose; reduce dose by 25%–30% if an opioid analgesic is also given *Induction of anesthesia:* IV 0.3–0.35 mg/kg initially, then reduce dose as above for maintenance; reduce initial dose to 0.15–0.3 mg/kg if a narcotic is also given	Preoperative or preprocedure sedation, induction of anesthesia: PO syrup 0.25–1 mg/kg (maximum dose, 20 mg) as a single dose
Oxazepam (Serax)	Anxiety Acute alcohol withdrawal	PO 10–30 mg 3–4 times daily *Older or debilitated adults:* PO 10 mg 3 times daily, gradually increased to 15 mg 3 times daily if necessary	
Quazepam (Doral)	Insomnia	PO 7.5–15 mg	Not for use in children < 18 years of age
Temazepam (Restoril)	Insomnia	PO 15–30 mg	Not for use in children < 18 years of age
Triazolam (Halcion)	Insomnia	PO 0.125–0.25 mg	Not for use in children < 18 years of age

IM, intramuscular; IV, intravenous; PO, oral.

Diazepam has been extensively studied and has more approved uses than others.

Contraindications to Use

Contraindications to benzodiazepines include severe respiratory disorders, severe liver or kidney disease, hypersensitivity reactions, and a history of alcohol or other drug abuse. The drugs must be used very cautiously when taken concurrently with any other CNS depressant drugs.

INDIVIDUAL DRUGS

Benzodiazepines

P **Diazepam** (Valium) is the prototype benzodiazepine. High-potency benzodiazepines such as **alprazolam** (Xanax), **lorazepam** (Ativan), and **clonazepam** (Klonopin) may be more commonly prescribed due to their greater therapeutic effects and rapid onset of action.

The trade names, indications for use, and dosage ranges of individual benzodiazepines are listed in Table 8-2.

Other Antianxiety and Sedative-Hypnotic Drugs

Several nonbenzodiazepine drugs of varied characteristics are also used as antianxiety and sedative-hypnotic agents. These include buspirone, clomipramine, and hydroxyzine as antianxiety agents, and chloral hydrate, dexmedetomidine, zaleplon, and zolpidem as sedative-hypnotics. Miscellaneous nonbenzodiazepines are listed in Table 8-3.

Buspirone (BuSpar) differs chemically and pharmacologically from other antianxiety drugs. Its mechanism of action is unclear, but it apparently interacts with serotonin and dopamine receptors in the brain. Compared with the benzodiazepines, buspirone lacks muscle relaxant and anticonvulsant effects; does not cause sedation or physical or psychological dependence; does not increase the CNS depression of alcohol and other drugs; and is not a controlled substance. Adverse effects include nervousness and excitement. Thus, clients wanting and accustomed to sedative effects may not like the drug or comply with instructions for its use. Its only clinical indication for use is the short-term treatment of anxiety. Although some beneficial effects may occur within 7 to 10 days, optimal effects may require 3 to 4 weeks. Because therapeutic effects may be delayed, buspirone is not considered beneficial for immediate effects or occasional (as-needed, or PRN) use. Buspirone is rapidly absorbed after oral administration. Peak plasma levels occur within 45 to 90 minutes. It is metabolized by the liver to inactive metabolites, which are then excreted in the urine and feces. Its elimination half-life is 2 to 3 hours.

Chloral hydrate (Noctec, Aquachloral), the oldest sedative-hypnotic drug, is relatively safe, effective, and inexpensive in usual therapeutic doses. It reportedly does not suppress REM sleep. Tolerance develops after approximately 2 weeks of continual use. It is a drug of abuse and may cause physical dependence.

Clomipramine (Anafranil), **fluoxetine** (Prozac, Sarafem), **fluvoxamine** (Luvox), **paroxetine** (Paxil), **sertraline** (Zoloft), and **venlafaxine** (Effexor, extended release only) are antidepressants (see Chap. 10) used for the treatment of one or more anxiety disorders.

Dexmedetomidine (Precedex) is a sedative that is approved only for short-term sedation (<24 hours) of clients in critical care settings who are being mechanically ventilated. It is given by continuous IV infusion and has a half-life of 2 hours. Dosage should be reduced in older adults, in clients with impaired liver function, and in patients who are receiving other CNS depressant drugs. Common adverse effects include bradycardia and hypotension.

Hydroxyzine (Vistaril) is an antihistamine with sedative and antiemetic properties. Clinical indications for use include anxiety, preoperative sedation, nausea and vomiting associated with surgery or motion sickness, and pruritus and urticaria associated with allergic dermatoses.

Zaleplon (Sonata) is an oral, nonbenzodiazepine hypnotic approved for the short-term treatment (7 to 10 days) of insomnia. It binds to the benzodiazepine BZ1 receptor and apparently enhances the inhibitory effects of GABA, as do the benzodiazepines. It is a Schedule IV controlled substance; a few studies indicate abuse potential similar to that associated with benzodiazepines.

Zaleplon is well absorbed, but bioavailability is only about 30% because of extensive presystemic or "first-pass" hepatic metabolism. Action onset is rapid and peaks in 1 hour. A high-fat, heavy meal slows absorption and may reduce the drug's effectiveness in inducing sleep. It is 60% bound to plasma proteins, and its half-life is 1 hour. The drug is metabolized mainly by aldehyde oxidase and slightly by the cytochrome P450 3A4 enzymes to inactive metabolites. The metabolites and a small amount of unchanged drug are excreted in the urine.

The drug is contraindicated in clients with hypersensitivity reactions and during lactation, and it should be used cautiously during pregnancy and in people who are depressed or have impaired hepatic or respiratory function. Adverse effects include depression, drowsiness, nausea, dizziness, headache, hypersensitivity, impaired coordination, and short-term memory impairment. To decrease risks of adverse effects, dosage should be reduced in clients with mild to moderate hepatic impairment and should be avoided in those with severe hepatic impairment. No dosage adjustment is needed with mild to moderate renal impairment; drug effects with severe renal impairment have not been studied. Dosage should also be reduced in older adults. Drug safety and effectiveness in children have not been established. Japanese clients may be at higher-than-average risk of adverse effects because these subjects had higher peak plasma levels and longer durations of action in clinical trials. These effects were attributed to differences in body weight or drug metabolizing enzymes resulting from dietary, environmental, or other factors.

Table 8-3 Drugs at a Glance: Miscellaneous Antianxiety and Sedative-Hypnotic Agents

GENERIC/TRADE NAME	MAJOR CLINICAL USE	ROUTES AND DOSAGE RANGES	
		Adults	Children
Antianxiety Agents			
Buspirone (BuSpar)	Anxiety	PO 5 mg 3 times daily, increased by 5 mg/d at 2- to 3-day intervals if necessary. Usual maintenance dose 20–30 mg/d in divided doses; maximum dose 60 mg/d.	Not recommended
Clomipramine (Anafranil)	Obsessive-compulsive disorder (OCD)	PO 25 mg/d initially; increase to 100 mg/d during the first 2 wk and to a maximum dose of 250 mg/d over several weeks if necessary.	PO 25 mg/d initially, gradually increased over 2 wk to a maximum of 3 mg/kg/d or 100 mg, whichever is smaller. Then increase to 3 mg/kg/d or 200 mg per day if necessary.
Hydroxyzine (Vistaril)	Anxiety, sedative, pruritus	PO 75–400 mg/d in 3 or 4 divided doses Pre- and postoperative and pre- and postpartum sedation, IM 25–100 mg in a single dose	PO 2 mg/kg per day in 4 divided doses. Pre- and postoperative sedation, IM 1 mg/kg in a single dose.
Sertraline (Zoloft)	Obsessive-compulsive disorder (OCD) Panic disorder Post-traumatic stress disorder (PTSD)	OCD, PO 50 mg once daily Panic disorder and PTSD, PO 25 mg once daily initially, increased after 1 wk to 50 mg once daily	OCD, 6–12 y: PO 25 mg once daily; 13–17 y, PO 50 mg once daily
Venlafaxine extended release (Effexor XR)	Generalized anxiety disorder	PO 37.5–75 mg once daily initially, increased up to 225 mg daily if necessary	Dosage not established
Sedative-Hypnotic Agents			
Chloral hydrate (Aquachloral, Noctec)	Sedative, hypnotic	Sedative: PO, rectal suppository 250 mg 3 times per day Hypnotic: PO, rectal suppository 500–1000 mg at bedtime; maximum dose, 2 g/d	Sedative: PO, rectal suppository 25 mg/kg per day, in 3 or 4 divided doses Hypnotic: PO, rectal suppository 50 mg/kg at bedtime; maximum single dose, 1 g
Dexmedetomidine (Precedex)	Sedation of intubated, mechanically ventilated patients in intensive care units	IV infusion 1 mcg/kg over 10 min initially, then 0.2–0.7 mcg/kg/h to maintain the desired level of sedation	Not recommended for children <18 years
Zaleplon (Sonata)	Hypnotic	PO 10 mg at bedtime; 5 mg for adults who are elderly, of low weight, or have mild to moderate hepatic impairment	Dosage not established
Zolpidem (Ambien)	Hypnotic	PO 10 mg at bedtime; 5 mg for older adults and those with hepatic impairment	Not recommended

IM, intramuscular; IV, intravenous; PO, oral.

Zaleplon should not be taken concurrently with alcohol or other CNS depressant drugs because of the increased risk of excessive sedation and respiratory depression. There is also a risk of increased serum zaleplon levels if the drug is taken concurrently with cimetidine (see Chap. 59). Cimetidine inhibits both the aldehyde oxidase and cytochrome P450 3A4 enzymes that metabolize zaleplon. If cimetidine is taken, zaleplon dosage should be reduced to 5 milligrams. It is very important that clients taking zaleplon be taught about this interaction because cimetidine is available without prescription, and the client may not inform the health care provider who prescribes zaleplon about taking cimetidine.

Overall, zaleplon is effective in helping a person get to sleep and has several advantages as a hypnotic, including the rapid onset; absence of active metabolites; absence of clinically significant cytochrome P450 drug interactions; rapid clearance from the body; and absence of major memory impairments. However, it may not increase total sleep time or decrease the number of awakenings during sleeping hours.

Zolpidem (Ambien) is a hypnotic that differs structurally from the benzodiazepines but produces similar effects. It is also similar to zaleplon. It is a Schedule IV drug approved for short-term treatment (7 to 10 days) of insomnia. Zolpidem should be given with caution to clients with signs and symptoms of major depression because of increased risk of intentional overdose.

Zolpidem is well absorbed with oral administration and has a rapid onset of action, usually within 20 to 30 minutes. Its half-life is 2.5 hours, and its hypnotic effects last 6 to 8 hours. It is 90% bound to plasma proteins. Bioavailability, peak plasma concentration, and half-life are increased in older adults and in clients with impaired hepatic function. Dosage should be reduced for these groups. Zolpidem is metabolized to inactive metabolites that are then eliminated by renal excretion. Dosage reductions are not required for clients with renal impairment, but these clients should be closely monitored.

Adverse effects are usually few and mild (eg, daytime drowsiness, dizziness, nausea, diarrhea), but rebound insomnia may occur for a night or two after stopping the drug, and withdrawal symptoms may occur if it is stopped abruptly after approximately a week of regular use. Zolpidem should not be taken concurrently with alcohol or other CNS depressant drugs because of the increased risk of excessive sedation and respiratory depression.

Herbal and Dietary Supplements

Numerous preparations have been used to relieve anxiety and insomnia. None has been adequately studied regarding dosage; effects; or interactions with prescribed drugs, over-the-counter drugs, or other supplements. Three products are commonly used.

Kava is derived from a shrub found in many South Pacific islands. It is claimed to be useful in numerous disorders, including anxiety, depression, insomnia, asthma, pain, rheumatism, muscle spasms, and seizures. It suppresses emotional excitability and may produce a mild euphoria. Effects include analgesia, sedation, diminished reflexes, impaired gait, and pupil dilation. Kava has been used or studied most often for treatment of anxiety, stress, and restlessness. It is thought to act similarly to the benzodiazepines by interacting with GABA receptors on nerve cell membranes. This action and limited evidence from a few small clinical trials may support use of the herb in the treatment of anxiety, insomnia, and seizure disorders. However, additional studies are needed to delineate therapeutic and adverse effects, dosing recommendations, and drug interactions when used for these conditions.

Adverse effects include impaired thinking, judgment, motor reflexes, and vision. Serious adverse effects may occur with long-term, heavy use, including decreased plasma proteins, decreased platelet and lymphocyte counts, dyspnea, and pulmonary hypertension. Kava should not be taken concurrently with other CNS depressant drugs (eg, benzodiazepines, ethanol), antiplatelet drugs, or levodopa (increases Parkinson symptoms). In addition, it should not be taken by women who are pregnant or lactating or by children under 12 years of age. Finally, it should be used cautiously by clients with renal disease, thrombocytopenia, or neutropenia. In December 2001, the Food and Drug Administration (FDA) issued a warning that products containing kava have been implicated in at least 25 cases of severe liver toxicity (eg, hepatitis, cirrhosis, liver failure).

Melatonin is a hormone produced by the pineal gland, an endocrine gland in the brain. Endogenous melatonin is derived from the amino acid tryptophan, which is converted to serotonin, which is then enzymatically converted to melatonin in the pineal gland. Exogenous preparations are produced synthetically and may contain other ingredients. Melatonin products are widely available. Recommended doses on product labels usually range from 0.3 to 5 milligrams.

Melatonin influences sleep–wake cycles; it is released during sleep, and serum levels are very low during waking hours. Prolonged intake of exogenous melatonin can reset the sleep–wake cycle. As a result, it is widely promoted for prevention and treatment of jet lag (considered a circadian rhythm disorder) and treatment of insomnia. It is thought to act similarly to the benzodiazepines in inducing sleep. In several studies of clients with sleep disturbances, those taking melatonin experienced modest improvement compared with those taking a placebo. Other studies suggest that melatonin supplements improve sleep in older adults with melatonin deficiency and decrease weight loss in people with cancer. Large, controlled studies are needed to determine the effects of long-term use and the most effective regimen when used for jet lag.

Melatonin supplements are contraindicated in clients with hepatic insufficiency because of reduced clearance. They are also contraindicated in people with a history of cerebrovascular disease, depression, or neurologic disorders. They should be used cautiously by people with renal impairment and those taking benzodiazepines or other CNS depressant drugs. Adverse effects include altered sleep patterns, confusion, headache, hypothermia, pruritus, sedation, and tachycardia.

Valerian is an herb used mainly as a sedative-hypnotic. It apparently increases the amount of GABA in the brain, probably by inhibiting the transaminase enzyme that normally metabolizes GABA. Increasing GABA, an inhibitory neurotransmitter, results in calming, sedative effects.

There are differences of opinion about the clinical usefulness of valerian; some practitioners say that studies indicate the herb's effectiveness as a sleep aid and mild antianxiety agent while other practitioners say that these studies were flawed by small samples, short durations, and poor definitions of client populations. An expert panel convened by the U.S. Pharmacopeia has advised that there is insufficient evidence to support the use of valerian for treating insomnia.

Adverse effects with acute overdose or chronic use include blurred vision, cardiac disturbance, excitability, headache, hypersensitivity reactions, insomnia, and nausea. There is a risk of hepatotoxicity from overdosage and from using combination herbal products containing valerian. Valerian should not be taken by people with hepatic impairment (risk of increased liver damage) or by pregnant or breast-feeding women (effects are unknown). The herb should not be taken concurrently with any other sedatives, hypnotics, alcohol, or CNS depressants because of the potential for additive CNS depression.

NURSING PROCESS

Assessment

Assess the client's need for antianxiety or sedative-hypnotic drugs, including intensity and duration of symptoms. Manifestations are more obvious with moderate to severe anxiety or insomnia. Some guidelines for assessment include the following:

- What is the client's statement of the problem? Does the problem interfere with usual activities of daily living? If so, how much and for how long?
- Try to identify factors that precipitate anxiety or insomnia in the client. Some common precursors are physical symptoms; feeling worried, tense, or nervous; factors such as illness, death of a friend or family member, divorce, or job stress; and excessive CNS stimulation from caffeine-containing beverages or drugs such as bronchodilators and nasal decongestants. In addition, excessive daytime sleep and too little exercise and activity may cause insomnia, especially in older clients.
- Observe for behavioral manifestations of anxiety, such as psychomotor agitation, facial grimaces, tense posture, and others.
- Observe for physiologic manifestations of anxiety. These signs may include increased blood pressure and pulse rate, increased rate and depth of respiration, increased muscle tension, and pale, cool skin.
- If behavioral or physiologic manifestations seem to indicate anxiety, try to determine whether this is actually the case. Because similar manifestations may indicate pain or other problems rather than anxiety, the observer's perceptions must be validated by the client before appropriate action can be taken.
- If insomnia is reported, observe for signs of sleep deprivation such as drowsiness, slow movements or speech, and difficulty concentrating or focusing attention.
- Obtain a careful drug history, including the use of alcohol and sedative-hypnotic drugs, and assess the likelihood of drug abuse and dependence. People who abuse other

drugs, including alcohol, are likely to abuse antianxiety and sedative-hypnotic drugs. Also, assess for use of CNS stimulant drugs (eg, appetite suppressants, bronchodilators, nasal decongestants, caffeine, cocaine) and herbs (eg, ephedra).
- Identify coping mechanisms used in managing previous situations of stress, anxiety, and insomnia. These are very individualized. Reading, watching television, listening to music, or talking to a friend are examples. Some people are quiet and inactive; others participate in strenuous activity. Some prefer to be alone; others prefer being with a friend, family member, or group.
- After drug therapy for anxiety or insomnia is begun, assess the client's level of consciousness and functional ability before each dose so that excessive sedation can be avoided.

Nursing Diagnoses

- Ineffective Individual Coping related to need for antianxiety or sedative-hypnotic drug
- Deficient Knowledge: Appropriate uses and effects of antianxiety or sedative-hypnotic drugs
- Deficient Knowledge: Nondrug measures for relieving anxiety and insomnia
- Noncompliance: Overuse
- Risk for Injury related to sedation, respiratory depression, impaired mobility, and other adverse effects
- Sleep Pattern Disturbance: Insomnia related to one or more causes (eg, anxiety, daytime sleep)

Planning/Goals

The client will
- Feel more calm, relaxed, and comfortable with anxiety; experience improved quantity and quality of sleep with insomnia
- Be monitored for excessive sedation and impaired mobility to prevent falls or other injuries (in health care settings)
- Verbalize and demonstrate nondrug activities to reduce or manage anxiety or insomnia
- Demonstrate safe, accurate drug usage
- Notify a health care provider if he or she wants to stop taking a benzodiazepine; agree to not stop taking a benzodiazepine abruptly
- Avoid preventable adverse effects, including abuse and dependence

Interventions

Use nondrug measures to relieve anxiety or to enhance the effectiveness of antianxiety drugs.
- Assist clients to identify and avoid or decrease situations that cause anxiety and insomnia, when possible.

In addition, help them to understand that medications do not solve underlying problems.

- Support the client's usual coping mechanisms when feasible. Provide the opportunity for reading, exercising, listening to music, or watching television; promote contact with significant others; or simply allow the client to be alone and uninterrupted for a while.
- Use interpersonal and communication techniques to help the client manage anxiety. The degree of anxiety and the clinical situation largely determine which techniques are appropriate. For example, staying with the client, showing interest, listening, and allowing him or her to verbalize concerns may be beneficial.
- Providing information may be a therapeutic technique when anxiety is related to medical conditions. People vary in the amount and kind of information they want, but usually the following topics should be included:
  - The overall treatment plan, including medical or surgical treatment, choice of outpatient care or hospitalization, expected length of treatment, and expected outcomes in terms of health and ability to function in activities of daily living
  - Specific diagnostic tests, including preparation; after-effects, if any; and how the client will be informed of results
  - Specific medication and treatment measures, including expected therapeutic results
  - What the client must do to carry out the plan of treatment
- When offering information and explanations, keep in mind that anxiety interferes with intellectual functioning. Thus, communication should be brief, clear, and repeated as necessary, because clients may misunderstand or forget what is said.
- Modify the environment to decrease anxiety-provoking stimuli. Modifications may involve altering temperature, light, and noise levels.
- Use measures to increase physical comfort. These may include a wide variety of activities, such as positioning, helping the client bathe or ambulate, giving back rubs, or providing fluids of the client's choice.
- Consult with other services and departments on the client's behalf. For example, if financial problems were identified as a cause of anxiety, social services may be able to help.
- When a benzodiazepine is used with diagnostic tests or minor surgery, provide instructions for postprocedure care to the client or to family members, preferably in written form.

Implement measures to decrease the need for or increase the effectiveness of sedative-hypnotic drugs, such as the following:

- Modify the environment to promote rest and sleep (eg, reduce noise and light).
- Plan care to allow uninterrupted periods of rest and sleep, when possible.
- Relieve symptoms that interfere with rest and sleep. Drugs such as analgesics for pain or antitussives for cough are usually safer and more effective than sedative-hypnotic drugs. Nondrug measures, such as positioning, exercise, and back rubs, may be helpful in relieving muscle tension and other discomforts. Allowing the client to verbalize concerns, providing information so that he or she knows what to expect, or consulting other personnel (eg, social worker, chaplain) may be useful in decreasing anxiety.
- Help the client modify lifestyle habits to promote rest and sleep (eg, limiting intake of caffeine-containing beverages, limiting intake of fluids during evening hours if nocturia interferes with sleep, avoiding daytime naps, having a regular schedule of rest and sleep periods, increasing physical activity, not trying to sleep unless tired or drowsy).

In addition, client teaching guidelines for antianxiety and sedative-hypnotic drugs are presented in the accompanying display.

Evaluation

- Decreased symptoms of anxiety or insomnia and increased rest and sleep are reported or observed.
- Excessive sedation and motor impairment are not observed.
- The client reports no serious adverse effects.
- Monitoring of prescriptions (eg, "pill counts") does not indicate excessive use.

APPLYING YOUR KNOWLEDGE 8-1:
LEGAL/ETHICAL DILEMMA

Mrs. Portman's daughter questions you about the medication her mother is receiving. She feels that her mother is too sedated and does not want her to receive any more medication. Without the medications, Mrs. Portman wanders away and is at risk to hurt herself. What would you do?

PRINCIPLES OF THERAPY

Drug Dosage

With benzodiazepines, dosage must be individualized and carefully titrated because requirements vary widely among clients. With antianxiety agents, the goal is to find the lowest effective dose that does not cause excessive daytime drowsiness or impaired mobility. In general, start with the smallest dose likely to be effective (eg, diazepam 2 mg three times daily or equivalent doses of others). Then, according to client response,

Antianxiety and Sedative-Hypnotic Drugs

General Considerations

☑ "Nerve pills" and "sleeping pills" can relieve symptoms temporarily, but they do not cure or solve the underlying problems. With rare exceptions, these drugs are recommended only for short-term use. For long-term relief, counseling or psychotherapy may be more beneficial because it can help you learn other ways to decrease your nervousness and difficulty in sleeping.

☑ Use nondrug measures to promote relaxation, rest, and sleep when possible. Physical exercise, reading, craft work, stress management, and relaxation techniques are safer than any drug.

☑ Try to identify and avoid factors that cause nervousness or insomnia, such as caffeine-containing beverages and stimulant drugs. This may prevent or decrease the severity of nervousness or insomnia so that sedative-type drugs are not needed. If the drugs are used, these factors can cancel or decrease the drugs' effects. Stimulant drugs include asthma and cold remedies and appetite suppressants.

☑ Most "nerve pills" and "sleeping pills" belong to the same chemical group and have similar effects, including the ability to decrease nervousness, cause drowsiness, and cause dependence. Thus, there is no logical reason to take a combination of the drugs for anxiety, or to take one drug for daytime sedation and another for sleep. Ativan, Xanax, Valium, and Restoril are commonly used examples of this group, but there are several others as well.

☑ Inform all health care providers when taking a sedative-type medication, preferably by the generic and trade names. This helps avoid multiple prescriptions of drugs with similar effects and reduces the risk of serious adverse effects from overdose.

☑ Do not perform tasks that require alertness if drowsy from medication. The drugs often impair mental and physical functioning, especially during the first several days of use, and thereby make routine activities potentially hazardous. Avoid smoking, ambulating without help, driving a car, operating machinery, and other potentially hazardous tasks. These activities may lead to falls or other injuries if undertaken while alertness is impaired.

☑ Avoid alcohol and other depressant drugs (eg, over-the-counter [OTC] antihistamines and sleeping pills, narcotic analgesics, sedating herbs such as kava and valerian, and the dietary supplement melatonin) while taking any antianxiety or sedative-hypnotic drugs (except buspirone). An antihistamine that causes drowsiness is the active ingredient in OTC sleep aids (eg, Compoz, Nytol, Sominex, Unisom) and in many pain reliever products with "PM" as part of their names (eg, Tylenol PM). Because these drugs depress brain functioning when taken alone, combining them produces additive depression and may lead to excessive drowsiness, difficulty breathing, traumatic injuries, and other potentially serious adverse drug effects.

☑ Store drugs safely, out of reach of children and adults who are confused or less than alert. Accidental or intentional ingestion may lead to serious adverse effects. Also, do not keep the drug container at the bedside, because a person sedated by a previous dose may take additional doses.

☑ Do not share these drugs with anyone else. These mind-altering, brain-depressant drugs should be taken only by those people for whom they are prescribed.

☑ Do not stop taking a Valium-related drug abruptly. Withdrawal symptoms can occur. When being discontinued, dosage should be gradually reduced, as directed by and with the supervision of a health care provider.

☑ Do not take "sleeping pills" every night. These drugs lose their effectiveness in 2–4 weeks if taken nightly, and cause sleep disturbances when stopped.

☑ Alprazolam (Xanax) is sometimes confused with ranitidine (Zantac), a drug for heartburn and peptic ulcers.

Self-Administration

☑ Follow instructions carefully about how much, how often, and how long to take the drugs. These drugs produce more beneficial effects and fewer adverse reactions when used in the smallest effective doses and for the shortest duration feasible in particular circumstances. All of the Valium-related drugs, zaleplon (Sonata), and zolpidem (Ambien) can cause physical dependence, which may eventually cause worse problems than the original anxiety or insomnia.

☑ Take sleeping pills just before going to bed so that you are lying down when the expected drowsiness occurs.

☑ Omit one or more doses if excessive drowsiness occurs to avoid difficulty breathing, falls, and other adverse drug effects.

☑ Take oral benzodiazepines with a glass of water; they may be taken with food if stomach upset occurs.

☑ Take buspirone on a daily schedule. It is not fully effective until after 3–4 weeks of regular use; it is ineffective for occasional use.

☑ Take zolpidem on an empty stomach, at bedtime, because the drug acts quickly to cause drowsiness.

☑ Take Xanax XR once daily, preferably in the morning. Take the tablet intact; do not crush, chew, or break it.

☑ Take Klonopin wafers (orally disintegrating tablets) by carefully peeling open the foil packaging and placing the tablet in the mouth. Disintegration quickly occurs in saliva, and the tablet can be swallowed with or without water.

doses can be titrated upward to relieve symptoms of anxiety and avoid adverse drug effects. The maximum daily dose of diazepam is 40 milligrams per day or (equivalent doses of other drugs). With hypnotics, the lowest effective doses should be taken on an intermittent basis, not every night. Additional guidelines include the following:

● Smaller-than-usual doses may be indicated in clients receiving cimetidine or other drugs that decrease the hepatic metabolism of benzodiazepines; in older adults; and in debilitated clients. With alprazolam, the most commonly prescribed benzodiazepine, the dose should be reduced by 50% if given concurrently with the antidepressant fluvoxamine.

  In older adults, most benzodiazepines are metabolized more slowly, and half-lives are longer than in younger adults. Exceptions are lorazepam and oxazepam, whose half-lives and dosages are the same for older adults as for younger ones. The recommended initial dose of zaleplon and zolpidem is 5 milligrams, one half of that recommended for younger adults.

● Larger-than-usual doses may be needed for clients who are severely anxious or agitated. Also, large doses are usually required to relax skeletal muscle; control muscle spasm; control seizures; and provide sedation before surgery, cardioversion, endoscopy, and angiography.

● When benzodiazepines are used with opioid analgesics, the analgesic dose should be reduced initially and increased gradually to avoid excessive CNS depression.

APPLYING YOUR KNOWLEDGE 8-2

Mrs. Portman is given 0.5 mg of alprazolam at 2:00 PM. You assess her at 6:00 PM and prepare her for her dinner. Mrs. Portman is very drowsy and has difficulty feeding herself. After dinner, Mrs. Portman begins to experience mild anxiety and you prepare to administer an appropriate dose of medication. What would you prepare and why?

Drug Administration

Frequency of Administration

The antianxiety benzodiazepines are often given in three or four daily doses. This is necessary for the short-acting agents, but there is no pharmacologic basis for multiple daily doses of the long-acting drugs. Because of their prolonged actions, all or most of the daily dose can be given at bedtime. This schedule promotes sleep, and there is usually enough residual sedation to maintain antianxiety effects throughout the next day. If necessary, one or two small supplemental doses may be given during the day. Although

the hypnotic benzodiazepines vary in their onset of action, they should be taken at bedtime because it is safer for clients to be recumbent when drowsiness occurs. Zaleplon and zolpidem also should be taken at bedtime because of their rapid onset of action.

Duration of Therapy

Benzodiazepines should be given for the shortest effective period to decrease the likelihood of drug abuse and physiologic and psychological dependence. Few problems develop with short-term use unless an overdose is taken or other CNS depressant drugs (eg, alcohol) are taken concurrently. Most problems occur with long-term use, especially of larger-than-usual doses. In general, an antianxiety benzodiazepine should not be taken for longer than 4 months and a hypnotic benzodiazepine should not be taken more than 3 or 4 nights a week for approximately 3 weeks.

For buspirone, recommendations for duration of therapy have not been established. For zaleplon and zolpidem, the recommended duration is no longer than 10 days.

Benzodiazepine Withdrawal: Prevention and Management

Physical dependence on benzodiazepines, which is associated with longer use and higher doses, is indicated by withdrawal symptoms when the drugs are stopped. Mild symptoms occur in approximately half the clients taking therapeutic doses for 6 to 12 weeks; severe symptoms are most likely to occur when high doses are taken regularly for more than 4 months and then abruptly discontinued. Although the drugs have not been proven effective for more than 4 months of regular use, this period is probably exceeded quite often in clinical practice.

Withdrawal symptoms may be caused by the abrupt separation of benzodiazepine molecules from their receptor sites and the resulting acute decrease in GABA neurotransmission. Because GABA is an inhibitory neurotransmitter, less GABA may produce a less inhibited CNS and therefore symptoms of hyperarousal or CNS stimulation. Common manifestations include increased anxiety, psychomotor agitation, insomnia, irritability, headache, tremor, and palpitations. Less common but more serious manifestations include confusion, abnormal perception of movement, depersonalization, psychosis, and seizures.

Severe symptoms are most likely to occur with short-acting drugs (eg, alprazolam, lorazepam, triazolam) unless they are discontinued very gradually. Symptoms may occur within 24 hours of stopping a short-acting drug, but they usually occur 4 to 5 days after stopping a long-acting drug such as diazepam. Symptoms can be relieved by administration of a benzodiazepine.

To prevent withdrawal symptoms, the drug should be tapered in dose and gradually discontinued. Reducing the dose by 10% to 25% every 1 or 2 weeks over 4 to 16 weeks usually is effective. However, the rate may need to be even slower with high doses or long-term use. After the drug is discontinued, the client should be monitored for a few weeks for symptoms of withdrawal or recurrence of symptoms for which the drug was originally prescribed.

Benzodiazepine Toxicity: Recognition and Management

Toxic effects of benzodiazepines include excessive sedation, respiratory depression, and coma. Flumazenil (Romazicon) is a specific antidote that competes with benzodiazepines for benzodiazepine receptors and reverses toxicity. Clinical indications for use include benzodiazepine overdose and reversal of sedation after diagnostic or therapeutic procedures. The degree of sedation reversal depends on the plasma concentration of the ingested benzodiazepine and the flumazenil dose and frequency of administration. The drug acts rapidly, with onset within 2 minutes and peak effects within 6 to 10 minutes. However, the duration of action is short (serum half-life is 60 to 90 minutes) compared with that of most benzodiazepines, so repeated doses are usually required. Adverse effects include precipitation of acute benzodiazepine withdrawal symptoms, agitation, confusion, and seizures. Re-sedation and hypoventilation may occur if flumazenil is not given long enough to coincide with the duration of action of the benzodiazepine.

The drug should be injected into a freely flowing IV line in a large vein. Dosage recommendations vary with use. For reversal of conscious sedation or general anesthesia, the initial dose is 0.2 milligrams over 15 seconds, then 0.2 milligrams every 60 seconds, if necessary, to a maximum of 1.0 milligrams (total of five doses). For overdose, the initial dose is 0.2 milligrams over 30 seconds, wait 30 seconds, then 0.3 milligrams over 30 seconds, then 0.5 milligrams every 60 seconds up to a total dose of 3 milligrams, if necessary, for the client to reach the desired level of consciousness. Slow administration and repeated doses are recommended to awaken the client gradually and decrease the risks of causing acute withdrawal symptoms. A client who does not respond within 5 minutes of administering the total recommended dose should be reassessed for other causes of sedation.

APPLYING YOUR KNOWLEDGE 8-3
Mrs. Portman continues to receive her medication for a few days and then is no longer given the alprazolam. She begins to experience anxiety, agitation, and irritability. What is the possible explanation for these symptoms?

Drug Therapy for Anxiety

Antianxiety drugs are not recommended for treating everyday stress and anxiety. Some authorities believe such use promotes reliance on drugs and decreases development of healthier coping mechanisms. For severe anxiety associated with a temporary stressful situation, an anxiolytic drug may be beneficial for short-term, PRN use; prolonged therapy is not recommended. These drugs are most clearly indicated when anxiety causes disability and interferes with job performance, interpersonal relationships, and other activities of daily living. Because anxiety often accompanies pain, antianxiety agents are sometimes used to treat pain. However, in the management of chronic pain, antianxiety drugs have not demonstrated a definite benefit. Anxiety about recurrence of pain is probably better controlled by adequate analgesia than by antianxiety drugs.

Physicians must consider the type of anxiety disorder before prescribing benzodiazepines. Benzodiazepines are considered superior to other medications in treating social anxiety disorders. They are effective in treating GAD; however, other drugs such as SSRIs may be more effective. In addition, benzodiazepines may be less beneficial for anxiety associated with posttraumatic stress disorder.

Because benzodiazepines are equally effective in relieving anxiety, other factors may assist the prescriber in choosing a particular drug for a particular client. For example, alprazolam, clorazepate, and diazepam decrease anxiety within 30 to 60 minutes. Thus, one of these drugs may be preferred when rapid onset of drug action is desired. Lorazepam, oxazepam, and prazepam have a slower onset of action and thus are not recommended for acute symptoms of anxiety. Because they have short half-lives and their elimination does not depend on the cytochrome P450 oxidizing enzymes in the liver, lorazepam and oxazepam are the drugs of choice for clients who are elderly, have liver disease, or are taking drugs that interfere with hepatic drug-metabolizing enzymes.

When benzodiazepines are used to treat GAD, clients often experience relief of symptoms within a few days. In addition, these clients rarely develop tolerance to anxiety-relieving effects or abuse the drugs. Persons most likely to abuse the drugs are those who have a history of drug abuse.

Buspirone is also an effective antianxiety agent, especially for clients with conditions (eg, chronic obstructive lung disease) that may be aggravated by the sedative and respiratory depressant effects of benzodiazepines. However, anxiety-relieving effects may be delayed for 2 to 4 weeks. Thus, buspirone is not useful for acute episodes of anxiety and it may be difficult to persuade some clients to take the drug long enough to be effective. Adverse effects are usually mild and can include nausea and dizziness. Buspirone should not be taken in combination with monoamine oxidase inhibitors; otherwise, buspirone has few drug–drug interactions. When used to treat GAD, some clinicians recommend relatively high doses of 30 to 60 milligrams daily (in two or three divided doses).

Antidepressant medications are increasingly being used as a first-line treatment for several anxiety disorders, including GAD. Although several others have been used, paroxetine and extended-release venlafaxine are approved by the FDA for treatment of GAD. Newer antidepressants such as mirtazapine (Remeron) are also used in the treatment of anxiety. In studies comparing the effects of antidepressants and benzodiazepines for treating GAD, it was concluded that benzodiazepines work faster (within a few days), but that antidepressants are more effective after 4 to 6 weeks. Some clinicians prescribe a combination of a benzodiazepine and an antidepressant. The benzodiazepine provides relief during the 2 to 3 weeks required for antidepressant effects, and then it is tapered and discontinued while the antidepressant is continued. Antidepressants do not cause cognitive impairment or dependence, as benzodiazepines do. In addition, clients with GAD often have depression as well. Thus, an antidepressant can relieve both anxiety and depression, but a benzodiazepine is not effective for treating depression.

One factor to consider in the use of antidepressants is that these drugs can increase the agitation and hyperarousal already present in the client with GAD. To minimize stimulation, initial doses of antidepressants should be about 50% less than the doses for depression. Then, the dose can be increased over 1 to 2 weeks. The optimal maintenance dose of an antidepressant for GAD is usually the same as for depression. Another factor is that patients may not be willing to take antidepressants long term because of the sexual dysfunction and weight gain associated with the drugs.

Overall, a combination of drug therapy and psychotherapy may be the most effective treatment for GAD. Benzodiazepines, buspirone, and antidepressants are the drugs of choice; cognitive behavioral therapy (CBT) is probably the nonpharmacologic treatment of choice. Drug therapy can relieve the symptoms; CBT can help clients learn to manage their anxiety and decrease their negative thinking. After anxiety is under control, some clinicians recommend continuing drug therapy for at least a year.

Drug Therapy for Insomnia

In general, sedative-hypnotic drugs should be used only when insomnia causes significant distress and resists management by nonpharmacologic means; they should not be used for occasional sleeplessness. The goal of treatment is to relieve anxiety or sleeplessness without permitting sensory perception, responsiveness to the environment, or alertness to drop below safe levels. The drugs of choice for most clients are the benzodiazepines and the BZ1 receptor–specific

drugs zaleplon and zolpidem. However, for clients with insomnia associated with major depression, antidepressants are preferred.

Sedative-hypnotic drugs should not be taken every night unless necessary. Intermittent administration helps maintain drug effectiveness and decreases the risks of drug abuse and dependence. It also decreases disturbances of normal sleep patterns. In chronic insomnia, no hypnotic drug is recommended for long-term treatment. Most benzodiazepine hypnotics lose their effectiveness in producing sleep after 4 weeks of daily use; triazolam loses effectiveness in 2 weeks. It is not helpful to switch from one drug to another because cross-tolerance develops. To restore the sleep-producing effect, administration of the hypnotic drug must be interrupted for 1 to 2 weeks.

When sedative-hypnotic drugs are prescribed for outpatients, the prescription should limit the number of doses dispensed and the number of refills. This is one way of decreasing the risk of abuse and suicide.

As with the antianxiety benzodiazepines, most hypnotic benzodiazepines are oxidized in the liver by the cytochrome P450 enzymes to metabolites that are then conjugated and excreted through the kidneys. An exception is temazepam (Restoril), which is eliminated only by conjugation with glucuronide. Thus, temazepam is the drug of choice for clients who are elderly, have liver disease, or are taking drugs that interfere with hepatic drug-metabolizing enzymes.

Use in Special Populations

Use in Children

Anxiety is a common disorder among children and adolescents. When given antianxiety and sedative-hypnotic drugs, they may have unanticipated or variable responses, including paradoxical CNS stimulation and excitement rather than CNS depression and calming. Few studies have been done in children. Thus, much clinical usage of these drugs is empiric, not approved by the FDA, and not supported by data. As with other populations, benzodiazepines should be given to children only when clearly indicated, in the lowest effective dose, and for the shortest effective time.

Drug pharmacodynamics and pharmacokinetics are likely to be different in children than in adults. Pharmacodynamic differences may stem from changes in neurotransmission systems in the brain as the child grows. Pharmacokinetic differences may stem from changes in distribution or metabolism of drugs; absorption seems similar to that in adults. In relation to distribution, children usually have a lesser percentage of body fat than adults. Thus, antianxiety and sedative-hypnotic drugs, which are usually highly lipid soluble, cannot be as readily stored in fat as they are in adults. This often leads to shorter half-lives and the need for more frequent administration. In relation to metabolism, young children (eg, preschoolers) usually have a faster rate than adults and may therefore require relatively high doses for their size and weight. In relation to excretion, renal function is usually similar to that of adults and most of the drugs are largely inactive. Thus, with normal renal function, excretion probably has little effect on blood levels of active drug or the child's response to the drug.

Oral and parenteral diazepam has been used extensively in children, in all age groups older than 6 months. Other benzodiazepines are not recommended for particular age groups (see Table 8-2). The effects of buspirone, zaleplon, and zolpidem in children are unknown, and these drugs are not recommended for use in children.

There is growing concern that SSRIs may make some children suicidal. Although these drugs are generally prescribed for depression, they may also be prescribed to treat some anxiety disorders. The FDA is currently studying this issue.

Use in Older Adults

Most antianxiety and sedative-hypnotic drugs are metabolized and excreted more slowly in older adults, so the effects of a given dose last longer. In addition, several of the benzodiazepines produce pharmacologically active metabolites, which prolong drug actions. Thus, the drugs may accumulate and increase adverse effects if dosages are not reduced. The initial dose of any antianxiety or sedative-hypnotic drug should be small, and any incremental increases should be made gradually to decrease the risks of adverse effects. Adverse effects include oversedation, dizziness, confusion, hypotension, and impaired mobility, which may contribute to falls and other injuries unless clients are carefully monitored and safeguarded. Benzodiazepines may produce paradoxical excitement and aggression in adults older than 50 years of age who have a history of psychosis. SSRIs are considered by some clinicians to be first-line interventions for anxiety in older patients because of their efficacy and relatively low incidence of side effects.

Benzodiazepines should be tapered rather than discontinued abruptly in older adults, as in other populations. Withdrawal symptoms may occur within 24 hours after abruptly stopping a short-acting drug but may not occur for several days after stopping a long-acting agent.

For anxiety, short-acting benzodiazepines, such as alprazolam or lorazepam, are preferred over long-acting agents, such as diazepam. Buspirone may be preferred over a benzodiazepine because it does not cause sedation, psychomotor impairment, or increased risk of falls. However, it must be taken on a regular schedule and is not effective for PRN use.

For insomnia, sedative-hypnotic drugs should usually be avoided or their use minimized in older adults. Finding and treating the causes and using nondrug measures to aid sleep are much safer. If a sedative-hypnotic is used, shorter-acting benzodiazepines are preferred because they are eliminated more rapidly and are therefore less likely to accumulate and cause adverse effects. In addition, dosages should be smaller than for younger adults; the drugs should not be used every night or for longer than a few days; and older adults should be monitored closely for adverse effects. If zaleplon or zolpidem is used, the recommended dose for older adults is half that of younger adults (5 mg).

Use in Clients With Hypoalbuminemia

Clients with hypoalbuminemia (eg, from malnutrition or liver disease) are at risk of adverse effects if they take drugs that are highly bound to plasma proteins, such as the benzodiazepines, buspirone, and zolpidem. If a benzodiazepine is given to clients with low serum albumin levels, alprazolam or lorazepam is preferred because these drugs are less extensively bound to plasma proteins and less likely to cause adverse effects. If buspirone or zolpidem is given, dosage may need to be reduced.

Use in Clients With Renal Impairment

Clients with renal impairment are often given sedatives to relieve anxiety and depression, and excessive sedation is the major adverse effect. It may be difficult to assess the client for excessive sedation because drowsiness, lethargy, and mental status changes are also common symptoms of uremia.

All benzodiazepines undergo hepatic metabolism and then elimination in urine. Several of the drugs produce active metabolites that are normally excreted by the kidneys. If renal excretion is impaired, the active metabolites may accumulate and cause excessive sedation and respiratory depression.

Buspirone is contraindicated in clients with severe renal impairment. Zaleplon and zolpidem may be used by these clients and do not require dosage reduction.

Use in Clients With Hepatic Impairment

Benzodiazepines undergo hepatic metabolism and then elimination in urine. In the presence of liver disease (eg, cirrhosis, hepatitis), the metabolism of most benzodiazepines is slowed, with resultant accumulation and increased risk of adverse effects. If a benzodiazepine is needed, lorazepam and oxazepam are preferred antianxiety agents, and temazepam is the preferred hypnotic. These drugs require only conjugation with glucuronide for elimination, and liver disease does not significantly affect this process. If other benzodiazepines are given to clients with advanced liver disease, small initial doses and slow, gradual increases are indicated. Buspirone is metabolized in the liver and should not be used by clients with severe hepatic impairment. Zaleplon and zolpidem are metabolized more slowly in clients with liver impairment; if used, dosage should be reduced to 5 milligrams. Zaleplon is not recommended for clients with severe liver impairment.

Use in Clients With Critical Illness

Antianxiety and sedative-hypnotic drugs are often used in critically ill clients to relieve stress, anxiety, and agitation. By their calming effects, they may also decrease cardiac workload (eg, heart rate, blood pressure, force of myocardial contraction, myocardial oxygen consumption) and respiratory effort. Additional benefits include improving tolerance of treatment measures (eg, mechanical ventilation); keeping confused clients from harming themselves by pulling out IV catheters, feeding or drainage tubes, wound drains, and other treatment devices; and allowing more rest or sleep. Dosage of sedative drugs can be titrated to some extent by assessing clients according to a sedation scale. For example, the Ramsay scale rates levels of sedation numerically, with 1 indicating a wide-awake and agitated client and 6 indicating an unresponsive client. The desirable level is usually 2 or 3, levels which indicate that the client is calm, drowsy, but easily aroused and responsive to commands. In addition to sedation, the drugs often induce amnesia, which may be a desirable effect in the critically ill.

Benzodiazepines are commonly used sedatives in critical care units. The drugs may be given orally or by gastrointestinal tube when the client is able to take medications enterally, needs a fairly stable sedative dose, and is expected to need prolonged sedation (eg, clients receiving mechanical ventilation). However, most clients receive IV sedatives, often in conjunction with opioid analgesics for pain control. IV drugs are usually given by infusion, sometimes by intermittent bolus injection. The infusions may be given on a short-term (eg, a few days) or long-term (eg, weeks) basis. Response to the benzodiazepines is somewhat unpredictable because most drug data were derived from short-term administration of the drugs to non–critically ill adults and may differ significantly with long-term infusions and administration to critically ill clients.

Lorazepam (Ativan) is probably the benzodiazepine of first choice. It has a slow onset of action (5 to 20 minutes) because of delayed brain penetration but an intermediate to prolonged duration. In addition, there is little accumulation and its elimination is not significantly affected by hepatic or renal disease. Because of the slow onset of action of lorazepam, an IV injection of diazepam or midazolam (Versed) is usually given to achieve rapid sedative effects. Midazolam is short acting when given in a single IV injection or for a short time to patients with normal hepatic, renal, and cardiac function. However, in the critical care setting, it is usually given by continuous IV infusion and both midazolam and an active metabolite may accu-

mulate. Overall, drug effects are less predictable in these clients because changes in protein binding, hepatic metabolism, and other factors lead to wide variations in drug elimination and duration of action. Some people (eg, those being mechanically ventilated, those who have had cardiac surgery, those with septic shock or acute renal failure) have continued to be sedated for days or hours after the drug is discontinued. In clients with renal failure, active metabolites may accumulate to high levels. For these reasons, plus its high cost, some clinicians recommend using midazolam for IV bolus dosing before starting lorazepam and for short-term periods of less than 48 hours.

Diazepam also may be given to clients who require rapid sedation (eg, those with extreme agitation). It acts within 1 to 5 minutes after IV injection and lasts about 30 to 100 minutes. However, diazepam should not be given long term because its metabolism forms an active metabolite with an extremely long half-life, which accumulates and may cause excessive sedation and respiratory depression.

Although the risk of adverse effects with a benzodiazepine is high in critically ill clients, routine use of flumazenil, the benzodiazepine antidote, is generally not recommended because it may cause seizures or cardiac arrest. These effects are most likely to occur in people with a history of seizures, cardiac arrest, head injury, cerebral hypoxia, or chronic benzodiazepine use.

Dexmedetomidine and propofol (Diprivan) are two non-benzodiazepines used for sedation in critical care units. Dexmedetomidine is a newer drug approved only for sedating intubated and mechanically ventilated patients in intensive care settings. It is recommended for short-term use of less than 24 hours and is given by continuous IV infusion. Dosage should be reduced in older clients and in those with impaired liver function. If given concurrently with other CNS depressant drugs (eg, propofol, alfentanil, midazolam), dosage of dexmedetomidine or the other drug should be reduced.

Use in Home Care

Although antianxiety and sedative-hypnotic drugs are not recommended for long-term use, they are often used at home. Previously described precautions and teaching needs related to safe use of the drugs apply in home care just as they do in other settings. The home care nurse should encourage clients to use nondrug methods of reducing anxiety and insomnia and should review the risks of injuries if mental and physical responses are slowed by the drugs. In addition, assess clients for signs and symptoms of overuse; withdrawal; and use of other sedating drugs, including alcohol, sedating antihistamines, and other prescription drugs. Although the home care nurse is more likely to encounter these drugs as legal prescriptions, they are also commonly abused street drugs.

N U R S I N G   A C T I O N S

Antianxiety and Sedative-Hypnotic Drugs

NURSING ACTIONS	RATIONALE/EXPLANATION
1. Administer accurately	To avoid excessive sedation and other adverse effects
a. If a client appears excessively sedated when a dose of an antianxiety or sedative-hypnotic drug is due, omit the dose and record the reason.	
b. For oral sedative-hypnotics:	
(1) Prepare the client for sleep before giving hypnotic doses of any drug.	Most of the drugs cause drowsiness within 15–30 minutes. The client should be in bed when he or she becomes drowsy to increase the therapeutic effectiveness of the drug and to decrease the likelihood of falls or other injuries.
(2) Give with a glass of water or other fluid.	The fluid enhances dissolution and absorption of the drug for a quicker onset of action.
(3) Raise bedrails and instruct the client to stay in bed or to ask for help if necessary to get out of bed.	To avoid falls and other injuries related to sedation and impaired mobility
c. For benzodiazepines:	
(1) Give orally, when feasible.	These drugs are well absorbed from the gastrointestinal (GI) tract, and onset of action occurs within a few minutes. Diazepam is better absorbed orally than intramuscularly (IM). When given IM, the drug crystallizes in tissue and is absorbed very slowly.
(2) Do not mix injectable diazepam with any other drug in a syringe or add to intravenous (IV) fluids.	Diazepam is physically incompatible with other drugs and solutions.
(3) Give IM benzodiazepines undiluted, deeply, into large muscle masses, such as the gluteus muscle of the hip.	These drugs are irritating to tissues and may cause pain at injection sites.
(4) With IV benzodiazepines, be very careful to avoid intra-arterial injection or extravasation into surrounding tissues. Have equipment available for respiratory assistance.	These drugs are very irritating to tissues and may cause venous thrombosis, phlebitis, local irritation, edema, and vascular impairment. They may also cause respiratory depression and apnea.
(5) Give IV **diazepam** slowly, over at least 1 minute for 5 mg (1 mL); into large veins (not hand or wrist veins); by direct injection into the vein or into IV infusion tubing as close as possible to the venipuncture site.	To avoid apnea and tissue irritation
(6) Give IV **lorazepam** slowly, over at least 1 minute for 2 mg, by direct injection into the vein or into IV infusion tubing. Immediately before injection, dilute with an equal volume of sterile water for injection, 0.9% sodium chloride injection, or 5% dextrose in water.	To avoid apnea, hypotension, and tissue irritation
(7) Give IV **midazolam** slowly, over approximately 2 minutes, after diluting the dose with 0.9% sodium chloride injection or 5% dextrose in water.	Rapid IV injection may cause severe respiratory depression and apnea; dilution facilitates slow injection.
(8) Midazolam may be mixed in the same syringe with morphine sulfate, and atropine sulfate.	No apparent chemical or physical incompatibilities occur with these substances.
(9) Do not crush, break, or allow patient to chew extended-release forms of **alprazolam.**	Increased drug absorption may lead to toxicity.
(10) Carefully peel open packaging of orally disintegrating tablets of **clonazepam** and place in the mouth. Be sure your hands are dry when handling tablets.	Tablets rapidly dissolve when moistened and can be swallowed with or without water.

(continued)

NURSING ACTIONS	RATIONALE/EXPLANATION
d. Give **hydroxyzine** orally or deep IM only. When given IM for preoperative sedation, it can be mixed in the same syringe with atropine, and most opioid analgesics likely to be ordered at the same time.	IM hydroxyzine is very irritating to tissues.
e. Give **clomipramine** in divided doses, with meals, initially; after titration to a stable dose, give the total daily dose at bedtime.	Giving with meals decreases adverse effects on the GI tract; giving the total dose once daily at bedtime decreases daytime sedation.
2. Observe for therapeutic effects	Therapeutic effects depend largely on the reason for use. With benzodiazepines, decreased anxiety and drowsiness may appear within a few minutes.
a. When a drug is given for antianxiety effects, observe for:	
(1) An appearance of being relaxed, perhaps drowsy, but easily aroused	With buspirone, antianxiety effects may occur within 7–10 days of regular use, with optimal effects in 3–4 weeks.
(2) Verbal statements such as "less worried," "more relaxed," "resting better"	
(3) Decrease in or absence of manifestations of anxiety, such as rigid posture, facial grimaces, crying, elevated blood pressure and heart rate	
(4) Less time spent in worrying or compulsive behaviors	
b. When a drug is given for hypnotic effects, drowsiness should be evident within approximately 30 minutes, and the client usually sleeps for several hours.	
c. When diazepam or lorazepam is given IV for control of acute convulsive disorders, seizure activity should decrease or stop almost immediately. When a drug is given for chronic anticonvulsant effects, lack of seizure activity is a therapeutic effect.	
d. When hydroxyzine is given for nausea and vomiting, absence of vomiting and verbal statements of relief indicate therapeutic effects.	
e. When hydroxyzine is given for antihistaminic effects in skin disorders, observe for decreased itching and fewer statements of discomfort.	
3. Observe for adverse effects	Most adverse effects are caused by central nervous system (CNS) depression.
a. Excessive sedation—drowsiness, stupor, difficult to arouse, impaired mental processes, impaired mobility, respiratory depression, confusion	These effects are more likely to occur with large doses or if the recipient is elderly, debilitated, or has liver disease that slows drug metabolism. Respiratory depression and apnea stem from depression of the respiratory center in the medulla oblongata; they are most likely to occur with large doses or rapid IV administration of diazepam, lorazepam, or midazolam. Excessive drowsiness is more likely to occur when drug therapy is begun, and it usually decreases within a week.
b. Hypotension	Hypotension probably results from depression of the vasomotor center in the brain and is more likely to occur with large doses or rapid IV administration of diazepam, lorazepam, or midazolam.
c. Pain and induration at injection sites	Parenteral solutions are irritating to tissues.
d. Paradoxical excitement, anger, aggression, and hallucinations	
e. Chronic intoxication—sedation, confusion, emotional lability, muscular incoordination, impaired mental processes, mental depression, GI problems, weight loss	These signs and symptoms may occur with benzodiazepines and are similar to those occurring with chronic alcohol abuse (see Chap. 14).
f. Withdrawal or abstinence syndrome—anxiety, insomnia, restlessness, irritability, tremors, postural hypotension, seizures	These signs and symptoms may occur when benzodiazepines are discontinued abruptly, especially after high doses or long-term use.

NURSING ACTIONS	RATIONALE/EXPLANATION
g. With buspirone, the most common adverse effects are headache, dizziness, nausea, nervousness, fatigue, and excitement. Less frequent effects include dry mouth, chest pain, tachycardia, palpitations, drowsiness, confusion, and depression.	
h. With zaleplon and zolpidem, common adverse effects include daytime drowsiness, dizziness, headache, nausea and diarrhea. Less frequent effects include ataxia, confusion, paradoxical excitation.	
4. Observe for drug interactions	
a. Drugs that *increase* effects of antianxiety and sedative-hypnotic drugs:	
(1) CNS depressants—alcohol, opioid analgesics, tricyclic antidepressants, sedating antihistamines, phenothiazine and other antipsychotic agents	All these drugs produce CNS depression when given alone. Any combination increases CNS depression, sedation, and respiratory depression. Combinations of these drugs are hazardous and should be avoided. Ingesting alcohol with antianxiety or sedative-hypnotic drugs may cause respiratory depression, coma, and convulsions. Although buspirone does not appear to cause additive CNS depression, concurrent use with other CNS depressants is best avoided.
(2) Amprenavir, clarithromycin, cimetidine, diltiazem, erythromycin, fluoxetine, fluvoxamine, itraconazole, ketoconazole, metoprolol, nefazodone, omeprazole, oral contraceptives, propranolol, ritonavir, valproic acid	These drugs inhibit cytochrome P450 3A4 enzymes that metabolize most benzodiazepines. Midazolam should be avoided in patients receiving a CYP3A4 inhibitor drug; lorazepam or propofol may be used for sedation. These drugs do not affect elimination of lorazepam or temazepam.
b. Drugs that *decrease* effects of antianxiety and sedative-hypnotic agents:	
(1) CNS stimulants—antiasthma drugs, appetite suppressants, bronchodilators (eg, albuterol, theophylline), nasal decongestants (eg, phenylephrine, pseudoephedrine), and lifestyle drugs (eg, caffeine, nicotine)	Phenylephrine and pseudoephedrine are available alone or in multi-symptom cold remedies.
(2) Enzyme inducers (eg, carbamazepine, isoniazid, phenytoin, rifampin)	With chronic use, these drugs antagonize their own actions and the actions of other drugs metabolized by the same enzymes in the liver. They increase the rate of drug metabolism and elimination from the body.
c. Drug that *increases* effects of zaleplon:	
(1) Cimetidine	Inhibits both aldehyde oxidase and CYP3A4 enzymes that metabolize zaleplon, thereby greatly increasing serum levels and risks of toxicity
d. Drug that *increases* effects of zolpidem:	
(1) Ritonavir	Inhibits hepatic metabolism of zolpidem and may cause severe sedation and respiratory depression. **These drugs should not be given concurrently.**

APPLYING YOUR KNOWLEDGE: ANSWERS

8-1 Help Mrs. Portman's daughter understand how the drugs help to manage her mother's anxiety and symptoms of agitation. The concern for the patient's safety needs to be emphasized. Perhaps a team meeting of the health care professionals involved in her mother's care would help her to accept the plan to care for her mother.

8-2 Prepare 0.25mg of Alprazolam, the smaller ordered dose. Daytime drowsiness or impaired mobility are signs of too much medication. Also, Mrs. Portman is elderly, so one half of the adult dose is recommended.

8-3 These symptoms are typical for withdrawal of benzodiazepines. Tapering the drug may reduce the likelihood of withdrawal symptoms or Mrs. Portman may need to continue on the medication for a longer period of time.

Review and Application Exercises

Short Answer Exercises

1. What is anxiety, and how may it be manifested?

2. How do benzodiazepines act to relieve anxiety?

3. What are some nonpharmacologic interventions to decrease anxiety?

4. When assessing a client before giving an antianxiety benzodiazepine, what assessment data would cause the nurse to omit the dose?

5. Why is sleep necessary? What functions does sleep fulfill?

6. Why are nonpharmacologic interventions to promote relaxation and sleep usually preferred over the use of sedative-hypnotic drugs?

7. What is the main difference between sedatives and hypnotics?

8. In terms of nursing care, what difference does it make whether a benzodiazepine is metabolized to active or inactive metabolites?

9. What are drug dependence, tolerance, and withdrawal symptoms in relation to the benzodiazepines?

10. What are some special precautions for using sedatives and hypnotics in older adults and those with renal or hepatic impairment or critical illness?

11. For an ambulatory client beginning a prescription for a benzodiazepine antianxiety or hypnotic agent, what instructions must be emphasized for safe, effective, and rational drug use?

12. When assisting in home care of a client taking a benzodiazepine, what kinds of data would the nurse collect to evaluate whether the client is using the drug appropriately or abusing it?

NCLEX-Style Questions

13. When using flumazenil (Romazicon) as an antidote for benzodiazepine overdose, the nurse should
    a. Administer the antidote IM into a large muscle.
    b. Inject the antidote IV push over 5 seconds.
    c. Observe for re-sedation after administration of the antidote.
    d. Administer the antidote one time only.

14. When administering benzodiazepines to clients with malnutrition or liver disease, the nurse should monitor carefully for
    a. toxicity
    b. withdrawal
    c. paradoxical excitation
    d. seizures

15. Which statement would indicate to the nurse the need for further client teaching?
    a. "I only use my medication when I really need it."
    b. "I avoid smoking after taking my sleeping pill."
    c. "I skip my evening glass of wine when I take my sleeping pill."
    d. "My sister often has a sleep problem similar to mine."

Selected References

American Psychiatric Association. (2000). *Diagnostic and statistical manual of mental disorders* (4th ed., text revision). Washington, DC: American Psychiatric Association.

Arikian, S., & Gorman, J. (2001). A review of the diagnosis, pharmacologic treatment, and economic aspects of anxiety disorders. *Primary Care Companion, Journal of Clinical Psychiatry, 3*(3), 110–117.

Chouinard, G. (2004). Issues in the clinical use of benzodiazepines: Potency, withdrawal, and rebound. *Journal of Clinical Psychiatry, 65*(Suppl. 5), 7–12.

Davidson, J. (2004). Use of benzodiazepines in social anxiety disorder, generalized anxiety disorder, and posttraumatic stress disorder. *Journal of Clinical Psychiatry, 65*(Suppl. 5), 29–33.

Dresser, G. K., Spence, J. D., & Bailey, D. G. (2000). Pharmacokinetic-pharmacodynamic consequences and clinical relevance of cytochrome P450 3A4 inhibition. *Clinical Pharmacokinetics, 38*(1), 41–57.

Drug Facts and Comparisons. (Updated monthly). St. Louis: Facts and Comparisons.

Fetrow, C. W., & Avila, J. R. (2001). *Professional's handbook of complementary & alternative medicines* (2nd ed.). Springhouse, PA: Springhouse.

Gordon, J., & Hen, R. (2004). The serotonergic system and anxiety. *Neuromolecular Medicine, 5*(1), 27–40.

Hadbavny, A. M., & Hoyt, J. W. (2000). Sedatives and analgesics in critical care. In A. Grenvik, S. M. Ayres, P. R. Holbrook, & W. C. Shoemaker (Eds.), *Textbook of critical care* (4th ed., pp. 961–971). Philadelphia: W. B. Saunders.

Holden, C. (2004). FDA weighs suicide risk in children on antidepressants. *Science, 303*(5659), 745.

Lauderdale, S., & Sheikh, J. (2003). Anxiety disorders in older adults. *Clinical Geriatric Medicine, 19*(4), 721–741.

Moroz, G. (2004). High-potency benzodiazepines: Recent clinical results. *Journal of Clinical Psychiatry, 65*(Suppl. 5), 13–18.

Waddell, D. L., Hummel, M. E., & Sumners, A. D. (2001). Three herbs you should get to know. *American Journal of Nursing, 101*(4), 48–53.

Antipsychotic Drugs

OBJECTIVES

After studying this chapter, you will be able to:

1. Discuss common manifestations of psychotic disorders, including schizophrenia.
2. Discuss characteristics of phenothiazines and related antipsychotics.
3. Compare characteristics of "atypical" antipsychotic drugs with those of "typical" phenothiazines and related antipsychotic drugs.
4. Describe the main elements of acute and long-term treatment of psychotic disorders.
5. State interventions to decrease adverse effects of antipsychotic drugs.
6. State interventions to promote compliance with outpatient use of antipsychotic drugs.

APPLYING YOUR KNOWLEDGE

Caroline Jones is brought to the mental health clinic by a friend. The friend says that Caroline has been seeing things that are not there and has become more withdrawn. Caroline has not taken care of her personal hygiene for some time. She is diagnosed with acute psychosis and is treated with psychotherapy and the medications haloperidol and risperidone.

INTRODUCTION

Psychosis

Antipsychotic drugs are used mainly for the treatment of *psychosis,* a severe mental disorder characterized by disordered thought processes (disorganized and often bizarre thinking); blunted or inappropriate emotional responses; bizarre behavior ranging from hypoactivity to hyperactivity with agitation, aggressiveness, hostility, and combativeness; social withdrawal in which a person pays less-than-normal attention to the environment and other people; deterioration from previous levels of occupational and social functioning (poor self-care and interpersonal skills); hallucinations; and paranoid delusions. *Hallucinations* are sensory perceptions of people or objects that are not present in the external environment. More specifically, people see, hear, or feel stimuli that are not visible to external observers, and they cannot distinguish between these false perceptions and reality. Hallucinations occur in delirium, dementias, schizophrenia, and other psychotic states. In schizophrenia or bipolar affective disorder, they are usually auditory; in delirium, they are usually visual or tactile; and in dementia, they are usually visual. *Delusions* are false beliefs that persist in the absence of rea-son or evidence. Deluded people often believe that other people control their thoughts, feelings, and behaviors or seek to harm them (*paranoia*). Delusions indicate severe mental illness. Although they are commonly associated with schizophrenia, delusions also occur with delirium, dementias, and other psychotic disorders.

Psychosis may be acute or chronic. Acute episodes, also called *confusion* or *delirium,* have a sudden onset over hours to days and may be precipitated by physical disorders (eg, brain damage related to cerebrovascular disease or head injury; metabolic disorders; infections); drug intoxication with adrenergics, antidepressants, some anticonvulsants, amphetamines, cocaine, and others; and drug withdrawal after chronic use (eg, alcohol; benzodiazepine antianxiety or sedative-hypnotic agents). In addition, acute psychotic episodes may be superimposed on chronic dementias and psychoses, such as schizophrenia. This chapter focuses primarily on schizophrenia as a chronic psychosis.

Schizophrenia

Although *schizophrenia* is often referred to as a single disease, it includes a variety of related disorders. Risk factors include a genetic predisposition and environmental stresses.

Symptoms may begin gradually or suddenly, usually during adolescence or early adulthood. According to the American Psychiatric Association's *Diagnostic and Statistical Manual of Mental Disorders, 4th edition, Text Revision* overt psychotic symptoms must be present for 6 months before schizophrenia can be diagnosed.

Behavioral manifestations of schizophrenia are categorized as positive and negative symptoms. *Positive symptoms* are characterized by central nervous system (CNS) stimulation and include agitation, behavioral disturbances, delusions, disorganized speech, hallucinations, insomnia, and paranoia. *Negative symptoms* are characterized by lack of pleasure (anhedonia), lack of motivation, blunted affect, poor grooming and hygiene, poor social skills, poverty of speech, and social withdrawal. However, all of these symptoms may occur in other disorders.

The etiology of schizophrenia is unclear. However, there is evidence that it results from abnormal neurotransmission systems in the brain, especially in the dopaminergic, serotonergic, and glutamatergic systems. There is also evidence of extensive interactions among neurotransmission systems. For example, the serotonergic and glutamatergic systems can alter dopaminergic activity, and drugs that may cause psychosis affect several systems (eg, adrenergics increase norepinephrine; antidepressants increase norepinephrine, serotonin, or both). Thus, schizophrenia probably results from imbalances and abnormal integration among several neurotransmission systems. In addition, illnesses or drugs that alter neurotransmission in one system are likely to alter neurotransmission in other systems. The dopaminergic, serotoninergic, and glutamatergic systems have been studied most.

The dopaminergic system has been more extensively studied than other systems, because schizophrenia has long been attributed to increased dopamine activity in the brain. Stimulation of dopamine can initiate psychotic symptoms or exacerbate an existing psychotic disorder. The importance of dopamine is further supported by two findings: (1) antipsychotic drugs exert their therapeutic effects by decreasing dopamine activity (ie, blocking dopamine receptors), and (2) drugs that increase dopamine levels in the brain (eg, bromocriptine, cocaine, levodopa) can cause signs and symptoms of psychosis.

In addition to the increased amount of dopamine, dopamine receptors are also involved. Two groups of dopamine receptors have been differentiated, mainly by the effects of the dopamine–receptor complex on intracellular functions. The first group stimulates cellular functions, whereas the second group decreases cellular functions and alters the movement of calcium and potassium ions across neuronal cell membranes. The second group (D_2 receptors) is considered important in the pathophysiology of schizophrenia. Thus, at the cellular level, dopamine activity is determined by its interaction with various receptors and the simultaneous actions of other neurotransmitters at the same target neurons. In general, overactivity of dopamine in some parts of the brain is thought to account for the positive symptoms of schizophrenia, and underactiv-

ity in another part of the brain is thought to account for the negative symptoms.

The serotonergic system, which is widespread in the brain, is mainly inhibitory in nature. In schizophrenia, serotonin apparently decreases dopamine activity in the part of the brain associated with negative symptoms, causing or aggravating these symptoms.

The glutamatergic neurotransmission system involves glutamate, the major excitatory neurotransmitter in the CNS. Glutamate receptors are widespread and possibly located on every neuron in the brain. They are also diverse, and their functions may vary according to subtypes and their locations in particular parts of the brain. When glutamate binds to its receptors, the resulting neuronal depolarization activates signaling molecules (eg, calcium, nitric oxide) within and between brain cells. Thus, glutamatergic transmission may affect every CNS neuron and is considered essential for all mental, sensory, motor, and affective functions. Dysfunction of glutamatergic neurotransmission has been implicated in the development of psychosis.

In addition, the glutamatergic system interacts with the dopaminergic and gamma-aminobutyric acid systems, and possibly other neurotransmission systems. In people with schizophrenia, evidence indicates the presence of abnormalities in the number, density, composition, and function of glutamate receptors. In addition, glutamate receptors are genetically encoded and can interact with environmental factors (eg, stress; alcohol and other drugs) during brain development. Thus, glutamatergic dysfunction may account for the roles of genetic and environmental risk factors in the development of schizophrenia as well as the cognitive impairments and negative symptoms associated with the disorder.

GENERAL CHARACTERISTICS OF ANTIPSYCHOTIC DRUGS

Antipsychotic drugs are derived from several chemical groups. These drugs may be broadly categorized as "typical," *conventional,* or *first-generation* agents (phenothiazines and older nonphenothiazines, such as haloperidol [Haldol], with similar pharmacologic actions, clinical uses, and adverse effects), or as "atypical" or *second-generation* agents, which can also be called *newer nonphenothiazines.*

Mechanism of Action

Most antipsychotic drugs bind to D_2 dopamine receptors and block the action of dopamine (Fig. 9-1). However, drug binding to the receptors does not account for antipsychotic effects because binding occurs within a few hours after a drug dose, and antipsychotic effects may not occur until the drugs have been given for a few weeks. Manifestations of hyperarousal (eg, anxiety, agitation, hyperactivity, insomnia, aggressive or combative behavior) are relieved more quickly than halluci-

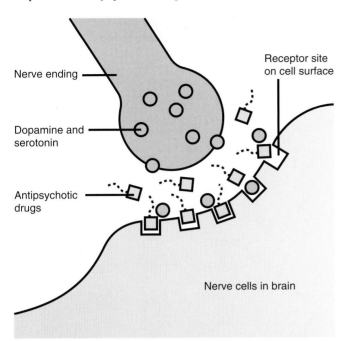

FIGURE 9-1 Antipsychotic drugs prevent dopamine and serotonin from occupying receptor sites on neuronal cell membranes and exerting their effects on cellular functions. This action leads to changes in receptors and cell functions that account for therapeutic effects (ie, relief of psychotic symptoms). Other neurotransmitters and receptors may also be involved.

nations, delusions, and thought disorders. One view of the delayed effects is that the blockade of dopamine receptors leads to changes in the receptors and postreceptor effects on cell metabolism and function. With chronic drug administration (ie, chronic blockade of dopamine receptors), there is an increased number of dopamine receptors on postsynaptic and possibly presynaptic nerve cell membranes (up-regulation). Clozapine (Clozaril) and other atypical agents interact with dopamine, serotonin, and glutamate receptors. Overall, the drugs re-regulate the abnormal neurotransmission systems associated with psychosis.

Indications for Use

The major clinical indication for use of antipsychotic drugs is schizophrenia. The drugs also are used to treat psychotic symptoms associated with brain impairment induced by head injury, tumor, stroke, alcohol withdrawal, overdoses of CNS stimulant drugs, and other disorders. They may be useful in the manic phase of bipolar affective disorder to control manic behavior until lithium, the drug of choice, becomes effective.

The phenothiazines are also used for clinical indications not associated with psychiatric illness. These include treatment of nausea, vomiting, and intractable hiccups. The drugs relieve nausea and vomiting by blocking dopamine receptors in the chemoreceptor trigger zone, a group of neurons in the medulla oblongata that causes nausea and vomiting when

activated by physical or psychological stimuli. The mechanism by which the drugs relieve hiccups is unclear.

Promethazine (Phenergan) is not used for antipsychotic effects, but is often used for antiemetic, sedative, and antihistaminic effects.

Contraindications to Use

Because of their wide-ranging adverse effects, antipsychotic drugs may cause or aggravate a number of conditions. They are contraindicated in clients with liver damage, coronary artery disease, cerebrovascular disease, parkinsonism, bone marrow depression, severe hypotension or hypertension, coma, or severely depressed states. They should be used cautiously in people with seizure disorders, diabetes mellitus, glaucoma, prostatic hypertrophy, peptic ulcer disease, and chronic respiratory disorders.

INDIVIDUAL DRUGS

Phenothiazines

These drugs are historically important because **P chlorpromazine** (Thorazine), the first drug to effectively treat psychotic disorders, belongs to this group. These drugs have been used since the 1950s, but their usage and clinical importance have waned in recent years.

The phenothiazines are well absorbed after oral and parenteral administration. They are distributed to most body tissues and reach high concentrations in the brain. They are metabolized in the liver by the cytochrome P450 enzyme system; several produce pharmacologically active metabolites. Metabolites are excreted in urine. These drugs do not cause psychological dependence, but they may cause physical dependence manifested by withdrawal symptoms (eg, lethargy, difficulty sleeping) if they are abruptly discontinued. Pharmacokinetics of various antipsychotics are presented in Table 9-1.

Phenothiazines have many effects, including CNS depression, autonomic nervous system depression (antiadrenergic and anticholinergic effects), antiemetic effects, lowering of body temperature, hypersensitivity reactions, and others. Phenothiazines differ mainly in potency and adverse effects: Some are as effective in doses of a few milligrams as others are in doses of several hundred milligrams. All phenothiazines produce the same kinds of adverse effects, but individual drugs differ in the incidence and severity of particular adverse effects. Information about administration, dosage, and other characteristics of individual phenothiazine drugs are listed in Table 9-2.

Nonphenothiazines

Nonphenothiazines include first-generation "typical" antipsychotics, which share many similarities to phenothiazines,

TABLE 9-1 Pharmacokinetics of Antipsychotic Drugs

| GENERIC NAME | ROUTE | ACTION | | | HALF-LIFE (HOURS) |
		Onset	Peak	Duration	
Aripiprazole	PO	Varies	3–5 h	24 h	75–146
Chlorpromazine	PO	30–60 min	2–4 h	4–6 h (10–12 h for extended release)	3–40
	IM	Unknown	2–3 h	4–18 h	3–40
Clozapine	PO	Unknown	1–6 h	4–12 h	9–17
Fluphenazine decanoate	IM	24–72 h	24 h	1–3 wks	7–10 days
Fluphenazine enanthate	IM	24–72 h	48 h	>4 wks	4 days
Fluphenazine hydrochloride	PO	60 min	3–5 h	6–8 h	5–15
Haloperidol	PO	2 h	2–6 h	8–12 h	21–24
	IM	20–30 min	30–45 min	4–8 h	
Haloperidol decanoate	IM	3–9 days	Unknown	1 month	3 wk
Loxapine	PO	30 min	1.5–3 h	12 h	3–4
Molindone	PO	Varies	30–90 min	24–36 h	1.5–6
Olanzapine	PO	Varies	4–5 h	weeks	20–27
Perphenazine	PO	Varies	Unknown	Unknown	Unknown
	IM/IV	5–10 min	1–2 h	6 h	
Quetiapine	PO	Varies	2–4 h	8–10 h	6
Risperidone	PO	1–2 h	3–17 h	weeks	20–30
Thiothixene	PO	Slow	1–3 h	12 h	3–4
Trifluoperazine	PO	Varies	2–4 h	<12 h	3–40
	IM	Rapid	1–2 h	<12 h	3–40
Ziprasidone	PO	Varies	1 h	6–8 h	3

IM, intramuscular; IV, intravenous; PO, oral.

and second-generation "atypical" antipsychotics, which vary in relation to typical drugs and to each other. Details about administration, dosage, and other characteristics of selected nonphenothiazines are listed in Table 9-3.

First-Generation "Typical" Antipsychotics

Haloperidol (Haldol) is a butyrophenone used in psychiatric disorders. A related drug, droperidol, is used in anaesthesia and as an antiemetic. Haloperidol is a frequently used, potent, long-acting drug. It is well absorbed after oral or intramuscular (IM) administration, is metabolized in the liver, and is excreted in urine and bile. It may cause adverse effects similar to those of the phenothiazines. Usually, it produces a relatively low incidence of hypotension and sedation and a high incidence of extrapyramidal effects.

Haloperidol may be used as the initial drug for treating psychotic disorders or as a substitute in clients who are hypersensitive or refractory to the phenothiazines. It also is used to treat some conditions in which other antipsychotic drugs are not used, including mental retardation with hyper-

kinesia (abnormally increased motor activity), Tourette's syndrome (a rare disorder characterized by involuntary movements and vocalizations), and Huntington's disease (a rare genetic disorder that involves progressive psychiatric symptoms and involuntary movements). For clients who are unable or unwilling to take the oral drug as prescribed, a slowly absorbed, long-acting formulation (haloperidol decanoate) may be given IM, once monthly.

Loxapine (Loxitane) is similar to phenothiazines and related drugs. It is recommended for use in only the treatment of schizophrenia.

Molindone (Moban) differs chemically from other agents but has similar pharmacologic actions.

Pimozide (Orap) is approved only for the treatment of Tourette's syndrome in clients who fail to respond to haloperidol. Potentially serious adverse effects include tardive dyskinesia, major motor seizures, and sudden death.

Thiothixene (Navane) is used only for antipsychotic effects, although it produces other effects similar to those of the phenothiazines.

(text continues on page 160)

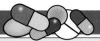

Table 9-2 Drugs at a Glance: Phenothiazine Antipsychotic Drugs

GENERIC/TRADE NAME	ROUTES OF ADMINISTRATION AND DOSAGE RANGES	MAJOR SIDE EFFECTS (INCIDENCE)		
		Sedation	Extrapyramidal Reactions	Hypotension
P Chlorpro-mazine (Thorazine)	*Adults:* PO 200–600 mg daily in divided doses. Dose may be increased by 100 mg daily q2–3 days until symptoms are controlled, adverse effects occur, or a maximum daily dose of 2 g is reached. IM 25–100 mg initially for acute psychotic symptoms, repeated in 1–4 hours PRN until control is achieved. *Elderly or debilitated adults:* PO one third to one half usual adult dose, increased by 25 mg daily q2–3 days if necessary. IM 10 mg q6–8h until acute symptoms are controlled. *Children:* PO, IM 0.5 mg/kg q4–8h. Maximum IM dose, 40 mg daily in children under 5 y of age and 75 mg for older children.	High	Moderate	Moderate to high
Fluphenazine decanoate and enanthate (Prolixin Decanoate; Prolixin Enanthate)	*Adults under 50 y:* IM; Sub-Q 12.5 mg initially followed by 25 mg every 2 weeks. Dosage requirements rarely exceed 100 mg q2–6 wk. *Adults over 50 y, debilitated clients, or clients with a history of extrapyramidal reactions:* 2.5 mg initially followed by 2.5–5 mg q10–14 days *Children:* No dosage established	Low to moderate	High	Low
Fluphenazine hydrochloride (Prolixin, Permitil)	*Adults:* PO 2.5–10 mg initially, gradually reduced to maintenance dose of 1–5 mg (doses above 3 mg are rarely necessary). Acute psychosis: 1.25 mg initially, increased gradually to 2.5–10 mg daily in 3–4 divided doses. *Elderly or debilitated adults:* PO 1–2.5 mg daily; IM one third to one half the usual adult dose *Children:* PO 0.75–10 mg daily in children 5 to 12 y. IM no dosage established.	Low to moderate	High	Low
Perphenazine (Trilafon)	*Adults:* PO 16–64 mg daily in divided doses. Acute psychoses: IM 5–10 mg initially, then 5 mg q6h if necessary. Maximum daily dose, 15 mg for ambulatory clients and 30 mg for hospitalized clients. *Elderly or debilitated adults:* PO, IM one third to one half usual adult dose *Children:* PO dosages not established, but the following amounts have been given in divided doses: ages 1–6 y, 4–6 mg daily; 6–12 y, 6 mg daily; over 12 y, 6–12 mg daily	Low to moderate	High	Low
Prochlorperazine (Compazine)	*Adults:* PO 10 mg 3–4 times daily, increased gradually (usual daily dose, 100–150 mg). IM 10–20 mg; may be repeated in 2–4 h. Switch to oral form as soon as possible. *Children over 2 y:* PO, rectal 2.5 mg 2–3 times daily; IM 0.06 mg/lb	Moderate	High	Low

(continued)

Table 9-2 Drugs at a Glance: Phenothiazine Antipsychotic Drugs (continued)

		MAJOR SIDE EFFECTS (INCIDENCE)		
GENERIC/TRADE NAME	ROUTES OF ADMINISTRATION AND DOSAGE RANGES	Sedation	Extrapyramidal Reactions	Hypotension
Trifluoperazine (Stelazine)	*Adults:* Outpatients PO 2–4 mg daily in divided doses. Hospitalized clients, PO 4–10 mg daily in divided doses. Acute psychoses: IM 1–2 mg q4–5h, maximum of 10 mg daily. *Elderly or debilitated adults:* PO, IM one third to one half usual adult dose. If given IM, give at less frequent intervals than above. *Children 6 y and over:* PO, IM 1–2 mg daily, maximum daily dose 15 mg *Children under 6 y:* no dosage established	Moderate	High	Low

IM, intramuscular; IV, intravenous; PO, oral.

Table 9-3 Drugs at a Glance: Nonphenothiazine Antipsychotic Drugs

	ROUTES AND DOSAGE RANGES	
GENERIC/TRADE NAME	Adults	Children
First-Generation, "Typical" Drugs		
Haloperidol (Haldol)	Acute psychosis, PO 1–15 mg/d initially in divided doses, gradually increased to 100 mg/d, if necessary; usual maintenance dose, 2–8 mg daily; IM 2–10 mg q1–8h until symptoms are controlled (usually within 72 h) Chronic schizophrenia, PO 6–15 mg/d; maximum 100 mg/d; dosage is reduced for maintenance, usually 15–20 mg/d Haloperidol decanoate IM, initial dose up to 100 mg, depending on the previous dose of oral drug, then titrated according to response. Usually given every 4 weeks. Tourette's syndrome, PO 6–15 mg/d; maximum 100 mg/d; usual maintenance dose, 9 mg/d Mental retardation with hyperkinesia, PO 80–120 mg/d, gradually reduced to a maintenance dose of approximately 60 mg/d; IM 20 mg/d in divided doses, gradually increased to 60 mg/d if necessary. Oral administration should be substituted after symptoms are controlled. *Elderly or debilitated adults:* Same as for children <12 y	*12 y and older:* Acute psychosis, chronic refractory schizophrenia, Tourette's syndrome, mental retardation with hyperkinesia: same as for adults *<12 y:* Acute psychosis, PO 0.5–1.5 mg/d initially, gradually increased in increments of 0.5 mg; usual maintenance dose, 2–4 mg/d. IM dosage not established. Chronic refractory schizophrenia, dosage not established Tourette's syndrome, PO 1.5–6 mg/d initially in divided doses; usual maintenance dose, 1.5 mg/d Mental retardation with hyperkinesia, PO 1.5 mg/d initially, in divided doses, gradually increased to a maximum of 15 mg/d, if necessary. When symptoms are controlled, dosage is gradually reduced to the minimum effective level. IM dosage not established.

(continued)

Table 9-3 Drugs at a Glance: Nonphenothiazine Antipsychotic Drugs (continued)

	ROUTES AND DOSAGE RANGES	
GENERIC/TRADE NAME	**Adults**	**Children**
Loxapine (Loxitane)	PO 10 mg twice a day initially, may be increased to 50 mg/d in severe psychoses; usual maintenance dose 20–60 mg/d; maximum dose, 250 mg/d IM 12.5–50 mg q4–6h or longer, depending on response. Change to oral drug when symptoms controlled. Elderly or debilitated adults: One third to one half the usual adult dosage	*16 y and older:* Same as adults *<16 y:* Not recommended
Molindone (Moban)	PO 50–75 mg/d, increased gradually if necessary up to 225 mg/d, then reduced for maintenance; usual maintenance dose, 15–40 mg/d Elderly or debilitated adults: One third to one half the usual adult dosage	*<12 y:* Dosage not established
Pimozide (Orap)	PO 1–2 mg/d in divided doses initially, increased if necessary; usual maintenance dose, approximately 10 mg/d; maximum dose, 20 mg/d	
Thiothixene (Navane)	PO 6–10 mg/d in divided doses; maximum 60 mg/d Acute psychosis, IM 8–16 mg/d in divided doses; maximum 30 mg/d *Elderly or debilitated adults:* PO, IM one third to one half the usual adult dosage	*12 y and older:* Same as adults *<12 y:* Dosage not established
Second-Generation, "Atypical" Drugs		
Aripiprazole (Abilify)	PO 10–15 mg once daily; maximum dose 30 mg/d	Dosage not established
P **Clozapine** (Clozaril)	PO 25 mg once or twice daily initially, increased by 25–50 mg/d, if tolerated, to 300–450 mg/d by end of 2nd wk	Dosage not established
Olanzapine (Zyprexa)	PO 5–10 mg/d initially; given once daily at bedtime; increased over several weeks to 20 mg/d, if necessary	Dosage not established
Quetiapine (Seroquel)	PO 25 mg bid initially; increased by 25–50 mg two or three times daily on second and third days, as tolerated, to 300–400 mg, in two or three divided doses on the fourth day Additional increments or decrements can be made at 2-day intervals; maximum dose 800 mg/d Elderly or debilitated adults: Use lower initial doses and increase more gradually, to a lower target dose than for other adults. Hepatic impairment: PO, same as for elderly or debilitated adults	Dosage not established

(continued)

Table 9-3 Drugs at a Glance: Nonphenothiazine Antipsychotic Drugs (continued)

	ROUTES AND DOSAGE RANGES	
GENERIC/TRADE NAME	Adults	Children
Risperidone (Risperdal)	PO, initially 1 mg twice daily (2 mg/d); increase to 2 mg twice daily on the second day (4 mg/d); increase to 3 mg twice daily on the third day (6 mg/d), if necessary. Usual maintenance dose, 4 to 8 mg/d. After initial titration, dosage increases or decreases should be made at a rate of 1 mg/wk. *Elderly or debilitated adults:* PO, initially 0.5 mg twice daily (1 mg/d); increase in 0.5-mg increments to 1.5 mg twice daily (3 mg/d) *Renal or hepatic impairment:* PO, same as for elderly or debilitated adults	*<12 y:* Dosage not established
(Risperdal Consta)	IM 25 mg every 2 wk; maximum dose not to exceed 50 mg/2 wk. Oral Risperdal should be continued for first 3 weeks of therapy to ensure adequate blood levels are maintained.	*< 18 y:* Dosage not established
Ziprasidone (Geodon)	PO 20 mg twice daily with food, initially; gradually increased up to 80 mg twice daily, if necessary	

IM, intramuscular; IV, intravenous; PO, oral.

Second-Generation "Atypical" Antipsychotics

In recent years, the "atypical" or newer nonphenothiazines have become the drugs of first choice. They have virtually replaced phenothiazines and related drugs except in clients doing well on older drugs and in the treatment of acute psychotic episodes. The atypical drugs have both similarities and differences when compared with other antipsychotic drugs and with each other. The main similarity is their effectiveness in treating the positive symptoms of psychosis; the main differences are greater effectiveness in relieving negative symptoms of schizophrenia and fewer resulting movement disorders (ie, extrapyramidal symptoms such as acute dystonia, parkinsonism, akathisia, and tardive dyskinesia). Although adverse effects are generally milder and more tolerable than with older drugs, clozapine may cause life-threatening agranulocytosis, and some of these drugs have been associated with weight gain, hyperglycemia, diabetes, and neuroleptic malignant syndrome.

P **Clozapine** (Clozaril), the prototype of the atypical agents, is chemically different from the older antipsychotic drugs. It blocks both dopamine and serotonin receptors in the brain. Clozapine is indicated for clients with schizophrenia, including those who have exhibited recurrent suicidal behavior.

Advantages of clozapine include improvement of negative symptoms, without causing the extrapyramidal effects associated with older antipsychotic drugs. However, despite these advantages, it is a second-line drug, recommended only for clients who have not responded to treatment with at least two other antipsychotic drugs or who have disabling tardive dyskinesia. The reason for the second-line status of clozapine is its association with agranulocytosis, a life-threatening decrease in white blood cells (WBCs), which usually occurs during the first 3 months of therapy. Weekly WBC counts are required during the first 6 months of therapy; if acceptable WBC counts are maintained, then WBC counts can be monitored every other week. In addition, clozapine is reportedly more likely to cause constipation, dizziness, drowsiness, hypotension, seizures, and weight gain than other atypical drugs.

Olanzapine (Zyprexa) has therapeutic effects similar to those of clozapine, but adverse effects may differ. Compared with clozapine, olanzapine is more likely to cause extrapyramidal effects and less likely to cause agranulocytosis. Compared with the typical antipsychotics, olanzapine reportedly causes less sedation, extrapyramidal symptoms, anticholinergic effects, and orthostatic hypotension. However, it has been associated with weight gain, hyperglycemia, and initiation or aggravation of diabetes mellitus.

The drug is well absorbed after oral administration; its absorption is not affected by food. A steady-state concentration is reached after approximately 1 week of once-daily administration. Olanzapine is metabolized in the liver and excreted in urine and feces.

Quetiapine (Seroquel), like the other atypical agents, blocks both dopamine and serotonin receptors and relieves both positive and negative symptoms of psychosis. After oral administration, quetiapine is well absorbed and may be taken without regard to meals. It is extensively metabolized in the liver by the cytochrome P450 enzyme system. Clinically significant drug interactions may occur with drugs that induce or inhibit the liver enzymes, and dosage of quetiapine may need to be increased in clients taking enzyme inducers (eg, carbamazepine, phenytoin, rifampin) or decreased in clients taking enzyme inhibitors (eg, cimetidine, erythromycin). Common adverse effects include drowsiness, headache, orthostatic hypotension, and weight gain.

Risperidone (Risperdal) also blocks both dopamine and serotonin receptors and relieves both positive and negative symptoms of psychosis. It is a frequently prescribed, first-choice agent that is usually well tolerated. In a study that compared risperidone and olanzapine, researchers concluded that both drugs were well tolerated and effective in treating schizophrenia, but risperidone relieved positive symptoms, anxiety, and depression to a greater degree and caused less weight gain than olanzapine.

Risperidone is well absorbed with oral administration. Peak blood levels occur in 1 to 2 hours, but therapeutic effects are delayed for 1 to 2 weeks. Risperidone is metabolized mainly in the liver by the cytochrome P450 2D6 enzymes and produces an active metabolite. Effects are attributed approximately equally to risperidone and the metabolite. Most (70%) of the drug is excreted in urine and some (14%) in feces. Adverse effects include agitation, anxiety, headache, insomnia, dizziness, and hypotension. Risperidone may also cause parkinsonism and other movement disorders, especially at higher doses, but is less likely to do so than the typical antipsychotic drugs.

Ziprasidone (Geodon) is another atypical agent used to treat schizophrenia. It is effective in suppressing many of the negative symptoms such as blunted affect, lack of motivation, and social withdrawal. It is contraindicated in people who are allergic to the drug; who are pregnant or lactating; who have a prolonged QT/QTc interval on electrocardiogram (ECG); or who have a history of severe heart disease. It must be used cautiously in people with impaired renal or hepatic function and cardiovascular disease. Because it may prolong the QT/QTc interval and cause torsades de pointes, a potentially fatal type of ventricular tachycardia, ziprasidone is probably not a drug of first choice.

Ziprasidone is metabolized in the liver and excreted in urine. Adverse effects include cardiac dysrhythmias, drowsiness, headache, and nausea; weight gain is less likely than with other antipsychotic drugs.

Aripiprazole (Abilify), the newest atypical drug, is approved for the treatment of schizophrenia and is the first in a new category of drugs called *partial dopamine agonists.* A *partial agonist* is a drug that has the ability to block a receptor if it is overstimulated and to stimulate a receptor if it is understimulated. The beneficial effect of aripiprazole in patients with schizophrenia is proposed to involve a combination of partial agonist activity at D_2 and serotonin 5-HT$_{1A}$ receptors and antagonist activity at serotonin 5-HT$_{2A}$ receptors. Aripiprazole also affects alpha$_1$ adrenergic receptors and histamine (H$_1$) receptors. Antagonism of alpha$_1$ adrenergic receptors may account for the occurrence of adverse effects such as orthostatic hypotension. Aripiprazole may also cause neuroleptic malignant syndrome, tardive dyskinesia, weight gain, hyperglycemia, and diabetes mellitus.

Aripiprazole is well absorbed orally, with or without food. It is 99% protein bound. It is metabolized in the liver by the CYP3A4 and CYP2D6 enzyme systems and has an active metabolite. Generally, no dosage adjustment for aripiprazole is required on the basis of hepatic or renal impairment. About 8% of the Caucasian population lacks the capacity to metabolize CYP2D6 substrates and therefore requires significantly lower doses of aripiprazole to avoid drug toxicity.

APPLYING YOUR KNOWLEDGE 9-1

After 6 weeks of therapy, Ms. Jones has far fewer symptoms; however, she has been observed to have a gradual loss of muscle movement. What adverse reaction is likely to be occurring?

NURSING PROCESS

Assessment

Assess the client's mental health status, need for antipsychotic drugs, and response to drug therapy. There is a wide variation in response to drug therapy. Close observation of physical and behavioral reactions is necessary to evaluate effectiveness and to individualize dosage schedules. Accurate assessment is especially important when starting drug therapy and when increasing or decreasing dosage. Some assessment factors include the following:

● Interview the client and family members. Attempts to interview an acutely psychotic person yield little useful information because of the client's distorted perception of reality. The nurse may be able to assess the client's level of orientation and delusional and hallucinatory activity. If possible, try to determine from family members or others what the client was doing or experiencing when the acute episode began (ie, predisposing factors, such as increased environmental stress or alcohol or drug ingestion); whether this is a first or a repeated episode of psychotic behavior; whether the person has physical illnesses, takes any drugs, or uses alcohol; whether the client seems to be a hazard to self or others; and some description of pre-illness personality traits, level of social interaction, and ability to function in usual activities of daily living.

● Observe the client for the presence or absence of psychotic symptoms such as agitation, hyperactivity, combativeness, and bizarre behavior.

● Obtain baseline data to help monitor the client's response to drug therapy. Some authorities advocate initial and periodic laboratory tests of liver, kidney, and blood functions, as well as electrocardiograms. Such tests may assist in early detection and treatment of adverse drug effects. Baseline blood pressure readings also may be helpful.

● Continue assessing the client's response to drug therapy and his or her ability to function in activities of daily living, whether the client is hospitalized or receiving outpatient treatment.

Nursing Diagnoses

● Altered Thought Processes related to psychosis
● Self-Care Deficit related to the disease process or drug-induced sedation
● Impaired Physical Mobility related to sedation
● Altered Tissue Perfusion related to hypotension
● Risk for Injury related to excessive sedation and movement disorders (extrapyramidal effects)
● Risk for Violence: Self-Directed or Directed at Others
● Noncompliance related to underuse of prescribed drugs

Planning/Goals

The client will
● Become less agitated within a few hours of the start of drug therapy, and less psychotic within 1–3 weeks
● Be kept safe while sedated from drug therapy
● Be cared for by staff in areas of nutrition, hygiene, exercise, and social interactions when unable to provide self-care
● Improve in ability to participate in self-care activities
● Avoid preventable adverse drug effects, especially those that impair safety
● Be helped to take medications as prescribed and return for follow-up appointments with health care providers

Interventions

Use nondrug measures when appropriate to increase the effectiveness of drug therapy and to decrease adverse reactions.

● Drug therapy is ineffective if the client does not receive sufficient medication; many people are unable or unwilling to take medications as prescribed. Any nursing action aimed toward more accurate drug administration increases the effectiveness of drug therapy.

Specific nursing actions must be individualized to the client and/or caregiver. Some general nursing actions that may be helpful include emphasizing the therapeutic benefits expected from drug therapy; answering questions or providing information about drug therapy and other aspects of the treatment plan; devising a schedule of administration times that is as convenient as possible for the client; and assisting the client or caregiver in preventing or managing adverse drug effects (see accompanying client teaching guidelines). Most adverse effects are less likely to occur or be severe with the newer atypical drugs than with phenothiazines and other older drugs.

● Supervise ambulation to prevent falls or other injuries if the client is drowsy or elderly or has postural hypotension.

● Several measures can help prevent or minimize hypotension, such as having the client lie down for approximately an hour after a large oral dose or an injection of antipsychotic medication; applying elastic stockings; and instructing the client to change positions gradually, elevate legs when sitting, avoid standing for prolonged periods, and avoid hot baths (hot baths cause vasodilation and increase the incidence of hypotension). In addition, the daily dose can be decreased or divided into smaller amounts.

● Dry mouth and oral infections can be decreased by frequently brushing the teeth; rinsing the mouth with water; chewing sugarless gum or candy; and ensuring an adequate fluid intake. Excessive water intake should be discouraged because it may lead to serum electrolyte deficiencies.

● The usual measures of increasing fluid intake, dietary fiber, and exercise can help prevent constipation.

● Support caregivers in efforts to maintain contact with inpatients and provide care for outpatients. One way is to provide caregivers with telephone numbers of health care providers and to make periodic telephone calls to caregivers.

● Provide client teaching regarding drug therapy (see accompanying display).

APPLYING YOUR KNOWLEDGE 9-2
Ms. Jones says she is dizzy when she gets up. What nursing measures can be implemented to prevent injury?

Evaluation

● Interview the client to determine the presence and extent of hallucinations and delusions.
● Observe the client for decreased signs and symptoms.
● Document abilities and limitations in self-care.
● Note whether any injuries have occurred during drug therapy.
● Interview the caregiver about the client's behavior and medication response (ie, during a home visit or telephone call).

CLIENT TEACHING GUIDELINES

Antipsychotic Drugs

Antipsychotic drugs are given to clients with schizophrenia, a chronic mental illness. Because of the nature of the disease, a responsible adult caregiver is needed to prompt a client about taking particular doses and to manage other aspects of the drug therapy regimen, as follows.

General Considerations

- ✔ Ask about the planned drug therapy regimen, including the desired results, when results can be expected, and the tentative length of drug therapy.
- ✔ Maintain an adequate supply of medication to ensure regular administration. Consistent blood levels are necessary to control symptoms and to prevent recurring episodes of acute illness and hospitalization.
- ✔ Do not allow the client to drive a car, operate machinery, or perform activities that require alertness when drowsy from medication. Drowsiness, slowed thinking, and impaired muscle coordination are especially likely during the first 2 weeks of drug therapy but tend to decrease with time.
- ✔ Report unusual side effects and all physical illnesses, because changes in drug therapy may be indicated.
- ✔ Try to prevent the client from taking unprescribed medications, including those available without prescription or those prescribed for another person, to prevent undesirable drug interactions. Alcohol and sleeping pills should be avoided because they may cause excessive drowsiness and decreased awareness of safety hazards in the environment.
- ✔ Keep all physicians informed about all the medications being taken by the client, to decrease risks of undesirable drug interactions.

- ✔ These drugs should be tapered in dosage and discontinued gradually; they should not be stopped abruptly.
- ✔ Notify your physician if you become pregnant or intend to become pregnant

Medication Administration

Assist or prompt the client to:
- ✔ Take medications in the correct doses and at the correct times, to maintain blood levels and beneficial effects.
- ✔ Avoid taking these medications with antacids. If an antacid is needed (eg, for heartburn), it should be taken 1 hour before or 2 hours after the antipsychotic drug. Antacids decrease absorption of these drugs from the intestine.
- ✔ Lie down for approximately an hour after receiving medication, if dizziness and faintness occur.
- ✔ Take the medication at bedtime, if able, so that drowsiness aids sleep and is minimized during waking hours.
- ✔ Practice good oral hygiene, including dental checkups, thorough and frequent toothbrushing, drinking fluids, and frequent mouth rinsing. Mouth dryness is a common side effect of the drugs. Although it is usually not serious, dry mouth can lead to mouth infections and dental cavities.
- ✔ Minimize exposure to sunlight, wear protective clothing, and use sunscreen lotions. Sensitivity to sunlight occurs with some of the drugs and may produce a sunburn type of skin reaction.
- ✔ Avoid exposure to excessive heat. Some of these medications may cause fever and heat prostration with high environmental temperatures. In hot weather or climates, keep the client indoors and use air conditioning or fans during the hours of highest heat levels.

PRINCIPLES OF THERAPY

Goals of Therapy

Overall, the goal of treatment is to relieve symptoms with minimal or tolerable adverse drug effects. In clients with acute psychosis, the goal during the first week of treatment is to decrease symptoms (eg, aggression, agitation, combativeness, hostility) and normalize patterns of sleeping and eating. The next goals may be increased ability for self-care and increased socialization. Therapeutic effects usually occur gradually, over 1 to 2 months. Long-term goals include increasing the client's ability to cope with the environment, promoting optimal functioning in self-care and activities of daily living, and preventing acute episodes and hospitalizations. With drug therapy, clients often can participate in psychotherapy, group therapy, or other treatment modalities; return to community settings; and return to their pre-illness level of functioning.

Drug Selection

The physician caring for a client with psychosis has a greater choice of drugs than ever before. Some general factors to consider include the client's age and physical condition, the severity and duration of illness, the frequency and severity of adverse effects produced by each drug, the client's use of and response to antipsychotic drugs in the past, the supervision available, and the physician's experience with a particular drug.

The atypical drugs (eg, risperidone) are the drugs of choice, especially for clients who are newly diagnosed with schizophrenia, because these drugs may be more effective in relieving some symptoms; they usually produce milder adverse effects; and clients seem to take them more consistently. The ability of the atypical antipsychotics to reduce adverse effects is seen as a significant advantage, because clients are more likely to take the drugs. Better compliance with drug therapy helps prevent acute episodes of psychosis and repeated hospitalizations, thereby reducing the overall cost of care, according to studies. A major drawback is the high cost of these drugs, which may preclude their use in some clients.

An additional drawback and concern is weight gain and abnormal glucose metabolism. Most of the drugs in the atypical group have been associated with weight gain, especially with the chronic use required for treatment of schizophrenia. Recent reports also associate clozapine, olanzapine, quetiapine, and aripiprazole with changes in blood glucose levels, including hyperglycemia and diabetes mellitus. In some extreme cases, ketoacidosis, hyperosmolar coma, and death have been reported. A causal relationship between use of these drugs and onset of diabetes has not been established. However, before starting one of the drugs, clients should be assessed for diabetes or risk factors related to the development of diabetes (eg, obesity; personal or family history of diabetes; symptoms of diabetes such as polyuria, polydipsia, or polyphagia). If symptoms or risk factors are identified, blood glucose levels should be checked before starting the drug and periodically during treatment.

When compared with atypical antipsychotic drugs, traditional or typical antipsychotic drugs are apparently equally effective, but some clients who do not respond well to one of them may respond to another. Because the typical drugs are similarly effective, some physicians base their choice on a drug's adverse effects. In addition, some physicians use a phenothiazine first and prescribe a nonphenothiazine as a second-line drug for clients with chronic schizophrenia whose symptoms have not been controlled by the phenothiazines and for clients with hypersensitivity reactions to the phenothiazines. Thioridazine (Mellaril), formerly a commonly used drug, is now indicated only when other drugs are ineffective because of its association with serious cardiac dysrhythmias.

Clients who are unable or unwilling to take daily doses of a maintenance antipsychotic drug may be given periodic injections of a long-acting form of fluphenazine, haloperidol, or risperidone. Extrapyramidal symptoms may be more problematic with depot injections of antipsychotic drugs.

Any person who has had an allergic or hypersensitivity reaction to an antipsychotic drug usually should not be given that drug (or any drug in the same chemical group) again. Cross-sensitivity occurs, and the likelihood of another allergic reaction is high.

There is no logical basis for giving more than one antipsychotic drug at a time. There is no therapeutic advantage, and the risk of serious adverse reactions is increased.

Dosage and Administration

Dosage and route of administration must be individualized according to the client's condition and response. Oral drugs undergo extensive first-pass metabolism in the liver so that a significant portion of a dose does not reach the systemic circulation and low serum drug levels are produced. In contrast, IM doses avoid first-pass metabolism and produce serum drug levels approximately double those of oral doses. Thus, usual IM doses are approximately half the oral doses.

Initial drug therapy for acute psychotic episodes may require IM administration and hospitalization; symptoms are usually controlled within 48 to 72 hours, after which oral drugs can be given. When treatment is initiated with oral drugs, divided daily doses are recommended. For maintenance therapy, once-daily dosing is usually preferred. A single bedtime dose is effective for most clients. This schedule increases compliance with prescribed drug therapy, allows better nighttime sleep, and decreases hypotension and daytime sedation. Effective maintenance therapy requires close supervision and contact with the client and family members.

Duration of Therapy

In schizophrenia, antipsychotic drugs are usually given for years because there is a high rate of relapse (acute psychotic episodes) when drug therapy is discontinued, most often by clients who become unwilling or unable to continue their medication regimen. Drug therapy usually is indicated for at least 1 year after an initial psychotic episode and for at least 5 years, perhaps for life, after multiple episodes. Several studies indicate that low-dose, continuous maintenance therapy is effective in long-term prevention of recurrent psychosis. With wider use of maintenance therapy and the newer, better-tolerated antipsychotic drugs, clients may experience fewer psychotic episodes and hospitalizations.

Drug Withdrawal: Recognition and Treatment

Antipsychotic drugs can cause symptoms of withdrawal when suddenly or rapidly discontinued. Specific symptoms are related to drug potency, extent of dopaminergic blockade, and anticholinergic effects. Low-potency drugs (eg, chlorpromazine), for example, have strong anticholinergic effects, and sudden withdrawal can cause cholinergic effects such as diarrhea, drooling, and insomnia. To prevent withdrawal symptoms, drugs should be tapered in dosage and gradually discontinued over several weeks.

Treatment of Extrapyramidal Symptoms

Extrapyramidal effects (ie, abnormal movements) are more likely to occur with usage of older antipsychotic drugs than with the newer atypical agents. If they do occur, an anticholinergic antiparkinson drug (see Chap. 12) can be given. Such neuromuscular symptoms appear in fewer than half of the clients taking traditional antipsychotic drugs and are better handled by reducing dosage, if this does not cause recurrence of psychotic symptoms. If antiparkinson drugs are given, they should be gradually discontinued in about 3 months. Extrapyramidal symptoms do not usually recur despite continued administration of the same antipsychotic drug at the same dosage.

Perioperative Use

A major concern about giving traditional antipsychotic drugs perioperatively is their potential for adverse interactions with other drugs. For example, the drugs potentiate the effects of general anesthetics and other CNS depressants that are often used before, during, and after surgery. As a result, risks of hypotension and excessive sedation are increased unless doses of other drugs are reduced. If hypotension occurs and requires vasopressor drugs, phenylephrine or norepinephrine should be used rather than epinephrine because antipsychotic drugs inhibit the vasoconstrictive (blood pressure–raising) effects of epinephrine. Guidelines for perioperative use of the newer, atypical drugs have not been developed. Cautious use is indicated because they may also cause hypotension, sedation, and other adverse effects.

Use in Special Populations

Use in Children

Antipsychotic drugs are used mainly for childhood schizophrenia, which is often characterized by more severe symptoms and a more chronic course than adult schizophrenia. Drug therapy is largely empiric, because few studies have been conducted in children and adolescents. Guidelines for the use of antipsychotic drugs have been published by the American Academy of Child and Adolescent Psychiatry. Major recommendations are listed in Box 9-1.

It is not clear which antipsychotics are safest and most effective in children and adolescents. Factors to consider include the following:

● Drug pharmacodynamics and pharmacokinetics are likely to be different in children compared with adults. Pharmacodynamic differences may stem from changes in neurotransmission systems in the brain as children grow. Pharmacokinetic differences may stem from changes in distribution or metabolism of drugs; absorption seems similar to that of adults. In relation to distribution, children usually have a lesser percentage of body fat than adults. Thus, antipsychotic drugs, which are highly lipid soluble, cannot be as readily stored in fat as they are in adults. This often leads to shorter half-lives and the need for more frequent administration. In relation to metabolism, children usually have a faster rate than adults and may therefore require relatively high doses for their size and weight. In relation to excretion, children's renal function is usually similar to that of adults and most of the drugs are largely inactivated by liver metabolism. Thus, with normal renal function, excretion probably has little effect on blood levels of active drug or a child's response to the drug.

● Although the newer drugs are being used, children's dosages have not been established and long-term effects are unknown. Traditional drugs are not usually recommended for children younger than 12 years of age. However, prochlorperazine (Compazine), trifluoperazine (Stelazine), and haloperidol (Haldol) may be used in children aged 2 to 12 years.

● Dosage regulation is difficult because children may require lower plasma levels for therapeutic effects, but

Box 9-1 Guidelines for the Use of Antipsychotic Drugs by the American Academy of Child and Adolescent Psychiatry

- Give a thorough psychiatric and physical examination before starting drug therapy.
- Choose a medication based on potency, adverse effects, and the client's medication response history, if available. A newer, atypical drug is probably the drug of first choice.
- Give the chosen drug at least 4–6 weeks before evaluating its effectiveness. If an inadequate response is then evident, a new antipsychotic drug should be tried.
- After an adequate response is obtained, continue drug therapy for at least several months. For newly diagnosed children who are symptom free for 6–12 months, it may be feasible to stop the drug for a trial period to reassess condition and drug dosage. In general, the lowest effective dose is recommended.

- Use psychosocial and psychotherapeutic interventions along with antipsychotic drugs.
- Have the physician or another health care provider maintain contact with the child and his or her parents or guardian and monitor responses to the medication. For example, weight charts and calculations of body mass index should be maintained with the atypical drugs because most are associated with weight gain and some are associated with the development of diabetes.
- Conduct more controlled studies of drug effects in children and adolescents.

From the American Academy of Child and Adolescent Psychiatry's *Practice Parameter for the Assessment and Treatment of Children and Adolescents with Schizophrenia.*

they also metabolize antipsychotic drugs more rapidly than adults. A conservative approach is to begin with a low dose and increase it gradually (no more than once or twice a week), if necessary. Divided doses may be useful initially, with later conversion to once daily at bedtime. Older adolescents may require doses comparable with those of adults.

● Adverse effects may be different in children. For example, extrapyramidal symptoms with conventional drugs are more likely to occur in children than in adults. If they do occur, dosage reduction is more effective in alleviating them than are the anticholinergic antiparkinson drugs commonly used in adults. In addition, hypotension is more likely to develop in children. Blood pressure should be closely monitored during initial dosage titration.

Use in Older Adults

Antipsychotic drugs should be used cautiously in older adults. Before they are started, a thorough assessment is necessary, because psychiatric symptoms are often caused by organic disease or other drugs. If this is the case, treating the disease or stopping the offending drug may eliminate the need for an antipsychotic drug. In addition, older adults are more likely to have problems for which the drugs are contraindicated (eg, severe cardiovascular disease, liver damage, Parkinson's disease) or must be used very cautiously (diabetes mellitus, glaucoma, prostatic hypertrophy, peptic ulcer disease, chronic respiratory disorders).

If antipsychotic drugs are used to control acute agitation in older adults, they should be used in the lowest effective dose for the shortest effective duration. If the drugs are used to treat dementia, they may relieve some symptoms (eg, agitation, hallucinations, hostility, suspiciousness, uncooperativeness), but they do not improve memory loss and may further impair cognitive functioning.

For older adults in long-term care facilities, there is concern that antipsychotic drugs may be overused to control agitated or disruptive behavior caused by nonpsychotic disorders and for which other treatments are preferable. For example, clients with dementia may become agitated because of environmental or medical problems. Alleviating such causes, when possible, is safer and more effective than administering antipsychotic drugs. Inappropriate use of antipsychotic drugs exposes clients to adverse drug effects and does not resolve underlying problems.

Because of the many implications for client safety and welfare, federal regulations have been established for the use of antipsychotics in facilities receiving Medicare and Medicaid funds. These regulations include appropriate (eg, psychotic disorders; delusions; schizophrenia; dementia and delirium that meet certain criteria) and inappropriate (eg, agitation not thought to indicate potential harm to the resident or others; anxiety; depression; uncooperativeness; wandering) indications. When antipsychotics are required in older adults, several issues should be considered (Box 9-2).

Box 9-2 Considerations Regarding Use of Antipsychotic Drugs in Older Adults

Drug Selection

With traditional antipsychotic drugs, haloperidol and fluphenazine may be better tolerated, but they cause a high incidence of extrapyramidal symptoms. With atypical drugs, clozapine is a second-line agent because it produces many adverse effects. Olanzapine, quetiapine, risperidone, ziprasidone, or aripiprazole may be useful, but little information is available about their use in older adults. Ziprasidone should not be used in older adults with cardiac dysrhythmias or severe cardiovascular disease.

Dosage

When the drugs are required, the recommended starting dosage is 25%–33% of the dosage recommended for younger adults. Dosage should also be increased more gradually, if necessary, and according to clinical response. The basic principle of "start low, go slow" is especially applicable. After symptoms are controlled, dosage should be reduced to the lowest effective level. Some specific drugs and dosage ranges include haloperidol 0.25–1.5 mg qd to qid; clozapine 6.25 mg qd, initially; risperidone 0.5 mg qd, initially; quetiapine, a lower initial dose, slower dose titration, and a lower target dose in older adults. No reduction of dosage is required based on age for aripiprazole.

As in other populations, antipsychotic drugs should be tapered in dosage and discontinued gradually rather than discontinued abruptly.

Adverse Effects

Older adults are at high risk of adverse effects because metabolism and excretion are usually slower or more likely to be impaired than in younger adults. With traditional antipsychotic drugs, anticholinergic effects (eg, confusion, memory impairment, hallucinations, urinary retention, constipation, heat stroke) may be especially problematic. In addition, cardiovascular effects (eg, hypotension, dysrhythmias) may be especially dangerous in older adults, who often have underlying cardiovascular diseases. Tardive dyskinesia, which may occur with long-term use of the typical antipsychotic drugs, may develop more rapidly and at lower drug dosages in older adults than in younger clients. There is also a risk of neuroleptic malignant syndrome, a rare but serious disorder characterized by confusion, dizziness, fever, and rigidity. Other adverse effects include oversedation, dizziness, confusion, and impaired mobility, which may contribute to falls and other injuries unless clients are carefully monitored and safeguarded. With atypical drugs, many of these adverse effects are less likely to occur, especially at the reduced dosages recommended for older adults.

Use in Various Ethnic Groups

Antipsychotic drug therapy for nonwhite populations in the United States is based primarily on dosage recommendations, pharmacokinetic data, adverse effects, and other characteristics of antipsychotic drugs derived from white recipients. However, some groups respond differently. Most of the differences are attributed to variations in hepatic drug-metabolizing enzymes. Those with strong enzyme activity are known as *extensive* or *fast metabolizers,* whereas those with slower rates of enzyme activity are *poor* or *slow metabolizers.* Fast metabolizers eliminate drugs rapidly and may need a larger-than-usual dose to achieve therapeutic effects, and poor metabolizers eliminate drugs slowly and therefore are at risk of drug accumulation and adverse effects. For example, in extensive metabolizers, risperidone has a half-life of 3 hours and its active metabolite has a half-life of 21 hours. In slow metabolizers, risperidone has a half-life of 20 hours and its active metabolite has a half-life of 30 hours. About 6% to 8% of white people are thought to be slow metabolizers. Although little research has been done, especially with the atypical drugs, and other factors may be involved, several studies document differences in antipsychotic drug effects in non-Caucasian populations:

African Americans tend to respond more rapidly; experience a higher incidence of adverse effects, including tardive dyskinesia; and metabolize antipsychotic drugs more slowly than whites.

In addition, compared with whites with psychotic disorders, African Americans may be given higher doses and more frequent injections of long-acting antipsychotic drugs, both of which may increase the incidence and severity of adverse effects.

Asians generally metabolize antipsychotic drugs slowly and therefore have higher plasma drug levels for a given dose than whites. Most studies have been done with haloperidol and in a limited number of Asian subgroups. Thus, it cannot be assumed that all antipsychotic drugs and all people of Asian heritage respond in the same way. To avoid drug toxicity, initial doses should be approximately half the usual doses given to whites and later doses should be titrated according to clinical response and serum drug levels.

Hispanics' responses to antipsychotic drugs are largely unknown. Some are extremely fast metabolizers who may have low plasma drug levels in relation to a given dose.

Use in Clients With Renal Impairment

Because most antipsychotic drugs are extensively metabolized in the liver and the metabolites are excreted through the kidneys, the drugs should be used cautiously in clients with impaired renal function. Renal function should be monitored periodically during long-term therapy. If renal function test results (eg, blood urea nitrogen) become abnormal, the drug may need to be lowered in dosage or discontinued. Because risperidone is metabolized to an active metabolite, recommended dosage reductions and titrations for clients with renal impairment are the same as those for older adults.

With highly sedating antipsychotic drugs, it may be difficult to assess the client for excessive sedation because drowsiness, lethargy, and mental status changes may also occur with renal impairment.

Use in Clients With Hepatic Impairment

Antipsychotic drugs undergo extensive hepatic metabolism and then elimination in urine. In the presence of liver disease (eg, cirrhosis, hepatitis), metabolism may be slowed and drug elimination half-lives prolonged, with resultant accumulation and increased risk of adverse effects. Thus, the drugs should be used cautiously in clients with hepatic impairment.

Jaundice has been associated with phenothiazines, usually after 2 to 4 weeks of therapy. It is considered a hypersensitivity reaction, and clients should not be re-exposed to a phenothiazine. If antipsychotic drug therapy is required in these clients, a drug from a different chemical group should be given. Overall, there is no conclusive evidence that pre-existing liver impairment increases the risk of jaundice, and clients with alcoholic cirrhosis have been treated without complications. With risperidone, recommended dosage reductions and titrations for clients with hepatic impairment are the same as those for older adults. With quetiapine, higher plasma levels occur in clients with hepatic impairment and a slower rate of dose titration and a lower target dose are recommended.

Periodic liver function tests (eg, gamma-glutamyl transpeptidase, alkaline phosphatase, bilirubin) are probably indicated, especially with long-term therapy or the use of clozapine, haloperidol, thiothixene, or a phenothiazine.

Use in Clients With Critical Illness

Antipsychotic drugs are infrequently used in clients who are critically ill. Some clients become acutely agitated or delirious and need sedation to prevent their injuring themselves by thrashing about, removing tubes and intravenous (IV) catheters, and so forth. Some physicians prefer a benzodiazepine-type of sedative, whereas others may use haloperidol. Before giving either drug, causes of delirium (eg, drug intoxication or withdrawal) should be identified and eliminated if possible.

If haloperidol is used, it is usually given IV, by bolus injection. The initial dose is 0.5 to 10 milligrams, depending on the severity of the agitation. It should be injected at a rate no faster than 5 milligrams per minute; the dose can be repeated every 30 to 60 minutes, up to a total amount of 30 milligrams, if necessary. Haloperidol has relatively weak sedative effects and does not cause respiratory depression. However, it can cause hypotension in clients who are volume depleted or receiving antihypertensive drugs. It can also cause cardiac dysrhythmias, including life-threatening torsades de pointes, in clients who are receiving large doses (>50 mg/day) or who have abnormal serum electrolyte levels (eg, calcium, potassium, magnesium). Clients should be on a cardiac monitor and the ECG should be checked for a prolonged QT interval.

For clients with chronic schizophrenia who are stabilized on an antipsychotic drug when they experience a critical illness, either continuing or stopping the drug may cause difficulties. Continuing the drug may worsen signs and symptoms of the critical illness (eg, hypotension). Stopping it may cause symptoms of withdrawal.

Little information is available about the newer drugs. If quetiapine is used, very low doses are recommended in older adults, clients with hepatic impairment, debilitated clients, and those predisposed to hypotension. A critically ill client could have all of these conditions.

Use in Home Care

Chronically mentally ill clients, such as those with schizophrenia, are among the most challenging in the caseload of the home care nurse. Major recurring problems include failure to take antipsychotic medications as prescribed and the concurrent use of alcohol and other drugs of abuse. Either problem is likely to lead to acute psychotic episodes and hospitalizations. The home care nurse must assist and support caregivers' efforts to maintain medications and manage adverse drug effects, other aspects of daily care, and follow-up psychiatric care. In addition, the home care nurse may need to coordinate the efforts of several health and social service agencies or providers.

NURSING ACTIONS

Antipsychotic Drugs

NURSING ACTIONS	RATIONALE/EXPLANATION
1. Administer accurately	
a. Check doses carefully, especially when starting or stopping an antipsychotic drug, or substituting one for another.	Doses are often changed. When a drug is started, initial doses are usually titrated upward over days or weeks, then reduced for maintenance; when the drug is stopped, doses are gradually reduced; when substituting, dosage of one may be increased while dosage of the other is decreased.
b. With older, typical drugs:	
(1) Give once daily, 1–2 hours before bedtime, when feasible.	Peak sedation occurs in about 2 hours and aids sleep. Also, adverse effects such as dry mouth and hypotension are less bothersome.
(2) When preparing solutions, try to avoid skin contact. If contact is made, wash the area immediately.	These solutions are irritating to the skin and many cause contact dermatitis.
(3) Mix liquid concentrates with at least 60 mL of fruit juice or water just before administration.	To mask the taste. If the client does not like juice or water, check the package insert for other diluents. Some of the drugs may be mixed with coffee, tea, milk, or carbonated beverages.
(4) For intramuscular injections, give only those preparations labeled for IM use; do not mix with any other drugs in a syringe; change the needle after filling the syringe; inject slowly and deeply into gluteal muscles; and have the client lie down for 30–60 minutes after the injection.	These drugs are physically incompatible with many other drugs, and a precipitate may occur; parenteral solutions are irritating to body tissues and changing needles helps protect the tissues of the injection tract from unnecessary contact with the drug; injecting into a large muscle mass decreases tissue irritation; lying down helps to prevent orthostatic hypotension.
(5) With parenteral fluphenazine, give the hydrochloride salt IM only; give the decanoate and enanthate salts IM or subcutaneously (Sub-Q).	To decrease tissue irritation
c. With newer, atypical drugs:	
(1) Give aripiprazole once daily, without regard to meals.	Manufacturer's recommendation
(2) Give olanzapine once daily, without regard to meals; with oral disintegrating tablets, peel back foil covering, transfer tablet to dry cup or fingers, and place the tablet into the mouth.	Manufacturer's recommendation. The disintegrating tablet does not require fluid.
(3) Give quetiapine in 2 or 3 daily doses.	
(4) Give risperidone twice daily; mix the oral solution with 3–4 oz of water, coffee, orange juice, or low-fat milk; do not mix with cola drinks or tea.	Manufacturer's recommendation

NURSING ACTIONS	RATIONALE/EXPLANATION

(5) Give Risperdal Consta deep IM into gluteal muscles.

Manufacturer's recommendation

(6) Give ziprasidone twice daily with food.

Manufacturer's recommendation

2. **Observe for therapeutic effects**

  a. When the drug is given for acute psychotic episodes, observe for decreased agitation, combativeness, and psychomotor activity.

The sedative effects of antipsychotic drugs are exerted within 48–72 hours. Sedation that occurs with treatment of acute psychotic episodes is a therapeutic effect. Sedation that occurs with treatment of nonacute psychotic disorders, or excessive sedation at any time, is an adverse reaction.

  b. When the drug is given for acute or chronic psychosis, observe for decreased psychotic behavior, such as:

These therapeutic effects may not be evident for 3–6 weeks after drug therapy is begun.

    (1) Decreased auditory and visual hallucinations

    (2) Decreased delusions

    (3) Continued decrease in or absence of agitation, hostility, hyperactivity, and other behavior associated with acute psychosis

    (4) Increased socialization

    (5) Increased ability in self-care activities

    (6) Increased ability to participate in other therapeutic modalities along with drug therapy.

  c. When the drug is given for antiemetic effects, observe for decreased or absent nausea or vomiting.

3. **Observe for adverse effects**

  a. With phenothiazines and related drugs, observe for:

    (1) Excessive sedation—drowsiness, lethargy, fatigue, slurred speech, impaired mobility, and impaired mental processes

Excessive sedation is most likely to occur during the first few days of treatment of an acute psychotic episode, when large doses are usually given. Psychotic clients also seem sedated because the drug lets them catch up on psychosis-induced sleep deprivation. Sedation is more likely to occur in elderly or debilitated people. Tolerance to the drugs' sedative effects develops, and sedation tends to decrease with continued drug therapy.

    (2) Extrapyramidal reactions

    Akathisia—compulsive, involuntary restlessness and body movements

Akathisia is the most common extrapyramidal reaction, and it may occur about 5–60 days after the start of antipsychotic drug therapy. The motor restlessness may be erroneously interpreted as psychotic agitation necessitating increased drug dosage. This condition can sometimes be controlled by substituting an antipsychotic drug that is less likely to cause extrapyramidal effects or by giving an anticholinergic antiparkinson drug.

    Parkinsonism—loss of muscle movement (akinesia), muscular rigidity and tremors, shuffling gait, postural abnormalities, mask-like facial expression, hypersalivation, and drooling

These symptoms are the same as those occurring with idiopathic Parkinson's disease. They can be controlled with anticholinergic antiparkinson drugs, given along with the antipsychotic drug for about 3 months, then discontinued. This reaction may occur about 5–30 days after antipsychotic drug therapy is begun.

    Dyskinesias (involuntary, rhythmic body movements) and *dystonias* (uncoordinated, bizarre movements of the neck, face, eyes, tongue, trunk, or extremities)

These are less common extrapyramidal reactions, but they may occur suddenly, approximately 1–5 days after drug therapy is started, and be very frightening to the client and health care personnel. The movements are caused by muscle spasms and result in exaggerated posture and facial distortions. These symptoms are sometimes misinterpreted as seizures, hysteria, or other disorders. Antiparkinson drugs are given parenterally during acute dystonic reactions, but continued administration is not usually required. These reactions occur most often in younger people.

(continued)

NURSING ACTIONS	RATIONALE/EXPLANATION
Tardive dyskinesia—hyperkinetic movements of the face (sucking and smacking of lips, tongue protrusion, and facial grimaces) and choreiform movements of the trunk and limbs	This syndrome occurs after months or years of high-dose antipsychotic drug therapy. The drugs may mask the symptoms so that the syndrome is more likely to be diagnosed when dosage is decreased or the drug is discontinued for a few days. It occurs gradually and at any age but is more common in older people, women, and people with organic brain disorders. The condition is usually irreversible, and there is no effective treatment. Symptoms are not controlled and may be worsened by antiparkinson drugs. Low dosage and short-term use of antipsychotic drugs help prevent tardive dyskinesia; drug-free periods may aid early detection.
(3) Antiadrenergic effects—hypotension, tachycardia, dizziness, faintness, fatigue	Hypotension is potentially one of the most serious adverse reactions to the antipsychotic drugs. It is most likely to occur when the client assumes an upright position after sitting or lying down (orthostatic or postural hypotension) but it does occur in the recumbent position. It is caused by peripheral vasodilation. Orthostatic hypotension can be assessed by comparing blood pressure readings taken with the client in supine and standing positions.
	Tachycardia occurs as a compensatory mechanism in response to hypotension and as an anticholinergic effect in which the normal vagus nerve action of slowing the heart rate is blocked.
(4) Anticholinergic effects—dry mouth, dental caries, blurred vision, constipation, paralytic ileus, urinary retention	These atropine-like effects are common with therapeutic doses and are increased with large doses of phenothiazines.
(5) Respiratory depression—slow, shallow breathing and decreased ability to breathe deeply, cough, and remove secretions from the respiratory tract	This stems from general central nervous system (CNS) depression, which causes drowsiness and decreased movement. It may cause pneumonia or other respiratory problems, especially in people with hypercarbia and chronic lung disease.
(6) Endocrine effects—menstrual irregularities, possibly impotence and decreased libido in the male client, weight gain	These apparently result from drug-induced changes in pituitary and hypothalamic functions.
(7) Hypothermia or hyperthermia	Antipsychotic drugs may impair the temperature-regulating center in the hypothalamus. Hypothermia is more likely to occur. Hyperthermia occurs with high doses and warm environmental temperatures.
(8) Hypersensitivity reactions:	
Cholestatic hepatitis—may begin with fever and influenza-like symptoms followed in approximately 1 week by jaundice	Cholestatic hepatitis results from drug-induced edema of the bile ducts and obstruction of the bile flow. It occurs most often in women and after 2–4 weeks of receiving the drug. It is usually reversible if the drug is discontinued.
Blood dyscrasias—leukopenia, agranulocytosis (fever, sore throat, weakness)	Some degree of leukopenia occurs rather often and does not seem to be serious. Agranulocytosis, on the other hand, occurs rarely but is life threatening. Agranulocytosis is most likely to occur during the first 4–10 weeks of drug therapy, in women, and in older people.
Skin reactions—photosensitivity, dermatoses	Skin pigmentation and discoloration may occur with exposure to sunlight.
(9) Electrocardiogram (ECG) changes, cardiac dysrhythmias	ECG changes may portend dysrhythmias, especially in people with underlying heart disease. Ziprasidone may prolong the QT/QTc interval, an ECG change associated with torsades de pointes, a life-threatening dysrhythmia.
(10) Neuroleptic malignant syndrome—fever (may be confused with heat stroke), muscle rigidity, agitation, confusion, delirium, dyspnea, tachycardia, respiratory failure, acute renal failure	A rare but potentially fatal reaction that may occur hours to months after initial drug use. Symptoms usually develop rapidly over 24–72 hours. Treatment includes stopping the antipsychotic drug, giving supportive care related to fever and other symptoms, and drug therapy (dantrolene, a skeletal muscle relaxant, and amantadine or bromocriptine, dopamine-stimulating drugs).

NURSING ACTIONS	RATIONALE/EXPLANATION

b. With aripiprazole, observe for:

   (1) CNS effects—anxiety, headache, somnolence, blurred vision, akathisia, tardive dyskinesia, neuroleptic malignant syndrome

   (2) GI effects—nausea, vomiting, constipation, dysphagia

   (3) Cardiovascular effects—orthostatic hypotension

   (4) Other—weight gain, hyperglycemia

c. With clozapine, observe for:

   (1) CNS effects—drowsiness, dizziness, headache, seizures

   (2) Gastrointestinal (GI) effects—nausea, vomiting, constipation

   (3) Cardiovascular effects—hypotension, tachycardia

   (4) Hematologic effects—agranulocytosis

> This is the most life-threatening adverse effect of clozapine. Clients' white blood cell (WBC) counts must be checked before starting clozapine, every week during the first six months of therapy, then every 2 weeks as long as WBC counts are satisfactory. WBC levels should be monitored weekly for 4 weeks after the drug is discontinued.

d. With olanzapine, observe for:

   (1) CNS effects—drowsiness, dizziness, akathisia, tardive dyskinesia, neuroleptic malignant syndrome

   (2) GI effects—constipation

   (3) Cardiovascular effects—hypotension, tachycardia

   (4) Other—weight gain, hyperglycemia, diabetes, hyperlipidemia

e. With quetiapine, observe for:

   (1) CNS effects—drowsiness, dizziness, headache, tardive dyskinesia, neuroleptic malignant syndrome

   (2) GI effects—anorexia, nausea, vomiting

   (3) Cardiovascular effects—orthostatic hypotension, tachycardia

   (4) Other—weight gain, hyperglycemia, diabetes

f. With risperidone, observe for:

   (1) CNS effects—agitation, anxiety, drowsiness, dizziness, headache, insomnia, tardive dyskinesia, neuroleptic malignant syndrome

   (2) GI effects—nausea, vomiting, constipation

   (3) Cardiovascular effects—orthostatic hypotension, dysrhythmias

   (4) Other—photosensitivity

g. With ziprasidone, observe for:

   (1) CNS effects—drowsiness, headache, extrapyramidal reactions

   (2) GI effects—nausea, constipation

   (3) Cardiovascular effects—dysrhythmias, hypotension, ECG changes

   (4) Other—fever

4. Observe for drug interactions

a. Drugs that *increase* effects of antipsychotic drugs:

   (1) Anticholinergics (eg, atropine)   Additive anticholinergic effects

(continued)

NURSING ACTIONS	RATIONALE/EXPLANATION
(2) Antidepressants, tricyclic	Potentiation of sedative and anticholinergic effects. Additive CNS depression, sedation, orthostatic hypotension, urinary retention, and glaucoma may occur unless dosages are decreased. Apparently these two drug groups inhibit the metabolism of each other, thus prolonging the actions of both groups if they are given concurrently.
(3) Antihistamines	Additive CNS depression and sedation
(4) CNS depressants—alcohol, opioid analgesics, antianxiety agents, sedative-hypnotics	Additive CNS depression. Also, severe hypotension, urinary retention, seizures, severe atropine-like reactions, and other adverse effects may occur, depending on which group of CNS depressant drugs is given.
(5) Propranolol	Additive hypotensive and ECG effects
(6) Thiazide diuretics, such as hydrochlorothiazide	Additive hypotension
(7) Lithium	Acute encephalopathy, including irreversible brain damage and dyskinesias, has been reported.
b. Drugs that *decrease* effects of antipsychotic drugs:	
(1) Antacids	Oral antacids, especially aluminum hydroxide and magnesium trisilicate, may inhibit gastrointestinal absorption of antipsychotic drugs.
(2) Carbamazepine, phenytoin, rifampin	By induction of drug-metabolizing enzymes in the liver
(3) Norepinephrine, phenylephrine	Antagonize the hypotensive effects of antipsychotic drugs
c. Drugs that alter effects of quetiapine and aripiprazole:	
(1) Cimetidine, erythromycin, itraconazole, and ketoconazole *increase* effects.	These drugs inhibit cytochrome CYP3A4 enzymes and slow the metabolism of quetiapine.
(2) Quinidine, fluoxetine, and paroxetine *increase* effect of aripiprazole only.	These drugs inhibit cytochrome CYP2D6 and slow the metabolism of aripiprazole.
(3) Carbamazepine, phenytoin, and rifampin *decrease* effects of both drugs.	These drugs induce cytochrome CYP3A4 enzymes and speed up the metabolism of both drugs.

APPLYING YOUR KNOWLEDGE: ANSWERS

9-1 Parkinsonism is a common side effect of antipsychotic medication. Notify the physician; antiparkinson drugs may be given along with the antipsychotic drugs.

9-2 The dizziness is most likely due to orthostatic hypotension as a side effect of the risperidone. Have Ms. Jones change position gradually, lie down for an hour after taking her medication, elevate her legs when in a sitting position, and avoid hot baths.

9-3 These symptoms are typical of neuroleptic malignant syndrome. This is a rare but potentially fatal reaction that requires rapid treatment.

Review and Application Exercises

Short Answer Exercises

1. How do antipsychotic drugs act to relieve psychotic symptoms?

2. What are some uses of antipsychotic drugs other than the treatment of schizophrenia?

3. What are major adverse effects of older antipsychotic drugs?

4. When instructing a client to rise slowly from a sitting or lying position, which adverse effect of an antipsychotic drug is the nurse trying to prevent?

5. In a client receiving an antipsychotic drug, what appearances or behaviors would lead the nurse to suspect an extrapyramidal reaction?

6. Are antipsychotic drugs likely to be overused and abused? Why or why not?

7. In an older client taking an antipsychotic drug, what special safety measures are needed? Why?

8. How do clozapine, olanzapine, quetiapine, risperidone, ziprasidone, and aripiprazole compare with older antipsychotic drugs in terms of therapeutic and adverse effects?

9. What can the home care nurse do to prevent acute psychotic episodes and hospitalization of chronically mentally ill clients?

NCLEX-Style Questions

10. For clients taking clozapine, the nurse should assess which of the following laboratory values weekly?
    a. complete blood count
    b. hemoglobin and hematocrit
    c. blood urea nitrogen and creatinine
    d. liver enzyme studies

11. Patients taking ziprasidone (Geodon) may have prolonged QT intervals, placing them at risk for which of the following?
    a. atrial fibrillation
    b. torsades de pointes
    c. complete heart block
    d. atrial tachycardia

12. The nurse should administer long-acting injections of antipsychotic drugs in which of the following ways?
    a. intramuscularly into the deltoid muscle
    b. subcutaneously into the abdomen
    c. intramuscularly into the gluteal muscle
    d. intravenously into a large vein

13. When administering atypical antipsychotics, the nurse should be alert to possible
    a. renal failure
    b. liver failure
    c. diabetes mellitus
    d. hypertension

14. An adverse effect of long-term use of phenothiazine antipsychotics is the development of which of the following?
    a. glaucoma
    b. tardive dyskinesia
    c. hypertension
    d. diabetes

Selected References

Alexopoulos, G., Streim, J., Carpenter, D., & Docherty, J. (2004). Expert consensus panel for using antipsychotic drugs in older patients. *Journal of Clinical Psychiatry, 65*(2), 5–99, 100–102.

American Academy of Child and Adolescent Psychiatry, Work Group on Quality Issues. (2001). The practice parameter for the assessment and treatment of children and adolescents with schizophrenia. *Journal of the American Academy of Child & Adolescent Psychiatry, 40*(7), 4S–23S.

American Psychiatric Association. (2000). *Diagnostic and statistical manual of mental disorders* (4th ed., text revision). Washington, DC: American Psychiatric Association.

Bhanji, N., Chouinard, G., & Margolese, H. (2004). A review of compliance, depot intramuscular antipsychotics and the new long-acting injectable atypical antipsychotic risperidone in schizophrenia. *European Neuropsychopharmacology, 14*(2), 87–92.

Conley, R. R., & Mahmoud, R. (2001). A randomized double-blind study of risperidone and olanzapine in the treatment of schizophrenia or schizoaffective disorder. *American Journal of Psychiatry, 158,* 765–774.

Correll, C., Leucht, S., & Kane, J. (2004). Lower risk for tardive dyskinesia associated with second-generation antipsychotics: A systematic review of 1-year studies. *American Journal of Psychiatry, 161*(3), 414–425.

Drug facts and comparisons. (Updated monthly). St. Louis: Facts and Comparisons.

Freeman, R. (2003). Schizophrenia. *New England Journal of Medicine, 349*(18), 1738–1749.

Glassman, A. H., & Bigger, J. T., Jr. (2001). Antipsychotic drugs: Prolonged QTc interval, torsades de pointes, and sudden death. *American Journal of Psychiatry, 158*(11), 1774–1782.

Goff, D. C., & Coyle, J. T. (2001). The emerging role of glutamate in the pathophysiology and treatment of schizophrenia. *American Journal of Psychiatry, 158*(9), 1367–1375.

Antidepressants and Mood Stabilizers

OBJECTIVES

After studying this chapter, you will be able to:

1. Describe major features of depression and bipolar disorder.
2. Discuss characteristics of antidepressants in terms of mechanism of action, indications for use, adverse effects, principles of therapy, and nursing process implications.
3. Compare and contrast selective serotonin reuptake inhibitors with tricyclic antidepressants.
4. Discuss selected characteristics of bupropion, mirtazapine, and venlafaxine.
5. Describe the use of lithium in bipolar disorder.
6. Discuss interventions to increase safety of lithium therapy.
7. Describe the nursing role in preventing, recognizing, and treating overdoses of antidepressant drugs and lithium.
8. Analyze important factors in using antidepressant drugs and lithium in special populations.

APPLYING YOUR KNOWLEDGE

While in the hospital, Carl Mehring, age 70, is diagnosed with chronic depression secondary to his chronic heart failure, hypertension, diabetes mellitus, and renal insufficiency. As Mr. Mehring's health has declined, so has his interest in his family, friends, and hobbies. His physician prescribes sertraline 50 mg PO twice a day.

INTRODUCTION

Mood disorders include depression, dysthymia, bipolar disorder, and cyclothymia (Box 10-1). Depression is estimated to affect 5% to 10% of adults in the United States and to be increasing in children and adolescents. It is associated with impaired ability to function in usual activities and relationships. The average depressive episode lasts about 5 months, and having one episode is a risk factor for developing another episode. Depression and antidepressant drug therapy are emphasized in this chapter, and bipolar disorder and mood-stabilizing drugs are also discussed.

Etiology of Depression

Despite extensive study and identification of numerous potential contributory factors, the etiology of depression is unclear. It is likely that depression results from interactions among several complex factors. Two of the major theories of depression pathogenesis are described in the following sections.

Monoamine Neurotransmitter Dysfunction

Depression is thought to result from a deficiency of norepinephrine and/or serotonin. This hypothesis stemmed from studies demonstrating that antidepressant drugs increase the amounts of one or both of these neurotransmitters in the central nervous system (CNS) synapse by inhibiting their reuptake into the presynaptic neuron. Serotonin received increased attention after the selective serotonin reuptake inhibitor (SSRI) antidepressants were marketed. Serotonin helps regulate several behaviors that are disturbed in depression, such as mood, sleep, appetite, energy level, and cognitive and psychomotor functions.

Emphasis shifted toward receptors because the neurotransmitter view did not explain why the amounts of neurotransmitter increased within hours after single doses of a drug, but relief of depression occurred only after weeks of drug therapy. Researchers identified changes in norepinephrine and serotonin receptors with chronic antidepressant drug therapy. Studies demonstrated that chronic drug administration (ie, increased neurotransmitter in the synapse for several weeks) results in fewer receptors on the postsynaptic mem-

Box 10-1 Types of Mood Disorders

Depression

Depression, often described as the most common mental illness, is characterized by depressed mood, feelings of sadness, or emotional upset, and it occurs in all age groups. Mild depression occurs in everyone as a normal response to life stresses and losses and usually does not require treatment; severe or major depression is a psychiatric illness and requires treatment. Major depression also is categorized as unipolar, in which people of usually normal moods experience recurrent episodes of depression.

Major Depression

The American Psychiatric Association's *Diagnostic and Statistical Manual of Mental Disorders,* 4th edition, lists criteria for a major depressive episode as a depressed mood plus at least five of the following symptoms for at least 2 weeks:

Loss of energy, fatigue
Indecisiveness
Difficulty thinking and concentrating
Loss of interest in appearance, work, and leisure and sexual activities
Inappropriate feelings of guilt and worthlessness
Loss of appetite and weight loss, or excessive eating and weight gain
Sleep disorders (hypersomnia or insomnia)
Somatic symptoms (eg, constipation, headache, atypical pain)

Obsession with death, thoughts of suicide
Psychotic symptoms, such as hallucinations and delusions

Dysthymia

Dysthymia involves a chronically depressed mood and at least two other symptoms (eg, anorexia, overeating, insomnia, hypersomnia, low energy, low self-esteem, poor concentration, feelings of hopelessness) for 2 years. Although the symptoms may cause significant social and work-related impairments, they are not severe enough to meet the criteria for major depression.

Bipolar Disorder

Bipolar disorder involves episodes of depression alternating with episodes of mania. *Mania* is characterized by excessive CNS stimulation with physical and mental hyperactivity (eg, agitation, constant talking, constant movement, grandiose ideas, impulsiveness, inflated self-esteem, little need for sleep, poor concentration, racing thoughts, short attention span) for at least 1 week. Symptoms are similar to those of acute psychosis or schizophrenia. *Hypomania* involves the same symptoms, but they are less severe, indicate less CNS stimulation and hyperactivity, and last 3 or 4 days.

Cyclothymia

Cyclothymia is a mild type of bipolar disorder that involves periods of hypomania and depression that do not meet the criteria for mania and major depression. Symptoms must be present for at least 2 years. It does not usually require drug therapy.

---

brane. This down-regulation of receptors, first noted with beta-adrenergic receptors, corresponds with therapeutic drug effects. All known treatments for depression lead to the down-regulation of beta receptors and occur in the same period as the behavioral changes associated with antidepressant drug therapy.

Alpha$_2$-adrenergic receptors (called *autoreceptors*), located on presynaptic nerve terminals, may also play a role. When these receptors are stimulated, they inhibit the release of norepinephrine. There is evidence that alpha$_2$ receptors are also down-regulated by antidepressant drugs, thus allowing increased norepinephrine release. With serotonin receptors, available antidepressants may increase the sensitivity of postsynaptic receptors and decrease the sensitivity of presynaptic receptors.

Physiologically, presynaptic receptors regulate the release and reuptake of neurotransmitters; postsynaptic receptors participate in the transmission of nerve impulses to target tissues. It seems apparent that long-term administration of antidepressant drugs produces complex changes in the sensitivities of both presynaptic and postsynaptic receptor sites.

Overall, there is increasing awareness that balance, integration, and interactions among norepinephrine, serotonin, and possibly other neurotransmission systems (eg, dopamine, acetylcholine) are probably more important etiologic factors than single neurotransmitter or receptor alterations. For example, animal studies indicate that serotonin is required for optimal functioning of the neurons that produce norepinephrine. Changes in neurons may also play a major role.

Neuroendocrine Factors

In addition to monoamine neurotransmission systems, researchers have identified nonmonoamine systems that influence neurotransmission and are significantly altered in depression. A major nonmonoamine is corticotropin-releasing factor or hormone (CRF or CRH), whose secretion is increased in people with depression. CRF-secreting neurons are widespread in the CNS, and CRF apparently functions as a neurotransmitter and mediator of the endocrine, autonomic, immune, and behavioral responses to stress as well as a releasing factor for corticotropin. Hypothalamic CRF is part of the hypothalamic–pituitary–adrenal (HPA) axis, which becomes hyperactive in depression. As a result, there is increased secretion of CRF by the hypothalamus; adrenocorticotropic hormone (ACTH) by the anterior pituitary; and cortisol by the adrenal cortex. The increased cortisol (part of the normal physiologic response to stress) is thought to decrease the numbers or sensitivity of cortisol receptors (down-regulation) and lead to depression. This view is supported by animal studies indicating that antidepressant drugs restore the ability of cortisol receptors to bind with cortisol. This alteration of cortisol receptors takes about 2 weeks, the approximate time interval required for the drugs to improve symptoms of depression. Extrahypothalamic CRF is also increased in depression. Secretion of both hypothalamic and extrahypothalamic CRF apparently returns to normal with recovery from depression.

Other neuroendocrine factors in clients with depression are thought to include abnormalities in the secretion and function of thyroid and growth hormones.

Additional Factors

Additional factors thought to play a role in the etiology of depression include the immune system, genetic factors, and environmental factors.

Immune cells (eg, T lymphocytes, B lymphocytes) produce cytokines (eg, interleukins, interferons, tumor necrosis factor), which affect neurotransmission. Possible mechanisms of cytokine-induced depression include increased CRF and activation of the HPA axis; alteration of monoamine neurotransmitters in several areas of the brain; or cytokines functioning as neurotransmitters and exerting direct effects on brain function.

Genetic factors are considered important mainly because close relatives of a depressed person are more likely to experience depression.

Environmental factors include stressful life events, which apparently change brain structure and function and contribute to the development of depression in some people. Changes have been identified in CRF, the HPA axis, and the noradrenergic neurotransmission system, all of which are activated as part of the stress response. These changes are thought to cause a hypersensitive or exaggerated response to later stressful events, including mild stress or daily life events. Most studies have involved early life trauma such as physical or sexual abuse in childhood.

Etiology of Bipolar Disorder

Like depression, mania and hypomania may result from abnormal functioning of neurotransmitters or receptors, such as a relative excess of excitatory neurotransmitters (eg, norepinephrine) or a relative deficiency of inhibitory neurotransmitters (eg, gamma-aminobutyric acid [GABA]). Drugs that stimulate the CNS can cause manic and hypomanic behaviors that are easily confused with schizophreniform psychoses.

GENERAL CHARACTERISTICS OF ANTIDEPRESSANT DRUGS

Drugs used in the pharmacologic management of depressive disorders are derived from several chemical groups. Older antidepressants include the tricyclic antidepressants (TCAs) and the monoamine oxidase (MAO) inhibitors. Newer drugs include the SSRIs and several individual drugs that differ from TCAs, MAO inhibitors, and SSRIs. General characteristics of antidepressants include the following:

- All are effective in relieving depression, but they differ in their adverse effects.
- All must be taken for 2 to 4 weeks before depressive symptoms improve.
- They are given orally, absorbed from the small bowel, enter the portal circulation, and circulate through the liver, where they undergo extensive first-pass metabolism before reaching the systemic circulation.
- They are metabolized by the cytochrome P450 enzymes in the liver. Many antidepressants and other drugs are metabolized by the 2D6 or 3A4 subgroup of the enzymes. Thus, antidepressants may interact with each other and with a wide variety of drugs that are normally metabolized by the same subgroups of enzymes.

Mechanisms of Action

Although the actions of antidepressant drugs are still being studied in relation to newer information about brain function and the etiology of mood disorders, these drugs apparently normalize abnormal neurotransmission systems in the brain by altering the amounts of neurotransmitters and the number or sensitivity of receptors. They may also modify interactions among neurotransmission systems and affect endocrine function (eg, the HPA axis and cortisol activity).

After neurotransmitters are released from presynaptic nerve endings, the molecules that are not bound to receptors are normally inactivated by reuptake into the presynaptic nerve fibers that released them or metabolized by MAO. Most antidepressants prevent the reuptake of multiple neurotransmitters; SSRIs selectively inhibit the reuptake of serotonin, and MAO inhibitors prevent the metabolism of neurotransmitter molecules. These mechanisms thereby increase the amount of neurotransmitter available to bind to receptors.

With chronic drug administration, receptors adapt to the presence of increased neurotransmitter by decreasing their number or sensitivity to the neurotransmitter. More specifically, norepinephrine receptors, especially postsynaptic beta receptors and presynaptic alpha$_2$ receptors, are downregulated. The serotonin$_2$ receptor, a postsynaptic receptor, and cortisol (glucocorticoid) receptors may also be downregulated.

Thus, antidepressant effects are attributed to changes in receptors rather than changes in neurotransmitters. Although some of the drugs act more selectively on one neurotransmission system than another initially, this selectivity seems to be lost with chronic administration.

With lithium, the exact mechanism of action is unknown. However, it is known to affect the synthesis, release, and reuptake of several neurotransmitters in the brain, including acetylcholine, dopamine, GABA, and norepinephrine. For example, the drug may increase the activity of GABA, an inhibitory neurotransmitter. It also stabilizes postsynaptic receptor sensitivity to neurotransmitters, probably by competing with calcium, magnesium, potassium, and sodium ions for binding sites.

Indications for Use

Antidepressant therapy may be indicated if depressive symptoms persist at least 2 weeks, impair social relationships or work performance, and occur independently of life events. In addition, antidepressants are increasingly being used for treatment of anxiety disorders. TCAs may be used in children and adolescents in the management of enuresis (bed-wetting or involuntary urination resulting from a physical or psychological disorder). In this setting, TCAs may be given after physical causes (eg, urethral irritation, excessive intake of fluids) have been ruled out. TCAs are also commonly used in the treatment of neuropathic pain. MAO inhibitors are considered third-line drugs, largely because of their potential for serious interactions with certain foods and other drugs.

Contraindications to Use

Antidepressants are contraindicated or must be used with caution in clients with acute schizophrenia; mixed mania and depression; suicidal tendencies; severe renal, hepatic, or cardiovascular disease; narrow-angle glaucoma; and seizure disorders.

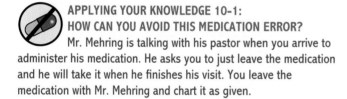

APPLYING YOUR KNOWLEDGE 10-1:
HOW CAN YOU AVOID THIS MEDICATION ERROR?
Mr. Mehring is talking with his pastor when you arrive to administer his medication. He asks you to just leave the medication and he will take it when he finishes his visit. You leave the medication with Mr. Mehring and chart it as given.

TYPES OF ANTIDEPRESSANTS AND INDIVIDUAL DRUGS

Additional characteristics of antidepressants and lithium are described in the following sections. Names, indications for use, and dosage ranges of individual drugs are listed in Table 10-1.

Tricyclic Antidepressants

TCAs, of which **P** **imipramine** is the prototype, are similar drugs that produce a high incidence of adverse effects such as sedation, orthostatic hypotension, cardiac dysrhythmias, anticholinergic effects (eg, blurred vision, dry mouth, constipation, urinary retention), and weight gain. They are well absorbed after oral administration, but first-pass metabolism by the liver results in blood level variations of 10- to 30-fold

among people given identical doses. After they are absorbed, these drugs are widely distributed in body tissues and metabolized by the liver to active and inactive metabolites. Because of adverse effects on the heart, especially in overdose, baseline and follow-up electrocardiograms (ECGs) are recommended for all clients. **Amitriptyline** (Elavil) is a commonly used TCA.

Selective Serotonin Reuptake Inhibitors

SSRIs, of which **P** **fluoxetine** (Prozac, Sarafem) is the prototype, produce fewer serious adverse effects than the TCAs. They are well absorbed with oral administration, undergo extensive first-pass metabolism in the liver, are highly protein bound (56%–95%), and have a half-life of 24 to 72 hours, which may lead to accumulation with chronic administration. Fluoxetine also forms an active metabolite with a half-life of 7 to 9 days. Thus, steady-state blood levels are achieved slowly, over several weeks, and drug effects decrease slowly (over 2 to 3 months) when fluoxetine is discontinued. Sertraline (Zoloft) and citalopram (Celexa) also have active metabolites, but fluoxetine and paroxetine (Paxil) are more likely to accumulate. Escitalopram (Lexapro), paroxetine, sertraline, and fluvoxamine (Luvox) reach steady-state concentrations in 1 to 2 weeks. SSRIs are usually given once daily.

Because SSRIs are highly bound to plasma proteins, they compete with endogenous compounds and other medications for binding sites. Because the drugs are highly lipid soluble, they accumulate in the CNS and other adipose-rich tissue.

Adverse effects include a high incidence of gastrointestinal (GI) symptoms (eg, nausea, diarrhea, weight loss) and sexual dysfunction (eg, delayed ejaculation in men, impaired orgasmic ability in women). Most SSRIs also cause some degree of CNS stimulation (eg, anxiety, nervousness, insomnia), which is most prominent with fluoxetine. Because serotonin release from platelets is essential for hemostasis and psychotropic drugs interfere with serotonin reuptake, these agents are associated with increased risk of GI bleeding. Concomitant use of nonsteroidal anti-inflammatory drugs (NSAIDS), aspirin, or warfarin increases this risk.

Serious, sometimes fatal, reactions have occurred due to combined therapy with an SSRI and an MAO inhibitor, and an SSRI and an MAO inhibitor should not be given concurrently or within 2 weeks of each other. In most cases, if a client taking an SSRI is to be transferred to an MAO inhibitor, the SSRI should be discontinued at least 14 days before starting the MAO inhibitor. However, fluoxetine should be discontinued at least 5 weeks before starting an MAO inhibitor.

APPLYING YOUR KNOWLEDGE 10-2
On his return visit to the physician 2 weeks later, Mr. Mehring's wife complains that she sees no improvement in her husband's mood and that he is taking too much medication. How would you respond?

(text continues on page 180)

Table 10-1 Drugs at a Glance: Antidepressant Agents

GENERIC/TRADE NAME	CLINICAL INDICATIONS	ROUTES AND DOSAGE RANGES
Tricyclic Antidepressants		
Amitriptyline (Elavil)	Depression	PO 50–100 mg once daily at bedtime, gradually increased to 150 mg daily if necessary; IM 80–120 mg daily in 4 divided doses *Adolescents and older adults:* PO 10 mg 3 times daily and 20 mg at bedtime
Amoxapine (Asendin)	Depression	PO 50 mg 2 or 3 times daily, increased to 100 mg 2 or 3 times daily by end of 1 wk. Give maintenance dose in a single dose at bedtime. *Older adults:* PO 25 mg 2 or 3 times daily, increased to 50 mg 2 or 3 times daily by end of 1 wk. Give maintenance dose in a single dose at bedtime.
Clomipramine (Anafranil)	Obsessive-compulsive disorder	PO 25 mg daily, increased to 100 mg daily by end of 2 wk, in divided doses, with meals. Give maintenance dose in a single dose at bedtime. Maximum dose, 250 mg daily. *Children and adolescents:* PO 25 mg daily, increased to 3 mg/kg or 100 mg, whichever is smaller, over 2 wk. Give maintenance dose in a single dose at bedtime. Maximum dose, 3 mg/kg or 200 mg, whichever is smaller.
Desipramine (Norpramin)	Depression	PO 100–200 mg daily in divided doses or as a single daily dose. Give maintenance dose once daily. Maximum dose, 300 mg/d. *Adolescents and older adults:* PO 25–100 mg daily in divided doses or as a single daily dose. Maximum dose, 150 mg/d.
Doxepin (Sinequan)	Depression	PO 75–150 mg daily, in divided doses or a single dose at bedtime. Maximum dose, 300 mg/d.
P **Imipramine** (Tofranil)	Depression Childhood enuresis	PO 75 mg daily in 3 divided doses, gradually increased to 200 mg daily if necessary. Maintenance dose, 75–150 mg daily. *Adolescents and older adults:* PO 30–40 mg daily in divided doses, increased to 100 mg daily if necessary. *Children >6 y:* Enuresis, PO 25–50 mg 1 h before bedtime
Nortriptyline (Aventyl, Pamelor)	Depression	PO 25 mg 3 or 4 times daily or in a single dose (75–100 mg) at bedtime. Maximum dose, 150 mg/d. *Adolescents and older adults:* 30–50 mg/d, in divided doses or a single dose once daily.
Protriptyline (Vivactil)	Depression	PO 15–40 mg daily in 3 or 4 divided doses. Maximum dose, 60 mg. *Adolescents and older adults:* PO 5 mg 3 times daily; increase gradually if necessary
Trimipramine maleate (Surmontil)	Depression	PO 75 mg daily, in divided doses or a single dose at bedtime, increased to 150 mg/d if necessary. Maximum dose, 200 mg/d. *Adolescents and older adults:* PO 50 mg daily, increased to 100 mg/d if necessary
Selective Serotonin Reuptake Inhibitors (SSRIs)		
Citalopram (Celexa)	Depression	PO 20 mg once daily, morning or evening, increased to 40 mg daily in 1 wk, if necessary *Elderly/hepatic impairment:* PO 20 mg daily
Escitalopram (Lexapro)	Depression Generalized anxiety disorder	PO 10 mg once daily. May increase to maximum dose of 20 mg after minimum of 1 wk of therapy
Fluoxetine (Prozac, Prozac Weekly, Sarafem)	Depression Obsessive-compulsive disorder Bulimia nervosa Premenstrual dysphoric disorder (Sarafem)	PO 20 mg once daily in the morning, increased after several weeks if necessary. Give doses larger than 20 mg once in the morning or in 2 divided doses, morning and noon; maximum daily dose 80 mg. Prozac Weekly (delayed-release capsules), PO 90 mg once each wk, starting 7 days after the last 20-mg dose *Children and adolescents 8–17 y for depression:* PO 10 mg/d. May increase to 20 mg/d if necessary.

Table 10-1 Drugs at a Glance: Antidepressant Agents (continued)

GENERIC/TRADE NAME	CLINICAL INDICATIONS	ROUTES AND DOSAGE RANGES
Fluvoxamine (Luvox)	Obsessive-compulsive disorder	PO 50 mg once daily at bedtime, increased in 50-mg increments every 4–7 d if necessary. For daily amounts above 100 mg, give in 2 divided doses. Maximum dose, 300 mg/d. *Children 8–17 y:* PO 25 mg once daily at bedtime, increased in 25-mg increments every 4–7 days if necessary. For daily amounts above 50 mg, give in 2 divided doses. Maximum dose 200 mg/d.
Paroxetine (Paxil, Paxil CR)	Depression Generalized anxiety disorder Obsessive-compulsive disorder Panic disorder Social anxiety disorder	PO 20 mg once daily in the morning, increased at 1 wk or longer intervals, if necessary; usual range, 20–50 mg/d; maximum dose, 60 mg/d. Controlled-release (CR) tablets, PO 25 mg once daily in the morning, increased up to 62.5 mg/d if necessary *Elderly or debilitated adults:* PO 10 mg once daily, increased if necessary. Maximum dose, 40 mg. *Severe renal or hepatic impairment:* Same as for older adults
Sertraline (Zoloft)	Depression Obsessive-compulsive disorder (OCD) Panic disorder Post-traumatic stress disorder (PTSD)	Depression, OCD, PO 50 mg once daily morning or evening, increased at 1-wk or longer intervals to a maximum daily dose of 200 mg Panic, PTSD, PO 25 mg once daily, increased after 1 wk to 50 mg once daily *Children:* OCD, 6–12 y, 25 mg once daily; 13–17 y, 50 mg once daily

Monoamine Oxidase (MAO) Inhibitors

GENERIC/TRADE NAME	CLINICAL INDICATIONS	ROUTES AND DOSAGE RANGES
Isocarboxazid (Marplan)	Depression	PO 10 mg twice daily
Phenelzine (Nardil)	Depression	PO 15 mg 3 times daily
Tranylcypromine (Parnate)	Depression	PO 30 mg daily in divided doses

Other Antidepressants

GENERIC/TRADE NAME	CLINICAL INDICATIONS	ROUTES AND DOSAGE RANGES
Bupropion (Wellbutrin, Wellbutrin SR, Wellbutrin XL, Zyban)	Depression (Wellbutrin) Smoking cessation (Zyban)	Immediate-release tablets, PO 100 mg twice daily, increased to 100 mg 3 times daily (at least 6 h apart) if necessary. Maximum single dose, 150 mg. Sustained-release (SR) tablets, PO 150 mg once daily in the morning, increased to 150 mg twice daily (at least 8 h apart). Maximum single dose, 150 mg. Wellbutrin XL: PO 150 mg once daily in the morning. May increase to target dose of 300 mg on or after fourth day of therapy. Maximum single dose, 450 mg.
Maprotiline	Depression	PO 75 mg daily in single or divided doses
Mirtazapine (Remeron)	Depression	PO 15 mg/d
Trazodone (Desyrel)	Depression	PO 100–300 mg daily, increased to a maximum dose of 600 mg daily if necessary
Venlafaxine (Effexor, Effexor XR)	Depression, Generalized anxiety disorder (XR form)	Immediate-release tablets, PO initially 75 mg/d in 2 or 3 divided doses, with food. Increase by 75 mg/d (4 d or longer between increments) up to 225 mg/d if necessary. Extended-release (XR) capsules, PO initially 37.5 or 75 mg/d in a single dose morning or evening. Increase by 75 mg/d (4 d or longer between increments) up to 225 mg/d if necessary. *Hepatic or renal impairment:* Reduce dose by 50% and increase very slowly.

Mood-Stabilizing Agent

GENERIC/TRADE NAME	CLINICAL INDICATIONS	ROUTES AND DOSAGE RANGES
Lithium carbonate (Eskalith, Lithobid)	Bipolar disorder (mania)	PO 600 mg 3 times daily or 900 mg twice daily (slow-release forms) Maintenance dose, PO 300 mg 3 or 4 times daily to maintain a serum lithium level of 0.6–1.2 mEq/L

PO, oral.

Monoamine Oxidase Inhibitors

MAO inhibitors are infrequently used, mainly because they may interact with some foods and drugs to produce severe hypertension and possible heart attack or stroke. Foods that interact contain tyramine, a monoamine precursor of norepinephrine. Normally, tyramine is deactivated in the GI tract and liver so that large amounts do not reach the systemic circulation. When deactivation is blocked by MAO inhibitors, tyramine is absorbed systemically and transported to adrenergic nerve terminals, where it causes a sudden release of large amounts of norepinephrine. Foods that should be avoided include aged cheeses and meats, concentrated yeast extracts, sauerkraut, and fava beans. Drugs that should be avoided include CNS stimulants (eg, amphetamines, cocaine), adrenergics (eg, pseudoephedrine), antidepressants (SSRIs, venlafaxine), buspirone, levodopa, and meperidine.

Other Antidepressants

Bupropion (Wellbutrin, Zyban) inhibits the reuptake of dopamine, norepinephrine, and serotonin. It was marketed with warnings related to seizure activity. Seizures are most likely to occur with doses above 450 milligrams per day and in clients known to have a seizure disorder.

After an oral dose, peak plasma levels are reached in about 2 hours. The average drug half-life is about 14 hours. The drug is metabolized in the liver and excreted primarily in the urine. Several metabolites are pharmacologically active. Dosage should be reduced in clients with impaired hepatic or renal function. Acute episodes of depression usually require several months of drug therapy. Bupropion is also used as a smoking cessation aid.

Bupropion has few adverse effects on cardiac function and does not cause orthostatic hypotension or sexual dysfunction. However, in addition to seizures, the drug has CNS stimulant effects (agitation, anxiety, excitement, increased motor activity, insomnia, restlessness) that may require a sedative during the first few days of administration. These effects may increase the risk of abuse. Other common adverse effects include dry mouth, headache, nausea and vomiting, and constipation.

Maprotiline is similar to the TCAs in therapeutic and adverse effects.

Mirtazapine (Remeron) blocks presynaptic alpha$_2$-adrenergic receptors (which increases the release of norepinephrine), serotonin receptors, and histamine H$_1$ receptors. Consequently, the drug decreases anxiety, agitation, insomnia, and migraine headaches as well as depression.

Mirtazapine is well absorbed after oral administration, and peak plasma levels occur within 2 hours after an oral dose. It is metabolized in the liver, mainly to inactive metabolites. Common adverse effects include drowsiness (with accompanying cognitive and motor impairment), increased appetite, weight gain, dizziness, dry mouth, and constipation. It does not cause sexual dysfunction.

Mirtazapine should not be taken concurrently with other CNS depressants (eg, alcohol, benzodiazepine antianxiety or hypnotic agents) because of additive sedation. In addition, it should not be taken concurrently with an MAO inhibitor or for 14 days after an MAO inhibitor is stopped. An MAO inhibitor should not be started until at least 14 days after mirtazapine is stopped.

Trazodone (Desyrel) is used more often for sedation and sleep than for depression because high doses (>300 mg/day) are required for antidepressant effects and these amounts cause excessive sedation in many clients. The drug is often given concurrently with a stimulating antidepressant, such as bupropion, fluoxetine, sertraline, or venlafaxine.

Trazodone is well absorbed with oral administration, and peak plasma concentrations are obtained within 30 minutes to 2 hours. It is metabolized by the liver and excreted primarily by the kidneys. Adverse effects include sedation, dizziness, edema, cardiac dysrhythmias, and priapism (prolonged and painful penile erection).

Venlafaxine (Effexor) inhibits the reuptake of norepinephrine, serotonin, and dopamine, thereby increasing the activity of these neurotransmitters in the brain. The drug crosses the placenta and may enter breast milk. It is metabolized in the liver and excreted in urine. It is contraindicated during pregnancy, and women should use effective birth control methods while taking this drug. Adverse effects include CNS (anxiety, dizziness, dreams, insomnia, nervousness, somnolence, tremors), GI (anorexia, nausea, vomiting, constipation, diarrhea), cardiovascular (hypertension, tachycardia, vasodilation), genitourinary (abnormal ejaculation, impotence, urinary frequency), and dermatologic (sweating, rash, pruritus) symptoms. Venlafaxine does not interact with drugs metabolized by the cytochrome P450 system, but it should not be taken concurrently with MAO inhibitors because of increased serum levels and risks of toxicity. If a client taking venlafaxine is to be transferred to an MAO inhibitor, the venlafaxine should be discontinued at least 7 days before starting the MAO inhibitor. If a client taking an MAO inhibitor is to be transferred to venlafaxine, the MAO inhibitor should be discontinued at least 14 days before starting venlafaxine.

Mood-Stabilizing Agents

Lithium carbonate (Eskalith) is a naturally occurring metallic salt that is used in clients with bipolar disorder, mainly to treat and prevent manic episodes. It is well absorbed after oral administration, with peak serum levels in 1 to 3 hours after a dose and steady-state concentrations in 5 to 7 days. Serum lithium concentrations should be monitored frequently because they vary widely among clients taking similar doses and because of the narrow range between therapeutic and toxic levels.

Lithium is not metabolized by the body; it is entirely excreted by the kidneys, so adequate renal function is a prerequisite for lithium therapy. Approximately 80% of a lithium dose is reabsorbed in the proximal renal tubules. The amount of reabsorption depends on the concentration of sodium in the proximal renal tubules. A sodium deficit causes more lithium to be reabsorbed and increases the risk of lithium toxicity. A sodium excess causes more lithium to be excreted (ie, lithium diuresis) and may lower serum lithium levels to nontherapeutic ranges.

Before lithium therapy is begun, baseline studies of renal, cardiac, and thyroid status should be obtained because adverse drug effects involve these organ systems. Baseline electrolyte studies are also necessary.

Anticonvulsants (see Chap. 11) are also used as mood-stabilizing agents in bipolar disorder because they modify nerve cell function. Carbamazepine (Tegretol) and valproate (Depakene) are commonly used. Newer drugs (eg, gabapentin, lamotrigine, topiramate, oxcarbazepine) are being used and studied regarding their effects in bipolar disorder, but none are approved by the Food and Drug Administration (FDA) for this purpose. Thus far, most of the drugs seem to have some beneficial effects but additional studies are needed.

Antipsychotics (see Chap. 9) are increasingly being used to treat bipolar disorder. Currently, quetiapine, risperidone, and olanzapine in combination with fluoxetine are approved by the FDA for this indication.

Herbal Supplement

St. John's wort (*Hypericum perforatum*) is an herb that is widely self-prescribed for depression. Several studies, most of which used about 900 milligrams daily of a standardized extract, indicate its usefulness in mild to moderate depression, with fewer adverse effects than antidepressant drugs. A 3-year, multicenter study by the National Institutes of Health concluded that the herb is not effective in major depression.

Antidepressant effects are attributed mainly to hypericin, although several other active components have also been identified. The mechanism of action is unknown, but the herb is thought to act similarly to antidepressant drugs. Some herbalists refer to St. John's wort as "natural Prozac."

Adverse effects, which are usually infrequent and mild, include constipation, dizziness, dry mouth, fatigue, GI distress, nausea, photosensitivity, restlessness, skin rash, and sleep disturbances. These symptoms are relieved by stopping the herb.

Drug interactions may be extensive. St. John's wort should not be combined with alcohol, antidepressant drugs (eg, MAO inhibitors, SSRIs, TCAs), nasal decongestants or other over-the-counter cold and flu medications, bronchodilators, opioid analgesics, or amino acid supplements containing phenylalanine and tyrosine. All of these interactions may result in hypertension, possibly severe.

Most authorities agree that there is insufficient evidence to support the use of St. John's wort for mild to moderate depression and that more studies are needed to confirm the safety and effectiveness of this herb. Most of the previous studies were considered flawed.

Overall, both consumers and health care professionals seem to underestimate the risks of taking this herbal supplement. For clients who report use of St. John's wort, teach them to purchase products from reputable sources because the amount and type of herbal content may vary among manufacturers; to avoid taking antidepressant drugs, alcohol, and cold and flu medications while taking St. John's wort; to avoid the herb during pregnancy because effects are unknown; and to use sunscreen lotions and clothing to protect themselves from sun exposure.

NURSING PROCESS

Assessment

Assess the client's condition in relation to depressive disorders.

- Identify clients at risk for current or potential depression. Areas to assess include health status, family and social relationships, and work status. Severe or prolonged illness, impaired interpersonal relationships, inability to work, and job dissatisfaction may precipitate depression. Depression also occurs without an identifiable cause.
- Observe for signs and symptoms of depression. Clinical manifestations are nonspecific and vary in severity. For example, fatigue and insomnia may be caused by a variety of disorders and range from mild to severe. When symptoms are present, try to determine their frequency, duration, and severity.
- When a client appears depressed or has a history of depression, assess for suicidal thoughts and behaviors. Statements indicating a detailed plan, accompanied by the intent, ability, and method for carrying out the plan, place the client at high risk for suicide.
- Identify the client's usual coping mechanisms for stressful situations. Coping mechanisms vary widely, and behavior that may be helpful to one client may not be helpful to another. For example, one person may prefer being alone or having decreased contact with family and friends, whereas another may find increased contact desirable.

Nursing Diagnoses

- Dysfunctional Grieving related to loss (of health, ability to perform usual tasks, job, significant other, and so forth)
- Self-Care Deficit related to fatigue and self-esteem disturbance with depression or sedation with antidepressant drugs

- Sleep Pattern Disturbance related to mood disorder or drug therapy
- Risk for Injury related to adverse drug effects
- Risk for Violence: Self-Directed or Directed at Others
- Deficient Knowledge: Effects and appropriate use of antidepressant and mood-stabilizing drugs

Planning/Goals

The client will

- Experience improvement of mood and depressive state
- Receive or self-administer the drugs correctly
- Be kept safe while sedated during therapy with the TCAs and related drugs
- Be assessed regularly for suicidal tendencies. If present, caretakers will implement safety measures.
- Be cared for by staff in areas of nutrition, hygiene, exercise, and social interactions when unable to provide self-care
- Resume self-care and other usual activities
- Avoid preventable adverse drug effects

Interventions

Use measures to prevent or decrease the severity of depression. General measures include supportive psychotherapy and reduction of environmental stress. Specific measures include the following:

- Support the client's usual mechanisms for handling stressful situations, when feasible. Helpful actions may involve relieving pain or insomnia, scheduling rest periods, and increasing or decreasing socialization.
- Call the client by name, encourage self-care activities, allow him or her to participate in setting goals and making decisions, and praise efforts to accomplish tasks. These actions promote a positive self-image.
- When signs and symptoms of depression are observed, initiate treatment before depression becomes severe. Institute suicide precautions for clients at risk. These usually involve close observation, often on a one-to-one basis, and removal of potential weapons from the environment. For clients hospitalized on medical-surgical units, transfer to a psychiatric unit may be needed.
- Provide client teaching regarding drug therapy (see accompanying display).

Evaluation

- Observe for behaviors indicating lessened depression.
- Interview regarding feelings and mood.
- Observe and interview regarding adverse drug effects.
- Observe and interview regarding suicidal thoughts and behaviors.

PRINCIPLES OF THERAPY

Drug Selection

Because the available drugs seem similarly effective, the choice of an antidepressant depends on the client's age; medical conditions; previous history of drug response, if any; and the specific drug's adverse effects. Cost also needs to be considered. Although the newer drugs are much more expensive than the TCAs, they may be more cost effective overall because TCAs are more likely to cause serious adverse effects; they require monitoring of plasma drug levels and ECGs; and clients are more likely to stop taking them. The SSRIs are the drugs of first choice. These drugs are effective and usually produce fewer and milder adverse effects than other drugs. Guidelines for choosing one SSRI over another have not been established.

TCAs are second-line drugs for the treatment of depression. Initial selection of TCAs may be based on the client's previous response or susceptibility to adverse effects. For example, if a client (or a close family member) responded well to a particular drug in the past, that is probably the drug of choice for repeated episodes of depression. The response of family members to individual drugs may be significant because there is a strong genetic component to depression and drug response. If therapeutic effects do not occur within 4 weeks, the TCA probably should be discontinued or changed, because some clients tolerate or respond better to one TCA than to another. For potentially suicidal clients, an SSRI or another newer drug is preferred over a TCA because the TCAs are much more toxic in overdoses.

MAO inhibitors are third-line drugs for the treatment of depression because of their potential interactions with other drugs and certain foods. An MAO inhibitor is most likely to be prescribed when the client does not respond to other antidepressant drugs or when electroconvulsive therapy is refused or contraindicated.

Criteria for choosing bupropion, mirtazapine, and venlafaxine are not clearly defined. Bupropion does not cause orthostatic hypotension or sexual dysfunction. Mirtazapine decreases anxiety, agitation, migraines, and insomnia, as well as depression. In addition, it does not cause sexual dysfunction or clinically significant drug–drug interactions. Venlafaxine has stimulant effects, increases blood pressure, and causes sexual dysfunction, but it does not cause significant drug–drug interactions.

For clients with certain concurrent medical conditions, antidepressants may have adverse effects. For clients with cardiovascular disorders, most antidepressants can cause hypotension, but the SSRIs, bupropion, and venlafaxine are rarely associated with cardiac dysrhythmias. Venlafaxine and MAO inhibitors can increase blood pressure. For clients with seizure disorders, bupropion, clomipramine, and maprotiline should be avoided. SSRIs, MAO inhibitors, and desipramine are less likely to cause seizures. For clients with diabetes

(text continues on page 184)

CLIENT TEACHING GUIDELINES

Antidepressants and Lithium

General Considerations

☑ Take antidepressants as directed to maximize therapeutic benefits and minimize adverse effects. Do not alter doses when symptoms subside. Antidepressants are usually given for several months, perhaps years. Lithium therapy may be lifelong.

☑ Therapeutic effects (relief of symptoms) may not occur for 2–4 weeks after drug therapy is started. As a result, it is very important not to think the drug is ineffective and stop taking it prematurely.

☑ Do not take other prescription or over-the-counter drugs without consulting a health care provider, including over-the-counter cold remedies. Potentially serious drug interactions may occur.

☑ Do not take the herbal supplement St. John's wort while taking a prescription antidepressant drug. Serious interactions may occur.

☑ Inform any physician, surgeon, dentist, or nurse practitioner about the antidepressant drugs being taken. Potentially serious adverse effects or drug interactions may occur if certain other drugs are prescribed.

☑ Avoid activities that require alertness and physical coordination (eg, driving a car, operating other machinery) until reasonably sure the medication does not make you drowsy or impair your ability to perform the activities safely.

☑ Avoid alcohol and other central nervous system depressants (eg, any drugs that cause drowsiness). Excessive drowsiness, dizziness, difficulty breathing, and low blood pressure may occur, with potentially serious consequences.

☑ Learn the name and type of a prescribed antidepressant drug to help avoid undesirable interactions with other drugs or a physician prescribing other drugs with similar effects. There are several different types of antidepressant drugs, with different characteristics and precautions for safe and effective usage.

☑ Escitalopram (Lexapro) is a derivative of citalopram (Celexa), and the two medications should not be taken concomitantly.

☑ Bupropion is a unique drug prescribed for depression (brand name Wellbutrin) and for smoking cessation (brand name Zyban). It is extremely important not to increase the dose or take the two brand names at the same time (as might happen with different physicians or filling prescriptions at different pharmacies). Overdoses may cause seizures, as well as other adverse effects. When used for smoking cessation, Zyban is recommended for up to 12 weeks if progress is being made. If significant progress is not made by approximately 7 weeks, it is considered unlikely that longer drug use will be helpful.

☑ Do not stop taking any antidepressant drug without discussing it with a health care provider. If a problem occurs, the type of drug, the dose, or other aspects may be changed to solve the problem and allow continued use of the medication.

☑ Counseling, support groups, relaxation techniques, and other non-medication treatments are recommended along with drug therapy.

☑ Notify your physician if you become pregnant or intend to become pregnant during therapy with antidepressant drugs.

Self-Administration

☑ With a selective serotonin reuptake inhibitor (eg, Celexa, Lexapro, Luvox, Paxil, Prozac, Zoloft), take in the morning because the drug may interfere with sleep if taken at bedtime. In addition, notify a health care provider if a skin rash or other allergic reaction occurs. Allergic reactions are uncommon but may require that the drug be discontinued.

☑ With a tricyclic antidepressant (eg, amitriptyline), take at bedtime to aid sleep and decrease adverse effects. Also, report urinary retention, fainting, irregular heartbeat, seizures, restlessness, and mental confusion. These are potentially serious adverse drug effects.

☑ With venlafaxine (Effexor), take as directed or ask for instructions. This drug is often taken twice daily. Notify a health care provider if a skin rash or other allergic reaction occurs. An allergic reaction may require that the drug be discontinued.

☑ There are short-, intermediate-, and long-acting forms of bupropion that are taken 3 times, 2 times, or 1 time per day, respectively. Be sure to take your medication as prescribed by your physician.

☑ With lithium, several precautions are needed for safe use:
   1. Take with food or milk or soon after a meal to decrease stomach upset.
   2. Do not alter dietary salt intake. Decreased salt intake (eg, low-salt diet) increases risk of adverse effects from lithium. Increased intake may decrease therapeutic effects.
   3. Drink 8–12 glasses of fluids daily; avoid excessive intake of caffeine-containing beverages. Caffeine has a diuretic effect and dehydration increases lithium toxicity.
   4. Do not take diuretic medications without consulting a health care provider. Diuretics cause loss of sodium and water, which increases lithium toxicity.
   5. Minimize activities that cause excessive perspiration, such as sweating during heavy exercise, sauna use, or outdoor activities during hot summer days. Loss of salt in sweat increases the risk of adverse effects from lithium.
   6. Report for measurements of lithium blood levels as instructed, and do not take the morning dose of lithium until the blood sample has been obtained. Regular measurements of blood lithium levels are necessary for safe and effective lithium therapy. Accurate measurement of serum drug levels requires that blood be drawn approximately 12 hours after the previous dose of lithium.
   7. If signs of overdose occur (eg, vomiting, diarrhea, unsteady walking, tremor, drowsiness, muscle weakness), stop taking lithium and contact the prescribing physician or other health care provider.

mellitus, SSRIs may have a hypoglycemic effect. Bupropion and venlafaxine have little effect on blood sugar levels.

Lithium is the drug of choice for clients with bipolar disorder. When used therapeutically, lithium is effective in controlling mania in 65% to 80% of clients. When used prophylactically, the drug decreases the frequency and intensity of manic cycles. Carbamazepine (Tegretol), an anticonvulsant, may be as effective as lithium as a mood-stabilizing agent. It is often used in clients who do not respond to lithium, although it is not approved by the FDA for this purpose.

Drug Dosage and Administration

Dosage of antidepressant drugs should be individualized according to clinical response. Antidepressant drug therapy is usually initiated with small, divided doses that are gradually increased until therapeutic or adverse effects occur.

With SSRIs and venlafaxine, therapy is begun with once-daily oral administration of the manufacturer's recommended dosage. Dosage may be increased after 3 or 4 weeks if depression is not relieved. As with most other drugs, smaller doses may be indicated in older adults and in clients taking multiple medications.

APPLYING YOUR KNOWLEDGE 10-3
Mr. Mehring reports he is having difficulty sleeping. What measures should be initiated?

With TCAs, therapy is begun with small doses, which are increased to the desired dose over 1 to 2 weeks. Minimal effective doses are approximately 150 milligrams per day of imipramine (Tofranil) or its equivalent. TCAs can be administered once or twice daily because they have long elimination half-lives. After dosage is established, TCAs are often given once daily at bedtime. This regimen is effective and well tolerated by most clients. Elderly clients may experience fewer adverse reactions if divided doses are continued. With TCAs, measurement of plasma levels is helpful in adjusting dosages.

With bupropion, seizures are more likely to occur with large single doses, large total doses, and large or abrupt increases in dosage. Recommendations to avoid these risk factors are as follows:

- Give bupropion in equally divided doses, three times daily (at least 6 hours apart) for immediate-release tablets, twice daily for sustained-release tablets, and once a day for extended-release forms of bupropion XL.
- The maximal single dose of immediate-release tablets is 150 mg (sustained-release, 200 mg; XL, 450 mg).
- The recommended initial dose is 200 mg, gradually increased to 300 mg. If no clinical improvement occurs after several weeks of 300 mg/day, the dosage may be increased to 450 mg, the maximal daily dose for immediate-release tablets (sustained-release, 400 mg; XL, 450 mg).
- The recommended maintenance dose is the lowest amount that maintains remission.

With lithium, dosage should be based on serum lithium levels, control of symptoms, and occurrence of adverse effects. Measurements of serum levels are required because therapeutic doses are only slightly lower than toxic doses and because clients vary widely in rates of lithium absorption and excretion. Thus, a dose that is therapeutic in one client may be toxic in another. Lower doses are indicated for older adults and for clients with conditions that impair lithium excretion (eg, diuretic drug therapy, dehydration, low-salt diet, renal impairment, decreased cardiac output).

When lithium therapy is being initiated, the serum drug concentration should be measured two or three times weekly in the morning, 12 hours after the last dose of lithium. For most clients, the therapeutic range of serum drug levels is 0.5 to 1.2 milliequivalents per liter (mEq/L; SI units, 0.5 to 1.2 mmol/L). Serum lithium levels should not exceed 1.5 milliequivalents per liter, because the risk of serious toxicity is increased at higher levels.

After symptoms of mania are controlled, lithium doses should be lowered. Serum lithium levels should be measured at least every 3 months during long-term maintenance therapy.

Duration of Drug Therapy

Guidelines for the duration of antidepressant drug therapy are not well established, and there are differences of opinion. Some authorities recommend 9 months of treatment after symptoms subside for a first episode of depression; 5 years after symptoms subside for a second episode; and long-term therapy after a third episode. One argument for long-term maintenance therapy is that depression tends to relapse or recur, and successive episodes often are more severe and more difficult to treat.

Maintenance therapy for depression requires close supervision and periodic reassessment of the client's condition and response. With the use of TCAs for acute depression, low doses have been given for several months, followed by gradual tapering of the dose and then drug discontinuation. However, recent studies indicate that full therapeutic doses (if clients can tolerate the adverse effects) for as long as 5 years are effective in preventing recurrent episodes. The long-term effects of SSRIs and newer agents have not been studied.

With lithium, long-term therapy is the usual practice because of a high recurrence rate if the drug is discontinued. When lithium is discontinued, most often because of adverse effects or the client's lack of adherence to the prescribed regimen, gradually tapering the dose over 2 to 4 weeks delays recurrence of symptoms.

Effects of Antidepressants on Other Drugs

The SSRIs are strong inhibitors of the cytochrome P450 enzyme system, which metabolizes many drugs, especially those metabolized by the 1A2, 2D6, and 3A4 groups of enzymes. Inhibiting the enzymes that normally metabolize or inactivate a drug produces the same effect as an excessive dose of the inhibited drug. As a result, serum drug levels and risks of adverse effects are greatly increased. Specific interactions include the following:

- Fluvoxamine inhibits both 1A2 and 3A4 enzymes. Inhibition of 1A2 enzymes slows metabolism of acetaminophen, caffeine, clozapine, haloperidol, olanzapine, tacrine, theophylline, TCAs, and warfarin. Inhibition of 3A4 enzymes slows metabolism of benzodiazepines (alprazolam, midazolam, triazolam), calcium channel blockers (diltiazem, nifedipine, verapamil), cyclosporine, erythromycin, protease inhibitors (antiacquired immunodeficiency syndrome (AIDS) drugs, indinavir, ritonavir, saquinavir), steroids, tamoxifen, warfarin, and zolpidem.
- Fluoxetine, paroxetine, and sertraline inhibit 2D6 enzymes and slow metabolism of bupropion, codeine, desipramine, dextromethorphan, flecainide, metoprolol, nortriptyline, phenothiazines, propranolol, risperidone, and timolol.
- TCAs are metabolized by 2D6 enzymes and may inhibit the metabolism of other drugs metabolized by the 2D6 group (other antidepressants, phenothiazines, carbamazepine, flecainide, propafenone). Lower-than-usual doses of both the TCA and the other drug may be needed.
- Mirtazapine and venlafaxine are not thought to have clinically significant effects on cytochrome P450 enzymes, but few studies have been done and effects are unknown.

Antidepressants and Suicide

In 2004, the FDA issued a public health advisory regarding worsening depression and suicidality in pediatric and adult clients taking antidepressant medications. The drugs that are the focus of this warning are the SSRIs citalopram (Celexa), escitalopram (Lexapro), fluoxetine (Prozac), fluvoxamine (Luvox), paroxetine (Paxil), and sertraline (Zoloft), and the other antidepressants bupropion (Wellbutrin), mirtazapine (Remeron), and venlafaxine (Effexor). Although the FDA has not presently concluded that these antidepressants worsen depression or cause suicidality, a warning statement recommending observation of adult and pediatric clients treated with these agents for worsening depression or the emergence of suicidality (especially at the onset of drug therapy, or when dosages are increased or decreased) has been added to product labeling. Health care providers should be aware that worsening symptoms could be a result of underlying disease or drug therapy. Symptoms of concern include anxiety, agitation, panic attacks, insomnia, irritability, hostility, impulsivity, akathisia, hypomania, and mania. The presence of these symptoms, especially if new (ie, not part of the client's presenting symptoms), severe, or abrupt in onset should prompt evaluation of drug therapy and possible discontinuation of

medications. If the decision is made to discontinue antidepressant therapy, it is important that medications be tapered rather than abruptly discontinued.

The FDA plans to continue to review data from clinical trials on antidepressant medications, data from drug manufacturers, and recommendations from groups such as the Psychopharmacological Drugs Advisory Committee and the Pediatric Subcommittee of the Anti-Infective Drugs Advisory Committee to try to determine whether there is significant evidence that some or all antidepressants increase the risk of suicidality.

Toxicity: Recognition and Management

Some antidepressant drugs are highly toxic and potentially lethal when taken in large doses. Toxicity is most likely to occur in depressed clients who intentionally ingest large amounts of drug in suicide attempts and in young children who accidentally gain access to medication containers. Measures to prevent acute poisoning from drug overdose include dispensing only a few days' supply (ie, 5 to 7 days) to clients with suicidal tendencies and storing the drugs in places inaccessible to young children. General measures to treat acute poisoning include early detection of signs and symptoms, stopping the drug, and instituting treatment if indicated. Specific symptoms and signs of overdose and treatment measures include the following:

- **SSRIs:** Symptoms include nausea, vomiting, agitation, restlessness, hypomania, and other signs of CNS stimulation. Management includes symptomatic and supportive treatment, such as maintaining an adequate airway and ventilation and administering activated charcoal.
- **TCAs:** Symptoms occur 1 to 4 hours after drug ingestion and consist primarily of CNS depression and cardiovascular effects (eg, nystagmus, tremor, restlessness, seizures, hypotension, dysrhythmias, myocardial depression). Death usually results from cardiac, respiratory, and circulatory failure. Management of TCA toxicity consists of performing gastric lavage and giving activated charcoal to reduce drug absorption; establishing and maintaining a patent airway; performing continuous ECG monitoring of comatose clients or those with respiratory insufficiency or wide QRS intervals; giving intravenous fluids and vasopressors for severe hypotension; and giving intravenous phenytoin (Dilantin) or fosphenytoin (Cerebyx), or a parenteral benzodiazepine (eg, lorazepam) if seizures occur.
- **MAO inhibitors:** Symptoms occur 12 hours or more after drug ingestion and consist primarily of adrenergic effects (eg, tachycardia, increased rate of respiration, agitation, tremors, convulsive seizures, sweating, heart block, hypotension, delirium, coma). Management consists of diuresis, acidification of urine, or hemodialysis to remove the drug from the body.

● **Bupropion:** Symptoms include agitation and other mental status changes, nausea and vomiting, and seizures. General treatment measures include hospitalization, decreasing absorption (eg, giving activated charcoal to conscious clients), and supporting vital functions. If seizures occur, an intravenous benzodiazepine (eg, lorazepam) is the drug of first choice.

● **Venlafaxine:** Symptoms include increased incidence or severity of adverse effects, with nausea, vomiting, and drowsiness most often reported. Seizures and diastolic hypertension may also occur. There are no specific antidotes; treatment is symptomatic and supportive.

● **Lithium:** Toxic manifestations occur at serum lithium levels greater than 2.5 mEq/L and include nystagmus, tremors, oliguria, confusion, impaired consciousness, visual or tactile hallucinations, choreiform movements, convulsions, coma, and death. Treatment involves supportive care to maintain vital functions, including correction of fluid and electrolyte imbalances. With severe overdoses, hemodialysis is preferred because it removes lithium from the body.

Antidepressant Withdrawal: Prevention and Management

Withdrawal symptoms have been reported with sudden discontinuation of most antidepressant drugs. In general, symptoms occur more rapidly and may be more intense with drugs that have a short half-life. As with other psychotropic drugs, these antidepressant drugs should be tapered in dosage and discontinued gradually unless severe drug toxicity, anaphylactic reactions, or other life-threatening conditions are present. Most antidepressants may be tapered and discontinued over approximately 1 week without serious withdrawal symptoms. For a client on maintenance drug therapy, the occurrence of withdrawal symptoms may indicate that the client has omitted doses or stopped taking the drug.

The most clearly defined withdrawal syndromes are associated with SSRIs and TCAs. With SSRIs, withdrawal symptoms include dizziness, nausea, and headache and last from several days to several weeks. More serious symptoms may include aggression, hypomania, mood disturbances, and suicidal tendencies. Fluoxetine has a long half-life and has not been associated with withdrawal symptoms. Other SSRIs have short half-lives and may cause withdrawal reactions if stopped abruptly. Paroxetine, which has a half-life of approximately 24 hours and does not produce active metabolites, may be associated with relatively severe withdrawal symptoms even when discontinued gradually, over 7 to 10 days. Symptoms may include a flu-like syndrome with nausea, vomiting, fatigue, muscle aches, dizziness, headache, and insomnia. The short-acting SSRIs should be tapered in dosage and gradually discontinued to prevent or minimize withdrawal reactions.

With TCAs, the main concern is strong anticholinergic effects. When stopped abruptly, especially with high doses, these drugs can cause symptoms of excessive cholinergic activity (ie, hypersalivation, diarrhea, urinary urgency, abdominal cramping, and sweating). A recommended rate for tapering TCAs is approximately 25 to 50 milligrams every 2 to 3 days.

Perioperative Use

Antidepressants must be used very cautiously, if at all, perioperatively because of the risk of serious adverse effects and adverse interactions with anesthetics and other commonly used drugs. It is usually recommended that antidepressants be tapered in dosage and gradually discontinued. MAO inhibitors are contraindicated and should be discontinued at least 10 days before elective surgery. TCAs should be discontinued several days before elective surgery and resumed several days after surgery. SSRIs and other antidepressants have not been studied in relation to perioperative use; however, it seems reasonable to discontinue the drugs when feasible because of potential adverse effects, especially on the cardiovascular system and CNS.

Lithium should be stopped 1 to 2 days before surgery and resumed when full oral intake of food and fluids is allowed. Lithium may prolong the effects of anesthetics and neuromuscular blocking drugs.

Use in Special Populations

Use in Various Ethnic Groups

Antidepressant drug therapy for nonwhite populations in the United States is based primarily on dosage recommendations, pharmacokinetic data, and adverse effects derived from white recipients. However, several studies document differences in drug effects in nonwhite populations. The differences are mainly attributed to genetic or ethnic variations in drug-metabolizing enzymes in the liver. Although all ethnic groups are genetically heterogeneous and individual members may respond differently, health care providers must consider potential differences in responses to drug therapy.

African Americans tend to have higher plasma drug levels for a given dose, respond more rapidly, experience a higher incidence of adverse effects, and metabolize TCAs more slowly than whites. To decrease adverse effects, initial doses may need to be lower than those given to whites, and later doses should be titrated according to clinical response and serum drug levels. In addition, baseline and periodic ECGs are recommended to detect adverse drug effects on the heart. Studies have not been done with newer antidepressants. With lithium, African Americans report more adverse reactions than whites and may need smaller doses.

Asians tend to metabolize antidepressant drugs slowly and therefore have higher plasma drug levels for a given dose than whites. Most studies have been done with TCAs and a limited number of Asian subgroups. Thus, it cannot be assumed that all antidepressant drugs and all people of Asian heritage respond the same. To avoid drug toxicity, initial doses should be approximately half the usual doses given to whites, and later doses should be titrated according to clinical response and serum drug levels. This recommendation is supported by a survey from several Asian countries that reported the use of much smaller doses of TCAs than in the United States. In addition, baseline and periodic ECGs are also recommended for Asian clients to detect adverse drug effects on the heart. Studies have not been done with newer antidepressants. With lithium, there are no apparent differences between effects in Asians and whites.

Hispanics' reactions to antidepressant drugs is largely unknown. Few studies have been performed; some report a need for lower doses of TCAs and greater susceptibility to anticholinergic effects, whereas others report no differences between Hispanics and whites.

Use in Children

Antidepressant drugs are widely prescribed in children and adolescents, in whom depression commonly occurs. However, only a few drugs are actually approved for use in the pediatric population. There is growing concern about a possibility that some antidepressant medications may worsen depression and suicidality in the pediatric population (see "Antidepressants and Suicidality"). These concerns are currently under investigation by the FDA. Overall, there are few reliable data or guidelines for the use of antidepressants in children and adolescents. Clinical trials are currently underway to address these concerns.

For most children and adolescents, it is probably best to reserve drug therapy for those who do not respond to non-pharmacologic treatment and those whose depression is persistent or severe enough to impair function in usual activities of daily living. The long-term effects of antidepressant drugs on the developing brain are unknown. FDA-approved SSRIs are considered first-line antidepressants and safer than TCAs and MAO inhibitors for children with depression. Fluoxetine is approved for treatment of pediatric major depression. (In addition, fluoxetine, sertraline, and fluvoxamine are approved for treatment of obsessive-compulsive disorder in children.) Common adverse effects include sedation and activation; it is often difficult to distinguish therapeutic effects (improvement of mood, increased energy and motivation) from the adverse effects of behavioral activation (agitation, hypomania, restlessness).

Safety and effectiveness have not been established for amoxapine and MAO inhibitors in children younger than 16 years of age or for bupropion, mirtazapine, and venlafaxine in children younger than 18 years of age.

TCAs are not recommended for use in children younger than 12 years of age except for short-term treatment of enuresis in children older than 6 years of age. Amitriptyline,

desipramine, imipramine, and nortriptyline are the TCAs most commonly prescribed to treat depression in children older than 12 years of age. Because of potentially serious adverse effects, blood pressure, ECGs, and plasma drug levels should be monitored. There is evidence that children metabolize TCAs faster than adults, and withdrawal symptoms (eg, increased GI motility, malaise, headache) are more common in children than in adults. Several TCAs are approved for treatment of depression in adolescents. (Clomipramine is approved for treatment of obsessive-compulsive disorder in children, and imipramine is also approved for treating childhood enuresis in children older than 6 years of age.)

Divided doses may be better tolerated and minimize withdrawal symptoms. When a TCA is used for enuresis, effectiveness may decrease over time, and no residual benefits continue after the drug is stopped. Common adverse effects include sedation, fatigue, nervousness, and sleep disorders. A TCA probably is not a drug of first choice for adolescents because TCAs are more toxic in overdose than other antidepressants, and suicide is a leading cause of death in adolescents.

For adolescents, it may be important to discuss sexual effects because the SSRIs and venlafaxine cause a high incidence of sexual dysfunction (eg, anorgasmia, decreased libido, erectile dysfunction). Bupropion and mirtazapine are unlikely to cause sexual dysfunction.

Lithium is not approved for use in children younger than 12 years of age, but it has been used to treat bipolar disorder and aggressiveness. Children normally excrete lithium more rapidly than adults. As with adults, initial doses should be relatively low and gradually increased according to regular measurements of serum drug levels.

Use in Older Adults

SSRIs are the drugs of choice in older adults as in younger ones because they produce fewer sedative, anticholinergic, cardiotoxic, and psychomotor adverse effects than the TCAs and related antidepressants. These drugs produce similar adverse effects in older adults as in younger adults. Although their effects in older adults are not well delineated, SSRIs may be eliminated more slowly, and smaller or less frequent doses may be prudent. The weight loss often associated with SSRIs may be undesirable in older adults. Venlafaxine may also be used in older adults, with smaller initial doses and increments recommended.

TCAs may cause or aggravate conditions that are common in older adults (eg, cardiac conduction abnormalities, urinary retention, narrow-angle glaucoma). In addition, impaired compensatory mechanisms make older adults more likely to experience anticholinergic effects, confusion, hypotension, and sedation. If a TCA is chosen for an older adult, nortriptyline or desipramine is preferred. In addition, any TCA should be given in small doses initially and gradually increased over several weeks, if necessary, to achieve therapeutic effects. Initial and maintenance doses should be small because the drugs are metabolized and excreted more slowly than in younger adults. Initial dosage should be decreased by 30% to 50% to avoid serious adverse reactions; increments should be small. Vital signs, serum drug levels, and ECGs should be monitored regularly.

MAO inhibitors may be more likely to cause hypertensive crises in older adults because cardiovascular, renal, and hepatic functions are often diminished.

With lithium, initial doses should be low and increased gradually, according to regular measurements of serum drug levels.

Use in Clients With Renal Impairment

Antidepressants should be used cautiously in the presence of severe renal impairment. Mild or moderate impairment contributes to few adverse effects, but severe impairment may increase plasma drug levels and adverse effects of virtually all antidepressants. Thus, small initial doses, slow increases, and less frequent dosing are indicated.

Lithium is eliminated only by the kidneys and it has a very narrow therapeutic range. If given to a client with renal impairment or unstable renal function, the dose must be markedly reduced and plasma lithium levels must be closely monitored.

Use in Clients With Hepatic Impairment

Hepatic impairment leads to reduced first-pass metabolism of most antidepressant drugs, resulting in higher plasma levels. The drugs should be used cautiously in clients with severe liver impairment. Cautious use means lower doses, longer intervals between doses, and slower dose increases than usual.

Fluoxetine and sertraline are less readily metabolized to their active metabolites in clients with hepatic impairment. For example, in clients with cirrhosis, the average half-life of fluoxetine may increase from 2 to 3 days to more than 7 days and that of norfluoxetine, the active metabolite, from 7 to 9 days to 12 days. Clearance of sertraline is also decreased in clients with cirrhosis. Paroxetine has a short half-life and no active metabolites, but increased plasma levels can occur with severe hepatic impairment.

TCAs are also less readily metabolized in people with severe hepatic impairment (eg, severe cirrhosis). This increases the risk of adverse effects such as sedation and hypotension.

Use in Clients With Critical Illness

Critically ill clients may be receiving an antidepressant when the critical illness develops or may need a drug to combat the depression that often develops with major illness. The decision to continue or start an antidepressant should be based on a thorough assessment of the client's condition, other drugs being given, potential adverse drug effects, and other factors. If an antidepressant is given, its use must be cautious and slow and the client's responses carefully monitored because critically ill clients are often frail and unstable, with multiple organ dysfunctions.

Use in Home Care

Whatever the primary problem for which a home care nurse is visiting a client, he or she must be vigilant for signs and symptoms of major depression. Depression often accompanies any serious physical illness and may occur in many other circumstances as well. The main role of the nurse may be recognizing depressive states and referring clients for treatment. If an antidepressant medication was recently started, the nurse may need to remind the client that it usually takes 2 to 4 weeks to take effect. The nurse should encourage the client to continue taking the medication. In addition, the nurse should observe the client's response and assess for suicidal thoughts or plans, especially at the beginning of therapy or when dosages are increased or decreased. The family should be taught to report any change in the client's behavior, especially anxiety, agitation, panic attacks, insomnia, irritability, hostility, impulsivity, akathisia, hypomania, and mania. A client who has one or more of these symptoms may be at greater risk for worsening depression or suicidality.

N U R S I N G   A C T I O N S

Antidepressants

NURSING ACTIONS	RATIONALE/EXPLANATION
1. Administer accurately	
a. Give most selective serotonin reuptake inhibitors (SSRIs) once daily in the morning; citalopram, escitalopram, and sertraline may be given morning or evening.	To prevent insomnia
b. Mix sertraline oral concentrate (20 mg/mL) in 4 oz of water, ginger ale, lemon/lime soda, lemonade, or orange juice only; give immediately after mixing.	Manufacturer's recommendations

NURSING ACTIONS	RATIONALE/EXPLANATION
c. Give tricyclic antidepressants (TCAs) and mirtazapine at bedtime.	To aid sleep and decrease daytime sedation
d. Give venlafaxine and lithium with food.	To decrease gastrointestinal (GI) effects (eg, nausea and vomiting)
2. Observe for therapeutic effects	
a. With antidepressants for depression, observe for statements of feeling better or less depressed; increased appetite, physical activity, and interest in surroundings; improved sleep patterns; improved appearance; decreased anxiety; decreased somatic complaints.	Therapeutic effects occur 2–4 weeks after drug therapy is started.
b. With antidepressants for anxiety disorders, observe for decreased symptoms of the disorders (see Chap. 8).	
c. With lithium, observe for decreases in manic behavior and mood swings.	Therapeutic effects do not occur until approximately 7–10 days after therapeutic serum drug levels (1–1.5 mEq/L with acute mania; 0.6–1.2 mEq/L for maintenance therapy) are attained. In mania, a benzodiazepine or an antipsychotic drug is usually given to reduce agitation and control behavior until the lithium takes effect.
3. Observe for adverse effects	
a. With SSRIs and venlafaxine, observe for dizziness, headache, nervousness, insomnia, nausea, diarrhea, dizziness, dry mouth, sedation, skin rash, sexual dysfunction.	GI upset and diarrhea are common with SSRIs; GI upset, diarrhea, agitation, and insomnia are common with venlafaxine. Although numerous adverse effects may occur, they are usually less serious than those occurring with most other antidepressants. Compared with the TCAs, SSRIs and other newer drugs are less likely to cause significant sedation, hypotension, and cardiac dysrhythmias, but they are more likely to cause nausea, nervousness, and insomnia.
b. With TCAs, observe for:	Most adverse effects result from anticholinergic or antiadrenergic activity. Cardiovascular effects are most serious in overdose.
(1) Central nervous system (CNS) effects—drowsiness, dizziness, confusion, poor memory	
(2) GI effects—nausea, dry mouth, constipation	
(3) Cardiovascular effects—cardiac dysrhythmias, tachycardia, orthostatic hypotension	
(4) Other effects—blurred vision, urinary retention, sexual dysfunction, weight gain or loss	
c. With monoamine oxidase (MAO) inhibitors, observe for blurred vision, constipation, dizziness, dry mouth, hypotension, urinary retention, hypoglycemia.	Anticholinergic effects are common. Hypoglycemia results from a drug-induced reduction in blood sugar.
d. With bupropion, observe for seizure activity, CNS stimulation (agitation, insomnia, hyperactivity, hallucinations, delusions), headache, nausea and vomiting, weight loss.	Adverse effects are most likely to occur if recommended doses are exceeded. Note that bupropion has few, if any, effects on cardiac conduction and does not cause orthostatic hypotension.
e. With mirtazapine, observe for sedation, confusion, dry mouth, constipation, nausea and vomiting, hypotension, tachycardia, urinary retention, photosensitivity, skin rash, weight gain.	Common effects are drowsiness, dizziness, and weight gain. Has CNS depressant and anticholinergic effects.
f. With lithium, observe for:	Most clients who take lithium experience adverse effects. Symptoms listed in (1) are common, occur at therapeutic serum drug levels (0.6–1.2 mEq/L), and usually subside during the first few weeks of drug therapy. Symptoms listed in (2) occur at higher serum drug levels (1.5–2.5 mEq/L). Nausea may be decreased by giving lithium with meals. Propranolol (Inderal), 20–120 mg daily, may be given to control tremors. Severe adverse effects may be managed by decreasing lithium dosage, omitting a few doses, or discontinuing the drug temporarily. Toxic symptoms occur at serum drug levels above 2.5 mEq/L.
(1) Metallic taste, hand tremors, nausea, polyuria, polydipsia, diarrhea, muscular weakness, fatigue, edema, weight gain	
(2) More severe nausea and diarrhea, vomiting, ataxia, incoordination, dizziness, slurred speech, blurred vision, tinnitus, muscle twitching and tremors, increased muscle tone	
(3) Leukocytosis	Lithium mobilizes white blood cells (WBCs) from bone marrow to the bloodstream. Maximum increase in WBCs occurs in 7–10 days.

(continued)

NURSING ACTIONS	RATIONALE/EXPLANATION
4. Observe for drug interactions	
a. Drugs that *increase* effects of SSRIs:	Drug interactions with the SSRIs vary with individual drugs.
(1) Cimetidine	May increase serum drug levels of SSRIs by slowing their metabolism
(2) MAO inhibitors	**SSRIs and MAO inhibitors should not be given concurrently or close together because serious and fatal reactions have occurred.** The reaction, attributed to excess serotonin and called the serotonin syndrome, may cause hyperthermia, muscle spasm, agitation, delirium, and coma. To avoid this reaction, an SSRI should not be started for at least 2 weeks after an MAO inhibitor is discontinued, and an MAO inhibitor should not be started for at least 2 weeks after an SSRI has been discontinued (5 weeks with fluoxetine, because of its long half-life).
(3) Linezolid	The antibiotic linezolid is a reversible nonselective MAO inhibitor (see above).
(4) Sumatriptan	Postmarketing studies report concomitant use of SSRIs and sumatriptan may result in weakness, hyperreflexia, and incoordination.
(5) Nonsteroidal anti-inflammatory drugs (NSAIDs), aspirin, warfarin	Serotonin release by platelets plays a role in hemostasis, and SSRIs may interfere with this release, resulting in an increased incidence of GI bleeding. Concomitant use of NSAIDs, aspirin, or warfarin potentiates this risk.
b. Drugs that *decrease* effects of SSRIs:	
(1) Carbamazepine, phenytoin, rifampin	These drugs induce liver enzymes that accelerate the metabolism of the SSRIs.
(2) Cyproheptadine	This is an antihistamine with antiserotonin effects.
c. Drugs that *increase* effects of mirtazapine and venlafaxine:	
(1) MAO inhibitors	See SSRIs, above. **These drugs and MAO inhibitors should not be given concurrently or close together because serious and fatal reactions have occurred.** Mirtazapine should be stopped at least 14 days and venlafaxine at least 7 days before starting an MAO inhibitor, and an MAO inhibitor should be stopped at least 14 days before starting mirtazapine or venlafaxine.
d. Drugs that *increase* effects of TCAs:	
(1) Antidysrhythmics (eg, quinidine, disopyramide, procainamide)	Additive effects on cardiac conduction, increasing risk of heart block
(2) Antihistamines, atropine, and other drugs with anticholinergic effects	Additive anticholinergic effects (eg, dry mouth, blurred vision, urinary retention, constipation)
(3) Antihypertensives	Additive hypotension
(4) Cimetidine	Increases risks of toxicity by decreasing hepatic metabolism and increasing blood levels of TCAs
(5) CNS depressants (eg, alcohol, benzodiazepine antianxiety and hypnotic agents, opioid analgesics)	Additive sedation and CNS depression
(6) MAO inhibitors	**TCAs should not be given with MAO inhibitors or within 2 weeks after an MAO inhibitor drug;** hyperpyrexia, convulsions, and death have occurred with concurrent use.
(7) SSRIs	Inhibit metabolism of TCAs
e. Drugs that *decrease* effects of TCAs:	
(1) Carbamazepine, phenytoin, rifampin, nicotine (cigarette smoking)	These drugs induce drug-metabolizing enzymes in the liver, which increases the rate of TCA metabolism and elimination from the body.

NURSING ACTIONS	RATIONALE/EXPLANATION
f. Drugs that *increase* effects of MAO inhibitors:	
(1) Anticholinergic drugs (eg, atropine, antipsychotic agents, TCAs)	Additive anticholinergic effects
(2) Adrenergic agents (eg, epinephrine, phenylephrine), alcohol (some beers and wines), levodopa, meperidine	Hypertensive crisis and stroke may occur.
g. Drugs that *increase* effects of lithium:	
(1) Angiotensin-converting enzyme inhibitors (eg, captopril)	Decrease renal clearance of lithium and thus increase serum lithium levels and risks of toxicity.
(2) Diuretics (eg, furosemide, hydrochlorothiazide)	Increase neurotoxicity and cardiotoxicity of lithium by increasing excretion of sodium and potassium and thereby decreasing excretion of lithium.
(3) NSAIDs	Decrease renal clearance of lithium and thus increase serum levels and risks of lithium toxicity.
(4) Phenothiazines	Increased risk of hyperglycemia
(5) TCAs	May increase effects of lithium and are sometimes combined with lithium for this purpose. These drugs also may precipitate a manic episode and increase risks of hypothyroidism.
h. Drugs that *decrease* effects of lithium:	
(1) Acetazolamide, sodium chloride (in excessive amounts), drugs with a high sodium content (eg, ticarcillin), theophylline	Increase excretion of lithium

APPLYING YOUR KNOWLEDGE: ANSWERS

10-1 The nurse should never leave an antidepressant at the bedside. Charting the medication as given when it has not yet been taken by the client is not truthful, and the client may forget to take the medication or may hold the medication for a later time and save up multiple doses. This is especially problematic with a client suffering from depression because he or she may have suicidal ideations.

10-2 Some antidepressant medications, such as sertraline, are in the class of selective serotonin reuptake inhibitors (SSRIs), which may not reach a therapeutic effect for up to 2 to 4 weeks. Provide appropriate teaching for both the client and his wife regarding therapeutic effect. Check to make sure that Mr. Mehring is taking the right dosage. Encourage him to continue taking the medication.

10-3 Check with the physician to see if Mr. Mehring's dose can be taken once a day in the morning. If this is not possible, then check to see if a different SSRI can be given that has once-a-day dosing. Taking the dose in the morning may solve Mr. Mehring's sleeping difficulty if the problem is due to the drug and not due to the depression.

Review and Application Exercises

Short Answer Exercises

1. During the initial assessment of any client, what kinds of appearances or behaviors may indicate depression?

2. Is antidepressant drug therapy indicated for most episodes of temporary sadness? Why or why not?

3. What are the major groups of antidepressant drugs?

4. How do the drugs act to relieve depression?

5. When a client begins antidepressant drug therapy, why is it important to explain that relief of depression may not occur for a few weeks?

6. What are common adverse effects of TCAs, and how may they be minimized?

7. What is the advantage of giving a TCA at bedtime rather than in the morning?

8. For a client taking an MAO inhibitor, what information would you provide for preventing a hypertensive crisis?

9. How do the SSRIs differ from TCAs?

10. How do the newer drugs, including mirtazapine and venlafaxine, compare with the SSRIs in terms of adverse effects and adverse drug–drug interactions?

11. List the main elements of treatment of antidepressant overdoses.

12. What are common adverse effects of lithium, and how may they be minimized?

13. What is the nurse's role in assessing and managing depression in special populations? In the home setting?

NCLEX-Style Questions

14. A nurse is teaching the importance of proper diet to a client taking tranylcypromine (Parnate) for depression. Which of the following food selections by the client indicates that further teaching is needed?
    a. a tossed salad and a bowl of vegetable soup
    b. a sandwich with salami and Swiss cheese
    c. a hamburger and french fries
    d. a cold plate with cottage cheese, chicken salad, and grapes

15. A client taking lithium is having problems with coordination and unstable gait. The client's lithium level is 2.3 mEq/L. The nurse should do which of the following?
    a. Continue to administer the lithium three times per day.
    b. Skip a dose of lithium and then resume the regular medication schedule.
    c. Administer an extra dose of lithium.
    d. Withhold the lithium and notify the physician of the lithium level.

16. Today your client begins a new drug regimen of escitalopram (Lexapro) for depression. Before administering this medication, you should assess for which of the following?
    a. prior recent use of monoamine oxidase inhibitor antidepressants (MAO inhibitors)
    b. prior diet high in tyramine-containing foods
    c. history of cigarette use
    d. history of seizure disorders

17. Your client has been taking imipramine (Tofranil) for 1 week for depression. He tells you he is going to stop taking this medication because it isn't working. Your best response is which of the following?
    a. "Contact your physician about taking a different antidepressant medication."
    b. "It may take up to 4 weeks before this medication makes you feel better."
    c. "You should slowly taper rather than suddenly discontinue this medication."
    d. "You should take an extra dose today to build up your blood level and get faster results."

Selected References

American Psychiatric Association. (2000). *Diagnostic and statistical manual of mental disorders* (4th ed., text revision). Washington, DC: American Psychiatric Association.

Drug facts and comparisons. (Updated monthly). St. Louis: Facts and Comparisons.

Fetrow, C. W., & Avila, J. R. (2001). *Professional's handbook of complementary & alternative medicines* (2nd ed.). Springhouse, PA: Springhouse.

Food and Drug Administration. (2004, October 15). *FDA launches a multipronged strategy to strengthen safeguards for children treated with antidepressant medications.* Retrieved September 1, 2005, from http://www.fda.gov/bbs/topics/news/2004/NEW01124.html

Holden, C. (2004). Psychopharmacology: FDA weighs suicide risk in children on antidepressants. *Science, 303*(5659), 745.

Kim, R. B. (Ed.). (2001). *Handbook of adverse drug interactions.* New Rochelle, NY: Medical Letter.

Nasrallah, H. A., & Korn, M. L. (2004). *The expanding role of antipsychotic pharmacotherapy in bipolar disorder.* Retrieved March 9, 2004, from Medscape CME Activities: http://www.medscape.com/viewprogram/2953

Stimmel, G. L. (2000). Mood disorders. In E. T. Herfindal & D. R. Gourley (Eds.), *Textbook of therapeutics: Drug and disease management* (7th ed., pp. 1203–1216). Philadelphia: Lippincott Williams & Wilkins.

Waddell, D. L., Hummel, M. E., & Sumners, A. D. (2001). Three herbs you should get to know: Kava, St. John's wort, ginkgo. *American Journal of Nursing, 101*(4), 48–54.

Yamada, M., & Yasuhara, H. (2004). Clinical pharmacology and MAO inhibitors: Safety and future. *Neurotoxicology, 25*(1–2). 215–221.

Antiseizure Drugs

OBJECTIVES

After studying this chapter, you will be able to:

1. Identify types and potential causes of seizures.
2. Discuss major factors that influence choice of an antiseizure drug for a client with a seizure disorder.
3. Give characteristics and effects of commonly used antiseizure drugs.
4. Differentiate between older and more recent antiseizure drugs.
5. Compare advantages and disadvantages between monotherapy and combination drug therapy for seizure disorders.
6. Apply the nursing process with clients receiving antiseizure drugs.
7. Describe strategies for prevention and treatment of status epilepticus.
8. Discuss the use of antiseizure drugs in special populations.

APPLYING YOUR KNOWLEDGE

Frank DeLaney is an 18-year-old college freshman who has been diagnosed with generalized and partial seizures. He has experienced at least three tonic-clonic seizures in the past 6 months and was started on phenytoin 1 month ago. The phenytoin has decreased the number of seizures but has not been successful at controlling the seizures to the degree the client would like. The physician at the student health center has added carbamazepine to the antiseizure regimen. You are working in the student health center and are counseling Frank about his disease process and medical regimen.

INTRODUCTION

Seizure Disorders

The terms *seizure* and *convulsion* are often used interchangeably, although they are not the same. A *seizure* involves a brief episode of abnormal electrical activity in nerve cells of the brain that may or may not be accompanied by visible changes in appearance or behavior. A *convulsion* is a tonic-clonic type of seizure characterized by spasmodic contractions of involuntary muscles.

Seizures may occur as single events in response to hypoglycemia, fever, electrolyte imbalances, overdoses of numerous drugs (eg, amphetamine, cocaine, isoniazid, lidocaine, lithium, methylphenidate, antipsychotics, theophylline), and withdrawal of alcohol or sedative-hypnotic drugs. Treatment of the underlying problem or temporary use of an antiseizure drug may relieve the seizures. An antiseizure drug is also called an *antiepileptic drug* (AED) or an *anticonvulsant*.

Epilepsy

When seizures occur in a chronic, recurrent pattern, they characterize a disorder known as *epilepsy,* which usually requires drug therapy. *Epilepsy* is characterized by abnormal and excessive electrical discharges of nerve cells. It is diagnosed by clinical signs and symptoms of seizure activity and by the presence of abnormal brain wave patterns on the electroencephalogram. The cause is unknown in 60% to 80% of children and adolescents and 50% of older adults. When epilepsy begins in infancy, causes include developmental defects, metabolic disease, or birth injury. Fever is a common cause during late infancy and early childhood, and inherited forms usually begin in childhood or adolescence. When epilepsy begins in adulthood, it is often caused by an acquired neurologic disorder (eg, head injury, stroke, brain tumor) or alcohol and other drug effects. The incidence of epilepsy is higher in young children and older adults than in other age groups.

Seizures are broadly classified as partial or generalized. *Partial seizures* begin in a specific area of the brain and often indicate a localized brain lesion such as birth injury, trauma, stroke, or tumor. They produce symptoms ranging from simple motor and sensory manifestations to more complex abnormal movements and bizarre behavior. Movements are usually automatic, repetitive, and inappropriate to the situation, such as chewing, swallowing, or aversive movements. Behavior is sometimes so bizarre that the person is diagnosed as psychotic or schizophrenic. In simple partial seizures, consciousness is not impaired; in complex partial seizures, the level of consciousness is decreased.

Generalized seizures are bilateral and symmetric and have no discernible point of origin in the brain. The most common type is the *tonic-clonic* or *major motor seizure*. The *tonic* phase involves sustained contraction of skeletal muscles; abnormal postures, such as opisthotonos; and absence of respiration, during which the person becomes cyanotic. The *clonic* phase is characterized by rapid rhythmic and symmetric jerking movements of the body. Tonic-clonic seizures are sometimes preceded by an aura—a brief warning, such as a flash of light or a specific sound or smell. In children, *febrile seizures* (ie, tonic-clonic seizures that occur in the absence of other identifiable causes) are the most common form of epilepsy.

Another type of generalized seizure is the *absence seizure,* characterized by abrupt alterations in consciousness that last only a few seconds. The person may have a blank, staring expression with or without blinking of the eyelids; twitching of the head or arms; and other motor movements. Other types of generalized seizures include the *myoclonic* type (contraction of a muscle or group of muscles) and the *akinetic* type (absence of movement). Some people are subject to *mixed seizures.*

Status epilepticus is a life-threatening emergency characterized by generalized tonic-clonic convulsions lasting for several minutes or occurring at close intervals during which the client does not regain consciousness. Hypotension, hypoxia, and cardiac dysrhythmias may also occur. There is a high risk of permanent brain damage and death unless prompt, appropriate treatment is instituted. In a person taking medications for a diagnosed seizure disorder, the most common cause of status epilepticus is abruptly stopping AEDs. In other clients, regardless of whether they have a diagnosed seizure disorder, causes of status epilepticus include brain trauma or tumors, systemic or central nervous system (CNS) infections, alcohol withdrawal, and overdoses of drugs (eg, cocaine, theophylline).

GENERAL CHARACTERISTICS OF ANTISEIZURE DRUGS

Antiseizure drugs can usually control seizure activity but do not cure the underlying disorder. Numerous difficulties, for both clinicians and clients, have been associated with AED therapy, including trials of different drugs; consideration of monotherapy versus combination therapy using two or more drugs; the need to titrate dosage over time; lack of seizure control while drugs are being selected and dosages adjusted; social stigma and adverse drug effects, often leading to poor client compliance; and undesirable drug interactions among AEDs and between AEDs and other medications. Attempts to overcome these difficulties have led to the development of several new drugs in recent years.

Drug therapy for epilepsy is rapidly evolving as older, more toxic drugs are virtually eliminated from clinical use and are being replaced by newer drugs. In this chapter, older

drugs that are still commonly used (phenytoin, carbamazepine, ethosuximide, phenobarbital, valproate) as well as newer drugs (gabapentin, lamotrigine, levetiracetam, oxcarbazepine, tiagabine, topiramate, zonisamide) are discussed.

Mechanism of Action

Although the exact mechanism of action of most AEDs is unknown, the drugs are thought to suppress seizures in one of the following ways: by decreasing movement of ions into nerve cells, by altering the activity of neurotransmitters (eg, gamma-aminobutyric acid [GABA], glutamate), or by a combination of these mechanisms. Because movement of sodium and calcium ions is required for normal conduction of nerve impulses, blocking these ions decreases responsiveness to stimuli and results in stabilized, less excitable cell membranes. Increasing the activity of GABA, the major inhibitory neurotransmitter in the brain, and decreasing the activity of glutamate, the major excitatory neurotransmitter, also decrease nerve cell excitability. The actions of both sodium channel blockers (eg, phenytoin, oxcarbazine) and GABA enhancers (eg, benzodiazepines, most of the newer AEDs) increase the amount of stimulation required to produce a seizure (called the *seizure threshold*). Overall, the AEDs are thought to stabilize neuronal membranes and decrease neuronal firing in response to stimuli. Some seem able to suppress abnormal neuronal firing without suppressing normal neurotransmission.

Indications for Use

The major clinical indication for AEDs is the prevention or treatment of seizures, especially the chronic recurring seizures of epilepsy. Indications for particular drugs depend on the types and severity of seizures involved. For example, most of the newer drugs are indicated for use with one or two other AEDs to treat more severe seizure disorders that do not respond to a single drug. However, oxcarbazepine is approved for monotherapy, and studies indicate that most of the other newer drugs may be effective as monotherapy in some types of seizures.

In addition to maintenance treatment of epilepsy, AEDs are used to stop acute, tonic-clonic convulsions and status epilepticus. The drug of choice is an intravenous (IV) benzodiazepine, usually lorazepam. After acute seizure activity is controlled, a longer-acting drug, such as phenytoin or fosphenytoin, is given to prevent recurrence. AEDs also are used prophylactically in clients with brain trauma from injury or surgery.

In addition to seizure disorders, AEDs are used to treat bipolar disorder (eg, carbamazepine, valproate). The Food and Drug Administration (FDA) has recently approved valproate for the treatment of acute mania. Carbamazepine has also been found useful, especially in more refractory bipolar episodes. Often these medications are combined with lithium for maximum effect. Both drugs are also used in the management of chronic neuropathic pain. Carbamazepine is approved for treatment of the pain associated with trigeminal neuralgia.

Gabapentin is the first oral medication approved by the FDA for the management of postherpetic neuralgia. Studies indicate that clients receiving gabapentin experienced significant pain relief, improvement in sleep, and improved overall quality of life. Some of the other, newer AEDs are being tested for effectiveness in relation to bipolar, neuropathic pain, and other disorders. Because the drugs are being used for other indications than seizure disorders, some people suggest they be called *neuromodulators* or *neurostabilizers* rather than AEDs or anticonvulsants.

Contraindications to Use

AEDs are contraindicated or must be used with caution in clients with CNS depression. Phenytoin, carbamazepine, gabapentin, lamotrigine, levetiracetam, oxcarbazepine, tiagabine, topiramate, and valproate are contraindicated in clients who have experienced a hypersensitivity reaction to the particular drug (usually manifested by a skin rash, arthralgia, and other symptoms). Phenytoin, carbamazepine, ethosuximide, lamotrigine, topiramate, and zonisamide are contraindicated or must be used cautiously in clients with hepatic or renal impairment. Additional contraindications include phenytoin in clients with sinus bradycardia or heart block; carbamazepine in those with bone marrow depression (eg, leukopenia, agranulocytosis); and tiagabine and valproic acid in people with liver disease. All of the drugs must be used cautiously during pregnancy because they are teratogenic in animals.

INDIVIDUAL DRUGS

Most AEDs are well absorbed with oral administration and are usually given by this route. Most are metabolized in the liver, and a few are eliminated mainly through the kidneys. The large majority commonly produce adverse effects such as ataxia (impaired muscular coordination such as a staggering gait when trying to walk), confusion, dizziness, and drowsiness. Some may cause serious or life-threatening adverse effects such as cardiac dysrhythmias, bone marrow depression, or pancreatitis. Because AEDs are so diverse, they cannot be adequately discussed as groups. Consequently, the drugs are described individually. Types of seizures for which the drugs are used and specific dosages are listed in Table 11-1.

P **Phenytoin** (Dilantin), the prototype, is one of the oldest and most widely used AEDs. It is often the initial drug of choice, especially in adults. In addition to treatment of seizure disorders, it is sometimes used to treat cardiac dysrhythmias.

With oral phenytoin, the rate and extent of absorption vary with the drug formulation. Peak plasma drug levels occur in 2 to 3 hours with prompt-acting forms and in about 12 hours in long-acting forms. Intramuscular (IM) phenytoin is poorly absorbed and not recommended. It is metabolized in the liver to inactive metabolites that are excreted in the urine.

Phenytoin is highly bound (90%) to plasma proteins, and only the free drug (the fraction not bound to plasma albumin) is active therapeutically. For most people, dosage is calculated on the basis of the total phenytoin value. The recognized therapeutic range, assuming a normal plasma albumin level, reflects the amount of phenytoin that is bound to albumin along with the unbound (free) portion. Monitoring the free phenytoin serum level (normal levels 0.8 to 2.0 mcg/mL) should be done in clients with altered albumin levels (elderly persons or those with cirrhosis, burns, malnutrition, cachexia, or nephrotic syndrome) and with factors that may decrease the affinity of phenytoin for albumin or cause displacement of the drug (eg, renal failure, interacting drugs [warfarin, salicylate, valproate], or increased bilirubin). Conditions or factors that decrease binding increase the available free portion of the drug and therefore these clients require lower-than-normal total plasma levels to achieve the normal therapeutic effects.

The most common adverse effects of phenytoin affect the CNS (eg, ataxia, drowsiness, lethargy) and gastrointestinal (GI) tract (eg, nausea, vomiting). Gingival hyperplasia, an overgrowth of gum tissue, is also common, especially in children. Long-term use may lead to an increased risk of osteoporosis because of its effect on vitamin D metabolism. Serious reactions are uncommon but may include allergic reactions, hepatitis, nephritis, bone marrow depression, and mental confusion.

Phenytoin may interact with many other drugs, mainly because it induces drug-metabolizing enzymes in the liver. Thus, it can increase the metabolism of itself and many other drugs, both AEDs and non-AEDs. In addition, many other drugs can affect phenytoin metabolism and protein binding.

Phenytoin is available as a capsule (generic and brand name), chewable tablet, oral suspension, and injectable solution. The injectable solution is highly irritating to tissues, and special techniques are required when the drug is given IV. *Clients should not switch between generic and trade name formulations of phenytoin because of differences in absorption and bioavailability. If a client is stabilized on a generic formulation and switches to Dilantin, there is a risk of higher serum phenytoin levels and toxicity. If a client takes Dilantin and switches to a generic form, there is a risk of lower serum phenytoin levels; loss of therapeutic effectiveness; and seizures. There may also be differences in bioavailability among generic formulations manufactured by different companies.*

APPLYING YOUR KNOWLEDGE 11-1
How do you determine if Frank is receiving an adequate dosage of phenytoin?

Fosphenytoin (Cerebyx) is a prodrug formulation that is rapidly hydrolyzed to phenytoin after IV or IM injection. It is approved for treatment of status epilepticus and for short-term use in clients who cannot take oral phenytoin. In contrast to other preparations of injectable phenytoin, fosphenytoin causes

(text continues on page 200)

Table 11-1 Drugs at a Glance: Antiseizure Drugs

GENERIC/TRADE NAME	TYPES OF SEIZURES USED TO TREAT	ROUTES AND DOSAGE RANGES		Remarks
		Adults	Children	
Carbamazepine (Tegretol)	Partial, generalized tonic-clonic, and mixed seizures	Epilepsy, PO 200 mg twice daily, increased gradually to 600–1200 mg daily if needed, in 3 or 4 divided doses Trigeminal neuralgia, PO 200 mg daily, increased gradually to 1200 mg if necessary	>12 y: PO 200 mg twice daily; may increase to 1000 mg daily for children 12–15 years and 1200 mg for children over 15 y, if necessary 6–12 y: PO 100 mg twice daily (tablet) or 50 mg 4 times daily (suspension), increase to 1000 mg daily if necessary, in 3 or 4 divided doses	• Available in oral and chewable tablets, extended-release tablets and capsules, and a suspension of 100 mg/5 mL • The suspension is absorbed more rapidly and produces higher peak drug levels than tablets. • Therapeutic serum drug level is 4 to 12 mcg/mL (SI units, 17–51 μmol/L).
Clonazepam (Klonopin)	Myoclonic or akinetic seizures, alone or with other AEDs; possibly effective in generalized tonic-clonic and psychomotor seizures	PO 1.5 mg/d, increased by 0.5 mg/d every 3–7 d if necessary; maximum dose, 20 mg/d	PO 0.01–0.03 mg/ kg/d, increased by 0.25–0.5 mg/d every 3–7 days if necessary; maximum dose, 0.2 mg/kg/d	Schedule IV drug
Clorazepate (Tranxene)	Partial seizures, with other AEDs	PO maximal initial dose 7.5 mg 3 times daily; increased by 7.5 mg every week, if necessary; maximum dose, 90 mg/d	>12 y: PO same as adults 9–12 y: PO maximal initial dose 7.5 mg two times daily; increased by 7.5 mg every week, if necessary; maximum dose, 60 mg/d	Schedule IV drug
Diazepam (Valium)	Acute convulsive seizures, status epilepticus	IV 5–10 mg no faster than 2 mg/min; repeat every 5–10 min if needed; maximum dose, 30 mg. Repeat in 2–4 h if necessary; maximum dose, 100 mg/24 h	>30 d and <5 y of age: IV 0.2–0.5 mg over 2–3 min, every 2–5 min up to a maximum of 5 mg 5 y and older: IV 1 mg every 2–5 min up to a maximum of 10 mg. Repeat in 2–4 h if necessary.	Schedule IV drug
Ethosuximide (Zarontin)	Absence seizures; also may be effective in myoclonic and akinetic epilepsy	PO initially 500 mg/d, increased by 250 mg weekly until seizures are controlled or toxicity occurs; maximum dose, 1500 mg/d	PO initially 250 mg/d, increased at weekly intervals until seizures are controlled or toxicity occurs; maximum dose, approximately 750–1000 mg/d	Available in oral capsules and syrup Therapeutic serum drug level is 40–80 mcg/mL.
Fosphenytoin (Cerebyx)	Status epilepticus and short-term use in clients who cannot take oral phenytoin	Nonemergent seizures, IV, IM loading dose 10–20 mg PE/kg; maintenance dose 4–6 mg PE/kg/d;	Dosage not established	Much easier to give IV than phenytoin; can also be given IM

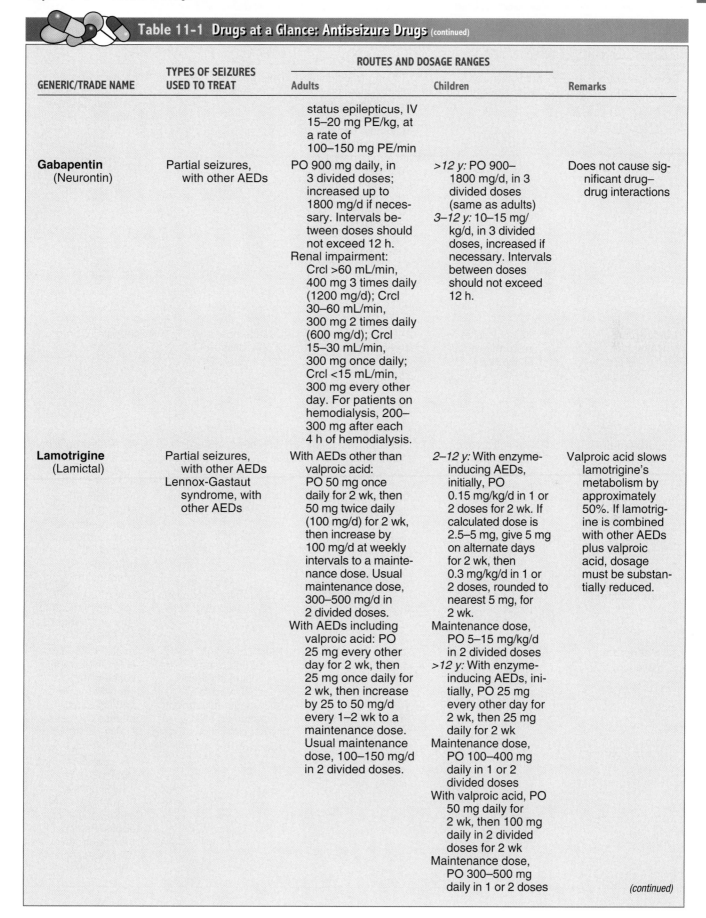

Table 11-1 Drugs at a Glance: Antiseizure Drugs (continued)

| GENERIC/TRADE NAME | TYPES OF SEIZURES USED TO TREAT | ROUTES AND DOSAGE RANGES | | Remarks |
		Adults	Children	
		status epilepticus, IV 15–20 mg PE/kg, at a rate of 100–150 mg PE/min		
Gabapentin (Neurontin)	Partial seizures, with other AEDs	PO 900 mg daily, in 3 divided doses; increased up to 1800 mg/d if necessary. Intervals between doses should not exceed 12 h. Renal impairment: Crcl >60 mL/min, 400 mg 3 times daily (1200 mg/d); Crcl 30–60 mL/min, 300 mg 2 times daily (600 mg/d); Crcl 15–30 mL/min, 300 mg once daily; Crcl <15 mL/min, 300 mg every other day. For patients on hemodialysis, 200–300 mg after each 4 h of hemodialysis.	*>12 y:* PO 900–1800 mg/d, in 3 divided doses (same as adults) *3–12 y:* 10–15 mg/ kg/d, in 3 divided doses, increased if necessary. Intervals between doses should not exceed 12 h.	Does not cause significant drug–drug interactions
Lamotrigine (Lamictal)	Partial seizures, with other AEDs Lennox-Gastaut syndrome, with other AEDs	With AEDs other than valproic acid: PO 50 mg once daily for 2 wk, then 50 mg twice daily (100 mg/d) for 2 wk, then increase by 100 mg/d at weekly intervals to a maintenance dose. Usual maintenance dose, 300–500 mg/d in 2 divided doses. With AEDs including valproic acid: PO 25 mg every other day for 2 wk, then 25 mg once daily for 2 wk, then increase by 25 to 50 mg/d every 1–2 wk to a maintenance dose. Usual maintenance dose, 100–150 mg/d in 2 divided doses.	*2–12 y:* With enzyme-inducing AEDs, initially, PO 0.15 mg/kg/d in 1 or 2 doses for 2 wk. If calculated dose is 2.5–5 mg, give 5 mg on alternate days for 2 wk, then 0.3 mg/kg/d in 1 or 2 doses, rounded to nearest 5 mg, for 2 wk. Maintenance dose, PO 5–15 mg/kg/d in 2 divided doses *>12 y:* With enzyme-inducing AEDs, initially, PO 25 mg every other day for 2 wk, then 25 mg daily for 2 wk Maintenance dose, PO 100–400 mg daily in 1 or 2 divided doses With valproic acid, PO 50 mg daily for 2 wk, then 100 mg daily in 2 divided doses for 2 wk Maintenance dose, PO 300–500 mg daily in 1 or 2 doses	Valproic acid slows lamotrigine's metabolism by approximately 50%. If lamotrigine is combined with other AEDs plus valproic acid, dosage must be substantially reduced.

(continued)

Table 11-1 Drugs at a Glance: Antiseizure Drugs (continued)

GENERIC/TRADE NAME	TYPES OF SEIZURES USED TO TREAT	ROUTES AND DOSAGE RANGES		
		Adults	Children	Remarks
Levetiracetam (Keppra)	Partial seizures, with other AEDs	PO 500 mg twice daily initially, increased by 1000 mg/d every 2 wk, if necessary. Maximum dose, 3000 mg daily. *Renal Impairment:* Crcl >80, 500–1500 mg; Crcl 50–80, 500–1000 mg; Crcl 30–50, 250–750 mg; Crcl <30, 250–500 mg End-stage renal disease, on hemodialysis, 500–1000 mg, with a supplemental dose of half the total daily dose (250–500 mg)	Dosage not established	A newer drug that may have several advantages over older agents
Lorazepam (Ativan)	Acute convulsive seizures, status epilepticus	IV 2–10 mg, diluted in an equal amount of sterile water for injection, 0.9% sodium chloride injection, or 5% dextrose in water, and injected over 2 min	Dosage not established	Schedule IV drug
Oxcarbazepine (Trileptal)	Partial seizures, as monotherapy or with other AEDs in adults, with other AEDs in children 4–16 years old	PO 600 mg twice daily (1200 mg/d) Severe renal impairment (Crcl <30 mL/min), PO 300 mg twice daily (600 mg/d) and increased slowly until response achieved	With other AEDs, PO 8–10 mg/kg/d, not to exceed 600 mg twice daily. Titrate to reach target dose over 2 wk.	• A newer drug with possible advantages over older drugs • Available in 150-, 300-, and 600-mg scored tablets and a 60 mg/mL fruit-flavored suspension
Phenobarbital	Generalized tonic-clonic and partial seizures	PO 100–300 mg daily in 2–3 divided doses	PO 5 mg/kg per day in 2–3 divided doses	Serum drug levels of 10–25 mcg/mL are in the therapeutic range.
P Phenytoin (Dilantin)	Generalized tonic-clonic and some partial seizures Prevention and treatment of seizures occurring during or after neurosurgery	PO 100 mg three times daily initially; 300 mg (long-acting) once daily as maintenance IV 100 mg q6–8h; maximum 50 mg/min	PO 4–7 mg/kg/d in divided doses. Dosing children is highly variable; dosage adjustment based on serum concentrations.	• Available in chewable tablets, oral suspension, immediate-release and extended-release capsules, and solution for injection • Therapeutic serum level is 5–20 mcg/mL (SI units 40–80 μmol/L). Concentrations at or above the upper therapeutic level may be associated with toxicity.

Table 11-1 Drugs at a Glance: Antiseizure Drugs (continued)

GENERIC/TRADE NAME	TYPES OF SEIZURES USED TO TREAT	ROUTES AND DOSAGE RANGES		Remarks
		Adults	Children	
Tiagabine (Gabitril)	Partial seizures, with other AEDs	PO 4 mg daily for 1 wk, increased by 4–8 mg/wk until desired effect; maximum dose 56 mg/d in 2–4 divided doses.	*12–18 y:* PO 4 mg daily for 1 wk, increased to 8 mg/d in 2 divided doses for 1 wk; then increased by 4–8 mg/wk up to a maximum of 32 mg/d in 2 to 4 divided doses *<12 y:* not recommended.	Most experience obtained in patients receiving at least one concomitant enzyme-inducing AED. Use in non-induced patients (eg, those receiving valproate monotherapy) may require lower doses or a slower dose titration.
Topiramate (Topamax)	Partial seizures, with other AEDs	PO 25–50 mg daily, increased by 25–50 mg per week until response. Usual dose, 400 mg daily in 2 divided doses.	*2–16 y:* PO wk 1, 25 mg every P.M., increase by 1–3 mg/kg/d at 1- or 2-wk intervals until response. Usual dose 5–9 mg/kg/d, in 2 divided doses.	
Valproic acid (Depakene capsules); **Sodium valproate** (Depakene syrup, Depacon injection); **Divalproex sodium** (Depakote enteric-coated tablets)	Absence, mixed, and complex partial seizures	PO 10–15 mg/kg/d, increase weekly by 5–10 mg/kg/d, until seizures controlled, adverse effects occur, or the maximum dose (60 mg/kg/d) is reached. Give amounts >250 mg/d in divided doses. Usual daily dose, 1000–1600 mg, in divided doses. IV client's usual dose, diluted in 5% dextrose or 0.9% sodium chloride injection	PO 15–30 mg/kg/d	• Therapeutic serum levels are 50–100 mcg/mL (SI units 350–700 μmol/L) • *Note:* Dosage ranges are the same for the different formulations; doses are in valproic acid equivalents. • Do not give IV >14 d; switch to oral product when possible. Several formulations of valproic acid are available in the United States. These products may contain valproic acid as the acid, as the sodium salt (sodium valproate), or a combination of the two (divalproex sodium).
Zonisamide (Zonegran)	Partial seizures, with other AEDs	PO 100–200 mg daily as a single dose or as 2–3 divided doses; increase by 100 mg/d every 1–2 wk if necessary; maximum dose, 600 mg daily	*<16 y:* not recommended	

AED, antiepileptic drug; Crcl, creatinine clearance; IV, intravenous; μmol/L, micromol/L; PE, phenytoin equivalent; PO, oral.

minimal tissue irritation, can be diluted with 5% dextrose or 0.9% sodium chloride solution, and can be given IV more rapidly. The manufacturer recommends that all dosages be expressed in phenytoin equivalents (PE). Fosphenytoin is available in 2-mL and 10-mL vials with 50 mg PE/mL (fosphenytoin 50 mg PE = phenytoin 50 mg). For IV administration, fosphenytoin can be diluted to a concentration of 1.5 to 25 mg PE/mL, and infused at a maximal rate of 150 mg PE/minute.

Carbamazepine (Tegretol) is used to treat seizure disorders as well as trigeminal neuralgia and bipolar disorder. It is given orally, and peak blood levels are reached in about 1.5 hours with the liquid suspension, in 4 to 5 hours with conventional tablets, and in 3 to 12 hours with extended-release forms (tablets and capsules). Carbamazepine is metabolized in the liver to an active metabolite. Because it induces its own metabolism, its half-life shortens with chronic administration. It is contraindicated in clients with previous bone marrow depression or hypersensitivity to carbamazepine and in those taking monoamine oxidase (MAO) inhibitors. MAO inhibitors should be discontinued at least 14 days before carbamazepine is started.

APPLYING YOUR KNOWLEDGE 11-2

Even though Frank has not indicated a history of a psychiatric disorder, what question should you ask before Frank begins treatment with the carbamazepine?

Clonazepam (Klonopin), **clorazepate** (Tranxene), **diazepam** (Valium), and **lorazepam** (Ativan) are benzodiazepines (see Chap. 8) used in seizure disorders. Clonazepam and clorazepate are used in long-term treatment of seizure disorders, alone or with other AEDs. Tolerance to antiseizure effects develops with long-term use. Clonazepam has a long half-life and may require weeks of continued administration to achieve therapeutic serum blood levels. As with other benzodiazepines, clonazepam produces physical dependence and withdrawal symptoms. Because of clonazepam's long half-life, withdrawal symptoms may appear several days after administration is stopped. Abrupt withdrawal may precipitate seizure activity or status epilepticus.

Diazepam and lorazepam are used to terminate acute convulsive seizures, especially the life-threatening seizures of status epilepticus. Diazepam has a short duration of action and must be given in repeated doses. Lorazepam has become the drug of choice to treat status epilepticus because its effects last longer than those of diazepam.

Ethosuximide (Zarontin) is the AED of choice for absence seizures and may be used with other AEDs for treatment of mixed types of seizures. It is well absorbed after oral administration and reaches peak serum levels in 3 to 7 hours; a steady-state serum concentration is reached in about 5 days. It is eliminated mainly by hepatic metabolism to inactive metabolites, and about 20% is excreted unchanged through the kidneys. Its elimination half-life is approximately 30 hours in children and 60 hours in adults.

Gabapentin (Neurontin) is used with other AEDs for treatment of partial seizures. In addition, it is commonly used to treat postherpetic neuralgia and other conditions such as chronic pain syndromes, including neuropathies (ie, diabetic and others). Gabapentin is 60% absorbed with usual doses, circulates largely in a free state because of minimal binding to plasma proteins, is not appreciably metabolized, and is eliminated by the kidneys as unchanged drug. Its elimination half-life is 5 to 7 hours in clients with normal renal function and as much as 50 hours in clients with impaired renal function, depending on creatinine clearance.

Adverse effects of gabapentin include dizziness, drowsiness, fatigue, loss of muscle coordination, tremor, nausea, vomiting, abnormal vision, gingivitis, and pruritus. Most adverse effects subside spontaneously or with dosage reduction. However, the first dose of gabapentin should be administered at bedtime, because the drug can cause significant somnolence and dizziness with the first dose. Gabapentin reportedly does not cause significant drug–drug interactions. Because the drug is eliminated only by the kidneys, dosage must be reduced in clients with renal impairment.

Lamotrigine (Lamictal) is used with other AEDs for treatment of partial seizures. It is thought to reduce the release of glutamate, an excitatory neurotransmitter, in the brain. It is well absorbed after oral administration, with peak plasma levels reached in 1.5 to 4.5 hours. Lamotrigine is about 55% bound to plasma proteins. It is metabolized in the liver to an inactive metabolite and eliminated mainly in the urine.

Adverse effects of lamotrigine include dizziness, drowsiness, headache, ataxia, blurred or double vision, nausea and vomiting, and weakness. Because a serious skin rash may occur, especially in children, lamotrigine should not be given to children younger than 16 years of age and should be discontinued at the first sign of skin rash in an adult. Skin rash is more likely to occur with concomitant valproic acid therapy, high lamotrigine starting dose, and rapid titration rate. It may resolve if lamotrigine is discontinued, but it progresses in some clients to a more severe form, such as Stevens-Johnson syndrome.

Lamotrigine has little effect on the metabolism of other AEDs, but other AEDs affect its metabolism. Phenytoin, carbamazepine, and phenobarbital induce drug-metabolizing enzymes in the liver and accelerate its metabolism. Valproic acid inhibits those enzymes and thereby slows its metabolism by approximately 50%. If lamotrigine is combined with other AEDs plus valproic acid, dosage must be substantially reduced. To discontinue, dosage should be tapered over at least 2 weeks.

Levetiracetam (Keppra) is a newer drug approved for treatment of partial seizures, in combination with other AEDs. It is chemically unrelated to other AEDs and its mechanism of action is unknown. It inhibits abnormal neuronal firing but does not affect normal neuronal excitability or function.

Levetiracetam is well and rapidly absorbed with oral administration; peak plasma levels occur in about 1 hour. Food reduces peak plasma levels by 20%, and these levels do not occur until 1.5 hours; however, this does not affect the extent of drug absorption. The drug is minimally bound (10%) to plasma proteins and reaches steady-state plasma concentrations after 2 days of twice-daily administration. This rapid attainment of therapeutic effects is especially useful for clients with frequent or severe seizures. The majority of a dose (66%) is eliminated by the kidneys as unchanged drug, and the dose must be reduced in clients with impaired renal function. The drug is not metabolized by the liver and does not affect the hepatic metabolism of other drugs. Thus, it has a low potential for drug interactions.

Levetiracetam was well tolerated in clinical trials, and the incidence of adverse events was similar to that of placebo. Common adverse effects include drowsiness, dizziness, and fatigue. Others include decreases in red and white blood cell counts, double vision, amnesia, anxiety, ataxia, emotional lability, hostility, nervousness, paresthesia, pharyngitis, and rhinitis.

Overall, levetiracetam has pharmacokinetic and other characteristics that may make it especially useful in clients who require combination AED therapy, who take drugs with increased potential for drug interactions, or who have impaired liver function.

Oxcarbazepine (Trileptal) is a newer drug that is structurally related to carbamazepine. It is approved for both monotherapy and adjunctive (with other AEDs) therapy in adults with partial seizures and for adjunctive therapy only in children. For clients receiving carbamazepine or oxcarbazepine, either drug may be substituted for the other without tapering the dose of one or gradually increasing the dose of the other. However, the equivalent dosage of oxcarbazepine is 50% higher than the carbamazepine dosage. In older adults, the recommended equivalent oxcarbazepine dosage is 20% higher than the carbamazepine dosage.

Oxcarbazepine is well absorbed after oral administration, with peak plasma levels occurring in about 5 hours. Most effects are attributed to an active metabolite produced during first-pass metabolism in the liver; the metabolite is 40% protein bound. The elimination half-life is 2 hours for oxcarbazepine and 9 hours for the metabolite. The metabolite is conjugated with glucuronic acid in the liver and excreted in the urine, along with a small amount of unchanged drug. Dosage must be reduced in clients with severe renal impairment (ie, creatinine clearance <30 mL/min).

In clinical trials, adverse effects were similar in adult and pediatric clients and when oxcarbazepine was used alone or with other AEDs. They included cardiac dysrhythmias, drowsiness, dizziness, hypotension, nausea, vomiting, skin rash, and hyponatremia. Because of the risk of hyponatremia, oxcarbazepine should be used with caution in clients taking other drugs that decrease serum sodium levels, and serum sodium levels should be monitored periodically during maintenance therapy. Some studies indicate that skin reactions occur less often with oxcarbazepine than with carbamazepine.

Several drug–drug interactions may occur with oxcarbazepine. The drug inhibits cytochrome P450 2C19 enzymes and induces 3A4 enzymes to influence the metabolism of other drugs metabolized by these enzymes. For example, oxcarbazepine increases metabolism of estrogens and may decrease the effectiveness of oral contraceptives and postmenopausal estrogen replacement therapy. In addition, other drugs that induce cytochrome P450 enzymes, including phenytoin, may reduce plasma levels of the active metabolite by about one third. Drugs that inhibit these enzymes (eg, cimetidine, erythromycin) do not significantly affect the elimination of oxcarbazepine or its metabolite.

Phenobarbital is a long-acting barbiturate that is used alone or with another AED (most often phenytoin). Its use has declined with the advent of other AEDs that cause less sedation and cognitive impairment. CNS depression and other adverse effects associated with barbiturates may occur, but drug dependence and barbiturate intoxication are unlikely with usual antiepileptic doses. Because phenobarbital has a long half-life (50 to 140 hours), it takes 2 to 3 weeks to reach therapeutic serum levels and 3 to 4 weeks to reach a steady-state concentration. It is metabolized in the liver; about 25% is eliminated unchanged in the urine. It induces drug-metabolizing enzymes in the liver and thereby accelerates the metabolism of most AEDs when given with them. Effects on other drugs begin 1 or 2 weeks after phenobarbital therapy is started.

Tiagabine (Gabitril), which may increase GABA levels in the brain, is used with other AEDs in clients with partial seizures. After oral administration, tiagabine is well absorbed; peak plasma levels occur in about 45 minutes if taken on an empty stomach and 2.5 hours if taken with food. It is highly protein bound (96%) and is extensively metabolized in the liver by the cytochrome P450 3A family of enzymes. Only 1% of the drug is excreted unchanged in the urine, and the metabolites are excreted in urine and feces. The elimination half-life is 4 to 7 hours in clients receiving enzyme-inducing AEDs (eg, phenytoin, carbamazepine). Clients with impaired liver function may need smaller doses because the drug is cleared more slowly. CNS effects (eg, confusion, drowsiness, impaired concentration or speech) are the most common adverse effects. GI upset and a serious skin rash may also occur.

Topiramate (Topamax), which has a broad spectrum of antiseizure activity, may act by increasing the effects of GABA and other mechanisms. It is rapidly absorbed and produces peak plasma levels about 2 hours after oral administration. The average elimination half-life is about 21 hours, and steady-state concentrations are reached in about 4 days with normal renal function. It is 20% bound to plasma proteins. Topiramate is not extensively metabolized and is primarily eliminated unchanged through the kidneys. For clients with a creatinine clearance below 70 milliliters per minute, dosage should be reduced by one half.

The most common adverse effects are ataxia, drowsiness, dizziness, and nausea. Renal stones may also occur. Interventions to help prevent renal stones include maintaining an adequate fluid intake, avoiding concurrent use of topiramate with other drugs associated with renal stone formation or increased urinary pH (eg, triamterene, zonisamide), and avoiding topiramate in people with conditions requiring fluid restriction (eg, heart failure) or a history of renal stones. Additive CNS depression may occur with alcohol and other CNS depressant drugs.

Valproic acid preparations (Depakene, Depakote, Depacon) are chemically unrelated to other AEDs. They are thought to enhance the effects of GABA in the brain and are also used to treat manic reactions in bipolar disorder and to prevent migraine headache.

Valproic acid preparations are well absorbed after oral administration and produce peak plasma levels in 1 to 4 hours (15 minutes to 2 hours with the syrup). They are highly bound (90%) to plasma proteins. They are primarily metabolized in the liver, and metabolites are excreted through the kidneys. Valproic acid (Depakene) is available in capsules, and sodium valproate is a syrup formulation. Divalproex sodium (Depakote) contains equal parts of valproic acid and sodium valproate and is available as delayed-release tablets and sprinkle capsules. Depacon is an injectable formulation of valproate. Dosages of all formulations are expressed in valproic acid equivalents.

Depakene, Depakote, and Depacon all produce less sedation and cognitive impairment than phenytoin and phenobarbital. Potentially serious adverse effects, although uncommon, include hepatotoxicity and pancreatitis. The drugs are contraindicated in people who have had hypersensitivity reactions to any of the preparations and people with hepatic disease or impaired hepatic function.

Zonisamide (Zonegran) is chemically a sulfonamide. (It is contraindicated for use in clients who are allergic to sulfonamides.) It is approved for adjunctive treatment of partial seizures and may also be effective for monotherapy and generalized seizures. It is thought to act by inhibiting the entry of sodium and calcium ions into nerve cells.

Zonisamide is well absorbed with oral administration and produces peak plasma levels in 2 to 6 hours. It is 40% bound to plasma proteins and also binds extensively to red blood cells. Its elimination half-life is about 63 hours in plasma and more than 100 hours in red blood cells. It is metabolized by the cytochrome P450 3A enzymes and perhaps other pathways. It is excreted in the urine as unchanged drug (35%) and metabolites (65%). Clients with impaired renal function may require lower doses or a slower titration schedule.

Adverse effects of zonisamide include drowsiness, dizziness, ataxia, confusion, abnormal thinking, nervousness, and fatigue, which can be reduced by increasing the dosage gradually, over several weeks. There is also a risk of kidney stones, which is higher in clients with an inadequate fluid intake or who also take topiramate or triamterene. Skin rash, including the life-threatening Stevens-Johnson syndrome, has been observed.

Drugs that induce the cytochrome P450 enzymes (eg, carbamazepine, phenytoin) increase the metabolism of zonisamide and reduce its half-life. However, administration with cimetidine, which inhibits the cytochrome P450 enzymes, does not seem to inhibit zonisamide metabolism or increase its half-life. Zonisamide apparently does not induce or inhibit cytochrome P450 enzymes and therefore has little effect on the metabolism of other drugs.

NURSING PROCESS

Assessment

Assess client status in relation to seizure activity and other factors:

- If the client has a known seizure disorder and is taking antiseizure drugs, helpful assessment data can be obtained by interviewing the client. Some questions and guidelines include the following:
  - How long has the client had the seizure disorder?
  - How long has it been since seizure activity occurred, or what is the frequency of seizures?
  - Does any particular situation or activity precipitate a seizure?
  - How does the seizure affect the client? For example, what parts of the body are involved? Does he or she lose consciousness? Is he or she drowsy and tired afterward?
  - Which antiseizure drugs are taken? How do they affect the client? How long has the client taken the drugs? Is the currently ordered dosage the same as what the client has been taking? Does the client usually take the drugs as prescribed, or does he or she find it difficult to do so?
  - What other drugs are taken? This includes both prescription and nonprescription drugs, as well as those taken regularly or periodically. This information is necessary because many drugs interact with antiseizure drugs to decrease seizure control or increase drug toxicity.
  - What is the client's attitude toward the seizure disorder? Clues to attitude may include terminology, willingness or reluctance to discuss the seizure disorder, compliance or rejection of drug therapy, and others.
- Check reports of serum drug levels for abnormal values.
- Identify risk factors for seizure disorders. In people without previous seizure activity, seizure disorders may develop with brain surgery, head injury, hypoxia, hypoglycemia, drug overdosage (CNS stimulants, such as amphetamines or cocaine, or local anesthetics, such as lidocaine), and withdrawal from CNS depressants, such as alcohol and barbiturates.
- To observe and record seizure activity accurately, note the location (localized or generalized); specific characteristics of abnormal movements or behavior; dura-

tion; concomitant events, such as loss of consciousness and loss of bowel or bladder control; and postseizure behavior.

● Assess for risk of status epilepticus. Risk factors include recent changes in antiseizure drug therapy, chronic alcohol ingestion, use of drugs known to cause seizures, and infection.

Nursing Diagnoses

● Ineffective Coping related to denial of the disease process and need for long-term drug therapy
● Deficient Knowledge: Disease process
● Deficient Knowledge: Drug effects
● Risk for Injury: Trauma related to ataxia, dizziness, confusion
● Risk for Injury: Seizure activity or drug toxicity
● Ineffective Management of Therapeutic Regimen: Individual: Underuse of Medications

Planning/Goals

The client will
● Take medications as prescribed
● Experience control of seizures
● Avoid serious adverse drug effects
● Verbalize knowledge of the disease process and treatment regimen
● Avoid discontinuing antiseizure medications abruptly
● Keep follow-up appointments with health care providers

Interventions

Use measures to minimize seizure activity. Guidelines include the following:
● Help the client identify conditions under which seizures are likely to occur. These precipitating factors, to be avoided or decreased when possible, may include ingestion of alcoholic beverages or stimulant drugs; fever; severe physical or emotional stress; and sensory stimuli, such as flashing lights and loud noises. Identification of precipitating factors is important because lifestyle changes (eg, reducing stress, reducing alcohol and caffeine intake, increasing exercise, improving sleep and diet) and treatment of existing disorders can reduce the frequency of seizures.
● Assist the client in planning how to get enough rest and exercise and eat a balanced diet, if needed.
● Discuss the seizure disorder, the plan for treatment, and the importance of complying with prescribed drug therapy with the client and family members (see accompanying client teaching display).
● Involve the client in decision making when possible.

● Inform the client and family that seizure control is not gained immediately when drug therapy is started. The goal is to avoid unrealistic expectations and excessive frustration while drugs and dosages are being changed in an effort to determine the best regimen for the client.
● Discuss social and economic factors that promote or prevent compliance.
● Protect a client experiencing a generalized tonic-clonic seizure by
  ● Placing a small pillow or piece of clothing under the head if injury could be sustained from the ground or floor
  ● Not restraining the client's movements; fractures may result
  ● Loosening tight clothing, especially around the neck and chest, to promote respiration
  ● Turning the client to one side so that accumulated secretions can drain from the mouth and throat when convulsive movements stop. The cyanosis, abnormal movements, and loss of consciousness that characterize a generalized tonic-clonic seizure can be quite alarming to witnesses. Most of these seizures, however, subside within 3 or 4 minutes, and the person starts responding and regaining normal skin color. If the person has one seizure after another (status epilepticus), has trouble breathing or continued cyanosis, or has sustained an injury, further care is needed, and a physician should be notified immediately.
● When risk factors for seizures, especially status epilepticus, are identified, try to prevent or minimize their occurrence.

Evaluation

● Interview and observe for decrease in or absence of seizure activity.
● Interview and observe for avoidance of adverse drug effects, especially those that impair safety.
● When available, check laboratory reports of serum drug levels for therapeutic ranges or evidence of underdosing or overdosing.

PRINCIPLES OF THERAPY

Goal of Therapy

Drug therapy is the main treatment of epilepsy for clients of all ages. The goal is to control seizure activity with minimal adverse drug effects. To meet this goal, therapy must be individualized. In most clients, treatment with a single AED is sufficient to meet this goal. However, in 20% to 30% of clients, two or more AEDs are required. In general, combination therapy is associated with more severe adverse

CLIENT TEACHING GUIDELINES

Antiseizure Medications

General Considerations

☑ Take the medications as prescribed. This is extremely important. These drugs must be taken regularly to maintain blood levels adequate to control seizure activity. At the same time, additional doses must not be taken because of increased risks of serious adverse reactions.

☑ Do not suddenly stop taking any antiseizure medication. Severe, even life-threatening, seizures may occur if the drugs are stopped abruptly.

☑ Discuss any problems (eg, seizure activity, excessive drowsiness, other adverse effects) associated with an antiseizure medication with the prescribing physician or other health care professional. Adjusting dose or time of administration may relieve the problems.

☑ Do not drive a car, operate machinery, or perform other activities requiring physical and mental alertness when drowsy from antiseizure medications. Excessive drowsiness, decreased physical coordination, and decreased mental alertness increase the likelihood of injury.

☑ Do not take other drugs without the physician's knowledge and inform any other physician or dentist about taking antiseizure medications. There are many potential drug interactions in which the effects of the antiseizure drug or other drugs may be altered when drugs are given concomitantly.

☑ Do not take any other drugs that cause drowsiness, including over-the-counter antihistamines and sleep aids.

☑ Carry identification, such as a MedicAlert device, with the name and dose of the medication being taken. This is necessary for rapid and appropriate treatment in the event of a seizure, accidental injury, or other emergency situation.

☑ Notify your physician if you become pregnant or intend to become pregnant during therapy. Oxcarbazepine (Trileptal) decreases the effectiveness of oral contraceptive drugs.

☑ Notify your physician if you are breast-feeding or intend to breast-feed during therapy.

Self-Administration

☑ Take most antiseizure medications with food or a full glass of fluid. This will prevent or decrease nausea, vomiting, and gastric distress, which are adverse reactions to most of these drugs. Levetiracetam (Keppra), oxcarbazepine (Trileptal), topiramate (Topamax), and zonisamide (Zonegran) may be taken with or without food.

☑ When taking generic phenytoin or the Dilantin brand of phenytoin:
  1. Do not switch from a generic to Dilantin, or vice versa, without discussing with the prescribing physician. There are differences

in formulations that may upset seizure control and cause adverse effects.
  2. Ask your physician if you should take (or give a child) supplements of folic acid, calcium, vitamin D, or vitamin K. These supplements may help to prevent some adverse effects of phenytoin.
  3. Brush and floss your teeth and have regular dental care to prevent or delay a gum disorder called *gingival hyperplasia*.
  4. If you have diabetes, you may need to check your blood sugar more often or take a higher dose of your antidiabetic medication. Phenytoin may inhibit the release of insulin and increase blood sugar.
  5. Notify your physician or another health care professional if you develop a skin rash, severe nausea and vomiting, swollen glands, bleeding, swollen or tender gums, yellowish skin or eyes, joint pain, unexplained fever, sore throat, unusual bleeding or bruising, persistent headache, or any indication of infection or bleeding, and if you become pregnant.
  6. If you are taking phenytoin liquid suspension or giving it to a child, mix it thoroughly immediately before use and measure it with a calibrated medicine cup or a measuring teaspoon. Do not use regular teaspoons because they hold varying amounts of medication.

☑ If you are taking oxcarbazepine liquid suspension or giving it to a child, mix it thoroughly immediately before use. Measure it with the syringe supplied by the manufacturer and squirt the medication directly into the mouth. Store the suspension at room temperature and use the bottle within 7 weeks or discard the amount remaining. It is helpful to write the date opened and the expiration date on the container.

☑ With valproic acid, the regular capsule should not be opened and the tablet should not be crushed for administration. The sprinkle capsule may be opened and the contents sprinkled on soft food for administration. The syrup formulation may be diluted in water or milk but should not be mixed in carbonated beverages.

☑ Swallow tablets or capsules of valproic acid (Depakene or Depakote) whole; chewing or crushing may cause irritation of the mouth and throat.

☑ Taking valproic acid at bedtime may reduce dizziness and drowsiness.

☑ Lamotrigine may cause photosensitivity. When outdoors, wear protective clothing and sunscreen.

☑ If taking lamotrigine, notify the physician immediately if a skin rash or decreased seizure control develops.

---

effects, interactions among AEDs, poor compliance, and higher costs.

Drug Selection

Several factors should be considered when developing a therapeutic regimen using one or more AEDs.

Seizure Type

Type of seizure is a major factor in drug selection. Therefore, an accurate diagnosis is essential before drug therapy is started. In general, for activity against both partial and generalized seizures, the AEDs lamotrigine, levetiracetam, topiramate, valproic acid, and zonisamide are used. For partial seizures, carbamazepine, gabapentin, oxcarbazepine, phenobarbital, phenytoin, and tiagabine are considered most useful. For absence seizures, ethosuximide is the drug of choice, and clonazepam and valproate are also effective. For mixed seizures, a combination of drugs is usually necessary.

Guidelines for newer drugs are evolving as research studies are performed and clinical experience with their use increases. Most of these agents are approved for combination therapy with other AEDs in clients whose seizures are not adequately controlled with a single drug. However, oxcarbazepine is approved for monotherapy of partial seizures, and some other drugs are also thought to be effective as monotherapy (eg, lamotrigine, valproate).

Adverse Effects

Adverse effects may be the deciding factor in choosing an AED because most types of seizures can be treated effectively by a variety of drugs. The use of carbamazepine and valproic acid increased largely because they cause less sedation and cognitive and psychomotor impairment than phenobarbital and phenytoin. Most of the newer AEDs reportedly cause fewer adverse effects and are better tolerated than the older drugs, even though these newer drugs may also cause potentially serious adverse effects. Fewer and milder adverse effects may greatly increase a client's willingness to comply with the prescribed regimen and attain seizure control.

Monotherapy Versus Combination Therapy

A single drug (monotherapy) is recommended when possible. If effective in controlling seizures, monotherapy has the advantages of fewer adverse drug effects, fewer drug–drug interactions, lower cost, and usually greater client compliance. If the first drug, in adequate dosage, fails to control seizures or causes unacceptable adverse effects, then another agent should be tried as monotherapy. Most practitioners recommend sequential trials of two to three agents as monotherapy before considering combination therapy.

When substituting one AED for another, the second drug should be added and allowed to reach therapeutic blood levels before the first drug is gradually decreased in dosage and discontinued. This is not necessary when substituting oxcarbazepine for carbamazepine or vice versa, because the drugs are similar.

When monotherapy is ineffective, a second, and sometimes a third, drug may be added. If combination therapy is ineffective, the clinician may need to reassess the client for type of seizure; medical conditions or drug–drug interactions that aggravate the seizure disorder or decrease the effectiveness of AEDs; and compliance with the prescribed drug therapy regimen.

Dosage Form

Dosage forms may increase seizure control, client convenience, and compliance. For example, extended-release or long-acting dosage forms can maintain more consistent serum drug levels and decrease frequency of administration. Most of the AEDs are available in oral tablets or capsules, and a few are available as oral liquids or injectable solutions.

Cost

Cost should be considered because it may be a major factor in client compliance. Although the newer drugs are generally effective and better tolerated than older agents, they are also quite expensive. Costs, which depend on manufacturers' wholesale prices and pharmacies' markups as well as prescribed dose amounts and other factors, may vary among pharmacies and change over time. When possible, prescribers can encourage compliance by choosing drugs that are covered by clients' insurance plans or, for uninsured clients, choosing less expensive drug therapy regimens or facilitating enrollment of the client in manufacturer or state drug discount programs.

Pregnancy Risk

Sexually active adolescent girls and women of childbearing potential who require an AED must be evaluated and monitored very closely because all of the AEDs are considered teratogenic. In general, infants exposed to one AED have a significantly higher risk of birth defects than those who are not exposed, and infants exposed to two or more AEDs have a significantly higher risk than those exposed to one AED.

Drug Dosage

The dosage of most drugs is determined empirically by observation of seizure control and adverse effects.

- Usually, larger doses are needed for a single drug than for multiple drugs; for clients with a large body mass (assuming normal liver and kidney function); and in cases of trauma, surgery, and emotional stress.
- Smaller doses are usually required for clients with liver disease and for clients who are taking multiple drugs. Smaller doses of gabapentin, levetiracetam, and topiramate must be given in the presence of renal impairment, and smaller doses of lamotrigine must be given when combined with valproic acid and another AED.
- For most drugs, initial doses are relatively low, and doses are gradually increased until seizures are controlled or adverse effects occur. Then doses may be lowered to the minimum effective level, to decrease adverse effects. Adverse effects are more likely to occur during initiation of treatment. If treatment is started too aggressively, clients may be unwilling to continue a particular medication even if doses are reduced in amount or frequency of administration.
  - When one AED is being substituted for another, dosage of the one being added is gradually increased

while the one being discontinued is gradually decreased. The first drug is usually stopped when therapeutic effects or therapeutic serum drug levels of the second drug are attained.

- When an AED is being discontinued, its dosage should always be tapered gradually, usually over 1 to 3 months. Abruptly stopping an AED may exacerbate seizures or cause status epilepticus.
- When fosphenytoin is substituted for oral phenytoin, the same total daily dosage (in phenytoin equivalents) may be given IV or IM.
- For clients receiving carbamazepine or oxcarbazepine, either agent may be substituted for the other without gradual reduction or titration of the dose. For most clients, the equivalent oxcarbazepine dosage is 50% higher than the carbamazepine dosage. When switching between agents in older adults, the recommended equivalent oxcarbazepine dosage is 20% higher than the carbamazepine dosage.

Monitoring Antiepileptic Drug Therapy

The effectiveness of drug therapy is evaluated primarily by client response in terms of therapeutic or adverse effects. Periodic measurements of serum drug levels are recommended, especially when multiple AEDs are being given. This strategy helps to

- Document blood levels associated with particular drug dosages, seizure control, or adverse drug effects
- Assess and document therapeutic failures
- Assess for drug malabsorption or client noncompliance
- Guide dosage adjustments
- Evaluate possible drug-related adverse effects

To be useful, serum drug levels must be interpreted in relation to clinical responses, because there are wide variations among clients receiving similar doses, probably due to differences in hepatic metabolism. In other words, doses should not be increased or decreased solely to maintain a certain serum drug level. In addition, the timing of collection of blood samples in relation to drug administration is important. For routine monitoring, blood samples should generally be obtained in the morning, before the first daily dose of an AED.

Several antiseizure drugs have the potential to cause blood, liver, or kidney disorders. For this reason, it is usually recommended that baseline blood studies (eg, complete blood count, platelet count) and liver function tests (eg, bilirubin, serum protein, aspartate aminotransferase) be performed before drug therapy starts and periodically thereafter.

When drug therapy fails to control seizures, there are several possible causes. A common one is the client's failure to take the antiseizure drug as prescribed. Other causes include incorrect diagnosis of the type of seizure, use of the wrong drug for the type of seizure, inadequate drug dosage, and too-frequent changes or premature withdrawal of drugs. Addi-

tional causes may include drug overdoses (eg, theophylline), severe electrolyte imbalances (eg, hyponatremia), or use of alcohol or recreational drugs.

Duration and Discontinuation of Therapy

Antiseizure drug therapy may be discontinued for some clients, usually after a seizure-free period of at least 2 years. Although opinions differ about whether, when, and how the drugs should be discontinued, studies indicate that medications can be stopped in approximately two thirds of clients whose epilepsy is completely controlled with drug therapy. Advantages of discontinuation include avoiding adverse drug effects and decreasing costs; disadvantages include recurrence of seizures, with possible status epilepticus. Even if drugs cannot be stopped completely, periodic attempts to decrease the number or dosage of drugs are probably desirable to minimize adverse reactions. Discontinuing drugs, changing drugs, or changing dosage must be done gradually over 2 to 3 months for each drug and with close medical supervision because sudden withdrawal or dosage decreases may cause status epilepticus. Only one drug should be reduced in dosage or gradually discontinued at a time.

Toxicity: Recognition and Management

Signs and symptoms of overdose and toxicity are usually extensions of known adverse effects. Severe overdoses disturb vital functions (eg, CNS depression with confusion, impaired consciousness and possible coma, respiratory depression; cardiovascular problems such as dysrhythmias and hypotension) and are life threatening. Fatalities have been reported with most antiseizure drugs.

If toxicity is suspected, serum drug levels should be assessed in clients taking those drugs with established therapeutic ranges. There are no specific antidotes, and treatment is symptomatic and supportive. For example, gastric lavage and activated charcoal may be indicated to prevent absorption of additional drug; an endotracheal tube should be inserted prior to lavage, to prevent aspiration. (Activated charcoal is not effective in adsorbing topiramate and is not recommended for topiramate overdose.) Hemodialysis is effective in removing drugs that are poorly bound to plasma proteins and that are excreted mainly or partly by the kidneys (eg, gabapentin, levetiracetam, topiramate, valproate). Vital signs, electrocardiogram, level of consciousness, pupillary reflexes, and urine output should be monitored.

Effects of Antiepileptic Drugs on Nonantiepileptic Drugs

Interactions between AEDs and many non-AEDs may be clinically significant. Because AEDs depress the CNS and cause drowsiness, their combination with any other CNS depressants may cause excessive sedation and other adverse CNS effects. AEDs may also decrease the effects of numerous other drugs, mainly by inducing drug-metabolizing enzymes in the liver. Enzyme induction means that the affected drugs are metabolized and eliminated more quickly. In some cases, larger doses of the affected drugs are needed to achieve therapeutic effects.

The older AEDs produce more effects on non-AEDs than newer agents. *Phenytoin* reduces the effects of cardiovascular drugs (eg, amiodarone, digoxin, disopyramide, dopamine, mexiletine, quinidine), female sex hormones (ie, estrogens, oral contraceptives, levonorgestrel), adrenal corticosteroids, antipsychotic drugs (eg, phenothiazines, haloperidol), oral antidiabetic agents (eg, sulfonylureas), doxycycline, furosemide, levodopa, methadone, and theophylline. The consequence of increasing metabolism of oral contraceptives may be unintended pregnancy. The consequence of decreasing the effects of sulfonylureas may be greater difficulty in controlling blood sugar levels in diabetic clients who require both drugs. Phenytoin decreases the therapeutic effects of acetaminophen but may increase the risk of hepatotoxicity by accelerating production of the metabolite that damages the liver. *Carbamazepine* reduces the effects of tricyclic antidepressants, oral anticoagulants, oral contraceptives, bupropion, cyclosporine, doxycycline, felodipine, and haloperidol. Carbamazepine has the same effects on acetaminophen as phenytoin.

Few interactions have been reported with the newer drugs. *Topiramate* decreases effects of digoxin and oral contraceptives. *Levetiracetam* does not induce or inhibit hepatic metabolism of drugs, and risks of interactions are minimal. *Oxcarbazepine* decreases effectiveness of felodipine and oral contraceptives (a barrier type of contraception is recommended during oxcarbazepine therapy). *Zonisamide* interacts with other AEDs, but no interactions have been reported with non-AEDs. More interactions with these drugs may be observed with longer clinical use.

Treatment of Status Epilepticus

An IV benzodiazepine (eg, lorazepam 0.1 mg/kg at 2 mg/minute) is the drug of choice for rapid control of tonic-clonic seizures. However, seizures often recur unless the benzodiazepine is repeated or another, longer-acting drug, such as IV phenytoin (20 mg/kg at 50 mg/minute) or fosphenytoin (20 mg/kg phenytoin equivalents at 150 mg/minute), is given. Further treatment is based on the client's response to these medications. Because there is a risk of significant respiratory depression with IV benzodiazepines, personnel and supplies for emergency resuscitation must be readily available.

Use in Special Populations

Use in Children

Oral drugs are absorbed slowly and inefficiently in newborns. If an antiseizure drug is necessary during the first 7 to 10 days

of life, IM phenobarbital is effective. Metabolism and excretion also are delayed during the first 2 weeks of life, but rates become more rapid than those of adults by 2 to 3 months of age. In infants and children, oral drugs are rapidly absorbed and have short half-lives. This produces therapeutic serum drug levels earlier in children than in adults. Rates of metabolism and excretion also are increased. Consequently, children require higher doses per kilogram of body weight than adults.

The rapid rate of drug elimination persists until approximately 6 years of age, then decreases until it stabilizes at around the adult rate by 10 to 14 years of age. AEDs must be used cautiously to avoid excessive sedation and interference with learning and social development.

There is little information about the effects of the newer AEDs in children. Most of the drugs are approved for use in children (ie, gabapentin, lamotrigine, oxcarbazepine, tiagabine, and topiramate, but not levetiracetam and zonisamide). Oxcarbazepine is metabolized faster in children younger than 8 years of age, and the rate of metabolism is similar to that in adults after 8 years of age. Several studies indicated that oxcarbazepine is effective in monotherapy and combination therapy, with relatively few and mild adverse effects.

Use in Older Adults

Seizure disorders commonly occur in older adults and require drug therapy. Older adults often have multiple medical conditions, take multiple drugs, and have decreases in protein binding and liver and kidney function. As a result, older adults are at high risk of adverse drug effects and adverse drug–drug interactions with AEDs. For example, reduced levels of serum albumin may increase the active portion of highly protein bound AEDs (eg, phenytoin, valproic acid) and increase risks for adverse effects even when total serum drug concentrations are normal. Similarly, decreased elimination by the liver and kidneys may lead to drug accumulation, with subsequent risks of dizziness, impaired coordination, and injuries due to falls.

In addition to the ataxia, confusion, dizziness, and drowsiness that may occur with most AEDs, older adults are also more likely to develop some adverse effects associated with specific drugs. For example, with carbamazepine, they may develop hyponatremia, especially if they also take sodium-losing diuretics (eg, furosemide, hydrochlorothiazide); or cardiac dysrhythmias, especially if they have underlying heart disease. Older adults with pre-existing heart disease should have a thorough cardiac evaluation before starting carbamazepine therapy. These effects may also occur with oxcarbazepine. With valproic acid, older adults may develop a tremor that is difficult to diagnose because of its gradual onset and similarity to the tremor occurring with Parkinson's disease. The tremor is often dose-related and reverses when the drug is reduced in dosage or discontinued.

Most of these potential problems can be averted or minimized by using AEDs very cautiously in older adults. In general, small initial doses, slow titration to desired doses, and small maintenance doses are needed. Using controlled-release formulations to minimize peak plasma concentrations may also be helpful. In addition, frequent assessment of clients for adverse effects and periodic monitoring of serum drug levels, liver function, and kidney function are indicated.

Use in Clients With Renal Impairment

Phenytoin is often used to prevent or treat seizure disorders in clients who are seriously ill. With renal impairment, protein binding is decreased and the amount of free, active drug is higher than in clients with normal renal function. Total phenytoin levels are still more commonly obtained in routine clinical practice; however, free levels are more relevant in the setting of renal failure. The use of *phenobarbital* in clients with severe renal impairment requires markedly reduced dosage, close monitoring of plasma drug levels, and frequent observation for toxic effects. Smaller doses of *gabapentin, levetiracetam, oxcarbazepine, topiramate,* and *zonisamide* must be given in the presence of renal impairment because these drugs are eliminated primarily through the kidneys. Dosage of oxcarbazepine should be decreased by 50% in clients with creatinine clearance of less than 30 milliliters per minute. Zonisamide should not be given to clients with renal failure and should be discontinued in clients who develop acute renal failure or increased serum creatinine and blood urea nitrogen levels during therapy. Elimination of *tiagabine* is not significantly affected by renal insufficiency, renal failure, or hemodialysis, and dose adjustment for renal dysfunction is not necessary. Renal stones have been reported with topiramate and zonisamide.

Use in Clients With Hepatic Impairment

Most AEDs are metabolized in the liver and may accumulate in the presence of liver disease or impaired liver function. The drugs should be used cautiously. *Tiagabine* is cleared more slowly in clients with liver impairment. Increased plasma levels of unbound tiagabine, increased elimination half-life, and increased frequency of neurologic adverse effects (eg, ataxia, dizziness, drowsiness, tremor) have been observed in clients with mild and moderate hepatic insufficiency. Doses may need to be reduced or given at less frequent intervals. *Topiramate* may also be cleared more slowly even though it is eliminated mainly through the kidneys and does not undergo significant hepatic metabolism. It should be used with caution in the presence of hepatic impairment.

 Valproic acid is a hepatotoxic drug and contraindicated for use in clients with hepatic impairment. No dosage adjustment is indicated with levetiracetam, oxcarbazepine, or zonisamide.

Use in Clients With Critical Illness

Phenytoin is often used to prevent or treat seizure disorders in critically ill clients, including those with head injuries. Phenytoin therapy can best be monitored by measuring free serum phenytoin concentrations, but laboratories usually report the total serum drug concentration. In some clients, a low total phenytoin level may still be therapeutic, and a dosage increase is not indicated. The occurrence of nystagmus (abnormal movements of the eyeball) indicates phenytoin toxicity; the drug should be reduced in dosage or discontinued until serum levels decrease. Because phenytoin is extensively metabolized in the liver, clients with severe illnesses may metabolize the drug more slowly and therefore experience toxicity.

For clients in critical care units for other disorders, a history of long-term antiepileptic therapy may be a risk factor for seizures, including status epilepticus, if the AED is stopped abruptly. At the same time, the use of continuous nasogastric enteral feedings may decrease the absorption of phenytoin administered through the same route, predisposing the client to the risk of seizure activity. In addition, continuing an AED may complicate drug therapy for other conditions because of adverse effects and potential drug–drug interactions. For example, phenytoin decreases ventricular automaticity and should not be used in critically ill clients with sinus bradycardia or heart block.

Use in Home Care

The home care nurse must work with clients and family members to implement and monitor AED therapy. When an AED is started, a few weeks may be required to titrate the dosage and determine whether the chosen drug is effective in controlling seizures. The nurse can play an important role in clinical assessment of the client in three ways: (1) interviewing the family about the occurrence of seizures (a log of date, time, duration, and characteristics of seizures can be very helpful), (2) ensuring that the client keeps appointments for serum drug level testing and follow-up care, and (3) encouraging compliance with the prescribed regimen. With long-term use of the drugs, the nurse must monitor the client for therapeutic and adverse drug effects, especially with changes in drugs or dosages. The nurse can also play a role in drawing the blood for levels of anticonvulsants to ensure appropriate dosing. With any evidence that the client is not taking medication as directed, the nurse may need to review the potential loss of seizure control and potential for status epilepticus.

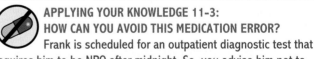

APPLYING YOUR KNOWLEDGE 11-3:
HOW CAN YOU AVOID THIS MEDICATION ERROR?
Frank is scheduled for an outpatient diagnostic test that requires him to be NPO after midnight. So, you advise him not to eat or drink anything after midnight, including medication, the night before his procedure. The next morning, before Frank has his procedure, he experiences a tonic-clonic seizure.

Antiseizure Drugs

NURSING ACTIONS	RATIONALE/EXPLANATION

1. **Administer accurately**

   a. Give on a regular schedule about the same time each day.

   To maintain therapeutic blood levels of drugs

   b. Give most oral antiseizure drugs after meals or with a full glass of water or other fluid; levetiracetam, oxcarbazepine, topiramate, and zonisamide may be taken with or without food.

   Most antiseizure drugs cause some gastric irritation, nausea, or vomiting. Taking the drugs with food or fluid helps decrease gastrointestinal side effects.

   c. To give phenytoin:

      (1) Shake oral suspensions of the drug vigorously before pouring and always use the same measuring equipment.

      In suspensions, particles of drug are suspended in water or other liquid. On standing, drug particles settle to the bottom of the container. Shaking the container is necessary to distribute drug particles in the liquid vehicle. If the contents are not mixed well every time a dose is given, the liquid vehicle will be given initially, and the concentrated drug will be given later. That is, underdosage will occur at first, and little if any therapeutic benefit will result. Overdosage will follow, and the risks of serious toxicity are greatly increased. Using the same measuring container ensures consistent dosage. Calibrated medication cups or measuring teaspoons or tablespoons are acceptable. Regular household teaspoons and tablespoons used for eating and serving are not acceptable because sizes vary widely.

      (2) Do not mix parenteral phenytoin in the same syringe with any other drug.

      Phenytoin solution is highly alkaline (pH approximately 12) and physically incompatible with other drugs. A precipitate occurs if mixing is attempted.

      (3) Give phenytoin as an undiluted intravenous (IV) bolus injection at a rate not exceeding 50 mg/min, then flush the IV line with normal saline or dilute in 50–100 mL of normal saline (0.9% NaCl) and administer over approximately 30–60 minutes. If piggybacked into a primary IV line, the primary IV solution must be normal saline or the line must be flushed with normal saline before and after administration of phenytoin. An in-line filter is recommended.

      Phenytoin cannot be diluted or given in IV fluids other than normal saline because it precipitates within minutes. Slow administration and dilution decrease local venous irritation from the highly alkaline drug solution. Rapid administration must be avoided because it may produce myocardial depression, hypotension, cardiac dysrhythmias, and even cardiac arrest.

   d. To give IV fosphenytoin:

      (1) Check the physician's order and the drug concentration carefully.

      The dose is expressed in phenytoin equivalents (PE; fosphenytoin 50 mg PE = phenytoin 50 mg).

      (2) Dilute the dose in 5% dextrose or 0.9% sodium chloride solution to a concentration of 1.5 mg PE/mL to 25 mg PE/mL and infuse no faster than 150 mg PE/min.

      The drug is preferably diluted in the pharmacy and labeled with the concentration and duration of the infusion. For a 100-mg PE dose, diluting with 4 mL yields the maximum concentration of 25 mg PE/mL; this amount could be infused in about 1 min at the maximal recommended rate. A 1-g loading dose could be added to 50 mL of 0.9% sodium chloride and infused in approximately 10 min at the maximal recommended rate.

      (3) Consult a pharmacist or the manufacturer's literature if any aspect of the dose or instructions for administration are unclear.

      To avoid error

   e. To give carbamazepine and phenytoin suspensions by nasogastric (NG) feeding tube, dilute with an equal amount of water, and rinse the NG tube before and after administration.

   Absorption is slow and decreased, possibly because of drug adherence to the NG tube. Dilution and tube irrigation decrease such adherence.

   f. To give oxcarbazepine suspension, use the 10-mL oral dosing syringe provided by the manufacturer with each bottle. Also check expiration date.

   For accurate measurement and a reminder that the suspension is given orally only. The suspension is stored at room temperature and must be used within 7 weeks after opening the bottle.

(continued)

NURSING ACTIONS	RATIONALE/EXPLANATION
2. Observe for therapeutic effects	
a. When the drug is given on a long-term basis to prevent seizures, observe for a decrease in or absence of seizure activity.	Therapeutic effects begin later with antiseizure drugs than with most other drug groups because the antiseizure drugs have relatively long half-lives. Optimum therapeutic benefits of phenytoin occur approximately 7–10 days after drug therapy is started.
b. When the drug is given to stop an acute convulsive seizure, seizure activity usually slows or stops within a few minutes.	Intravenous lorazepam is the drug of choice for controlling an acute convulsion.
3. Observe for adverse effects	
a. Central nervous system (CNS) effects—ataxia, dizziness, drowsiness, double vision	These effects are common, especially during the first week or two of drug therapy.
b. Gastrointestinal effects—anorexia, nausea, vomiting	These common effects of oral drugs can be reduced by taking the drugs with food or a full glass of water.
c. Hypersensitivity reactions—often manifested by skin disorders such as rash, urticaria, exfoliative dermatitis, Stevens-Johnson syndrome (a severe reaction accompanied by headache, arthralgia, and other symptoms in addition to skin lesions)	These may occur with almost all the antiseizure drugs. Some are mild; some are potentially serious but rare. These skin reactions are usually sufficient reason to discontinue the drug. About 25%–30% of patients with allergic reactions to carbamazepine are likely to be allergic to oxcarbazepine.
d. Blood dyscrasias—anemia, leukopenia, thrombocytopenia, agranulocytosis	Most antiseizure drugs decrease blood levels of folic acid, which may progress to megaloblastic anemia. The other disorders indicate bone marrow depression and are potentially life threatening. They do not usually occur with phenytoin, but may infrequently occur with most other antiseizure drugs.
e. Respiratory depression	This is not likely to be a significant adverse reaction except when a depressant drug, such as lorazepam, is given IV to control acute seizures, such as status epilepticus. Even then, respiratory depression can be minimized by avoiding overdosage and rapid administration.
f. Liver damage—hepatitis symptoms, jaundice, abnormal liver function test results	Hepatic damage may occur with phenytoin, and fatal hepatotoxicity has been reported with valproic acid.
g. Gingival hyperplasia	Occurs often with phenytoin, especially in children. It may be prevented or delayed by vigorous oral hygiene.
h. Hypocalcemia	May occur when antiseizure drugs are taken in high doses and over long periods
i. Hyponatremia	May occur with carbamazepine and oxcarbazepine, especially if taken concurrently with sodium-losing diuretics (eg, furosemide, hydrochlorothiazide). Usually transient and levels return to normal with fluid restriction or dose reduction.
j. Lymphadenopathy resembling malignant lymphoma	This reaction has occurred with several antiseizure drugs, most often with phenytoin.
k. Pancreatitis	Life-threatening pancreatitis has occurred after short- and long-term therapy with valproic acid. Patients should be monitored for the development of acute abdominal pain, nausea, and vomiting.
l. Kidney stones	May occur with topiramate and zonisamide. Inadequate fluid intake or concurrent administration of triamterene may increase risk.
4. Observe for drug interactions	
a. Drugs that *increase* effects of antiseizure drugs:	
(1) CNS depressants—alcohol, sedating antihistamines, benzodiazepines, opioid analgesics, sedatives	Additive CNS depression
(2) Most other antiseizure drugs	Additive or synergistic effects. The drugs are often given in combination, to increase therapeutic effects.

NURSING ACTIONS	RATIONALE/EXPLANATION
b. Drugs that *decrease* effects of antiseizure drugs:	
(1) Tricyclic antidepressants, antipsychotic drugs	These drugs may lower the seizure threshold and precipitate seizures. Dosage of antiseizure drugs may need to be increased.
(2) Carbamazepine, phenytoin, and other enzyme inducers	These drugs inhibit themselves and other antiseizure drugs by activating liver enzymes and accelerating the rate of drug metabolism.
c. Additional drugs that alter effects of phenytoin and fosphenytoin:	
(1) Alcohol (acute ingestion), allopurinol, amiodarone, benzodiazepines, chlorpheniramine, cimetidine, fluconazole, fluoxetine, isoniazid, metronidazole, miconazole, omeprazole, paroxetine, sertraline, and trimethoprim increase effects.	These drugs increase phenytoin toxicity by inhibiting hepatic metabolism of phenytoin or by displacing it from plasma protein-binding sites.
(2) Alcohol (chronic ingestion), antacids, antineoplastics, folic acid, pyridoxine, rifampin, sucralfate, and theophylline decrease effects.	These drugs decrease effects of phenytoin by decreasing absorption, accelerating metabolism, or by unknown mechanisms.
(3) Phenobarbital has variable interactions with phenytoin.	Phenytoin and phenobarbital have complex interactions with unpredictable effects. Although phenobarbital induces drug metabolism in the liver and may increase the rate of metabolism of other anticonvulsant drugs, its interaction with phenytoin differs. Phenobarbital apparently decreases serum levels of phenytoin and perhaps its half-life. Still, the anticonvulsant effects of the two drugs together are greater than those of either drug given alone. The interaction apparently varies with dosage, route, time of administration, the degree of liver enzyme induction already present, and other factors. Thus, whether a significant interaction will occur in a client is unpredictable. Probably the most important clinical implication is that close observation of the client is necessary when either drug is being added or withdrawn.
d. Additional drugs that alter effects of carbamazepine:	
(1) Cimetidine, clarithromycin, diltiazem, erythromycin, isoniazid, valproic acid, and verapamil increase effects.	Most of these drugs inhibit the cytochrome P450 enzymes (1A2, 2C8, and/or 3A4 groups) that normally metabolize carbamazepine, thereby increasing blood levels of carbamazepine. Valproic acid inhibits an epoxide hydrolase enzyme and causes an active metabolite to accumulate. Toxicity may result even if carbamazepine blood levels are at therapeutic concentrations.
(2) Alcohol, phenytoin, and phenobarbital decrease effects.	These drugs increase activity of hepatic drug-metabolizing enzymes, thereby decreasing blood levels of carbamazepine.
e. Drugs that alter the effects of gabapentin:	
(1) Antacids	Reduce absorption of gabapentin. Gabapentin should be given at least 2 hours after a dose of an antacid to decrease interference with absorption.
f. Drugs that alter effects of lamotrigine:	
(1) Valproic acid increases effects.	Valproic acid inhibits the liver enzymes that metabolize lamotrigine, thereby increasing blood levels and slowing metabolism of lamotrigine. As a result, lamotrigine dosage must be substantially reduced when the drug is given in a multidrug regimen that includes valproic acid.
(2) Carbamazepine, phenytoin, and phenobarbital decrease effects.	These drugs induce drug-metabolizing enzymes in the liver and thereby increase the rate of metabolism of themselves and of lamotrigine.
g. Drugs that *decrease* effects of oxcarbazepine:	
(1) Phenobarbital, phenytoin, valproic acid, verapamil	These drugs induce drug-metabolizing enzymes in the liver and thereby increase the metabolism and hasten the elimination of oxcarbazepine.

(continued)

NURSING ACTIONS	RATIONALE/EXPLANATION
h. Drug that *increases* effects of phenobarbital:	
(1) Valproic acid	May increase plasma levels of phenobarbital as much as 40%, probably by inhibiting liver metabolizing enzymes.
i. Additional drugs that *increases* effects of valproate:	
(1) Cimetidine	Inhibits drug-metabolizing enzymes, thereby slowing elimination from the body and increasing blood levels of valproic acid
(2) Salicylates	Displace valproic acid from binding sites on plasma proteins, thereby increasing the serum level of unbound valproic acid
j. Drugs that *decrease* effects of zonisamide:	
(1) Carbamazepine, phenytoin, phenobarbital	These drugs induce drug-metabolizing enzymes in the liver and thereby increase the metabolism and hasten the elimination of zonisamide.
k. Interactions with clonazepam, lorazepam, and diazepam	These drugs are benzodiazepines, discussed in Chapter 8.

APPLYING YOUR KNOWLEDGE: ANSWERS

11-1 Monitor the phenytoin level. The normal free phenytoin level is 0.8 to 2 mcg/mL. Adequate serum levels are needed for seizure control.

11-2 Ask if Frank is taking a monoamine oxidase (MAO) inhibitor, which may be used to treat depression. Carbamazepine should not be taken within 14 days of an MAO inhibitor.

11-3 The client must always taper the dosage of an AED gradually, or the seizures may exacerbate.

Review and Application Exercises

Short Answer Exercises

1. For a client with a newly developed seizure disorder, why is it important to verify the type of seizure by electroencephalogram before starting AEDs?

2. What are the indications for use of the major AEDs?

3. What are the major adverse effects of commonly used AEDs, and how can they be minimized?

4. What are the advantages and disadvantages of treatment with a single drug and of treatment with multiple drugs?

5. Which of the benzodiazepines are used as AEDs?

6. What are the advantages of carbamazepine and valproic acid compared with the benzodiazepines, phenytoin, and phenobarbital?

7. How are the newer drugs similar to or different from phenytoin?

8. What is the treatment of choice for an acute convulsion or status epilepticus?

9. Why is it important when teaching clients to emphasize that none of the AEDs should be stopped abruptly?

10. How can a home care nurse monitor AED therapy during a home visit?

NCLEX-Style Questions

11. An 18-year-old client presents to the clinic with complaints of breast tenderness, nausea, vomiting, and absence of menses for 2 months. She has a history of a seizure disorder that is well controlled with oxcarbazepine (Trileptal). She believes that she has been taking her oral contraceptives as directed but asks if she could be pregnant. The nurse recognizes that the best response to the client's question is which of the following?
   a. "Oxcarbazepine can decreases the effectiveness of oral contraceptive drugs, so we need to do a pregnancy test."
   b. "You can't be pregnant if you have been taking your pills correctly."
   c. "Don't worry; birth control pills are very effective."
   d. "Taking antiseizure drugs with oral contraceptives significantly decreases your risk of pregnancy."

12. A client scheduled for her next dose of phenytoin (Dilantin) has a serum plasma phenytoin level of 16 mcg/mL. Based on this information, the nurse should do which of the following?
   a. Administer the drug.

b. Hold the dose and obtain another plasma drug level before the next dose.

c. Hold the drug and notify the prescriber.

d. Administer half of the prescribed dose.

13. A client taking gabapentin (Neurontin) begins to exhibit tremors, dizziness, and abnormal vision. The nurse should assess the client for signs of which of the following?
   a. additional adverse effects of gabapentin
   b. liver dysfunction
   c. impending seizure activity
   d. cardiac toxicity and dysrhythmias

14. A client is started on phenytoin (Dilantin). A teaching plan for the client should include strategies to minimize which of the following common side effects?
   a. hypoglycemia
   b. photosensitivity
   c. gingival hyperplasia
   d. hyponatremia

15. A client is brought to the emergency department with ongoing tonic-clonic seizure activity. The health care provider orders lorazepam (Ativan) 4 mg IV. Lorazepam is the drug of choice for which of the following types of seizures?
   a. partial seizures
   b. tonic-clonic seizures
   c. absence seizures
   d. status epilepticus

Selected References

Alldredge, B. K. (2000). Seizure disorders. In E. T. Herfindal & D. R. Gourley (Eds.), *Textbook of therapeutics: Drug and disease management* (7th ed., pp. 1107–1137). Philadelphia: Lippincott Williams & Wilkins.

Bourdet, S. V., Gidal, B. E., & Alldredge, B. K. (2001). Pharmacologic management of epilepsy in the elderly. *Journal of the American Pharmaceutical Association, 41*(3), 421–436.

Buck, M. L. (2001). Oxcarbazepine use in children and adolescents [Electronic version]. *Pediatric Pharmacotherapy, 7*(11), 711–716.

Drug facts and comparisons. (Updated monthly). St. Louis: Facts and Comparisons.

Gidal, B. E., Garnett, W. R., & Graves, N. (2002). Epilepsy. In J. T. DiPiro, R. L. Talbert, G. C. Yee, G. R. Matzke, B. G. Wells, & L. M. Posey (Eds.), *Pharmacotherapy: A pathophysiologic approach* (5th ed., pp. 1817–1829). New York: McGraw-Hill.

Hovinga, C. A. (2001). Levetiracetam: A novel antiepileptic drug. *Pharmacotherapy, 21*(11), 1375–1388.

Kim, R. B. (Ed.). (2001). *Handbook of adverse drug interactions.* New Rochelle, NY: Medical Letter.

Lacy, C. F., Armstrong, L. L., Goldman, M. P., & Lance, L. L. (2003). *Lexi-Comp's drug information handbook* (11th ed.). Hudson, Ohio: American Pharmaceutical Association.

Mellegers, M. A., Furlan, A. D., & Mailis, A. (2001). Gabapentin for neuropathic pain: Systematic review of controlled and uncontrolled literature. *Clinical Journal of Pain, 17,* 284–295.

Sachdeo, R., Beydoun, A., Schachter, S., et al. (2001). Oxcarbazepine (Trileptal) as monotherapy in patients with partial seizures. *Neurology, 57*(5): 864–871.

Serpell, M. G., & Neuropathic Pain Study Group. (2002). Gabapentin in neuropathic pain syndromes: A randomised, double-blind, placebo-controlled trial. *Pain, 99*(3): 557–566.

Sirven, J. I., & Waterhouse, E. (2003). Management of status epilepticus. *American Family Physician, 68*(3), 469–476.

Antiparkinson Drugs

OBJECTIVES

After studying this chapter, you will be able to:

1. Describe major characteristics of Parkinson's disease.
2. Differentiate the types of commonly used antiparkinson drugs.
3. Discuss therapeutic and adverse effects of dopaminergic and anticholinergic drugs.
4. Discuss the use of antiparkinson drugs in special populations.
5. Apply the nursing process with clients experiencing parkinsonism.

APPLYING YOUR KNOWLEDGE

Emma Holt is an 81-year-old female who had been experiencing hand tremors, slow movement, a shuffling gait, and excessive salivation. Her physician diagnosed her with Parkinson's disease and started her on levodopa/carbidopa 25/100 four times a day and benztropine at bedtime. Following a fall, she is admitted for evaluation.

INTRODUCTION

Parkinson's disease (also called *parkinsonism*) is a chronic, progressive, degenerative disorder of the central nervous system (CNS) characterized by abnormalities in movement and posture (tremor, bradykinesia, joint and muscular rigidity, postural instability). It occurs more often in men, usually between 50 and 80 years of age. Classic parkinsonism results from destruction of or degenerative changes in dopamine-producing nerve cells in an area of the brain that controls movement. The cause of the nerve-cell damage is unknown; age-related degeneration, genetics, and exposure to toxins (eg, organophosphate pesticides) are possible etiologic factors. Early-onset parkinsonism (before 45 years of age) is considered genetic in origin. Signs and symptoms of Parkinson's disease also may occur with other CNS diseases, brain tumors, and head injuries and with the use of older antipsychotic drugs (eg, phenothiazines).

The basal ganglia in the brain normally contain substantial amounts of the neurotransmitters dopamine and acetylcholine. The correct balance of dopamine and acetylcholine is important in regulating posture, muscle tone, and voluntary movement. People with Parkinson's disease have an imbalance in these neurotransmitters, resulting in a decrease in inhibitory brain dopamine and a relative increase in excitatory acetylcholine. Although the imbalance between dopamine and acetylcholine is considered a major factor, research also indicates imbalances of other neurotransmitters (eg, gamma-aminobutyric acid [GABA], glutamate, norepinephrine, serotonin). The roles of the other imbalances in parkinsonism are still being investigated.

The first symptom of Parkinson's disease is often a tremor that begins in one hand or on one side of the body. Other common symptoms include slow movement (bradykinesia), inability to move (akinesia), rigid limbs, shuffling gait, stooped posture, reduced facial expression, and a soft speaking voice. Less common symptoms include depression, personality changes, dementia, sleep disturbances, speech impairment, or sexual difficulty. Symptom severity usually worsens over time. However, disease progression is often quite gradual, and clients may retain near-normal functional abilities for several years.

GENERAL CHARACTERISTICS OF ANTIPARKINSON DRUGS

Drugs used in Parkinson's disease increase levels of dopamine (levodopa, dopamine agonists, monoamine oxidase [MAO] inhibitors, catechol-*O*-methyltransferase [COMT] inhibitors) or inhibit the actions of acetylcholine (anticholinergic agents) in the brain. Thus, the drugs help adjust the balance of neurotransmitters.

Dopaminergic Drugs

Levodopa, carbidopa, amantadine, bromocriptine, entacapone, pergolide, pramipexole, ropinirole, selegiline, and tolcapone increase dopamine concentrations in the brain and exert dopaminergic activity, directly or indirectly. **Levodopa** (L-dopa) is the mainstay of drug therapy for idiopathic parkinsonism. Carbidopa is used only in conjunction with levodopa. The other drugs are used as adjunctive agents, usually with levodopa.

Mechanism of Action

Dopaminergic drugs increase the amount of dopamine in the brain by various mechanisms (Fig. 12-1). Amantadine increases dopamine release and decreases dopamine reuptake by presynaptic nerve fibers. Bromocriptine, pergolide, pramipexole, and ropinirole are dopamine agonists that directly stimulate postsynaptic dopamine receptors. Levodopa is a precursor substance that is converted to dopamine. Selegiline blocks one of the enzymes (MAO-B) that normally inactivates dopamine. Entacapone and tolcapone block another enzyme (COMT) that normally inactivates dopamine and levodopa.

Indications for Use

Entacapone, levodopa, pergolide, pramipexole, ropinirole, selegiline, and tolcapone are indicated for the treatment of idiopathic or acquired parkinsonism. Carbidopa is used only to decrease peripheral breakdown of levodopa and allow more to reach the brain. Some of the other drugs have additional uses. Amantadine is also used to prevent and treat influenza A viral infections. Bromocriptine is also used in the treatment of amenorrhea and galactorrhea associated with hyperprolactinemia.

Contraindications to Use

Levodopa is contraindicated in clients with narrow-angle glaucoma, hemolytic anemia, angina pectoris, transient ischemic attacks, or a history of melanoma or undiagnosed skin disorders, and in clients taking MAO inhibitor drugs (eg, phenelzine). In addition, levodopa must be used with caution in clients with severe cardiovascular, pulmonary, renal, hepatic, or endocrine disorders. Bromocriptine and pergolide are ergot derivatives and therefore are contraindicated in people who are hypersensitive to ergot alkaloids or who have uncontrolled hypertension. Selegiline, entacapone, and tolcapone are contraindicated in people with hypersensitivity reactions to the drugs. Tolcapone is contraindicated in people with impaired liver function.

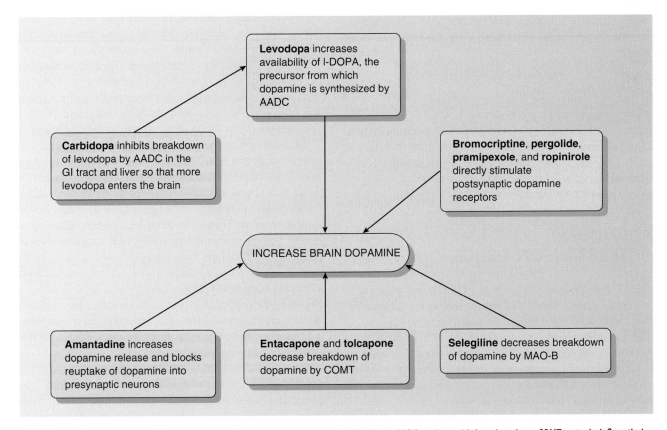

FIGURE 12-1 Mechanisms by which dopaminergic drugs increase dopamine in the brain. AADC, amino acid decarboxylase; COMT, catechol-*O*-methyltransferase; MAO-B, monoamine oxidase B.

Anticholinergic Drugs

Anticholinergic drugs are discussed in Chapter 20 and are described here only in relation to their use in the treatment of Parkinson's disease. Only anticholinergic drugs that are centrally active (ie, those that penetrate the blood–brain barrier) are useful in treating parkinsonism. Atropine and scopolamine are centrally active but are not used because of a high incidence of adverse reactions. In addition to the primary anticholinergic drugs, an antihistamine (diphenhydramine) is used for parkinsonism because of its strong anticholinergic effects.

Mechanism of Action

Anticholinergic drugs decrease the effects of acetylcholine. This decreases the apparent excess of acetylcholine in relation to the amount of dopamine.

Indications for Use

Anticholinergic drugs are used in idiopathic parkinsonism to decrease salivation, spasticity, and tremors. They are used primarily in people who have minimal symptoms or who cannot tolerate levodopa, or in combination with other antiparkinson drugs. Anticholinergic agents also are used to relieve symptoms of parkinsonism that can occur with the use of antipsychotic drugs. If used for this purpose, a course of therapy of approximately 3 months is recommended because symptoms usually subside by then, even if the antipsychotic drug is continued.

Contraindications to Use

Anticholinergic drugs are contraindicated in clients with glaucoma, gastrointestinal (GI) obstruction, prostatic hypertrophy, urinary bladder-neck obstruction, and myasthenia gravis. The drugs must be used cautiously in clients with cardiovascular disorders (eg, tachycardia, dysrhythmias, hypertension) and liver or kidney disease.

INDIVIDUAL ANTIPARKINSON DRUGS

Dopaminergic antiparkinson drugs are described in this section. Trade names, routes, and dosage ranges for dopaminergic and anticholinergic agents are listed in Table 12-1.

P **Levodopa** (Larodopa, Dopar) is the most effective drug available for the treatment of Parkinson's disease. It relieves all major symptoms, especially bradykinesia and rigidity. Levodopa does not alter the underlying disease process, but it may improve a client's quality of life.

Levodopa acts to replace dopamine in the basal ganglia of the brain. Dopamine cannot be used for replacement therapy because it does not penetrate the blood–brain barrier. Levo-

dopa readily penetrates the CNS and is converted to dopamine by the enzyme amino acid decarboxylase (AADC). The dopamine is stored in presynaptic dopaminergic neurons and functions like endogenous dopamine. In advanced stages of Parkinson's disease, there are fewer dopaminergic neurons and thus less storage capacity for dopamine derived from levodopa. As a result, levodopa has a shorter duration of action and drug effects "wear off" between doses.

In peripheral tissues (eg, GI tract, liver), levodopa is metabolized extensively by AADC and to a lesser extent by COMT. Because most levodopa is metabolized in peripheral tissues, large doses are required to obtain therapeutic levels of dopamine in the brain. These large amounts increase adverse drug effects. To reduce levodopa dosage and decrease adverse effects, carbidopa, an AADC inhibitor, is given to decrease the peripheral metabolism of levodopa. The combination of levodopa and carbidopa greatly increases the amount of available levodopa, so that levodopa dosage can be reduced by approximately 70%. The two drugs are usually given together in a fixed-dose formulation called *Sinemet*. When carbidopa inhibits the decarboxylase pathway of levodopa metabolism, the COMT pathway becomes more important (see entacapone and tolcapone, COMT inhibitors, below). A newer product, Stalevo, combines levodopa, carbidopa, and entacapone to further decrease metabolism of levodopa.

Levodopa is well absorbed from the small intestine after oral administration, reaches peak serum levels within 30 to 90 minutes, and has a short serum half-life (1–3 hours). Absorption is decreased by delayed gastric emptying, hyperacidity of gastric secretions, and competition with amino acids (from digestion of protein foods) for sites of absorption in the small intestine. Levodopa is metabolized to 30 or more metabolites, some of which are pharmacologically active and probably contribute to drug toxicity; the metabolites are excreted primarily in the urine, usually within 24 hours.

Because of adverse effects and recurrence of parkinsonian symptoms after a few years of levodopa therapy, levodopa is usually reserved for clients with significant symptoms and functional disabilities. In addition to treating Parkinson's disease, levodopa also may be useful in other CNS disorders in which symptoms of parkinsonism occur (eg, juvenile Huntington's chorea, chronic manganese poisoning). Levodopa relieves only parkinsonian symptoms in these conditions.

APPLYING YOUR KNOWLEDGE 12-1

Mrs. Holt tells you that she has a friend who takes her medication for Parkinson's disease once a day, and questions you why she must take her medication more than once a day. What is the most appropriate response?

Carbidopa (Lodosyn) inhibits the enzyme AADC. As a result, less levodopa is decarboxylated in peripheral tissues; more levodopa reaches the brain, where it is decarboxylated to dopamine; and much smaller doses of levodopa can be given. Carbidopa does not penetrate the blood–brain barrier.

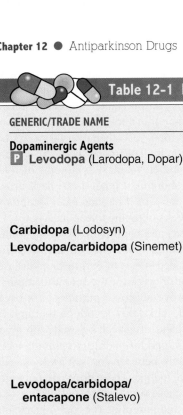

Table 12-1 Drugs at a Glance: Antiparkinson Drugs

GENERIC/TRADE NAME	ROUTES AND DOSAGE RANGES
Dopaminergic Agents	
P Levodopa (Larodopa, Dopar)	PO 0.5–1 g/d initially in 3 or 4 divided doses, increase gradually by no more than 0.75 g/d, every 3–7 d. The rate of dosage increase depends mainly on the client's tolerance of adverse effects, especially nausea and vomiting. Average maintenance dose, 3–6 g/d; maximum dose, 8 g/d. Dosage must be reduced when carbidopa is also given (see carbidopa, below).
Carbidopa (Lodosyn)	PO 70–100 mg/d, depending on dosage of levodopa; maximum dose, 200 mg/d
Levodopa/carbidopa (Sinemet)	*Clients not receiving levodopa:* PO 1 tablet of 25 mg carbidopa/100 mg levodopa 3 times daily or 1 tablet of 10 mg carbidopa/100 mg levodopa 3 or 4 times daily, increased by 1 tablet every day or every other day until a dosage of 8 tablets daily is reached Sinemet CR PO 1 tablet twice daily at least 6 h apart initially, increased up to 8 tablets daily and q4h intervals if necessary *Clients receiving levodopa:* Discontinue levodopa at least 8 h before starting Sinemet. PO 1 tablet of 25 mg carbidopa/250 mg levodopa 3 or 4 times daily for clients taking >1500 mg levodopa or 1 tablet of 25 mg carbidopa/100 mg levodopa for clients taking <1500 mg levodopa
Levodopa/carbidopa/ entacapone (Stalevo)	Patients already taking the drugs separately can be switched to the combination tablet containing an equivalent amount of each drug. For patients taking >600 mg levodopa daily when starting entacapone, dosage should be titrated and stabilized with the individual drugs before using the combination product. Patients taking <600 mg levodopa daily may be started directly on the corresponding dosage of Stalevo, but levodopa dosage may need to be reduced.
Amantadine (Symmetrel)	PO 100 mg twice a day
Bromocriptine (Parlodel)	PO 1.25 mg twice a day with meals, increased by 2.5 mg/d every 2–4 wk if necessary for therapeutic benefit. Reduce dose gradually if severe adverse effects occur.
Entacapone (Comtan)	PO 200 mg with each dose of levodopa/carbidopa, up to 8 times (1600 mg) daily
Pergolide (Permax)	PO 0.05–0.1 mg/d at bedtime, increased by 0.05–0.15 mg every 3 d to a maximum dose of 6 mg/d if necessary
Pramipexole (Mirapex)	PO wk 1, 0.125 mg 3 times daily; wk 2, 0.25 mg 3 times daily; wk 3, 0.5 mg 3 times daily; wk 4, 0.75 mg 3 times daily; wk 5, 1 mg 3 times daily; wk 6, 1.25 mg 3 times daily; wk 7, 1.5 mg 3 times daily Renal impairment: Creatinine clearance (Crcl) > 60 mL/min, 0.125 mg 3 times daily initially, up to a maximum of 1.5 mg 3 times daily; Crcl 35–59 mL/min, 0.125 mg 2 times daily initially, up to a maximum of 1.5 mg 2 times daily; Crcl 15–34 mL/min, 0.125 mg once daily, up to a maximum of 1.5 mg once daily
Ropinirole (Requip)	PO wk 1, 0.25 mg 3 times daily; wk 2, 0.5 mg 3 times daily; wk 3, 0.75 mg 3 times daily; wk 4, 1 mg 3 times daily
Selegiline (Eldepryl)	PO 5 mg twice daily, morning and noon
Tolcapone (Tasmar)	PO 100–200 mg 3 times daily; maximum dose, 600 mg daily
Anticholinergic Agents **Benztropine** (Cogentin)	PO 0.5–1 mg at bedtime initially, gradually increased to 4–6 mg daily if necessary
Diphenhydramine (Benadryl)	PO 25 mg 3 times daily, gradually increased to 50 mg 4 times daily if necessary Adults: Drug-induced extrapyramidal reactions, IM, IV 10–50 mg; maximal single dose, 100 mg; maximal daily dose, 400 mg Children: Drug-induced extrapyramidal reactions, IM 5 mg/kg per day; maximal daily dose, 300 mg
Trihexyphenidyl (Trihexy)	PO 1–2 mg daily initially, gradually increased to 12–15 mg daily, until therapeutic or adverse effects occur Adults: Drug-induced extrapyramidal reactions, PO 1 mg initially, gradually increased to 5–15 mg daily if necessary

IM, intramuscular; IV, intravenous; PO, oral.

Although carbidopa is available alone, it is most often given in the levodopa/carbidopa fixed-dose combination product, Sinemet.

Amantadine (Symmetrel) is a synthetic antiviral agent initially used to prevent infection from influenza A virus. Amantadine increases the release and inhibits the reuptake of dopamine in the brain, thereby increasing dopamine levels. The drug relieves symptoms rapidly, within 1 to 5 days, but it loses efficacy with 6 to 8 weeks of continuous administration. Consequently, it is usually given for 2- to 3-week periods during initiation of drug therapy with longer-acting agents (eg, levodopa), or when symptoms worsen. Amantadine is often given with levodopa. Compared with other antiparkinson drugs, amantadine is considered less effective than levodopa but more effective than anticholinergic agents.

Amantadine is well absorbed from the GI tract and has a relatively long duration of action. It is excreted unchanged in the urine. Dosage must be reduced with impaired renal function to avoid drug accumulation.

Bromocriptine (Parlodel) and **pergolide** (Permax) are ergot derivatives that directly stimulate dopamine receptors in the brain. They are used in the treatment of idiopathic Parkinson's disease, with levodopa/carbidopa, to prolong effectiveness and allow reduced dosage of levodopa. Pergolide has a longer duration of action than bromocriptine and may be effective in some clients unresponsive to bromocriptine. Adverse effects are similar for the two drugs.

Entacapone (Comtan) and **tolcapone** (Tasmar) are COMT inhibitors. COMT plays a role in brain metabolism of dopamine and metabolizes approximately 10% of peripheral levodopa. By inhibiting COMT, entacapone and tolcapone increase levels of dopamine in the brain and relieve symptoms more effectively and consistently. Although the main mechanism of action seems to be inhibiting the metabolism of levodopa in the bloodstream, the drugs may also inhibit COMT in the brain and prolong the activity of dopamine at the synapse. These drugs are used only in conjunction with levodopa/carbidopa, and dosage of levodopa must be reduced.

Entacapone is well absorbed with oral administration and reaches a peak plasma level in 1 hour. It is highly protein bound (98%), has a half-life of about 2.5 hours, and is metabolized in the liver to an inactive metabolite. Dosage must be reduced by 50% in the presence of impaired liver function. The parent drug and the metabolite are 90% excreted through the biliary tract and feces; 10% is excreted in the urine. Adverse effects include confusion, dizziness, drowsiness, hallucinations, nausea, and vomiting. These can be reduced by lowering the dose of either levodopa or entacapone. Although there were few instances of liver enzyme elevation or hemoglobin decreases during clinical trials, it is recommended that liver enzymes and red blood cell counts be done periodically.

Tolcapone is also well absorbed with oral administration. Its elimination half-life is 2 to 3 hours and it is metabolized in the liver. During clinical trials, diarrhea was a common adverse effect. Because of several reports of liver damage and deaths from liver failure, tolcapone should be used only in clients who do not respond to other drugs. When used, liver aminotransferase enzymes (serum alanine aminotransferase [ALT] and aspartate aminotransferase [AST]) should be monitored every 2 weeks for 1 year, then every 4 weeks for 6 months, then every 2 months. Tolcapone should be discontinued if ALT and AST are elevated, if symptoms of liver failure occur (anorexia, abdominal tenderness, dark urine, jaundice, clay-colored stools), or if parkinsonian symptoms do not improve after 3 weeks of taking tolcapone.

Pramipexole (Mirapex) and **ropinirole** (Requip) stimulate dopamine receptors in the brain. They are approved for both beginning and advanced stages of Parkinson's disease. In early stages, one of these drugs can be used alone to improve motor performance, improve ability to participate in usual activities of daily living, and delay levodopa therapy. In advanced stages, one of these drugs can be used with levodopa and perhaps other antiparkinson drugs to provide more consistent relief of symptoms between doses of levodopa and allow reduced dosage of levodopa. These drugs are not ergot derivatives and may not cause some adverse effects associated with bromocriptine and pergolide (eg, pulmonary and peritoneal fibrosis, constriction of coronary arteries).

Pramipexole is rapidly absorbed with oral administration. Peak serum levels are reached in 1 to 3 hours after a dose and steady-state concentrations in about 2 days. It is less than 20% bound to plasma proteins and has an elimination half-life of 8 to 12 hours. Most of the drug is excreted unchanged in the urine; only 10% of the drug is metabolized. As a result, renal failure may cause higher-than-usual plasma levels and possible toxicity, but hepatic disease is unlikely to alter drug effects.

Ropinirole is also well absorbed with oral administration. It reaches peak serum levels in 1 to 2 hours and steady-state concentrations within 2 days. It is 40% bound to plasma proteins and has an elimination half-life of 6 hours. It is metabolized by the cytochrome P450 enzymes in the liver to inactive metabolites, which are excreted through the kidneys. Less than 10% of ropinirole is excreted unchanged in the urine. Thus, liver failure may decrease metabolism, allow drug accumulation, and increase adverse effects. Renal failure does not appear to alter drug effects.

Selegiline (Eldepryl) inhibits metabolism of dopamine by MAO, which exists in two types, MAO-A and MAO-B, both of which are found in the CNS and peripheral tissues. They are differentiated by their relative specificities for individual catecholamines. MAO-A acts more specifically on tyramine, norepinephrine, epinephrine, and serotonin. This enzyme is the main subtype in GI mucosa and in the liver and is responsible for metabolizing dietary tyramine. If MAO-A is inhibited in the intestine, tyramine in various foods is absorbed systemically rather than deactivated. As a result, there is excessive stimulation of the sympathetic nervous system and severe hypertension and stroke can occur. This life-threatening reaction can also occur with medications that are normally metabolized by MAO.

MAO-B metabolizes dopamine; in the brain, most MAO activity is due to type B. At oral dosages of 10 milligrams per day or less, selegiline inhibits MAO-B selectively and is unlikely to cause severe hypertension and stroke. However, at dosages greater than 10 milligrams per day, selectivity is lost and metabolism of both MAO-A and MAO-B is inhibited. Dosages greater than 10 milligrams per day should be avoided in clients with Parkinson's disease. Selegiline inhibition of MAO-B is irreversible, and drug effects persist until more MAO is synthesized in the brain, which may take several months.

In early Parkinson's disease, selegiline may be effective as monotherapy. In advanced disease, it is given to enhance the effects of levodopa. Its addition aids symptom control and allows the dosage of levodopa/carbidopa to be reduced.

NURSING PROCESS

Assessment

Assess for signs and symptoms of Parkinson's disease and drug-induced extrapyramidal reactions. These may include the following, depending on the severity and stage of progression.

- Slow movements (bradykinesia) and difficulty in changing positions, assuming an upright position, eating, dressing, and other self-care activities
- Stooped posture
- Accelerating gait with short steps
- Tremor at rest (eg, "pill rolling" movements of fingers)
- Rigidity of arms, legs, and neck
- Mask-like, immobile facial expression
- Speech problems (eg, low volume, monotonous tone, rapid, difficult to understand)
- Excessive salivation and drooling
- Dysphagia
- Excessive sweating
- Constipation from decreased intestinal motility
- Mental depression from self-consciousness and embarrassment over physical appearance and activity limitations. The intellect is usually intact until the late stages of the disease process.

Nursing Diagnoses

- Bathing/Grooming Self-Care Deficit related to tremors and impaired motor function
- Impaired Physical Mobility related to alterations in balance and coordination
- Deficient Knowledge: Safe usage and effects of antiparkinson drugs
- Imbalanced Nutrition: Less Than Body Requirements related to difficulty in chewing and swallowing food

Planning/Goals

The client will
- Experience relief of excessive salivation, muscle rigidity, spasticity, and tremors
- Experience improved motor function, mobility, and self-care abilities
- Increase knowledge of the disease process and drug therapy
- Take medications as instructed
- Avoid falls and other injuries from the disease process or drug therapy.

Interventions

Use measures to assist the client and family in coping with symptoms and maintaining function. These include the following:
- Provide physical therapy for heel-to-toe gait training; widening stance to increase balance and base of support; other exercises.
- Encourage ambulation and frequent changes of position, assisted if necessary.
- Help with active and passive range-of-motion exercises.
- Encourage self-care as much as possible. Cutting meat; opening cartons; giving frequent, small meals; and allowing privacy during mealtime may be helpful. If the client has difficulty chewing or swallowing, chopped or soft foods may be necessary. Hook-and-loop-type fasteners or zippers are easier to handle than buttons. Slip-on shoes are easier to manage than laced ones.
- Spend time with the client and encourage socialization with other people. Victims of Parkinson's disease tend to become withdrawn, isolated, and depressed.
- Schedule rest periods. Tremor and rigidity are aggravated by fatigue and emotional stress.
- Provide facial tissues if drooling is a problem.
- Provide appropriate client teaching related to drug therapy (see accompanying display).

Evaluation

- Interview and observe for relief of symptoms.
- Interview and observe for increased mobility and participation in activities of daily living.
- Interview and observe regarding correct usage of medications.

APPLYING YOUR KNOWLEDGE 12-2

Because Mrs. Holt was admitted following a fall and is experiencing many of the typical symptoms of a person with Parkinson's disease, she may have difficulty with ambulation. What referral should you initiate to improve her safety?

CLIENT TEACHING GUIDELINES

Antiparkinson Drugs

General Considerations

✔ Beneficial effects of antiparkinson drugs may not occur for a few weeks; do not stop taking the drugs before they have had a chance to work.

✔ Do not take other drugs without the physician's knowledge and consent. This is necessary to avoid adverse drug interactions. Prescription and nonprescription drugs may interact with antiparkinson drugs to increase or decrease effects.

✔ Avoid driving an automobile or operating other potentially hazardous machinery if vision is blurred or drowsiness occurs with levodopa.

✔ Change positions slowly, especially when assuming an upright position, and wear elastic stockings, if needed, to prevent dizziness from a drop in blood pressure.

Self- or Caregiver Administration

✔ Take antiparkinson drugs with or just after food to prevent or reduce anorexia, nausea, and vomiting.

✔ Do not crush or chew Sinemet CR. It is formulated to be released slowly; crushing or chewing destroys this feature.

✔ Take or give selegiline in the morning and at noon. This schedule decreases stimulating effects that may interfere with sleep if the drug is taken in the evening.

✔ Take or give entacapone with each dose of levodopa/carbidopa, up to 8 times daily.

✔ Decrease excessive mouth dryness by maintaining an adequate fluid intake (2000–3000 mL daily if not contraindicated) and using sugarless chewing gum and hard candies. Both anticholinergics and levodopa may cause mouth dryness. This is usually a therapeutic effect in Parkinson's disease. However, excessive mouth dryness causes discomfort and dental caries.

✔ Report adverse effects. Adverse effects can often be reduced by changing drugs or dosages. However, some adverse effects usually must be tolerated for control of disease symptoms.

PRINCIPLES OF THERAPY

Goals of Therapy

Antiparkinson drugs aim to control symptoms, maintain functional ability in activities of daily living, minimize adverse drug effects, and slow disease progression.

Drug Selection

Choices of antiparkinson drugs depend largely on the type of parkinsonism (eg, idiopathic or drug induced) and the severity of symptoms. In addition, because of difficulties with levodopa therapy (eg, adverse effects, loss of effectiveness in a few years, possible acceleration of the loss of dopaminergic neurons in the brain), several drug therapy strategies and combinations are used to delay the start of levodopa therapy and, after it is started, to reduce levodopa dosage.

- For drug-induced parkinsonism or extrapyramidal symptoms, an anticholinergic agent is the drug of choice.
- For early idiopathic parkinsonism, when symptoms and functional disability are relatively mild, several drugs may be used in monotherapy.
  - An anticholinergic agent may be the initial drug of choice in clients younger than 60 years of age, especially when tremor is the major symptom. An anticholinergic drug relieves tremor in approximately 50% of clients.
  - Amantadine may be useful in relieving bradykinesia or tremor.
  - A dopamine agonist may improve functional disability related to bradykinesia, rigidity, impaired physical dexterity, impaired speech, shuffling gait, and tremor.

- For advanced idiopathic parkinsonism, a combination of medications is used. Two advantages of combination therapy are better control of symptoms and reduced dosage of individual drugs.
  - An anticholinergic agent may be given with levodopa alone or with a levodopa/carbidopa combination.
  - Amantadine may be given in combination with levodopa or other antiparkinson agents.
  - A dopamine agonist is usually given with levodopa/carbidopa. The combination provides more effective relief of symptoms and allows lower dosage of levodopa. Although available dopamine agonists are similarly effective, pramipexole and ropinirole cause less severe adverse effects than bromocriptine and pergolide.
  - The levodopa/carbidopa combination is probably the most effective drug when bradykinesia and rigidity become prominent. However, because levodopa becomes less effective after approximately 5 to 7 years, many clinicians use other drugs first and reserve levodopa for use when symptoms become more severe.
  - Selegiline may be given with levodopa/carbidopa and with entacapone, because selegiline acts in the brain and entacapone acts peripherally.
  - Entacapone is used only with levodopa/carbidopa; simultaneous administration of carbidopa and entacapone significantly increases the plasma half-life of levodopa. (Stalevo is a newer product that combines levodopa, carbidopa, and entacapone.) Tolcapone should be used only when other drugs are ineffective, because of its association with liver failure.

- When changes are made in a drug therapy regimen, one change at a time is recommended so that effects of the change are clear.
- A recent study shows that rasagiline may improve movement in clients with Parkinson's disease (see Research Brief).

Drug Dosage

The dosage of antiparkinson drugs is highly individualized. The general rule is to start with low initial dosage and gradually increase it until therapeutic effects, adverse effects, or maximum drug dosage is achieved. Additional guidelines include the following:

- The optimal dose is the lowest one that allows the client to function adequately. Optimal dosage may not be established for 6 to 8 weeks with levodopa.

RESEARCH BRIEF

Rasagiline (Agilect), A New Antiparkinson Drug

SOURCE:

Schwid, S. R. (2005). Rasagiline improves movement in Parkinson's. *Archives of Neurology, 62,* 241–248.

SUMMARY:

This study involved 472 people with Parkinson's disease who were taking levodopa. Participants were experiencing at least 2 ½ hours daily of "off time," when their movements were poorly controlled. Researchers compared the effects of adding rasagiline to the effects of adding a placebo to the levodopa regimen. During 26 weeks of treatment, clients who received rasagiline had a decrease in daily "off time" of almost 2 hours while those who received placebo had a less than 1 hour decrease in "off time." The researchers concluded that rasagiline reduced fluctuations in movement control in levodopa-treated clients, improved ability to perform activities of daily living, and caused minimal adverse effects. In addition, the drug was considered safe and effective alone in treating clients with early disease (indicated by previous studies) and in combination with other anti-Parkinson drugs in treating clients with more advanced disease.

NURSING IMPLICATIONS:

Rasagiline seems to be a promising addition to drug therapy for Parkinson's disease. Increasing functional ability with minimal adverse drug effects would be a significant development for clients and helpful to health care providers and caregivers as well.

- Dosages need to be adjusted as parkinsonism progresses.
- Dosage must be individualized for levodopa and carbidopa. Only 5% to 10% of a dose of levodopa reaches the CNS, even with the addition of carbidopa. When carbidopa is given with levodopa, the dosage of levodopa must be reduced by approximately 75%. A daily dose of approximately 70 to 100 mg of carbidopa is required to saturate peripheral AADC.
- A levodopa/carbidopa combination is available in three dosage formulations (10 mg carbidopa/100 mg levodopa, 25 mg carbidopa/100 mg levodopa, and 25 mg carbidopa/250 mg levodopa) of immediate-release tablets (Sinemet) and two dosage formulations (25 mg carbidopa/100 mg levodopa, 50 mg carbidopa/200 mg levodopa) of sustained-release tablets (Sinemet CR). Various preparations can be mixed to administer optimal amounts of each ingredient. Sinemet CR is not as well absorbed as the short-acting form, and a client being transferred to Sinemet CR needs a dosage increase of approximately one third.
- With levodopa, dosage should be gradually increased to the desired therapeutic level. In addition, therapeutic effects may be increased and adverse effects decreased by frequent administration of small doses.
- With pramipexole and ropinirole, dosage is started at low levels and gradually increased over several weeks. When the drugs are discontinued, they should be tapered in dosage over 1 week. With pramipexole, lower doses are indicated in older adults and those with renal impairment; with ropinirole, lower doses may be needed with hepatic impairment.
- Entacapone (200 mg) should be taken with each dose of levodopa (up to 8 times per day). Each tablet of Stalevo contains 200 mg of entacapone along with various amounts of levodopa and carbidopa.
- When combinations of drugs are used, dosage adjustments of individual components are often necessary. When levodopa is added to a regimen of anticholinergic drug therapy, for example, the anticholinergic drug need not be discontinued or reduced in dosage. However, when a dopaminergic drug is added to a regimen containing levodopa/carbidopa, dosage of levodopa/carbidopa must be reduced.

 APPLYING YOUR KNOWLEDGE 12-3:
HOW CAN YOU AVOID THIS MEDICATION ERROR?
The physician writes a drug order for levodopa/carbidopa 25/100. The pharmacy supplies Sinemet CR 25/100 and you administer the medication.

Use in Special Populations

Use in Children

Safety and effectiveness for use in children have not been established for most antiparkinson drugs, including the centrally acting anticholinergics (all ages), levodopa (<12 years), and bromocriptine (<15 years). However, anticholinergics are sometimes given to children who have drug-induced extrapyramidal reactions.

Because parkinsonism is a degenerative disorder of adults, antiparkinson drugs are most likely to be used in children for other purposes. Amantadine for influenza A prevention or treatment is not recommended for neonates or infants younger than 1 year of age, but may be given to children 9 to 12 years of age.

Use in Older Adults

Dosage of amantadine may need to be reduced because the drug is excreted mainly through the kidneys, and renal function is usually decreased in older adults. Dosage of levodopa/carbidopa may need to be reduced because of an age-related decrease in peripheral AADC, the enzyme that carbidopa inhibits.

Anticholinergic drugs may cause blurred vision, dry mouth, tachycardia, and urinary retention. They also decrease sweating and may cause fever or heatstroke. Fever may occur in any age group, but heatstroke is more likely to occur in older adults, especially with cardiovascular disease, strenuous activity, and high environmental temperatures. When centrally active anticholinergics are given for Parkinson's disease, agitation, mental confusion, hallucinations, and psychosis may occur. Many other drugs in addition to the primary anticholinergics have significant anticholinergic activity, such as some antihistamines in over-the-counter cold remedies and sleep aids; tricyclic antidepressants; and phenothiazine antipsychotic drugs. When anticholinergic drugs are needed in older adults, dosage should be minimized, combinations of drugs with anticholinergic effects should be avoided, and clients should be closely monitored for adverse drug effects.

Older clients are at increased risk of having hallucinations with dopamine agonist drugs. In addition, pramipexole dosage may need to be reduced in older adults with impaired renal function.

Use in Clients With Renal Impairment

With amantadine, excretion is primarily via the kidneys, and the drug should be used with caution in clients with renal failure. With pramipexole, clearance is reduced in clients with moderate or severe renal impairment, and lower initial and maintenance doses are recommended. With ropinirole and entacapone, no dosage adjustments are needed for renal impairment.

Use in Clients With Hepatic Impairment

With ropinirole, cautious use in clients with hepatic impairment is warranted, and dosage may need to be reduced. With tolcapone, elevated liver enzymes and a few deaths from liver failure have been reported. In clients with noncirrhotic liver disease, dosage reductions are not needed. However, tolcapone metabolism is impaired in clients with hepatic cirrhosis, and plasma drug levels are high. Dosage should be reduced, and maintenance dosage should be less than the daily 600 milligrams recommended for clients with noncirrhotic liver disease. In addition, liver transaminase enzymes should be monitored frequently. With entacapone, periodic measurements of liver transaminase enzymes are recommended, although liver failure has not been associated with this drug.

Use in Home Care

The home care nurse can help clients and caregivers understand that the purpose of drug therapy is to control symptoms and that noticeable improvement may not occur for several weeks. Also, the nurse can encourage clients to consult physical therapists, speech therapists, and dietitians to help maintain their ability to perform activities of daily living. In addition, teaching about preventing or managing adverse drug effects may be necessary. Caregivers may need to be informed that most activities (eg, eating, dressing) take longer and require considerable effort by clients with parkinsonism.

NURSING ACTIONS

Antiparkinson Drugs

NURSING ACTIONS	RATIONALE/EXPLANATION
1. Administer accurately	
a. Give most antiparkinson drugs with or just after food; entacapone can be given without regard to meals.	To prevent or reduce nausea and vomiting
b. Do not crush Sinemet CR and instruct clients not to chew the tablet.	Crushing and chewing destroys the controlled-release feature of the formulation.
c. Do not give levodopa with iron preparations or multivitamin–mineral preparations containing iron.	Iron decreases absorption of levodopa.

NURSING ACTIONS	RATIONALE/EXPLANATION
d. Give selegiline in the morning and at noon.	To decrease central nervous system (CNS) stimulating effects that may interfere with sleep if the drug is taken in the evening
e. Give entacapone with each dose of levodopa/carbidopa, up to 8 times daily.	
2. Observe for therapeutic effects	
a. With anticholinergic agents, observe for decreased tremor, salivation, drooling, and sweating.	Decreased salivation and sweating are therapeutic effects when these drugs are used in Parkinson's disease, but they are adverse effects when the drugs are used in other disorders.
b. With levodopa and dopaminergic agents, observe for improvement in mobility, balance, posture, gait, speech, handwriting, and self-care ability. Drooling and seborrhea may be abolished, and mood may be elevated.	Therapeutic effects are usually evident within 2–3 weeks, as levodopa dosage approaches 2–3 g/d, but may not reach optimum levels for 6 months.
3. Observe for adverse effects	
a. With anticholinergic drugs, observe for atropine-like effects, such as:	
(1) Tachycardia and palpitations	These effects may occur with usual therapeutic doses but are not likely to be serious except in people with underlying heart disease.
(2) Excessive CNS stimulation (tremor, restlessness, confusion, hallucinations, delirium)	This effect is most likely to occur with large doses of trihexyphenidyl (Trihexy) or benztropine (Cogentin). It may occur with levodopa.
(3) Sedation and drowsiness	These are most likely to occur with benztropine. The drug has antihistaminic and anticholinergic properties, and sedation is attributed to the antihistamine effect.
(4) Constipation, impaction, paralytic ileus	These effects result from decreased gastrointestinal motility and muscle tone. They may be severe because decreased intestinal motility and constipation also are characteristics of Parkinson's disease; thus, additive effects may occur.
(5) Urinary retention	This reaction is caused by loss of muscle tone in the bladder and is most likely to occur in elderly men who have enlarged prostate glands.
(6) Dilated pupils (mydriasis), blurred vision, photophobia	Ocular effects are due to paralysis of accommodation and relaxation of the ciliary muscle and the sphincter muscle of the iris.
b. With levodopa, observe for:	
(1) Anorexia, nausea, and vomiting	These symptoms usually disappear after a few months of drug therapy. They may be minimized by giving levodopa with food, gradually increasing dosage, administering smaller doses more frequently or adding carbidopa so that dosage of levodopa can be reduced.
(2) Orthostatic hypotension—check blood pressure in both sitting and standing positions q4h while the client is awake.	This effect is common during the first few weeks but usually subsides eventually. It can be minimized by arising slowly from supine or sitting positions and by wearing elastic stockings.
(3) Cardiac dysrhythmias (tachycardia, premature ventricular contractions) and increased myocardial contractility	Levodopa and its metabolites stimulate beta-adrenergic receptors in the heart. People with pre-existing coronary artery disease may need a beta-adrenergic blocking agent (eg, propranolol) to counteract these effects.
(4) Dyskinesia—involuntary movements that may involve only the tongue, mouth, and face or the whole body	Dyskinesia eventually develops in most people who take levodopa. It is related to duration of levodopa therapy rather than dosage. Carbidopa may heighten this adverse effect, and there is no way to prevent it except by decreasing levodopa dosage. Many people prefer dyskinesia to lowering drug dosage and subsequent return of the parkinsonism symptoms.

(continued)

NURSING ACTIONS	RATIONALE/EXPLANATION
(5) CNS stimulation—restlessness, agitation, confusion, delirium	This is more likely to occur with levodopa/carbidopa combination drug therapy.
(6) Abrupt swings in motor function (on–off phenomenon)	This fluctuation may indicate progression of the disease process. It often occurs after long-term levodopa use.
c. With amantadine, observe for:	
(1) CNS stimulation—insomnia, hyperexcitability, ataxia, dizziness, slurred speech, mental confusion, hallucinations	Compared with other antiparkinson drugs, amantadine produces few adverse effects. The ones that occur are mild, transient, and reversible. However, adverse effects increase if daily dosage exceeds 200 mg.
(2) Livedo reticularis—patchy, bluish discoloration of skin on the legs	This is a benign but cosmetically unappealing condition. It usually occurs with long-term use of amantadine and disappears when the drug is discontinued.
d. With bromocriptine and pergolide, observe for:	
(1) Nausea	These symptoms are usually mild and can be minimized by starting with low doses and increasing the dose gradually until the desired effect is achieved. If adverse effects do occur, they usually disappear with a decrease in dosage.
(2) Confusion and hallucinations	
(3) Hypotension	
e. With pramipexole and ropinirole, observe for:	These effects occurred more commonly than others during clinical trials.
(1) Nausea	
(2) Confusion, hallucinations	
(3) Dizziness, drowsiness	
(4) Dyskinesias	
(5) Orthostatic hypotension	
f. With selegiline, observe for:	
(1) CNS effects—agitation, ataxia, bradykinesia, confusion, dizziness, dyskinesias, hallucinations, insomnia	
(2) Nausea, abdominal pain	
g. With entacapone and tolcapone, observe for:	These effects occurred more commonly than others during clinical trials.
(1) Anorexia, nausea, vomiting, diarrhea, constipation	
(2) Dizziness, drowsiness	
(3) Dyskinesias and dystonias	
(4) Hallucinations	
(5) Orthostatic hypotension	
4. **Observe for drug interactions**	
a. Drugs that *increase* effects of anticholinergic drugs:	
(1) Antihistamines, disopyramide (Norpace), thiothixene (Navane), phenothiazines, and tricyclic antidepressants	These drugs have anticholinergic properties and produce additive anticholinergic effects.
b. Drugs that *decrease* effects of anticholinergic drugs:	
(1) Cholinergic agents	These drugs counteract the inhibition of gastrointestinal motility and tone, which is a side effect of anticholinergic drug therapy.
c. Drugs that *increase* effects of levodopa:	
(1) Amantadine, anticholinergic agents, bromocriptine, carbidopa, entacapone, pergolide, pramipexole, ropinirole, selegiline, tolcapone	These drugs are often used in combination for treatment of Parkinson's disease.

NURSING ACTIONS	RATIONALE/EXPLANATION
(2) Tricyclic antidepressants	These drugs potentiate levodopa effects and increase the risk of cardiac arrhythmias in people with heart disease.
(3) Monoamine oxidase type A (MAO-A) inhibitors, including isocarboxazid (Marplan), phenelzine (Nardil), and tranyl-cypromine (Parnate)	The combination of a catecholamine precursor (levodopa) and MAO-A inhibitors that decrease metabolism of catecholamines can result in excessive amounts of dopamine, epinephrine, and norepinephrine. Heart palpitations, headache, hypertensive crisis, and stroke may occur. Levodopa and MAO-A inhibitors should not be given concurrently. Also, levodopa should not be started within 3 weeks after an MAO-A inhibitor is discontinued. Effects of MAO-A inhibitors persist for 1–3 weeks after their discontinuation.
	These effects are unlikely to occur with selegiline, an MAO-B inhibitor, which more selectively inhibits the metabolism of dopamine. However, selectivity may be lost at doses higher than the recommended 10 mg/d. Selegiline is used with levodopa.
d. Drugs that *decrease* effects of levodopa:	
(1) Anticholinergics	Although anticholinergics are often given with levodopa for increased antiparkinson effects, they also may decrease effects of levodopa by delaying gastric emptying. This causes more levodopa to be metabolized in the stomach and decreases the amount available for absorption from the intestine.
(2) Alcohol; benzodiazepines (eg, diazepam [Valium]); antiemetics; antipsychotics such as phenothiazines, haloperidol (Haldol), and thiothixene (Navane)	The mechanisms by which most of these drugs decrease effects of levodopa are not clear. Phenothiazines block dopamine receptors in the basal ganglia.
(3) Oral iron preparations	Iron binds with levodopa and reduces levodopa absorption, possibly by as much as 50%.
(4) Pyridoxine (vitamin B_6)	Pyridoxine stimulates decarboxylase, the enzyme that converts levodopa to dopamine. As a result, more levodopa is metabolized in peripheral tissues, and less reaches the CNS, where antiparkinson effects occur.
e. Drugs that *decrease* effects of dopaminergic antiparkinson drugs:	
(1) Antipsychotic drugs	These drugs are dopamine antagonists and therefore inhibit the effects of dopamine agonists.
(2) Metoclopramide (Reglan)	

APPLYING YOUR KNOWLEDGE: ANSWERS

12-1 Provide client teaching and inform Mrs. Holt that the drug she is taking acts quickly and must be taken several times a day in order to provide relief of her symptoms. The half-life of levodopa/carbidopa is only 1 to 3 hours.

12-2 A referral for physical therapy is most appropriate. Gait training and a widened stance will provide Mrs. Holt with increased balance and a better base of support.

12-3 The pharmacy provided the correct drug and the correct strength; however, it provided the extended-release form of the drug when the immediate-release form was ordered. In addition to checking the drug name and strength, you must check the dosage form.

Review and Application Exercises

Short Answer Exercises

1. Which neurotransmitter is deficient in idiopathic and drug-induced parkinsonism?

2. How do the antiparkinson drugs act to alter the level of the deficient neurotransmitter?

3. What are the advantages and disadvantages of the various drugs used to treat parkinsonism?

4. Why is it desirable to delay the start of levodopa therapy and, after it is started, to reduce dosage as much as possible?

5. What is the rationale for various combinations of antiparkinson drugs?

6. What are the major adverse effects of antiparkinson drugs, and how can they be minimized?

NCLEX-Style Questions

7. Parkinson's disease is attributed to an imbalance of neurotransmitters in which of the following structures?
a. basal ganglia
b. cerebral cortex
c. limbic system
d. reticular activating system

8. The main pathophysiology of Parkinson's disease is a decrease in the brain content of which of the following substances?
a. acetylcholine
b. serotonin
c. glutamate
d. dopamine

9. Periodic assessment of a client with parkinsonism should include which of the following?
a. blood tests of liver function
b. blood tests of kidney function
c. evaluation of mental status
d. evaluation of responses to drug therapy

10. The main purpose of combination drug therapy for parkinsonism is to
a. stop disease progression
b. relieve adverse effects of other drugs
c. reduce dosage of levodopa
d. delay the need for drug therapy

11. Carbidopa is usually given along with levodopa because it
a. crosses the blood–brain barrier and acts centrally
b. inhibits peripheral breakdown of levodopa
c. directly stimulates dopamine receptors in the brain
d. decreases adverse effects of anticholinergic antiparkinson drugs

Selected References

Drug facts and comparisons. (Updated monthly). St. Louis: Facts and Comparisons.

Jankovic, J. (2004). Parkinsonism. In L. Goldman & D. Ausiello (Eds.), *Cecil textbook of medicine* (22nd ed., pp. 2306–2310). Philadelphia: W. B. Saunders.

Nelson, M. V., Berchou, R. C., & LeWitt, P. A. (2002). Parkinson's disease. In J. T. DiPiro, R. L. Talbert, G. C. Yee, G. R. Matzke, B. G. Wells, & L. M. Posey (Eds.), *Pharmacotherapy: A pathophysiologic approach* (5th ed., pp. 1089–1102). New York: McGraw-Hill.

Porth, C. M., & Curtis, R. L. (2005). Disorders of motor function. In C. M. Porth, *Pathophysiology: Concepts of altered health states* (7th ed., pp. 1193–1226). Philadelphia: Lippincott Williams & Wilkins.

Smeltzer, S. C., & Bare, B. G. (2004). *Brunner & Suddarth's textbook of medical-surgical nursing* (10th ed., pp. 1979–1986). Philadelphia: Lippincott Williams & Wilkins.

Skeletal Muscle Relaxants

OBJECTIVES

After studying this chapter, you will be able to:

1. Discuss common symptoms and disorders for which skeletal muscle relaxants are used.
2. Differentiate uses and effects of selected skeletal muscle relaxants.
3. Describe nonpharmacologic interventions to relieve muscle spasm and spasticity.
4. Apply the nursing process with clients experiencing muscle spasm or spasticity.

APPLYING YOUR KNOWLEDGE

Annette Milewski, age 52, has had multiple sclerosis since she was 33 years of age. She is prescribed baclofen (Lioresal) 15 mg PO, tid to control spasticity. Her family and a home health aide provide the care she requires. You are the home health nurse visiting for her monthly evaluation.

INTRODUCTION

Skeletal muscle relaxants are used to decrease muscle spasm or spasticity that occurs in certain neurologic and musculoskeletal disorders. (Neuromuscular blocking agents used as adjuncts to general anesthesia for surgery are included in Appendix F.)

Muscle Spasm

Muscle spasm or cramp is a sudden, involuntary, painful muscle contraction that occurs with trauma or an irritant. Spasms may involve alternating contraction and relaxation (clonic) or sustained contraction (tonic). Muscle spasm may occur with musculoskeletal trauma or inflammation (eg, sprains, strains, bursitis, arthritis). It is also encountered with acute or chronic low back pain, a common condition that is primarily a disorder of posture.

Spasticity

Spasticity involves increased muscle tone or contraction and stiff, awkward movements. It occurs in neurologic disorders such as spinal cord injury and multiple sclerosis (MS).

In clients with spinal cord injury, spasticity requires treatment when it impairs safety, mobility, and the ability to per-form activities of daily living (eg, self-care in hygiene, eating, dressing, and work or recreational activities). Stimuli that precipitate spasms vary from one individual to another and may include muscle stretching, bladder infections or stones, constipation and bowel distention, or infections. Each person should be assessed for personal precipitating factors, so that these factors can be avoided if possible. Treatment measures include passive range-of-motion and muscle-stretching exercises and antispasmodic medications (eg, baclofen, dantrolene).

MS is a major cause of neurologic disability among young and middle-aged adults; occurs more often in women than in men; and has a pattern of exacerbations and remissions. It is considered an autoimmune disorder that occurs in genetically susceptible individuals, and its cause is unknown. MS involves destruction of portions of the myelin sheath that covers nerves in the brain, spinal cord, and optic nerve. Myelin normally insulates the neuron from electrical activity and conducts electrical impulses rapidly along nerve fibers. When myelin is destroyed (a process called *demyelination,* which probably results from inflammation), fibrotic lesions are formed and nerve conduction is slowed or blocked around the lesions. Lesions in various states of development (eg, acute, subacute, chronic) often occur at multiple sites in the central nervous system (CNS). Muscle weakness and other symptoms vary according to the location and duration of the myelin damage.

In recent years, researchers have discovered that nerve cells can be repaired (remyelinated) if the process that damaged the myelin is stopped before the oligodendrocytes (the cells that form myelin) are destroyed. Other researchers are trying to develop methods for enhancing nerve conduction velocity in demyelinated nerves. For example, exposure to cold by wearing a cooling vest or exercising in cool water temporarily increases the rate of nerve conduction and improves symptoms in some people. Avoiding environmental heat and conditions that cause fever may also help, because elevated body temperature slows nerve conduction and often aggravates MS symptoms.

People with minimal symptoms do not require treatment but should be encouraged to maintain a healthy lifestyle. Those with more extensive symptoms should try to avoid emotional stress, extremes of environmental temperature, infections, and excessive fatigue. Physical therapy may help maintain muscle tone, and occupational therapy may help maintain ability to perform activities of daily living.

Drug therapy for MS may involve several types of medications for different types and stages of the disease. Corticosteroids are used to treat acute exacerbations (see Chap. 23); interferon beta or glatiramer is given to prevent relapses; immunosuppressive drugs (eg, methotrexate) are used to treat progressive disease; and a variety of drugs, including antidepressants for depression and skeletal muscle relaxants for spasticity, are used to treat symptoms. Baclofen, tizanidine, or dantrolene may be used to control spasticity. In some cases, decreasing spasticity may not be desirable, because clients with severe leg weakness may require some degree of spasticity to ambulate. In cases of severe spasticity, baclofen may be given intrathecally through an implanted subcutaneous pump.

APPLYING YOUR KNOWLEDGE 13-1
What general teaching points should you emphasize with Mrs. Milewski and her caregivers to prevent exacerbation of symptoms?

GENERAL CHARACTERISTICS OF SKELETAL MUSCLE RELAXANTS

Mechanism of Action

All skeletal muscle relaxants except dantrolene are centrally active drugs. Pharmacologic action is usually attributed to general depression of the CNS but may involve blockage of nerve impulses that cause increased muscle tone and contraction. It is unclear whether relief of pain results from sedative effects, muscular relaxation, or a placebo effect. In addition, although parenteral administration of some drugs (eg, diazepam, methocarbamol) relieves pain associated with

acute musculoskeletal trauma or inflammation, it is uncertain whether oral administration of usual doses exerts a beneficial effect in acute or chronic disorders.

Baclofen and diazepam increase the effects of gamma-aminobutyric acid, an inhibitory neurotransmitter. Tizanidine inhibits motor neurons in the brain. Dantrolene is the only skeletal muscle relaxant that acts peripherally on the muscle itself; it inhibits the release of calcium in skeletal muscle cells, thereby decreasing the strength of muscle contraction.

Indications for Use

Skeletal muscle relaxants are used primarily as adjuncts to other treatment measures such as physical therapy. Occasionally, parenteral agents are given to facilitate orthopedic procedures and examinations. In spastic disorders, skeletal muscle relaxants are indicated when spasticity causes severe pain or inability to tolerate physical therapy, sit in a wheelchair, or participate in self-care activities of daily living (eg, eating, dressing). The drugs should not be given if they cause excessive muscle weakness and impair rather than facilitate mobility and function. Dantrolene also is indicated for prevention and treatment of malignant hyperthermia (see "Individual Drugs").

Contraindications to Use

Most skeletal muscle relaxants cause CNS depression and have the same contraindications as other CNS depressants. They should be used cautiously in clients with impaired renal or hepatic function or respiratory depression and in clients who must be alert for activities of daily living (eg, driving a car, operating potentially hazardous machinery). Orphenadrine and cyclobenzaprine have high levels of anticholinergic activity and therefore should be used cautiously in clients with glaucoma, urinary retention, cardiac dysrhythmias, or tachycardia.

APPLYING YOUR KNOWLEDGE 13-2
During your assessment, you note that Mrs. Milewski is having more weakness in her lower extremities during this visit as compared with your visit 1 month ago. You also note that the physician has recently increased the dose of baclofen from 10 to 15 mg. How would you respond?

INDIVIDUAL DRUGS

Individual skeletal muscle relaxants are described below. Routes and dosage ranges are listed in Table 13-1.

Baclofen (Lioresal) is used mainly to treat spasticity in MS and spinal cord injuries. It is contraindicated in people with hypersensitivity reactions and in those with muscle spasm from rheumatic disorders. It can be given orally and intrathecally through an implanted subcutaneous pump. Check the literature from the pump manufacturer for information about pump implantation and drug infusion techniques.

Table 13-1 Drugs at a Glance: Skeletal Muscle Relaxants

GENERIC/TRADE NAME	ROUTES AND DOSAGE RANGES	
	Adults	Children
Baclofen (Lioresal)	PO 5 mg 3 times daily for 3 d; 10 mg 3 times daily for 3 d; 15 mg 3 times daily for 3 d; then 20 mg 3 times daily, if necessary Intrathecal via implanted pump: Dosage varies widely; see manufacturer's recommendations.	*<12 years:* Safety not established
Carisoprodol (Soma)	PO 350 mg 3 or 4 times daily, with the last dose at bedtime	*<12 years:* Not recommended
Cyclobenzaprine (Flexeril)	PO 10 mg 3 times daily. Maximal recommended duration, 3 weeks; maximal recommended dose, 60 mg daily	*<15 years:* Safety and effectiveness have not been established.
Dantrolene (Dantrium)	PO 25 mg daily initially, gradually increased weekly (by increments of 50–100 mg/d) to a maximal dose of 400 mg daily in 4 divided doses Preoperative prophylaxis of malignant hyperthermia: PO 4–8 mg/kg/d in 3–4 divided doses for 1 or 2 days before surgery Intraoperative malignant hyperthermia: IV push 1 mg/kg initially, continued until symptoms are relieved or a maximum total dose of 10 mg/kg has been given Postcrisis follow-up treatment: PO 4–8 mg/kg/d in 4 divided doses for 1–3 days	Spasticity: PO 1 mg/kg/d initially, gradually increased to a maximal dose of 3 mg/kg 4 times daily, not to exceed 400 mg daily Malignant hyperthermia: Same as adult
Diazepam (Valium)	PO 2–10 mg 3 or 4 times daily IM, IV 5–10 mg repeated in 3–4 hours if necessary	PO 0.12–0.8 mg/kg/d in 3 or 4 divided doses IM, IV 0.04–0.2 mg/kg in a single dose, not to exceed 0.6 mg/kg within an 8-h period
Metaxalone (Skelaxin)	PO 800 mg 3 or 4 times daily	*>12 years:* Same as adult *<12 years:* Safety and effectiveness have not been established.
Methocarbamol (Robaxin)	PO 1.5–2 g 4 times daily for 48–72 hours, reduced to 1 g 4 times daily for maintenance IM 500 mg q8h IV 1–3 g daily at a rate not to exceed 300 mg/min (3 mL of 10% injection). Do not give IV more than 3 days.	Safety and effectiveness have not been established except for treatment of tetanus (IV 15 mg/kg every 6 h as indicated).
Orphenadrine citrate (Norflex)	PO 100 mg twice daily IM, IV 60 mg twice daily	Not recommended
Tizanidine (Zanaflex)	PO 4 mg q6–8h initially, increased gradually if needed. Maximum of 3 doses and 36 mg in 24 h	Safety and effectiveness have not been established.

IM, intramuscular; IV, intravenous; PO, oral.

Oral baclofen begins to act in 1 hour, peaks in 2 hours, and lasts 4 to 8 hours. It is metabolized in the liver and excreted in urine; its half-life is 3 to 4 hours. Dosage must be reduced in clients with impaired renal function. Common adverse effects include drowsiness, dizziness, confusion, constipation, fatigue, headache, hypotension, insomnia, nausea, and weakness. When discontinued, dosage should be tapered and the drug withdrawn over 1 to 2 weeks.

Carisoprodol (Soma) is used to relieve discomfort from acute, painful musculoskeletal disorders. It is not recommended for long-term use. If used long term or in high doses, it can cause physical dependence, and it may cause symptoms of withdrawal if stopped abruptly. The drug is contraindicated in clients with intermittent porphyria, a rare metabolic disorder characterized by acute abdominal pain and neurologic symptoms. Oral drug acts within 30 minutes, peaks in 1 to 2 hours, and lasts 4 to 6 hours. It is metabolized in the liver and has a half-life of 8 hours. Common adverse effects include drowsiness, dizziness, and impaired motor coordination.

Cyclobenzaprine (Flexeril) has the same indication for use as carisoprodol. It is contraindicated in clients with cardiovascular disorders (eg, recent myocardial infarction, dysrhythmias, heart block) or hyperthyroidism. The oral drug acts in 1 hour, peaks in 4 to 6 hours, and lasts 12 to 24 hours. The half-life is 1 to 3 days. Duration of use should not exceed 3 weeks. Common adverse effects are drowsiness, dizziness, and anticholinergic effects (eg, dry mouth, constipation, urinary retention, tachycardia).

Dantrolene (Dantrium) acts directly on skeletal muscle to inhibit muscle contraction. It is used to relieve spasticity in neurologic disorders (eg, MS, spinal cord injury) and to prevent or treat malignant hyperthermia, a rare but life-threatening complication of anesthesia characterized by hypercarbia, metabolic acidosis, skeletal muscle rigidity, fever, and cyanosis. For preoperative prophylaxis in people with previous episodes of malignant hyperthermia, the drug is given orally for 1 to 2 days before surgery. For intraoperative malignant hyperthermia, the drug is given intravenously (IV). After an occurrence during surgery, the drug is given orally for 1 to 3 days to prevent recurrence of symptoms.

Oral dantrolene acts slowly, peaking in 4 to 6 hours and lasting 8 to 10 hours, whereas IV drug acts rapidly, peaking in about 5 hours and lasting 6 to 8 hours. Common adverse effects include drowsiness, dizziness, diarrhea, and fatigue. The most serious adverse effect is potentially fatal hepatitis, with jaundice and other symptoms that usually occur within 1 month of starting drug therapy. Liver function tests should be monitored periodically in all clients receiving dantrolene. These adverse effects do not occur with short-term use of IV drug for malignant hyperthermia.

Metaxalone (Skelaxin) is used to relieve discomfort from acute, painful musculoskeletal disorders. It is contraindicated in clients with anemias or severe renal or hepatic impairment. Oral drug acts within 60 minutes, peaks in 2 hours, and lasts 4 to 6 hours. It has a half-life of 2 to 3 hours, is metabolized in the liver, and is excreted in urine. Common adverse effects include drowsiness, dizziness, and nausea; hepatotoxicity and hemolytic anemia may also occur. Liver function should be monitored during therapy.

Methocarbamol (Robaxin) is used to relieve discomfort from acute, painful musculoskeletal disorders. It may also be used to treat tetanus. The parenteral form is contraindicated in clients with renal impairment, because the solution contains polyethylene glycol. The oral drug acts within 30 minutes and peaks in 2 hours, and the parenteral drug acts rapidly but peak and duration of action are unknown. Methocarbamol has a half-life of 1 to 2 hours. It is metabolized in the liver and excreted in urine and feces. Common adverse effects with oral drug include drowsiness, dizziness, nausea, and urticaria; effects with injected drug also include fainting, incoordination, and hypotension. The drug may also give urine a green, brown, or black color. This is considered a harmless effect, but clients should be informed about it.

Orphenadrine (Norflex) is used to relieve discomfort from acute, painful musculoskeletal disorders. Because of its strong anticholinergic effects, the drug is contraindicated in glaucoma, duodenal obstruction, prostatic hypertrophy, urinary bladder-neck obstruction, and myasthenia gravis. It should be used cautiously in clients with cardiovascular disease (eg, heart failure, coronary insufficiency, dysrhythmias) and renal or hepatic impairment. The action of both oral and parenteral drug peaks in 2 hours and lasts 4 to 6 hours. The drug has a half-life of 14 hours, is metabolized in the liver, and is excreted in urine and feces. Common adverse effects include drowsiness, dizziness, constipation, dry mouth, nausea, tachycardia, and urinary retention.

Tizanidine (Zanaflex) is an alpha$_2$ adrenergic agonist, similar to clonidine, that is used to treat spasticity in clients with MS, spinal cord injury, or brain trauma. It should be used cautiously in clients with renal or hepatic impairment and hypotension. It is given orally, and it begins to act within 30 to 60 minutes, peaks in 1 to 2 hours, and lasts 3 to 4 hours. Its half-life is 3 to 4 hours. It is metabolized in the liver and excreted in urine. Common adverse effects include drowsiness, dizziness, constipation, dry mouth, and hypotension. Hypotension may be significant and occur at usual doses. The drug may also cause psychotic symptoms, including hallucinations.

NURSING PROCESS

Assessment

Assess for muscle spasm and spasticity.
● With muscle spasm, assess for:
  ● **Pain.** This is a prominent symptom of muscle spasm and is usually aggravated by movement. Try to determine the location as specifically as possible, as well as the intensity, duration, and precipitating factors (eg, traumatic injury, strenuous exercise).

● **Accompanying signs and symptoms,** such as bruises (ecchymoses), edema, or signs of inflammation (redness, heat, edema, tenderness to touch)
● With spasticity, assess for pain and impaired functional ability in self-care (eg, eating, dressing). In addition, severe spasticity interferes with ambulation and other movement as well as exercises to maintain joint and muscle mobility.

Nursing Diagnoses

● Pain related to muscle spasm
● Impaired Physical Mobility related to spasm and pain
● Bathing/Hygiene Self-Care Deficit related to spasm and pain
● Deficient Knowledge: Nondrug measures to relieve muscle spasm, pain, and spasticity and safe usage of skeletal muscle relaxants
● Risk for Injury: Dizziness, sedation related to CNS depression

Planning/Goals

The client will
● Experience relief of pain and spasm
● Experience improved motor function
● Increase self-care abilities in activities of daily living
● Take medications as instructed
● Use nondrug measures appropriately
● Be safeguarded when sedated from drug therapy

Interventions

Use adjunctive measures for muscle spasm and spasticity.
● Physical therapy (massage, moist heat, exercises)

● Relaxation techniques
● Correct posture and lifting techniques (eg, stooping rather than bending to lift objects, holding heavy objects close to the body, *not* lifting excessive amounts of weight)
● Regular exercise and use of warm-up exercises. Strenuous exercise performed on an occasional basis (eg, weekly or monthly) is more likely to cause acute muscle spasm.

Provide appropriate teaching related to drug therapy (see accompanying display).

Evaluation

● Interview and observe for relief of symptoms.
● Interview and observe regarding correct usage of medications and nondrug therapeutic measures.

APPLYING YOUR KNOWLEDGE 13-3
Mrs. Milewski's family gives her all her morning medications as soon as she wakes up. Mrs. Milewski is complaining about an upset stomach. What should be changed?

PRINCIPLES OF THERAPY

Goals of Therapy

Skeletal muscle relaxants aim to relieve pain, muscle spasm, and muscle spasticity without impairing the ability to perform self-care activities of daily living.

CLIENT TEACHING GUIDELINES
Skeletal Muscle Relaxants

General Considerations

✔ Use nondrug measures, such as exercises and applications of heat and cold, to decrease muscle spasm and spasticity.
✔ Avoid activities that require mental alertness or physical coordination (eg, driving an automobile, operating potentially dangerous machinery) if drowsy from medication.
✔ Do not take other drugs without the physician's knowledge, including nonprescription drugs. The major risk occurs with concurrent use of alcohol, antihistamines, sleeping aids, or other drugs that cause drowsiness.
✔ Avoid herbal preparations that cause drowsiness or sleep, including kava and valerian.

Self-Administration

✔ Take the drugs with milk or food, to avoid nausea and stomach irritation.
✔ Do not stop drugs abruptly. Dosage should be decreased gradually, especially with baclofen (Lioresal), carisoprodol (Soma), and cyclobenzaprine (Flexeril). Suddenly stopping baclofen may cause hallucinations; stopping the other drugs may cause fatigue, headache, and nausea.

Drug Selection

Choice of a skeletal muscle relaxant depends mainly on the disorder being treated.

- For acute muscle spasm and pain, oral or parenteral drugs may be used. These drugs cause sedation and other adverse effects and are recommended for short-term use. Cyclobenzaprine should not be used longer than 3 weeks.
- For orthopedic procedures, parenteral agents are preferred because they have greater sedative and pain-relieving effects.
- For spasticity in people with MS, baclofen (Lioresal) is approved. It is variably effective, and its clinical usefulness may be limited by adverse effects.
- None of the skeletal muscle relaxants has been established as safe for use during pregnancy and lactation.
- For children, the drug should be chosen from those with established pediatric dosages.

Use in Special Populations

Use in Children

For most of the skeletal muscle relaxants, safety and effectiveness for use in children 12 years of age and younger have not been established. The drugs should be used only when clearly indicated; for short periods; when close supervision is available for monitoring drug effects (especially sedation); and when mobility and alertness are not required.

Use in Older Adults

Any CNS depressant or sedating drug should be used cautiously in older adults. Risks of falls, mental confusion, and other adverse effects are higher because of impaired drug metabolism and excretion.

Use in Clients With Renal Impairment

The skeletal muscle relaxants should be used cautiously in clients with renal impairment. Dosage of baclofen must be reduced.

Use in Clients With Hepatic Impairment

Dantrolene may cause potentially fatal hepatitis, with jaundice and other symptoms that usually occur within 1 month of starting drug therapy. Liver function tests should be monitored periodically in all clients receiving dantrolene.

Metaxalone and tizanidine can cause liver damage. Thus, liver function should be assessed before starting either drug and periodically during treatment. If liver damage occurs, the drugs should be stopped. The drugs should not be given to clients with pre-existing liver disease.

Use in Home Care

The home care nurse is likely to be involved with the use of baclofen, dantrolene, or tizanidine in chronic spastic disorders. Clients may need continued assessment of drug effects, monitoring of functional abilities, assistance in arranging blood tests of liver function, and other care. Caregivers may need instruction about nonpharmacologic interventions to help prevent or relieve spasticity.

NURSING ACTIONS

Skeletal Muscle Relaxants

NURSING ACTIONS	RATIONALE/EXPLANATION
1. Administer accurately	
a. Give baclofen and metaxalone with milk or food.	To decrease gastrointestinal distress
b. Do not mix parenteral diazepam in a syringe with any other drugs.	Diazepam is physically incompatible with other drugs.
c. Inject intravenous (IV) diazepam directly into a vein or the injection site nearest the vein (during continuous IV infusions) at a rate of approximately 2 mg/min.	Diazepam may cause a precipitate if diluted. Avoid contact with IV solutions as much as possible. A slow rate of injection minimizes the risks of respiratory depression and apnea.
d. Avoid extravasation with IV diazepam, and inject intramuscular (IM) diazepam deeply into a gluteal muscle.	To prevent or reduce tissue irritation
e. With IV methocarbamol, inject or infuse slowly, no more than 3 mL/min.	Rapid administration may cause bradycardia, hypotension, and dizziness.

NURSING ACTIONS	RATIONALE/EXPLANATION
f. With IV methocarbamol, have the client lie down during and at least 15 minutes after administration.	To minimize orthostatic hypotension and other adverse drug effects
g. Avoid extravasation with IV methocarbamol, and give IM methocarbamol deeply into a gluteal muscle (no more than 5mL per site).	Parenteral methocarbamol is a hypertonic solution that is very irritating to tissues. Thrombophlebitis may occur at IV injection sites, and sloughing of tissue may occur at sites of extravasation or IM injections.
2. Observe for therapeutic effects	
a. When the drug is given for acute muscle spasm, observe for:	Therapeutic effects usually occur within 30 minutes after IV injection of diazepam or methocarbamol.
(1) Decreased pain and tenderness	
(2) Increased mobility	
(3) Increased ability to participate in activities of daily living	
b. When the drug is given for spasticity in chronic neurologic disorders, observe for:	
(1) Increased ability to maintain posture and balance	
(2) Increased ability for self-care (eg, eating and dressing)	
(3) Increased tolerance for physical therapy and exercises	
3. Observe for adverse effects	
a. With centrally active agents, observe for:	
(1) Drowsiness and dizziness	These are the most common adverse effects.
(2) Blurred vision, lethargy, flushing	These effects occur more often with IV administration of drugs. They are usually transient.
(3) Nausea, vomiting, abdominal distress, constipation or diarrhea, ataxia, areflexia, flaccid paralysis, respiratory depression, tachycardia, hypotension	These effects are most likely to occur with large oral doses.
(4) Hypersensitivity—skin rash, pruritus	The drug should be discontinued if hypersensitivity reactions occur. Serious allergic reactions (eg, anaphylaxis) are rare.
(5) Psychological or physical dependence with diazepam and other antianxiety agents	Most likely to occur with long-term use of large doses
b. With a peripherally active agent (dantrolene), observe for:	Adverse effects are usually transient.
(1) Drowsiness, fatigue, lethargy, weakness, nausea, vomiting	These effects are the most common.
(2) Headache, anorexia, nervousness	Less common effects
(3) Hepatotoxicity	This potentially serious adverse effect is most likely to occur in people older than 35 years of age who have taken the drug 60 days or longer. Women older than 35 years of age who take estrogens have the highest risk. Hepatotoxicity can be prevented or minimized by administering the lowest effective dose, monitoring liver enzymes (aspartate aminotransferase [AST] and alanine aminotransferase [ALT]) during therapy, and discontinuing the drug if no beneficial effects occur within 45 days.
4. Observe for drug interactions	
a. Drugs that *increase* effects of skeletal muscle relaxants:	
(1) Central nervous system (CNS) depressants (alcohol, antianxiety agents, antidepressants, antihistamines, antipsychotic drugs, sedative-hypnotics)	Additive CNS depression with increased risks of excessive sedation and respiratory depression or apnea
(2) Monoamine oxidase inhibitors	May potentiate effects by inhibiting metabolism of muscle relaxants
(3) Antihypertensive agents	Increased hypotension, especially with tizanidine

APPLYING YOUR KNOWLEDGE: ANSWERS

13-1 Clients with MS should be encouraged to avoid emotional stress; exposure to extremes in environmental temperature; infection; and excessive fatigue.

13-2 Baclofen should not be given if it causes excessive muscle weakness and impairs rather than facilitates mobility and function. Contact Mrs. Milewski's physician.

13-3 Provide client/caregiver teaching. Baclofen should be given with milk or food to reduce gastrointestinal irritation.

Review and Application Exercises

Short Answer Exercises

1. How do skeletal muscle relaxants act to relieve spasm and pain?

2. What are the indications for the use of skeletal muscle relaxants?

3. What are the contraindications to the use of skeletal muscle relaxants?

4. What are the major adverse effects of skeletal muscle relaxants, and how can they be minimized?

5. What are some nonpharmacologic interventions to use instead of, or along with, skeletal muscle relaxants?

NCLEX-Style Questions

6. Adverse effects of centrally active skeletal muscle relaxants include which of the following?
   a. muscle spasms
   b. insomnia
   c. nervousness
   d. hypotension

7. Which of the following muscle relaxants is the only one that acts peripherally on muscles?
   a. dantrolene (Dantrium)
   b. baclofen (Lioresal)
   c. methocarbamol (Robaxin)
   d. diazepam (Valium)

8. For a client with MS receiving baclofen (Lioresal), the main therapeutic effect is
   a. increased drowsiness
   b. improved appetite
   c. decreased muscle spasticity
   d. improved renal function

Selected References

Bainbridge, J. L., Corboy, J. R., & Gidal, B. E. (2002). Multiple sclerosis. In J. T. DiPiro, R. L. Talbert, G. C. Yee, G. R. Matzke, B. G. Wells, & L. M. Posey (Eds.), *Pharmacotherapy: A pathophysiologic approach* (5th ed., pp. 1019–1030). New York: McGraw-Hill.

Drug facts and comparisons. (Updated monthly). St. Louis: Facts and Comparisons.

Porth, C. M., & Curtis, R. L. (2005). Disorders of motor function. In C. M. Porth, *Pathophysiology: Concepts of altered health states* (7th ed., pp. 1193–1226). Philadelphia: Lippincott Williams & Wilkins.

Substance Abuse Disorders

OBJECTIVES

After studying this chapter, you will be able to:

1. Identify risk factors for development of drug dependence.
2. Describe the effects of alcohol, cocaine, marijuana, and nicotine on selected body organs.
3. Compare and contrast characteristics of dependence associated with alcohol, benzodiazepines, cocaine, and opiates.
4. Describe specific antidotes for overdoses of central nervous system (CNS) depressant drugs and the circumstances indicating their use.
5. Outline major elements of treatment for overdoses of commonly abused drugs that do not have antidotes.
6. Describe interventions to prevent or manage withdrawal reactions associated with alcohol, benzodiazepines, cocaine and other CNS stimulants, and opiates.

APPLYING YOUR KNOWLEDGE

Bryan Wilson is a 24-year-old man who regularly uses marijuana, alcohol, and tobacco. He also occasionally uses cocaine as a recreational drug. He is seen in the ER in acute intoxication. He is admitted for withdrawal and treatment.

INTRODUCTION

Substance abuse is a significant health, social, economic, and legal problem. It is often associated with substantial damage to the abuser and society (eg, crime, child and spouse abuse, traumatic injury, chronic health problems, death). In this chapter, *substance abuse* is defined as self-administration of a drug for prolonged periods or in excessive amounts to the point of producing physical or psychological dependence; impairing functions of body organs; reducing the ability to function in usual activities of daily living; and decreasing the ability and motivation to function as a productive member of society.

Most drugs of abuse are those that affect the CNS and alter the state of consciousness. These include prescription and nonprescription and legal and illegal drugs. Commonly abused drugs include CNS depressants (eg, alcohol, antianxiety and sedative-hypnotic agents, opioid analgesics), CNS stimulants (eg, amphetamines and derivatives, cocaine, nicotine), and other mind-altering drugs (eg, marijuana, "ecstasy"). Although these drugs produce different effects, they are associated with feelings of pleasure, positive reinforcement, and compulsive self-administration. Most are also associated with tolerance if used repeatedly. This means that the body adjusts to the drugs

so that higher doses are needed to achieve feelings of pleasure ("reward") or stave off withdrawal symptoms ("punishment"). Both reward and punishment serve to reinforce continued substance abuse.

Drugs of abuse seem to be readily available. Internet websites have become an important source of the drugs. In some instances, instructions for manufacturing particular drugs are available. Although patterns of drug abuse vary in particular populations and in geographic areas, continuing trends seem to include increased use of methamphetamine, "club drugs," prescription drugs, and multiple drugs.

Dependence

Characteristics of drug dependence include craving a drug, often with unsuccessful attempts to decrease its use; compulsive drug-seeking behavior; physical dependence (withdrawal symptoms if drug use is decreased or stopped); and continuing to take a drug despite adverse consequences (eg, drug-related illnesses, mental or legal problems, job loss or decreased ability to function in an occupation, impaired family relationships).

Psychological dependence involves feelings of satisfaction and pleasure from taking the drug. These feelings, perceived as extremely desirable by the drug-dependent person, contribute to acute intoxication, development and maintenance of drug-abuse patterns, and return to drug-taking behavior after periods of abstinence.

Physical dependence involves physiologic adaptation to chronic use of a drug so that unpleasant symptoms occur when the drug is stopped, when its action is antagonized by another drug, or when its dosage is decreased. The withdrawal or abstinence syndrome produces specific manifestations according to the type of drug and does not occur as long as adequate dosage is maintained. Attempts to avoid withdrawal symptoms reinforce psychological dependence and promote continuing drug use and relapses to drug-taking behavior. Tolerance is often an element of drug dependence, and increasing doses are therefore required to obtain psychological effects or avoid physical withdrawal symptoms. A person may be dependent on several drugs; most substance abusers use multiple drugs.

Drug dependence is a complex phenomenon. Although the cause is unknown, one theory is that drugs stimulate or inhibit neurotransmitters in the brain to produce pleasure and euphoria or to decrease unpleasant feelings such as anxiety. For example, dopaminergic neurons in the limbic system are associated with the brain's reward system and are thought to be sites of action of alcohol, amphetamines, cocaine, nicotine, and opiates. These major drugs of abuse increase dopaminergic transmission and the availability of dopamine. For example, amphetamines promote dopamine release and inhibit its reuptake, and cocaine inhibits dopamine reuptake. These actions are believed to stimulate the brain's reward system and lead to compulsive drug administration and abuse.

The noradrenergic neurotransmission system, which uses norepinephrine as its neurotransmitter, is often involved as well as the dopaminergic system. Noradrenergic neurons innervate the limbic system and cerebral cortex and are important in setting mood and affect. Drugs that alter noradrenergic transmission have profound effects on mood and affect. Amphetamines and cocaine increase noradrenergic transmission as with dopaminergic transmission, by promoting the release of norepinephrine and/or inhibiting its reuptake. Increased norepinephrine leads to mood elevation and euphoria, which promotes continued drug abuse. Increased norepinephrine also leads to major adverse effects of amphetamines and cocaine, including myocardial infarction, severe hypertension, and stroke, as well as profound mood swings from euphoria to depression.

Other factors important in developing drug dependence include the specific drug; the amount, frequency, and route of administration; the person's psychological and physiologic characteristics; and environmental or circumstantial characteristics. Peer pressure is often an important factor in initial and continuing drug ingestion. A genetic factor seems evident in alcohol abuse: Studies indicate that children of abusers are at risk of becoming abusers themselves, even if reared away from the abusing parent. Additional general characteristics of substance abuse and dependence include the following:

- Substance abuse involves all socioeconomic levels and affects all age groups. It is especially prevalent among adolescents and young adults. Patterns of abuse may vary by age group. For example, adolescents and young adults are more likely to use illicit drugs and older adults are more likely to abuse alcohol and prescription drugs. Health care professionals (eg, physicians, pharmacists, nurses) are also considered at high risk for development of substance abuse disorders, at least partly because of easy access.
- A person who abuses one drug is likely to abuse others.
- Multiple drugs are often abused concurrently. Alcohol, for example, is often used with other drugs of abuse, probably because it is legal and readily available. In addition, alcohol, marijuana, opioids, and sedatives are often used to combat the anxiety and nervousness induced by cocaine, methamphetamine, and other CNS stimulants.
- Drug effects vary according to the type of substance being abused, the amount, route of administration, duration of use, and phase of substance abuse (eg, acute intoxication, withdrawal syndromes, organ damage, medical illness). Thus, acute intoxication often produces profound behavioral changes and chronic abuse often leads to serious organ damage and impaired ability to function in work, family, or social settings. Withdrawal symptoms are characteristic of particular types of drugs and are usually opposite to the effects originally produced. For example, withdrawal symptoms of alcohol and sedative-type drugs are mainly agitation, nervousness, and hyperactivity.
- Abusers of alcohol and other drugs are not reliable sources of information about the types or amounts of drugs used. Most abusers understate the amount and frequency of substance use; heroin addicts may overstate the amount used in attempts to obtain higher doses of methadone. In addition, those who use illegal street drugs may not know what they have taken because of varying purity, potency, additives, contaminants, names, and substitutions of one drug for another.
- Substance abusers rarely seek health care unless circumstances force the issue. Thus, most substance abuse comes to the attention of health care professionals when the abuser experiences a complication such as acute intoxication, withdrawal, or serious medical problems resulting from chronic drug overuse, misuse, or abuse.
- Smoking or inhaling drug vapors is a preferred route of administration for cocaine, marijuana, and nicotine because the drugs are rapidly absorbed from the large surface area of the lungs. Then, they rapidly circulate to the heart and brain without dilution by the systemic circulation or metabolism by enzymes.
- Substance abusers who inject drugs intravenously (IV) are prey to serious problems because they use impure drugs of unknown potency, contaminated needles, poor

hygiene, and other dangerous practices. Specific problems include overdoses, death, and numerous infections (eg, hepatitis, human immunodeficiency virus infection, endocarditis, phlebitis, cellulitis at injection sites).

Many drugs abused for their mind-altering properties have clinical usefulness and are discussed elsewhere: "Antianxiety and Sedative-Hypnotic Drugs" (Chap. 8), "Opioid Analgesics and Opioid Antagonists" (Chap. 6), and "Central Nervous System Stimulants" (Chap. 15). This chapter describes commonly abused substances, characteristics and treatment of substance-related disorders, and drugs used to treat substance-related disorders (see Table 14-1).

CENTRAL NERVOUS SYSTEM DEPRESSANTS

CNS depressants are drugs that slow down or "depress" brain activity. They include alcohol, antianxiety and sedative-hypnotic agents, and opiates.

Alcohol (Ethanol)

Alcohol is commonly abused around the world. It is legal and readily available, and its use is accepted in most societies. There is no clear dividing line between use and abuse, but rather a continuum of progression over several years. Alcohol exerts profound metabolic and physiologic effects on all organ systems (Box 14-1). Some of these effects are evident with acute alcohol intake, whereas others become evident with chronic intake of substantial amounts. Alcohol is thought to exert its effects on the CNS by enhancing the activity of gamma-aminobutyric acid, an inhibitory neurotransmitter, or by inhibiting the activity of glutamate, an excitatory neurotransmitter.

When alcohol is ingested orally, a portion is inactivated in the stomach (by the enzyme alcohol dehydrogenase) and not absorbed systemically. Women have less enzyme activity than men and therefore absorb approximately 30% more alcohol than men when comparable amounts are ingested according to weight and size. As a result, women are especially vulnerable to adverse effects of alcohol, including more rapid intoxication from smaller amounts of alcohol and earlier development of hepatic cirrhosis and other complications of alcohol abuse.

In men and women, alcohol is absorbed partly from the stomach but mostly from the upper small intestine. It is rapidly absorbed when the stomach and small intestine are empty. Food delays absorption by diluting the alcohol and delaying gastric emptying. After it is absorbed, alcohol is quickly distributed to all body tissues, partly because it is lipid soluble and crosses cell membranes easily. The alcohol concentration in the brain rapidly approaches that in the blood, and CNS effects usually occur within a few minutes. These effects depend on the amount ingested, how rapidly it was ingested, whether the stomach was empty, and other factors. Effects with acute intox-

ication usually progress from a feeling of relaxation to impaired mental and motor functions to stupor and sleep. Excited behavior may occur because of depression of the cerebral cortex, which normally controls behavior. The person may seem more relaxed, talkative, and outgoing, or more impulsive and aggressive because inhibitions have been lessened.

The rate of alcohol metabolism largely determines the duration of CNS effects. Most alcohol is oxidized in the liver to acetaldehyde, which can be used for energy or converted to fat and stored. When metabolized to acetaldehyde, alcohol no longer exerts depressant effects on the CNS. Although the rate of metabolism differs with acute ingestion or chronic intake and some other factors, it is approximately 120 milligrams per kilogram of body weight or 10 milliliters per hour. This is the amount of alcohol contained in approximately $\frac{2}{3}$ ounce of whiskey, 3 to 4 ounces of wine, or 8 to 12 ounces of beer. *Alcohol is metabolized at the same rate regardless of the amount present in body tissues.*

In older adults, the pharmacokinetics of alcohol are essentially the same as in younger adults. However, equivalent amounts of alcohol produce higher blood levels in older adults because of changes in body composition (eg, a greater proportion of fatty tissue).

Alcohol Interactions With Other Drugs

Alcohol may cause significant interactions when used with other drugs. These interactions often differ between acute and chronic ingestion. *Acute ingestion* inhibits drug-metabolizing enzymes. This slows the metabolism of some drugs, thereby increasing their effects and the likelihood of toxicity. *Chronic ingestion* induces metabolizing enzymes. This increases the rate of metabolism and decreases drug effects. Long-term ingestion of large amounts of alcohol, however, causes liver damage and impaired ability to metabolize drugs.

Because so many variables influence alcohol's interactions with other drugs, it is difficult to predict effects of interactions in particular people. However, some important interactions include those with other CNS depressants, antihypertensive agents, antidiabetic agents, oral anticoagulants, and disulfiram. These are summarized as follows:

- With other CNS depressants (eg, sedative-hypnotics, opioid analgesics, antianxiety agents, antipsychotic agents, general anesthetics, tricyclic antidepressants), alcohol potentiates CNS depression and increases risks of excessive sedation, respiratory depression, and impaired mental and physical functioning. Combining alcohol with these drugs may be lethal and should be avoided.
- With antihypertensive agents, alcohol potentiates vasodilation and hypotensive effects.
- With oral antidiabetic drugs, alcohol potentiates hypoglycemic effects.
- With oral anticoagulants (eg, warfarin), alcohol interactions vary. Acute ingestion increases anticoagulant effects and the risk of bleeding. Chronic ingestion

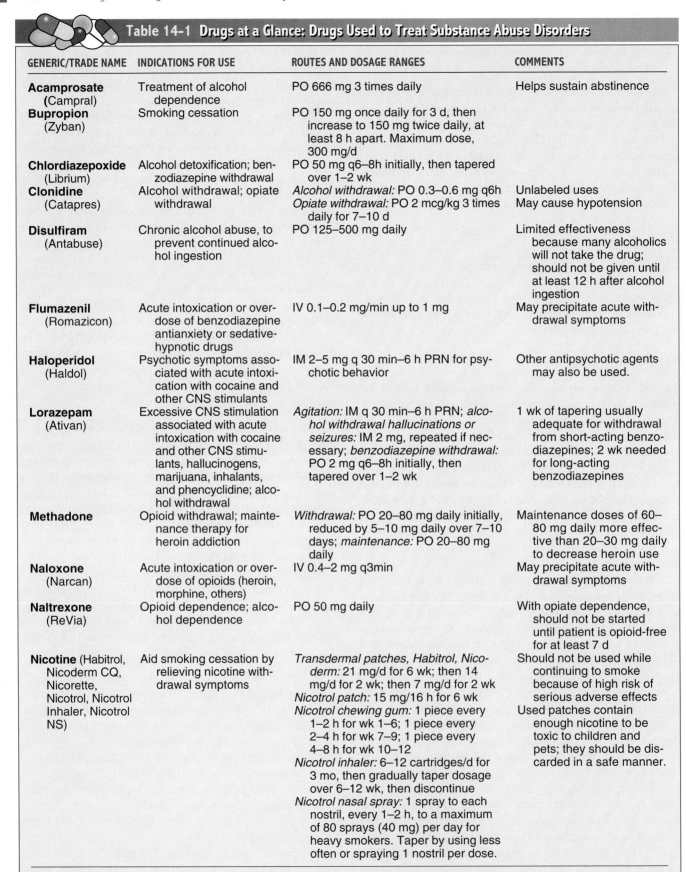

Table 14-1 Drugs at a Glance: Drugs Used to Treat Substance Abuse Disorders

GENERIC/TRADE NAME	INDICATIONS FOR USE	ROUTES AND DOSAGE RANGES	COMMENTS
Acamprosate (Campral)	Treatment of alcohol dependence	PO 666 mg 3 times daily	Helps sustain abstinence
Bupropion (Zyban)	Smoking cessation	PO 150 mg once daily for 3 d, then increase to 150 mg twice daily, at least 8 h apart. Maximum dose, 300 mg/d	
Chlordiazepoxide (Librium)	Alcohol detoxification; benzodiazepine withdrawal	PO 50 mg q6–8h initially, then tapered over 1–2 wk	
Clonidine (Catapres)	Alcohol withdrawal; opiate withdrawal	*Alcohol withdrawal:* PO 0.3–0.6 mg q6h *Opiate withdrawal:* PO 2 mcg/kg 3 times daily for 7–10 d	Unlabeled uses May cause hypotension
Disulfiram (Antabuse)	Chronic alcohol abuse, to prevent continued alcohol ingestion	PO 125–500 mg daily	Limited effectiveness because many alcoholics will not take the drug; should not be given until at least 12 h after alcohol ingestion
Flumazenil (Romazicon)	Acute intoxication or overdose of benzodiazepine antianxiety or sedative-hypnotic drugs	IV 0.1–0.2 mg/min up to 1 mg	May precipitate acute withdrawal symptoms
Haloperidol (Haldol)	Psychotic symptoms associated with acute intoxication with cocaine and other CNS stimulants	IM 2–5 mg q 30 min–6 h PRN for psychotic behavior	Other antipsychotic agents may also be used.
Lorazepam (Ativan)	Excessive CNS stimulation associated with acute intoxication with cocaine and other CNS stimulants, hallucinogens, marijuana, inhalants, and phencyclidine; alcohol withdrawal	*Agitation:* IM q 30 min–6 h PRN; *alcohol withdrawal hallucinations or seizures:* IM 2 mg, repeated if necessary; *benzodiazepine withdrawal:* PO 2 mg q6–8h initially, then tapered over 1–2 wk	1 wk of tapering usually adequate for withdrawal from short-acting benzodiazepines; 2 wk needed for long-acting benzodiazepines
Methadone	Opioid withdrawal; maintenance therapy for heroin addiction	*Withdrawal:* PO 20–80 mg daily initially, reduced by 5–10 mg daily over 7–10 days; *maintenance:* PO 20–80 mg daily	Maintenance doses of 60–80 mg daily more effective than 20–30 mg daily to decrease heroin use
Naloxone (Narcan)	Acute intoxication or overdose of opioids (heroin, morphine, others)	IV 0.4–2 mg q3min	May precipitate acute withdrawal symptoms
Naltrexone (ReVia)	Opioid dependence; alcohol dependence	PO 50 mg daily	With opiate dependence, should not be started until patient is opioid-free for at least 7 d
Nicotine (Habitrol, Nicoderm CQ, Nicorette, Nicotrol, Nicotrol Inhaler, Nicotrol NS)	Aid smoking cessation by relieving nicotine withdrawal symptoms	*Transdermal patches, Habitrol, Nicoderm:* 21 mg/d for 6 wk; then 14 mg/d for 2 wk; then 7 mg/d for 2 wk *Nicotrol patch:* 15 mg/16 h for 6 wk *Nicotrol chewing gum:* 1 piece every 1–2 h for wk 1–6; 1 piece every 2–4 h for wk 7–9; 1 piece every 4–8 h for wk 10–12 *Nicotrol inhaler:* 6–12 cartridges/d for 3 mo, then gradually taper dosage over 6–12 wk, then discontinue *Nicotrol nasal spray:* 1 spray to each nostril, every 1–2 h, to a maximum of 80 sprays (40 mg) per day for heavy smokers. Taper by using less often or spraying 1 nostril per dose.	Should not be used while continuing to smoke because of high risk of serious adverse effects Used patches contain enough nicotine to be toxic to children and pets; they should be discarded in a safe manner.

CNS, central nervous system; IM, intramuscular; IV, intravenous; PO, oral.

Box 14-1 Effects of Alcohol Abuse

Central and Peripheral Nervous System Effects

Sedation ranging from drowsiness to coma; impaired memory, learning, and thinking processes; impaired motor coordination, with ataxia or staggering gait, altered speech patterns, poor task performance, and hypoactivity or hyperactivity; mental depression, anxiety, insomnia; impaired interpersonal relationships; brain damage, polyneuritis, and Wernicke-Korsakoff syndrome.

Hepatic Effects

Induces drug-metabolizing enzymes that accelerate metabolism of alcohol and many other drugs and produce tolerance and cross-tolerance; eventually damages the liver enough to impair drug metabolism, leading to accumulation and toxic effects; decreases use and increases production of lactate, leading to lactic acidosis, decreased renal excretion of uric acid, and secondary hyperuricemia; decreases use and increases production of lipids, leading to hyperlipidemia and fatty liver. Fatty liver causes accumulation of fat and protein, leading to hepatomegaly; eventually produces severe liver injury characterized by necrosis and inflammation (alcoholic hepatitis) or by fibrous bands of scar tissue that irreversibly alter structure and function (cirrhosis).

The incidence of liver disease correlates with the amount of alcohol consumed and the progression of liver damage is attributed directly to ethanol or indirectly to the metabolic changes produced by ethanol.

Gastrointestinal Effects

Slowed gastric emptying time; increased intestinal motility, which probably contributes to the diarrhea that often occurs with alcoholism; damage to the epithelial cells of the intestinal mucosa; multiple nutritional deficiencies, including protein and water-soluble vitamins, such as thiamine, folic acid, and vitamin B_{12}; pancreatic disease, which contributes to malabsorption of fat, nitrogen, and vitamin B_{12}.

Cardiovascular Effects

Damage to myocardial cells; cardiomyopathy manifested by cardiomegaly, edema, dyspnea, abnormal heart sounds, and electrocardiographic changes indicating left ventricular hypertrophy, abnormal T waves, and conduction disturbances; possible impairment of coronary blood flow and myocardial contractility.

Hematologic Effects

Bone marrow depression due to alcohol or associated conditions, such as malnutrition, infection, and liver disease; several types of anemia including *megaloblastic anemia* from folic acid deficiency, *sideroblastic anemia* (sideroblasts are precursors of red blood cells) probably from nutritional deficiency, *hemolytic anemia* from abnormalities in the structure of red blood cells, *iron deficiency anemia* usually from gastrointestinal bleeding, and anemias from hemodilution, chronic infection, and fatty liver and bone marrow failure associated with cirrhosis; thrombocytopenia and decreased platelet aggregation from folic acid deficiency, hypersplenism, and other factors; decreased numbers and impaired function of white blood cells, which lead to decreased resistance to infection.

Endocrine Effects

Increased release of cortisol and catecholamines and decreased release of aldosterone from the adrenal glands; hypogonadism, gynecomastia, and feminization in men with cirrhosis due to decreased secretion of male sex hormones; degenerative changes in the anterior pituitary gland; decreased secretion of antidiuretic hormone from the posterior pituitary; hypoglycemia due to impaired glucose synthesis or hyperglycemia due to glycogenolysis.

Skeletal Effects

Impaired growth and development, which is most apparent in children born to alcoholic mothers. Fetal alcohol syndrome is characterized by low birth weight and length and by birth defects, such as cleft palate and cardiac septal defects. Impairment of growth and motor development persists in the postnatal period, and mental retardation becomes apparent. Other effects include decreased bone density, osteoporosis, and increased susceptibility to fractures; osteonecrosis due to obstructed blood supply; hypocalcemia, which leads to bone resorption and decreased skeletal mass; hypomagnesemia, which may further stimulate bone resorption; hypophosphatemia, probably from inadequate dietary intake of phosphorus.

Muscular Effects

Acute myopathy, which may be manifested by acute pain, tenderness, edema, and hyperkalemia; chronic myopathy, which may involve muscle weakness, atrophy, episodes of acute myopathy associated with a drinking spree, and elevated creatine phosphokinase.

---

decreases anticoagulant effects by inducing drug-metabolizing enzymes in the liver and increasing the rate of warfarin metabolism. However, if chronic ingestion has caused liver damage, metabolism of warfarin may be slowed. This increases the risk of excessive anticoagulant effect and bleeding.

● With disulfiram (Antabuse), alcohol produces significant distress (flushing, tachycardia, bronchospasm, sweating, nausea and vomiting). This reaction may be used to treat alcohol dependence.

● A disulfiram-like reaction also may occur with other drugs, including cefoperazone (Cefobid), cefotetan (Cefotan), chlorpropamide (Diabinese), tolbutamide (Orinase), and metronidazole (Flagyl).

Alcohol Dependence

Alcohol dependence involves acute or chronic consumption of alcohol in excess of the limits accepted by the person's culture, at times considered inappropriate by that culture, and to the extent that physical health and social relationships are impaired. Psychological dependence, physical dependence, tolerance, and cross-tolerance (with other CNS depressants) are prominent characteristics.

Acute intoxication impairs thinking, judgment, and psychomotor coordination. These impairments lead to poor work performance, accidents, and disturbed relationships with other people. Conscious control of behavior is lost, and exhibitionism, aggressiveness, and assaultiveness often result. Chronic ingestion affects essentially all body systems and may cause severe organ damage and mental problems. Effects are summarized in Box 14-1.

Signs and symptoms of alcohol withdrawal include agitation, anxiety, tremors, sweating, nausea, tachycardia, fever, hyperreflexia, postural hypotension, and, if severe, convulsions and delirium. Delirium tremens, the most serious form of alcohol withdrawal, is characterized by confusion, disorientation, delusions, visual hallucinations, and other signs of acute psychosis. The intensity of the alcohol withdrawal syndrome varies with the duration and amount of alcohol ingestion. Withdrawal symptoms start within a few hours after a person's last drink and last for several days.

Treatment of Alcohol Dependence

Alcohol dependence is a progressive illness, and early recognition and treatment are desirable. The alcohol-dependent person is unlikely to seek treatment for alcohol abuse unless an acute situation forces the issue. He or she is likely, however, to seek treatment for other disorders, such as nervousness, anxiety, depression, insomnia, and gastroenteritis. Thus, health professionals may recognize alcohol abuse in its early stages if they are aware of indicative assessment data.

If the first step of treatment is recognition of alcohol abuse, the second step is probably confronting the client with evidence of alcohol abuse and trying to elicit cooperation. Unless the client admits that alcohol abuse is a problem and agrees to participate in a treatment program, success is unlikely. The client may fail to make return visits or may seek treatment elsewhere. If the client agrees to treatment, the three primary approaches are psychological counseling, referral to a self-help group such as Alcoholics Anonymous, and drug therapy.

APPLYING YOUR KNOWLEDGE 14-1
For Mr. Wilson's treatment to be successful, what are the primary approaches that should be used?

Acute intoxication with alcohol does not usually require treatment. If the client is hyperactive and combative, a sedative-type drug may be given. The client must be closely observed because sedatives potentiate alcohol, and excessive CNS depression may occur. If the client is already sedated and stuporous, he or she can be allowed to sleep off the alcohol effects. If the client is comatose, supportive measures are indicated. For example, respiratory depression may require insertion of an artificial airway and mechanical ventilation.

Benzodiazepine antianxiety agents are the drugs of choice for treating alcohol withdrawal syndromes. They can help the client participate in rehabilitation programs and can be gradually reduced in dosage and discontinued. They provide adequate sedation and have a significant anticonvulsant effect. Some physicians prefer a benzodiazepine with a long half-life (eg, diazepam [Valium] or **chlordiazepoxide** [Librium]) whereas others prefer one with a short half-life (eg, **lorazepam** [Ativan] or oxazepam). Lorazepam and oxazepam are less likely to accumulate and may be best for older adults or clients with hepatic disease. Alcoholic clients usually require high doses of benzodiazepines because of the drugs' cross-tolerance with alcohol.

Seizures require treatment if they are repeated or continuous. Antiseizure drugs need not be given for more than a few days unless the person has a pre-existing seizure disorder. **Clonidine** (Catapres) may be given to reduce symptoms (eg, hyperactivity, tremors) associated with excessive stimulation of the sympathetic nervous system. Midazolam or propofol may be useful for treating delirium tremens because their doses can be easily titrated to manage the symptoms.

APPLYING YOUR KNOWLEDGE 14-2
Although Mr. Wilson's acute intoxication may not require treatment, his chronic abuse of alcohol will result in the need for treatment of alcohol withdrawal symptoms. The physician prescribes a benzodiazepine. Why?

Drug therapy for maintenance of sobriety is limited, mainly because of poor compliance. The three drugs approved for this purpose are **acamprosate** (Campral), **disulfiram** (Antabuse), and **naltrexone** (ReVia). Acamprosate (Campral) helps to maintain abstinence in alcohol-dependent persons. It should be started as soon as possible after withdrawal has occurred and abstinence has been achieved. The drug is thought to act by decreasing the activity of glutamate, an excitatory neurotransmitter in the brain, and increasing the activity of gamma aminobutyric acid (GABA), an inhibitory neurotransmitter. It is excreted in urine as an unchanged drug. Dosage should be reduced with moderate renal impairment (creatine clearance 30–50 mL/minute) and is contraindicated with severe renal impairment (CrCl <30 mL/minute). Diarrhea is the most common adverse effect; most other effects (eg, insomnia, depression, anxiety) may also occur with alcohol withdrawal. Severe adverse effects are rare (<1%) and no significant drug–drug interactions have been identified. The drug may be taken without regard to food intake.

Disulfiram interferes with hepatic metabolism of alcohol and allows accumulation of acetaldehyde. If alcohol is ingested during disulfiram therapy, acetaldehyde causes nausea and vomiting, dyspnea, hypotension, tachycardia, syncope, blurred vision, headache, and confusion. Severe reactions include respiratory depression, cardiovascular collapse, cardiac dysrhythmias, myocardial infarction, congestive heart failure, unconsciousness, convulsions, and death. The reaction lasts as long as alcohol is present in the blood. Ingestion of prescription and over-the-counter medications that contain alcohol may cause a reaction in the disulfiram-treated alcoholic. Disulfiram alone may produce adverse reactions of drowsiness, fatigue, impotence, headache, and dermatitis. Disulfiram also interferes with the metabolism of phenytoin and warfarin, which may increase blood levels of the drugs and increase their toxicity. Because of these reactions, disulfiram must be given only with the client's full consent, cooperation, and knowledge.

Naltrexone is an opiate antagonist that reduces craving for alcohol and increases abstinence rates when combined with psychosocial treatment. A possible mechanism is blockade of the endogenous opioid system, which is thought to reinforce alcohol craving and consumption. The most common adverse effect is nausea; others include anxiety, dizziness, drowsiness, headache, insomnia, nervousness, and vomiting. Naltrexone is hepatotoxic in high doses and contraindicated in clients with acute hepatitis or liver failure.

In addition to drug therapy to treat withdrawal and maintain sobriety, alcohol abusers often need treatment of coexisting psychiatric disorders, such as depression. Antidepressant drugs seem to decrease alcohol intake as well as relieve depression.

APPLYING YOUR KNOWLEDGE 14-3

Preparations are being made for Mr. Wilson's discharge and outpatient therapy. He is prescribed Antabuse. Why is he given this drug, and what will he experience if he consumes alcohol while taking it?

Barbiturates and Benzodiazepines

Barbiturates are old drugs that are rarely used therapeutically but remain drugs of abuse. Overdoses may cause respiratory depression, coma, and death. Withdrawal is similar to alcohol withdrawal and may be more severe. Seizures and death can occur. With short-acting barbiturates such as pentobarbital (Nembutal) and secobarbital (Seconal), withdrawal symptoms begin 12 to 24 hours after the last dose and peak at 24 to 72 hours. With phenobarbital, symptoms begin 24 to 48 hours after the last dose and peak in 5 to 8 days.

Benzodiazepines are widely used for antianxiety and sedative-hypnotic effects (see Chap. 8) and are also widely abused, mainly by people who also abuse alcohol and/or other drugs. Benzodiazepines rarely cause respiratory depression or death, even in overdose, unless taken with alcohol or other drugs. They may, however, cause oversedation, memory impairment, poor motor coordination, and confusion. Withdrawal reactions can be extremely uncomfortable. Symptoms begin 12 to 24 hours after the last dose of a short-acting drug such as alprazolam (Xanax), and peak at 24 to 72 hours. With long-acting drugs such as diazepam and chlordiazepoxide, symptoms begin 24 to 48 hours after the last dose and peak within 5 to 8 days.

Combining any of these drugs with each other or with alcohol can cause serious depression of vital functions and death. Unfortunately, abusers often combine drugs in their quest for a greater "high" or to relieve the unpleasant effects of CNS stimulants and other street drugs.

Barbiturate or Benzodiazepine Dependence

This type of dependence resembles alcohol dependence in symptoms of intoxication and withdrawal. Other characteristics include physical dependence, psychological dependence, tolerance, and cross-tolerance. Signs and symptoms of withdrawal include anxiety, tremors and muscle twitching, weakness, dizziness, distorted visual perceptions, nausea and vomiting, insomnia, nightmares, tachycardia, weight loss, postural hypotension, generalized tonic-clonic seizures, and delirium that resembles the delirium tremens of alcoholism or a major psychotic episode. Convulsions are more likely to occur during the first 48 hours of withdrawal and delirium after 48 to 72 hours. Signs and symptoms of withdrawal are less severe with the benzodiazepines than with the barbiturates.

Treatment of Barbiturate or Benzodiazepine Dependence

Treatment may involve overdose and withdrawal syndromes. Overdose produces intoxication similar to that produced by alcohol. There may be a period of excitement and emotional lability followed by progressively increasing signs of CNS depression (eg, impaired mental function, muscular incoordination, sedation). Treatment is unnecessary for mild overdose if vital functions are adequate. The client usually sleeps off the effects of the drug. The rate of recovery depends primarily on the amount of drug ingested and its rate of metabolism. More severe overdoses cause respiratory depression and coma.

There is no antidote for barbiturate overdose; treatment is symptomatic and supportive. The goals of treatment are to maintain vital functions until the drug is metabolized and eliminated from the body. Insertion of an artificial airway and mechanical ventilation often are necessary.

For benzodiazepine overdose, a specific antidote is available to reverse sedation, coma, and respiratory depression. **Flumazenil** (Romazicon) competes with benzodiazepines for benzodiazepine receptors. The drug has a short duration of action, and repeated IV injections are usually needed. Recipients must be closely observed because symptoms of overdose may recur when the effects of a dose of flumazenil subside and because the drug may precipitate acute withdrawal symptoms (eg, agitation, confusion, seizures) in benzodiazepine abusers.

Treatment of withdrawal may involve administration of a benzodiazepine or phenobarbital to relieve acute signs and symptoms, then tapering the dose until the drug can be discontinued. Barbiturate and benzodiazepine withdrawal syndromes can be life threatening. The person may experience cardiovascular collapse, generalized tonic-clonic seizures, and acute psychotic episodes. These can be prevented by gradually withdrawing the offending drug. If they do occur, each situation requires specific drug therapy and supportive measures. Withdrawal reactions should be supervised and managed by experienced people, such as health care professionals or staff at detoxification centers.

Opioids

Opioids are potent analgesics and extensively used in pain management (see Chap. 6). They are also commonly abused. Legal opioid analgesics are increasingly being diverted from their appropriate use and bought and sold as street drugs. Because therapeutic opioids are discussed elsewhere, the focus here is heroin. Heroin, a semisynthetic derivative of morphine, is a common drug of abuse. It is a Schedule I drug in the United States and is not used therapeutically.

Heroin may be taken by IV injection, smoking, or nasal application (snorting). IV injection produces intense euphoria, which occurs within seconds, lasts a few minutes, and is followed by a period of sedation. Effects diminish over approximately 4 hours, depending on the dose. Addicts may inject several times daily, cycling between desired effects and symptoms of withdrawal. Tolerance to euphoric effects develops rapidly, leading to dosage escalation and continued use to avoid withdrawal. Like other opioids, heroin causes severe respiratory depression with overdose and produces a characteristic abstinence syndrome.

Opioid Dependence

Opioids produce tolerance and high degrees of psychological and physical dependence. Most other drugs that produce dependence do so with prolonged usage of large doses, but morphine-like drugs produce dependence with repeated administration of small doses. Medical usage of these drugs produces physical dependence and tolerance but rarely leads to use or abuse for mind-altering effects. Thus, "addiction" should not be an issue when the drugs are needed for pain management in clients with cancer or other severe illnesses.

Acute effects of opioid administration vary according to dosage, route of administration, and physical and mental characteristics of the user. They may produce euphoria, sedation, analgesia, respiratory depression, postural hypotension, vasodilation, pupil constriction, and constipation.

Treatment of Opioid Dependence

Treatment may be needed for overdose or withdrawal syndromes. Overdose may produce severe respiratory depression and coma. Insertion of an endotracheal tube and mechanical ventilation may be required. Drug therapy consists of an opioid antagonist to reverse opioid effects. Giving an opioid antagonist (eg, naloxone) can precipitate withdrawal symptoms. If there is no response to the opioid antagonist, the symptoms may be caused by depressant drugs other than opioids. In addition to profound respiratory depression, pulmonary edema, hypoglycemia, pneumonia, cellulitis, and other infections often accompany opioid overdose and require specific treatment measures.

Signs and symptoms of withdrawal can be reversed immediately by giving the drug producing the dependence. Therapeutic withdrawal, which is more comfortable and safer, can be managed by gradually reducing dosage over several days. Clonidine, a drug used mainly for hypertension, is sometimes used to relieve withdrawal symptoms associated with excessive stimulation of the sympathetic nervous system.

Ideally, the goal of treatment for opioid abuse is abstinence from further opioid usage. Because this goal is rarely met, long-term drug therapy may be used to treat heroin dependence. One method uses opioid substitutes to prevent withdrawal symptoms and improve a lifestyle that revolves around obtaining, using, and recovering from a drug. **Methadone** has long been used for this purpose, usually a single, daily oral dose given in a methadone clinic. Proponents say that methadone blocks euphoria produced by heroin, acts longer, and reduces preoccupation with drug use. This allows a more normal lifestyle for the client and reduces morbidity and mortality associated with the use of illegal and injected drugs. Also, because methadone is free, the heroin addict does not commit crimes to obtain drugs. Opponents say that methadone maintenance only substitutes one type of drug dependence for another. In addition, a substantial percentage of those receiving methadone maintenance therapy abuse other drugs, including cocaine.

A second treatment option is **naltrexone** (ReVia), an opioid antagonist that prevents opioids from occupying receptor sites and thereby prevents their physiologic effects. Used to maintain opioid-free states in the opioid addict, it is recommended for use in conjunction with psychological counseling to promote client motivation and compliance. If the client taking naltrexone has mild or moderate pain, nonopioid analgesics (eg, acetaminophen or a nonsteroidal anti-inflammatory drug) should be given. If the client has severe pain and requires an opioid, it should be given in a setting staffed and equipped for cardiopulmonary resuscitation because respiratory depression may be deeper and more prolonged than usual. In addition, clients needing elective surgery and opioid analgesics should be instructed to stop taking naltrexone at least 72 hours before the scheduled procedure.

CENTRAL NERVOUS SYSTEM STIMULANTS

Amphetamines and Related Drugs

Amphetamines and some related drugs (see Chap. 15) are used therapeutically for narcolepsy and attention deficit-hyperactivity disorder (ADHD). However, except for the use of methylphenidate (Ritalin) in treating ADHD, amphetamines are more important as drugs of abuse than therapeutic agents. The effects of amphetamines, including methamphetamine, are similar to those of cocaine. The drugs increase the activity of norepinephrine and dopamine by increasing their release, blocking their reuptake, and inhibiting the enzyme (monoamine oxidase) that normally metabolizes catecholamine neurotransmitters.

Methamphetamine is a widely available and abused amphetamine. It is often manufactured in illegal "meth labs." Ingredients for its manufacture were formerly readily available, but laws now restrict their purchase and possession. Methamphetamine is taken orally, by IV injection, and by inhalation (after chemical treatment to produce crystals, which are then heated and the vapors smoked or inhaled.). Inhalation or IV injection produces an intense, pleasurable sensation that lasts only a few minutes. Methamphetamine may be preferred over cocaine by many users because it has a longer duration of action.

Amphetamine-Type Dependence

Amphetamines and related drugs produce stimulation and euphoria; users often increase the amount and frequency of administration to reach or continue the state of stimulation. Psychological effects are similar to those produced by cocaine and are largely dose related. Small amounts produce mental alertness, wakefulness, and increased energy. Large amounts may cause psychosis (eg, hallucinations, paranoid delusions). Tolerance develops to amphetamines.

Acute ingestion of these drugs masks underlying fatigue or depression; withdrawal allows these conditions to emerge in an exaggerated form. The resulting exhaustion and depression reinforce the compulsion to continue using the drugs. Users may take them alone or to counteract the effects of other drugs. In the latter case, these drugs may be part of a pattern of polydrug use in which CNS depressants such as alcohol or sedative-type drugs ("downers") are alternated with CNS stimulants, such as amphetamines ("uppers").

Treatment of Amphetamine-Type Dependence

Treatment of amphetamine-type abuse is mainly concerned with overdosage because these drugs do not produce physical dependence and withdrawal as alcohol, opioids, and sedative-hypnotic drugs do. The client is likely to be hyperactive, agitated, and hallucinating (toxic psychosis) and may have tachycardia, fever, and other symptoms. Symptomatic treatment includes sedation, lowering of body temperature, and administration of an antipsychotic drug. Sedative-type drugs must be used with great caution, however, because depression and sleep usually follow amphetamine use, and these after-effects can be aggravated by sedative administration.

Cocaine

Cocaine is a popular drug of abuse. It produces strong CNS stimulation by preventing reuptake of catecholamine neurotransmitters (eg, dopamine, norepinephrine), which increases

and prolongs neurotransmitter effects. Its two main forms are cocaine hydrochloride powder and "crack." Crack is strong, inexpensive, and extremely addicting. It is prepared by altering cocaine hydrochloride with chemicals and heat to form rock-like formations of cocaine base. The process removes impurities and results in a very potent drug. Cocaine powder is commonly inhaled (snorted) through the nose; "crack" is heated and the vapors inhaled. Both forms are rapidly absorbed; peak blood levels are higher with "crack" than with cocaine powder. The effects of cocaine use are very short. The euphoria from smoking "crack" lasts about 5 to 10 minutes and that from snorting the powder may last 15 to 30 minutes. Cocaine is also metabolized and eliminated rapidly; the elimination half-life is about 1 hour.

In addition to intense euphoria, acute use of cocaine or "crack" produces increased energy and alertness, sexual arousal, tachycardia, increased blood pressure, and restlessness. High doses can cause cardiac dysrhythmias, convulsions, myocardial infarction, respiratory failure, stroke, and death, even in young, healthy adults and even with initial exposure. Either acute or chronic use produces numerous physiologic effects (Box 14-2). Cocaine withdrawal begins within hours of stopping drug use and lasts up to several days. Symptoms include depression (which may be profound), drowsiness, fatigue, and sleep disturbances (eg, nightmares).

Cocaine Dependence

Cocaine is not thought to produce physical dependence. However, the euphoria associated with intake and the depression and fatigue associated with stopping intake are believed to induce psychological dependence and compulsive use. Because cocaine effects are very brief, users often ingest the drug every few minutes as long as it is available. Crack cocaine reportedly can cause psychological dependence with one use.

Treatment of Cocaine Dependence

Drug therapy is largely symptomatic. Thus, agitation and hyperactivity may be treated with a benzodiazepine antianxiety agent; psychosis may be treated with **haloperidol** (Haldol) or another antipsychotic agent; cardiac dysrhythmias may be treated with usual antidysrhythmic drugs; myocardial infarction may be treated by standard methods; and so forth. Initial detoxification and long-term treatment are best accomplished in centers or units that specialize in substance-abuse disorders.

Long-term treatment of cocaine abuse usually involves psychotherapy, behavioral therapy, and 12-step programs. In addition, many clients need treatment for coexisting psychiatric disorders.

Nicotine

Nicotine, one of many active ingredients in tobacco products, is the ingredient that promotes compulsive use, abuse, and dependence. Inhaling smoke from a cigarette produces CNS

Box 14-2 Physiologic and Behavioral Effects of Cocaine Abuse

Central Nervous System Effects

Cerebral infarct, subarachnoid and other hemorrhages; excessive central nervous system stimulation, manifested by anxiety, agitation, delirium, hyperactivity, irritability, insomnia, anorexia, and weight loss; psychosis with paranoid delusions and hallucinations that may be indistinguishable from schizophrenia; seizures.

Cardiovascular Effects

Dysrhythmias, including tachycardia, premature ventricular contractions, ventricular tachycardia and fibrillation, and asystole; cardiomyopathy; myocardial ischemia and acute myocardial infarction; hypertension; stroke; rupture of the aorta; constriction of coronary and peripheral arteries.

Respiratory Effects

With snorting of cocaine, rhinitis, rhinorrhea, and damage (ulceration, perforation, necrosis) of the nasal septum from vasoconstriction and ischemia. With inhalation of crack cocaine vapors, respiratory symptoms occur in up to 25% of users and may include bronchitis, bronchospasm, cough, dyspnea, pneumonia, pulmonary edema, and fatal lung hemorrhage.

Gastrointestinal Effects

Nausea; weight loss; intestinal ischemia, possible necrosis.

Genitourinary Effects

Delayed orgasm for men and women; difficulty in maintaining erection.

---

stimulation in a few seconds. The average cigarette contains approximately 6 to 8 milligrams of nicotine and delivers approximately 1 milligram of nicotine systemically to the smoker (most is burned or dissipated as "sidestream" smoke). Nicotine obtained from chewing tobacco produces longer-lasting effects because it is more slowly absorbed than inhaled nicotine. Nicotine produces its effects by increasing levels of dopamine and other substances in the brain.

Nicotine is readily absorbed through the lungs, skin, and mucous membranes. It is extensively metabolized, mainly in the liver, and its metabolites are eliminated by the kidneys. It is also excreted in breast milk of nursing mothers. Adverse effects include nausea in new smokers at low blood levels and in experienced smokers at blood levels higher than their accustomed levels. Nicotine poisoning can occur in infants and children from ingestion of tobacco products, skin contact with used nicotine transdermal patches, or chewing nicotine gum. Poisoning may also occur with accidental ingestion of insecticide sprays containing nicotine. Oral ingestion usually causes vomiting, which limits the amount of nicotine absorbed. Toxic effects of a large dose may include hypertension, cardiac dysrhythmias, convulsions, coma, respiratory arrest, and paralysis of skeletal muscle. With chronic tobacco use, nicotine is implicated in the vascular disease and sudden cardiac death associated with smoking. However, the role of nicotine in the etiology of other disorders (eg, cancer, pulmonary disease) associated with chronic use of tobacco is unknown. Effects are summarized in Box 14-3.

Nicotine Dependence

Like alcohol and opiate dependence, nicotine dependence is characterized by compulsive use and the development of tolerance and physical dependence. Mental depression is also associated with nicotine dependence. It is unknown whether depression leads to smoking or develops concomitantly with nicotine dependence. Cigarette smokers may smoke to obtain the perceived pleasure of nicotine's effects, avoid the discomfort of nicotine withdrawal, or both. Evidence indicates a compulsion to smoke when blood levels of nicotine become low. Abstinence from smoking leads to signs and symptoms of withdrawal (eg, anxiety, irritability, difficulty concentrating, restlessness, headache, increased appetite, weight gain, sleep disturbances), which usually begin within 24 hours of the last exposure to nicotine.

Treatment of Nicotine Dependence

Most tobacco users who quit do so on their own. For those who are strongly dependent and unable or unwilling to quit on their own, there are two main methods of treatment. One method is the use of **bupropion,** an antidepressant (see Chap. 10). The antidepressant formulation is marketed as Wellbutrin; the smoking-cessation formulation is Zyban,

Box 14-3 Effects of Nicotine

Central Nervous System Effects

Central nervous system stimulation with increased alertness; possibly feelings of enjoyment; decreased appetite; tremors; convulsions at high doses.

Cardiovascular Effects

Cardiac stimulation with tachycardia, vasoconstriction, increased blood pressure, increased force of myocardial contraction, and increased cardiac workload.

Gastrointestinal Effects

Increases secretion of gastric acid; increases muscle tone and motility; nausea and vomiting; aggravates gastroesophageal and peptic ulcer disease.

a sustained-release tablet. The other method is nicotine replacement therapy with drug formulations of nicotine. These products prevent or reduce withdrawal symptoms, but they do not produce the subjective effects or peak blood levels seen with cigarettes.

Nicotine is available in transdermal patches, chewing gum, an oral inhaler, and a nasal spray. The gum, inhaler, and spray are used intermittently during the day; the transdermal patch is applied once daily. Transdermal patches produce a steady blood level of nicotine and clients seem to use them more consistently than they use the other products. The patches and gum are available over the counter; the inhaler and nasal spray require a prescription. The products are contraindicated in people with significant cardiovascular disease (angina pectoris, dysrhythmias, or recent myocardial infarction). Adverse effects include soreness of mouth and throat (with gum), nausea, vomiting, dizziness, hypertension, dysrhythmias, confusion, and skin irritation at sites of transdermal patch application.

Nicotine products are intended to be used for limited periods of 3 to 6 months, with tapering of dosage and discontinuation. Although they are effective in helping smokers achieve abstinence, many users resume smoking.

Overall, treatment regimens that combine counseling and behavioral therapy with drug therapy are more successful than those using drug therapy alone. In addition, a combination of Zyban and nicotine transdermal patches is sometimes used and may be more effective than either drug alone.

**APPLYING YOUR KNOWLEDGE 14-4:
HOW CAN THE NURSE AVOID THIS MEDICATION ERROR BY THE CLIENT?**

Mr. Wilson is given Zyban 150 mg PO for smoking cessation. He has been taken off the benzodiazepine and is on Antabuse 250 mg daily. After he no longer craves cigarettes, he stops taking all his medications.

Marijuana

Marijuana and other cannabis preparations are obtained from *Cannabis sativa,* the hemp plant, which grows in most parts of the world, including the entire United States. Marijuana and hashish are the two cannabis preparations used in the United States. Marijuana is obtained from leaves and stems; hashish, prepared from plant resin, is 5 to 10 times as potent as commonly available marijuana. These cannabis preparations contain several related compounds called *cannabinoids*. Delta-9-tetrahydrocannabinol (Δ-9-THC) is the main psychoactive ingredient, but metabolites and other constituents also may exert pharmacologic activity. The mechanism of action is unknown, although specific cannabinoid receptors have been identified in several regions of the brain. The endogenous substances that react with these receptors have not been determined.

Cannabis preparations are difficult to classify. Some people call them depressants; some call them stimulants; and others label them as mind-altering, hallucinogenic, psychotomimetic, or unique in terms of fitting into drug categories. It is also difficult to predict the effects of these drugs. Many factors apparently influence a person's response. One factor is the amount of active ingredients, which varies with the climate and soil where the plants are grown and with the method of preparation. Other factors include dose, route of administration, personality variables, and the environment in which the drug is taken.

Marijuana can be taken orally but is more often smoked and inhaled through the lungs. It is more potent and more rapid in its actions when inhaled. After smoking, subjective effects begin in minutes, peak in approximately 30 minutes, and last 2 to 3 hours. Low doses are mildly intoxicating and similar to small amounts of alcohol. Large doses can produce panic reactions and hallucinations similar to acute psychosis. Effects wear off as THC is metabolized to inactive products. Many physiologic effects (Box 14-4) and adverse reactions have been reported with marijuana use, including impaired ability to drive an automobile and perform other common tasks of everyday life.

Except for dronabinol (Marinol), marijuana and other cannabis preparations are illegal and not used therapeutically in most of the United States. Dronabinol, a formulation of Δ-9-THC, is used to treat nausea and vomiting associated

---

Box 14-4 Effects of Marijuana

Central Nervous System Effects
Impaired memory; perceptual and sensory distortions; disturbances in time perception; mood alteration; restlessness; depersonalization; panic reactions; paranoid ideation; impaired performance on cognitive, perceptual, and psychomotor tasks; drowsiness with high doses.

Cardiovascular Effects
Hypertension; bradycardia; peripheral vasoconstriction; orthostatic hypotension and tachycardia at high doses.

Respiratory Effects
Irritation and cellular changes in bronchial mucosa; bronchospasm; impaired gas exchange; aspergillosis in immunocompromised people; possibly increased risk of mouth, throat, and lung cancer (some known carcinogens are much higher in marijuana smoke than in tobacco smoke).

Musculoskeletal Effects
Ataxia; impaired coordination; increased reaction time.

Miscellaneous Effects
Constipation; decreased libido; thirst; decreased intraocular pressure.

with anticancer drugs and to stimulate appetite in clients with acquired immunodeficiency syndrome (AIDS). The risks of abuse are high, and the drug may cause physical and psychological dependence. It is a Schedule III controlled drug. Cannabinoids can also decrease intraocular pressure and may be useful in treating glaucoma. Some people promote legalization of marijuana for medical uses. However, clinicians state that such usage is no more effective than available legal treatments that have less abuse potential.

Marijuana Dependence and Treatment

Tolerance and psychological dependence do not usually develop with occasional use but may occur with chronic use; physical dependence rarely occurs. There is no specific treatment other than abstinence.

Hallucinogens

Hallucinogenic drugs include a variety of substances that cause mood changes, anxiety, distorted sensory perceptions, hallucinations, delusions, depersonalization, pupil dilation, elevated body temperature, and elevated blood pressure.

LSD

LSD (lysergic acid diethylamide) is a synthetic derivative of lysergic acid, a compound in ergot and some varieties of morning glory seeds. It is very potent, and small doses can alter normal brain functioning. LSD is usually distributed as a soluble powder and ingested in capsule, tablet, or liquid form. The exact mechanism of action is unknown, and effects cannot be predicted accurately. LSD alters sensory perceptions and thought processes; impairs most intellectual functions, such as memory and problem-solving ability; distorts perception of time and space; and produces sympathomimetic reactions, including increased blood pressure, heart rate, and body temperature, as well as pupil dilation. Adverse reactions include self-injury and possibly suicide, violent behavior, psychotic episodes, "flashbacks" (a phenomenon characterized by psychological effects and hallucinations that may recur days, weeks, or months after the drug is taken), and possible chromosomal damage resulting in birth defects.

Mescaline

Mescaline is an alkaloid of the peyote cactus. It is the least active of the commonly used psychotomimetic agents but produces effects similar to those of LSD. It is usually ingested in the form of a soluble powder or capsule.

Phencyclidine

Phencyclidine (PCP) produces excitement, delirium, hallucinations, and other profound psychological and physiologic effects, including a state of intoxication similar to that produced by alcohol; altered sensory perceptions; impaired thought processes; impaired motor skills; psychotic reactions; sedation and analgesia; nystagmus and diplopia; and pressor effects that can cause hypertensive crisis, cerebral hemorrhage, convulsions, coma, and death. Death from overdose also has occurred as a result of respiratory depression. Bizarre murders, suicides, and self-mutilations have been attributed to the schizophrenic reaction induced by PCP, especially in high doses. The drug also produces flashbacks.

PCP is usually distributed in liquid or crystal form and can be ingested, inhaled, or injected. It is usually sprayed or sprinkled on marijuana or herbs and smoked. Probably because it is cheap, easily synthesized, and readily available, PCP is often sold as LSD, mescaline, cocaine, or THC (the active ingredient in marijuana). It is also added to low-potency marijuana without the user's knowledge. Consequently, the drug user may experience severe and unexpected reactions, including death.

Hallucinogen Dependence

Tolerance develops, but there is no apparent physical dependence or abstinence syndrome. Psychological dependence probably occurs but is usually not intense. Users may prefer one of these drugs, but they apparently do without or substitute another drug if the one they favor is unavailable. A major danger with these drugs is their ability to impair judgment and insight, which can lead to panic reactions in which users may try to injure themselves (eg, by running into traffic).

Treatment of Hallucinogen Dependence

There is no specific treatment for hallucinogen dependence. Those who experience severe panic reactions may be kept in a safe, supportive environment until drug effects wear off, or may be given a sedative-type drug.

"Club" and "Date-Rape" Drugs

"Ecstasy," flunitrazepam (Rohypnol), gamma-hydroxybutyrate (GHB), and ketamine are reported to be widely and increasingly used, mainly by adolescents and young adults. The "club drug" designation stems from use at all-night dance parties called "raves"; the "date-rape drug" designation stems from reported use of these drugs in unaware females to facilitate sexual conquest.

Ecstasy

Ecstasy (3,4 methylenedioxy-methamphetamine or MDMA) is an illegal, Schedule I derivative of amphetamine. It is structurally similar to methamphetamine and mescaline and produces stimulant and hallucinogenic effects. MDMA first became popular with adolescents and young adults at "raves," but its use has spread to a variety of settings and age groups. It is usually taken orally, as a tablet, but it may be crushed and snorted or injected. Users report increased energy and perception, euphoria, and feelings of closeness to others. These effects occur within an hour after oral ingestion and last 4 to 6 hours.

Although users apparently think this is a safe drug, evidence indicates it is extremely dangerous. Adverse effects include acute psychiatric symptoms (eg, anxiety, panic, depression, paranoid thinking), cardiac dysrhythmias, coma, dehydration, delirium, hypertension, hyperthermia, hyponatremia, rhabdomyolysis, seizures, tachycardia, and death. These effects have occurred with a single use. Another major concern is the drug's neurotoxicity. Early effects include spasmodic jerking, involuntary jaw clenching, and teeth grinding. Long-term or permanent changes may result from damage to the nerve cells in the brain that use serotonin as a neurotransmitter. MDMA increases the release and inhibits reuptake of serotonin. This action floods the brain with high amounts of serotonin, which is important in emotion, mood, and memory. Chronic use of MDMA may deplete serotonin and lead to sadness or depression, insomnia, memory impairment, low energy or passivity, and a decreased ability to feel emotions or pleasure.

In addition to the many adverse effects of MDMA, users also need to be concerned about the actual product they are taking. There have been numerous reports of other drugs (eg, LSD, methamphetamine, ketamine, PCP) being sold as ecstasy. All of these drugs may have serious adverse effects as well.

MDMA is not thought to cause dependence or withdrawal syndromes. Emergency treatment of MDMA abuse usually involves decreasing the high body temperature, replacing fluids and electrolytes, and monitoring for cardiovascular complications.

Flunitrazepam (Rohypnol)

Flunitrazepam is a benzodiazepine (see Chap. 8) that is manufactured and used in Europe and other parts of the world. It is a Schedule I drug in the United States and has never been approved for any therapeutic use. The drug is usually taken orally, but the tablets are sometimes ground into a powder and snorted. Flunitrazepam is often taken with other drugs, including alcohol, cocaine, heroin, or marijuana. In addition to intentional use, the odorless and colorless drug has reportedly been added to punch and other drinks at fraternity parties and other social events, leading to its designation as a "date-rape" drug.

Even when flunitrazepam is taken alone in relatively low doses, the drug can cause muscle relaxation, general sedative and hypnotic effects, and the appearance of intoxication, with slurred speech, poor coordination, swaying, and bloodshot eyes. These effects begin within 30 minutes, peak within 2 hours, and may last 8 hours or longer, depending on dosage.

Other adverse effects include confusion, dizziness, drowsiness, hypotension, memory impairment, and visual disturbances. In high doses, flunitrazepam causes a loss of muscle control, loss of consciousness, and partial amnesia. Combining the drug with alcohol increases its adverse effects.

As with other benzodiazepines, flunitrazepam causes dependence. After dependence has developed, stopping the drug induces withdrawal symptoms such as extreme anxiety, confusion, headache, irritability, muscle pain, and restlessness. Cardiovascular collapse, convulsions, delirium, hallucinations, numbness and tingling of the extremities, and shock also may occur. Withdrawal seizures can occur a week or longer after stopping the drug. The main treatment for flunitrazepam dependence is gradually tapering and discontinuing the drug.

Gamma-Hydroxybutyrate (GHB)

GHB is a Schedule I controlled drug whose only approved use in the United States is for research. It is a CNS depressant that is structurally related to the inhibitory neurotransmitter, gamma-aminobutyric acid (GABA). Usage of GHB has increased in recent years, mainly in the party or dance-club setting, and is increasingly involved in poisonings, overdoses, date rapes, and fatalities. Some users admit they took the drug intentionally; some say the drug was added to their drinks without their knowledge or consent.

GHB is available in an odorless, colorless liquid or as a white powder and is taken orally, often combined with alcohol. Effects include drowsiness, respiratory depression, seizures, unconsciousness, and vomiting. As with other sedative drugs, respiratory depression leading to hypoxia and death is the most serious adverse effect. Treatment of acute toxicity is mainly symptomatic and supportive. Stopping the drug after chronic use causes withdrawal symptoms of severe agitation, mental status changes, elevated blood pressure, and tachycardia within hours of the last dose.

In addition to its use as a "club" or "date-rape" drug, GHB is sometimes used by body builders for alleged anabolic effects. Formerly sold in health food stores as a nutritional supplement with numerous claims of beneficial effects, the drug became a controlled drug in 2000 after serious illnesses and deaths were reported. However, precursor substances (that are converted to GHB in the body) are reportedly still available in gyms and health food stores as dietary supplements.

Ketamine

Ketamine is an anesthetic that is chemically related to PCP and used mainly by veterinarians. It has become a "recreational" drug and its effects are similar to those of PCP and LSD (eg, distorted senses and perceptions, dissociative reactions). The hallucinations produced by ketamine last about an hour, but the user's senses, judgment, coordination, and self-control may be impaired as long as 24 hours after the initial use of the drug. These effects produce a high risk of injuries.

Other effects include respiratory depression, heart rate abnormalities, and a withdrawal syndrome. Ketamine became a Schedule III controlled substance in 1999.

Ketamine is usually injected, but it may be taken orally, smoked, or swallowed. It is sometimes added to marijuana cigarettes. Effects include increased blood pressure, tachycardia, respiratory depression, airway obstruction, apnea, hypertonic muscles and movement disorders, and psychosis. With overdoses, seizures, polyneuropathy, increased intracranial pressure, respiratory arrest, and cardiac arrest may occur. With chronic use, flashbacks and other effects may last up to 2 years after stopping the drug. Long-term effects include tolerance and possibly physical and/or psychological dependence.

Volatile Solvents (Inhalants)

These drugs include acetone, toluene, and gasoline. These solvents may be constituents of some types of glue, plastic cements, aerosol sprays, and other products. Some general inhalation anesthetics, such as nitrous oxide, have also been abused to the point of dependence. Volatile solvents are most often abused by preadolescents and adolescents who squeeze glue into a plastic bag, for example, and sniff the fumes. Suffocation sometimes occurs when the sniffer loses consciousness while the bag covers the face.

These substances produce symptoms comparable with those of acute alcohol intoxication, including initial mild euphoria followed by ataxia, confusion, and disorientation. Some substances in gasoline and toluene also may produce symptoms similar to those produced by the hallucinogens, including euphoria, hallucinations, recklessness, and loss of self-control. Large doses may cause convulsions, coma, and death. Substances containing gasoline, benzene, or carbon tetrachloride are especially likely to cause serious damage to the liver, kidneys, and bone marrow.

These substances produce psychological dependence, and some produce tolerance. There is some question about whether physical dependence occurs. If it does occur, it is considered less intense than the physical dependence associated with alcohol, barbiturates, and opiates.

NURSING PROCESS

Assessment

Assess clients for signs of alcohol and other drug abuse, including abuse of prescription drugs such as antianxiety agents, opioids, and sedative-hypnotics. Some general screening-type questions are appropriate for any initial nursing assessment. The overall purpose of these questions is to determine whether a current or potential problem exists and whether additional information is needed. Some clients may refuse to answer or give answers that contradict other assessment data. Denial of excessive drinking and of problems resulting from alcohol use is a prominent characteristic of alcoholism; underreporting the extent of drug use is common in other types of drug abuse as well. Useful information includes each specific drug, the amount, the frequency of administration, and the duration of administration. If answers to general questions reveal problem areas, such as long-term use of alcohol or psychotropic drugs, more specific questions can be formulated to assess the scope and depth of the problem. It may be especially difficult to obtain needed information about illegal "street drugs," most of which have numerous, frequently changed names. For nurses who often encounter substance abusers, efforts to keep up with drug names and terminology may be helpful.

- Interview the client regarding alcohol and other drug use to help determine immediate and long-term nursing care needs. For example, information may be obtained that would indicate the likelihood of a withdrawal reaction; the risk of increased or decreased effects of a variety of drugs; and the client's susceptibility to drug abuse. People who abuse one drug are likely to abuse others, and abuse of multiple drugs is a more common pattern than abuse of a single drug. These and other factors aid effective planning of nursing care.
- Assess behavior that may indicate drug abuse, such as alcohol on the breath, altered speech patterns, staggering gait, hyperactivity or hypoactivity, and other signs of excessive CNS depression or stimulation. Impairments in work performance and in interpersonal relationships also may be behavioral clues.
- Assess for disorders that may be caused by substance abuse. These disorders may include infections, liver disease, accidental injuries, and psychiatric problems of anxiety or depression. These disorders may be caused by other factors, of course, and are nonspecific.
- Check laboratory reports, when available, for abnormal liver function test results, indications of anemia, abnormal white blood cell counts, abnormal electrolytes (hypocalcemia, hypomagnesemia, and acidosis are common in alcoholics), and alcohol and drug levels in the blood.

Nursing Diagnoses

Related nursing diagnoses may include

- Ineffective Coping related to reliance on alcohol or other drugs
- Risk for Injury: Adverse effects of abused drug(s)
- Disturbed Thought Processes related to use of psychoactive drugs
- Risk for Other- or Self-Directed Violence related to disturbed thought processes, impaired judgment, and impulsive behavior
- Imbalanced Nutrition: Less Than Body Requirements related to drug effects and drug-seeking behavior

- Dysfunctional Family Processes: Alcoholism
- Risk for Injury: Infection, hepatitis, or AIDS related to use of contaminated needles and syringes for IV drugs

Planning/Goals

- Safety will be maintained for clients impaired by alcohol and drug abuse.
- Information will be provided regarding drug effects and treatment resources.
- The client's efforts toward stopping drug usage will be recognized and reinforced.

Interventions

- Administer prescribed drugs correctly during acute intoxication or withdrawal.
- Decrease environmental stimuli for the person undergoing drug withdrawal.
- Record vital signs; cardiovascular, respiratory, and neurologic functions; mental status; and behavior at regular intervals.
- Support use of resources for stopping drug abuse (psychotherapy, treatment programs).
- Request client referrals to psychiatric/mental health physicians, nurse clinical specialists, or self-help programs when indicated.
- Use therapeutic communication skills to discuss alcohol or other drug-related health problems, health-related benefits of stopping substance use or abuse, and available services or treatment options (see Research Brief for smoking cessation information).
- Teach nondrug techniques for coping with stress and anxiety.
- Provide positive reinforcement for efforts toward quitting substance abuse.
- Inform smokers with young children in the home that cigarette smoke can precipitate or aggravate asthma and upper respiratory disorders in children.
- Inform smokers with nonsmoking spouses or other members of the household that secondhand smoke can increase the risks of cancer and lung disease in the nonsmokers as well as the smoker.
- For smokers who are concerned about weight gain if they quit smoking, emphasize that the health benefits of quitting far outweigh the disadvantages of gaining a few pounds, and discuss ways to control weight without smoking.

Evaluation

- Observe for improved behavior (eg, less impulsiveness, improved judgment and thought processes, commits no injury to self or others).

- Observe for use or avoidance of nonprescribed drugs while hospitalized.
- Interview to determine the client's insight into personal problems stemming from drug abuse.
- Verify enrollment in a treatment program.
- Observe for appropriate use of drugs to decrease abuse of other drugs.

RESEARCH BRIEF

Smoking Cessation

SOURCE:

Anthonisen, N. R., Skeans, M. A., Wise, R. A., et al. (2005). The effects of a smoking cessation intervention on 14.5 year mortality: A randomized clinical trial. *Annals of Internal Medicine, 142,* 233–239.

SUMMARY:

This study was part of the Lung Health Study, which involved 5887 volunteers at 10 sites in the United States and Canada. Subjects were smokers, 35 to 60 years of age, with mild to moderate airway obstruction. Individuals with serious disease, hypertension, obesity, or excessive alcohol intake were excluded. The intervention was a 10-week smoking cessation program that included physician encouragement and 12 group sessions using behavior modification and nicotine gum. The intervention group was compared with participants who received usual care. After 5 years, 21.7% of the intervention participants had stopped smoking, compared with 5.4% of the usual-care participants. After as long as 14.5 years of follow-up, all-cause mortality was significantly lower in the intervention group. The leading causes of death in the Lung Health Study were lung cancer and coronary heart disease (CHD), and smoking cessation was beneficial in both conditions. With CHD, studies have indicated reduced mortality rates within 2 years of smoking cessation; the mechanisms by which smoking contributes to CHD are apparently reversible to some extent in the short term. With lung cancer, smoking is thought to cause potentially irreversible genetic changes in epithelial cells; the effects of smoking cessation probably stem from the absence of further damage rather than from reversal of existing disease.

NURSING IMPLICATIONS:

This study provides additional evidence that nurses and other health care providers should themselves refrain from smoking, discourage adolescents and others from starting to smoke, and support smoking cessation efforts in any practice setting.

PRINCIPLES OF THERAPY

Prevention of Alcohol and Other Drug Abuse

Use measures to prevent substance abuse. Although there are difficulties in trying to prevent conditions for which causes are not known, some of the following community-wide and individual measures may be helpful:

- Decrease the supply or availability of commonly abused drugs. Most efforts at prevention have tried to reduce the supply of drugs. For example, laws designate certain drugs as illegal and provide penalties for possession or use of these drugs. Other laws regulate circumstances in which legal drugs, such as opioid analgesics, may be used. Also, laws regulate the sale of alcoholic beverages.

- Decrease the demand for drugs. Because this involves changing attitudes, it is very difficult but more effective in the long run. Many current attitudes seem to promote drug use, misuse, and abuse, including:
    - The belief that a drug is available for every mental and physical discomfort and should be taken in preference to tolerating even minor discomfort. Consequently, society has a permissive attitude toward taking drugs. Of course, there are many appropriate uses of drugs, and clients certainly should not be denied their benefits. The difficulties emerge when there is excessive reliance on drugs as chemical solutions to personal or social problems that are not amenable to chemical solutions.
    - The widespread acceptance and use of alcohol. In some groups, every social occasion is accompanied by alcoholic beverages of some kind.
    - The apparently prevalent view that drug abuse refers only to the use of illegal drugs and that using alcohol or prescription drugs, however inappropriately, does not constitute drug abuse.
    - The acceptance and use of illegal drugs in certain subgroups of the population. This is especially prevalent in high school and college students.

- Efforts to change attitudes and decrease demand for drugs can be made through education and counseling about such topics as drug effects and nondrug ways to cope with the stresses and problems of daily life.

- Each person must take personal responsibility for drinking alcoholic beverages and taking mind-altering drugs for the purpose of "getting high." Initially, conscious, voluntary choices are made to drink or not to drink, to take a drug or not to take it. This period varies somewhat, but drug dependence develops in most instances only after prolonged use. When mind-altering drugs are prescribed for a legitimate reason, the client must use them in prescribed doses and preferably for a short time.

- Physicians can help prevent drug abuse by prescribing drugs appropriately, prescribing mind-altering drugs in limited amounts and for limited periods, using nondrug measures when they are likely to be effective, educating clients about the drugs prescribed for them, participating in drug education programs, and recognizing, as early as possible, clients who are abusing or who are likely to abuse drugs. Some authorities recommend that physicians question all clients about smoking cigarettes and offer treatment when indicated.

- Nurses can help prevent drug abuse by administering drugs appropriately, using nondrug measures when possible, teaching clients about drugs prescribed for them, and participating in drug education programs. Some resources for information and educational materials include the following:

    National Institute on Drug Abuse
    6001 Executive Blvd
    Bethesda, MD 20892-9561
    Phone: (301) 443-1124
    www.nida.nih.gov
    National Clearinghouse for Alcohol and Drug
      Abuse Information (NCADI)
    Center for Substance Abuse Prevention
    5600 Fishers Lane
    Rockwall II
    Rockville, MD 20857
    Phone: (301) 443-0365
    E-Mail: nnadal@samhsa.gov
    www.health.org

- Parents can help prevent drug abuse in their children by minimizing their own use of drugs and by avoiding heavy cigarette smoking. Children are more likely to use illegal drugs if their parents have a generally permissive attitude about drug taking; if either parent takes mind-altering drugs regularly; and if either parent is a heavy cigarette smoker.

- Pregnant women should avoid alcohol, nicotine, and other drugs of abuse because of potentially harmful effects on the fetus.

Goals of Therapy

The major goals of treatment for substance abuse are detoxification, initiation of abstinence, and prevention of relapse. Clients who are likely to benefit from treatment are those who admit that substance abuse is causing significant problems in their ability to function in activities of daily living. Despite advances in treatment and the many adverse consequences of substance abuse, relapses to drug-taking behavior are common among those who have been detoxified or even abstinent for varying periods of time.

Treatment Measures for Substance Abuse

Treatment measures for alcohol and other drugs of abuse are not very successful. Even people who have been institutionalized and achieved a drug-free state for prolonged periods are apt to resume their drug-taking behavior when released from the institution. So far, voluntary self-help groups, such as Alcoholics Anonymous and Narcotics Anonymous, have been more successful than health professionals in dealing with drug abuse. Health professionals are more likely to be involved in acute situations, such as intoxication or overdose, withdrawal syndromes, or various medical-surgical conditions. As a general rule, treatment depends on the type, extent, and duration of drug-taking behavior and the particular situation for which treatment is needed. Some general management principles include the following:

- Psychological rehabilitation efforts should be part of any treatment program for a drug-dependent person. Several approaches may be useful, including psychotherapy, voluntary groups, and other types of emotional support and counseling. Substance abusers are assisted and encouraged to develop more healthful coping skills to deal with life stresses and to alter the environment or relationships in which substance use occurs. Much of this counseling is done by health care providers who specialize in treatment of drug dependence.
- Drug therapy is limited in treating drug dependence for several reasons. First, specific antidotes are available only for benzodiazepines (flumazenil) and opioid narcotics (naloxone). Second, there is a high risk of substituting one abused drug for another. Third, there are significant drawbacks to giving CNS stimulants to reverse effects of CNS depressants, and vice versa. Fourth, there is often inadequate information about the types and amounts of drugs taken.
- Despite these drawbacks, however, there are some clinical indications for drug therapy, including treatment of overdose or withdrawal syndromes. Even when drug therapy is indicated, there are few guidelines for optimal use. Doses, for example, must often be estimated initially and then titrated according to response. Drug therapy may be provided by primary care prescribers or prescribers who specialize in treatment of drug dependence.
- General care of clients with drug overdose is primarily symptomatic and supportive. The aim of treatment is usually to support vital functions, such as respiration and circulation, until the drug is metabolized and eliminated from the body. For example, respiratory depression from an overdose of a CNS depressant drug may be treated by inserting an artificial airway and mechanical ventilation. Removal of some drugs can be hastened by hemodialysis.
- Treatment of substance abuse may be complicated by the presence of other disorders. For example, depression and other psychiatric disorders are common.

APPLYING YOUR KNOWLEDGE: ANSWERS

14-1 The first step is for Mr. Wilson to realize he is abusing alcohol and other drugs. His cooperation in the treatment program is critical to his success. The program should consist of psychological counseling, referral to a self-help group, and drug therapy.

14-2 A benzodiazepine antianxiety agent is the drug of choice. This drug will help Mr. Wilson participate in his rehabilitation program and can be gradually reduced in dosage. Taking a benzodiazepine will provide Mr. Wilson with adequate sedation and will also have a significant anticonvulsant effect.

14-3 Antabuse is a drug that interferes with the metabolism of alcohol. If Mr. Wilson drinks alcohol while on Antabuse, he will experience nausea and vomiting, dyspnea, hypotension, tachycardia, syncope, blurred vision, headache, and confusion. Mr. Wilson must know what he is taking and cooperate with the treatment plan.

14-4 Mr. Wilson needs further instruction regarding his medication. He can stop taking the Zyban when he no longer craves nicotine; however, he must continue to take the Antabuse.

Review and Application Exercises

Short Answer Exercises

1. Why is it important to assess each client in relation to alcohol and other substance abuse?

2. What are the signs and symptoms of overdose with alcohol, benzodiazepine antianxiety or sedative-hypnotic agents, cocaine, and opiates?

3. What are general interventions for treatment of drug overdoses?

4. What are specific antidotes for opioid and benzodiazepine overdoses, and how are they administered?

5. Which commonly abused drugs may produce life-threatening withdrawal reactions if stopped abruptly?

6. How can severe withdrawal syndromes be prevented, minimized, or safely managed?

7. What are the advantages of treating substance abuse disorders in centers established for that purpose?

NCLEX-Style Questions

8. With CNS depressants, withdrawal symptoms include
   a. sleep
   b. muscle relaxation

c. euphoria

d. agitation

9. Compulsive drug use is attributed mainly to
   a. drug stimulation of the "reward" center in the brain
   b. a belief that the drugs are not harmful
   c. parental pressure to do well in school
   d. a permissive attitude toward taking drugs by parents and society

10. Flumazenil (Romazicon) is an antidote for over-doses of
    a. alcohol
    b. benzodiazepines
    c. opioids
    d. amphetamines

11. Overdosage of cocaine can cause
    a. severe lung damage
    b. anaphylaxis
    c. life-threatening cardiac dysrhythmias
    d. hypotension

12. Which of the following drug products can be used to aid smoking cessation?
    a. naltrexone (ReVia)
    b. disulfiram (Antabuse)
    c. bupropion (Zyban)
    d. clonidine (Catapres)

Selected References

Acute reactions to drugs of abuse. (2002, March 4). *The Medical Letter on Drugs and Therapeutics, 44*(1125), 21–24.

DerMarderosian, A. (Ed.). (2001). Marijuana. In *The review of natural products* (pp. 391–393). St. Louis: Facts and Comparisons.

Doering, P. L. (2002). Substance-related disorders: Alcohol, nicotine, and caffeine. In J. T. DiPiro, R. L. Talbert, G. C. Yee, G. R. Matzke, B. G. Wells, & L. M. Posey (Eds.), *Pharmacotherapy: A pathophysiologic approach* (5th ed., pp. 1203–1218). New York: McGraw-Hill.

Doering, P. L. (2002). Substance-related disorders: Overview and depressants, stimulants and hallucinogens. In J. T. DiPiro, R. L. Talbert, G. C. Yee, G. R. Matzke, B. G. Wells, & L. M. Posey (Eds.), *Pharmacotherapy: A pathophysiologic approach* (5th ed., pp. 1183–1202). New York: McGraw-Hill.

Enoch, M. A., & Goldman, D. (2002). Problem drinking and alcoholism: Diagnosis and treatment. *American Family Physician, 65*(3), 441–450.

Kenna, G. A., McGeary, J. E., & Swift, R. M. (2004). Pharmacotherapy, pharmacogenomics, and the future of alcohol dependence and treatment. *American Journal of Health-System Pharmacy, 61*(21), 2272–2279.

Lange, R. A., & Hillis, L. D. (2001). Cardiovascular complications of cocaine use. *New England Journal of Medicine, 345*(5), 351–358.

National Institute of Drug Abuse. (2004). *Research report series: MDMA abuse (Ecstasy).* Retrieved August 13, 2005, from http://www.drugabuse.gov

Porth, C. M. (2005). *Pathophysiology: Concepts of altered health states* (7th ed.). Philadelphia: Lippincott Williams & Wilkins.

Reynolds, E. W., & Bada, H. S. (2003). Pharmacology of drugs of abuse. *Obstetric & Gynecology Clinics of North America, 30,* 501–522.

Rhoades, R. A., & Tanner, G. A. (2003). *Medical physiology* (2nd ed.). Philadelphia: Lippincott Williams & Wilkins.

Samet, J. H. (2004). Drug abuse and dependence. In L. Goldman & D. Ausiello (Eds.), *Cecil textbook of medicine* (22nd ed., pp. 145–152). Philadelphia: W. B. Saunders.

Schwartz, R. H. (2002). Marijuana: A decade and a half later, still a crude drug with underappreciated toxicity. *Pediatrics, 109*(2), 284–289.

Smeltzer, S. C., & Bare, B. G. (2004). *Brunner & Suddarth's textbook of medical-surgical nursing* (10th ed.). Philadelphia: Lippincott Williams & Wilkins.

Central Nervous System Stimulants

After studying this chapter, you will be able to:

1. Describe general characteristics of central nervous system (CNS) stimulants.
2. Discuss reasons for decreased use of amphetamines for therapeutic purposes.
3. Discuss the rationale for treating attention deficit-hyperactivity disorder with CNS stimulants.
4. Identify effects and sources of caffeine.
5. Identify nursing interventions to prevent, recognize, and treat stimulant overdose.

APPLYING YOUR KNOWLEDGE

Kevin Granata was diagnosed with attention deficit-hyperactivity disorder at age 8. He is now 11 years old and a student at the school where you are the school nurse. As a result of taking methylphenidate (Ritalin) 15 mg daily and receiving individual counseling, Kevin's attention span and school performance improved.

Part of the annual school physical examination for all children is to track height and weight. Kevin's height is less than normal for his age group and he has lost weight since his examination last year. When you talk with his teachers, they report that he is restless in class and has an extremely short attention span. He has had more difficulty getting along with his classmates.

INTRODUCTION

Many drugs stimulate the central nervous system (CNS), but only a few are used therapeutically, and their indications for use are limited. Two disorders treated with CNS stimulants are narcolepsy and attention deficit-hyperactivity disorder (ADHD).

Narcolepsy

Narcolepsy is a sleep disorder characterized by daytime "sleep attacks" in which the person goes to sleep at any place or at any time. Signs and symptoms also include excessive daytime drowsiness, fatigue, muscle weakness and hallucinations at onset of sleep, and disturbances of nighttime sleep patterns. The hazards of drowsiness during normal waking hours and suddenly going to sleep in unsafe environments restrict activities of daily living.

Narcolepsy affects men and women equally and usually begins during the teenage or young-adult years. Its cause is unknown, and sleep studies are required for an accurate diagnosis. In addition to drug therapy, prevention of sleep deprivation, regular sleeping and waking times, avoiding shift work, and short naps may be helpful in reducing daytime sleepiness.

However, even apparently adequate amounts of nighttime sleep do not produce full alertness.

Attention Deficit-Hyperactivity Disorder

ADHD is reportedly the most common psychiatric or neurobehavioral disorder in children. It occurs before 7 years of age and is characterized by persistent hyperactivity, a short attention span, difficulty completing assigned tasks or schoolwork, restlessness, and impulsiveness. Such behaviors make it difficult for the child to get along with others (eg, family members, peer groups, teachers) and to function in situations requiring more controlled behavior (eg, classrooms).

Formerly, ADHD was thought to disappear with adolescence, but it is now believed to continue into adolescence and adulthood in one third to two thirds of clients. In adolescents and adults, impulsiveness and inattention continue, but hyperactivity is not a prominent feature. A major criterion for diagnosing later ADHD is a previous diagnosis of childhood ADHD. Some studies indicate that children with ADHD are more likely to have learning disabilities, mood disorders, and substance-abuse disorders as adolescents and adults. In addition, difficulties in structured settings such as school or work may continue.

GENERAL CHARACTERISTICS OF STIMULANTS

Most CNS stimulants act by facilitating initiation and transmission of nerve impulses that excite other cells. The drugs are somewhat selective in their actions at lower doses, but tend to involve the entire CNS at higher doses. The major groups are amphetamines and related drugs; analeptics; and xanthines. In addition, *atomoxetine* is a newer drug that acts selectively to inhibit reuptake of norepinephrine in nerve synapses. It is used in the treatment of ADHD.

Amphetamines increase the amounts of norepinephrine, dopamine, and possibly serotonin in the brain, thereby producing mood elevation or euphoria, increasing mental alertness and capacity for work, decreasing fatigue and drowsiness, and prolonging wakefulness. However, larger doses produce signs of excessive CNS stimulation, such as restlessness, hyperactivity, agitation, nervousness, difficulty concentrating on tasks, and confusion. Overdoses can produce convulsions and psychotic behavior. Amphetamines also stimulate the sympathetic nervous system, resulting in increased heart rate and blood pressure, pupil dilation (mydriasis), slowed gastrointestinal (GI) motility, and other symptoms. In ADHD, the drugs reduce behavioral symptoms and may improve cognitive performance.

Amphetamines are Schedule II drugs under the Controlled Substances Act and have a high potential for drug abuse and dependence. These drugs are widely sold on the street and commonly abused (see Chap. 14). *Amphetamine-related drugs* (methylphenidate and dexmethylphenidate) have essentially the same effects as the amphetamines and are also Schedule II drugs.

Analeptics are used infrequently (see doxapram and modafinil, below).

Xanthines stimulate the cerebral cortex, increasing mental alertness and decreasing drowsiness and fatigue. Other effects include myocardial stimulation with increased cardiac output and heart rate; diuresis; and increased secretion of pepsin and hydrochloric acid. Large doses can impair mental and physical functions by producing restlessness, nervousness, anxiety, agitation, insomnia, cardiac dysrhythmias, and gastritis.

Indications for Use

Amphetamines and methylphenidate are used in the treatment of narcolepsy and ADHD. Atomoxetine and dexmethylphenidate are indicated only for ADHD. Of the two analeptics, doxapram is used occasionally to treat respiratory depression, and modafinil is approved only for treatment of narcolepsy. Caffeine (a xanthine) is an ingredient in nonprescription analgesics and stimulants that promote wakefulness (eg, NoDoz). A combination of caffeine and sodium benzoate is occasionally used as a respiratory stimulant in neonates.

Contraindications to Use

CNS stimulants cause cardiac stimulation and thus are contraindicated in clients with cardiovascular disorders (eg, angina, dysrhythmias, hypertension) that are likely to be aggravated by the drugs. They also are contraindicated in clients with anxiety or agitation, glaucoma, or hyperthyroidism. They are usually contraindicated in clients with a history of drug abuse.

INDIVIDUAL DRUGS

Individual drugs are described below. Dosages are listed in Table 15-1.

Amphetamines and Related Drugs

P **Amphetamine, dextroamphetamine** (Dexedrine), and **methamphetamine** (Desoxyn) are closely related drugs that share characteristics of the amphetamines as a group. They are more important as drugs of abuse than as therapeutic agents.

Methylphenidate (eg, Ritalin) is chemically related to amphetamines and produces similar actions and adverse effects. It is well absorbed after oral administration. In children, peak plasma levels occur in about 2 hours with immediate-release tablets and in about 5 hours with extended-release tablets. Half-life is 1 to 3 hours, but pharmacologic effects last 4 to 6 hours. The drug is mostly metabolized in the liver and excreted in the urine.

Dexmethylphenidate (Focalin) is very similar to methylphenidate and the amphetamines. It is well absorbed after oral administration and reaches peak plasma levels in 1 to 1.5 hours. It is metabolized in the liver and excreted in urine.

Analeptics

Doxapram (Dopram) is occasionally used by anesthesiologists and pulmonary specialists as a respiratory stimulant. Although it increases tidal volume and respiratory rate, it also increases oxygen consumption and carbon dioxide production. Limitations include a short duration of action (5–10 minutes after a single intravenous [IV] dose) and therapeutic dosages near or the same as those that produce convulsions. Endotracheal intubation and mechanical ventilation are safer and more effective in relieving respiratory depression from depressant drugs or other causes.

Modafinil (Provigil) is used to treat narcolepsy. Its ability to promote wakefulness is similar to that of amphetamines and methylphenidate, but its mechanism of action is unknown. Like other CNS stimulants, it also has psychoactive and euphoric effects that alter mood, perception, and thinking. It is a Schedule IV controlled drug. It is rapidly absorbed (food may delay absorption), reaches peak plasma levels in 2 to 4 hours, is 60% bound to plasma proteins, and is 90% metabolized by the liver to metabolites that are then excreted in

Table 15-1 Drugs at a Glance: Central Nervous System Stimulants

GENERIC/TRADE NAME	INDICATIONS FOR USE	ROUTES AND DOSAGE RANGES	
		Adults	Children
Amphetamines			
P Amphetamine	Narcolepsy ADHD	Narcolepsy: PO 5–60 mg/d in divided doses	Narcolepsy: ≥6 y: PO 5 mg/d initially, increased by 5 mg/d at weekly intervals to effective dose ADHD: 3–5 y: PO 2.5 mg/d initially, increased by 2.5 mg/d at weekly intervals until response; ≥6 y: PO 5 mg once or twice daily initially, increased by 5 mg/d at weekly intervals until optimal response (usually no more than 40 mg/d)
Dextroamphetamine (Dexedrine)	Narcolepsy ADHD	Narcolepsy: PO 5–60 mg/d in divided doses	Narcolepsy: ≥6 y: PO 5 mg/d initially, increased by 5 mg/d at weekly intervals to effective dose ADHD: 3–5 y: PO 2.5 mg/d initially, increased by 2.5 mg/d at weekly intervals until optimal response; ≥6 y: PO 5 mg once or twice daily initially, increased by 5 mg/d at weekly intervals until optimal response (usually no more than 40 mg/d)
Methamphetamine (Desoxyn)	ADHD in children		PO 5–10 mg daily initially. Usual dose, 15–25 mg daily, in 2 divided doses
Amphetamine mixture (Adderall)	ADHD Narcolepsy	Narcolepsy: PO 10 mg/d initially, increased if necessary	≥6y: ADHD, PO 5 mg 1–2 times daily, increased if necessary
Amphetamine-Related Drugs			
Dexmethylphenidate (Focalin)	ADHD		PO 2.5–10 mg twice daily
Methylphenidate (Ritalin, Ritalin SR, Concerta, Metadate, Metadate CD, Metadate ER)	ADHD Narcolepsy	Narcolepsy: PO 10–60 mg/d in 2 or 3 divided doses	≥6 y: ADHD, PO 5 mg twice a day initially, increase by 5–10 mg at weekly intervals to a maximum of 60 mg/d if necessary
Analeptics			
Doxapram (Dopram)		IV 0.5–1.5 mg/kg in single or divided doses; IV continuous infusion 5 mg/min initially, decreased to 2.5 mg/min or more. Dose by infusion should not exceed 3 g.	
Modafinil (Provigil)	Narcolepsy	PO 200 mg once daily, in the morning. Dosage should be reduced by 50% with severe hepatic impairment.	Dosage not established for children <16 years of age

(continued)

Table 15-1 Drugs at a Glance: Central Nervous System Stimulants (continued)

GENERIC/TRADE NAME	INDICATIONS FOR USE	ROUTES AND DOSAGE RANGES	
		Adults	Children
Other			
Atomoxetine (Strattera)	ADHD	PO 40 mg/d initially, increased after 3 d to 80 mg daily; given as a single dose in the morning or as 2 divided doses in morning and early evening	Weight ≤70 kg: PO 0.5 mg/ kg/d, increased after 3 d to approximately 1.2 mg/ kg/d; given as a single dose in the morning or as 2 divided doses in morn- ing and early evening

ADHD, attention deficit-hyperactivity disorder; IV, intravenous; PO, oral.

urine. Steady-state concentrations are reached in 2 to 4 days, and half-life with chronic use is about 15 hours.

Modafinil is not recommended for clients with a history of left ventricular hypertrophy or ischemic changes on electro-cardiograms. Adverse effects include anxiety, chest pain, dizziness, dyspnea, dysrhythmias, headache, nausea, nervous-ness, and palpitations. Dosage should be reduced by 50% in clients with severe hepatic impairment. The effects of severe renal impairment are unknown.

Xanthines

Caffeine has numerous pharmacologic actions, including CNS stimulation, diuresis, hyperglycemia, cardiac stimulation, coronary and peripheral vasodilation, cerebrovascular vaso-constriction, skeletal muscle stimulation, increased secretion of gastric acid and pepsin, and bronchodilation from relaxation of smooth muscle. In low to moderate amounts, caffeine increases alertness and capacity for work and decreases fatigue. Large amounts cause excessive CNS stimulation with anxiety, agita-tion, diarrhea, insomnia, irritability, nausea, nervousness, pre-mature ventricular contractions, hyperactivity and restlessness, tachycardia, tremors, and vomiting. Toxic amounts may cause delirium and seizures. With large amounts or chronic use, caf-feine has been implicated as a causative or aggravating factor in cardiovascular disease (hypertension, dysrhythmias); GI dis-orders (esophageal reflux, peptic ulcers); reproductive dis-orders; osteoporosis (may increase loss of calcium in urine); carcinogenicity; psychiatric disturbances; and drug-abuse lia-bility. Caffeine produces tolerance to its stimulating effects, and psychological dependence or habituation occurs.

Pharmaceutical preparations include an oral preparation and a solution for injection. Caffeine is usually prescribed as caffeine citrate for oral use and as caffeine and sodium ben-zoate for parenteral use because these forms are more soluble than caffeine itself. Caffeine is an ingredient in some nonpre-scription analgesic preparations and may increase analgesia. It is combined with an ergot alkaloid to treat migraine head-aches (eg, Cafergot) and is the active ingredient in nonpre-scription stimulant (antisleep) preparations. A combination of caffeine and sodium benzoate is used as a respiratory stimu-lant in neonatal apnea unresponsive to other therapies.

Caffeine is a frequently consumed CNS stimulant world-wide, and most is consumed from dietary sources (eg, coffee, tea, soft drinks). The caffeine content of coffee and tea bever-ages is determined by the particular coffee bean or tea leaf and the method of preparation. Caffeine is added to about 70% of the soft drinks ingested in the United States. Oral caffeine is rapidly absorbed from the GI tract; it produces peak blood lev-els within 30 to 45 minutes and crosses the blood–brain bar-rier easily. Its half-life is about 3.5 to 5 hours. It is extensively metabolized in the liver and excreted mainly in urine.

Because of the widespread ingestion of caffeine-containing beverages and the wide availability of over-the-counter prod-ucts that contain caffeine, toxicity may result from concomitant consumption of caffeine from several sources. Some authorities recommend that normal, healthy, nonpregnant adults consume no more than 250 milligrams of caffeine daily. Sources and amounts of caffeine are summarized in Table 15-2.

Theophylline preparations are xanthines used in the treat-ment of respiratory disorders, such as asthma and bronchitis. In these conditions, the desired effect is bronchodilation and improvement of breathing; CNS stimulation is then an adverse effect (see Chap. 44).

Atomoxetine

Atomoxetine (Strattera) is approved only for the treatment of ADHD. It has a low risk of abuse and dependence compared with the other drugs used for ADHD. It is not a controlled drug. Atomoxetine is rapidly absorbed with oral administration, with peak plasma levels in 1 to 2 hours. It is highly protein bound (98%) and elimination half-life is about 5 hours. Atomoxetine is metabolized in the liver by cytochrome P450 enzymes 2D6 and 2C19, and is excreted mainly in urine. Dosage should be reduced by 50% with moderate hepatic insufficiency and by 75% with severe hepatic insufficiency. The drug may be taken with or without food. Adverse effects that reportedly occur in more than 10% of users include abdominal pain, anorexia, cough, dry mouth, headache, insomnia, nausea, and vomiting.

TABLE 15-2 Sources of Caffeine

SOURCE	AMOUNT (oz)	CAFFEINE (mg)	REMARKS
Coffee			
Brewed, regular	5–8	40–180	Caffeine content varies with product and preparation.
Instant	5–8	30–120	
Espresso	2	120	
Tea			
Brewed, leaf or bag	8	80	Caffeine content varies with product and preparation.
Instant	8	50	
Iced	12	70	
Soft Drinks			
Coke, Diet Coke	12	45	Most other cola drinks contain 35–45 mg/12 oz.
Pepsi, Diet Pepsi	12	38	
Mountain Dew	12	54	
OTC Analgesics			
Anacin, Vanquish	1 tablet or caplet	32–33	
APAP-Plus, Excedrin, Midol	1 tablet, caplet, or geltab	60–65	
OTC Antisleep Products			
Caffedrine, NoDoz, Vivarin	1 tablet or capsule	200	
OTC Diuretic			
Aqua-Ban	1 tablet	100	Recommended dosage: 2 tablets 3 times daily (600 mg/d)
Prescription Drugs			
Cafergot	1 tablet	100	Recommended dosage: 2 tablets at onset of migraine, then 1 tablet every hour if needed, up to 6 tablets (600 mg/attack)
Fiorinal	1 capsule	40	Recommended dosage: 1–2 capsules every 4 hours, up to 6 capsules/d (240 mg/d) Also contains butalbital, a barbiturate, and is a Schedule III controlled drug

OTC = over-the-counter.

Herbal and Dietary Supplements

Guarana is made from the seeds of a South American shrub. The main active ingredient is caffeine, which is present in greater amounts than in coffee beans or dried tea leaves. Guarana is widely used as a source of caffeine by soft-drink manufacturers. It is also used as a flavoring agent and is an ingredient in herbal stimulant and weight-loss products, energy drinks, vitamin supplements, candies, and chewing gums. The product, which may also contain theophylline and theobromine, is also available in teas, extracts, elixirs, capsules, and tablets of various strengths. In general, the caffeine content of a guarana product is unknown, and guarana may not be listed as an ingredient. As a result, consumers may not know how much caffeine they are ingesting in products containing guarana.

As with caffeine from other sources, guarana may cause excessive nervousness and insomnia. It is contraindicated during pregnancy and lactation and should be used cautiously, if at all, in people who are sensitive to the effects of caffeine or who have cardiovascular disease. Overall, the use of guarana as a CNS stimulant and weight-loss aid is not recommended and should be discouraged.

NURSING PROCESS

Assessment

- Assess use of stimulant and depressant drugs (prescribed, over-the-counter, or street drugs).
- Assess caffeine intake as a possible cause of nervousness, insomnia, or tachycardia, alone or in combination with other CNS stimulants.
- Try to identify potentially significant sources of caffeine.

- Assess for conditions that are aggravated by CNS stimulants.
- For a child with possible ADHD, assess behavior as specifically and thoroughly as possible.
- For any client receiving amphetamines or methylphenidate, assess behavior for signs of tolerance and abuse.

Nursing Diagnoses

- Sleep Pattern Disturbance related to hyperactivity, nervousness, insomnia
- Risk for Injury: Adverse drug effects (excessive cardiac and CNS stimulation, drug dependence)
- Deficient Knowledge: Drug effects on children and adults
- Noncompliance: Overuse of drug

Planning/Goals

The client will
- Take drugs safely and accurately
- Improve attention span and task performance (children and adults with ADHD) and decrease hyperactivity (children with ADHD)
- Have fewer sleep episodes during normal waking hours (for clients with narcolepsy)

Interventions

- For a child receiving a CNS stimulant, assist parents in scheduling drug administration and drug holidays (eg, weekends, summers) to increase beneficial effects and help prevent drug dependence and stunted growth.
- Record weight at least weekly.
- Promote nutrition to avoid excessive weight loss.
- Provide information about the condition for which a stimulant drug is being given and the potential consequences of overusing the drug (see accompanying Client Teaching Guidelines).

Evaluation

- Ask parents and teachers of children with ADHD to report on behavior and academic performance.
- For adolescents and adults with ADHD, ask the client or family about the client's ability to function in work, school, or social environments.
- Assess for decreased inappropriate sleep episodes in clients with narcolepsy.

PRINCIPLES OF THERAPY

Goals of Therapy

The main goal of therapy with CNS stimulants is to relieve symptoms of the disorders for which they are given. A secondary goal is to have clients use the drugs appropriately. Stimulants are often misused and abused by people who want to combat fatigue and delay sleep, such as long-distance drivers, students, and athletes. Use of amphetamines or other

---

CLIENT TEACHING GUIDELINES

Methylphenidate and Dexmethylphenidate

General Considerations

✔ These drugs may mask symptoms of fatigue, impair physical coordination, and cause dizziness or drowsiness. Use caution while driving or performing other tasks requiring alertness.

✔ Notify a health care provider of nervousness, insomnia, heart palpitations, vomiting, fever, or skin rash. These are adverse drug effects and dosage may need to be reduced.

✔ Avoid other central nervous system stimulants, including caffeine.

✔ Record weight at least weekly; report excessive losses.

✔ The drugs may cause weight loss; caloric intake (of nutritional foods) may need to be increased, especially in children.

✔ Take these drugs only as prescribed. These drugs have a high potential for abuse. The risks of drug dependence are lessened if they are taken correctly.

✔ Get adequate rest and sleep. Do not take stimulant drugs to delay fatigue and sleep; these are normal, necessary resting mechanisms for the body.

✔ Prevent nervousness, anxiety, tremors, and insomnia from excessive caffeine intake by decreasing consumption of coffee and other caffeine-containing beverages or by drinking decaffeinated coffee, tea, and cola. Sprite and 7-Up have no caffeine.

Self-Administration and Administration to Children

✔ Take regular tablets approximately 30 to 45 minutes before meals. Take the last dose of the day in the afternoon, before 6 P.M., to avoid interference with sleep.

✔ Ritalin SR, Concerta, Metadate CD, and Metadate ER are long-acting forms of methylphenidate. They should be swallowed whole, without crushing or chewing.

✔ If excessive weight loss, nervousness, or insomnia develops, ask the prescribing physician if the dose can be reduced or taken on a different schedule to relieve these adverse effects.

stimulants for this purpose is not justified. These drugs are dangerous for drivers and those involved in similar activities, and have no legitimate use in athletics. Methylphenidate has become a drug of abuse.

APPLYING YOUR KNOWLEDGE 15-1
A teacher comes to the health office and tells to you that he has observed Kevin selling his methylphenidate to the star soccer player for the school. What advice will you give to this teacher, and what obligation do you have regarding Kevin's personal health information?

Drug Dosage

When any CNS stimulant is prescribed, the smallest effective dose should be given, and the number of doses that can be obtained with one prescription should be limited. This action reduces the likelihood of drug dependence or diversion (drug use by people for whom the drug is not prescribed).

Toxicity: Recognition and Management

Overdoses may occur with acute or chronic ingestion of large amounts of a single stimulant; combinations of stimulants; or concurrent ingestion of a stimulant and another drug that slows the metabolism of the stimulant. Signs of toxicity may include severe agitation, cardiac dysrhythmias, combativeness, confusion, delirium, hallucinations, high body temperature, hyperactivity, hypertension, insomnia, irritability, nervousness, panic states, restlessness, tremors, seizures, coma, circulatory collapse, and death.

Treatment is largely symptomatic and supportive. In general, place the client in a cool room, monitor cardiac function and body temperature, and minimize external stimulation. Activated charcoal (1 g/kg body weight) may be given. With amphetamines, urinary acidification, IV fluids, and IV diuretics (eg, furosemide, mannitol) hasten drug excretion. IV diazepam or lorazepam may be given to control agitation, hyperactivity, or seizures, and haloperidol may be given to control symptoms of psychosis. If cardiovascular collapse occurs, fluid replacement and vasopressors may be used. If a long-acting form of the stimulant drug has been ingested, saline cathartics may be useful to remove undissolved drug granules.

With caffeine, ingestion of 15 to 30 milligrams per kilogram of body weight (eg, 1–2 g for a person weighing 70 kg [150 lb]) may cause myocardial irritability, muscle tremors or spasms, and vomiting. Oral doses of 5 grams or more may cause death. Signs of toxicity are correlated with serum levels of caffeine. Several cups of coffee may produce levels of 5 to 10 micrograms per milliliter and symptoms of agitation and tremors. Cardiac dysrhythmias and seizures occur at higher levels. Additional manifestations of caffeine toxicity include opisthotonus, decerebrate posturing, muscle hypertonicity, rhabdomyolysis with subsequent renal failure, pul-

monary edema, hyperglycemia, hypokalemia, leukocytosis, ketosis, and metabolic acidosis.

Treatment is symptomatic and supportive, with activated charcoal if indicated. IV diazepam or lorazepam may be used to control seizures. Hemodialysis is indicated if the serum caffeine concentration is >100 micrograms per milliliter or if life-threatening seizures or cardiac dysrhythmias occur.

APPLYING YOUR KNOWLEDGE 15-2
Kevin comes to the health office complaining that his heart is racing. He is very agitated and has tremors of his hands. What action should you initiate?

Effects of Central Nervous System Stimulants on Other Drugs

Caffeine may increase adverse effects of clozapine and theophylline by decreasing their metabolism and increasing their blood levels. It may increase effects of aspirin by increasing aspirin absorption. It may decrease effects of lithium by increasing lithium clearance. **Dexmethylphenidate** and **methylphenidate** may increase effects of phenytoin and antidepressants (selective serotonin reuptake inhibitors and tricyclics), and they may decrease effects of antihypertensive drugs. **Modafinil** may increase effects of clomipramine, phenytoin, tricyclic antidepressants, and warfarin. It may decrease effects of cyclosporine and oral contraceptives. **Atomoxetine** may increase the effects of drugs that stimulate cardiovascular function (eg, increase heart rate and blood pressure).

Use in Special Populations

Use in Children

CNS stimulants are not recommended for ADHD in children younger than 3 years of age. When used, dosage should be carefully titrated and monitored to avoid excessive CNS stimulation, anorexia, and insomnia. Suppression of weight and height has been reported, and growth should be monitored at regular intervals during drug therapy. In children with psychosis or Tourette's syndrome, CNS stimulants may exacerbate symptoms.

In ADHD, careful documentation of baseline symptoms over approximately 1 month is necessary to establish the diagnosis and evaluate outcomes of treatment. This can be done with videotapes of behavior, observations and ratings by clinicians familiar with ADHD, and by interviewing the child, parents, or caretakers. Some authorities believe that this condition is overdiagnosed and that stimulant drugs are prescribed unnecessarily. Guidelines for treatment of ADHD include the following:

- Counseling and psychotherapy (eg, parental counseling, family therapy) are recommended along with drug therapy for effective treatment and realistic expectations of outcomes.

- Young children may not require treatment until starting school. Then, the goal of drug therapy is to control symptoms, facilitate learning, and promote social development.

- Drug therapy is indicated when symptoms are moderate to severe; are present for several months; and interfere in social, academic, or behavioral functioning. When possible, drug therapy should be omitted or reduced in dosage when children are not in school (eg, weekends, vacations).

- Methylphenidate has been the most commonly used drug; the roles of dexmethylphenidate and atomoxetine are not clearly delineated. Methylphenidate is usually given daily, including weekends, for the first 3 to 4 weeks of treatment to allow caregivers to assess beneficial and adverse effects. Desirable effects may include improvement in behavior, attention span, and quality and quantity of school work, and better relationships with other children and family members. Adverse effects include appetite suppression and weight loss, which may be worse during the first 6 months of therapy.

- Drug holidays (stopping drug administration) are controversial. Some clinicians say they are indicated only if no significant problems occur during the drug-free period and that drug holidays are not recommended for most children. Other clinicians believe they are desirable when children are not in school (eg, summer) and are necessary periodically to re-evaluate the child's condition. Dosage adjustments are often needed at least annually as the child grows and hepatic metabolism slows. In addition, the drug-free periods decrease weight loss and growth suppression.

APPLYING YOUR KNOWLEDGE 15-3
What might be a drug-related reason for Kevin's weight loss? How would you instruct Kevin on the appropriate way to take his medication?

Use in Older Adults

CNS stimulants should be used cautiously in older adults. As with most other drugs, slowed metabolism and excretion increase the risks of accumulation and toxicity. Older adults are likely to experience anxiety, nervousness, insomnia, and mental confusion from excessive CNS stimulation. In addition, older adults often have cardiovascular disorders (eg, angina, dysrhythmias, hypertension) that may be aggravated by the cardiac-stimulating effects of the drugs, including dietary caffeine. In general, reduced doses are safer in older adults.

N U R S I N G   A C T I O N S

Central Nervous System Stimulants

NURSING ACTIONS	RATIONALE/EXPLANATION
1. Administer accurately	
a. Give amphetamines and methylphenidate early in the day, at least 6 hours before bedtime.	To avoid interference with sleep. If insomnia occurs, give the last dose of the day at an earlier time or decrease the dose.
b. For children with attention deficit-hyperactivity disorder (ADHD), give amphetamines and methylphenidate about 30 minutes before meals.	To minimize the drugs' appetite-suppressing effects and risks of interference with nutrition and growth
c. Do not crush or open and instruct clients not to bite or chew long-acting forms of methylphenidate (Concerta, Metadate CD, Metadate ER, Ritalin SR).	Breaking the tablets or capsules destroys the extended-release feature and allows the drug to be absorbed faster. An overdose may result.
d. Give atomoxetine with or without food.	
2. Observe for therapeutic effects	Therapeutic effects depend on the reason for use.
a. Fewer "sleep attacks" with narcolepsy	
b. Improved behavior and performance of cognitive and psycho-motor tasks with ADHD	
c. Increased mental alertness and decreased fatigue	
3. Observe for adverse effects	Adverse effects may occur with acute or chronic ingestion of any CNS stimulant drugs.
a. Excessive central nervous system (CNS) stimulation— hyperactivity, nervousness, insomnia, anxiety, tremors, convulsions, psychotic behavior	These reactions are more likely to occur with large doses.

NURSING ACTIONS	RATIONALE/EXPLANATION
b. Cardiovascular effects—tachycardia, other dysrhythmias, hypertension	These reactions are caused by the sympathomimetic effects of the drugs.
c. Gastrointestinal effects—anorexia, gastritis, weight loss, nausea, diarrhea, constipation	
4. Observe for drug interactions	
a. Drugs that *increase* the effects of CNS stimulants:	
(1) Other CNS stimulant drugs	Such combinations are potentially dangerous and should be avoided or minimized.
(2) Albuterol and related antiasthmatic drugs, pseudo-ephedrine	These drugs cause CNS- and cardiac-stimulating effects.
b. Drugs that *decrease* effects of CNS stimulants:	
(1) CNS depressants	IV diazepam or lorazepam may be used to decrease agitation, hyper-activity, and seizures occurring with stimulant overdose.
c. Drugs that *increase* effects of amphetamines:	
(1) Alkalinizing agents (eg, antacids)	Drugs that increase the alkalinity of the gastrointestinal tract increase intestinal absorption of amphetamines, and urinary alkalinizers decrease urinary excretion. Increased absorption and decreased excretion serve to potentiate drug effects.
(2) Monoamine oxidase (MAO) inhibitors	Potentiate amphetamines by slowing drug metabolism. These drugs thereby increase the risks of headache, subarachnoid hemorrhage, and other signs of a hypertensive crisis. The combination may cause death and should be avoided.
d. Drugs that *decrease* effects of amphetamines:	
(1) Acidifying agents	Urinary acidifying agents (eg, ammonium chloride) increase urinary excretion and lower blood levels of amphetamines. Decreased absorption and increased excretion serve to decrease drug effects.
(2) Antipsychotic agents	Decrease or antagonize the excessive CNS stimulation produced by amphetamines. Chlorpromazine (Thorazine) or haloperidol (Haldol) is sometimes used in treating amphetamine overdose.
e. Drugs that *increase* effects of modafinil:	
(1) Itraconazole, ketoconazole	These drugs inhibit cytochrome P450 3A4 enzymes that partly metab-olize modafinil.
f. Drugs that *decrease* effects of modafinil:	
(1) Carbamazepine, phenytoin, rifampin	These drugs induce cytochrome P450 3A4 enzymes that partly metab-olize modafinil.
g. Drugs that *increase* effects of caffeine:	
(1) Fluvoxamine, mexiletine, theophylline	These drugs inhibit the cytochrome P450 1A2 enzymes that partici-pate in the metabolism of caffeine. Decreased metabolism may increase adverse effects.
(2) Cimetidine, oral contraceptives	May impair caffeine metabolism
h. Drugs that *decrease* effects of caffeine:	
(1) Carbamazepine, phenytoin, rifampin	These drugs induce drug-metabolizing enzymes, thereby decreasing blood levels and increasing clearance of caffeine.

APPLYING YOUR KNOWLEDGE: ANSWERS

15-1 Inform the teacher that there is no legitimate use of this drug by athletes. Kevin, his parents, and the principal of the school should be informed of the behavior. There is no need to disclose any of Kevin's personal health information.

15-2 Kevin is most likely having a toxicity reaction. Place him in a cool room that has minimal external stimulation. Monitor Kevin's heart rate, blood pressure, and temperature.

15-3 Losing weight is a common adverse effect of methylphenidate. Evaluate how well Kevin is eating. Provide tips on taking drugs safely and accurately. Instruct Kevin to take his medication 30 to 45 minutes before meals and to take his last dose of the day before 6 P.M. Taking the drugs before meals will minimize the drug's appetite-suppressing effects, and taking this medication before 6 P.M. will avoid interference with sleep.

Review and Application Exercises

Short Answer Exercises

1. What kinds of behaviors may indicate narcolepsy?

2. What kinds of behaviors may indicate ADHD?

3. What is the rationale for treating narcolepsy and ADHD with CNS stimulants?

4. What are the major adverse effects of CNS stimulants, and how may they be minimized?

5. Do you think children taking CNS stimulants for ADHD should have drug-free periods? Justify your answer.

NCLEX-Style Questions

6. When a CNS stimulant is used to treat a child with ADHD, which of the following outcomes is expected?

a. increased behavioral problems
b. improved performance in schoolwork
c. decreased ability to complete a task
d. increased hyperactivity

7. A child receiving a CNS stimulant for ADHD should be monitored for which of the following?
a. abnormal liver function
b. weight loss
c. fever
d. seizure activity

8. Caffeine and other CNS stimulants may cause which of the following adverse effects?
a. increased appetite
b. respiratory depression
c. sedation
d. cardiac dysrhythmias

Selected References

Carillo, J. A., & Benitez, J. (2000). Clinically significant pharmacokinetic interactions between dietary caffeine and medications. *Clinical Pharmacokinetics, 39*(2), 127–153.

Doering, P. L. (2002). Substance-related disorders: Alcohol, nicotine, and caffeine. In J. T. DiPiro, R. L. Talbert, G. C. Yee, G. R. Matzke, B. G. Wells, & L. M. Posey (Eds.), *Pharmacotherapy: A pathophysiologic approach* (5th ed., pp. 1203–1218). New York: McGraw-Hill.

Dopheide, J. A., & Theesen, K. A. (2002). Childhood disorders. In J. T. DiPiro, R. L. Talbert, G. C. Yee, G. R. Matzke, B. G. Wells, & L. M. Posey (Eds.), *Pharmacotherapy: A pathophysiologic approach* (5th ed., pp. 1145–1154). New York: McGraw-Hill.

Drug facts and comparisons. (Updated monthly). St. Louis: Facts and Comparisons.

Kehoe, W. A. (2001). Treatment of attention deficit hyperactivity disorder in children. *The Annals of Pharmacotherapy, 35*(9), 1130–1134.

Kim, R. B. (Ed.). (2001). *Handbook of adverse drug interactions.* New Rochelle, NY: Medical Letter.

Lacy, C. F., Armstrong, L. L., Goldman, M. P., et al. (2004). *Lexi-Comp's drug information handbook* (12th ed.). Hudson, OH: Lexi-Comp.

Porth, C. M. (2005). Sleep and sleep disorders. *Pathophysiology: Concepts of altered health states* (7th ed., pp. 268–270). Philadelphia: Lippincott Williams & Wilkins.

Simon, R. P., & Sunseri, M. J. (2004). Disorders of sleep and arousal. In L. Goldman & D. Ausiello (Eds.), *Cecil textbook of medicine* (22nd ed., pp. 2277–2280). Philadelphia: W. B. Saunders.

Spencer, T., Biederman, J., Wilens, T., et al. (2001). Efficacy of a mixed amphetamine salts compound in adults with attention-deficit/hyperactivity disorder. *Archives of General Psychiatry, 58*(8), 775–782.

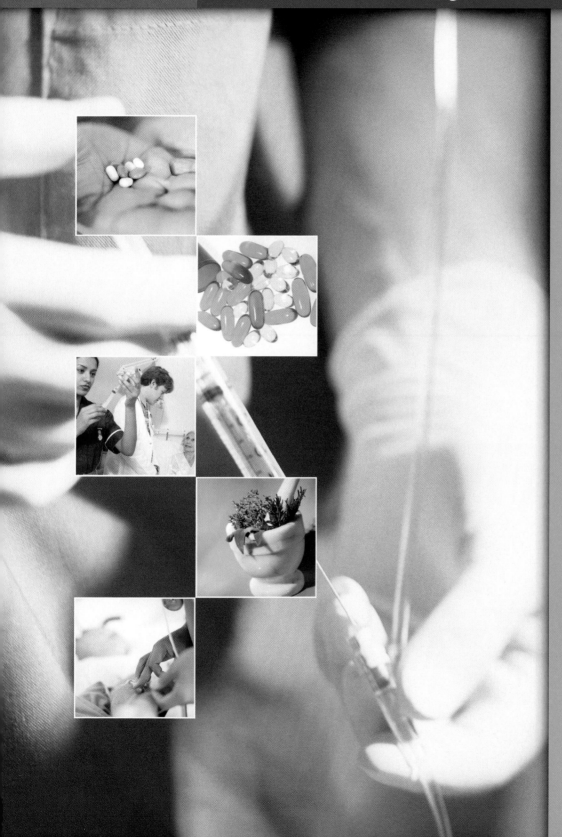

CHAPTER OUTLINE

16 Physiology of the Autonomic Nervous System

17 Adrenergic Drugs

18 Antiadrenergic Drugs

19 Cholinergic Drugs

20 Anticholinergic Drugs

Physiology of the Autonomic Nervous System

OBJECTIVES

After studying this chapter, you will be able to:

1. Identify physiologic effects of the sympathetic nervous system.
2. Differentiate subtypes and functions of sympathetic nervous system receptors.
3. Identify physiologic effects of the parasympathetic nervous system.
4. Differentiate subtypes and functions of parasympathetic nervous system receptors.
5. Describe signal transduction and the intracellular events that occur when receptors of the autonomic nervous system are stimulated.
6. State names and general characteristics of drugs affecting the autonomic nervous system.

INTRODUCTION

The nervous system is composed of two main divisions, the central nervous system (CNS) and the peripheral nervous system (PNS) (Fig. 16-1). The CNS includes the brain and spinal cord. It receives and processes incoming sensory information and responds by sending out signals that initiate or modify body processes.

The PNS includes all the neurons and ganglia found outside the CNS. The PNS includes afferent (sensory) neurons and efferent motor neurons. Afferent neurons carry sensory input from the periphery to the CNS and modify motor output through the action of reflex arcs. Efferent neurons carry motor signals from the CNS to the peripheral areas of the body.

The efferent portion of the PNS is further subdivided into the somatic nervous system and the autonomic nervous system (ANS). The somatic nervous system innervates skeletal muscles and controls voluntary movement. The ANS, without conscious thought or effort, controls involuntary activities in smooth muscle, secretory glands, and in the visceral organs of the body such as the heart.

The functions of the ANS can be broadly described as activities designed to maintain a constant internal environment (homeostasis), to respond to stress or emergencies, and

to repair body tissues. The ANS is regulated by centers in the CNS, including the hypothalamus, brain stem, and spinal cord. It is subdivided into the sympathetic nervous system and the parasympathetic nervous system.

STRUCTURE AND FUNCTION OF THE AUTONOMIC NERVOUS SYSTEM

Nerve impulses are generated and transmitted to body tissues in the sympathetic and parasympathetic nervous systems as they are in the CNS (see Chap. 5). Preganglionic nerve impulses travel from the CNS along the presynaptic nerves to ganglia. *Ganglia* are bundles of nerve tissue composed of the terminal end of the presynaptic neuron and clusters of postsynaptic neuron cell bodies. A neurotransmitter is released from the terminal end of the presynaptic neuron, allowing the nervous impulse to bridge the synapse between the presynaptic and postsynaptic nerve. The postganglionic impulses travel from the ganglia to target or *effector* tissues of the heart, blood vessels, glands, other visceral organs, and smooth muscle. A neurotransmitter is released from the terminal end of the postsynaptic neuron, allowing the impulse

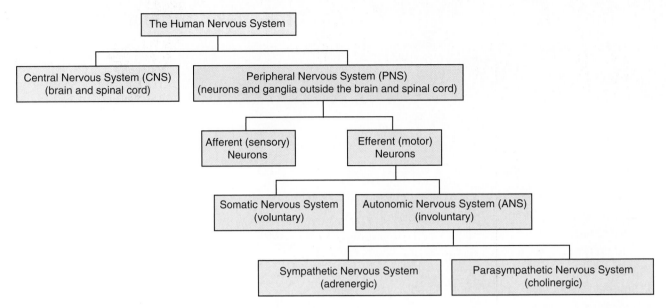

FIGURE 16-1 Divisions of the human nervous system.

to reach the effector tissue, stimulate a receptor, and bring about a response (Fig. 16-2).

The main neurotransmitters of the ANS are acetylcholine and norepinephrine (see Chap. 5). Acetylcholine is synthesized from acetylcoenzyme A and choline. It is released at *preganglionic fibers* of both the sympathetic nervous system and parasympathetic nervous system and at *postganglionic fibers* of the parasympathetic nervous system. Acetylcholine is also released from postganglionic sympathetic neurons that innervate the sweat glands and from motor neurons of the somatic nervous system that innervate the skeletal muscles. The nerve fibers that secrete acetylcholine are called *cholinergic fibers*. Acetylcholine acts on receptors in body organs and tissues to cause parasympathetic effects.

Norepinephrine is synthesized from the amino acid tyrosine by a series of enzymatic conversions that also produce dopamine and epinephrine (ie, tyrosine → dopamine → norepinephrine → epinephrine). Norepinephrine is the end product of this chemical reaction, except in the adrenal medulla, where most of the norepinephrine is converted to epinephrine. Norepinephrine is released at most postganglionic fibers of the sympathetic nervous system. Nerve fibers secreting norepinephrine are called *adrenergic fibers*. Norepinephrine acts on receptors in body organs and tissues to cause sympathetic effects.

Neurotransmitters, such as acetylcholine and norepinephrine, as well as medications and hormones that can bind to receptors in the ANS, are collectively called *ligands*. When receptors located on target tissues are stimulated by a ligand, a cascade of intracellular events known as *signal transduction* is initiated. The ligand that binds the receptor is the *first messenger*. In most cases, this ligand–receptor interaction activates a cell membrane–bound G protein and an effector enzyme,

which then activate a molecule inside the cell called a *second messenger*. This second messenger is the link between events that are occurring outside the cell (ie, receptor activation by the ligand) and resulting events that will occur inside the cell, such as opening ion channels, stimulating other enzymes, and increasing intracellular calcium levels. These intracellular events ultimately produce the physiologic responses to neurotransmitter and hormone release or drug administration. Figure 16-3 illustrates the intracellular events of signal transduction that occur when an adrenergic beta receptor is stimulated by epinephrine.

Involuntary organs and tissues in the body are innervated by both divisions of the ANS; however, most organs are predominantly controlled by one system. For example in the gastrointestinal tract, the parasympathetic nervous system predominates and stimulation of the parasympathetic nervous system regulates the routine activities of digestion and elimination.

The two divisions of the ANS are usually antagonistic in their actions on a particular organ. When the sympathetic system excites a particular organ, the parasympathetic system often inhibits it and vice versa. Stimulation of the ANS causes excitatory effects in some organs but inhibitory effects in others. For example, sympathetic stimulation of the heart causes an increased rate and force of myocardial contraction; parasympathetic stimulation decreases rate and force of contraction, thereby resting the heart. In the gastrointestinal tract, stimulation of the parasympathetic nervous system promotes digestion; sympathetic stimulation decreases blood flow and impairs digestion. Exceptions to this antagonistic action include sweating and regulation of arteriolar blood-vessel diameter, which is controlled by the sympathetic nervous system.

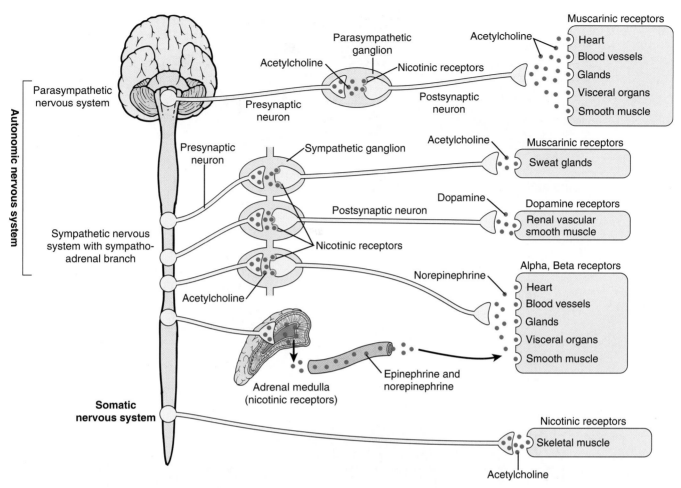

FIGURE 16-2 Organization of the autonomic and somatic nervous systems.

Sympathetic Nervous System

The sympathetic nervous system is stimulated by physical or emotional stress, such as strenuous exercise or work, pain, hemorrhage, intense emotions, and temperature extremes. Increased capacity for vigorous muscle activity in response to a perceived threat, whether real or imaginary, is often called the *fight-or-flight* reaction. Specific body responses include:

- Increased arterial blood pressure and cardiac output
- Increased blood flow to the brain, heart, and skeletal muscles; decreased blood flow to viscera, skin, and other organs not needed for fight-or-flight
- Increased rate of cellular metabolism—increased oxygen consumption and carbon dioxide production
- Increased breakdown of muscle glycogen for energy
- Increased blood sugar
- Increased mental activity and ability to think clearly
- Increased muscle strength
- Increased rate of blood coagulation
- Increased rate and depth of respiration
- Pupil dilation to aid vision

- Increased sweating. (Note that acetylcholine is the neurotransmitter for this sympathetic response. This is a deviation from the normal postganglionic neurotransmitter, which is norepinephrine.)

These responses are protective mechanisms designed to help the person cope with the stress or get away from it. The intensity and duration of the sympathetic response depends on the amounts of norepinephrine and epinephrine present.

Norepinephrine is synthesized in adrenergic nerve endings and released into the synapse when adrenergic nerve endings are stimulated. It exerts intense but brief effects on presynaptic and postsynaptic adrenergic receptors. The effects of norepinephrine are terminated by reuptake of most of the neurotransmitter back into the nerve endings, where it is packaged into vesicles for reuse as a neurotransmitter. This reuptake and termination process can be inhibited by cocaine and tricyclic antidepressant medications, and is responsible for the activation of the sympathetic nervous system seen with these drugs. The remainder of the norepinephrine, which was not taken back into the nerve endings,

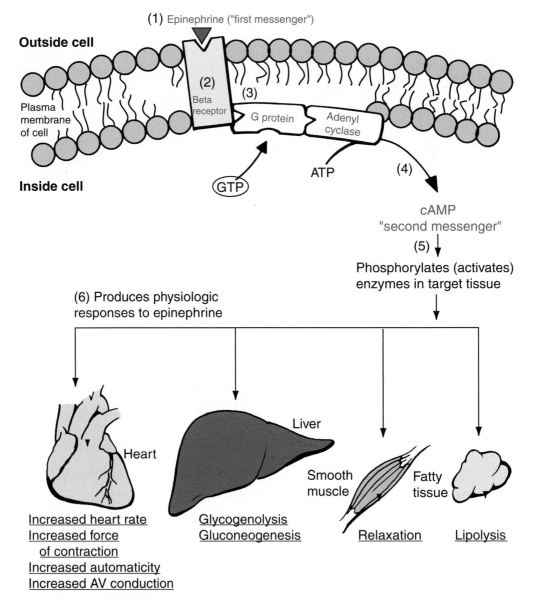

FIGURE 16-3 Signal transduction mechanism for an adrenergic beta receptor. Epinephrine (1), the "first messenger," interacts with a beta receptor (2). This hormone–receptor complex activates a G protein, which reacts with a guanosine triphosphate (GTP) (3). The activated G protein then activates the enzyme adenyl cyclase, which (4) catalyzes the conversion of adenosine triphosphate (ATP) to cyclic adenosine monophosphate (cAMP), the "second messenger." (5) cAMP activates enzymes, which bring about the biologic responses to epinephrine (6).

diffuses into surrounding tissue fluids and blood, or it is metabolized by monoamine oxidase (MAO) or catechol-*O*-methyltransferase (COMT).

Norepinephrine also functions as a circulating neurohormone, along with epinephrine. In response to adrenergic nerve stimulation, norepinephrine and epinephrine are secreted into the bloodstream by the adrenal medullae and transported to all body tissues. They are continually present in arterial blood in amounts that vary according to the degree of stress present and the ability of the adrenal medullae to respond to stimuli. The larger proportion of the circulating hormones (approximately 80%) is epinephrine. These catecholamines exert the same effects on target tissues as those caused by direct stimulation of the sympathetic nervous system. However, the effects last longer because the hormones are removed from the blood more slowly. These hormones are metabolized mainly in the liver by the enzymes MAO and COMT.

Dopamine is also an adrenergic neurotransmitter and catecholamine. In the brain, dopamine is essential for normal function (see Chap. 5). In peripheral tissues, its main effects are on the heart and blood vessels of the renal system and viscera, where it produces vasodilation.

Adrenergic Receptors

When norepinephrine and epinephrine act on body cells that respond to sympathetic nerve or catecholamine stimulation, they interact with two distinct adrenergic receptors, alpha and beta. Norepinephrine acts mainly on alpha receptors; epinephrine acts on both alpha and beta receptors. These receptors have been further subdivided into alpha$_1$, alpha$_2$, beta$_1$, and beta$_2$ receptors. A beta$_3$ receptor has been identified, and studies suggest that stimulation of this receptor may augment heat production, produce lipolysis (thermogenesis), and increase energy expenditure. Several compounds are being tested to treat obesity, hyperglycemia, and the problem of insulin resistance in diabetes. Currently, there are no beta$_3$ agonist drugs approved by the Food and Drug Administration for human use.

When dopamine acts on body cells that respond to adrenergic stimulation, it can activate alpha$_1$ and beta$_1$ receptors as well as dopaminergic receptors. Only dopamine can activate dopaminergic receptors. Dopamine receptors are located in the brain, in blood vessels of the kidneys and other viscera, and probably in presynaptic sympathetic nerve terminals. Activation (agonism) of these receptors may result in stimulation or inhibition of cellular function. Like alpha and beta receptors, dopamine receptors are divided into several subtypes (D$_1$ to D$_5$), and specific effects depend on which subtype of receptor is activated. Table 16-1 describes the locations of adrenergic receptors in the body and the response that occurs when each receptor is stimulated.

The intracellular events resulting from signal transduction after stimulation of adrenergic receptors are thought to include the following mechanisms:

● *Alpha$_1$ receptors:* The binding of adrenergic substances to receptor proteins in the cell membrane of smooth muscle cells is thought to open ion channels, allow calcium ions to move into the cell, and produce muscle contraction (eg, vasoconstriction, gastrointestinal and bladder-sphincter contraction).

● *Alpha$_2$ receptors:* In the brain, some of the norepinephrine released into the synaptic cleft between neurons returns to the nerve endings from which it was released and stimulates presynaptic alpha$_2$ receptors. This negative feedback causes less norepinephrine to be released by subsequent nerve impulses. The result is decreased sympathetic outflow and an antiadrenergic effect. The probable mechanism is that the calcium required for neurotransmitter release from storage vesicles is prevented from entering the presynaptic nerve cell. Also, cyclic adenosine monophosphate (cAMP) is decreased.

● *Beta$_1$, beta$_2$, and beta$_3$ receptors:* Activation of these receptors stimulates activity of adenyl cyclase, an enzyme in cell membranes. Adenyl cyclase, in turn, stimulates formation of cyclic adenosine monophos-

TABLE 16-1 Adrenergic Receptors

TYPE	LOCATION	EFFECTS OF STIMULATION
Alpha$_1$	Blood vessels	Vasoconstriction
	Kidney	Decreased renin secretion
	Intestinal smooth muscle	Relaxation
	Liver	Glycogenolysis, gluconeo-genesis
	Genitourinary smooth muscle	Contraction
	Eye (radial muscle)	Blinking, mydriasis
	Pregnant uterus	Uterine contraction
	Male sexual organs	Ejaculation
Alpha$_2$	Nerve endings	Inhibit release of norepinephrine
	Vascular smooth muscle	Vasoconstriction
	Pancreatic beta cells	Inhibit insulin secretion
	Platelets	Aggregation
Beta$_1$	Heart	Increased heart rate, force of contraction, automaticity, and rate of atrioventricular conduction
	Kidney	Increased renin release
Beta$_2$	Bronchioles	Bronchodilation
	Blood vessels	Vasodilation
	Gastrointestinal tract	Decreased motility and tone
	Liver	Glycogenolysis, gluconeo-genesis
	Urinary bladder	Relaxed detrusor muscle
	Pregnant uterus	Relaxation
Dopamine	Blood vessels of kidney, heart, other viscera	Vasodilation

phate (cAMP). cAMP serves as a second messenger and can initiate several different intracellular actions, with specific actions depending on the type of cell. cAMP is rapidly degraded by an enzyme called phosphodiesterase to 5′ adenosine monophosphate (AMP). Drugs such as theophylline inhibit phosphodiesterase and increase cAMP concentrations, resulting in bronchodilation (see Chap. 44).

● *Dopaminergic receptors D$_1$ and D$_5$:* Activation of these receptors is thought to stimulate the production of cAMP, as does activation of beta$_1$ and beta$_2$ receptors.

● *Dopaminergic receptor D₂:* Activation of this receptor is thought to inhibit formation of cAMP and to alter calcium- and potassium-ion currents. D_3 and D_4 receptors are subgrouped with D_2 receptors, but the effects of their activation have not been clearly delineated.

The number of receptors and the binding activity of receptors to target organs and tissues is dynamic and may be altered. These phenomena are most clearly understood with beta receptors. For example, when chronically exposed to high concentrations of substances that stimulate their function, the beta receptors decrease in number and become less efficient in stimulating adenyl cyclase. The resulting decrease in beta-adrenergic responsiveness is called *desensitization* or *down-regulation* of receptors. Conversely, when chronically exposed to substances that block their function, the receptors may increase in number and become more efficient in stimulating adenyl cyclase. The resulting increase in beta-adrenergic responsiveness, called *hypersensitization* or *up-regulation,* may lead to an exaggerated response when the blocking substance is withdrawn.

Parasympathetic Nervous System

Functions stimulated by the parasympathetic nervous system are often described as resting, reparative, or vegetative functions. They include digestion, excretion, cardiac deceleration, anabolism, and near vision.

Approximately 75% of all parasympathetic nerve fibers are in the vagus nerves. These nerves supply the thoracic and abdominal organs; their branches go to the heart, lungs, esophagus, stomach, small intestine, the proximal half of the colon, the liver, gallbladder, pancreas, and the upper portions of the ureters. Other parasympathetic fibers supply pupillary sphincters and circular muscles of the eye; lacrimal, nasal, submaxillary, and parotid glands; descending colon and rectum; lower portions of the ureters and bladder; and genitalia.

Specific body responses to parasympathetic stimulation include:

● Dilation of blood vessels in the skin
● Decreased heart rate, possibly bradycardia
● Increased secretion of digestive enzymes and motility of the gastrointestinal tract
● Constriction of smooth muscle of bronchi
● Increased secretions from glands in the lungs, stomach, intestines, and skin (sweat glands)
● Constricted pupils (from contraction of the circular muscle of the iris) and accommodation to near vision (from contraction of the ciliary muscle of the eye)
● Contraction of smooth muscle in the urinary bladder
● Contraction of skeletal muscle
● Release of nitrous oxide from the endothelium of blood vessels, resulting in decreased platelet aggregation, decreased inflammation, relaxation of vascular smooth muscle, and dilation of blood vessels.

Parasympathetic responses are regulated by acetylcholine, a neurotransmitter in the brain, ANS, and neuromuscular junctions. Acetylcholine is formed in cholinergic nerve endings from choline and acetylcoenzyme A, in a chemical reaction catalyzed by choline acetyltransferase. After its release from the nerve ending, the effect of acetylcholine on receptors of the parasympathetic nervous system is brief and measured in milliseconds. The action of acetylcholine on receptors is terminated due to rapid metabolism by acetylcholinesterase, an enzyme present in the nerve ending and on the surface of the receptor organ. Acetylcholinesterase splits the active acetylcholine into inactive acetate and choline. The choline is taken up again by the presynaptic nerve terminal and reused to form more acetylcholine. Acetylcholine exerts excitatory effects at nerve synapses and neuromuscular junctions and inhibitory effects at some peripheral sites such as the heart.

Cholinergic Receptors

When acetylcholine acts on body cells that respond to parasympathetic nerve stimulation, it interacts with two types of cholinergic receptors: nicotinic and muscarinic. Nicotinic receptors are located in motor nerves and skeletal muscle. When they are activated by acetylcholine, the cell membrane depolarizes and produces muscle contraction. Muscarinic receptors are located in most internal organs, including the cardiovascular, respiratory, gastrointestinal, and genitourinary systems. When muscarinic receptors are activated by acetylcholine, the affected cells may be excited or inhibited in their functions.

Nicotinic and muscarinic receptors have been further subdivided, with two types of nicotinic and five types of muscarinic receptors identified. Although the subtypes of cholinergic receptors have not been as well characterized as those of the adrenergic receptors, the intracellular events resulting from signal transduction after receptor stimulation are thought to include the following mechanisms:

● *Muscarinic₁ receptors:* Activation of these receptors results in a series of processes during which phospholipids in the cell membrane and inside the cell are broken down. One of the products of phospholipid metabolism is inositol phosphate. Inositol phosphate acts as a second messenger to increase the intracellular concentration of calcium. Calcium also acts as a second messenger and functions to activate several intracellular enzymes; initiate contraction of smooth muscle cells; and increase secretions of exocrine glands.
● *Muscarinic₂ receptors:* Activation of these receptors results in inhibition of adenyl cyclase in the heart, smooth muscle, and brain. As a result, less cAMP is formed to act as a second messenger and stimulate intracellular activity. Receptor stimulation also results in activation of potassium channels in cell membranes of the heart. The overall consequence of M_2 activation is inhibition of affected cells.

● *Muscarinic₃ receptors:* Activation apparently causes the same cascade of intracellular processes as with activation of the M_1 receptors. In addition, nitrous oxide is generated from vascular endothelial cells, resulting in dilation of vessels.

● *Muscarinic₄ receptors:* Activation results in a molecular response similar to M_2 receptor activation. Their location and function have not yet been delineated.

● *Muscarinic₅ receptors:* Receptor activation results in a molecular response similar to M_1 receptor activation. The receptor has been identified in central nervous system tissues; however, its function has not been delineated.

Although five muscarinic receptor subtypes have been identified, currently available drug therapies do not selectively differentiate among the various receptor subtypes.

● *Nicotinic_n receptors:* These receptors are located on autonomic ganglia and the adrenal medulla. Activation results in enhanced transmission of nerve impulses at all parasympathetic and sympathetic ganglia, and release of epinephrine from the adrenal medullae.

● *Nicotinic_m receptors:* These are located at neuromuscular junctions in skeletal muscle. Their activation causes muscle contraction.

● *Nicotinic_CNS receptors:* These receptors are located on presynaptic nerve fibers in the brain and spinal cord. Their activation promotes the release of acetylcholine in the cerebral cortex.

Nicotinic receptors are composed of five different protein subunits. The protein subunits that make up a *nicotinic_n* receptor vary from those that make up a *nicotinic_m* receptor, thus allowing the development of medications that are more selective in their actions. For example, neuromuscular blocking medications such as pancuronium, which act selectively at *nicotinic_m* receptors, can paralyze skeletal muscles in clients when limiting movement is therapeutic (such as in the ventilated client or during surgery), without adversely affecting the other functions of the ANS.

CHARACTERISTICS OF AUTONOMIC DRUGS

Many drugs are used clinically because of their ability to stimulate or block activity of the sympathetic nervous system or parasympathetic nervous system. Drugs that stimulate activity act like endogenous neurotransmitter substances; drugs that block activity prevent the actions of both endogenous substances and stimulating drugs.

Because ANS receptors are widespread throughout the body, drugs that act on the ANS usually affect the entire body rather than certain organs and tissues. Drug effects depend on which branch of the ANS is involved and whether it is stimulated or inhibited by drug therapy. Thus, knowledge of the physiology of the ANS is required if drug effects are to be understood and predicted. In addition, it is becoming increasingly important to understand receptor activity and the consequences of stimulation or inhibition. More drugs are being developed to stimulate or inhibit particular subtypes of receptors. This is part of the continuing effort to design drugs that act more selectively on particular body tissues and decrease adverse effects on other body tissues. For example, drugs such as terbutaline have been developed to stimulate beta₂ receptors in the respiratory tract and produce bronchodilation (a desired effect) with decreased stimulation of beta₁ receptors in the heart (an adverse effect).

The terminology used to describe autonomic drugs is often confusing because different terms are used to refer to the same phenomenon. Thus, *sympathomimetic, adrenergic,* and *alpha-* and *beta-adrenergic agonists* are used to describe a drug that has the same effects on the human body as stimulation of the sympathetic nervous system. *Parasympathomimetic, cholinomimetic,* and *cholinergic* are used to describe a drug that has the same effects on the body as stimulation of the parasympathetic nervous system. There are also drugs that oppose or block stimulation of these systems. *Sympatholytic, antiadrenergic,* and *alpha-* and *beta-adrenergic blocking drugs* inhibit sympathetic stimulation. *Parasympatholytic, anticholinergic,* and *cholinergic blocking drugs* inhibit parasympathetic stimulation. This book uses the terms *adrenergic, antiadrenergic, cholinergic,* and *anticholinergic* when describing medications.

Review and Application Exercises

Short Answer Exercises

1. What are the major differences between the sympathetic and parasympathetic branches of the ANS?

2. What are the major sympathetic nervous system and parasympathetic nervous system neurotransmitters?

3. What are the locations and functions of sympathetic nervous system receptors?

4. What is meant when drugs are described as adrenergic, sympathomimetic, antiadrenergic, sympatholytic, cholinergic, or anticholinergic?

Selected References

Hoffman, B. R., & Taylor, P. (2001). Neurotransmission: The autonomic and somatic motor nervous systems. In J. G. Hardman & L. E. Limbird (Eds.), *Goodman & Gilman's The pharmacological basis of therapeutics* (10th ed., pp. 115–153). New York: McGraw-Hill.

Katzung, B. G. (2001). Introduction to autonomic pharmacology. In B. G. Katzung (Ed.), *Basic and clinical pharmacology* (8th ed., pp. 75–91). New York: McGraw-Hill.

Piano, M. R., & Huether, S. E. (2002). Mechanisms of hormonal regulation. In K. L. McCance & S. E. Huether (Eds.), *Pathophysiology: The biologic basis for disease in adults and children* (4th ed., pp. 597–623). St. Louis: Mosby.

Adrenergic Drugs

OBJECTIVES

After studying this chapter, you will be able to:

1. Identify effects produced by stimulation of alpha- and beta-adrenergic receptors.
2. List characteristics of adrenergic drugs in terms of effects on body tissues, indications for use, adverse effects, nursing process implications, principles of therapy, and observation of client responses.
3. Discuss use of epinephrine to treat anaphylactic shock, acute bronchospasm, and cardiac arrest.
4. Identify clients at risk for the adverse effects associated with adrenergic drugs.
5. List commonly used over-the-counter preparations and herbal preparations that contain adrenergic drugs.
6. Discuss principles of therapy and nursing process for using adrenergic drugs in special populations.
7. Describe signs and symptoms of toxicity due to noncatecholamine adrenergic drugs.
8. Discuss treatment of overdose with noncatecholamine adrenergic drugs.
9. Teach the client about safe, effective use of adrenergic drugs.

APPLYING YOUR KNOWLEDGE

Larry Rich is a 71-year-old male with chronic obstructive pulmonary disease (COPD). He has had asthma for all of his adult life and is admitted to the acute care department with respiratory distress secondary to pneumonia. He has a very modest pension and is covered by Medicare, which sometimes makes it difficult for him to pay for medical supplies and medication. Although Mr. Rich has never been a smoker, he did work as a welder for 45 years. Due to his acute bronchospasm, his physician orders epinephrine 1:10,000 IV stat.

INTRODUCTION

Adrenergic drugs produce effects similar to those produced by stimulation of the sympathetic nervous system and therefore have widespread effects on body tissues (see Chap. 16). Major therapeutic uses and adverse effects of adrenergic medications derive from drug action on the heart, blood vessels, and lungs. Some adrenergic drugs are exogenous formulations of naturally occurring neurotransmitters and hormones, such as norepinephrine, epinephrine, and dopamine. Other adrenergic medications, such as phenylephrine, pseudoephedrine, and isoproterenol, are synthetic chemical relatives of naturally occurring neurotransmitters and hormones.

Specific effects of adrenergic medications depend mainly on the type of adrenergic receptor activated by the drug. The drugs discussed in this chapter (epinephrine, ephedrine, pseudoephedrine, isoproterenol, and phenylephrine) affect multiple adrenergic receptors and have many clinical uses. Other adrenergic drugs are more selective for specific adrenergic receptors

or are given topically to produce more localized therapeutic effects and fewer systemic adverse effects. These drugs have relatively restricted clinical indications and are discussed more extensively elsewhere ("Drugs Used in Hypotension and Shock," Chap. 51; "Drugs for Asthma and Other Bronchoconstrictive Disorders," Chap. 44; "Nasal Decongestants, Antitussives, and Cold Remedies," Chap. 46; and "Drugs Used in Ophthalmic Conditions," Chap. 63). Table 17-1 groups commonly used adrenergic drugs by adrenergic receptor activity and gives their clinical use.

GENERAL CHARACTERISTICS OF ADRENERGIC DRUGS

Mechanisms of Action

Adrenergic drugs have three mechanisms of action. For the most part, adrenergic drugs interact directly with *postsynaptic* alpha$_1$- or beta-adrenergic receptors on the surface membrane

TABLE 17-1 Commonly Used Adrenergic Drugs

GENERIC/TRADE NAME	MAJOR CLINICAL USES
Alpha and Beta Activity	
Dopamine	Hypotension and shock
Epinephrine (Adrenalin)	Allergic reactions, cardiac arrest, hypotension and shock, local vaso-constriction, broncho-dilation, cardiac stimulation, ophthalmic conditions
Ephedrine	Bronchodilation, cardiac stimulation, nasal decongestion
Pseudoephedrine (Sudafed)	Nasal decongestion
Norepinephrine (Levophed)	Hypotension and shock
Alpha Activity	
Metaraminol (Aramine)	Hypotension and shock
Naphazoline hydrochloride (Privine)	Nasal decongestion
Oxymetazoline hydrochloride (Afrin)	Nasal decongestion
Phenylephrine (Neo-Synephrine)	Hypotension and shock, nasal decongestion, ophthalmic conditions
Propylhexedrine (Benzedrex)	Nasal decongestion
Tetrahydrozoline hydrochloride (Tyzine, Visine)	Nasal decongestion, local vasoconstriction in the eye
Tuaminoheptane (Tuamine)	Nasal decongestion
Xylometazoline hydrochloride (Otrivin)	Nasal decongestion
Beta Activity	
Albuterol (Proventil)	Bronchodilation
Bitolterol (Tornalate)	Bronchodilation
Dobutamine (Dobutrex)	Cardiac stimulation
Isoproterenol (Isuprel)	Bronchodilation, cardiac stimulation
Isoetharine	Bronchodilation
Metaproterenol (Alupent)	Bronchodilation
Pirbuterol (Maxair)	Bronchodilation
Salmeterol (Serevent)	Bronchodilation
Terbutaline (Brethine)	Bronchodilation, preterm labor inhibition

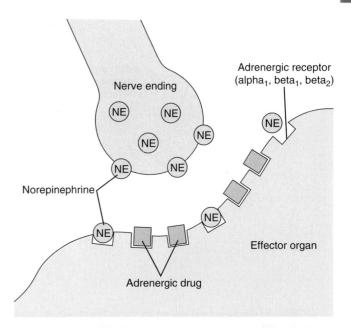

FIGURE 17-1 Mechanism of direct adrenergic drug action. Adrenergic drugs interact directly with postsynaptic alpha$_1$ and beta receptors on target effector organs, activating the organ in a similar fashion as the neurotransmitter norepinephrine. NE, norepinephrine.

Some adrenergic drugs exert indirect effects on *postsynaptic* adrenergic receptors. Indirect adrenergic effects may be produced by drugs such as amphetamines, which increase the amount of norepinephrine released into the synapse from storage sites in nerve endings (Fig. 17-2A). Norepinephrine then stimulates the alpha and beta receptors, producing sympathetic effects in the body. Inhibition of norepinephrine reuptake from the synapse is another mechanism that produces indirect adrenergic effects. Remember that norepinephrine reuptake is the major way that sympathetic nerve transmission is terminated. Drugs such as tricyclic antidepressants and cocaine block norepinephrine reuptake, resulting in stimulation of alpha- and beta-adrenergic receptors (Fig. 17-2B).

The third mechanism of adrenergic drug action is called *mixed acting* and is a combination of direct and indirect receptor stimulation. Mixed-acting drugs directly stimulate adrenergic receptors by binding to them and indirectly stimulate adrenergic receptors by increasing the release of norepinephrine into synapses. Ephedrine and pseudoephedrine are examples of mixed-acting adrenergic drugs.

Because many body tissues have both alpha and beta receptors, the effect produced by an adrenergic drug depends on the type of receptor activated and the number of affected receptors in a particular body tissue. Some adrenergic drugs are nonselective, acting on both alpha and beta receptors. Other medications are more selective, acting only on certain subtypes of receptors (see Table 17-1).

The predominant effect in response to activation of alpha$_1$ receptors by an adrenergic drug is vasoconstriction of blood vessels, which increases the blood pressure. This is sometimes

of target organs and tissues (Fig. 17-1). The drug–receptor complex then alters the permeability of the cell membrane to ions or extracellular enzymes. The influx of these molecules stimulates intracellular metabolism and production of other enzymes, structural proteins, energy, and other products required for cell function and reproduction. Epinephrine, isoproterenol, norepinephrine, and phenylephrine are examples of direct-acting adrenergic drugs.

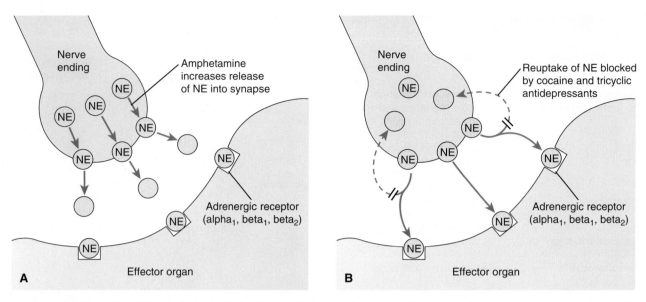

FIGURE 17-2 Mechanisms of indirect adrenergic drug action. Stimulation of postsynaptic alpha$_1$, beta$_1$, and beta$_2$ receptors results from adrenergic medications that act indirectly, increasing the release of norepinephrine (NE) into the synapse (**A**) or inhibiting the reuptake of norepinephrine from the synapse (**B**).

referred to as a *pressor* (or *vasopressor*) effect. Alpha$_1$-activated vasoconstriction of blood vessels in nasal mucous membranes decreases nasal congestion, resulting in a decongestant effect. Other adrenergic effects resulting from alpha$_1$ activation include mydriasis, contraction of gastrointestinal (GI) and genitourinary sphincters, and elevated blood glucose.

The predominant effect in response to activation of beta$_1$ receptors in the heart is cardiac stimulation. Beta$_1$ activation results in increased force of myocardial contraction, or a positive inotropic effect; increased heart rate, or a positive chronotropic effect; and increased speed of electrical conduction in the heart, or a positive dromotropic effect. Another adrenergic effect resulting from beta$_1$ activation is increased renin secretion from the kidneys.

The predominant clinical effect in response to activation of beta$_2$ receptors is bronchodilation. Activation of beta$_2$ receptors in blood vessels results in vasodilation and increased blood flow to the heart, brain, and skeletal muscles; tissues needed for the "fight-or-flight" sympathetic response. Beta$_2$ activation also results in hepatic glycogenolysis and gluconeogenesis, and decreased pancreatic insulin secretion, resulting in hyperglycemia. Other adrenergic effects resulting from beta$_2$ activation include relaxation of smooth muscle in the uterus, urinary bladder, and GI tract.

Activation of beta$_3$ adrenergic receptors produces lipolysis and increased release of free fatty acids into the blood.

It is interesting to note that drugs that activate alpha$_2$ receptors on *presynaptic* nerve fibers do not produce a sympathetic effect. These drugs inhibit the release of the neurotransmitter norepinephrine into synapses of the sympathetic nervous system, thus exerting an antiadrenergic response in the body. Although activation of presynaptic alpha$_2$ receptors in the

periphery is not of clinical significance, activation of these receptors in the central nervous system (CNS) by medications is useful in treating hypertension (see Chaps. 18 and 52).

Indications for Use

Clinical indications for the use of adrenergic drugs stem mainly from their effects on the heart, blood vessels, and bronchi. They are often used as emergency drugs in the treatment of acute cardiovascular, respiratory, and allergic disorders.

In cardiac arrest, Stokes-Adams syndrome (sudden attacks of unconsciousness caused by heart block), and profound bradycardia, they may be used as cardiac stimulants. In hypotension and shock, they may be used to increase blood pressure. In hemorrhagic or hypovolemic shock, the drugs are second-line agents that may be used if adequate fluid volume replacement does not restore sufficient blood pressure and circulation to maintain organ perfusion.

In bronchial asthma and other obstructive pulmonary diseases, the drugs are used as bronchodilators to relieve bronchoconstriction and bronchospasm. In upper respiratory infections, including the common cold and sinusitis, they may be given orally or applied topically to the nasal mucosa for decongestant effects.

Adrenergic drugs are useful in treating a variety of symptoms of allergic disorders. Severe allergic reactions are characterized by hypotension, bronchoconstriction, and laryngoedema. As vasoconstrictors, the drugs are useful in correcting the hypotension that often accompanies severe allergic reactions. The drug-induced vasoconstriction of blood vessels in mucous membranes produces a decongestant effect to relieve edema in the respiratory tract, skin, and other tissues.

As bronchodilators, the drugs also help relieve the bronchospasm of severe allergic reactions. Adrenergic drugs may be used to treat allergic rhinitis; acute hypersensitivity (anaphylactoid reactions to drugs, animal serums, insect stings, and other allergens); serum sickness; urticaria; and angioneurotic edema.

Other clinical uses of adrenergic drugs include relaxation of uterine musculature and inhibition of uterine contractions in preterm labor. They also may be added to local anesthetics for their vasoconstrictive effect, thus preventing unwanted systemic absorption of the anesthetic; prolonging anesthesia; and reducing bleeding. Topical uses include application to skin and mucous membranes for vasoconstriction and hemostatic effects, and to the eyes for vasoconstriction and mydriasis.

Contraindications to Use

Contraindications to using adrenergic drugs include cardiac dysrhythmias, angina pectoris, hypertension, hyperthyroidism, and cerebrovascular disease; stimulation of the sympathetic nervous system worsens these conditions. Narrow-angle glaucoma is a contraindication, because the drugs result in mydriasis, closure of the filtration angle of the eye, and increased intraocular pressure. Hypersensitivity to an adrenergic drug or any component is also a contraindication. For example, some adrenergic preparations contain sulfites, to which some people are allergic.

Adrenergic drugs are contraindicated with local anesthesia of distal areas with a single blood supply (eg, fingers, toes, nose, ears) because of potential tissue damage and sloughing from vasoconstriction. They should not be given during the second stage of labor because they may delay progression. They should be used with caution in clients with anxiety, insomnia, and psychiatric disorders because of their stimulant effects on the CNS and in older adults because of their cardiac- and CNS-stimulating effects.

INDIVIDUAL DRUGS

Adrenergic drugs are described in this section. Generic and trade names, routes, and dosages are listed in Table 17-2.

Epinephrine and Other Adrenergic Drugs

P **Epinephrine** (Adrenalin) is the prototype of the adrenergic drugs. When it is given systemically, the effects may be therapeutic or adverse, depending on the reason for use, dosage, and route of administration. Epinephrine stimulates alpha$_1$ and all beta receptors. At usual doses, beta-adrenergic effects on the heart and vascular and other smooth muscles predominate. However, at high doses, alpha$_1$-adrenergic effects (eg, vasoconstriction) predominate.

The effects and clinical indications for epinephrine are the same as for most adrenergic drugs. Epinephrine is the adrenergic drug of choice for relieving the acute bronchospasm and laryngeal edema of anaphylactic shock, the most serious allergic reaction. It is used in cardiac arrest for its cardiac stimulant and peripheral vasoconstrictive effects. Peripheral vasoconstriction allows shunting of blood to the heart and brain, with increased perfusion pressure in the coronary and cerebral circulations. This action is thought to be the main beneficial effect in cardiac arrest and cardiopulmonary resuscitation (CPR). Epinephrine is also added to local anesthetics for vasoconstrictive effects, which include prolonging the action of the local anesthetic drug, preventing systemic absorption, and minimizing bleeding.

Epinephrine is the active ingredient in many over-the-counter (OTC) inhalation products for asthma (eg, Micro-Nefrin, Primatene Mist, others); here it produces bronchodilation. People who have heart disease or are elderly should not use these products on a regular basis. These epinephrine preparations have a short duration of action, which promotes frequent and excessive use. Prolonged use may cause adverse effects and result in the development of tolerance to the therapeutic effects of the drug. Parenteral epinephrine should be used with caution in infants and children, because syncope has occurred with use in asthmatic children.

Epinephrine is not given orally, because enzymes in the GI tract and liver destroy it. It may be given by inhalation, injection, or topical application. Numerous epinephrine solutions are available for various routes of administration (Table 17-3). Solutions vary widely in the amount of drug they contain. They must be used correctly to avoid potentially serious hazards.

Epinephrine crosses the placenta but not the blood–brain barrier. When given by injection, it acts rapidly but has a short duration of action. Intravenous (IV) epinephrine acts almost immediately to produce an increase in blood pressure; a positive inotropic and positive chronotropic effect on the myocardium; hyperglycemia; bronchodilation; and vasoconstriction of arterioles in the skin, mucosa, and most viscera. For acute asthma attacks, subcutaneous (Sub-Q) administration usually produces bronchodilation within 5 to 10 minutes; maximal effects may occur within 20 minutes. Most epinephrine is rapidly metabolized in the liver to inactive metabolites, which are then excreted in the urine. The remaining epinephrine is deactivated by reuptake at synaptic receptor sites. Epinephrine is excreted in breast milk.

Ephedrine is a mixed-acting adrenergic drug that acts by stimulating alpha$_1$ and beta receptors and causing release of norepinephrine from presynaptic terminals. Its actions are less potent but longer lasting than those of epinephrine. Ephedrine produces more CNS stimulation than other adrenergic drugs. It may be used in the treatment of bronchial asthma to prevent bronchospasm, but it is less effective than epinephrine for acute bronchospasm and respiratory distress.

Ephedrine can be given orally or parenterally. When given orally, therapeutic effects occur within 1 hour and last 3 to

(text continues on page 278)

Table 17-2 Drugs at a Glance: Selected Adrenergic Drugs

GENERIC/TRADE NAME	USE	PREPARATIONS, ROUTES AND DOSAGE RANGES	
		Adults	**Children**
Epinephrine (Adrenalin)	Bronchodilator	*Aqueous epinephrine 1 mg/mL **(1:1000)**:* IM, Sub-Q: 0.1–0.5 mg q 15 min to q 4h if needed. Do not exceed 1 mg in a single dose *IV injection **(1:1000)**:* Dilute 1 mg with 10 mL NaCl injection for a final concentration of 1:10,000 or 0.1 mg/mL. Give 0.1–2.25 mg (1–2.5 mL) of this solution. Single-dose maximum: 1 mg (10 mL) *Epinephrine 1% aqueous solution **(1:100)** for inhalation (nebulization):* Instill 8–15 drops into nebulizer reservoir. Administer 1–3 inhalations 4–6 times/d. *Epinephrine by metered dose inhaler (MDI) (~200– 275 mcg/puff):* 1 puff at onset of bronchospasm. Repeat if needed after 1–5 min. Dose is individualized to patient's needs.	*Aqueous epinephrine 1 mg/mL **(1:1000)**:* Sub-Q: 0.01 mg/kg q 20 min to 4h if needed. Do not exceed 0.5 mg in a single dose.
	Profound bradycardia/ hypotension	*Aqueous epinephrine 1 mg/mL **(1:1000)**: Continuous infusion:* Add 1 mg epinephrine to 500 mL D5W, administer at 1–5 mL/min, and titrate to response.	
	Cardiac arrest	Aqueous epinephrine 1 mg/mL **(1:1000)**: *IV injection:* 1 mg q 3–5 min. Higher doses (up to 0.2 mg/kg) may be used if 1-mg dose fails. *Continuous infusion:* Add 30 mg epinephrine to 250 mL NS or D5W, run at 100 mL/h, and titrate to response. *Endotracheally:* 2.0–2.5 mg of **1:1000** solution diluted in 10 mL NS	*Aqueous epinephrine 0.1 mg/mL **(1:10,000)**: IV injection:* Give 0.01 mg/kg (0.1 mL/kg) q 3–5 min. *Subsequent doses: Aqueous epinephrine 1 mg/mL **(1:1000)**:* Give 0.1 mg/kg (0.1 mL/kg) up to 0.2 mg/kg (0.2 ml/kg) *Endotracheally:* 0.1 mg/kg of **1:1000** solution q 3–5 min until IV access is established
	Allergic reaction/ anaphylaxis	*Aqueous epinephrine 1 mg/mL **(1:1000)**:* IM, Sub-Q: 0.1–0.5 mg q 20 min to q4h. Do not exceed 1 mg in a single dose.	*Aqueous epinephrine 1 mg/mL: **(1:1000)**:* IV: 0.01 mg q20 min to q4h. Do not exceed 0.5 mg in a single dose.
	Ophthalmic agent	*Epinephrine HCl 0.1%, 0.5%, 1%, and 2%* 1–2 drops in eyes 1–2 times/day	
	Nasal agent for hemostasis	*Epinephrine nasal solution 0.1% **(1:1000)**:* 1–2 drops per nostril q4–6h	

(continued)

Table 17-2 Drugs at a Glance: Selected Adrenergic Drugs (continued)

GENERIC/TRADE NAME	USE	PREPARATIONS, ROUTES AND DOSAGE RANGES	
		Adults	Children
Ephedrine	Asthma	*PO:* 12.5–25 mg q4h. Do not exceed 150 mg/24h	*6–12 y:* PO 6.25–12.5 mg q4–6h. *2–6 y:* PO 0.3–0.5 mg/kg q4–6h
	Hypotension	*IM, Sub-Q:* 25–50 mg *IV push:* 5–25 mg/dose slowly, repeated q 5–10 min as needed then q3–4h. Do not exceed 150 mg/24h.	
	Nasal congestion	*PO:* 25–50 mg q4h *0.25% nasal spray or 1% nasal jelly*	
Pseudoephedrine (Sudafed)	Nasal congestion	Give 30–60 mg PO q4–6h or 120 mg sustained-release formula q12h. Do not exceed 240 mg/24h.	*6–12 y:* PO 30 mg q6h. Do not exceed 120 mg/24h. *2–5 y:* PO 15 mg q6h. Do not exceed 60 mg/24h.
Isoproterenol (Isuprel)	Bronchodilator	*Aerosol solutions: 0.2% **(1:500)**, 0.25% **(1:400)**:* 1–2 metered doses 4–6 times/d. Second inhalation is given 2–5 min after the first. *Nebulization solution: 0.031%, 0.062%, 0.25%. 0.5%, and 1%* 5–15 inhalations, repeated once in 10–30 min if needed. Treatments can be given up to 5 times/d. *Glossets: 10 and 15 mg* SL 10–20 mg q3–4h, not to exceed 60 mg/d.	Generally same as adult. Generally same as adult. *Glossets: 10 mg* SL 5–10 mg 3 times daily not to exceed 30 mg/d. Not a preferred route due to erratic absorption.
	Cardiac dysrhythmias	*IV:* 20–60 mcg bolus initially, followed by IV infusion. Dilute 1 mg/250 mL D5W, NS, or LR. Titrate to patient response: 2–10 mcg/min.	
	Shock	Dilute 1 mg/250 mL D5W, NS, or LR and infuse at 0.05–5 mcg/min. Titrate to patient response.	
Phenylephrine (Neo-Synephrine, others)	Hypotension/shock	*IM, Sub-Q:* 2–5 mg q1–2h. Initial dose not to exceed 5 mg. *IV bolus:* 0.1–0.5 mg, diluted in NaCl injection, given slowly q 10–15 min as needed. Initial dose not to exceed 0.5 mg *IV infusion:* 10 mg in 250 mL D5W or NS. Infuse at 100–180 mcg/min initially. When BP stable, reduce to maintenance rate of 40–60 mcg/min.	
	Nasal congestion	*Nasal decongestants: 0.25%, 0.5%, 1.0% solutions* 1–2 drops or sprays q4h. Therapy should not exceed 5 days.	
	Ophthalmic agent/ mydriatic agent	*Ophthalmic preparations: 2.5% or 10% solutions* Instill one drop. May be repeated in 10–60 min	

BP, blood pressure; D5W, dextrose 5% in water; IM, intramuscular; IV, intravenous; LR, lactated Ringer's; NS, 0.9% sodium chloride; PO, oral; SL, sublingual; Sub-Q, subcutaneous.

TABLE 17-3 Epinephrine Concentrations and Administration Routes

FINAL CONCENTRATION	ROUTE
1% (1:100)	Inhalation
0.5% (1:200)	Subcutaneous
0.1% (1:1000)	Subcutaneous
	Intramuscular
0.01% (1:10,000)	Intravenous
0.001% (1:100,000)	Intradermal (in combination with local anesthetics)

5 hours. When given Sub-Q, it acts in approximately 20 minutes, and its effects last approximately 60 minutes. When given intramuscularly, it acts in approximately 10 to 20 minutes, and its effects last less than 60 minutes. Ephedrine is excreted unchanged in the urine. Acidic urine increases the rate of drug elimination.

Ephedrine is a common ingredient in OTC antiasthma tablets (eg, Bronkaid, Primatene, others). The tablets contain 12.5 to 25 milligrams of ephedrine and 100 to 130 milligrams of theophylline, a xanthine bronchodilator. Other clinical uses include shock associated with spinal or epidural anesthesia, Stokes-Adams syndrome, allergic disorders, nasal congestion, and eye disorders.

APPLYING YOUR KNOWLEDGE 17-1
Review Mr. Rich's drug order. Why did the physician order this medication IV instead of PO?

Pseudoephedrine (Sudafed) is a related drug, stimulating alpha$_1$ and beta receptors. It is used as a bronchodilator and nasal decongestant. Pseudoephedrine is given orally and is available OTC alone and as an ingredient in several multi-ingredient sinus, allergy, and cold remedies. Pseudoephedrine is eliminated primarily in the urine. Its elimination may be slowed by alkaline urine, which promotes drug reabsorption in the renal tubules.

Isoproterenol (Isuprel) is a synthetic catecholamine that acts on beta$_1$- and beta$_2$-adrenergic receptors. Its main actions are to stimulate the heart, dilate blood vessels in skeletal muscle, and relax bronchial smooth muscle. Compared with epinephrine, isoproterenol has similar cardiac stimulant effects, but it does not affect alpha receptors and therefore does not cause vasoconstriction. It is well absorbed when given by injection or as an aerosol. However, absorption is unreliable with sublingual and oral preparations, so their use is not recommended. It is metabolized more slowly than epinephrine by the enzyme catechol-O-methyltransferase (COMT). It is not well metabolized by monoamine oxidase (MAO), which may account for its slightly longer duration of action than epinephrine.

Isoproterenol may be used as a cardiac stimulant in heart block and cardiogenic shock and as a bronchodilator in respiratory conditions characterized by bronchospasm. However, beta$_2$-selective agonists (eg, albuterol, others) are preferred for bronchodilating effects because they cause less cardiac stimulation. Too-frequent use of inhaled isoproterenol may lead to tolerance and decreased bronchodilating effects.

Phenylephrine (eg, Neo-Synephrine, others) is a synthetic drug that acts on alpha-adrenergic receptors to produce vasoconstriction. Vasoconstriction decreases cardiac output and renal perfusion and increases peripheral vascular resistance and blood pressure. There is little cardiac stimulation because phenylephrine does not activate beta$_1$ receptors in the heart or beta$_2$ receptors in blood vessels.

Phenylephrine may be given to increase blood pressure in hypotension and shock. Compared with epinephrine, phenylephrine produces longer-lasting elevation of blood pressure (20–50 minutes with injection). When given systemically, phenylephrine produces a reflex bradycardia. This effect may be used therapeutically to relieve paroxysmal atrial tachycardia. However, other medications such as calcium channel blockers (see Chaps. 49 and 50) are more likely to be used for this purpose. Other uses of phenylephrine include local application for nasal decongestant and mydriatic effects. Various preparations are available for different uses. Phenylephrine is often an ingredient in prescription and nonprescription cold and allergy remedies. It is excreted primarily in the urine.

 Herbal and Dietary Supplements

Ephedra (**ma huang**) is an OTC dietary supplement used for weight control, boosting sports performance, and increasing energy levels. Ephedra is a plant source of ephedrine alkaloids, including ephedrine and pseudoephedrine. The OTC use of ephedra has been linked to increased risk of hypertension, heart attack, stroke, and death. The Dietary Supplement Health and Education Act of 1994 grants the Food and Drug Administration (FDA) the authority to remove a dietary supplement from the market if it "presents a significant or unreasonable risk of illness or injury when used according to its labeling or under ordinary conditions of use." In 2004, using this law, the FDA prohibited the sale of any dietary supplements containing ephedrine alkaloids (ie, ephedra).

NURSING PROCESS

Assessment

Assess the client's status in relation to the following conditions.

● **Allergic disorders.** It is standard procedure to question a client about allergies on initial contact or admission to a health care agency. If the client reports a previous allergic reaction, try to determine what caused it and what specific symptoms occurred. It may be helpful to ask if swelling, breathing difficulty, or hives (urticaria) occurred. With anaphylactic reactions, severe respiratory distress (from bronchospasm and laryngeal edema) and profound hypotension (from vasodilation) may occur.

- **Asthma.** If the client is known to have asthma, assess the frequency of attacks, the specific signs and symptoms experienced, the precipitating factors, the actions taken to obtain relief, and the use of bronchodilators or other medications on a long-term basis. With acute bronchospasm, respiratory distress is clearly evidenced by loud, rapid, gasping, wheezing respirations. Acute asthma attacks may be precipitated by exposure to allergens or respiratory infections. When available, check arterial blood gas reports for the adequacy of oxygen–carbon dioxide gas exchange. Hypoxemia ($\downarrow$Po$_2$), hypercarbia ($\uparrow$Pco$_2$), and acidosis ($\downarrow$pH) may occur with acute bronchospasm.

- **Chronic obstructive pulmonary disorders.** Emphysema and chronic bronchitis are characterized by bronchoconstriction and dyspnea with exercise or at rest. Check arterial blood gas reports when available. Hypoxemia, hypercarbia, and acidosis are likely with chronic bronchoconstriction. Acute bronchospasm may be superimposed on the chronic bronchoconstrictive disorder, especially with a respiratory infection.

- **Cardiovascular status.** Assess for conditions that are caused or aggravated by adrenergic drugs (eg, angina, hypertension, tachydysrhythmias).

Nursing Diagnoses

- Impaired Gas Exchange related to bronchoconstriction
- Ineffective Tissue Perfusion related to hypotension and shock or vasoconstriction with drug therapy
- Imbalanced Nutrition: Less than Body Requirements related to anorexia
- Disturbed Sleep Pattern: Insomnia, nervousness
- Noncompliance: Overuse
- Risk for Injury related to cardiac stimulation (dysrhythmias, hypertension)
- Deficient Knowledge: Drug effects and safe usage

Planning/Goals

The client will

- Receive or self-administer drugs accurately
- Experience relief of symptoms for which adrenergic drugs are given
- Comply with instructions for safe drug use
- Demonstrate knowledge of adverse drug effects to be reported
- Avoid preventable adverse drug effects
- Avoid combinations of adrenergic drugs

Interventions

Use measures to prevent or minimize conditions for which adrenergic drugs are required.

- Decrease exposure to allergens. Allergens include cigarette smoke, foods, drugs, air pollutants, plant pollens, insect venoms, and animal dander. Specific allergens must be determined for each person.
- For clients with chronic lung disease, use measures to prevent respiratory infections. These include interventions to aid removal of respiratory secretions, such as adequate hydration, ambulation, deep-breathing and coughing exercises, and chest physiotherapy. Immunizations with pneumococcal pneumonia vaccine (a single dose) and influenza vaccine (annually) are also strongly recommended.
- When administering substances known to produce hypersensitivity reactions (penicillin and other antibiotics, allergy extracts, vaccines, local anesthetics), observe the recipient carefully for at least 30 minutes after administration. Have adrenergic and other emergency drugs and equipment readily available in case a reaction occurs.
- Use noninvasive interventions in addition to adrenergic medications when treating shock and hypotension. These include applying external pressure over a bleeding site to control hemorrhage and placing the client in a recumbent position to improve venous return and blood pressure.

Provide appropriate teaching for drug therapy (see accompanying client teaching display).

Evaluation

- Observe for increased blood pressure and improved tissue perfusion when a drug is given for hypotension and shock or anaphylaxis.
- Interview and observe for improved breathing and arterial blood gas reports when a drug is given for bronchoconstriction or anaphylaxis.
- Interview and observe for decreased nasal congestion.

PRINCIPLES OF THERAPY

Drug Selection and Administration

The choice of drug, dosage, and route of administration depends largely on the reason for use (see Table 17–1). Adrenergic drugs are given IV only for emergencies, such as cardiac arrest, severe arterial hypotension, circulatory shock, and anaphylactic shock. IV or Sub-Q epinephrine is the drug of choice in anaphylactic shock. No standard doses of individual adrenergic drugs are always effective; the dose must be individualized or titrated to the client's response. This is especially true in emergencies, but it also applies to long-term use.

C L I E N T   T E A C H I N G   G U I D E L I N E S

Adrenergic Drugs

General Considerations

☑ Take no other medications without the physician's knowledge and approval. Many over-the-counter (OTC) cold remedies and appetite suppressants contain adrenergic drugs. Use of these along with pre-scribed adrenergic drugs can result in overdose and serious cardio-vascular or central nervous system problems. In addition, adrenergic drugs interact with numerous other drugs to increase or decrease effects; some of these interactions may be life threatening.

☑ Herbal preparations of ephedra or ma huang contain derivatives of ephedrine and should not be taken with other adrenergic medica-tions. Excessive central nervous system and cardiovascular stimu-lation may result. (Sale of supplements containing ephedra was banned by the FDA in 2003.)

☑ Tell your health care provider if you are pregnant, breast-feeding, taking any other prescription or OTC drugs, or if you are allergic to sulfite preservatives.

☑ Use these drugs only as directed. The potential for abuse is high, especially for the client with asthma or other chronic lung disease who is seeking relief from labored breathing. Some of these drugs are prescribed for long-term use, but excessive use does not increase therapeutic effects. Instead, it causes tolerance and decreased benefit from usual doses and increases the incidence and severity of adverse reactions.

☑ Frequent cardiac monitoring and checks of flow rate, blood pres-sure, and urine output are necessary if you are receiving intra-venous adrenergic drugs to stimulate your heart or raise your blood pressure. These measures increase the safety and benefits of drug therapy rather than indicate the presence of a critical con-dition. Ask your nurse if you have concerns about your condition.

☑ You may feel anxious or tense; have difficulty sleeping; and expe-rience palpitations, blurred vision, headache, tremor, dizziness,

and pallor. These are effects of the medication. Use of relaxation techniques to promote rest and decrease muscle tension may be helpful.

☑ Use caution when driving or performing activities requiring alert-ness, dexterity, and good vision.

☑ Report adverse reactions such as fast pulse, palpitations, and chest pain so that drug dosage can be re-evaluated and therapy changed if needed.

Self-Administration

☑ Do not use topical decongestants longer than 3 to 5 days. Long-term use may be habit forming. Burning on use and rebound con-gestion after the dose wears off are common. Stop using the medication gradually.

☑ Stinging may occur when using ophthalmic preparations. Do not let the tip of the applicator touch your eye or anything else during administration of the medication, to avoid contamination. Do not wear soft contact lenses while using ophthalmic adrenergic drugs; discoloration of the lenses may occur. Report blurred vision, headache, palpitations, and muscle tremors to your health care provider.

☑ Follow guidelines for use of your inhaler. Do not increase the dosage or frequency; tolerance may occur. Report chest pain, dizziness, or failure to obtain relief of symptoms. Saliva and sputum may be discolored pink with isoproterenol.

☑ Learn to self-administer an injection of epinephrine if you have severe allergies. Always carry your injection kit with you. Seek immediate medical care after self-injection of epinephrine.

☑ If you are diabetic, monitor your glucose levels carefully because adrenergic medications may elevate them.

APPLYING YOUR KNOWLEDGE 17-2:
HOW CAN YOU AVOID THIS MEDICATION ERROR?
Epinephrine 1 mg is ordered to be given in a 1:10,000 dilution. You add 1 mL of normal saline and administer the drug.

Treatment of Specific Disorders

Because adrenergic drugs are often used in crises, they must be readily available in all health care settings (eg, hospitals, long-term care facilities, physicians' offices). All health care personnel should know where emergency drugs are stored.

Anaphylaxis

Epinephrine is the drug of choice for the treatment of ana-phylaxis. It relieves bronchospasm, laryngeal edema, and hypotension. In conjunction with its alpha (vasoconstriction)

and beta (cardiac stimulation, bronchodilation) effects, epi-nephrine acts as a physiologic antagonist of histamine and other bronchoconstricting and vasodilating substances released during anaphylactic reactions. People susceptible to severe allergic responses should carry a syringe of epinephrine at all times. Epipen and Epipen Jr. are prefilled, autoinjection syringes for self-administration of epinephrine in emergency situations.

Victims of anaphylaxis who have been taking beta-adrenergic blocking drugs (eg, propranolol [Inderal]) do not respond as readily to epinephrine as those not taking beta blockers. Larger doses of epinephrine and large amounts of IV fluids may be required. Adjunct medications that may be useful in treating severe cases of anaphylaxis include corti-costeroids, norepinephrine, and aminophylline. Antihista-mines are not very useful because histamine plays a minor role in causing anaphylaxis, compared with leukotrienes and other inflammatory mediators.

APPLYING YOUR KNOWLEDGE 17-3
The physician orders piperacillin/tazobactam, a beta-lactam antibiotic, to treat Mr. Rich's pneumonia. Within 15 minutes of the start of the antibiotic infusion, Mr. Rich begins an anaphylactic reaction. He is agitated and flushed and complains of palpitations. He is having severe difficulty breathing due to bronchospasm. The physician orders epinephrine. What are the nursing implications for Mr. Rich's reaction to the antibiotic, and what assessment is needed relative to the adverse effects of epinephrine?

Cardiopulmonary Resuscitation

Epinephrine is often administered during CPR. The most important action of epinephrine during cardiac arrest is constriction of peripheral blood vessels, which shunts blood to the central circulation and increases blood flow to the heart and brain. This beneficial effect comes at the expense of increased oxygen consumption by the myocardium, ventricular dysrhythmias and myocardial dysfunction after resuscitation. Epinephrine was once considered the drug of choice in the treatment of cardiac arrest. The most recent Advanced Cardiac Life Support (ACLS) guidelines for health professionals (2000) continue to support epinephrine for first use, classifying it as class *indeterminate* for the treatment of defibrillation-resistant ventricular tachycardia and ventricular fibrillation during cardiac arrest. Class *indeterminate* refers to a promising treatment that lacks research evidence of benefit.

Vasopressin may be used in this situation as an alternative pressor. An advantage of vasopressin over epinephrine is the ability of vasopressin to increase coronary blood flow and the availability of oxygen to the myocardium during resuscitation efforts. Vasopressin is classified as class *IIb*, which means that the usefulness of the drug is supported by fair-to-good research. Class *IIb* drugs are considered optional or alternative interventions by the majority of experts in treatment of cardiac arrest; recent evidence suggests that vasopressin may be superior to epinephrine for treatment of asystolic cardiac arrest (see Research Brief). When used during resuscitation efforts, vasopressin is given as a single dose of 40 units IV (see Chap. 22). Epinephrine is still considered the drug of choice for the treatment of cardiac arrest in cases of nonventricular tachycardia/fibrillation such as pulseless electrical activity. Epinephrine is beneficial in these situations because it stimulates electrical and mechanical activity and produces myocardial contraction.

The specific effects of epinephrine depend largely on the dose and route of administration. The optimal dose in CPR has not been established. ACLS guidelines recommend epinephrine 1 milligram IV every 3 to 5 minutes. If this fails, higher doses of epinephrine (up to 0.2 mg/kg) are acceptable but not recommended. In fact, there is growing evidence that higher doses of epinephrine may be harmful to both adults and children (see Research Brief).

RESEARCH BRIEF

Epinephrine vs. Vasopressin: A Look at Selected Current Research

SOURCES:
1. Gueugniaud, P., Mols, P., Goldstein, P., Pham, E., Dubien, P., Deweerdt, C., Vergnion, M., Petit, P., & Carli, P. (2004). A comparison of repeated high doses and repeated standard doses of epinephrine for cardiac arrest outside the hospital. *New England Journal of Medicine, 339*(22), 1595–1601.

2. Perondi, M., Reis, A., Paiva, E., Nadkarni, V., & Berg, R. (2004). A comparison of high-dose and standard-dose epinephrine in children with cardiac arrest. *New England Journal of Medicine, 350*(17), 1722–1730.

3. Wenzel, V., Kismer, A., Arntz, R., Sitter, H., Stadlbauer, K., & Lindner, K., European Resuscitation Council During Cardiopulmonary Resuscitation Study Group. (2004). A comparison of vasopressin and epinephrine for out-of-hospital cardiopulmonary resuscitation. *New England Journal of Medicine, 350*(2), 105–113.

SUMMARY:
There is ongoing debate and research regarding the pharmacologic approach to cardiac arrest that will produce the highest rate of restoration of spontaneous circulation and the highest survival rates post-resuscitation. Results of the studies cited above are as follows:

1. More than 3300 clients in a prospective multi-center study of out-of-hospital cardiac arrest *incidents* were randomly assigned to receive either high-dose epinephrine (5 mg) or standard-dose epinephrine (1 mg) during resuscitation efforts. Spontaneous circulation returned to 40.4% of clients in the high-dose group, compared with 36.4% in the standard-dose group. However, only 2.3% of the clients in the high-dose group survived to be discharged from the hospital, compared with 2.8% in the standard-dose group. There was no difference in the neurologic status between the two groups of survivors. The researchers concluded that high doses of epinephrine produced significantly higher rates of resuscitation, but did not have beneficial effects on long-term survival or neurologic outcome.

2. The 68 children in a prospective, double-blind study of in-hospital cardiac arrest *incidents* were randomly assigned to receive either high-dose epinephrine (0.1 mg/kg) or standard-dose epinephrine (0.01 mg/kg) after failure of an initial, standard dose of epinephrine. The two groups did not differ significantly in rate of return to spontaneous circulation. However, survival at 24 hours post-resuscitation was significantly

(Continued)

**Epinephrine vs. Vasopressin:
A Look at Selected Current Research (*Continued*)**

lower in the high-dose epinephrine group (1 of 34) than in the standard-dose group (7 of 34). None of the children in the high-dose group survived to hospital discharge, and 4 in the standard-dose group were discharged. In addition, in the 30 children whose cardiac arrest was a result of respiratory arrest, none in the high-dose epinephrine group (12) were alive at 24 hours, compared with 7 in the standard-dose group (18). The researchers concluded that there was no benefit to high-dose epinephrine for in-hospital resuscitation in children after failure of a standard dose of epinephrine, and that high-dose epinephrine therapy may be detrimental to the desired outcome.

3. More than 1180 clients experiencing out-of-hospital cardiac arrest were randomly assigned to receive either two injections of vasopressin (40 IU) or two injections of epinephrine (1 mg), followed by additional treatment with epinephrine if needed. There were no significant differences between the two treatment groups with regard to survival to hospital admission for clients experiencing ventricular fibrillation or pulseless electrical activity (PEA). However, for clients with asystole, survival to hospital admission (29% vs. 30.3%) and survival to hospital discharge (4.7% vs. 1.5%) were significantly improved in the vasopressin group. Among the clients for whom spontaneous circulation was not initially restored with the two injections of epinephrine or vasopressin, additional treatment with epinephrine was beneficial in the vasopressin group but did not improve survival in the epinephrine group. There was no difference in the neurologic status of survivors in either group. The researchers concluded that the effects of vasopressin were similar to epinephrine in the management of cardiac arrest due to ventricular fibrillation or PEA; however, vasopressin was superior to epinephrine in the treatment of asystole. In addition, vasopressin followed by epinephrine may be more effective than epinephrine alone in treatment of refractory cardiac arrest.

NURSING IMPLICATIONS: It is imperative that nurses in critical care areas maintain current Advanced Cardiac Life Support (ACLS) certification and stay alert to research findings that may influence ACLS protocols for resuscitation in the future.

Hypotension and Shock

In hypotension and shock, initial efforts involve identifying and treating the cause when possible. Such treatments include placing the client in the recumbent position; blood transfusions; fluid and electrolyte replacement; treatment of infection; and use of positive inotropic drugs to treat heart failure. If these measures are ineffective in raising the blood pressure enough to maintain perfusion to vital organs such as the brain, kidneys, and heart, vasopressor drugs may be used. The usual goal of vasopressor drug therapy is to maintain tissue perfusion and a mean arterial pressure of at least 80 to 100 mm Hg.

Nasal Congestion

Adrenergic drugs are given topically and systemically to constrict blood vessels in nasal mucosa and decrease the nasal congestion associated with the common cold, allergic rhinitis, and sinusitis. Topical agents are effective, undergo little systemic absorption, are available OTC, and are widely used. However, overuse leads to decreased effectiveness (tolerance); irritation and ischemic changes in the nasal mucosa; and rebound congestion. These effects can be minimized by using small doses only when necessary and for no longer than 3 to 5 days.

Oral drugs have a slower onset of action than topical ones but may last longer. They also may cause more adverse effects, which may occur with usual therapeutic doses and are especially likely with high doses. The most problematic adverse effects are cardiac and CNS stimulation. Commonly used oral agents are pseudoephedrine and ephedrine. Pseudoephedrine seems to be the safest in relation to risks of hypertension and cerebral hemorrhage (stroke). Ephedrine may cause hypertension even in normotensive people, and risks are higher risks in hypertensive people. Hypertensive clients should avoid these drugs if possible.

Toxicity of Adrenergics: Recognition and Management

Unlike catecholamines, which are quickly cleared from the body, excessive use of noncatecholamine adrenergic drugs (phenylephrine, ephedrine, and pseudoephedrine) can lead to overdose and toxicity. These drugs are an ingredient in OTC products such as nasal decongestants, cold preparations, and appetite suppressants. Phenylephrine and ephedrine have a narrow therapeutic index; toxic doses are only two to three times greater than the therapeutic dose. Pseudoephedrine toxicity occurs with doses four to five times greater than the normal therapeutic dose. Ephedrine and ephedra-containing herbal preparations (eg, ma huang, herbal ecstasy) are often abused as an alternative to amphetamines. These substances were banned in the U.S. in 2003.

The primary clinical manifestation of noncatecholamine adrenergic drug toxicity is severe hypertension, which may lead to headache, confusion, seizures, and intracranial hemorrhage. Reflex bradycardia and atrioventricular block also have been associated with phenylephrine toxicity.

Treatment involves maintaining an airway and assisting with ventilation if needed. Activated charcoal may be administered early in treatment. Hypertension is aggressively treated with vasodilators such as phentolamine or nitroprusside. Beta blockers are not used alone to treat hypertension without first administering a vasodilator, to avoid a paradoxical increase in blood pressure. Dialysis and hemoperfusion are not effective in clearing these drugs from the body. Urinary acidification may enhance elimination of ephedrine and pseudoephedrine; however, this technique is not routinely used because of the risk of renal damage from myoglobin deposition in the kidney.

Use in Special Populations

Use in Children

Adrenergic agents are used to treat asthma, hypotension, shock, cardiac arrest, and anaphylaxis in children. However, guidelines for safe and effective use of adrenergic drugs in children are not well established. Children are very sensitive to drug effects, including cardiac and CNS stimulation, and recommended doses usually should not be exceeded.

Epinephrine is mainly used in children for treatment of bronchospasm due to asthma or allergic reactions. Parenteral epinephrine may cause syncope when given to asthmatic children. Isoproterenol is rarely given parenterally to children, but if it is, the first dose should be approximately half the adult dose, and later doses should be based on the response to the first dose. There is little reason to use the inhalation route, because in children, as in adults, selective beta$_2$ agonists such as albuterol are preferred for bronchodilation in asthma.

Phenylephrine is most often used to relieve congestion of the upper respiratory tract and may be given topically, as nose drops. Doses must be carefully measured. Rebound nasal congestion occurs with overuse.

Use in Older Adults

Adrenergic agents are used to treat asthma, hypotension, shock, cardiac arrest, and anaphylaxis in older adults. These drugs stimulate the heart to increase rate and force of contraction and blood pressure. Because older adults often have chronic cardiovascular conditions (eg, angina, dysrhythmias, congestive heart failure, coronary artery disease, hypertension, peripheral vascular disease) that are aggravated by adrenergic drugs, careful monitoring by the nurse is required.

Adrenergic drugs are often prescribed as bronchodilators and decongestants in older adults. Therapeutic doses increase the workload of the heart and may cause symptoms of impaired cardiovascular function. Overdoses may cause severe cardiovascular dysfunction, including life-threatening dysrhythmias. The drugs also cause CNS stimulation. With therapeutic doses, anxiety, restlessness, nervousness, and insomnia often occur in older adults. Overdoses may cause hallucinations, convulsions, CNS depression, and death.

Adrenergics are ingredients in OTC asthma remedies, cold remedies, nasal decongestants, and appetite suppressants. Cau-

tious use of these preparations is required in older adults. The drugs should not be taken concurrently with prescription adrenergic drugs because of the high risk of overdose and toxicity.

Ophthalmic preparations of adrenergic drugs also should be used cautiously. For example, phenylephrine is used as a vasoconstrictor and mydriatic. Applying larger-than-recommended doses to the normal eye or usual doses to the traumatized, inflamed, or diseased eye may result in sufficient systemic absorption of the drug to cause increased blood pressure and other adverse effects.

Use in Clients With Renal Impairment

Adrenergic drugs exert effects on the renal system that may cause problems for clients with renal impairment. For example, adrenergic drugs with alpha$_1$ activity cause constriction of renal arteries, thereby diminishing renal blood flow and urine production. These drugs also constrict urinary sphincters, causing urinary retention and painful urination, especially in men with prostatic hyperplasia.

Many adrenergic drugs and their metabolites are eliminated by the renal system. In the presence of renal disease, these compounds may accumulate and cause increased adverse effects.

Use in Clients With Hepatic Impairment

The liver is rich in the enzymes MAO and COMT, which are responsible for metabolism of circulating epinephrine and other adrenergic drugs (eg, norepinephrine, dopamine, isoproterenol). However, other tissues in the body also possess these enzymes and are capable of metabolizing natural and synthetic catecholamines. Any unchanged drug can be excreted in the urine. Many noncatecholamine adrenergic drugs are excreted largely unchanged in the urine. Therefore, liver disease is not usually considered a contraindication to administering adrenergic drugs.

Use in Clients With Critical Illness

Adrenergic drugs are an important component of the emergency drug box. They are essential for treating hypotension; shock; asystole and other dysrhythmias; acute bronchospasm; and anaphylaxis. Although they may save the life of a critically ill client, use of adrenergic drugs may result in secondary health problems that require monitoring and intervention. These health problems include:

- Potential for the vasopressor action of adrenergic drugs to result in diminished renal perfusion and decreased urine output
- Potential for adrenergic drugs with beta$_1$ activity to induce irritable cardiac dysrhythmias
- Potential for adrenergic drugs with beta$_1$ activity to increase myocardial oxygen requirement
- Potential for adrenergic drugs with vasopressor action to decrease perfusion to the liver, with subsequent liver damage

- Hyperglycemia, hypokalemia, and hypophosphatemia due to beta$_1$-adrenergic effects
- Severe hypertension and reflex bradycardia
- Tissue necrosis after extravasation

Occurrence of any of these adverse effects may complicate the already complex care of critically ill clients. Careful assessment and prompt nursing intervention are essential.

Use in Home Care

Adrenergic drugs are often used in the home setting. Frequently prescribed drugs include bronchodilators and nasal decongestants. OTC drugs with the same effects are also commonly used to treat asthma, allergic rhinitis, cold symptoms, and appetite suppression for weight control. A major function of the home care nurse is to teach clients to use the drugs correctly (especially metered-dose inhalers); to report excessive CNS or cardiac stimulation to a health care provider; and not to take OTC drugs or herbal preparations with the same or similar ingredients as prescription drugs.

Excessive adverse effects are probably most likely to occur in children and older adults. Older adults often have other illnesses that may be aggravated by adrenergic drugs or they may take other drugs whose effects may be altered by concomitant use of adrenergics.

NURSING ACTIONS

Adrenergic Drugs

NURSING ACTIONS	RATIONALE/EXPLANATION
1. Administer accurately	
a. Check package inserts or other references if not absolutely sure about the preparation, concentration, or method of administration for an adrenergic drug.	The many different preparations and concentrations available for various routes of administration increase the risk of medication error unless extreme caution is used. Preparations for intravenous (IV), subcutaneous, inhalation, ophthalmic, or nasal routes must be used by the designated route only.
b. To give epinephrine subcutaneously, use a tuberculin syringe, aspirate, and massage the injection site.	The tuberculin syringe is necessary for accurate measurement of the small doses usually given (often less than 0.5 mL). Aspiration is necessary to avoid inadvertent IV administration of the larger, undiluted amount of drug intended for subcutaneous use. Massaging the injection site accelerates drug absorption and thus relief of symptoms.
c. For inhalation, be sure to use the correct drug concentration, and use the nebulizing device properly.	Inhalation medications are often administered by clients themselves or by respiratory therapists if intermittent positive-pressure breathing is used. The nurse may need to demonstrate and supervise self-administration initially.
d. Do *not* give epinephrine and isoproterenol at the same time or within 4 hours of each other.	Both of these drugs are potent cardiac stimulants, and the combination could cause serious cardiac dysrhythmias. However, they have synergistic bronchodilating effects, and doses can be alternated and given safely if the drugs are given no more closely together than 4 hours.
e. Follow package insert guidelines carefully when diluting epinephrine for IV injection or IV infusion. Administer in an intensive care unit, when possible, using an infusion pump and a central IV line. Use parenteral solutions of epinephrine only if clear. Epinephrine is unstable in alkaline solutions.	Dilution increases safety of administration. A solution that is brown or contains a precipitate should not be used. Discoloration indicates chemical deterioration of epinephrine. Do not administer at the same time that sodium bicarbonate is being administered.
f. For IV infusion of isoproterenol and phenylephrine:	
(1) Administer in an intensive care unit when possible.	These drugs are given IV in emergencies, during which the client's condition must be carefully monitored. Frequent recording of blood pressure and pulse and continuous electrocardiographic monitoring are needed.

NURSING ACTIONS	RATIONALE/EXPLANATION
(2) Use only clear drug solutions.	A brownish color or precipitate indicates deterioration, and such solutions should not be used.
(3) Dilute isoproterenol in 500 mL of 5% dextrose injection. Phenylephrine can be diluted in 5% dextrose injection or 0.9% sodium chloride solution. Do not add the drug until ready to use.	Mixing solutions when ready for use helps to ensure drug stability. Note that drug concentration varies with the amount of drug and the amount of IV solution to which it is added.
(4) Use an infusion device to regulate flow rate accurately.	Flow rate usually requires frequent adjustment according to blood pressure measurements. An infusion device helps to regulate drug administration, so wide fluctuations in blood pressure are avoided.
(5) Use a "piggyback" IV apparatus.	Only one bottle contains an adrenergic drug, and it can be regulated or discontinued without disruption of the primary IV line.
(6) Start the adrenergic drug solution slowly and increase flow rate according to the client's response (eg, blood pressure, color, mental status). Slow or discontinue the solution gradually as well.	To avoid abrupt changes in circulation and blood pressure
g. When giving adrenergic drugs as eye drops or nose drops, do not touch the dropper to the eye or nose.	Contaminated droppers can be a source of bacterial infection.
2. Observe for therapeutic effects	These depend on the reason for use.
a. When the drug is used as a bronchodilator, observe for absence or reduction of wheezing, less labored breathing, and decreased rate of respirations.	Indicates prevention or relief of bronchospasm. Acute bronchospasm is usually relieved within 5 minutes by injected or inhaled epinephrine or inhaled isoproterenol.
b. When epinephrine is given in anaphylactic shock, observe for decreased tissue edema and improved breathing and circulation.	Epinephrine injection usually relieves laryngeal edema and bronchospasm within 5 minutes and lasts for approximately 20 minutes.
c. When isoproterenol or phenylephrine is given in hypotension and shock, observe for increased blood pressure, stronger pulse, and improved urine output, level of consciousness, and color.	These are indicators of improved circulation.
d. When a drug is given nasally for decongestant effects, observe for decreased nasal congestion and ability to breathe through the nose.	The drugs act as vasoconstrictors to reduce engorgement of nasal mucosa.
e. When given as eye drops for vasoconstrictor effects, observe for decreased redness. When giving for mydriatic effects, observe for pupil dilation.	
3. Observe for adverse effects	Adverse effects depend to some extent on the reason for use. For example, cardiovascular effects are considered adverse reactions when the drugs are given for bronchodilation. Adverse effects occur with usual therapeutic doses and are more likely to occur with higher doses.
a. Cardiovascular effects—cardiac dysrhythmias, hypertension	Tachycardia and hypertension are common; if severe or prolonged, myocardial ischemia or heart failure may occur. Premature ventricular contractions and other serious dysrhythmias may occur. Propranolol (Inderal) or another beta blocker may be given to decrease heart rate and hypertension resulting from overdosage of adrenergic drugs. Phentolamine may be used to decrease severe hypertension.
b. Excessive central nervous system (CNS) stimulation— nervousness, anxiety, tremor, insomnia	These effects are more likely to occur with ephedrine or high doses of other adrenergic drugs. Sometimes, a sedative-type drug is given concomitantly to offset these effects.
c. Rebound nasal congestion, rhinitis, possible ulceration of nasal mucosa	These effects occur with excessive use of nasal decongestant drugs.

(continued)

NURSING ACTIONS	RATIONALE/EXPLANATION
4. Observe for drug interactions	
a. Drugs that *increase* effects of adrenergic drugs:	Most of these drugs increase incidence or severity of adverse reactions.
(1) Anesthetics, general (eg, halothane)	Increased risk of cardiac dysrhythmias. Potentially hazardous.
(2) Anticholinergics (eg, atropine)	Increased bronchial relaxation. Also increased mydriasis and therefore contraindicated with narrow-angle glaucoma.
(3) Antidepressants, tricyclic (eg, amitriptyline [Elavil])	Increased pressor response with IV epinephrine
(4) Antihistamines	May increase pressor effects
(5) Cocaine	Increases pressor and mydriatic effects by inhibiting uptake of norepinephrine by nerve endings. Cardiac dysrhythmias, convulsions, and acute glaucoma may occur.
(6) Digoxin	Sympathomimetics, especially beta-adrenergics like epinephrine and isoproterenol, increase the likelihood of cardiac dysrhythmias due to ectopic pacemaker activity.
(7) Doxapram (Dopram)	Increased pressor effect
(8) Ergot alkaloids	Increased vasoconstriction. Extremely high blood pressure may occur. There also may be decreased perfusion of fingers and toes.
(9) Monoamine oxidase (MAO) inhibitors (eg, isocarboxazid [Marplan])	**CONTRAINDICATED. THE COMBINATION MAY CAUSE DEATH.** When these drugs are given concurrently with adrenergic drugs, there is danger of cardiac dysrhythmias, respiratory depression, and acute hypertensive crisis with possible intracranial hemorrhage, convulsions, coma, and death. Effects of a MAO inhibitor may not occur for several weeks after treatment is started and may last up to 3 weeks after the drug is stopped. Every client taking a MAO inhibitor should be warned against taking any other medication without the advice of a physician or pharmacist.
(10) Methylphenidate (Ritalin)	Increased pressor and mydriatic effects. The combination may be hazardous in glaucoma.
(11) Thyroid preparations (eg, Synthroid)	Increased adrenergic effects, resulting in increased likelihood of dysrhythmias
(12) Xanthines (in caffeine-containing substances, such as coffee, tea, cola drinks; theophylline)	Synergistic bronchodilating effect. Sympathomimetics with CNS-stimulating properties (eg, ephedrine, isoproterenol) may produce excessive CNS stimulation with cardiac dysrhythmias, emotional disturbances, and insomnia.
(13) Beta-adrenergic blocking agents (eg, propranolol [Inderal])	May augment hypertensive response to epinephrine (see also b[4] below)
b. Drugs that *decrease* effects of adrenergics drugs:	
(1) Anticholinesterases (eg, neostigmine [Prostigmin], pyridostigmine [Mestinon]) and other cholinergic drugs	Decrease mydriatic effects of adrenergics; thus, the two groups should not be given concurrently in ophthalmic conditions.
(2) Antihypertensives (eg, methyldopa)	Generally antagonize pressor effects of adrenergics, which act to increase blood pressure while antihypertensives act to lower it.
(3) Antipsychotic drugs (eg, haloperidol [Haldol])	Block the vasopressor action of epinephrine. Therefore, epinephrine should not be used to treat hypotension induced by these drugs.
(4) Beta-adrenergic blocking agents (eg, propranolol [Inderal])	Decrease bronchodilating effects of adrenergics and may exacerbate asthma. Contraindicated with asthma.
(5) Phentolamine (Regitine)	Antagonizes vasopressor effects of adrenergics

APPLYING YOUR KNOWLEDGE: ANSWERS

17-1 Epinephrine is not given orally because the enzymes in the GI tract and liver destroy it.

17-2 Epinephrine 1:1000 has a 1 mg/1 mL concentration. To yield a 1:10,000 solution, 10 mL of normal saline should have been used. Read drug-mixing instructions carefully.

17-3 Mr. Rich has had an anaphylactic reaction to an antibiotic. Make sure to advise Mr. Rich of his allergy and note it on his chart. Observe the client for increased blood pressure, tachycardia, and hyperglycemia (adverse effects of epinephrine).

Review and Application Exercises

Short Answer Exercises

1. How do adrenergic drugs act to relieve symptoms of acute bronchospasm, anaphylaxis, cardiac arrest, hypotension and shock, and nasal congestion?

2. Which adrenergic receptors are stimulated by administration of epinephrine?

3. Why is it important to have epinephrine and other adrenergic drugs readily available in all health care settings?

4. Which adrenergic drug is the drug of choice to treat acute anaphylactic reactions?

5. Why is inhaled epinephrine not a drug of choice for long-term treatment of asthma and other bronchoconstrictive disorders?

6. What are the major adverse effects of adrenergic drugs?

7. Why are clients with cardiac dysrhythmias, angina pectoris, hypertension, or diabetes mellitus especially likely to experience adverse reactions to adrenergic drugs?

8. For a client who reports frequent use of OTC asthma remedies and cold remedies, what teaching is needed to increase client safety?

9. Mentally rehearse nursing interventions for various emergency situations (anaphylaxis, acute respiratory distress, cardiac arrest) in terms of medications and equipment needed and how to obtain them promptly.

10. What signs and symptoms occur with overdose of noncatecholamine adrenergic drugs? What interventions are needed to treat the toxicity?

NCLEX-Style Questions

11. The medical history of a client with nasal congestion includes depression. Which of the following medications would contraindicate the use of pseudoephedrine (Sudafed) to treat the nasal congestion?
    a. fluoxetine (Prozac)
    b. amitriptyline (Elavil)
    c. isocarboxazid (Marplan)
    d. lithium (Lithotab)

12. Which of the following is the main therapeutic benefit of administering drugs with beta$_2$ agonist activity?
    a. vasoconstriction and elevation of the blood pressure
    b. relaxation of bronchial smooth muscle and bronchodilation
    c. elevated heart rate and improved force of myocardial contraction
    d. uterine contraction and induction of labor

13. A client with asthma tells the nurse he is using his metered-dose inhaler of epinephrine more frequently than prescribed, to control wheezing. The nurse is concerned because this behavior may result in
    a. drug tolerance
    b. heart failure
    c. drug toxicity
    d. diabetes mellitus

14. The nurse teaches the diabetic client using adrenergic medications to anticipate
    a. no change in blood glucose levels
    b. a decrease in blood glucose levels
    c. an increase in blood glucose levels
    d. more fluctuation in blood glucose levels

15. When responding to hypotension due to hypovolemic shock, which of the following should be administered first?
    a. epinephrine (Adrenalin)
    b. isoproterenol (Isuprel)
    c. normal saline IV
    d. ephedrine

16. Which of the following drugs is first administered by the nurse to treat an anaphylactic reaction to penicillin?
    a. diphenhydramine (Benadryl)
    b. epinephrine (Adrenalin)
    c. isoproterenol (Isuprel)
    d. dexamethasone (Decadron)

Selected References

Drug facts and comparisons. (Updated monthly). St. Louis: Facts and Comparisons.

Fetrow, C. W., & Avila, J. R. (2001). *Complementary and alternative medicines* (2nd ed.). Springhouse, PA: Springhouse.

Gueugniaud, P., Mols, P., Goldstein, P., Pham, E., Dubien, P., Deweerdt, C., Vergnion, M., Petit, P., & Carli, P. (2004). A comparison of repeated high doses and repeated standard doses of epinephrine for cardiac arrest outside the hospital. *New England Journal of Medicine, 339*(22), 1595–1601.

Hazinski, M. F., Cummings, R. O., & Field, J. M. (Eds.). (2000). *Handbook of emergency cardiovascular care for health care providers.* Dallas: American Heart Association.

Hoffman, B. B. (2001). Adrenoreceptor-activating and other sympathomimetic drugs. In B. G. Katzung (Ed.), *Basic and clinical pharmacology* (8th ed., pp. 120–137). New York: McGraw-Hill.

Hoffman, B. B. (2001). Catecholamines, sympathomimetic drugs, and adrenergic receptor antagonists. In J. G. Hardman & L. E. Limbird (Eds.), *Goodman and Gilman's The pharmacological basis of therapeutics* (10th ed., pp. 215–268). New York: McGraw-Hill.

Hoffman, B. B., & Taylor, P. (2001). Neurotransmission: The autonomic and somatic motor nervous systems. In J. G. Hardman & L. E. Limbird (Eds.), *Goodman & Gilman's The pharmacological basis of therapeutics* (10th ed., pp. 115–153). New York: McGraw-Hill.

Lister, G., & Fontan, J. (2004). Can resuscitation jeopardize survival? *The New England Journal of Medicine 350* (17), 1708–1709.

Olson, K. R. (Ed.). (1999). *Poisoning and drug overdose* (3rd ed.). Stamford, CT: Appleton & Lange.

Perondi, M., Reis, A., Paiva, E., Nadkarni, V., & Berg, R. (2004). A comparison of high-dose and standard-dose epinephrine in children with cardiac arrest. *New England Journal of Medicine, 350*(17), 1722–1730.

Piano, M. R., & Huether, S. E. (2002). Mechanisms of hormonal regulation. In K. L. McCance & S. E. Huether (Eds.), *Pathophysiology: The biologic basis for disease in adults and children* (4th ed., pp. 597–623). St. Louis: Mosby.

Wenzel, V., Kismer, A., Arntz, R., Sitter, H., Stadlbauer, K., & Lindner, K., European Resuscitation Council During Cardiopulmonary Resuscitation Study Group. (2004). A comparison of vasopressin and epinephrine for out-of-hospital cardiopulmonary resuscitation. *New England Journal of Medicine, 350*(2), 105–113.

Antiadrenergic Drugs

OBJECTIVES

After studying this chapter, you will be able to:

1. List characteristics of antiadrenergic drugs in terms of effects on body tissues, indications for use, nursing process implications, principles of therapy, and observation of client response.
2. Discuss alpha$_1$-adrenergic blocking drugs and alpha$_2$-adrenergic agonists in terms of indications for use, adverse effects, and other selected characteristics.
3. Compare and contrast beta-adrenergic blocking drugs in terms of cardioselectivity, indications for use, adverse effects, and other selected characteristics.
4. Teach clients about safe, effective use of antiadrenergic drugs.
5. Discuss principles of therapy and nursing process for using antiadrenergic drugs in special populations.

APPLYING YOUR KNOWLEDGE

William Jones is a 58-year-old Caucasian male with a long history of hypertension. He has hyperlipidemia, type II diabetes mellitus, and coronary artery disease with a history of a myocardial infarction (MI) and triple coronary artery bypass graft. He is prescribed Lopressor 100 mg daily and clonidine transdermal patch every 7 days.

INTRODUCTION

Antiadrenergic drugs decrease or block the effects of sympathetic nerve stimulation, endogenous catecholamines (eg, epinephrine), and adrenergic drugs. The drugs are chemically diverse and have a wide spectrum of pharmacologic activity. Specific effects depend mainly on the client's health status when a drug is given, and the drug's binding with particular adrenergic receptors. Included in this chapter are centrally active antiadrenergic drugs such as clonidine, which are used primarily in the treatment of hypertension, and peripherally active alpha- and beta-adrenergic blocking agents, which are used to treat various cardiovascular and other disorders. A few uncommonly used antiadrenergic drugs for hypertension are included in Chapter 52.

A basal level of sympathetic tone is necessary to maintain normal body functioning, including regulation of blood pressure, blood glucose levels, and stress response. Therefore, the goal of antiadrenergic drug therapy is to suppress pathologic stimulation—not the normal physiologic response to activity, stress, and other stimuli.

GENERAL CHARACTERISTICS OF ANTIADRENERGIC DRUGS

Mechanisms of Action

Antiadrenergic effects can occur either when alpha$_1$ or beta receptors are blocked by adrenergic antagonists or when presynaptic alpha$_2$ receptors are stimulated by agonist drugs. Most antiadrenergic drugs have *antagonist* or *blocking effects* when they bind with alpha$_1$, beta$_1$, beta$_2$, or a combination of receptors in peripheral tissues, thus preventing adrenergic effects. Antiadrenergic drugs may be nonselective, exerting antiadrenergic effects on several adrenergic receptors simultaneously; or they may act selectively, blocking only one adrenergic receptor.

Clonidine and related drugs have *agonist effects* at presynaptic alpha$_2$ receptors in the brain. As stated in Chapter 17, this agonist effect results in a negative feedback type of mechanism that decreases the release of additional norepinephrine. Thus, the overall effect is decreased sympathetic outflow from the brain and decreased activation of alpha and beta receptors by norepinephrine throughout the body.

Alpha-Adrenergic Agonists and Blocking Drugs

Alpha₂-adrenergic agonists such as clonidine (Catapres) inhibit the release of norepinephrine in the brain, thereby decreasing the effects of sympathetic nervous system stimulation throughout the body. A major clinical effect is decreased blood pressure. Although clinical effects are attributed mainly to drug action at presynaptic alpha₂ receptors in the brain, postsynaptic alpha₂ receptors in the brain and peripheral tissues (eg, vascular smooth muscle) may also be involved. Activation of alpha₂ receptors in the pancreatic islets suppresses insulin secretion.

Some *alpha-adrenergic blocking drugs* may be selective for alpha₁ receptors in peripheral tissues such as smooth muscles and glands innervated by sympathetic nerve fibers. These drugs act primarily in the skin, mucosa, intestines, lungs, and kidneys to block or prevent alpha-mediated vasoconstriction. Specific effects of alpha₁-adrenergic blocking drugs include dilation of arterioles and veins, increased local blood flow, decreased blood pressure, constriction of pupils, and increased motility of the gastrointestinal (GI) tract. Alpha-adrenergic antagonists often activate reflexes that oppose the decrease in blood pressure by increasing heart rate and cardiac output and by causing fluid retention.

Alpha₁-adrenergic blocking drugs such as tamsulosin also can prevent alpha-mediated contraction of smooth muscle in nonvascular tissues. This action makes these drugs useful in the treatment of benign prostatic hyperplasia (BPH), a condition characterized by obstructed urine flow as the enlarged prostate gland presses on the urethra. Alpha₁-blocking agents can decrease urinary retention and improve urine flow by relaxing muscles in the prostate and urinary bladder. Clients diagnosed with BPH should be evaluated for prostatic cancer before starting drug therapy because the signs and symptoms of BPH and prostatic cancer are similar. The two conditions may also coexist.

Nonselective alpha-adrenergic blocking drugs such as phentolamine occupy peripheral alpha₁ receptors, causing vasodilation, and presynaptic alpha₂ receptors, causing cardiac stimulation. Consequently, decreased blood pressure is accompanied by tachycardia and perhaps other dysrhythmias.

Beta-Adrenergic Blocking Drugs

Beta-adrenergic blocking agents occupy beta-adrenergic receptor sites and prevent the receptors from responding to sympathetic nerve impulses, circulating catecholamines, and beta-adrenergic drugs (Fig. 18-1).

Beta₁ receptor blockade has an inhibitory effect on the cardiovascular system resulting in decreased heart rate (negative chronotropy); decreased force of myocardial contraction (negative inotropy); slowed conduction through the atrioventricular (AV) node (negative dromotropy); decreased automaticity of ectopic pacemakers; decreased cardiac output at rest and with exercise; and decreased blood pressure in supine and standing positions, especially in people with hypertension. Chronic use of beta blockers is associated with increased very–low-density

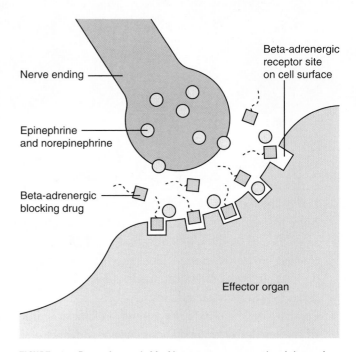

FIGURE 18-1 Beta-adrenergic blocking agents prevent epinephrine and norepinephrine from occupying receptor sites on cell membranes. This action alters cell functions normally stimulated by epinephrine and norepinephrine, according to the number of receptor sites occupied by the beta-blocking drugs. (Adapted by J. Harley from *Encyclopedia Britannica Medical and Health Annual.* [1983]. Chicago, Encyclopedia Britannica.)

lipoprotein (VLDL) and decreased high-density lipoprotein (HDL) cholesterol. These changes pose a potential risk for clients with cardiovascular disease. Beta₁ receptor blockade also results in decreased renin secretion from the kidneys; decreased production of aqueous humor in the eye; and diminished portal vein pressure in clients with cirrhosis.

Beta₂ receptor blockade produces bronchoconstriction of the smooth muscles in the respiratory tract, especially in people with asthma or other chronic lung diseases. Beta₂ receptor blockade also results in less effective metabolism of glucose (decreased glycogenolysis) when needed by the body, especially in people taking beta-blocking agents along with antidiabetic drugs. These diabetic clients may experience more severe and prolonged hypoglycemia. In addition, tachycardia, the early warning symptom of hypoglycemia, may be blocked by the medication, thereby delaying recognition and treatment. Beta₂ receptor blockade also increases the tone of smooth muscles in the GI tract, urinary bladder, and uterus.

Indications for Use

Alpha-Adrenergic Agonists and Blocking Drugs

Alpha₂ agonists are used in the treatment of hypertension. Clonidine, administered by the epidural route, is also approved for the relief of severe pain in cancer clients. Investigational uses of clonidine include the treatment of tic disorders, postmenopausal hot flashes, migraine, attention deficit-hyperactivity disorder, drug-induced akathisia, and alcohol withdrawal and opioid dependence, as well as use as adjunct medication during anesthesia. Clonidine has not received approval by the Food and Drug Administration (FDA) for these purposes.

Selective alpha$_1$-adrenergic blocking drugs are used in the treatment of hypertension, BPH, vasospastic disorders, and persistent pulmonary hypertension in the newborn. Nonselective alpha-blocking drugs are not used as antihypertensive drugs except in hypertension caused by excessive catecholamines. Excessive catecholamines may result from overdoses of adrenergic drugs or from pheochromocytoma, a rare tumor of the adrenal medulla that secretes epinephrine and norepinephrine and causes hypertension, tachycardia, and cardiac dysrhythmias. Although the treatment of choice for pheochromocytoma is surgical excision, alpha-adrenergic blocking drugs are useful adjuncts. They are given before and during surgery, usually in conjunction with beta blockers to block the sympathetic effect of excessive catecholamine secretion. Nonselective alpha blockers also are used in vascular diseases characterized by vasospasm, such as Raynaud's disease and frostbite, in which they improve blood flow. Phentolamine also can be used to prevent tissue necrosis due to extravasation of potent vasoconstrictors such as norepinephrine and dopamine into subcutaneous tissues.

APPLYING YOUR KNOWLEDGE 18-1

What explanation do you give Mr. Jones when he asks what the patch does for his condition?

Beta-Adrenergic Blocking Drugs

Clinical indications for use of beta-blocking agents are mainly cardiovascular disorders (eg, angina pectoris, cardiac tachydysrhythmias, hypertension, myocardial infarction [MI], heart failure [HF]) and glaucoma.

In angina, beta blockers decrease myocardial contractility, cardiac output, heart rate, and blood pressure. These effects decrease myocardial oxygen demand (cardiac workload), especially in response to activity, exercise, and stress. In dysrhythmias, the drugs slow the sinus rate and prolong conduction through the AV node, thereby slowing the ventricular response rate to supraventricular tachydysrhythmias. In hypertension, the actions of beta blockers are unclear. Possible mechanisms include reduced cardiac output, inhibition of renin, and inhibition of sympathetic nervous system stimulation in the brain. However, the drugs effective in hypertension do not consistently demonstrate these effects; for example, a drug may lower blood pressure without reducing cardiac output or inhibiting renin.

After MI, beta blockers help protect the heart from reinfarction and decrease mortality rates over several years. A possible mechanism is preventing or decreasing the incidence of catecholamine-induced dysrhythmias. In HF, beta blockers play an important role but require careful monitoring on the part of the physician and the nurse. Administration of beta blockers may potentially worsen the condition of people with HF by blocking the sympathetic stimulation that helps maintain cardiac output. However, in many clients with HF, even those of advanced age and with advanced disease, the drugs are beneficial. For these clients, beta blockers decrease the risk of sudden cardiac death and may reduce ventricular remodeling that accompanies HF and leads to further deterioration of cardiac function.

In glaucoma, the drugs reduce intraocular pressure by binding to beta-adrenergic receptors in the ciliary body of the eye and decreasing formation of aqueous humor.

Contraindications to Use

Alpha$_2$ agonists are contraindicated in clients with hypersensitivity to the drugs, and methyldopa is also contraindicated in clients with active liver disease. Alpha-adrenergic blocking agents are contraindicated in angina pectoris, MI, HF, and stroke.

Beta-adrenergic blocking agents are contraindicated in bradycardia and heart block. Nonselective beta blockers are contraindicated with asthma and other allergic or pulmonary conditions characterized by bronchoconstriction; however, the selective beta$_1$ blockers may be used in people with these disorders. Research has shown that beta blockers can be beneficial in selected clients with mild to moderate chronic HF; however, the drugs have not been proven safe for people older than 80 years of age or those with severe HF.

INDIVIDUAL DRUGS

Selected antiadrenergic medications are described in the following sections. Trade names, clinical indications, and dosage ranges are presented in Table 18-1 for alpha-adrenergic agonists and blocking drugs and in Table 18-2 for beta-adrenergic blocking drugs.

Alpha-Adrenergic Agonists and Blocking Drugs

Alpha$_2$-adrenergic agonists include clonidine, guanabenz, guanfacine, and methyldopa. These drugs produce similar therapeutic and adverse effects but differ in their pharmacokinetics and frequency of administration. Oral **clonidine** (Catapres) reduces blood pressure within 1 hour, reaches peak plasma levels in 3 to 5 hours, and has a plasma half-life of approximately 12 to 16 hours (longer with renal impairment). Approximately half the oral dose is metabolized in the liver, and the remainder is excreted unchanged in urine. When transdermal clonidine is given, therapeutic plasma levels are reached in 2 to 3 days and last 1 week.

(text continues on page 294)

Table 18-1 Drugs at a Glance: Alpha-Adrenergic Agonists and Blocking Drugs

GENERIC/TRADE NAME	CLINICAL INDICATIONS	ROUTES AND DOSAGE RANGES
Alpha$_2$ Agonists		
Clonidine (Catapres)	Hypertension	PO 0.1 mg 2 times daily initially, gradually increased if necessary. Average maintenance dose, 0.2–0.8 mg/d. Transdermal 0.1-mg patch every 7 d initially; increase every 7–14 d to 0.2 mg or 0.3 mg if necessary. Maximum dose, two 0.3-mg patches every 7 d
Guanabenz (Wytensin)	Hypertension	PO 4 mg twice daily, increased by 4–8 mg/d every 1–2 wk if necessary to a maximal dose of 32 mg twice daily
Guanfacine (Tenex)	Hypertension	PO 1 mg daily at bedtime, increased to 2 mg after 3–4 wk, then to 3 mg if necessary
Methyldopa	Hypertension	*Adults:* PO 250 mg 2 or 3 times daily initially, increased gradually at intervals of not less than 2 d until blood pressure is controlled or a daily dose of 3 g is reached *Children:* PO 10 mg/kg/d in 2 to 4 divided doses initially, increased or decreased according to response. Maximal dose, 65 mg/kg/d or 3 g daily, whichever is less
Selective Alpha$_1$-Blocking Drugs		
Alfuzosin (UroXatral)	BPH	PO 10 mg daily after same meal each day
Doxazosin (Cardura)	Hypertension BPH	PO 1 mg once daily initially, increased to 2 mg, then to 4, 8, and 16 mg if necessary
Prazosin (Minipress)	Hypertension BPH	PO 1 mg 2 to 3 times daily initially, increased if necessary to a total daily dose of 20 mg in divided doses. Average maintenance dose, 6–15 mg/d
Tamsulosin HCl (Flomax)	BPH	PO 0.4 mg/d after same meal each day. Dose may be increased if needed after 2–4 wk trial period.
Terazosin (Hytrin)	Hypertension	PO 1 mg at bedtime initially, increased gradually to maintenance dose, usually 1–5 mg once daily
	BPH	1–5 mg once daily
Nonselective Alpha-Blocking Drugs		
Phentolamine	Hypertension caused by pheochromocytoma	*Before and during surgery for pheochromocytoma:* IV, IM 5–20 mg as needed to control blood pressure
	Prevention of tissue necrosis from extravasation of vasoconstrictive drugs	*Prevention of tissue necrosis:* IV 10 mg in each liter of IV solution containing a potent vasoconstrictor *Treatment of extravasation:* Sub-Q 5–10 mg in 10 mL saline, infiltrated into the area within 12 h

BPH, benign prostatic hyperplasia; IM, intramuscular; IV, intravenous; PO, oral; Sub-Q, subcutaneous.

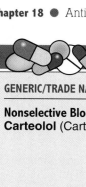

Table 18-2 Drugs at a Glance: Beta-Adrenergic Blocking Agents

GENERIC/TRADE NAME	CLINICAL INDICATIONS	ROUTES AND DOSAGE RANGES
Nonselective Blocking Agents		
Carteolol (Cartrol)*	Hypertension Glaucoma	PO: Initially, 2.5 mg once daily, gradually increased to a maximum daily dose of 10 mg if necessary. Usual maintenance dose, 2.5–5 mg once daily. Extend dosage interval to 48 h for a creatinine clearance of 20–60 mL/min and to 72 h for a creatinine clearance below 20 mL/min.
Levobunolol (Betagan)	Glaucoma	Topically to affected eye, 1 drop twice daily
Metipranolol (OptiPranolol)	Glaucoma	Topically to each eye, 1 drop once or twice daily
Penbutolol (Levatol)*	Hypertension	PO 20 mg once daily
Propranolol (Inderal)	Hypertension	PO 40 mg twice daily initially, may be increased to 120–240 mg daily in divided doses Sustained-release capsules, PO 80 mg once daily, may be increased to 120–160 mg once daily Maximal daily dose, 640 mg
	Angina pectoris	PO 80–320 mg in 2–4 divided doses Sustained release, PO 80–160 mg once daily Maximal daily dose, 320 mg
	Dysrhythmias	PO 10–30 mg, q6–8h Life-threatening dysrhythmias, IV 1–3 mg at a rate not to exceed 1 mg/min with electrocardiographic and blood-pressure monitoring
	Myocardial infarction	PO 180–240 mg daily in 3 or 4 divided doses Maximal daily dose, 240 mg
	Hypertrophic subaortic stenosis	PO 20–40 mg daily in 3 or 4 divided doses Sustained release, PO 80–160 mg once daily
	Migraine prophylaxis	PO 80–240 mg daily in divided doses Sustained release, PO 80 mg once daily
Pindolol (Visken)*	Hypertension	PO 5 mg twice daily initially, increased by 10 mg every 3–4 wk, to a maximal daily dose of 60 mg if necessary
Nadolol (Corgard)	Hypertension Angina pectoris	Hypertension, PO 40 mg once daily initially, gradually increased. Usual daily maintenance dose, 80–320 mg Angina, PO 40 mg once daily initially, increased by 40–80 mg at 3- to 7-d intervals. Usual daily maintenance dose, 80–240 mg
Sotalol (Betapace)	Cardiac dysrhythmias	PO 80–160 mg twice daily
Timolol (Blocadren, Timoptic)	Hypertension Myocardial infarction Glaucoma	Hypertension, PO 10 mg twice daily initially, increased at 7-d intervals to a maximum of 60 mg/d in 2 divided doses; usual maintenance dose, 20–40 mg daily Myocardial infarction, PO 10 mg twice daily Glaucoma, topically to eye, 1 drop of 0.25% or 0.5% solution (Timoptic) in each eye twice daily
Cardioselective Blocking Agents		
Acebutolol (Sectral)*	Hypertension Ventricular dysrhythmias	Hypertension, PO 400 mg daily in 1 or 2 doses; usual maintenance dose, 400–800 mg daily Dysrhythmias, PO 400 mg daily in 2 divided doses; usual maintenance dose, 600–1200 mg daily
Atenolol (Tenormin)	Hypertension Angina pectoris Myocardial infarction	Hypertension, PO 50–100 mg daily Angina, PO 50–100 mg daily, increased to 200 mg daily if necessary Myocardial infarction, IV 5 mg over 5 min, then 5 mg 10 min later, then 50 mg PO 10 min later, then 50 mg 12 h later. Thereafter, PO 100 mg daily, in 1 or 2 doses, for 6–9 d or until discharge from hospital

(continued)

Table 18-2 Drugs at a Glance: Beta-Adrenergic Blocking Agents (continued)

GENERIC/TRADE NAME	CLINICAL INDICATIONS	ROUTES AND DOSAGE RANGES
Betaxolol (Betoptic, Kerlone)	Glaucoma Hypertension	Topically to each eye, 1 drop twice daily Hypertension, PO 10–20 mg daily
Bisoprolol (Zebeta)	Hypertension	PO 5–20 mg once daily
Esmolol (Brevibloc)	Supraventricular tachy-arrhythmias	IV 50–200 mcg/kg/min; average dose, 100 mcg/kg/min, titrated to effect with close monitoring of client's condition
Metoprolol (Lopressor)	Hypertension Myocardial infarction	Hypertension, PO 100 mg daily in single or divided doses, increased at 7-d or longer intervals; usual maintenance dose, 100–450 mg/d Myocardial infarction, early treatment, IV 5 mg every 2 min for total of 3 doses (15 mg), then 50 mg PO q6h for 48 h, then 100 mg PO twice daily. Myocardial infarction, late treatment, PO 100 mg twice daily, for at least 3 months, up to 1–3 y
Alpha–Beta-Blocking Agents		
Carvedilol (Coreg)*	Hypertension Congestive heart failure	PO 6.25 mg twice daily for 7–14 d, then increase to 12.5 mg twice daily if necessary for 7–14 d, then increase to 25 mg twice daily if necessary (maximum dose)
Labetalol (Trandate, Normodyne)	Hypertension, including hypertensive emergencies	PO 100 mg twice daily IV 20 mg over 2 min then 40–80 mg every 10 min until desired blood pressure achieved or 300 mg given IV infusion 2 mg/min (eg, add 200 mg of drug to 250 mL 5% dextrose solution for a 2 mg/3 mL concentration)

* These drugs also have intrinsic sympathomimetic activity (ISA).
IV, intravenous; PO, oral.

Guanabenz (Wytensin) action occurs within 1 hour, peaks within 2 to 4 hours, and lasts 6 to 8 hours. It is metabolized extensively; very little unchanged drug is excreted in urine. **Guanfacine** (Tenex) is well absorbed and widely distributed, with approximately 70% bound to plasma proteins. Peak plasma levels occur in 1 to 4 hours, and the half-life is 10 to 30 hours. Approximately half of the drug is metabolized, and the metabolites and unchanged drug are excreted in urine. Because of its longer half-life, guanfacine can be given once daily.

Methyldopa (Aldomet) is an older drug with low to moderate absorption. With oral drug, peak plasma levels are reached in 2 to 4 hours, and peak antihypertensive effects occur in approximately 2 days. When discontinued, blood pressure increases in approximately 2 days. Intravenous (IV) administration reduces blood pressure in 4 to 6 hours and lasts 10 to 16 hours. Methyldopa is metabolized to some extent in the liver but is largely excreted in urine. In clients with renal impairment, blood pressure–lowering effects may be pronounced and prolonged because of slower excretion. In addition to the adverse effects that occur with all these drugs, methyldopa also may cause hemolytic anemia and hepatotoxicity (eg, jaundice, hepatitis).

Alpha$_1$-adrenergic antagonists include alfuzosin, doxazosin, prazosin, terazosin, tamsulosin, and tolazoline. P **Prazosin** (Minipress), the prototype, is well absorbed after oral administration and reaches peak plasma concentrations in 1 to 3 hours; action lasts approximately 4 to 6 hours. The drug is highly bound to plasma proteins, and the plasma half-life is approximately 2 to 3 hours. It is extensively metabolized in the liver, and its metabolites are excreted by the kidneys. **Doxazosin** (Cardura) and **terazosin** (Hytrin) are similar to prazosin but have longer half-lives (doxazosin, 10–20 hours; terazosin, approximately 12 hours) and durations of action (doxazosin, up to 36 hours; terazosin, 18 hours or longer). Prazosin must be taken in multiple doses. Doxazosin and terazosin may usually be taken once daily to control hypertension or symptoms of BPH.

Tamsulosin (Flomax) is the first alpha$_1$ antagonist designed specifically to treat BPH. Tamsulosin blocks alpha$_1$ receptors in the male genitourinary system, producing smooth-muscle relaxation in the prostate gland and urinary bladder neck. Urinary flow rate is improved, and symptoms of BPH are reduced. Because of the specificity of tamsulosin for receptors in the genitourinary system, this drug causes less orthostatic hypotension than other alpha$_1$ antagonists.

After oral administration, more than 90% of tamsulosin is absorbed. Administration with food decreases bioavailability by 30%. Tamsulosin is highly protein bound and is metabolized by the liver. Approximately 10% of the drug is excreted unchanged in the urine. An advantage of tamsulosin is the ability to start the drug at the recommended dosage. Most of the alpha$_1$ antagonists must be gradually increased to the recommended dosage. Common adverse effects include abnormal ejaculation and dizziness.

Alfuzosin (UroXatral) is another alpha$_1$-blocking drug specifically indicated for BPH. This moderately protein bound, extended-release medication is similar to prazosin but has the advantage of once-a-day dosing. It has a half-life of 10 hours and a duration of action of 24 hours. Alfuzosin should be taken after meals to promote absorption. It is metabolized extensively in the liver by cytochrome P450 3A4 enzymes and should not be given with potent inhibitors of this enzyme such as ketoconazole, itraconazole, or ritonavir, or in the presence of moderate to severe liver insufficiency, because drug toxicity will occur. In addition, alfuzosin can prolong the Q–T interval and therefore should be used with caution in people with congenital or acquired Q–T prolongation. Common adverse effects include dizziness, headache, fatigue, and increased incidence of upper respiratory infections.

Of the alpha-adrenergic blocking drugs, phenoxybenzamine (Dibenzyline) is an old drug that exerts its action by binding permanently to alpha receptors and producing drug effects until the body builds new receptors. Therefore, the drug action of phenoxybenzamine is long acting, persisting for 3 to 4 days. *Phenoxybenzamine has been withdrawn from the United States market because of its irreversible long-lasting effect.* **Phentolamine** (Regitine) is similar to phenoxybenzamine but more useful clinically. Phentolamine acts competitively at alpha receptors, and is therefore short acting; effects last only a few hours and can be reversed by an alpha-adrenergic stimulant drug such as norepinephrine.

Beta-Adrenergic Blocking Drugs

Numerous beta-blocking drugs are marketed in the United States. Although they produce similar effects, they differ from the prototype ⓟ **propranolol** (Inderal) with respect to several properties.

Clinical Indications

Propranolol is the oldest and most extensively studied beta blocker. In addition to its use in the treatment of hypertension, dysrhythmias, angina pectoris, and MI, propranolol is used to treat a wide variety of other conditions. In hypertrophic obstructive cardiomyopathy, it is used to improve exercise tolerance by increasing stroke volume. In pheochromocytoma, it is used in conjunction with an alpha-blocking drug to counter the effect of excessive catecholamine secretion, thereby preventing tachycardia and dysrhythmias. In dissecting aortic aneurysms, it is used to decrease systolic blood pressure. In hyperthyroidism, it decreases heart rate, cardiac output, and tremor.

Propranolol is also useful, by an unknown mechanism, for the prevention of migraine headache. However, it is not helpful in acute attacks of migraine headache. It also relieves palpitation and tremor associated with anxiety and stage fright, but it is not approved for clinical use as an antianxiety drug. Some people experiencing alcohol withdrawal may also benefit from administration of propranolol.

Research indicates that propranolol may be useful in treating cirrhosis of the liver. The drug may decrease the incidence of the initial episode of bleeding esophageal varices; prevent rebleeding episodes; and decrease the mortality rate due to hemorrhage.

Most beta blockers are approved for the treatment of hypertension. A beta blocker may be used alone or with another antihypertensive drug, such as a diuretic. Labetalol (Trandate, Normodyne) is also approved for treatment of hypertensive emergencies. Atenolol (Tenormin), metoprolol (Lopressor), nadolol (Corgard), and propranolol are approved as antianginal agents. Acebutolol (Sectral), esmolol (Brevibloc), propranolol, and sotalol (Betapace) are approved as antidysrhythmic agents. Atenolol, metoprolol, propranolol, and timolol (Blocadren, Timoptic) are used to prevent MI or reinfarction. Betaxolol (Betoptic, Kerlone), carteolol (Cartrol), and timolol are used for hypertension and glaucoma. Levobunolol (Betagan) and metipranolol (OptiPranolol) are used only for glaucoma.

A growing number of studies demonstrate that **carvedilol** (Coreg), a cardioselective beta blocker, is useful not only in treating mild to moderate cases of chronic HF but also in reducing the risk of sudden death. Carvedilol has been shown to reduce risk of death or hospitalization in clients with mild to moderate HF by 38%. Despite concern that people who have severe HF or are more advanced in age would not be able to tolerate beta blockers, carvedilol appears to be well tolerated, even if the HF is advanced. Exactly how beta blockers benefit clients with HF is unclear. Possible mechanisms of action include blockade of the damaging effects of sympathetic stimulation on the heart; beta receptor up-regulation; decreased sympathetic stimulation due to decreased plasma norepinephrine and antidysrhythmic effects; and improved diastolic function by lengthening diastolic filling time. Research has shown that carvedilol demonstrates antioxidant activity. The clinical significance of this finding for clients with HF is not yet clear.

APPLYING YOUR KNOWLEDGE 18-2
What is the potential benefit of using Lopressor for Mr. Jones's hypertension and his coronary history?

Receptor Selectivity

Carteolol, levobunolol, metipranolol, penbutolol, nadolol, pindolol, propranolol, sotalol, and timolol are nonselective beta blockers. The term *nonselective* means that the drugs block both beta$_1$ (cardiac) and beta$_2$ (mainly smooth muscle in the bronchi and blood vessels) receptors. Blockade of beta$_2$ receptors is associated with adverse effects such as bronchoconstriction, peripheral vasoconstriction, and interference with glycogenolysis.

Acebutolol, atenolol, betaxolol, bisoprolol, esmolol, and metoprolol are *cardioselective* agents, which means that they have more effect on beta$_1$ receptors than on beta$_2$ receptors. As a result, they may cause less bronchospasm, less impairment of glucose metabolism, and less peripheral vascular insufficiency. These drugs are preferred when beta blockers are needed by clients with diabetes mellitus, peripheral vascular disorders, or asthma or other bronchospastic pulmonary disorders (see Research Brief). However, cardioselectivity is lost at higher doses because most organs have both beta$_1$ and beta$_2$ receptors rather than one or the other exclusively.

Labetalol and carvedilol block alpha$_1$ receptors to cause vasodilation and beta$_1$ and beta$_2$ receptors to cause all the effects of the nonselective agents. Both alpha- and beta-adrenergic blocking actions contribute to antihypertensive effects, but it is unclear whether these drugs have any definite advantage over other beta blockers. They may cause less bradycardia but more postural hypotension than other beta-blocking agents, and they may cause less reflex tachycardia than other vasodilators.

Intrinsic Sympathomimetic Activity

Drugs with this characteristic (acebutolol, carteolol, carvedilol, penbutolol, and pindolol) have a chemical structure similar to that of catecholamines. As a result, they can block some beta receptors and stimulate others. It was once thought that these drugs would produce fewer adverse effects than other beta blockers; however, this has not occurred clinically. The primary use for medications with intrinsic sympathomimetic activity is to treat people who experience bradycardia with other beta blockers. These medications should not be used to prevent recurrent MI because of their potential to increase dysrhythmias and oxygen consumption by the myocardium.

Membrane-Stabilizing Activity

Several beta blockers have a membrane-stabilizing effect that is sometimes described as quinidine-like (ie, producing myocardial depression). Because the doses required to produce this effect are much higher than those used for therapeutic effects, this characteristic is considered clinically insignificant.

RESEARCH BRIEF

Use of Cardioselective Beta Blockers in Clients With Chronic Obstructive Pulmonary Disease

SOURCE:

Salpeter, S., Ormiston, T., Salpeter, E., Poole, P., & Cates C. (2003). Cardioselective beta-blockers for chronic obstructive pulmonary disease: A meta-analysis. *Respiratory Medicine, 97*(10), 1094–1101.

SUMMARY:

Beta blockers have been shown to benefit clients with hypertension, heart failure, and myocardial infarction. However, they have traditionally been considered contraindicated in clients with obstructive airway disorders because of the bronchoconstrictive effects of beta blockade. This meta-analysis of 19 randomized, blinded, controlled trials sought to assess the effect of cardioselective beta blockers on respiratory function in clients with chronic obstructive pulmonary disease (COPD) by assessing the effect of the beta blocker on the forced expiratory volume in 1 second (FEV$_1$). Cardioselective beta blockers produced no significant change in FEV$_1$ or respiratory symptoms compared with a placebo when given as a single dose or for longer duration. In view of their results and the demonstrated benefits of beta blockers in conditions such as heart failure, coronary artery disease, and hypertension, the researchers concluded that cardioselective beta blockers should be considered for clients with COPD.

NURSING IMPLICATIONS:

Nurses should be prepared to explain the benefits of beta blockers to clients with COPD and teach clients about their proper home monitoring and use.

Potassium Channel Blockade

Unique among beta blockers, sotalol exerts an antidysrhythmic effect by blocking potassium channels in cell membranes, thereby prolonging repolarization and the refractory period of the heart. At low doses, beta-blocking effects predominate and at high doses, antidysrhythmic effects predominate. Sotalol is used to treat life-threatening ventricular dysrhythmias and to maintain normal sinus rhythm in clients who frequently reconvert to atrial fibrillation/flutter (see Chap. 49).

Lipid Solubility

The more lipid-soluble beta blockers were thought to penetrate the central nervous system (CNS) more extensively and cause adverse effects such as confusion, depression, hallucinations, and insomnia. Some clinicians state that this characteristic is important only in terms of drug usage and excretion in certain disease states. Thus, a water-soluble, renally excreted beta blocker may be preferred in clients with liver disease, and a lipid-soluble, hepatically metabolized drug may be preferred in clients with renal disease.

Routes of Elimination

Most beta-blocking drugs are metabolized in the liver. Atenolol, carteolol, nadolol, and an active metabolite of acebutolol are excreted by the kidneys; dosage must be reduced in the presence of renal failure.

Routes of Administration

Most beta blockers can be given orally. Atenolol, esmolol, labetalol, metoprolol, and propranolol also can be given IV, and ophthalmic solutions are applied topically to the eye. Betaxolol, carteolol, and timolol are available in oral and ophthalmic forms.

Duration of Action

Acebutolol, atenolol, bisoprolol, carteolol, penbutolol, and nadolol have long serum half-lives and can usually be given once daily. Carvedilol, labetalol, metoprolol, pindolol, sotalol, and timolol are usually given twice daily. Propranolol required administration several times daily until development of a sustained-release capsule allowed once-daily dosing.

NURSING PROCESS

Assessment

● Assess the client's condition in relation to disorders in which antiadrenergic drugs are used. Because most of the drugs are used to treat hypertension, assess blood-pressure patterns over time, when possible, including antihypertensive drugs used and the response obtained. With other cardiovascular disorders, check blood pressure for elevation and pulse for tachycardia or dysrhythmia, and determine the presence or absence of chest pain, migraine headache, or hyperthyroidism. If the client reports or medical records indicate one or more of these disorders, assess for specific signs and symptoms. With BPH, assess for signs and symptoms of urinary retention and difficulty voiding.
● Assess for conditions that contraindicate the use of antiadrenergic drugs.
● Assess vital signs to establish a baseline for later comparisons.
● Assess for use of prescription and nonprescription drugs that are likely to increase or decrease effects of antiadrenergic drugs.

● Assess for lifestyle habits that are likely to increase or decrease effects of antiadrenergic drugs (eg, ingestion of caffeine or nicotine).

Nursing Diagnoses

● Decreased Cardiac Output related to drug-induced postural hypotension (alpha$_2$ agonists, alpha$_1$-blocking agents, nonselective alpha-blocking agents, and beta blockers) and worsening HF (beta blockers)
● Impaired Gas Exchange related to drug-induced bronchoconstriction with beta blockers
● Sexual Dysfunction in men related to impotence and decreased libido
● Fatigue related to decreased cardiac output
● Noncompliance with drug therapy related to adverse drug effects or inadequate understanding of drug regimen
● Risk for Injury related to hypotension, dizziness, sedation
● Deficient Knowledge of drug effects and safe usage

Planning/Goals

The client will
● Receive or self-administer drugs accurately
● Experience relief of symptoms for which antiadrenergic drugs are given
● Comply with instructions for safe drug usage
● Avoid stopping antiadrenergic drugs abruptly
● Demonstrate knowledge of adverse drug effects to be reported
● Avoid preventable adverse drug effects
● Keep appointments for blood pressure monitoring and other follow-up activities

Interventions

Use measures to prevent or decrease the need for antiadrenergic drugs. Because the sympathetic nervous system is stimulated by physical and emotional stress, efforts to decrease stress may indirectly decrease the need for drugs to antagonize sympathetic effects. Such efforts may include the following:
● Helping the client stop or decrease cigarette smoking. Nicotine stimulates the CNS and the sympathetic nervous system to cause tremors, tachycardia, and elevated blood pressure.
● Teaching measures to relieve pain, anxiety, and other stresses
● Counseling regarding relaxation techniques
● Helping the client avoid temperature extremes
● Helping the client avoid excessive caffeine in coffee or other beverages
● Helping the client develop a reasonable balance among rest, exercise, work, and recreation

- Recording vital signs at regular intervals in hospitalized clients to monitor for adverse effects
- Helping with activity or ambulation as needed to prevent injury from dizziness

In addition, teaching guidelines are included in the accompanying display.

Evaluation

- Observe for decreased blood pressure when antiadrenergic drugs are given for hypertension.
- Interview regarding decreased chest pain when beta blockers are given for angina.
- Interview and observe for signs and symptoms of adverse drug effects (eg, edema, tachycardia with alpha agonists and blocking agents; bradycardia, congestive HF, bronchoconstriction with beta blockers).
- Interview regarding knowledge and use of drugs.

PRINCIPLES OF THERAPY

Drug Selection and Administration

Alpha-Adrenergic Agonists and Blocking Drugs

When an alpha$_1$-blocking agent (doxazosin, prazosin, terazosin) is given for hypertension, "first-dose syncope" may occur due to hypotension. This reaction can be prevented or minimized by starting with a low dose, increasing the dose gradually, and giving the first dose at bedtime. The decreased blood pressure also stimulates reflex mechanisms to raise blood pressure (increase heart rate and cardiac output, fluid retention), and a diuretic may be necessary.

When an alpha$_2$ agonist is given for hypertension, it is very important not to stop the drug abruptly because of the risk of rebound hypertension. For example, to discontinue clonidine, the dosage should be gradually reduced over 2 to 4 days.

Beta-Adrenergic Blocking Drugs

For most people, a nonselective beta blocker that can be taken once or twice daily is acceptable. For others, the choice of a beta blocker depends largely on the client's condition and response to the drugs. For example, cardioselective drugs are preferred for clients who have pulmonary disorders and diabetes mellitus, and drugs with intrinsic sympathomimetic activity may be preferred for those who experience significant bradycardia with beta blockers lacking this property.

Dosage of beta blockers must be individualized because of wide variations in plasma levels from comparable doses. Variations are attributed to the initial metabolism in the liver, the extent of binding to plasma proteins, and the degree of beta-adrenergic stimulation that the drugs must overcome. In general, low doses should be used initially and increased gradually until therapeutic or adverse effects occur. Adequacy of dosage or extent of beta blockade can be assessed

---

CLIENT TEACHING GUIDELINES

Alpha$_2$ Agonists and Alpha-Blocking Drugs

General Considerations

- ✔ Have your blood pressure checked regularly. Report high or low values to your health care provider.
- ✔ The adverse reactions of palpitations, weakness, and dizziness usually disappear with continued use. However, they may recur with conditions promoting vasodilation (dosage increase, exercise, high environmental temperatures, ingesting alcohol or a large meal).
- ✔ To prevent falls and injuries, if the above reactions occur, sit down or lie down immediately and flex arms and legs. Change positions slowly, especially from supine to standing.
- ✔ Do not drive a car or operate machinery if drowsy or dizzy from medication.
- ✔ Do not stop the drugs abruptly. Hypertension, possibly severe, may develop.
- ✔ With methyldopa, report any signs of abdominal pain, nausea, vomiting, diarrhea, or jaundice to your health care provider. Regular blood tests are needed to make sure the medication is working as it should.

- ✔ Do not take over-the-counter or other medications without the physician's knowledge. Many drugs interact to increase or decrease the effects of antiadrenergic drugs.

Self-Administration

- ✔ Sedation and first-dose syncope may be minimized by taking all or most of the prescribed dose at bedtime.
- ✔ When using the clonidine transdermal patch, select a hairless area on the upper arm or torso for the application. The patch is changed once a week.
- ✔ Avoid alcohol use with these medications because excessive drowsiness may occur.
- ✔ With extended-release medications such as alfuzosin (UroXatral), do not crush, split, or chew the tablets, because overdose may occur.
- ✔ Take alfuzosin (UroXatral) and tamsulosin (Flomax) after a meal.

CLIENT TEACHING GUIDELINES

Beta-Blocking Drugs

General Considerations

✔ Count your pulse daily and report to a health care provider if under 50 for several days in succession. This information helps to determine if the drug therapy needs to be altered to avoid more serious adverse effects.

✔ Report weight gain (more than 2 lb within a week), ankle edema, shortness of breath, or excessive fatigue. These are signs of heart failure. If they occur, the drug may be stopped.

✔ Report fainting spells, excessive weakness, or difficulty in breathing. Beta-blocking drugs decrease the usual adaptive responses to exercise or stress. Syncope may result from hypotension, bradycardia, or heart block; its occurrence probably indicates stopping or decreasing the dose of the drug.

✔ Do not stop taking the drugs abruptly. Stopping the drugs suddenly may cause or aggravate chest pain (angina).

✔ Do not take over-the-counter or other medications without the physician's knowledge. Many drugs interact to increase or decrease the effects of beta-blocking agents.

Self-Administration

✔ Consistently take the drug at the same time each day with or without food. This maintains consistent therapeutic blood levels.

✔ Do not crush or chew long-acting forms of these medications.

---

by determining whether the heart rate increases in response to exercise.

The only beta blocker approved by the FDA to treat HF is carvedilol. Treatment should begin with a low dose of the beta blocker, often administered concurrently with an angiotensin-converting enzyme (ACE) inhibitor. The purpose of the ACE inhibitor is to counteract any initial aggravation of the HF symptoms due to the carvedilol. The client should be closely monitored for adverse effects such as worsening HF.

A beta blocker used to prevent MI should be started as soon as the client is hemodynamically stable after a definite or suspected acute MI. The drug should be continued for at least 2 years. (A beta blocker with intrinsic sympathomimetic activity should not be used for this purpose.) Studies have shown that such use of a beta blocker may reduce mortality by as much as 25%. However, many post-MI clients still do not receive a prescription for this medication.

Beta blockers should not be discontinued abruptly. Long-term blockade of beta-adrenergic receptors increases the receptors' sensitivity to epinephrine and norepinephrine when the drugs are discontinued. There is a risk of severe hypertension, angina, dysrhythmias, and MI from the increased or excessive sympathetic nervous system stimulation. Thus, the dosage should be tapered and gradually discontinued to allow beta-adrenergic receptors to return to predrug density and sensitivity. An optimal tapering period has not been defined. Some authorities recommend 1 to 2 weeks, and others recommend reducing the dosage over approximately 10 days to 30 milligrams per day of propranolol (or an equivalent amount of other drugs), and continuing this amount at least 2 weeks before the drug is stopped completely.

Beta blockers are indicated to reduce hemodynamic complications during the perioperative period. Esmolol is often the beta blocker of choice in this situation because it is cardioselective, can be given IV, and has a rapid onset of action. Cardiac output may be an important factor in determining the amount of IV anesthetic needed for induction, and esmolol is known to reduce cardiac output. A recent study found that propofol requirements for induction were reduced by 25% after pretreatment with esmolol. During the intraoperative and postoperative periods, esmolol is useful for controlling tachycardia and hypertension. With some types of anesthesia such as desflurane, intraoperative administration of esmolol promotes more rapid awakening after anesthesia and reduced need for opioid analgesics. Postoperatively, esmolol may also be useful in preventing myocardial ischemia.

Various drugs may be used to treat adverse effects of beta blockers. Atropine can be given for bradycardia; digoxin and diuretics for HF; vasopressors for hypotension; and bronchodilator drugs for bronchoconstriction.

It is important to note that bronchodilation does not occur in a client taking beta blockers when given epinephrine to treat an allergic reaction to an allergen or during allergy testing. This absence of the nornal response to epinephrine is due to drug-induced beta$_2$ blockade.

Use in Special Populations

Use in Children

Most alpha-adrenergic agonists and blocking agents have not been established as safe and effective in children.

Beta-adrenergic blocking drugs are used in children for disorders similar to those in adults. However, safety and effectiveness have not been established, and manufacturers of most of the drugs do not recommend pediatric use or suggest dosages. The drugs are probably contraindicated in young children with resting heart rates of less than 60 beats per minute.

When beta blockers are given, general guidelines include the following:

- Adjust dosage for body weight.
- Monitor responses closely. Children are more sensitive to adverse drug effects than adults.
- Remember that if beta blockers are given to infants (up to 1 year of age) with immature liver function, blood levels may be higher and accumulation is more likely even when doses are based on weight.
- When monitoring responses, remember that heart rate and blood pressure vary among children according to age and level of growth and development. They also differ from those of adults.
- Recall that children are more likely to have asthma than adults. Thus, they may be at greater risk of drug-induced bronchoconstriction.

Propranolol is probably the most frequently used beta blocker in children. The drug is given orally for hypertension, and dosage should be individualized. The usual dosage range is 2 to 4 milligrams per kilogram of body weight per day, in two equal doses. Calculation of the dosage on the basis of body surface area is not recommended because of possible excessive blood levels of drug and greater risk of toxicity. As with adults, the drug should not be stopped abruptly and should be tapered gradually over 1 to 3 weeks.

Use in Older Adults

Alpha$_2$-adrenergic agonists (clonidine and related drugs) may be used to treat hypertension in older adults, and alpha$_1$-adrenergic antagonists (prazosin and related drugs) may be used to treat hypertension and BPH. Dosage of these drugs should be reduced because older adults are more likely to experience adverse drug effects, especially with impaired renal or hepatic function. As with other populations, these drugs should not be stopped suddenly. Instead, they should be tapered in dosage and discontinued gradually, over 1 to 2 weeks.

Beta-adrenergic blocking drugs are commonly used in older adults for angina, dysrhythmias, hypertension, HF, prevention of recurrent MI, and glaucoma. Several recent clinical trials and research studies, including the Metoprolol CR/XL Randomized Intervention trial in Congestive Heart Failure, the U.S. Carvedilol Heart Failure Trials Program, and the Carvedilol Prospective Randomized Cumulative Survival (COPERNICUS) trial, demonstrated that older adults can tolerate and benefit from use of beta blockers in

the treatment of HF. In hypertension, beta blockers are not recommended for monotherapy because older adults may be less responsive than younger adults. Thus, the drugs are probably most useful as second drugs (with diuretics) in clients who require multidrug therapy and clients who also have angina pectoris or another disorder for which a beta blocker is indicated.

Whatever the indications for beta blockers in older adults, the drugs should be used cautiously and clients' responses should be monitored closely. Older adults are likely to have disorders that put them at higher risk of adverse drug effects, such as HF and other cardiovascular conditions; renal or hepatic impairment; and chronic pulmonary disease. Thus, they may experience bradycardia, bronchoconstriction, and hypotension to a greater degree than younger adults. Dosage usually should be reduced because of decreased hepatic blood flow and subsequent slowing of drug metabolism. As in other populations, beta blockers should be tapered in dosage and discontinued over 1 to 3 weeks to avoid myocardial ischemia and other potentially serious adverse cardiovascular effects.

APPLYING YOUR KNOWLEDGE 18-3:
HOW CAN YOU AVOID THIS MEDICATION ERROR?
You are preparing medication for Mr. Jones. The pharmacy has substituted Lopressor with a generic drug. Mr. Jones informs you that he cannot take another form of the drug, so you hold the dose and do not administer today's metoprolol.

Use in Various Ethnic Groups

Most studies involve adults with hypertension and compare drug therapy responses between African Americans and Caucasians. Findings indicate that monotherapy with alpha$_1$ blockers and combination therapy with alpha and beta blockers is equally effective in the two groups. However, monotherapy with beta blockers is less effective in African Americans than in Caucasians. When beta blockers are used in African Americans, they should usually be part of a multidrug treatment regimen, and higher doses may be required. In addition, labetalol, an alpha and beta blocker, has been shown to be more effective in the African-American population than propranolol, timolol, or metoprolol. According to the U.S. Carvedilol Heart Failure Trials Program and the COPERNICUS trials, African Americans with HF responded favorably to a combination of carvedilol plus ACE inhibitors, even when their condition was advanced.

Several studies indicate that Asians achieve higher blood levels of beta blockers with given doses and, in general, need much smaller doses than Caucasians. This increased sensitivity to the drugs may result from slower metabolism and excretion.

Use in Clients With Renal Impairment

Centrally acting alpha$_2$ agonists such as clonidine, guanabenz, and methyldopa are eliminated by a combination of liver metabolism and renal excretion. Renal impairment may result in slower excretion of these medications, with subsequent accumulation and increased adverse effects.

Alpha$_1$-adrenergic antagonists such as prazosin, terazosin, alfuzosin, doxazosin, and tamsulosin are eliminated primarily by liver metabolism and biliary excretion. Therefore, renal impairment is not a contraindication to use of these medications. However, tolazoline is excreted by the kidneys, and reduced dosage should be considered in the presence of renal impairment.

Many beta blockers are eliminated primarily in the urine and pose potentially serious problems for clients with renal failure. In renal failure, dosage of acebutolol, atenolol, carteolol, and nadolol must be reduced because they are eliminated mainly through the kidneys. The dosage of acebutolol and nadolol should be reduced if creatinine clearance is less than 50 milliliters per minute, and the dosage of atenolol should be reduced if the creatinine clearance is less than 35 milliliters per minute. With carteolol, the same amount is given per dose, but the interval between doses is extended to 48 hours for a creatinine clearance of 20 to 60 milliliters per minute, and to 72 hours for a creatinine clearance of less than 20 milliliters per minute.

Use in Clients With Liver Impairment

Caution must be used when administering centrally acting alpha$_2$-adrenergic agonists such as clonidine, guanabenz, and methyldopa to clients with liver impairment. These medications rely on hepatic metabolism as well as renal elimination to clear the body. Furthermore, methyldopa has been associated with liver disorders such as hepatitis and hepatic necrosis.

Alpha$_1$-adrenergic medications such as prazosin, alfuzosin, terazosin, doxazosin, and tamsulosin rely heavily on liver metabolism and biliary excretion to clear the body. Liver impairment may result in increased drug levels and adverse effects.

In the presence of hepatic disease (eg, cirrhosis) or impaired blood flow to the liver (eg, reduced cardiac output from any cause), dosage of some beta blockers such as propranolol, metoprolol, and timolol should be substantially reduced because these drugs are extensively metabolized in the liver. The use of atenolol or nadolol is preferred in liver disease because both are eliminated primarily by the kidneys.

Use in Clients With Critical Illness

Antiadrenergic drugs are one of several families of medications that may be used to treat urgent or malignant hypertension. An alpha$_2$ agonist such as clonidine might be prescribed under such conditions. A loading dose of clonidine 0.2 milligram, followed by 0.1 milligram hourly until the diastolic pressure falls below 110 mm Hg, may be administered. A dose of 0.7 mg should not be exceeded when using clonidine to treat malignant hypertension.

Beta blockers may be used in the treatment of acute MI. Early administration of a beta blocker after an acute MI results in a lower incidence of reinfarction, ventricular dysrhythmias, and mortality. These results have been demonstrated with several different agents; however, those with intrinsic sympathomimetic activity are not prescribed for this purpose. Clients must be carefully monitored for hypotension and HF when receiving beta blockers after an MI.

Use in Home Care

Antiadrenergic drugs are commonly used in the home setting, mainly to treat chronic disorders in adults. With alpha$_1$-adrenergic blocking drugs, the home care nurse may need to teach clients ways to avoid orthostatic hypotension. Most clients probably take these medications for hypertension. However, some older men with BPH take one of these drugs to aid urinary elimination. For an older man taking one of these drugs, the home care nurse must assess the reason for use to teach the client and monitor for drug effects.

With beta-adrenergic blocking drugs, the home care nurse may need to assist clients and caregivers in assessing for therapeutic and adverse drug effects. It is helpful to have the client or someone else in the household count and record the radial pulse daily, preferably about the same time interval before or after taking a beta blocker. Several days of a slow pulse should probably be reported to the health care provider who prescribed the beta blocker, especially if the client also has excessive fatigue or signs of HF.

If wheezing respirations (indicating bronchoconstriction) develop in a client taking a nonselective beta blocker, the client or the home care nurse must consult the prescribing physician about changing to a cardioselective beta blocker. If a client has diabetes mellitus, the home care nurse must interview and observe the client for alterations in blood sugar control, especially increased episodes of hypoglycemia. If a client has hypertension, the home care nurse must teach the client to avoid over-the-counter (OTC) asthma and cold remedies, decongestants, appetite suppressants, and herbal preparations such as ma huang, black cohosh, and St. John's wort because these drugs act to increase blood pressure and may reduce the benefits of antiadrenergic medications. In addition, OTC analgesics such as ibuprofen, ketoprofen, and naproxen may raise blood pressure by causing retention of sodium and water.

APPLYING YOUR KNOWLEDGE 18-4

Mr. Jones has diabetes and is therefore at increased risk of what complication from Lopresser?

N U R S I N G   A C T I O N S

Antiadrenergic Drugs

NURSING ACTIONS	RATIONALE/EXPLANATION

1. Administer accurately

  a. With alpha$_2$ agonists:

    (1) Give all or most of a dose at bedtime, when possible. — To minimize daytime drowsiness and sedation

    (2) Apply the clonidine skin patch to a hairless, intact area on the upper arm or torso; then apply adhesive overlay securely. Do not cut or alter the patch. Remove a used patch and fold its adhesive edges together before discarding. Apply a new patch in a new site. — To promote effectiveness and safe usage

  b. With alpha$_1$-blocking drugs:

    (1) Give the first dose of doxazosin, prazosin, or terazosin at bedtime. — To prevent fainting from severe orthostatic hypotension

    (2) Give alfuzosin and tamsulosin after the same meal each day. — Drug absorption is delayed in fasting conditions.

  c. With beta-adrenergic blocking drugs:

    (1) Check blood pressure and pulse frequently, especially when dosage is being increased. — To monitor therapeutic effects and the occurrence of adverse reactions. Some clients with heart rates between 50 and 60 beats per minute may be continued on a beta blocker if hypotension or escape dysrhythmias do not develop.

    (2) See Table 18–2 and manufacturers' literature regarding intravenous (IV) administration. — Specific instructions vary with individual drugs.

2. Observe for therapeutic effects

  a. With alpha$_2$ agonists and alpha-blocking drugs:

    (1) With hypertension, observe for decreased blood pressure. — With most of the drugs, blood pressure decreases within a few hours. However, antihypertensive effects with clonidine skin patches occur 2–3 days after initial application (overlap with oral clonidine or other antihypertensive drugs may be needed) and persist 2–3 days when discontinued.

    (2) With benign prostatic hyperplasia, observe for improved urination. — The client may report a larger stream, less nocturnal voiding, and more complete emptying of the bladder.

    (3) In pheochromocytoma, observe for decreased pulse rate, blood pressure, sweating, palpitations, and blood sugar. — Because symptoms of pheochromocytoma are caused by excessive sympathetic nervous system stimulation, blocking stimulation with these drugs produces a decrease or absence of symptoms.

    (4) In Raynaud's disease or frostbite, observe affected areas for improvement in skin color and temperature and in the quality of peripheral pulses. — These conditions are characterized by vasospasm, which diminishes blood flow to the affected part. The drugs improve blood flow by vasodilation.

  b. With beta-blocking drugs:

    (1) With hypertension, observe for decreasing blood pressure. — Blood pressure is lowered when sympathetic nervous system activity is inhibited.

    (2) With angina, observe for absence of chest pain, nausea, vomiting, sweating, and anxiety. — Angina is characterized by inadequate blood flow and oxygenation to the myocardium. The drugs reduce cardiac workload and therefore reduce oxygen demand.

    (3) With dysrhythmias, observe for regular pulse and signs of adequate cardiac output. — Rhythm disturbances decrease cardiac output.

NURSING ACTIONS	RATIONALE/EXPLANATION
3. **Observe for adverse effects**	Adverse effects are usually extensions of therapeutic effects.
a. With alpha$_2$ agonists and alpha-blocking drugs:	
(1) Hypotension	Hypotension may range from transient postural hypotension to a more severe hypotensive state resembling shock. "First-dose syncope" may occur with prazosin and related drugs.
(2) Sedation, drowsiness	Sedation can be minimized by increasing dosage slowly and giving all or most of the daily dose at bedtime.
(3) Tachycardia	Tachycardia occurs as a reflex mechanism to increase blood supply to body tissues in hypotensive states.
(4) Edema	These drugs promote retention of sodium and water. Concomitant diuretic therapy may be needed to maintain antihypertensive effects with long-term use.
(5) Impaired ejaculation	Blockade of the sympathetic nervous system impedes efferent nerve conduction to the seminal vesicles.
(6) Prolonged Q–T interval and dysrhythmias with alfuzosin	Prolongation of the Q–T interval increases the risk of ventricular dysrhythmias such as torsades de pointes.
b. With beta-blocking drugs:	
(1) Bradycardia and heart block	These are extensions of the therapeutic effects, which slow conduction of electrical impulses through the atrioventricular node, particularly in clients with compromised cardiac function.
(2) Congestive heart failure—edema, dyspnea, fatigue	Caused by reduced force of myocardial contraction
(3) Bronchospasm—dyspnea, wheezing	Caused by drug-induced constriction of bronchi and bronchioles. It is more likely to occur in people with bronchial asthma or other obstructive lung disease.
(4) Fatigue and dizziness, especially with activity or exercise	These symptoms occur because the usual sympathetic nervous system stimulation in response to activity or stress is blocked by drug action.
(5) Central nervous system (CNS) effects—depression, insomnia, vivid dreams, and hallucinations	The mechanism by which these effects are produced is unknown.
4. **Observe for drug interactions**	
a. Drugs that *increase* effects of alpha-antiadrenergic drugs:	
(1) Other antihypertensive drugs	Additive antihypertensive effects
(2) CNS depressants	Additive sedation and drowsiness
(3) Nonsteroidal anti-inflammatory drugs	Additive sodium and water retention, possible edema
(4) Epinephrine	Epinephrine increases the hypotensive effects of phentolamine and should not be given to treat shock caused by these drugs. Because epinephrine stimulates both alpha- and beta-adrenergic receptors, the net effect is vasodilation and a further drop in blood pressure.
(5) Ketoconazole, itraconazole, and ritonavir (with alfuzosin)	These drugs inhibit the enzyme CYP3A4, which is responsible for the metabolism of alfuzosin.
b. Drugs that *decrease* effects of alpha-antiadrenergic drugs:	
(1) Alpha adrenergics (eg, norepinephrine)	Norepinephrine is a strong vasoconstricting agent and is the drug of choice for treating shock caused by overdosage of, or hypersensitivity to, phenoxybenzamine or phentolamine.
(2) Estrogens, oral contraceptives, nonsteroidal anti-inflammatory drugs	These drugs may cause sodium and fluid retention and thereby decrease antihypertensive effects of alpha-antiadrenergic drugs.

(continued)

NURSING ACTIONS	RATIONALE/EXPLANATION
c. Drugs that *increase* effects of beta-adrenergic blocking drugs (eg, propranolol):	
(1) Other antihypertensives	Synergistic antihypertensive effects. Clients who do not respond to beta blockers or vasodilators alone may respond well to the combination. Also, beta blockers prevent reflex tachycardia, which usually occurs with vasodilator antihypertensive drugs.
(2) Phentolamine	Synergistic effects to prevent excessive hypertension before and during surgical excision of pheochromocytoma
(3) Cimetidine, furosemide	Increase plasma levels by slowing hepatic metabolism
(4) Digoxin	Additive bradycardia, heart block
(5) Phenytoin	Potentiates cardiac depressant effects of propranolol
(6) Quinidine	The combination may be synergistic in treating cardiac arrhythmias. However, additive cardiac depressant effects also may occur (bradycardia, decreased force of myocardial contraction [negative inotropy], decreased cardiac output).
(7) Verapamil, IV	IV verapamil and IV propranolol should never be used in combination because of additive bradycardia and hypotension.
d. Drugs that *decrease* effects of beta-adrenergic blocking drugs:	
(1) Antacids	Decrease absorption of several oral beta blockers
(2) Atropine	Increases heart rate and may be used to counteract excessive bradycardia caused by beta blockers
(3) Isoproterenol	Stimulates beta-adrenergic receptors and therefore antagonizes effects of beta-blocking agents. Isoproterenol also can be used to counteract excessive bradycardia.
(4) Cocaine	May reduce or cancel the effects of beta-blocking drugs

---

APPLYING YOUR KNOWLEDGE: ANSWERS

18-1 Clonidine is effective in reducing blood pressure. It works by reducing central nervous system outflow, which raises blood pressure.

18-2 Lopressor will act as an antianginal and antihypertensive drug for Mr. Jones. It also may protect the heart from reinfarction.

18-3 Beta-blocking medication should be discontinued slowly, over 1 to 3 weeks. Notify the physician and pharmacy if the client cannot/will not take the substituted drug; do not stop the drug abruptly.

18-4 Diabetic clients are prone to hypoglycemia as an adverse effect of their antidiabetic medication. Mr. Jones is at risk for more severe and prolonged hypoglycemia because he is taking Lopressor (metoprolol).

Review and Application Exercises

Short Answer Exercises

1. How do alpha$_2$ agonists and alpha$_1$-blocking drugs decrease blood pressure?

2. What are safety factors in administering and monitoring the effects of alpha$_2$ agonists and alpha$_1$-blocking drugs?

3. Why should a client be cautioned against stopping alpha$_2$ agonists and alpha$_1$-blocking drugs abruptly?

4. What are the main mechanisms by which beta blockers relieve angina pectoris?

5. How are beta blockers thought to be "cardioprotective" in preventing repeat MIs?

6. What are some noncardiovascular indications for the use of propranolol?

7. What are the main differences between cardioselective and nonselective beta blockers?

8. Why are cardioselective beta blockers preferred for clients with asthma or diabetes mellitus?

9. List at least five adverse effects of beta blockers.

10. Explain the drug effects that contribute to each adverse reaction.

11. What signs, symptoms, or behaviors would lead you to suspect adverse drug effects?

12. Do the same adverse effects occur with betablocker eye drops that occur with systemic drugs? If so, how may they be prevented or minimized?

13. What information needs to be included in teaching clients about beta-blocker therapy?

14. What is the risk of abruptly stopping a beta-blocker drug rather than tapering the dose and gradually discontinuing the drug, as recommended?

15. How can beta blockers be both therapeutic and nontherapeutic for HF?

NCLEX-Style Questions

16. A client with a history of emphysema is prescribed propanolol (Inderal) to treat hypertension. In this situation, the nurse should assess for the presence of
    a. hyperglycemia
    b. tachycardia
    c. bronchoconstriction
    d. respiratory depression

17. Your diabetic client requires a beta blocker to treat a tachydysrhythmia. Due to the beta-blocker therapy, you should teach this client not to rely on which of the following signs of developing hypoglycemia?
    a. increased thirst
    b. irritability
    c. tachycardia
    d. hunger

18. A client is taking clonidine (Catapres) for hypertension. It is important for the nurse to give this client which of the following instructions?
    a. Change from lying to standing positions slowly.
    b. Rest often to avoid exercise intolerance.

c. Promptly report episodes of wheezing and difficulty breathing.
d. Take the medication in the morning to avoid insomnia.

19. The nurse should anticipate administering which of the following medications if a vasoconstrictor such as dopamine (Intropin) extravasates?
    a. phentolamine (Regitine)
    b. propranolol (Inderal)
    c. esmolol (Brevibloc)
    d. tamsulosin (Flomax)

20. The nurse should monitor which of the following tests in a hypertensive client taking methyldopa (Aldomet)?
    a. prostate-specific antigen
    b. serum electrolytes
    c. blood glucose
    d. liver studies

21. Which of the following instructions should be given to the client with benign prostatic hyperplasia before taking his first dose of prazosin (Minipress)?
    a. Take your medication in the morning after meals.
    b. Take your medication at bedtime.
    c. Take your medication on an empty stomach.
    d. Take your medication with a glass of milk.

Selected References

Coloma, M., Chiu, J., White, P., & Armbruster, S. (2001). The use of esmolol as an alternative to remifentanil during desflurane anesthesia for fast-track outpatient gynecologic laparoscopic surgery. *Anesthesia and Analgesia, 92*(2), 352–357.

Colucci, W. (2004). Landmark study: The carvedilol post-infarction survival control in left ventricular dysfunction study (CAPRICORN). *The American Journal of Cardiology, 93*(9, Suppl. 1), 13–16.

Dargie, H. S., & Lechat, P. C. (1999). The cardiac insufficiency bisoprolol study II (CIBIS-II): A randomised trial. *Lancet, 353*(2), 9–13.

Drug facts and comparisons. (Updated monthly). St. Louis: Facts and Comparisons.

Fetrow, C. W., & Avila, J. R. (2001). *Complementary and alternative medicines* (2nd ed.). Springhouse, PA: Springhouse.

Harwood, T., Butterworth, J., Prielipp, R., Royster, R., Hansen, K., Plonl, G., & Dean, R. (1999). The safety and effectiveness of esmolol in the perioperative period in patients undergoing abdominal aortic surgery. *Journal of Cardiothoracic and Vascular Anesthesia, 13*(5), 555–561.

Hoffman, B. B. (2001). Adrenoreceptor antagonist drugs. In B. G. Katzung (Ed.), *Basic and clinical pharmacology* (8th ed., pp. 138–154). New York: McGraw-Hill.

Hoffman, B. B. (2001). Catecholamines, sympathomimetic drugs, and adrenergic receptor antagonists. In J. G. Hardman & L. E. Limbird (Eds.), *Goodman and Gilman's The pharmacological basis of therapeutics* (10th ed., pp. 215–268). New York: McGraw-Hill.

Kudzma, E. C. (1999). Culturally competent drug administration. *American Journal of Nursing, 99*(8), 46–51.

Kurm, H. (2004). Tolerability of carvedilol in heart failure: Clinical trials experience. The *American Journal of Cardiology, 93*(9, Suppl. 1), 58–63.

Ormiston, T., & Salpeter, R. (2003). Beta-blocker use in patients with congestive heart failure and concomitant obstructive airway disease: Moving from myth to evidence-based practice. *Heart Failure Monitoring, 4*(2), 45–54.

Piano, M. R., & Huether, S. E. (2002). Mechanisms of hormonal regulation. In K. L. McCance & S. E. Huether (Eds.), *Pathophysiology: The biologic basis for disease in adults and children* (4th ed., pp. 597–623). St. Louis: Mosby.

Robinson, K. M., & McCance, K. L. (2002). Alterations of the reproductive system. In K. L. McCance & S. E. Huether (Eds.), *Pathophysiology: The biologic basis for disease in adults and children* (4th ed., pp. 597–623). St. Louis: Mosby.

Salpeter, S., Ormiston, T., Salpeter, E., Poole, P., & Cates C. (2003). Cardioselective beta-blockers for chronic obstructive pulmonary disease: A meta-analysis. *Respiratory Medicine, 97*(10), 1094–1101.

Urban, M., Markowitz, S., Gordon, M., Urquhart, B., & Kligfield, P. (2000). Postoperative prophylactic administration of beta-adrenergic blockers in patients at risk for myocardial ischemia. *Anesthesia and Analgesia, 90*(6), 1257–1261.

White, P., Wang, B., Tang, J., Wender, R., Naruse, R., & Sloninsky, A. (2003). The effect of intraoperative use of esmolol and nicardipine on recovery after ambulatory surgery. *Anesthesia and Analgesia, 97*(6), 1633–1638.

Wilson, E., McKinlay, S., Crawford, J., & Robb, H. (2004). The influence of esmolol on the dose of propofol required for induction of anaesthesia. *Anaesthesia, 59*(2), 122–126.

Yancy, C. (2004). Special considerations for carvedilol use in heart failure. *The American Journal of Cardiology, 93*(9, Suppl. 1), 64–68.

Cholinergic Drugs

OBJECTIVES

After studying this chapter, you will be able to:

1. Describe effects and indications for use of selected cholinergic drugs.
2. Discuss drug therapy for myasthenia gravis.
3. Discuss the use of cholinergic drug therapy for paralytic ileus and urinary retention.
4. Discuss drug therapy for Alzheimer's disease.
5. Describe major nursing care needs of clients receiving cholinergic drugs.
6. Describe signs, symptoms, and treatment of overdose with cholinergic drugs.
7. Discuss atropine and pralidoxime as antidotes for cholinergic drugs.
8. Discuss principles of therapy for using cholinergic drugs in special populations.
9. Teach clients about safe, effective use of cholinergic drugs.

APPLYING YOUR KNOWLEDGE

Betty Humbarger is a 39-year-old female who has myasthenia gravis. The use of neostigmine 30 mg three to four times a day has controlled her symptoms.

INTRODUCTION

Cholinergic drugs stimulate the parasympathetic nervous system in the same manner as acetylcholine (see Chap. 16). Some drugs act directly to stimulate cholinergic receptors; others act indirectly by inhibiting the enzyme acetylcholinesterase, thereby slowing acetylcholine metabolism at autonomic nerve synapses. Selected drugs are discussed here in relation to their use in myasthenia gravis, Alzheimer's disease, and atony of the smooth muscle of the gastrointestinal (GI) and urinary systems, which results in paralytic ileus and urinary retention, respectively.

In normal neuromuscular function, acetylcholine is released from nerve endings and binds to nicotinic receptors on cell membranes of muscle cells to cause muscle contraction. Myasthenia gravis is an autoimmune disorder in which autoantibodies are thought to destroy nicotinic receptors for acetylcholine on skeletal muscle. As a result, acetylcholine is less able to stimulate muscle contraction, and muscle weakness occurs.

In normal brain function, acetylcholine is an essential neurotransmitter and plays an important role in cognitive functions, including memory storage and retrieval. Alzheimer's disease, the most common type of dementia in adults, is characterized by abnormalities in the cholinergic, serotonergic, noradrenergic, and glutamatergic neurotransmission systems (see Chap. 5). In the cholinergic system, there is a substantial loss of neurons that secrete acetylcholine in the brain, and decreased activity of choline acetyltransferase, the enzyme required for synthesis of acetylcholine.

Acetylcholine stimulates cholinergic receptors in the gut to promote normal secretory and motor activity. Cholinergic stimulation results in increased peristalsis and relaxation of the smooth muscle in sphincters to facilitate movement of flatus and feces. The secretory functions of the salivary and gastric glands are also stimulated.

Acetylcholine stimulates cholinergic receptors in the urinary system to promote normal urination. Cholinergic stimulation results in contraction of the detrusor muscle and relaxation of the urinary sphincter to facilitate emptying the urinary bladder.

GENERAL CHARACTERISTICS OF CHOLINERGIC DRUGS

Mechanisms of Action and Effects

Direct-acting cholinergic drugs are synthetic derivatives of choline. Most direct-acting cholinergic drugs are quaternary amines, carry a positive charge, and are lipid insoluble. They do not readily enter the central nervous system; thus, their effects occur primarily in the periphery. Direct-acting cholinergic drugs are highly resistant to metabolism by acetylcholinesterase, the enzyme that normally metabolizes acetylcholine. This allows the drugs to have a longer duration of action than acetylcholine would produce. Direct-acting cholinergic drugs have widespread systemic effects when they activate muscarinic receptors in cardiac muscle, smooth muscle, exocrine glands, and the eye (Fig. 19-1).

Specific effects of direct-acting cholinergic drugs include:

- Decreased heart rate, vasodilation, and unpredictable changes in blood pressure
- Increased tone and contractility in GI smooth muscle, relaxation of sphincters, and increased salivary-gland and GI secretions
- Increased tone and contractility of smooth muscle (detrusor) in the urinary bladder and relaxation of the sphincter
- Increased tone and contractility of bronchial smooth muscle
- Increased respiratory secretions
- Constriction of pupils (miosis) and contraction of ciliary muscle, resulting in accommodation for near vision

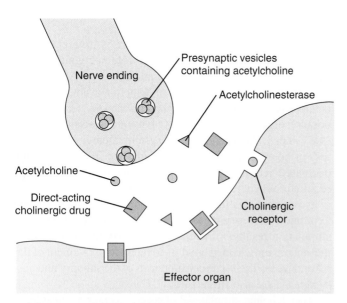

FIGURE 19-1 Mechanism of direct cholinergic drug action. Direct-acting cholinergic drugs interact with postsynaptic cholinergic receptors on target effector organs, activating the organ in a similar fashion as the neurotransmitter acetylcholine.

Indirect-acting cholinergic or anticholinesterase drugs decrease the inactivation of acetylcholine in the synapse by the enzyme acetylcholinesterase. Acetylcholine can then accumulate in the synapse and enhance the activation of postsynaptic muscarinic as well as nicotinic receptors (Fig. 19-2). In addition to the cholinergic drug effects described above, the added effect of indirect-acting cholinergic drugs on nicotinic receptors in skeletal muscles results in improved skeletal muscle tone and strength. Indirect-acting cholinergic medications for Alzheimer's disease are widely distributed, including to the central nervous system. Thus indirect-acting cholinergic drugs are able to improve cholinergic neurotransmission in the brain.

Anticholinesterase drugs are classified as either reversible or irreversible inhibitors of acetylcholinesterase. The reversible inhibitors exhibit a moderate duration of action and have several therapeutic uses, such as for Alzheimer's disease and myesthenia gravis, as described later. The irreversible inhibitors produce prolonged effects and are highly toxic. These agents are used primarily as poisons (ie, insecticides and nerve gases); management of the toxicity caused by these agents is discussed later in this chapter. The only therapeutic use of these drugs is in the treatment of glaucoma (see Chap. 63).

Indications for Use

Cholinergic drugs have limited but varied uses. A direct-acting drug, bethanechol, is used to treat urinary retention due to urinary bladder atony and postoperative abdominal distention due to paralytic ileus. The anticholinesterase agents are used in the diagnosis and treatment of myasthenia gravis. They are also used to reverse the action of nondepolarizing neuromuscular blocking agents, such as tubocurarine, used in surgery (see Appendix F). Anticholinesterase agents do not reverse the neuromuscular blockade produced by depolarizing neuromuscular blocking agents, such as succinylcholine. In addition, tacrine, donepezil, rivastigmine, and galantamine are anticholinesterase agents approved for treatment of Alzheimer's disease. Cholinergic drugs may also be used to treat glaucoma (see Chap. 63).

Contraindications to Use

Cholinergic drugs are contraindicated in urinary or GI tract obstruction because they increase the contractility of smooth muscle in the urinary and GI systems and may result in injury to structures proximal to the obstruction. Cholinergic drugs are contraindicated in individuals with asthma because they may cause bronchoconstriction and increased respiratory secretions. Individuals with peptic ulcer disease should not use cholinergic drugs because they increase gastric acid secretion. These drugs are also contraindicated in clients with

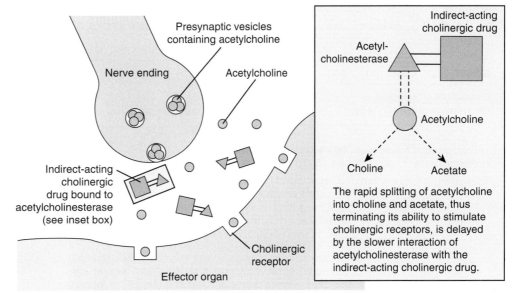

FIGURE 19-2 Mechanism of indirect cholinergic drug action. Indirect-acting cholinergic drugs prevent the enzymatic breakdown of the neurotransmitter acetylcholine. The acetylcholine remains in the synapse and continues to interact with cholinergic receptors on target effector organs, producing a cholinergic response.

inflammatory abdominal conditions and recent bowel surgery, because the drugs cause increased tone and motility of the intestinal smooth muscle and may lead to rupture of the bowel. Individuals with coronary artery disease should not take cholinergics because they can result in bradycardia, vasodilation, and hypotension.

Clients with hyperthyroidism should avoid cholinergic drugs. In the individual with hyperthyroidism, the initial response to cholinergic medications (bradycardia and hypotension) triggers the baroreceptor reflex. As this reflex attempts to resolve the hypotension, norepinephrine is secreted from sympathetic nerves regulating the heart. Norepinephrine may trigger reflex tachycardia and other cardiac dysrhythmias.

Pregnant women should not take cholinergic medications. Tacrine is also contraindicated in previous users who developed jaundice or a serum bilirubin level above 3 milligrams per deciliter.

INDIVIDUAL DRUGS

Cholinergic drugs are described in the following sections. Trade names, clinical indications, and dosage ranges are listed in Table 19-1.

Direct-Acting Cholinergics

Bethanechol (Urecholine) is a synthetic derivative of choline. Because the drug produces smooth-muscle contractions, it should not be used in obstructive conditions of the urinary or GI tracts.

Reversible Indirect-Acting Cholinergics (Anticholinesterases)

P **Neostigmine** (Prostigmin) is the prototype anticholinesterase agent. It is used for long-term treatment of myasthenia gravis and as an antidote for tubocurarine and other nondepolarizing skeletal muscle relaxants used in surgery. Neostigmine, like bethanechol, is a quaternary amine and carries a positive charge. This reduces its lipid solubility and results in poor absorption from the GI tract. Consequently, oral doses are much larger than parenteral doses. When it is used for long-term treatment of myasthenia gravis, resistance to its action may occur and larger doses may be required.

Edrophonium (Tensilon) is a short-acting cholinergic drug used to diagnose myasthenia gravis, to differentiate between myasthenic crisis and cholinergic crisis, and to reverse the neuromuscular blockade produced by nondepolarizing skeletal muscle relaxants. It is given IM or IV by a physician who remains in attendance. Atropine, an antidote, and life-support equipment, such as ventilators and endotracheal tubes, must be available when the drug is given.

Ambenonium (Mytelase) is a long-acting drug used for the treatment of myasthenia gravis. It is used less often than neostigmine and pyridostigmine. It may be useful in clients who are allergic to bromides, however, because the other drugs are both bromide salts. Ambenonium may be useful for myasthenic clients on ventilators because it is less likely to increase respiratory secretions than other anticholinesterase drugs.

Physostigmine salicylate (Antilirium) is the only anticholinesterase capable of crossing the blood–brain barrier. Unlike other drugs in this group, physostigmine is not a quaternary amine, does not carry a positive charge, and therefore is more lipid soluble. It is sometimes used as an antidote for overdosage of anticholinergic drugs, including atropine,

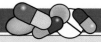

Table 19-1 Drugs at a Glance: Selected Cholinergic Drugs

GENERIC/TRADE NAME	ROUTES AND DOSAGE RANGES	
	Adults	**Children**
Direct-Acting Cholinergics		
Bethanechol (Urecholine)	PO 10–50 mg 2 to 4 times daily, maximum single dose not to exceed 50 mg	Safety and efficacy not established <8 y. PO: 0.6 mg/kg 3 to 4 times daily.
Indirect-Acting Cholinergics (Anticholinesterase Drugs)		
Ambenonium (Mytelase)	PO 5–25 mg 3 or 4 times daily	Safety and efficacy not established.
Edrophonium (Tensilon)	*Diagnosis of myasthenia gravis:* *IV route preferred:* 2 mg IV over 15–30 sec; 8 mg IV given 45 seconds later if no response Test dose may be repeated in 30 min. *IM route:* 10 mg; may follow up with an additional 2 mg 30 min later if no response *Differentiation of myasthenic crisis from cholinergic crisis:* 2 mg IV, observe response for 60 s. May repeat with subsequent doses of 3 mg and 5 mg if no response to initial dose. BE PREPARED to intubate.	*Diagnosis of myasthenia gravis:* *Infants:* 0.5 mg IV. *<34 kg:* 1 mg IV; may titrate up to 5 mg if no response. >34 kg: 2 mg IV; may titrate up to 10 mg if no response *Children <34 kg:* 2 mg IM. *Children >34 kg:* 5 mg, IM.
Neostigmine (Prostigmin)	*Prevention/treatment of postoperative distention and urinary retention:* 0.25–0.5 mg IM or Sub-Q q 4–6 h for 2–3 d. *Treatment of myasthenia gravis:* Dosage individualized to patient needs. PO 15–375 mg/day in 3 or 4 divided doses. Sub-Q, IV, or IM 0.5 mg initially. Individualize subsequent doses. *Diagnosis of myasthenia gravis:* 0.022 mg/kg IM *Antidote for nondepolarizing neuromuscular blockers:* Give atropine sulfate 0.6–1.2 mg IV several min before slow IV injection of neostigmine 0.5–2 mg. Repeat as needed; total dose not to exceed 5 mg	*Prevention/treatment of post-operative distention and urinary retention* Safety and efficacy not established *Treatment of myasthenia gravis:* PO 0.3–0.6 mg/kg q3–4h Sub-Q, IV, IM 0.01–0.04 mg/kg/dose q2–3h as needed *Diagnosis of myasthenia gravis:* 0.04 mg/kg IM *Antidote for nondepolarizing neuro-muscular blockers* Give 0.008–0.025 mg/kg atropine sulfate IV several min before slow IV injection of neostigmine 0.07–0.08 mg/kg.
Physostigmine (Antilirium)	IM, IV 0.5–2 mg. Give IV slowly, no faster than 1 mg/min to avoid adverse effects of bradycardia, respiratory distress, and seizures.	
Pyridostigmine (Mestinon)	PO 60 mg 3 times daily initially; individualize dose to control symptoms. Average dose in 24 h: 600 mg. Range in 24 h: 60–1500 mg. IM, IV slowly: 1/30th the oral dose	PO 7 mg/kg/d divided into 5 or 6 doses *Neonates of mothers with myasthenia gravis, who have difficulty with sucking/breathing/swallowing:* 0.05–0.15 mg/kg IM. Change to syrup as soon as possible.
Indirect-Acting Cholinergics for Alzheimer's Disease (Anticholinesterase Drugs)		
Donepezil (Aricept)	PO 5 mg daily at bedtime for 4–6 wk, then increase to 10 mg daily if needed.	
Galantamine (Razadyne)	PO 8 mg/d initially, with food; increase to 16 mg/d after 4 wks if needed. May continue to increase q 4 wk up to maximum dose of 24 mg/d.	
Rivastigmine (Exelon)	PO 1.5 mg twice daily with food initially. May titrate to higher doses at 1.5-mg intervals q 2 wk to a maximum dose of 12 mg/d.	
Tacrine (Cognex)	PO 40 mg/d (10 mg 4 times daily) for 6 wk. If amino-transferase levels are satisfactory after weekly monitoring, may increase the dose to 80 mg/d (20 mg 4 times daily). If liver function remains nor-mal, may increase daily dose by 10 mg q 6 wk to a total of 120–160 mg/d	

IM, intramuscular; IV, intravenous; PO, oral; Sub-Q, subcutaneous.

antihistamines, tricyclic antidepressants, and phenothiazine antipsychotics. However, its potential for causing serious adverse effects limits its usefulness. Some preparations of physostigmine are also used in the treatment of glaucoma (see Chap. 63).

Pyridostigmine (Mestinon) is similar to neostigmine in actions, uses, and adverse effects. It may have a longer duration of action than neostigmine and is the maintenance drug of choice for clients with myasthenia gravis. An added advantage is the availability of a slow-release form, which is effective for 8 to 12 hours. When this form is taken at bedtime, the client does not have to take other medications during the night and does not awaken too weak to swallow.

Reversible Indirect-Acting Cholinergics (Anticholinesterases) for Alzheimer's Disease

Donepezil (Aricept) is used to treat mild to moderate Alzheimer's disease. In long-term studies, donepezil delayed the progression of the disease for up to 55 weeks. Donepezil increases acetylcholine in the brain by inhibiting its metabolism. Donepezil is well absorbed after oral administration and absorption is unaffected by food. The drug is highly bound (96%) to plasma proteins. It is metabolized in the liver to several metabolites, some of which are pharmacologically active; metabolites and some unchanged drug are excreted mainly in urine. Adverse effects include nausea, vomiting, diarrhea, bradycardia, and possible aggravation of asthma, peptic ulcer disease, and chronic obstructive pulmonary disease. Unlike tacrine, donepezil does not cause liver toxicity.

Galantamine (Razadyne) is a newer long-acting anticholinesterase agent approved by the Food and Drug Administration for the treatment of Alzheimer's disease. Its pharmacokinetics and adverse-effect profile are similar to donepezil and rivastigimine.

Rivastigmine (Exelon) is a long-acting central anticholinesterase agent approved for the treatment of Alzheimer's disease. It lasts 12 hours, making twice-a-day dosing possible. Like other drugs in this class, it is not a cure for Alzheimer's disease but does slow the progression of symptoms. Rivastigmine is metabolized by the liver and excreted in the feces. It has an adverse-effect profile similar to donepezil. It may be taken with food to decrease GI distress.

Tacrine (Cognex) is a centrally acting anticholinesterase agent approved for treatment of clients with mild to moderate Alzheimer's disease. The drug does not cure the disease, but it may delay progression in some clients. Tacrine is well absorbed after oral administration and reaches peak plasma levels in 1 to 2 hours. It is approximately 50% protein bound, is extensively metabolized in the liver, is excreted in the urine, and has an elimination half-life of 2 to 4 hours. The initial enthusiasm for tacrine has declined because of inconsistent results of clinical trials and the occurrence of hepatotoxicity. Although tacrine is still available, it is no longer actively marketed by the drug manufacturer. Approximately 20% to 50% of clients receiving low-dose tacrine therapy experience elevated alanine aminotransferase (ALT) values of three times normal. Ninety percent of these clients return to normal liver function values when the drug is discontinued.

NURSING PROCESS

Assessment

Assess the client's condition in relation to disorders for which cholinergic drugs are used.

● In clients known to have myasthenia gravis, assess for muscle weakness. This may be manifested by ptosis (drooping) of the upper eyelid and diplopia (double vision) caused by weakness of the eye muscles. More severe disease may be indicated by difficulty in chewing, swallowing, and speaking; accumulation of oral secretions, which the client may be unable to expectorate or swallow; decreased skeletal muscle activity, including impaired chest expansion; and eventual respiratory failure.
● In clients with possible urinary retention, assess for bladder distention, time and amount of previous urination, and fluid intake.
● In clients with possible paralytic ileus, assess for presence of bowel sounds, abdominal distention, and elimination pattern.
● In clients with Alzheimer's disease, assess for abilities and limitations in relation to memory, cognitive functioning, self-care activities, and pre-existing conditions that may be aggravated by a cholinergic drug.

Nursing Diagnoses

● Impaired gas exchange related to increased respiratory secretions, bronchospasm, and/or respiratory paralysis
● Ineffective Breathing Pattern related to bronchoconstriction
● Ineffective Airway Clearance related to increased respiratory secretions
● Self-Care Deficit related to muscle weakness, cognitive impairment, or diplopia
● Deficient Knowledge: Drug administration and effects

Planning/Goals

The client will
● Verbalize or demonstrate correct drug administration
● Improve in self-care abilities
● Regain usual patterns of urinary and bowel elimination
● Maintain effective oxygenation of tissues
● Report adverse drug effects
● For clients with myasthenia gravis, at least one family member will verbalize or demonstrate correct drug

administration, symptoms of too much or too little drug, and emergency care procedures.

● For clients with dementia, a caregiver will verbalize or demonstrate correct drug administration and knowledge of adverse effects to be reported to a health care provider.

Interventions

● Use measures to prevent or decrease the need for cholinergic drugs. Ambulation, adequate fluid intake, and judicious use of opioid analgesics or other sedative-type drugs help prevent postoperative urinary retention. In myasthenia gravis, muscle weakness is aggravated by exercise and improved by rest. Therefore, scheduling activities to avoid excessive fatigue and to allow adequate rest periods may be beneficial.
● With drug therapy for Alzheimer's disease, assist and teach caregivers to:
  ● Maintain a quiet, stable environment and daily routines to decrease confusion (eg, verbal or written reminders, simple directions, adequate lighting, calendars, personal objects within view and reach).
  ● Avoid altering dosage or stopping the drug without consulting the prescribing physician.
  ● Be sure that the client keeps appointments for supervision and blood tests.
  ● Report signs and symptoms (ie, skin rash, jaundice, light-colored stools) that may indicate hepatotoxicity for clients taking tacrine.
  ● Notify surgeons about tacrine therapy. Exaggerated muscle relaxation may occur if succinylcholine-type drugs are given.
● Do not give cholinergic drugs for bladder atony and urinary retention or for paralytic ileus in the presence of an obstruction.
● For long-term use, assist clients and families to establish a schedule of drug administration that best meets the client's needs.
● With myasthenia gravis, recommend that one or more family members be trained in cardiopulmonary resuscitation.

In addition, teaching guidelines are given in the accompanying display.

Evaluation

● Observe and interview about the adequacy of urinary elimination.
● Observe abilities and limitations in self-care.
● Question the client and at least one family member of the client with myasthenia gravis about correct drug usage, symptoms of underdosage and overdosage, and emergency care procedures.
● Question caregivers of clients with dementia about the client's level of functioning and response to medication.

PRINCIPLES OF THERAPY

Use in Myasthenia Gravis

Guidelines for the use of anticholinesterase drugs in myasthenia gravis include the following:

● Drug dosage should be increased gradually until maximal benefit is obtained. Larger doses are often required with increased physical activity, emotional stress, and infections, and sometimes premenstrually.
● Some clients with myasthenia gravis cannot tolerate optimal doses of anticholinesterase drugs unless atropine is given to decrease the severity of adverse reactions due to muscarinic activation. However, atropine should be given only if necessary because it may mask the sudden increase of adverse effects. Such an increase is the first sign of overdose.
● Drug dosage in excess of the amount needed to maintain muscle strength and function can produce a cholinergic crisis. A cholinergic crisis is characterized by excessive stimulation of the parasympathetic nervous system. If early symptoms are not treated, hypotension and respiratory failure may occur. At high doses, anticholinesterase drugs weaken rather than strengthen skeletal muscle contraction because excessive amounts of acetylcholine accumulate at motor endplates and reduce nerve impulse transmission to muscle tissue.
● Some people acquire partial or total resistance to anticholinesterase drugs after taking them for months or years. Therefore, do not assume that drug therapy that is effective initially will continue to be effective over the long-term course of the disease.
● All anticholinesterase drugs should be taken with food or milk to decrease the risk of gastric distress and ulceration.

APPLYING YOUR KNOWLEDGE 19-1
Ms. Humbarger tells you that she usually increases the dose of her medication according to her symptoms, and that she usually requires less medication when she is in the hospital. What is your most appropriate action/response?

Cholinergic vs. Myasthenic Crisis: Recognition and Management

Differentiating myasthenic crisis from cholinergic crisis may be difficult because both are characterized by respiratory difficulty or failure. It is necessary to differentiate between them, however, because they require opposite treatment measures. Myasthenic crisis requires more anticholinesterase drug, whereas cholinergic crisis requires discontinuing any anticholinesterase drug that the client has been receiving.

The physician may be able to make an accurate diagnosis from signs and symptoms and their timing in relation to medication; that is, signs and symptoms having their onset within

CLIENT TEACHING GUIDELINES

Cholinergic Drugs

General Considerations

✔ Because cholinergic drugs used for urinary retention usually act within 60 minutes after administration, be sure bathroom facilities are available.

✔ Wear a medical alert identification device if taking long-term cholinergic drug therapy for myasthenia gravis, hypotonic bladder, or Alzheimer's disease.

✔ Atropine 0.6 mg IV may be administered for overdose of cholinergic drugs.

✔ Record symptoms of myasthenia gravis and effects of drug therapy, especially when drug therapy is initiated and medication doses are being titrated. The amount of medication required to control symptoms of myasthenia gravis varies greatly and the physician needs this information to adjust the dosage correctly.

✔ Do not overexert yourself if you have myasthenia gravis. Rest between activities. Although the dose of medication may be increased during periods of increased activity, it is desirable to space activities to obtain optimal benefit from the drug, at the lowest possible dose, with the fewest adverse effects.

✔ Report increased muscle weakness, difficulty breathing, or recurrence of myasthenic symptoms to the physician. These are signs of drug underdosage (myasthenic crisis) and indicate a need to increase or change drug therapy.

✔ Report adverse reactions, including abdominal cramps, diarrhea, excessive oral secretions, difficulty in breathing, and muscle weakness. These are signs of drug overdosage (cholinergic crisis) and require immediate discontinuation of drugs and treatment by the physician. Respiratory failure can result if this condition is not recognized and treated properly.

✔ Clients taking tacrine need weekly monitoring of liver aminotransferase levels for 18 weeks when initiating therapy and weekly monitoring for 6 weeks after any increase in dose. Caregivers should report any signs or symptoms of adverse drug reactions such as nausea, vomiting, diarrhea, rash, jaundice, or change in the color of stools. The drug should not be suddenly discontinued.

✔ If dizziness or syncope occurs when taking tacrine, donepezil, or other anticholinesterase drugs, ambulation should be supervised to avoid injury.

✔ Caregivers should record observed effects of anticholinesterase medications given to treat Alzheimer's disease. These medications are often titrated upward to improve cognitive function and delay symptom progression, and this information will be helpful to the prescriber.

Self- or Caregiver Administration

✔ Take drugs as directed on a regular schedule to maintain consistent blood levels and control of symptoms.

✔ Do not chew or crush sustained-release medications.

✔ Take oral cholinergics on an empty stomach to lessen nausea and vomiting. Also, food decreases absorption of tacrine by up to 40%.

✔ Ensure adequate fluid intake if vomiting or diarrhea occurs as a side effect of cholinergic medications.

✔ Avoid taking St. John's wort because concurrent use may reduce blood levels of donepezil.

---

approximately 1 hour after a dose of anticholinesterase drug are more likely to be caused by cholinergic crisis (too much drug). Signs and symptoms beginning 3 hours or more after a drug dose are more likely to be caused by myasthenic crisis (too little drug).

If the differential diagnosis cannot be made on the basis of signs and symptoms, the client can be intubated, mechanically ventilated, and observed closely until a diagnosis is possible. Still another way to differentiate between the two conditions is for the physician to inject a small dose of IV edrophonium (Tensilon). The ideal test dose if edrophonium has not been determined. An incremental dosing schedule begins with 2 milligrams IV, followed by a 60-second period of time during which the response of the individual is observed. Subsequent doses of 3 and 5 milligrams may be given if indicated by a lack of response. If the edrophonium test causes a dramatic improvement in breathing, the test is considered positive and the diagnosis is myasthenic crisis. If the edrophonium test makes the client even weaker, the diagnosis is cholinergic crisis. Edrophonium or any other diagnostic pharmacologic agent should be administered only after endotracheal intubation and controlled ventilation have been instituted.

Treatment for cholinergic crisis includes withdrawal of anticholinesterase drugs; administration of atropine, an anticholinergic drug (see Chap. 20); and measures to maintain respiration. It is important to understand that atropine will reverse only the muscarinic effects of cholinergic crisis, having no effect on reversing nicotinic receptor–mediated skeletal muscle weakness. Endotracheal intubation and mechanical ventilation may be necessary due to this profound skeletal muscle weakness, including muscles of respiration.

Treatment for myasthenic crisis includes administration of additional anticholinesterase medications and measures to maintain respirations until the medications are effective in improving muscle strength.

Use in Alzheimer's Disease

The goal of drug therapy for Alzheimer's disease is to slow the loss of memory and cognition, thus preserving the independence of the individual for as long as possible. Practice guidelines developed by the American Academy of Neurology (2001) recommend early diagnosis and treatment of Alzheimer's disease with cholinesterase inhibitors for all clients with mild to moderate symptoms. Although these drugs do not cure Alzheimer's disease, they do delay the onset of the disease somewhat and bring about a slight improvement in cognition and function.

Additional medications that may be beneficial in slowing the progression of Alzheimer's disease include high-dose vitamin E therapy; and memantine (Namenda), an N-methyl D-aspartate (NMDA) antagonist. Estrogen is not recommended as a treatment for Alzheimer's disease.

There is research evidence that the long-term use of nonsteroidal anti-inflammatory drugs (NSAIDs) such as ibuprofen, naproxen, and aspirin prior to the onset of symptoms of Alzheimer's disease may help prevent the disorder. Studies are underway to determine if NSAIDs are beneficial in treating the disease after the onset of symptoms.

Toxicity of Cholinergic Drugs: Recognition and Management

Atropine, an anticholinergic, antimuscarinic drug, is a specific antidote to cholinergic agents. The drug and equipment for its injection should be readily available whenever cholinergic drugs are given. It is important to note that atropine reverses only the muscarinic effects of cholinergic drugs, primarily in the heart, smooth muscle, and glands. Atropine does not interact with nicotinic receptors and therefore cannot reverse the nicotinic effects of skeletal-muscle weakness or paralysis due to overdose of the indirect cholinergic drugs.

Management of Mushroom Poisoning

Muscarinic receptors in the parasympathetic nervous system were given their name because they can be stimulated by muscarine, an alkaloid that is found in small quantities in the Amanita muscaria mushroom. Some mushrooms found in North America, such as the Clitocybe and Inocybe mushrooms, however, contain much larger quantities of muscarine. Accidental or intentional ingestion of these mushrooms results in intense cholinergic stimulation (cholinergic crisis) and is potentially fatal. Atropine is the specific antidote for mushroom poisoning.

Toxicity of Irreversible Anticholinesterase Agents: Recognition and Management

Most irreversible anticholinesterase agents are highly lipid soluble and can enter the body by a variety of routes including the eye, skin, respiratory system, and GI tract. Because they readily cross the blood–brain barrier, their effects are seen peripherally as well as centrally.

Exposure to toxic doses of irreversible anticholinesterase agents, such as organophosphate insecticides (malathion, parathion) or nerve gases (sarin, tabun, soman), produces a cholinergic crisis characterized by excessive cholinergic (muscarinic) stimulation and neuromuscular blockade. This cholinergic crisis occurs because the irreversible anticholinesterase poison binds to the enzyme acetylcholinesterase and inactivates it. Consequently, acetylcholine remains in cholinergic synapses and causes excessive stimulation of muscarinic and nicotinic receptors.

Emergency treatment includes decontamination procedures such as removing contaminated clothing, flushing the poison from skin and eyes, and using activated charcoal and lavage to remove ingested poison from the GI tract. Pharmacologic treatment includes administering atropine to counteract the muscarinic effects of the poison (eg, salivation, urination, defecation, bronchial secretions, laryngospasm, bronchospasm).

To relieve the neuromuscular blockade produced by nicotinic effects of the poison, a second drug, pralidoxime, is needed. Pralidoxime (Protopam), a cholinesterase reactivator, is a specific antidote for overdose with irreversible anticholinesterase agents. Pralidoxime treats toxicity by causing the anticholinesterase poison to release the enzyme acetylcholinesterase. The reactivated acetylcholinesterase can then degrade excess acetylcholine at the cholinergic synapses, including the neuromuscular junction. Because pralidoxime cannot cross the blood–brain barrier, it is effective only in the peripheral areas of the body. Pralidoxime must be given as soon after the poisoning as possible. If too much time passes, the bond between the irreversible anticholinesterase agent and acetylcholinesterase becomes stronger and pralidoxime is unable to release the enzyme from the poison.

Treatment of anticholinesterase overdose may also require diazepam or lorazepam to control seizures. Mechanical ventilation may be necessary to treat respiratory paralysis.

Use in Special Populations

Use in Children

Bethanechol is occasionally used to treat urinary retention and paralytic ileus, but safety and effectiveness for children younger than 8 years of age have not been established. Neostigmine is used to treat myasthenia gravis and to reverse neuromuscular blockade after general anesthesia but is not recommended for urinary retention. Pyridostigmine may be used in the neonate of a mother with myasthenia gravis to treat difficulties with sucking, swallowing, and breathing.

Although galantamine and donepezil are approved only for the treatment of Alzheimer's disease, these medications are currently under investigation to treat attention deficit-hyperactivity disorder (ADHD). Some studies have shown that these medications may be useful in treating the child with ADHD by improving cognition relative to executive functioning, including planning, time-management, and organizational skills.

Precautions and adverse effects for cholinergic drugs are the same for children as for adults.

Use in Older Adults

Indirect-acting cholinergic drugs may be used in clients with myasthenia gravis or Alzheimer's disease, or to treat overdoses of atropine and other centrally acting anticholinergic drugs (eg, those used for parkinsonism). Older adults are more likely to experience adverse drug effects because of age-related physiologic changes and superimposed pathologic conditions.

Use in Clients With Renal Impairment

Because bethanechol and other cholinergic drugs increase pressure in the urinary tract by stimulating detrusor muscle contraction and relaxation of urinary sphincters, they are contraindicated for clients with urinary tract obstructions or weaknesses in the bladder wall. Administering a cholinergic drug to these people might result in rupture of the bladder.

Some aspects of the pharmacokinetics of cholinergic drugs are unknown. Many of the drugs are degraded enzymatically by cholinesterases. However, a few (eg, neostigmine, pyridostigmine) undergo hepatic metabolism and tubular excretion in the kidneys. Renal impairment may result in accumulation and increased adverse effects, especially with chronic use.

Use in Clients With Hepatic Impairment

The hepatic metabolism of neostigmine and pyridostigmine may be impaired by liver disease, resulting in increased adverse effects.

The use of tacrine is contraindicated in clients with liver disease. Approximately 20% to 50% of all clients experience an increase in liver ALT levels after beginning therapy with tacrine. Most enzyme elevation occurs in the first 18 weeks of therapy and is more common in female clients. When tacrine is started, serum ALT should be monitored weekly for 18 weeks. Then, if values are within normal limits and signs of liver damage do not occur, the test can be done every 3 months.

Immediate withdrawal of the medication usually restores liver enzymes to normal levels with no permanent liver injury.

Use in Critical Illness

Cholinergic drugs have several specific uses in critical illness. These include:

- Neostigmine, pyridostigmine, and edrophonium to reverse neuromuscular blockade (skeletal muscle paralysis) caused by nondepolarizing muscle relaxants.
- Anticholinesterase drugs to treat myasthenic crisis and improve muscle strength.
- Physostigmine in severe cases as an antidote to anticholinergic poisoning with drugs such as atropine or tricyclic antidepressants.

Use in Home Care

Medications to treat long-term conditions such as myasthenia gravis or Alzheimer's disease are often administered in the home setting. The person using the drugs may have difficulty with self-administration. The client with myasthenia gravis may have diplopia or diminished muscle strength that makes it difficult to self-administer medications. The client with Alzheimer's disease may have problems with remembering to take medications and may easily underdose or overdose him- or herself. It is important to work with responsible family members in such cases to ensure accurate drug administration.

APPLYING YOUR KNOWLEDGE 19-2:
HOW CAN YOU AVOID THIS MEDICATION ERROR?
After administering her medication, you leave Ms. Humbarger's room to tend to other clients. When you return 4 hours later, Ms. Humbarger complains that she is having increased difficulty breathing. You recognize this as a cholinergic crisis and prepare to administer the antidote atropine.

N U R S I N G   A C T I O N S

Cholinergic Drugs

NURSING ACTIONS	RATIONALE/EXPLANATION
1. Administer accurately	
a. Give oral bethanechol before meals.	If these drugs are given after meals, nausea and vomiting may occur because the drug stimulates contraction of muscles in the gastrointestinal (GI) tract.
b. With pyridostigmine and other drugs for myasthenia gravis, give at regularly scheduled intervals with food or milk.	For consistent blood levels and control of symptoms. These drugs increase the risk of GI distress and ulceration.

(continued)

NURSING ACTIONS	RATIONALE/EXPLANATION
c. Give tacrine on an empty stomach, 1 hour before or 2 hours after a meal, if possible, at regular intervals around the clock (eg, q6h). Give with meals if GI upset occurs.	Food decreases absorption and decreases serum drug levels by 30% or more. Regular intervals increase therapeutic effects and decrease adverse effects.
d. Give donepezil at bedtime.	Manufacturer's recommendation.
e. Give galantamine and rivastigmine with food.	To decrease GI distress
2. Observe for therapeutic effects	
a. When the drug is given for postoperative hypoperistalsis, observe for bowel sounds, passage of flatus through the rectum, or a bowel movement.	These are indicators of increased GI muscle tone and motility.
b. When bethanechol or neostigmine is given for urinary retention, micturition usually occurs within approximately 60 minutes. If it does not, urinary catheterization may be necessary.	
c. When the drug is given to clients with myasthenia gravis, observe for increased muscle strength as shown by:	
(1) Decreased or absent ptosis of eyelids	With neostigmine, onset of action is 2–4 hours after oral administration and 10–30 minutes after injection. Duration is approximately 3–4 hours. With pyridostigmine, onset of action is approximately 30–45 minutes after oral use, 15 minutes after IM injection, and 2–5 minutes after IV injection. Duration is approximately 4–6 hours. The long-acting form of pyridostigmine lasts 8–12 hours.
(2) Decreased difficulty with chewing, swallowing, and speech	
(3) Increased skeletal muscle strength, increased tolerance of activity, less fatigue	
d. With cholinergic drugs to treat Alzheimer's disease (tacrine, donepezil, galantamine, and rivastigmine) observe for improvement in memory and cognitive functioning in activities of daily living.	Improved functioning is most likely to occur in patients with mild to moderate dementia.
3. Observe for adverse effects	Adverse effects occur with usual therapeutic doses but are more likely with large doses. They are caused by stimulation of the parasympathetic nervous system.
a. Central nervous system effects—convulsions, dizziness, drowsiness, headache, loss of consciousness	
b. Respiratory effects—increased secretions, bronchospasm, laryngospasm, respiratory failure	
c. Cardiovascular effects—dysrhythmias (bradycardia, tachycardia, atrioventricular block), cardiac arrest, hypotension, syncope	These may be detected early by regular assessment of blood pressure and heart rate. Bradycardia is probably the most likely dysrhythmia to occur.
d. GI effects—nausea and vomiting, diarrhea, increased peristalsis, abdominal cramping, increased secretions (ie, saliva, gastric and intestinal secretions). With tacrine, observe for signs of hepatotoxicity (eg, jaundice, elevated liver enzymes).	GI effects commonly occur. Tacrine may be hepatotoxic.
e. Other effects—increased frequency and urgency of urination, increased sweating, miosis, skin rash	Skin rashes are most likely to occur from formulations of neostigmine or pyridostigmine that contain bromide.
4. Observe for drug interactions	
a. Drugs that *increase* effects of direct-acting cholinergics such as bethanechol:	
(1) Other cholinergic drugs	Have additive cholinergic effect
(2) Cholinesterase inhibitors	Prevent degradation of cholinesterase and prolong cholinergic response

NURSING ACTIONS	RATIONALE/EXPLANATION
b. Drugs that *decrease* effects of cholinergic agents:	
(1) Anticholinergic drugs (eg, atropine)	Antagonize effects of cholinergic drugs (miosis; increased tone and motility in smooth muscle of GI tract, bronchi, and urinary bladder; bradycardia). Atropine is the specific antidote for overdosage with cholinergic drugs.
(2) Antihistamines	Most antihistamines have anticholinergic properties that antagonize effects of cholinergic drugs.
c. Drugs that *decrease* effects of anticholinesterase agents:	
(1) Corticosteroids	May antagonize anticholinesterase agents and increase muscle weakness in myasthenia gravis. However, corticosteroids are often prescribed for their anti-immune effect.
(2) Aminoglycoside antibiotics (eg, gentamicin)	Can produce neuromuscular blockade that antagonizes effects of anticholinesterase drugs and causes muscle weakness in myasthenia gravis
(3) Succinylcholine	Increased and prolonged neuromuscular blockade occurs when indirect-acting cholinergics and succinylcholine are given concurrently.
d. Drug that *increases* effects of tacrine:	
(1) Cimetidine	Slows metabolism of tacrine in the liver, thereby increasing risks of accumulation and adverse effects

APPLYING YOUR KNOWLEDGE: ANSWERS

19-1 You should do as the client requests regarding her medication dosage. Many clients with myasthenia gravis require a higher dose of their medication with physical activity. Ms. Humbarger is not as active in the hospital.

19-2 Ms. Humbarger is experiencing a myasthenic crisis. Signs and symptoms having onset within approximately 1 hour after a dose of an anticholinesterase drug are more likely to be caused by cholinergic crisis (too much drug). Signs and symptoms beginning 3 hours or more after a drug dose are more likely to be caused by myasthenic crisis (too little drug). Ms. Humbarger received her medication 4 hours ago. You should respond to myasthenic crisis by administering more anticholinesterase drug.

Review and Application Exercises

Short Answer Exercises

1. What are the actions of cholinergic drugs?

2. Which neurotransmitter is involved in cholinergic (parasympathetic) stimulation?

3. When a cholinergic drug is given to treat myasthenia gravis, what is the expected effect?

4. What is the difference between cholinergic crisis and myasthenic crisis? How are they treated?

5. When indirect-acting cholinergic drugs are used to treat Alzheimer's disease, what is the desired effect?

6. Is a cholinergic drug the usual treatment of choice for urinary bladder atony? Why or why not?

7. What are the adverse effects of cholinergic drugs?

8. How are overdoses of cholinergic drugs treated?

NCLEX-Style Questions

9. A client with myasthenia gravis is admitted to the emergency department with complaints of muscle weakness and respiratory distress. A test dose of edrophonium (Tensilon) is given and the client ceases to breathe, requiring mechanical ventilation. The results of this test indicate
   a. The client is underdosed on his medications and is in myasthenic crisis.

b. The client is allergic to edrophonium and is having an anaphylactic reaction.

c. The client is overdosed on his medications and is in cholinergic crisis.

d. The client's condition is not due to myasthenia gravis because edrophonium did not improve the symptoms.

10. A 65-year-old client has been admitted with a diagnosis of benign prostatic hyperplasia. How should the nurse respond to an order for bethanechol (Urecholine) to treat urinary retention in this situation?

a. Give the medication as ordered.

b. Insert a foley catheter before administering the medication.

c. Provide a urinal because urinary frequency will increase after drug administration.

d. Question this order because the client's urinary retention is due to an obstructive process.

11. The nurse should be prepared to administer which of the following drugs as an antidote to cholinergic drug overdose?

a. epinephrine (Adrenalin)

b. diphenhydramine (Benadryl)

c. atropine (AtroPen)

d. propanolol (Inderal)

12. You are teaching family members how to administer galantamine for Alzheimer's disease. Your instructions should include

a. Take this medication with food.

b. Take this medication on an empty stomach.

c. Take this medication at bedtime.

d. Take this medication at the start of each day.

13. When treating a client in cholinergic crisis due to exposure to an organophosphate insecticide, the nurse must be prepared to administer which drug to relieve neuromuscular blockade?

a. atropine (AtroPen)

b. pralidoxime (Protopam)

c. epinephrine (Adrenalin)

d. physostigmine (Antilirium)

Selected References

American Academy of Neurology. (2001). *Practice guidelines.* Retrieved August 31, 2005, from www.aan.com/professionals/practice/guidelines.cfm

Brown, J. H., & Taylor, P. (2001). Muscarinic receptor agonists and antagonists. In J. G. Hardman & L. E. Limbird (Eds.), *Goodman and Gilman's The pharmacological basis of therapeutics* (10th ed., pp. 155–173). New York: McGraw-Hill.

Drug facts and comparisons. (Updated monthly). St. Louis: Facts and Comparisons.

Karch, A. M. (2005). *2006 Lippincott's nursing drug guide.* Philadelphia: Lippincott Williams & Wilkins.

Lehmann, C. (2003). ADHD symptoms respond to cholinergic drugs. *Psychiatric News, 38*(22), 25.

Myasthenia Gravis Foundation of America. (2001). *Emergency management of myasthenia gravis.* Retrieved August 31, 2005, from http://www.myasthenia.org/information/EmergencyMgmt.htm

Myasthenia Gravis Foundation of America. (2001). *Facts about autoimmune myasthenia gravis for patients and families.* Retrieved August 31, 2005, from http://www.myasthenia.org/information/EmergencyMgmt.htm

National Institute on Aging. (2002). *Medications fact sheet, Alzheimer's Disease Education & Referral Center.* Retrieved August 31, 2005, from http://www.alzheimers.org/pubs/medications.htm

Olson, K. R. (Ed.). (1999). *Poisoning and drug overdose* (3rd ed.). Stamford, CT: Appleton & Lange.

Pappano, A. J. (2001). Cholinoceptor-activating and cholinesterase-inhibiting drugs. In B. G. Katzung (Ed.)., *Basic and clinical pharmacology* (8th ed., pp. 92–106). New York: McGraw-Hill.

Taylor, P. (2001). Anticholinesterase agents. In J. G. Hardman & L. E. Limbird (Eds.), *Goodman and Gilman's The pharmacological basis of therapeutics* (10th ed., pp. 175–191). New York: McGraw-Hill.

Anticholinergic Drugs

OBJECTIVES

After studying this chapter, you will be able to:

1. List characteristics of anticholinergic drugs in terms of effects on body tissues, indications for use, nursing process implications, observation of client response, and teaching clients.
2. Discuss atropine as the prototype of anticholinergic drugs.
3. Discuss clinical disorders or symptoms for which anticholinergic drugs are used.
4. Describe the mechanism by which atropine relieves bradycardia.
5. Review anticholinergic effects of antipsychotics, tricyclic antidepressants, and antihistamines.
6. Discuss principles of therapy and nursing process for using anticholinergic drugs in special populations.
7. Describe the signs and symptoms of atropine or anticholinergic drug overdose and its treatment.
8. Teach clients about the safe, effective use of anticholinergic drugs.

APPLYING YOUR KNOWLEDGE

Glen Downes is a 77-year-old male who has chronic obstructive pulmonary disease and experiences a syncopal episode. He is admitted to your unit with stable vital signs. The physician orders ipratropium two puffs four times a day and places Mr. Downes on a cardiac monitor.

INTRODUCTION

Anticholinergic drugs block the action of acetylcholine on the parasympathetic nervous system. Most anticholinergic drugs interact with muscarinic cholinergic receptors in the brain, secretory glands, heart, and smooth muscle and are sometimes called *antimuscarinic drugs.* When given at high doses, a few anticholinergic drugs are also able to block nicotinic receptors in autonomic ganglia and skeletal muscles. Glycopyrrolate is an example of such a medication. This drug class includes belladonna alkaloids and their derivatives, such as atropine, and many synthetic substitutes.

Most anticholinergic medications are either tertiary amines or quaternary amines (Table 20-1). *Tertiary amines* are uncharged lipid-soluble molecules. Atropine and scopolamine are tertiary amines and therefore are able to cross cell membranes readily. They are well absorbed from the gastrointestinal (GI) tract and conjunctiva, and they cross the blood–brain barrier. Tertiary amines are excreted in the urine.

Some belladonna derivatives and synthetic anticholinergics are *quaternary amines.* These drugs carry a positive charge and are lipid insoluble. Consequently, they do not readily cross cell membranes. They are poorly absorbed from the GI tract and do not cross the blood–brain barrier. Quaternary amines are excreted largely in the feces.

GENERAL CHARACTERISTICS OF ANTICHOLINERGIC DRUGS

Mechanism of Action and Effects

These drugs act by occupying receptor sites on target organs innervated by the parasympathetic nervous system, thereby leaving fewer receptor sites free to respond to acetylcholine (Fig. 20-1). Parasympathetic response is absent or decreased, depending on the number of receptors blocked by anticholinergic drugs and the underlying degree of parasympathetic activity. Because cholinergic muscarinic receptors are widely

TABLE 20-1 Common Tertiary Amine and Quaternary Amine Anticholinergic Drugs

TERTIARY AMINES	QUATERNARY AMINES
Atropine	Glycopyrrolate (Robinul)
Benztropine (Cogentin)	Ipratropium (Atrovent)
Biperiden (Akineton)	Mepenzolate (Cantil)
Dicyclomine hydrochloride (Bentyl)	Methscopolamine (Pamine)
Flavoxate (Urispas)	Propantheline bromide (Pro-Banthine)
l-Hyoscyamine (Anaspaz)	Tiotropium (Spiriva)
Oxybutynin (Ditropan)	Trospium chloride (Sanctura)
Procyclidine (Kemadrin)	
Scopolamine	
Tolterodine (Detrol and Detrol LA)	
Trihexyphenidyl (Trihexy)	

distributed in the body, anticholinergic drugs produce effects in a variety of locations, including the central nervous system (CNS), heart, smooth muscle, glands, and the eye.

Specific effects on body tissues and organs include:

- **CNS stimulation followed by depression,** which may result in coma and death. This is most likely to occur with large doses of anticholinergic drugs that cross the blood–brain barrier (atropine, scopolamine, and antiparkinson agents).
- **Decreased cardiovascular response to parasympathetic (vagal) stimulation that slows heart rate.**

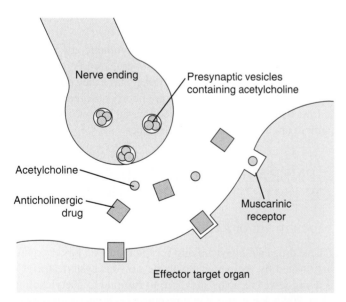

FIGURE 20-1 Mechanism of action of anticholinergic drugs. Anticholinergic (antimuscarinic) drugs prevent acetylcholine from interacting with muscarinic receptors on target effector organs, thus blocking or decreasing a parasympathetic response in these organs.

Atropine is the anticholinergic drug most often used for its cardiovascular effects. According to Advanced Cardiac Life Support (ACLS) protocol, atropine is the drug of choice to treat symptomatic sinus bradycardia. Low doses (<0.5 mg) may produce a slight and temporary decrease in heart rate; however, moderate to large doses (0.5–1 mg) increase heart rate by blocking parasympathetic vagal stimulation. Although the increase in heart rate may be therapeutic in bradycardia, it can be an adverse effect in clients with other types of heart disease because atropine increases the myocardial oxygen demand. Atropine usually has little or no effect on blood pressure. Large doses cause facial flushing because of dilation of blood vessels in the neck.

- **Bronchodilation and decreased respiratory-tract secretions.** Anticholinergics block the action of acetylcholine in bronchial smooth muscle when given by inhalation. This action reduces intracellular GMP, a bronchoconstrictive substance. When anticholinergic drugs are given systemically, respiratory secretions decrease and may become viscous, resulting in mucous plugging of small respiratory passages. Administering the medications by inhalation decreases this effect while preserving the beneficial bronchodilation effect.
- **Antispasmodic effects in the GI tract due to decreased muscle tone and motility.** The drugs have little inhibitory effect on gastric acid secretion with usual doses and insignificant effects on pancreatic and intestinal secretions.
- **Mydriasis and cycloplegia in the eye.** Normally, anticholinergics do not change intraocular pressure, but with narrow-angle glaucoma, they may increase intraocular pressure and precipitate an episode of acute glaucoma. When the pupil is fully dilated, photophobia may be uncomfortable, and reflexes to light and accommodation may disappear.
- **Miscellaneous effects** include decreased secretions from salivary and sweat glands; relaxation of ureters, urinary bladder, and the detrusor muscle; and relaxation of smooth muscle in the gallbladder and bile ducts.

The clinical usefulness of anticholinergic drugs is limited by their widespread effects. Consequently, several synthetic drugs have been developed in an effort to increase selectivity of action on particular body tissues, especially to retain the antispasmodic and antisecretory effects of atropine while eliminating its adverse effects. This effort has been less than successful—all the synthetic drugs produce atropine-like adverse effects when given in sufficient dosage.

One group of synthetic drugs is used for antispasmodic effects in GI disorders. Another group of synthetic drugs includes centrally active anticholinergics used in the treatment of Parkinson's disease (see Chap. 12). They balance the relative cholinergic dominance that causes the movement disorders associated with parkinsonism.

Indications for Use

Anticholinergic drugs are used for disorders in many body systems. Clinical indications include the following:

- **GI disorders.** Anticholinergics have been used for peptic ulcer disease, gastritis, pylorospasm, and diverticulitis. These conditions are often characterized by excessive gastric acid and abdominal pain because of increased motility and spasm of GI smooth muscle. However, anticholinergics are weak inhibitors of gastric acid secretion, even in maximal doses that usually produce intolerable adverse effects, making them a second choice for treatment of peptic ulcers. Although the drugs do not heal peptic ulcers, they may relieve abdominal pain by relaxing GI smooth muscle. In addition, anticholinergics may be helpful in reducing the frequency of bowel movements and abdominal discomfort associated with irritable colon or colitis. Anticholinergics are not usually prescribed for chronic inflammatory disorders (eg, diverticulitis, ulcerative colitis) or acute intestinal infections (eg, bacterial, viral, amebic). Other drugs are more useful in treating the diarrhea and increased intestinal motility that occurs in these conditions.
- **Genitourinary disorders.** Anticholinergic drugs may be given for their antispasmodic effects on smooth muscle to relieve the symptoms of urinary incontinence and frequency that accompany an overactive bladder. In infections such as cystitis, urethritis, and prostatitis, the drugs decrease the frequency and pain of urination. The drugs are also given to increase bladder capacity in enuresis, paraplegia, or neurogenic bladder.
- **Ophthalmology.** Anticholinergic drugs are applied topically for mydriatic and cycloplegic effects to aid examination or surgery. They are also used to treat some inflammatory disorders. Anticholinergic preparations used in ophthalmology are discussed further in Chapter 63.
- **Respiratory disorders** characterized by bronchoconstriction (ie, asthma, chronic bronchitis). Ipratropium or tiotropium bromide may be given by inhalation for bronchodilating effects (see Chap. 44).
- **Cardiac disorders.** Atropine may be given to increase heart rate in bradycardia and heart block characterized by hypotension and shock.
- **Parkinson's disease.** Anticholinergic drugs are given for their central effects in decreasing salivation, spasticity, and tremors. They are used mainly in clients who have minimal symptoms, who do not respond to levodopa, or who cannot tolerate levodopa because of adverse reactions or contraindications. An additional use of anticholinergic drugs is to relieve parkinson-like symptoms that occur with older antipsychotic drugs.
- **Preoperative use.** Anticholinergics are given to prevent vagal stimulation and potential bradycardia, hypotension, and cardiac arrest. They are also given to reduce respiratory tract secretions, especially in head and neck surgery and bronchoscopy.
- **Anticholinesterase toxicity, mushroom poisoning, or organophosphate pesticide poisoning** (see Chap. 19). Atropine is given to treat excessive cholinergic stimulation.

Contraindications to Use

Contraindications to the use of anticholinergic drugs include any condition characterized by symptoms that would be aggravated by the drugs. Some of these are prostatic hypertrophy, myasthenia gravis, hyperthyroidism, glaucoma, tachydysrhythmias, myocardial infarction, and heart failure unless bradycardia is present. Anticholinergic drugs should not be given in hiatal hernia or other conditions contributing to reflux esophagitis because the drugs delay gastric emptying, relax the cardioesophageal sphincter, and increase esophageal reflux.

INDIVIDUAL DRUGS

The therapeutic uses, dosages, and routes of administration for selected anticholinergic drugs are presented in Table 20-2.

Belladonna Alkaloids and Derivatives

🅿 **Atropine,** the prototype of anticholinergic drugs, is a naturally occurring belladonna alkaloid that can be extracted from the belladonna plant or prepared synthetically. It is usually prepared as atropine sulfate, a salt that is very soluble in water. It is well absorbed from the GI tract and distributed throughout the body. It crosses the blood–brain barrier to enter the CNS, where large doses produce stimulant effects and toxic doses produce depressant effects. Atropine is also absorbed systemically when applied locally to mucous membranes. The drug is rapidly excreted in the urine. Pharmacologic effects are of short duration except for ocular effects, which may last for several days.

Belladonna tincture is a mixture of alkaloids in an aqueous–alcohol solution. It is most often used in GI disorders because of its antispasmodic effect. It is an ingredient in several drug mixtures.

Homatropine hydrobromide is a semisynthetic derivative of atropine used as eye drops to produce mydriasis and cycloplegia. Compared with atropine, homatropine may be preferable, because ocular effects do not last as long.

Hyoscyamine (Anaspaz) is a belladonna alkaloid used in GI and genitourinary disorders characterized by spasm, increased secretion, and increased motility. It has the same effects as other atropine-like drugs.

Ipratropium (Atrovent) is an anticholinergic drug chemically related to atropine. When given as a nasal spray, it is useful in treating rhinorrhea due to allergy or the common cold.

(text continues on page 324)

Table 20-2 Drugs at a Glance: Selected Anticholinergic Drugs

GENERIC/TRADE NAME	USE	ROUTES AND DOSAGE RANGES	
		Adults	**Children**
Belladonna Alkaloids and Derivatives			
Atropine	Systemic use	PO, IM, Sub-Q, IV 0.4–0.6 mg	PO, IM, Sub-Q, IV: 7–16 lb: 0.1 mg 16–24 lb: 0.15 mg 24–40 lb: 0.2 mg 40–65 lb: 0.3 mg 65–90 lb: 0.4 mg >90 lb: 0.4–0.6 mg
	Surgery	IM, Sub-Q, or IV 0.4–0.6 mg prior to induction. Use 0.4-mg dose with cyclopropane anesthesia.	0.1 mg (newborn) to 0.6 mg (12 y) given Sub-Q 30 min prior to surgery
	Bradyarrhythmias	IV 0.4–1 mg (up to 2 mg) q1–2h PRN	
	Antidote for cholinergic poisoning	IV Titrate large doses of 2–3 mg as needed until signs of atropine toxicity appear and cholinergic crisis is controlled.	
Ophthalmic atropine (Isopto-Atropine)	Mydriatic/cycloplegia/ inflammation of uveal tract	*For refraction:* Instill 1 or 2 drops of 1% solution into eye(s) 1 h before refraction. *For uveitis:* Instill 1–2 drops of 1% solution into eye(s) 4 times daily.	*For refraction:* Instill 1–2 drops of 0.5% solution twice daily for 1–3 d before procedure.
Homatropine (Isopto-Homatropine)	Mydriatic/cycloplegia/ inflammation of uveal tract	*For refraction:* Instill 1–2 drops of 2% solution or 1 drop of 5% solution into eye before procedure. May repeat at 5–10 min intervals as needed. *For uveitis:* Instill 1 or 2 drops of 2% or 5% solution 2–4 times daily or every 3–4 h as needed.	*For refraction:* Instill 1 drop of 2% solution into eye before procedure. May repeat q 10 min as needed. *For uveitis:* Instill 1 drop of 2% solution 2–4 times daily
Hyoscyamine (Anaspaz)	Antispasmodic/anti-secretory for gastro-intestinal (GI) and genitourinary (GU) disorders	PO, SL 0.125–0.25 mg 3 or 4 times daily before meals and at bedtime. PO (timed-release formula): 0.375–0.75 q12h. IM, IV, Sub-Q: 0.25–0.5 mg q6h	*Children 2–10 y:* PO 0.062–0.125 mg q 6–8h. *Children <2 y:* half of the previous dose
Ipratropium (Atrovent)	Bronchodilation	2 puffs (36 mcg) of aerosol 4 times daily. Additional inhalations may be needed. Do not exceed 12 puffs/24h. Solution for inhalation: 500 mcg, 3 or 4 times daily.	
	Nasal spray for rhinorrhea	2 sprays/nostril of 0.03% spray 2 or 3 times daily. 2 sprays/nostril of 0.06% spray 3–4 times daily.	2 sprays/nostril of 0.03% spray 2 or 3 times daily
Scopolamine	Systemic use	PO 0.4–0.8 mg daily. Sub-Q, IM 0.32–0.65 mg IV 0.32–0.65 mg diluted in sterile water for injection	Not approved for PO use <6 y *Parenteral:* 0.006 mg/kg *Maximum dose:* 0.3 mg
	Antiemetic	*Transdermal:* Apply disk 4 h before antiemetic effect is needed. Replace q3d.	Not approved in children

Table 20-2   Drugs at a Glance: Selected Anticholinergic Drugs (continued)

GENERIC/TRADE NAME	USE	ROUTES AND DOSAGE RANGES	
		Adults	**Children**
	Mydriatic/cycloplegia/ inflammation of uveal tract	*For refraction:* Instill 1 or 2 drops into eye 1 h before refracting. *For uveitis:* Instill 1 or 2 drops into eye(s) up to 3 times daily.	Same as adult dose
Tiotropium bromide (Spiriva)	Bronchodilation	Inhalation of contents of one capsule (18mcg) daily using the HandiHaler inhalation device	Safety and efficacy not established
Antisecretory/Antispasmodic Anticholinergics for Gastrointestinal Disorders			
Dicyclomine hydrochloride (Bentyl)	Antisecretory/ antispasmodic	PO 20–40 mg before meals and at bedtime IM 20 mg before meals and at bedtime	
Glycopyrrolate (Robinul)	Antisecretory/ antispasmodic Preanesthetic	PO 1–2 mg 2 or 3 times daily IM, IV 0.1–0.2 mg IM 0.004 mg/kg 30–60 min before anesthesia	*< 12 y:* Not recommended *<2 y:* 0.004 mg/lb IM 30–60 min before anesthesia *2–12 y:* 0.002–0.004 mg/lb IM 30–60 min before anesthesia
Mepenzolate	Antisecretory/ antispasmodic	PO 25–50 mg 4 times daily before meals and at bedtime	
Propantheline bromide (Pro-Banthine)	Antisecretory/ antispasmodic	PO 7.5–15 mg 30 min before meals and at bedtime	
Anticholinergics Used in Parkinson's Disease			
Benztropine (Cogentin)	Parkinsonism	PO, IM, IV 0.5–1 mg at bedtime. May increase up to 6 mg given at bedtime or in 2–4 divided doses.	
	Drug-induced extrapyramidal symptoms	*For acute dystonia: IM, IV* 1–2 mg. May repeat if needed. For prevention: PO 1–2 mg.	
Biperiden (Akineton)	Parkinsonism	PO 2 mg 3 or 4 times daily. Maximum dose 16 mg/d.	
	Drug-induced extrapyramidal symptoms	PO 2 mg 3 or 4 times daily	
Procyclidine (Kemadrin)	Parkinsonism	PO 2.5 mg 3 times daily after meals. May increase to 5 mg 3 times daily after meals.	
	Drug-induced extrapyramidal symptoms	PO 2.5 mg 3 times daily. Increase by 2.5-mg increments until symptoms are resolved. Usual maximum dose 10–20 mg daily.	
Trihexyphenidyl (Trihexy)	Parkinsonism	PO 1–2 mg. Increase by 2-mg increments at 3- to 5-d intervals until a total of 6–10 mg is given daily in divided doses 3–4 times daily at mealtimes and bedtimes.	

(continued)

Table 20-2 Drugs at a Glance: Selected Anticholinergic Drugs (continued)

GENERIC/TRADE NAME	USE	ROUTES AND DOSAGE RANGES	
		Adults	**Children**
	Drug-induced extrapyramidal symptoms	PO 1 mg initially. Increase as needed to control symptoms.	
Urinary Antispasmodics **Flavoxate** (Urispas)	Overactive bladder	PO 100–200 mg 3 or 4 times daily. Reduce when symptoms improve.	*<12 y:* Safety and efficacy not established
Oxybutynin (Ditropan and Ditropan XL)	Overactive bladder	PO 5 mg 2 or 3 times daily. Maximum dose 5 mg 4 times daily. *Extended-release* 5 mg PO daily up to 30 mg/daily.	*>5 y:* 5 mg PO twice daily. Maximum dose 5 mg 3 times daily
Tolterodine (Detrol and Detrol LA)	Overactive bladder	PO 2 mg twice daily. May decrease to 1 mg when symptoms improve. Reduce doses to 1 mg PO twice daily in presence of hepatic impairment.	Safety and efficacy not established
Trospium chloride (Sanctura)	Overactive bladder	PO 20 mg twice daily at least 1 h before meals or on an empty stomach	Safety and efficacy not established

IM, intramuscular; IV, intravenous; PO, oral; PRN, as needed; SL, sublingual; Sub-Q, subcutaneous.

When given as an inhalation treatment or aerosol to clients with chronic obstructive pulmonary disease (COPD), it is beneficial as a bronchodilator. An advantage of administration of anticholinergic drugs by the respiratory route over the systemic route is less thickening of respiratory secretions and therefore a reduced incidence of mucus-plugged airways.

Scopolamine is similar to atropine in terms of uses, adverse effects, and peripheral effects, but different in central effects. When it is given parenterally, scopolamine depresses the CNS and causes amnesia, drowsiness, euphoria, relaxation, and sleep. Effects of the drug appear more quickly and disappear more readily than those of atropine. Scopolamine also is used in motion sickness. It is available as oral tablets and as a transdermal adhesive disk that is placed behind the ear. The disk (Transderm-V) protects against motion sickness for 72 hours.

Tiotropium bromide (Spiriva HandiHaler) is a dry powder in capsule form intended for oral inhalation with the HandiHaler inhalation device. This long-acting, antimuscarinic, anticholinergic, quaternary ammonium compound inhibits M_3 receptors in smooth muscle, resulting in bronchodilation. Tiotropium is indicated for daily maintenance treatment of bronchospasm associated with COPD. It is not indicated for acute episodes of bronchospasm (ie, rescue therapy). Tiotropium is eliminated via the renal system, and clients with moderate to severe renal dysfunction should be carefully monitored for drug toxicity. No dosage adjustments are required for older clients or clients with hepatic impairment or mild renal impairment.

Antisecretory/Antispasmodic Anticholinergics Used in Gastrointestinal Disorders

Dicyclomine, glycopyrrolate, mepenzolate, and propantheline are older medications, previously commonly used to treat peptic ulcer disease. With the introduction of medications such as proton pump inhibitors and other drugs that more effectively treat hyperacidity with fewer adverse effects (see Chap. 59), anticholinergics are infrequently prescribed today.

Dicyclomine is also useful as an antispasmodic agent for treatment of irritable bowel syndrome.

Centrally Acting Anticholinergics Used in Parkinson's Disease

Older anticholinergic drugs such as atropine are rarely used to treat Parkinson's disease because of their undesirable peripheral effects (eg, dry mouth, blurred vision, photophobia, constipation, urinary retention, tachycardia). Newer, centrally acting synthetic anticholinergic drugs are more selective for muscarinic receptors in the CNS and are designed to produce fewer adverse effects.

Trihexyphenidyl (Trihexy) is used in the treatment of parkinsonism and extrapyramidal reactions caused by some antipsychotic drugs. Trihexyphenidyl relieves smooth muscle spasm by a direct action on the muscle and by inhibiting the parasympathetic nervous system. The drug supposedly has fewer adverse effects than atropine, but approximately half the recipients report mouth dryness, blurring of vision, and other adverse effects common to anticholinergic drugs. Trihexyphenidyl requires the same precautions as other anticholinergic drugs and is contraindicated in glaucoma. **Biperiden** (Akineton) and **procyclidine** (Kemadrin) are chemical derivatives of trihexyphenidyl and have similar actions.

Benztropine (Cogentin) is a synthetic drug with both anticholinergic and antihistaminic effects. Its anticholinergic activity approximates that of atropine. A major clinical use is to treat acute dystonic reactions caused by antipsychotic drugs, and to prevent their recurrence in clients receiving long-term antipsychotic drug therapy. It also may be given in small doses to supplement other antiparkinson drugs. In full dosage, adverse reactions are common.

Urinary Antispasmodics

Flavoxate (Urispas) was developed specifically to counteract spasm in smooth muscle tissue of the urinary tract. It has anticholinergic, local anesthetic, and analgesic effects. Thus, the drug relieves dysuria, urgency, frequency, and pain with genitourinary infections, such as cystitis and prostatitis.

Oxybutynin (Ditropan and Ditropan XL) has direct antispasmodic effects on smooth muscle and anticholinergic effects. It increases bladder capacity and decreases frequency of voiding in clients with neurogenic bladder. Oxybutynin is now available in an extended-release form for once-daily dosing.

Tolterodine (Detrol and Detrol LA) is a competitive antimuscarinic, anticholinergic agent that inhibits bladder contraction, decreases detrusor muscle pressure, and delays the urge to void. It is used to treat urinary frequency, urgency, and urge incontinence. Tolterodine is more selective for muscarinic receptors in the urinary bladder than in other areas of the body, such as the salivary glands, and therefore anticholinergic adverse effects are less marked. Reduced doses (1 mg) are recommended for clients with hepatic dysfunction. Tolterodine is also available in an extended-release form.

Trospium chloride (Sanctura) is a newer antimuscarinic, anticholinergic drug for treatment of urgency, urge incontinence, and urinary frequency associated with overactive bladder. Trospium reduces the tone of smooth muscle in the bladder, exerting an antispasmodic effect. Because of its quaternary structure, less than 10% of an orally administered dose is absorbed, and food further delays absorption. Therefore, it is recommended that the medication be taken at least 1 hour before meals or on an empty stomach. Absorbed trospium is eliminated by a combination of glomerular filtration and active tubular secretion. Trospium has the potential for interaction with other drugs that are eliminated by active tubular secretion

(eg, digoxin, procainamide, pancuronium, morphine, vancomycin, metformin, tenofovir), resulting in increased serum concentration of either trospium or the co-administered drug because of competition for the urinary tubular pump. Reduced dosages of trospium are recommended for clients with renal insufficiency and those older than 75 years of age who may be less able to tolerate the adverse effects of anticholinergic drugs.

NURSING PROCESS

Assessment

● Assess the client's condition in relation to disorders for which anticholinergic drugs are used (ie, check for bradycardia or heart block, diarrhea, dysuria, abdominal pain, and other disorders). If the client reports or medical records indicate a specific disorder, assess for signs and symptoms of that disorder (eg, Parkinson's disease).
● Assess for disorders in which anticholinergic drugs are contraindicated (eg, glaucoma, prostatic hypertrophy, reflux esophagitis, myasthenia gravis, hyperthyroidism).
● Assess use of other drugs with anticholinergic effects, such as antihistamines (histamine$_1$ receptor antagonists [see Chap. 45]), antipsychotic agents, and tricyclic antidepressants.

Nursing Diagnoses

● Impaired Urinary Elimination: Decreased bladder tone and urine retention
● Constipation related to slowed GI function
● Disturbed Thought Processes: Confusion, disorientation, especially in older adults
● Deficient Knowledge: Drug effects and accurate usage
● Risk for Injury related to drug-induced blurred vision and photophobia
● Risk for Noncompliance related to adverse drug effects
● Risk for Altered Body Temperature: Hyperthermia

Planning/Goals

The client will
● Receive or self-administer the drugs correctly
● Experience relief of symptoms for which anticholinergic drugs are given
● Be assisted to avoid or cope with adverse drug effects on vision, thought processes, bowel and bladder elimination, and heat dissipation

Interventions

Use measures to decrease the need for anticholinergic drugs. For example, with peptic ulcer disease, teach the client to avoid factors known to increase gastric secretion and GI motility (alcohol; cigarette smoking; caffeine-containing beverages, such as coffee, tea, and cola drinks;

ulcerogenic drugs, such as aspirin). Late evening snacks also should be avoided because increased gastric acid secretion occurs approximately 90 minutes after eating and may cause pain and awakening from sleep. Although milk was previously considered an "ulcer food," it contains protein and calcium, which promote acid secretion, and is a poor buffer of gastric acid. Thus, drinking large amounts of milk should be avoided.

Client Teaching Guidelines for Anticholinergic Drugs are presented in the accompanying display.

Evaluation

- Interview and observe in relation to safe, accurate drug administration.
- Interview and observe for relief of symptoms for which the drugs are given.
- Interview and observe for adverse drug effects.

PRINCIPLES OF THERAPY

Treatment of Specific Disorders

Renal or Biliary Colic

Atropine is sometimes given with morphine or meperidine to relieve the severe pain of renal or biliary colic. It acts mainly to decrease the spasm-producing effects of the opioid analgesics. It has little antispasmodic effect on the involved muscles and is not used alone for this purpose.

CLIENT TEACHING GUIDELINES
Anticholinergic Drugs

General Considerations

- Do not take other drugs without the physician's knowledge. In addition to some prescribed antiparkinson drugs, antidepressants, antihistamines, and antipsychotic drugs with anticholinergic properties, over-the-counter sleeping pills and antihistamines have anticholinergic effects. Taking any of these concurrently could cause overdosage or excessive anticholinergic effects.
- Use measures to minimize risks of heat exhaustion and heat stroke:
  - Wear light, cool clothing in warm climates or environments.
  - Maintain fluid and salt intake if not contraindicated.
  - Limit exposure to direct sunlight.
  - Limit physical activity.
  - Take frequent cool baths.
  - Ensure adequate ventilation, with fans or air conditioners if necessary.
  - Avoid alcoholic beverages.
- Use sugarless chewing gum and hard candy, if not contraindicated, to relieve mouth dryness.
- Carry out good dental hygiene practices (eg, regular brushing of teeth) to prevent dental caries and loss of teeth that may result from drug-induced xerostomia (dry mouth from decreased saliva production). This is more likely to occur with long-term use of these drugs.
- To prevent injury due to blurring of vision or drowsiness, avoid potentially hazardous activities (eg, driving or operating machinery).
- To reduce sensitivity to light (photophobia), dark glasses can be worn outdoors in strong light.

- If you wear contact lenses and experience dry eyes, use an ophthalmic lubricating solution.
- When using anticholinergic ophthalmic preparations, if eye pain occurs, stop using the medication and contact your physician or health care provider. This may be a warning sign of undiagnosed glaucoma.
- Notify your physician or health care provider if urinary retention or constipation occurs.
- Tell your physician or health care provider if you are pregnant or breast-feeding or allergic to sulfite preservatives or any other atropine compound.

Self-Administration

- Take anticholinergic drugs for gastrointestinal disorders 30 minutes before meals and at bedtime.
- Safeguard anticholinergic medications from children because they are especially sensitive to atropine poisoning.
- To prevent constipation, eat a diet high in fiber. Include whole grains, fruits, and vegetables in your daily menu. Also, drink 2 to 3 quarts of fluid a day and exercise regularly.
- Take trospium at least 1 hour before meals or on an empty stomach.
- To take tiotropium, follow the manufacturer's guidelines for using the HandiHaler to self-administer the drug by inhalation. Place a capsule into the center of the HandiHaler inhalation device. Pierce the capsule by pressing and releasing the button on the side of the inhalation device. Inhale through the mouthpiece to disperse the drug. **Do not** swallow tiotropium capsules. Avoid allowing tiotropium powder to enter the eyes.

Overactive Urinary Bladder

Urinary antispasmodics are useful in relieving the urgency, frequency, and urge incontinence associated with overactive bladder. Although these medications are formulated to be more selective for the muscarinic receptors in the smooth muscle of the urinary bladder, unwanted anticholinergic effects such as dry mouth, constipation, and mydriasis may occur.

Preoperative Use in Clients With Glaucoma

Glaucoma is usually listed as a contraindication to anticholinergic drugs because the drugs impair outflow of aqueous humor and may cause an acute attack of glaucoma (increased intraocular pressure). However, anticholinergic drugs can be given safely before surgery to clients with open-angle glaucoma (80% of clients with primary glaucoma) if they are receiving miotic drugs such as pilocarpine. If anticholinergic preoperative medication is needed in clients predisposed to angle closure, the hazard of causing acute glaucoma can be minimized by also giving pilocarpine eye drops and acetazolamide.

Gastrointestinal Disorders

In peptic ulcer disease, more effective drugs have been developed, and anticholinergics are rarely used. When anticholinergic drugs are given for GI disorders, larger doses may be given at bedtime to prevent pain and awakening during sleep.

Parkinson's Disease

When anticholinergic drugs are used in parkinsonism, small doses are given initially and gradually increased. This regimen decreases adverse reactions.

Extrapyramidal Reactions

When anticholinergic drugs are used in drug-induced extrapyramidal reactions (parkinson-like symptoms), they should be prescribed only if symptoms occur. They should not be used routinely to prevent extrapyramidal reactions, because fewer than half of clients taking antipsychotic drugs experience such reactions. Most drug-induced reactions last approximately 3 months and do not recur if anticholinergic drugs are discontinued at that time. (An exception is tardive dyskinesia, which does not respond to anticholinergic drugs and may be aggravated by them.)

Muscarinic Agonist Poisoning

Atropine is the antidote for poisoning by cholinergic (muscarinic) agonists such as certain species of mushrooms, cholinergic agonist drugs, cholinesterase inhibitor drugs, and insecticides containing organophosphates. Symptoms of muscarinic poisoning include salivation, lacrimation, visual disturbances, bronchospasm, diarrhea, bradycardia, and hypotension. Atropine prevents the poison from interacting with the muscarinic receptor, thus reversing the toxic effects.

Asthma and Other Chronic Obstructive Lung Diseases

Oral anticholinergics are not used to treat asthma and other COPDs because of the possibility of thickened respiratory secretions and formation of mucus plugs in airways. Administration of ipratropium or tiotropium by inhalation causes the beneficial bronchodilating effect.

Toxicity of Anticholinergics: Recognition and Management

Overdose of atropine or other anticholinergic drugs produces the usual pharmacologic effects in a severe and exaggerated form. The anticholinergic overdose syndrome is characterized by hyperthermia; hot, dry, flushed skin; dry mouth; mydriasis; delirium; tachycardia; paralytic ileus; and urinary retention. Myoclonic movements and choreoathetosis may be seen. Seizures, coma, and respiratory arrest may also occur. Treatment involves use of activated charcoal to absorb ingested poison. Hemodialysis, hemoperfusion, peritoneal dialysis, and repeated doses of charcoal are not effective.

Physostigmine salicylate (Antilirium), an acetylcholinesterase inhibitor, is a specific antidote for overdose of anticholinergics. It is usually given intravenously (IV) at a slow rate of injection, because rapid administration may cause bradycardia, hypersalivation (with subsequent respiratory distress), and seizures. The adult dose is 2 milligrams (no more than 1 mg/minute), and the pediatric dose is 0.5 to 1 milligrams (no more than 0.5 mg/minute). Repeated doses may be given if life-threatening dysrhythmias, convulsions, or coma occur with anticholinergic overdose. However, the benefit of repeat dosing must be balanced against the risk of physostigmine overdose. Excessive administration of physostigmine can precipitate a cholinergic crisis, leading to seizures and dysrhythmias. Atropine is the antidote for physostigmine overdose.

Diazepam or a similar drug may be given for excessive CNS stimulation (eg, delirium, excitement) that accompanies anticholinergic toxicity. Ice bags, cooling blankets, and tepid sponge baths may help reduce fever. Artificial ventilation and cardiopulmonary resuscitative measures are used if excessive depression of the CNS causes coma and respiratory failure. Infants, children, and the elderly are especially susceptible to the toxic effects of anticholinergic drugs.

Anticholinergic drugs have potential intoxicating effects. Abuse of these drugs may produce euphoria, disorientation, hallucinations, and paranoia in addition to the classic anticholinergic adverse reactions.

Use in Special Populations

Use in Children

Systemic anticholinergics, including atropine, glycopyrrolate, and scopolamine, are given to children of all ages for essentially the same effects as for adults. Most of the antisecretory, antispasmodic drugs for GI disorders are not recommended for children. With the urinary antispasmodics, flavoxate is not recommended for children younger than 12 years of age; oxybutynin is not recommended for children younger than 5 years of age; and the safety and efficacy of tolterodine and trospium are not established in children. Similarly, the safety and efficacy of ipratropium and tiotropium, which are used for bronchodilation in chronic lung disorders, are not established in children.

Anticholinergic drugs cause the same adverse effects in children as in adults. However, the effects may be more severe in children, who are especially sensitive to these drugs. Facial flushing is common, and skin rashes may occur.

Ophthalmic anticholinergic drugs should be used only with close medical supervision. Cyclopentolate and tropicamide have been associated with behavioral disturbances and psychotic reactions in children. Tropicamide also has been associated with cardiopulmonary collapse.

Use in Older Adults

Anticholinergic drugs are given in older adults for the same purposes as in younger adults. In addition to the primary anticholinergic drugs, many others that are commonly prescribed for older adults have high anticholinergic activity, including many antihistamines (histamine$_1$ receptor antagonists), tricyclic antidepressants, and antipsychotic drugs.

Older adults are especially likely to have significant adverse reactions because of slowed drug metabolism and the frequent presence of several disease processes. Some common adverse effects, with suggestions for reducing their impact, are:

- **Blurred vision.** Clients may need help with ambulation, especially with stairs or in other potentially hazardous environments. Remove obstacles and hazards when possible.
- **Confusion.** Provide whatever assistance is needed to prevent falls and other injuries.
- **Heat stroke.** Help avoid precipitating factors, such as strenuous activity and high environmental temperatures.
- **Constipation.** Encourage or assist with an adequate intake of high-fiber foods and fluids and adequate exercise when feasible.
- **Urinary retention.** Encourage adequate fluid intake and avoid high doses of the drugs. Men should be examined for prostatic hypertrophy.
- **Hallucinations and other psychotic symptoms.** These are most likely to occur with the centrally active anticholinergics given for Parkinson's disease or drug-induced extrapyramidal effects, such as trihexyphenidyl or benztropine. Regulate and supervise dosage of these drugs carefully.

APPLYING YOUR KNOWLEDGE 20-2
Mr. Downes complains about being unable to move his bowels and having difficulty with urination. How do you respond?

Use in Clients With Renal Impairment

Anticholinergic drugs that have a tertiary amine structure, such as atropine, are eliminated by a combination of hepatic metabolism and renal excretion. In the presence of renal impairment, they may accumulate and cause increased adverse effects. Quaternary amines are eliminated largely in the feces and are less affected by renal impairment.

Use in Clients With Hepatic Impairment

Some anticholinergic drugs are metabolized by the liver. Therefore, in the presence of hepatic impairment, they may accumulate and cause adverse effects. Tolterodine is an example of such a medication. Dosages should be reduced and given less frequently in the presence of liver impairment.

Use in Clients With Critical Illness

Atropine is an important drug in the emergency drug box. According to ACLS guidelines, atropine is the first drug to be administered in the emergency treatment of bradydysrhythmias. Atropine 0.5 to 1 milligram should be administered IV every 5 minutes, and may be repeated up to 2 to 3 milligrams (0.03–0.04 mg/kg total dose). For clients with asystole, 1 milligram of atropine is administered IV and repeated every 3 to 5 minutes if asystole persists, up to 0.04 milligrams per kilogram of body weight. Administration of atropine in doses less than 0.5 milligram should be avoided, because this may result in a paradoxical bradycardia. Atropine may be administered by endotracheal tube in clients without IV access. The recommended dose is 2 to 3 milligrams diluted in 10 milliliters of normal saline.

Use in Home Care

Anticholinergic drugs are commonly used in home care with children and adults. Children and older adults are probably most likely to experience adverse effects of these drugs and should be monitored carefully. With older clients, the home care nurse needs to assess medication regimens for combinations of drugs with anticholinergic effects, especially if mental confusion develops or worsens. The home care nurse may also need to teach older clients or caregivers that the drugs prevent sweating and heat loss and increase risks of heat stroke, if precautions to avoid overheating are not taken.

APPLYING YOUR KNOWLEDGE 20-3:
HOW CAN YOU AVOID THIS MEDICATION ERROR?
Mr. Bing is another client of yours on the unit. He is a 50-year-old man with a medical history of cholelithiasis, glaucoma, and hypertension. He has had surgery today to remove his gallbladder. You assess Mr. Bing and find that he is experiencing nausea. The resident on call orders a scopolamine patch. You follow the order and apply the patch.

Anticholinergic Drugs

NURSING ACTIONS	RATIONALE/EXPLANATION

1. Administer accurately

a. For gastrointestinal disorders, give most oral anticholinergic drugs approximately 30 min before meals and at bedtime.

To allow the drugs to reach peak antisecretory effects by the time ingested food is stimulating gastric acid secretion. Bedtime administration helps prevent awakening with abdominal pain.

b. When given before surgery, parenteral preparations of atropine can be mixed in the same syringe with several other common preoperative medications, such as meperidine (Demerol), morphine, oxymorphone (Numorphan), and promethazine (Phenergan).

The primary reason for mixing medications in the same syringe is to decrease the number of injections and thus decrease client discomfort. Note, however, that extra caution is required when mixing drugs to be sure that the dosage of each drug is accurate. Also, if any question exists regarding compatibility with another drug, it is safer not to mix the drugs, even if two or three injections are required.

c. When applying topical atropine solutions or ointment to the eye, be sure to use the correct concentration and blot any excess from the inner canthus.

Atropine ophthalmic preparations are available in several concentrations (usually 1%, 2%, and 3%). Excess medication should be removed so the drug will not enter the nasolacrimal (tear) ducts and be absorbed systemically through the mucous membrane of the nasopharynx or be carried to the throat and swallowed.

d. If propantheline is to be given intravenously, dissolve the 30-mg dose of powder in no less than 10 mL of sterile water for injection.

Parenteral administration is reserved for clients who cannot take the drug orally.

e. Instruct clients to swallow oral propantheline tablets, not to chew them.

The tablets have a hard sugar coating to mask the bitter taste of the drug.

f. Parenteral glycopyrrolate can be given through the tubing of a running intravenous infusion of physiologic saline or lactated Ringer's solution.

g. Do not crush extended-release forms of anticholinergic drugs such as Detrol LA and Ditropan XL.

Crushing long-acting medications may result in high blood levels of the medication and increased adverse effects.

h. Take trospium (Sanctura) on an empty stomach.

Food interferes with absorption.

i. Follow the manufacturer's guidelines for administration of tiotropium using the HandiHaler inhalation device. Use the drug immediately after opening. Do not allow the powder to enter the eyes.

This ensures proper dosage and prevents reduced effectiveness.

Drug powder in the eyes may caused blurred vision and pupil dilation.

2. Observe for therapeutic effects

Therapeutic effects depend primarily on the reason for use. Thus, a therapeutic effect in one condition may be an adverse effect in another condition.

a. When a drug is given for *peptic ulcer disease* or other gastrointestinal disorders, observe for decreased abdominal pain.

Relief of abdominal pain is due to the smooth muscle relaxant or antispasmodic effect of the drug.

b. When the drug is given for *diagnosing or treating eye disorders,* observe for pupil dilation (mydriasis) and blurring of vision (cycloplegia).

Note that these ocular effects are considered adverse effects when the drugs are given for problems not related to the eyes.

c. When the drug is given for *symptomatic bradycardia,* observe for increased pulse rate.

These drugs increase heart rate by blocking action of the vagus nerve.

d. When the drug is given for *urinary-tract disorders,* such as cystitis or enuresis, observe for decreased frequency of urination. When the drug is given for *renal colic due to stones,* observe for decreased pain. When the drug is given for *overactive bladder,* observe for fewer symptoms of urgency, urge incontinence, and frequency.

Anticholinergic drugs decrease muscle tone and spasm in the smooth muscle of the ureters and urinary bladder.

e. When the centrally acting anticholinergics are given for *Parkinson's disease,* observe for decrease in tremor, salivation, and drooling.

Decreased salivation is a therapeutic effect with parkinsonism but an adverse reaction in most other conditions.

(continued)

NURSING ACTIONS	RATIONALE/EXPLANATION
3. Observe for adverse effects	These depend on reasons for use and are dose related.
a. Tachycardia	Tachycardia may occur with usual therapeutic doses because anticholinergic drugs block vagal action, which normally slows heart rate. Tachycardia is not likely to be serious except in clients with underlying heart disease. For example, in clients with angina pectoris, prolonged or severe tachycardia may increase myocardial ischemia to the point of causing an acute attack of angina (chest pain) or even myocardial infarction. In clients with congestive heart failure, severe or prolonged tachycardia can increase the workload of the heart to the point of causing acute heart failure or pulmonary edema.
b. Excessive central nervous system (CNS) stimulation (tremor, restlessness, confusion, hallucinations, delirium) followed by excessive CNS depression (coma, respiratory depression)	These effects are more likely to occur with large doses of atropine because atropine crosses the blood-brain barrier. Large doses of trihexyphenidyl (Trihexy) also may cause CNS stimulation.
c. Sedation and amnesia with scopolamine or benztropine (Cogentin)	This may be a therapeutic effect but becomes an adverse reaction if severe or if the drug is given for another purpose. Benztropine has anticholinergic and antihistaminic properties. Apparently, drowsiness and sedation are caused by the antihistaminic component.
d. Constipation or paralytic ileus	These effects are the result of decreased gastrointestinal motility and muscle tone. Constipation is more likely with large doses or parenteral administration. Paralytic ileus is not likely unless the drugs are given to clients who already have decreased gastrointestinal motility.
e. Decreased oral and respiratory tract secretions, which cause mouth dryness and thick respiratory secretions	Mouth dryness is more annoying than serious in most cases and is caused by decreased salivation. However, clients with chronic lung disease, who usually have excessive secretions, tend to retain them with the consequence of frequent respiratory tract infections.
f. Paradoxical bronchospasm	This effect is detrimental and requires that the drug be discontinued.
g. Urinary retention	This reaction is caused by loss of bladder tone and is most likely to occur in elderly men with enlarged prostate glands. Thus, the drugs are usually contraindicated with prostatic hypertrophy.
h. Hot, dry skin; fever; heat stroke	These effects are due to decreased sweating and impairment of the normal heat-loss mechanism. Fever may occur with any age group. Heat stroke is more likely to occur with cardiovascular disease, strenuous physical activity, and high environmental temperatures, especially in older people.
i. Ocular effects—mydriasis, blurred vision, photophobia	These are adverse effects when anticholinergic drugs are given for conditions not related to the eyes.
j. Angioedema with tiotropium	This effect requires that the drug be discontinued.
4. Observe for drug interactions	
a. Drugs that *increase* effects of anticholinergic drugs: antihistamines, disopyramide, phenothiazines, thioxanthene agents, tricyclic antidepressants, amantadine	These drugs have anticholinergic properties and produce additive anticholinergic effects.
b. Drugs that *decrease* effects of anticholinergic drugs: cholinergic drugs	These drugs counteract the inhibition of gastrointestinal motility and tone induced by atropine. They are sometimes used in atropine overdose.
c. For trospium, use caution when administering concurrently with drugs that are eliminated by active tubular secretion (eg, digoxin, metformin, morphine, pancuronium, procainamide, tenofovir, vancomycin).	As these drugs compete for urinary tubular pumps, increased serum concentration of trospium or the co-administered drug may occur.

APPLYING YOUR KNOWLEDGE: ANSWERS

20-1 Observe for increased heart rate. These drugs work by blocking the action of the vagus nerve.

20-2 Encourage the client to increase the fiber in his diet and to drink 2 to 3 quarts of fluid a day to help with the constipation. Notify the physician of Mr. Downes's constipation and urinary retention.

20-3 Mr. Bing has a history of glaucoma. Scopolamine is an anticholinergic medication and is contraindicated for a client with glaucoma.

Review and Application Exercises

Short Answer Exercises

1. How do anticholinergic drugs exert their therapeutic effects?

2. What are the indications and contraindications for use of anticholinergic drugs?

3. What is the effect of anticholinergic drugs on heart rate, and what is the mechanism for this effect?

4. Under what circumstances is it desirable to administer atropine before surgery, and why?

5. What are adverse effects of anticholinergic drugs?

6. What treatment measures are indicated for a client with an overdose of a drug with anticholinergic effects?

7. Name two other commonly used drug groups that have anticholinergic effects.

8. What nursing observations and interventions are needed to increase client safety and comfort during anticholinergic drug therapy?

NCLEX-Style Questions

9. Your 62-year-old client has a sinus bradycardia with a rate of 48 beats per minute. He is confused and his skin is cool and clammy. What is the drug of choice in this situation?
   a. atropine sulfate
   b. epinephrine (Adrenalin)
   c. isoproterenol (Isuprel)
   d. dopamine (Intropin)

10. Your client is taking an anticholinergic medication. Which of the following instructions would be appropriate for this client?
    a. Limit oral intake because these medications cause fluid retention.
    b. Be sure a bathroom is near because these medications may cause diarrhea.
    c. Avoid overheating and wear cool, loose clothing because these medications impair sweating.
    d. Change positions slowly because these medications may cause orthostatic hypotension.

11. Shortly after administration of the first dose of atropine, your client complains of acute eye pain. The nurse should
    a. Administer a PRN (as needed) dose of analgesic, such as acetaminophen.
    b. Place a cool, damp cloth over the client's eyes for comfort.
    c. Hold further doses of atropine and notify the physician immediately.
    d. Prepare to treat an allergic reaction to atropine with epinephrine (Adrenalin).

12. Your client with chronic lung disease is in respiratory distress due to acute bronchospasm. Which of the following orders for treatment of this condition would you question?
    a. epinephrine (Adrenalin)
    b. albuterol (Ventolin)
    c. aminophylline (Truphylline)
    d. tiotropium (Spiriva)

Selected References

Brown, J. H., & Taylor, P. (2001). Muscarinic receptor agonists and antagonists. In J. G. Hardman & L. E. Limbird (Eds.), *Goodman & Gilman's The pharmacological basis of therapeutics* (10th ed., pp. 155–173). New York: McGraw-Hill.

Drug facts and comparisons. (Updated monthly). St. Louis: Facts and Comparisons.

Hazinski, M. F., Cummins, R. O., & Field, J. M. (Eds.). (2000). *Handbook of emergency cardiovascular care for health care providers.* Dallas: American Heart Association.

Karch, A. M. (2005). *2006 Lippincott's nursing drug guide.* Philadelphia: Lippincott Williams & Wilkins.

Olson, K. R. (Ed.). (1999). *Poisoning and drug overdose* (3rd ed). Stamford, CT: Appleton & Lange.

Pappano, A. J., & Katzung, B. G. (2001) Cholinoceptor-blocking drugs. In B. G. Katzung (Ed.), *Basic and clinical pharmacology* (8th ed., pp 107–119). New York: McGraw-Hill.

Piano, M. R. & Huether, S. E. (2002). Mechanisms of hormonal regulation. In K. L. McCance & S. E. Huether (Eds.), *Pathophysiology: The biologic basis for disease in adults and children* (4th ed., pp. 597–623). St. Louis: Mosby.

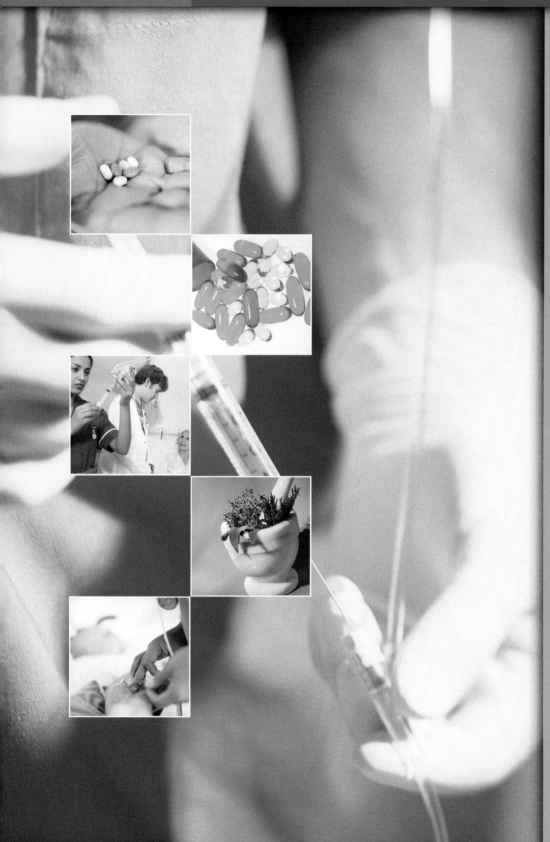

SECTION 4

Drugs Affecting the Endocrine System

CHAPTER OUTLINE

21 Physiology of the Endocrine System

22 Hypothalamic and Pituitary Hormones

23 Corticosteroids

24 Thyroid and Antithyroid Drugs

25 Hormones That Regulate Calcium and Bone Metabolism

26 Antidiabetic Drugs

27 Estrogens, Progestins, and Hormonal Contraceptives

28 Androgens and Anabolic Steroids

Physiology of the Endocrine System

OBJECTIVES

After studying this chapter, you will be able to:

1. Discuss the relationship between the endocrine system and the central nervous system.
2. Describe general characteristics and functions of hormones.
3. Differentiate steroid and protein hormones in relation to site of action and pharmacokinetics.
4. Discuss hormonal action at the cellular level.
5. Describe the second-messenger roles of cyclic adenosine monophosphate and calcium within body cells.
6. Differentiate between physiologic and pharmacologic doses of hormonal drugs.

INTRODUCTION

The endocrine system participates in the regulation of essentially all body activities, including metabolism of nutrients and water, reproduction, growth and development, and adapting to changes in internal and external environments. The major elements of the endocrine system are the hypothalamus of the brain, pituitary gland, thyroid gland, parathyroid glands, pancreas, adrenal glands, ovaries, and testes. These tissues function through *hormones,* substances that are synthesized and secreted into body fluids by one group of cells and have physiologic effects on other body cells. Hormones act as chemical messengers to transmit information between body cells and organs. Most hormones from the traditional endocrine glands are secreted into the bloodstream and act on distant organs.

In addition to the major endocrine organs, other tissues also produce hormones. These endocrine-like cells intermingle with nonendocrine cells in various organs. Their hormones are secreted into tissue fluids and act locally on nearby cells, as in the following examples:

- The gastrointestinal mucosa produces hormones that are important in the digestive process (eg, gastrin, enterogastrone, secretin, cholecystokinin).
- The kidneys produce erythropoietin, a hormone that stimulates the bone marrow to produce red blood cells.
- White blood cells produce cytokines that function as messengers among leukocytes in inflammatory and immune processes.
- Many body tissues produce prostaglandins and leukotrienes, which have a variety of physiologic effects.

Neoplasms also may produce hormones. In endocrine tissues, neoplasms may be an added source of the hormone normally produced by the organ. In nonendocrine tissues, various hormones may be produced. For example, lung tumors may produce corticotropin (adrenocorticotropic hormone [ACTH]), antidiuretic hormone, or parathyroid hormone; kidney tumors may produce parathyroid hormone. The usual effects are those of excess hormone secretion.

This chapter focuses on the traditional endocrine organs and their hormones. Specific organs are discussed in the following chapters; general characteristics of the endocrine system and hormones are described in the following sections and in Box 21-1.

ENDOCRINE SYSTEM–NERVOUS SYSTEM INTERACTIONS

The endocrine and nervous systems are closely connected, anatomically and physiologically, and work in harmony to integrate and regulate body functions. In general, the nervous system regulates rapid muscular and sensory activities by secreting substances that act as neurotransmitters, circulating hormones, and local hormones (eg, norepinephrine, epinephrine). The endocrine system regulates slow metabolic activities by secreting hormones that control cellular metabolism, transport of substances across cell membranes, and other functions (eg, reproduction, growth and development, secretion).

The main connecting link between the nervous system and the endocrine system is the hypothalamus, which responds to nervous system stimulation by producing hormones. Secretion of almost all hormones from the pituitary gland is controlled by the hypothalamus. Special nerve fibers originating in the hypothalamus and ending in the posterior pituitary gland control secretions of the posterior pituitary. The hypothalamus secretes hormones called *releasing* and *inhibitory factors,* which regulate functions of the anterior pituitary. The anterior pituitary, in turn, secretes hormones that act on target tissues, usually to stimulate production of other hormones. For example, hypothalamic corticotropin-releasing hormone stimulates the anterior pituitary to produce corticotropin, and corticotropin, in turn, stimulates the adrenal cortex to produce cortisol. This complex interrelationship is often referred to as the *hypothalamic–pituitary–adrenocortical axis.* It functions by a *negative feedback* system, in which hormone secretion is stimulated when hormones are needed and inhibited when they are not needed. The hypothalamic–pituitary–thyroid axis also functions by a negative feedback mechanism.

GENERAL CHARACTERISTICS OF HORMONES

Hormones are extremely important in regulating body activities. Their normal secretion and function help to maintain the internal environment and determine response and adaptation to the external environment. Hormones participate in complex interactions with other hormones and nonhormone chemical substances in the body to influence every aspect of life. Although hormones are usually studied individually, virtually all endocrine functions are complex processes that are influenced by more than one hormone.

Although hormones circulating in the bloodstream reach essentially all body cells, some (eg, growth hormone, thyroid hormone) affect almost all cells, whereas others affect specific "target" tissues (eg, corticotropin stimulates the adrenal cortex). In addition, *one hormone can affect different tissues* (eg, ovarian estrogen can act on ovarian follicles to promote their maturation; on the endometrial lining of the uterus to stimulate its growth and cyclic changes; on breast tissue to stimulate growth of milk ducts; and on the hypothalamic–pituitary system to regulate its own secretion), or *several hormones can affect a single tissue or function* (eg, catecholamines, glucagon, secretin, and prolactin regulate lipolysis [release of fatty acids from adipose tissue]).

Several hormones are secreted in cyclic patterns. For example, ACTH, cortisol, and growth hormone are secreted

---

Box 21-1 Major Hormones and Their General Functions

Anterior pituitary hormones are growth hormone (also called somatotropin), corticotropin, thyroid-stimulating hormone, follicle-stimulating hormone, luteinizing hormone, and prolactin. Most of these hormones function by stimulating secretion of other hormones.

Posterior pituitary hormones are antidiuretic hormone (ADH or vasopressin) and oxytocin. ADH helps maintain fluid balance; oxytocin stimulates uterine contractions during childbirth.

Adrenal cortex hormones, commonly called corticosteroids, include the glucocorticoids, such as cortisol, and the mineralocorticoids, such as aldosterone. Glucocorticoids influence carbohydrate storage, exert anti-inflammatory effects, suppress corticotropin secretion, and increase protein catabolism. Mineralocorticoids help regulate electrolyte balance, mainly by promoting sodium retention and potassium loss. The adrenal cortex also produces sex hormones. The adrenal medulla hormones are epinephrine and norepinephrine (see Chap. 17).

Thyroid hormones include triiodothyronine (T_3 or liothyronine) and tetraiodothyronine (T_4 or thyroxine). These hormones regulate the metabolic rate of the body and greatly influence growth and development.

Parathyroid hormone, also called parathormone or PTH, regulates calcium and phosphate metabolism.

Pancreatic hormones are insulin and glucagon, which regulate the metabolism of glucose, lipids, and proteins.

Ovarian hormones (female sex hormones) are estrogens and progesterone. Estrogens promote growth of specific body cells and development of most female secondary sexual characteristics. Progesterone helps prepare the uterus for pregnancy and the mammary glands for lactation.

Testicular hormone (male sex hormone) is testosterone, which regulates development of masculine characteristics.

Placental hormones are chorionic gonadotropin, estrogen, progesterone, and human placental lactogen, all of which are concerned with reproductive functions.

in 24-hour (circadian) cycles, whereas estrogen and progestin secretion are related to the 28-day menstrual cycle.

Hormone Pharmacokinetics

Protein-derived hormones (amines, amino acids, peptides, and polypeptides) are synthesized, stored, and released into the bloodstream in response to a stimulus. The steroid hormones, which are synthesized in the adrenal cortex and gonads from cholesterol, are released as they are synthesized. Most hormones are constantly present in the blood; plasma concentrations vary according to body needs, the rate of synthesis and release, and the rate of metabolism and excretion.

Protein-derived hormones usually circulate in an unbound, active form. Steroid and thyroid hormones are transported by specific carrier proteins synthesized in the liver. (Some drugs may compete with a hormone for binding sites on the carrier protein. If this occurs, hormone effects are enhanced because more unbound, active molecules are available to act on body cells.)

Hormones must be continuously inactivated to prevent their accumulation and excessive effects. Several mechanisms operate to eliminate hormones from the body. The water-soluble, protein-derived hormones have a short duration of action and are inactivated by enzymes mainly in the liver and kidneys. The lipid-soluble steroid and thyroid hormones have a longer duration of action because they are bound to plasma proteins. After they are released by the plasma proteins, these hormones are conjugated in the liver to inactive forms and then excreted in bile or urine. A third, less common mechanism is inactivation by enzymes at receptor sites on target cells.

Hormone Action at the Cellular Level

Hormones modify rather than initiate cellular reactions and functions. After hormone molecules reach a responsive cell, they bind with receptors in the cell membrane (eg, catecholamines and protein hormones) or inside the cell (eg, steroid and thyroid hormones). The number of hormone receptors and the affinity of the receptors for the hormone are the major determinants of target-cell response to hormone action.

The main target organs for a given hormone contain large numbers of receptors. However, the number of receptors may be altered by various conditions. For example, receptors may be increased (called *up-regulation*) when there are low levels of hormone. This allows the cell to obtain more of the needed hormone than it can obtain with fewer receptors. Receptors may be decreased (called *down-regulation*) when there are excessive amounts of hormone. This mechanism protects the cell by making it less responsive to excessive hormone levels. Receptor up-regulation and down-regulation occur with chronic exposure to abnormal levels of hormones. In addition, receptor proteins may be decreased by inadequate formation or antibodies that destroy them. Thus, receptors are

constantly being synthesized and degraded, so the number of receptors may change within hours. Receptor affinity for binding with hormone molecules probably changes as well.

After binding occurs, the resulting hormone–receptor complex initiates intracellular biochemical reactions, depending on the particular hormone and the type of cell. Many hormones act as a "first messenger" to the cell, and the hormone–receptor complex activates a "second messenger." The second messenger then activates intracellular structures to produce characteristic cellular functions and products. Steroid hormones from the adrenal cortex, ovaries, and testes stimulate target cells to synthesize various proteins (eg, enzymes, transport and structural proteins) needed for normal cellular function.

Second-Messenger Systems

Three major second-messenger systems, cyclic adenosine monophosphate (cAMP), calcium–calmodulin, and phospholipid products, are described in this section.

Cyclic AMP is the second messenger for many hormones, including corticotropin, catecholamines, glucagon, thyroid-stimulating hormone, follicle-stimulating hormone, luteinizing hormone, parathyroid hormone, secretin, and antidiuretic hormone. It is formed by the action of the enzyme *adenyl cyclase* on adenosine triphosphate, a component of all cells and the main source of energy for cellular metabolism. After it is formed, cAMP activates a series of enzyme reactions that alter cell function. The amount of intracellular cAMP is increased by hormones that activate adenyl cyclase (eg, the pituitary hormones, calcitonin, glucagon, parathyroid hormone) and decreased by hormones that inactivate adenyl cyclase (eg, angiotensin, somatostatin). Cyclic AMP is inactivated by phosphodiesterase enzymes.

Calcium is the second messenger for angiotensin II, a strong vasoconstrictor that participates in control of arterial blood pressure, and for gonadotropin-releasing hormone. The postulated sequence of events is that hormone binding to receptors increases intracellular calcium. The calcium binds with an intracellular regulatory protein called *calmodulin*. The calcium–calmodulin complex activates protein kinases, which then regulate contractile structures of the cell, cell membrane permeability, and intracellular enzyme activity. Specific effects include contraction of smooth muscle, changes in the secretions produced by secreting cells, and changes in ciliary action in the lungs.

Phospholipid products are mainly involved with local hormones. Phospholipids are major components of the cell membrane portion of all body cells. Some local hormones activate cell membrane receptors and transform them into phospholipase C, an enzyme that causes some of the phospholipids in cell membranes to split into smaller molecules (eg, inositol triphosphate and diacylglycerol). These products then act as second messengers to intracellular structures. Inositol triphosphate mobilizes intracellular calcium ions and the calcium ions then fulfill their functions as second messengers, as described previously. Diacylglycerol activates protein kinase C, an enzyme important in cell reproduction. Also, the lipid component of diacylglycerol is arachidonic acid, the precursor for prostaglandins, leukotrienes, and other local hormones with extensive effects.

Steroid Stimulation of Protein Synthesis

Steroid hormones are lipid soluble and therefore cross cell membranes easily. Inside the cell cytoplasm, the hormone molecules bind with specific receptor proteins. The hormone–receptor complex then enters the nucleus of the cell, where it activates nucleic acids (DNA and RNA) and the genetic code to synthesize new proteins.

Hormonal Disorders

Abnormal secretion and function of hormones, even minor alterations, can impair physical and mental health. Malfunction of an endocrine organ is usually associated with hyposecretion, hypersecretion, or inappropriate secretion of its hormones. Any malfunction can produce serious disease or death.

Glandular Hypofunction

Hypofunction may be associated with a variety of circumstances, including the following:

1. A congenital defect may result in the absence of an endocrine gland, the presence of an abnormally developed gland, or the absence of an enzyme required for glandular synthesis of its specific hormone.
2. The endocrine gland may be damaged or destroyed by impaired blood flow, infection or inflammation, autoimmune disorders, or neoplasms.
3. The endocrine gland may atrophy and become less able to produce its hormone because of aging, drug therapy, disease, or unknown reasons.
4. The endocrine gland may produce adequate hormone, but the hormone may not be able to function normally because of receptor defects (not enough receptors or the receptors present are unable to bind with the hormone).
5. Even if there is adequate hormone and adequate binding to receptors, intracellular metabolic processes (eg, enzyme function, protein synthesis, energy production) may not respond appropriately.

Glandular Hyperfunction

Hyperfunction is usually characterized by excessive hormone production. Excessive amounts of hormone may occur from excessive stimulation and enlargement of the endocrine gland, from a hormone-producing tumor of the gland, or from a hormone-producing tumor of nonendocrine tissues

(eg, some primary lung tumors produce antidiuretic hormone and ACTH).

USE OF HORMONAL DRUGS

Hormonal drugs are powerful drugs that produce widespread therapeutic and adverse effects. Hormones given for therapeutic purposes may be natural hormones from human or animal sources or synthetic. Many of the most important hormones have been synthesized, and synthetic preparations may have more potent and prolonged effects than naturally occurring hormones. Administration of one hormone may alter effects of other hormones. These alterations result from the complex interactions among hormones.

Hormones are given for physiologic or pharmacologic effects, and they are more often given for disorders resulting from endocrine gland hypofunction than for those related to hyperfunction. *Physiologic* use involves giving small doses as a replacement or substitute for the amount secreted by a normally functioning endocrine gland. Such use is indicated only when a gland cannot secrete an adequate amount of hormone. Examples of physiologic use include insulin administration in diabetes mellitus and adrenal corticosteroid administration in Addison's disease. *Pharmacologic* use involves relatively large doses for effects greater than physiologic effects. For example, adrenal corticosteroids are widely used for anti-inflammatory effects in endocrine and nonendocrine disorders.

Review and Application Exercises

Short Answer Exercises

1. How do hormones function in maintaining homeostasis?

2. What is the connection between the nervous system and the endocrine system?

3. What is meant by a negative feedback system?

4. Because classic hormones are secreted into blood and circulated to essentially all body cells, why do they not affect all body cells?

5. What are the functions and characteristics of the pituitary gland?

Selected References

Guyton, A. C., & Hall, J. E. (2000). *Textbook of medical physiology* (10th ed.). Philadelphia: W. B. Saunders.

Matfin, G., Kuenzi, J. A., & Guven, S. (2004). Mechanisms of endocrine control. In C. M. Porth, *Pathophysiology: Concepts of altered health states* (7th ed., pp. 951–960). Philadelphia: Lippincott Williams & Wilkins.

Hypothalamic and Pituitary Hormones

OBJECTIVES

After studying this chapter, you will be able to:

1. Describe clinical uses of selected hormones.
2. Differentiate characteristics and functions of anterior and posterior pituitary hormones.
3. Discuss limitations of hypothalamic and pituitary hormones as therapeutic agents.
4. State major nursing considerations in the care of clients receiving specific hypothalamic and pituitary hormones.

APPLYING YOUR KNOWLEDGE

Jose Rojas is a 24-year-old Hispanic man who has suffered a head injury while riding his motorcycle without a helmet. He has been admitted for observation, with multiple abrasions and a blow to the head. Mr. Rojas begins to produce massive amounts of clear, pale-yellow urine. The physician diagnoses him with diabetes insipidus and orders desmopressin 0.2 mL in two divided doses intranasally.

INTRODUCTION

The hypothalamus of the brain and the pituitary gland interact to control most metabolic functions of the body and to maintain homeostasis (Fig. 22-1). They are anatomically connected by the hypophyseal stalk. The hypothalamus controls secretions of the pituitary gland. The pituitary gland, in turn, regulates secretions or functions of other body tissues, called *target* tissues. The pituitary gland is actually two glands, each with different structures and functions. The *anterior pituitary* is composed of different types of glandular cells that synthesize and secrete different hormones. The *posterior pituitary* is anatomically an extension of the hypothalamus and is composed mainly of nerve fibers. Although it does not manufacture any hormones itself, it stores and releases hormones synthesized in the hypothalamus.

TYPES OF HORMONES

Hypothalamic Hormones

The hypothalamus produces a releasing hormone or an inhibiting hormone that corresponds to each of the major hormones of the anterior pituitary gland.

Corticotropin-releasing hormone or **factor** (CRH or CRF) causes release of corticotropin (also called *adrenocorticotropic hormone* [ACTH]) in response to stress and threatening stimuli. CRH is secreted most often during sleep and its secretion is influenced by several neurotransmitters. Acetylcholine and serotonin stimulate secretion, and gamma-aminobutyric acid (GABA) and norepinephrine inhibit secretion. The ability of CRH to stimulate corticotropin secretion is increased by vasopressin and decreased or prevented by somatostatin and elevated levels of glucocorticoids. CRH can be used in the diagnosis of Cushing's disease, a disorder characterized by excess cortisol.

Growth hormone–releasing hormone (GHRH) causes release of growth hormone (GH) in response to low blood levels of GH. Found in the pancreas as well as the hypothalamus, GHRH structurally resembles a group of hormones that includes glucagon, secretin, vasoactive intestinal peptide, and gastric inhibitory peptide. Secretion of hypothalamic GHRH is stimulated by dopamine, norepinephrine, epinephrine, GABA, acetylcholine, and serotonin. The stimulatory effect of GHRH on secretion of GH is blocked by somatostatin. GHRH may be used to test pituitary function and to stimulate growth in children with GHRH deficiency.

Growth hormone release–inhibiting hormone (somatostatin) inhibits release of GH. Although originally discovered

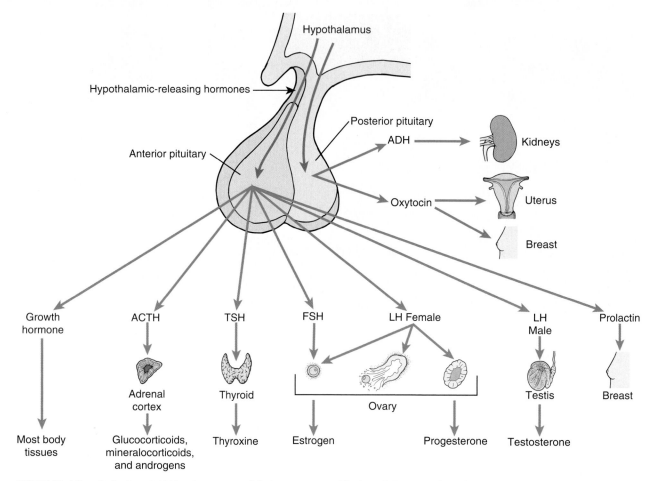

FIGURE 22-1 Hypothalamic and pituitary hormones and their target organs. The hypothalamus produces hormones that act on the anterior pituitary or are stored in the posterior pituitary. The anterior pituitary produces hormones that act on various body tissues and stimulate production of other hormones. ACTH, adrenocorticotropic hormone; ADH, antidiuretic hormone; FSH, follicle-stimulating hormone; LH, luteinizing hormone; TSH, thyroid-stimulating hormone.

from the hypothalamus, it is found in many tissues. It is distributed throughout the brain and spinal cord, where it functions as a neurotransmitter. It is also found in the intestines and the pancreas, where it regulates secretion of insulin and glucagon. Somatostatin secretion is increased by several neurotransmitters, including acetylcholine, dopamine, epinephrine, GABA, and norepinephrine.

In addition to inhibiting GH, somatostatin also inhibits other functions, including secretion of corticotrophin, thyroid-stimulating hormone (TSH or thyrotropin), prolactin, pancreatic secretions (eg, insulin, glucagon), and gastrointestinal (GI) secretions (gastrin, cholecystokinin, secretin, vasoactive intestinal peptide); as well as GI motility, bile flow, and mesenteric blood flow. Hypothalamic somatostatin blocks the action of GHRH and decreases thyrotropin-releasing hormone (TRH)–induced release of TSH. GH stimulates secretion of somatostatin, and the effects of somatostatin on TSH may contribute to TSH deficiency in children being treated with GH. A long-acting somatostatin analog, octreotide (Sando-

statin), may be used to treat acromegaly and TSH-secreting pituitary tumors.

Thyrotropin-releasing hormone (TRH) causes release of TSH in response to stress, such as exposure to cold. TRH may be used in diagnostic tests of pituitary function and hyperthyroidism.

Gonadotropin-releasing hormone (GnRH) causes release of follicle-stimulating hormone (FSH) and luteinizing hormone (LH). Several synthetic equivalents of GnRH are used clinically.

Prolactin-releasing factor is active during lactation after childbirth.

Prolactin-inhibitory factor (PIF) is active at times other than during lactation.

Anterior Pituitary Hormones

The anterior pituitary gland produces seven hormones. Two of these, GH and prolactin, act directly on their target tissues;

the other five act indirectly by stimulating target tissues to produce other hormones.

Corticotropin, also called *ACTH,* stimulates the adrenal cortex to produce corticosteroids. Secretion is controlled by the hypothalamus and by plasma levels of cortisol, the major corticosteroid. When plasma levels are adequate for body needs, the anterior pituitary does not release corticotropin (negative feedback mechanism). Although manufacturers recommend corticotropin for treatment of disorders that respond to glucocorticoids, corticotropin is less predictable and less convenient than glucocorticoids and has no apparent advantages.

GH, also called *somatotropin,* stimulates growth of body tissues. It regulates cell division and protein synthesis required for normal growth and promotes an increase in cell size and number, including growth of muscle cells and lengthening of bone. These effects occur mainly via altered metabolism of carbohydrate, protein, and fat by direct and indirect effects. GH is one of a battery of hormones that affects carbohydrate metabolism by maintaining blood glucose within a normal range. It is often considered an insulin antagonist because it suppresses the abilities of insulin to stimulate uptake of glucose in peripheral tissues and enhance glucose synthesis in the liver. Paradoxically, administration of GH produces hyperinsulinemia by stimulating insulin secretion. In addition, GH stimulates protein anabolism in many tissues. The hormone also enhances fat utilization by stimulating triglyceride breakdown and oxidation in fat-storing cells.

In children, levels of GH rise rapidly during adolescence, peak in the 20s, and then start to decline. Deficient GH in children produces dwarfism, a condition marked by severely decreased linear growth and, frequently, severely delayed mental, emotional, dental, and sexual growth as well. If untreated, excessive GH in preadolescents produces gigantism, resulting in heights of 8 or 9 feet.

In adults, deficient GH (less than expected for age) can cause increased fat; reduced skeletal and heart muscle mass; reduced strength; reduced ability to exercise; and worsened cholesterol levels (ie, increased low-density lipoprotein cholesterol and decreased high-density lipoprotein cholesterol), which increase risk factors for cardiovascular disease. Excessive GH in adults produces acromegaly, which distorts facial features and is associated with an increased incidence of diabetes mellitus and hypertension.

Thyrotropin (also called *TSH*) regulates secretion of thyroid hormones. Thyrotropin secretion is controlled by a negative feedback mechanism in proportion to metabolic needs. Thus, increased thyroid hormones in body fluids inhibit secretion of thyrotropin by the anterior pituitary and of TRH by the hypothalamus.

FSH, one of the gonadotropins, stimulates functions of sex glands. FSH is produced by the anterior pituitary gland of both sexes, beginning at puberty. It acts on the ovaries in a cyclical fashion during the reproductive years, stimulating growth of ovarian follicles. These follicles then produce estrogen, which prepares the endometrium for implantation of a fertilized ovum. FSH acts on the testes to stimulate the production and growth of sperm (spermatogenesis), but it does not stimulate secretion of male sex hormones.

LH (also called *interstitial cell-stimulating hormone*) is another gonadotropin that stimulates hormone production by the gonads of both sexes. In women, LH is important in the maturation and rupture of the ovarian follicle (ovulation). After ovulation, LH acts on the cells of the collapsed follicular sac to produce the corpus luteum, which then produces progesterone during the last half of the menstrual cycle. When blood progesterone levels rise, a negative feedback effect is exerted on hypothalamic and anterior pituitary secretion of gonadotropins. Decreased pituitary secretion of LH causes the corpus luteum to die and stop producing progesterone. Lack of progesterone causes slough and discharge of the endometrial lining as menstrual flow. (Of course, if the ovum has been fertilized and attached to the endometrium, menstruation does not occur.) In men, LH stimulates the Leydig's cells in the spaces between the seminiferous tubules. These cells then secrete androgens, mainly testosterone.

Prolactin plays a part in milk production by nursing mothers. It is not usually secreted in nonpregnant women because of the hypothalamic hormone PIF. During late pregnancy and lactation, various stimuli, including suckling, inhibit the production of PIF, and thus prolactin is synthesized and released.

Melanocyte-stimulating hormone plays a role in skin pigmentation, but its function in humans is not clearly delineated.

Posterior Pituitary Hormones

The posterior pituitary gland stores and releases two hormones that are synthesized by nerve cells in the hypothalamus.

Antidiuretic hormone (ADH), also called *vasopressin,* functions to regulate water balance. When ADH is secreted, it makes renal tubules more permeable to water. This allows water in renal tubules to be reabsorbed into the plasma and so conserves body water. In the absence of ADH, little water is reabsorbed, and large amounts are lost in the urine.

ADH is secreted when body fluids become concentrated (high amounts of electrolytes in proportion to the amount of water) and when blood volume is low. In the first instance, ADH causes reabsorption of water, dilution of extracellular fluids, and restoration of normal osmotic pressure. In the second instance, ADH raises blood volume and arterial blood pressure toward homeostatic levels.

Oxytocin functions in childbirth and lactation. It initiates uterine contractions at the end of gestation to induce childbirth, and it causes milk to move from breast glands to nipples so the infant can obtain the milk by suckling.

INDIVIDUAL DRUGS

Although hypothalamic hormones and pituitary hormones have few therapeutic uses, they have important functions when used in certain circumstances, and drug formulations of most hormones have been synthesized. Selected drugs are described below. Indications for use, routes, and dosage ranges are listed in Table 22-1.

Hypothalamic Hormones

Gonadorelin (Factrel), **goserelin** (Zoladex), **histrelin** (Vantas), **leuprolide** (Lupron), **nafarelin** (Synarel), and **triptorelin** (Trelstar) are equivalent to GnRH. After initial stimulation of LH and FSH secretion, chronic administration of therapeutic doses inhibits gonadotropin secretion. This action results in decreased production of testosterone and estrogen, which is reversible when administration is stopped. In males, testosterone is reduced to castrate levels. In premenopausal females, estrogens are reduced to postmenopausal levels. These effects occur within 2 to 4 weeks after drug therapy is begun. In children with central precocious puberty, gonadotropins (testosterone in males; estrogen in females) are reduced to prepubertal levels.

These GnRH equivalents cannot be given orally, because they would be destroyed by enzymes in the GI tract. Most are given by injection and are available in depot preparations that can be given once monthly or less often. Adverse effects are basically those of testosterone or estrogen deficiency. When given for prostate cancer, the drugs may cause increased bone pain and increased difficulty in urinating during the first few weeks of treatment. The drugs may also cause or aggravate depression.

Octreotide (Sandostatin) has pharmacologic actions similar to those of somatostatin. Indications for use include acromegaly, in which it reduces blood levels of GH and insulin-like growth factor-1 (IGF-1); carcinoid tumors, in which it inhibits diarrhea and flushing; and vasoactive intestinal peptide tumors, in which it relieves diarrhea (by decreasing GI secretions and motility). It is also used to treat diarrhea in acquired immunodeficiency syndrome (AIDS) and other conditions. The drug is most often given subcutaneously and may be self-administered. The long-acting formulation (Sandostatin LAR Depot) must be given intramuscularly in a gluteal muscle. Dosage should be reduced for older adults.

Anterior Pituitary Hormones

Abarelix (Plenaxis) is a GnRH antagonist indicated for the palliative treatment of advanced symptomatic prostate cancer in men who are not candidates for therapy with LH-releasing hormone, refuse surgical castration, and have one or more of the following: (1) risk of neurologic compromise due to metastatic disease, (2) ureteral or bladder-outlet obstruction due to local encroachment or metastasis, or (3) severe bone pain from skeletal metastases that persists despite narcotic analgesia. Abarelix reduces the amount of testosterone produced in the body by inhibiting gonadotropin and related androgen production by directly and competitively blocking GnRH receptors in the anterior pituitary gland. Treatment

failure can be detected by measuring total serum testosterone concentrations just prior to administration on day 29 and every 8 weeks thereafter. Effectiveness beyond 12 months has not been established.

Corticotropin (ACTH, Acthar Gel), which is obtained from animal pituitary glands, is mainly of historical interest. For therapeutic purposes, it has been replaced by adrenal corticosteroids. It may be used occasionally as a diagnostic test to differentiate primary adrenal insufficiency (Addison's disease, which is associated with atrophy of the adrenal gland) from secondary adrenal insufficiency caused by inadequate pituitary secretion of corticotropin. However, **cosyntropin** (Cortrosyn), a synthetic formulation, is more commonly used to test for suspected adrenal insufficiency.

Growth hormone is synthesized from bacteria by recombinant DNA technology. **Somatropin** (eg, Humatrope) is therapeutically equivalent to endogenous GH produced by the pituitary gland. The main clinical use of GH is for children whose growth is impaired by a deficiency of endogenous hormone. The drugs are ineffective when impaired growth results from other causes or after puberty, when epiphyses of the long bones have closed. GH is also used to treat short stature in children that is associated with chronic renal failure or Turner's syndrome (a genetic disorder that occurs in girls). In adults, the drugs may be used to treat deficiency states (eg, those caused by disease, surgery, or radiation of the pituitary gland) or the tissue wasting associated with AIDS. In general, dosage should be individualized according to response. Excessive administration can cause gigantism.

Human chorionic gonadotropin (HCG; eg, Chorex) produces physiologic effects similar to those of naturally occurring LH. In males, it is used to evaluate the ability of Leydig's cells to produce testosterone; to treat hypogonadism due to pituitary deficiency; and to treat cryptorchidism (undescended testicle) in preadolescent boys. In women, recombinant HCG **choriogonadotropin alpha** (Ovidrel), is used in combination with menotropins to induce ovulation in the treatment of infertility. Excessive doses or prolonged administration can lead to sexual precocity, edema, and breast enlargement caused by oversecretion of testosterone and estrogen.

Menotropins (Pergonal), a gonadotropin preparation obtained from the urine of postmenopausal women, contains both FSH and LH. It is usually combined with HCG to induce ovulation in the treatment of infertility caused by lack of pituitary gonadotropins.

Pegvisomant (Somavert) is a GH receptor antagonist used in the treatment of acromegaly in adults who are unable to tolerate or are resistant to other management strategies. The drug selectively binds to GH receptors, blocking the binding of endogenous GH. In general, dosage should be individualized according to response. Dosage reduction of hypoglycemic agents may be required because the drug may increase glucose tolerance. Increased dosages of pegvisomant may be necessary when administered with narcotics. The drug should be used with caution in the elderly and in people with renal or hepatic disease.

Table 22-1 Drugs at a Glance: Hypothalamic and Pituitary Drugs

GENERIC/TRADE NAME	INDICATIONS FOR USE	ROUTES AND DOSAGE RANGES	
		Adults	Children
Hypothalamic Hormones			
Gonadorelin (Factrel)	Diagnostic test of gonadotropic functions of the anterior pituitary	Sub-Q, IV 100 mcg	
Goserelin (Zoladex)	Endometriosis Metastatic breast cancer Prostate cancer	Sub-Q implant into upper abdominal wall, 3.6 mg every 28 days or 10.8 mg every 3 mo	
Histrelin (Vantas)	CPP in children (<18 y, girls; <9.5 y, boys)		10 mcg/kg Sub-Q once a day
Leuprolide (Lupron)	Advanced prostatic cancer CPP in children Endometriosis Uterine fibroid tumors	Endometriosis, uterine fibroids, IM depot injection, 3.75 mg every mo or 11.25 mg every 3 mo for 6 mo Prostate cancer, Sub-Q 1 mg daily; IM depot 7.5 mg every mo, 22.5 mg every 3 mo, or 30 mg every 4 mo; implant (Viadur) one (72 mg) every 12 mo	CPP, Sub-Q 50 mcg/kg/d; IM Depot-Ped, weight 25 kg or less, 7.5 mg; >25 to 37.5 kg, 11.25 mg; >37.5 kg, 15 mg every mo
Nafarelin (Synarel)	Endometriosis CPP in children	1 spray (200 mcg) in one nostril in the morning and 1 spray in the other nostril in the evening (400 mcg/d), starting between the 2nd and 4th days of the menstrual cycle	2 sprays (400 mcg) in each nostril morning and evening (1600 mcg/d), until resumption of puberty is desired
Octreotide (Sandostatin; LAR Depot [long-acting])	Acromegaly Carcinoid tumors Vasoactive intestinal peptide tumors Diarrhea	Acromegaly, Sub-Q 50–100 mcg 3 times daily; long-acting: 100 mcg–200 mcg 3 times daily, may be adjusted up to 500 mcg 3 times daily Carcinoid tumors, Sub-Q 100–600 mcg daily (average 300 mcg) in 2–4 divided doses Intestinal tumors, Sub-Q 200–300 mcg daily in 2–4 divided doses Diarrhea, IV, Sub-Q 50 mcg 2 or 3 times daily initially, then adjusted according to response	Dosage not established but 1–10 mcg/kg reportedly well tolerated in young clients
Triptorelin (Trelstar)	Advanced prostatic cancer	3.75 mg depot injection IM	
Anterior Pituitary Hormones			
Abaralix (Plenaxis)	Advanced prostatic cancer	100 mg IM to buttock on days 15, 29, q4wk thereafter	

(continued)

Table 22-1 Drugs at a Glance: Hypothalamic and Pituitary Drugs (continued)

GENERIC/TRADE NAME	INDICATIONS FOR USE	ROUTES AND DOSAGE RANGES Adults	Children
Corticotropin (ACTH, Acthar Gel)	Stimulate synthesis of hormones by the adrenal cortex Diagnostic test of adrenal function	Therapeutic use, IM, Sub-Q 20 units 4 times daily Diagnostic use, IV infusion, 10–25 units in 500 mL of 5% dextrose or 0.9% sodium chloride solution, over 8 h Acthar Gel, IM 40–80 units q24–72h	
Cosyntropin (Cortrosyn)	Diagnostic test in suspected adrenal insufficiency	IM, IV 0.25 mg (equivalent to 25 units ACTH)	
Growth hormone: Somatrem (Protropin) **Somatropin** (Genotropin, Humatrope, Norditropin, Nutropin, Serostim)	Promote growth in children whose growth is impaired by a deficiency of endogenous growth hormone		*Somatrem,* IM up to 0.1 mg/kg 3 times per wk *Somatropin,* IM up to 0.06 mg/kg 3 times per wk
HCG (Chorex, Choron, Pregnyl)	Cryptorchidism Induce ovulation in the treatment of infertility	Cryptorchidism and male hypogonadism, IM 500–4000 units 2–3 times per wk for several wk To induce ovulation, IM 5000–10,000 units in 1 dose, 1 d after treatment with menotropins	*Preadolescent boys:* Cryptorchidism and hypogonadism, IM 500–4000 units 2–3 times per wk for several wk
Choriogonadotropin alpha (Ovidrel)	Induce ovulation in the treatment of infertility	250 mcg Sub-Q in 1 dose, 1 d after treatment with menotropins	
Follitropin alfa (Gonal-F, Gonal-F RFF pen)	Stimulate ovulation	Sub-Q 75 IU of FSH to maximum daily dose of 300 IU Prefilled pen: 300–900 IV of FSH as individualized dosage	
Follitropin beta (Follistim)	Stimulate ovulation	Sub-Q 75 IU of FSH to maximum daily dose of 300 IU	
Menotropins (Pergonal)	Combined with HCG to induce ovulation in treatment of infertility caused by lack of pituitary gonadotropins	IM 1 ampule (75 units FSH and 75 units LH) daily for 9–12 d, followed by HCG to induce ovulation	
Pegvisomant (Somavert)	Acromegaly unresponsive to other management strategies	Load: 40 mg Sub-Q Maintenance: 10 mg Sub-Q; titrate by 5 mg increments q4–6 wk according to IGF-1 levels to maximum of 30 mg/d	
Thyrotropin alfa (Thyrogen)	Diagnostic test of thyroid function	IM 0.9 mg every 24 h for 2 doses or every 72 h for 3 doses	*<16 y:* Dosage not established

Table 22-1 Drugs at a Glance: Hypothalamic and Pituitary Drugs (continued)

		ROUTES AND DOSAGE RANGES	
GENERIC/TRADE NAME	**INDICATIONS FOR USE**	**Adults**	**Children**
Urofollitropin (Bravelle)	Stimulate ovulation	Sub-Q 150 IU of FSH daily for the first 5 d to maximum daily dose of 450 IU	
Posterior Pituitary Hormones			
Desmopressin (DDAVP, Stimate)	Neurogenic diabetes insipidus Hemostasis (parenteral only) in spontaneous, trauma-induced, and perioperative bleeding	Diabetes insipidus, intranasally 0.1–0.4 mL/d, usually in 2 divided doses Hemophilia A, von Willebrand's disease, IV 0.3 mcg/kg in 50 mL sterile saline, infused over 15–30 min	*3 mo–2 y:* Diabetes insipidus, intranasally 0.05–0.3 mL/d in 1–2 doses *Weight >10 kg:* Hemophilia A, von Willebrand's disease, same as adult dosage *Weight ≤10 kg:* Hemophilia A, von Willebrand's disease, IV 0.3 mcg/kg in 10 mL of sterile saline
Vasopressin (Pitressin)	Diabetes insipidus	IM, Sub-Q, intranasally on cotton pledgets, 0.25–0.5 mL (5–10 units) 2–3 times daily	IM, Sub-Q, intranasally on cotton pledgets, 0.125–0.5 mL (2.5–10 units) 3–4 times daily
Oxytocin (Pitocin)	Induce labor Control postpartum bleeding	Induction of labor, IV 1-mL ampule (10 units) in 1000 mL of 5% dextrose injection (10 units/1000 mL = 10 milliunits/mL), infused at 0.2–2 milliunits/min initially, then regulated according to frequency and strength of uterine contractions Prevention or treatment of postpartum bleeding, IV 10–40 units in 1000 mL of 5% dextrose injection, infused at 125 mL/h (40 milliunits/min) or 0.6–1.8 units (0.06–0.18 mL) diluted in 3–5 mL sodium chloride injection and injected slowly; IM 0.3–1 mL (3–10 units)	

ACTH, adrenocorticotropic hormone; CPP, central precocious puberty; FSH, follicle-stimulating hormone; HCG, human chorionic gonadotropin; IGF-1, insulin-like growth factor-1; IV, intravenous; IM, intramuscular; LH, luteinizing hormone; Sub-Q, subcutaneous.

Thyrotropin alfa (Thyrogen) is a synthetic formulation of TSH used as a diagnostic adjunct for serum thyroglobin (Tg) testing in individuals with well-differentiated thyroid cancer. The testing can be performed with or without radioiodine imaging. Because there is a risk of missing the diagnosis of thyroid cancer or predicting the extent of the disease, thyroid hormone withdrawal Tg testing radioactive imaging is the standard test for evaluating the presence, extent, and location of thyroid cancer. Thyrotropin alfa must be used cautiously in clients with coronary artery disease and with a large amount of residual thyroid tissue as the drug produces a temporary rise of thyroid hormone concentration in the blood.

Urofollitropin (Bravelle), **follitropin alfa** (Gonal-F), and **follitropin beta** (Follistim) are drug preparations of FSH.

These drugs are used to stimulate ovarian function in the treatment of infertility and are used sequentially with HCG. Urofollitropin is extracted from the urine of postmenopausal women and acts directly on the ovaries to stimulate follicular ovulation. The development of follitropin alfa and follitropin beta as recombinant products advances the treatment of infertility, appears to be well tolerated, and has similar efficacy. A new liquid formulation of follitropin alfa (Gonal-F RFF Pen) is available in a prefilled and ready-to-use multidose FSH injection.

Posterior Pituitary Hormones

Desmopressin (DDAVP, Stimate), and **vasopressin** Pitressin) are synthetic equivalents of ADH. A major clinical use is the treatment of neurogenic diabetes insipidus, a disorder characterized by a deficiency of ADH and the excretion of large amounts of dilute urine. Diabetes insipidus may be idiopathic, hereditary, or acquired as a result of trauma, surgery, tumor, infection, or other conditions that impair the function of the hypothalamus or posterior pituitary.

Parenteral desmopressin is also used as a hemostatic in clients with hemophilia A or mild to moderate von Willebrand's disease (type 1). The drug is effective in controlling spontaneous or trauma-induced bleeding and intraoperative and postoperative bleeding when given 30 minutes before the procedure. Vasopressin is also used in the treatment of bleeding esophageal varices because of its vasoconstrictive effects. Desmopressin may be inhaled intranasally; vasopressin must be injected.

Oxytocin (Pitocin) is a synthetic drug that exerts the same physiologic effects as the posterior pituitary hormone. Thus, it promotes uterine contractility and is used clinically to induce labor and in the postpartum period to control bleeding. Oxytocin must be used only when clearly indicated and when the recipient can be supervised by well-trained personnel, as in a hospital.

APPLYING YOUR KNOWLEDGE 22-1:
HOW CAN YOU AVOID THIS MEDICATION ERROR?
You prepare Mr. Rojas's medication and administer 0.2 mL of desmopressin intranasally.

NURSING PROCESS

Assessment

Assess for disorders for which hypothalamic and pituitary hormones are given.
- For children with impaired growth, assess height and weight (actual and compared with growth charts) and diagnostic radiographic reports of bone age.

- For clients with diabetes insipidus, assess baseline blood pressure, weight, ratio of fluid intake to urine output, urine specific gravity, and laboratory reports of serum electrolytes.
- For clients with diarrhea, assess the number and consistency of stools per day as well as hydration status.
- For clients with infertility, assess drug-specific adverse effects (dizziness, nausea, headache and abdominal cramps, hot flashes/flushes, ovarian enlargement, blurring of vision and other visual symptoms).

Nursing Diagnoses

- Deficient Knowledge: Drug administration and effects
- Altered Growth and Development
- Anxiety related to multiple injections
- Risk for Injury: Adverse drug effects
- Ineffective Coping related to frustration with difficulty with conception

Planning/Goals

The client will
- Experience relief of symptoms without serious adverse effects
- Take or receive the drug accurately
- Comply with procedures for monitoring and follow-up
- Cope effectively and acknowledge feelings of grief, disappointment, and failure

Interventions

- For children receiving GH, help the family set reasonable goals for increased height and weight and comply with accurate drug administration and follow-up procedures (eg, periodic radiographs to determine bone growth and progress toward epiphyseal closure; recording height and weight at least weekly). Client Teaching Guidelines for Growth Hormone are given in the accompanying display.
- For clients with diabetes insipidus, help them develop a daily routine to monitor their response to drug therapy (eg, weigh themselves; monitor fluid intake and urine output for approximately equal amounts; check urine specific gravity [should be at least 1.015] and replace fluids accordingly).
- For clients with infertility, reinforce teaching about potential risks and benefits of drug therapy and about proper self-administration techniques of preparation, injection, and disposal of medication and supplies. Educate about evaluating basal body temperature patterns and continuing medical supervision as long as the drugs are being taken, and alert the couple about the risk of multiple births. Refer to local support groups, and acknowledge feelings of grief, disappointment, and failure. Client Teaching Guidelines for Fertility Drugs are given in the accompanying display.

C L I E N T   T E A C H I N G   G U I D E L I N E S

Growth Hormone

General Considerations

☑ Growth hormone (GH) is taken to normalize growth and development in children with a GH deficiency, not for people merely desiring an increase in stature. The drugs are contraindicated in children after epiphyseal closure occurs.

☑ GH is taken until a satisfactory height has been achieved, epiphyseal closure occurs, or until no further stimulation of growth occurs.

☑ Periodic tests of growth curve, bone age, serum glucose levels, thyroid function, and somatomedin levels are necessary, as well as funduscopic eye examinations.

☑ Children who have GH deficiency may develop slipped capital femoral epiphysis more frequently, and those with scoliosis may see a progression of the condition.

Self-Administration

☑ Take GH only if prescribed and as prescribed.

☑ Continue with medical supervision as long as GH is being taken.

☑ Ask a health care provider if you are uncertain about how to administer GH.

☑ Report severe hip or knee pain or the development of a limp to the prescriber immediately, because this may indicate slipped capital femoral epiphysis. In addition, report any signs of severe headache or acute visual changes, because they may indicate the complication of increased intracranial pressure.

Evaluation

● Interview and observe for compliance with instructions for taking the drug(s).

● Observe for relief of symptoms for which pituitary hormones were prescribed.

● Observe for effective coping with the underlying condition and the effects of treatment.

APPLYING YOUR KNOWLEDGE 22-2

What nursing measures should be implemented to appropriately monitor Mr. Rojas?

PRINCIPLES OF THERAPY

Hypothalamic hormones and pituitary hormones have few therapeutic uses. Most hypothalamic hormones are used to diagnose pituitary insufficiency. Pituitary hormones are not used extensively because most conditions in which they are indicated are uncommon; other effective agents are available for some uses; and deficiencies of target-gland hormones (eg, corticosteroids, thyroid hormones, male or female sex hormones) are usually more effectively treated with those hormones than with anterior pituitary hormones that stimulate their secretion. However, the hormones perform important functions when used in particular circumstances, and

C L I E N T   T E A C H I N G   G U I D E L I N E S

Fertility Drugs

General Considerations

☑ Fertility drugs stimulate ovulation and fertility. Pregnancy typically may occur within 4–6 weeks of therapy.

☑ These drugs are contraindicated in pregnant women. If pregnancy is suspected, the drugs should be discontinued, and the physician who prescribed them should be notified.

☑ These drugs should not be used by women who are breast-feeding or by children.

☑ In many cases, couples who are infertile experience feelings of grief, disappointment, and failure. Often they can benefit from participation in local support groups.

Self-Administration

☑ Take fertility drugs only if prescribed and as prescribed.

☑ Continue with medical supervision as long as the drugs are being taken.

☑ Ask the health care provider if you are uncertain about how the drug is administered; proper use of infusion devices; and how to monitor basal body temperature patterns.

☑ Monitor ovulation and discontinue the drug, if instructed, when ovulation is suspected.

☑ Recognize that the risk of multiple births is increased with the use of these drugs.

☑ Report adverse effects, such as dizziness, nausea, headache and abdominal cramps, hot flashes/flushes, and blurring of vision and other visual symptoms.

☑ For maximum desired response, have intercourse daily beginning the day before human chorionic gonadotropin therapy until ovulation occurs.

drug formulations of most hormones have been synthesized for these purposes.

Because the hormones are proteins, they must be given by injection or nasal inhalation. If taken orally, they would be destroyed by proteolytic enzymes in the GI tract.

Hypothalamic Hormones

Hypothalamic hormones are rarely used in most clinical practice settings. The drugs should be prescribed by health care providers who are knowledgeable about endocrinology and should be administered according to the manufacturers' literature.

APPLYING YOUR KNOWLEDGE 22-3
You return to Mr. Rojas's room to assess the client. Mr. Rojas has an elevated blood pressure of 190/100. His sodium level is low at 117 mEq/L, and his urine osmolality is below normal. How do you respond?

Pituitary Hormones

Most drug therapy with pituitary hormones is given to replace or supplement naturally occurring hormones in situations involving inadequate function of the pituitary gland (hypopituitarism). Conditions resulting from excessive amounts of pituitary hormones (hyperpituitarism) are more often treated with surgery or radiation. Diagnosis of suspected pituitary disorders should be thorough to promote more effective treatment, including drug therapy. Dosage of all pituitary hormones must be individualized, because the responsiveness of affected tissues varies.

Toxicity: Abuse of Growth Hormone

Inappropriate use of GH is an increasing concern. Young athletes may use the drug for body building and to enhance athletic performance. If so, they are likely to use relatively high doses. In addition, the highest levels of physiologic hormone are secreted during adolescence. The combination of high pharmacologic and high physiologic amounts increases risks of health problems from excessive hormone. Also, there is little evidence that hormone use increases muscle mass or strength beyond that achieved with exercise alone.

Middle-aged and older adults may use GH to combat the effects of aging, such as decreased energy, weaker muscles and joints, and wrinkled skin. One source of the product is apparently "anti-aging" clinics. Although it is not illegal for health care providers to prescribe GH for these populations, such use is unproven in safety and effectiveness. Endocrinologists emphasize that optimal adult levels of GH are unknown, and use of GH to slow aging is unproven and potentially dangerous because the long-term effects are unknown.

Possible adverse effects associated with GH, especially with high doses or chronic use, include acromegaly, diabetes, hypertension, and increased risk of serious cardiovascular disease (eg, heart failure). There is also concern about a possible link between GH, which stimulates tumor growth, and cancer. GH stimulates the release of IGF-1 (also called *somatomedin*), a substance that circulates in the blood and stimulates cell division. Most tumor cells have receptors that recognize IGF-1, bind it, and allow it to enter the cell, where it could trigger uncontrolled cell division. This concern may be greater for middle-aged and older adults, because malignancies are more common in these groups than in adolescents and young adults.

APPLYING YOUR KNOWLEDGE 22-4: LEGAL/ETHICAL DILEMMA
During his stay, Mr. Rojas's family comes to visit him often. You meet his mother and his two younger brothers. After one of their visits, Mr. Rojas confides that Juan, age 13, is taking GH because he is in the 35th height percentile for his age. His other brother Miguel, age 15, plays basketball and wants to be taller. Miguel has convinced his brother Juan to share his drug with him. What action should you take and why?

N U R S I N G   A C T I O N S

Hypothalamic and Pituitary Hormones

NURSING ACTIONS	RATIONALE/EXPLANATION
1. **Administer accurately**	
a. Read the manufacturer's instructions and drug labels carefully before drug preparation and administration.	These hormone preparations are given infrequently and often require special techniques of administration.
2. **Observe for therapeutic effects**	Therapeutic effects vary widely, depending on the particular pituitary hormone given and the reason for use.
a. With gonadorelin and related drugs, observe for ovulation or decreased symptoms of endometriosis and absence of menstruation.	Therapeutic effects depend on the reason for use. Note that different formulations are used to stimulate ovulation and treat endometriosis.

NURSING ACTIONS	RATIONALE/EXPLANATION
b. With corticotropin, therapeutic effects stem largely from increased secretion of adrenal cortex hormones, especially the glucocorticoids, and include anti-inflammatory effects (see Chap. 23).	Corticotropin is usually not recommended for the numerous non-endocrine inflammatory disorders that respond to glucocorticoids. Administration of glucocorticoids is more convenient and effective than administration of corticotropin.
c. With chorionic gonadotropin, menotropins, follitropin alpha, and follitropin beta given in cases of female infertility, ovulation and conception are therapeutic effects.	
d. With chorionic gonadotropin given in cryptorchidism, the therapeutic effect is descent of the testicles from the abdomen to the scrotum.	
e. With growth hormone, observe for increased skeletal growth and development.	Indicated by appropriate increases in height and weight
f. With antidiuretics (desmopressin and vasopressin), observe for decreased urine output, increased urine specific gravity, decreased signs of dehydration, decreased thirst.	These effects indicate control of diabetes insipidus.
g. With oxytocin given to induce labor, observe for the beginning or the intensifying of uterine contractions.	
h. With oxytocin given to control postpartum bleeding, observe for a firm uterine fundus and decreased vaginal bleeding.	
i. With octreotide given for diarrhea, observe for decreased number and fluidity of stools.	Octreotide is often used to control diarrhea associated with a number of conditions.
3. Observe for adverse effects	
a. With gonadorelin, observe for headache, nausea, lightheadedness, and local edema, pain, and pruritus after subcutaneous injections.	Systemic reactions occur infrequently.
b. With aberelix, observe for hot flushes, sleep disturbance, breast enlargement, and back pain.	Most of these adverse effects are due to the reduction of testosterone secretion by the testes.
c. With corticotropin, observe for sodium and fluid retention, edema, hypokalemia, hyperglycemia, osteoporosis, increased susceptibility to infection, myopathy, behavioral changes.	These adverse reactions are in general the same as those produced by adrenal cortex hormones. Severity of adverse reactions tends to increase with dosage and duration of corticotropin administration.
d. With human chorionic gonadotropin given to preadolescent boys, observe for sexual precocity, breast enlargement, and edema.	Sexual precocity results from stimulation of excessive testosterone secretion at an early age.
e. With growth hormone, observe for mild edema, headache, localized muscle pain, weakness, and hyperglycemia.	Adverse effects are not common. Another adverse effect may be development of antibodies to the drug, but this does not prevent its growth-stimulating effects.
f. With menotropins, observe for symptoms of ovarian hyperstimulation, such as abdominal discomfort, weight gain, ascites, pleural effusion, oliguria, and hypotension.	Adverse effects can be minimized by frequent pelvic examinations to check for ovarian enlargement and by laboratory measurement of estrogen levels. Multiple gestation (mostly twins) is a possibility and is related to ovarian overstimulation.
g. With desmopressin, observe for headache, nasal congestion, nausea, and increased blood pressure. A more serious adverse reaction is water retention and hyponatremia.	Adverse reactions usually occur only with high dosages and tend to be relatively mild. Water intoxication (headache, nausea, vomiting, confusion, lethargy, coma, convulsions) may occur with any antidiuretic therapy if excessive fluids are ingested.
h. With pegvisomant, observe for pain, injection site reaction, nausea, flu syndrome, and diarrhea.	Adverse effects are usually mild or occur infrequently.
i. With vasopressin, observe for water intoxication; chest pain, myocardial infarction, increased blood pressure; abdominal cramps, nausea, and diarrhea.	With high doses, vasopressin constricts blood vessels, especially coronary arteries, and stimulates smooth muscle of the gastrointestinal tract. Special caution is necessary in clients with heart disease, asthma, or epilepsy.

(continued)

NURSING ACTIONS	RATIONALE/EXPLANATION
j. With oxytocin, observe for excessive stimulation or contractility of the uterus, uterine rupture, and cervical and perineal lacerations.	Severe adverse reactions are most likely to occur when oxytocin is given to induce labor and delivery.
k. With octreotide, observe for dysrhythmias, bradycardia, diarrhea, headache, hyperglycemia, injection-site pain, and symptoms of gallstones.	These are more common effects, especially in those receiving octreotide for acromegaly.
l. With triptorelin, observe for hot flushes, skeletal pain, impotence, headache, and hypertension.	Adverse reactions due to decreased levels of LH and FSH
4. **Observe for drug interactions**	
a. Drugs that *increase* effects of vasopressin:	Potentiate vasopressin
(1) General anesthetics, chlorpropamide (Diabinese)	
b. Drug that *decreases* effects of vasopressin:	
(1) Lithium	Inhibits the renal tubular reabsorption of water normally stimulated by vasopressin
c. Drugs that *increase* effects of oxytocin:	
(1) Estrogens	With adequate estrogen levels, oxytocin increases uterine contractility. When estrogen levels are low, the effect of oxytocin is reduced.
(2) Vasoconstrictors or vasopressors (eg, ephedrine, epinephrine, norepinephrine)	Severe, persistent hypertension with rupture of cerebral blood vessels may occur because of additive vasoconstrictor effects. This is a potentially lethal interaction and should be avoided.

APPLYING YOUR KNOWLEDGE: ANSWERS

22-1 The dose is to be given in two divided doses. You should have administered 0.1 mL in the first dose and the other 0.1 mL in the second dose. The total dose is what is ordered.

22-2 Monitor Mr. Rojas's daily weight, intake and output, and when available, the urine specific gravity. A client with diabetes insipidus will lose 8 to 10 L of urine a day or more. You must monitor the fluid status of the client.

22-3 Mr. Rojas is most likely having a serious adverse reaction to the desmopressin. Hyponatremia and water retention should be reported to the physician and you should continue to monitor the client.

22-4 The nurse has a professional responsibility to discuss the situation with the boys' mother. Excessive hormone increases the risk of health problems for Juan and Miguel.

Review and Application Exercises

Short Answer Exercises

1. What hormones are secreted by the hypothalamus and pituitary, and what are their functions?

2. What are the functions and clinical uses of ADH and GH?

3. What are adverse effects of the hypothalamic and pituitary hormones used in clinical practice?

NCLEX-Style Questions

4. Because GH is an insulin antagonist, administration of GH to a person with type 1 diabetes mellitus may result in which of the following?
   a. hyperglycemia
   b. an increase in insulin production
   c. a decreased need for insulin
   d. no significant effect

5. The father of an 11-year-old boy is concerned because his son is shorter than his friends. He asks the nurse whether the boy should be taking GH so that he can be competitive when playing basketball in middle school. Both of the boy's parents are of short stature. Which of the following is the best response on the part of the nurse?
   a. "The treatment is very expensive so we need to check and see if your insurance will cover it."

b. "Don't worry, many basketball players who are short in stature are successful."

c. "Short stature is not the only requirement for treatment with GH. Let's spend some time discussing how we can determine your son's need for GH."

d. "GH will not increase your child's stature, because you and your wife are also very short."

6. Cosyntropin (Cortrosyn) is commonly used to test for which of the following conditions?

a. hypothalamic dysfunction

b. thyroid cancer

c. pituitary dysfunction

d. adrenal insufficiency

7. A client taking high doses of vasopressin has a blood pressure of 188/96 mm Hg and complains of abdominal cramps, nausea, and diarrhea. The nurse recognizes that these GI symptoms result from which of the following conditions?

a. smooth-muscle stimulation of the GI tract

b. neurologic toxicity

c. gastroparesis

d. drug interaction with a nutrient

Selected References

Drug facts and comparisons. (Updated monthly). St. Louis: Facts and Comparisons.

Guyton, A. C., & Hall, J. E. (2000). *Textbook of medical physiology* (10th ed.). Philadelphia: W. B. Saunders.

Lacy, C. F., Armstrong, L. L., Goldman, M. P., & Lance, L. L. (2004). *Lexi-Comp's drug information handbook* (12th ed.). Hudson, OH: Lexi-Comp.

Marshall, J. C., & Barkan, A. L. (2000). Disorders of the hypothalamus and anterior pituitary. In H. D. Humes (Ed.), *Kelley's Textbook of internal medicine* (4th ed., pp. 2663–2683). Philadelphia: Lippincott Williams & Wilkins.

Porth, C. M. (2005). *Pathophysiology: Concepts of altered health states* (7th ed.). Philadelphia: Lippincott Williams & Wilkins.

Robinson, A. G. (2000). Disorders of posterior pituitary function. In H. D. Humes (Ed.), *Kelley's Textbook of internal medicine* (4th ed., pp. 2684–2691). Philadelphia: Lippincott Williams & Wilkins.

Corticosteroids

OBJECTIVES

After studying this chapter, you will be able to:

1. Review physiologic effects of endogenous corticosteroids.
2. Discuss clinical indications for use of exogenous corticosteroids.
3. Differentiate between physiologic and pharmacologic doses of corticosteroids.
4. Differentiate between short-term and long-term corticosteroid therapy.
5. List at least 10 adverse effects of long-term corticosteroid therapy.
6. Explain the pathophysiologic basis of adverse effects.
7. State the rationale for giving corticosteroids topically when possible rather than systemically.
8. Use other drugs and interventions to decrease the need for corticosteroids.
9. Discuss the use of corticosteroids in selected populations and conditions.
10. Apply the nursing process with a client receiving long-term systemic corticosteroid therapy, including teaching needs.

APPLYING YOUR KNOWLEDGE

Sue Hubble is a 70-year-old African-American female. She is 5 feet 9 inches tall and weighs 275 pounds. She has type 2 diabetes mellitus, and, as a result of lifelong smoking, has been diagnosed with chronic obstructive pulmonary disease (COPD). In her home, she uses oxygen. In addition to her respiratory drugs and her drugs for diabetes, she has been taking prednisone 20 mg PO daily for the past month. You are Ms. Hubble's home care nurse.

INTRODUCTION

Corticosteroids, also called *glucocorticoids* or *steroids*, are hormones produced by the adrenal cortex, part of the adrenal glands. These hormones affect almost all body organs and are extremely important in maintaining homeostasis when secreted in normal amounts. Disease results from inadequate or excessive secretion. Exogenous corticosteroids are used as drugs in a variety of disorders. Their use must be closely monitored, because they have profound therapeutic and adverse effects. To understand the effects of corticosteroids used as drugs (exogenous corticosteroids), it is necessary to understand the physiologic effects and other characteristics of the endogenous hormones.

Secretion of Endogenous Corticosteroids

Corticosteroid secretion is controlled by the hypothalamus, the anterior pituitary, and adrenal cortex (the hypothalamic–pituitary–adrenal, or HPA, axis). Various stimuli (eg, low plasma levels of corticosteroids; pain; anxiety; trauma; illness; anesthesia) activate the system. These stimuli cause the hypothalamus of the brain to secrete corticotropin-releasing hormone or factor (CRH or CRF), which stimulates the anterior pituitary gland to secrete corticotropin, and corticotropin then stimulates the adrenal cortex to secrete corticosteroids.

The rate of corticosteroid secretion is usually maintained within relatively narrow limits but changes according to need. When plasma corticosteroid levels rise to an adequate level, secretion of corticosteroids slows or stops. The mechanism by which the hypothalamus and anterior pituitary "learn" that no more corticosteroids are needed is called a *negative feedback mechanism.*

This negative feedback mechanism is normally very important, but it does not work during stress responses. The stress response activates the sympathetic nervous system (SNS) to produce more epinephrine and norepinephrine and the adrenal cortex to produce as much as 10 times the normal amount of cortisol. The synergistic interaction of these hormones increases the person's ability to respond to stress. However, the increased

SNS activity continues to stimulate cortisol production and overrules the negative feedback mechanism. Excessive and prolonged corticosteroid secretion damages body tissues.

Corticosteroids are secreted directly into the bloodstream. Cortisol is approximately 90% bound to plasma proteins (80% to an alpha globulin called *transcortin* or *cortisol-binding globulin* and 10% to albumin). This high degree of protein binding slows cortisol movement out of the plasma, so that it has a relatively long plasma half-life of 60 to 90 minutes. The remaining 10% is unbound and biologically active. In contrast, aldosterone is only 60% bound to plasma proteins and has a short half-life of 20 minutes. In general, protein binding functions as a storage area from which the hormones are released as needed. This promotes more consistent blood levels and more uniform distribution to the tissues.

Types of Endogenous Corticosteroids

The adrenal cortex produces approximately 30 steroid hormones, which are divided into glucocorticoids, mineralocorticoids, and adrenal sex hormones. Chemically, all corticosteroids are derived from cholesterol and have similar chemical structures. Despite their similarities, however, slight differences cause them to have different functions.

Glucocorticoids

The term *corticosteroids* actually refers to all secretions of the adrenal cortex, but it is most often used to designate the glucocorticoids, which are important in metabolic, inflammatory, and immune processes. Glucocorticoids include cortisol, corticosterone, and cortisone. Cortisol accounts for at least 95% of glucocorticoid activity, and approximately 15 to 20 milligrams of glucocorticoids are secreted daily. Corticosterone accounts for a small amount of activity, and approximately 1.5 to 4 milligrams of corticosterone are secreted daily. Cortisone accounts for little activity and is secreted in minute quantities. Glucocorticoids are secreted cyclically, with the largest amount being produced in the early morning and the smallest amount during the evening hours (in people with a normal day–night schedule). At the cellular level, glucocorticoids account for most of the characteristics and physiologic effects of the corticosteroids (Box 23-1).

Mineralocorticoids

Mineralocorticoids play a vital role in the maintenance of fluid and electrolyte balance. Aldosterone is the main mineralocorticoid and is responsible for approximately 90% of mineralocorticoid activity. Characteristics and physiologic effects of mineralcorticoids are summarized in Box 23-2.

Adrenal Sex Hormones

The adrenal cortex secretes male (androgens) and female (estrogens and progesterone) sex hormones. Compared with the effect of hormones produced by the testes and ovaries, the adrenal sex hormones have an insignificant effect on normal body function. Adrenal androgens, secreted continuously in small quantities by both sexes, are responsible for most of the physiologic effects exerted by the adrenal sex hormones. They increase protein synthesis (anabolism), which increases the mass and strength of muscle and bone tissue; they affect development of male secondary sex characteristics; and they increase hair growth and libido in women. Excessive secretion of adrenal androgens in women causes masculinizing effects (eg, hirsutism, acne, breast atrophy, deepening of the voice, amenorrhea). Female sex hormones are secreted in small amounts and normally exert few physiologic effects. Excessive secretion may produce feminizing effects in men (eg, breast enlargement, decreased hair growth, voice changes).

Disorders of the Adrenal Cortex

Disorders of the adrenal cortex involve increased or decreased production of corticosteroids, especially cortisol as the primary glucocorticoid and aldosterone as the primary mineralocorticoid. These disorders include the following:

- **Primary adrenocortical insufficiency (Addison's disease)** is associated with destruction of the adrenal cortex by disorders such as tuberculosis, cancer, or hemorrhage; with atrophy of the adrenal cortex caused by autoimmune disease or prolonged administration of exogenous corticosteroids; and with surgical excision of the adrenal glands. In primary adrenocortical insufficiency, there is inadequate production of both cortisol and aldosterone.
- **Secondary adrenocortical insufficiency,** produced by inadequate secretion of corticotropin, is most often caused by prolonged administration of corticosteroids. This condition is largely a glucocorticoid deficiency; mineralocorticoid secretion is not significantly impaired.
- **Congenital adrenogenital syndromes and adrenal hyperplasia** result from deficiencies in one or more enzymes required for cortisol production. Low plasma levels of cortisol lead to excessive corticotropin secretion, which then leads to excessive adrenal secretion of androgens and hyperplasia (abnormal increase in number of cells).
- **Androgen-producing tumors** of the adrenal cortex, which are usually benign, produce masculinizing effects.
- **Adrenocortical hyperfunction** (Cushing's disease) may result from excessive corticotropin or a primary adrenal tumor. Adrenal tumors may be benign or malignant. Benign tumors often produce one corticosteroid normally secreted by the adrenal cortex, but malignant tumors often secrete several corticosteroids.
- **Hyperaldosteronism** is a rare disorder caused by adenoma (a benign tissue from glandular tissue) or hyperplasia of the adrenal cortex cells that produce aldosterone. It is characterized by hypokalemia, hypernatremia, hypertension, thirst, and polyuria.

Box 23-1 Effects of Glucocorticoids on Body Processes and Systems

Carbohydrate Metabolism

- ↑Formation of glucose (gluconeogenesis) by breaking down protein into amino acids. The amino acids are then transported to the liver, where they are acted on by enzymes that convert them to glucose. The glucose is then returned to the circulation for use by body tissues or storage in the liver as glycogen.
- ↓Cellular use of glucose, especially in muscle cells. This is attributed to a ↓effect of insulin on the proteins that normally transport glucose into cells and by ↓numbers and functional capacity of insulin receptors.
- Both the ↑production and ↓use of glucose promote higher levels of glucose in the blood (hyperglycemia) and may lead to diabetes mellitus. These actions also increase the amount of glucose stored as glycogen in the liver, skeletal muscles, and other tissues.

Protein Metabolism

- ↑Breakdown of protein into amino acids (catabolic effect); ↑rate of amino acid transport to the liver and conversion to glucose
- ↓Rate of new protein formation from dietary and other amino acids (antianabolic effect)
- The combination of ↑breakdown of cell protein and ↓protein synthesis leads to protein depletion in virtually all body cells except those of the liver. Thus, glycogen stores in the body are ↑ and protein stores are ↓.

Lipid Metabolism

- ↑Breakdown of adipose tissue into fatty acids; the fatty acids are transported in the plasma and used as a source of energy by body cells.
- ↑Oxidation of fatty acids within body cells

Inflammatory and Immune Responses

- ↓Inflammatory response. Inflammation is the normal bodily response to tissue damage and involves three stages. First, a large amount of plasma-like fluid leaks out of capillaries into the damaged area and becomes clotted. Second, leukocytes migrate into the area. Third, tissue healing occurs, largely by growth of fibrous scar tissue. Normal or physiologic amounts of glucocorticoids probably do not significantly affect inflammation and healing, but large amounts of glucocorticoids inhibit all three stages of the inflammatory process.

  More specifically, corticosteroids stabilize lysosomal membranes (and thereby prevent the release of inflammatory proteolytic enzymes); ↓capillary permeability (and thereby ↓leakage of fluid and proteins into the damaged tissue); ↓the accumulation of neutrophils and macrophages at sites of inflammation (and thereby impair phagocytosis of pathogenic microorganisms and waste products of cellular metabolism);

and ↓production of inflammatory chemicals, such as interleukin-1, prostaglandins, and leukotrienes, by injured cells.
- ↓Immune response. The immune system normally protects the body from foreign invaders, and several immune responses overlap inflammatory responses, including phagocytosis. In addition, the immune response stimulates the production of antibodies and activated lymphocytes to destroy the foreign substance. Glucocorticoids impair protein synthesis, including the production of antibodies; ↓the numbers of circulating lymphocytes, eosinophils, and macrophages; and ↓amounts of lymphoid tissue. These effects help to account for the immunosuppressive and antiallergic actions of the glucocorticoids.

Cardiovascular System

- Help to regulate arterial blood pressure by modifying vascular smooth muscle tone, by modifying myocardial contractility, and by stimulating renal mineralocorticoid and glucocorticoid receptors
- ↑The response of vascular smooth muscle to the pressor effects of catecholamines and other vasoconstrictive agents

Nervous System

- Physiologic amounts help to *maintain normal nerve excitability;* pharmacologic amounts ↓nerve excitability, slow activity in the cerebral cortex, and alter brain wave patterns.
- ↓Secretion of corticotropin-releasing hormone by the hypothalamus and of corticotropin by the anterior pituitary gland. This results in suppression of further glucocorticoid secretion by the adrenal cortex (negative feedback system).

Musculoskeletal System

- Maintain muscle strength when present in physiologic amounts but cause muscle atrophy (from protein breakdown) when present in excessive amounts
- ↓Bone formation and growth and ↑bone breakdown. Glucocorticoids also ↓intestinal absorption and ↑renal excretion of calcium. These effects contribute to bone demineralization (osteoporosis) in adults and to ↓linear growth in children.

Respiratory System

- Maintain open airways. Glucocorticoids do not have direct bronchodilating effects, but help to maintain and restore responsiveness to the bronchodilating effects of endogenous catecholamines, such as epinephrine.
- Stabilize mast cells and other cells to inhibit the release of bronchoconstrictive and inflammatory substances, such as histamine.

Gastrointestinal System

- ↓Viscosity of gastric mucus. This effect may ↓protective properties of the mucus and contribute to the development of peptic ulcer disease.

↑, increase/increased; ↓, decrease/decreased;

Box 23-2 Effects of Mineralocorticoids on Body Processes and Systems

- The overall physiologic effects are to conserve sodium and water and eliminate potassium. Aldosterone increases sodium reabsorption from kidney tubules, and water is reabsorbed along with the sodium. When sodium is conserved, another cation must be excreted to maintain electrical neutrality of body fluids; thus, potassium is excreted. This is the only potent mechanism for controlling the concentration of potassium ions in extracellular fluids.
- Secretion of aldosterone is controlled by several factors, most of which are related to kidney function. In general, secretion is increased when the potassium level of extra-

cellular fluid is high, the sodium level of extracellular fluid is low, the renin–angiotensin system of the kidneys is activated, or the anterior pituitary gland secretes corticotropin.
- Inadequate secretion of aldosterone causes hyperkalemia, hyponatremia, and extracellular fluid volume deficit (dehydration). Hypotension and shock may result from decreased cardiac output. Absence of mineralocorticoids causes death.
- Excessive secretion of aldosterone produces hypokalemia, hypernatremia, and extracellular fluid volume excess (water intoxication). Edema and hypertension may result.

GENERAL CHARACTERISTICS OF EXOGENOUS CORTICOSTEROIDS

Mechanisms of Action

Like endogenous glucocorticoids, exogenous drug molecules act at the cellular level by binding to glucocorticoid receptors in target tissues. The drugs are lipid soluble and easily diffuse through the cell membranes of target cells. Inside the cell, they bind with receptors in intracellular cytoplasm. The drug–receptor complex then moves to the cell nucleus, where it interacts with DNA to stimulate or suppress gene transcription.

Glucocorticoids increase or decrease transcription of many genes to alter the synthesis of proteins that regulate their many physiologic effects (eg, enzymes, transport proteins, structural proteins). Metabolic effects do not occur for at least 45 to 60 minutes because of the time required for protein synthesis. Several hours or days may be needed for full production of proteins.

Because the genes vary in different types of body cells, glucocorticoid effects also vary, depending on the specific cells being targeted. For example, supraphysiologic concentrations of glucocorticoids induce the synthesis of lipolytic and proteolytic enzymes and other specific proteins in various tissues. Overall, corticosteroids have multiple mechanisms of action and effects (Fig. 23-1), including the following:

- **Inhibiting arachidonic acid metabolism.** Normally, when a body cell is injured or activated by various stimuli, the enzyme phospholipase A_2 causes the phospholipids in cell membranes to release arachidonic acid. Free arachidonic acid is then metabolized to produce proinflammatory prostaglandins (see Chap. 7) and leukotrienes. At sites of tissue injury or inflammation, corticosteroids induce the synthesis of proteins that suppress the activation of phospholipase A_2. This action, in turn, decreases the release of arachidonic acid and the formation of prostaglandins and leukotrienes.

- **Strengthening or stabilizing biologic membranes.** Two biologic membranes are especially important in inflammatory processes. Stabilization of *cell membranes* inhibits the release of arachidonic acid and production of prostaglandins and leukotrienes, as described above. Stabilization of *lysosomal membranes* inhibits release of bradykinin, histamine, enzymes, and perhaps other substances from lysosomes. (Lysosomes are intracellular structures that contain inflammatory chemical mediators and enzymes that destroy cellular debris and phagocytized pathogens.) This reduces capillary permeability and thus prevents leakage of fluid into the injured area and development of edema. It also reduces the chemicals that normally cause vasodilation and tissue irritation.

- **Inhibiting the production of interleukin-1, tumor necrosis factor, and other cytokines.** This action also contributes to the anti-inflammatory and immunosuppressant effects of glucocorticoids.

- **Impairing phagocytosis.** The drugs inhibit the ability of phagocytic cells to leave the bloodstream and move into the injured or inflamed tissue.

- **Impairing lymphocytes.** The drugs inhibit the ability of these immune cells to increase in number and perform their functions.

- **Inhibiting tissue repair.** The drugs inhibit the growth of new capillaries, fibroblasts, and collagen needed for tissue repair.

Indications for Use

Corticosteroids are extensively used to treat many different disorders. Except for replacement therapy in deficiency states, the use of corticosteroids is largely empiric. Because the drugs affect virtually every aspect of inflammatory and immune responses, they are used in the treatment of a broad spectrum of diseases with an inflammatory or immunologic component.

Corticosteroid preparations applied topically in ophthalmic and dermatologic disorders are discussed in Chapters 63

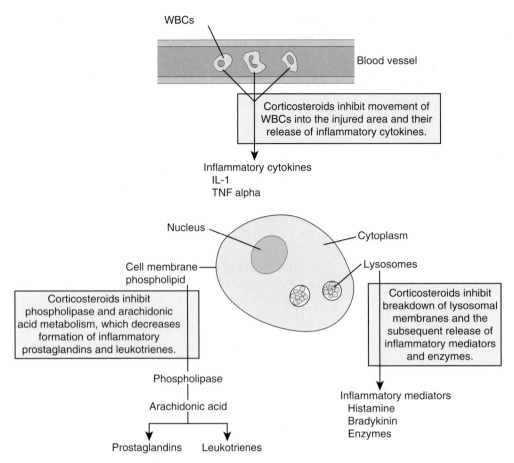

FIGURE 23-1 Inflammatory processes and anti-inflammatory actions of corticosteroids. Cellular responses to injury include the following: Phospholipid in the cell membrane is acted on by phospholipase to release arachidonic acid. Metabolism of arachidonic acid produces the inflammatory mediators prostaglandins and leukotrienes; Lysosomal membrane breaks down and releases inflammatory chemicals (eg, histamine, bradykinin, intracellular digestive enzymes). White blood cells (WBCs) are drawn to the area and release inflammatory cytokines (eg, interleukin-1 [IL-1], tumor necrosis factor [TNF] alpha). Overall, corticosteroid drugs act to inhibit the release, formation, or activation of various inflammatory mediators.

and 64, respectively. The corticosteroids discussed in this chapter are used to treat potentially serious or disabling disorders. These disorders include the following:

- **Allergic** or hypersensitivity disorders, such as allergic reactions to drugs, serum and blood transfusions, and dermatoses with an allergic component
- **Collagen** disorders, such as systemic lupus erythematosus, scleroderma, and periarteritis nodosa. Collagen is the basic structural protein of connective tissue, tendons, cartilage, and bone, and it is therefore present in almost all body tissues and organ systems. The collagen disorders are characterized by inflammation of various body tissues. Signs and symptoms depend on which body tissues or organs are affected and the severity of the inflammatory process.
- **Dermatologic** disorders that may be treated with systemic corticosteroids include acute contact dermatitis, erythema multiforme, herpes zoster (prophylaxis of postherpetic neuralgia), lichen planus, pemphigus, skin rashes caused by drugs, and toxic epidermal necrolysis.
- **Endocrine** disorders, such as adrenocortical insufficiency and congenital adrenal hyperplasia. Corticosteroids are given to replace or substitute for the natural hormones (both glucocorticoids and mineralocorticoids)

in cases of insufficiency and to suppress corticotropin when excess secretion causes adrenal hyperplasia. These conditions are rare and account for a small percentage of corticosteroid usage.

- **Gastrointestinal** disorders, such as ulcerative colitis and regional enteritis (Crohn's disease)
- **Hematologic** disorders, such as idiopathic thrombocytopenic purpura or acquired hemolytic anemia
- **Hepatic** disorders characterized by edema, such as cirrhosis and ascites
- **Neoplastic** disease, such as acute and chronic leukemias, Hodgkin's disease, other lymphomas, and multiple myeloma. The effectiveness of corticosteroids in these conditions probably stems from their ability to suppress lymphocytes and other lymphoid tissue.
- **Neurologic** conditions, such as cerebral edema, brain tumor, acute spinal cord injury, and myasthenia gravis
- **Ophthalmic** disorders, such as optic neuritis, sympathetic ophthalmia, and chorioretinitis
- **Organ or tissue transplants and grafts** (eg, kidney, heart, bone marrow). Corticosteroids suppress cellular and humoral immune responses (see Chap. 41) and help prevent rejection of transplanted tissue. Drug therapy is usually continued as long as the transplanted tissue is in place.

- **Renal** disorders characterized by edema, such as the nephrotic syndrome
- **Respiratory** disorders, such as asthma, status asthmaticus, chronic obstructive pulmonary disease (COPD), and inflammatory disorders of nasal mucosa (rhinitis). In asthma, corticosteroids increase the number of beta-adrenergic receptors and increase or restore responsiveness of beta receptors to beta-adrenergic bronchodilating drugs. In asthma, COPD, and rhinitis, the drugs decrease mucus secretion and inflammation.
- **Rheumatic** disorders, such as ankylosing spondylitis, acute and chronic bursitis, acute gouty arthritis, rheumatoid arthritis, and osteoarthritis
- **Shock.** Corticosteroids are clearly indicated only for shock resulting from adrenocortical insufficiency (Addisonian or adrenal crisis), which may mimic hypovolemic or septic shock. The use of corticosteroids in septic shock has been highly controversial, and randomized studies and meta-analyses have indicated that corticosteroids are not beneficial in treating septic shock. However, more recent small studies indicate possible clinical usefulness in septic shock, because this form of shock may be associated with relative adrenal insufficiency. In anaphylactic shock resulting from an allergic reaction, corticosteroids may increase or restore cardiovascular responsiveness to adrenergic drugs.

Indications for use, routes and dosage ranges are given in Table 23-1.

Contraindications to Use

Corticosteroids are contraindicated in systemic fungal infections and in people who are hypersensitive to drug formulations. They should be used with caution in clients at risk for infections (they may decrease resistance), clients with infections (they may mask signs and symptoms so that infections become more severe before they are recognized and treated), diabetes mellitus (they cause or increase hyperglycemia), peptic ulcer disease, inflammatory bowel disorders, hypertension, congestive heart failure, and renal insufficiency.

APPLYING YOUR KNOWLEDGE 23-1
You arrive at Ms. Hubble's home and begin your assessment of the client. You notice the appearance of white patches on Ms. Hubble's mouth. What action do you take?

All adrenal corticosteroids are available as drug preparations, as are many synthetic derivatives developed by altering the basic steroid molecule in efforts to increase therapeutic effects while minimizing adverse effects. When corticosteroids are administered from sources outside the body, they are given mainly for replacement or therapeutic purposes. Replacement involves small doses to correct a

deficiency state and restore normal function (physiologic effects). Therapeutic purposes require relatively large doses to exert pharmacologic effects. Drug effects involve extension of the physiologic effects of endogenous corticosteroids and new effects that do not occur with small, physiologic doses. The most frequently desired pharmacologic effects are anti-inflammatory, immunosuppressive, antiallergic, and antistress. These are glucocorticoid effects. Mineralocorticoid and androgenic effects are usually considered adverse reactions.

- The drugs are palliative; they control many symptoms but do not cure underlying disease processes. In chronic disorders, they may enable clients to continue the usual activities of daily living and delay disability. However, the disease may continue to progress, and long-term use of systemic corticosteroids inevitably produces serious adverse effects.
- Drug effects vary, so a specific effect may be considered therapeutic in one client but adverse in another. For example, an increased blood sugar level is therapeutic for the client with adrenocortical insufficiency or an islet-cell adenoma of the pancreas, but is an adverse reaction for most clients, especially those with diabetes mellitus. In addition, some clients respond more favorably or experience adverse reactions more readily than others taking equivalent doses. This is partly caused by individual differences in the rate at which corticosteroids are metabolized.
- Administration of exogenous corticosteroids suppresses the HPA axis. This decreases secretion of corticotropin, which, in turn, causes atrophy of the adrenal cortex and decreased production of endogenous adrenal corticosteroids.
- P **Hydrocortisone**, the exogenous equivalent of endogenous cortisol, is the prototype of corticosteroid drugs. When a new corticosteroid is developed, it is compared with hydrocortisone to determine its potency in producing anti-inflammatory and antiallergic responses, increasing deposition of liver glycogen, and suppressing secretion of corticotropin. Daily administration of physiologic doses (15–20 mg of hydrocortisone or its equivalent) or administration of pharmacologic doses (more than 15–20 mg of hydrocortisone or its equivalent) for approximately 2 weeks suppresses the HPA axis. HPA recovery usually occurs within a few weeks or months after corticosteroids are discontinued, but may take 9 to 12 months. During that time, supplemental corticosteroids are usually needed during stressful situations (eg, fever, illness, surgical procedures) to improve the client's ability to respond to stress and prevent acute adrenocortical insufficiency.
- Anti-inflammatory activity of glucocorticoids is approximately equal when the drugs are given in equivalent

(text continues on page 360)

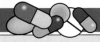 **Table 23-1 Drugs at a Glance: Corticosteroids***

	ROUTES AND DOSAGE RANGES	
GENERIC/TRADE NAME	**Adults**	**Children**
Glucocorticoids		
Beclamethasone oral inhalation (QVAR)	1–2 inhalations (40–80 mcg) 2 times daily (maximum daily dose 320 mcg)	
Nasal inhalation (Beconase AQ)	1–2 inhalations (42–84 mcg in each nostril) 2 times daily; as maintenance, 1 inhalation each nostril	*>6 y:* 1–2 inhalations (42–84 mcg) each nostril daily
Betamethasone (Celestone)	PO 0.6–7.2 mg daily initially, gradually reduced to lowest effective dose	
Betamethasone acetate and sodium phosphate (Celestone Soluspan)	IM 0.5–9 mg daily Intra-articular injection 0.25–2 mL	
Budesonide oral inhalation (Pulmicort Terbuhaler, Pulmicort Respules)	Turbuhaler, 200–400 mcg twice daily	Turbuhaler, *>6 y:* 200 mcg twice daily Respules, *12 mo–8 y:* 0.5 mg daily in 1 single or 2 divided doses
Nasal inhalation (Rhinocort)	256 mcg daily initially (2 sprays each nostril morning and evening or 4 sprays each nostril every morning). When symptoms are controlled, reduce dosage to lowest effective maintenance dose.	*> 6 y:* Same as adults
Oral capsule (Entocort EC)	Crohn's disease, PO 9 mg once daily in the morning, for up to 8 wk	
Cortisone (Cortone)	PO 25–300 mg daily, individualized for condition and response	
Dexamethasone (Decadron)	PO 0.75–9 mg daily in 2–4 doses; higher ranges for serious diseases	
Dexamethasone acetate	IM 8–16 mg (1–2 mL) in single dose, repeated every 1–3 wk if necessary	
Dexamethasone sodium phosphate	IM, IV 0.5–9 mg, depending on severity of disease	
Flunisolide oral inhalation (AeroBid)	2 inhalations (500 mcg) twice daily	*6–15 y:* Same as adults
Nasal inhalation (Nasarel)	2 sprays in each nostril twice daily; maximal daily dose 8 sprays in each nostril	*6–14 y:* 1 spray in each nostril 3 times daily or 2 sprays in each nostril 2 times daily; maximal daily dose 4 sprays in each nostril
Fluticasone (Flovent) oral inhalation	2 inhalations (88 mcg) 2 times daily (maximum daily dose 440 mcg inhaled 2 times daily)	*<12 y:* not recommended
(Flonase) nasal inhalation	200 mcg daily initially (2 sprays each nostril once daily or 1 spray each nostril twice daily). After a few days, reduce dosage to 100 mcg daily (1 spray each nostril once daily) for maintenance therapy.	*≥12 y:* 100 mcg daily (1 spray per nostril once daily)
Hydrocortisone (Hydrocortone, Cortef)	PO 20–240 mg daily, depending on condition and response	
Hydrocortisone sodium phosphate	IV, IM, Sub-Q 15–240 mg daily in 2 divided doses	
Hydrocortisone sodium succinate	IV, IM 100–400 mg initially, repeated at 2, 4, or 6 hour intervals if necessary	

Table 23-1 Drugs at a Glance: Corticosteroids* (continued)

GENERIC/TRADE NAME	ROUTES AND DOSAGE RANGES	
	Adults	Children
Hydrocortisone retention enema (Cortenema)	Rectally, one enema (100 mg) nightly for 21 d or until optimal response	
Hydrocortisone acetate intrarectal foam (Cortifoam)	1 applicatorful 1–2 times daily for 2–3 wk, then once every 2–3 d if needed	
Methylprednisolone (Medrol)	PO 4–48 mg daily initially, gradually reduced to lowest effective level	
Methylprednisolone sodium succinate (Solu-Medrol)	IV, IM 10–40 mg initially, adjusted to condition and response	Infants and children: IV, IM not less than 0.5 mg/kg/24 hours
Methylprednisolone acetate (Depo-Medrol)	IM 40–120 mg once daily	
Mometasone (Nasonex)	2 sprays (50 mcg/spray) in each nostril once daily (200 mcg/d)	*>12 y:* Same as adults *3–11 y:* 1 spray (50 mcg) in each nostril once daily (100 mcg/d)
Prednisolone (Delta-Cortef)	PO 5–60 mg daily initially, adjusted for maintenance	
Prednisolone acetate	IM 4–60 mg daily initially, adjusted for maintenance	
Prednisone (Deltasone)	PO 5–60 mg daily initially, reduced for maintenance	
Triamcinolone (Aristocort, Kenacort)	PO 4–48 mg daily initially, reduced for maintenance	
Triamcinolone acetonide (Kenalog-40)	IM 2.5–60 mg daily, depending on the disease. Reduce dosage and start oral therapy when feasible.	
Oral inhalation (Azmacort)	2 inhalations (200 mcg) 3–4 times daily or 4 inhalations (400 mcg) 2 times daily	*6–12 y:* 1–2 inhalations (100–200 mcg) 3–4 times daily or 2–4 inhalations (200–400 mcg) 2 times daily. Maximum daily dose, 12 inhalations (1200 mcg)
Nasal inhalation (Nasacort)	2 sprays (110 mcg) in each nostril once daily (total dose 220 mcg/d). May increase to maximal daily dose of 440 mcg if indicated	*≥6 y:* 2 sprays (110 mcg) in each nostril once daily (220 mcg/d) initially; reduce to 1 spray per nostril once daily (110 mcg/d)
Triamcinolone diacetate (Aristocort Forte)	IM 20–80 mg initially	
Mineralocorticoid **Fludrocortisone** (Florinef)	Chronic adrenocortical insufficiency, PO 0.1 mg daily Salt-losing adrenogenital syndromes, PO 0.1–0.2 mg daily	PO 0.05–0.1 mg daily

*Ophthalmic and dermatologic preparations are discussed in Chapters 63 and 64, respectively.

IM, intramuscular; IV, intravenous; PO, oral; Sub-Q, subcutaneous.

doses (hydrocortisone 20 mg; prednisone and prednisolone 5 mg; methylprednisolone and triamcinolone 4 mg; dexamethasone 0.75 mg; and betamethasone 0.6 mg). Mineralocorticoid activity is high in cortisone (which is rarely used); intermediate in hydrocortisone, prednisolone, and prednisone; and low in newer agents.

- Duration of action also varies and is only known for oral drugs. Betamethasone and dexamethasone last 48 hours; methylprednisolone, prednisolone, prednisone, and triamcinolone last 18 to 36 hours; and hydrocortisone lasts 18 hours.

- Corticosteroids are metabolized in the liver (mainly by cytochrome P450 3A4 enzymes) and conjugated to inactive metabolites. About 25% of the metabolites are excreted in the bile, then in the feces. The other 75% enter the circulation and are excreted by the kidneys. Metabolism is slowed by hepatic disease, and excretion is slowed by renal disease. In these conditions, corticosteroids may accumulate and cause signs and symptoms of hypercorticism.

APPLYING YOUR KNOWLEDGE 23-2

Ms. Hubble asks you why she has to take the prednisone because it has not made her COPD go away. How should you respond?

NURSING PROCESS

Assessment

Initiation of Corticosteroid Therapy

- For a client expected to receive short-term corticosteroid therapy, the major focus of assessment is the extent and severity of symptoms. Such data can then be used to evaluate the effectiveness of drug therapy.

- For a client expected to receive long-term, systemic corticosteroid therapy, a thorough assessment is needed. This may include diagnostic tests for diabetes mellitus, tuberculosis, and peptic ulcer disease, because these conditions may develop from or be exacerbated by administration of corticosteroid drugs. If one of these conditions is present, corticosteroid therapy must be altered and other drugs given concomitantly.

- If acute infection is found on initial assessment, it should be treated with appropriate antibiotics either before corticosteroid drugs are started or concomitantly with corticosteroid therapy. This is necessary because corticosteroids may mask symptoms of infection and impair healing. Thus, even minor infections can become serious if left untreated during corticosteroid therapy. If infection occurs during long-term corticosteroid therapy, appropriate antibiotic therapy (as determined by culture of the causative microorganism and antibiotic

sensitivity studies) is again indicated. Also, increased doses of corticosteroids are usually indicated to cope with the added stress of the infection.

Previous or Current Corticosteroid Therapy

Initial assessment of every client should include information about previous or current treatment with systemic corticosteroids. This can usually be determined by questioning the client or reviewing medical records.

- If the nurse determines that the client has taken corticosteroids in the past, additional information is needed about the specific drug and dosage taken, the purpose and length of therapy, and when therapy was stopped. Such information is necessary for planning nursing care. If the client had an acute illness and received an oral or injected corticosteroid for approximately 1 week or received corticosteroids by local injection or application to skin lesions, no special nursing care is likely to be required. However, if the client took systemic corticosteroids for 2 weeks or longer during the past year, nursing observations must be especially vigilant. Such a client may be at higher risk for acute adrenocortical insufficiency during stressful situations. If the client has surgery, corticosteroid therapy is restarted either before or on the day of surgery and continued, in decreasing dosage, for a few days after surgery. In addition to anesthesia and surgery, potentially significant sources of stress include hospitalization, various diagnostic tests, concurrent infection or other illnesses, and family problems.

  If the client is currently taking a systemic corticosteroid drug, again the nurse must identify the drug, the dosage and schedule of administration, the purpose for which the drug is being taken, and the length of time involved. After this basic information is obtained, the nurse can further assess client status and plan nursing care. Some specific factors include the following:

- If the client undergoes anesthesia and surgery, expect that higher doses of corticosteroids will be given for several days. This may be done by changing the drug, the route of administration, and the dosage. Specific regimens vary according to type of anesthesia, surgical procedure, client condition, prescriber preference, and other variables. A client having major abdominal surgery may be given 300 to 400 mg of hydrocortisone (or the equivalent dosage of other drugs) on the day of surgery and then be tapered back to maintenance dosage within a few days.

- Note that additional corticosteroids may be given in other situations as well. One extra dose may be adequate for a short-term stress situation, such as an angiogram or other invasive diagnostic test.

- Using all available data, assess the likelihood of the client's having acute adrenal insufficiency.

- Assess for signs and symptoms of adrenocortical excess and adverse drug effects.
- Assess for signs and symptoms of the disease for which long-term corticosteroid therapy is being given.

Nursing Diagnoses

- Disturbed Body Image related to cushingoid changes in appearance
- Imbalanced Nutrition: Less Than Body Requirements related to protein and potassium losses
- Imbalanced Nutrition: More Than Body Requirements related to sodium and water retention and hyperglycemia
- Excess Fluid Volume related to sodium and water retention
- Risk for Injury related to adverse drug effects of impaired wound healing, increased susceptibility to infection, weakening of skin and muscles, osteoporosis, gastrointestinal ulceration, diabetes mellitus, hypertension, and acute adrenocortical insufficiency
- Ineffective Coping related to chronic illness; long-term drug therapy and drug-induced mood changes, irritability and insomnia
- Deficient Knowledge related to disease process and corticosteroid drug therapy

Planning/Goals

The client will

- Take the drug correctly
- Practice measures to decrease the need for corticosteroids and minimize adverse effects
- Be monitored regularly for adverse drug effects
- Keep appointments for follow-up care
- Be assisted to cope with body image changes
- Verbalize or demonstrate essential drug information

Interventions

For clients on long-term, systemic corticosteroid therapy, use supplementary drugs as ordered and nondrug measures to decrease dosage and adverse effects of corticosteroid drugs. Specific measures include the following:

- Help clients set reasonable goals of drug therapy. For example, partial relief of symptoms may be better than complete relief if the latter requires larger doses or longer periods of treatment with systemic drugs.
- In clients with bronchial asthma and COPD, other treatment measures should be continued during corticosteroid therapy. With asthma, the corticosteroid needs to be given on a regular schedule; inhaled bronchodilators can usually be taken as needed.
- In clients with rheumatoid arthritis, rest, physical therapy, and salicylates or other nonsteroid anti-inflammatory drugs are continued. Systemic corticosteroid therapy is reserved for severe, acute exacerbations when possible.

- Help clients identify stressors and find ways to modify or avoid stressful situations when possible. For example, most clients probably do not think of extreme heat or cold or minor infections as significant stressors. However, they can be for people taking corticosteroids. This assessment of potential stressors must be individualized because a situation viewed as stressful by one client may not be stressful to another.
- Encourage activity, if not contraindicated, to slow demineralization of bone (osteoporosis). This is especially important in postmenopausal women who are not taking replacement estrogens, because they are very susceptible to osteoporosis. Walking is preferred if the client is able. Range-of-motion exercises are indicated in immobilized or bedridden people. Also, bedridden clients taking corticosteroids should have their positions changed frequently because these drugs thin the skin and increase the risk of pressure ulcers. This risk is further increased if edema also is present.
- Dietary changes may be beneficial in some clients. Salt restriction may help prevent hypernatremia, fluid retention, and edema. Foods high in potassium may help prevent hypokalemia. A diet high in protein, calcium, and vitamin D may help prevent osteoporosis. Increased intake of vitamin C may help decrease bleeding in the skin and soft tissues.
- Avoid exposing the client to potential sources of infection by washing hands frequently; using aseptic technique when changing dressings; keeping health care personnel and visitors with colds or other infections away from the client; and following other appropriate measures. Reverse or protective isolation is sometimes indicated, commonly for those clients who have had organ transplantation and are receiving corticosteroids to help prevent rejection of the transplanted organ.
- Handle tissues very gently during any procedures (eg, bathing, assisting out of bed, venipunctures). Because long-term corticosteroid therapy weakens the skin and bones, there are risks of skin damage and fractures with even minor trauma.

Client Teaching Guidelines for Long-Term Corticosteroid Therapy are presented in the accompanying display.

Evaluation

- Interview and observe for relief of symptoms for which corticosteroids were prescribed.
- Interview and observe for accurate drug administration.
- Interview and observe for use of nondrug measures indicated for the condition being treated.
- Interview and observe for adverse drug effects on a regular basis.
- Interview regarding drug knowledge and effects to be reported to health care providers.

CLIENT TEACHING GUIDELINES

Long-Term Corticosteroid Therapy

General Considerations

☑ In most instances, corticosteroids are used to relieve symptoms; they do not cure the underlying disease process. However, they can improve comfort and quality of life.

☑ When taking an oral corticosteroid (eg, prednisone) for longer than 2 weeks, it is extremely important to take the drug as directed. Missing a dose or two, stopping the drug, changing the amount or time of administration, taking extra drug (except as specifically directed during stress situations), or any other alterations may result in complications. Some complications are relatively minor; several are serious, even life threatening. When these drugs are being discontinued, the dosage is gradually reduced over several weeks. They must not be stopped abruptly.

☑ Wear a special medical alert bracelet or tag or carry an identification card stating the drug being taken; the dosage; the prescriber's name, address, and telephone number; and instructions for emergency treatment. If an accident or emergency situation occurs, health care providers must know about corticosteroid drug therapy to give additional amounts during the stress of the emergency.

☑ Report to all health care providers consulted that corticosteroid drugs are being taken or have been taken within the past year. Current or previous corticosteroid therapy can influence treatment measures, and such knowledge increases the ability to provide appropriate treatment.

☑ Maintain regular medical supervision. This is extremely important so that the prescriber can detect adverse reactions, evaluate disease status, and evaluate drug response and indications for dosage change, as well as other responsibilities that can be carried out only with personal contact between the prescriber and the client. Periodic blood tests, x-ray studies, and other tests may be performed during long-term corticosteroid therapy.

☑ Take no other drugs, prescription or nonprescription, without notifying the prescriber who is supervising corticosteroid therapy. Corticosteroid drugs influence reactions to other drugs, and some other drugs interact with corticosteroids either to increase or decrease their effects. Thus, taking other drugs can decrease the expected therapeutic benefits or increase the incidence or severity of adverse effects.

☑ Avoid exposure to infection when possible. Avoid crowds and people known to have an infection. Also, wash hands frequently and thoroughly. These drugs increase the likelihood of infection, so preventive measures are necessary. Also, if infection does occur, healing is likely to be slow.

☑ Practice safety measures to avoid accidents (eg, falls and possible fractures due to osteoporosis, cuts or other injuries because of delayed wound healing, soft tissue trauma because of increased tendency to bruise easily).

☑ Weigh frequently when starting corticosteroid therapy and at least weekly during long-term maintenance. An initial weight gain is likely to occur and is usually attributed to increased appetite. Later weight gains may be caused by fluid retention.

☑ Ask the prescriber about the amount and kind of activity or exercise needed. As a general rule, being as active as possible helps to prevent or delay osteoporosis, a common adverse effect. However, increased activity may not be desirable for everyone. A client with rheumatoid arthritis, for example, may become too active when drug therapy relieves joint pain and increases mobility.

☑ Follow instructions for other measures used in treatment of the particular condition (eg, other drugs and physical therapy for rheumatoid arthritis). Such measures may allow smaller doses of corticosteroids and decrease adverse effects.

☑ Because the corticosteroid impairs the ability to respond to stress, dosage may need to be temporarily increased with illness, surgery, or other stressful situations. Clarify with the prescriber predictable sources of stress and the amount of drug to be taken if the stress cannot be avoided.

☑ In addition to stressful situations, report sore throat, fever, or other signs of infection; weight gain of 5 pounds or more in a week; or swelling in the ankles or elsewhere. These symptoms may indicate adverse drug effects and changes in corticosteroid therapy may be indicated.

☑ Muscle weakness and fatigue or disease symptoms may occur when drug dosage is reduced, withdrawn, or omitted (eg, the non-drug day of alternate-day therapy). Although these symptoms may cause some discomfort, they should be tolerated if possible rather than increasing the corticosteroid dose. If severe, of course, dosage or time of administration may have to be changed.

☑ Dietary changes may be helpful in reducing some adverse effects of corticosteroid therapy. Decreasing salt intake (eg, by not adding table salt to foods and avoiding obviously salty foods, such as many snack foods and prepared sandwich meats) may help decrease swelling. Eating high-potassium foods, such as citrus fruits and juices or bananas, may help prevent potassium loss. An adequate intake of calcium, protein, and vitamin D (meat and dairy products are good sources) may help to prevent or delay osteoporosis. Vitamin C (eg, from citrus fruits) may help to prevent excessive bruising.

☑ Do not object when your prescriber reduces your dose of oral corticosteroid, with the goal of stopping the drug entirely or continuing with a smaller dose. Long-term therapy should be used only when necessary because of the potential for serious adverse effects, and the lowest effective dose should be given.

☑ With local applications of corticosteroids, there is usually little systemic absorption and few adverse effects, compared with oral or injected drugs. When effective in relieving symptoms, it is better to use a local than a systemic corticosteroid. In some instances, combined systemic and local application allows administration of a lesser dose of the systemic drug.

Commonly used local applications are applied topically for skin disorders; by oral inhalation for asthma; and by nasal inhalation for allergic rhinitis. Although long-term use is usually well tolerated, systemic toxicity can occur if excess corticosteroid is inhaled or if occlusive dressings are used over skin lesions. Thus, a corticosteroid for local application must be applied correctly and not overused.

CLIENT TEACHING GUIDELINES

Long-Term Corticosteroid Therapy (Continued)

☑ Corticosteroids are not the same as the steroids often abused by athletes and body builders. Those are anabolic steroids derived from testosterone, the male sex hormone.

Self- or Caregiver Administration

☑ Take an oral corticosteroid with a meal or snack to decrease gastrointestinal upset.

☑ If taking the medication once a day or every other day, take before 9 AM; if taking multiple doses, take at evenly spaced intervals throughout the day.

☑ Report to the prescriber if unable to take a dose orally because of vomiting or some other problem. In some circumstances, the dose may need to be given by injection.

☑ If taking an oral corticosteroid in tapering doses, be sure to follow instructions exactly to avoid adverse effects.

☑ When applying a corticosteroid to skin lesions, do not apply more often than ordered and do not cover with an occlusive dressing unless specifically instructed to do so.

☑ With an intranasal corticosteroid, use on a regular basis (usually once or twice daily) for the best anti-inflammatory effects.

☑ With an oral-inhalation corticosteroid, use on a regular schedule for anti-inflammatory effects. The drugs are *not* effective in relieving acute asthma attacks or shortness of breath and should not be used "as needed" for that purpose. Use metered-dose inhalers as follows (unless instructed otherwise by a health care provider):

1. Shake canister thoroughly.
2. Place canister between lips (both open and pursed lips have been recommended) or outside lips.
3. Exhale completely.
4. Activate canister while taking a slow, deep breath.
5. Hold breath for 10 seconds or as long as possible.
6. Wait at least 1 minute before taking additional inhalations.
7. Rinse mouth after inhalations to decrease the incidence of oral thrush (a fungal infection).
8. Rinse mouthpiece at least once per day.

APPLYING YOUR KNOWLEDGE 23-3

You test Ms. Hubble's blood glucose level and it is 345 mg/dL. Why is this client hyperglycemic, and what action should you take?

PRINCIPLES OF THERAPY

Goal of Therapy

The goal of corticosteroid therapy is usually to reduce symptoms to a tolerable level. Total suppression of symptoms may require excessively large doses and produce excessive adverse effects. Because systemic corticosteroids can cause serious adverse reactions, indications for their clinical use should be as clear-cut as possible.

Drug Selection

Choice of corticosteroid drug is influenced by many factors, including the purpose for use, characteristics of specific drugs, desired route of administration, characteristics of individual clients, and expected adverse effects. Some guidelines for rational drug choice include the following:

● Hydrocortisone and cortisone are usually the drugs of choice in adrenocortical insufficiency which requires replacement of both glucocorticoids and mineralocorticoids whether caused by Addison's disease, adrenalectomy, or inadequate corticotropin. These drugs have greater mineralocorticoid activity compared with other corticosteroids. If additional mineralocor-

ticoid activity is required, fludrocortisone can be given.

● Prednisone is often the glucocorticoid of choice in nonendocrine disorders in which anti-inflammatory, antiallergic, antistress, and immunosuppressive effects are desired. A corticosteroid drug with primarily glucocorticoid activity is necessary.

● Beclomethasone (QVAR, Beconase AQ), budesonide (Pulmicort, Rhinocort), flunisolide (AeroBid), fluticasone (Flonase, Flovent), mometasone (Nasonex), and triamcinolone (Azmacort, Nasacort) are corticosteroids formulated to be given by oral or nasal inhalation in respiratory disorders. Their use replaces, prevents, delays, or decreases use of systemic drugs and thereby decreases risks of serious adverse effects. However, high doses or frequent use may suppress adrenocortical function.

● Dexamethasone (parenterally or orally) is considered the corticosteroid of choice for cerebral edema associated with brain tumors, craniotomy, or head injury, because dexamethasone is thought to penetrate the blood–brain barrier more readily and achieve higher concentrations in cerebrospinal fluids and tissues. It also has minimal sodium- and water-retaining properties. With brain tumors, the drug is more effective in metastatic lesions and glioblastomas than astrocytomas and meningiomas.

● Hydrocortisone, dexamethasone, and methylprednisolone are among those drugs that may be given parenterally and are useful in acute, life-threatening situations that require such administration, usually intravenously (IV). This requirement limits the choice of drugs, because not all corticosteroids are available in injectable preparations.

Drug Dosage

Many factors have an effect on drug dosage, such as the specific drug to be given, the desired route of administration, the reason for use, expected adverse effects, and client characteristics. In general, the smallest effective dose should be given for the shortest effective time. The dosage must be individualized according to the severity of the disorder being treated, whether the disease is acute or chronic, and the client's response to drug therapy. (Dosage for children is calculated according to severity of disease rather than weight.) If life-threatening disease is present, high doses are usually given until acute symptoms subside. Then the dose is gradually reduced until a maintenance dose is determined or the drug is discontinued. If life-threatening disease is not present, relatively high doses may still be given initially and then lowered. Doses should be gradually reduced (tapered) over several days. With long-term corticosteroid therapy, periodic attempts to reduce dosage are desirable to decrease adverse effects. One way is to reduce the dose gradually until symptoms worsen, indicating the minimally effective dose.

Physiologic doses (approximately 15–20 mg of hydrocortisone or its equivalent daily) are given to replace or substitute for endogenous adrenocortical hormone. Pharmacologic doses (supraphysiologic amounts) are usually required for anti-inflammatory, antiallergic, antistress, and immunosuppressive effects.

Compared with hydrocortisone, newer corticosteroids are more potent on a weight basis but are equipotent in anti-inflammatory effects when given in equivalent doses. Statements of equivalency with hydrocortisone are helpful in evaluating new drugs, comparing different drugs, and changing drugs or dosages. However, dosage equivalents apply only to drugs given orally or IV.

Drug Administration

Routes of Administration

Corticosteroids can be given by several different routes, based on the clinical problem, to produce local or systemic effects. If feasible, these drugs should be given locally rather than systemically to prevent or decrease systemic toxicity. In recent years there have been several formulations developed for oral inhalation in the treatment of asthma and for nasal inhalation in the treatment of allergic rhinitis. When these drugs must be given systemically, the oral route is preferred. Parenteral administration is indicated only for clients who are seriously ill or unable to take oral medications.

For intramuscular or IV injections, sodium phosphate or sodium succinate salts are used because they are most soluble in water. For intra-articular or intralesional injections, acetate salts are used because they have low solubility in water and provide prolonged local action.

Frequency of Administration

Scheduling of drug administration is more important with corticosteroids than with most other drug classes. Most adverse effects occur with long-term administration of high doses. A major adverse reaction is suppression of the HPA axis and subsequent loss of adrenocortical function. Certain schedules are often recommended to prevent or minimize HPA suppression.

Corticosteroids can be given in relatively large, divided doses for approximately 48 to 72 hours in acute situations until the condition has been brought under control. After acute symptoms subside or 48 to 72 hours have passed, the dosage is tapered so that a slightly smaller dose is given each day until the drug can be discontinued completely (total period of use: approximately 1 week). Such a regimen may be useful in allergic reactions, contact dermatitis, exacerbations of chronic conditions (eg, bronchial asthma), and stressful situations such as surgery.

Daily administration is required in cases of chronic adrenocortical insufficiency. The entire daily dose can be taken each morning, between 6 and 9 A.M. This schedule simulates normal endogenous corticosteroid secretion.

Alternate-day therapy (ADT), in which a double dose is taken every other morning, is usually preferred for other chronic conditions. This schedule allows rest periods so that adverse effects are decreased while anti-inflammatory effects continue. ADT seems to be as effective as more frequent administration in most clients with bronchial asthma, ulcerative colitis, and other conditions for which long-term corticosteroid therapy is prescribed. ADT is used only for maintenance therapy (ie, clinical signs and symptoms are controlled initially with more frequent drug administration). ADT can be started after symptoms have subsided and stabilized.

Intermediate-acting glucocorticoids (eg, prednisone, prednisolone, methylprednisolone) are the drugs of choice for ADT. Long-acting drugs (eg, betamethasone, dexamethasone) are not recommended because of their prolonged suppression of adrenocortical function.

ADT has other advantages. It probably decreases susceptibility to infection and does not retard growth in children, as do other schedules.

ADT is not usually indicated in clients who have previously received corticosteroids on a long-term basis. First, these clients already have maximal HPA suppression, so a major advantage of ADT is lost. Second, if these clients begin ADT, recurrence of symptoms and considerable discomfort may occur on days when drugs are omitted. Clients with severe disease and very painful or disabling symptoms also may experience severe discomfort with ADT.

Stress Dosage Corticosteroid Therapy

Long-term use of pharmacologic doses (eg, more than 5 mg of prednisone daily) produces adverse reactions. For this reason, long-term corticosteroid therapy should be reserved for life-threatening conditions or severe, disabling symptoms that do not respond to treatment with more benign drugs or other measures. For people receiving chronic corticosteroid therapy, dosage must be increased during periods of stress or illness. Some common sources of stress for most people include surgery and anesthesia, infections, anxiety, and extremes of temperature. Note that events that are stressful for one client may not be stressful for another. Some guidelines for corticosteroid dosage during stress include the following:

- During minor or relatively mild illness (eg, viral upper respiratory infection; any febrile illness; strenuous exercise; gastroenteritis with vomiting and diarrhea; minor surgery), doubling the daily maintenance dose is usually adequate. After the stress period is over, dosage may be reduced abruptly to the usual maintenance dose.
- During major stress or severe illness, even larger doses are necessary. For example, a client undergoing abdominal surgery may require 300 to 400 mg of hydrocortisone on the day of surgery. This dose can gradually be reduced to usual maintenance doses within approximately 5 days if postoperative recovery is uncomplicated. As a general rule, it is better to administer excessive doses temporarily than to risk inadequate doses and adrenal insufficiency. The client also may require sodium chloride and fluid replacement, antibiotic therapy if infection is present, and supportive measures if shock occurs.
- During acute stress situations of short duration, such as traumatic injury or invasive diagnostic tests (eg, angiography), a single dose of approximately 100 mg of hydrocortisone immediately after the injury or before the diagnostic test is usually sufficient.
- Many chronic diseases that require long-term corticosteroid therapy are characterized by exacerbations and remissions. Dosage of corticosteroids usually must be increased during acute flare-ups of disease symptoms but can then be decreased gradually to maintenance levels.

Treatment of Specific Disorders

Allergic Rhinitis

Allergic rhinitis (also called *seasonal rhinitis, hay fever,* and *perennial rhinitis*) is a common problem for which corticosteroids are given by nasal spray, once or twice daily. Therapeutic effects usually occur within a few days with regular use. Systemic adverse effects are minimal with recommended doses but may occur with higher doses, including adrenocortical insufficiency from HPA suppression.

Arthritis

Corticosteroids are the most effective drugs for rapid relief of the pain, edema, and restricted mobility associated with acute episodes of joint inflammation. They are usually given on a short-term basis. When inflammation is limited to three or fewer joints, the preferred route of drug administration is by injection directly into the joint. Intra-articular injections relieve symptoms in approximately 2 to 8 weeks, and several formulations are available for this route. However, corticosteroids do not prevent disease progression and joint destruction. As a general rule, a joint should not be injected more often than three times yearly because of risks of infection and damage to intra-articular structures from the injections and from overuse when pain is relieved.

Asthma

Corticosteroids are commonly used in the treatment of asthma because of their anti-inflammatory effects. In addition, corticosteroids increase the effects of adrenergic bronchodilators to prevent or treat bronchoconstriction and bronchospasm. The drugs work by increasing the number and responsiveness of beta-adrenergic receptors and preventing the tolerance usually associated with chronic administration of these bronchodilators. Research studies indicate that responsiveness to beta-adrenergic bronchodilators increases within 2 hours and that numbers of beta receptors increase within 4 hours.

In acute asthma or status asthmaticus unrelieved by inhaled beta-adrenergic bronchodilators, high doses of systemic corticosteroids are given orally or IV along with bronchodilators for approximately 5 to 10 days. Although these high doses suppress the HPA axis, the suppression lasts for only 1 to 3 days, and other serious adverse effects are avoided. Thus, systemic corticosteroids are used for short-term therapy, as needed, and not for long-term treatment. People who regularly use inhaled corticosteroids also require high doses of systemic drugs during acute attacks because aerosols are not effective. As soon as acute symptoms subside, the dose should be tapered; the lowest effective maintenance dose should be used, or the drug should be discontinued.

In chronic asthma, inhaled corticosteroids are the drugs of first choice. This recommendation evolved from increased knowledge about the importance of inflammation in the pathophysiology of asthma and the development of aerosol corticosteroids that are effective with minimal adverse effects. Inhaled drugs may be given alone or with systemic drugs. In general, inhaled corticosteroids can replace oral drugs when daily dosage of the oral drug has been tapered to 10 to 15 milligrams of prednisone or the equivalent. When a client is being switched from an oral to an inhaled corticosteroid, the inhaled drug should be started during tapering of the oral drug, approximately 1 or 2 weeks before discontinuing or reaching the lowest anticipated dose of the oral drug. When a client requires a systemic corticosteroid, co-administration of an aerosol allows smaller doses of the systemic corticosteroid. Although the inhaled drugs can cause suppression of the HPA axis and adrenocortical function, especially at higher doses, they are much less likely to do so than systemic drugs.

Cancer

Corticosteroids are commonly used in the treatment of lymphomas, lymphocytic leukemias, and multiple myeloma. In these disorders, corticosteroids inhibit cell reproduction and are cytotoxic to lymphocytes. In addition to their anticancer effects in hematologic malignancies, corticosteroids are beneficial in treatment of several signs and symptoms that often accompany cancer, although the mechanisms of action are unknown and drug/dosage regimens vary widely. Corticosteroids are used to treat anorexia; nausea and vomiting; cerebral edema and inflammation associated with brain metastases or radiation of the head; spinal cord compression; pain and edema related to pressure on nerves or bone metastases; graft-versus-host disease after bone marrow transplantation; and other disorders that occur in clients with cancer. Clients tend to feel better when taking corticosteroids, although the basic disease process may be unchanged.

Primary Central Nervous System Lymphomas

Formerly considered rare tumors of older adults, central nervous system lymphomas are being diagnosed more frequently in younger clients. They are usually associated with chronic immunosuppression caused by immunosuppressant drugs or acquired immunodeficiency syndrome (AIDS). Many of these lymphomas are very sensitive to corticosteroids, and therapy is indicated when the diagnosis is established.

Other Central Nervous System Tumors

Corticosteroid therapy may be useful in both supportive and definitive treatment of brain and spinal cord tumors, and neurologic signs and symptoms often improve dramatically within 24 to 48 hours. Corticosteroids help relieve symptoms by controlling edema around the tumor, at operative sites, and at sites receiving radiation therapy. Some clients no longer require corticosteroids after surgical or radiation therapy, whereas others require continued therapy to manage neurologic symptoms. Adverse effects of long-term corticosteroid therapy may include mental changes ranging from mild agitation to psychosis, and steroid myopathy (muscle weakness and atrophy) that may be confused with tumor progression. Mental symptoms usually improve if drug dosage is reduced and resolve if the drug is discontinued; steroid myopathy may persist for weeks or months.

Chemotherapy-Induced Emesis

Corticosteroids have strong antiemetic effects; the mechanism is unknown. One effective regimen is a combination of an oral or IV dose of dexamethasone (10–20 mg) and a serotonin antagonist or metoclopramide given immediately before the chemotherapeutic drug. This regimen is the treatment of choice for chemotherapy with cisplatin, which is a strongly emetic drug.

Chronic Obstructive Pulmonary Disease

Corticosteroids are more helpful in acute exacerbations than in stable COPD. However, oral corticosteroids may improve pulmonary function and symptoms in some clients. For example, for a client with inadequate relief from a bronchodilator, a trial of a corticosteroid (eg, prednisone 20–40 mg each morning for 5–7 days) may be justified. Treatment should be continued only if there is significant improvement. As in other conditions, the lowest effective dose is needed to minimize adverse drug effects.

Inhaled corticosteroids can also be tried. They produce minimal adverse effects, but their effectiveness in COPD has not been clearly demonstrated.

Inflammatory Bowel Disease

Crohn's disease and ulcerative colitis often require periodic corticosteroid therapy.

In moderate Crohn's disease, oral prednisone, 40 milligrams daily, is usually given until symptoms subside. With severe disease, clients often require hospitalization, IV fluids for hydration, and parenteral corticosteroids until symptoms subside. An oral form of budesonide (Entocort EC) may be used for Crohn's disease. The capsule dissolves in the small intestine and acts locally before being absorbed into the bloodstream and transported to the liver for metabolism. It has fewer adverse effects than systemic corticosteroids, but is also less effective and more expensive.

In ulcerative colitis, corticosteroids are usually used when aminosalicylates (eg, mesalamine) are not effective or when symptoms are more severe. Initially, hydrocortisone enemas may be effective. If not effective, oral prednisone (20–60 mg daily) may be given until symptoms subside. In severe disease, oral prednisone may be required initially. After remission of symptoms is achieved, the dose can be tapered by 2.5 to 5 milligrams per day each week to a dose of 20 milligrams. Then, tapering may be slowed to 2.5 to 5 milligrams per day every other week. As in Crohn's disease, clients with severe ulcerative colitis often require hospitalization and parenteral corticosteroids. One regimen uses IV hydrocortisone 300 milligrams per day or the equivalent dose of another drug. When the client's condition improves, oral prednisone can replace the IV corticosteroid.

Spinal Cord Injury

High-dose corticosteroid therapy to treat spinal cord injury is a common practice in clinical settings, although controversy exists regarding its use. Data suggest that methylprednisolone may be effective in acute spinal cord injury when given in high doses within 8 hours of the injury. Methylprednisolone improves neurologic recovery, although it does not improve mortality, and its use is unlikely to result in normal neurologic function. In addition, severe adverse outcomes including wound and systemic infections, gastrointestinal hemorrhage, and pneumonia have been reported.

Prevention of Acute Adrenocortical Insufficiency

Suppression of the HPA axis may occur with corticosteroid therapy and may lead to life-threatening inability to increase cortisol secretion when needed to cope with stress. It is most likely to occur with abrupt withdrawal of systemic corticosteroid drugs. The risk of HPA suppression is high with systemic drugs given for more than a few days, although clients vary in degree and duration of suppression with comparable doses, and the minimum dose and duration of therapy that cause suppression are unknown.

When corticosteroids are given for replacement therapy, adrenal insufficiency is lifelong, and drug administration must be continued. When the drugs are given for purposes other than replacement and then discontinued, the HPA axis usually recovers within several weeks to months, but recovery may take a year. Several strategies have been developed to minimize HPA suppression and risks of acute adrenal insufficiency, including:

- Administering a systemic corticosteroid during high-stress situations (eg, moderate or severe illness, trauma, surgery) to clients who have received pharmacologic doses for 2 weeks within the previous year or who receive long-term systemic therapy (ie, are steroid dependent)
- Giving short courses of systemic therapy for acute disorders, such as asthma attacks, then decreasing the dose or stopping the drug within a few days
- Gradually tapering the dose of any systemic corticosteroid. Although specific guidelines for tapering dosage have not been developed, higher doses and longer durations of administration in general require slower tapering, possibly over several weeks. The goal of tapering may be to stop the drug or to decrease the dosage to the lowest effective amount.
- Using local rather than systemic therapy when possible, alone or in combination with low doses of systemic drugs. Numerous preparations are available for local application, including aerosols for oral or nasal inhalation; formulations for topical application to the skin, eyes, and ears; and drugs for intra-articular injections.
- Using ADT, which involves titrating the daily dose to the lowest effective maintenance level, then giving a double dose every other day

Use in Special Populations

Use in Children

Corticosteroids are used for the same conditions in children as in adults; a common indication is for treatment of asthma. With severe asthma, continual corticosteroid therapy may be required. A major concern with children is growth retardation, which can occur with small doses and administration by inhalation. Many children have a growth spurt when the corticosteroid is discontinued. Drug effects on adult stature are unknown.

Parents and prescribers can monitor drug effects by recording height and weight weekly. ADT is less likely to impair normal growth and development than daily administration. In addition, for both systemic and inhaled corticosteroids, each child's dose should be titrated to the lowest effective amount.

Use in Older Adults

Corticosteroids are used for the same conditions in older adults as in younger ones. Older adults are especially likely to have conditions that are aggravated by the drugs (eg, congestive heart failure, hypertension, diabetes mellitus, arthritis, osteoporosis, increased susceptibility to infection, concomitant drug therapy that increases risks of gastrointestinal ulceration and bleeding). Consequently, risk–benefit ratios of systemic corticosteroid therapy should be carefully considered, especially for long-term therapy.

When used, lower doses are usually indicated because of decreased muscle mass, plasma volume, hepatic metabolism, and renal excretion in older adults. In addition, therapeutic and adverse responses should be monitored regularly by a health care provider (eg, blood pressure, serum electrolytes, and blood glucose levels at least every 6 months). As in other populations, adverse effects are less likely to occur with oral or nasal inhalations than with oral drugs.

Use in Clients With Renal Impairment

Systemic corticosteroids should be used with caution because of slowed excretion, with possible accumulation and signs and symptoms of hypercorticism. In renal transplantation, corticosteroids are extensively used, along with other immunosuppressive drugs, to prevent or treat rejection reactions. In these clients, as in others, adverse effects of systemic corticosteroids may include infections, hypertension, glucose intolerance, obesity, cosmetic changes, bone loss, growth retardation in children, cataracts, pancreatitis, peptic ulcerations, and psychiatric disturbances. Doses should be minimized, and eventually the drugs can be withdrawn in some clients.

Use in Clients With Hepatic Impairment

Metabolism of corticosteroids is slowed by severe hepatic disease, and corticosteroids may accumulate and cause signs and symptoms of hypercorticism. In addition, clients with liver disease should be given prednisolone rather than prednisone. Liver metabolism of prednisone is required to convert it to its active form, prednisolone.

Use in Clients With Critical Illness

Corticosteroids have been extensively used in the treatment of serious illness, with much empiric usage.

Adrenal Insufficiency

Adrenal insufficiency is the most clear-cut indication for use of a corticosteroid, and even a slight impairment of the adrenal response during severe illness can be lethal if corticosteroid therapy is not instituted. For example, hypotension is a common symptom in critically ill clients, and hypotension caused by adrenal insufficiency may mimic either hypovolemic or septic shock. If adrenal insufficiency is the cause of the hypotension, administration of corticosteroids can eliminate the need for vasopressor drugs to maintain adequate tissue perfusion.

However, adrenal insufficiency may not be recognized because hypotension and other symptoms also occur with many illnesses. The normal response to critical illness (eg, pain, hypovolemia) is an increased and prolonged secretion of cortisol. If this does not occur, or if too little cortisol is produced, a state of adrenal insufficiency exists. One way to evaluate a client for adrenal insufficiency is a test in which a baseline serum cortisol level is measured, after which corticotropin is given IV to stimulate cortisol production, and the serum cortisol level is measured again in approximately 30 to 60 minutes. Test results are hard to interpret in seriously ill clients, though, because serum cortisol concentrations that would be normal in normal subjects may be low in this population. In addition, a lower-than-expected rise in serum cortisol levels may indicate a normal HPA axis that is already maximally stimulated, or interference with the ability of the adrenal cortex to synthesize cortisol. Thus, a critically ill client may have a limited ability to increase cortisol production in response to stress.

In any client suspected of having adrenal insufficiency, a single IV dose of corticosteroid seems justified. If the client does have adrenal insufficiency, the corticosteroid may prevent immediate death and allow time for other diagnostic and therapeutic measures. If the client does not have adrenal insufficiency, the single dose is not harmful.

Acute Respiratory Failure in Chronic Obstructive Pulmonary Disease

Some studies support the use of IV methylprednisolone. Thus, if other medications do not produce adequate bronchodilation, it seems reasonable to try an IV corticosteroid during the first 72 hours of the illness. However, corticosteroid therapy increases the risks of pulmonary infection.

Adult Respiratory Distress Syndrome

Although corticosteroids have been widely used, several well-controlled studies demonstrate that the drugs are not beneficial in early treatment or in prevention of adult respiratory distress syndrome (ARDS). Thus, corticosteroids should be used in these clients only if there are other specific indications.

Sepsis

Large, well-controlled, multicenter studies have shown that the use of corticosteroids in gram-negative bacteremia, sepsis, or septic shock has no beneficial effect. In addition, the drugs do not prevent development of ARDS or multiple organ dysfunction syndrome or decrease mortality in clients with sepsis. In addition, clients receiving corticosteroids for other conditions are at risk of sepsis, because the drugs impair the ability of white blood cells to leave the bloodstream and reach a site of infection.

Acquired Immunodeficiency Syndrome

Adrenal insufficiency is being increasingly recognized in clients with AIDS, who should be assessed and treated for it, if indicated. In addition, corticosteroids improve survival and decrease risks of respiratory failure with pneumocystosis, a common cause of death in clients with AIDS. The recommended regimen is prednisone 40 milligrams twice daily for 5 days, then 40 milligrams once daily for 5 days, then 20 milligrams daily until completion of treatment for pneumocystosis. The effect of corticosteroids on risks of other opportunistic infections or neoplasms is unknown.

Use in Home Care

Corticosteroids are extensively used in the home setting, by all age groups, for a wide variety of disorders, and by most routes of administration. Because of potentially serious adverse effects, especially with oral drugs, it is extremely important that these drugs be used as prescribed. A major responsibility of home care nurses is to teach, demonstrate, supervise, monitor, or do whatever is needed to facilitate correct use. In addition, home care nurses must teach clients and caregivers interventions to minimize adverse effects of these drugs.

APPLYING YOUR KNOWLEDGE 23-4

Long-term therapy with corticosteroids involves multiple teaching opportunities for the nurse. What should you include as priorities when providing a teaching plan for Ms. Hubble?

N   U   R   S   I   N   G   A   C   T   I   O   N   S

Corticosteroids

NURSING ACTIONS	RATIONALE/EXPLANATION

1. Administer accurately

a. Read the drug label carefully to be certain of having the correct preparation for the intended route of administration.

Many corticosteroid drugs are available in several different preparations. For example, hydrocortisone is available in formulations for intravenous (IV) or intramuscular (IM) administration, for intra-articular injection, and for topical application in creams and ointments of several different strengths. These preparations cannot be used interchangeably without causing potentially serious adverse reactions and decreasing therapeutic effects. Some drugs are available for only one use. For example, several preparations are for topical use only; beclomethasone is prepared only for oral and nasal inhalation.

b. With oral corticosteroids:

(1) Give single daily doses or alternate day doses between 6 and 9 A.M.

Early-morning administration causes less suppression of hypothalamic–pituitary–adrenal (HPA) function.

(2) Give multiple doses at evenly spaced intervals.

(3) If dosage is being tapered, follow the exact schedule.

To avoid adverse effects

(4) Give with meals or snacks.

To decrease gastrointestinal (GI) upset

(5) With oral budesonide (Entocort EC), ask the client to swallow the drug whole, without biting or chewing.

This drug is formulated to dissolve in the intestine and have local anti-inflammatory effects. Biting or chewing allows it to dissolve in the stomach.

(6) Do *not* give these drugs with an antacid containing aluminum or magnesium (eg, Maalox, Mylanta).

The antacids decrease absorption of corticosteroids, with possible reduction of therapeutic effects.

c. For IV or IM administration:

(1) Shake the medication vial well before withdrawing medication.

Most of the injectable formulations are suspensions, which need to be mixed well for accurate dosage.

(2) Give a direct IV injection over at least 1 minute.

To increase safety of administration

d. For oral or nasal inhalation of a corticosteroid, check the instruction leaflet that accompanies the inhaler.

These drugs are given by metered-dose inhalers or nasal sprays, and correct usage of the devices is essential to drug administration and therapeutic effects.

2. Observe for therapeutic effects

The primary objective of corticosteroid therapy is to relieve signs and symptoms, because the drugs are not curative. Therefore, therapeutic effects depend largely on the reason for use.

a. With adrenocortical insufficiency, observe for absence or decrease of weakness, weight loss, anorexia, nausea, vomiting, hyperpigmentation, hypotension, hypoglycemia, hyponatremia, and hyperkalemia.

These signs and symptoms of impaired metabolism do not occur with adequate replacement of corticosteroids.

b. With rheumatoid arthritis, observe for decreased pain and edema in joints, greater capacity for movement, and increased ability to perform usual activities of daily living.

c. With asthma and chronic obstructive pulmonary disease, observe for decrease in respiratory distress and increased tolerance of activity.

d. With skin lesions, observe for decreasing inflammation.

(continued)

NURSING ACTIONS	RATIONALE/EXPLANATION
e. When the drug is given to suppress the immune response to organ transplants, therapeutic effect is the absence of signs and symptoms indicating rejection of the transplanted tissue.	
3. Observe for adverse effects	These are uncommon with replacement therapy but common with long-term administration of the pharmacologic doses used for many disease processes. Adverse reactions may affect every body tissue and organ.
a. Adrenocortical insufficiency—fainting, weakness, anorexia, nausea, vomiting, hypotension, shock, and if untreated, death	This reaction is likely to occur in clients receiving daily corticosteroid drugs who encounter stressful situations. It is caused by drug-induced suppression of the HPA axis, which makes the client unable to respond to stress by increasing adrenocortical hormone secretion.
b. Adrenocortical excess (hypercorticism or Cushing's disease)	Most adverse effects result from excessive corticosteroids.
(1) "Moon face," "buffalo hump" contour of shoulders, obese trunk, thin extremities	This appearance is caused by abnormal fat deposits in cheeks, shoulders, breasts, abdomen, and buttocks. These changes are more cosmetic than physiologically significant. However, the alterations in self-image can lead to psychological problems. These changes cannot be prevented, but they may be partially reversed if corticosteroid therapy is discontinued or reduced in dosage.
(2) Diabetes mellitus—glycosuria, hyperglycemia, polyuria, polydipsia, polyphagia, impaired healing, and other signs and symptoms	Corticosteroid drugs can cause hyperglycemia and diabetes mellitus or aggravate pre-existing diabetes mellitus by their effects on carbohydrate metabolism.
(3) Central nervous system effects—euphoria, psychological dependence, nervousness, insomnia, depression, personality and behavioral changes, aggravation of pre-existing psychiatric disorders	Some clients enjoy the drug-induced euphoria so much that they resist attempts to withdraw the drug or decrease its dosage.
(4) Musculoskeletal effects—osteoporosis, pathologic fractures, muscle weakness and atrophy, decreased linear growth in children	Demineralization of bone produces thin, weak bones that fracture easily. Fractures of vertebrae, long bones, and ribs are relatively common, especially in postmenopausal women and immobilized clients. Myopathy results from abnormal protein metabolism. Decreased growth in children results from impaired bone formation and protein metabolism.
(5) Cardiovascular, fluid, and electrolyte effects—fluid retention, edema, hypertension, congestive heart failure, hypernatremia, hypokalemia, metabolic alkalosis	These effects result largely from mineralocorticoid activity, which causes retention of sodium and water. They are more likely to occur with older corticosteroids, such as hydrocortisone and prednisone.
(6) Gastrointestinal effects—nausea, vomiting, possible peptic ulcer disease, increased appetite, obesity	
(7) Increased susceptibility to infection and delayed wound healing	Caused by suppression of normal inflammatory and immune processes and impaired protein metabolism
(8) Menstrual irregularities, acne, excessive facial hair	Caused by excessive sex hormones, primarily androgens
(9) Ocular effects—increased intraocular pressure, glaucoma, cataracts	
(10) Integumentary effects—skin becomes reddened, thinner, has stretch marks, and is easily injured	
4. Observe for drug interactions	
a. Drugs that *increase* effects of corticosteroids:	
(1) Estrogens, oral contraceptives, ketoconazole, macrolide antibiotics (eg, erythromycin)	These drugs apparently inhibit the enzymes that normally metabolize corticosteroids in the liver.
(2) Diuretics (eg, furosemide, thiazides)	Increase hypokalemia

NURSING ACTIONS	RATIONALE/EXPLANATION
b. Drugs that *decrease* effects of corticosteroids:	
(1) Antacids, cholestyramine	Decrease absorption
(2) Carbamazepine, phenytoin, rifampin	These drugs induce microsomal enzymes in the liver and increase the rate at which corticosteroids are metabolized or deactivated.

APPLYING YOUR KNOWLEDGE: ANSWERS

23-1 Notify Ms. Hubble's physician. This is a sign of thrush or oral candidiasis, a fungal infection. The client requires immediate treatment and may not be able to continue on the prednisone if the infection becomes systemic. Systemic fungal infections are a contraindication to the administration of corticosteroids.

23-2 Prednisone is a drug that will treat the symptoms of COPD, but it is not designed to cure the underlying disease process. Because the drug reduces respiratory inflammation, Ms. Hubble will have less difficulty with breathing.

23-3 Prednisone causes hyperglycemia in many clients and especially in clients with diabetes mellitus. The physician should be notified for a change in Ms. Hubble's diabetic medication. Also, the nurse should review Ms. Hubble's diet.

23-4 The teaching plan should include taking the drug as ordered, carrying medical alert identification that includes the drugs taken, taking measures to avoid infection, and observing for any signs of infection or delayed wound healing. The nurse should encourage activity as tolerated to prevent osteoporosis, and teach the client when to seek medical attention.

Review and Application Exercises

Short Answer Exercises

1. What are the main characteristics and functions of cortisol?

2. What is the difference between glucocorticoid and mineralocorticoid components of corticosteroids?

3. How do glucocorticoids affect body metabolism?

4. What is meant by the HPA axis?

5. What are the mechanisms by which exogenous corticosteroids may cause adrenocortical insufficiency and excess?

6. What adverse effects are associated with chronic use of systemic corticosteroids?

7. What are the main differences between administering corticosteroids in adrenal insufficiency versus in other disorders?

8. When a corticosteroid is given by inhalation to clients with asthma, what is the expected effect?

NCLEX-Style Questions

9. It is important to taper the dose in long-term systemic corticosteroid therapy rather than stopping the drug abruptly because tapering results in which of the following?
   a. less suppression of hypothalamic–pituitary–adrenal function
   b. increased client compliance with drug therapy
   c. greater tolerance of adverse effects
   d. significantly increased anti-inflammatory effect

10. A nurse is instructing a client regarding the correct way follow the order, "prednisone 10 mg PO once daily." The nurse should tell the client to take
    a. the entire dose once a day at bedtime
    b. the entire dose once a day on arising
    c. half of the dose in the morning and half at bedtime
    d. one third of the dose in the morning and two thirds in the afternoon

11. A client who has been on long-term corticosteroid therapy begins to gain weight and complains that her rings no longer fit on her hands. She asks the nurse why she is gaining weight. The nurse tells the client that the most likely cause of later weight gain when undergoing corticosteroid therapy is
    a. increased appetite
    b. hyperglycemia
    c. muscle hypertrophy
    d. fluid retention

12. A client taking an inhaled steroid should be instructed to rinse her mouth after administration of the drug to avoid development of which of the following conditions?
a. anorexia
b. nausea and vomiting
c. thrush
d. gingival hyperplasia

13. Clients taking glucocorticoids have an increased risk for which of the following conditions?
a. allergic reaction
b. hypotension
c. hypoglycemia
d. infection

Selected References

Abraham, E., & Evans, T. (2002, August). Corticosteroids and septic shock. *Journal of the American Medical Association, 288*(7), 886–887.

Annane, D., Sébille, V., Charpentier, C., et. al. (2002, August). Effect of treatment with low doses of hydrocortisone and fludrocortisone on mortality in patients with septic shock. *Journal of the American Medical Association, 288*(7), 862–871.

Budesonide (Entocort EC) for Crohn's disease. (2002). *Medical Letter on Drugs and Therapeutics, 44,* 6–8.

Carson, P. P. (2000). Emergency: Adrenal crisis. *American Journal of Nursing, 100*(7), 49–50.

De Benedictis, F. M., Teper, A., Green, R. J., et al. (2001). Effects of 2 inhaled corticosteroids on growth. *Archives of Pediatric and Adolescent Medicine, 155*(11), 1248–1254.

Drug facts and comparisons. (Updated monthly). St. Louis: Facts and Comparisons.

Guyton, A. C., & Hall, J. E. (2000). *Textbook of medical physiology* (10th ed.). Philadelphia: W. B. Saunders.

Hoffmeister, A. M., & Tietze, K. J. (2000). Adrenocortical dysfunction and clinical use of steroids. In E. T. Herfindal & D. R. Gourley (Eds.), *Textbook of therapeutics: Drug and disease management* (7th ed., pp. 305–324). Philadelphia: Lippincott Williams & Wilkins.

Humes, H. D. (Ed.). (2000). *Kelley's Textbook of internal medicine* (4th ed.). Philadelphia: Lippincott Williams & Wilkins.

Lacy, C. F., Armstrong, L. L., Goldman, M. P., & Lance, L. L. (2004). *Lexi-Comp's drug information handbook* (12th ed.). Hudson, OH: Lexi-Comp.

Matfin, G., Kuenzi, J. A, & Guven, S. (2005). Disorders of endocrine control of growth and metabolism. In C. M. Porth, *Pathophysiology: Concepts of altered health states* (7th ed., pp. 961–985). Philadelphia: Lippincott Williams & Wilkins.

Sin, D. D., Man, J., Sharpe, H., Gan, W. Q., & Paul Man, S. F. (2004, July). Pharmacological management to reduce exacerbations in adults with asthma: A systematic review and meta-analysis. *Journal of the American Medical Association, 292*(3), 367–376.

Spencer, M. T., & Bazarian, J. J. (2003). Are corticosteroids effective in traumatic spinal cord injury? *Annals of Emergency Medicine, 41*(3), 410–413.

Togger, D. A., & Brenner, P. S. (2001). Metered dose inhalers. *American Journal of Nursing, 101*(10), 26–32.

Thyroid and Antithyroid Drugs

OBJECTIVES

After studying this chapter, you will be able to:

1. Describe physiologic effects of thyroid hormone.
2. Identify subclinical, symptomatic, and severe effects of inadequate or excessive thyroid hormone.
3. Describe characteristics, uses, and effects of thyroid drugs.
4. Describe characteristics, uses, and effects of antithyroid drugs.
5. Discuss the influence of thyroid and antithyroid drugs on the metabolism of other drugs.
6. Teach clients self-care activities related to the use of thyroid and antithyroid drugs.

APPLYING YOUR KNOWLEDGE

Brenda Zalewski is a 45-year-old woman who had a goiter as a child and a thyroidectomy at age 12. She has been taking a synthetic thyroid preparation since that time. Ms. Zalewski takes a maintenance dose of Synthroid 0.1 mg PO daily. She is 5 feet 8 inches tall and weighs 215 pounds.

INTRODUCTION

The thyroid gland produces three hormones: thyroxine, triiodothyronine, and calcitonin. Thyroxine (also called T_4) contains four atoms of iodine, and triiodothyronine (also called T_3) contains three atoms of iodine. T_3 is more potent than T_4 and has a more rapid onset but a shorter duration of action. Despite these minor differences, the two hormones produce the same physiologic effects and have the same actions and uses. Calcitonin functions in calcium metabolism and is discussed in Chapter 25.

Production of T_3 and T_4 depends on the presence of iodine and tyrosine in the thyroid gland. Plasma iodide is derived from dietary sources and from the metabolic breakdown of thyroid hormone, which allows some iodine to be reused. The thyroid gland extracts iodide from the circulating blood, concentrates it, and secretes enzymes that change the chemically inactive iodide to free iodine atoms. In a series of chemical reactions, iodine atoms become attached to tyrosine, an amino acid derived from dietary protein, to form the thyroid hormones T_3 and T_4. After they are formed, the hormones are stored within the chemically inactive thyroglobulin molecule. Tyrosine forms the basic structure of thyroglobulin.

Thyroid hormones are released into the circulation when the thyroid gland is stimulated by thyroid-stimulating hormone (thyrotropin or TSH) from the anterior pituitary gland. Because the thyroglobulin molecule is too large to cross cell membranes, proteolytic enzymes break down the molecule so the active hormones can be released. After their release from thyroglobulin, the hormones become largely bound to plasma proteins. Only the small amounts left unbound are biologically active. The bound thyroid hormones are released to tissue cells very slowly. In tissue cells, the hormones combine with intracellular proteins so they are again stored. They are released slowly within the cell and used over a period of days or weeks. When they are used by the cells, the thyroid hormones release iodine atoms. Most of the iodine is reabsorbed and used to produce new thyroid hormones; the remainder is excreted in the urine.

Thyroid hormones control the rate of cellular metabolism and thereby influence the functioning of virtually every cell in the body. The heart, skeletal muscle, liver, and kidneys are especially responsive to the stimulating effects of thyroid hormones. The brain, spleen, and gonads are less responsive. Thyroid hormones are required for normal growth and development and are considered especially critical for brain and skeletal development and maturation. These hormones are thought to act mainly by controlling intracellular protein synthesis. Some specific physiologic effects include:

- Increased rate of cellular metabolism and oxygen consumption with a resultant increase in heat production
- Increased heart rate, force of contraction, and cardiac output (increased cardiac workload)
- Increased carbohydrate metabolism
- Increased fat metabolism, including increased lipolytic effects of other hormones and metabolism of cholesterol to bile acids
- Inhibition of pituitary secretion of TSH

Two types of thyroid disorders requiring drug therapy are hypothyroidism and hyperthyroidism. These disorders produce opposing effects on body tissues, depending on the levels of circulating thyroid hormone. Specific effects and clinical manifestations are listed in Table 24-1.

Hypothyroidism

Primary hypothyroidism occurs when disease or destruction of thyroid gland tissue causes inadequate production of thyroid hormones. Common causes of primary hypothyroidism include chronic (Hashimoto's) thyroiditis, an autoimmune disorder, and treatment of hyperthyroidism with antithyroid drugs, radiation therapy, or surgery. Other causes include previous radiation to the thyroid area of the neck and treatment with amiodarone, lithium, or iodine preparations. Secondary hypothyroidism occurs when there is decreased TSH from the anterior pituitary gland or decreased thyrotropin-releasing hormone (TRH) secreted from the hypothalamus.

Congenital hypothyroidism (cretinism) occurs when a child is born without a thyroid gland or with a poorly functioning gland. Cretinism is uncommon in the United States but may occur with a lack of iodine in the mother's diet. Symptoms are rarely present at birth but develop gradually during infancy and early childhood, and they include poor growth and development, lethargy and inactivity, feeding problems, slow pulse, subnormal temperature, and constipation. If cretinism is untreated until the child is several months old, permanent mental retardation is likely to result.

Adult hypothyroidism (myxedema) may be subclinical or clinical and occurs much more often in women than in men. Subclinical hypothyroidism, the most common thyroid disorder, involves a mildly elevated serum TSH and normal serum thyroxine levels. It is usually asymptomatic. If the thyroid gland cannot secrete enough hormone despite excessive release of TSH, hypothyroidism occurs, and a goiter (thyroid enlargement) may occur from the overstimulation. Clinical hypothyroidism produces variable signs and symptoms, depending on the amount of circulating thyroid hormone. Initially, manifestations (see Table 24-1) are mild and vague. They usually increase in incidence and severity over time as the thyroid gland gradually atrophies and functioning glandular tissue is replaced by nonfunctioning fibrous connective tissue.

Myxedema coma is severe, life-threatening hypothyroidism characterized by coma, hypothermia, cardiovascular collapse, hypoventilation, and severe metabolic disorders such as hyponatremia, hypoglycemia, and lactic acidosis. Predisposing factors include exposure to cold, infection, trauma, respiratory disease, and administration of central nervous system depressants (eg, anesthetics, analgesics, sedatives). A person with severe hypothyroidism cannot metabolize and excrete the drugs.

Hyperthyroidism

Hyperthyroidism is characterized by excessive secretion of thyroid hormone and usually involves an enlarged thyroid gland that has an increased number of cells and an increased rate of secretion. It may be associated with Graves' disease, nodular goiter, thyroiditis, overtreatment with thyroid drugs, functioning thyroid carcinoma, and pituitary adenoma that secretes excessive amounts of TSH. The hyperplastic thyroid gland may secrete 5 to 15 times the normal amount of thyroid hormone. As a result, body metabolism is greatly increased. Specific physiologic effects and clinical manifestations of hyperthyroidism are listed in Table 24-1. These effects vary, depending on the amount of circulating thyroid hormone, and they usually increase in incidence and severity with time if hyperthyroidism is not treated.

Subclinical hyperthyroidism is defined as a reduced TSH (less than 0.1 microunit/L) and normal T_3 and T_4 levels. The most common cause is excess thyroid hormone therapy. Subclinical hyperthyroidism is a risk factor for osteoporosis in postmenopausal women who do not take estrogen replacement therapy, because it leads to reduced bone mineral density. It also greatly increases the risk of atrial fibrillation in clients older than 60 years of age.

Thyroid storm or thyrotoxic crisis is a rare but severe complication characterized by extreme symptoms of hyperthyroidism, such as severe tachycardia, fever, dehydration, heart failure, and coma. It is most likely to occur in clients with hyperthyroidism that has been inadequately treated, especially when stressful situations occur (eg, trauma, infection, surgery, emotional upset).

It should be noted that iodine is present in foods (especially seafood) and in contrast dyes used for gallbladder and other radiologic procedures. Ingestion of large amounts of iodine from these sources may result in goiter and hyperthyroidism.

GENERAL CHARACTERISTICS OF THYROID AND ANTITHYROID DRUGS

Mechanism of Action

Thyroid drugs such as the synthetic drug levothyroxine provide an exogenous source of thyroid hormone. Antithyroid drugs act by decreasing production or release of thyroid

Chapter 24 ● Thyroid and Antithyroid Drugs

TABLE 24-1 Thyroid Disorders and Their Effects on Body Systems

HYPOTHYROIDISM	HYPERTHYROIDISM
Cardiovascular Effects	
Increased capillary fragility	Tachycardia
Decreased cardiac output	Increased cardiac output
Decreased blood pressure	Increased blood volume
Decreased heart rate	Increased systolic blood pressure
Cardiac enlargement	Cardiac dysrhythmias
Congestive heart failure	Congestive heart failure
Anemia	
More rapid development of atherosclerosis and its complications (eg, coronary artery and peripheral vascular disease)	
Central Nervous System Effects	
Apathy and lethargy	Nervousness
Emotional dullness	Emotional instability
Slow speech, perhaps slurring and hoarseness as well	Restlessness
Hypoactive reflexes	Anxiety
Forgetfulness and mental sluggishness	Insomnia
Excessive drowsiness and sleeping	Hyperactive reflexes
Metabolic Effects	
Intolerance of cold	Intolerance of heat
Subnormal temperature	Low-grade fever
Increased serum cholesterol	Weight loss despite increased appetite
Weight gain	
Gastrointestinal Effects	
Decreased appetite	Increased appetite
Constipation	Abdominal cramps
	Diarrhea
	Nausea and vomiting
Muscular Effects	
Weakness	Weakness
Fatigue	Fatigue
Vague aches and pains	Muscle atrophy
	Tremors
Integumentary Effects	
Dry, coarse, and thickened skin	Moist, warm, flushed skin due to vasodilation and increased sweating
Puffy appearance of face and eyelids	Hair and nails soft
Dry and thinned hair	
Thick and hard nails	
Reproductive Effects	
Prolonged menstrual periods	Amenorrhea or oligomenorrhea
Infertility or sterility	
Decreased libido	
Miscellaneous Effects	
Increased susceptibility to infection	Dyspnea
Increased sensitivity to narcotics, barbiturates, and anesthetics due to slowed metabolism of these drugs	Polyuria
	Hoarse, rapid speech
	Increased susceptibility to infection
	Excessive perspiration
	Localized edema around the eyeballs, which produces characteristic eye changes, including exophthalmos

hormones. The thioamide drugs inhibit synthesis of thyroid hormone. Iodine preparations inhibit the release of thyroid hormones and cause them to be stored within the thyroid gland. Radioactive iodine emits rays that destroy the thyroid gland tissue.

Indications for Use

Thyroid drugs are indicated for primary or secondary hypothyroidism, cretinism, and myxedema. Antithyroid drugs may be necessary for hyperthyroidism associated with Graves' disease, nodular goiter, thyroiditis, overtreatment with thyroid drugs, functioning thyroid carcinoma, and pituitary adenoma that secretes excessive amounts of TSH. Antithyroid drugs may also be indicated for thyroid storm.

Contraindications to Use

Iodine preparations and thioamide antithyroid drugs are contraindicated in pregnancy, because they can lead to goiter and hypothyroidism in the fetus or newborn. Radioactive iodine is contraindicated during lactation as well. Because radioactive iodine may cause cancer and chromosome damage in children it should be used only for hyperthyroidism that cannot be controlled by other drugs or surgery.

INDIVIDUAL DRUGS

Thyroid and antithyroid drugs are described in the following section. Dosages are listed in Table 24-2.

Thyroid Drugs (Used in Hypothyroidism)

P **Levothyroxine** (Synthroid, Levothroid), a synthetic preparation of T_4, is the drug of choice for long-term treatment of hypothyroidism and serves as the prototype. This potent form of T_4 contains a uniform amount of hormone and can be given parenterally. Absorption with oral administration varies from 48% to 79% of the dose administered. Taking the medication on an empty stomach increases absorption; malabsorption syndromes cause excessive fecal loss. Most (99%) of the circulating levothyroxine is bound to serum proteins, including thyroid-binding globulin as well as thyroid-binding prealbumin and albumin. Levothyroxine has a long half-life of about 6 to 7 days in euthyroidism, (normal thyroid function), but is prolonged to 9 to 10 days in hypothyroidism and shortened to 3 to 4 days in hyperthyroidism.

Much of the levothyroxine is converted to liothyronine (T_3; see below) in peripheral tissues. This conversion (ie, removal of an iodine atom, called *deiodination*) occurs at several locations, including the liver, kidneys, and other tissues. Some of the hormone is conjugated with glucuronide or sulfate and excreted in the bile and intestine.

Liothyronine (Cytomel, Triostat) is a synthetic preparation of T_3. Compared with levothyroxine, liothyronine

has a more rapid onset and a shorter duration of action. Consequently, it may be more likely to produce high concentrations in blood and tissues and cause adverse reactions. Also, it requires more frequent administration if used for long-term treatment of hypothyroidism. Only the intravenous formulation (Triostat) is used in treating myxedema coma.

Liotrix (Thyrolar) contains levothyroxine and liothyronine in a 4:1 ratio, resembling the composition of natural thyroid hormone. Thyrolar is available in strengths ranging from 15 to 180 milligrams in thyroid equivalency.

APPLYING YOUR KNOWLEDGE 24-1
While Ms. Zalewski is in the hospital, you are administering her daily medications. Hospital routine is to administer all once-daily medications at 9:00 A.M. When reviewing the medication administration sheets, you note Ms. Zalewski is to receive Synthroid at 9:00 A.M. Breakfast trays are usually served to patients between 8:00 and 8:30 A.M. What action should you take with regard to administration of the Synthroid?

Antithyroid Drugs (Used in Hyperthyroidism)

P **Propylthiouracil** (PTU) is the prototype of the thioamide antithyroid drugs. It can be used alone to treat hyperthyroidism; as part of the preoperative preparation for thyroidectomy; before or after radioactive iodine therapy; and in the treatment of thyroid storm. PTU acts by inhibiting production of thyroid hormones and peripheral conversion of T_4 to the more active T_3. It does not interfere with release of thyroid hormones previously produced and stored. Thus, therapeutic effects do not occur for several days or weeks until the stored hormones have been used.

PTU is well absorbed with oral administration, and peak plasma levels occur within 30 minutes. Plasma half-life is 1 to 2 hours. However, duration of action depends on the half-life within the thyroid gland rather than plasma half-life. Because this time is relatively short, PTU must be given every 8 hours. The drug is metabolized in the liver and excreted in urine.

Methimazole (Tapazole) is similar to PTU in actions, uses, and adverse reactions. It is also well absorbed with oral administration and rapidly reaches peak plasma levels.

Strong iodine solution (Lugol's solution) and **saturated solution of potassium iodide** (SSKI) are iodine preparations sometimes used in short-term treatment of hyperthyroidism. The drugs inhibit release of thyroid hormones, causing them to accumulate in the thyroid gland. Lugol's solution is usually used to treat thyrotoxic crisis and to decrease the size and vascularity of the thyroid gland before thyroidectomy. SSKI is more often used as an expectorant but may be given as preparation for thyroidectomy. Iodine preparations should not be followed by propylthiouracil, methimazole, or radioactive iodine because the latter drugs

Table 24-2 Drugs at a Glance: Drugs for Hypothyroidism and Hyperthyroidism

GENERIC/TRADE NAME	ROUTES AND DOSAGE RANGES	
	Adults	Children
Drugs for Hypothyroidism		
P **Levothyroxine** (Synthroid, Levothroid)	PO 0.05 mg/d initially, increased by 0.025 mg every 2–3 wk until desired response obtained; usual maintenance dose, 0.1–0.2 mg/d (100–200 mcg/d) Myxedema coma, IV 0.4 mg in a single dose; then 0.1–0.2 mg daily Thyroid-stimulating hormone (TSH) suppression in thyroid cancer, nodules, and euthyroid goiters, PO 2.6 mcg/kg/d for 7–10 d *Older adults, clients with cardiac disorders, and clients with hypothyroidism of long duration:* PO 0.0125–0.025 mg/d for 6 wk, then dose is doubled every 6–8 wk until the desired response is obtained Myxedema coma, same as adult dosage	Congenital hypothyroidism, PO as follows: *>12 y:* >150 mcg/d (or 2–3 mcg/kg/d) *6–12 y:* 100–150 mcg/d (or 4–5 mcg/kg/d) *1–5 y:* 75–100 mcg/d (or 5–6 mcg/kg/d) *6–12 mo:* 50–75 mcg/d (or 6–8 mcg/kg/d) *Birth–6 mo:* 25–50 mcg/d (or 8–10 mcg/kg/d)
Liothyronine (Cytomel, Triostat)	PO 25 mcg/d initially, increased by 12.5–25 mcg every 1–2 wk until desired response Myxedema coma, IV 25–50 mcg initially, then adjust dosage according to clinical response. Usual dosage, 65–100 mcg/d, with doses at least 4 h apart and no more than 12 h apart *Older adults:* PO 2.5–5 mcg/d for 3–6 wk, then doubled every 6 wk until desired response Myxedema coma, IV 10–20 mcg initially, then adjusted according to clinical response	PO 5 mcg/d initially, increased by 5 mcg/d every 3–4 d until desired response. Doses as high as 20–80 mcg/d may be required in congenital hypothyroidism.
Liotrix (Thyrolar)	PO 15–30 mg/d initially, increased gradually every 2–3 wk until response is obtained. Usual maintenance dose, 60–120 mg/d *Older adults,* clients with cardiac disorders, and clients with hypothyroidism of long duration: PO one fourth to one half the usual adult dose initially, doubled every 8 wk if necessary	
Drugs for Hyperthyroidism		
P **Propylthiouracil**	PO 300–400 mg/d in divided doses q8h, until the client is euthyroid; then 100–150 mg/d in 3 divided doses, for maintenance	*>10 y:* PO 150–300 mg/d in divided doses q8h; usual maintenance dose, 100–300 mg/d in 2 divided doses, q12h *6–10 y:* 50–150 mg/d in divided doses q8h
Methimazole (Tapazole)	PO 15–60 mg/d initially, in divided doses q8h until the client is euthyroid; maintenance, 5–15 mg/d in 2 or 3 doses	PO 0.4 mg/kg/d initially, in divided doses q8h; maintenance dose, one half initial dose
Strong iodine solution (Lugol's solution)	PO 2–6 drops 3 times per day for 10 d before thyroidectomy	PO 2–6 drops 3 times per day for 10 d before thyroidectomy
Saturated solution of potassium iodide (SSKI)	PO 5 drops 3 times per day for 10 d before thyroidectomy	PO 5 drops 3 times per day for 10 d before thyroidectomy
Sodium iodide [131]**I** (Iodotope)	PO, IV, dosage as calculated by a radiologist trained in nuclear medicine	PO, IV, dosage as calculated by a radiologist trained in nuclear medicine
Propranolol (Inderal)	PO 40–160 mg/d in divided doses	

IV, intravenous; PO, oral.

cause release of stored thyroid hormone and may precipitate acute hyperthyroidism.

Sodium iodide [131]I (Iodotope) is a radioactive isotope of iodine. The thyroid gland cannot differentiate between regular iodide and radioactive iodide, so it picks up the radioactive iodide from the circulating blood. As a result, small amounts of radioactive iodide can be used as a diagnostic test of thyroid function, and larger doses are used therapeutically to treat hyperthyroidism. Therapeutic doses act by emitting beta and gamma rays, which destroy thyroid tissue and thereby decrease production of thyroid hormones. It is also used to treat thyroid cancer.

Propranolol (Inderal) is an antiadrenergic, not an antithyroid, drug. It does not affect thyroid function, hormone secretion, or hormone metabolism. It is most often used to treat cardiovascular conditions, such as dysrhythmias, angina pectoris, and hypertension. When given to clients with hyperthyroidism, propranolol blocks beta-adrenergic receptors in various organs and thereby controls symptoms of hyperthyroidism resulting from excessive stimulation of the sympathetic nervous system. These symptoms include tachycardia, palpitations, excessive sweating, tremors, and nervousness. Propranolol is useful for controlling symptoms during the delayed response to thioamide drugs and radioactive iodine; before thyroidectomy; and in treating thyrotoxic crisis. When the client becomes euthyroid and hyperthyroid symptoms are controlled by definitive treatment measures, propranolol should be discontinued.

NURSING PROCESS

Assessment

● Assess for signs and symptoms of thyroid disorders (see Table 24-1). During the course of treatment with thyroid or antithyroid drugs, the client's blood level of thyroid hormone may range from low to normal to high. At either end of the continuum, signs and symptoms may be dramatic and obvious. As blood levels change toward normal as a result of treatment, signs and symptoms become less obvious. If presenting signs and symptoms are treated too aggressively, they may change toward the opposite end of the continuum and indicate adverse drug effects. Thus, *each client receiving a drug that alters thyroid function must be assessed for indicators of hypothyroidism, euthyroidism, and hyperthyroidism.*

● Check laboratory reports for serum TSH (normal = 0.5 to 4.1 µU/mL) when available. An elevated serum TSH is the first indication of primary hypothyroidism and commonly occurs in middle-aged women, even in the absence of other signs and symptoms. Serum TSH is used to monitor response to drugs that alter thyroid function.

Nursing Diagnoses

● Decreased Cardiac Output related to disease- or drug-induced thyroid disorders
● Imbalanced Nutrition: Less Than Body Requirements with hyperthyroidism
● Imbalanced Nutrition: More Than Body Requirements with hypothyroidism
● Ineffective Thermoregulation related to changes in metabolism rate and body heat production
● Deficient Knowledge: Disease process and drug therapy

Planning/Goals

The client will
● Achieve normal blood levels of thyroid hormone
● Receive or take drugs accurately
● Experience relief of symptoms of hypothyroidism or hyperthyroidism
● Be assisted to cope with symptoms until therapy becomes effective
● Avoid preventable adverse drug effects
● Maintain the therapeutic and avoid the adverse effects of drug therapy

Interventions

Use nondrug measures to control symptoms, increase effectiveness of drug therapy, and decrease adverse reactions. Some areas for intervention include the following:

● **Environmental temperature.** Regulate for the client's comfort, when possible. Clients with *hypothyroidism* are very intolerant of cold, due to their slow metabolism rate. Chilling and shivering should be prevented because of added strain on the heart. Provide blankets and warm clothing as needed. Clients with *hyperthyroidism* are very intolerant of heat and perspire excessively, due to their rapid metabolism rate. Provide cooling baths and lightweight clothing as needed.
● **Diet.** Despite a poor appetite, *hypothyroid* clients are often overweight because of a slow metabolism rate. Thus, a low-calorie, weight-reduction diet may be indicated. In addition, an increased intake of high-fiber foods is usually needed to prevent constipation as a result of decreased gastrointestinal secretions and motility. Despite a good appetite, *hyperthyroid* clients are often underweight because of a rapid metabolism rate. They often need extra calories and nutrients to prevent tissue breakdown. These can be provided by extra meals and snacks. The client may wish to avoid highly seasoned and high-fiber foods because they may increase diarrhea.
● **Fluids.** With *hypothyroidism,* clients need an adequate intake of low-calorie fluids to prevent constipation. With

hyperthyroidism, clients need large amounts of fluids (3000–4000 mL/day) unless contraindicated by cardiac or renal disease. The fluids are needed to eliminate heat and waste products produced by the hypermetabolic state. Much of the client's fluid loss is visible as excessive perspiration and urine output.

● **Activity.** With *hypothyroidism,* encourage activity to maintain cardiovascular, respiratory, gastrointestinal, and musculoskeletal function. With *hyperthyroidism,* encourage rest and quiet, nonstrenuous activity. Because clients differ in what they find restful, this must be determined with each client. A quiet room, reading, and soft music may be helpful. Mild sedatives are often given. The client is caught in the dilemma of needing rest because of the high metabolic rate but being unable to rest because of nervousness and excitement.

● **Skin care.** *Hypothyroid* clients are likely to have edema and dry skin. When edema is present, inspect pressure points, turn often, and avoid trauma when possible. Edema increases risks of skin breakdown and decubitus ulcer formation. Also, increased capillary fragility increases the likelihood of bruising from seemingly minor trauma. When skin is dry, use soap sparingly and lotions and other lubricants freely.

● **Eye care.** *Hyperthyroid* clients may have exophthalmos. In mild cases, use measures to protect the eye. For example, dark glasses, local lubricants, and patching of the eyes at night may be needed. Diuretic drugs and elevating the head of the bed may help reduce periorbital edema and eyeball protrusion. If the eyelids cannot close, they are sometimes taped shut to avoid corneal abrasion. In severe exophthalmos, the preceding measures are taken and large doses of corticosteroids are usually given.

Client Teaching Guidelines for Levothyroxine and for Propylthiouracil or Methimazole are presented in the accompanying displays.

Evaluation

● Interview and observe for compliance with instructions for taking medications.
● Observe for relief of symptoms.
● Check laboratory reports for normal blood levels of TSH or thyroid hormones.
● Interview and observe for adverse drug effects.
● Check appointment records for compliance with follow-up procedures.

APPLYING YOUR KNOWLEDGE 24-2
You are preparing a teaching plan for Ms. Zalewski. Considering her height and weight, what should you include for this client?

PRINCIPLES OF THERAPY

Goals of Therapy

The goal of treatment with thyroid drugs is to restore euthyroidism and normal metabolism. In hypothyroidism,

---

CLIENT TEACHING GUIDELINES

Levothyroxine

General Considerations

✔ Thyroid hormone is required for normal body functioning and for life. When a person's thyroid gland is unable to produce enough thyroid hormone, levothyroxine is used as a synthetic substitute. Thus, levothyroxine therapy for hypothyroidism is lifelong; stopping it may lead to life-threatening illness.
✔ Periodic tests of thyroid function are needed.
✔ Dosage adjustments are made according to clinical response and results of thyroid function tests.
✔ Do not switch from one brand name to another; effects may be different.
✔ Levothyroxine stimulates the central nervous system and the heart; excessive stimulation may occur if it is taken with other stimulating drugs. Thus, you should consult a health care provider before taking over-the-counter drugs that stimulate the heart or cause nervousness (eg, asthma remedies, cold remedies, decon-

gestants). In addition, you should probably limit your intake of caffeine-containing beverages to 2 to 3 servings daily.

Self-Administration

✔ Take every morning, on an empty stomach, for best absorption. Also, do not take the drug with an antacid (eg, Tums, Maalox), an iron preparation, or sucralfate (Carafate). These drugs decrease absorption of levothyroxine. If it is necessary to take one of these drugs, take levothyroxine 2 hours before or 4 to 6 hours after the other drug.
✔ Take at about the same time each day for more consistent blood levels and more normal body metabolism.
✔ Report chest pain, heart palpitations, nervousness, or insomnia. These adverse effects result from excessive stimulation and may indicate that drug dosage or intake of other stimulants needs to be reduced.

CLIENT TEACHING GUIDELINES

Propylthiouracil or Methimazole

General Considerations

✔ These drugs are sometimes called *antithyroid drugs* because they are given to decrease the production of thyroid hormone by an overactive thyroid gland.

✔ These drugs must be taken for 1 year or longer to decrease thyroid hormone levels to normal.

✔ Periodic tests of thyroid function and drug dosage adjustments are needed.

✔ Ask the prescribing physician if it is necessary to avoid or restrict amounts of seafood or iodized salt. These sources of iodide may need to be reduced or omitted during antithyroid drug therapy.

Self-Administration

✔ Take at regular intervals around the clock, usually every 8 hours.

✔ Report fever, sore throat, unusual bleeding or bruising, headache, skin rash, yellowing of the skin, or vomiting. If these adverse effects occur, drug dosage may need to be reduced or the drug may need to be discontinued.

✔ Consult a health care provider before taking over-the-counter drugs. Some drugs contain iodide, which can increase the likelihood of goiter and the risk of adverse effects from excessive doses of iodide (eg, some cough syrups, asthma medications, and multivitamins may contain iodide).

---

the goal of thyroid replacement therapy is to administer a dosage in sufficient amounts to compensate for the thyroid deficit, so as to resolve symptoms and restore serum TSH and thyroid hormone to normal. In hyperthyroidism, the goals are to reduce thyroid hormone production to relieve symptoms; return serum TSH and thyroid hormone levels to normal; and avoid complete destruction of the thyroid gland.

APPLYING YOUR KNOWLEDGE 24-3

You are performing the assessment of Ms. Zalewski and observe tachycardia, increased systolic blood pressure, nervousness, insomnia, hunger, and fatigue. What laboratory test should be assessed and what action should you take?

Thyroid Drugs

Drug Selection

Regardless of the cause of hypothyroidism and the age at which it occurs, the specific treatment is replacement of thyroid hormone from an exogenous source. Synthetic levothyroxine is the drug of choice for thyroid hormone replacement because of uniform potency, once-daily dosing, and low cost. In clients with subclinical hypothyroidism, levothyroxine should be given if the serum TSH level is higher than 10 microunits per liter. There is some difference of opinion about treatment for TSH values between 5 and 10 microunits per liter. Two arguments for treatment of subclinical hypothyroidism are the high rate of progression to symptomatic hypothyroidism and improvement of cholesterol metabolism (eg, low-density lipoprotein, or "bad" cholesterol, is reduced with treatment).

In clients with symptomatic hypothyroidism, levothyroxine therapy is definitely indicated. In addition to improve-

ment of metabolism, treatment may also improve cardiac function, energy level, mood, muscle function, and fertility. In myxedema coma, levothyroxine or liothyronine is given intravenously, along with interventions to relieve precipitating factors and to support vital functions until the thyroid hormone becomes effective, often within 24 hours.

Drug Dosage

Dosage is influenced by the choice of drug, the client's age and general condition, severity and duration of hypothyroidism, and clinical response to drug therapy. The dosage must be individualized to approximate the amount of thyroid hormone needed to make up the deficit in endogenous hormone production. As a general rule, initial dosage is relatively small. Dosage is gradually increased at approximately 2-week intervals until symptoms are relieved and a normal serum TSH level (0.5–4.2 microunits/L) is reestablished. Maintenance dosage for long-term therapy is based on the client's clinical status and periodic measurement of serum TSH.

Duration of Therapy

Thyroid replacement therapy in the client with hypothyroidism is lifelong. Medical supervision is needed frequently during early treatment and at least annually after the client's condition has stabilized and maintenance dosage has been determined.

Hypothyroid and the Metabolism of Other Drugs

Changes in the rate of body metabolism affect the metabolism of many drugs. Most drugs given to clients with hypothyroidism have a prolonged effect, because drug metabolism in the liver is delayed and the glomerular filtration rate of the kidneys is decreased. Drug absorption from the intestine or a parenteral injection site also may be slowed. As a result, dosage of many other drugs should be reduced, including digoxin and insulin. In addition, people with hypothyroidism are especially likely to experience respiratory depression and myxedema coma with opioid analgesics and other sedating drugs. These drugs should be avoided when possible. However, when necessary, they are given very cautiously and in dosages of approximately one third to one half the usual dose. Even then, clients must be observed very closely for respiratory depression.

After thyroid replacement therapy is started and stabilized, the client becomes euthyroid; has a normal rate of metabolism; and can tolerate usual doses of most drugs if other influencing factors are not present. On the other hand, excessive doses of thyroid drugs may produce hyperthyroidism and a greatly increased rate of metabolism. In this situation, larger doses of most other drugs are necessary to produce the same effects. However, rather than increasing dosage of other drugs, dosage of thyroid drugs should be reduced so the client is euthyroid again.

Adrenal Insufficiency

When hypothyroidism and adrenal insufficiency coexist, the adrenal insufficiency should be treated with a corticosteroid drug before starting thyroid replacement. Thyroid hormones increase tissue metabolism and tissue demands for adrenocortical hormones. If adrenal insufficiency is not treated first, administration of thyroid hormone may cause acute adrenocortical insufficiency, a life-threatening condition.

Antithyroid Drugs

Treatment of hyperthyroidism depends on the cause. If the cause is an adenoma or multinodular goiter, surgery or radioactive iodine therapy is recommended, especially in older clients. If the cause is excessive levothyroxine (for hypothyroidism), the dose of levothyroxine should be reduced. If the cause is Graves' disease, antithyroid drugs, radioactive iodine, surgery, or a combination of these methods may be warranted. All these methods reduce the amount of thyroid hormones circulating in the bloodstream.

Drug Selection

The antithyroid drugs include the thioamide derivatives (propylthiouracil and methimazole) and iodine preparations (Lugol's solution and SSKI). The thioamide drugs are inexpensive and relatively safe, and they do not damage the thyroid gland. These drugs may be used as the primary treatment (for which they may be given 6 months to 2 years) or to decrease blood levels of thyroid hormone before radioactive iodine therapy or surgery.

Radioactive iodine is a frequently used treatment. It is safe, effective, inexpensive, and convenient. One disadvantage is hypothyroidism, which usually develops within a few months and requires lifelong thyroid hormone replacement therapy. Another disadvantage is the delay in therapeutic benefits. Results may not be apparent for 3 months or longer, during which time severe hyperthyroidism must be brought under control with one of the thioamide antithyroid drugs.

Other iodine preparations are not used in long-term treatment of hyperthyroidism. They are indicated when a rapid clinical response is needed, as in thyroid storm and acute hyperthyroidism, or to prepare a hyperthyroid person for thyroidectomy. A thioamide drug is given to produce a euthyroid state, and an iodine preparation is given to reduce the size and vascularity of the thyroid gland to reduce the risk of excessive bleeding. Maximal effects are reached in approximately 10 to 15 days of continuous therapy, and this is probably the primary advantage. Disadvantages of this combination of drugs include the following:

● They may produce goiter, hyperthyroidism, or both.
● They cannot be used alone. Therapeutic benefits are temporary, and symptoms of hyperthyroidism may reappear and even be intensified if other treatment methods are not also used.
● Radioactive iodine cannot be used effectively for a prolonged period in a client who has received iodine preparations. Even if the iodine preparation is discontinued, the thyroid gland is saturated with iodine and does not attract enough radioactive iodine for treatment to be effective. Also, if radioactive iodine is given later, acute hyperthyroidism is likely to result because the radioactive iodine causes the stored hormones to be released into the circulation.
● Although giving a thioamide drug followed by an iodine preparation is standard preparation for thyroidectomy, the opposite sequence of administration is unsafe. If the iodine preparation is given first and followed by PTU or methimazole, the client is likely to experience acute hyperthyroidism because the thioamide causes release of the stored thyroid hormones.

Drug Dosage

Dosage of the thioamide antithyroid drugs is relatively large until a euthyroid state is reached, usually in 6 to 8 weeks. A maintenance dose, in the smallest amount that prevents recurrent symptoms of hyperthyroidism, is then given for 1 year or longer. Dosage should be decreased if the thyroid gland enlarges or signs and symptoms of hypothyroidism occur.

Radioactive iodide is usually given in a single dose to middle-aged and elderly people on an outpatient basis. For most clients, no special radiation precautions are necessary. If a very large dose is given, the client may be isolated for 8 days, which is the half-life of radioactive iodide.

Duration of Therapy

No clear-cut guidelines exist regarding duration of antithyroid drug therapy because exacerbations and remissions occur. It is usually continued until the client is euthyroid for 6 to 12 months. Diagnostic tests to evaluate thyroid function or a trial withdrawal then may be implemented to determine whether the client is likely to remain euthyroid without further drug therapy. If a drug is to be discontinued, this is usually done gradually over weeks or months.

The therapeutic effects of radioactive iodide are delayed for several weeks or as long as 6 months. During this time, symptoms may be controlled with thioamide drugs or propranolol.

Hyperthyroidism and the Metabolism of Other Drugs

Treatment of hyperthyroidism changes the rate of body metabolism, including the rate of metabolism of many drugs. In the hyperthyroid state, drug metabolism may be very rapid, and higher doses of most drugs may be necessary to achieve therapeutic results. When the client becomes euthyroid, the rate of drug metabolism is decreased. Consequently, doses of all medications should be evaluated and probably reduced to avoid severe adverse effects.

Use in Special Populations

Use in Children

For *hypothyroidism,* replacement therapy is required because thyroid hormone is essential for normal growth and development. As in adults, levothyroxine is the drug of choice in children and dosage needs may change with growth. For congenital hypothyroidism (cretinism), drug therapy should be started within 6 weeks of birth and continued for life. Initially, the recommended dose is 10 to 15 micrograms per kilogram of body weight per day. Delay in replacement therapy may result in permanent retardation despite resolution of the symptoms that resulted from thyroid deficit. Then, maintenance doses for long-term therapy vary with the child's age and weight, usually decreasing over time to a typical adult dose at 11 to 20 years of age. Infants requiring thyroid hormone replacement need relatively large doses. After thyroid drugs are started, the maintenance dosage is determined by periodic radioimmunoassay of serum thy-

roxine levels and by periodic radiographs to follow bone development.

To monitor drug effects on growth in children, height and weight should be recorded and compared with growth charts at regular intervals. Children should be monitored closely for adverse drug effects, which are similar to those seen in adults.

For *hyperthyroidism,* PTU or methimazole is used. Potential risks for adverse effects are similar to those in adults. Radioactive iodine may cause cancer and chromosome damage in children; therefore, this agent should be used only for hyperthyroidism that cannot be controlled by other antithyroid drugs or surgery.

Use in Older Adults

Signs and symptoms of thyroid disorders may mimic those of other disorders that often occur in older adults (eg, congestive heart failure). Therefore, a thorough physical examination and diagnostic tests of thyroid function are necessary before starting any type of treatment.

For *hypothyroidism,* levothyroxine is given. Thyroid hormone replacement increases the workload of the heart and may cause serious adverse effects in older adults, especially those with cardiovascular disease. Cardiac effects also may be increased in clients receiving bronchodilators or other cardiac stimulants. Clients who are older or who have cardiovascular disease require cautious treatment because of a high risk of adverse effects on the cardiovascular system. Thus, these clients are given smaller initial dosages and smaller increments at longer intervals than younger adults. For example, the drugs should be given in small initial dosages (eg, 25 mcg/day) and increased by 25 micrograms per day at monthly intervals until euthyroidism is attained and a maintenance dose established. Periodic measurements of serum TSH levels are indicated to monitor drug therapy, and doses can be adjusted when indicated.

Blood pressure and pulse should be monitored regularly. As a general rule, the drug should not be given if the resting heart rate is more than 100 beats per minute.

For *hyperthyroidism,* PTU or methimazole may be used, but radioactive iodine is often preferred because it is associated with fewer adverse effects than other antithyroid drugs or surgery. Clients should be monitored closely for hypothyroidism, which usually develops within a year after receiving treatment for hyperthyroidism.

 APPLYING YOUR KNOWLEDGE 24-4:
HOW CAN YOU AVOID THIS MEDICATION ERROR?
Ms. Zalewski complains about acid indigestion. You notice that Maalox has been ordered for her, and give a dose with her morning medication.

N U R S I N G   A C T I O N S

Thyroid and Antithyroid Drugs

NURSING ACTIONS	RATIONALE/EXPLANATION
1. Administer accurately	
a. With thyroid drugs:	
(1) Administer in a single daily dose, on an empty stomach (eg, before breakfast).	Fasting increases drug absorption; early administration allows peak activity during daytime hours and is less likely to interfere with sleep.
(2) Check the pulse rate before giving the drug. If the rate is over 100 per minute or if any changes in cardiac rhythm are noted, consult the physician before giving the dose.	Tachycardia or other cardiac dysrhythmias may indicate adverse cardiac effects. Dosage may need to be reduced or the drug stopped temporarily.
(3) To give levothyroxine to an infant or young child, the tablet may be crushed and a small amount of formula or water added. After it is mixed, administer it soon, by spoon or dropper. Do *not* store the liquid very long. The crushed tablet may also be sprinkled on a small amount of food (eg, cereal, applesauce).	Accurate and consistent administration is vital to promoting normal growth and development.
(4) Do not switch among various brands or generic forms of the drug.	Differences in bioavailability have been identified among products. Changes in preparations may alter dosage and therefore symptom control.
b. With antithyroid and iodine drugs:	
(1) Administer q8h.	All these drugs have rather short half-lives and must be given frequently and regularly to maintain therapeutic blood levels. In addition, if iodine preparations are not given every 8 hours, symptoms of hyperthyroidism may recur.
(2) Dilute iodine solutions in a full glass of fruit juice or milk, if possible, and have the client drink the medication through a straw.	Dilution of the drug reduces gastric irritation and masks the unpleasant taste. Using a straw prevents staining the teeth.
2. Observe for therapeutic effects	
a. With thyroid drugs, observe for:	
(1) Increased energy and activity level, less lethargy and fatigue	Therapeutic effects result from a return to normal metabolic activities and relief of the symptoms of hypothyroidism. Therapeutic effects may be evident as early as 2 or 3 days after drug therapy is started or delayed up to approximately 2 weeks. All signs and symptoms of myxedema should disappear in approximately 3 to 12 weeks.
(2) Increased alertness and interest in surroundings	
(3) Increased appetite	
(4) Increased pulse rate and temperature	
(5) Decreased constipation	
(6) Reversal of coarseness and other changes in skin and hair	
(7) With cretinism, increased growth rate (record height periodically)	
(8) With myxedema, diuresis, weight loss, and decreased edema	
(9) Decreased serum cholesterol and possibly decreased creatine phosphokinase, lactate dehydrogenase, and aspartate aminotransferase levels	These serum levels are often elevated with myxedema and may return to normal when thyroid replacement therapy is begun.
b. With antithyroid and iodine drugs, observe for:	
(1) Slower pulse rate	With propylthiouracil and methimazole, some therapeutic effects are apparent in 1 or 2 weeks, but euthyroidism may not occur for 6 or 8 weeks.
(2) Slower speech	

(continued)

NURSING ACTIONS	RATIONALE/EXPLANATION
(3) More normal activity level (slowing of hyperactivity)	With iodine solutions, therapeutic effects may be apparent within 24 hours. Maximal effects occur in approximately 10 to 15 days. However, therapeutic effects may not be sustained. Symptoms may reappear if the drug is given longer than a few weeks, and they may be more severe than initially.
(4) Decreased nervousness	
(5) Decreased tremors	
(6) Improved ability to sleep and rest	
(7) Weight gain	

3. **Observe for adverse effects**

a. With thyroid drugs, observe for tachycardia and other cardiac dysrhythmias, angina pectoris, myocardial infarction, congestive heart failure, nervousness, hyperactivity, insomnia, diarrhea, abdominal cramps, nausea and vomiting, weight loss, fever, intolerance to heat.

Most adverse reactions stem from excessive doses, and signs and symptoms produced are the same as those occurring with hyperthyroidism. Excessive thyroid hormones make the heart work very hard and fast in attempting to meet tissue demands for oxygenated blood and nutrients. Symptoms of myocardial ischemia occur when the myocardium does not get an adequate supply of oxygenated blood. Symptoms of congestive heart failure occur when the increased cardiac workload is prolonged. Cardiovascular problems are more likely to occur in clients who are elderly or who already have heart disease.

b. With propylthiouracil and methimazole, observe for:

   (1) Hypothyroidism—bradycardia, congestive heart failure, anemia, coronary artery and peripheral vascular disease, slow speech and movements, emotional and mental dullness, excessive sleeping, weight gain, constipation, skin changes, and others

   (2) Blood disorders—leukopenia, agranulocytosis, hypoprothrombinemia

   Leukopenia may be difficult to evaluate because it may occur with hyperthyroidism and with antithyroid drugs. Agranulocytosis occurs rarely but is the most severe adverse reaction; the earliest symptoms are likely to be sore throat and fever. If these occur, report them to the physician immediately.

   (3) Integumentary system—skin rash, pruritus, alopecia

   (4) Central nervous system (CNS)—headache, dizziness, loss of sense of taste, drowsiness, paresthesias

   (5) Gastrointestinal system—nausea, vomiting, abdominal discomfort, gastric irritation, cholestatic hepatitis

   (6) Other—lymphadenopathy, edema, joint pain, drug fever

c. With iodine preparations, observe for:

   Adverse effects are uncommon with short-term use.

   (1) Iodism—metallic taste, burning in mouth, soreness of gums, excessive salivation, gastric or respiratory irritation, rhinitis, headache, redness of conjunctiva, edema of eyelids

   (2) Hypersensitivity—acneiform skin rash, pruritus, fever, jaundice, angioedema, serum sickness

   Allergic reactions rarely occur.

   (3) Goiter with hypothyroidism

   Uncommon but may occur in adults and newborns whose mothers have taken iodides for long periods

4. **Observe for drug interactions**

a. Drugs that *increase* effects of thyroid hormones:

   (1) *Activating antidepressants* (eg, bupropion, venlafaxine), adrenergic antiasthmatic drugs (eg, albuterol, epinephrine), nasal decongestants

   These drugs may cause CNS and cardiovascular stimulation when taken alone. When combined with thyroid hormones, excessive cardiovascular stimulation may occur and cause myocardial ischemia, cardiac dysrhythmias, hypertension, and other adverse cardiovascular effects. Excessive CNS stimulation may produce anxiety, nervousness, hyperactivity, and insomnia.

NURSING ACTIONS	RATIONALE/EXPLANATION
b. Drugs that *decrease* effects of thyroid hormones:	
(1) Antacids, cholestyramine, iron, sucralfate	Decrease absorption of levothyroxine; give levothyroxine 2 hours before or 4 to 6 hours after one of these drugs.
(2) Antihypertensives	Decrease cardiac-stimulating effects
(3) Estrogens, including oral contraceptives containing estrogens	Estrogens increase thyroxine-binding globulin, thereby increasing the amount of bound, inactive levothyroxine in clients with hypo-thyroidism. This decreased effect does not occur in clients with adequate thyroid-hormone secretion because the increased binding is offset by increased T4 production. Women taking oral contraceptives may need larger doses of thyroid hormone replacement than would otherwise be needed.
(4) Propranolol (Inderal)	This drug decreases cardiac effects of thyroid hormones. It is used in hyperthyroidism to reduce tachycardia and other symptoms of excessive cardiovascular stimulation.
(5) Phenytoin, rifampin	Induce enzymes that metabolize (inactivate) levothyroxine more rapidly
c. Drug that *increases* effects of antithyroid drugs:	
(1) Lithium	Acts synergistically to produce hypothyroidism

APPLYING YOUR KNOWLEDGE: ANSWERS

24-1 Change the medication time to 7:30 A.M. to assure that Synthroid is given on an empty stomach. Taking the drug on an empty stomach will increase its absorption.

24-2 Teach Ms. Zalewski to maintain a diet that is low in fat and calories and high in fiber, and to monitor for variations in weight.

24-3 Evaluate Ms. Zalewski's TSH level. The normal range is 0.5–4.2 microunits/L. Her symptoms are typical of a client with hyperthyroidism. Notify the prescriber of these symptoms.

24-4 Synthroid should not be given with an antacid, iron preparation, or sucralfate. These drugs decrease the absorption of Synthroid. If the client requires an antacid, the antacid should be given 2 hours before or 4 to 6 hours after the dose of Synthroid.

Review and Application Exercises

Short Answer Exercises

1. Where is TSH produced, and what is its function?

2. What is the role of thyroid hormones in maintaining body functions?

3. What signs and symptoms are associated with hypothyroidism?

4. In primary hypothyroidism, are blood levels of TSH increased or decreased?

5. What are adverse effects of drug therapy for hypothyroidism?

6. What signs and symptoms are associated with hyperthyroidism?

7. Which drugs reduce blood levels of thyroid hormone in hyperthyroidism, and how do they act?

8. What are adverse effects of drug therapy for hyperthyroidism?

9. When propranolol is used in the treatment of hyperthyroidism, what are its expected effects?

10. What is the effect of thyroid disorders on metabolism of other drugs?

NCLEX-Style Questions

11. A male client asks a nurse when he should take his daily dose of levothyroxine. The nurse recommends that the client take the drug
    a. before breakfast on an empty stomach
    b. with meals in divided doses

c. at bedtime with a snack

d. whenever it is convenient

12. Which of the following agents is the drug of first choice for treatment of hypothyroidism?
    a. propranolol (Inderal)
    b. levothyroxine (Synthroid, Levothroid)
    c. liothyronine (Cytomel, Triostat)
    d. propylthiouracil

13. Which of the following clients with Graves' disease would be an appropriate candidate for sodium iodide ^{131}I therapy?
    a. an 8-year-old boy
    b. a 28-year-old breast-feeding mother
    c. a 35-year-old pregnant woman
    d. a 40-year-old man

14. Propranolol is useful in the treatment of hyperthyroidism to relieve which of the following symptoms?
    a. heat intolerance
    b. exophthalmos
    c. dry skin
    d. tachycardia

15. Which of the following orders should a nurse question in a client with hypothyroidism?
    a. psyllium seed (Metamucil)
    b. levothyroxine (Synthroid)
    c. morphine sulfate
    d. liothyronine (Cytomel)

Selected References

Dong, B. J. (2000). Thyroid disorders. E. T. In Herfindal & D. R. Gourley (Eds.), *Textbook of therapeutics: Drug and disease management* (7th ed., pp. 325–358). Philadelphia: Lippincott Williams & Wilkins.

Drug facts and comparisons. (Updated monthly). St. Louis: Facts and Comparisons.

Fatourechi, V. (2001). Subclinical thyroid disease. *Mayo Clinic Proceedings, 76*(4), 413–417.

Guyton, A. C., & Hall, J. E. (2000). *Textbook of medical physiology* (10th ed.). Philadelphia: W. B. Saunders.

Lacy, C. F., Armstrong, L. L., Goldman, M. P., Lance, L. L. (2004). *Lexi-Comp's drug information handbook* (12th ed.). Hudson, OH: Lexi-Comp.

Matfin, G., Kuenzi, J. A., & Guven, S. (2005). Disorders of endocrine control of growth and metabolism. In C. M. Porth, *Pathophysiology: Concepts of altered health states* (7th ed., pp. 961–985). Philadelphia: Lippincott Williams & Wilkins.

Wartofsky, L. (2000). Disorders of the thyroid gland. In H. D. Humes (Ed.), *Kelley's Textbook of internal medicine* (4th ed., pp. 2693–2719). Philadelphia: Lippincott Williams & Wilkins.

Hormones That Regulate Calcium and Bone Metabolism

OBJECTIVES

After studying this chapter, you will be able to:

1. Describe the roles of parathyroid hormone, calcitonin, and vitamin D in regulating calcium metabolism.
2. Identify populations at risk for hypocalcemia.
3. Discuss prevention and treatment of hypocalcemia and osteoporosis.
4. Identify clients at risk for hypercalcemia.
5. Discuss recognition and management of hypercalcemia as a medical emergency.
6. Discuss the use of calcium and vitamin D supplements, calcitonin, and bisphosphonate drugs in the treatment of osteoporosis.

APPLYING YOUR KNOWLEDGE

Carolyn Taylor is a 68-year-old retired teacher. She has chronic venous insufficiency and osteoporosis. Ms. Taylor has suffered two fractures from falls in recent years. She has been menopausal for 16 years and has not been on estrogen replacement therapy due to her vascular disease. Her physician prescribes alendronate in the once-weekly dose.

INTRODUCTION

Calcium and bone metabolism are regulated by three hormones: parathyroid hormone (PTH), calcitonin, and vitamin D, which act to maintain normal serum levels of calcium. When serum calcium levels are decreased, hormonal mechanisms are activated to raise them; when they are elevated, mechanisms act to lower them (Fig. 25-1). Overall, the hormones alter absorption of dietary calcium from the gastrointestinal tract, movement of calcium from bone to serum, and excretion of calcium through the kidneys.

Disorders of calcium and bone metabolism include hypocalcemia, hypercalcemia, osteoporosis, Paget's disease, and bone breakdown associated with breast cancer and multiple myeloma. Drugs used to treat these disorders mainly alter serum calcium levels or strengthen bone. This chapter describes the characteristics of the hormones, calcium, phosphorus, and some associated disorders.

Hormones Involved in Calcium Metabolism

Parathyroid Hormone

PTH secretion is stimulated by low serum calcium levels and inhibited by normal or high levels (a negative feedback system). Because phosphate is closely related to calcium in body functions, PTH also regulates phosphate metabolism. In general, when serum calcium levels increase, serum phosphate levels decrease, and vice versa. Thus, an inverse relationship exists between calcium and phosphate.

When the serum calcium level falls below the normal range, PTH raises the level by acting on bone, intestines, and kidneys. In bone, breakdown is increased, so that calcium moves from bone into the serum. In the intestines, there is increased absorption of calcium ingested in food (PTH activates vitamin D, which increases intestinal absorption). In the kidneys, there is increased reabsorption of calcium in the renal tubules and less urinary excretion. The opposite effects occur with phosphate (ie, PTH decreases serum phosphate and increases urinary phosphate excretion).

Disorders of parathyroid function are related to insufficient production of PTH (hypoparathyroidism) or excessive production of PTH (hyperparathyroidism). Hypoparathyroidism is most often caused by removal of or damage to the parathyroid glands during neck surgery. Hyperparathyroidism is most often caused by a tumor or hyperplasia of a parathyroid gland. It also may result from ectopic secretion of PTH by malignant tumors (eg, carcinomas of the lung, pancreas, kidney, ovary, prostate gland, or bladder). Clinical manifestations and treatment of hypoparathyroidism are the same as those of hypocalcemia. Clinical manifestations and treatment of hyperparathyroidism are the same as those of hypercalcemia.

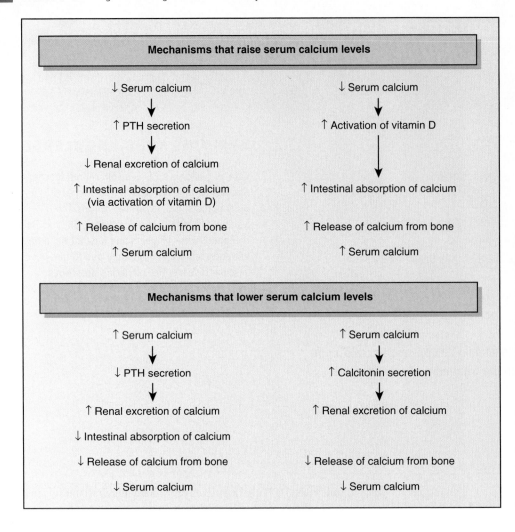

FIGURE 25-1 Hormonal regulation of serum calcium levels. When serum calcium levels are low (hypocalcemia), there is increased secretion of parathyroid hormone (PTH) and increased activation of vitamin D. These mechanisms lead to decreased loss of calcium in the urine, increased absorption of calcium from the intestine, and increased resorption of calcium from bone. These mechanisms work together to raise serum calcium levels to normal.

When serum calcium levels are high (hypercalcemia), there is decreased secretion of PTH and increased secretion of calcitonin. These mechanisms lead to increased loss of calcium in the urine, decreased absorption of calcium from the intestine, and decreased resorption of calcium from bone. These mechanisms lower serum calcium levels to normal.

Calcitonin

Calcitonin is a hormone from the thyroid gland whose secretion is controlled by the concentration of ionized calcium in the blood flowing through the thyroid gland. When the serum level of ionized calcium is increased, secretion of calcitonin is increased. The function of calcitonin is to lower serum calcium in the presence of hypercalcemia, which it does by decreasing movement of calcium from bone to serum and increasing urinary excretion of calcium. The action of calcitonin is rapid but of short duration. Thus, this hormone has little effect on long-term calcium metabolism.

Vitamin D (Calciferol)

Vitamin D is a fat-soluble vitamin that includes both ergocalciferol (obtained from foods) and cholecalciferol (formed by exposure of skin to sunlight). It functions as a hormone and plays an important role in calcium and bone metabolism. The main action of vitamin D is to raise serum calcium levels by increasing intestinal absorption of calcium and mobilizing calcium from bone. It also promotes bone formation by providing adequate serum concentrations of minerals. Vita-

min D is not physiologically active in the body. It must be converted to an intermediate metabolite in the liver, then to an active metabolite (1,25-dihydroxyvitamin D or calcitriol) in the kidneys. PTH and adequate hepatic and renal function are required to produce the active metabolite.

Deficiency of vitamin D causes inadequate absorption of calcium and phosphorus. This, in turn, leads to low levels of serum calcium and stimulation of PTH secretion. In children, this sequence of events produces inadequate mineralization of bone (rickets), a rare condition in the United States. In adults, vitamin D deficiency causes osteomalacia, a condition characterized by decreased bone density and strength.

Calcium and Phosphorus

Calcium and phosphorus are discussed together because they are closely related physiologically. These mineral nutrients are found in many of the same foods, from which they are absorbed together. They are regulated by PTH and excreted through the kidneys. They are both required in cellular structure and function and, as calcium phosphate, in formation and maintenance of bones and teeth. Their characteristics and functions are summarized in Box 25-1.

Box 25-1 Characteristics and Functions of Calcium and Phosphorus

Calcium

Calcium is the most abundant cation in the body. Approximately 99% is located in the bones and teeth; the rest is in the extracellular fluid and soft tissues. Approximately half of serum calcium is bound, mostly to serum proteins, and is physiologically inactive. The other half is ionized and physiologically active. Ionized calcium can leave the vascular compartment and enter cells, where it participates in intracellular functions. An adequate amount of free (ionized) calcium is required for normal function of all body cells.

Calcium is obtained from the diet, but only 30% to 50% is absorbed from the small intestine; the rest is lost in feces. Absorption is increased in the presence of vitamin D, lactose, moderate amounts of fat, and high protein intake; increased acidity of gastric secretions; and a physiologic need. Absorption is inhibited by vitamin D deficiency; a high-fat diet; the presence of oxalic acid (from beet greens, chard), which combines with calcium to form insoluble calcium oxalate in the intestine; alkalinity of intestinal secretions, which leads to formation of insoluble calcium phosphate; diarrhea or other conditions of rapid intestinal motility, which do not allow sufficient time for absorption; and immobilization.

Calcium is lost from the body in feces, urine, and sweat. Even when there is deficient intake, approximately 150 mg are lost daily through the intestines (in mucosal and biliary secretions and sloughed intestinal cells). In lactating women, relatively large amounts are lost in breast milk.

Functions

- Calcium participates in many metabolic processes, including the regulation of:
  - Cell membrane permeability and function
  - Nerve-cell excitability and transmission of impulses (eg, it is required for release of neurotransmitters at synapses)
  - Contraction of cardiac, skeletal, and smooth muscle
  - Conduction of electrical impulses in the heart
  - Blood coagulation and platelet adhesion processes
  - Hormone secretion
  - Enzyme activity
  - Catecholamine release from the adrenal medulla
  - Release of chemical mediators (eg, histamine from mast cells)
- Calcium is required for building and maintaining bones and teeth. Bone calcium is composed mainly of calcium phosphate and calcium carbonate. In addition to these bound forms, a small amount of calcium is available for exchange with serum. This acts as a reserve supply of calcium. Calcium is constantly shifting between bone and serum as bone is formed and broken down. When serum calcium levels become low, calcium moves into serum.

Requirements and Sources

The calcium requirement of normal adults is approximately 1000 mg daily. Increased daily amounts are needed by growing children (1200 mg), pregnant or lactating women (1200 mg), and postmenopausal women who do not take replacement estrogens (1500 mg to prevent osteoporosis).

The best sources of calcium are milk and milk products. Three 8-oz glasses of milk daily contain approximately the amount needed by healthy adults. Calcium in milk is readily used by the body because milk also contains lactose and vitamin D, both of which are involved in calcium absorption. Other sources of calcium include vegetables (eg, broccoli, spinach, kale, mustard greens) and seafood (eg, clams, oysters).

Phosphorus

Phosphorus is one of the most important elements in normal body function. Most phosphorus is combined with calcium in bones and teeth as calcium phosphate (approximately 80%). The remainder is distributed in every body cell and in extracellular fluid. It is combined with carbohydrates, lipids, proteins, and various other compounds.

Phosphorus is obtained from the diet, and approximately 70% of dietary phosphorus is absorbed from the gastrointestinal (GI) tract. The most efficient absorption occurs when calcium and phosphorus are ingested in approximately equal amounts. Because this equal ratio is present in milk, milk is probably the best source of phosphorus. In general, factors that increase or decrease calcium absorption act the same way on phosphorus absorption. Vitamin D enhances, but is not essential for, phosphorus absorption. Large amounts of calcium or aluminum in the GI tract may combine with phosphate to form insoluble compounds and thereby decrease absorption of phosphorus.

Phosphorus is lost from the body primarily in urine. In people with acute or chronic renal failure, phosphorus intake is restricted because excretion is impaired.

Functions

Phosphorus, most of which is located intracellularly as the phosphate ion, performs many metabolic functions:

- It is an essential component of deoxyribonucleic acid, ribonucleic acid, and other nucleic acids in body cells. Thus, it is required for cell reproduction and body growth.
- It combines with fatty acids to form phospholipids, which are components of all cell membranes in the body. This reaction also prevents buildup of excessive amounts of free fatty acids.
- It forms a phosphate buffer system, which helps to maintain acid–base balance. When excess hydrogen ions are present in kidney tubules, phosphate combines with them and allows their excretion in urine. At the same time, bicarbonate is retained by the kidneys and contributes to alkalinity of body fluids. Although there are other buffering systems in the body, failure of the phosphate system leads to metabolic acidosis (retained hydrogen ions or acid and lost bicarbonate ions or base).
- It is necessary for cellular use of glucose and production of energy.
- It is necessary for proper function of several B vitamins (ie, the vitamins function as coenzymes in various chemical reactions only when combined with phosphate).

Requirements and Sources

Daily requirements for phosphorus are approximately 800 mg for normal adults and 1200 mg for growing children and pregnant or lactating women. Phosphorus is widely available in foods. Good sources are milk and other dairy products, meat, poultry, fish, eggs, and nuts. There is little risk of phosphorus deficiency with an adequate intake of calcium and protein.

Calcium Disorders and Bone Metabolism

The calcium disorders are hypocalcemia and hypercalcemia, either of which can be life threatening. The bone disorders discussed in this chapter are those characterized by increased resorption of calcium and loss of bone mass. These disorders weaken bone and lead to fractures, pain, and disability. Selected calcium and bone disorders are described in Box 25-2.

Bone is mineralized connective tissue that functions as structural support and a reservoir for calcium, phosphorus, magnesium, sodium, and carbonate. The role of bone in maintaining serum calcium levels takes precedence over its structural function (ie, bone may be weakened or destroyed as calcium leaves bone and enters serum). Bone tissue is constantly being formed and broken down in a process called *remodeling*. During childhood, adolescence, and early adulthood, formation usually exceeds breakdown (resorption) as the person attains adult height and peak bone mass. After approximately 35 years of age, resorption is greater than formation. Hormonal deficiencies, some diseases, and some medications (eg, glucocorticoids) can also increase resorption, resulting in loss of bone mass and osteoporosis.

INDIVIDUAL DRUGS

Calcium and Vitamin D Preparations

Calcium and vitamin D supplements are used to treat hypocalcemia and to prevent and treat osteoporosis. These drugs are described in the following sections, and names and dosages of individual drug preparations are listed in Table 25-1.

Calcium Preparations

An intravenous (IV) calcium salt (usually **calcium gluconate**) is given for acute, symptomatic hypocalcemia. An oral preparation (eg, **calcium carbonate** or **citrate**) is given for asymptomatic, less severe, or chronic hypocalcemia. These preparations differ mainly in the amounts of calcium they contain and the routes by which they are given.

Even when serum calcium levels are normal, calcium supplements may be needed by people who do not get enough calcium in their diets. Most diets in people of all ages, especially in young women and older adults, are thought to be deficient in calcium. Calcium supplements are also used in the prevention and treatment of osteoporosis.

Vitamin D Preparations

Vitamin D is used in chronic hypocalcemia if calcium supplements alone cannot maintain serum calcium levels within a normal range. It is also used to prevent deficiency states and treat hypoparathyroidism and osteoporosis. Although authorities agree that dietary intake is better than supplements, some suggest a vitamin D supplement for people who ingest less than the

recommended amount (400 IU daily for those 6 months to 24 years of age; 200 IU for those 25 years of age and older). In addition, the recommended amount for older adults may be too low, especially for those who receive little exposure to sunlight, and dosage needs for all age groups may be greater during winter, when there is less sunlight. If used, vitamin D supplements should be taken cautiously and not overused; excessive amounts can cause serious problems, including hypercalcemia.

Drugs Used in Hypercalcemia and Selected Bone Disorders

Drugs used for hypercalcemia include bisphosphonates, calcitonin, corticosteroids, 0.9% sodium chloride IV infusion, and others. Drugs used for osteoporosis inhibit bone breakdown and demineralization and include bisphosphonates, calcitonin, estrogens, and antiestrogens. These drugs are described in the following sections, and most indications for use and dosages are listed in Table 25-2.

Bisphosphonates

Alendronate (Fosamax), **etidronate** (Didronel), **ibandronate** (Boniva), **pamidronate** (Aredia), **risedronate** (Actonel), **tiludronate** (Skelid), and **zoledronate** (Zometa) are drugs that bind to bone and inhibit calcium resorption from bone. Although indications for use vary among the drugs, they are used mainly in the treatment of hypercalcemia and osteoporosis. Etidronate also inhibits bone mineralization and may cause osteomalacia. Newer bisphosphonates do not have this effect.

Bisphosphonates are poorly absorbed from the intestinal tract and must be taken on an empty stomach, with water, at least 30 minutes before any other fluid, food, or medication. The drugs are not metabolized. The drug bound to bone is slowly released into the bloodstream. Most of the drug that is not bound to bone is excreted in the urine.

Calcitonin-salmon (Calcimar, Miacalcin) is used in the treatment of hypercalcemia, Paget's disease, and osteoporosis. In hypercalcemia, calcitonin lowers serum calcium levels by inhibiting bone resorption. Calcitonin is most likely to be effective in hypercalcemia caused by hyperparathyroidism, prolonged immobilization, or certain malignant neoplasms. In acute hypercalcemia, calcitonin may be used along with other measures to lower serum calcium levels rapidly. A single injection of calcitonin decreases serum calcium levels in approximately 2 hours, and its effects last approximately 6 to 8 hours.

In Paget's disease, calcitonin slows the rate of bone turnover, improves bone lesions on radiologic examination, and relieves bone pain. In osteoporosis, calcitonin prevents further bone loss in the presence of adequate calcium and vitamin D. In addition, calcitonin helps control pain in clients with osteoporosis or metastatic bone disease. Both subcutaneous injections and intranasal administration relieve pain within 1 to 12 weeks. The drug is given daily initially, then two to three times a week. The mechanism by which pain is reduced is unknown.

Box 25-2 Calcium and Bone Disorders

Hypocalcemia

Hypocalcemia is an abnormally low blood calcium level (ie, <8.5 mg/dL). It may be caused by inadequate intake of calcium and vitamin D, numerous disorders (eg, diarrhea or malabsorption syndromes that cause inadequate absorption of calcium and vitamin D, hypoparathyroidism, renal failure, severe hypomagnesemia, hypermagnesemia, acute pancreatitis, rhabdomyolysis, tumor lysis syndrome, vitamin D deficiency), and several drugs (eg, cisplatin, cytosine arabinoside, foscarnet, ketoconazole, pentamidine, agents used to treat hypercalcemia). Calcium deficits caused by inadequate dietary intake affect bone tissue rather than serum calcium levels. Hypocalcemia associated with renal failure is caused by two mechanisms. First, inability to excrete phosphate in urine leads to accumulation of phosphate in the blood (hyperphosphatemia). Because phosphate levels are inversely related to calcium levels, hyperphosphatemia induces hypocalcemia. Second, when kidney function is impaired, vitamin D conversion to its active metabolite is impaired. This results in decreased intestinal absorption of calcium.

Clinical manifestations are characterized by increased neuromuscular irritability, which may progress to tetany. Tetany is characterized by numbness and tingling of the lips, fingers, and toes; twitching of facial muscles; spasms of skeletal muscle; carpopedal spasm; laryngospasm; and convulsions. In young children, hypocalcemia may be manifested by convulsions rather than tetany and erroneously diagnosed as epilepsy. This may be a serious error because anticonvulsant drugs used for epilepsy may further decrease serum calcium levels. Severe hypocalcemia may cause lethargy or confusion.

Hypercalcemia

Hypercalcemia is an abnormally high blood calcium level (ie, >10.5 mg/dL). It may be caused by hyperparathyroidism, hyperthyroidism, malignant neoplasms, vitamin D or vitamin A intoxication, aluminum intoxication, prolonged immobilization, adrenocortical insufficiency, and ingestion of thiazide diuretics, estrogens, and lithium. Cancer is a common cause, especially carcinomas (of the breast, lung, head and neck, or kidney) and multiple myeloma. Cancer stimulates bone breakdown, which increases serum calcium levels. Increased urine output leads to fluid volume deficit. This leads, in turn, to increased reabsorption of calcium in renal tubules and decreased renal excretion of calcium. Decreased renal excretion potentiates hypercalcemia. Clients at risk for hypercalcemia should be monitored for early signs and symptoms so treatment can be started before severe hypercalcemia develops.

Clinical manifestations are caused by the decreased ability of nerves to respond to stimuli and the decreased ability of muscles to contract and relax. Hypercalcemia has a depressant effect on nerve and muscle function. Gastrointestinal problems with hypercalcemia include anorexia, nausea, vomiting, constipation, and abdominal pain. Central nervous system problems include apathy, depression, poor memory, headache, and drowsiness. Severe hypercalcemia may produce lethargy, syncope, disorientation, hallucinations, coma, and death. Other signs and symptoms include weakness and decreased tone in skeletal and smooth muscle, dysphagia, polyuria, polyphagia, and cardiac dysrhythmias. In addition, calcium may be deposited in various tissues, such as the conjunctiva, cornea, and kidneys. Calcium deposits in the kidneys (renal calculi) may lead to irreversible damage and impairment of function.

Osteoporosis

Osteoporosis is characterized by decreased bone density (osteopenia) and weak, fragile bones that often lead to fractures, pain, and disability. Although any bones may be affected, common fracture sites are the vertebrae of the lower dorsal and lumbar spines, wrists, and hips. Risk factors include female sex, advanced age, small stature, lean body mass, white or Asian race, positive family history, low calcium intake, menopause, sedentary lifestyle, nulliparity, smoking, excessive ingestion of alcohol or caffeine, high protein intake, high phosphate intake, hyperthyroidism, and chronic use of certain medications (eg, corticosteroids, phenytoin). Postmenopausal women who do not take estrogen replacement therapy are at high risk because of estrogen deficiency, age-related bone loss, and a low peak bone mass. Osteoporosis occurs in men but less often than in women. Both men and women who take high doses of corticosteroids are at high risk because the drugs demineralize bone. In addition, renal transplant recipients can acquire osteoporosis from corticosteroid therapy, decreased renal function, increased parathyroid hormone secretion, and cyclosporine immunosuppressant therapy.

Osteopenia or early osteoporosis may be present and undetected unless radiography or a bone density measurement is done. If detected, treatment is needed to slow bone loss. If undetected or untreated, clinical manifestations of osteoporosis include shortened stature (a measurable loss of height), back pain, spinal deformity, or a fracture. Fractures often occur with common bending or lifting movements or falling.

Paget's Disease

Paget's disease is an inflammatory skeletal disease that affects older people. Its etiology is unknown. It is characterized by a high rate of bone turnover and results in bone deformity and pain. It is treated with non-narcotic analgesics and drugs that decrease bone resorption (eg, bisphosphonates, calcitonin).

Estrogens and Antiestrogens

Estrogens are discussed here in relation to osteoporosis; see Chapter 27 for other uses and dosages. Estrogen replacement therapy (ERT) is beneficial for preventing postmenopausal osteoporosis. ERT is most beneficial immediately after menopause, when a period of accelerated bone loss occurs. Mechanisms by which ERT protects against bone loss and fractures are thought to include decreased bone breakdown, increased calcium absorption from the intestine, and increased calcitriol (active form of vitamin D that promotes absorption and use of

(text continues on page 394)

Table 25-1 Drugs at a Glance: Calcium and Vitamin D Preparations

GENERIC/TRADE NAME	ROUTES AND DOSAGE RANGES	
	Adults	Children
Oral Calcium Products		
Calcium acetate (25% calcium) (PhosLo)	PO 2–4 tablets with each meal	Dosage not established
Calcium carbonate precipitated (40% calcium) (Os-Cal, Tums)	PO 1–1.5 g 3 times daily with meals (maximal dose, 8 g daily)	
Calcium citrate (21% calcium) (Citracal)	PO 1–2 tablets (200 mg calcium per tablet) 2–4 times daily	
Calcium gluconate (9% calcium)	PO 1–2 g 3 or 4 times daily	PO 500 mg/kg/d in divided doses
Calcium lactate (13% calcium)	PO 1 g 3 times daily with meals	PO 500 mg/kg/d in divided doses
Tricalcium phosphate (39% calcium) (Posture)	PO 1–2 tablets (600 mg calcium per tablet) 2–4 times daily	
Parenteral Calcium Products		
Calcium chloride (10 mL of 10% solution contains 273 mg [13.6 mEq] of calcium)	IV 500 mg–1 g (5–10 mL of 10% solution) every 1–3 d, depending on clinical response or serum calcium measurements	2.7–5 mg/kg/dose every 4–6 h depending on clinical response or serum calcium measurements
Calcium gluconate (10 mL of 10% solution contains 93 mg [4.65 mEq] of calcium)	IV 5–20 mL of 10% solution	IV 500 mg/kg/d in divided doses
Vitamin D Preparations		
Calcitriol (Rocaltrol, Calcijex)	Dialysis patients, hypoparathyroidism, PO 0.25 mcg daily initially, then adjusted according to serum calcium levels (usual daily maintenance dose, 0.5–1 mcg)	Hypoparathyroidism, ≥6 y: PO 0.5–2 mcg daily 1–5 y: PO 0.25–0.75 mcg daily
Cholecalciferol (Delta-D)	PO 400–1000 IU daily	
Dihydrotachysterol (Hytakerol)	PO 0.75–2.5 mg daily for several days, then decreased (average daily maintenance dose, 0.6 mg)	
Doxercalciferol (Hectorol)	Dialysis patients, PO 10 mcg 3 times weekly initially, increased if necessary. Maximum dose, 20 mcg 3 times weekly	
Ergocalciferol (Calciferol, Drisdol)	Hypoparathyroidism, PO 50,000–200,000 units daily initially (average daily maintenance dose, 25,000–100,000 units)	
Paricalcitol (Zemplar)	Dialysis patients, 0.04–0.1 mcg/kg every other d initially; increased by 2–4 mcg at 2- to 4-week intervals, if necessary. Reduce dosage or stop therapy if hypercalcemia occurs.	

IV, intravenous; PO, oral.

GENERIC/TRADE NAME	INDICATIONS FOR USE	ROUTES AND DOSAGE RANGES
Bisphosphonates		
Alendronate (Fosamax)	Osteoporosis: Prevention and treatment in postmenopausal women	Osteoporosis: *Postmenopausal women*: Prevention, PO 5 mg once daily or 35 mg once weekly; treatment, PO 10 mg once daily or 70 mg once weekly.
	Treatment in men and women with glucocorticoid-induced osteoporosis	*Men*: 10 mg once daily Glucocorticoid-induced, 5 mg once daily
	Paget's disease	Paget's disease, PO 40 mg daily for 6 mo; repeated if necessary
Etidronate (Didronel)	Paget's disease	Paget's disease, PO 5–10 mg/kg/d up to 6 mo or 11–20 mg/kg/d up to 3 mo; may be repeated after 3 mo if symptoms recur
	Heterotopic ossification	Heterotopic ossification: With spinal cord injury, PO 20 mg/kg/d for 2 wk, then 10 mg/kg/d for 10 wk; with total hip replacement, PO 20 mg/kg/d for 1 mo before and 3 mo after surgery
	Hypercalcemia of malignancy	Hypercalcemia of malignancy, IV 7.5 mg/kg/d, in at least 250 mL of 0.9% sodium chloride solution and infused over at least 2 h, daily for 3–7 d
Ibandronate (Boniva)	Treatment and prevention of osteoporosis in postmenopausal women	PO 2.5 mg once daily or 150 mg every month
Pamidronate (Aredia)	Hypercalcemia of malignancy	Hypercalcemia, if IV 60 mg give over 4 h; if 90 mg give over 24 h
	Osteolytic lesions of breast cancer metastases or multiple myeloma	Osteolytic bone lesions; Breast cancer, IV 90 mg over 2 h every 3–4 wk; multiple myeloma, IV 90 mg over 4 h once monthly
	Paget's disease	Paget's disease, IV 30 mg over 4 h, daily for 3 doses
Risedronate (Actonel)	Osteoporosis, postmenopausal and glucocorticoid-induced, prevention and treatment	Prevention and treatment of osteoporosis, PO 5 mg once daily or 35 mg once weekly
	Paget's disease	Paget's disease, PO 30 mg once daily for 2 mo
Tiludronate (Skelid)	Paget's disease	PO 400 mg once daily for 3 mo
Zoledronate (Zometa)	Hypercalcemia of malignancy	IV 4 mg over 15 min or longer
Calcitonin		
Calcitonin-salmon (Calcimar, Miacalcin)	Hypercalcemia	Hypercalcemia, Sub-Q, IM 4 IU/kg q12h; can be increased after 1 or 2 d to 8 IU/kg q12h; maximum dose, 8 IU/kg q6h
	Paget's disease	Paget's disease, Sub-Q, IM 50–100 IU/d
	Postmenopausal osteoporosis	Postmenopausal osteoporosis, Sub-Q, IM 100 IU/d; nasal spray (Miacalcin) 200 IU/d
Parathyroid Hormone		
Teriparatide (Forteo)	Osteoporosis	Sub-Q 20 mcg daily
Miscellaneous Agents		
Furosemide (Lasix)	Hypercalcemia	*Adults:* IV 80–100 mg q2h until a diuretic response is obtained or other treatment measures are initiated *Children:* IV 20–40 mg q4h until a diuretic response is obtained or other treatment measures are initiated
Phosphate salts (Neutra-Phos)	Hypercalcemia	PO 1–2 tablets 3 or 4 times daily, or contents of 1 capsule mixed with 75 mL of water 4 times daily
Prednisone or hydrocortisone	Hypercalcemia	Prednisone PO 20–50 mg twice daily (or equivalent dose of another glucocorticoid) for 5–10 d, then tapered to the minimum dose required to prevent hypercalcemia Hydrocortisone IM, IV 100–500 mg/d
0.9% Sodium chloride injection	Acute hypercalcemia	4–6 L/d

IM, intramuscular; IV, intravenous; PO, oral; Sub-Q, subcutaneous.

calcium in bone building) concentration. Progestins have been used with estrogens in women with an intact uterus because of the increased risk of endometrial cancer with estrogen therapy alone. However, estrogen and estrogen–progestin combinations are no longer recommended because adverse effects are thought to outweigh benefits.

In postmenopausal osteoporosis, other drugs may be used instead of estrogen. Raloxifene (Evista) and tamoxifen (Nolvadex) act like estrogen in some body tissues and prevent the action of estrogen in other body tissues. Raloxifene is classified as a selective estrogen receptor modulator and is approved for prevention of postmenopausal osteoporosis. It has estrogenic effects in bone tissue, thereby decreasing bone breakdown and increasing bone mass density. It has antiestrogen effects in uterine and breast tissue. Tamoxifen, which is classified as an antiestrogen, is used to prevent and treat breast cancer. It also has estrogenic effects and can be used to prevent osteoporosis and cardiovascular disease, although it is not approved for these uses. Tamoxifen may help prevent osteoporosis in clients with breast cancer.

Parathyroid Hormone

Teriparatide (Forteo) is a recombinant DNA version of PTH. It is approved for the treatment of osteoporosis in women. Other drugs for osteoporosis slow bone loss, whereas teriparatide increases bone formation by increasing the number of bone-building cells (osteoblasts). Teriparatide also increases serum levels of calcium and calcitriol. In clinical trials, the drug increased vertebral bone mineral density and decreased vertebral fractures. It is recommended for use in clients with severe osteoporosis or those who have not responded adequately to other treatments, partly because osteosarcoma developed in some animals given high doses for long periods. No osteosarcoma developed in humans during clinical trials, but the longest of these trials was 2 years.

Teriparatide is rapidly and well absorbed following subcutaneous injection. Bioavailability is 95%, and peak serum levels occur in 30 minutes. The drug is metabolized and excreted through the liver, kidneys, and bone. It is not expected to accumulate in bone or other tissues, to interact significantly with other drugs, or to require dosage adjustment with renal or hepatic impairment. Adverse effects include nausea, headache, back pain, dizziness, syncope, and leg cramps.

Corticosteroids

Glucocorticoids (see Chap. 23) are used in the treatment of hypercalcemia due to malignancies or vitamin D intoxication. These drugs lower serum calcium levels by inhibiting cytokine release; by direct cytolytic effects on some tumor cells; by inhibiting calcium absorption from the intestine; and by increasing calcium excretion in the urine. **Hydrocortisone** or **prednisone** is often used. The serum calcium level

decreases in approximately 5 to 10 days, and after it stabilizes, the dosage should be gradually reduced to the minimum needed to control symptoms of hypercalcemia. High dosage or prolonged administration leads to serious adverse effects.

Other Drugs for Hypercalcemia

Furosemide (Lasix) is a loop diuretic (see Chap. 53) that increases calcium excretion in urine by preventing its reabsorption in renal tubules. It can be given via the IV route for rapid effects in acute hypercalcemia, but authorities do not agree about its use. Some recommend furosemide after extracellular fluid volume has been restored and saline diuresis occurs with IV infusion of several liters of 0.9% sodium chloride. Others recommend furosemide only if evidence of fluid overload is found or if heart failure occurs. Thiazide diuretics are contraindicated in clients with hypercalcemia because they *decrease* urinary excretion of calcium.

Phosphate salts (Neutra-Phos) inhibit intestinal absorption of calcium and increase deposition of calcium in bone. (Neutra-Phos is an oral combination of sodium phosphate and potassium phosphate.) Oral salts are effective in the treatment of hypercalcemia due to any cause. A potential adverse effect of phosphates is calcification of soft tissues due to deposition of calcium phosphate, which can lead to severe impairment of function in the kidneys and other organs. Phosphates should be given only when hypercalcemia is accompanied by hypophosphatemia (serum phosphorus <3 mg/dL) and renal function is normal, to minimize the risk of soft tissue calcification. Serum calcium, phosphorus, and creatinine levels should be monitored frequently, and the dose should be reduced if serum phosphorus exceeds 4.5 milligrams per deciliter or the product of serum calcium and phosphorus exceeds 60 milligrams per deciliter.

Sodium chloride (0.9%) injection (normal saline) is an IV solution that contains water, sodium, and chloride. It is included here because it is the treatment of choice for hypercalcemia and is usually effective. The sodium contained in the solution inhibits the reabsorption of calcium in renal tubules and thereby increases urinary excretion of calcium. The solution relieves the dehydration caused by vomiting and polyuria, and it dilutes the calcium concentration of serum and urine. Several liters are given daily. Clients should be monitored closely for signs of fluid overload, and serum calcium, magnesium, and potassium levels should be measured every 6 to 12 hours. Large amounts of magnesium and potassium are lost in the urine, and adequate replacement is essential.

APPLYING YOUR KNOWLEDGE 25-1

You are giving instructions to Ms. Taylor on the proper administration method for taking her alendronate. In addition to instructing Ms. Taylor to take this medication with water, what important instruction must you include for this client?

NURSING PROCESS

Assessment

- Assess for risk factors and manifestations of hypocalcemia and calcium deficiency:
  - Assess dietary intake of dairy products, other calcium-containing foods, and vitamin D.
  - Check serum calcium reports for abnormal values. The normal total serum calcium level is approximately 8.5 to 10.5 mg/dL (SI units 2.2–2.6 mmol/L). Approximately half of the total serum calcium (eg, 4–5 mg/dL) should be free ionized calcium, the physiologically active form. To interpret serum calcium levels accurately, serum albumin levels and acid–base status must be considered. Low serum albumin decreases the total serum level of calcium by decreasing the amount of calcium that is bound to protein; however, the ionized concentration is unaffected by serum albumin levels. Metabolic and respiratory alkalosis increase binding of calcium to serum proteins, thereby maintaining normal total serum calcium but decreasing the ionized values. Conversely, metabolic and respiratory acidosis decrease binding and therefore increase the concentration of ionized calcium.
  - Check for *Chvostek's sign:* Tap the facial nerve just below the temple, in front of the ear. If facial muscles twitch, hyperirritability of the nerve is present, and tetany may occur.
  - Check for *Trousseau's sign:* Constrict blood circulation in an arm (usually with a blood-pressure cuff) for 3 to 5 minutes. This produces ischemia and increased irritability of peripheral nerves, which causes spasms of the lower arm and hand muscles (carpopedal spasm) if tetany is present.
- Assess for conditions in which hypercalcemia is likely to occur (eg, cancer, prolonged immobilization, vitamin D overdose).
- Observe for signs and symptoms of hypercalcemia in clients at risk. Electrocardiographic changes indicative of hypercalcemia include a shortened Q–T interval and an inverted T wave.
- Assess for risk factors and manifestations of osteoporosis, especially in postmenopausal women and men and women on chronic corticosteroid therapy.
  - If risk factors are identified, ask if preventive measures are being used (eg, increasing calcium intake, exercise, medications).
  - If the client is known to have osteoporosis, ask about duration and severity of symptoms, age of onset, location, whether fractures have occurred, what treatments have been performed, and response to treatments.
- If Paget's disease is suspected, assess for an elevated serum alkaline phosphatase level and abnormal bone scan reports.

Nursing Diagnoses

- Deficient Knowledge: Recommended daily amounts and dietary sources of calcium and vitamin D
- Deficient Knowledge: Disease process and drug therapy for osteoporosis
- Risk for Injury: Tetany, sedation, seizures from hypocalcemia
- Risk for Injury: Hypercalcemia related to overuse of supplements; hypocalcemia from aggressive treatment of hypercalcemia

Planning/Goals

The client will
- Achieve and maintain normal serum levels of calcium
- Increase dietary intake of calcium-containing foods to prevent or treat osteoporosis
- Use calcium or vitamin D supplements in recommended amounts
- Comply with instructions for safe drug use
- Be monitored closely for therapeutic and adverse effects of drugs used to treat hypercalcemia
- Comply with procedures for follow-up treatment of hypocalcemia, hypercalcemia, or osteoporosis
- Avoid preventable adverse effects of treatment for acute hypocalcemia or hypercalcemia

Interventions

Assist all clients in meeting the recommended daily requirements of calcium and vitamin D. With an adequate protein and calcium intake, enough phosphorus also is obtained.

- The best dietary source is milk and other dairy products, including yogurt.
- Unless contraindicated by the client's condition, recommend that adults drink at least two 8-oz glasses of milk daily. This furnishes approximately half the daily calcium requirement; the remainder will probably be obtained from other foods.
- Children need approximately four glasses of milk or an equivalent amount of calcium in milk and other foods to support normal growth and development.
- Pregnant and lactating women also need approximately four glasses of milk or the equivalent to meet increased needs. Vitamin and mineral supplements are often prescribed during these periods.
- Postmenopausal women who take estrogens need at least 1000 mg daily. Those who do not take estrogens need at least 1500 mg.
- For clients who avoid or minimize their intake of dairy products because of the calories, identify low-calorie sources, such as skim milk and low-fat yogurt.

- Milk that has been fortified with vitamin D is the best food source. Exposure of skin to sunlight is also needed to supply adequate amounts of vitamin D.
- For people who are unable or unwilling to ingest sufficient calcium, a supplement may be needed to prevent osteoporosis.

Assist clients with hypercalcemia to decrease formation of renal calculi by forcing fluids to approximately 3000 to 4000 milliliters per day and preventing urinary tract infections.

Client Teaching Guidelines for Drugs for Osteoporosis are presented in the accompanying display.

Evaluation

- Check laboratory reports of serum calcium levels for normal values.
- Interview and observe for relief of symptoms of hypocalcemia, hypercalcemia, or osteoporosis.
- Interview and observe intake of calcium-containing foods.

- Question about normal calcium requirements and how to meet them.
- Interview and observe for accurate drug usage and compliance with follow-up procedures.
- Interview and observe for therapeutic and adverse drug effects.

APPLYING YOUR KNOWLEDGE 25-2

Clients like Ms. Taylor who has osteoporosis should take preventive measures in addition to taking their prescribed medication. One important measure is to increase the intake of foods that contain high levels of calcium. What dietary recommendations would you make to Ms. Taylor?

PRINCIPLES OF THERAPY

Goal of Therapy

The goal of therapy is to restore normal calcium balance in the body. Drugs used for hypocalcemia help correct calcium

---

C L I E N T   T E A C H I N G   G U I D E L I N E S

Drugs for Osteoporosis

General Considerations

☑ Osteoporosis involves weak bones that fracture easily and may cause pain and disability.

☑ Important factors in prevention and treatment include an adequate intake of calcium and vitamin D (from the diet, from supplements, or from a combination of both sources), regular weight-bearing exercise, and drugs that can slow bone loss.

☑ It is better to obtain calcium and vitamin D from foods such as milk and other dairy products. Approximately 1000 to 1500 milligrams of calcium and 400 IU of vitamin D are recommended daily.

☑ If unable to get sufficient dietary calcium and vitamin D, consider supplements of these nutrients. Consult a health care provider about the types and amounts. For example, a daily multivitamin and mineral supplement may contain adequate amounts when added to dietary intake. If taking other supplements, avoid those containing bone meal because they may contain lead and other contaminants that are toxic to the human body. Do not take more than the recommended amounts of supplements; overuse can cause serious, life-threatening problems.

☑ The main drugs approved for prevention and treatment of osteoporosis are the bisphosphonates (eg, Fosamax, Actonel). These drugs help prevent the loss of calcium from bone, thereby strengthening bone and reducing the risks of fractures.

☑ For people at high risk for development of osteoporosis (eg, postmenopausal women, men and women who take an oral or inhaled corticosteroid such as prednisone or fluticasone [Flonase]), or

those being treated for osteoporosis, a baseline measurement of bone mineral density and periodic follow-up measurements are needed. This is a noninvasive test that does not involve any injections or device insertions.

Self-Administration

☑ If taking a calcium supplement, calcium carbonate 500 milligrams twice daily is often recommended. This can be obtained with the inexpensive over-the-counter antacid Tums, which contains 200 milligrams of calcium per tablet.

☑ Do not take a calcium supplement with an iron preparation, tetracycline, ciprofloxacin, or phenytoin. Instead, take the drugs at least 2 hours apart to avoid calcium interference with absorption of the other drugs.

☑ If taking both a calcium supplement and a bisphosphonate, take the calcium at least 2 hours after the bisphosphonate. Calcium, antacids, and other drugs interfere with absorption of bisphosphonate.

☑ Take bisphosphonates with 6 to 8 ounces of water at least 30 minutes before any food, other fluid, or other medication. Beverages other than water and foods decrease absorption and effectiveness.

☑ Take a bisphosphonate in an upright position and do not lie down for at least 30 minutes. This helps prevent esophageal irritation and stomach upset.

☑ If taking a bisphosphonate, report new or worsening dysphagia, retrosternal pain, or heartburn to your health care provider. This may be an indication of esophageal irritation due to the bisphosphonate.

deficit, reduce the risk of tetany, and slow development of osteoporosis. Drugs used for hypercalcemia support treatment of the underlying condition and control serum calcium levels.

Drugs Used for Hypocalcemia

Drug Dosage and Administration

Calcium preparations and perhaps vitamin D are used to treat hypocalcemia. IV administration of calcium, usually 10 to 20 milliliters of 10% calcium gluconate (1–2 g of calcium), is necessary to treat acute, severe hypocalcemia, which is a medical emergency. Doses may be repeated, a continuous infusion may be given, or oral supplements may be used to avoid symptoms of hypocalcemia and maintain normal serum calcium levels (as measured every 4–6 hours). Once the hypocalcemia is stabilized, treatment is aimed at management of the underlying cause or prevention of recurrence. If hypocalcemia is caused by diarrhea or malabsorption, treatment of the underlying condition decreases loss of calcium from the body and increases absorption. Serum magnesium levels should also be measured, and, if hypomagnesemia is present, it must be treated before treatment of hypocalcemia can be effective.

Oral calcium supplements are preferred for less acute situations or for long-term treatment of chronic hypocalcemia. Vitamin D is given also if a calcium preparation alone cannot maintain serum calcium levels within a normal range. When vitamin D is given to treat hypocalcemia, dosage is determined by frequent measurement of serum calcium levels. Usually, higher doses are given initially, and lower doses are given for maintenance therapy. Calcium salts and vitamin D are combined in many over-the-counter preparations promoted as dietary supplements (Table 25-3). These preparations contain variable amounts of calcium and vitamin D. In general, intake of calcium should not exceed 2500 milligrams daily, from all sources, and intake of vitamin D should not exceed 400 IU daily. These mixtures are not indicated for maintenance therapy in chronic hypocalcemia.

Calcium supplements can decrease bone loss and fractures, especially in women. Calcium carbonate contains the most elemental calcium by weight (40%). It is inexpensive and available in a nonprescription form as the antacid Tums. Calcium citrate is reportedly better absorbed than calcium carbonate.

Effects of Calcium Preparations on Other Drugs

Calcium preparations and digoxin have similar effects on the myocardium. Therefore, if calcium is given to a client taking digoxin, the risks of digitalis toxicity and cardiac dysrhythmias are increased. This combination must be used very cautiously. Oral calcium preparations decrease effects of oral tetracycline drugs by combining with the antibiotic and preventing its absorption. They should not be given at the same time or within 2 to 3 hours of each other.

Drugs Used for Hypercalcemia

Treatment of hypercalcemia depends largely on the cause and severity. When the cause is a tumor of parathyroid tissue, surgical excision is commonly used. When the cause is a malignant tumor, treatment of the tumor with surgery, radiation, or chemotherapy may reduce production of PTH. When the cause is excessive intake of vitamin D, the vitamin D preparation should be stopped immediately. Serum calcium levels should be measured periodically to monitor effects of therapy.

Drug Dosage and Administration

Acute hypercalcemia (ie, severe symptoms or a serum calcium level >12 mg/dL), is a medical emergency and rehydration is a priority. An IV saline infusion (0.9% or 0.45% NaCl) 4000 milliliters per day (or more if kidney function is adequate) is effective. After rehydration, furosemide may be given IV to increase renal excretion of calcium and prevent fluid overload. Because sodium, potassium, and water are also lost in the urine, these must be replaced in the IV fluids.

In mild hypercalcemia, further drug therapy is usually not necessary; most clients respond to the aforementioned treatment. In moderate to severe hypercalcemia, pamidronate or zoledronate may be the drug of choice. When pamidronate is given in a single IV infusion containing 60 or 90 milligrams, serum calcium levels decrease within 2 days, reach their lowest levels in approximately 7 days, and remain lower for 2 weeks or longer. Treatment can be repeated if hypercalcemia recurs. Zoledronate can be

TABLE 25-3 Selected Calcium/Vitamin D Combination Products

GENERIC/ TRADE NAME	CALCIUM (MG)*/ TABLET OR CAPSULE	VITAMIN D (IU)†/ TABLET
Caltrate 600 + D and Caltrate Plus	600	200
Citracal caplets + D	315	200
Dical-D tablets	117	133
Dical-D wafers	233	200
Os-Cal 250 + D	250	125
Os-Cal 500 + D	500	125
Posture-D	600	125

*mg of elemental calcium; †IU, international units.

given over 15 minutes and effects may last longer than those of pamidronate. Adverse effects of the two drugs are similar. Phosphates should not be used, unless hypophosphatemia is present. They are also contraindicated in clients with persistent urinary tract infections and an alkaline urine, because kidney stones composed of calcium phosphate are likely to form in such cases.

In chronic hypercalcemia, treatment of the underlying disease process and measures to control serum calcium levels (eg, a high fluid intake and mobilization to help retain calcium in bone) are necessary. Oral phosphate administration may help if other measures are ineffective.

For clients receiving a calcium channel blocker (see Chap. 50), the drugs may be less effective in the presence of hypercalcemia. For calcium channel blocker overdose, replacement may require an hourly infusion after a bolus dose.

Drugs Used for Osteoporosis

To avoid or slow bone loss, preventive measures should be implemented in people of all ages, including a consistently adequate dietary intake of calcium to promote normal bone development and maintenance. In children, adolescents, and young adults, an adequate calcium intake promotes bone growth and peak bone mass. A well-stocked "reservoir" means that in later years, when bone loss exceeds formation, more bone can be lost before osteoporosis develops. Measures to prevent osteoporosis include the following:

- Adequate calcium intake, which may slow the development of osteoporosis and fractures in postmenopausal women and men older than 40 years of age. Although dietary intake is much preferred, a supplement may be needed to ensure a daily intake of 1000 to 1500 mg, especially in adolescent girls, frail older adults, and those receiving corticosteroids.
- Use of alendronate (Fosamax) and risedronate (Actonel), which are approved by the Food and Drug Administration for prevention of osteoporosis. (With alendronate, recommended dosage is smaller for prevention than for treatment.) Raloxifene (Evista) is approved for prevention of postmenopausal osteoporosis in women who are unable or unwilling to take ERT.
- Adequate intake of vitamin D. However, supplementation is probably not indicated unless a deficiency can be demonstrated. Serum calcitriol can be measured in clients at risk for vitamin D deficiency, including older adults and those on chronic corticosteroid therapy.
- Lifestyle changes, including regular exercise and smoking cessation. Numerous studies indicate that vigorous, weight-bearing exercise helps promote and maintain strong bone, and inactivity promotes bone weakening and loss. Smoking decreases the amount

of active estrogen in the body and thus accelerates bone loss.

Preventive measures are necessary for clients on chronic corticosteroid therapy (eg, prednisone 7.5 mg daily; equivalent amounts of other systemic drugs; high doses of inhaled drugs). For both men and women, most of the preceding guidelines apply (eg, calcium supplements, regular exercise, a bisphosphonate drug). In addition, low doses and nonsystemic routes help prevent osteoporosis and other adverse effects. For men, corticosteroids decrease testosterone levels by approximately one half, and replacement therapy may be needed.

Preventive measures are also necessary for clients taking phenytoin (Dilantin) and phenobarbital, because these drugs may contribute to osteoporosis through their effects on calcium metabolism. These anticonvulsant medications increase hepatic metabolism of vitamin D, which leads to a decrease in calcium absorption in the intestine. Supplemental calcium and vitamin D as well as specific drugs for osteoporosis should be considered if bone density is low.

When bone loss is evident (from diagnostic tests of bone density or occurrence of fractures), several interventions may help slow further skeletal bone loss or prevent fractures. Most drugs used to treat osteoporosis decrease the rate of bone breakdown and thus slow the rate of bone loss. Alendronate (Fosamax) 10 milligrams daily or 70 milligrams weekly and risedronate (Actonel) 5 milligrams daily can increase bone mineral density, reduce risks of vertebral fractures, and slow progression of vertebral deformities and loss of height. One of these drugs is often used in combination with estrogen and calcium and vitamin D supplements. The drug teriparatide (Forteo) actually increases bone formation.

Clients diagnosed with osteoporosis require adequate calcium and vitamin D (at least the recommended dietary allowance), whether obtained from the diet or from supplements. Calcium 600 milligrams and vitamin D 200 IU once or twice daily are often recommended for postmenopausal women with osteoporosis, and pharmacologic doses of vitamin D are sometimes used to treat clients with serious osteoporosis. If such doses are used, caution should be exercised, because excessive amounts of vitamin D can cause hypercalcemia and hypercalciuria.

In addition, regular exercise and smoking cessation may be necessary. Treatment of men is similar to that of women, except that testosterone replacement may be required. In corticosteroid-induced osteoporosis, multiple treatment measures may be necessary, including increased dietary and supplemental calcium and possibly vitamin D supplementation; hormone replacement; corticosteroid dosage reduction; exercise; and a bisphosphonate or calcitonin to slow skeletal bone loss.

Use in Special Populations

Use in Children

Hypocalcemia is uncommon in children. However, inadequate calcium in the diet is thought to be common, especially in girls. Both inadequate calcium and exercise in children are risk factors for eventual osteoporosis. If hypocalcemia or dietary calcium deficiency develops, principles of using calcium or vitamin D supplements are the same as those in adults. Children should be monitored closely for signs and symptoms of adverse effects, including hypercalcemia. Hypercalcemia is probably most likely to occur in children with a malignant tumor. Guidelines for treating hypercalcemia in children are essentially the same as those for adults, with drug dosages adjusted. Safety, effectiveness, and dosage of etidronate, pamidronate, and zoledronate have not been established.

Use in Older Adults

Hypocalcemia is uncommon, because calcium moves from bone to blood to maintain normal serum levels. However, calcium deficiency commonly occurs because of long-term dietary deficiencies of calcium and vitamin D; impaired absorption of calcium from the intestine; lack of exposure to sunlight; and impaired liver or kidney metabolism of vitamin D to its active form. These and other factors lead to demineralization and weakening of bone (osteoporosis) and an increased risk of fractures. Postmenopausal women are at high risk for osteoporosis. Although osteoporosis also develops in older men, it occurs less often, at a later age, and to a lesser extent than in older women. Both men and women who take corticosteroids are at risk for osteoporosis. The risk is higher with systemic corticosteroids but may also occur with oral or inhaled drugs, especially at higher doses. In general, all older adults must continue their dietary intake of dairy products and other calcium-containing foods. Older adults with osteoporosis or risk factors for osteoporosis may need calcium supplements and a bisphosphonate or calcitonin to prevent or treat the disorder.

Hypercalcemia usually requires large amounts of IV 0.9% sodium chloride (eg, 150–200 mL/hour). Older adults often have chronic cardiovascular disorders that may be aggravated by this treatment, and they should be monitored closely for signs of fluid overload, congestive heart failure, pulmonary edema, and hypertension.

Use in Clients With Renal Impairment

Clients with renal impairment or failure often have disturbances in calcium and bone metabolism. If hypercalcemia develops in clients with severely impaired renal function, hemodialysis or peritoneal dialysis with calcium-free solution is effective and safe. Calcium acetate may be used to prevent or treat hyperphosphatemia. The calcium reduces blood levels of phosphate by reducing its absorption from foods. That is, calcium binds with dietary phosphate to produce calcium phosphate, which is insoluble and excreted in feces. If vitamin D therapy is needed to treat osteomalacia associated with renal impairment, calcitriol (eg, Rocaltrol) or dihydrotachysterol (Hytakerol) is preferred (see Table 25-1). Calcitriol is the active form of vitamin D and thus requires no metabolism; dihydrotachysterol is a synthetic compound that is metabolized in the liver but not in the kidneys.

None of the bisphosphonate drugs is recommended for use in severe renal impairment (eg, serum creatinine >5 mg/dL or creatinine clearance <30 mL/minute). With alendronate, dosage does not need to be reduced in mild to moderate impairment (eg, creatinine clearance 35–60 mL/minute). Etidronate should be used cautiously with mild renal impairment and is contraindicated with severe renal impairment. Pamidronate and zoledronate are nephrotoxic and renal function should be closely monitored during their use.

Teriparatide (Forteo), a form of PTH, apparently does not require dosage adjustment in renal impairment.

Use in Clients With Hepatic Impairment

The bisphosphonates are not metabolized in the liver and are unlikely to affect liver function. Teriparatide (Forteo), a form of PTH, apparently does not require dosage adjustment in hepatic impairment.

Use in Home Care

Home care nurses have an excellent opportunity to promote health and prevent illness related to calcium and bone disorders. Nurses who assist in the care of any seriously ill client should also be able to recognize and obtain immediate treatment for hypocalcemia or hypercalcemia. For example, hypercalcemia may occur in clients with cancer, especially cancers involving bone.

All members of a household should be assessed in relation to calcium and vitamin D intake because an adequate amount of these nutrients is needed throughout life. Intake of both calcium and vitamin D is often inadequate in children and adolescent girls, who may risk developing osteoporosis. It may be necessary to teach about dietary and supplemental sources of these nutrients, as well as adverse effects of excessive amounts. Clients who are taking medications to prevent or treat osteoporosis may also require teaching or other assistance.

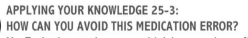 **APPLYING YOUR KNOWLEDGE 25-3:**
HOW CAN YOU AVOID THIS MEDICATION ERROR?
Ms. Taylor knows she cannot drink her morning coffee or eat her breakfast for 30 minutes after taking her alendronate. You tell her to get up and take her medication then go back to bed for half an hour.

N U R S I N G   A C T I O N S

Drugs Used in Calcium and Bone Disorders

NURSING ACTIONS	RATIONALE/EXPLANATION
1. Administer accurately	
a. With calcium preparations:	
(1) Give oral preparations with or after meals.	To increase absorption
(2) Give intravenous (IV) preparations slowly (0.5–2 mL/min), check pulse and blood pressure closely, and monitor the electrocardiogram (ECG) if possible.	These solutions may cause dysrhythmias and hypotension if injected rapidly. They are also irritating to tissues.
(3) Do not mix IV preparations with any other drug in the same syringe.	Calcium reacts with some other drugs and forms a precipitate.
b. With bisphosphonates:	
(1) Give alendronate, ibandronate, and risedronate with 6–8 ounces of plain water, at least 30 minutes before the first food, beverage, or medication of the day.	To promote absorption and decrease esophageal and gastric irritation
(2) Give etidronate on an empty stomach, as a single dose or in divided doses. Avoid giving within 2 hours of ingesting dairy products, antacids, or vitamin or mineral preparations.	If gastrointestinal (GI) symptoms occur with the single dose, divided doses may relieve them. Substances containing calcium or other minerals decrease absorption of etidronate.
(3) Give IV pamidronate and zoledronate according to the manufacturers' instructions.	These drugs require reconstitution, diluting with IV fluids, and specific time intervals of administration.
c. Give calcitonin at bedtime.	To decrease nausea and discomfort from flushing
d. With phosphate salts, mix powder forms with water for oral administration. See package inserts for specific instructions.	
2. Observe for therapeutic effects	
a. With calcium preparations, observe for:	
(1) Relief of symptoms of neuromuscular irritability and tetany, such as decreased muscle spasms and decreased paresthesias	
(2) Serum calcium levels within the normal range (8.5–10.5 mg/dL)	
(3) Absence of Chvostek's and Trousseau's signs	
b. With alendronate or risedronate for osteoporosis, observe for improved bone mass density and absence of fractures.	Early osteopenia and osteoporosis are asymptomatic. Measurement of bone mass density is the only way to quantify bone loss.
c. With calcitonin, corticosteroids, pamidronate, or zoledronate for hypercalcemia, observe for:	
(1) Decreased serum calcium level	Calcitonin lowers serum calcium levels in about 2 hours after injection and effects last 6–8 hours. Corticosteroids require 10–14 days to lower serum calcium. Bisphosphonates lower serum calcium levels within 2 days, but may require a week or more to produce normal serum calcium levels.
(2) Decreased signs and symptoms of hypercalcemia	
3. Observe for adverse effects	
a. With calcium preparations, observe for hypercalcemia:	
(1) GI effects—anorexia, nausea, vomiting, abdominal pain, constipation	

NURSING ACTIONS	RATIONALE/EXPLANATION
(2) Central nervous system effects—apathy, poor memory, depression, drowsiness, disorientation	
(3) Other effects—weakness and decreased tone in skeletal and smooth muscles, dysphagia, polyuria, polydipsia, cardiac dysrhythmias	
(4) Serum calcium >10.5 mg/dL	
(5) ECG changes indicating hypercalcemia (a prolonged Q–T interval and an inverted T wave)	
b. With vitamin D preparations, observe for hypervitaminosis D and hypercalcemia (see above).	This is most likely to occur with chronic ingestion of high doses daily. In children, accidental ingestion may lead to acute toxicity.
c. With alendronate, ibandronate, and risedronate, observe for:	
(1) GI effects—abdominal distention, acid regurgitation, dysphagia, esophagitis, flatulence	Adverse effects are usually minor with the doses taken for prevention or treatment of osteoporosis, if the drugs are taken as directed. More severe effects may occur with the higher doses taken for Paget's disease.
(2) Other effects—headache, musculoskeletal pain, decreased serum calcium and phosphate	
d. With calcitonin, observe for nausea, vomiting, tissue irritation at administration sites, and allergic reactions.	Adverse effects are usually mild and transient. Nasal administration produces greater client compliance than injections, with few adverse effects.
e. With drug therapy for hypercalcemia, observe for hypocalcemia.	Hypocalcemia may occur with vigorous treatment of hypercalcemia. This can be minimized by monitoring serum calcium levels frequently and adjusting drug dosages and other treatments.
f. With pamidronate and zoledronate, observe for:	
(1) GI effects—anorexia, nausea, vomiting, constipation	
(2) Cardiovascular effects—fluid overload, hypertension	
(3) Electrolyte imbalances—hypokalemia, hypomagnesemia, hypophosphatemia	
(4) Musculoskeletal effects—muscle and joint pain	
(5) Miscellaneous effects—fever, tissue irritation at IV insertion site, pain, anemia	
g. With etidronate, observe for anorexia, nausea, diarrhea, bone pain, fever, fluid overload, and increased serum creatinine.	Adverse effects are more frequent and more severe at higher doses. The drug is nephrotoxic and should not be used in clients with renal failure.
h. With phosphates, observe for nausea, vomiting, and diarrhea.	
4. Observe for drug interactions	
a. Drugs that *increase* effects of calcium:	
(1) Vitamin D	Increases intestinal absorption of calcium from both dietary and supplemental drug sources
(2) Thiazide diuretics	Reduce calcium losses in urine
b. Drugs that *decrease* effects of calcium:	
(1) Corticosteroids (prednisone, others), calcitonin, and phosphates	These drugs lower serum calcium levels by various mechanisms. They are used in the treatment of hypercalcemia.
c. Drugs that *increase* effects of vitamin D:	
(1) Thiazide diuretics	Thiazide diuretics administered to hypoparathyroid clients may cause hypercalcemia (potentiate vitamin D effects).

(continued)

NURSING ACTIONS	RATIONALE/EXPLANATION
d. Drugs that *decrease* effects of vitamin D:	
(1) Phenytoin	Accelerates metabolism of vitamin D in the liver and may cause vitamin D deficiency, hypocalcemia, and rickets or osteomalacia. Increased intake of vitamin D may be needed.
(2) Cholestyramine resin (Questran)	May decrease intestinal absorption of vitamin D preparations
(3) Mineral oil	Mineral oil is a fat and therefore combines with fat-soluble vitamins, such as vitamin D, and prevents their absorption from the gastro-intestinal tract.
e. Drugs that *decrease* effects of oral bisphosphonates:	
(1) Antacids and calcium supplements	These drugs interfere with absorption of bisphosphonates and should be taken at least 2 hours after a bisphosphonate.
f. Drug that *decreases* the effects of tiludronate:	
(1) Aspirin	Aspirin decreases the bioavailability of tiludronate by up to 50% when taken within 2 hours of tiludronate.
g. Drugs that alter effects of calcitonin:	
(1) Testosterone and other androgens *increase* effects.	Androgens and calcitonin have additive effects on calcium retention and inhibition of bone resorption (movement of calcium from bone to serum).
(2) Parathyroid hormone *decreases* effects.	Parathyroid hormone antagonizes or opposes calcitonin.
h. Drugs that *decrease* effects of phosphate salts:	
(1) Antacids containing aluminum and magnesium	Aluminum and magnesium may combine with phosphate and thereby prevent its absorption and therapeutic effect.

APPLYING YOUR KNOWLEDGE: ANSWERS

25-1 Alendronate must be taken 30 minutes prior to any intake of food, fluid, or other medication. Alendronate is very poorly absorbed from the gastrointestinal tract and any other substance will diminish the absorption of this medication.

25-2 For most individuals, a daily intake of between 1000 to 1500 mg of calcium is recommended. Milk and dairy products contain high levels of calcium. Two 8-oz glasses of milk provide one half of the daily calcium requirement (600 mg). Postmenopausal women should increase their calcium intake to 1500 mg per day.

25-3 Any client taking alendronate needs to be instructed to remain in an upright position for at least 30 minutes after taking this medication. Avoiding the supine position reduces the risk of esophageal irritation.

Review and Application Exercises

Short Answer Exercises

1. What are the major physiologic functions of calcium?

2. What is the normal serum level of calcium?

3. What are some nursing interventions to prevent hypocalcemia?

4. What signs and symptoms may indicate hypocalcemia?

5. How is hypocalcemia treated?

6. What signs and symptoms may indicate hypercalcemia?

7. How is hypercalcemia treated?

8. Why is it important to have an adequate intake of calcium and vitamin D throughout life?

9. What are the main elements of prevention and treatment of osteoporosis?

NCLEX-Style Questions

10. To decrease nausea and discomfort from flushing with calcitonin, the nurse should instruct the client to take the drug in which of the following ways?
    a. with a warm beverage
    b. with a glass of orange juice

   c. with breakfast

   d. at bedtime

11. Rapid administration of IV calcium may result in which of the following conditions?

   a. cardiac dysrhythmias

   b. nephrotoxicity

   c. ototoxicity

   d. pathologic fractures

12. Which of the following drugs is used to treat osteoporosis and can actually increase bone formation?

   a. teriparatide (Forteo)

   b. phosphate salts (Neutra-Phos)

   c. furosemide (Lasix)

   d. calcitriol (Rocaltrol)

13. If oral calcium preparations are given at the same time or within 2 to 3 hours of each other, they prevent absorption of which of the following antibiotics?

   a. penicillin

   b. cephalosporin

   c. tetracycline

   d. erythromycin

14. Alendronate acts primarily to decrease plasma calcium levels by

   a. inhibiting calcium resorption from bone

   b. binding calcium in the blood

   c. promoting renal excretion of calcium

   d. limiting intestinal absorption of calcium

Selected References

Drug facts and comparisons. (Updated monthly). St. Louis: Facts and Comparisons.

Hackley, B., & Rousseau, M. E. (2004). Managing menopausal symptoms after the Women's Health Initiative. *Journal of Midwifery and Women's Health, 49*(2), 87–95.

Lacy, C. F., Armstrong, L. L., Goldman, M. P., & Lance, L. L. (2004). Lexi-Comp's drug information handbook (12th ed.). Hudson, OH: Lexi-Comp.

Lobaugh, B. L., & Drezner, M. K. (2000). Approach to hypercalemia and hypocalcemia. In H. D. Humes (Ed.), *Kelley's Textbook of internal medicine* (4th ed., pp. 2652–2662). Philadelphia: Lippincott Williams & Wilkins.

Parent-Stevens, L. (2000). Osteoporosis and osteomalacia. In E. T. Herfindal & D. R. Gourley (Eds.), *Textbook of therapeutics: Drug and disease management* (7th ed., pp. 709–723). Philadelphia: Lippincott Williams & Wilkins.

Porth, C. M. (2004). *Pathophysiology: Concepts of altered health states* (7th ed.). Philadelphia: Lippincott Williams & Wilkins.

Prestwood, K. M. (2000). Diagnosis and management of osteoporosis in older adults. In H. D. Humes (Ed.), *Kelley's Textbook of internal medicine* (4th ed., pp. 3074–3082). Philadelphia: Lippincott Williams & Wilkins.

Shoback, D., & Gross, C. (2000). Metabolic bone disease. In H. D. Humes (Ed.), *Kelley's Textbook of internal medicine* (4th ed., pp. 2769–2784). Philadelphia: Lippincott Williams & Wilkins.

Singh, R. F., & Dong, B. J. (2000). Parathyroid disorders. In E. T. Herfindal & D. R. Gourley (Eds.), *Textbook of therapeutics: Drug and disease management* (7th ed., pp. 359–375). Philadelphia: Lippincott Williams & Wilkins.

Zoledronate (Zometa). (2001, December 10). *Medical Letter on Drugs and Therapeutics, 43*(1120), 110–111.

Antidiabetic Drugs

OBJECTIVES

After studying this chapter, you will be able to:

1. Describe major effects of endogenous insulin on body tissues.
2. Discuss insulins and insulin analogs in terms of characteristics and uses.
3. Discuss the relationships among diet, exercise, and drug therapy in controlling diabetes.
4. Differentiate types of oral antidiabetic agents in terms of mechanisms of action, indications for use, adverse effects, and nursing process implications.
5. Explain the benefits of maintaining glycemic control in preventing complications of diabetes.
6. State reasons for combinations of insulin and oral agents or different types of oral agents.
7. Assist clients or caregivers in learning how to manage diabetes care, including administration of antidiabetic medications.
8. Collaborate with nurse diabetes educators, dietitians, and others in teaching self-care activities to clients with diabetes.
9. Assess and monitor clients' conditions in relation to diabetes and their compliance with prescribed management strategies.
10. Discuss dietary and herbal supplements that affect blood sugar and diabetes control.

APPLYING YOUR KNOWLEDGE

David Furgeson is a 44-year-old man with type 2 diabetes. He is overweight and requires insulin in addition to his oral medication to control his fasting blood glucose level. Mr. Furgeson's current medications include:

Novolin 70/30 insulin 15 units every morning
Glimepiride 4 mg PO daily
Metformin 500 mg PO twice daily

INTRODUCTION

Insulin and oral agents are the two types of drugs used to lower blood glucose in diabetes mellitus. To assist readers in understanding the clinical use of these drugs, characteristics of endogenous insulin, diabetes, and the drugs are described.

Endogenous Insulin

Insulin is a protein hormone secreted by beta cells in the pancreas. The average adult pancreas secretes 40 to 60 units of insulin daily. This includes a basal amount of 1 to 2 units per hour and additional amounts (4–6 units/hour) after meals or when the blood sugar level exceeds 100 milligrams per deciliter. In a fasting state, serum insulin levels are low and stored glucose and amino acids are used for energy needs of tissues that require glucose. After a meal, serum insulin levels increase and peak in a few minutes, then decrease to baseline levels in 2 to 3 hours.

Insulin is secreted into the portal circulation and transported to the liver, where about half is used or degraded. The other half reaches the systemic circulation, where it circulates mainly in an unbound form and is transported to body cells.

At the cellular level (Fig. 26-1), insulin binds with and activates receptors on the cell membranes of about 80% of body cells. Liver, muscle, and fat cells have many insulin receptors and are primary tissues for insulin action. After insulin–receptor binding occurs, cell membranes become highly permeable to glucose and allow rapid entry of glucose into the cells. The cell membranes also become more permeable to amino acids, fatty acids, and electrolytes such as potassium, magnesium, and phosphate ions. Cellular metabolism is altered by the movement of these substances into the cells; activation of some enzymes and inactivation of others; movement of proteins between intracellular compartments; changes in the amounts of proteins produced; and perhaps other mechanisms. Overall, the changes in cellular metabo-

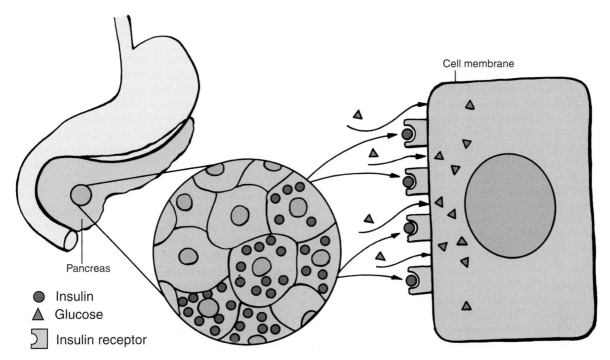

FIGURE 26-1 Normal glucose metabolism. After insulin binds with receptors on the cell membrane, glucose can move into the cell, promoting cellular metabolism and energy production.

Insulin ● Insulin

Glucose ▲ Glucose

⊃ Insulin receptor

lism stimulate anabolic effects (eg, utilization and storage of glucose, amino acids, and fatty acids) and inhibit catabolic processes (eg, breakdown of glycogen, fat, and protein). After binding to insulin and entering the cell, receptors may be degraded or recycled back to the cell surface.

Insulin is cleared from circulating blood in 10 to 15 minutes because of rapid binding to peripheral tissues or metabolic breakdown. The insulin that does not combine with receptors is metabolized in the liver, kidneys, plasma, and muscles. In the kidneys, insulin is filtered by the glomeruli and reabsorbed by the tubules, which also degrade it. Severe renal impairment slows the clearance of insulin from the blood.

Insulin plays a major role in metabolism of carbohydrate, fat, and protein (Box 26-1). These foodstuffs are broken down into molecules of glucose, lipids, and amino acids, respectively. The molecules enter the cells and are converted to energy for cellular activities. The energy can be used immediately or converted to storage forms for later use. When carrying out its metabolic functions, the overall effect of insulin is to lower blood glucose levels, primarily by the following mechanisms:

● In the liver, insulin acts to *decrease* breakdown of glycogen (glycogenolysis); form new glucose from fatty acids and amino acids (gluconeogenesis); and form ketone bodies (ketogenesis). At the same time, it acts to *increase* synthesis and storage of glycogen and fatty acids.
● In adipose tissue, insulin acts to *decrease* breakdown of fat (lipolysis) and to *increase* production of glycerol and fatty acids.

● In muscle tissue, insulin acts to *decrease* protein breakdown and amino acid output and to *increase* amino acid uptake, protein synthesis, and glycogen synthesis.

Regulation of Insulin Secretion

Insulin decreases blood sugar and regulates the amount of glucose available for cellular metabolism and energy needs, during both fasting and feeding. Insulin secretion involves coordination of various nutrients, hormones, the autonomic nervous system, and other factors.

Glucose is the major stimulus of insulin secretion; others include amino acids, fatty acids, ketone bodies, and stimulation of beta$_2$-adrenergic receptors or vagal nerves. Oral glucose is more effective than intravenous (IV) glucose because glucose or food in the digestive tract stimulates vagal activity and induces the release of gastrointestinal (GI) hormones called incretins. Incretin hormones stimulate the release of insulin when glucose levels are normal or elevated. In addition, incretin hormones reduce glucagon production and delay gastric emptying. Two incretin hormones have been identified: glucose-dependent insulinotropic peptide (GIP) and glucagon-like peptide-1 (GLP-1). GLP-1 also appears to improve insulin sensitivity and may increase the formation of new beta cells in the pancreas. The therapeutic uses of incretin hormones are currently being investigated for the development of new drugs to treat type 2 diabetes.

Other hormones that raise blood glucose levels and stimulate insulin secretion include cortisol, glucagon, growth hormone, epinephrine, estrogen, and progesterone. Excessive,

Box 26-1 Effects of Insulin on Metabolism

Carbohydrate Metabolism
- Insulin increases glucose transport into the liver, skeletal muscle, adipose tissue, the heart, and some smooth muscle organs (such as the uterus); it must be present for muscle and fat tissues to use glucose for energy.
- Insulin regulates glucose metabolism to produce energy for cellular functions. If excess glucose is present after this need is met, it is converted to glycogen and stored for future energy needs or converted to fat and stored. The excess glucose transported to liver cells is converted to fat only after glycogen stores are saturated. When insulin is absent or blood glucose levels are low, these stored forms of glucose can be reconverted. The liver is especially important in restoring blood sugar levels by breaking down glycogen or by forming new glucose.

Fat Metabolism
- Insulin promotes transport of glucose into fat cells, where it is broken down. One of the breakdown products is alpha-glycerophosphate, which combines with fatty acids to form triglycerides. This is the mechanism by which insulin promotes fat storage.

- When insulin is lacking, fat is released into the bloodstream as free fatty acids. Blood concentrations of triglycerides, cholesterol, and phospholipids are also increased. The high blood lipid concentration probably accounts for the atherosclerosis that tends to develop early and progress more rapidly in people with diabetes mellitus. Also, when more fatty acids are released than the body can use as fuel, some fatty acids are converted into ketones. Excessive amounts of ketones produce acidosis and coma.

Protein Metabolism
- Insulin increases the total amount of body protein by increasing transport of amino acids into cells and synthesis of protein within the cells. The basic mechanism of these effects is unknown.
- Insulin potentiates the effects of growth hormone.
- Lack of insulin causes protein breakdown into amino acids, which are released into the bloodstream and transported to the liver for energy or gluconeogenesis. The lost proteins are not replaced by synthesis of new proteins and protein wasting causes abnormal functioning of many body organs, severe weakness, and weight loss.

---

prolonged endogenous secretion or administration of pharmacologic preparations of these hormones can exhaust the ability of pancreatic beta cells to produce insulin and thereby cause or aggravate diabetes mellitus.

Factors that inhibit insulin secretion include stimulation of pancreatic alpha$_2$-adrenergic receptors and stress conditions such as hypoxia, hypothermia, surgery, or severe burns.

Diabetes Mellitus

Diabetes mellitus is a chronic systemic disease characterized by metabolic and vascular abnormalities. Metabolic problems occur early in the disease process and are related to changes in the metabolism of carbohydrate, fat, and protein. A major clinical manifestation of disordered metabolism is hyperglycemia.

Vascular problems include atherosclerosis throughout the body and changes in small blood vessels, which especially affect the retina and kidney. Clinical manifestations of vascular disorders may include hypertension, myocardial infarction, stroke, retinopathy, blindness, nephropathy, and peripheral vascular disease.

Classifications

The two major classifications are type 1 and type 2. Although both are characterized by hyperglycemia, they differ in onset, course, pathology, and treatment. Other types of diabetes may be induced by disease processes, certain drugs, and pregnancy.

Type 1

Type 1 diabetes, a common chronic disorder of childhood, results from an autoimmune disorder that destroys pancreatic beta cells. Symptoms usually develop when 10% to 20% of functioning beta cells remain, but may occur at any time if acute illness or stress increases the body's demand for insulin beyond the capacity of the remaining beta cells to secrete insulin. Eventually, all the beta cells are destroyed and no insulin is produced.

Type 1 may occur at any age but usually starts between 4 and 20 years of age. The peak incidence for girls is 10 to 12 years, for boys, 12 to 14 years. Type 1 usually has a sudden onset; produces severe symptoms; is difficult to control; produces a high incidence of complications, such as diabetic ketoacidosis (DKA) and renal failure; and requires administration of exogenous insulin. About 10% of people with diabetes have type 1.

Type 2

Type 2 is characterized by hyperglycemia and insulin resistance. The hyperglycemia results from increased production of glucose by the liver and decreased uptake of glucose in liver, muscle, and fat cells. *Insulin resistance* means that higher-than-usual concentrations of insulin are required. Thus, insulin is present but unable to work effectively (ie, inhibit hepatic production of glucose and cause glucose to move from the bloodstream into liver, muscle, and fat cells). Most insulin resistance is attributed to impaired insulin action at the cellular level, possibly related to postreceptor, intracellular mechanisms.

Type 2 may occur at any age but usually starts after 40 years. Compared with type 1, it usually has a gradual onset; produces less severe symptoms initially; is easier to control; causes less DKA and renal failure but more myocardial infarctions and strokes; and does not necessarily require exogenous insulin because endogenous insulin is still produced. About 90% of people with diabetes have type 2; 20% to 30% of them require exogenous insulin.

Type 2 is a heterogenous disease, and etiology probably involves multiple factors such as a genetic predisposition and environmental factors. Obesity is a major cause. With obesity and chronic ingestion of excess calories, along with a sedentary lifestyle, more insulin is required. The increased need leads to prolonged stimulation and eventual "fatigue" of pancreatic beta cells. As a result, the cells become less responsive to elevated blood glucose levels and less able to produce enough insulin to meet metabolic needs. Thus, insulin is secreted but is inadequate or ineffective, especially when insulin demand is increased by obesity, pregnancy, aging, or other factors.

In the United States, African Americans, Hispanics, Native Americans, and some Asian Americans and Pacific Islanders are at high risk for development of type 2 diabetes. Prevalence rates are about 9.6% in African Americans and 10.9% in Hispanic Americans, compared with 6.2% in Caucasians. Undiagnosed diabetes is reportedly common in Mexican Americans.

Signs and Symptoms

Most signs and symptoms stem from a lack of effective insulin and the subsequent metabolic abnormalities. Their incidence and severity depend on the amount of effective insulin and they may be precipitated by infection, rapid growth, pregnancy, or other factors that increase demand for insulin. Most early symptoms result from disordered carbohydrate metabolism, which causes excess glucose to accumulate in the blood (hyperglycemia). Hyperglycemia produces glucosuria, which, in turn, produces polydipsia, polyuria, dehydration, and polyphagia.

Glucosuria usually appears when the blood glucose level is approximately twice the normal value and the kidneys receive more glucose than can be reabsorbed. However, renal threshold varies, and the amount of glucose lost in the urine does not accurately reflect blood glucose. In children, glucose tends to appear in urine at much lower or even normal blood glucose levels. In older people, the kidneys may be less able to excrete excess glucose from the blood. As a result, blood glucose levels may be high with little or no glucose in the urine.

When large amounts of glucose are present, water is pulled into the renal tubule. This results in a greatly increased urine output (polyuria). The excessive loss of fluid in urine leads to increased thirst (polydipsia) and, if fluid intake is inadequate, to dehydration. Dehydration also occurs because high blood glucose levels increase osmotic pressure in the bloodstream, and fluid is pulled out of the cells in the body's attempt to regain homeostasis.

Polyphagia (increased appetite) occurs because the body cannot use ingested foods. People with uncontrolled diabetes lose weight because of abnormal metabolism.

Complications

Complications of diabetes mellitus are common and potentially disabling or life threatening. Diabetes is a leading cause of myocardial infarction, stroke, blindness, leg amputation, and kidney failure. These complications result from hyperglycemia and other metabolic abnormalities that accompany a lack of effective insulin. The metabolic abnormalities associated with hyperglycemia can cause early, acute complications, such as DKA or hyperosmolar hyperglycemic nonketotic coma (HHNC; Box 26-2). Eventually, metabolic abnormalities lead to damage in blood vessels and other body tissues. For example, atherosclerosis develops earlier, progresses more rapidly, and becomes more severe in people with diabetes. Microvascular changes lead to nephropathy, retinopathy, and peripheral neuropathy. Other complications include musculoskeletal disorders, increased numbers and severity of infections, and complications of pregnancy.

HYPOGLYCEMIC DRUGS

Insulin

Insulin is described in this section, and individual insulins are listed in Table 26-1.

- Exogenous insulin used to replace endogenous insulin has the same effects as the pancreatic hormone.
- Insulin and its analogs (structurally similar chemicals) lower blood glucose levels by increasing glucose uptake by body cells, especially skeletal muscle and fat cells, and by decreasing glucose production in the liver.
- The main clinical indication for insulin is treatment of diabetes mellitus. Insulin is the only effective treatment for type 1 diabetes because pancreatic beta cells are unable to secrete endogenous insulin and metabolism is severely impaired. Insulin is required for clients with type 2 diabetes who cannot control their disease with diet, weight control, and oral agents. It may be needed by anyone with diabetes during times of stress, such as illness, infection, or surgery. Insulin also is used to control diabetes induced by chronic pancreatitis, surgical excision of pancreatic tissue, hormones and other drugs, and pregnancy (gestational diabetes). In nondiabetic clients, insulin is used to prevent or treat hyperglycemia induced by IV parenteral nutrition and to treat hyperkalemia. In hyperkalemia, an IV infusion of insulin and dextrose solution causes potassium to move from the blood into the cells; it does not eliminate potassium from the body.

Box 26-2 Acute Complications of Diabetes Mellitus

Diabetic Ketoacidosis (DKA)

This life-threatening complication occurs with severe insulin deficiency. In the absence of insulin, glucose cannot be used by body cells for energy and fat is mobilized from adipose tissue to furnish a fuel source. The mobilized fat circulates in the bloodstream, from which it is extracted by the liver and broken down into glycerol and fatty acids. The fatty acids are further changed in the liver to ketones (eg, acetoacetic acid, acetone), which then enter the bloodstream and are circulated to body cells for metabolic conversion to energy, carbon dioxide, and water.

The ketones are produced more rapidly than body cells can use them and their accumulation produces acidemia (a drop in blood pH and an increase in blood hydrogen ions). The body attempts to buffer the acidic hydrogen ions by exchanging them for intracellular potassium ions. Hydrogen ions enter body cells, and potassium ions leave the cells to be excreted in the urine. Another attempt to remove excess acid involves the lungs. Deep, labored respirations, called *Kussmaul's respirations*, eliminate more carbon dioxide and prevent formation of carbonic acid. A third attempt to regain homeostasis involves the kidneys, which excrete some of the ketones, thereby producing acetone in the urine.

DKA worsens as the compensatory mechanisms fail. Clinical signs and symptoms become progressively more severe. Early ones include blurred vision, anorexia, nausea and vomiting, thirst, and polyuria. Later ones include drowsiness, which progresses to stupor and coma, Kussmaul's respirations, dehydration and other signs of fluid and electrolyte imbalances, and decreased blood pressure, increased pulse, and other signs of shock.

Two major causes of DKA are omission of insulin and illnesses such as infection, trauma, myocardial infarction, or stroke.

Hyperosmolar Hyperglycemic Nonketotic Coma (HHNC)

HHNC is another type of diabetic coma that is potentially life threatening. It is relatively rare and carries a high mortality rate. The term *hyperosmolar* refers to an excessive amount of glucose, electrolytes, and other solutes in the blood in relation to the amount of water.

Like DKA, HHNC is characterized by hyperglycemia, which leads to osmotic diuresis and resultant thirst, polyuria, dehydration, and electrolyte losses, as well as neurologic signs ranging from drowsiness to stupor to coma. Additional clinical problems may include hypovolemic shock, thrombosis, renal problems, or stroke. In contrast with DKA, hyperosmolar coma occurs in people with previously unknown or mild diabetes, usually after an illness; occurs in hyperglycemic conditions other than diabetes (eg, severe burns, corticosteroid drug therapy); and does not cause ketosis.

- The only clear-cut contraindication to the use of insulin is hypoglycemia, because of the risk of brain damage (Box 26-3). Pork insulin is contraindicated in clients allergic to the animal protein.

- Available insulins are pork insulin and human insulin. Pork insulin differs from human insulin by one amino acid. Human insulin is synthesized in the laboratory with recombinant DNA techniques using strains of *Escherichia coli* or by modifying pork insulin to replace the single different amino acid. The name *human insulin* means that the synthetic product is identical to endogenous insulin (ie, has the same number and sequence of amino acids). It is not derived from the human pancreas.

  Insulin analogs are synthesized in the laboratory by altering the type or sequence of amino acids in insulin molecules. *Insulin lispro* (Humalog), *insulin aspart* (Novolog), and *insulin glulisine* (Apidra) are short-acting products. Lispro, the first analog to be marketed, is identical to human insulin except for the reversal of two amino acids (lysine and proline). It is absorbed more rapidly and has a shorter half-life after subcutaneous (Sub-Q) injection than regular (short-acting) human insulin. As a result, it is similar to physiologic insulin secretion after a meal; more effective at decreasing postprandial hyperglycemia; and less likely to cause hypoglycemia before the next meal. Injection just before a meal produces hypoglycemic effects similar to those of an injection of conventional regular insulin given 30 minutes before a meal. *Aspart* has an even more rapid onset

and shorter duration of action. The newest short-acting insulin analog, *glulisine,* has the shortest onset time (5–10 minutes). In contrast, *insulin glargine* is a long-acting preparation used to provide a basal amount of insulin through 24 hours, similar to normal, endogenous insulin secretion.

- Insulin cannot be given orally because it is a protein that is destroyed by proteolytic enzymes in the GI tract. It is given only parenterally, most often Sub-Q. However, a nasal spray formulation is being developed.

- Rapid-acting insulin analogs are appropriate insulins for continuous Sub-Q insulin infusion using external insulin pumps (Fig. 26-2). Advantages of this method of insulin delivery include improved lifestyle flexibility and better control of blood glucose levels. Disadvantages include undetected interruptions in insulin delivery, resulting in the development of hyperglycemia and ketosis, and infection at the needle site. Hypoglycemia can also occur in pump users as with those administering insulin via Sub-Q injection. Insulin mixtures and intermediate/long-acting insulins are not approved for use in continuous Sub-Q infusion pumps.

- Insulins differ in onset and duration of action. They are usually categorized as short-, intermediate-, or long-acting. Short-acting insulins have a rapid onset and a short duration of action. Intermediate- and long-acting insulins (except for insulin glargine) are modified by

(text continues on page 412)

Table 26-1 Drugs at a Glance: Insulins

GENERIC/TRADE NAME	CHARACTERISTICS	ROUTES AND DOSAGE RANGES	ACTION (H)		
			Onset	Peak	Duration
Short-Acting Insulin **Insulin injection** (Regular Iletin II, Humulin R, Novolin R)	• A clear liquid solution with the appearance of water • The hypoglycemic drug of choice for diabetic clients experiencing acute or emergency situations, diabetic ketoacidosis, hyperosmolar nonketotic coma, severe infections or other illnesses, major surgery, and pregnancy • The only insulin preparation that can be given IV	Sub-Q, dosage individualized according to blood glucose levels. For sliding scale, 5–20 units before meals and bedtime, depending on blood glucose levels IV, dosage individualized. For ketoacidosis, regular insulin may be given by direct injection, intermittent infusion, or continuous infusion. One regimen involves an initial bolus injection of 10–20 units followed by a continuous low-dose infusion of 2–10 units/h, based on hourly blood and urine glucose levels.	½–1	2–3	5–7

Intermediate-Acting Insulins
Isophane insulin
   suspension (NPH,
   NPH Iletin II,
   Humulin N,
   Novolin N)
	• Commonly used for long-term administration
	• Modified by addition of protamine (a protein) and zinc
	• A suspension with a cloudy appearance when correctly mixed in the drug vial
	• Given *only* Sub-Q
	• Not recommended for use in acute situations
	• Hypoglycemic reactions are more likely to occur during mid to late afternoon
		Sub-Q, dosage individualized. Initially, 7–26 units may be given once or twice daily.	1–1½	8–12	18–24

Insulin zinc
   suspension
   (Lente Iletin II,
   Lente L,
   Humulin L)
	• Modified by addition of zinc
	• May be used interchangeably with NPH insulin
	• A suspension with a cloudy appearance when correctly mixed in the drug vial
	• Given only Sub-Q
		Sub-Q, dosage individualized. Initially, 7–26 units may be given once or twice daily.	1–2	8–12	18–24

Long-Acting Insulin **Extended insulin zinc** **suspension** (Humulin U, Ultralente)	• Modified by addition of zinc and formation of large crystals, which are slowly absorbed • Hypoglycemic reactions are frequent and likely to occur during sleep.	Sub-Q, dosage individualized. Initially, 7–26 units may be given once daily.	4–8	10–30	36 plus

Table 26-1 Drugs at a Glance: Insulins (continued)

GENERIC/TRADE NAME	CHARACTERISTICS	ROUTES AND DOSAGE RANGES	ACTION (H)		
			Onset	Peak	Duration
Insulin Mixtures **NPH 70%** **Regular 30%** (Humulin 70/30, Novolin 70/30) **NPH 50%** **Regular 50%** (Humulin 50/50)	• Stable mixture • Onset, peak, and duration of action same as individual components See Humulin 70/30, above	Sub-Q, dosage individualized Sub-Q, dosage individualized			
Insulin Analogs **Insulin lispro** (Humalog)	• A synthetic insulin of recombinant DNA origin, created by reversing two amino acids • Has a faster onset and a shorter duration of action than human regular insulin • Intended for use with a longer-acting insulin	Sub-Q, dosage individualized, 15 min before meals. May also be given in external insulin pumps	$\frac{1}{4}$	$\frac{1}{2}$–$1\frac{1}{2}$	6–8
Insulin aspart (NovoLog)	Similar to lispro	Sub-Q, dosage individualized	$\frac{1}{4}$	1–3	3–5
Insulin glargine (Lantus)	• Long acting • Provides basal amount of insulin • Must *not* be diluted or mixed with any other insulin or solutions	Sub-Q, dosage individualized, once daily at bedtime	1.1	None	24
Insulin glulisine (Apidra)	• Clear, colorless solution • More rapid onset of action and shorter duration of action than regular human insulin • Should be used in regimens that include a longer-acting insulin or basal insulin analog • May be mixed with NPH insulin for injection only. Draw up Apidra first, then NPH insulin. Do NOT mix Apidra with other insulins in Sub-Q infusion pumps.	Sub-Q by injection or continuous infusion pump, dosage individualized. When used as a mealtime insulin, give up to 15 min before or within 20 min of beginning the meal.	$\frac{1}{12}$–$\frac{1}{6}$ (5–10 min)	1	4
Analog Mixture **Insulin lispro** **protamine 75%** **Insulin lispro 25%** (Humalog Mix 75/25)	• Same onset, peak, and duration as individual components	Sub-Q, dosage individualized			

IV, intravenous; NPH, isophane; Sub-Q, subcutaneous.

Box 26-3 Hypoglycemia: Characteristics and Management

Hypoglycemia may occur with insulin, meglitinides, or oral sulfonylureas. When hypoglycemia is suspected, the blood glucose level should be measured if possible, although signs and symptoms and the plasma glucose level at which they occur vary from person to person. Hypoglycemia is a blood glucose below 60 to 70 mg/dL and is especially dangerous at approximately 40 mg/dL or below. Central nervous system effects may lead to accidental injury or permanent brain damage; cardiovascular effects may lead to cardiac dysrhythmias or myocardial infarction. Causes of hypoglycemia include:

- Intensive insulin therapy (ie, continuous subcutaneous [Sub-Q] infusion or three or more injections daily)
- Omitting or delaying meals
- An excessive or incorrect dose of insulin or an oral agent that causes hypoglycemia
- Altered sensitivity to insulin
- Decreased clearance of insulin or an oral agent (eg, with renal insufficiency)
- Decreased glucose intake
- Decreased production of glucose in the liver
- Giving an insulin injection intramuscularly (IM) rather than Sub-Q
- Drug interactions that decrease blood glucose levels
- Increased physical exertion
- Ethanol ingestion

Hormones That Raise Blood Sugar

Normally, when hypoglycemia occurs, several hormones (glucagon, epinephrine, growth hormone, and cortisol) work to restore and maintain blood glucose levels. Glucagon and epinephrine, the dominant counter-regulatory hormones, act rapidly because they are activated as soon as blood glucose levels start declining. Growth hormone and cortisol act more slowly, about 2 hours after hypoglycemia occurs.

People with diabetes who develop hypoglycemia may have impaired secretion of these hormones, especially those clients with type 1 diabetes. Decreased secretion of glucagon is often evident in clients who have had diabetes for 5 years or longer. Decreased secretion of epinephrine also occurs in people who have been treated with insulin for several years. Decreased epinephrine decreases tachycardia, a common sign of hypoglycemia, and may delay recognition and treatment.

The Conscious Client

Treatment of hypoglycemic reactions consists of immediate administration of a rapidly absorbed carbohydrate. For the conscious client who is able to swallow, the carbohydrate is given orally. Foods and fluids that provide approximately 15 grams of carbohydrate include:

- Two sugar cubes or 1 to 2 teaspoons of sugar, syrup, honey, or jelly
- Two or three small pieces of candy or eight Lifesaver candies
- 4 oz of fruit juice, such as orange, apple, or grape
- 4 oz of ginger ale

- Coffee or tea with 2 teaspoons of sugar added
- Commercial glucose products (eg, Glutose, B-D Glucose). These products must be swallowed to be effective.

Symptoms usually subside within 15 to 20 minutes. If they do not subside, the client should take another 10 to 15 grams of oral carbohydrate. *If acarbose or miglitol has been taken with insulin or a sulfonylurea and a hypoglycemic reaction occurs, glucose (oral or intravenous [IV]) or glucagon must be given for treatment.* Sucrose (table sugar) and other oral carbohydrates do not relieve hypoglycemia because the presence of acarbose or miglitol prevents their digestion and absorption from the gastrointestinal tract.

The Unconscious Client

For the unconscious client, carbohydrate cannot be given orally because of the risks of aspiration. Therefore, the treatment choices are parenteral glucose or glucagon.

If the client is in a health care facility where medical help is readily available, IV glucose in a 25% or 50% solution is the treatment of choice. It acts rapidly to raise blood glucose levels and arouse the client. If the client is at home or elsewhere, glucagon may be given if available and there is someone to inject it. A family member or roommate may be taught to give glucagon Sub-Q or IM. It can also be given IV. The usual adult dose is 0.5 to 1 milligram. Glucagon is a pancreatic hormone that increases blood sugar by converting liver glycogen to glucose. It is effective only when liver glycogen is present. Some clients cannot respond to glucagon because glycogen stores are depleted by conditions such as starvation, adrenal insufficiency, or chronic hypoglycemia. The hyperglycemic effect of glucagon occurs more slowly than that of IV glucose and is of relatively brief duration. If the client does not respond to one or two doses of glucagon within 20 minutes, IV glucose is indicated.

Avoid Overtreatment

Caution is needed in the treatment of hypoglycemia. Although the main goal of treatment is to relieve hypoglycemia and restore the brain's supply of glucose, a secondary goal is to avoid overtreatment and excessive hyperglycemia. The client having a hypoglycemic reaction should not use it as an excuse to eat high-caloric foods or large amounts of food. Health care personnel caring for the client should avoid giving excessive amounts of glucose.

Posthypoglycemia Care

Once hypoglycemia is relieved, the person should have a snack or a meal. Slowly absorbed carbohydrate and protein foods, such as milk, cheese, and bread, are needed to replace glycogen stores in the liver and to prevent secondary hypoglycemia from rapid use of the carbohydrates given earlier. In addition, the episode needs to be evaluated for precipitating factors so that these can be minimized to prevent future episodes. Repeated episodes mean that the therapeutic regimen and client compliance must be re-evaluated and adjusted if indicated.

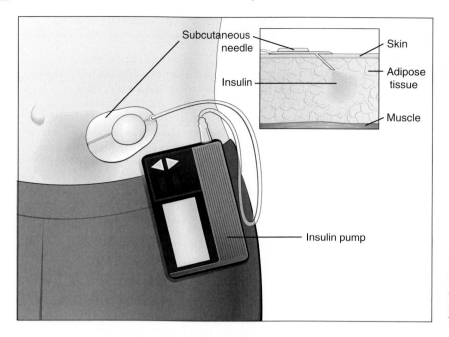

Subcutaneous needle

Insulin

Skin

Adipose tissue

Muscle

Insulin pump

FIGURE 26-2 Continuous subcutaneous (Sub-Q) insulin infusion pump. The insulin dosage is programmed into the pump's computer and the appropriate amount of insulin is injected into the adipose tissue through a needle inserted into the Sub-Q area.

adding protamine (a large, insoluble protein), zinc, or both to slow absorption and prolong drug action. Several mixtures of an intermediate- and a short-acting insulin are available and commonly used.

- U-100, the main insulin concentration in the United States, contains 100 units of insulin per milliliter of solution. *It can be accurately measured only in a syringe designed for use with U-100 insulin.*

- Sub-Q insulin is absorbed most rapidly when injected into the abdomen, followed by the upper arm, thigh, and buttocks. Absorption is delayed or decreased by injection into Sub-Q tissue with lipodystrophy or other lesions; by circulatory problems such as edema or hypotension; by insulin-binding antibodies (which develop after 2 or 3 months of insulin administration); and by injecting cold (ie, refrigerated) insulin.

- Temperature extremes can cause loss of potency. Insulin retains potency up to 36 months under refrigeration and 18 to 24 months at room temperature. At high temperatures (eg, 100°F or 37.8°C), insulin loses potency in about 2 months. If frozen, insulin clumps or precipitates, cannot be measured accurately, and should be discarded.

APPLYING YOUR KNOWLEDGE 26-1

The main adverse effect of insulin 70/30 is hypoglycemia. At what time during a 24-hour period should you be especially alert to assess for the effects of hypoglycemia in Mr. Furgeson?

Oral Hypoglycemic Drugs

There are five types of oral antidiabetic agents, all of which may be used to treat type 2 diabetes when diet and exercise alone fail to control the disorder. The drugs lower blood sugar by different mechanisms (Fig. 26-3) and may be used in var-

ious combinations for additive effects. Some are also combined with insulin. These drugs are further described below and in Table 26-2.

Sulfonylureas

- The sulfonylureas are the oldest and largest group of oral agents. They lower blood glucose mainly by increasing secretion of insulin. They may also increase peripheral use of glucose, decrease production of glucose in the liver, increase the number of insulin receptors, or alter postreceptor actions to increase tissue responsiveness to insulin. Because the drugs stimulate pancreatic beta cells to produce more insulin, they are effective only when functioning pancreatic beta cells are present.

- First-generation drugs (eg, acetohexamide, chlorpropamide, tolazamide, tolbutamide) have largely been replaced by the second generation and are not discussed further. The second-generation drugs, glipizide, glyburide, and glimepiride, are similar in therapeutic and adverse effects. The main adverse effect is hypoglycemia (see Box 26-3).

- The sulfonylureas are chemically related to sulfonamide antibacterial drugs; well absorbed with oral administration; more than 90% bound to plasma proteins; and metabolized in the liver to inactive metabolites, which are excreted mainly by the kidneys (except for glyburide, which is excreted about equally in urine and bile).

- A sulfonylurea may be given alone or with most other antidiabetic drugs in the treatment of type 2 diabetes, including insulin, acarbose, miglitol, metformin, pioglitazone, or rosiglitazone.

- Sulfonylureas are contraindicated in clients with hypersensitivity to them; with severe renal or hepatic impair-

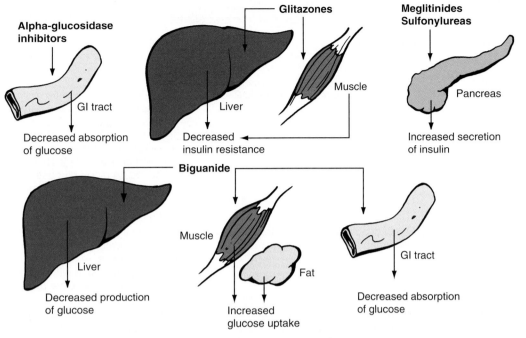

FIGURE 26-3 Actions of oral antidiabetic drugs. The drugs lower blood sugar by decreasing absorption or production of glucose, by increasing secretion of insulin, or by increasing the effectiveness of available insulin (decreasing insulin resistance).

ment; and during pregnancy. They are unlikely to be effective during periods of stress, such as major surgery, severe illness, or infection. Insulin is usually required in these circumstances.

Alpha-Glucosidase Inhibitors

- Acarbose and miglitol inhibit alpha-glucosidase enzymes (eg, sucrase, maltase, amylase) in the GI tract and thereby delay digestion of complex carbohydrates into glucose and other simple sugars. As a result, glucose absorption is delayed and there is a smaller increase in blood glucose levels after a meal.
- The drugs are metabolized in the GI tract by digestive enzymes and intestinal bacteria. Some of the metabolites are absorbed systemically and excreted in urine; plasma concentrations are increased in the presence of renal impairment.
- One of the drugs may be combined with insulin or an oral agent, usually a sulfonylurea.
- These drugs are contraindicated in clients with hypersensitivity, DKA, hepatic cirrhosis, inflammatory or malabsorptive intestinal disorders, and severe renal impairment.

Biguanide

- Metformin increases the use of glucose by muscle and fat cells, decreases hepatic glucose production, and decreases intestinal absorption of glucose. It is prefer-

ably called an *antihyperglycemic* rather than a *hypoglycemic* agent because it does not cause hypoglycemia, even in large doses, when used alone.
- It is absorbed from the small intestine, circulates without binding to plasma proteins, and has a serum half-life of 1.3 to 4.5 hours. It is not metabolized in the liver and is excreted unchanged in the urine.
- Metformin may be used alone or in combination with insulin or other oral agents. It is widely prescribed as the initial drug in obese clients with newly diagnosed type 2 diabetes, mainly because it does not cause weight gain as most other oral agents do.
- It is contraindicated in clients with diabetes complicated by fever, severe infections, severe trauma, major surgery, acidosis, or pregnancy (insulin is indicated in these conditions). It is also contraindicated in clients with serious hepatic or renal impairment, cardiac or respiratory insufficiency, hypoxia, or a history of lactic acidosis because these conditions may increase production of lactate and the risk of potentially fatal lactic acidosis.

Glitazones

- These drugs, pioglitazone and rosiglitazone, are also called *thiazolidinediones* (*TZDs*) and *insulin sensitizers*.
- They decrease insulin resistance, a major factor in the pathophysiology of type 2 diabetes. The drugs stimulate receptors on muscle, fat, and liver cells. This stimulation increases or restores the effectiveness of circulating insulin

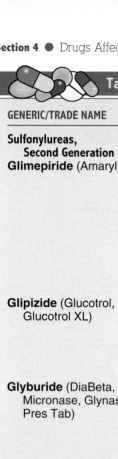

Table 26-2 Drugs at a Glance: Oral Drugs for Diabetes Mellitus

GENERIC/TRADE NAME	CHARACTERISTICS	ROUTES AND DOSAGE RANGES
Sulfonylureas, Second Generation **Glimepiride** (Amaryl)	Onset of action, about 1 h; peak, 2–3 h	PO, initially 1–2 mg once daily, with breakfast or first main meal. Maximum starting dose 2 mg or less. Maintenance dose 1–4 mg once daily. After a dose of 2 mg is reached, increase dose in increments of 2 mg or less at 1- to 2-week intervals, based on blood glucose levels. Maximum recommended dose, 8 mg once daily In combination with insulin, PO 8 mg once daily with first main meal
Glipizide (Glucotrol, Glucotrol XL)	Onset of action, approximately 1–1.5 h; duration, 10–16 h	PO, initially 5 mg daily in a single dose, 30 min before breakfast Maximum dose, 40 mg daily In elderly, may start with 2.5 mg daily Extended-release: Give once daily with breakfast.
Glyburide (DiaBeta, Micronase, Glynase Pres Tab)	Onset of action, approximately 2–4 h; duration, 24 h. Glynase is better absorbed, acts faster (onset, about 1 h; duration, 24 h), and is given in smaller doses than other forms of glyburide.	PO, initially 2.5–5 mg daily in a single dose, with breakfast Maximum dose, 20 mg daily Glynase: PO, initially 1.5–3 mg daily with breakfast. Maximum dose, 12 mg daily
Alpha-Glucosidase Inhibitors **Acarbose** (Precose)	Delays digestion of carbohydrate foods when acarbose and food are present in GI tract at the same time	PO, initially 25 mg, 3 times daily with first bite of main meals; increase at 4- to 8-week intervals to a maximum dose of 50 mg 3 times daily (for patients weighing under 60 kg) if necessary, depending on 1-h postprandial blood glucose levels and tolerance. Clients weighing more than 60 kg may need doses up to 100 mg 3 times daily (the maximum dose).
Miglitol (Glyset)	Delays digestion of carbohydrates in the GI tract	PO, initially 25 mg 3 times daily with the first bite of each main meal, gradually increased if necessary Maximum dose, 100 mg 3 times daily
Biguanide **Metformin** (Glucophage, Glucophage XR))	Older adults are at higher risk for development of lactic acidosis, a rare but potentially fatal reaction. Thus, smaller doses and monitoring of renal function are recommended.	PO, initially 500 mg twice daily, with morning and evening meals; increase dose in increments of 500 mg/d every 2–3 wk if necessary, up to a maximum of 3000 mg daily, based on patient tolerance and blood glucose levels. In older patients, do not increase to maximum dose. Extended-release: PO once daily with the evening meal.
Glitazones **Pioglitazone** (Actos)	Increases effects of insulin; may be used alone or with insulin, metformin, or a sulfonylurea	PO 15–30 mg once daily
Rosiglitazone (Avandia)	Increases effects of insulin; may be used alone or with metformin	PO 4–8 mg once daily, in 1 dose or 2 divided doses

Table 26-2 Drugs at a Glance: Oral Drugs for Diabetes Mellitus (continued)

GENERIC/TRADE NAME	CHARACTERISTICS	ROUTES AND DOSAGE RANGES
Meglitinides **Nateglinide** (Starlix)	• Onset of action, within 20 min; peak, 1 h; duration, 3–4 h	PO 120 mg 3 times daily, 1–30 min before meals. Omit dose if skip a meal.
Repaglinide (Prandin)	• Onset of action, within 30 min; peak, 1 h; duration, approximately 3–4 h	PO 1–2 mg 15–30 min before each meal, increased to 4 mg before meals if necessary. Maximum dose, 16 mg daily. Omit a dose if skip a meal; add a dose if add a meal.
Combination Drugs* **Glyburide/metformin** (Glucovance)	• Available in preparations containing 1.25 mg glyburide and 250 mg metformin; 2.5 mg glyburide and 500 mg metformin; or 5 mg glyburide and 500 mg metformin	Initially, PO 1.25 mg/250 mg once or twice daily with meals. *Clients previously treated with glyburide or other sulfonylurea plus metformin:* Initially, PO 2.5 or 5 mg/500 mg twice daily with meals, not to exceed previous doses of separate drugs
Metformin/glipizide (Metaglip)	• Available as tablets containing metformin 250 or 500 mg and glipizide 2.5 or 5 mg	PO 2.5/250 mg once daily, increased if necessary
Rosiglitazone/ **metformin** (Avandamet)	• Available in tablets containing 1, 2, or 4 mg rosiglitazone and 500 mg metformin and 2 or 4 mg rosiglitazone and 1000 mg metformin	PO, variable dose; maximum daily dose, 8 mg rosiglitazone and 2000 mg metformin

*See Appendix A for additional combination drugs.
GI, gastrointestinal; PO, oral.

and results in increased uptake of glucose by peripheral tissues and decreased production of glucose by the liver.

● The drugs may be used as monotherapy with diet and exercise or in combination with insulin, metformin, or a sulfonylurea.

● The drugs are contraindicated in clients with active liver disease or a serum alanine aminotransferase (ALT) level more than 2.5 times the upper limit of normal. They are also contraindicated in clients who are hypersensitive to them.

● The drugs should be used very cautiously, if at all, in clients at risk of developing congestive heart failure. Glitazones increase plasma volume and may cause fluid retention and heart failure. In one study, heart failure developed in 4.5% of glitazone users within 10 months and in 12.4% of users within 36 months. In people who did not take a glitazone, 2.6% developed heart failure within 10 months and 8.4% within 36 months.

Meglitinides

● Nateglinide and repaglinide are nonsulfonylureas that lower blood sugar by stimulating pancreatic secretion of insulin.

● They can be used as monotherapy with diet and exercise or in combination with metformin.

● The drugs are well absorbed from the GI tract; peak plasma level occurs within 1 hour. They have a plasma

half-life of 1 to 1.5 hours and are highly bound (>98%) to plasma proteins. They are metabolized in the liver; metabolites are excreted in urine and feces.

● Repaglinide is metabolized and removed from the bloodstream within 3 to 4 hours after a dose, nateglinide within about 6 hours. This decreases the workload of pancreatic beta cells (ie, decreases duration of beta-cell stimulation); allows serum insulin levels to return to normal before the next meal; and decreases risks of hypoglycemic episodes.

● These drugs should be taken just before or up to 30 minutes before a meal. If a meal is skipped, the drug dose should be skipped; if a meal is added, a drug dose should be added.

Herbal and Dietary Supplements

Increasing numbers of people are choosing alternative medications to complement or in some cases to replace prescription medications (see Research Brief). With most herbs and dietary supplements, even the commonly used ones (eg, echinacea, St. John's wort), the effects on blood glucose levels are unknown; well-controlled, long-term studies of effects have not been done; and interactions with antidiabetic drugs are unknown. Thus, anyone with diabetes who wishes to take an herbal or dietary supplement should consult a health care provider, read product labels carefully, seek the most authoritative information available,

RESEARCH BRIEF

Use of Alternative Medicines in Diabetes Mellitus

SOURCE:

Ryan A. E., & Marceau C. (2001). Use of alternative medicines in diabetes mellitus. *Diabetic Medicine, 18*(3), 242.

SUMMARY:

Five hundred and two diabetic subjects and 201 control subjects were interviewed about their use of prescribed medications, alternative medications, and over-the-counter supplements.

In the group with diabetes, 78% were taking prescribed antidiabetic medications, 44% reported taking over-the-counter supplements, and 31% were taking alternative medications. Use of alternative medications for the purpose of reducing blood glucose levels was not a common practice among diabetic subjects. The most commonly used complementary therapies included vitamins, calcium, aspirin, garlic, echinacea, herbal mixtures, and glucosamine. In the control group, 63% were taking prescribed medications, 51% were taking over-the-counter supplements, and 37% were taking alternative medications. Even though subjects rated the effectiveness of the alternative medications lower than prescribed medications, they still reported some beneficial effect. Diabetic subjects reported spending almost as much money on complementary therapies as they did on prescription drugs.

NURSING IMPLICATIONS:

Use of complementary therapies by diabetic clients is comparable to the level of use in nondiabetic people. Because complementary therapies have the potential for impacting blood glucose levels of diabetic clients, nurses should take careful drug histories, including questions about use of herbal and over-the-counter supplements. Nurses should also educate diabetic clients about the potential impact of complementary therapies on blood glucose levels when this information is available.

and monitor blood glucose closely when starting the supplement. Described below are some products that reportedly affect blood sugar and that should be used cautiously, if at all, by clients with diabetes.

Supplements That May Increase Blood Glucose Levels

Bee pollen may cause hyperglycemia and decrease the effects of antidiabetic medications. It should *not* be used by people with diabetes.

Ginkgo biloba extract is thought to increase blood sugar in clients with diabetes by increasing hepatic metabolism of insulin and oral hypoglycemic drugs, thereby making the drugs less effective. It is not recommended for use.

Glucosamine, as indicated by animal studies, may cause impaired beta-cell function and insulin secretion similar to that observed in humans with type 2 diabetes. Long-term effects in humans are unknown, but the product is considered potentially harmful to people with diabetes or impaired glucose tolerance (prediabetes). Adverse effects on blood sugar and drug interactions with antidiabetic medications have not been reported. However, blood sugar should be monitored carefully. With chondroitin, which is often taken with glucosamine for osteoarthritis, there is no information about effects on blood sugar, use by diabetic clients, or interactions with antidiabetic drugs.

Supplements That May Decrease Blood Glucose Levels

Basil, which is commonly used in cooking, is also available as an herbal supplement. The amounts used in cooking are unlikely to affect blood sugar, but larger amounts may cause hypoglycemia or increase the hypoglycemic effects of insulin and oral antidiabetic drugs. The use of supplemental amounts should probably be avoided by people with diabetes. If used, blood glucose levels should be closely monitored.

Bay leaf is commonly used in cooking (it should be removed from the food before eating) and is also available as an extract made with ground leaves. It increases the effects of insulin and is sometimes recommended by nutritionists for diabetic diets. If used, blood glucose levels should be monitored closely.

Chromium is a trace mineral required for normal glucose metabolism. It may increase production of insulin receptors and insulin binding to the receptors, thereby increasing insulin effectiveness, lowering blood glucose levels, and decreasing insulin requirements in people with diabetes. It also may have beneficial effects on serum cholesterol levels. However, evidence for these effects is inconsistent, with some supporting and some negating the use of chromium supplements.

Chromium deficiency, considered rare in the United States, may play a role in the development of diabetes and atherosclerosis. If so, beneficial effects of a supplement may be more evident in a deficiency state. In one study of pregnant women and older adults with marginal levels of chromium, administration of a supplement improved glucose tolerance. At present, there is insufficient evidence to recommend routine chromium supplementation in diabetic clients. In nondiabetic clients, chromium supplements do not have hypoglycemic effects.

Echinacea. Some clinical trials have been done, but people with diabetes were excluded. It was concluded that diabetics should not take echinacea.

Garlic. Some sources report no known effects on blood glucose; others report a decrease in animals and humans. Some researchers also reported increased serum insulin and improvement in liver glycogen storage after garlic administration. There is a potential for additive hypoglycemic effects with antidiabetic drugs, although no apparent interactions have been reported.

Ginseng. Several studies (generally small and not well designed) indicate that ginseng lowers blood glucose levels in both diabetic and nondiabetic subjects. It may be useful in preventing diabetes or complications of diabetes. However, larger and longer studies are needed before general use can be recommended for diabetic or nondiabetic clients. For nondiabetic clients who use ginseng, the herb may need to be taken with a meal to prevent unintentional hypoglycemia. For diabetic clients, use of ginseng should be very cautious (if at all), with frequent monitoring of blood glucose and signs of hypoglycemia, because of possible additive effects with antidiabetic medications. Its use should also be accompanied by proper diet, physical activity, and antidiabetic medication.

Glucomannan, which is promoted as a diet aid and laxative, has hypoglycemic effects and should be avoided or used very cautiously by people with diabetes. If used, blood sugar levels should be monitored closely and lower doses of antidiabetic drugs may be needed.

Guar gum is a type of fiber that becomes gel-like upon contact with liquids (eg, like Metamucil). It is used as a thickening agent in foods and drugs and is an ingredient in some over-the-counter weight-loss products. It should be used cautiously, if at all, by people with diabetes because it has hypoglycemic effects and slows GI motility. Several cases of esophageal and intestinal obstruction have been reported with weight-loss products.

APPLYING YOUR KNOWLEDGE 26-2
Mr. Furgeson complains about feeling weak and confused. Your assessment reveals he is sweating and has tremors of his upper extremities. What action should you take?

NURSING PROCESS

Assessment

Assess the client's knowledge, attitude, and condition in relation to diabetes, the prescribed treatment plan, and complications. Assessment data should include past man-

ifestations of the disease process and the client's response to them; present status; and potential problem areas.

● *Historic data* include age at onset of diabetes, prescribed control measures and their effectiveness, the ease or difficulty of complying with the prescribed treatment, occurrence of complications such as ketoacidosis, and whether other disease processes have interfered with diabetes control.

● *Assess the client's current status,* in relation to the following areas:

● **Diet.** Ask about the prescribed nutritional plan, who prepares the food, what factors help in following the diet, what factors interfere with following the diet, the current weight, and whether there has been a recent weight change. Also ask if herbal or other dietary supplements are used. If so, list each one by name and frequency of use. If a nutritionist is available, ask one to assess the client's dietary practice and needs.

● **Activity.** Ask the client to describe usual activities of daily living, including those related to work, home, and recreation, and whether he or she participates in a regular exercise program. If so, ask for more information about what, how often, how long, and so forth. If not, teaching is needed because exercise is extremely important in diabetes management.

● **Medication.** If the client takes insulin, ask what kind; how much; who administers it; usual time of administration; sites used for injections; and if a hypoglycemic reaction to insulin has ever been experienced, how it was handled. This information helps to assess knowledge, usual practices, and teaching needs. If the client takes an oral antidiabetic drug, ask the name, dosage, and time taken.

● **Monitoring methods.** Testing the blood for glucose and the urine for ketones (eg, when blood sugar is elevated, when ill and unable to eat) are the two main methods of self-monitoring glycemic control. Ask about the method used, the frequency of testing, and the pattern of results. If possible, observe the client performing and interpreting an actual test to assess accuracy.

● **Skin and mucous membranes.** Inspect for signs of infection and other lesions. Infections often occur in the axillary and groin areas because these areas have large numbers of microorganisms. Periodontal disease (pyorrhea) may be manifested by inflammation and bleeding of the gums. Women with diabetes are susceptible to monilial vaginitis and infections under the breasts. Check the sites of insulin injection for atrophy (dimpling or indentation), hypertrophy (nodules or lumps), and fibrosis (hardened areas). Check the lower leg for brown spots; these are caused by small hemorrhages into the skin and may indicate widespread changes in the blood vessels.

Problems are especially likely to develop in the feet from infection, trauma, pressure, vascular insufficiency, and neuropathy. Therefore, inspect the feet for calluses, ulcers, and signs of infection. When such problems develop, sensory impairment from neuropathy may delay detection and impaired circulation may delay healing. Check pedal pulses, color, and temperature in both feet to evaluate arterial blood flow. Ankle edema may indicate venous insufficiency or impaired cardiac function.

- **Eyes.** Ask about difficulties with vision and if eyes are examined regularly. Diabetic clients are prone to development of retinopathy, cataracts, and possibly glaucoma.
- **Cardiovascular system.** Clients with diabetes have a high incidence of atherosclerosis, which makes them susceptible to hypertension, angina pectoris, myocardial infarction, peripheral vascular disease, and stroke. Therefore, check blood pressure and ask about chest pain and pain in the legs with exercise (intermittent claudication).
- **Genitourinary system.** People with diabetes often have kidney and bladder problems. Assess for signs of urinary tract infection; albumin, white blood cells, or blood in urine; edema; increased urination at night; difficulty voiding; generalized itching; fatigue; and muscular weakness. Impotence may develop in men and is attributed to neuropathy.

- Assess blood sugar reports for abnormal levels. Two or more fasting blood glucose levels greater than 126 mg/dL or two random levels greater than 200 mg/dL are diagnostic of diabetes. Decreased blood sugar levels are especially dangerous at 40 mg/dL or below.
- Assess the glycosylated hemoglobin (also called *glycated hemoglobin* and *HbA_{1c}*) level when available. This test indicates glucose bound to hemoglobin in red blood cells (RBCs) when RBCs are exposed to hyperglycemia. The binding is irreversible and lasts for the lifespan of RBCs (approximately 120 days). The test reflects the average blood sugar during the previous 2 to 3 months. The goal is usually less than 7% (the range for people without diabetes is approximately 4%–6%). The test should be done every 3 to 6 months.

  Test results are not affected by several factors that alter blood sugar levels, such as time of day, food intake, exercise, recently administered antidiabetic drugs, emotional stress, or client cooperation. The test is especially useful with children; those whose diabetes is poorly controlled; those who do not test blood glucose regularly; and those who change their usual habits before a scheduled appointment with a health care provider so that their blood sugar control appears better than it actually is.

Nursing Diagnoses

- Ineffective Tissue Perfusion, peripheral, related to atherosclerosis and vascular impairment
- Disturbed Sensory Perception, visual and tactile, related to impaired vision or neuropathy
- Ineffective Coping related to chronic illness and required treatment
- Anxiety: Managing a chronic illness, finger sticks, insulin injections
- Risk for Injury: Trauma, infection, hypoglycemia, hyperglycemia
- Noncompliance related to inability or unwillingness to manage the disease process and required treatment
- Deficient Knowledge: Disease process and management; administration and effects of antidiabetic drugs; interrelationships among diet, exercise, and antidiabetic drugs; and management of hypoglycemia, "sick days," and other complications

Planning/Goals

The client will
- Learn self-care activities
- Manage drug therapy to prevent or minimize hypoglycemia and other adverse effects
- Develop a consistent pattern of diet and exercise
- Use available resources to learn about the disease process and how to manage it
- Take antidiabetic drugs accurately
- Self-monitor blood glucose and urine ketones appropriately
- Keep appointments for follow-up and monitoring procedures by a health care provider

Interventions

Use nondrug measures to improve control of diabetes and to help prevent complications.

- Assist the client in maintaining the prescribed diet. Specific measures vary but may include teaching the client and family about the importance of diet; referring the client to a dietitian; and helping the client identify and modify factors that decrease compliance with the diet. If the client is obese, assist in developing a program to lose weight and then maintain weight at a more nearly normal level.
- Assist the client to develop and maintain a regular exercise program.
- Perform and interpret blood tests for glucose accurately, and assist clients and family members to do so. Self-monitoring of blood glucose levels allows the client to see the effects of diet, exercise, and hypoglycemic medications on blood glucose levels and may promote compliance.

Several products are available for home glucose monitoring. All involve obtaining a drop of capillary blood from a finger or forearm with a sterile lancet. The blood is placed on a semipermeable membrane that contains a reagent. The amount of blood glucose can be read with various machines (eg, glucometers).

- Test urine for ketones when the client is sick, when blood glucose levels are above 200 mg/dL, and when episodes of nocturnal hypoglycemia are suspected. Also teach clients and family members to test urine when indicated.
- Promote early recognition and treatment of problems by observing for signs and symptoms of urinary tract infection, peripheral vascular disease, vision changes, ketoacidosis, hypoglycemia, and others. Teach clients and families to observe for these conditions and report their occurrence.
- Discuss the importance of regular visits to health care facilities for blood sugar measurements, weights, blood pressure measurements, and eye examinations.
- Perform and teach correct foot care. Have the client observe the following safeguards: avoid going barefoot, to prevent trauma to the feet; wear correctly fitted shoes; wash the feet daily with warm water, dry well, inspect for any lesions or pressure areas, and apply lanolin if the skin is dry; wear cotton or wool socks because they are more absorbent than synthetic materials; cut toenails straight across and only after the feet have been soaked in warm water and washed thoroughly. Teach the client to avoid use of hot water bottles or electric heating pads; cutting toenails if vision is impaired; use of strong antiseptics on the feet; and cutting corns or calluses. Also teach the client to report any lesions on the feet to the physician.
- Help clients keep up with newer developments in diabetes care by providing information, sources of information, consultations with specialists, and other resources. However, do not overwhelm a newly diagnosed diabetic client with excessive information or assume that a long-term diabetic client does not need information.

Provide appropriate client teaching for any drug therapy (see accompanying display).

Evaluation

- Check blood sugar reports regularly for normal or abnormal values.
- Check glycosylated hemoglobin reports when available.
- Interview and observe for therapeutic and adverse responses to antidiabetic drugs.
- Interview and observe for compliance with prescribed treatment.
- Interview clients and family members about the frequency and length of hospitalizations for diabetes mellitus.

APPLYING YOUR KNOWLEDGE 26-3
Mr. Furgeson does not follow a prescribed diet. Even though he tells you that he gives himself his own insulin, he does not seem to be very knowledgeable about the use of the syringe and injection sites. He has not attended diabetic education classes because the time of the class interferes with his work schedule. What nursing diagnosis would be appropriate for Mr. Furgeson?

PRINCIPLES OF THERAPY

Goals of Therapy

For most clients, the goals of treatment are to maintain blood glucose at normal or near-normal levels; promote normal metabolism of carbohydrate, fat, and protein; prevent acute and long-term complications; and prevent hypoglycemic episodes.

There is strong evidence that strict control of blood sugar delays the onset and slows progression of complications of diabetes. In addition to glycemic control, other measures can be used to help prevent complications of diabetes. Administration of angiotensin-converting enzyme (ACE) inhibitors (eg, captopril) has protective effects on the kidneys in both type 1 and type 2 diabetes and in both normotensive and hypertensive people. Although ACE inhibitors are also used in the treatment of hypertension, their ability to delay nephropathy seems to be independent of antihypertensive effects. Additional measures to preserve renal function include effective treatment of hypertension, limited intake of dietary protein, prompt treatment of urinary tract infections, and avoidance of nephrotoxic drugs when possible.

Current research suggests a number of treatment strategies may be beneficial in reducing the cardiovascular disease risk associated with type 2 diabetes mellitus. Some clinicians are recommending the routine use of statins such as simvastatin to reduce the risk of occlusive arterial disease in all clients with diabetes regardless of cholesterol level. In addition, there is evidence that reducing insulin resistance through the use of glitazones may significantly reduce the incidence of cardiovascular disease risk factors in clients with type 2 diabetes. Additional measures to reduce cardiovascular disease risk include reducing weight; controlling hypertension with an ACE inhibitor or angiotensin receptor blocker; use of aspirin therapy; and smoking cessation.

Treatment Regimens

When possible, it is desirable to have an interdisciplinary diabetes care team (eg, physician, nurse diabetes educator, dietitian, perhaps others) work with the client to design, monitor, and revise an individualized treatment plan. This is especially important for clients with newly diagnosed diabetes to assist them in learning to manage their disease and make appropriate lifestyle changes.

(text continues on page 422)

General Considerations

☑ Wear or carry diabetic identification (eg, a Medic-Alert necklace or bracelet) at all times, to aid treatment if needed.

☑ Learn as much as you can about diabetes and its management. Few other diseases require as much adaptation in activities of daily living, and you must be well informed to control the disease, minimize complications, and achieve an optimal quality of life. Although much information is available from health care providers (physicians, nurses, nurse diabetes educators, nutritionists), an additional major resource is the

American Diabetes Association
1660 Duke St.
Alexandria, VA 22314
1-800-ADA-DISC
http://www.diabetes.org

☑ In general, a consistent schedule of diet, exercise, and medication produces the best control of blood sugar levels and the least risk of complications.

☑ Diet, weight control, and exercise are extremely important in managing diabetes. Maintaining normal weight and avoiding excessive caloric intake decrease the need for medication and decrease the workload of the pancreas. Exercise helps body tissues use insulin better, which means that glucose moves out of the bloodstream and into muscles and other body tissues. This promotes more normal blood glucose levels and decreases long-term complications of diabetes.

☑ Take any antidiabetic medication as prescribed. If unable to take a medication, notify a health care provider. To control blood sugar most effectively, medications are balanced with diet and exercise. If you take insulin, you need to know what type(s) you are taking, how to obtain more, and how to store it. Unopened vials of insulin should be refrigerated. An opened vial may be stored at room temperature for 28 days. DO NOT freeze insulin. Regular and isophane (NPH) insulins and mixtures (eg, Humulin) are available over-the-counter; Humalog, NovoLog, Lantus, and Apidra require a prescription. Keep several days' supply of insulin and syringes on hand to allow for weather or other conditions that might prevent replacement of insulin or other supplies when needed.

☑ You need to know the signs and symptoms of high blood sugar (hyperglycemia): increased blood glucose and excessive thirst, hunger, and urine output. Persistent hyperglycemia may indicate a need to change some aspect of the treatment program, such as diet or medication.

☑ You need to know the symptoms of low blood sugar (hypoglycemia): sweating, nervousness, hunger, weakness, tremors, and mental confusion. Hypoglycemia may indicate too much medication or exercise or too little food. Treatment is a rapidly absorbed source of sugar, which usually reverses symptoms within 10 to 20 minutes. If you are alert and able to swallow, take 4 ounces of fruit juice, 4 to 6 ounces of a sugar-containing soft drink, a piece of fruit or $\frac{1}{3}$ cup of raisins, two to three glucose tablets (5 grams each), a tube of glucose gel, 1 cup of skim milk, tea or coffee with 2 teaspoons of sugar, or eight Life-

saver candies. Avoid taking so much sugar that hyperglycemia occurs.

If you take acarbose (Precose) or miglitol (Glyset) along with insulin; glimepiride (Amaryl); glipizide (Glucotrol); or glyburide (DiaBeta, Glynase, Micronase) and a hypoglycemic reaction occurs, you must take some form of glucose (or glucagon) for treatment. Sucrose (table sugar) and other oral carbohydrates do not relieve hypoglycemia because the presence of acarbose or miglitol prevents their digestion and absorption from the gastrointestinal (GI) tract.

☑ You need to have a family member or another person who is able to recognize and manage hypoglycemia in case you are unable to obtain or swallow a source of glucose. If you take insulin, glucagon should be available in the home and a caregiver should know how to give it.

☑ The best way to prevent, delay, or decrease the severity of diabetes complications is to maintain blood sugar at a normal or near-normal level. Other measures include regular visits to health care providers, preferably a team of specialists in diabetes care; regular vision and glaucoma testing; and special foot care. In addition, if you have hypertension or elevated lipid levels, treatment can help prevent heart attacks and strokes.

☑ Take only drugs prescribed by a physician who knows you have diabetes. Avoid other prescriptions and over-the-counter drugs unless these are discussed with the physician treating the diabetes because adverse reactions and interactions may occur. For example, nasal decongestants (alone or in cold remedies) and asthma medications may cause tachycardia and nervousness, which may be interpreted as hypoglycemia. In addition, liquid cold remedies and cough syrups may contain sugar and raise blood glucose levels.

☑ If you wish to take any kind of herbal or dietary supplement, you should discuss this with the health care provider who is managing your diabetes. There has been little study of these preparations in relation to diabetes; many can increase or decrease blood sugar and alter diabetes control. If you start a supplement, you need to check your blood sugar frequently to see how it affects your blood glucose level.

☑ Test blood regularly for glucose. A schedule individualized to your needs is best. Testing should be done more often when medication dosages are changed or when you are ill. Current blood glucose technology allows the selection of the fingertip or or other location such as the forearm to obtain the blood sample. Glucose-concentrations measured at different sites may vary. The fingertips are the most accurate site and should be the preferred test site if hypoglycemia is suspected.

☑ Reduce insulin dosage or eat extra food if you expect to exercise more than usual. Specific recommendations should be individualized and worked out with health care providers in relation to the type of exercise.

☑ Ask for written instructions about managing "sick days" and call your physician if unsure about what you need to do. Although each person needs individualized instructions, some general guidelines include the following:

CLIENT TEACHING GUIDELINES

Antidiabetic Drugs (Continued)

☑ Continue your antidiabetic medications unless instructed otherwise. Additional insulin also may be needed, especially if ketosis develops. Ketones (acetone) in the urine indicate insulin deficiency or insulin resistance.

☑ Check blood glucose levels at least four times daily; test urine for ketones when the blood glucose level exceeds 250 mg/dL or with each urination. If unable to test urine, have someone else do it.

☑ Rest, keep warm, do not exercise, and keep someone with you if possible.

☑ If unable to eat solid food, take easily digested liquids or semiliquid foods. About 15 grams of carbohydrate every 1 to 2 hours is usually enough and can be provided by ½ cup of apple juice, applesauce, cola, cranberry juice, eggnog, Cream of Wheat cereal, custard, vanilla ice cream, regular gelatin, or frozen yogurt.

☑ Drink 2 to 3 quarts of fluids daily, especially if you have a fever. Water, tea, broths, clear soups, diet soda, or carbohydrate-containing fluids are acceptable.

☑ Record the amount of fluid intake as well as the number of times you urinate, vomit, or have loose stools.

☑ Seek medical attention if a pre-meal blood glucose level is more than 250 mg/dL, if urine acetone is present, if you have fever above 100°F, if you have several episodes of vomiting or diarrhea, or if you have difficulty in breathing, chest pain, severe abdominal pain, or severe dehydration.

Self-Administration

☑ Use correct techniques for injecting insulin:

☑ Follow instructions for times of administration as nearly as possible. Different types of insulin have different onsets, peaks, and durations of action. Accurate timing (eg, in relation to meals), can increase beneficial effects and decrease risks of hypoglycemic reactions.

☑ Wash hands; wash injection site, if needed.

☑ Draw up insulin in a good light, being very careful to draw up the correct dose. If you have trouble seeing the syringe markers, get a magnifier or ask someone else to draw up the insulin. Prefilled syringes or cartridges for pen devices are also available.

☑ Instructions may vary about cleaning the top of the insulin vial and the injection site with an alcohol swab and about pulling back on the plunger after injection to see if any blood enters the syringe. These techniques have been commonly used, but many diabetes experts do not believe they are necessary.

☑ Inject straight into the fat layer under the skin, at a 90-degree angle. If very thin, pinch up a skinfold and inject at a 45-degree angle.

☑ Rotate injection sites. Your health care provider may suggest a rotation plan. Many people rotate between the abdomen and the thighs. Insulin is absorbed fastest from the abdomen. Do not inject insulin within 2 inches of the "belly button" or into any skin lesions.

☑ If it is necessary to mix two insulin preparations, ask for specific instructions about the technique and then follow it consistently. There is a risk of inaccurate dosage of both insulins unless measured very carefully. Commercial mixtures are also available for some combinations.

☑ Change insulin dosage only if instructed to do so and the circumstances are specified.

☑ Carry sugar, candy, or a commercial glucose preparation for immediate use if a hypoglycemic reaction occurs.

☑ Take oral drugs as directed. Recommendations usually include the following:

☑ Take glipizide or glyburide approximately 30 minutes before meals; take glimepiride with breakfast or the first main meal. Take Glucotrol XL with breakfast.

☑ Take acarbose or miglitol with the first bite of each main meal. The drugs need to be in the GI tract with food because they act by decreasing absorption of sugar in the food. Starting with a small dose and increasing it gradually helps to prevent bloating, "gas pains," and diarrhea.

☑ Take metformin (Glucophage) with meals to decrease stomach upset. Take Glucophage XR with the evening meal.

☑ Take repaglinide (Prandin) or nateglinide (Starlix) about 15 to 30 minutes before meals (2, 3, or 4 times daily). Doses may vary from 0.5 to 4.0 milligrams, depending on fasting blood glucose levels. Dosage changes should be at least 1 week apart. If you skip a meal, you should skip that dose of repaglinide or nateglinide; if you eat an extra meal, you should take an extra dose.

☑ Take pioglitazone (Actos) and rosiglitazone (Avandia) without regard to meals.

☑ If you take glimepiride, glipizide, glyburide, repaglinide or nateglinide, alone or in combination with other antidiabetic drugs, be prepared to handle hypoglycemic reactions (as with insulin, above). Acarbose, miglitol, metformin, pioglitazone, and rosiglitazone do not cause hypoglycemia when taken alone. Do not skip meals and snacks. This increases the risk of hypoglycemic reactions.

☑ If you exercise vigorously, you may need to decrease your dose of antidiabetic drug or eat more. Ask for specific instructions related to the type and frequency of the exercise.

The best regimen for a particular client depends on the type of diabetes, the client's age and general condition, and the client's ability and willingness to comply with the prescribed therapy. In type 1 diabetes, the only effective treatment measures are insulin, diet, and exercise. In type 2, the initial treatment of choice is diet, exercise, and weight control. If this regimen is ineffective, oral agents or insulin may be added.

Guidelines for Insulin Therapy

Choice of Insulin

When insulin therapy is indicated, the physician may choose from several preparations that vary in composition, onset, duration of action, and other characteristics. Some factors to be considered include the following:

- Human insulin is preferred for newly diagnosed type 1 diabetes, gestational diabetes, poorly controlled diabetes, clients having surgery or an illness that requires short-term insulin therapy, and clients with insulin allergy.
- Regular insulin (insulin injection) has a rapid onset of action and can be given IV. Therefore, it is the insulin of choice during acute situations, such as DKA, severe infection or other illness, and surgical procedures.
- Isophane insulin (NPH) is often used for long-term insulin therapy. For many clients, a combination of NPH and a short-acting insulin provides more consistent control of blood glucose levels. Although several regimens are used, a common one is a mixture of regular and NPH insulins administered before the morning and evening meals. A commercial mixture is more convenient and probably more accurate than a mixture prepared by a client or caregiver, if the proportions of insulins are appropriate for the client.
- Insulin lispro, aspart, or glulisine may be used instead of Sub-Q regular insulin in most situations, but safe usage requires both health care providers and clients to be aware of differences. Regular insulin, insulin aspart, and insulin glulisine are also approved for use in external insulin pumps that administer a Sub-Q continuous infusion.
- Insulin glargine may be used to provide a basal amount of insulin over 24 hours, with a short-acting insulin or short-acting insulin analog at meal times.

Drug Dosage

Dosage of insulin must be individualized according to blood glucose levels. The goal is to alleviate symptoms of hyperglycemia and re-establish metabolic balance without causing hypoglycemia. An initial dose of 0.5 to 1 unit per kilogram of body weight per day may be started and then adjusted to maintain blood glucose levels (tested before meals and at bedtime) of 90 to 130 milligrams per deciliter in adults (100–200 mg/dL in children younger than 5 years of age). However, many fac-

tors influence blood glucose response to exogenous insulin and therefore influence insulin requirements.

- Factors that increase insulin requirements include weight gain; increased caloric intake; pregnancy; decreased activity; acute infections; hyperadrenocorticism (Cushing's disease); primary hyperparathyroidism; acromegaly; hypokalemia; and drugs such as corticosteroids, epinephrine, levothyroxine, and thiazide diuretics. Clients who are obese may require 2 units/kg/day because of resistance to insulin in peripheral tissues.
- Factors that decrease insulin requirements include weight reduction; decreased caloric intake; increased physical activity; development of renal insufficiency; stopping administration of corticosteroids, epinephrine, levothyroxine, and diuretics; hypothyroidism; hypopituitarism; recovery from hyperthyroidism; recovery from acute infections; and the "honeymoon period" (see below), which may occur with type 1 diabetes.

  People who need less than 0.5 unit/kg/day may produce some endogenous insulin or their tissues may be more responsive to insulin because of exercise and good physical conditioning. Renal insufficiency decreases dosage requirements because less insulin is metabolized in the kidneys than with normal renal function. The "honeymoon period," characterized by temporary recovery of beta-cell function and production of insulin, may occur after diabetes is first diagnosed. Insulin requirements may decrease rapidly, and if the dosage is not decreased, severe hypoglycemic reactions may occur.

- In acute situations, dosage of regular insulin needs frequent adjustments based on measurements of blood glucose. When insulin is given IV in a continuous infusion, 20% to 30% binds to the IV fluid container and the infusion tubing.
- Dosage of insulin for long-term therapy is determined by blood glucose levels at various times of the day and is adjusted when indicated (eg, because of illness or changes in physical activity). Titrating insulin dosage may be difficult and time consuming; it requires cooperation and collaboration between clients and health care providers.
- Insulin pumps are being increasingly used, especially by adolescents and young adults who want flexibility in diet and exercise. These devices allow continuous Sub-Q administration of regular insulin, insulin aspart, or insulin glulisine. A basal amount of insulin is injected (eg, 1 unit/hour or a calculated fraction of the dose used previously) continuously, with bolus injections before meals. This method of insulin administration maintains more normal blood glucose levels and avoids wide fluctuations. Candidates for insulin pumps include clients with diabetes that is poorly controlled with other methods and those who are able and willing to care for the devices properly.

Drug Administration

Timing of Insulin Administration

Many clients who take insulin need at least two injections daily to control hyperglycemia. A common regimen is one half to two thirds of the total daily dose in the morning before breakfast, and the remaining one half or one third before the evening meal or at bedtime. With regular insulin before meals, it is very important that the medication be injected 30 to 45 minutes before meals so that the insulin will be available when blood sugar increases after meals. With insulin lispro, aspart, or glulisine before meals, it is important to inject the medication about 15 minutes before eating. If the client does not eat within 15 minutes, hypoglycemia may occur. Insulin glargine should be given at bedtime.

Selection of Subcutaneous Sites for Insulin Injections

Several factors affect insulin absorption from injection sites, including the site location; environmental temperature; and exercise or massage. Studies indicate that insulin is absorbed fastest from the abdomen, followed by the deltoid, thigh, and hip. Because of these differences, many clinicians recommend rotating injection sites *within* areas. This technique decreases rotations *between* areas and promotes more consistent blood glucose levels. With regard to temperature, insulin is absorbed more rapidly in warmer sites and environments. In relation to exercise, people who exercise should avoid injecting insulin into Sub-Q tissue near the muscles to be used. The increased blood flow that accompanies exercise promotes rapid absorption and may lead to hypoglycemia.

Timing of Food Intake

Clients receiving insulin need food at the peak action time of the insulin and at bedtime. The food is usually taken as a between-meal and a bedtime snack. These snacks help prevent hypoglycemic reactions between meals and at night. When hypoglycemia occurs during sleep, recognition and treatment may be delayed. This delay may allow the reaction to become more severe.

Use With Oral Antidiabetic Drugs

Insulin has been used successfully with all currently available types of oral agents (alpha-glucosidase inhibitors, biguanide, glitazones, meglitinides, and sulfonylureas).

Management of Diabetic Ketoacidosis

Insulin therapy is a major component of any treatment for DKA. Clients with DKA have a deficiency in the total amount of insulin in the body and a resistance to the action of the insulin that is available, probably due to acidosis, hyperosmolality, infection, and other factors. To be effective, insulin therapy must be individualized according to frequent measurements of blood glucose. Low doses, given by continuous IV infusion, are preferred in most circumstances.

Additional measures include identification and treatment of conditions that precipitate DKA; administration of IV fluids to correct hyperosmolality and dehydration; administration of potassium supplements to restore and maintain normal serum potassium levels; and administration of sodium bicarbonate to correct metabolic acidosis. Infection is one of the most common causes of DKA. If no obvious source of infection is identified, cultures of blood, urine, and throat swabs are recommended. When infection is identified, antimicrobial drug therapy may be indicated.

IV fluids, the first step in treating DKA, usually consist of 0.9% sodium chloride, an isotonic solution. Hypotonic solutions are usually avoided because they allow intracellular fluid shifts and may cause cerebral, pulmonary, and peripheral edema.

Although serum potassium levels may be normal at first, they fall rapidly after insulin and IV fluid therapy are begun. Decreased serum potassium levels are caused by expansion of extracellular fluid volume, movement of potassium into cells, and continued loss of potassium in the urine as long as hyperglycemia persists. For these reasons, potassium supplements are usually added to IV fluids. Because both hypokalemia and hyperkalemia can cause serious cardiovascular disturbances, dosage of potassium supplements must be based on frequent measurements of serum potassium levels. Also, continuous or frequent electrocardiogram monitoring is recommended.

Severe acidosis can cause serious cardiovascular disturbances, which usually stem from peripheral vasodilation and decreased cardiac output with hypotension and shock. Acidosis usually can be corrected by giving fluids and insulin; sodium bicarbonate may be given if the pH is less than 7.2. If used, sodium bicarbonate should be given slowly and cautiously. Rapid alkalinization can cause potassium to move into body cells faster than it can be replaced IV. The result may be severe hypokalemia and cardiac dysrhythmias. Also, giving excessive amounts of sodium bicarbonate can produce alkalosis.

Treatment of the Unconscious Client

When a person with diabetes becomes unconscious and it is unknown whether the unconsciousness is caused by DKA or by hypoglycemia, the client should be treated for hypoglycemia. If hypoglycemia is the cause, giving glucose may avert brain damage. If DKA is the cause, giving glucose does not harm the client. Sudden unconsciousness in a client who takes insulin is most likely to result from an insulin reaction producing hypoglycemia; DKA usually develops gradually over several days or weeks.

Hyperosmolar Hyperglycemic Nonketotic Coma (HHNC)

Treatment of HHNC is similar to that of DKA in that insulin, IV fluids, and potassium supplements are major components. Regular insulin is given by continuous IV infusion, and dosage is individualized according to frequent measurements of blood glucose levels. IV fluids are given to correct the profound dehydration and hyperosmolality, and potassium is given IV to replace the large amounts lost in urine during a hyperglycemic state.

Perioperative Insulin Therapy

Clients with diabetes who undergo major surgery have increased risks of both surgical and diabetic complications. Risks associated with surgery and anesthesia are greater if diabetes is not well controlled and complications of diabetes (eg, hypertension, nephropathy, vascular damage) are already evident. Hyperglycemia and poor metabolic control are associated with increased susceptibility to infection, poor wound healing, and fluid and electrolyte imbalances. Risks of diabetic complications are increased because the stress of surgery increases insulin requirements and may precipitate DKA. Metabolic responses to stress include increased secretion of catecholamines, cortisol, glucagon, and growth hormone, all of which increase blood glucose levels. In addition to hyperglycemia, protein breakdown, lipolysis, ketogenesis, and insulin resistance occur. The risk of hypoglycemia is also increased.

The goals of treatment are to avoid hypoglycemia, severe hyperglycemia, ketoacidosis, and fluid and electrolyte imbalances. Maintenance of blood glucose levels between 120 and 180 milligrams per deciliter during the perioperative period is desirable. In general, mild hyperglycemia (eg, blood glucose levels between 150 and 250 mg/dL) is considered safer for the client than hypoglycemia, which may go unrecognized during anesthesia and surgery. Because surgery is a stressful event that increases blood glucose levels and the body's need for insulin, insulin therapy is usually required.

The goal of insulin therapy is to avoid ketosis from inadequate insulin and hypoglycemia from excessive insulin. Specific actions depend largely on the severity of diabetes and the type of surgical procedure. Diabetes should be well controlled before any type of surgery. Minor procedures usually require little change in the usual treatment program; major operations usually require a different medication regimen.

In general, regular, short-acting insulin is used with major surgery or surgery requiring general anesthesia. IV administration of insulin is preferred because it provides more predictable absorption than Sub-Q injections. For clients who use an intermediate-acting insulin, a different regimen using regular insulin in doses approximating the usual daily requirement is needed. For clients who usually manage their diabetes with diet alone or with diet and oral medications, insulin therapy may be started. Human insulin is preferred for temporary use to minimize formation of insulin antibodies. Small doses are usually required.

For elective major surgery, clients should be scheduled early in the day to avoid prolonged fasting. In addition, most authorities recommend omitting usual doses of insulin on the day of surgery and oral antidiabetic medications for 1 or 2 days before surgery. While the client is NPO (nothing by mouth), before and during surgery, IV insulin is usually given. Along with the insulin, clients need adequate sources of carbohydrate. This is usually supplied by IV solutions of 5% or 10% dextrose at a rate of 5 grams of glucose per hour (D_5W at a rate of 100 mL per hour provides 5 g of glucose).

After surgery, IV insulin and dextrose may be continued until the client is able to eat and drink. Several protocols exist for postoperative glucose control. Most involve continuous infusions of insulin with frequent blood glucose monitoring and subsequent titration of the insulin infusion to maintain a predetermined goal. Regular insulin can also be given Sub-Q every 4 to 6 hours, with frequent blood glucose measurements. Oral fluids and foods that contain carbohydrate should be resumed as soon as possible. When meals are fully tolerated, the preoperative insulin or oral medication regimen can be resumed. Additional regular insulin can be given for elevated blood glucose and ketone levels, if indicated.

Guidelines for Oral Antidiabetic Drug Therapy

Sulfonylureas

- Sulfonylureas are not effective in all clients with type 2 diabetes and many clients experience primary or secondary treatment failure. *Primary failure* involves a lack of initial response to the drugs. *Secondary failure* means that a therapeutic response occurs when the drugs are first given, but the drugs eventually become ineffective. Reasons for secondary failure may include decreased compliance with diet and exercise instructions, failure to take the drugs as prescribed, or decreased ability of the pancreatic beta cells to produce more insulin in response to the drugs.
- These drugs must be used cautiously in clients with impaired renal or hepatic function.
- Dosage of sulfonylureas is usually started low and increased gradually until the fasting blood glucose level is 110 mg/dL or less. The lowest dose that achieves normal fasting and postprandial blood sugar levels is recommended.
- Sulfonylureas are not recommended for use during pregnancy because of risks of fetal hypoglycemia and death, congenital anomalies, and overt diabetes in women with gestational diabetes (because the drugs stimulate an already overstimulated pancreas).

Alpha-Glucosidase Inhibitors

- These drugs do not alter insulin secretion or cause hypoglycemia.
- Acarbose and miglitol should be taken at the beginning of a meal so they will be present in the GI tract with food and able to delay digestion of carbohydrates.
- Low initial doses and gradual increases decrease GI upset (eg, bloating, diarrhea) and promote client compliance.

● Clients taking acarbose or miglitol should continue their diet, exercise, and blood glucose testing routines.

Biguanide

● Renal function should be assessed before starting metformin and at least annually during long-term therapy. The drug should not be given initially if renal impairment is present; it should be stopped if renal impairment occurs during treatment.

● As with other antidiabetic drugs, clients taking metformin should continue their diet, exercise, and blood glucose testing regimens.

● Parenteral radiographic contrast media containing iodine (eg, Cholografin, Hypaque) may cause renal failure, and they have been associated with lactic acidosis in clients receiving metformin. Metformin should be discontinued at least 48 hours before diagnostic tests are performed with these materials and should not be resumed for at least 48 hours after the tests are done and tests indicate renal function is normal.

Glitazones

● Liver function tests (eg, serum aminotransferase enzymes) should be checked before starting therapy and periodically thereafter.

● In addition, clients should be monitored closely for edema and other signs of congestive heart failure.

Meglitinides

● As with other antidiabetic drugs, clients taking one of these drugs should continue their diet, exercise, and blood glucose testing regimens.

● Dosage is flexible, depending on food intake, but clients should eat within a few minutes after taking a dose, to avoid hypoglycemia.

Use With Insulin

All of the currently available types of oral agents (alpha-glucosidase inhibitors, biguanide, glitazones, meglitinides, and sulfonylureas) have been used successfully with insulin.

APPLYING YOUR KNOWLEDGE 26-4:
HOW CAN YOU AVOID THIS MEDICATION ERROR?
Mr. Furgeson is scheduled for a renal arteriogram. You tell him to take his antidiabetic medication as usual.

Combination Drug Therapy for Type 2 Diabetes

Combination drug therapy is an increasing trend in type 2 diabetes that is not controlled by diet, exercise, and single-drug therapy. Useful combinations include drugs with different mechanisms of action, and several rational combinations are currently available. Most studies have involved combinations of two drugs; some three-drug combinations are also being used. All combination therapy should be monitored with periodic measurements of fasting plasma glucose and glycosylated hemoglobin levels. If adequate glycemic control is not achieved, oral drugs may need to be discontinued and insulin therapy started. Two-drug combinations include the following:

● **Insulin plus a sulfonylurea.** Advantages include lower fasting blood glucose levels, decreased glycosylated hemoglobin levels, increased secretion of endogenous insulin, smaller daily doses of insulin, and no significant change in body weight. The role of insulin analogs in combination therapy is not clear. One regimen, called BIDS, uses bedtime insulin, usually NPH, with a daytime sulfonylurea, usually glyburide.

● **Insulin plus a glitazone.** Glitazones increase the effectiveness of insulin, whether endogenous or exogenous.

● **Sulfonylurea plus acarbose or miglitol.** This combination is Food and Drug Administration (FDA) approved for clients who do not achieve adequate glycemic control with one of the drugs alone.

● **Sulfonylurea plus metformin.** Glimepiride is FDA approved for this combination.

● **Sulfonylurea plus a glitazone.** The sulfonylurea increases insulin and the glitazone increases insulin effectiveness.

● **Metformin plus a meglitinide.** If one of the drugs alone does not produce adequate glycemic control, the other one may be added. Dosage of each drug should be titrated to the minimal dose required to achieve the desired effects.

Use in Special Populations

Use in Diabetic Clients Who Are Ill

Illness may affect diabetes control in several ways. First, it causes a stress response. Part of the stress response is increased secretion of glucagon, epinephrine, growth hormone, and cortisol, hormones that raise blood glucose levels (by stimulating gluconeogenesis and inhibiting insulin action) and cause ketosis (by stimulating lipolysis and ketogenesis). Second, if the illness makes a person unable or unwilling to eat, hypoglycemia can occur. Third, if the illness affects GI function (eg, causes vomiting or diarrhea), the person may be unable to drink enough fluids to prevent dehydration and electrolyte imbalance. In addition, hyperglycemia induces an osmotic diuresis that increases dehydration and electrolyte imbalances.

As a result of these potentially serious effects, an illness that would be minor in people without diabetes may become a major illness or medical emergency in people with diabetes. Everyone involved should be vigilant about recognizing and seeking prompt treatment for any illness. In addition, clients with diabetes (or their caregivers) should be taught how to adjust their usual regimens to maintain metabolic balance and prevent severe complications. The main goal during illness is to prevent complications such as severe hyperglycemia, dehydration, and DKA.

Use in Children

Diabetes, one of the most common chronic disorders of childhood, usually appears after 4 years of age and peaks in incidence at 10 to 12 years for girls and 12 to 14 years for boys. Approximately 75% of all newly diagnosed cases of type 1 diabetes occur in people under the age of 18.

The incidence of type 2 diabetes in children and adolescents, especially in ethnic minority populations, is increasing. Many experts refer to this increased incidence as an emerging epidemic. Estimates of type 2 diabetes incidence range from 4.1 cases per 1000 12- to 19-year-olds across the United States, to 50.9 per 1000 15- to 19-year-old Pima Indians of Arizona. Somewhere between 8% and 45% of recently diagnosed cases of diabetes among children and adolescents in the United States is type 2.

Type 1 Diabetes
Insulin is the only drug indicated for use; it is required as replacement therapy because affected children cannot produce insulin. Factors that influence management and insulin therapy include the following:

- Effective management requires a consistent schedule of meals, snacks, blood glucose monitoring, insulin injections and dose adjustments, and exercise. Insulin injections must be given three or four times per day. A healthful, varied diet, rich in whole grains, fruits, and vegetables and limited in simple sugars, is recommended. In addition, food intake must be synchronized with insulin injections and usually involves three meals and three snacks, all at regularly scheduled times.

  Such a schedule is difficult to maintain in children, but extremely important in promoting normal growth and development. A major factor in optimal treatment is a supportive family in which at least one member is thoroughly educated about the disease and its management. Less-than-optimal treatment can lead to stunted growth; delayed puberty; and early development of complications such as retinopathy, nephropathy, or neuropathy.

- Infections and other illnesses may cause wide fluctuations in blood glucose levels and interfere with metabolic control. For example, some infections cause hypoglycemia; others, especially chronic infections, may cause hyperglycemia and insulin resistance and may precipitate ketoacidosis. As a result, insulin requirements may vary widely during illness episodes and should be based on blood glucose and urine ketone levels. Hypoglycemia often develops in young chil-

dren, partly because of anorexia and smaller glycogen reserves.

- During illness, children are highly susceptible to dehydration, and an adequate fluid intake is very important. Many clinicians recommend sugar-containing liquids (eg, regular sodas, clear juices, regular gelatin desserts) if blood glucose values are lower than 250 mg/dL. When blood glucose values are above 250 mg/dL, diet soda, unsweetened tea, and other fluids without sugar should be given.

- For infants and toddlers who weigh less than 10 kg or require less than 5 units of insulin per day, a diluted insulin can be used because such small doses are hard to measure in a U-100 syringe. The most common dilution is U-10, and a diluent is available from insulin manufacturers. Vials of diluted insulin should be clearly labeled and discarded after 1 month.

- Rotation of injection sites is important in infants and young children because of the relatively small areas for injection at each anatomic site and to prevent lipodystrophy.

- Young children usually adjust to injections and blood glucose monitoring better when the parents express less anxiety about these vital procedures.

- Avoiding hypoglycemia is a major goal in infants and young children because of potentially damaging effects on growth and development. For example, the brain and spinal cord do not develop normally without an adequate supply of glucose. Animal studies indicate that prolonged hypoglycemia results in decreased brain weight, numbers of neurons, and protein content. Myelinization of nerve cells is also decreased. Because complex motor and intellectual functions require an intact central nervous system, frequent, severe, or prolonged hypoglycemia can be a serious problem in infants, toddlers, and preschoolers. In addition, recognition of hypoglycemia may be delayed because signs and symptoms are vague and the children may be unable to communicate them to parents or caregivers. Because of these difficulties, most pediatric diabetologists recommend maintaining blood glucose levels between 100 and 200 mg/dL to prevent hypoglycemia. In addition, *the bedtime snack and blood glucose measurement should never be skipped.*

- Signs and symptoms of hypoglycemia in older children are similar to those in adults (eg, hunger, sweating, tachycardia). In young children, hypoglycemia may be manifested by changes in behavior, including severe hunger, irritability, and lethargy. In addition, mental functioning may be impaired in all age groups, even with mild hypoglycemia. Anytime hypoglycemia is suspected, blood glucose should be tested.

- Adolescents may resist adhering to their prescribed treatment regimens, and effective management may be especially difficult during this developmental period.

Adolescents and young adults may delay, omit, or decrease dosage of insulin to fit in socially (eg, by eating more, sleeping in, drinking alcohol) or to control their weight. Omitting or decreasing insulin dosage may lead to repeated episodes of ketoacidosis. Also, adolescent females may develop eating disorders.
● A good resource is the Juvenile Diabetes Foundation (JDF), a not-for-profit health agency with support groups and other activities for families affected by diabetes.
> Juvenile Diabetes Foundation International
> 120 Wall Street
> New York, NY 10005-4001
> 1-800-JDF-CURE
> 1-800-223-1138

Type 2 Diabetes

Type 2 diabetes is being increasingly identified in children. This trend is attributed mainly to obesity and inadequate exercise because most children with type 2 are seriously overweight and have poor eating habits. In addition, most are members of high-risk ethnic groups (eg, African American, Native American, Hispanic) and have relatives with diabetes. These children are at high risk for development of serious complications during early adulthood, such as myocardial infarction during their fourth decade. Management involves exercise, weight loss, a more healthful diet, and in some cases drug therapy including insulin may be indicated. Attention must also be given to treating comorbid conditions such as hypertension and hyperlipidemia.

Use in Older Adults

It is estimated that at least 20% of people over the age of 65 have diabetes. General precautions for safe and effective use of antidiabetic drugs apply to older adults, including close monitoring of blood glucose levels; however, control of cardiovascular risk factors may play a greater role in reducing morbidity and mortality in this population. In addition, older adults may have impaired vision or other problems that decrease their ability to perform needed tasks (eg, self-administration of insulin; monitoring blood glucose levels; managing diet and exercise). They also may have other disorders and may take other drugs that complicate management of diabetes. For example, renal insufficiency may increase risks of adverse effects with antidiabetic drugs; and treatment with thiazide diuretics, corticosteroids, estrogens, and other drugs may cause hyperglycemia, thereby increasing dosage requirements for antidiabetic drugs.

With oral sulfonylureas, hypoglycemia is a concern for the older person. Drugs with a short duration of action and inactive metabolites are considered safer, especially with impaired liver or kidney function. Therapy usually should start with a low dose, which is then increased or decreased according to blood glucose levels and clinical response.

Few guidelines have been developed for the use of newer antidiabetic drugs in older adults. Insulin analogs appear to have some advantages over conventional insulin. Acarbose, miglitol, and metformin may not be as useful in older adults as in younger ones because of the high prevalence of impaired renal function. These drugs are relatively contraindicated in clients with renal insufficiency because they have a longer half-life and may accumulate. With metformin, dosage should be based on periodic tests of renal function and the drug should be stopped if renal impairment occurs or if serum lactate increases. In addition, dosage should not be titrated to the maximum amount recommended for younger adults. Use of glitazones and metformin is often contraindicated in older adults who are more likely to have cardiovascular disorders that increase risks of fluid retention and congestive heart failure. With meglitinides, effects were similar in younger and older adults during clinical trials.

Use in Clients With Renal Impairment

Insulin. Frequent monitoring of blood glucose levels and dosage adjustments may be needed. It is difficult to predict dosage needs because, on the one hand, less insulin is degraded by the kidneys (normally about 25%) and this may lead to higher blood levels of insulin if dosage is not reduced. On the other hand, muscles and possibly other tissues are less sensitive to insulin, and this insulin resistance may result in an increased blood glucose level if dosage is not increased. Overall, vigilance is required to prevent dangerous hypoglycemia, especially in clients whose renal function is unstable or worsening.

Oral drugs. Sulfonylureas and their metabolites are excreted mainly by the kidneys; renal impairment may lead to accumulation and hypoglycemia. They should be used cautiously, with close monitoring of renal function, in clients with mild to moderate renal impairment, and are contraindicated in severe renal impairment. **Alpha-glucosidase inhibitors** are excreted by the kidneys and accumulate in clients with renal impairment. However, dosage reduction is not helpful because the drugs act locally, within the GI tract. **Metformin** requires assessment of renal function before starting and at least annually during long-term therapy. It should not be given initially if renal impairment is present; it should be stopped if renal impairment occurs during treatment. **Meglitinides** do not require initial dosage adjustments, but increments should be made cautiously in clients with renal impairment or renal failure requiring hemodialysis.

Use in Clients With Hepatic Impairment

Insulin. There may be higher blood levels of insulin in clients with hepatic impairment because less insulin may be degraded. Careful monitoring of blood glucose levels and insulin dosage reductions may be needed to prevent hypoglycemia.

Oral drugs. Sulfonylureas should be used cautiously and liver function should be monitored. They are metabolized in the liver and hepatic impairment may result in higher serum drug levels and inadequate release of hepatic glucose in response to hypoglycemia. With glipizide, initial dosage should be reduced in clients with liver failure. Glyburide may cause hypoglycemia in clients with liver disease. **Alpha-glucosidase inhibitors** require no precautions with hepatic impairment because acarbose is metabolized in the GI tract and miglitol is not metabolized. **Metformin** is not recommended for use in clients with clinical or laboratory evidence of hepatic impairment because risks of lactic acidosis may be increased. **Meglitinides** should be used cautiously and dosage increments should be made very slowly, because serum drug levels are higher, for a longer period of time, in clients with moderate to severe hepatic impairment. **Glitazones** have been associated with hepatotoxicity and require monitoring of liver enzymes. The drugs should not be given to clients with active liver disease or a serum ALT more than 2.5 times the upper limit of normal. After glitazone therapy is initiated, liver enzymes should be measured every 2 months for 1 year, then periodically.

Use in Clients With Critical Illness

Critically ill clients, with and without diabetes mellitus, often experience hyperglycemia associated with insulin resistance. Hyperglycemia may complicate the progress of the critically ill client, resulting in increased complications such as postoperative infections, poor recovery, and increased mortality. Tight glycemic control is a key factor in preventing complications and improving mortality in the intensive-care–unit patient.

Insulin is more likely to be used in critical illness than any of the oral agents. Reasons include the greater ability to titrate dosage needs in clients who are often debilitated and unstable, with varying degrees of cardiovascular, liver, and kidney impairment. One important consideration with IV insulin therapy is that 30% or more of a dose may adsorb into containers of IV fluid or infusion sets. In addition, many critically ill clients are unable to take oral drugs.

Some critically ill clients are also at risk for serious hypoglycemia, especially if they are debilitated, sedated, or unable to recognize and communicate symptoms. Vigilant monitoring is essential for any client who has diabetes and a critical illness.

Use in Home Care

Most diabetes care is delivered in ambulatory care settings or in the home, and any client with diabetes may need home care. Hospitalization usually occurs only for complications, and clients are quickly discharged if possible. The home care nurse may need to assist clients of multiple age groups to learn self-care and assist caregivers to support clients' efforts or actively participate in diabetes management. Some aspects of the nursing role include mobilizing and coordinating health care providers and community resources; teaching and supporting clients and caregivers; monitoring the client's health status and progress in disease management; and preventing or solving problems.

The person with diabetes has a tremendous amount of information to learn about living with this disease on a day-to-day basis. For most clients, the goal of diabetes education is self-care in terms of diet, exercise, medication administration, blood glucose monitoring, and prevention, recognition, and treatment of complications. For some clients, a parent or caregiver may assume most of the responsibility for diabetes management. Because of the amount and complexity of information, a multidisciplinary health care team that includes a nurse diabetes educator is preferred in home care as in other settings. The role of the home care nurse may include initial teaching or reinforcement and follow-up of teaching done by others.

N U R S I N G   A C T I O N S

Antidiabetic Drugs

NURSING ACTIONS	RATIONALE/EXPLANATION
1. Administer accurately	
a. With insulin:	
(1) Store the insulin vial in current use and administer insulin at room temperature. Refrigerate extra vials.	Cold insulin is more likely to cause lipodystrophy, local sensitivity reactions, discomfort, and delayed absorption. Insulin preparations are stable for months at room temperature if temperature extremes are avoided.
(2) Avoid freezing temperatures (32°F) or high temperatures (95°F or above).	Extremes of temperature decrease insulin potency and cause clumping of the suspended particles of modified insulins. This clumping phenomenon causes inaccurate dosage even if the volume is accurately measured.

NURSING ACTIONS	RATIONALE/EXPLANATION
(3) Discard insulin that has become discolored, turbid, or unusually viscous.	These changes suggest deterioration or contamination of the insulin.
(4) Use only an insulin syringe calibrated to measure U-100 insulin.	For accurate measurement of the prescribed dose
(5) With isophane (NPH) and Lente insulins, be sure they are mixed to a uniform cloudy appearance before drawing up a dose.	These insulin preparations are suspensions, and the components separate on standing. Unless the particles are resuspended in the solution and distributed evenly, dosage will be inaccurate.
(6) When short-acting and NPH insulins must be mixed, prepare as follows:	The insulins must be drawn up in the same sequence every time. Short-acting insulin should *always* be drawn up first, to avoid contamination of the short-acting insulin with the NPH. Because short-acting insulin combines with excess protamine in NPH, the concentration of short-acting insulin is changed when they are mixed. Following the same sequence also leaves the same type of insulin in the needle and syringe (dead space) every time. Although dead space is not usually a significant factor with available insulin syringes, it may be with small doses.
(a) Draw into the insulin syringe the amount of air equal to the total amount of both insulins.	
(b) Draw up the short-acting insulin first. Inject the equivalent portion of air, and aspirate the ordered dose.	
(c) With the NPH vial, insert the remaining air (avoid injecting short-acting insulin into the NPH vial), and aspirate the ordered dose.	
(d) Expel air bubbles, if present, and verify that the correct dosage is in the syringe.	
(e) Administer combined insulins *consistently* within 15 minutes of mixing or after a longer period; that is, do not give one dose within 15 minutes of mixing and another 2 hours or days after mixing.	Short-acting insulin combines with excess protamine when mixed with NPH insulin. This reaction occurs within 15 minutes of mixing and alters the amount of short-acting insulin present. After 15 minutes, the mixture is stable for approximately 1 month at room temperature and 3 months when refrigerated. Thus, to administer the same dose consistently, the mixture must be given at approximately the same time interval after mixing.
(7) Rotate injection sites systematically, within the same anatomic area (eg, abdomen) until all sites are used. Avoid random rotation between the abdomen and thigh or arm, for example.	Frequent injection in the same site can cause tissue fibrosis, erratic absorption, and deposits of unabsorbed insulin. Also, if insulin is usually injected into fibrotic tissue where absorption is slow, injection into healthy tissue may result in hypoglycemia because of more rapid absorption. Further, deposits of unabsorbed insulin may initially lead to hyperglycemia. If dosage is increased to control the apparent hyperglycemia, hypoglycemia may occur. Rates of absorption differ among anatomic sites, and random rotation increases risks of hypoglycemic reactions.
(8) Inject insulin at a 90-degree angle into a subcutaneous pocket created by raising subcutaneous tissue away from muscle tissue. Avoid intramuscular injection.	Injection into a subcutaneous pocket is thought to produce less tissue irritation and better absorption than injection into subcutaneous tissue. Intramuscular injection should not be used because of rapid absorption.
(9) With insulin analogs, give aspart within 5 to 10 minutes of starting a meal; give lispro within 15 minutes before or immediately after a meal; give glulisine 15 minutes before meals or within 20 minutes of beginning the meal; give glargine once daily at bedtime.	Manufacturers' recommendations. Aspart, lispro and glulisine act rapidly; glargine is long acting.
b. With oral sulfonylureas: Give glipizide or glyburide 30 minutes before breakfast and the evening meal. Give glimepiride and Glucotrol XL with breakfast.	To promote absorption and effective plasma levels. Most of these drugs are given once or twice daily.
c. With acarbose and miglitol: Give at the beginning of each main meal, three times daily.	These drugs must be in the gastrointestinal (GI) tract when carbohydrate foods are ingested because they act by decreasing absorption of sugar in the foods.

(continued)

NURSING ACTIONS	RATIONALE/EXPLANATION
d. With metformin: Give with meals. Give Glucophage XR with evening meal	To decrease GI upset
e. With pioglitazone and rosiglitazone: Give once daily, without regard to meals.	Manufacturers' recommendations
f. With repaglinide and nateglinide: Give 15 to 30 minutes before meals (2, 3, or 4 times daily). If the client does not eat a meal, omit that dose; if the client eats an extra meal, give an extra dose.	Dosage is individualized according to the levels of fasting blood glucose and glycosylated hemoglobin.
2. Observe for therapeutic effects	
a. Improved blood glucose levels (fasting, preprandial, and postprandial) and glycosylated hemoglobin levels	The general goal is normal or near-normal blood glucose levels. However, specific targeted levels for individuals vary depending on intensity of treatment, risks of hypoglycemia, and other factors. Improved metabolic control can prevent or delay complications.
b. Absent or decreased ketones in urine (N = none)	In diabetes, ketonuria indicates insulin deficiency and impending diabetic ketoacidosis if preventive measures are not taken. Thus, always report the presence of ketones. In addition, when adequate insulin is given, ketonuria decreases. Ketonuria does not often occur with type 2 diabetes.
c. Absent or decreased pruritus, polyuria, polydipsia, polyphagia, and fatigue	These signs and symptoms occur in the presence of hyperglycemia. When blood sugar levels are lowered with antidiabetic drugs, they tend to subside.
d. Decreased complications of diabetes	
3. Observe for adverse effects	
a. With insulin, sulfonylureas, and meglitinides:	
(1) Hypoglycemia	Hypoglycemia is more likely to occur with insulin than with oral agents and at peak action times of the insulin being used (eg, ½–1½ h after injection of lispro; 1 h after injection of glulisine; 1–3 h after injection of aspart; 2 to 3 h after injection of regular insulin; 8 to 12 h after injection of NPH or Lente insulin).
(a) Sympathetic nervous system (SNS) activation— tachycardia, palpitations, nervousness, weakness, hunger, perspiration	The SNS is activated as part of the stress response to low blood glucose levels. Epinephrine and other hormones act to raise blood glucose levels.
(b) Central nervous system impairment—mental confusion, incoherent speech, blurred or double vision, headache, convulsions, coma	There is an inadequate supply of glucose for normal brain function.
(2) Weight gain	This effect may decrease compliance with drug therapy, especially in adolescent and young-adult females.
b. With insulin:	
(1) Local insulin allergy—erythema, induration, itching at injection sites	Uncommon with human insulin
(2) Systemic allergic reactions—skin rash, dyspnea, tachycardia, hypotension, angioedema, anaphylaxis	Uncommon; if a severe systemic reaction occurs, skin testing and desensitization are usually required.
(3) Lipodystrophy—atrophy and "dimpling" at injection site; hypertrophy at injection site	These changes in subcutaneous fat occur from too-frequent injections into the same site. They are uncommon with human insulin.
c. With sulfonylureas:	
(1) Hypoglycemia and weight gain—see above	Hypoglycemia occurs less often with oral agents than with insulin. It is more likely to occur in patients who are elderly, debilitated, or who have impaired renal and hepatic function.

NURSING ACTIONS	RATIONALE/EXPLANATION
(2) Allergic skin reactions—skin rash, urticaria, erythema, pruritus	These reactions may subside with continued use of the drug. If they do not subside, the drug should be discontinued.
(3) GI upset—nausea, heartburn	These are the most commonly reported adverse effects. If severe, reducing drug dosage usually relieves them.
(4) Miscellaneous—fluid retention and hyponatremia; facial flushing if alcohol is ingested; hematologic disorders (hemolytic or aplastic anemia, leukopenia, thrombocytopenia, others)	These are less common adverse effects.
d. With acarbose and miglitol: GI symptoms—bloating, flatulence, diarrhea, abdominal pain	These are commonly reported. They are caused by the presence of undigested carbohydrate in the lower GI tract. They can be decreased by low doses initially and gradual increases.
e. With metformin:	
(1) GI effects—anorexia, nausea, vomiting, diarrhea, abdominal discomfort, decreased intestinal absorption of folate and vitamin B_{12}	GI symptoms are common adverse effects. They may be minimized by taking the drug with meals and increasing dosage slowly.
(2) Allergic skin reactions—eczema, pruritus, erythema, urticaria	
(3) Lactic acidosis—drowsiness, malaise, respiratory distress, bradycardia and hypotension (if severe), blood lactate levels above 5 mmol/L, blood pH below 7.35	A rare but serious adverse effect (approximately 50% *fatal*). Most likely with renal or hepatic impairment, advanced age, or hypoxia. This is a medical emergency that requires hospitalization for treatment.
	Hemodialysis is effective in correcting acidosis and removing metformin.
	Lactic acidosis may be prevented by monitoring plasma lactate levels and stopping the drug if they exceed 3 mmol/L. Other reasons to stop the drug include decreased renal or hepatic function, a prolonged fast, or a very–low-calorie diet. The drug should be stopped immediately if a patient has a myocardial infarction or septicemia.
f. With pioglitazone and rosiglitazone:	
(1) Upper respiratory infections—pharyngitis, sinusitis	
(2) Liver damage or failure	Few cases of liver failure have been reported, but the drugs are related to troglitazone (Rezulin), a drug that was taken off the market because of hepatotoxicity. Monitoring of liver enzymes is recommended during therapy.
(3) Fluid retention, edema, and congestive heart failure	Several reports indicate increased risks of developing or worsening heart failure.
(4) Weight gain	
(5) Headache	
(6) Anemia	
g. With nateglinide and repaglinide:	
(1) Hypoglycemia	If occurs, usually of mild to moderate intensity
(2) Rhinitis, respiratory infection, influenza symptoms	These were the most commonly reported during clinical drug trials.
4. Observe for drug interactions	
a. Drugs that *increase* effects of insulin:	
(1) Angiotensin-converting enzyme (ACE) inhibitors (eg, captopril)	

(continued)

NURSING ACTIONS	RATIONALE/EXPLANATION
(2) Alcohol	Increased hypoglycemia. Ethanol inhibits gluconeogenesis (in people with or without diabetes).
(3) Anabolic steroids	
(4) Antidiabetic drugs, oral	Oral agents are increasingly being used with insulin in the treatment of type 2 diabetes. The risks of hypoglycemia are greater with the combination but depend on the dosage of each drug and other factors that affect blood glucose levels.
(5) Antimicrobials (sulfonamides, tetracyclines)	
(6) Beta-adrenergic blocking agents (eg, propranolol)	Increase hypoglycemia by inhibiting the effects of catecholamines on gluconeogenesis and glycogenolysis (effects that normally raise blood glucose levels in response to hypoglycemia). They also may mask signs and symptoms of hypoglycemia (eg, tachycardia, tremors) that normally occur with a hypoglycemia-induced activation of the SNS.
b. Drugs that *decrease* effects of insulin:	These *diabetogenic* drugs may cause or aggravate diabetes because they raise blood sugar levels. Insulin dosage may need to be increased. Except with glucagon, hyperglycemia is an adverse effect of the drugs. Phenytoin and propranolol raise blood sugar by inhibiting insulin secretion; glucagon, a treatment for hypoglycemia, raises blood glucose by converting liver glycogen to glucose.
(1) Adrenergics (eg, albuterol, epinephrine, others)	
(2) Corticosteroids (eg, prednisone)	
(3) Estrogens and oral contraceptives	
(4) Glucagon	
(5) Levothyroxine (Synthroid)	
(6) Phenytoin (Dilantin)	
(7) Propranolol (Inderal)	
(8) Thiazide diuretics (eg, hydrochlorothiazide)	
c. Drugs that *increase* effects of sulfonylureas:	
(1) Acarbose, miglitol, metformin, pioglitazone, rosiglitazone	One of these drugs may be used concomitantly with a sulfonylurea to improve glycemic control in patients with type 2 diabetes. There is an increased risk of hypoglycemia with the combinations.
(2) Alcohol (acute ingestion)	Additive hypoglycemia
(3) Cimetidine (Tagamet)	May inhibit metabolism of sulfonylureas, thereby increasing and prolonging hypoglycemic effects
(4) Insulin	Additive hypoglycemia
d. Drugs that *decrease* effects of sulfonylureas:	
(1) Alcohol	Heavy, chronic intake of alcohol induces metabolizing enzymes in the liver. This accelerates metabolism of sulfonylureas, shortens their half-lives, and may produce hyperglycemia.
(2) Beta-blocking agents	Decrease hypoglycemic effects, possibly by decreasing release of insulin in the pancreas
(3) Corticosteroids, diuretics, epinephrine, estrogens, and oral contraceptives	These drugs have hyperglycemic effects.
(4) Glucagon	Raises blood glucose levels. It is used to treat severe hypoglycemia induced by insulin or oral antidiabetic agents.
(5) Nicotinic acid	Large doses have a hyperglycemic effect.
(6) Phenytoin (Dilantin)	Inhibits insulin secretion and has hyperglycemic effects
(7) Rifampin	Increases the rate of metabolism of sulfonylureas by inducing liver-metabolizing enzymes
(8) Thyroid preparations	Antagonize the hypoglycemic effects of oral antidiabetic drugs

NURSING ACTIONS	RATIONALE/EXPLANATION
e. Drugs that *decrease* effects of acarbose and miglitol:	
(1) Digestive enzymes	Decrease effects and should not be used concomitantly
(2) Intestinal adsorbents (eg, charcoal)	Decrease effects and should not be used concomitantly
f. Drugs that *increase* effects of metformin:	
(1) Alcohol	Increases risk of hypoglycemia and lactic acidosis. Patients should avoid acute and chronic ingestion of excessive alcohol.
(2) Cimetidine	Increases risk of hypoglycemia. Cimetidine interferes with metabolism and increases blood levels of metformin.
(3) Furosemide	Increases blood levels of metformin
(4) Sulfonylurea hypoglycemic agents	The combination of these drugs is used to improve control of hyperglycemia in type 2 diabetes but it also increases risk of hypoglycemia.
g. Drugs that *increase* effects of pioglitazone:	
(1) Erythromycin, ketoconazole and related drugs	Inhibit cytochrome P450 3A4 enzymes that partially metabolize pioglitazone and may increase adverse effects. This interaction not reported with rosiglitazone, which is metabolized mainly by 2C8 and 2C9 enzymes.
h. Drugs that *increase* effects of nateglinide and repaglinide:	
(1) Nonsteroidal anti-inflammatory drugs and other agents that are highly bound to plasma proteins	May displace drugs from binding sites, therefore increasing their blood levels
(2) Beta blockers	
(3) Cimetidine, erythromycin, ketoconazole, miconazole	May inhibit hepatic metabolism of repaglinide and nateglinide and increase their blood levels
(4) Sulfonamides	
i. Drugs that *decrease* effects of nateglinide and repaglinide:	
(1) Adrenergics, corticosteroids, estrogens, niacin, oral contraceptives, thiazide diuretics	May cause hyperglycemia
(2) Carbamazepine, rifampin	Induce drug-metabolizing enzymes in the liver, which leads to faster inactivation

APPLYING YOUR KNOWLEDGE: ANSWERS

26-1 This insulin is a mixed type composed of both regular and NPH insulins. The peak times for both of these insulins would be when Mr. Furgeson is most likely to experience hypoglycemia. The nurse should be especially watchful for the signs and symptoms of hypoglycemia at 2 to 3 hours after insulin administration and again at 8 to 12 hours after administration.

26-2 Measure Mr. Furgeson's blood glucose level if possible. Also, give the client 15 grams of carbohydrate. This would include sugar, candy, fruit juice, or 4 ounces of regular soda.

26-3 Deficient Knowledge: Antidiabetic drugs and administration, diet and management of hypoglycemia and other complications. Based on assessment data, this is a priority diagnosis and nursing interventions are necessary.

26-4 You should hold the metformin for 48 hours prior to any diagnostic test involving radiographic contrast media. Mr. Furgeson will be NPO the morning of the test and should not take his medication until the test is over and he is able to eat. The metformin will continue on hold for 48 hours after the test. The combination of metformin and contrast media containing iodine may lead to renal failure and/or lactic acidosis.

Review and Application Exercises

Short Answer Exercises

1. What is the function of insulin in normal cellular metabolism?

2. What are the effects of insulin, cortisol, epinephrine, glucagon, and growth hormone on blood glucose levels?

3. What are the major differences between type 1 and type 2 diabetes?

4. What is the rationale for maintaining near-normal blood glucose levels? What is the major risk?

5. At what blood glucose range is brain damage most likely to occur?

6. Compare regular, NPH, and Lente insulins in terms of onset, peak, and duration of action.

7. Describe major characteristics and uses of insulin analogs.

8. In a diabetic client with typical signs and symptoms, distinguish between manifestations of hyperglycemia and hypoglycemia.

9. Contrast the five types of oral hypoglycemic agents in terms of mechanisms of action, indications for use, contraindications to use, and adverse effects.

10. For an adult client newly diagnosed with type 2 diabetes, outline interventions to assist the client in learning self-care.

11. Prepare a teaching plan for a client starting insulin therapy and for a client starting an oral hypoglycemic drug.

12. For a diabetic client who reports using dietary and herbal supplements, analyze specific supplements in relation to their potential impact on blood sugar control.

NCLEX-Style Questions

13. Your client is NPO for surgery at 10:00 A.M. He routinely receives 30 units of Humulin 70/30 every morning at 7:00 A.M. What is the appropriate nursing action in this situation?
    a. Administer 30 units of Humulin 70/30 Sub-Q.
    b. Hold the insulin because the client is NPO.
    c. Give the client a light breakfast and administer the insulin as ordered.
    d. Contact the physician for a pre-surgery insulin order.

14. Which of the following insulins cannot be administered in a continuous Sub-Q insulin infusion pump?
    a. regular insulin (Humulin R)
    b. insulin aspart (Novolog)
    c. insulin glulisine (Apidra)
    d. insulin glargine (Lantus)

15. When teaching a newly diagnosed diabetic client how to self-administer short- and intermediate-acting insulin Sub-Q, which of the following instructions is correct?
    a. The order of drawing up the two insulins into the syringe does not matter.
    b. Draw the short-acting insulin into the syringe first, followed by the intermediate-acting insulin.
    c. Draw the intermediate-acting insulin into the syringe first, followed by the short-acting insulin.
    d. You will need to give yourself two injections because mixing these insulins together is unsafe.

16. An older person with type 2 diabetes who takes metformin presents to the emergency department with symptoms of drowsiness, malaise, respiratory distress, and bradycardia. You suspect
    a. hypoglycemia
    b. hyperglycemia
    c. lactic acidosis
    d. metabolic alkalosis

17. The nurse should be especially alert to the adverse effect of hypoglycemia in a type-2 diabetic client taking which of the following oral hypoglycemics?
    a. sulfonylureas
    b. alpha-glucosidase inhibitors
    c. biguanide
    d. glitazones

Selected References

American Diabetes Association. (2004). Continuous subcutaneous insulin infusion. *Diabetes Care, 27*(Suppl. 1, Position Statement 2004), S110.

American Diabetes Association. (2004). Insulin administration. *Diabetes Care, 27*(Suppl. 1, Position Statement 2004), S106–S107.

American Diabetes Association. (2004). Standards of medical care in diabetes. *Diabetes Care, 27*(Suppl. 1, Position Statement 2004), S15–S35.

Baggio, L. L., & Drucker, D. J. (2004). *Incretin hormones and the treatment of type 2 diabetes. American Diabetes Association 64th Scientific Sessions.* Retrieved September 16, 2005, from http://www.medscape.com/viewarticle/482591

Bloomgarden, Z. T. (2003). *Blood glucose monitoring. 18th International Diabetes Federation Congress.* Retrieved September 16, 2005, from http://www.medscape.com/viewarticle/462885

Bloomgarden, Z. T. (2004). *New technologies in insulin delivery: Inhaled insulin. American Diabetes Association 64th Scientific Sessions.* Retrieved September 16, 2005, from http://www.medscape.com/viewarticle/482592

Buse, J. (2004). *The incretin hormones in the treatment of type 2 diabetes: An expert interview with John Buse, MD, PhD.* Retrieved September 16, 2005, from http://www.medscape.com/viewarticle/480545

DerMarderosian, A. (Ed.) (2001). *The review of natural products.* St. Louis: Facts and Comparisons.

Drug facts and comparisons. (Updated monthly). St Louis: Facts and Comparisons.

Fagot-Campagna, A., & Narayan, K. M. V. (2001). Editorial: Type 2 diabetes in children. *British Medical Journal, 322,* 377–378.

Fetrow, C. W., Avila, J. R., & Margolis, S. (2003). *Professional's handbook of complementary & alternative medicines.* Springhouse, PA: Springhouse.

Fink, M. P. (2004, May 6). The role of maintaining tight control of blood glucose in the ICU. *ACS Surgery: Principles and Practice.* Retrieved September 16, 2005, from http://www.medscape.com/viewarticle/474745

Guven, S., Kuenzi, J. A., & Matfin, G. (2005). Diabetes mellitus and the metabolic syndrome. In C. M. Porth, *Pathophysiology: Concepts of altered health states* (7th ed., pp. 987–1015). Philadelphia: Lippincott Williams & Wilkins.

Guyton, A. C., & Hall, J. E. (2000). *Textbook of medical physiology* (10th ed.). Philadelphia: W. B. Saunders.

Harmel, A. P. (2004). *Changing guidelines: Should all patients with type 2 diabetes be on a statin? American Diabetes Association 64th Scientific Sessions.* Retrieved September 16, 2005, from http://www.medscape.com/viewarticle/482450

Harmel, A. P. (2004). *Macrovascular disease risk in patients with type 2 diabetes: Beyond statin use. American Diabetes Association 64th Scientific Sessions.* Retrieved September 16, 2005, from http://www.medscape.com/viewarticle/482451

Hoffman, R. P. (2001). Eating disorders in adolescents with type 1 diabetes. *Postgraduate Medicine, 109*(4), 67–69, 73–74.

Hu, F. B., Manson, J. E., Stampfer, M. J., et al. (2001). Diet, lifestyle, and the risk of type 2 diabetes mellitus in women. *New England Journal of Medicine, 345*(11), 790–797.

Inzucchi, S. E. (2002). Oral antihyperglycemic therapy for type 2 diabetes. *Journal of the American Medical Association, 287*(3), 360–372.

Kendall, D. M. (2004). *Targeting insulin resistance: Diabetes prevention, cardiovascular disease risk and the thiazlidinediones. American Diabetes Association 64th Scientific Sessions.* Retrieved September 16, 2005, from http://www.medscape.com/viewarticle/482449.

Kudolo, G. B. (2001). The effect of 3-month ingestion of ginkgo biloba extract (EGb761) on pancreatic beta-cell function in response to glucose loading in individuals with non-insulin-dependent diabetes mellitus. *Journal of Clinical Pharmacology, 41*(6), 600–611.

Ludwig, D. S., & Ebbeling, C. B. (2001). Type 2 diabetes mellitus in children. *Journal of the American Medical Association, 286*(12), 1427–1430.

Marks, J. B. (2003, January 1). Perioperative management of diabetes. *American Family Physician.* Retrieved September 16, 2005, from htpp://www.aafp.org/afp 20030101/93.html

Massey, P. B. (2002). Dietary supplements. *Medical Clinics of North America, 86*(1), 127–147.

Mautz, H. (2001). Undiagnosed diabetes common among Mexican-Americans. *Diabetes Care, 24*(7), 1204–1209.

Rocchini, A. P. (2002). Childhood obesity and a diabetes epidemic (Editorial). *New England Journal of Medicine, 346*(11), 854–855.

Ryan, A. E., & Marceau, C. (2001). Use of alternative medicines in diabetes mellitus. *Diabetic Medicine, 18*(3), 242.

Sinha, R., Fisch, G., Teague, B., et al. (2002). Prevalence of impaired glucose tolerance among children and adolescents with marked obesity. *New England Journal of Medicine, 346*(11), 802–810.

Estrogens, Progestins, and Hormonal Contraceptives

OBJECTIVES

After studying this chapter, you will be able to:

1. Discuss the effects of endogenous estrogens and progestins.
2. Describe the benefits and risks of postmenopausal hormone replacement therapy.
3. Describe adverse effects associated with estrogens, progestins, and hormonal contraceptives.
4. Apply nursing process with clients taking estrogens, progestins, and hormonal contraceptives.

APPLYING YOUR KNOWLEDGE

Vickie Dalquist is a 21-year-old student. She has chosen to use oral contraceptives to prevent unwanted pregnancy. Vickie takes Ortho Tri-Cyclen. You are the nurse at the student health clinic.

INTRODUCTION

Estrogens and progestins are female sex hormones produced primarily by the ovaries and secondarily by the adrenal cortex in nonpregnant women. Small amounts of estrogens are also synthesized in the liver, kidney, brain, skeletal muscle, testes, and adipose tissue. In normal premenopausal women, estrogen synthesis in adipose tissue may be a significant source of the hormone. Some evidence indicates that a minimum body weight (about 105 lb) and fat content (16%–24%) are required for initiation and maintenance of the menstrual cycle. This view is supported by the observation that women with anorexia nervosa, chronic disease, or malnutrition and those who are long-distance runners usually have amenorrhea. With anorexia nervosa, regaining weight and body mass usually re-establishes normal menstrual patterns.

Small amounts of progesterone, a progestin concerned almost entirely with reproduction, are secreted by the testes and adrenal glands. In men and in postmenopausal women, the peripheral sites produce all endogenous (naturally occur-

ring) estrogen. Almost no progesterone is synthesized in postmenopausal women.

As with other steroid hormones, estrogens and progestins are synthesized from cholesterol. The ovaries and adrenal glands can manufacture cholesterol or extract it from the blood. Through a series of chemical reactions, cholesterol is converted to progesterone and then to androgens, testosterone, and androstenedione. The ovaries use these male sex hormones to produce estrogens. After formation, the hormones are secreted into the bloodstream in response to stimulation by the anterior pituitary gonadotropic hormones, follicle-stimulating hormone (FSH), and luteinizing hormone (LH). In the bloodstream, the hormones combine with serum proteins and are transported to target tissues where they enter body cells. They cross cell membranes easily because of their steroid structure and lipid solubility. Inside the cells, the hormones bind to estrogen or progestin receptors and regulate intracellular protein synthesis. Estrogen can enhance target-tissue responses to progesterone by increasing progesterone receptors. Progesterone seems to inhibit tissue responses to estrogen by decreasing estrogen receptors.

Estrogens

Three ovarian estrogens (estradiol, estrone, and estriol) are secreted in significant amounts. Estradiol is the major estrogen because it exerts more estrogenic activity than the other two estrogens combined. The main function of the estrogens is to promote growth in tissues related to reproduction and sexual characteristics in women. More specific effects of estrogens on body tissues are described in Box 27-1.

In nonpregnant women, between puberty and menopause, estrogens are secreted in a monthly cycle called the *menstrual cycle.* During the first half of the cycle, before ovulation, estrogens are secreted in progressively larger amounts. During the second half of the cycle, estrogens and progesterone are secreted in increasing amounts until 2 to 3 days before the onset of menstruation. At that time, secretion of both hormones decreases abruptly. When the endometrial lining of the uterus loses its hormonal stimulation, it is discharged vaginally as menstrual flow.

During pregnancy, the placenta produces large amounts of estrogen, mainly estriol. The increased estrogen causes enlargement of the uterus and breasts, growth of glandular tissue in the breasts, and relaxation of ligaments and joints in the pelvis. All these changes are necessary for the growth and birth of the fetus.

Finally, estrogens are deactivated in the liver, partly or mainly by cytochrome P450 3A4 enzymes. The estrogens are then conjugated with glucuronic acid or sulfuric acid, which makes them water soluble and readily excreted through the kidneys. Metabolites are also formed in the gastrointestinal tract, brain, skin, and other steroid target tissues. Most of the conjugates are excreted in urine, and some are excreted in bile and recirculated to the liver or excreted in feces.

Progesterone

In the nonpregnant woman, progesterone is secreted by the corpus luteum during the last half of the menstrual cycle, which occurs after ovulation. This hormone continues the changes in the endometrial lining of the uterus begun by estrogens during the first half of the menstrual cycle. These changes provide for implantation and nourishment of a fertilized ovum. When fertilization does not take place, the estrogen and progesterone levels decrease and menstruation occurs.

Box 27-1 Effects of Endogenous Estrogens

Breasts
- Stimulate growth at puberty by causing deposition of fat, formation of connective tissue, and construction of ducts. These ducts become part of the milk-producing apparatus after additional stimulation by progesterone.

Sexual Organs
- Enlarge the fallopian tubes, uterus, vagina, and external genitalia at puberty, when estrogen secretion increases greatly
- Cause the endometrial lining of the uterus to proliferate and develop glands that later nourish the implanted ovum when pregnancy occurs
- Increase resistance of the epithelial lining of the vagina to trauma and infection

Skeleton
- Stimulate skeletal growth so that, beginning at puberty, height increases rapidly for several years. Estrogen then causes the epiphyses to unite with the shafts of the long bones, and linear growth is halted. This effect of estrogen is stronger than the similar effect of testosterone in the male. Consequently, women stop growing in height several years earlier than men and on the average are shorter than men.
- Conserve calcium and phosphorus for healthy bones and teeth. This action promotes bone formation and decreases bone loss.
- Broaden the pelvis in preparation for childbirth

Skin and Subcutaneous Tissue
- Increase vascularity in the skin. This leads to greater skin warmth and likelihood of bleeding in women.
- Cause deposition of fat in subcutaneous tissue, especially in the breasts, thighs, and buttocks, which produces the characteristic female figure

Anterior Pituitary Gland
- Decrease pituitary secretion of follicle-stimulating hormone and increase secretion of luteinizing hormone when blood levels are sufficiently high (negative feedback mechanism)

Metabolism
- Affect metabolism of both reproductive and nonreproductive tissues. Estrogen receptors are found in female reproductive organs, breast tissue, bone, the brain, liver, heart, and blood vessels. They are also found in various tissues in men.
- Increase protein anabolism, bone growth, and epiphyseal closure in young girls
- Decrease bone resorption
- Increase sodium and water retention, serum triglycerides, and high-density lipoproteins (HDL or "good" cholesterol)
- Decrease low-density lipoproteins (LDL or "bad" cholesterol)
- Increase the amount of cholesterol in bile and thereby increase gallstone formation

Blood Coagulation
- Enhance coagulation by increasing blood levels of several clotting factors, including prothrombin and factors VII, IX, and X, and probably increase platelet aggregation

If the ovum is fertilized, progesterone acts to maintain the pregnancy. The corpus luteum produces progesterone during the first few weeks of gestation. Then, the placenta produces the progesterone needed to maintain the endometrial lining of the uterus. In addition to its effects on the uterus, progesterone prepares the breasts for lactation by promoting development of milk-producing cells. Milk is not secreted, however, until the cells are further stimulated by prolactin from the anterior pituitary gland. Progesterone also may help maintain pregnancy by decreasing uterine contractility. This, in turn, decreases the risk of spontaneous abortion.

Progesterone, in general, has opposite effects on lipid metabolism compared with estrogen. That is, progestins decrease high-density lipoprotein cholesterol and increase low-density lipoprotein cholesterol, both of which increase risks of cardiovascular disease. Physiologic progesterone increases insulin levels but does not usually impair glucose tolerance. However, long-term administration of potent synthetic exogenous progestins, such as norgestrel, may decrease glucose tolerance and make diabetes mellitus more difficult to control. Like estrogen, progesterone is metabolized in the liver.

GENERAL CHARACTERISTICS OF ESTROGENS, PROGESTINS, AND HORMONAL CONTRACEPTIVES

Mechanisms of Action

The precise mechanisms by which estrogens and progestins produce their effects are unknown. Estrogens circulate in the bloodstream to target cells, where they enter cells and combine with receptor proteins in cell cytoplasm. The estrogen–receptor complex is then transported to the cell nucleus where it interacts with DNA to produce RNA and new DNA. These substances stimulate cell reproduction and production of various proteins. Progestins also diffuse freely into cells, where they bind to progesterone receptors.

Hormonal contraceptives act by several mechanisms. First, they inhibit hypothalamic secretion of gonadotropin-releasing hormone, which inhibits pituitary secretion of FSH and LH. When these gonadotropic hormones are absent, ovulation and therefore conception cannot occur. Second, the drugs produce cervical mucus that resists penetration of spermatozoa into the upper reproductive tract. Third, the drugs interfere with endometrial maturation and reception of ova that are released and fertilized. These overlapping mechanisms make the drugs highly effective in preventing pregnancy.

Indications for Use

Estrogens

Indications for use of exogenous estrogens include the following:

● **As replacement therapy in deficiency states.** Deficiency states usually result from hypofunction of the pituitary gland or the ovaries and may occur anytime during the life cycle. For example, in the adolescent girl with delayed sexual development, estrogen can be given to produce the changes that normally occur at puberty. In the woman of reproductive age (approximately 12 to 45 years of age), estrogens are occasionally used in menstrual disorders, including amenorrhea and abnormal uterine bleeding due to estrogen deficiency.

● **As a component in birth control pills and other contraceptive preparations.** An estrogen, when combined with a progestin, is used widely in females in the 12-to-45 age range to control fertility. If pregnancy does occur, estrogens are contraindicated because their use during pregnancy has been associated with the occurrence of vaginal cancer in female offspring and possible harmful effects on male offspring.

● **Menopause.** Estrogens are prescribed to relieve symptoms of estrogen deficiency (eg, atrophic vaginitis and vasomotor instability, which produces "hot flashes") and to prevent or treat osteoporosis. Such use is usually called estrogen replacement therapy (ERT). When estrogen is prescribed for women with an intact uterus, a progestin is also given to prevent endometrial cancer. Both drug therapies are commonly referred to as hormone replacement therapy (HRT), a term used to describe the administration of one or more female hormones.

In addition, ERT and HRT have been used long-term for cardioprotective effects because it was believed that the drugs decreased myocardial infarctions and deaths from cardiovascular disease. This view was based largely on observational studies that indicated that postmenopausal women had a much higher risk of heart disease than did premenopausal women. The difference was attributed to decreased hormone production at menopause. The drugs, if prescribed, should be limited to short-term use (eg, 2 years) to relieve menopausal symptoms but not for long-term use for cardioprotective effects. A recent well-done study indicated that for estrogen-only and combined estrogen–progestin therapy, risks are greater than benefits (Box 27-2).

Progestins

Progestins are most often used in combination with an estrogen in contraceptive products. They also are used to suppress ovarian function in dysmenorrhea, endometriosis, endometrial cancer, and uterine bleeding. These uses of progestins are extensions of the physiologic actions of progesterone on the neuroendocrine control of ovarian function

Box 27-2 Hormone Replacement Therapy in Postmenopausal Women

Background

For many years, estrogen replacement therapy (ERT) has been used in postmenopausal women to manage symptoms of menopause. Estrogen was thought to have cardioprotective effects, partly because the incidence of heart attacks in women increased substantially after menopause and became similar to the incidence in men. Several studies also indicated beneficial effects in preventing osteoporosis, a common disorder in postmenopausal women. As a result of these observations, the use of ERT evolved from management of menopausal symptoms to prevention of cardiovascular disease and osteoporosis. Other benefits were also attributed to ERT. Because estrogen alone increases risks of endometrial cancer in women with an intact uterus, a progestin was added.

Estrogen–Progestin Combinations

Combined estrogen–progestin hormone replacement therapy became the standard of care for women with an intact uterus and was widely prescribed for its perceived benefits in maintaining women's health. In 2002, the prevailing opinion changed dramatically to indicate that combined estrogen–progestin therapy should *not* be used to prevent cardiovascular disease in healthy postmenopausal women, because risks were greater than benefits.

This opinion resulted largely from the Women's Health Initiative (WHI), a clinical trial and observational study that enrolled postmenopausal women 50 to 79 years of age. The WHI study was conducted in healthy women to determine if an estrogen–progestin combination (in women with an intact uterus) or estrogen alone (in postmenopausal women who have had a hysterectomy) would prevent the development of coronary heart disease (CHD). The published report of the Writing Group for the WHI Investigators revealed that risks from long-term use of an estrogen–progestin combination (Prempro) outweighed its benefits. This part of the study in women with an intact uterus was stopped after an average follow-up period of 5 years (8 years planned), because of a higher incidence of invasive breast cancer. Results also indicated increased risks of heart attacks, strokes, and blood-clotting disorders and decreased risks of osteoporotic fractures and colon cancers.

Analysis of data indicated that in 10,000 women taking the estrogen–progestin combination, there would be seven more CHD events, eight more strokes, eight more pulmonary emboli, eight more invasive breast cancers, six fewer colorectal cancers, and five fewer hip fractures. Although these numbers

are not large and the risk is relatively small, the investigators concluded that the drug combination produced more harm than benefit and should not be started or continued to prevent CHD in healthy women.

The Heart and Estrogen–Progestin Replacement Studies, HERS and HERS II, involved postmenopausal women with an intact uterus who already had CHD. Results indicated that the drug combination (estrogen 0.625 mg and medroxyprogesterone 2.5 mg) conferred no benefit in relation to preventing serious cardiovascular events and actually increased risks during the first year of therapy. As with healthy women, the conclusion was that the hormones should not be started or continued for preventive purposes in women with CHD.

For individual women, the benefits in reducing symptoms of menopause, fractures from osteoporosis, and colon cancer must be weighed against the increased risks of CHD, thromboembolic stroke, venous thromboembolism, breast cancer, and cholecystitis. Thromboembolic disorders are most likely to occur during the first year of use; risks of developing breast cancer and gallbladder disease increase with the duration of drug use. If an estrogen–progestin combination is prescribed to relieve menopausal symptoms in women who have not had a hysterectomy, the drug combination should probably be used for 1 to 2 years, then be discontinued.

Estrogen Alone

For postmenopausal women who have had a hysterectomy and thus do not need a progestin to prevent endometrial cancer, estrogen alone has been used to prevent or treat symptoms of menopause. The arm of the WHI study that explored the use of estrogen-only therapy in post-hysterectomy women was stopped in the interest of safety in 2004, a year early, because no overall benefit was found during 6.8 years of follow-up. The consensus was that the hormone increased the risk of stroke and offered no protection against heart disease. The increased risk was small, estimated at about eight extra strokes per year for every 10,000 women taking estrogen. The study also found that estrogen-only therapy significantly increased the hazard of deep vein thrombosis and had no significant effect on the risk of colorectal or breast cancer. A reduced risk of hip and other fractures was reported. A related study also found that the hormone might also increase the risk of dementia and mild cognitive impairment in older women. As recommended for the estrogen–progestin combinations group, individual women and their health care providers must weigh risks versus benefits.

and on the endometrium. For approximately 20 to 25 years, progestins were used in combination with estrogen for long-term HRT in postmenopausal women with an intact uterus. With HRT, the purpose of a progestin is to prevent endometrial cancer, which can occur with unopposed estrogenic stimulation. Currently, however, the combination is not recommended for long-term use because a major clinical trial

indicated that the adverse effects outweigh the beneficial effects (see Box 27-2).

Hormonal Contraceptives

The primary clinical indication for the use of hormonal contraceptives is to control fertility and prevent pregnancy. Some products are used for contraception after unprotected sexual intercourse. These preparations also are used to treat menstrual disorders (eg, amenorrhea, dysmenorrhea).

Contraindications to Use

Because of their widespread effects on body tissues and reported adverse reactions, estrogens, progestins, and hormonal contraceptives are contraindicated in:

- Known or suspected pregnancy, because teratogenic effects to the fetus may result
- Thromboembolic disorders, such as thrombophlebitis, deep vein thrombosis, or pulmonary embolism
- Known or suspected cancers of breast or genital tissues, because the drugs may stimulate tumor growth. An exception is the use of estrogens for treatment of metastatic breast cancer in women at least 5 years postmenopause.
- Undiagnosed vaginal or uterine bleeding
- Fibroid tumors of the uterus
- Active liver disease or impaired liver function
- History of cerebrovascular disease, coronary artery disease, thrombophlebitis, hypertension, or conditions predisposing to these disease processes
- Women older than 35 years of age who smoke cigarettes. These women have a greater risk of thromboembolic disorders if they take hormonal contraceptives, possibly because of increased platelet aggregation with estrogen ingestion and cigarette smoking. In addition, estrogen increases hepatic production of blood clotting factors.
- Family history of breast or reproductive system cancer

INDIVIDUAL DRUGS

When exogenous estrogens and progestins are administered for therapeutic purposes, they produce the same effects as endogenous hormones. Multiple preparations of estrogens and progestins are available for various purposes and routes of administration. Clinical indications, routes of administration, and dosages are discussed in the estrogens and progestins Drugs at a Glance tables.

Estrogens

Table 27-1 summarizes important drug information about estrogens. The most widely used synthetic steroidal estrogen is **ethinyl estradiol** (Estinyl), which is used in hormonal contraceptives. Ethinyl estradiol is well absorbed with oral administration and reaches peak plasma levels within 2 hours. It is 98% bound to plasma proteins and its half-life varies from 6 to 20 hours. Ethinyl estradiol undergoes extensive first-pass hepatic metabolism and is further metabolized and conjugated in the liver; the conjugates are then excreted in bile and urine.

Transdermal estradiol patches (eg, Climara, Estraderm, Vivelle) allow for absorption of estrogen through the skin to the bloodstream. The patches are applied weekly or biweekly depending on the preparation. Serum levels produced through transdermal application more closely mimic premenopausal estrogen levels compared with serum levels with oral estrogens. Rates of absorption vary, depending on the type of patch applied. The total amount of drug absorbed and the resulting plasma drug concentrations from transdermal estrogen can increase during exposure to heat; so clients should be advised to avoid prolonged sun exposure in the area of the patch. Transdermal estradiol gel (Estrogel) also allow for absorption of estrogen through the skin to the bloodstream. The gel is applied topically daily, usually to the forearm, and has been shown to be effective with a lower frequency of skin reactions than transdermal patch therapy.

Conjugated estrogens (Premarin) and some synthetic derivatives of natural estrogens (eg, ethinyl estradiol) are chemically modified to be effective with oral administration. Conjugated estrogens are used to treat moderate to severe vasomotor and atrophic symptoms associated with menopause; to prevent postmenopausal osteoporosis; and as palliative treatment for metastatic breast carcinoma and advanced androgen-dependent prostatic cancer. Intravenous injection is used, in the absence of organic pathology, for the treatment of abnormal uterine bleeding caused by hormonal imbalance. Conjugated estrogens are well absorbed with oral administration and are released slowly over several hours. Degradation occurs very slowly in the liver, allowing for high intrinsic potency with these preparations.

Along with several cream formulations, a vaginal tablet (Vagifem) and a vaginal ring (Estring) of estrogen are available for topical application in treating atrophic vaginitis.

Nonsteroidal synthetic preparations are chemically altered to slow their metabolism in the liver. They are also less bound to serum proteins than naturally occurring hormones. As with conjugated estrogens, nonsteroidal synthetic preparations are well absorbed with oral administration and are released slowly over several hours. Degradation occurs very slowly in the liver, allowing for high intrinsic potency with these preparations.

Progestins

Progestins (Table 27-2) are used as non-contraceptives and as oral contraceptives, both as estrogen–progestin combinations and as progestin-only preparations ("minipills"). The choice of a combination contraceptive product may be determined by the progestin component. Progestins with minimal androgenic activity are **desogestrel** and **norgestimate;** those with intermediate activity include **norethindrone** and **ethynodiol;** and those with high androgenic effects include **norgestrel.** Progestins are rapidly absorbed after oral administration and go through prompt hepatic degradation. The drug can reach maximum concentration in 1 to 2 hours. Drug half-life varies. Dur-

Table 27-1 Drugs at a Glance: Estrogens

GENERIC/TRADE NAME	ROUTES AND DOSAGE RANGES FOR VARIOUS INDICATIONS			
	Menopausal Symptoms	Female Hypogonadism	Prevention of Osteoporosis	Other
Conjugated estrogens (synthetic) (Cenestin)	PO 0.625–1.25 mg daily			
Conjugated estrogens (Premarin)	PO 0.3–1.25 mg daily for 21 d followed by 7 d without the drug	PO 2.5–7.5 mg daily in divided doses, cyclically, 20 d on, 10 d off the drug	PO 0.625 mg daily for 21 d, then 7 d without the drug	Dysfunctional uterine bleeding: IM or IV for emergency use, 25 mg, repeated in 6–12 h if necessary Atrophic vaginitis: Topically, 2.4 g of vaginal cream inserted daily
Dienestrol (DV)				Atrophic or senile vaginitis: Topically, vaginal cream applied 2 or 3 times daily for approximately 2 wk, then reduced to 3 times weekly
Esterified estrogens (Estratab)	PO 0.3–1.25 mg daily for 21 d, then 7 d without the drug	PO 2.5–7.5 mg daily in divided doses, for 21 d, then 7 d without the drug		
Estradiol (Estrace, Estring)	PO 1–2 mg daily for 3 wk, then 1 wk off or daily Monday through Friday, none on Saturday or Sunday as prescribed		PO 0.5 mg daily for 23 d and no drug for 5 d each month	Atrophic vaginitis: Cream, 2–4 g daily for 2 wk, then 1–2 g daily for 2 wk, then 1 g 1–3 times weekly; vaginal ring (Estring), 1 every 3 mo
Estradiol cypionate (Depo-Estradiol)	IM 1–5 mg every 3–4 wk	IM 1.5–2 mg at monthly intervals		
Estradiol hemihydrate (Vagifem)				Atrophic vaginitis: 1 tablet, inserted into vagina, daily for 2 wk, then twice weekly
Estradiol transdermal gel (Estrogel)	Topically to skin; one complete pump depression daily to clean, dry skin			
Estradiol transdermal system (Estraderm, Climara, Vivelle)	Topically to skin, 1 patch 1 or 2 times per wk			
Estradiol valerate (Delestrogen)	IM 10–20 mg every 4 wk	IM 10–20 mg every 4 wk		

(continued)

Table 27-1 Drugs at a Glance: Estrogens (continued)

GENERIC/TRADE NAME	ROUTES AND DOSAGE RANGES FOR VARIOUS INDICATIONS			
	Menopausal Symptoms	Female Hypogonadism	Prevention of Osteoporosis	Other
Estrone	IM 0.1–0.5 mg weekly in single or divided doses	IM 0.1–2 mg weekly		Dysfunctional uterine bleeding: IM 2–4 mg daily for several days until bleeding is controlled, followed by progestin for 1 wk
Estropipate (Ogen)	PO 0.625–5 mg daily, cyclically	PO 1.25–7.5 mg daily for 3 wk, followed by an 8- to 10-d rest period. Repeat as needed.	PO 0.625 mg daily for 25 d and no drug for 6 d each month	Ovarian failure: Same dosage as for female hypogonadism Atrophic vaginitis: Topically, 1–2 g vaginal cream daily
Ethinyl estradiol (Estinyl)	PO 0.02–0.05 mg daily, cyclically	PO 0.05 mg 1 to 3 times daily for 2 wk with addition of progestin for last 2 wk of month		

IM, intramuscular; IV, intravenous; PO, oral.

Table 27-2 Drugs at a Glance: Progestins

GENERIC/TRADE NAME	ROUTES AND DOSAGE RANGES FOR VARIOUS INDICATIONS			
	Menstrual Disorders	Endometriosis	Endometrial Cancer	Other
Hydroxyprogesterone caproate (Hylutin)	Amenorrhea, dysfunctional uterine bleeding: IM 375 mg. With amenorrhea, if no bleeding after 21 d, begin cyclic therapy with estradiol and repeat every 4 wk for 4 cycles.			Uterine adenocarcinoma: IM 1 g or more initially; repeat one or more times each wk (maximum, 7 g/wk). Stop when relapse occurs or after 12 wk with no response. Test for endogenous estrogen production: IM 250 mg, repeated in 4 wk. Bleeding 7–14 d after injection indicates endogenous estrogen.
Medroxyprogesterone acetate (Depo-Provera, Provera)	Dysfunctional uterine bleeding: PO 5–10 mg daily for 5–10 d, beginning on 16th or 21st d of cycle		IM 400–1000 mg weekly until improvement, then 400 mg monthly	

Table 27-2 Drugs at a Glance: Progestins (continued)

	ROUTES AND DOSAGE RANGES FOR VARIOUS INDICATIONS			
GENERIC/TRADE NAME	**Menstrual Disorders**	**Endometriosis**	**Endometrial Cancer**	**Other**
Megestrol acetate (Megace)	Amenorrhea: PO 5–10 mg daily for 5–10 d		PO 40–320 mg daily in 4 divided doses for at least 2 mo	Breast cancer: PO 160 mg daily in 4 divided doses for at least 2 mo
Norethindrone acetate (Aygestin)	Amenorrhea, dysfunctional uterine bleeding: PO 2.5–10 mg daily, starting on 5th d of menstrual cycle and ending on 25th d	PO 5 mg daily for 2 wk, increased by 2.5 mg daily every 2 wk to dose of 15 mg. Then give 10–15 mg daily for maintenance.		
Progesterone	Amenorrhea, dysfunctional uterine bleeding: IM 5–10 mg for 6–8 consecutive d			

IM, intramuscular; PO, oral.

ing the first 6 hours, half-life is about 2 to 3 hours; thereafter, half-life extends to 8 to 9 hours. Metabolites are excreted primarily in the urine. Progestins administered intramuscularly are also rapidly absorbed, with a half-life of just a few minutes. Long-acting forms can maintain effective concentrations for 3 to 6 months; maximum concentrations can be achieved in 24 hours with a half-life of about 10 weeks. Gel preparations have sustained-release properties and absorption is prolonged with half-lives of 1 to 2 days.

There is no evidence to suggest that use of progestins in the first trimester of pregnancy to prevent habitual abortion is safe. There is evidence that when the drug is given during the first 4 months of pregnancy that fetal harm is possible.

Table 27-3 provides information about noncontraceptive estrogen–progestin combinations. Several noncontraceptive combination oral tablets are available for treatment of menopausal symptoms and osteoporosis. Two combination products (Combi-Patch and Ortho Evra) are available in transdermal patches for topical application.

Hormonal Contraceptives

Most hormonal contraceptives consist of a synthetic estrogen (eg, ethinyl estradiol) and a synthetic progestin (eg, norethindrone) (Table 27-4). Norethindrone undergoes first-pass metabolism so that it is only 65% bioavailable. It reaches peak plasma levels in 0.5 to 4 hours and has a half-life of 5 to 14 hours. It is metabolized in the liver and excreted in urine and feces. Monophasic contraceptives contain fixed amounts of both estrogen and progestin components. Biphasics and triphasics contain either fixed amounts of estrogen and varied amounts of progestin or varied amounts of both estrogen and progestin. Biphasic and triphasic preparations mimic normal variations of hormone secretion, decrease the total dosage of hormones, and may decrease adverse effects. These contraceptives are dispensed in containers with color-coded tablets that must be taken in the correct sequence. Dispensers with 28 tablets contain seven inactive or placebo tablets of a third color. A few contraceptives are progestin-only products. These are not widely used because they are less effective in preventing pregnancy and are more likely to cause vaginal bleeding, which makes them less acceptable to many women. Several combination products and alternative dosage forms are available to help individualize treatment and promote compliance.

APPLYING YOUR KNOWLEDGE 27-1

Vickie comes to the clinic for a routine visit. You review her medication history. Vickie asks about the different-colored pills in her contraceptive container. What is the best response?

Herbal and Dietary Supplement

Black cohosh is an herb used to self-treat symptoms of menopause. It is reportedly effective in relieving vasomotor instability. Most information is derived from small German studies using Remifemin, the brand name of a standardized extract that is marketed as an alternative to estrogen therapy for menopausal symptoms. The product apparently does not affect the endometrium or estrogen-dependent cancers, and its effects on bone and osteoporosis are unknown. Animal

Table 27-3 Drugs at a Glance: Noncontraceptive Estrogen–Progestin Combination

TRADE NAME	ESTROGEN	PROGESTIN	INDICATIONS FOR USE	ROUTES AND DOSAGE RANGES
Activelle	Estradiol 1 mg	Norethindrone 0.5 mg	Menopausal symptoms; prevention of osteoporosis	PO 1 tablet daily
Combi-Patch	Estradiol 0.05 mg	Norethindrone 0.14 or 0.25 mg	Estrogen deficiency states due to menopause, hypogonadism, castration, or primary ovarian failure	1 transdermal patch twice weekly
Femhrt	Ethinyl estradiol 5 mcg	Norethindrone 1 mg	Menopausal symptoms; prevention of osteoporosis	PO 1 tablet daily
Ortho-Prefest	Estradiol 1 mg*	Norgestimate 0.09 mg	Menopausal symptoms; prevention of osteoporosis	PO 1 tablet estrogen-only (pink) daily for 3 d, then 1 combination tablet (white) daily for 3 d. Repeat this 6-d regimen continuously, without interruption.
Premphase	Conjugated estrogens 0.625 mg*	Medroxyprogesterone 5 mg	Menopausal symptoms; prevention of osteoporosis	PO 1 tablet of estrogen-only once daily on d 1–14, then 1 combination tablet once daily on d 15–28
Prempro	Conjugated estrogens 0.3, 0.45, 0.625 mg	Medroxyprogesterone 1.5. 2.5, or 5 mg	Menopausal symptoms; prevention of osteoporosis	PO 1 tablet once daily in dial packs 28s

*Also available with estrogen only.
PO, oral.

studies indicate binding to estrogen receptors and suppression of LH. Other trade names include Estroven, Femtrol, and GNC Menopause Formula.

Adverse effects may include nausea, vomiting, dizziness, hypotension, and visual disturbances. Blood pressure should be monitored closely in hypertensive clients, because the herb may increase the hypotensive effects of antihypertensive drugs. Black cohosh is contraindicated in pregnancy and not recommended for use longer than 6 months for menopausal symptoms.

Overall, this herb may be considered in clients who refuse estrogen therapy recommended by a prescriber or have conditions in which estrogen is contraindicated. If Remifemin is taken, the recommended dosage is 1 tablet (standardized to contain 20 mg of herbal drug) twice daily. Other dosage forms are available, and dosage depends on the method of preparation.

APPLYING YOUR KNOWLEDGE 27-2

Vickie comes back to the clinic and tells you that she has not had a menstrual period this past month. Further assessment reveals that Vickie may not have taken all of her pills in sequence and that she has been sexually active. She is about 3 weeks overdue for her period. What action would you take?

NURSING PROCESS

Assessment

Before drug therapy is started, clients need a thorough history and physical examination, including measurements of blood pressure, serum cholesterol, and triglycerides.

TABLE 27-4 Hormonal Contraceptives

TRADE NAME	PHASE	ESTROGEN (MCG)	PROGESTIN (MG)
Monophasics			
Alesse		Ethinyl estradiol 20	Levonorgestrel 0.1
Apri		Ethinyl estradiol 30	Desogestrel 0.15
Aviane		Ethinyl estradiol 20	Levonorgestrel 0.1
Brevicon		Ethinyl estradiol 35	Norethindrone 0.5
Demulen 1/35		Ethinyl estradiol 35	Ethynodiol 1
Demulen 1/50		Ethinyl estradiol 50	Ethynodiol 1
Desogen		Ethinyl estradiol 30	Desogestrel 0.15
Levlen		Ethinyl estradiol 30	Levonorgestrel 0.15
Levlite		Ethinyl estradiol 20	Levonorgestrel 0.1
Levora		Ethinyl estradiol 30	Levonorgestrel 0.15
Loestrin 21 1.5/30		Ethinyl estradiol 30	Norethindrone 1.5
Loestrin Fe 1/20		Ethinyl estradiol 20	Norethindrone 1
Loestrin Fe 1.5/30		Ethinyl estradiol 30	Norethindrone 1.5
Lo/Ovral		Ethinyl estradiol 30	Norgestrel 0.3
Low-Orgestrel		Ethinyl estradiol 30	Norgestrel 0.3
Microgestin Fe 1/20		Ethinyl estradiol 20	Norethindrone 1
Microgestin Fe 1.5/30		Ethinyl estradiol 30	Norethindrone 1.5
Modicon		Ethinyl estradiol 35	Norethindrone 0.5
Necon 0.5/35		Ethinyl estradiol 35	Norethindrone 0.5
Necon 1/35		Ethinyl estradiol 35	Norethindrone 1
Necon 1/50		Mestranol 50	Norethindrone 1
Nordette		Ethinyl estradiol 30	Levonorgestrel 0.15
Norinyl 1 + 35		Ethinyl estradiol 35	Norethindrone 1
Norinyl 1 + 50		Mestranol 50	Norethindrone 1
Nortrel 0.5/35		Ethinyl estradiol 35	Norethindrone 0.5
Nortrel 1/35		Ethinyl estradiol 35	Norethindrone 1
Ogestrel		Ethinyl estradiol 50	Norgestrel 0.5
Ortho-Cept		Ethinyl estradiol 30	Desogestrel 0.15
Ortho-Cyclen		Ethinyl estradiol 35	Norgestimate 0.25
Ortho-Novum 1/35		Ethinyl estradiol 35	Norethindrone 1
Ortho-Novum 1/50		Mestranol 50	Norethindrone 1
Ovcon-35		Ethinyl estradiol 35	Norethindrone 0.4
Ovcon-50		Ethinyl estradiol 50	Norethindrone 1
Ovral-28		Ethinyl estradiol 50	Norgestrel 0.5
Yasmin		Ethinyl estradiol 30	Drospirenone 3
Zovia 1/35E		Ethinyl estradiol 35	Ethynodiol 1
Zovia 1/50E		Ethinyl estradiol 50	Ethynodiol 1
Biphasics			
Jenest-28	*I:* 10 d	Ethinyl estradiol 35	Norethindrone 0.5
	II: 11 d	Ethinyl estradiol 35	Norethindrone 1
Mircette	*I:* 21 d	Ethinyl estradiol 20	Desogestrel 0.15
	II: 5 d	Ethinyl estradiol 10	
Necon 10/11	*I:* 10 d	Ethinyl estradiol 35	Norethindrone 0.5
	II: 11 d	Ethinyl estradiol 35	Norethindrone 1
Ortho-Novum 10/11	*I:* 10 d	Ethinyl estradiol 35	Norethindrone 0.5
	II: 11 d	Ethinyl estradiol 35	Norethindrone 1
Triphasics			
Estrostep 21	*I:* 5 d	Ethinyl estradiol 20	Norethindrone 1
	II: 7 d	Ethinyl estradiol 30	Norethindrone 1
	III: 9 d	Ethinyl estradiol 35	Norethindrone 1
Estrostep Fe	*I:* 5 d	Ethinyl estradiol 20	Norethindrone 1
	II: 7 d	Ethinyl estradiol 30	Norethindrone 1
	III: 9 d	Ethinyl estradiol 35	Norethindrone 1
Ortho-Novum 7/7/7	*I:* 7 d	Ethinyl estradiol 35	Norethindrone 0.5
	II: 7 d	Ethinyl estradiol 35	Norethindrone 0.75
	III: 7 d	Ethinyl estradiol 35	Norethindrone 1

(continued)

TABLE 27-4 Hormonal Contraceptives (continued)

TRADE NAME	PHASE	ESTROGEN (MCG)	PROGESTIN (MG)
Ortho Tri-Cyclen	I: 7 d	Ethinyl estradiol 35	Norgestimate 0.18
	II: 9 d	Ethinyl estradiol 35	Norgestimate 0.215
	III: 5 d	Ethinyl estradiol 35	Norgestimate 0.25
Tri-Levlen	I: 6 d	Ethinyl estradiol 30	Levonorgestrel 0.05
	II: 5 d	Ethinyl estradiol 40	Levonorgestrel 0.075
	III: 10 d	Ethinyl estradiol 30	Levonorgestrel 0.125
Tri-Norinyl	I: 7 d	Ethinyl estradiol 35	Norethindrone 0.5
	II: 9 d	Ethinyl estradiol 35	Norethindrone 1
	III: 5 d	Ethinyl estradiol 35	Norethindrone 0.5
Triphasil	I: 6 d	Ethinyl estradiol 30	Levonorgestrel 0.05
	II: 5 d	Ethinyl estradiol 40	Levonorgestrel 0.075
	III: 10 d	Ethinyl estradiol 30	Levonorgestrel 0.125
Trivora-28	I: 6 d	Ethinyl estradiol 30	Levonorgestrel 0.05
	II: 5 d	Ethinyl estradiol 40	Levonorgestrel 0.075
	III: 10 d	Ethinyl estradiol 30	Levonorgestrel 0.125
Progestin-Only Products			
Depo-Provera			Medroxyprogesterone 1.5
Micronor			Norethindrone 0.35
Norplant Subdermal System			Levonorgestrel 216
Nor-QD			Norethindrone 0.35
Ovrette			Norgestrel 0.075
Progestasert intrauterine			Progesterone 38
Transdermal Preparation			
Ortho Evra		Ethinyl estradiol 0.02 mg/ 24 h (0.75 mg/wk)	Norelgestromin 0.15 mg/ 24 h (6 mg/wk)
Emergency Contraceptive			
Preven		Ethinyl estradiol 0.05 mg/ tablet	Levonorgestrel 0.25 mg/ tablet

These parameters must be monitored periodically as long as the drugs are taken.

- Assess for conditions in which estrogens and progestins are used (eg, menstrual disorders, menopausal symptoms).
- Assess for conditions that increase risks of adverse effects or are contraindications for hormonal therapy (eg, thromboembolic disorders, pregnancy).
- Record blood pressure with each outpatient contact or regularly with hospitalized clients. Increases are likely in premenopausal women, especially with oral contraceptives, but are unlikely in women who are postmenopausal who are receiving physiologic replacement doses.
- Check laboratory reports of cholesterol and triglyceride levels when available.
- Assess diet and presence of cigarette smoking. A high-fat diet increases the risks of gallbladder disease and perhaps other problems; cigarette smoking increases risks of thromboembolic disorders in women older than 35 years of age who take oral contraceptives.

- Assess the client's willingness to comply with instructions about drug therapy and follow-up procedures.
- Assess for signs and symptoms of thromboembolic disorders regularly. These are most likely to occur in women older than 35 years of age who take oral contraceptives, women who are postmenopausal who receive combined estrogen–progestin HRT, and women or men who take large doses for cancer.

Nursing Diagnoses

- Disturbed Body Image in women, related to effects of hormone deficiency states
- Disturbed Body Image in men, related to feminizing effects and impotence from female hormones
- Excess Fluid Volume related to sodium and water retention
- Deficient Knowledge: Effects of hormonal therapy
- Risk for Injury related to increased risks of hypertension and gallbladder disease

Planning/Goals

The client will

- Be assisted to cope with self-concept and body image changes
- Take the drugs accurately, for the length of time prescribed
- Experience relief of symptoms for which the drugs are given
- Avoid preventable adverse drug effects
- Keep appointments for monitoring of drug effects

Interventions

- Assist clients of childbearing age to choose an appropriate contraceptive method. If the choice is an estrogen–progestin combination, help the client take it accurately.
- Help postmenopausal women plan for adequate calcium and vitamin D in the diet and adequate weight-bearing exercise to maintain bone strength and prevent osteoporosis.
- Assist clients in obtaining follow-up health care when indicated.
- Provide client teaching for drug therapy (see accompanying displays).

Evaluation

- Interview and observe for compliance with instructions for taking the drugs.
- Interview and observe for therapeutic and adverse drug effects.

APPLYING YOUR KNOWLEDGE 27-3

Vickie is not pregnant and she decides to remain on oral contraceptives. She explains to you that she sometimes does not take her pill because they make her sick to her stomach. How do you respond?

PRINCIPLES OF THERAPY

Need for Continuous Supervision

Because estrogens, progestins, and hormonal contraceptives are often taken for years and may cause adverse reactions, clients taking these drugs need continued supervision by a health care provider. Before the drugs are prescribed, a complete medical history; a physical examination including breast and pelvic examinations and a Papanicolaou (Pap) test; urinalysis; and weight and blood

---

CLIENT TEACHING GUIDELINES

Hormone Replacement Therapy

General Considerations

☑ Hormone replacement therapy (HRT) relieves symptoms of menopause and helps to prevent or treat osteoporosis.

☑ Women receiving HRT should be under medical supervision and should have a physical examination at least annually to check blood pressure and breasts, pelvis, and other areas for possible adverse reactions when these drugs are taken for long periods.

☑ Women who have not had a hysterectomy should take both estrogen and progestin; the progestin component (eg, Provera) prevents endometrial cancer, an adverse effect of estrogen-only therapy. Post-hysterectomy, women should take estrogen-only medications. However, the Women's Health Initiative study concluded that risks of adverse effects with estrogen-only therapy and estrogen–progestin combinations are greater than previously believed (see Box 27-2). Women who are considering HRT (eg, for severe symptoms of menopause) should discuss their individual risks and potential benefits with their health care providers.

☑ Combined estrogen–progestin therapy may increase blood sugar levels in women with diabetes. This effect is attributed to progestin and is unlikely to occur with estrogen-only therapy.

☑ Women with diabetes should report increased blood glucose levels.

Self-Administration

☑ Take estrogens and progestins with food or at bedtime to decrease nausea, a common adverse reaction.

☑ Apply transdermal estrogen patches (Climara, Estraderm, Vivelle) to clean, dry skin, preferably the abdomen. Press the patch tightly for 10 seconds to get a good seal and rotate sites so that at least a week passes between applications to a site; avoid prolonged sun exposure to the area of the patch.

☑ Apply transdermal estrogen gel (Estrogel) to clean, dry skin, avoiding the breast; avoid fire, flame, or smoking until gel has dried because it is flammable.

☑ Weigh weekly and report sudden weight gain. Fluid retention and edema may occur and produce weight gain.

☑ Report any unusual vaginal bleeding.

CLIENT TEACHING GUIDELINES

General Considerations

☑ Seek information about the use of oral contraceptives.

☑ Oral contraceptives are very effective at preventing pregnancy, but they *do not* prevent transmission of sexually transmitted diseases (eg, acquired immunodeficiency syndrome, chlamydia, gonorrhea).

☑ See a health care provider every 6 to 12 months for blood-pressure measurement, breast and pelvic examinations, and other care as indicated. This is very important to monitor for adverse drug effects such as high blood pressure, gallbladder disease, and blood-clotting disorders.

☑ Do not smoke cigarettes. Cigarette smoking increases risks of blood clots in the legs, lungs, heart, or brain. The blood clots may cause heart attack, stroke, or other serious diseases.

☑ Several medications may reduce the effectiveness of oral contraceptives (ie, increase the likelihood of pregnancy). These include several antibiotics (eg, ampicillin, clarithromycin and similar drugs, rifampin, penicillin V, sulfonamides [eg, Bactrim], tetracyclines, and antiseizure medications (eg, carbamazepine, oxcarbazepine, phenytoin, topiramate). Inform all health care providers who prescribe medications for you that you are taking a birth control pill.

☑ Be prepared to use an additional or alternative method of birth control if a dose is missed, if you are unable to take the oral contraceptive because of illness, or if you have an infection for which an antibiotic is prescribed. For example, use a different method of birth control while taking an antibiotic and for the remainder of that cycle.

☑ Avoid pregnancy for approximately 3 to 6 months after the drugs are stopped.

Self-Administration

☑ Read, keep, and follow instructions in the package inserts that are dispensed with the drugs. These inserts provide information about safe and effective use of the drugs.

☑ Take oral contraceptives with meals or food or at bedtime to decrease nausea. (If using Ortho Evra, a contraceptive skin patch that lasts a week, follow package instructions for correct application.)

☑ Take at about the same time every day to maintain effective blood levels and establish a routine so that missed doses are less likely. Missing one dose may allow pregnancy to occur. If you forget to take one pill, take it as soon as you remember. If you do not remember until the next scheduled pill, you can take two pills at once. If you miss two pills in a row, you may take two pills for the next 2 days. If you miss more than two pills, notify your health care provider.

☑ Use sunscreen and protective clothing when outdoors. The drugs may cause photosensitivity, with increased likelihood of sunburn after short periods of exposure.

☑ Weigh weekly and report sudden weight gain. The drugs may cause fluid retention; decreasing salt intake may be helpful.

☑ Report any unusual vaginal bleeding; calf tenderness, redness, or swelling; chest pain; weakness or numbness in an arm or leg; or sudden difficulty with seeing or talking.

---

pressure measurements are recommended. These examinations should be repeated at least annually as long as the client is taking the drugs.

Drug Selection

Choice of preparation depends on the reason for use, desired route of administration, and duration of action. Conjugated estrogen (eg, Premarin) is a commonly used oral estrogen, and medroxyprogesterone (eg, Provera) is a commonly used oral progestin. Transdermal estradiol (eg, Climara, Estraderm, Vivelle) allows for absorption of estrogen through the skin to the bloodstream. Two advantages have been recognized with this form of administration. Because the liver is bypassed, the total dose of estrogen is reduced. Additionally, the serum levels produced through transdermal application more closely mimic

premenopausal estrogen levels compared with serum levels with oral estrogens.

The choice of a combination contraceptive product may be determined by the progestin component. Some progestins are more likely to cause weight gain, acne, and changes in blood lipids that increase risks of myocardial infarction or stroke. These adverse effects are attributed mainly to the androgenic activity of the progestin, and some progestins have more androgenic effects than others. Duration of action may also be a factor. Some crystalline suspensions of estrogens and oil solutions of both estrogens and progesterone prolong drug action by slowing absorption. Long-acting progestin contraceptive preparations such as the intramuscular depot medroxyprogesterone (Depo-Provera) last 3 months per injection; intrauterine progesterone lasts 1 year; and levonorgestrel subcutaneous implants (Norplant) last 5 years.

Drug Dosage

Although dosage needs vary with clients and the conditions for which the drugs are prescribed, a general rule is to use the smallest effective dose for the shortest effective time. Estrogens are often given cyclically. In one regimen, the drug is taken for 3 weeks and then omitted for 1 week; in another, it is omitted the first 5 days of each month. These regimens more closely resemble normal secretion of estrogen and avoid prolonged stimulation of body tissues. A progestin may be added for 10 days each month.

Drug Administration

Naturally occurring, nonconjugated estrogens (estradiol, estrone) and *natural progesterone* are given intramuscularly because they are rapidly metabolized if administered orally. *Nonsteroidal synthetic preparations* are usually administered orally or topically.

Drug Interactions

These drugs may interact with several drugs or drug groups to increase or decrease their effects. Most interactions have been reported with oral contraceptives.

Estrogens may *decrease* the effectiveness of sulfonylurea antidiabetic drugs (probably by increasing their metabolism); warfarin, an oral anticoagulant (by increasing hepatic production of several clotting factors); and phenytoin, an anticonvulsant (possibly by increasing fluid retention). Estrogens may *increase* the adverse effects and risks of toxicity with corticosteroids, ropinirole, and tacrine by inhibiting their metabolism. Ropinirole and tacrine should not be used concurrently with an estrogen.

Oral contraceptives *decrease* effects of some benzodiazepines (eg, lorazepam, oxazepam, temazepam), insulin, sulfonylurea antidiabetic drugs, and warfarin. If one of these drugs is taken concurrently with an oral contraceptive, increased dosage may be needed for therapeutic effects. Contraceptives *increase* effects of several drugs by inhibiting their metabolism. These include alcohol, some benzodiazepines (eg, alprazolam, triazolam), tricyclic antidepressants, beta blockers (eg, metoprolol), caffeine, corticosteroids, and theophylline (a xanthine bronchodilator). If one of these drugs is taken concurrently with an oral contraceptive, the drug may accumulate to toxic levels. Dosage may need to be reduced.

Use for Specific Indications

Contraception

The most effective and widely used contraceptives are estrogen–progestin combinations (see Table 27-4). Estrogen–progestin contraceptive preparations are nearly 100% effective in preventing pregnancy when taken correctly.

Numerous preparations are available, with different components and different doses of components, so that a preparation can be chosen to meet individual needs. Most oral contraceptives contain an estrogen and a progestin. The estrogen dose is usually 30 to 35 micrograms. Smaller amounts (eg, 20 mcg) may be adequate for small or underweight women; larger amounts (eg, 50 mcg) may be needed for large or overweight women. Effects of estrogen components are similar when prescribed in equipotent doses, but progestins differ in progestogenic, estrogenic, antiestrogenic, and androgenic activity. Consequently, adverse effects may differ to some extent, and a client may be able to tolerate one contraceptive better than another.

Current products contain small amounts of estrogen and cause fewer adverse effects than previous products. Despite the decreased estrogen dosage, oral contraceptives may still be safest when administered to nonsmoking women younger than 35 years of age who do not have a history of thromboembolic problems, diabetes mellitus, hypertension, or migraine. When estrogen is contraindicated, a progestin-only contraceptive may be used.

It is necessary to assess each client's need and desire for contraception, as well as her willingness to comply with the prescribed regimen. Assessment includes determining a client's knowledge about birth control, both pharmacologic and nonpharmacologic, and identifying clients in whom hormonal contraceptives are contraindicated or who are at increased risk for adverse drug effects. Compliance involves the willingness to take the drugs as prescribed and to have breast and pelvic examinations and blood pressure measurements every 6 to 12 months.

Emergency (Postcoital) Contraception

Emergency contraception (ie, high doses of estrogen and progestin) may be used to avoid pregnancy after unprotected sexual intercourse, especially for victims of rape or incest or for women whose physical or mental health is threatened by pregnancy. Emergency contraception is most effective if started within 24 hours and no later than 72 hours after exposure. The drugs are believed to act mainly by inhibiting ovulation.

Although Preven (levonorgestrel 0.25 mg and ethinyl estradiol 0.05 mg) is the only drug approved by the Food and Drug Administration for postcoital contraception, multiple tablets of several birth control pills are also effective. The drugs are given in two doses, 12 hours apart. Amounts include four tablets of Levlen, Lo/Ovral, Nordette, Triphasil, or Tri-Levlen; two tablets of Ovral; and five tablets of Alesse. These are high doses, and common adverse effects are nausea and vomiting. Antiemetic medication or repeating vomited doses may be needed. Women who take a hormonal contraceptive should probably ask the prescriber about possible postcoital use.

Menopause

Menopause usually occurs in women who are 48 to 55 years of age. A woman who has not menstruated for a full year is considered menopausal, although symptoms of estrogen deficiency and irregular periods start approximately 4 years before final cessation. Physiologic menopause results from the gradual cessation of ovarian function and the resultant decrease in estrogen levels. Surgical menopause results from excision of both ovaries and the sudden loss of ovarian estrogen. Although estrogens from the adrenal cortex and other sites are still produced, the amount is insufficient to prevent estrogen deficiency.

ERT prevents vasomotor instability ("hot flashes" or "hot flushes") and other menopausal symptoms. A commonly prescribed regimen is a conjugated estrogen (Premarin) 0.625 to 1.25 milligrams daily for 25 days of each month, with a progestin, such as Provera, 10 milligrams daily for 10 days of each month, on days 15 to 25 of the cycle. The main function of the progestin is to decrease the risk of endometrial cancer; thus, women who have had a hysterectomy do not need it. Another regimen uses estradiol as a transdermal patch (eg, Climara, Estraderm, Vivelle), which releases the drug slowly; provides more consistent blood levels than oral formulations; and is applied weekly or biweekly, depending on the formulation. A newer synthetic conjugated estrogen (Cenestin) is also approved for short-term treatment of hot flashes and sweating; it is not approved for long-term use in preventing osteoporosis in postmenopausal women. In addition, selective serotonin reuptake inhibitors (see Chapter 10) have shown great potential in reducing vasomotor symptoms. In randomized clinical trials, venlafaxine (Effexor), paroxetine (Paxil), and fluoxetine (Prozac) have been shown to reduce hot flashes significantly.

Osteoporosis: Prevention and Treatment

Estrogen or estrogen–progestin therapy is effective and has been widely used to prevent or treat osteoporosis and prevent fractures in postmenopausal women (see Chap. 25). Estrogenic effects in preventing bone loss include decreased bone resorption (breakdown), increased intestinal absorption of calcium, and increased calcitriol concentration. Calcitriol is the active form of vitamin D, which is required for absorption of calcium.

Estrogen and progestin may be used less often for osteoporosis in future for two main reasons. First, recent evidence (see Box 27-2) indicates that the risks of estrogen–progestin and estrogen-only hormonal therapy outweigh the benefits. Second, there are other effective measures for prevention and treatment of osteoporosis, including calcium and vitamin D supplements, bisphosphonate drugs (eg, alendronate, risedronate), and weight-bearing exercise.

Use in Special Populations

Use in Children

There is little information about the effects of estrogens in children, and the drugs are not indicated for use. Because estrogens cause epiphyseal closure, they should be used with caution before completion of bone growth and attainment of adult height. When hormonal contraceptives are given to adolescent girls, as in other populations, the smallest effective doses should be used.

Use in Older Adults

The short-term use (1–2 years) of estrogens or estrogens and progestins in postmenopausal women may be indicated for management of menopausal symptoms. Long-term use of estrogen-only therapy and estrogen–progestin combinations is no longer recommended for most women, because of potentially serious adverse effects.

Use in Clients With Hepatic Impairment

Estrogens are contraindicated in impaired liver function, liver disease, or liver cancer. Impaired liver function may lead to impaired estrogen metabolism, with resultant accumulation and adverse effects. In addition, women who have had jaundice during pregnancy have an increased risk of recurrence if they take estrogen-containing contraceptives. Any client in whom jaundice develops when taking estrogen should stop taking the drug. Because jaundice may indicate liver damage, the cause should be investigated. Progestins are contraindicated in clients with impaired liver function or liver disease.

Use in Home Care

Estrogens, progestins, and hormonal contraceptives are usually self-administered. Home care nurses may encounter clients or family members taking one of the drugs when visiting the home for another purpose. It may be necessary to teach or assist clients to take the drugs as prescribed. In addition, clients may need encouragement to keep appointments for follow-up supervision and blood pressure monitoring. When visiting families that include adolescent girls or young women, home care nurses may need to teach about birth control measures or about preventing osteoporosis by improving diet and exercise patterns. In families that include postmenopausal women, home care nurses may need to teach about nonhormonal strategies for preventing or treating osteoporosis and cardiovascular disease.

 APPLYING YOUR KNOWLEDGE 27-4:
HOW CAN YOU AVOID THIS MEDICATION ERROR?
Vickie returns to the clinic for a urinary tract infection. The physician prescribes an antibiotic. You send Vickie to the school pharmacy and then home.

N U R S I N G   A C T I O N S

Estrogens, Progestins, and Hormonal Contraceptives

NURSING ACTIONS	RATIONALE/EXPLANATION
1. Administer accurately	
a. Give oral estrogens, progestins, and contraceptive preparations after meals or at bedtime.	To decrease nausea, a common adverse reaction
b. With aqueous suspensions to be given intramuscularly, roll the vial between the hands several times.	To be sure that drug particles are evenly distributed through the liquid vehicle
c. Give oil preparations deeply into a large muscle mass, preferably gluteal muscles.	
d. With estradiol skin patches, apply to clean, dry skin of the abdomen, buttocks, upper inner thigh, or upper arm. Avoid breasts, waistline areas, and areas exposed to sunlight. Press with palm of hand for about 10 seconds. Rotate sites.	To facilitate effective absorption and adherence to the skin and avoid skin irritation
e. With Combi-Patch, apply to clean, dry skin of the lower abdomen; rotate sites.	Manufacturer's recommendation. Rotating sites decreases skin irritation.
f. With Ortho Evra patch, apply to abdomen, buttocks, upper torso (except breasts), or upper outer arm.	Manufacturer's recommendation
2. Observe for therapeutic effects	
a. With estrogens:	Therapeutic effects vary, depending on the reason for use.
(1) When given for menopausal symptoms, observe for decrease in hot flashes and vaginal problems.	
(2) When given for amenorrhea, observe for menstruation.	
(3) When given for female hypogonadism, observe for menstruation, breast enlargement, axillary and pubic hair, and other secondary sexual characteristics.	
(4) When given to prevent or treat osteoporosis, observe for improved bone density tests and absence of fractures.	
b. With progestins:	
(1) When given for menstrual disorders, such as abnormal uterine bleeding, amenorrhea, dysmenorrhea, premenstrual discomfort, and endometriosis, observe for relief of symptoms.	
3. Observe for adverse effects	
a. With estrogens:	
(1) Menstrual disorders—breakthrough bleeding, dysmenorrhea, amenorrhea	Estrogen drugs may alter hormonal balance.
(2) Gastrointestinal system—nausea, vomiting, abdominal cramps, bloating	Nausea commonly occurs but usually subsides within 1 to 2 weeks of continued therapy. When high doses of estrogens are used as postcoital contraceptives, nausea and vomiting may be severe enough to require administration of antiemetic drugs.
(3) Gallbladder disease	Postmenopausal women taking an estrogen are 2 to 4 times more likely than non-users to require surgery for gallbladder disease.

(continued)

NURSING ACTIONS	RATIONALE/EXPLANATION
(4) Cardiovascular system—thromboembolic conditions such as thrombophlebitis, pulmonary embolism, cerebral thrombosis, and coronary thrombosis; edema and weight gain	Estrogens promote blood clotting by stimulating hepatic production of four clotting factors (II, VII, IX, X). Thromboembolic disorders are most likely to occur in women older than 35 years of age who take oral contraceptives and smoke cigarettes; postmenopausal women taking long-term estrogen and progestin therapy; and men or women who receive large doses of estrogens for cancer treatment. Edema and weight gain are caused by fluid retention.
(5) Central nervous system—headache, migraine headache, dizziness, mental depression	Estrogens may cause or aggravate migraine headache in some women; the mechanism is unknown.
(6) Cancer—endometrial and possibly breast cancer	When estrogens are used alone in postmenopausal women, they cause endometrial hyperplasia and may cause endometrial cancer. Women with an intact uterus should also be given a progestin, which opposes the effects of estrogen on the endometrium.
	Opinions differ regarding estrogens as a cause of breast cancer. Most studies indicate little risk; a few indicate some risk, especially with high doses for prolonged periods (ie, 10 y or longer). However, estrogens do stimulate growth in breast cancers that have estrogen receptors.
b. With progestins:	
(1) Menstrual disorders—breakthrough bleeding	Irregular vaginal bleeding is a common adverse effect that decreases during the first year of use. This is a major reason that some women do not want to take progestin-only contraceptives.
(2) Cardiovascular system—decreased high-density lipoprotein and increased low-density lipoprotein cholesterol	These adverse effects on plasma lipids potentially increase the risks of cardiovascular disease.
(3) Gastrointestinal system—nausea, increased or decreased weight	Nausea may be decreased by taking with food.
(4) Central nervous system—drowsiness, insomnia, mental depression	
(5) Miscellaneous effects—edema, weight gain	
c. Combined estrogen and progestin oral contraceptives:	
(1) Gastrointestinal effects—nausea, others	Nausea may be minimized by taking the drugs with food or at bedtime.
(2) Cardiovascular effects—thromboembolism, myocardial infarction, stroke, hypertension	These effects occurred with earlier oral contraceptives, which contained larger amounts of estrogen than those currently used, and are much less common in most people who take low-dose preparations. However, for women older than 35 years of age who smoke, there is an increased risk of myocardial infarction and other cardiovascular disorders, even with low-dose pills.
(3) Gallbladder disease—cholelithiasis and cholecystitis	Women who use oral contraceptives or estrogen–progestin hormone replacement therapy are several times more likely to develop gallbladder disease than non-users. This is attributed to increased concentration of cholesterol in bile acids, which leads to decreased solubility and increased precipitation of stones.
(4) Miscellaneous—edema, weight gain, headache	
4. Observe for drug interactions	
a. Drugs that *decrease* effects of estrogens, progestins, and oral contraceptives:	
(1) Anticonvulsants—carbamazepine, oxcarbazepine, phenytoin, topiramate	Decrease effects by inducing enzymes that accelerate metabolism of estrogens and progestins

NURSING ACTIONS	RATIONALE/EXPLANATION
(2) Antimicrobials (a) Antibacterials—ampicillin, macrolides (erythromycin, clarithromycin, dirithromycin), metronidazole, penicillin V, rifampin, sulfonamides, tetracyclines, trimethoprim (b) Antifungals—fluconazole, itraconazole, ketoconazole (c) Antivirals—efavirenz, ritonavir, lopinavir/ritonavir combination	Most interactions with antimicrobials have been reported with oral contraceptives. Rifampin induces drug-metabolizing enzymes that accelerate drug inactivation. Other antimicrobials act mainly by disrupting the normal bacterial flora of the gastrointestinal tract and decreasing enterohepatic recirculation of estrogens. This action may decrease effectiveness of contraceptives or cause breakthrough bleeding. To prevent pregnancy from occurring during antimicrobial therapy, a larger dose of oral contraceptive or an additional or alternative form of birth control is probably advisable.

APPLYING YOUR KNOWLEDGE: ANSWERS

27-1 Explain to Vickie that her color-coded tablets have different amounts of medication in them, making them more closely resemble the normal variations in hormones in the body. Emphasize the need to take the tablets in the correct sequence.

27-2 Vickie should stop taking the oral contraceptives and her pregnancy state should be evaluated. Pregnancy is a contraindication for continuation of the hormones. Damage may occur to the fetus if oral contraceptives are taken during pregnancy.

27-3 Instruct Vickie to take her pills with food or at bedtime to reduce nausea. If the nausea continues and she cannot take the pills in continued sequence, perhaps considering another form of contraception would be appropriate.

27-4 Vickie should have been instructed to use an alternate method of birth control while she is on antibiotics. Antibiotics decrease the effectiveness of oral contraceptives.

Review and Application Exercises

Short Answer Exercises

1. What are the reproductive and nonreproductive functions of estrogens?

2. What are the functions of progestins?

3. What is considered the major mechanism of action of hormonal contraceptives?

4. What are the adverse effects of hormonal contraceptives, and how can they be prevented or minimized?

5. Outline the points you would make for and against HRT for a postmenopausal woman.

6. Prepare a teaching plan for a perimenopausal or postmenopausal woman about nonpharmacologic measures to manage menopausal symptoms and prevent osteoporosis.

NCLEX-Style Questions

7. ERT prevents menopausal symptoms. Hot flushes/flashes are the result of which of the following?
   a. insufficient gonadotropin secretion
   b. vasomotor instability
   c. high levels of estrogen
   d. decreased progesterone

8. Progesterone is a progestin concerned almost entirely with reproduction. In the nonpregnant women, progesterone is secreted by which of the following?
   a. corpus luteum
   b. hypothalamus
   c. anterior pituitary
   d. adrenal cortex

9. Black cohosh has been used to self-treat symptoms of menopause. Due to the risk of adverse effects, clients should be monitored closely for which of the following conditions?
   a. dysrhythmias
   b. hypertension
   c. hypotension
   d. bradycardia

10. Client teaching for a client who will be using the transdermal estradiol patch Estraderm should include information about applying the patch to
   a. the skin daily
   b. clean and dry skin
   c. the same area for consistency
   d. the skin every 2 weeks

Selected References

Barbieri, R. L. (2000). Disorders of the reproductive cycle in women. In H. D. Humes (Ed.), *Kelley's Textbook of internal medicine* (4th ed., pp. 2740–2743). Philadelphia: Lippincott Williams & Wilkins.

DerMarderosian, A. (Ed.). (2001). *The review of natural products.* St. Louis: Facts and Comparisons.

Drug facts and comparisons. (Updated monthly). St. Louis: Facts and Comparisons.

Fletcher, S. W., & Colditz, G. A. (2002). Editorial. Failure of estrogen plus progestin therapy for prevention. *Journal of the American Medical Association, 288*(3), 366–367.

Grady, D. (2003). Postmenopausal hormones: Therapy for symptoms only. *New England Journal of Medicine, 348*(19), 1835–1837.

Gruber, C. J., Tschugguel, W., Schneeberger, C., & Huber, J. C. (2002). Production and actions of estrogens. *New England Journal of Medicine, 346*(5), 340–351.

Guyton, A. C., & Hall, J. E. (2000). *Textbook of medical physiology* (10th ed.). Philadelphia: W. B. Saunders.

Hackley, B., & Rousseau, M. E. (2004). Managing menopausal symptoms after the Women's Health Initiative. *Journal of Midwifery and Women's Health, 49*(2), 87–95.

Kim, R. B. (Ed.). (2001). *Handbook of adverse drug interactions.* New Rochelle, NY: Medical Letter.

Lacy, C. F., Armstrong, L. L., Goldman, M. P., Lance, L. L. (2004). *Lexi-Comp's drug information handbook* (12th ed.). Hudson, OH: Lexi-Comp.

Levine, J. (2003). Long-term estrogen and hormone replacement therapy for the prevention and treatment of osteoporosis. *Current Women's Health Reports, 3*(3), 181–186

Marcus, E. N. (2000). Principles of women's medicine. In H. D. Humes (Ed.), *Kelley's Textbook of internal medicine* (4th ed., pp. 299–303). Philadelphia: Lippincott Williams & Wilkins.

Mehring, P. M. (2005). The female reproductive system. In C. M. Porth, *Pathophysiology: Concepts of altered health states* (7th ed., pp. 1051–1064). Philadelphia: Lippincott Williams & Wilkins.

Morelli, V., & Naquin, C. (2002). Alternative therapies for traditional disease states: Menopause. *American Family Physician, 66*(1), 129–134.

Morris, B. J., & Young, C. (2000). Emergency contraception. *American Journal of Nursing, 100*(9), 46–48.

Nelson, H. D., Humphrey, L. L., Nygren, P., et al. (2002). Postmenopausal hormone replacement therapy. *Journal of the American Medical Association, 288*(7), 872–881.

Ortho Evra—A contraceptive patch. (2002, January 21). *Medical Letter on Drugs and Therapeutics, 44*(1122), 8.

Petitti, D. B. (2002). Editorial. Hormone replacement therapy for prevention: More evidence, more pessimism. *Journal of the American Medical Association, 288*(1), 99–101.

Scholtz, D., & Carmichael, J. M. (2000). Contraception. In E. T. Herfindal & D. R. Gourley (Eds.), *Textbook of therapeutics: Drug and disease management* (7th ed., pp. 2019–2036). Philadelphia: Lippincott Williams & Wilkins.

Women's Health Initiative Steering Committee. (2004). Effects of conjugated equine estrogen in postmenopausal women with hyterectomy. *Journal of the American Medical Association, 291*(14), 1701–1712.

Writing Group for the Women's Health Initiative Investigators. (2002). Risks and benefits of estrogen plus progestin in healthy postmenopausal women: Principal results from the Women's Health Initiative Randomized Controlled Trial. *Journal of the American Medical Association, 288*(3), 321–333.

Androgens and Anabolic Steroids

OBJECTIVES

After studying this chapter, you will be able to:

1. Discuss effects of endogenous androgens.
2. Discuss uses and effects of exogenous androgens and anabolic steroids.
3. Describe potential consequences of abusing androgens and anabolic steroids.
4. Counsel clients about the physiologic effects of the dietary supplements androstenedione and dehydroepiandrosterone (DHEA).

APPLYING YOUR KNOWLEDGE

Barbara Watson is a 35-year-old female. She has endometriosis. Ms. Watson is receiving danazol (Danocrine) 800 mg daily in two divided doses.

INTRODUCTION

Androgens are male sex hormones secreted by the testes in men, the ovaries in women, and the adrenal cortex of both sexes. Like the female sex hormones, the naturally occurring male sex hormones are steroids synthesized from cholesterol. The sex organs and adrenal glands can produce cholesterol or remove it from the blood. Cholesterol then undergoes a series of conversions to progesterone, androgenic prehormones, and testosterone. The androgens produced by the ovaries have little androgenic activity and are used mainly as precursor substances for the production of naturally occurring estrogens. The adrenal glands produce several androgens, including androstenedione and dehydroepiandrosterone (DHEA). Androstenedione and DHEA are weak androgens with little masculinizing effect that are mainly converted to estrogens.

Testosterone

Testosterone is normally the only important male sex hormone. It is secreted by the Leydig's cells in the testes in response to stimulation by luteinizing hormone from the anterior pituitary gland. The main functions of testosterone are related to the development of male sexual characteristics, reproduction, and metabolism (Box 28-1).

About 97% of the testosterone secreted by the testes binds to plasma albumin or to sex hormone–binding globulin and circulates in the blood for 30 minutes to several hours. The bound testosterone is either transferred to the tissues or broken down into inactive products that are excreted. Much of the testosterone that transfers to tissues undergoes intracellular conversion to dihydrotestosterone, especially in the external genitalia of the male fetus and the prostate gland in the adult male. The dihydrotestosterone combines with receptor proteins in the cytoplasm; the steroid–receptor combination then migrates to the cell nucleus where it induces transcription of DNA and RNA and stimulates production of proteins. Almost all testosterone effects result from the increased formation of proteins throughout the body, especially in the cells of target organs and tissues responsible for development of male sexual characteristics.

The portion of testosterone that does not become attached to tissues is converted into androsterone and DHEA by the liver. These are conjugated with glucuronic or sulfuric acid and excreted in the bile or urine.

Anabolic Steroids

Anabolic steroids are synthetic drugs with increased anabolic activity and decreased androgenic activity compared with testosterone. They were developed during attempts to modify

Box 28-1 Effects of Testosterone on Body Tissues

Fetal Development

Large amounts of chorionic gonadotropin are produced by the placenta during pregnancy. Chorionic gonadotropin is similar to luteinizing hormone (LH) from the anterior pituitary gland. It promotes development of the interstitial or Leydig's cells in fetal testes, which then secrete testosterone. Testosterone production begins in the second month of fetal life. When present, testosterone promotes development of male sexual characteristics (eg, penis, scrotum, prostate gland, seminal vesicles, and seminiferous tubules), and suppresses development of female sexual characteristics. In the absence of testosterone, the fetus develops female sexual characteristics.

Testosterone also provides the stimulus for the descent of the testes into the scrotum. This normally occurs after the seventh month of pregnancy, when the fetal testes are secreting relatively large amounts of testosterone. If the testes do not descend before birth, administration of testosterone or gonadotropic hormone, which stimulates testosterone secretion, produces descent in most cases.

Adult Development

Little testosterone is secreted in boys until 11 to 13 years of age. At the onset of puberty, testosterone secretion increases rapidly and remains at a relatively high level until about 50 years of age, after which it gradually declines.

- The testosterone secreted at puberty acts as a growth hormone to produce enlargement of the penis, testes, and scrotum until approximately 20 years of age. The prostate gland, seminal vesicles, seminiferous tubules, and vas deferens also increase in size and functional ability. Under the combined influence of testosterone and follicle-stimulating hormone (FSH) from the ante-

rior pituitary gland, sperm production is initiated and maintained throughout the man's reproductive life.
- **Skin.** Testosterone increases skin thickness and activity of the sebaceous glands. Acne in the male adolescent is attributed to the increased production of testosterone.
- **Voice.** The larynx enlarges and deepens the voice of the adult man.
- **Hair.** Testosterone produces the distribution of hair growth on the face, limbs, and trunk typical of the adult man. In men with a genetic trait toward baldness, large amounts of testosterone cause alopecia (baldness) of the scalp.
- **Skeletal muscles.** Testosterone is largely responsible for the larger, more powerful muscles of men. This characteristic is caused by the effects of testosterone on protein metabolism. Testosterone helps the body retain nitrogen, form new amino acids, and build new muscle protein. At the same time, it slows the loss of nitrogen and amino acids formed by the constant breakdown of body tissues. Overall, testosterone increases protein anabolism (buildup) and decreases protein catabolism (breakdown).
- **Bone.** Testosterone makes bones thicker and longer. After puberty, more protein and calcium are deposited and retained in bone matrix. This causes a rapid rate of bone growth. The height of a male adolescent increases rapidly for a time, then stops as epiphyseal closure occurs. This happens when the cartilage at the end of the long bones in the arms and legs becomes bone. Further lengthening of the bones is then prevented.

Anterior Pituitary Function

High blood levels of testosterone decrease secretion of FSH and LH from the anterior pituitary gland. This, in turn, decreases testosterone production.

---

testosterone so that its tissue-building and growth-stimulating effects could be retained while its masculinizing effects could be eliminated or reduced.

Abuse of Androgen and Anabolic Steroid Drugs

Androgens and anabolic steroids are widely abused in attempts to enhance muscle development, muscle strength, and athletic performance. Because of their abuse potential, the drugs are Schedule III controlled substances. Although nonprescription sales of the drugs are illegal, they apparently are easily obtained.

Athletes are considered a high-risk group because some start taking the drugs in their early teenage years and continue for years. The number of teens taking anabolic steroids is thought to be small in comparison with the number using marijuana, amphetamines, and other illegal drugs. However, the number is also thought to be increasing, and long-term effects may be as bad as the effects that occur with use of other illegal drugs. Although steroids have a reputation for

being dangerous to adult athletes, such as body builders and football players, they are considered even more dangerous for teens because teens are still growing. Anabolic steroids can stop bone growth and damage the heart, kidneys, and liver of adolescents. In addition to those who take steroids to enhance athletic performance, some males take the drugs to produce a more muscular appearance and impress females. Steroid abusers usually take massive doses and often take several drugs or combine injectable and oral drugs for maximum effects. The large doses produce potentially serious adverse effects in several body tissues:

- **Cardiovascular disorders** include hypertension, decreased high-density blood lipoproteins (HDL) and increased low-density lipoproteins (LDL), all of which promote heart attacks and strokes.
- **Liver disorders** include benign and malignant neoplasms, cholestatic hepatitis and jaundice, and peliosis hepatis, a disorder in which blood-filled cysts develop in the liver and may lead to hemorrhage or liver failure.

- **Central nervous system disorders** include aggression, hostility, combativeness, and dependence characterized by preoccupation with drug use, inability to stop taking the drugs, and withdrawal symptoms similar to those that occur with alcohol, cocaine, and narcotics. In some cases, psychosis may develop.
- **Reproductive system disorders** include decreased testicular function (eg, decreased secretion of endogenous testosterone, decreased formation of sperm), testicular atrophy, and impotence in men. They include amenorrhea in women.
- **Metabolic disorders** include atherosclerosis-promoting changes in cholesterol metabolism and retention of fluids, with edema and other imbalances. Fluid and electrolyte retention contribute to the increased weight associated with drug use.
- **Dermatologic disorders** include moderate to severe acne in both sexes, depending on drug dosage.

Many of these adverse effects persist several months after the drugs are stopped and may be irreversible. Names of anabolic steroids include oxandrolone (Oxandrin), oxymetholone (Anadrol-50), and stanazolol (Winstrol).

GENERAL CHARACTERISTICS OF ANDROGENS AND ANABOLIC STEROIDS USED AS DRUGS

- When male sex hormones or androgens are given from exogenous sources for therapeutic purposes, they produce the same effects as the naturally occurring hormones. These effects include inhibition of endogenous sex hormones and sperm formation through negative feedback of pituitary luteinizing hormone (LH) and follicle-stimulating hormone (FSH).
- Male sex hormones given to women antagonize or reduce the effects of female sex hormones. Thus, administration of androgenic or anabolic steroids to women suppresses menstruation and causes atrophy of the endometrial lining of the uterus.
- Several dosage forms of androgens are available; they differ mainly in route of administration and pharmacokinetics.
  - Naturally occurring androgens are given by injection because they are metabolized rapidly by the liver if given orally. Some esters of testosterone have been modified to slow the rate of metabolism and thus prolong action. For example, intramuscular (IM) testosterone cypionate and testosterone enanthate have slow onsets of action and last 2 to 4 weeks.
  - Oral testosterone is extensively metabolized in its first pass through the liver, so that nearly half of a dose is lost before it reaches the systemic circulation. As a result, doses as high as 400 mg/day may be needed to produce adequate blood levels for full replacement therapy. Methyltestosterone is a synthetic formulation that is less extensively metabolized by the liver and more suitable for oral administration.
  - Several transdermal formulations of testosterone are available. They have a rapid onset of action and last approximately 24 hours. A topical gel (a 10-g dose delivers 100 mg) produces normal serum testosterone levels within 4 hours after application, and absorption of testosterone into the blood continues for 24 hours. Steady-state serum concentrations occur by the second or third day of use. When the gel is discontinued, serum testosterone levels remain in the normal range for 24 to 48 hours, but decrease to pretreatment levels within about 5 days.

    Androderm is applied to nonscrotal skin, and testosterone is continuously absorbed for 24 hours, with normal blood levels achieved during the first day of drug use. Applying the patch at night produces serum testosterone levels similar to those in healthy young men (ie, higher concentrations in the morning and lower ones in the evening).
  - Like endogenous testosterone, drug molecules are highly bound (98%) to plasma proteins and serum half-life varies (eg, 8 days for IM testosterone cypionate, 9 hours for oral fluoxymesterone). The drugs are inactivated primarily in the liver. About 90% of a dose is excreted in urine as conjugates of testosterone and its metabolites. About 6% of a dose is excreted in feces.
- Danazol is a synthetic drug with weak androgenic activity. It is given orally, has a half-life of 4 to 5 hours, and is metabolized in the liver. Route of excretion is unknown.
- All synthetic anabolic steroids are weak androgens. Consequently, giving these drugs for anabolic effects also produces masculinizing effects. This characteristic limits the clinical usefulness of these drugs in women and children. Profound changes in growth and sexual development may occur if these drugs are given to young children.

Mechanism of Action

Like other steroid drugs, androgenic and anabolic drugs penetrate the cell membrane and bind to receptor proteins in the cell cytoplasm. The steroid–receptor complex is then transported to the nucleus, where it activates RNA and DNA production and stimulates cellular synthesis of protein.

Indications for Use

With male sex hormones, the most clear-cut indication for use is to treat androgen deficiency states (eg, hypogonadism, cryptorchidism, impotence, oligospermia) in boys and men. Hypogonadism may result from hypothalamic–pituitary or testicular dysfunction. In prepubertal boys, administration of the drugs stimulates the development of masculine characteristics. In postpubertal men who become androgen deficient, the hormones re-establish and maintain masculine characteristics and functions.

In women, danazol (Danocrine) may be used to prevent or treat endometriosis or fibrocystic breast disease. Anabolic steroids are more often abused for body-building purposes than used for therapeutic effects.

Although some drug literature still lists metastatic breast cancer and some types of anemia as indications for use, androgens have largely been replaced by newer drugs for these purposes. In breast cancer, for example, androgens are second-line hormonal agents, after anti-estrogens (eg, tamoxifen). In anemia associated with renal failure, synthetic erythropoietin is more effective and likely to be used.

Contraindications to Use

Androgens and anabolic steroids are contraindicated during pregnancy (because of possible masculinizing effects on a female fetus); in clients with pre-existing liver disease; and in men with prostate-gland disorders. Men with an enlarged prostate may have additional enlargement, and men with prostatic cancer may experience tumor growth. Although not contraindicated in children, these drugs must be used very cautiously and with x-ray studies performed approximately every 6 months to evaluate bone growth.

INDIVIDUAL DRUGS

Clinical indications, routes, and dosage ranges are listed in Table 28-1.

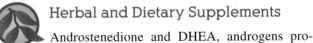

Herbal and Dietary Supplements

Androstenedione and DHEA, androgens produced by the adrenal cortex, are also available as over-the-counter (OTC) dietary supplements. They are marketed as safe, natural, alternative androgens for building muscles. These products, which have weak androgenic activity, act mainly as precursors for the production of sex hormones. Androstenedione, for example, may be converted to testosterone by way of an enzyme found in most body tissues. However, it may also be converted to estrogens and the testosterone that is produced may be further converted to estrogen (estradiol). In one study, young men

---

Table 28-1 Drugs at a Glance: Androgens

| GENERIC/TRADE NAME | ROUTES AND DOSAGE RANGES | |
	Hypogonadism	Other
Testosterone cypionate (Depo-Testosterone)	IM 50–200 mg every 2–4 wk	
Testosterone enanthate (Delatestryl)	IM 50–200 mg every 2–4 wk	
Testosterone gel (Androgel 1%)	5 g (50 mg of drug) once daily to skin of shoulders and upper arms or abdomen	
Testosterone pellets	Sub-Q 150–450 mg every 3–6 mo	*Delayed puberty:* Sub-Q lower dosage range, for a limited duration (eg, every 3 mo for 2–3 doses)
Testosterone transdermal systems (Androderm)	Apply 2 Androderm systems (dose of 5 mg) nightly to back, abdomen, upper arm, or thigh	
Testolactone (Teslac)		*Breast cancer:* PO 250 mg 4 times daily
Fluoxymesterone (Halotestin)	PO 5–20 mg daily	
Methyltestosterone (Android, Testred)		*Cryptorchidism:* PO 30 mg daily; buccal tablets, 15 mg daily
Danazol		*Endometriosis:* PO 800 mg daily in 2 divided doses for 3–9 mo
		Fibrocystic breast disease: PO 100–400 mg daily in 2 divided doses for 3–6 mo

IM, intramuscular; PO, oral; Sub-Q, subcutaneous.

with normal serum testosterone levels were given an androstenedione supplement for 8 weeks. The researchers found little effect on serum testosterone levels or muscle development with resistance training. They also found increased serum levels of estrone and estradiol, which indicate that a significant proportion of the androstenedione was converted to estrogens. Thus, taking a supplement for masculinizing effects may produce feminizing effects instead.

DHEA is available alone as oral capsules or tablets and in a topical cream with vitamins and herbs. Most DHEA products of plant origin are produced in Europe and China. They are marketed with numerous claims for health benefits, including inhibition of aging, atherosclerosis, cancer, diabetes mellitus, and osteoporosis. Most claims stem from laboratory and animal studies. A few small human studies have been done, most of which used a dose of 50 milligrams daily. Overall, there is no conclusive evidence that DHEA supplementation will prevent or treat such conditions. In addition, long-term effects in humans are unknown.

DHEA is contraindicated in men with prostate cancer or benign prostatic hypertrophy (BPH) and in women with estrogen-responsive breast or uterine cancer, because DHEA may stimulate growth of these tissues. Clients older than 40 years of age should be aggressively screened for hormonally sensitive cancers before taking DHEA.

Adverse effects of DHEA include aggressiveness, hirsutism, insomnia, and irritability. Whether large doses of the OTC products can produce some of the serious adverse effects associated with standard anabolic steroids is unknown.

NURSING PROCESS

Assessment

Before drug therapy is started, clients need a thorough history and physical examination. Periodic monitoring of the client's condition is needed throughout drug therapy.

- Assess for conditions in which androgens are used (eg, deficiency states).
- Assess for conditions that increase risks of adverse effects or are contraindications (eg, pregnancy, liver disease, prostatic hypertrophy).
- Check laboratory reports of liver function tests (the drugs may cause cholestatic jaundice and liver damage), serum electrolyte levels (the drugs may cause sodium and water retention), and serum lipid levels (the drugs may increase levels and aggravate atherosclerosis).
- Assess weight and blood pressure regularly. These may be elevated by retention of sodium and water with resultant edema, especially in clients with congestive heart failure.

- For children, check x-ray examination reports of bone growth status initially and approximately every 6 months while the drugs are being taken.
- Assess the client's attitude toward taking male sex hormones.
- Assess the client's willingness to comply with instructions for taking the drugs and follow-up procedures.

Nursing Diagnoses

- Disturbed Body Image related to masculinizing effects and menstrual irregularities
- Deficient Knowledge: Physiologic and psychological consequences of overuse and abuse of the drugs to enhance athletic performance
- Noncompliance: Overuse of drugs or dietary supplements
- Risk for Injury: Liver disease and other serious adverse drug effects

Planning/Goals

The client will
- Use the drugs for medical purposes only
- Receive or take the drugs as prescribed
- Avoid abuse of drugs or dietary supplements for body building
- Be counseled regarding effects of overuse and abuse if identified as being at risk (eg, athletes, especially weight lifters and football players)
- Avoid preventable adverse drug effects
- Comply with monitoring and follow-up procedures

Interventions

- Assist clients to use the drug correctly (see accompanying client teaching display).
- Assist clients to reduce sodium intake if edema develops.
- Record weight and blood pressure at regular intervals.
- Participate in school or community programs to inform children, parents, coaches, athletic trainers, and others of the risks of inappropriate use of androgens, anabolic steroids, and related dietary supplements.

Evaluation

- Interview and observe for compliance with instructions for taking prescribed drugs.
- Interview and observe for therapeutic and adverse drug effects.
- Question athletes about illegal use of the drugs.
- Observe athletes for increased weight and behavioral changes that may indicate drug abuse.

CLIENT TEACHING GUIDELINES

Androgens

General Considerations

✔ Take the drugs only if prescribed and as prescribed. Use by athletes for body building is inappropriate and, if not prescribed by a licensed prescriber, is illegal.

✔ Continue medical supervision as long as the drugs are being taken.

✔ Weigh once or twice weekly and record the amount. An increase may indicate fluid retention and edema.

✔ Practice frequent and thorough skin cleansing to decrease acne, which is most likely to occur in women and children.

Self-Administration

✔ Take oral preparations before or with meals, in divided doses.

✔ For buccal preparations:

✔ Take in divided doses.

✔ Place the tablet between the cheek and gum and allow to dissolve (do not swallow).

✔ Avoid eating, drinking, or smoking while the tablet is in place.

✔ With transdermal systems:

✔ Apply 2 Androderm systems nightly to clean, dry skin on back, abdomen, upper arm, or thigh. Do not apply to scrotum. Rotate sites, with 7 days between applications to a site. Press firmly into place for adherence.

✔ Apply the prescribed amount of gel to clean, dry, intact skin of the shoulders and upper arms or the abdomen (do **not** apply to the genital area), once daily, preferably in the morning. Wash hands after application and allow sites to dry before dressing. After application, wait at least 1 hour and preferably 4 to 6 hours before showering or swimming.

APPLYING YOUR KNOWLEDGE 28-1

You are counseling Ms. Watson. What teaching points do you cover?

PRINCIPLES OF THERAPY

Duration of Therapy

Drug therapy with androgens may be short or long term, depending on the condition in question, the client's response to treatment, and the incidence of adverse reactions. If feasible, intermittent rather than continuous therapy is recommended.

Effects of Androgens and Anabolic Steroids on Other Drugs

Androgens may increase effects of cyclosporine and warfarin, apparently by slowing their metabolism and increasing their concentrations in the blood. These combinations should be avoided if possible. However, if required, serum creatinine and cyclosporine levels should be monitored with cyclosporine and prothrombin time or international normalized ratio (INR) with warfarin.

Androgens also increase effects of sulfonylurea antidiabetic drugs. Concurrent use should be avoided if possible. If required, smaller doses of sulfonylureas may be needed, blood glucose levels should be monitored closely, and clients should be assessed for signs of hypoglycemia. Danazol inhibits metabolism of carbamazepine and increases risks of toxicity. Concurrent use should be avoided.

APPLYING YOUR KNOWLEDGE 28-2

You are assessing Ms. Watson for adverse effects of her danazol. What signs and symptoms do you assess?

Use in Special Populations

Use in Children

The main indication for use of androgens is for boys with established deficiency states. Because the drugs cause epiphyseal closure, hands and wrists should undergo x-ray examination every 6 months to detect bone maturation and prevent loss of adult height. Stimulation of skeletal growth continues for approximately 6 months after drug therapy is stopped. If premature puberty occurs (precocious sexual development, enlarged penis), the drug should be stopped. The drugs may cause or aggravate acne. Scrupulous skin care and other anti-acne treatment may be needed, especially in adolescent boys.

Use in Older Adults

The main indication for use of androgens is a deficiency state in men. Older adults often have hypertension and other cardiovascular disorders that may be aggravated by the sodium and water retention associated with androgens and anabolic steroids. In men, the drugs may increase prostate size and interfere with urination; increase risk of prostatic cancer; and cause excessive sexual stimulation and priapism.

Use in Clients With Hepatic Impairment

Androgens and anabolic steroids are contraindicated in clients with pre-existing liver disease. Prolonged use of high doses may cause potentially life-threatening conditions such as peliosis hepatis, hepatic neoplasms, and hepatocellular carcinoma. In addition, androgen therapy should be discontinued if cholestatic hepatitis with jaundice occurs, or if liver function tests become abnormal. Drug-induced jaundice is reversible when the medication is stopped.

APPLYING YOUR KNOWLEDGE 28-3

Ms. Watson's brother is visiting from out of town. Warren Watson is a 27-year-old body builder. He has an 11-year history of abusing a variety of anabolic steroids. Ms. Watson is worried about him and convinces him to come to the clinic for a checkup.

At the clinic, Mr. Watson states that he takes no medication. You measure his blood pressure to be 180/94 mm Hg. Mr. Watson says he has "white-coat syndrome" and that his blood pressure is never elevated except at the office. When approached about his high blood pressure, he refuses to be treated. What is your nursing responsibility?

N U R S I N G   A C T I O N S

Androgens and Anabolic Steroids

NURSING ACTIONS	RATIONALE/EXPLANATION
1. Administer accurately	
a. Give intramuscular preparations of testosterone, other androgens. and anabolic steroids deeply, preferably in the gluteal muscle.	
b. Give oral preparations before or with meals, in divided doses.	To decrease gastrointestinal disturbances
c. For buccal preparations:	
(1) Give in divided doses.	
(2) Place the tablet between the cheek and gum.	Buccal preparations must be absorbed through the mucous membranes.
(3) Instruct the client not to swallow the tablet and not to drink, chew, or smoke until the tablet is completely absorbed.	
d. With transdermal systems:	Correct site selection and application are necessary for therapeutic effects. Scrotal skin is more permeable to testosterone than other skin areas.
(1) Apply 2 Androderm systems nightly to clean, dry skin on back, abdomen, upper arm, or thigh. Do *not* apply to scrotum. Rotate sites, with 7 days between applications to a site. Press firmly into place for adherence.	
(2) Apply Androgel 1% to shoulders and upper arms or abdomen, once daily, preferably in the morning.	Manufacturer's recommendation. Clients may prefer self-application. Skin should be clean, dry, and intact; hands should be washed after application; and showering and swimming should be avoided for at least 1 hour and preferably 4 to 6 hours after application.
e. Inject testosterone pellets (Testopel) subcutaneously.	Manufacturer's recommendation
2. Observe for therapeutic effects	
a. When the drug is given for hypogonadism, observe for masculinizing effects, such as growth of sexual organs, deepening of voice, growth of body hair, and acne.	
b. When the drug is given for anabolic effects, observe for increased appetite, euphoria, or statements of feeling better.	
3. Observe for adverse reactions	
a. Virilism or masculinizing effects:	
(1) In adult men with adequate secretion of testosterone—priapism, increased sexual desire, reduced sperm count, and prostate enlargement	

(continued)

NURSING ACTIONS	RATIONALE/EXPLANATION
(2) In prepubertal boys—premature development of sex organs and secondary sexual characteristics, such as enlargement of the penis, priapism, pubic hair	
(3) In women—masculinizing effects include hirsutism, deepening of the voice, menstrual irregularities	
b. Jaundice—dark urine, yellow skin and sclera, itching	
c. Edema	More likely in clients who are elderly or who have heart or kidney disease
d. Hypercalcemia	More likely in women with advanced breast cancer
e. Difficulty voiding due to prostate enlargement	More likely in middle-aged or elderly men
f. Inadequate growth in height of children	
4. Observe for drug interactions	
a. Drugs that *decrease* effects of androgens:	
(1) Barbiturates	Increase enzyme induction and rate of metabolism
(2) Calcitonin	Decreases calcium retention and thus antagonizes calcium-retaining effects of androgens

APPLYING YOUR KNOWLEDGE: ANSWERS

28-1 Teach Ms. Watson to weigh herself and to have her blood pressure assessed regularly. She should call her physician immediately if she becomes pregnant.

28-2 Assess for hirsutism, deepening of the voice, and menstrual irregularities.

28-3 You have an obligation to explain the health risks of untreated hypertension. Client teaching guidelines would include discussing health habits that may be contributing to the problem.

Review and Application Exercises

Short Answer Exercises

1. How does testosterone promote development of male sexual characteristics?

2. What is the major clinical indication for therapeutic use of testosterone and related androgens?

3. What is the difference between androgenic activity and anabolic activity?

4. What are the adverse effects of using large doses of anabolic steroids in body-building efforts?

5. If your 14-year-old brother said some friends were telling him to take drugs to increase muscle development and athletic ability, how would you reply? Justify your answer.

NCLEX-Style Questions

6. The most clear-cut therapeutic indication for use of male sex hormones is
   a. to treat androgen deficiency states in boys and men
   b. for body-building purposes
   c. to treat metastatic breast cancer
   d. to treat anemia associated with renal failure

7. Four clients in an endocrine clinic are ordered to begin androgen therapy. The nurse reviews each client's current medications and identifies which client as able to begin androgen therapy without the risk of a known drug interaction?
   a. client 1, taking cyclosporine
   b. client 2, taking warfarin
   c. client 3, taking sulfonylureas
   d. client 4, taking heparin

8. What percentage of testosterone secreted by the testes binds to plasma albumin or to sex hormone–binding globulin and circulates in the blood?
   a. 26%
   b. 49%

c. 78%

d. 97%

9. A 19-year-old female athlete presents for her first prenatal visit and tells the nurse that she has been on androgen therapy to improve her distance running. She asks the nurse if she can continue taking the androgens to maintain her "competitive edge." The nurse should instruct the client that
   a. She can continue taking androgens, because the drugs pose no risk to the fetus.
   b. She can continue taking androgens, but a higher dose will be required due to increased drug metabolism during pregnancy.
   c. She can continue taking androgens until the third trimester, when they must be discontinued because androgens cause an increased risk of premature rupture of membranes.
   d. She must stop taking androgens immediately, because they pose a risk to the fetus; she should discuss this with her health care provider at today's visit.

10. Which of the following statements by a male client taking transdermal androgens indicates that further teaching is necessary?

a. "I need to weigh myself once or twice weekly and record the amount."

b. "I should wash my face and body thoroughly to decrease the risk of acne."

c. "The patch systems should be applied nightly to skin on my back, abdomen, upper arm, or thigh."

d. "I should apply the patch systems in the morning to the same site each and every day."

Selected References

Drug facts and comparisons. (Updated monthly). St. Louis: Facts and Comparisons.

Gooren, L. J. G., & Bunck, M. C. M. (2004). Androgen replacement therapy: Present and future. *Drugs, 64*(17), 1861–1891.

Guyton, A. C., & Hall, J. E. (2000). *Textbook of medical physiology* (10th ed.). Philadelphia: W. B. Saunders.

Lacy, C. F., Armstrong, L. L., Goldman, M. P., Lance, L. L. (2004). *Lexi-Comp's drug information handbook* (12th ed.). Hudson, OH: Lexi-Comp.

Porth, C. M. (2005). *Pathophysiology: Concepts of altered health states* (7th ed.). Philadelphia: Lippincott Williams & Wilkins.

Snyder, P. J. (2000). Disorders of gonadal function in men. In H. D. Humes (Ed.), *Kelley's Textbook of internal medicine* (4th ed., pp. 2743–2750). Philadelphia: Lippincott Williams & Wilkins.

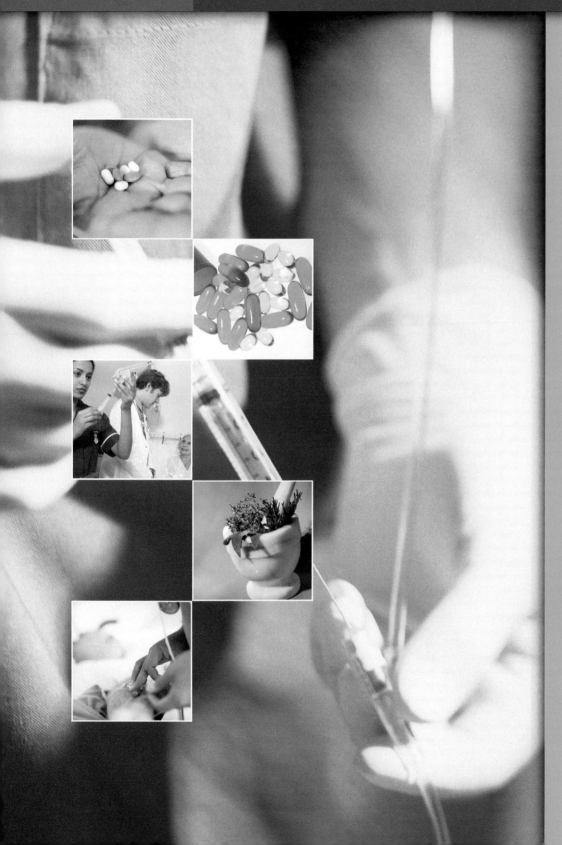

SECTION 5

Drugs Used to Treat Infections

CHAPTER OUTLINE

29 General Characteristics of Antimicrobial Drugs

30 Beta-Lactam Antibacterials: Penicillins, Cephalosporins, and Other Drugs

31 Aminoglycosides and Fluoroquinolones

32 Tetracyclines, Sulfonamides, and Urinary Agents

33 Macrolides, Ketolides, and Miscellaneous Antibacterials

34 Drugs for Tuberculosis and *Mycobacterium avium* Complex (MAC) Disease

35 Antiviral Drugs

36 Antifungal Drugs

37 Antiparasitics

General Characteristics of Antimicrobial Drugs

OBJECTIVES

After studying this chapter, you will be able to:

1. Identify populations who have an increased risk of infection.
2. Discuss common pathogens and methods of infection control.
3. Assess clients for local and systemic signs of infection.
4. Discuss common and potentially serious adverse effects of antimicrobial drugs.
5. Identify clients at increased risk for adverse drug reactions.
6. Discuss ways to increase benefits and decrease hazards of antimicrobial drug therapy.
7. Discuss ways to minimize emergence of drug-resistant microorganisms.
8. State appropriate nursing implications for a client receiving an antimicrobial drug.
9. Discuss important elements of using antimicrobial drugs in children, older adults, clients with renal or hepatic impairment, and clients with critical illness.

APPLYING YOUR KNOWLEDGE

Rosalie Kurth is a 72-year-old grandmother and retired factory worker. Her work in a dusty environment has led her to have chronic bronchitis. She has been treated multiple times over the years with antibiotic drugs for recurrent infections. Ms. Kurth cares for her two grandchildren, ages 3 and 5, while their mother works. Ms. Kurth's exposure to the multiple infective organisms of childhood has resulted in more frequent infections and the need for antibiotics.

INTRODUCTION

Antimicrobial drugs are used to prevent or treat infections caused by pathogenic (disease-producing) microorganisms. The human body and the environment contain many microorganisms, most of which live in a state of balance with the human host and do not cause disease. When the balance is upset and infection occurs, characteristics of the infecting microorganism(s) and the adequacy of host defense mechanisms are major factors in the severity of the infection and the person's ability to recover. Conditions that impair defense mechanisms increase the incidence and severity of infections and impede recovery. In addition, use of antimicrobial drugs may lead to serious infections caused by drug-resistant microorganisms. To help prevent infectious diseases and participate effectively in antimicrobial drug therapy, the nurse must be knowledgeable about microorganisms, host responses to microorganisms, and antimicrobial drugs.

MICROORGANISMS AND INFECTIONS

In an infection, microorganisms initially attach to host cell receptors (ie, proteins, carbohydrates, lipids). For example, some bacteria have hairlike structures that attach them to skin and mucous membranes. Most microorganisms preferentially attach themselves to particular body tissues. The microorganisms may then invade tissues, multiply, and produce infection. A major characteristic of microorganisms is their ability to survive in various environments. Bacteria, for example, may form mutant strains, alter their structures and functions, or become embedded in a layer of mucus. These adaptations help protect them from normal body defense mechanisms and antimicrobial drugs. Drug-resistant bacterial strains can be produced in the presence of antimicrobial drugs. Classifications, normal microbial flora, and common pathogenic microorganisms are described in the following sections.

Classifications

Bacteria are subclassified according to whether they are aerobic (require oxygen) or anaerobic (cannot live in the presence of oxygen), their reaction to Gram's stain (gram positive or gram negative), and their shape (eg, cocci, bacilli).

Viruses are intracellular parasites that survive only in living tissues. They are officially classified according to their structure, but are more commonly described according to origin and the disorders or symptoms they produce. Human pathogens include adenoviruses, herpesviruses, and retroviruses (see Chap. 35).

Fungi are plant-like organisms that live as parasites on living tissue or as saprophytes on decaying organic matter. Approximately 50 species are pathogenic in humans (see Chap. 36).

Normal Microbial Flora

The human body normally has areas that are sterile and areas that are colonized with microorganisms. Sterile areas are body fluids and cavities, the lower respiratory tract (trachea, bronchi, lungs), much of the gastrointestinal (GI) and genitourinary tracts, and the musculoskeletal system. Colonized areas include the skin, upper respiratory tract, and colon.

Normal skin flora includes staphylococci, streptococci, diphtheroids, and transient environmental organisms. The upper respiratory tract contains staphylococci, streptococci, pneumococci, diphtheroids, and *Haemophilus influenzae.* The external genitalia contain skin organisms; the vagina contains lactobacilli, *Candida,* and *Bacteroides.* The colon contains *Escherichia coli, Klebsiella, Enterobacter, Proteus, Pseudomonas, Bacteroides,* clostridia, lactobacilli, streptococci, and staphylococci. Microorganisms that are part of the normal flora and nonpathogenic in one area of the body may be pathogenic in other parts of the body; for example, *E. coli* often cause urinary tract infections.

Normal flora protects the human host by occupying space and consuming nutrients. This interferes with the ability of potential pathogens to establish residence and proliferate. If the normal flora is suppressed by antimicrobial drug therapy, potential pathogens may thrive. For example, the yeast *Candida albicans* is a normal resident of the vagina and the intestinal tract. An antibacterial drug may destroy the normal bacterial flora without affecting the fungal organism. As a result, *C. albicans* can proliferate and cause infection. Much of the normal flora can cause disease under certain conditions, especially in elderly, debilitated, or immunosuppressed people. Normal bowel flora also synthesizes vitamin K and vitamin B complex.

Infectious Diseases

Colonization involves the presence of normal microbial flora or transient environmental organisms that do not harm the host. Infectious disease involves the presence of a pathogen plus clinical signs and symptoms indicative of an infection.

These microorganisms are usually spread by direct contact with an infected person or contaminated hands, food, water, or objects. Box 29-1 describes common bacterial pathogens of humans. Accurate assessment and documentation of symptoms can aid diagnosis of infectious diseases.

Opportunistic Pathogens

Opportunistic microorganisms are usually normal endogenous or environmental flora and nonpathogenic. However, they become pathogens in hosts whose defense mechanisms are impaired. Opportunistic infections are likely to occur in people with severe burns, cancer, human immunodeficiency virus (HIV) infection, indwelling intravenous (IV) or urinary catheters, and antibiotic or corticosteroid drug therapy. Opportunistic bacterial infections, often caused by drug-resistant microorganisms, are usually serious and may be life threatening. Fungi of the *Candida* genus, especially *C. albicans,* may cause life-threatening bloodstream or deep-tissue infections, such as abdominal abscesses. Viral infections may cause fatal pneumonia in people with renal or cardiac disorders; in those with HIV infection; and in those who have received bone marrow transplants.

Laboratory Identification of Pathogens

Laboratory tests of infected fluids or tissues can identify probable pathogens. Bacteria can be identified based on Gram's stain and culture. *Gram's stain* identifies microscopic appearance, including shape and color of the organisms. *Culture* involves growing a microorganism in the laboratory. Growth on selective culture media characterizes color, shape, and texture of the growing colonies. Identification of other microorganisms (eg, intracellular pathogens such as chlamydiae and viruses) may require different techniques. *Serology* identifies infectious agents indirectly by measuring the antibody level (titer) in the serum of a diseased host. A tentative diagnosis can be made if the antibody level against a specific pathogen rises during the acute phase of the disease and falls during convalescence. *Detection of antigens* uses features of culture and serology but reduces the time required for diagnosis. Another technique to identify an organism involves polymerase chain reaction (PCR), which can detect whether *DNA* for a specific organism is present in a sample.

Community-Acquired Versus Nosocomial Infections

Infections are often categorized as community-acquired or nosocomial. Because the microbial environments differ, the two types of infections often have different causes and require different antimicrobial drugs. As a general rule, community-acquired infections are less severe and easier to treat, although drug-resistant strains are increasing (eg, methicillin-resistant

Box 29-1 Common Bacterial Pathogens

Gram-Positive Bacteria

Staphylococci

Staphylococcus aureus organisms are part of the normal microbial flora of the skin and upper respiratory tract and also are common pathogens. Some people carry (are colonized with) the organism in the anterior nares. The organisms are spread mainly by direct contact with people who are infected or who are carriers. The hands of health care workers are considered a major source of indirect spread and nosocomial infections. The organisms also survive on inanimate surfaces for long periods of time.

S. aureus organisms cause boils, carbuncles, burn and surgical-wound infections, and internal abscesses. Burns or surgical wounds often become infected from clients' own nasal carriage or from health care personnel. The organisms cannot penetrate intact skin or mucous membranes. However, they can penetrate damaged tissues and produce endotoxins that destroy erythrocytes, leukocytes, platelets, fibroblasts, and other human cells. Also, many strains produce enterotoxins that cause food poisoning when ingested. The enterotoxins survive heating at temperatures high enough to kill the organisms, so reheating foods does not prevent food poisoning.

High-risk groups for staphylococcal infections include newborns, the elderly, and those who are malnourished, have diabetes, or are obese. In children, staphylococcal infections of the respiratory tract are most common in those younger than 2 years of age. In adults, staphylococcal pneumonia often occurs in people with chronic lung disease or as a secondary bacterial infection after influenza. The influenza virus destroys the ciliated epithelium of the respiratory tract and thereby aids bacterial invasion.

Staphylococcus species, non-*aureus* (SSNA) describes a group of organisms that are also part of the normal microbial flora of the skin and mucosal surfaces and are increasingly common pathogens. The most common member of this group involved in infections is *Staphylococcus epidermidis*. However, not all laboratories routinely further identify the specific organism when SSNA is identified, and microbiology laboratory reports may just report SSNA. For this discussion, we will use the term *SSNA* unless a specific reference needs to be made to *S. epidermidis*.

Infections due to SSNA are associated with the use of treatment devices such as intravascular catheters, prosthetic heart valves, cardiac pacemakers, orthopedic prostheses, cerebrospinal fluid shunts, and peritoneal catheters. SSNA infections include endocarditis, bacteremia, and other serious infections and are especially hazardous to neutropenic and immunocompromised clients. Treatment usually requires removal of any infected medical device as well as appropriate antibiotic therapy.

Streptococci

Certain streptococci are part of the normal microbial flora of the throat and nasopharynx in many healthy people. Infections are usually spread by inhalation of droplets from the upper respiratory tract of carriers or people with infections. However, these organisms do not cause disease unless the mucosal barrier is damaged by trauma, previous infection, or surgical manipulation. Such damage allows the organisms to enter the bloodstream and gain access to other parts of the body. For example, the organisms may cause endocarditis if they reach damaged heart valves.

Streptococcus pneumoniae organisms, often called *pneumococci,* are common bacterial pathogens. They cause pneumonia, sinusitis, otitis media, and meningitis. Pneumococcal pneumonia usually develops when the mechanisms that normally expel organisms inhaled into the lower airway (ie, the mucociliary blanket and cough reflex) are impaired by viral infection, smoking, immobility, or other insults. When *S. pneumoniae* reach the alveoli, they proliferate, cause acute inflammation, and spread rapidly to involve one or more lobes. Alveoli fill with proteinaceous fluid, neutrophils, and bacteria. When the pneumonia resolves, there is usually no residual damage to the pulmonary parenchyma. Older adults have high rates of illness and death from pneumococcal pneumonia, which can often be prevented by pneumococcal vaccine. Pneumococcal vaccine (see Chap. 39) contains 23 strains of the pneumococci that cause most of the serious infections.

Pneumococcal sinusitis and otitis media usually follow a viral illness, such as the common cold. The viral infection injures the protective ciliated epithelium and fills the air spaces with nutrient-rich tissue fluid, in which the pneumococci thrive. *S. pneumoniae* is a common pathogen in bacterial sinusitis. In young children, upper respiratory tract infections may be complicated by acute sinusitis. With otitis media, most children have repeated episodes by 6 years of age and the pneumococcus causes approximately half of these cases. Recurrent otitis media during early childhood may result in reduced hearing acuity. Otitis media rarely occurs in adults.

Pneumococcal meningitis may develop from sinus or middle ear infections or an injury that allows organisms from the nasopharynx to enter the meninges. *S. pneumoniae* infection is a common cause of bacterial meningitis in adults. Other potential secondary complications include septicemia, endocarditis, pericarditis, and empyema.

Susceptible pneumococcal infections may be treated with penicillin G. For people who are allergic to penicillin, a cephalosporin or a macrolide may be effective. *S. pneumoniae* organisms are developing resistance such that empiric treatment must be based on the likelihood of multidrug-resistant *S. pneumoniae* (MDRSP). Rates of MDRSP vary by locale; if high, the organisms will be resistant to penicillin and also cross-resistant to other alternatives such as second- and third-generation cephalosporins and possibly macrolides. Alternatives include fluoroquinolones, vancomycin, telithromycin, or high doses of amoxicillin/clavulanate. Empiric treatment of meningitis where *S. pneumoniae* is known or suspected should include a third-generation cephalosporin (ceftriaxone or cefotaxime) plus vancomycin. Empiric treatment for pneumonia should include a fluoroquinolone or a macrolide in those areas with high penicillin and cephalosporin resistance rates.

(continued)

Box 29-1 Common Bacterial Pathogens (continued)

Streptococcus pyogenes (beta-hemolytic streptococcus) organisms are often part of the normal flora of the skin and oropharynx. The organisms spread from person to person by direct contact with oral or respiratory secretions. They cause severe pharyngitis ("strep throat"), scarlet fever, rheumatic fever, and endocarditis. With streptococcal pharyngitis, people remain infected with the organism for weeks after symptoms resolve and thus serve as a reservoir for infection.

Enterococci

Enterococci are normal flora in the human intestine but are also found in soil, food, water, and animals. Although the genus *Enterococcus* contains approximately 12 species, the main pathogens are *Enterococcus faecalis* and *Enterococcus faecium.* Most enterococcal infections occur in hospitalized clients, especially those in critical care units. Risk factors for nosocomial infections include serious underlying disease, prior surgery, renal impairment, and the presence of urinary or vascular catheters. These organisms, especially *E. faecalis,* are usually secondary invaders in urinary tract or wound infections. Enterococci may also cause endocarditis. This serious infection occurs most often in people with underlying heart disease, such as an injured valve. When the organisms reach a heart valve, they multiply and release emboli of foreign particles into the bloodstream. Symptoms of endocarditis include fever, heart murmurs, enlarged spleen, and anemia. This infection is diagnosed by isolating enterococci from blood cultures. If not treated promptly and appropriately, often with ampicillin and gentamicin, enterococcal endocarditis may be fatal. Antimicrobial resistance is increasing among the enterococci, as it is among other gram-positive bacteria.

Gram-Negative Bacteria

Bacteroides

Bacteroides are anaerobic bacteria normally found in the digestive, respiratory, and genital tracts. They are the most common bacteria in the colon, where they greatly outnumber *Escherichia coli. Bacteroides fragilis,* the major human pathogen, causes intra-abdominal and pelvic abscesses (eg, after surgery or trauma that allows fecal contamination of these tissues), brain abscesses (eg, from bacteremia or spread from a middle-ear or sinus infection), and bacteremia, which may spread the organisms throughout the body.

Escherichia coli

E. coli inhabit the intestinal tract of humans. They are normally nonpathogenic in the intestinal tract but are common pathogens in other parts of the body. They may be beneficial by synthesizing vitamins and by competitively discouraging growth of potential pathogens.

E. coli cause most urinary tract infections. They also cause pneumonia and sepsis in immunocompromised hosts and meningitis and sepsis in newborns. *E. coli* pneumonia often occurs in debilitated clients after colonization of the oropharynx with organisms from their endogenous microbial flora. In healthy people, the normal gram-positive organisms of oral cavities attach to material that coats the surface of oral mucosa and prevents transient *E. coli* from establishing residence. Debili-

tated or severely ill people produce an enzyme that destroys the material that allows gram-positive flora to adhere to oral mucosa. This allows *E. coli* (and other gram-negative enteric bacteria) to compete successfully with the normal gram-positive flora and colonize the oropharynx. Then, droplets of the oral flora are aspirated into the respiratory tract, where impaired protective mechanisms allow survival of the aspirated organisms.

E. coli also cause enteric gram-negative sepsis, which is acquired from the normal enteric bacterial flora. When *E. coli* and other enteric organisms reach the bloodstream of healthy people, host defenses eliminate the organisms. When the organisms reach the bloodstream of people with severe illnesses and conditions such as neutropenia, the host is unable to mount adequate defenses and sepsis occurs. In newborns, *E. coli* are the most common gram-negative organisms causing nosocomial septic shock and meningitis.

In addition, *E. coli* often cause diarrhea and dysentery. One strain, called *O157:H7,* causes hemorrhagic colitis, a disease characterized by severe abdominal cramps, copious bloody diarrhea, and hemolytic-uremic syndrome (hemolytic anemia, thrombocytopenia, and acute renal failure). Hemolytic-uremic syndrome occurs most often in children. The main reservoir of this strain is the intestinal tract of animals, especially cattle, and several epidemics have been associated with ingestion of undercooked ground beef. Other sources include contaminated water and milk and person-to-person spread. Because it cannot survive in nature, the presence of *E. coli* in milk or water indicates fecal contamination.

Treatment of *E. coli* infections is complicated by increasing resistance to cephalosporins, commonly used agents. Resistance is mediated by production of extended-spectrum beta-lactamases, which inactivates the antibiotic. Effective treatments may include aminoglycosides, fluoroquinolones, or trimethoprim-sulfamethoxazole.

Klebsiella

Klebsiella organisms, which are normal bowel flora, may infect the respiratory tract, urinary tract, bloodstream, burn wounds, and meninges, most often as opportunistic infections in debilitated persons. *Klebsiella pneumoniae* are a common cause of pneumonia, especially in people with pulmonary disease, bacteremia, and sepsis.

Proteus

Proteus organisms are normally found in the intestinal tract and in decaying matter. They most often cause urinary tract and wound infections but may infect any tissue, especially in debilitated people. Infection usually occurs with antibiotic therapy, which decreases drug-sensitive bacteria and allows drug-resistant bacteria to proliferate.

Pseudomonas

Pseudomonas organisms are found in water, soil, skin, and intestines. They are found in the stools of some healthy people and possibly 50% of inpatients. *Pseudomonas aeruginosa,* the species most often associated with human disease, can cause infections of the respiratory tract, urinary tract, wounds, burns,

Box 29-1 Common Bacterial Pathogens (continued)

meninges, eyes, and ears. Because of its resistance to many antibiotics, it can cause severe infections in people receiving antibiotic therapy for burns, wounds, and cystic fibrosis. *P. aeruginosa* colonizes the respiratory tract of most clients with cystic fibrosis and infects approximately 25% of burn clients. Infection is more likely to occur in hosts who are very young or very old or who have an impaired immune system. Sources of infection include catheterization of the urinary tract, trauma or procedures involving the brain or spinal cord, and contamination of respiratory ventilators.

Serratia

Serratia marcescens organisms are found in infected people, water, milk, feces, and soil. They cause serious nosocomial infections of the urinary tract, respiratory tract, skin, burn wounds, and bloodstream. They also may cause hospital epidemics and produce drug-resistant strains. High-risk clients include newborns, the debilitated, and the immunosuppressed.

Salmonella

Approximately 1400 *Salmonella* species have been identified; several are pathogenic to humans. The organisms cause gastro-

enteritis, typhoid fever, septicemia, and a severe, sometimes fatal type of food poisoning. The primary reservoir is the intestinal tract of many animals. Humans become infected through ingestion of contaminated water or food. Water becomes polluted by introduction of feces from any animal excreting salmonellae. Infection via food usually results from ingestion of contaminated meat or by hands transferring organisms from an infected source. In the United States, under-cooked poultry and eggs are common sources.

Salmonella enterocolitis is a common cause of foodborne outbreaks of gastroenteritis. Diarrhea usually begins several hours after ingesting contaminated food and may continue for several days, along with nausea, vomiting, headache, and abdominal pain.

Shigella

Shigella species cause gastrointestinal problems ranging from mild diarrhea to severe bacillary dysentery. Humans, who seem to be the only natural hosts, become infected after ingestion of contaminated food or water. Effects of shigellosis are attributed to loss of fluids, electrolytes, and nutrients and to the ulceration that occurs in the colon wall.

Staphylococcus aureus [MRSA]). Nosocomial infections may be more severe and difficult to manage because they often result from drug-resistant microorganisms and occur in people whose resistance to disease is impaired. Drug-resistant strains of staphylococci, *Pseudomonas,* and *Proteus* are common causes of nosocomial infections.

Antibiotic-Resistant Microorganisms

The increasing prevalence of bacteria resistant to the effects of antibiotic drugs is a major public health concern (Box 29-2). Antibiotic resistance occurs in most human pathogens. Infections caused by drug-resistant organisms often require more toxic and expensive drugs, lead to prolonged illness or hospitalization, and increase mortality rates.

Resistant microorganisms grow and multiply when susceptible organisms (eg, normal flora) are suppressed by antimicrobial drugs or when normal body defenses are impaired by immunosuppressive disorders or drugs. They may emerge during or after antimicrobial drug therapy. Contributing factors include:

- **Widespread use of antimicrobial drugs, especially broad-spectrum agents.** Antibiotics affect the bacteria for which they are prescribed, transient organisms, other pathogens, and normal flora. When the normal flora is suppressed, space and nutrients become available to support the growth of organisms resistant to the effects of that antibiotic. The resistant organisms soon become the predominant strain. After they are established, resistant

bacteria can cause superinfection in the original host, spread to other hosts, and even spread their resistance properties for that antibiotic to other species of bacteria. In addition to resistance to the effects of one antibiotic, cross-resistance to similar antibiotics also occurs because most antibiotics are variations of a few basic types.

- **Interrupted or inadequate antimicrobial treatment of infections.** Clients often stop taking a prescribed antibiotic when symptoms subside or they feel better. In such circumstances, only the most susceptible bacteria are affected and resistant organisms can become established residents.

- **Type of bacteria.** Both gram-positive and gram-negative bacteria are producing more antibiotic-resistant strains. Examples of gram-positive organisms with increasing antibiotic resistance include staphylococci, streptococci, and enterococci. Gram-negative bacteria associated with high rates of antibiotic resistance include *Pseudomonas aeruginosa* and *Serratia, Enterobacter,* and *Acinetobacter* species. These organisms are inherently resistant to penetration of antibiotics and acquire resistance by multiple mechanisms.

- **Type of infection.** Infections often associated with high rates of resistance include lower respiratory tract infections and those associated with cystic fibrosis or osteomyelitis. These infections are often difficult to treat because they tend to recur; involve multiple, gram-negative, or resistant organisms; and involve anatomic locations that antibiotics do not penetrate well.

Box 29-2 Antibiotic-Resistant Staphylococci, Streptococci, and Enterococci

Methicillin-Resistant and Vancomycin-Intermediate/Resistant *Staphylococcus* Species

Penicillin-resistant staphylococci developed in the early days of penicillin use because the organisms produced beta-lactamase enzymes (penicillinases) that destroyed penicillin. Methicillin was one of five drugs developed to resist the action of beta-lactamase enzymes and thus be effective in treating staphylococcal infections. Eventually, strains of *Staphylococcus aureus* became resistant to these drugs as well. The mechanism of resistance in methicillin-resistant *S. aureus* (MRSA) is alteration of penicillin-binding proteins (PBPs). PBPs, the target sites of penicillins and other beta-lactam antibiotics, are proteins required for maintaining integrity of bacterial cell walls. Susceptible *S. aureus* have five PBPs called 1, 2, 3, 3a or 3′, and 4. Beta-lactam antibiotics bind to these enzymes and produce defective bacterial cell walls, which kill the organisms. MRSA have an additional PBP called *2a* or *2′*. Methicillin cannot bind effectively to the PBPs and inhibit bacterial cell-wall synthesis except with very high drug concentrations. Consequently, minimum inhibitory concentrations (MICs) of methicillin increased to high levels that were difficult to achieve.

The term *MRSA* is commonly used but misleading because the organisms are widely resistant to penicillins (including all of the antistaphylococcal penicillins, not just methicillin) and cephalosporins. Many strains of MRSA are also resistant to erythromycin, clindamycin, tetracycline, and the aminoglycosides. MRSA frequently colonize nasal passages of health care workers and are increasing as a cause of nosocomial infections, especially in critical care units. In addition, the incidence of methicillin-resistant *Staphylococcus epidermidis* (MRSE, often reported as *methicillin-resistant SSNA*) isolates is increasing.

A major reason for concern about infections caused by MRSA and MRSE is that vancomycin is the drug of choice for treatment. However, vancomycin has been used extensively to treat or prevent infections caused by *S. aureus, S. epidermidis*, and enterococci, and vancomycin resistance is increasing in those species. In 1997, the first case of vancomycin-intermediate *S. aureus* (VISA) in the United States was detected. By 2002, the first cases of vancomycin-resistant *S. aureus* (VRSA) had been reported. Options to treat these infections are limited (linezolid, quinupristin-dalfopristin, daptomycin), and measures to reduce the incidence and prevent spread of the organisms are of paramount importance.

Penicillin-Resistant *Streptococcus pneumoniae* (Pneumococci)

Penicillin has long been the drug of choice for treating pneumococcal infections (eg, community-acquired pneumonia; bacteremia; meningitis; and otitis media in children). However, penicillin-resistant strains and multidrug-resistant strains are being identified with increasing frequency. Risk factors for the development of resistant strains include frequent antibiotic use and prophylactic antibiotics. After they have developed, resistant strains spread to other people, especially in children's daycare centers and in hospital settings. Children in daycare

centers are often colonized or infected with antibiotic-resistant *S. pneumoniae*. This is attributed to a high incidence of otitis media, which is often treated with a penicillin or cephalosporin. Resistant strains in adults and older clients are often associated with previous use of a penicillin or cephalosporin and hospitalization.

S. pneumoniae are thought to develop resistance to penicillin by decreasing the ability of their PBPs to bind with penicillin (and other beta-lactam antibiotics). Organisms displaying high-level penicillin resistance may be cross-resistant to second- and third-generation cephalosporins, amoxicillin/clavulanate, and the macrolides. In pneumococcal infections resistant to penicillins and cephalosporins, vancomycin, fluoroquinolones, macrolides, and telithromycin are drugs of choice. To decrease spread of resistant *S. pneumoniae,* the Centers for Disease Control and Prevention (CDC) have proposed:

- Improved surveillance to delineate prevalence by geographic area and assist clinicians in choosing appropriate antimicrobial therapy.
- Rational use of antimicrobials to reduce exposures to drug-resistant pneumococci. For example, prophylactic antibiotic therapy for otitis media may increase colonization and infection of young children with resistant organisms.
- Pneumococcal vaccination for people older than 2 years of age with increased risk of pneumococcal infection, and for all people older than 65 years of age.

Vancomycin-Resistant Enterococci (VRE)

Enterococci have intrinsic and acquired resistance to many antibacterial drugs. For example, penicillins and cephalosporins inhibit rather than kill the organisms at achievable concentrations, and aminoglycosides are ineffective if used alone. As a result, standard treatment of an enterococcal infection outside of the urinary tract has involved a combination of ampicillin and gentamicin. This combination is often successful because the ampicillin damages the bacterial cell wall and allows the aminoglycoside to penetrate the bacterial cell. For ampicillin-allergic clients, vancomycin is given with an aminoglycoside.

This treatment is becoming less effective because some strains of enterococci have developed resistance to ampicillin, gentamicin, and vancomycin. The incidence of multidrug-resistant enterococci and VRE has increased in recent years. Three major types (VanA, VanB, and VanC) of VRE have been described, with different patterns of antimicrobial susceptibility. Some strains remain susceptible to ampicillin, whereas others are only susceptible to linezolid, quinupristin-dalfopristin, chloramphenicol, or newer fluoroquinolones.

A major contributing factor to VRE is increased use of vancomycin to prevent or treat other infections such as staphylococcal (MRSA and MRSE) infections. Therefore, to decrease the spread of VRE, the CDC recommends limiting the use of vancomycin. Specific recommendations include avoiding or minimizing use in routine surgical prophylaxis; empiric therapy for febrile clients with neutropenia (unless the prevalence of MRSA or MRSE is high); systemic or local prophylaxis for

Box 29-2 Antibiotic-Resistant Staphylococci, Streptococci, and Enterococci (continued)

intravascular catheter infection or colonization; selective decontamination of the gastrointestinal tract; eradication of MRSA colonization; primary treatment of antibiotic-associated colitis; and routine prophylaxis for very low birth weight infants or clients on continuous ambulatory peritoneal dialysis. Thorough hand hygiene and environmental cleaning are also important,

because VRE can survive for long periods on hands, gloves, stethoscopes, and environmental surfaces. Personnel should remove or change gloves after contact with clients known to be colonized or infected with VRE. Stethoscopes should be used only with infected clients or cleaned thoroughly between clients if used for both VRE-infected and uninfected clients.

- **Condition of the host.** Clients who are malnourished, severely ill, immunosuppressed, or receiving mechanical ventilation are at high risk for infections, including those caused by antibiotic-resistant organisms.
- **Location or setting.** Resistant organisms are especially likely to emerge in critical care units and large teaching hospitals, where seriously ill clients often require extensive antibiotic therapy. The constant presence of antibiotics provides an environment conducive to selection and replication of resistant organisms. Clients in critical care units are more at risk for infection with antibiotic-resistant organisms because of person-to-person transmission by health care workers or equipment.

Resistant organisms and the antibiotics to which they develop resistance vary in geographic areas, communities, and hospitals according to the use of particular antibiotics. Nationally, resistant bacterial strains of major concern include penicillin-resistant *Streptococcus pneumoniae;* methicillin-resistant *S. aureus* and *Staphylococcus epidermidis;* vancomycin-resistant enterococcus (VRE); extended-spectrum beta-lactamase (ESBL)–producing gram-negative bacilli; and multidrug-resistant tuberculosis (MDR-TB). All of these organisms are resistant to multiple antibiotics. The first four are described in Box 29-2; MDR-TB is discussed in Chapter 34. Viruses and fungi also develop resistance to antimicrobial drugs, as discussed in Chapters 35 and 36.

Mechanisms of Resistance

Bacteria have developed numerous ways to acquire resistance to antimicrobial drugs, including

- Production of enzymes that inactivate the drugs. For example, beta-lactamase enzymes change the chemical structure of penicillins and cephalosporins by opening the beta-lactam ring and preventing the antibiotic from binding with its target site (called *penicillin-binding proteins*) in the bacterial cell wall.
- Modification of target sites for the antibiotic. This is a mechanism of resistance employed by bacteria against fluoroquinolones.
- Production of an alternative enzyme to bypass antibiotic activity (eg, methicillin-resistant staphylococci).
- Changing their cell wall structure to reduce permeability. An example would be alteration in porin channels among *P. aeruginosa* to produce imipenem resistance.

- Acquiring or increasing the ability to pump drug molecules out of the cell (efflux). Examples include some gram-positive cocci resistant to tetracyclines.
- Modification of a binding target for the antibiotic (eg, macrolides).

Bacteria have efficient mechanisms for exchange of genetic material (DNA or plasmids) that allow them to spread antibiotic resistance from one bacterial strain to another, including different species or types of bacteria. Thus, when a new antibiotic is used, resistance may rapidly appear and be disseminated to multiple bacteria.

Host Defense Mechanisms

Although the numbers and virulence of microorganisms help determine whether a person acquires an infection, another major factor is the host's ability to defend itself against the would-be invaders.

Major defense mechanisms of the human body are intact skin and mucous membranes; various anti-infective secretions; mechanical movements; phagocytic cells; and the immune and inflammatory processes. The skin prevents penetration of foreign particles, and its secretions and normal bacterial flora inhibit growth of pathogenic microorganisms. Secretions of the GI, respiratory, and genitourinary tracts (eg, gastric acid, mucus) kill, trap, or inhibit growth of microorganisms. Coughing, swallowing, and peristalsis help remove foreign particles and pathogens trapped in mucus, as does the movement of cilia. Phagocytic cells in various organs and tissues engulf and digest pathogens and cellular debris. The immune system produces lymphocytes and antibodies (see Chap. 38). The inflammatory process is the body's response to injury by microorganisms, foreign particles, chemical agents, or physical irritation of tissues. Inflammation localizes, destroys, dilutes, or removes the injurious agents so tissue healing can occur.

Many factors impair host defense mechanisms and predispose to infection by disease-producing microorganisms. These factors include the following:

- Breaks in the skin and mucous membranes related to trauma, inflammation, open lesions, or insertion of prosthetic devices, tubes, and catheters for diagnostic or therapeutic purposes
- Impaired blood supply

- Neutropenia and other blood disorders
- Malnutrition
- Poor personal hygiene
- Suppression of normal bacterial flora by antimicrobial drugs
- Suppression of the immune system and the inflammatory response by immunosuppressive drugs, cytotoxic antineoplastic drugs, and adrenal corticosteroids
- Diabetes mellitus and other chronic diseases
- Advanced age

CHARACTERISTICS OF ANTIMICROBIAL DRUGS

Terms and Concepts

Several terms are used to describe these drugs. *Anti-infective* and *antimicrobial* include antibacterial, antiviral, and antifungal drugs; *antibacterial* and *antibiotic* refer to drugs used in bacterial infections and are often used interchangeably. Most of the drugs in this section are antibacterials. Antiviral and antifungal drugs are discussed in Chapters 35 and 36, respectively.

Additional terms for antibacterial drugs include *broad spectrum,* for those effective against several groups of microorganisms, and *narrow spectrum,* for those effective against a few groups. The action of an antibacterial drug is usually described as *bactericidal* (kills the microorganism) or *bacteriostatic* (inhibits growth of the microorganism). Whether a drug is bactericidal or bacteriostatic often depends on its concentration at the infection site and the susceptibility of the microorganism to the drug. Successful treatment with bacteriostatic antibiotics depends on the ability of the host's immune system to eliminate the inhibited bacteria and an adequate duration of drug therapy. Stopping an antibiotic prematurely can result in rapid resumption of bacterial growth. Bactericidal drugs are preferred in serious infections, especially in people with impaired immune function.

Mechanisms of Action

Most antimicrobial drugs act on a specific target in the infecting organism (Fig. 29-1). Almost any structure unique to infecting organism, such as proteins or nucleic acids, can be a target for antibiotics. Specific mechanisms of action of antimicrobial drugs include the following:

- Inhibition of bacterial cell wall synthesis, or activation of enzymes that disrupt bacterial cell walls (eg, penicillins, cephalosporins, vancomycin)
- Inhibition of protein synthesis by bacteria or production of abnormal bacterial proteins (eg, aminoglycosides, clindamycin, macrolides, ketolides, tetracyclines). These drugs bind irreversibly to bacterial ribosomes, intracellular structures that synthesize proteins. When anti-

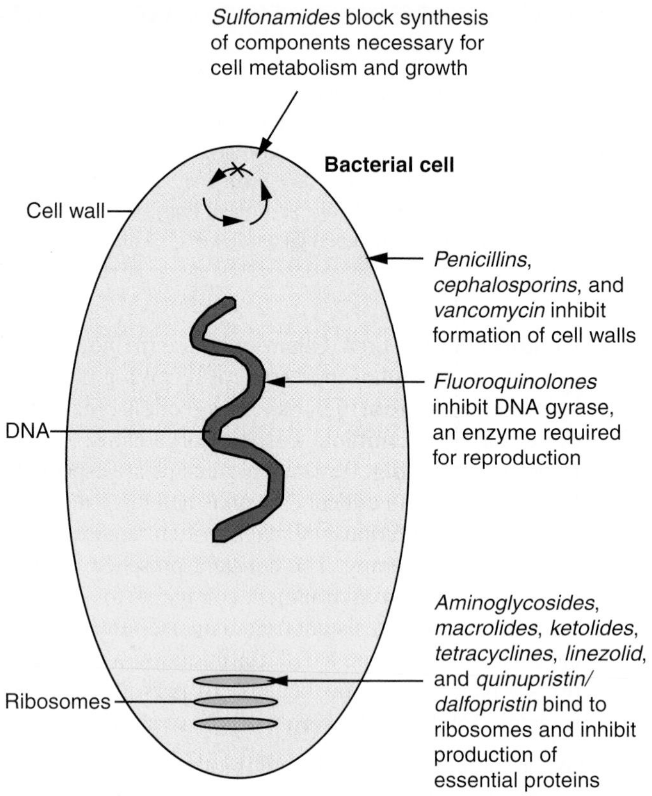

FIGURE 29-1 Actions of antibacterial drugs on bacterial cells.

microbial drugs are bound to the ribosomes, bacteria cannot synthesize the proteins necessary for cell walls and other structures.

- Disruption of microbial cell membranes (eg, antifungals)
- Inhibition of organism reproduction by interfering with nucleic acid synthesis (eg, fluoroquinolones, rifampin, anti–acquired immunodeficiency syndrome antivirals)
- Inhibition of cell metabolism and growth (eg, sulfonamides, trimethoprim)

Indications for Use

Antimicrobial drugs are used to treat and prevent infections. Because laboratory tests (except Gram's stain and a rapid test for group A streptococci) to identify causative organisms usually take 24 hours or longer, empiric therapy against the most likely pathogens is often begun. After organisms are identified, more specific therapy is instituted. Prophylactic therapy is recommended to prevent the following:

- Group A streptococcal infections and possibly rheumatic fever, rheumatic heart disease, and glomerulonephritis. Penicillin is commonly used.
- Bacterial endocarditis in clients with cardiac valvular disease who are having dental, surgical, or other invasive procedures. Amoxicillin or ampicillin, with or without an aminoglycoside, is usually recommended for at-risk persons undergoing certain types of procedures.

- Tuberculosis in clients with latent tuberculosis infection (see Chap. 34)
- Perioperative infections in high-risk clients (eg, those whose resistance to infection is lowered because of age, poor nutrition, disease, or drugs) and for high-risk surgical procedures (eg, cardiac or GI surgery, certain orthopedic procedures, organ transplants)
- Sexually transmitted diseases (eg, gonorrhea, syphilis, chlamydial infections) after exposure has occurred
- Recurrent urinary tract infections in premenopausal, sexually active women. A single dose of a fluoroquinolone or trimethoprim-sulfamethoxazole for two doses, taken after sexual intercourse is often effective.

NURSING PROCESS

Assessment

Assess for current or potential infection.

- General signs and symptoms of infection are the same as those of inflammation, although the terms are not synonymous. *Inflammation* is the normal response to any injury; *infection* requires the presence of a microorganism. The two often occur together. Inflammation may weaken tissue, allowing microorganisms to invade and cause infection. Infection (tissue injury by microorganisms) arouses inflammation. Local signs include redness, heat, edema, and pain; systemic signs include fever and leukocytosis. Specific manifestations depend on the site of infection. Common sites are the respiratory tract, surgical or other wounds, and the genitourinary tract.
- Assess each client for the presence of factors that increase risks of infection (see "Host Defense Mechanisms," earlier).
- Assess culture reports for causative organisms.
- Assess susceptibility reports for appropriate antibacterial drug therapy.
- Assess clients for drug allergies. If present, ask about specific signs and symptoms.
- Assess baseline data about renal and hepatic function and other factors that aid monitoring for therapeutic and adverse drug effects.
- Assess for characteristics that increase risks of adverse drug effects.

Nursing Diagnoses

- Fatigue related to infection
- Activity Intolerance related to fatigue
- Diarrhea related to antimicrobial therapy
- Imbalanced Nutrition: Less Than Body Requirements related to anorexia, nausea, and vomiting associated with antimicrobial therapy

- Risk for Injury related to infection or adverse drug effects
- Risk for Infection related to emergence of drug-resistant microorganisms
- Deficient Knowledge: Methods of preventing infections

Planning/Goals

The client will

- Receive antimicrobial drugs accurately when given by health care providers or caregivers
- Take drugs as prescribed and for the length of time prescribed when self-administered as an outpatient
- Experience decreased fever, white blood cell (WBC) count, and other signs and symptoms of infection
- Be monitored regularly for therapeutic and adverse drug effects
- Receive prompt recognition and treatment of potentially serious adverse effects
- Verbalize and practice measures to prevent future infections
- Be safeguarded against nosocomial infections by health care providers

Interventions

- Use measures to prevent and minimize the spread of infection.
- Wash hands thoroughly and often. This is probably the most effective method of preventing infections.
- Support natural defense mechanisms by promoting general health measures (eg, nutrition, adequate fluid intake, rest, exercise).
- Keep the client's skin clean and dry, especially the hands, underarms, groin, and perineum, because these areas harbor large numbers of microorganisms. Also, take care to prevent trauma to the skin and mucous membranes. Damaged tissues are susceptible to infection.
- Treat all body fluids (eg, blood, aspirates from abdomen or chest) and body substances (eg, sputum, feces, urine, wound drainage) as infectious. Major elements of standard precautions to prevent transmission of hepatitis B, HIV, and other pathogens include wearing gloves when likely to be exposed to any of these materials and thorough hand hygiene when the gloves are removed. Wear protective eyewear when a risk of spatter is present. Rigorous and consistent use of the recommended precautions helps to protect health care providers and clients.
- Implement isolation procedures appropriately.
- To prevent spread of respiratory infections, have clients wash hands after coughing, sneezing, or contact with infected people; cover mouth and nose with tissues when sneezing or coughing and dispose of tissues by placing them in a paper bag and burning it; expectorate

sputum (swallowing may cause reinfection); and avoid crowds when possible, especially during influenza season (approximately November through February). Recommend an annual influenza vaccine to high-risk populations (eg, people with chronic diseases such as diabetes and heart, lung, or renal problems; older adults; health care personnel who are likely to be exposed). Pneumococcal vaccine (see Chap. 39) is recommended for the same populations.

- Assist or instruct clients at risk about pulmonary hygiene measures to prevent accumulation or promote removal of respiratory secretions. These measures include ambulating; turning; coughing and deep-breathing exercises; and incentive spirometry. Retained secretions are good culture media for bacterial growth.
- Use sterile technique when changing any dressing. If a wound is not infected, sterile technique helps prevent infection. If the wound is already infected, sterile technique avoids introducing new bacteria. For all but the smallest of dressings without drainage, remove the dressing with clean gloves, discard it in a moisture-proof bag, and wash hands before putting on sterile gloves to apply the new dressing.
- To minimize spread of staphylococcal infections, infected clients should be isolated, and infected personnel with skin lesions should not work until their lesions are healed. Personnel with skin lesions probably spread more staphylococci than clients because personnel are more mobile.
- For clients with infections, monitor temperature for increased or decreased fever, and monitor WBC count for decrease.
- For clients receiving antimicrobial therapy, maintain a total fluid intake of approximately 3000 mL/24 hours, if not contraindicated by the client's condition. An adequate intake and avoidance of fluid volume deficit may help decrease drug toxicity, especially with aminoglycoside antibiotics. On the other hand, a client receiving IV antibiotics, with 50 to 100 mL of fluid per dose, may be at risk for fluid volume overload.
- Assist clients with hand hygiene; maintaining nutrition and fluid balance; getting adequate rest; and handling secretions correctly. These measures help the body to fight the infection, prevent further infection, and enhance the effectiveness of anti-infective drugs.
- Assist clients in using antimicrobial drugs safely and effectively. Provide appropriate client teaching (see accompanying display).

Evaluation

- Interview and observe for compliance with instructions for using antimicrobial drugs.
- Observe for adverse drug effects.
- Interview and observe for practices to prevent infection.

APPLYING YOUR KNOWLEDGE 29-1
Ms. Kurth tells you that she frequently takes her antibiotic for just long enough to feel better and then saves the rest of her medication for another illness. What teaching guidelines should you provide to her regarding safe and accurate self-administration of antibiotics?

PRINCIPLES OF THERAPY

Goal of Therapy for Infections

The goal of treatment is to eradicate the causative microorganism and return the host to full physiologic functioning. This differs from the goal of most drug therapy, which is to relieve signs and symptoms rather than cure the underlying disorder.

APPLYING YOUR KNOWLEDGE 29-2
Ms. Kurth is hospitalized for acute infection and is receiving IV antibiotic medication. What are the nurse's responsibilities for accurate antibiotic administration?

Rational Use of Antimicrobial Drugs

Antimicrobials are among the most frequently used drugs worldwide. Their success in saving lives and decreasing severity and duration of infectious diseases has encouraged their extensive use. Authorities believe that much antibiotic use involves overuse, misuse, or abuse of the drugs. That is, an antibiotic is not indicated at all or the wrong drug, dose, route, or duration is prescribed. Inappropriate use of antibiotics increases adverse drug effects, infections with drug-resistant microorganisms, and health care costs. In addition, it decreases the number of effective drugs for serious or antibiotic-resistant infections.

Guidelines to promote more appropriate use of antimicrobial drugs include the following:

- Avoid the use of broad-spectrum antibacterial drugs to treat trivial or viral infections; use narrow-spectrum agents if they are likely to be effective. Give antibacterial drugs only when a significant bacterial infection is diagnosed or strongly suspected or when there is an established indication for prophylaxis. Antibacterial drugs are ineffective in viral infections and should not be used to treat them.
- Collect specimens (eg, sputum, urine) for culture and Gram's stain before giving the first dose of an antibiotic. For best results, specimens must be collected accurately and taken directly to the laboratory. If analysis is delayed, contaminants may overgrow pathogenic microorganisms.
- Minimize antimicrobial drug therapy for fever unless other clinical manifestations or laboratory data indicate infection.

General Considerations

☑ Wash hands often and thoroughly, especially before preparing food or eating and after exposure to any body secretions (eg, urine, feces, sputum, nasal secretions). This is probably the most effective way to prevent infection and to avoid spreading an infection to others.

☑ A balanced diet and adequate fluid intake, rest, and exercise also help the body to fight infection, prevent further infection, and increase the effectiveness of antimicrobial drugs.

☑ Take all prescribed doses of an antimicrobial; do not stop when symptoms are relieved. If medication is stopped too soon, symptoms of the current infection may recur and new infections that are caused by antibiotic-resistant organisms and that are harder to treat may develop.

☑ If problems occur with taking an antimicrobial drug, report them to a health care provider rather than stopping the drug.

☑ Do not take antimicrobials left over from a previous illness or prescribed for someone else. Even if infection is present, the likelihood of having the appropriate drug on hand, and in adequate amounts, is extremely small. Thus, taking drugs not prescribed for the particular illness tends to maximize risks and minimize benefits. Also, if the infection is viral, antibacterial drugs are ineffective and should not be used.

☑ Report any other drugs being taken to the prescribing physician. Drug interactions may occur, and changes in drug therapy may be indicated.

☑ Report any drug allergies to all health care providers and wear a medical identification emblem that lists allergens.

☑ Some antibiotics (eg, ampicillin, nitrofurantoin, penicillin V, sulfonamides, tetracyclines) decrease the effectiveness of estrogens and oral contraceptives. Women taking these drugs should use another method of contraception. Inadequate blood levels of estrogen may be indicated by breakthrough bleeding.

Self-Administration

☑ Unless instructed otherwise, take antimicrobial drugs at evenly spaced intervals around the clock. This helps maintain beneficial blood levels of most drugs.

☑ Some oral antimicrobials should be taken on an empty stomach, approximately 1 hour before or 2 hours after meals. Food may decrease absorption and effectiveness. If the medication causes intolerable nausea or vomiting, a few bites of food may be taken.

☑ Store most liquid preparations in the refrigerator, check expiration dates, and discard them when indicated. These preparations are stable and effective for a limited time.

☑ Take the medications with a full glass of water. This helps tablets and capsules to dissolve better in the stomach and decreases stomach irritation.

☑ Report nausea, vomiting, diarrhea, skin rash, recurrence of symptoms for which the antimicrobial drug was prescribed, or signs of new infection (eg, fever, cough, sore mouth, drainage). These problems may indicate adverse effects of the drug, lack of therapeutic response to the drug, or another infection. Any of these requires evaluation and may indicate changes in drug therapy.

● Use antimicrobial drugs in combination with other interventions to decrease microbial proliferation, such as universal precautions, medical isolation techniques, frequent and thorough hand hygiene, and preoperative skin and bowel cleansing.

● Follow recommendations of the Centers for Disease Control and Prevention for prevention and treatment of infections, especially those caused by drug-resistant organisms (eg, gonorrhea, penicillin-resistant streptococcal infections, MRSA, VRE, MDR-TB).

● Consult infectious disease physicians, infection control nurses, and infectious disease pharmacists about local patterns of drug-resistant organisms and treatment of complicated infections.

Drug Selection

After an infection requiring treatment is diagnosed, numerous factors influence the choice of an antimicrobial drug or combination of drugs.

Empiric Therapy

Because most laboratory tests used to definitively identify causative organisms and to determine susceptibility to antibiotics require 48 to 72 hours, the physician usually prescribes for immediate administration a drug that is likely to be effective. This empiric therapy is based on an informed estimate of the most likely pathogen(s) given the client's signs and symptoms and apparent site of infection. A single broad-spectrum antibiotic or a combination of drugs is often chosen.

Culture and Susceptibility Studies

Culture identifies the causative organism, and susceptibility tests determine which drugs are likely to be effective against the organism. Therapists can then "match the drug to the bug." Culture and susceptibility studies are important in both suspected gram-positive and gram-negative infections because of the high incidence of drug-resistant microorganisms.

When a specific organism is identified by laboratory culture, tests can be performed to measure the organism's susceptibility to particular antibiotics. Laboratory reports indicate whether the organism is susceptible (S) or resistant (R) to the tested drugs. One indication of susceptibility is the minimum inhibitory concentration (MIC). The MIC is the lowest concentration of an antibiotic that prevents visible growth of microorganisms. Some laboratories report MIC instead of, or in addition to, S or R.

Susceptible organisms have low or moderate MICs that can be attained by giving usual doses of an antimicrobial agent. For the drug to be effective, its serum and tissue concentrations should usually exceed the MIC of an organism for a period of time. By how much and for how long drug concentrations need to exceed the MIC depend on the drug class and the bacterial species. With beta-lactam agents (eg, penicillins, cephalosporins), the drug concentration usually needs to be maintained above the MIC of the infecting organism for a majority of the dosing interval. With the aminoglycosides (eg, gentamicin, others), the drug concentration does not need to be maintained above the MIC of the organism for the entire dosing interval, because aminoglycosides have a postantibiotic effect. Postantibiotic effect is a persistent effect of an antimicrobial on bacterial growth after brief exposure of the organisms to a drug. Some studies demonstrate that large doses of aminoglycosides, given once daily, are as effective as more frequent dosing and may cause less nephrotoxicity.

Resistant organisms have high MICs and may require higher concentrations of drug than can be achieved in the body. In some cases the minimum bactericidal concentration (MBC) is reported, indicating no growth of the organism in the presence of a particular antibiotic. The MBC is especially desirable for infected hosts with impaired immune functions.

Clients' responses to antimicrobial therapy cannot always be correlated with the MIC of an infecting pathogen. Thus, reports of drug susceptibility testing must be applied in the context of the site of infection, the characteristics of the drug, and the clinical status of the client.

Antibiotic Resistance Patterns

Because these patterns of resistance change in the community and agencies, continuing efforts must be made. *P. aeruginosa* is resistant to many antibiotics, and those strains resistant to gentamicin may be susceptible to amikacin, ceftazidime, imipenem, or aztreonam. Some gram-negative organisms have become increasingly resistant to aminoglycosides, third-generation cephalosporins, and aztreonam, but they may be susceptible to carbapenems or cefepime.

Organism Most Likely to Infect a Particular Site
For example, urinary tract infections are often caused by *E. coli*. Thus, a drug effective against this organism is indicated.

Ability to Penetrate Infected Tissues
Several antimicrobials are effective in urinary tract infections because they are excreted in the urine. However, the choice of an effective antimicrobial drug may be limited in infections of the brain, eyes, gallbladder, or prostate gland because many drugs are unable to reach therapeutic concentrations in these tissues.

Toxicity and Risk-to-Benefit Ratio
In general, the least toxic drug should always be used. However, for serious infections, more toxic drugs may be necessary.

Cost
If an older, less expensive drug meets the criteria for rational drug selection and is likely to be effective in a given infection, it should be used instead of a more expensive agent. For hospitals and nursing homes, personnel costs relating to preparation and administration should be considered as well as purchasing costs.

Combination Therapy

Antimicrobial drugs are often used in combination. Indications for combination therapy may include the following:

- Infections caused by multiple microorganisms (eg, abdominal and pelvic infections)
- Nosocomial infections, which may be caused by many different organisms
- Serious infections in which a combination is synergistic (eg, an aminoglycoside and an antipseudomonal penicillin for pseudomonal infections)
- Likely emergence of drug-resistant organisms if a single drug is used (eg, in tuberculosis). Although drug combinations are widely used to prevent resistance, the only clearly effective use of combination therapy is for treatment of tuberculosis.
- Fever or other signs of infection in clients whose immune system is suppressed. Combinations of antibacterial plus antiviral and/or antifungal drugs may be needed.

Drug Dosage and Administration

Dosage (amount and frequency of administration) should be individualized according to characteristics of the causative organism, the chosen drug, and the client's size and condition (eg, type and severity of infection, ability to use and excrete the chosen drug). For example, dosage may need to be increased for more resistant organisms such as *P. aeruginosa* and for infections in which antibiotics have difficulty penetrating to the site of infection (eg, meningitis). Dosage often must be reduced if the client has renal impairment or other disorders that delay drug elimination.

Most antimicrobial drugs are given orally or IV for systemic infections. The route of administration depends on the client's condition (eg, location and severity of the infection, ability to take oral drugs) and the available drug dosage forms. In serious infections, the IV route is preferred for most drugs.

Duration of Therapy

Duration of therapy varies from a single dose to years, depending on the reason for use. For most acute infections, the average duration is approximately 7 to 10 days or until the recipient has been afebrile and asymptomatic for 48 to 72 hours.

Use in Special Populations

Perioperative Use

When used to prevent infections associated with surgery, a single dose of an antimicrobial medication is usually given within 1 hour of the first incision. This provides effective tissue concentrations during the procedure. If intraoperative contamination occurs, the client should be treated for an infection. The choice of drug depends on the pathogens most likely to colonize the operative area. For most surgeries involving an incision through the skin, a first-generation cephalosporin such as cefazolin (Kefzol) with activity against *S. aureus* or *Streptococcus* species is commonly used. Repeated doses may be given during surgery for procedures of long duration, procedures involving insertion of prosthetic materials, and contaminated or infected operative sites. Postoperative antimicrobials are indicated with intraoperative contamination, traumatic wounds, or ruptured viscera.

Use in Children

Antimicrobial drugs are commonly used in hospitals and ambulatory settings for respiratory infections, otitis media, and other infections. General principles of pediatric (see Chap. 4) and antimicrobial drug therapy apply. Other guidelines include the following:

- Penicillins and cephalosporins are considered safe for most age groups. However, they are eliminated more slowly in neonates because of immature renal function and must be used cautiously and dosed appropriately for age. As with other classes of drugs, many penicillins and cephalosporins do not have Food and Drug Administration (FDA) approval for use in children (usually younger than 12 years of age). However, pediatric specialty references reflect the growing body of experience in using these drugs in younger children.
- Erythromycin, azithromycin (Zithromax), and clarithromycin (Biaxin) are considered safe.
- Aminoglycosides (eg, gentamicin) may cause nephrotoxicity and ototoxicity in any client population. Neonates are at high risk because of immature renal function.
- Tetracyclines are contraindicated in children younger than 8 years of age because of drug effects on teeth and bone (see Chap. 32).
- Clindamycin (Cleocin) warrants monitoring liver and kidney function when it is given to neonates and infants.

- Fluoroquinolones (eg, ciprofloxacin [Cipro]) are contraindicated for use in children (<18 years of age) because weight-bearing joints have been impaired in young animals given the drugs. However, if fluoroquinolones are the only therapeutic option for a resistant pathogen, the prescriber may decide to use a fluoroquinolone in children.
- Trimethoprim-sulfamethoxazole (Bactrim) is used in children, although children younger than 2 months of age have not been evaluated.
- Linezolid (Zyvox) is considered safe for use in children.

Use in Older Adults

Antimicrobial drugs are commonly used in all health care settings for infections in older adults as in younger adults. General principles of geriatric (see Chap. 4) and antimicrobial drug therapy apply. Other guidelines include the following:

- Penicillins are usually safe. However, hyperkalemia may occur with large IV doses of penicillin G potassium (1.7 mEq potassium per 1 million units), and hypernatremia may occur with ticarcillin (Ticar), which contains 5.6 mEq sodium per gram. Hyperkalemia and hypernatremia are more likely to occur with impaired renal function.
- Cephalosporins (eg, cefazolin) are considered safe but may cause or aggravate renal impairment, especially when other nephrotoxic drugs are used concurrently. Dosage of most cephalosporins should be reduced in the presence of renal impairment (see Chap. 30).
- Macrolides and ketolides (eg, erythromycin, telithromycin) are usually safe. Dosage of clarithromycin should be reduced with severe renal impairment.
- Aminoglycosides (eg, gentamicin) are contraindicated in the presence of impaired renal function if less toxic drugs are effective against causative microorganisms. Older adults are at increased risk of nephrotoxicity and ototoxicity from these drugs. Interventions to decrease adverse drug effects are described in Chapter 31.
- Tetracyclines (except doxycycline) and nitrofurantoin (Macrodantin) are contraindicated in the presence of impaired renal function if less toxic drugs are effective against causative organisms.
- Clindamycin may cause diarrhea and should be used with caution in the presence of GI disease, especially colitis.
- Trimethoprim/sulfamethoxazole (Bactrim, Septra) may be associated with an increased risk of severe adverse effects in older adults, especially those with impaired liver or kidney function. Severe skin reactions and bone marrow depression are the most frequently reported severe reactions.
- Daptomycin (Cubicin), quinupristin-dalfopristin (Synercid), and linezolid (Zyvox) are newer agents that may be used in older adults.

Use in Clients With Renal Impairment

Antimicrobial drug therapy requires close monitoring in clients with renal impairment. Many drugs are excreted primarily by the kidneys; some are nephrotoxic and may further damage the kidneys. In the presence of renal impairment, drugs may accumulate and produce toxic effects. Thus, dosage reductions are necessary for some drugs. Methods of calculating dosage are usually based on rates of creatinine clearance (CrCl). For some antibiotics, such as the aminoglycosides and vancomycin, serum drug concentrations should also be used to individualize dosage.

The following formula may be used to estimate CrCl:

Male: Weight in kilograms × (140–age), divided by
72 × serum creatinine (in milligrams per 100 mL)
Female: 0.85 × above value

Dosage may be reduced by giving smaller individual doses, by increasing the time interval between doses, or both. Anti-infective drugs can be categorized as follows in relation to renal impairment:

- Drugs that should be avoided in severe renal impairment (ie, CrCl <15–30 mL/minute) unless the infecting organism is sensitive only to a particular drug. These drugs include the tetracyclines (except doxycycline) and flucytosine.
- Drugs that may exacerbate renal impairment and should not be used if safer alternatives are available. If used, dosage must be carefully adjusted, renal function must be closely monitored, and the client must be closely observed for adverse effects. These drugs include aminoglycosides, amphotericin B, and the fluoroquinolones. Monitoring serum drug concentrations is recommended when using aminoglycoside antibiotics.
- Drugs that require dosage reduction in severe renal impairment. These include penicillin G; ampicillin; most cephalosporins; fluoroquinolones; and trimethoprim-sulfamethoxazole.
- Drugs that require little or no dosage adjustment. These include chloramphenicol, clindamycin, doxycycline, erythromycin, isoniazid, nafcillin, and rifampin.

An additional factor is important in clients with acute or chronic renal failure who are receiving hemodialysis or peritoneal dialysis: Some drugs are removed by dialysis, and an extra dose may be needed during or after dialysis. Clients with acute renal failure receiving continuous renal replacement therapy (CRRT) may also require adjustments in drug doses. Generally, CRRT is more effective at removing drugs than hemodialysis and peritoneal dialysis. Reference texts or scientific articles should be consulted to determine appropriate doses of antibiotics in these clients.

Use in Clients With Hepatic Impairment

Antimicrobial therapy in clients with liver impairment is not well defined. Some drugs are metabolized by the liver (eg, cef-operazone, chloramphenicol, clindamycin, erythromycin), and dosage must be reduced in clients with severe liver impairment. Some are associated with elevations of liver enzymes and/or hepatotoxicity (eg, certain fluoroquinolones, tetracyclines, isoniazid, rifampin). Laboratory monitoring may be helpful in high-risk populations.

Penicillins and other beta-lactam drugs rarely cause jaundice, hepatitis, or liver failure. However, acute liver injuries have been reported with the combination of amoxicillin-clavulanate (Augmentin), and some cases of cholestatic jaundice have been reported with ticarcillin-clavulanate (Timentin). Hepatotoxicity is attributed to the clavulanate component. These drugs are contraindicated in clients who have had cholestatic jaundice or hepatic dysfunction associated with their use and must be used with caution in clients with hepatic impairment.

Some fluoroquinolones have been associated with liver enzyme abnormalities and hepatotoxicity (eg, hepatitis, liver impairment or failure). The drugs should be used cautiously in clients with or at risk for development of impaired liver function. The drug should be stopped if jaundice or any other symptoms of liver dysfunction develop.

Use in Clients With Critical Illness

Antimicrobials are frequently given in critical care units. Many clients have multiple organ impairments or chronic diseases with a superimposed acute illness or injury (eg, surgery, trauma, burns). Thus, antimicrobial therapy is often more aggressive, complex, and expensive in critically ill clients than in other clients. In addition, measurement of plasma drug levels and dosage adjustment are often necessary to accommodate the changing physiology of a critically ill client. Drug levels are usually measured after four or five doses are given so that steady-state concentrations have been reached.

Clients in critical care units are at high risk for acquiring nosocomial pneumonia because of the severity of their illness, duration of hospitalization, and antimicrobial drug therapy. The strongest predisposing factor is mechanical ventilation, which bypasses airway defenses against movement of microorganisms from the upper to the lower respiratory tract. Organisms often associated with nosocomial pneumonia are *S. aureus* and gram-negative bacilli. Bacterial pneumonia is usually treated with a broad-spectrum antibiotic until culture and susceptibility reports become available.

Selection of antibacterial drugs may be difficult because of frequent changes in antibiotic resistance patterns. Antibiotic rotation (ie, switching preferred antibiotic or antibiotic classes used to treat infections, on a scheduled basis) has been successful in reducing rates of ventilator-associated pneumonia and mortality.

Use in Home Care

Infections are among the most common illnesses in all age groups, and they are often treated by antibiotic therapy at home, with medications administered by the client or a family-member caregiver. If a home care nurse is involved, responsibilities may include teaching family members how to administer antibiotics (eg, teaching a parent how to store and measure a liquid antibiotic); how to care for the person with an infection; and how to protect other people in the environment from the infection. General infection-control practices include frequent and thorough hand hygiene, use of gloves when indicated, and appropriate handling and disposal of body substances (eg, blood, urine, feces, sputum, vomitus, wound drainage).

Increasingly, IV antibiotics are being given in the home. Any client who needs more than a few days of IV antibiotic therapy may be a candidate for home care. Some infections that require relatively long-term IV antibiotic therapy include endocarditis, osteomyelitis, and some surgical-wound infections. Numerous people and agencies may be involved in pro-

viding this service. First, the client and family need to be able and willing to manage some aspects of therapy and to provide space for necessary supplies. Second, arrangements must be made for procuring equipment, supplies, and medication. In some areas, nurses employed by equipment companies help families prepare and use IV infusion pumps. Medication is usually obtained from a local pharmacy in a unit-dose package ready for administration.

The role of the home care nurse includes teaching the client and caregiver how to store and administer the medication, monitor the IV site, monitor the infection, manage problems, and report client responses. Specific responsibilities may vary according to drug administration (intermittently or by continuous infusion), whether the client has a peripheral or central IV line, and other factors. The family should be provided with detailed instructions and emergency telephone numbers of the home care nurse, the pharmacy, and the supply company.

NURSING ACTIONS

Antimicrobial Drugs

NURSING ACTIONS	RATIONALE/EXPLANATION
1. Administer accurately	
a. Schedule at evenly spaced intervals around the clock.	To maintain therapeutic blood levels
b. Some oral antimicrobials should be given on an empty stomach, approximately 1 hour before or 2 hours after meals. Check specific recommendations.	To decrease binding to foods and inactivation by gastric acid
c. For oral and parenteral solutions from powder forms, follow label instructions for mixing and storing. Check expiration dates.	Several antimicrobial drugs are marketed in powder forms because they are unstable in solution. When mixed, measured amounts of diluent must be added for drug dissolution and the appropriate concentration. Parenteral solutions are usually prepared in the pharmacy. Many solutions require refrigeration to prolong stability. None of the solutions should be used after the expiration date because drug decomposition is likely.
d. Give parenteral antimicrobial solutions alone; do not mix with any other drug in a syringe or intravenous (IV) solution.	To avoid chemical and physical incompatibilities that may cause drug precipitation or inactivation
e. Give intramuscular (IM) antimicrobials deeply into large muscle masses (preferably gluteal muscles), and rotate injection sites.	To decrease tissue irritation
f. For IV administration, use dilute solutions, giving direct injections slowly and intermittent infusions over 30–60 minutes. After infusions, flush the IV tubing with at least 10 milliliters of IV solution. For children, check instructions for individual drugs to avoid excessive concentrations and excessive fluids.	Most antimicrobials that are given IV can be given by intermittent infusion. Although instructions vary with specific drugs, most reconstituted drugs can be further diluted with 50–100 milliliters of IV fluid (D_5W, NS, D_5-1/4%, or D_5-1/2% NaCl). Dilution and slow administration minimize vascular irritation and phlebitis. Flushing ensures that the entire dose is given and prevents contact between drugs in the tubing.
2. Observe for therapeutic effects	
a. With local infections, observe for decreased redness, edema, heat, and pain.	Signs and symptoms of inflammation and infection usually subside within approximately 48 hours after antimicrobial therapy is begun.
b. With systemic infections, observe for decreased fever and white blood cell count, increased appetite, and reports of feeling better.	Although systemic manifestations of infection are similar regardless of the cause, local manifestations vary with the type or location of the infection.

(continued)

NURSING ACTIONS	RATIONALE/EXPLANATION
c. With wound infections, observe for decreased signs of local inflammation and decreased drainage. Drainage also may change from purulent to serous.	
d. With respiratory infections, observe for decreased dyspnea, coughing, and secretions. Secretions may change from thick and colored to thin and white.	
e. With urinary tract infections, observe for decreased urgency, frequency, and dysuria. If urinalysis is done, check the laboratory report for decreased bacteria and white blood cells.	
f. Absence of signs and symptoms of infection when given prophylactically	
3. Observe for adverse effects	
a. Hypersensitivity	Reactions are more likely to occur in those with previous hypersensitivity reactions and those with a history of allergy, asthma, or hay fever.
(1) Anaphylaxis—hypotension, respiratory distress, urticaria, angioedema, vomiting, diarrhea	Hypersensitivity may occur with most antimicrobial drugs but is more common with penicillins. Anaphylaxis may occur with oral administration but is more likely with parenteral administration and may occur within 5–30 minutes of injection. Hypotension results from vasodilation and circulatory collapse. Respiratory distress results from bronchospasm or laryngeal edema.
(2) Serum sickness—chills, fever, vasculitis, generalized lymphadenopathy, joint edema and inflammation, bronchospasm, urticaria	This is a delayed allergic reaction, occurring 1 week or more after the drug is started. Signs and symptoms are caused by inflammation.
(3) Acute interstitial nephritis (AIN), hematuria, oliguria, proteinuria, pyuria	AIN is considered a hypersensitivity reaction that may occur with many antimicrobials, including penicillins, cephalosporins, aminoglycosides, sulfonamides, tetracyclines, and others. It is usually reversible if the causative agent is promptly stopped.
b. Superinfection	Superinfection is a new or secondary infection that occurs during antimicrobial therapy for a primary infection. Superinfections are common and potentially serious because responsible microorganisms are often drug-resistant staphylococci, gram-negative organisms (eg, *Pseudomonas aeruginosa*), or fungi (eg, *Candida*).
(1) Recurrence of systemic signs and symptoms (eg, fever, malaise)	
(2) New localized signs and symptoms—redness, heat, edema, pain, drainage, cough	
(3) Stomatitis or "thrush"—sore mouth; white patches on oral mucosa; black, furry tongue	From overgrowth of fungi
(4) Pseudomembranous colitis—severe diarrhea characterized by blood, pus, and mucus in stools	May occur with most antibiotics. Antibiotics suppress normal bacterial flora and allow the overgrowth of *Clostridium difficile*. The organism produces a toxin that kills mucosal cells and produces superficial ulcerations that are visible with sigmoidoscopy. Discontinuing antibiotics and giving metronidazole or oral vancomycin are curative measures. However, relapses may occur.
(5) Monilial vaginitis—rash in perineal area, itching, vaginal discharge	From overgrowth of yeast organisms
c. Phlebitis at IV sites; pain at IM sites	Many antimicrobial parenteral solutions are irritating to body tissues.
d. Nausea and vomiting	These often occur with oral antimicrobials, probably from irritation of gastric mucosa.

NURSING ACTIONS	RATIONALE/EXPLANATION
e. Diarrhea	Commonly occurs; is caused by irritation of gastrointestinal mucosa and changes in intestinal bacterial flora; and may range from mild to severe. Pseudomembranous colitis is one type of severe diarrhea.
f. Nephrotoxicity	
(1) See AIN, earlier	More likely to occur in clients who are elderly or who have impaired renal function.
(2) Acute tubular necrosis (ATN)—increased blood urea nitrogen and serum creatinine, decreased creatinine clearance, fluid and electrolyte imbalances	Aminoglycosides are the antimicrobial agents most often associated with ATN.
g. Neurotoxicity—confusion, hallucinations, neuromuscular irritability, convulsive seizures	More likely with large IV doses of penicillins or cephalosporins, especially in clients with impaired renal function.
h. Bleeding—hypoprothrombinemia, platelet dysfunction	Most often associated with penicillins and cephalosporins.
4. Observe for drug interactions	See following chapters. The most significant interactions are those that alter effectiveness or increase drug toxicity.

APPLYING YOUR KNOWLEDGE: ANSWERS

29-1 Teach all clients to take all of the prescribed doses and not to stop when their symptoms are relieved. Failure to take all of the medication may lead to an increased risk for a drug-resistant infection. Additionally, teach all clients not to take antibiotics left over from a previous illness. The likelihood of having the right drug in the right amount to adequately treat the infection is extremely small. This practice of taking leftover medication may also lead to an increased risk of developing a drug-resistant infection.

29-2 Collect specimens for culture before the first dose of an antibiotic is given, unless a life-threatening infection is present. Practice impeccable infection-control principles, including frequent and thorough hand hygiene, proper use of gloves, and proper handling and disposal of body fluids. Schedule antibiotics at evenly spaced intervals around the clock, to maintain therapeutic blood levels. Check specific recommendations with regard to the administration of the antibiotic with food and other medication to decrease binding to food and drugs and prevent inactivation. Follow all instructions for mixing and storing medication and check expiration dates. Give parenteral antibiotics alone; do not mix with any other drug, to avoid chemical and physical incompatibilities that may cause drug precipitation or inactivation. Flush the IV tubing after each dose to ensure the entire dose is administered.

Review and Application Exercises

Short Answer Exercises

1. How does the body defend itself against infection?

2. When assessing a client, what signs and symptoms may indicate an infectious process?

3. Do all infections require antimicrobial drug therapy? Why or why not?

4. With antimicrobial drug therapy, what is meant by the terms *bacteriostatic, bactericidal,* antimicrobial *spectrum* of activity, and *minimum inhibitory concentration?*

5. Why is it important to identify the organism causing an infection?

6. Why are infections of the brain, eye, and prostate gland more difficult to treat than infections of the GI, respiratory, and urinary tracts?

7. What factors promote the development of drug-resistant microorganisms, and how can they be prevented or minimized?

8. What are common adverse effects associated with antimicrobial drug therapy?

9. When teaching a client about a prescribed antibiotic, a common instruction is to take all the medicine and not to stop prematurely. Why is this information important?

10. When a dose of an antibiotic is prescribed to prevent postoperative infection, should it be given before, during, or after surgery? Why?

11. What special precautions are needed for clients with renal or hepatic impairment or critical illness?

NCLEX-Style Questions

12. When teaching a mother about the antibiotic liquid preparation for her child's acute bronchitis, the nurse should do which of the following?
   a. Instruct the mother to administer the antibiotic until the child is afebrile.
   b. Tell the mother to expect the child's respiratory secretions to become thicker and darker as the infection responds to treatment.
   c. Instruct the mother to keep any remaining antibiotic liquid preparation for the next episode of bronchitis.
   d. Remind the mother that frequent hand hygiene after handling respiratory secretions is one way to reduce spread of infections.

13. The nurse should give which of the following instructions to clients taking oral antibiotics?
   a. Take oral antibiotics with a full glass of water.
   b. Always take an oral antibiotic after a full meal.
   c. If stomach upset occurs, take the oral antibiotic with a full, fatty meal.
   d. Do not refrigerate oral liquid antibiotic preparations.

14. Critically ill clients are at increased risk of infections due to resistant organisms for all the following reasons except
   a. They may have multiple medical conditions.
   b. Health care workers may spread resistant organisms on their hands in the closed environment.
   c. They have increased host defenses.
   d. Equipment used in critical care units may be a fomite for spread between people.

15. A client is hospitalized with a large sacral wound and a urinary tract infection. The nurse should watch for which of the following signs that the client is not responding appropriately to antibiotic treatment?
   a. decreased drainage from the wound
   b. increased bacteria and WBC counts on urinalysis

   c. decreased pain at the wound site
   d. increased activity tolerance

16. To decrease the spread of vancomycin-resistant enterococcus (VRE), the nurse caring for a client with VRE should do all of the following except
   a. Use gloves when providing care involving direct client contact.
   b. Thoroughly wash hands after contact with the client.
   c. Clean equipment thoroughly after use by the client.
   d. Ensure the physician has prescribed vancomycin.

Selected References

Abate, B. J., & Barriere, S. L. (2002). Antimicrobial regimen selection. In J. T. DiPiro, R. L. Talbert, G. C. Yee, G. R. Matzke, B. G. Wells, & L. M. Posey (Eds.), *Pharmacotherapy: A pathophysiologic approach* (5th ed., pp. 1817–1829). New York: McGraw-Hill.

Centers for Disease Control and Prevention. (2002). *Staphylococcus aureus* resistant to vancomycin. *Morbidity and Mortality Weekly Report, 51,* 565–567.

Chambers, H. F. (2001). Antimicrobial agents: General considerations. In J. G. Hardman & L. E. Limbird (Eds.), *Goodman & Gilman's The pharmacological basis of therapeutics* (10th ed., pp. 1143–1170). New York: McGraw-Hill.

Garau, J. (2002). Treatment of drug-resistant pneumococcal pneumonia. *Lancet Infectious Diseases, 2*(7), 404–415.

Gill, V. J., Fedorko, D. P., & Witebsky, F. G. (2000). The clinician and the microbiology laboratory. In G. L. Mandell, J. E. Bennett, & R. Dolin (Eds.), *Principles and practice of infectious diseases* (5th ed., pp. 184–221). Philadelphia: Churchill Livingstone.

Mangram, A. J., Horan, T. C., Pearson, M. L., Silver, L. C., Jarvis, W. R., & The Hospital Infection Control Practices Advisory Committee. (1999). Guideline for the prevention of surgical site infection. *Infection Control and Hospital Epidemiology, 20*(4), 247–278.

Moellering, R. C. (2000). Principles of anti-infective therapy. In G. L. Mandell, J. E. Bennett, & R. Dolin (Eds.), *Principles and practice of infectious diseases* (5th ed., pp. 223–233). Philadelphia: Churchill Livingstone.

Nolin, T. D., Abraham, P. A., & Matzke, G. R. (2002). Drug-induced renal disease. In J. T. DiPiro, R. L. Talbert, G. C. Yee, G. R. Matzke, B. G. Wells, & L. M. Posey (Eds.), *Pharmacotherapy: A pathophysiologic approach* (5th ed., pp. 889–909). New York: McGraw-Hill.

Raymond, D. P., Pelletier, S. J., Crabtree, T. D., et al. (2001). Impact of a rotating empiric antibiotic schedule on infectious mortality in an intensive care unit. *Critical Care Medicine, 29,* 1101–1108.

Rybak, M. J., & Aeschlimann, J. R. (2002). Laboratory tests to direct antimicrobial pharmacotherapy. In J. T. DiPiro, R. L. Talbert, G. C. Yee, G. R. Matzke, B. G. Wells, & L. M. Posey (Eds.), *Pharmacotherapy: A pathophysiologic approach* (5th ed., pp. 1797–1815). New York: McGraw-Hill.

Schmitz, F., & Fluit, A. C. (2004). Mechanisms of antibacterial resistance. In J. Cohen, W. E. Powderly, S. F. Berkley, et al. (Eds.). *Infectious Diseases* (2nd ed., pp 1733–1747). New York: Mosby.

Silveira, F., Fujitani, S., & Paterson, D. L. (2004). Antibiotic-resistant infections in the critically ill adult. *Clinics in Laboratory Medicine, 24*(2), 329–341.

Beta-Lactam Antibacterials:
Penicillins, Cephalosporins, and Other Drugs

OBJECTIVES

After studying this chapter, you will be able to:

1. Describe general characteristics of beta-lactam antibiotics.
2. Discuss penicillins in relation to effectiveness, safety, spectrum of antibacterial activity, mechanism of action, indications for use, administration, observation of client response, and teaching of clients.
3. Differentiate among extended-spectrum penicillins.
4. Question clients about allergies before the initial dose of a penicillin.
5. Describe characteristics of beta-lactamase inhibitor drugs.
6. State the rationale for combining a penicillin and a beta-lactamase inhibitor drug.
7. Discuss similarities and differences between cephalosporins and penicillins.
8. Differentiate cephalosporins in relation to antibacterial spectrum, indications for use, and adverse effects.
9. Describe major characteristics of carbapenem and monobactam drugs.
10. Apply principles of using beta-lactam antibacterials in selected client situations.

APPLYING YOUR KNOWLEDGE

Carmen Nudson is a 44-year-old woman who is undergoing bronchoscopy to evaluate chronic hoarseness. The physician orders cefazolin 1 g IV just prior to the procedure.

INTRODUCTION

Beta-lactam antibacterials derive their name from the beta-lactam ring that is part of their chemical structure. An intact beta-lactam ring is essential for antibacterial activity. Several gram-positive and gram-negative bacteria produce beta-lactamase enzymes that disrupt the beta-lactam ring and in-activate the drugs. This is a major mechanism by which microorganisms acquire resistance to beta-lactam antibiotics. Penicillinase and cephalosporinase are beta-lactamase enzymes that act on penicillins and cephalosporins, respectively.

Despite the common element of a beta-lactam ring, characteristics of beta-lactam antibiotics differ widely because of variations in their chemical structures. The drugs may differ in antibacterial spectrum of activity, routes of administration, susceptibility to beta-lactamase enzymes, and adverse effects. Beta-lactam antibiotics include penicillins, cephalosporins, carbapenems, and monobactams, which are described in the following sections. Pharmacokinetic characteristics of selected drugs are listed in Table 30-1 and routes and usual dosage ranges are listed in the Drugs at a Glance tables.

Beta-lactam antibacterial drugs inhibit synthesis of bacterial cell walls by binding to proteins (penicillin-binding proteins) in bacterial cell membranes. This binding produces a defective cell wall that allows intracellular contents to leak out, destroying the microorganism. Beta-lactam antibiotics are most effective when bacterial cells are dividing.

PENICILLINS

The penicillins are effective, safe, and widely used anti-bacterial agents. The group includes natural extracts from the *Penicillium* mold and several semisynthetic derivatives. When **P** **penicillin,** the prototype, was introduced, it was effective against streptococci, staphylococci, gonococci, meningococci, *Treponema pallidum,* and other organisms. It had to be given parenterally because it was destroyed by gastric acid, and injec-

TABLE 30-1 Pharmacokinetics of Selected Beta-Lactam Drugs

GROUP/DRUG NAME	ROUTE OF ADMINISTRATION	PROTEIN BINDING (%)	HALF-LIFE (min) WITH NORMAL RENAL FUNCTION	MAIN ROUTE OF ELIMINATION	ACTION Onset	Peak	Duration (h)
Penicillins							
Penicillin G (aqueous)	IM, IV	60	30–60	Renal	Rapid	30 min	4–6
Penicillin V	PO	80	30	Renal	Varies	60 min	4–6
Amoxicillin	PO	20	60–90	Renal	30–60 min	1–2 h	6–8
Dicloxacillin	PO	98	30–60	Hepatic/renal	Varies	60–90 min	4–6
Nafcillin	IM, IV	87–90	60	Hepatic/renal	Rapid	60 min	4
Piperacillin	IM, IV	16	60	Renal	Rapid	30–60 min	4–6
Ticarcillin	IM, IV	45	60	Renal	Rapid	30–75 min	4–6
Cephalosporins							
Cefaclor	PO	25	35–54	Renal		30–60 min	8–12
Cefazolin	IM, IV	80–86	90–120	Renal	IM 30 min	0.5–2 h	6–8
					IV immediate	5 min	6–8
Cefepime	IM, IV	20	102–138	Renal	IM 30 min	1.5–2 h	10–12
					IV immediate	5 min	10–12
Cefixime	PO	65	180–240	Renal		2–6 h	
Cefoperazone	IM, IV	82–93	120	Biliary	IM 1 h	1–2 h	6–12
					IV 5–10 min	15–20 min	6–12
Cefotetan	IM, IV	88–90	180–276	Renal	IM 30–60 min	1.5–3 h	18–24
					IV 15–20 min	30 min	18–24
Ceftazidime	IM, IV	<10	114–120	Renal	IM 30 min	1 h	24–28
					IV rapid	1h	24–28
Ceftriaxone	IM, IV	85–95	348–522	Hepatic	IM 30 min	1.5–4 h	15–18
					IV rapid	Immediate	15–18
Cefuroxime	PO, IM, IV	50	80	Renal	PO varies	2 h	18–24
					IM 20 min	30 min	18–24
					IV rapid	Immediate	18–24
Cephalexin	PO	10	50–80	Renal		60 min	8–10
Cephradine	PO	8–17	48–80	Renal	Varies	1 h	6–8
Carbapenem							
Imipenem-cilastatin	IM, IV	20/40	60 (for each component)	Renal	Varies	2 h	6–8
Monobactam							
Aztreonam	IM, IV	56	90–120	Renal	IV rapid	30 min	6–8
					IM varies	60–90 min	6–8

IM, intramuscular; IV, intravenous; PO, oral.

tions were painful. With extensive use, strains of drug-resistant staphylococci appeared. Later penicillins were developed to increase gastric acid stability, beta-lactamase stability, and antimicrobial spectrum of activity, especially against gram-negative microorganisms. Semisynthetic derivatives are formed by adding side chains to the penicillin nucleus.

After absorption, penicillins are widely distributed and achieve therapeutic concentrations in most body fluids, including joint, pleural, and pericardial fluids and bile. Therapeutic levels are not usually obtained in intraocular and cerebrospinal fluids (CSF) unless inflammation is present because normal cell membranes act as barriers to drug penetration.

Penicillins are rapidly excreted by the kidneys and produce high drug concentrations in the urine (an exception is nafcillin, which is excreted by the liver).

Indications for Use

Clinical indications for use of penicillins include bacterial infections caused by susceptible microorganisms. As a class, penicillins usually are more effective in infections caused by gram-positive bacteria than those caused by gram-negative bacteria. However, their clinical uses vary significantly according to the subgroup or individual drug and microbial patterns of resistance. The drugs are often useful in skin/soft tissue, respiratory, gastrointestinal, and genitourinary infections. However, the incidence of resistance among streptococci, staphylococci, and other microorganisms continues to grow.

Contraindications to Use

Contraindications include hypersensitivity or allergic reactions to any penicillin preparation. An allergic reaction to one penicillin means the client is allergic to all members of the penicillin class. The potential for cross-allergenicity with cephalosporins and carbapenems exists, so other alternatives should be selected in penicillin-allergic clients when possible.

Subgroups and Individual Penicillins

Table 30-2 provides pertinent information about individual penicillins.

Penicillins G and V

Penicillin G (Pfizerpen, Bicillin, Wycillin) remains effective for a limited number of uses. Many strains of staphylococci and gonococci have acquired resistance to penicillin G, preventing its use for treatment of infections caused by these organisms. Some strains of streptococci have acquired resistance to penicillin G, although the drug is still effective in many streptococcal infections. It remains the drug of choice for the treatment of streptococcal pharyngitis; for prevention of recurrent attacks in clients who have had previous acute rheumatic fever due to group A streptococcus; and for treatment of neurosyphilis.

Several preparations of penicillin G are available for intravenous (IV) and intramuscular (IM) administration. They cannot be used interchangeably. Only aqueous preparations can be given IV. Preparations containing benzathine or procaine can be given only IM. Long-acting repository forms have additives that decrease their solubility in tissue fluids and delay their absorption.

Penicillin V (Veetids) is derived from penicillin G and has the same antibacterial spectrum. It is not destroyed by gastric acid and is given only by the oral route. It is well absorbed and produces therapeutic blood levels.

Penicillinase-Resistant (Antistaphylococcal) Penicillins

This group includes three drugs **dicloxacillin**, **nafcillin**, and **oxacillin**) that are effective in some infections caused by staphylococci resistant to penicillin G. An older member of this group, methicillin, is no longer marketed for clinical use. However, susceptibility of bacteria to the antistaphylococcal penicillins is determined by exposing the bacteria to methicillin (methicillin-susceptible or -resistant) or oxacillin (oxacillin-susceptible or -resistant) in bacteriology laboratories. Although called "methicillin-resistant," these staphylococcal microorganisms are also resistant to other antistaphylococcal penicillins.

These drugs are formulated to resist the penicillinases that inactivate other penicillins. They are recommended for use in known or suspected staphylococcal infections, except for methicillin-resistant *Staphylococcus aureus* (MRSA) infections.

Aminopenicillins

Ampicillin (Principin) is a broad-spectrum, semisynthetic penicillin that is bactericidal for several types of gram-positive and gram-negative bacteria. It has been effective against enterococci, *Proteus mirabilis*, *Salmonella*, *Shigella*, and *Escherichia coli*, but resistant forms of these organisms are increasing. It is ineffective against penicillinase-producing staphylococci and gonococci.

Ampicillin is excreted mainly by the kidneys; thus, it is useful in some urinary tract infections (UTI). Because some is excreted in bile, it is useful in biliary tract infections not caused by biliary obstruction. It is used in the treatment of bronchitis, sinusitis, and otitis media.

P **Amoxicillin** (Amoxil, Trimox) is similar to ampicillin except it is only available orally. It is better absorbed and produces therapeutic blood levels more rapidly than oral ampicillin. It also causes less gastrointestinal distress.

The aminopenicillins are drugs of choice for prevention of bacterial endocarditis due to procedures that produce transient bacteremia.

Extended-Spectrum (Antipseudomonal) Penicillins

The drugs in this group (**carbenicillin** [Geocillin], **ticarcillin** [Ticar], and **piperacillin**) have a broad spectrum of antimicrobial activity, especially against gram-negative organisms such as *Pseudomonas* and *Proteus* species and *E. coli*. For pseudomonal infections, one of these drugs is usually given concomitantly with an aminoglycoside or a fluoroquinolone (see Chap. 31). Carbenicillin is available as an oral formulation for UTI or prostatitis caused by susceptible pathogens. The other drugs are usually given by intermittent IV infusion, although most can be given IM.

Penicillin–Beta-Lactamase Inhibitor Combinations

Beta-lactamase inhibitors are drugs with a beta-lactam structure but little antibacterial activity. They bind with and inactivate the beta-lactamase enzymes produced by many bacteria (eg, *E. coli*; *Klebsiella*, *Enterobacter*, and *Bacteroides* species; *S. aureus*). When combined with a penicillin, the beta-lactamase inhibitor protects the penicillin from destruction by

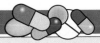

Table 30-2 Drugs at a Glance: Penicillins

GENERIC/TRADE NAME	ROUTES AND USUAL DOSAGE RANGES	
	Adults	Children
Penicillins G and V		
Penicillin G potassium and sodium (Pfizerpen)	IM 300,000–8 million U daily IV 6–20 million U daily by continuous or intermittent infusion q2–4h. Up to 60 million U daily have been given in certain serious infections.	IM, IV 50,000–300,000 U/kg/d in divided doses q4h
Penicillin G benzathine (Bicillin)	IM 1.2–2.4 million U in a single dose Prophylaxis of recurrent rheumatic fever, IM 1.2 million U every 3–4 wk Treatment of syphilis, IM 2.4 million U (1.2 million U in each buttock) in a single dose	IM 50,000 U/kg in 1 dose Prophylaxis of recurrent rheumatic fever, IM same as adult
Penicillin G procaine (Wycillin)	IM 600,000–2.4 million U daily in 1 or 2 doses	IM 300,000 U/day in divided doses q12h
Penicillin V (Veetids)	PO 125–500 mg 4–6 times daily	Same as adults *Infants:* PO 15–50 mg/kg/d in 3–6 divided doses
Penicillinase-Resistant (Antistaphylococcal) Penicillins		
Dicloxacillin	PO 250 mg q6h	*Weight ≥ 40 kg:* Same as adults *Weight < 40 kg:* 25 mg/kg/d in 4 divided doses q6h
Nafcillin	IM 500 mg q4–6h IV 500 mg–2 g in 15–30 mL sodium chloride injection, infused over 5–10 min, q4h; maximal daily dose, 18 g for serious infections	IM, IV 50–200 mg/kg/d in 4 to 6 divided doses q4–6h
Oxacillin	PO, IM, IV 500 mg–1 g q4–6h. For direct IV injection, the dose should be well diluted and given over 10–15 min.	*Weight > 40 kg:* Same as adults *Weight ≤ 40 kg:* PO, IM, IV 50–100 mg/kg/d in 4 divided doses q6h
Aminopenicillins		
Ampicillin (Principen)	PO, IM, IV 250–500 mg q6h. In severe infections, doses up to 2 g q4h may be given IV.	*Weight > 20 kg:* Same as adults *Weight ≤ 20 kg:* PO, IM, IV 50–200 mg/kg/d in divided doses q6h
Amoxicillin (Amoxil, Trimox)	PO 250–500 mg q8h	*Weight > 20 kg:* Same as adults *Weight ≤ 20 kg:* 20–40 mg/kg/d in divided doses q8h
Extended-Spectrum (Antipseudomonal) Penicillins		
Carbenicillin indanyl sodium (Geocillin)	PO 382–764 mg 4 times daily	PO 30–50 mg/kg/d in divided doses q6h
Ticarcillin (Ticar)	IM, IV 1–3 g q6h. IM injections should not exceed 2 g/injection.	*Weight < 40 kg:* 100–300 mg/kg/d q6–8h
Piperacillin (Pipracil)	IV, IM 200–300 mg/kg/d in divided doses q4–6h. Usual adult dosage, 3–4 g q4–6h; maximal daily dose, 24 g	*< 12 y:* Dosage not established
Penicillin/Beta-Lactamase Inhibitor Combinations		
Ampicillin-sulbactam (Unasyn)	IM, IV 1.5–3 g q6h	*Weight ≥ 40 kg:* same as adults *Weight < 40 kg:* 300 mg/kg/d in divided doses q6h
Amoxicillin clavulanate (Augmentin)	PO 250–500 mg q8h or 875 mg q12h	*Weight < 40 kg:* 20–40 mg/kg/d in divided doses q8h *Weight ≥ 40 kg:* same as adults
Piperacillin-tazobactam (Zosyn)	IV 2.25–4.5 g q6–8h	IV 100–300 mg/kg/d in divided doses q4–6h
Ticarcillin-clavulanate (Timentin)	IV 3.1 g q4–6h	*Weight < 60 kg:* 200–300 mg/kg/d in divided doses q4–6h

IM, intramuscular; IV, intravenous; PO, oral.

the enzymes and extends the penicillin's spectrum of antimicrobial activity. Thus, the combination drug may be effective in infections caused by bacteria that are resistant to a beta-lactam antibiotic alone. Clavulanate, sulbactam, and tazobactam are the beta-lactamase inhibitors available in combinations with penicillins.

Unasyn is a combination of ampicillin and sulbactam available in vials with 1 gram of ampicillin and 0.5 gram of sulbactam, or 2 grams of ampicillin and 1 gram of sulbactam. **Augmentin** contains amoxicillin and clavulanate. It is available in 250-, 500-, and 875-milligram tablets, each of which contains 125 milligrams of clavulanate. Thus, two 250-milligram tablets are not equivalent to one 500-milligram tablet. It is also available as 1000-milligram extended-release tablets containing 62.5 milligrams of clavulanate. **Timentin** is a combination of ticarcillin and clavulanate in an IV formulation containing 3 grams of ticarcillin and 100 milligrams of clavulanate. **Zosyn** is a combination of piperacillin and tazobactam in an IV formulation. Three dosage strengths are available, with 2 grams piperacillin and 0.25 gram tazobactam; 3 grams piperacillin and 0.375 gram tazobactam; or 4 grams piperacillin and 0.5 gram tazobactam.

CEPHALOSPORINS

Cephalosporins are a widely used group of drugs that are derived from a fungus. Although technically cefoxitin and cefotetan (cephamycins derived from a different fungus) and loracarbef (a carbacephem) are not cephalosporins, they are categorized with the cephalosporins because of their similarities to the group. Cephalosporins are broad-spectrum agents with activity against both gram-positive and gram-negative bacteria. Compared with penicillins, they are in general less active against gram-positive organisms but more active against gram-negative ones.

After they are absorbed, cephalosporins are widely distributed into most body fluids and tissues, with maximum concentrations in the liver and kidneys. Many cephalosporins do not reach therapeutic levels in CSF; exceptions are cefuroxime, a second-generation drug, and the third-generation agents. These drugs reach therapeutic levels when meninges are inflamed. Most cephalosporins are excreted through the kidneys. Exceptions include cefoperazone, which is excreted in bile, and ceftriaxone, which undergoes dual elimination via the biliary tract and kidneys. Cefotaxime is primarily metabolized in the liver to an active metabolite, desacetylcefotaxime, which is eliminated by the kidneys.

Indications for Use

Clinical indications for the use of cephalosporins include surgical prophylaxis and treatment of infections of the respiratory tract, skin and soft tissues, bones and joints, urinary tract, brain and spinal cord, and bloodstream (septicemia). In most infections with streptococci and staphylococci, penicillins are more effective and less expensive. In infections caused by MRSA, cephalosporins are not clinically effective even if in vitro testing indicates susceptibility. Infections caused by *Neisseria gonorrhoeae,* at one time susceptible to penicillin, are now treated with a third-generation cephalosporin such as ceftriaxone. Cefepime is indicated for use in sepsis; in severe infections of the lower respiratory and urinary tracts, skin and soft tissue, and female reproductive tract; and in febrile neutropenic clients. It may be used as monotherapy for all infections caused by susceptible organisms except *Pseudomonas aeruginosa;* a combination of drugs should be used for serious pseudomonal infections.

Contraindications to Use

A contraindication to the use of a cephalosporin is a previous severe anaphylactic reaction to a penicillin. Because cephalosporins are chemically similar to penicillins, there is a risk of cross-sensitivity. However, incidence of cross-sensitivity is low, especially in clients who have had delayed reactions (eg, skin rash) to penicillins. Another contraindication is cephalosporin allergy. Immediate allergic reactions with anaphylaxis, bronchospasm, and urticaria occur less often than delayed reactions with skin rash, drug fever, and eosinophilia.

Classification

Tables 30-3 and 30-4 provide important information about oral and parenteral cephalosporins.

First-Generation Cephalosporins

The first cephalosporin, cephalothin, is no longer available for clinical use. However, it is used for determining susceptibility to first-generation cephalosporins, which have essentially the same spectrum of antimicrobial activity. These drugs are effective against streptococci; staphylococci (except MRSA); *Neisseria, Salmonella, Shigella, Escherichia, Klebsiella,* and *Bacillus* species; *Corynebacterium diphtheriae; P. mirabilis;* and *Bacteroides* species (except *Bacteroides fragilis*). They are not effective against *Enterobacter, Pseudomonas,* and *Serratia* species. Cefazolin is the drug of choice for surgical prophylaxis in most surgical procedures.

Second-Generation Cephalosporins

Second-generation cephalosporins are more active against some gram-negative organisms and against anaerobic organisms than the first-generation drugs. Thus, they may be effective in infections resistant to other antibiotics, including

Table 30-3 Drugs at a Glance: Oral Cephalosporins

GENERIC/TRADE NAME	INDICATIONS FOR USE	ROUTES AND USUAL DOSAGE RANGES	
		Adults	Children
First Generation			
Cefadroxil (Duricef, Ultracef)	A derivative of cephalexin that has a longer half-life and can be given less often	PO 1–2 g twice daily	30 mg/kg/d in 2 doses q12h
Cephalexin (Keflex)	First oral cephalosporin; still used extensively	PO 250–500 mg q6h, increased to 4 g q6h if necessary in severe infections	PO 25–50 mg/kg/d in divided doses q6h
Cephradine (Velosef)	Essentially the same as cephalexin	PO 250–500 mg q6h, up to 4 g daily in severe infections	PO 25–50 mg/kg/d in divided doses q6h. In severe infections, up to 100 mg/kg/d may be given.
Second Generation			
Cefaclor (Ceclor)	More active against *Hemophilus influenzae* and *Escherichia coli* than first-generation drugs	PO 250–500 mg q8h	PO 20–40 mg/kg/d in 3 divided doses q8h
Cefprozil (Cefzil)	Similar to cefaclor	PO 250–500 mg q12–24h	PO 15 mg/kg q12h
Cefuroxime (Ceftin)	1. Can also be given parenterally 2. Available only in tablet form 3. The tablet may be crushed and added to a food (eg, applesauce), but the crushed tablet leaves a strong, bitter, persistent aftertaste.	PO 250 mg q12h; severe infections, 500 mg q12h; urinary tract infection, 125 mg q12h	*>12 y*, same as adults; *<12 y*, 125 mg q12h Otitis media, *>2 y*, 250 mg q12h, *<2 y*, 125 mg q12h
Loracarbef (Lorabid)	A synthetic drug similar to cefaclor	PO 200–400 mg q12h	PO 15–30 mg/kg/d in divided doses q12h
Third Generation			
Cefdinir (Omnicef)	Indicated for bronchitis, pharyngitis, and otitis media caused by streptococci or *H. influenzae*	PO 300 mg q12h or 600 mg q24h for 10 d	*≥13 y*, PO same as adults *6 mo–12 y*, PO 7 mg/kg q12h or 14 mg/kg q24h for 10 d
Cefditoren pivoxil (Spectracef)	Indicated for pharyngitis, bacterial exacerbations of chronic bronchitis, and skin/skin structure infections	Bronchitis or pharyngitis, PO 400 mg twice daily (q12h) for 10 d Skin infections, PO 200 mg twice daily for 10 d	*≥12 y*, same as adults
Cefixime (Suprax)	First oral third-generation drug	PO 200 mg q12h or 400 mg q24h	PO 4 mg/kg q12h or 8 mg/kg q24h; give adult dose to children 50 kg of weight or ≥12 y
Cefpodoxime (Vantin)	Similar to cefixime except has some activity against staphylococci (except methicillin-resistant *Staphylococcus aureus*)	PO 200–400 mg q12h	PO 5 mg/kg q12h Give 10 mg/kg (400 mg or adult dose) to children ≥13 y with skin and soft-tissue infections

Table 30-3 Drugs at a Glance: Oral Cephalosporins (continued)

GENERIC/TRADE NAME	INDICATIONS FOR USE	ROUTES AND USUAL DOSAGE RANGES	
		Adults	Children
Ceftibuten (Cedax)	1. Indicated for bronchitis, otitis media, pharyngitis, or tonsillitis caused by streptococci or *H. Influenzae* 2. Can be given once daily 3. Available in a capsule for oral use and an oral pediatric suspension that comes in two concentrations (90 mg/5 mL and 180 mg/5 mL)	PO 400 mg daily for 10 d	Oral suspension with 90 mg/5 mL *10 kg:* 5 mL daily *20 kg:* 10 mL daily *40 kg:* 20 mL daily *> 45 kg:* Same as adults Oral suspension with 180 mg/5 mL *10 kg:* 2.5 mL daily *20 kg:* 5 mL daily *40 kg:* 10 mL daily *> 45 kg:* Same as adults

PO, oral.

infections caused by *Hemophilus influenzae, Klebsiella* species, *E. coli,* and some strains of *Proteus.* Because each of these drugs has a different antimicrobial spectrum, susceptibility tests must be performed for each drug rather than for the entire group, as may be done with first-generation drugs. Cefoxitin (Mefoxin), for example, is active against *B. fragilis,* an anaerobic organism resistant to most drugs.

Third-Generation Cephalosporins

Third-generation cephalosporins further extend the spectrum of activity against gram-negative organisms. In addition to activity against the usual enteric pathogens (eg, *E. coli; Proteus* and *Klebsiella* species), they are also active against several strains resistant to other antibiotics and to first- and second-generation cephalosporins. Thus, they may be useful in infections caused by unusual strains of enteric organisms such as *Citrobacter, Serratia,* and *Providencia* species. Another difference is that third-generation cephalosporins penetrate inflamed meninges to reach therapeutic concentrations in CSF. Thus, they may be useful in meningeal infections caused by common pathogens, including *H. influenzae, Neisseria meningitidis,* and *Streptococcus pneumoniae.* Although some of the drugs are active against *Pseudomonas* organisms, drug-resistant strains may emerge when a cephalosporin is used alone for treatment of pseudomonal infection.

Overall, cephalosporins gain gram-negative activity and lose gram-positive activity as they move from the first to the third generation. The second- and third-generation drugs are more active against gram-negative organisms because they are more resistant to the beta-lactamase enzymes

(cephalosporinases) produced by some bacteria to inactivate cephalosporins.

Fourth-Generation Cephalosporins

Fourth-generation cephalosporins have a greater spectrum of antimicrobial activity and greater stability against breakdown by beta-lactamase enzymes compared with third-generation drugs. Cefepime is the first fourth-generation cephalosporin to be developed. It is active against both gram-positive and gram-negative organisms. With gram-positive organisms, it is active against streptococci and staphylococci (except for methicillin-resistant staphylococci). With gram-negative organisms, its activity against *P. aeruginosa* is similar to that of ceftazidime and its activity against Enterobacteriaceae is greater than that of third-generation cephalosporins. Moreover, cefepime retains activity against strains of Enterobacteriaceae and *P. aeruginosa* that have acquired resistance to third-generation agents.

APPLYING YOUR KNOWLEDGE 30-1

Why is cefazolin the drug of choice for Ms. Nudson's situation?

CARBAPENEMS

Carbapenems are broad-spectrum, bactericidal beta-lactam antimicrobials. Like other beta-lactam drugs, they inhibit synthesis of bacterial cell walls by binding with penicillin-binding proteins. The group consists of three drugs (Table 30-5).

Imipenem-cilastatin (Primaxin) is given parenterally and distributed in most body fluids. When given alone, the antibiotic imipenem is rapidly broken down by an enzyme

(text continues on page 494)

Table 30-4 Drugs at a Glance: Parenteral Cephalosporins

GENERIC/TRADE NAME	INDICATIONS FOR USE	ROUTES AND USUAL DOSAGE RANGES	
		Adults	Children
First Generation **Cefazolin** (Kefzol, Ancef)	Active against streptococci, staphylococci, *Neisseria, Salmonella, Shigella, Escherichia, Klebsiella, Listeria, Bacillus, Hemophilus influenzae, Corynebacterium diphtheriae, Proteus mirabilis,* and *Bacteroides* (except *B. fragilis*)	IM, IV 250 mg–1 g q6–8h	IM, IV 50–100 mg/kg/d in 3–4 divided doses
Second Generation **Cefotetan** (Cefotan)	1. Effective against most organisms except *Pseudomonas* 2. Highly resistant to beta-lactamase enzymes	IV, IM 1–2 g q12h for 5–10 d; maximum dose, 3 g q12h in life-threatening infections Surgical prophylaxis, IV 1–2 g 30–60 min before surgery	Dosage not established
Cefoxitin (Mefoxin)	1. The first cephamycin (derived from a different fungus than cephalosporins) 2. A major clinical use may stem from increased activity against *B. fragilis,* an organism resistant to most other antimicrobial drugs.	IV 1–2 g q4–6h Surgical prophylaxis, IV 1 or 2 g 30–60 min before surgery	IV 80–160 mg/kg/d in divided doses q4–6h. Do not exceed 12 g/d.
Cefuroxime (Kefurox, Zinacef)	1. Similar to other second-generation cephalosporins 2. Penetrates cerebrospinal fluid in presence of inflamed meninges	IV, IM, 750 mg–1.5 g q8h Surgical prophylaxis, IV 1.5 g 30–60 min before initial skin incision	*>3 mo:* IV, IM 50–100 mg/kg/d in divided doses q6–8h Bacterial meningitis, IV 200–240 mg/kg/d in divided doses q6–8h, reduced to 100 mg/kg/d on clinical improvement
Third Generation **Cefoperazone** (Cefobid)	1. Active against gram-negative and gram-positive organisms, including gram-negative organisms resistant to earlier cephalosporins 2. Excreted primarily in bile; half-life prolonged in hepatic failure	IV, IM 2–4 g/d in divided doses q8–12h	Dosage not established
Cefotaxime (Claforan)	1. Antibacterial activity against most gram-positive and gram-negative bacteria, including several strains resistant to other antibiotics 2. Recommended for serious infections caused by susceptible microorganisms	IV, IM 1 g q6–8h; maximum dose, 12 g/24h	*Weight >50 kg:* same as adults *Weight <50 kg* and *age > 1 mo:* IV, IM 50–180 mg/kg/d, in divided doses q4–6h *Neonates:* ≤ 1 wk, IV 50 mg/kg q12h; *1–4 wk,* IV 50 mg/kg q8h

Table 30-4 Drugs at a Glance: Parenteral Cephalosporins (continued)

GENERIC/TRADE NAME	INDICATIONS FOR USE	ROUTES AND USUAL DOSAGE RANGES	
		Adults	Children
Ceftazidime (Fortaz)	1. Active against gram-positive and gram-negative organisms 2. Especially effective against gram-negative organisms, including *Pseudomonas aeruginosa* and other bacterial strains resistant to aminoglycosides 3. Indicated for serious infections caused by susceptible organisms	IV, IM 1 g q8–12h	*1 mo–12 y:* IV 30–50 mg/kg q8h, not to exceed 6 g/d *<1 mo:* IV 30 mg/kg q12h
Ceftizoxime (Cefizox)	1. Broader gram-negative and anaerobic activity, especially against *B. fragilis* 2. More active against Enterobacteriaceae than cefoperazone 3. Dosage must be reduced with even mild renal insufficiency (CrCl < 80 mL/min).	IV, IM 1–2 g q8–12h	*>6 mo:* IV, IM 50 mg/kg q6–8h, increased to a total daily dose of 200 mg/kg if necessary
Ceftriaxone (Rocephin)	1. First third-generation cephalosporin approved for once-daily dosing 2. Antibacterial activity against most gram-positive and gram-negative bacteria, including several strains resistant to other antibiotics	IV, IM 1–2 g once daily (q24h)	IV, IM 50–75 mg/kg/d, not to exceed 2 g daily, in divided doses q12h Meningitis, IV, IM 100 mg/kg/d, not to exceed 4 g daily, in divided doses q12h
Fourth Generation **Cefepime** (Maxipime)	1. Indicated for urinary-tract infections caused by *Escherichia coli* or *Klebsiella pneumoniae;* skin and soft tissue infections caused by susceptible streptococci or staphylococci; pneumonia caused by *Streptococcus pneumoniae* or *P. aeruginosa;* complicated intra-abdominal infection and empiric therapy of febrile, neutropenic clients 2. Dosage must be reduced with renal impairment.	IV 0.5–2 g q12h IM 0.5–1 g q12h	*Weight ≤ 40 kg:* 50–150 mg/kg/day in 2–3 divided doses, not to exceed recommended adult dose

IM, intramuscular; IV, intravenous.

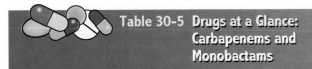

Table 30-5 Drugs at a Glance: Carbapenems and Monobactams

GENERIC/TRADE NAME	ROUTES AND USUAL DOSAGE RANGES	
	Adults	Children
Carbapenems		
Ertapenem (Invanz)	IV 1 g once daily over 15–30 min	Dosage not established
Imipenem-cilastatin (Primaxin)	IV 250–1,000 mg q6–8h. Maximum dose, 4 g/d IM 500–750 mg q12h	Weight >40 kg, same as adults Weight <40 kg, IV up to 10 mg/kg/d in divided doses. Maximum dose, 2 g/d
Meropenem (Merrem)	IV 1 g q8h, as a bolus injection over 3–5 min or infusion over 15–30 min	≥ 3 mo, IV 20–40 mg/kg q8h
Monobactam		
Aztreonam (Azactam)	IM, IV: UTI, 0.5–1.0 g q8–12h Moderate systemic infection, 1–2 g q8–12h Severe systemic infection, 2 g q6–8h	IM, IV 30 mg/kg q6–8h

IM, intramuscular; IV, intravenous; UTI, urinary tract infection.

(dehydropeptidase) in renal tubules and therefore reaches only low concentrations in the urine. Imipenem is formulated with cilastatin, which inhibits the destruction of imipenem by the enzyme. The addition of cilastatin increases the urinary concentration of imipenem, and reduces the potential renal toxicity of the antibacterial agent. Recommended doses indicate the amount of imipenem; the solution contains an equivalent amount of cilastatin.

The drug is effective in infections caused by a wide range of bacteria, including penicillinase-producing staphylococci, *E. coli*, *Proteus* species, *Enterobacter–Klebsiella–Serratia* species, *P. aeruginosa*, and *Enterococcus faecalis*. Its main use is treatment of infections caused by organisms resistant to other drugs. Adverse effects are similar to those of other beta-lactam antibiotics, including the risk of cross-sensitivity in clients with penicillin hypersensitivity. Central nervous

system toxicity, including seizures, has been reported. Seizures are more likely in clients with a seizure disorder or when recommended doses are exceeded; however, they have occurred in other clients as well. To prepare the solution for IM injection, lidocaine, a local anesthetic, is added to decrease pain. This solution is contraindicated in people allergic to this type of local anesthetic or who have severe shock or heart block.

Meropenem (Merrem) has a broad spectrum of antibacterial activity and may be used as a single drug for empiric therapy before causative microorganisms are identified. It is effective against penicillin-susceptible staphylococci and *S. pneumoniae;* most gram-negative aerobes (eg, *E. coli, H. influenzae, Klebsiella pneumoniae, P. aeruginosa*); and some anaerobes, including *B. fragilis*. It is indicated for use in intra-abdominal infections and bacterial meningitis caused by susceptible organisms. Adverse effects are similar to those of imipenem.

Ertapenem (Invanz) also has a broad spectrum of antibacterial activity, although more limited than imipenem and meropenem. It is approved for complicated intra-abdominal, skin and skin structure, acute pelvic, and urinary tract infections. It can be used to treat community-acquired pneumonia caused by penicillin-susceptible *S. pneumoniae*. Unlike imipenem and meropenem, ertapenem does not have in vitro activity against *P. aeruginosa* and *Acinetobacter baumannii*.

Ertapenem shares the adverse effect profile of the other carbapenems. Lidocaine is also used in preparation of the solution for IM injection, and the same cautions should be used as with imipenem.

MONOBACTAM

Aztreonam (Azactam) (see Table 30-5) is active against gram-negative bacteria, including Enterobacteriaceae and *P. aeruginosa*, and many strains that are resistant to multiple antibiotics. Activity against gram-negative bacteria is similar to that of the aminoglycosides, but the drug does not cause kidney damage or hearing loss. Aztreonam is stable in the presence of beta-lactamase enzymes. Because gram-positive and anaerobic bacteria are resistant to aztreonam, the drug's ability to preserve normal gram-positive and anaerobic flora may be an advantage over other antimicrobial agents.

Indications for use include infections of the urinary tract, skin and skin structures, and lower respiratory tract, as well as intra-abdominal and gynecologic infections and septicemia. Adverse effects are similar to those for penicillin, including possible hypersensitivity reactions.

NURSING PROCESS

General aspects of the nursing process in antimicrobial drug therapy, as described in Chapter 29, apply to the client receiving penicillins, cephalosporins, aztreonam, and carbapenems. In this chapter, only those aspects related specifically to these drugs are included.

Assessment

With penicillins, ask clients if they have ever taken a penicillin and, if so, whether they ever had a skin rash, hives, swelling, or difficulty breathing associated with the drug. With cephalosporins, ask clients if they have ever taken one of the drugs, as far as they know, and whether they ever had a severe reaction to penicillin. Naming a few cephalosporins (eg, Ceclor, Keflex, Rocephin, Suprax) may help the client identify previous usage.

Nursing Diagnoses

- Risk for Injury: Hypersensitivity reactions with penicillins or cephalosporins
- Risk for Injury: Renal impairment with cephalosporins
- Deficient Knowledge: Correct home care administration and usage of oral beta-lactams

Planning/Goals

The client will

- Take oral beta-lactam antibacterials as directed
- Receive parenteral beta-lactam drugs by appropriate techniques to minimize tissue irritation
- Receive prompt and appropriate treatment if hypersensitivity reactions occur

Interventions

- After giving a penicillin parenterally in an outpatient setting, keep the client in the area for at least 30 minutes. Anaphylactic reactions are more likely to occur with parenteral than oral use and within a few minutes after injection.
- In any client care setting, keep emergency equipment and supplies readily available.
- Monitor client response to beta-lactam drugs.
- Monitor dosages of beta-lactam drugs for clients with impaired renal function.
- Provide client teaching regarding drug therapy (see accompanying displays).

Evaluation

- Observe for improvement in signs of infection.
- Interview and observe for adverse drug effects.

PRINCIPLES OF THERAPY

Goal of Therapy

The goal of antimicrobial therapy is to prevent or treat infections caused by pathogenic microorganisms.

Drug Selection

Choice of a beta-lactam antibacterial depends on the organism causing the infection, severity of the infection, and other factors.

CLIENT TEACHING GUIDELINES

Oral Penicillins

General Considerations

☑ Do not take any penicillin if you have ever had an allergic reaction to penicillin in which you had difficulty breathing, swelling, or skin rash. However, some people call a minor stomach upset an allergic reaction and are not given penicillin when that is the best antibiotic in a given situation.

☑ Complete the full course of drug treatment for greater effectiveness and prevention of secondary infection with drug-resistant bacteria.

☑ Follow instructions carefully about the dose and how often it is taken. Drug effectiveness depends on maintaining adequate blood levels.

☑ Penicillins often need more frequent administration than some other antibiotics, because they are rapidly excreted by the kidneys.

Self- or Caregiver Administration

☑ Take most penicillins on an empty stomach, 1 hour before or 2 hours after a meal. Penicillin V, amoxicillin, and Augmentin can be taken without regard to meals.

☑ Take each dose with a full glass of water; do not take with orange juice or with other acidic fluids (they may destroy the drug).

☑ Take at even intervals, preferably around the clock.

☑ Shake liquid penicillins well, to mix thoroughly and measure the dose accurately.

☑ Discard liquid penicillin after 1 week if stored at room temperature or after 2 weeks if refrigerated. Liquid forms deteriorate and should not be taken after their expiration dates.

☑ Report skin rash, hives, itching, severe diarrhea, shortness of breath, fever, sore throat, black tongue, or any unusual bleeding. These symptoms may indicate a need to stop the penicillin.

General Considerations

✔ Inform your physician if you have ever had a severe allergic reaction to penicillin in which you had difficulty breathing, swelling, or skin rash. A small number of people are allergic to both penicillins and cephalosporins because the drugs are somewhat similar in their chemical structures.

✔ Also inform your physician if you have had a previous allergic reaction to a cephalosporin (eg, Ceclor, Keflex). If not sure whether a new prescription is a cephalosporin, ask the pharmacist before having the prescription filled.

✔ Complete the full course of drug treatment for greater effectiveness and prevention of secondary infection with drug-resistant bacteria.

✔ Follow instructions about dosing frequency; effectiveness depends on maintaining adequate blood levels.

Self- or Caregiver Administration

✔ Take most oral drugs with food or milk to prevent stomach upset.

✔ Take cefpodoxime (Vantin) and cefuroxime (Ceftin) with food to increase absorption.

✔ Do not take cefaclor (Ceclor), cefdinir (Omnicef), or cefpodoxime (Vantin) with antacids containing aluminum or magnesium (eg, Maalox, Mylanta) or with Pepcid, Tagamet, or Zantac. These drugs decrease absorption of these antibiotics and make them less effective. If necessary to take one of the drugs, take it 2 hours before or 2 hours after a dose of these antibiotics.

✔ Shake liquid preparations well to mix thoroughly and measure the dose accurately.

✔ Report the occurrence of diarrhea, especially if it is severe or contains blood, pus, or mucus. Cephalosporins can cause antibiotic-associated colitis and the drug may need to be stopped.

✔ Inform the prescribing physician if you are breast-feeding. These drugs enter breast milk.

Penicillins

Penicillin G or amoxicillin is the drug of choice in many infections. An antipseudomonal penicillin is indicated in *Pseudomonas* infections. An antistaphylococcal penicillin is indicated in staphylococcal infections; antistaphylococcal drugs of choice are nafcillin for IV use and dicloxacillin for oral use.

Cephalosporins

First-generation drugs are often used for surgical prophylaxis, especially with prosthetic implants, because gram-positive organisms such as staphylococci cause most infections of surgical sites. They may also be used alone for treatment of infections caused by susceptible organisms in body sites where drug penetration and host defenses are adequate. Cefazolin (Kefzol) is a frequently used parenteral agent. It reaches a higher serum concentration, is more protein bound, and has a slower rate of elimination than other first-generation drugs. These factors prolong serum half-life, so cefazolin can be given less frequently. Cefazolin may also be administered IM.

Second-generation cephalosporins are also often used for surgical prophylaxis, especially for gynecologic and colorectal surgery. They are also used for treatment of intra-abdominal infections such as pelvic inflammatory disease, diverticulitis, penetrating wounds of the abdomen, and other infections caused by organisms inhabiting pelvic and colorectal areas.

Third-generation cephalosporins are recommended for serious infections caused by susceptible organisms that are resistant to first- and second-generation cephalosporins. They are often used in the treatment of infections caused by *E. coli; Proteus, Klebsiella,* and *Serratia* species; and other Enterobacteriaceae, especially when the infections occur in body sites not readily reached by other drugs (eg, CSF, bone) and in clients with immunosuppression. Although effective against many *Pseudomonas* strains, these drugs should not be used alone in treating pseudomonal infections because drug resistance develops.

Fourth-generation drugs are most useful in serious gram-negative infections, especially infections caused by organisms resistant to third-generation drugs. Cefepime has the same indications for use as ceftazidime, a third-generation drug.

Drug Dosage and Administration

Choice of route and dosage depends mainly on the severity of the infection being treated. For serious infections, beta-lactam antibacterials are usually given IV in large doses. With penicillins, most must be given every 4 to 6 hours to maintain therapeutic blood levels, because the kidneys rapidly excrete them. The oral route is often used for less serious infections and for long-term prophylaxis of rheumatic fever. The IM route is rarely used in hospitalized clients but may be used in ambulatory settings. With cephalosporins, a few are sufficiently absorbed for oral administration; these are most often used in mild infections and UTI. Although some cephalosporins can be given IM, the injections cause pain and induration. Cefazolin is preferred for IM administration because it is less irritating to tissues.

Hypersensitivity to Penicillins

Before giving the initial dose of any penicillin preparation, ask the client if he or she has ever taken penicillin and, if so, whether an allergic reaction occurred. Penicillin is the most common cause of drug-induced anaphylaxis, a life-threatening hypersensitivity reaction, and a person known to be hypersensitive should be given another type of antibiotic.

In the rare instance in which penicillin is considered essential, a skin test may be helpful in assessing hypersensitivity. Benzylpenicilloyl polylysine (Pre-Pen) or a dilute solution of the penicillin to be administered (10,000 units/mL) may be applied topically to a skin scratch made with a sterile needle. If the scratch test is negative (no urticaria, erythema, or pruritus), the preparation may be injected intradermally. Allergic reactions, including fatal anaphylactic shock, have occurred with skin tests and after negative skin tests. If the scratch test is positive, desensitization may be accomplished by giving gradually increasing doses of penicillin.

Because anaphylactic shock may occur with administration of the penicillins, especially by parenteral routes, emergency drugs and equipment must be readily available. Treatment may require parenteral epinephrine, oxygen, and insertion of an endotracheal or tracheostomy tube if laryngeal edema occurs.

APPLYING YOUR KNOWLEDGE 30-2
The physician finds signs of infection during Ms. Nudson's bronchoscopy and orders the client to take amoxicillin 500 mg every 8 hours for 10 days, pending the results of the culture and susceptibility studies. Ms. Nudson has the prescription filled and starts taking the medication. What should members of the health care team assess before Ms. Nudson takes this medication?

Use of Penicillins in Specific Situations

Treatment of Streptococcal Infections

Clinicians should perform culture and susceptibility studies and be aware of local patterns of streptococcal susceptibility or resistance before prescribing penicillins for streptococcal infections. When used, penicillins should be given for the full prescribed course of treatment to prevent complications such as rheumatic fever, endocarditis, and glomerulonephritis.

Use in Combination With Probenecid

Probenecid (Benemid) can be given concurrently with penicillins to increase serum drug levels. Probenecid acts by blocking renal excretion of the penicillins. This action may be useful when high serum levels are needed with oral penicillins or when a single large dose is given IM for prevention or treatment of syphilis.

Use in Combination With Aminoglycosides

Aminoglycosides are often given concomitantly with penicillin for serious infections, such as those caused by *P. aeruginosa.*

The drugs should not be admixed in a syringe or in an IV solution, because the penicillin inactivates the aminoglycoside.

APPLYING YOUR KNOWLEDGE 30-3
Ms. Nudson has never before had a reaction to a medication and calls the office to report a skin rash and difficulty breathing. What action should you take?

Use in Special Populations

Perioperative Use of Cephalosporins

Some cephalosporins are used in surgical prophylaxis. The particular drug depends largely on the type of organism likely to be encountered in the operative area. First-generation drugs, mainly cefazolin, are used for procedures associated with gram-positive postoperative infections, such as prosthetic implant surgery. Second-generation cephalosporins (mainly cefotetan and cefoxitin) are often used for abdominal procedures, especially gynecologic and colorectal surgery, in which enteric gram-negative postoperative infections may occur. Third-generation drugs should not be used for surgical prophylaxis because they are less active against staphylococci than cefazolin; the gram-negative organisms they are most useful against are rarely encountered in elective surgery; widespread usage for prophylaxis promotes emergence of drug-resistant organisms; and they are very expensive.

When used perioperatively, cephalosporins should be given within 2 hours before the first skin incision is made so the drug has time to reach therapeutic serum and tissue concentrations. A single dose is usually sufficient, although repeat doses are necessary in clients undergoing a surgical procedure exceeding 4 hours or procedures involving major blood loss. Postoperative doses are rarely necessary, but, if used, should generally not exceed 24 hours.

Use in Children

Penicillins and cephalosporins are widely used to treat infections in children and are generally safe. They should be used cautiously in neonates because immature kidney function slows their elimination. Dosages should be based on age, weight, severity of the infection being treated, and renal function. Specialized pediatric dosing references can provide guidance to dosing of most beta-lactams based on the child's age and weight.

Use in Older Adults

Beta-lactam antibacterials are relatively safe, although decreased renal function, other disease processes, and concurrent drug therapies increase the risks of adverse effects in older adults. With penicillins, hyperkalemia may occur with large IV doses of penicillin G potassium and hypernatremia may occur with ticarcillin. Hypernatremia is less likely with other antipseudomonal penicillins such as piperacillin. Cephalosporins may aggravate renal impairment, especially when other nephrotoxic drugs are used concurrently. Dosage of most cephalosporins must be reduced in the presence of renal impairment, depending on creatinine clearance (CrCl).

With aztreonam, imipenem-cilastatin, meropenem, and ertapenem, dose and frequency of administration are determined by renal status as indicated by CrCl.

Use in Clients With Renal Impairment

Beta-lactam antimicrobials are excreted mainly by the kidneys and may accumulate in the presence of renal impairment. Dosage of many beta-lactams must be decreased according to CrCl. In addition, some of the drugs are nephrotoxic. References should be consulted to determine dosages recommended for various levels of CrCl. Additional considerations are included in the following sections.

Penicillins
- Dosage of penicillin G, carbenicillin, piperacillin, piperacillin-tazobactam, and ticarcillin should be reduced.
- Clients on hemodialysis usually require an additional dose after treatment because hemodialysis removes substantial amounts and produces subtherapeutic serum drug levels.
- Carbenicillin, which is used to treat UTI, does not reach therapeutic levels in urine in clients with severe renal impairment (CrCl <10 mL/minute).
- Nephropathy, such as interstitial nephritis, although infrequent, has occurred with all penicillins. It is most often associated with high doses of parenteral penicillins and is attributed to hypersensitivity reactions. Manifestations include fever, skin rash, eosinophilia, and possibly increased levels of blood urea nitrogen and serum creatinine.
- Electrolyte imbalances, mainly hypernatremia and hyperkalemia, may occur. Hypernatremia is most likely to occur when ticarcillin (5.6 mEq sodium/g) is given to clients with renal impairment or congestive heart failure. Hypokalemic metabolic acidosis may also occur with ticarcillin because potassium loss is enhanced by high sodium intake. Hyperkalemia may occur with large IV doses of penicillin G potassium (1.7 mEq/ 1 million units).

Cephalosporins
- Reduce dosage because usual doses may produce high and prolonged serum drug levels. In renal failure (CrCl <20 to 30 mL/minute), dosage of all cephalosporins except cefoperazone should be reduced. Cefoperazone is excreted primarily through the bile and therefore does not accumulate with renal failure.
- Cefotaxime is converted to active metabolites that are normally eliminated by the kidneys. These metabolites accumulate and may cause toxicity in clients with renal impairment.

Carbapenems
- Dosage of imipenem should be reduced in most clients with renal impairment and the drug is contraindicated in clients with severe renal impairment (CrCl of 5 mL/minute or less) unless hemodialysis is started within 48 hours. For clients already on hemodialysis, the drug may cause seizures and should be used very cautiously, if at all.
- Dosage of meropenem should be reduced with renal impairment (CrCl <50 mL/minute).
- Dosage of ertapenem should be reduced to 500 mg daily with renal impairment (CrCl <30 mL/minute). For clients on hemodialysis, administer the daily dose after dialysis.

Monobactam
- After an initial loading dose, the dosage of aztreonam should be reduced by 50% or more in clients with CrCl of 30 mL/minute or less. Give at the usual intervals of 6, 8, or 12 hours.
- For serious or life-threatening infections in clients on hemodialysis, give 12.5% of the initial dose after each hemodialysis session, in addition to maintenance doses.

Use in Clients With Hepatic Impairment

- A few beta-lactam antibiotics may cause or aggravate hepatic impairment.
- Amoxicillin-clavulanate (Augmentin) should be used with caution in clients with hepatic impairment. It is contraindicated in clients who have had cholestatic jaundice and hepatic dysfunction with previous use of the drug. Cholestatic liver impairment usually subsides when the drug is stopped. Hepatotoxicity is attributed to the clavulanate component and has also occurred with ticarcillin-clavulanate (Timentin).
- Cefoperazone is excreted mainly in bile and its serum half-life increases in clients with hepatic impairment or biliary obstruction. Adverse effects include cholestasis, jaundice, and hepatitis. Serum drug levels should be monitored if high doses are given (>4 g).
- Aztreonam, imipenem, meropenem, and ertapenem may cause abnormalities in liver function test results (ie, elevated alanine and aspartate aminotransferases [ALT and AST] and alkaline phosphatase), but hepatitis and jaundice rarely occur.

Use in Clients With Critical Illness

Beta-lactam antimicrobials are commonly used in critical care units to treat pneumonia, bloodstream, wound, and other infections. The beta-lactam drugs are frequently given concomitantly with other antimicrobial drugs because critically ill clients often have multiorganism or nosocomial infections. Renal, hepatic, and other organ functions should be monitored in critically ill clients and drug dosages should be reduced when indicated.

With penicillins, the extended-spectrum drugs (eg, piperacillin) and penicillin–beta-lactamase inhibitor combinations (eg, Unasyn) are most likely to be used. With cephalosporins, third- and fourth-generation drugs are commonly used and are usually given by intermittent IV infusions every 8 or 12 hours. Continuous infusions of beta-lactam antibiotics also may be used. Blood levels of cephalosporins and penicillins need to be maintained above the minimum inhibitory concentration (MIC) of the microorganisms causing the infection being treated. Thus, continuous infusions may be of benefit with serious infections, especially those caused by relatively resistant organisms such as *Pseudomonas* or *Acinetobacter*.

Use in Home Care

Many beta-lactam antibiotics are given in the home setting. With oral agents, the role of the home care nurse is mainly to teach accurate administration and observation for therapeutic and adverse effects. With liquid suspensions for children, shaking to re-suspend medication and measuring with a measuring spoon or calibrated device are required for safe dosing. Household spoons should *not* be used because they vary widely in capacity. General guidelines for IV therapy are discussed in Chapter 29; specific guidelines depend on the drug being given.

APPLYING YOUR KNOWLEDGE 30-4:
HOW CAN YOU AVOID THIS MEDICATION ERROR?

Ms. Nudson recovers from her allergic reaction to the penicillin. Her medical records now indicate that she is allergic to PCN. Her culture reports from the bronchoscopic examination have become available; her infection is caused by an organism sensitive to Zosyn. The nurse prepares the dose to be administered and starts the infusion. Ms. Nudson experiences anaphylaxis and has to be resuscitated.

N U R S I N G   A C T I O N S

Beta-Lactam Antibacterials

NURSING ACTIONS	RATIONALE/EXPLANATION
1. Administer accurately	
a. With penicillins:	
(1) Give most oral penicillins on an empty stomach, approximately 1 hour before or 2 hours after a meal. Penicillin V, amoxicillin, and amoxicillin/clavulanate may be given without regard to meals.	To decrease binding to foods and inactivation by gastric acid. The latter three drugs are not significantly affected by food.
(2) Give oral drugs with a full glass of water, preferably; do not give with orange juice or other acidic fluids.	To promote absorption and decrease inactivation, which may occur in an acidic environment
(3) Give intramuscular (IM) penicillins deeply into a large muscle mass.	To decrease tissue irritation
(4) For intravenous (IV) administration, usually dilute reconstituted penicillins in 50–100 milliliters of 5% dextrose or 0.9% sodium chloride injection and infuse over 30–60 minutes.	To minimize vascular irritation and phlebitis
(5) Give reconstituted ampicillin IV or IM within 1 hour.	The drug is stable in solution for a limited time, after which effectiveness is lost.
b. With cephalosporins:	
(1) Give most oral drugs with food or milk. Cefpodoxime and cefuroxime should be taken with food.	To decrease nausea and vomiting. Food delays absorption but does not affect the amount of drug absorbed. An exception is the pediatric suspension of ceftibuten, which must be given at least 2 hours before or 1 hour after a meal. Food increases the absorption of cefpodoxime and cefuroxime.
(2) Give IM drugs deeply into a large muscle mass.	The drugs are irritating to tissues and cause pain, induration, and possibly sterile abscess. The IM route is rarely used.
(3) For IV administration, usually dilute reconstituted drugs in 50–100 milliliters of 5% dextrose or 0.9% sodium chloride injection and infuse over 30 minutes.	These drugs are irritating to veins and cause thrombophlebitis. This can be minimized by using small IV catheters, large veins, adequate dilution, and slow infusion rates, and by changing venipuncture sites. Thrombophlebitis is more likely to occur with doses of more than 6 g/day for longer than 3 days.

(continued)

NURSING ACTIONS	RATIONALE/EXPLANATION
c. With carbapenems:	
(1) For IV imipenem, mix reconstituted solution in 100 milliliters of 0.9% NaCl or 5% dextrose injection. Give 250- to 500-mg doses over 20–30 minutes; give 750-mg to 1-g doses over 40–60 minutes.	Manufacturer's recommendations
(2) For IM imipenem and ertapenem, mix with 1% lidocaine without epinephrine and inject deeply into a large muscle mass with a 21-gauge, 2-inch needle.	To decrease pain of injection
(3) For IV meropenem, give as an injection over 3–5 minutes or as an infusion over 15–30 minutes.	
(4) For IV ertapenem, mix in 50 milliliters 0.9% sodium chloride and infuse over 30 minutes.	Manufacturer's recommendations
d. With aztreonam:	
(1) For IM administration, add 3 milliliters diluent per gram of drug, and inject into a large muscle mass.	
(2) For IV injection, add 6–10 milliliters sterile water, and inject into vein or IV tubing over 3–5 minutes.	
(3) For IV infusion, mix in at least 50 milliliters of 0.9% NaCl or 5% dextrose injection per gram of drug and give over 20–60 minutes.	
2. Observe for therapeutic effects	See Chapter 29.
a. Decreased signs of local and systemic infection	
b. Decreased signs and symptoms of the infection for which the drug is given	
c. Absence of signs and symptoms of infection when given prophylactically	
3. Observe for adverse effects	
a. Hypersensitivity—anaphylaxis, serum sickness, skin rash, urticaria	See Nursing Actions in Chapter 29 for signs and symptoms. Reactions are more likely to occur in those with previous hypersensitivity reactions and those with a history of allergy, asthma, or hay fever. Anaphylaxis is more likely with parenteral administration and may occur within 5–30 minutes of injection.
b. Phlebitis at IV sites and pain at IM sites	Parenteral solutions are irritating to body tissue.
c. Superinfection	See Chapter 29 for signs and symptoms.
d. Nausea and vomiting	May occur with all beta-lactam drugs, especially with high oral doses
e. Diarrhea, colitis, pseudomembranous colitis	Diarrhea commonly occurs with beta-lactam drugs and may range from mild to severe. The most severe form is pseudomembranous colitis, which is more often associated with ampicillin and the cephalosporins than other beta-lactams.
f. Nephrotoxicity	
(1) Acute interstitial nephritis (AIN)—hematuria, oliguria, proteinuria, pyuria	AIN may occur with any of the beta-lactams, especially with high parenteral doses of penicillins.
(2) Increased blood urea nitrogen and serum creatinine; casts in urine	More likely with cephalosporins, especially in clients who are older or who have impaired renal function, unless dosage is reduced
g. Neurotoxicity—confusion, hallucinations, neuromuscular irritability, convulsive seizures	More likely with large IV doses of penicillins, cephalosporins, or carbapenems, especially in clients with impaired renal function
h. Coagulation disorders and bleeding from hypoprothrombinemia or platelet dysfunction	Ticarcillin may cause decreased platelet aggregation. Cefoperazone and cefotetan may cause hypoprothrombinemia (by killing intestinal

NURSING ACTIONS	RATIONALE/EXPLANATION
	bacteria that normally produce vitamin K or a chemical structure that prevents activation of prothrombin) or platelet dysfunction. Bleeding can be treated by giving vitamin K. Vitamin K does not restore normal platelet function or normal bacterial flora in the intestines.
4. Observe for drug interactions	
a. Drugs that *increase* effects of penicillins:	
(1) Gentamicin and other aminoglycosides	Synergistic activity against *Pseudomonas* organisms when given concomitantly with extended-spectrum (antipseudomonal) penicillins
	Synergistic activity against enterococci that cause subacute bacterial endocarditis, brain abscess, meningitis, or urinary tract infection
	Synergistic activity against *Staphylococcus aureus* when used with nafcillin
(2) Probenecid (Benemid)	Decreases renal excretion of penicillins, thus elevating and prolonging penicillin blood levels
b. Drugs that *decrease* effects of penicillins:	
(1) Acidifying agents (ascorbic acid, cranberry juice, orange juice)	Most oral penicillins are destroyed by acids, including gastric acid. Amoxicillin and penicillin V are acid stable.
(2) Erythromycin	Erythromycin inhibits the bactericidal activity of penicillins against most organisms but potentiates activity against resistant strains of *S. aureus.*
(3) Tetracyclines	These bacteriostatic antibiotics slow multiplication of bacteria and thereby inhibit the penicillins, which act against rapidly multiplying bacteria.
(4) Aminoglycosides, if admixed	The penicillin will inactivate the aminoglycoside.
c. Drugs that *increase* effects of cephalosporins:	
(1) Loop diuretics (furosemide, ethacrynic acid)	Increased renal toxicity
(2) Probenecid	Increases blood levels by decreasing renal excretion of the cephalosporins. This may be a desirable interaction to increase blood levels and therapeutic effectiveness or allow smaller doses.
d. Drugs that *decrease* effects of cephalosporins:	
(1) Antacids containing aluminum or magnesium (eg, Mylanta) and histamine H_2 antagonists (eg, cimetidine, ranitidine)	These drugs decrease absorption of cefaclor, cefdinir, and cefpodoxime. Give the drugs at least 2 hours apart.
e. Drugs that *increase* effects of carbapenems:	
(1) Probenecid	Probenecid minimally increases serum drug levels of carbapenems, but it is not recommended for concomitant use with any of the drugs.
(2) Cyclosporine	May increase central nervous system adverse effects of imipenem
f. Drugs that *alter* effects of aztreonam	Few documented, clinically significant interactions reported, but potential interactions are those that occur with other beta-lactam antibiotics.

APPLYING YOUR KNOWLEDGE: ANSWERS

30-1 First-generation cephalosporins are the drug of choice for surgical prophylaxis. They are active against a large number of bacteria and have a low incidence of adverse effects.

30-2 The physician, pharmacist, and nurse should ask Ms. Nudson if she has ever taken penicillin and if she has ever had an allergic reaction to it. Penicillin is the most common cause of drug-induced anaphylaxis.

30-3 Tell Ms. Nudson to call 911. She should be transported to the nearest emergency facility immediately. This is most likely a severe reaction to the penicillin.

30-4 The nurse should recognize that piperacillin-tazobactam (Zosyn) is a combination of a penicillin and a beta-lactamase inhibitor. An allergy to any penicillin means that Ms. Nudson cannot receive *any other* penicillin-containing drug.

Review and Application Exercises

Short Answer Exercises

1. How do beta-lactam drugs act against bacteria?

2. What adverse effects are associated with beta-lactam drugs, and how may they be prevented or minimized?

3. What are beta-lactamase enzymes, and what do they do to beta-lactam antibacterial drugs?

4. How are penicillins and other beta-lactam drugs excreted?

5. What are the main differences between penicillin G or V and antistaphylococcal and antipseudomonal penicillins?

6. What is the reason for combining clavulanate, sulbactam, or tazobactam with a penicillin?

7. When giving injections of penicillin in an outpatient setting, it is recommended to keep clients in the area and observe them for at least 30 minutes. Why?

8. When probenecid is given concurrently with a penicillin, what is its purpose?

9. What are the signs and symptoms of anaphylaxis?

10. For clients with renal impairment, which drugs in this chapter require reduced dosage?

11. Which drugs in this chapter may cause pseudomembranous (antibiotic-associated) colitis?

12. What are the signs, symptoms, and treatment of pseudomembranous colitis?

NCLEX-Style Questions

13. A nurse is preparing to administer the first dose of piperacillin-tazobactam (Zosyn) to a client in an infusion clinic. The nurse should take which of the following precautions?

    a. Asking the client about past allergic reactions to penicillins.
    b. Asking the client about past allergic reactions to aminoglycosides.
    c. Mixing the piperacillin-tazobactam with lidocaine to reduce pain of infusion.
    d. Instructing the client to eat a snack to decrease stomach upset from piperacillin-tazobactam.

14. A woman is to receive Augmentin 500 mg PO q8h for bronchitis. The nurse retrieves two 250-mg tablets from the medication cart. This is incorrect for which of the following reasons?

    a. The amount of sulbactam in Augmentin 250 mg is 62.5 mg per tablet, twice the intended amount.
    b. This will provide twice the intended dose of clavulanate.
    c. The 250-mg tablets have less absorption than the 500-mg tablets.
    d. Augmentin can only be given IV, so giving tablets means that the wrong drug is being administered.

15. A nurse working in the neurointensive care unit is caring for a head-injury victim who has been experiencing seizures and now has *P. aeruginosa* pneumonia. The physician has prescribed imipenem 1 g IV q6h plus gentamicin for the pneumonia. Prior to administering the antibiotics, the nurse should do which of the following?

    a. Not admix the imipenem and gentamicin in the same IV bag to prevent inactivation of the gentamicin.
    b. Remind the physician of the client's seizures and inquire whether a different antibiotic might be safer.
    c. Suggest to the physician that imipenem is used to treat gram-positive infections and will not be effective in this client.
    d. Set the infusion pump to deliver the imipenem over 15 minutes.

16. In acute renal failure, doses of all of the following antibiotics must be reduced except
    a. nafcillin
    b. cefazolin
    c. meropenem
    d. aztreonam

17. Which of the following classes of cephalosporins has the best ac3tivity against gram-positive organisms?

a. first-generation cephalosporins
b. second-generation cephalosporins
c. third-generation cephalosporins
d. fourth-generation cephalosporins

Selected References

Bush, L. M., & Johnson, C. C. (2000). Antibacterial therapy: Ureido-penicillins and beta-lactam/beta-lactamase inhibitor combinations. *Infectious Disease Clinics of North America, 14*(2), 409–433.

Dancer, S. J. (2001). The problem with cephalosporins. *Journal of Antimicrobial Chemotherapy, 48,* 463–478.

Drug facts and comparisons. (Updated monthly). St. Louis: Facts and Comparisons.

Kendler, J. S., & Hartman, B. J. (2004). ß-lactam antibiotics. In J. Cohen, W. E. Powderly, S. F. Berkley, et al. (Eds.), *Infectious Diseases* (2nd ed., pp. 1773–1789). New York: Mosby.

Petri, W. A., Jr. (2001). Antimicrobial agents: Penicillins, cephalosporins, and other beta-lactam antibiotics. In J. G. Hardman & L. E. Limbird (Eds.), *Goodman & Gilman's The pharmacological basis of therapeutics* (10th ed., pp. 1189–1218). New York: McGraw-Hill.

Weed, J. G. (2003). Antimicrobial prophylaxis in the surgical patient. *Medical Clinics of North America, 87*(1), 59–75.

Aminoglycosides and Fluoroquinolones

OBJECTIVES

After studying this chapter, you will be able to:

1. Describe characteristics of aminoglycosides and fluoro-quinolones in relation to effectiveness, safety, spectrum of antimicrobial activity, indications for use, administration, and observation of client responses.
2. Discuss factors influencing selection and dosage of amino-glycosides and fluoroquinolones.
3. State the rationale for the increasing use of single daily doses of aminoglycosides.
4. Discuss the importance of measuring serum drug levels during aminoglycoside therapy.
5. Describe measures to decrease nephrotoxicity and ototoxicity with aminoglycosides.
6. Describe characteristics, uses, adverse effects, and nursing process implications of fluoroquinolones.
7. Discuss principles of using aminoglycosides and fluoro-quinolones in renal impairment and critical illness.

APPLYING YOUR KNOWLEDGE

Roger Dallas is an 84-year-old man who has been prescribed ciprofloxacin (Cipro) 500 mg PO every 12 hours to treat an infected leg wound. He has experienced arterial insufficiency to his lower extremities for many years, secondary to atherosclerosis. The medical plan is to clear the infection so that Mr. Dallas can have surgery to restore circulation to his lower extremities.

INTRODUCTION

The aminoglycosides have been widely used to treat serious gram-negative infections for many years. The quinolones are also older drugs originally used only for treatment of urinary tract infections (see Chap. 32). The fluoro-quinolones are synthesized by adding a fluorine molecule to the quinolone structure. This addition increases drug activity against gram-negative microorganisms, broadens the antimicrobial spectrum to include several other micro-organisms, and allows use of the drugs in treating systemic infections. General characteristics; mechanisms of action; indications for and contraindications to use; nursing process implications; and principles of therapy for these drugs are described in this chapter. Individual drugs, with routes of administration and dosage ranges, are listed in the Drugs at a Glance tables.

AMINOGLYCOSIDES

Aminoglycosides (Table 31-1) are bactericidal agents with similar pharmacologic, antimicrobial, and toxicologic characteristics. They are used to treat infections caused by gram-negative microorganisms such as *Pseudomonas* and *Proteus* species, *Escherichia coli,* and *Klebsiella, Enterobacter,* and *Serratia* species.

These drugs are poorly absorbed from the gastrointestinal (GI) tract. Thus, when given orally, they exert local effects in the GI tract. They are well absorbed from intramuscular injection sites and reach peak effects in 30 to 90 minutes if circulatory status is good. After intravenous (IV) administration, peak effects occur within 30 to 60 minutes. Plasma half-life is 2 to 4 hours with normal renal function.

After parenteral administration, aminoglycosides are widely distributed in extracellular fluid and reach therapeutic levels in

Table 31-1 Drugs at a Glance: Aminoglycosides

GENERIC/TRADE NAME	CHARACTERISTICS	ROUTES AND DOSAGE RANGES	
		Adults	Children
Amikacin (Amikin)	Retains a broader spectrum of antibacterial activity than other aminoglycosides because it resists degradation by most enzymes that inactivate gentamicin and tobramycin Major clinical use is in infections caused by organisms resistant to other aminoglycosides (eg, *Pseudomonas, Proteus, Escherichia coli, Klebsiella, Enterobacter, Serratia*), whether community or hospital acquired.	IM, IV 15 mg/kg q24h, 7.5 mg/kg q12h, or 5 mg/kg q8h	*Older children:* Same as adults *Neonates:* IM, IV 10 mg/kg initially, then 7.5 mg/kg q12h
Gentamicin (Garamycin)	Effective against several gram-negative organisms, although some strains have become resistant Acts synergistically with antipseudomonal penicillins against *Pseudomonas aeruginosa* and with ampicillin or vancomycin against enterococci	IV, IM 3–5 mg/kg q24h, 1.5–2.5 mg/kg q12h, or 1–1.7 mg/kg q8h	*Children:* IV, IM 6–7.5 mg/kg/d in 3 divided doses, q8h *Infants and neonates:* IV, IM 7.5 mg/kg/d in 3 divided doses, q8h *Premature infants and neonates <1 wk:* IV, IM 5 mg/kg/d in 2 divided doses, q12h
Kanamycin (Kantrex)	Occasionally used to decrease bowel organisms before surgery, treat hepatic coma, or treat multidrug-resistant tuberculosis	IV, IM 15 mg/kg/d, in 2 or 3 divided doses PO, suppression of intestinal bacteria, 1 g every h for 4 doses, then 1 g q6h for 36–72 h; hepatic coma, 8–12 g daily in divided doses	IV, IM same as adults
Neomycin	Given orally or topically only because too toxic for systemic use Although poorly absorbed from GI tract, toxic levels may accumulate in presence of renal failure. Used topically, often in combination with other drugs, to treat infections of the eye, ear, and skin (burns, wounds, ulcers, dermatoses) When used for wound or bladder irrigations, systemic absorption may occur if the area is large or if drug concentration exceeds 0.1%.	PO, suppression of intestinal bacteria (with erythromycin 1 g) 1 g at 19, 18, and 9 h before surgery (3 doses); hepatic coma, 4–12 g daily in divided doses	
Paromomycin (Humatin)	Acts against bacteria and amebae in the intestinal lumen Used to treat hepatic coma and intestinal amebiasis. It is not effective in amebic infections outside the intestine.	Intestinal amebiasis, PO 25–35 mg/kg/d, in 3 divided doses, with meals, for 5–10 d. Repeat after 2 wk, if necessary.	Intestinal amebiasis, same as adults

(continued)

Table 31-1 Drugs at a Glance: Aminoglycosides (continued)

GENERIC/TRADE NAME	CHARACTERICTICS	ROUTES AND DOSAGE RANGES	
		Adults	Children
	Usually not absorbed from GI tract and unlikely to cause ototoxicity and nephrotoxicity associated with systemically absorbed aminoglycosides. However, systemic absorption may occur in the presence of inflammatory or ulcerative bowel disease.	Hepatic coma, PO 4 g/d in divided doses for 5–6 d	
Streptomycin	May be used in a 4- to 6-drug regimen for treatment of multidrug-resistant tuberculosis	IM 15 mg/kg/d (maximum 1 g) or 25–30 mg/kg 2 or 3 times weekly (maximum 1.5 g per dose)	IM 20–40 mg/kg/d in 2 divided doses, q12h (maximum dose, 1 g/d) or 25–30 mg/kg 2–3 times weekly (maximum 1.5 g)
Tobramycin (Nebcin)	Similar to gentamicin in antibacterial spectrum, but may be more active against *Pseudomonas* organisms. Often used with other antibiotics for septicemia and infections of burn wounds, other soft tissues, bone, the urinary tract, and the central nervous system	IV, IM 3–5 mg/kg q24h, 1.5–2.5 mg/kg q12h, or 1–1.7 mg/kg q8h	IV, IM 6–7.5 mg/kg/d in 3 divided doses, q8h *Neonates (≤1 wk):* IV, IM up to 4 mg/kg/d in 2 divided doses, q12h

GI, gastrointestinal; IM, intramuscular; IV, intravenous; PO, oral.

blood, urine, bone, inflamed joints, and pleural and ascitic fluids. They accumulate in high concentrations in the kidney and inner ear. They are poorly distributed to the central nervous system, intraocular fluids, and respiratory tract secretions.

Injected drugs are not metabolized; they are excreted unchanged in the urine, primarily by glomerular filtration. Oral drugs are excreted in feces.

Mechanism of Action

Aminoglycosides penetrate the cell walls of susceptible bacteria and bind irreversibly to 30S ribosomes, intracellular structures that synthesize proteins. As a result, the bacteria cannot synthesize the proteins necessary for their function and replication.

Indications for Use

The major clinical use of parenteral aminoglycosides is to treat serious systemic infections caused by susceptible aerobic gram-negative organisms. Many hospital-acquired infections are caused by gram-positive cocci and gram-negative organisms. These infections have become more common with control of other types of infections; widespread use of

antimicrobial drugs; and diseases (eg, acquired immunodeficiency syndrome [AIDS]) or treatments (eg, radical surgery, therapy with antineoplastic or immunosuppressive drugs) that lower host resistance. Although they can occur anywhere, infections due to gram-negative organisms commonly involve the respiratory and genitourinary tracts, skin, wounds, bowel, and bloodstream. Any infection with gram-negative organisms may be serious and potentially life threatening. Management is difficult because the organisms are in general less susceptible to antibacterial drugs, and drug-resistant strains develop rapidly. In pseudomonal infections, an aminoglycoside is often given concurrently with an antipseudomonal penicillin (eg, piperacillin) for synergistic therapeutic effects. The penicillin-induced breakdown of the bacterial cell wall makes it easier for the aminoglycoside to reach its site of action inside the bacterial cell. Decreased mortality has been demonstrated from combination antibiotic therapy in treatment of infections due to *Pseudomonas aeruginosa* and other multidrug resistant gram-negative bacilli. However, routine use of combination antibiotic therapy containing an aminoglycoside has not been associated with decreased mortality in other gram-negative infections.

A second clinical use is for treatment of tuberculosis. Streptomycin may be used as part of a 4–6 drug regimen for treatment of multidrug-resistant tuberculosis (MDR-TR). However, it is considered a second-line agent because of increasing resistance and should only be used after susceptibility results confirm its usefulness. For clients who develop drug-induced hepatitis in response to first-line drugs, streptomycin or another second-line drug may be substituted until the hepatitis resolves or the causative antitubercular agent is identified.

A third clinical use is for synergistic action when combined with ampicillin, penicillin G, or vancomycin in the treatment of enterococcal and *Staphylococcus epidermidis* infections. Regimens for these infections, particularly meningitis or endocarditis, should include **gentamicin** in divided doses rather than once-daily dosing. Some strains are resistant to gentamicin, however, and microbiology results should be reviewed for each client.

A final clinical use is oral administration to suppress intestinal bacteria. Neomycin and kanamycin may be given before bowel surgery and to treat hepatic coma. In hepatic coma, intestinal bacteria produce ammonia, which enters the bloodstream and causes encephalopathy. Drug therapy to suppress intestinal bacteria decreases ammonia production. Paromomycin is used mainly in the treatment of acute and chronic intestinal amebiasis.

A few aminoglycosides are administered topically to the eye or to the skin. These are discussed in Chapters 63 and 64, respectively.

Contraindications to Use

Hypersensitivity to the aminoglycosides is a contraindication. Aminoglycosides are generally reserved for infections that have not responded to less toxic drugs. The drugs are nephrotoxic and ototoxic and must be used very cautiously in the presence of renal impairment. Dosages are adjusted according to serum drug levels and creatinine clearance. The drugs must also be used cautiously in clients with myasthenia gravis and other neuromuscular disorders because muscle weakness may be increased.

FLUOROQUINOLONES

Fluoroquinolones are synthetic bactericidal drugs with activity against gram-negative and gram-positive organisms. They may allow oral, ambulatory treatment of infections that previously required parenteral therapy and hospitalization. Most fluoroquinolones are given orally, after which they are well absorbed; achieve therapeutic concentrations in most body fluids; and are metabolized to some extent in the liver. The kidneys are the main route of elimination, with approximately 30% to 60% of an oral dose excreted unchanged in the urine. Dosage should be reduced in renal impairment.

Mechanism of Action

The drugs act by interfering with topoisomerase II (DNA gyrase) and topoisomerase IV, enzymes that are required for synthesis of bacterial DNA and therefore are required for bacterial growth and replication.

Indications for Use

Fluoroquinolones are indicated for various infections caused by aerobic gram-negative and other microorganisms. Thus, they may be used to treat infections of the respiratory, genitourinary, and GI tracts as well as infections of bones, joints, skin, and soft tissues. Fluoroquinolones are also useful in treating infections due to *Neisseria gonorrhoeae,* but resistance is becoming a problem. Although still effective in most cases of gonorrhea, fluoroquinolones should not be given to men who have sex with men or when infection likely occurred during travel, especially to Asia, the Pacific Islands, England, and Wales, because of increased rates of fluoroquinolone-resistant *N. gonorrhoeae.* Because recommendations for treatment of gonorrhea change as resistance becomes more prevalent, consult www.cdc.gov/std for the most current recommendations.

Fluoroquinolones, specifically ciprofloxacin, are currently recommended as the first-line treatment for suspected *Bacillus anthracis* infections (anthrax) until culture and susceptibility results are available. Additional uses include treatment of MDR-TR (see Chap. 34), *Mycobacterium avium* complex (MAC) infections in clients with acquired immune deficiency syndrome (AIDS; see Chap. 34), and fever in neutropenic cancer clients. Indications vary with individual drugs and are listed in Table 31-2.

Contraindications to Use

Fluoroquinolones are contraindicated in clients who have experienced a hypersensitivity reaction and in children younger than 18 years of age, if other alternatives are available. Limited data are available on the safety of fluoroquinolones in pregnant or lactating women; the drugs should not be used unless the benefits outweigh the potential risks.

NURSING PROCESS

General aspects of the nursing process as described in Chapter 29 apply to the client receiving aminoglycosides and fluoroquinolones. In this chapter, only those aspects related specifically to these drugs are included.

Assessment

With aminoglycosides, assess for the presence of factors that predispose to nephrotoxicity or ototoxicity.

● Check laboratory reports of renal function (eg, serum creatinine, creatinine clearance, blood urea nitrogen [BUN]) for abnormal values.

Table 31-2 Drugs at a Glance: Fluoroquinolones

GENERIC/TRADE NAME	CHARACTERISTICS	ROUTES AND DOSAGE RANGES
Ciprofloxacin (Cipro)	1. Effective in respiratory, urinary tract, gastrointestinal tract, and skin and soft-tissue infections as well as sexually transmitted diseases caused by chlamydiae and *Neisseria gonorrhoeae* organisms 2. Used as one of 4 to 6 drugs in treatment of multidrug-resistant tuberculosis	PO 250–750 mg q12h UTI/pyelonephritis; extended-release tablets 500 mg–1 g q24h IV 200–400 mg q8–12h
Gatifloxacin (Tequin)	Indicated for pneumonia, bronchitis, sinusitis, skin and soft tissue infections, urinary infections, pyelonephritis, and gonorrhea	PO, IV infusion 400 mg once daily. Give IV dose over 60 min; avoid rapid administration.
Gemifloxacin (Factive)	Indicated for acute bacterial exacerbation of chronic bronchitis and community-acquired pneumonia (mild to moderate severity)	PO 320 mg once daily for 5–7 d
Levofloxacin (Levaquin)	A broad-spectrum agent effective for treatment of bronchitis, cystitis, pneumonia, sinusitis, skin and skin-structure infections, and pyelonephritis	PO, IV 250–750 mg once daily. Infuse IV dose slowly over 60 min.
Lomefloxacin (Maxaquin)	Approved for bronchitis, urinary infections, and transurethral surgical procedures	PO 400 mg once daily Preoperatively, PO 400 mg as a single dose, 1–6 h before surgery
Moxifloxacin (Avelox)	Indicated for community-acquired pneumonia, sinusitis, bronchitis, skin and soft-tissue infections	PO, IV 400 mg once daily. Infuse IV dose slowly over 60 min.
Norfloxacin (Noroxin)	Used only for UTI and uncomplicated gonorrhea	PO 400 mg twice daily
Ofloxacin (Floxin)	See ciprofloxacin, above	PO, IV 200–400 mg q12h for 3–10 d Gonorrhea, PO 400 mg as a single dose

IV, intravenous; PO, oral; UTI, urinary tract infection.

- Assess for impairment of balance or hearing, including audiometry reports if available.
- Analyze current medications for drugs that interact with aminoglycosides to increase risks of nephrotoxicity or ototoxicity.
- With fluoroquinolones, assess for the presence of factors that increase risks of adverse drug effects (eg, impaired renal function, inadequate fluid intake, frequent or prolonged exposure to sunlight in usual activities of daily living).
- Assess laboratory tests (eg, complete blood counts, tests of renal and hepatic function) for abnormal values.

Planning/Goals

The client will

- Receive aminoglycoside dosages that are individualized by age, weight, renal function, and serum drug levels
- Have serum aminoglycoside levels monitored when indicated

- Have renal function tests performed regularly during aminoglycoside and fluoroquinolone therapy
- Be well hydrated during aminoglycoside and fluoroquinolone therapy
- Be observed regularly for adverse drug effects

Interventions

- With aminoglycosides, weigh clients accurately (dosage is based on weight) and monitor laboratory reports of BUN, serum creatinine levels, serum drug levels, and urinalysis for abnormal values.
- Force fluids to at least 2000 to 3000 mL daily if not contraindicated. Keeping the client well hydrated reduces risks of nephrotoxicity with aminoglycosides and crystalluria with fluoroquinolones.
- Avoid concurrent use of other nephrotoxic drugs when possible.
- Provide appropriate teaching (see accompanying Client Teaching Guidelines).

Evaluation

- Interview and observe for improvement in the infection being treated.
- Interview and observe for adverse drug effects.

APPLYING YOUR KNOWLEDGE 31-1

Mr. Dallas tells you that he is experiencing a moderate amount of indigestion and asks what he should use to treat it. What is the best response, taking into consideration Mr. Dallas's use of Cipro?

PRINCIPLES OF THERAPY

Drug Selection

The choice of aminoglycoside depends on local susceptibility patterns and specific organisms causing an infection. Gentamicin is often given for systemic infections if resistant microorganisms have not developed in the clinical setting. If gentamicin-resistant organisms have developed, amikacin or tobramycin may be given because they are usually less susceptible to drug-destroying enzymes. In terms of toxicity, the aminoglycosides cause similar effects.

The choice of fluoroquinolone is also determined by local susceptibility patterns and specific organisms because individual drugs differ somewhat in their antimicrobial spectra. The drugs cause similar adverse effects.

Drug Dosage: Aminoglycosides

Dosage of aminoglycosides must be carefully regulated because therapeutic doses are close to toxic doses. Two major dosing schedules are used, one involving multiple daily doses and one involving a single daily dose. The multiple-dose regimen has been used traditionally and guidelines are well defined. The single-dose regimen, which takes advantage of the pharmcodynamic properties of aminoglycosides, is being used increasingly. These two regimens are described in the following sections.

Multiple Daily Dosing

- An *initial loading dose,* based on client weight and the desired peak serum concentration, is given to achieve therapeutic serum concentrations rapidly. If the client is obese, lean or ideal body weight should be used because aminoglycosides are not significantly distributed in body fat. In clients with normal renal function, the recommended loading dose for gentamicin and tobramycin is 1.5 to 2 mg/kg of body weight; for amikacin the loading dose is 5 to 7.5 mg/kg.
- *Maintenance doses* are based on serum drug concentrations. Peak serum concentrations should be assessed 30 to 60 minutes after drug administration (5–8 mcg/mL for gentamicin and tobramycin, 20–30 mcg/mL for amikacin). Measurement of both peak and trough levels helps to maintain therapeutic serum levels without excessive toxicity. For gentamicin and tobramycin, peak levels above 10 to 12 mcg/mL and trough levels above 2 mcg/mL for prolonged periods have been

---

C L I E N T   T E A C H I N G   G U I D E L I N E S

Oral Fluoroquinolones

General Considerations

✔ Avoid exposure to sunlight during and for several days after taking one of these drugs. Stop taking the drug and notify the prescribing physician if skin burning, redness, swelling, rash, or itching occurs. Sunscreen lotions do not prevent photosensitivity reactions.

✔ Be very careful if driving or doing other tasks requiring alertness or physical coordination. These drugs may cause dizziness or lightheadedness.

Self-Administration

✔ Take norfloxacin (Noroxin) 1 hour before or 2 hours after meals. Ciprofloxacin (Cipro), gatifloxacin (Tequin), gemifloxacin (Fac-

tive), levofloxacin (Levaquin), lomefloxacin (Maxaquin), ofloxacin (Floxin), and moxifloxacin (Avelox) can be taken without regard to meals. Do not take ciprofloxacin alone with dairy products or calcium-fortified juices due to decreased drug absorption.

✔ Drink 2 to 3 quarts of fluid daily if able. This helps to prevent kidney problems.

✔ Do not take antacids containing magnesium or aluminum (eg, Mylanta or Maalox); any products containing iron, magnesium, calcium (eg, Tums), or zinc (eg, multivitamins); or buffered didanosine preparations at the same time, or for several hours before or after a dose of the fluoroquinolone. (Consult product-specific information for individual drug recommendations.)

associated with nephrotoxicity. For accuracy, blood samples must be drawn at the correct times and the timing of drug administration and blood sampling must be accurately documented.

- *With impaired renal function,* dosage of aminoglycosides must be reduced. Methods of adjusting dosage include lengthening the time between doses or reducing doses. References should be consulted for specific recommendations on adjusting aminoglycoside doses for renal impairment.

- *In urinary tract infections,* smaller doses can be used than in systemic infections because the aminoglycosides reach high concentrations in the urine.

Single Daily Dosing

The use of once-daily (or extended-interval) aminoglycoside dosing is increasing. This dosing method uses high doses (eg, gentamicin, 7 mg/kg) to produce high initial drug concentrations, but a repeat dose is not administered until the serum concentration is quite low. The rationale for this dosing approach is a potential increase in efficacy with a reduced incidence of nephrotoxicity. Most clients can be successfully treated with one daily dose using this approach. However, certain populations require more than one daily dose, but still require fewer daily doses than are necessary in multiple-dosing strategies (thus, extended-interval dosing).

This practice evolved from increased knowledge about the concentration-dependent bactericidal effects and postantibiotic effects of aminoglycosides. *Concentration-dependent bactericidal effects* mean that the drugs kill more microorganisms with a large dose and high peak serum concentrations. *Postantibiotic effects* mean that aminoglycosides continue killing microorganisms even with low serum concentrations. These characteristics allow administration of high doses to achieve high peak serum concentrations and optimal killing of microorganisms. The longer interval until the next dose allows the client to eliminate the drug to very low serum concentrations for approximately 6 hours. During this low-drug period, the postantibiotic effect is active while there is minimal drug accumulation in body tissues. Reported advantages of this regimen include increased bactericidal effects, less nephrotoxicity, reduced need for serum drug concentration data, and reduced nursing time for administration.

Guidelines for Reducing Toxicity of Aminoglycosides

In addition to the preceding recommendations, guidelines to decrease the incidence and severity of adverse effects include the following:

- Identify clients at high risk for adverse effects (eg, neonates, older adults, clients with renal impairment, clients

with disease processes or drug therapies that impair blood circulation and renal function).

- Keep clients well hydrated to decrease drug concentration in serum and body tissues. The drugs reach higher concentrations in the kidneys and inner ears than in other body tissues. This is a major factor in nephrotoxicity and ototoxicity. The goal of an adequate fluid intake is to decrease the incidence and severity of these adverse effects.

- Use caution with concurrent administration of diuretics. Diuretics may increase the risk of nephrotoxicity by decreasing fluid volume, thereby increasing drug concentration in serum and tissues. Dehydration is most likely to occur with loop diuretics such as furosemide.

- Give the drug for no longer than 10 days unless necessary for treatment of certain infections. Clients are most at risk when high doses are given for prolonged periods.

- Detect adverse effects early and reduce dosage or discontinue the drug. Changes in renal function tests that indicate nephrotoxicity may not occur until the client has received an aminoglycoside for several days. If nephrotoxicity occurs, it is usually reversible if the drug is stopped. Early ototoxicity is detectable only with audiometry and is generally not reversible.

APPLYING YOUR KNOWLEDGE 31–2

Mr. Dallas's wound is not responding to treatment. Due to his need for surgery, he is hospitalized for IV antibiotic therapy. His physician orders gentamicin IV once every 24 hours, to be dosed by the pharmacist. The medication is dosed and Mr. Dallas receives doses for 3 days. What assessments should you perform to observe for toxicity?

Drug Dosage: Fluoroquinolones

Recommended dosages of fluoroquinolones should not be exceeded in any clients, and dosages should be reduced in the presence of renal impairment.

Use in Special Populations

Use in Children

Aminoglycosides must be used cautiously in children as with adults. Dosage must be accurately calculated according to weight and renal function. Serum drug concentrations must be monitored and dosage adjusted as indicated to avoid toxicity. Neonates may have increased risk of nephrotoxicity and ototoxicity because of their immature renal function. Neomycin is not recommended for use in infants and children. Fluoroquinolones are not recommended for use in children if other alternatives are available because they have been associated with permanent damage in cartilage and joints in some animal studies.

Use in Older Adults

With aminoglycosides, advanced age is considered a major risk factor for development of toxicity. Because of impaired renal function, other disease processes (eg, diabetes), and multiple-drug therapy, older adults are at high risk for development of aminoglycoside-induced nephrotoxicity and ototoxicity. Aminoglycosides should not be given to older adults with impaired renal function if less toxic drugs are effective against causative organisms. When the drugs are given, extreme caution is required. Interventions to decrease the incidence and severity of adverse drug effects are listed earlier at "Guidelines for Reducing Toxicity of Aminoglycosides." These interventions are important with any client receiving an aminoglycoside, but are especially important with older adults. In addition, prolonged therapy (>1 week) increases risk of toxicity and should be avoided when possible.

Fluoroquinolones are commonly used in older adults for the same indications as in younger adults. In older adults with normal renal function, the drugs should be accompanied by an adequate fluid intake and urine output to prevent drug crystals from forming in the urinary tract. In addition, urinary alkalinizing agents should be avoided because drug crystals form more readily in alkaline urine. In those with impaired renal function, a common condition in older adults, the drugs should be used cautiously and in reduced dosage.

Use in Clients With Renal Impairment

Aminoglycosides are nephrotoxic and must be used very cautiously in clients with renal impairment. Both aminoglycosides and fluoroquinolones require dosage adjustments in renal impairment. Dosage guidelines have been established according to creatinine clearance and often involve lower dosages and prolonged intervals between doses (eg, 36–72 hours). Guidelines for reducing nephrotoxicity of aminoglycosides are as listed previously.

With fluoroquinolones, reported renal effects include azotemia, crystalluria, hematuria, interstitial nephritis, nephropathy, and renal failure. Nephrotoxicity occurs less often than with aminoglycosides, and most cases of acute renal failure have occurred in older adults. It is unknown whether renal failure is caused by hypersensitivity or is a direct toxic effect of fluoroquinolones. Crystalluria rarely occurs in acidic urine but may occur in alkaline urine. Guidelines for reducing nephrotoxicity include using lower dosages, having longer intervals between doses, receiving adequate hydration, and avoiding substances that alkalinize the urine.

Use in Clients With Hepatic Impairment

With aminoglycosides, hepatic impairment is not a significant factor because the drugs are excreted through the kidneys. With fluoroquinolones, however, hepatotoxicity has been observed with some of the drugs. Clinical manifestations range from abnormalities in liver enzyme test results to hepatitis, liver necrosis, or hepatic failure.

Use in Clients With Critical Illness

Aminoglycosides and fluoroquinolones are often used in critically ill clients because this population has a high incidence of serious and difficult-to-treat infections. Aminoglycosides are usually given with other antimicrobials to provide broad-spectrum activity. Because critically ill clients are at high risk for development of nephrotoxicity and ototoxicity with aminoglycosides, guidelines for safe drug usage should be strictly followed. Renal function should be monitored to assess for needed dosage reductions in clients with renal dysfunction receiving aminoglycosides or fluoroquinolones. Because fluoroquinolones may be hepatotoxic, hepatic function should be monitored during therapy.

Fluoroquinolones are usually infused IV in critically ill clients. However, administration orally or by GI tube (eg, nasogastric, gastrostomy, jejunostomy) may be feasible in some clients. Concomitant administration of antacids or enteral feedings decreases absorption.

Use in Clients With Diabetes

Fluoroquinolones are associated with hyperglycemia and hypoglycemia. Older clients may be more at risk for these glucose disturbances. Severe hypoglycemia has occurred in clients receiving concomitant glyburide and fluoroquinolones. Although most cases have occurred in diabetic clients, severe cases of hyperglycemia have occurred in clients not previously diagnosed as diabetic. Gatifloxacin has been associated with hypoglycemic and hyperglycemic events more commonly than other fluoroquinolones. The explanation for an increased association with gatifloxacin is not currently known.

Use in Home Care

Parenteral aminoglycosides are usually given in a hospital setting. Oral fluoroquinolones are often self-administered at home. The role of the home care nurse is primarily to teach clients or caregivers how to take the drugs effectively and to observe for adverse drug effects.

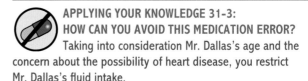 **APPLYING YOUR KNOWLEDGE 31-3:**
HOW CAN YOU AVOID THIS MEDICATION ERROR?
Taking into consideration Mr. Dallas's age and the concern about the possibility of heart disease, you restrict Mr. Dallas's fluid intake.

N U R S I N G   A C T I O N S

Aminoglycosides and Fluoroquinolones

NURSING ACTIONS	RATIONALE/EXPLANATION

1. **Administer accurately**

   a. With aminoglycosides:

   (1) For intravenous (IV) administration, dilute the drug in 50–100 milliliters of 5% dextrose or 0.9% sodium chloride injection and infuse over 30–60 minutes. The concentration of gentamicin solution should not exceed 1 mg/mL.

   To achieve therapeutic blood levels

   (2) Give intramuscular aminoglycosides in a large muscle mass, and rotate sites.

   To avoid local tissue irritation. This is less likely to occur with aminoglycosides than with most other antibiotics.

   b. With fluoroquinolones:

   (1) Give norfloxacin 1 hour before or 2 hours after a meal or milk or other dairy products. Do not give ciprofloxacin with dairy products alone. Ciprofloxacin, gatifloxacin, gemifloxacin, levofloxacin, lomefloxacin, ofloxacin, and moxifloxacin may be given without regard to food intake.

   To promote therapeutic plasma drug levels. Food in the gastrointestinal (GI) tract interferes with absorption of norfloxacin, and dairy products alone interfere with absorption of ciprofloxacin.

   (2) Give IV infusions over 60 minutes.

   To decrease vein irritation and phlebitis

   (3) When giving ciprofloxacin, gatifloxacin, or levofloxacin IV into a primary IV line (eg, using piggyback apparatus or Y connector), stop the primary solution until ciprofloxacin is infused.

   To avoid physical or chemical incompatibilities

2. **Observe for therapeutic effects**

   a. Decreased signs and symptoms of the infection for which the drug is being given

   See Chapter 29.

3. **Observe for adverse effects**

   a. With aminoglycosides, observe for:

   Adverse effects are more likely to occur with parenteral administration of large doses for prolonged periods. However, they may occur with oral administration in the presence of renal impairment and with usual therapeutic doses.

   (1) Nephrotoxicity—casts, albumin, red or white blood cells in urine; decreased creatinine clearance; increased serum creatinine; increased blood urea nitrogen

   Renal damage is most likely to occur in clients who are elderly; receive high doses or prolonged therapy; have prior renal damage; or receive other nephrotoxic drugs. This is the most serious adverse reaction. Risks of kidney damage can be minimized by using the drugs appropriately, detecting early signs of renal impairment, and keeping clients well hydrated.

   (2) Ototoxicity—deafness or decreased hearing, tinnitus, dizziness, ataxia

   This results from damage to the eighth cranial nerve. Incidence of ototoxicity is increased in older clients and in those with previous auditory damage; high doses or prolonged duration of therapy; and concurrent use of other ototoxic drugs.

   (3) Neurotoxicity—respiratory paralysis and apnea

   This is caused by neuromuscular blockade and is more likely to occur after rapid IV injection, administration to a client with myasthenia gravis, or concomitant administration of general anesthetics or neuromuscular blocking agents (eg, succinylcholine, tubocurarine). This effect also may occur if an aminoglycoside is administered shortly after surgery, due to the residual effects of anesthetics or neuromuscular blockers. Neostigmine or calcium may be given to counteract apnea.

   (4) Hypersensitivity—skin rash, urticaria

   This is an uncommon reaction except with topical neomycin, which may cause sensitization in as many as 10% of recipients.

NURSING ACTIONS	RATIONALE/EXPLANATION
(5) Nausea, vomiting, diarrhea, peripheral neuritis, paresthesias	Uncommon with parenteral aminoglycosides. Diarrhea often occurs with oral administration.
b. With fluoroquinolones, observe for:	The drugs are usually well tolerated.
(1) Hepatotoxicity (abnormal liver enzyme tests, hepatitis, hepatic failure)	Hepatotoxicity has been observed with most of the drugs.
(2) Allergic reactions (anaphylaxis, urticaria)	Uncommon, but some fatalities have been reported.
(3) Nausea, vomiting, diarrhea, pseudomembranous colitis	Nausea is the most common GI symptom.
(4) Headache, dizziness, confusion, tremors, hallucinations, depression, seizures	Uncommon, but may develop after first dose. Use caution in clients with known or suspected central nervous system disorders that lower seizure threshold.
(5) Crystalluria	Uncommon, but may occur with an inadequate fluid intake
(6) Photosensitivity (skin redness, rash, itching)	May occur with most fluoroquinolones with exposure to sunlight
(7) Glucose tolerance	Fluoroquinolones are associated with hyperglycemia and hypoglycemia. Older clients and those with diabetes are most at risk.
(8) Other	Adverse effects involving most body systems have been reported with one or more of the fluoroquinolones. Most have a low incidence (<1%) of occurrence.
4. Observe for drug interactions	
a. Drugs that *increase* effects of aminoglycosides:	The listed drugs increase toxicity.
(1) Amphotericin B, cephalosporins, cisplatin, cyclosporine, enflurane, vancomycin	These drugs are nephrotoxic alone and may increase nephrotoxicity of aminoglycosides.
(2) Loop diuretics (furosemide, bumetanide)	Increased ototoxicity
(3) Neuromuscular blocking agents (eg, pancuronium, vecuronium)	Increased neuromuscular blockade with possible paralysis of respiratory muscles and apnea
b. Drugs that *decrease* effects of aminoglycosides:	
(1) Penicillins, when admixed directly in same syringe with aminoglycosides	Chemical inactivation
c. Drugs that *increase* effects of fluoroquinolones:	
(1) Cimetidine, probenecid	Cimetidine inhibits hepatic metabolism and probenecid inhibits renal excretion of fluoroquinolones. These actions may increase serum drug levels.
d. Drugs that *decrease* effects of fluoroquinolones:	
(1) Antacids, iron preparations, sucralfate, zinc preparations, buffered didanosine preparations	These drugs interfere with absorption of fluoroquinolones from the GI tract.

APPLYING YOUR KNOWLEDGE: ANSWERS

31-1 Mr. Dallas should wait for 2 hours before or after he has taken the Cipro before taking an antacid for his indigestion. Antacids interfere with the absorption of fluoroquinolones from the GI tract.

31-2 Assess Mr. Dallas's hearing and his renal function because gentamicin is ototoxic and nephrotoxic.

31-3 The client should be encouraged to take 2 to 3 liters of fluid a day unless contraindicated. The intake of fluid will help prevent nephrotoxicity.

Review and Application Exercises

Short Answer Exercises

1. Why must aminoglycosides be given parenterally for systemic infections?

2. How are aminoglycosides excreted?

3. What are risk factors for aminoglycoside-induced nephrotoxicity and ototoxicity?

4. How would you assess a client for nephrotoxicity or ototoxicity?

5. What is the reason for giving an aminoglycoside and an antipseudomonal penicillin in the treatment of serious infections caused by *P. aeruginosa?*

6. Why should an aminoglycoside and an antipseudomonal penicillin *not* be combined in a syringe or IV fluid for administration?

7. Which laboratory tests need to be monitored regularly for a client receiving a systemic aminoglycoside?

8. What is the rationale for giving an oral aminoglycoside to treat hepatic coma?

9. What are the main clinical uses of fluoroquinolones?

10. What are adverse effects of fluoroquinolones, and how may they be prevented or minimized?

11. Why is it important to maintain an adequate fluid intake and urine output while taking a fluoroquinolone?

12. Why are fluoroquinolones not preferred drugs for children?

NCLEX-Style Questions

13. A hospitalized client is scheduled to receive levofloxacin 500 mg PO at 9:00 A.M. The medication administration record also indicates that Maalox 30 mL PO and hydrochlorothiazide 25 mg PO are due at 9:00 A.M. The nurse should
    a. Administer all the medications as scheduled.
    b. Hold the Maalox until 11:00 A.M.
    c. Ask the physician to discontinue hydrochlorothiazide because of increased risk of ototoxicity.
    d. Administer the Maalox and levofloxacin, but hold the hydrochlorothiazide.

14. A critically ill client is receiving tobramycin 1.5 mg/kg IV every 8 hours. The client has recently stopped making urine and the most recent laboratory results indicate that the creatinine level has risen from normal to 3.6 mg/dL. At the next scheduled administration time for tobramycin, the nurse should
    a. Administer half the prescribed dose.
    b. Hold the tobramycin and notify the physician.
    c. Administer tobramycin as prescribed.
    d. Draw a blood sample for testing the tobramycin level before the dose and then administer as prescribed.

15. A client has just been given a prescription for moxifloxacin 400 mg PO once daily for acute bronchitis. The nurse should teach the client
    a. not to take moxifloxacin with a meal
    b. to restrict fluid intake to avoid fluid overload

    c. to take moxifloxacin with an antacid (eg, Tums) to decrease the chance of stomach upset
    d. to avoid prolonged exposure to sunlight

16. A nursing home client is brought to the emergency department with acute pyelonephritis. The emergency room physician prescribes ciprofloxacin 500 mg PO twice daily. The client has a history of seizures and bradycardia. The nurse should
    a. Counsel the client's caregiver to avoid administering the ciprofloxacin with the client's anticonvulsant.
    b. Ask the physician to check blood levels of the client's anticonvulsant(s) before giving the first dose of ciprofloxacin.
    c. Call the client's seizure and dysrhythmia history to the physician's attention and inquire whether another type of antibiotic might be selected.
    d. Counsel the client's caregiver to discontinue the ciprofloxacin after the client's fever is gone.

17. A physician writes an order for gentamicin 7 mg/kg IV every 24 hours and ampicillin 500 mg IV every 6 hours. The client has a diagnosis of endocarditis. This is not an ideal antibiotic regimen for endocarditis because
    a. Gentamicin should be dosed using the multiple daily dosing method for endocarditis.
    b. The addition of gentamicin to ampicillin increases the risk of treatment failure in endocarditis.
    c. The appropriate single daily dose of gentamicin is 15 mg/kg once daily.
    d. Streptomycin is the recommended aminoglycoside for use in endocarditis.

Selected References

Centers for Disease Control and Prevention. (2004). Increases in fluoroquinolone-resistant *Neisseria gonorrhoeae* among men who have sex with men: United States, 2003, and revised recommendations for gonorrhea treatment, 2004. *Morbidity and Mortality Weekly Report, 53*(16), 335–338.

Chambers, H. F. (2001). Antimicrobial agents: The aminoglycosides. In J. G. Hardman & L. E. Limbird (Eds.), *Goodman & Gilman's The pharmacological basis of therapeutics* (10th ed., pp. 1219–1238). New York: McGraw-Hill.

Drug facts and comparisons. (Updated monthly). St. Louis: Facts and Comparisons.

Joint Committee of the American Thoracic Society, the Infectious Diseases Society of America, and the Centers for Disease Control and Prevention. (2003, June 20). Treatment of tuberculosis. *Morbidity and Mortality Weekly Report: Recommendations and Reports, 52*(RR-11), 1–77.

Kaye, D. (2004). Current use for old antibacterial agents: Polymyxins, rifampin, and aminoglycosides. *Infectious Disease Clinics of North America, 18*(3), 669–689.

Olsen, K. M., Rudis, M. I., Rebuck, J. A., et al. (2004). Effect of once-daily dosing vs. multiple daily dosing of tobramycin on enzyme markers of nephrotoxicity. *Critical Care Medicine, 32*(8), 1678–1682.

Safdar, N., Handelsman, J., & Maki, D. G. (2004). Does combination antimicrobial therapy reduce mortality in Gram-negative bacteraemia? A meta-analysis. *Lancet Infectious Diseases, 4*(8), 519–527.

Sprandel, K. A., & Rodvold, K. A. (2003). Safety and tolerability of fluoroquinolones. *Clinical Cornerstone* (Suppl. 3), S29–S36.

Tetracyclines, Sulfonamides, and Urinary Agents

OBJECTIVES

After studying this chapter, you will be able to:

1. Discuss major characteristics and clinical uses of tetracyclines.
2. Recognize doxycycline as the tetracycline of choice in renal failure.
3. Discuss characteristics, clinical uses, adverse effects, and nursing implications of selected sulfonamides.
4. Recognize trimethoprim-sulfamethoxazole as a combination drug that is commonly used for urinary tract and systemic infections.
5. Describe the use of urinary antiseptics in the treatment of urinary tract infections.
6. Teach clients strategies for preventing, recognizing, and treating urinary tract infections.

APPLYING YOUR KNOWLEDGE

Sharon Dee is an 18-year-old college student. She comes to the health clinic with complaints of urinary frequency and burning on urination. Her medication history includes ongoing, long-term treatment of acne with a tetracycline. She takes 250 mg of the drug PO daily. The physician diagnoses her with a urinary tract infection and prescribes trimethoprim-sulfamethoxazole (Bactrim) 160/800 mg PO every 12 hours for 10 days.

INTRODUCTION

Tetracyclines and sulfonamides are older, broad-spectrum, bacteriostatic drugs that are rarely used for systemic infections because of microbial resistance and the development of more effective or less toxic drugs. However, the drugs are useful in selected infections. Urinary antiseptics are used only in urinary tract infections (UTI). All of these drugs are described in this chapter and are listed in the Drugs at a Glance tables.

The **tetracyclines** are similar in pharmacologic properties and antimicrobial activity. They are effective against a wide range of gram-positive and gram-negative organisms, although they are usually not drugs of choice. Bacterial infections caused by *Brucella* and *Vibrio cholerae* are still treated by tetracyclines. The drugs also remain effective against rickettsiae, chlamydia, some protozoa, spirochetes, and others. Doxycycline (Vibramycin) is one of the drugs of choice for *Bacillus anthracis* (anthrax) and *Chlamydia trachomatis,* and is used in respiratory-tract infections due to *Mycoplasma pneumoniae.* Tetracyclines are widely distributed into most body tissues and fluids. The older tetracyclines are excreted mainly in urine; doxycycline is eliminated in urine and feces; and minocycline is eliminated mainly by the liver. Table 32-1 provides pertinent information about various tetracyclines.

Sulfonamides are bacteriostatic against a wide range of gram-positive and gram-negative bacteria, although increasing resistance is making them less useful. Susceptibility should be documented by culture and sensitivity testing, but sulfonamides may be active against *Streptococcus pyogenes,* some staphylococcal strains, *Haemophilus influenzae, Nocardia, C. trachomatis,* and toxoplasmosis. The combination of trimethoprim-sulfamethoxazole (Bactrim, Septra) is useful in bronchitis, UTIs due to Enterobacteriaceae, and *Pneumocystis jiroveci* infection (in high doses). Individual drugs vary in extent of systemic absorption and clinical indications. Some sulfonamides are well absorbed and can be used in systemic infections; others are poorly absorbed and exert more local effects. Table 32-2 summarizes key information about sulfonamides.

Urinary antiseptics may be bactericidal for sensitive organisms in the urinary tract because these drugs are concentrated in renal tubules and reach high levels in urine. They

Table 32-1 Drugs at a Glance: Tetracyclines

GENERIC/TRADE NAME	COMMENTS	ROUTES AND DOSAGE RANGES	
		Adults	Children
Tetracycline (Achromycin, others)	• Prototype drug • Marketed under generic and numerous trade names	PO 1–2 g/d in 2–4 equal doses	*>8 y:* PO 25–50 mg/kg/d in 4 divided doses
Demeclocycline (Declomycin)	• The tetracycline most likely to cause photosensitivity • Primarily used to treat inappropriate secretion of antidiuretic hormone • No longer recommended for treatment of gonorrhea	PO 150 mg q6h or 300 mg q12h	*>8 y:* PO 6–12 mg/kg/d in 2–4 divided doses
Doxycycline (Vibramycin)	• Well absorbed from the gastrointestinal tract. Oral administration yields serum drug levels equivalent to those obtained by parenteral administration. • Highly lipid soluble; therefore, reaches therapeutic levels in CSF, the eye, and the prostate gland • Can be given in smaller doses and less frequently than other tetracyclines because of long serum half-life (approximately 18 h) • Excreted by kidneys to a lesser extent than other tetracyclines and is considered safe for clients with impaired renal function	PO 100 mg q12h for 2 doses, then 100 mg once daily or in divided doses; severe infections, 100 mg q12h IV 200 mg the first d, then 100–200 mg daily in 1 or divided doses; give over 1–4 h.	*> 8 y:* PO, IV *Weight ≥45 kg:* same as adults *Weight <45 kg:* PO, IV 4.4 mg/kg/d divided q12h for 2 doses, then 2.2 mg/kg/d in 1 or 2 divided doses; severe infections, 4.4 mg/kg/d in divided doses q12h. Give IV doses over 1–4 h.
Minocycline (Minocin)	• Well absorbed after oral administration • Like doxycycline, readily penetrates CSF, the eye, and the prostate gland • Metabolized more than other tetracyclines, and smaller amounts are excreted in urine and feces	PO, IV 200 mg initially, then 100 mg q12h. IV, infuse over 6 h.	*>8 y:* PO, IV 4 mg/kg initially, then 2 mg/kg q12h

CSF, cerebrospinal fluid; IV, intravenous; PO, oral.

are not used in systemic infections because they do not attain therapeutic plasma levels. An additional drug, phenazopyridine, is given to relieve pain associated with UTI. It has no antibacterial activity.

Mechanisms of Action

Tetracyclines penetrate microbial cells by passive diffusion and an active transport system. Intracellularly, they bind to 30S ribosomes, like the aminoglycosides, and inhibit microbial protein synthesis. *Sulfonamides* act as antimetabolites of para-aminobenzoic acid (PABA), which microorganisms require to produce folic acid; folic acid, in turn, is required for the production of bacterial intracellular proteins. Sulfonamides enter into the reaction instead of PABA, compete for the enzyme involved, and cause formation of nonfunctional derivatives of folic acid. Thus, sulfonamides halt multiplication of new bacteria but do not kill mature, fully formed bacteria. With the exception of the topical sulfonamides used in burn therapy, the presence of pus, serum, or necrotic tissue interferes with sulfonamide action because these materials contain PABA. Some bacteria can change their metabolic pathways to use precursors or other forms of folic acid and thereby develop resistance to the antibacterial action of sul-

Table 32-2 Drugs at a Glance: Sulfonamides

GENERIC/TRADE NAME	CHARACTERISTICS	CLINICAL INDICATIONS	ROUTES AND DOSAGE RANGES	
			Adults	Children
Single Agents				
Sulfadiazine	• A short-acting, rapidly absorbed, rapidly excreted agent for systemic infections • The addition of folinic acid may be recommended.	• Nocardiosis • Toxoplasmosis	PO 2–4 g daily in 3–6 equally divided doses	*>2 mo:* PO 75 mg/kg initially, then 150 mg/kg/d in 4–6 divided doses: maximal daily dose, 6 g
Sulfasalazine (Azulfidine)	• Poorly absorbed • Does not alter normal bacterial flora in the intestine. Effectiveness in ulcerative colitis may be due to antibacterial (sulfapyridine) and anti-inflammatory (aminosalicylic acid) metabolites.	• Ulcerative colitis/Crohn's disease • Rheumatoid arthritis	Ulcerative colitis, PO 3–4 g daily in 4 divided doses initially; 2 g daily in 4 divided doses for maintenance; maximal daily dose, 4 g Rheumatoid arthritis, PO 2–3 g daily in divided doses, q12h	PO 30–60 mg/kg/d in 2–6 divided doses initially, followed by 30 mg/kg/d in 4 divided doses; maximum daily dose, 2 g
Sulfisoxazole	• Rapidly absorbed, rapidly excreted • Highly soluble and less likely to cause crystalluria than most other sulfonamides	• UTI • Ocular infections	PO 2–4 g initially, then 4–8 g daily in 4–6 divided doses	*>2 mo:* PO 75 mg/kg of body weight initially, then 150 mg/kg/d in 4–6 divided doses; maximal daily dose, 6 g
Combination Agent				
Trimethoprim-sulfamethoxazole (Bactrim, Septra, others)	• May exhibit synergistic effectiveness against many organisms (verify susceptibility first), including streptococci *(S. viridans)*, staphylococci *(S. epidermidis, S. aureus)*, *Escherichia coli, Salmonella, Shigella, Serratia, Klebsiella, Nocardia,* and others. Most strains of *Pseudomonas* are resistant. • The two drugs have additive antibacterial effects because they interfere with different steps in bacterial synthesis and activation of folic acid, an essential nutrient.	• Acute and chronic UTI • Acute exacerbations of chronic bronchitis • Acute otitis media caused by susceptible strains of *Hemophilus influenzae* and *Streptococcus pneumoniae* • Shigellosis • Infection by *Pneumocystis jiroveci* (prevention and treatment) • IV preparation indicated for *P. jiroveci* pneumonia, severe UTI, and shigellosis	UTI, trimethoprim 160 mg and sulfamethoxazole 800 mg PO q12h for 10–14 d Shigellosis, same dose as above for 5 d Severe UTI, IV 8–10 mg (trimethoprim component)/kg/d in 2–4 divided doses, up to 14 d *P. jiroveci* pneumonia, IV 15–20 mg (trimethoprim component)/kg/d in 3 or 4 divided doses, q6–8h up to 21 d; IV doses should be given over 60–90 min.	UTI and otitis media, PO 8 mg/kg trimethoprim and 40 mg/kg sulfamethoxazole in 2 divided doses q12h for 10 d Shigellosis, same dose as above for 5 d Severe UTI, IV 8–10 mg (trimethoprim component)/kg in 2–4 divided doses, q6–8h or q12h, up to 14 d *P. jiroveci* pneumonia, IV 15–20 mg (trimethoprim component)/kg/d in 3 or 4 divided doses, q6–8h up to 21 d

(continued)

Table 32-2   **Drugs at a Glance: Sulfonamides** (continued)

			ROUTES AND DOSAGE RANGES	
GENERIC/TRADE NAME	CHARACTERISTICS	CLINICAL INDICATIONS	Adults	Children

	• The combination is less likely to produce resistant bacteria than either agent alone.
	• Oral preparations contain different amounts of the two drugs, as follows:
	   – "Regular" tablets contain trimethoprim 80 mg and sulfamethoxazole 400 mg.
	   – Double-strength tablets (eg, Bactrim D.S., Septra D.S.) contain trimethoprim 160 mg and sulfamethoxazole 800 mg.
	   – Oral suspension contains trimethoprim 40 mg and sulfamethoxazole 200 mg in each 5 mL.
	• IV preparation contains trimethoprim 80 mg and sulfamethoxazole 400 mg in 5 mL.
	• Dosage must be reduced in renal insufficiency.
	• The preparation is contraindicated if creatinine clearance is <15 mL/min.			

Topical Sulfonamides				
Mafenide (Sulfamylon)	• Effective against most gram-negative and gram-positive organisms, especially *Pseudomonas aeruginosa* • Application causes pain and burning. • Mafenide is absorbed systemically and may produce metabolic acidosis.	Prevention of bacterial colonization and infection of severe burn wounds	Topical application to burned area, once or twice daily, in a thin layer	Same as adults

Table 32-2 Drugs at a Glance: Sulfonamides (continued)

| GENERIC/TRADE NAME | CHARACTERISTICS | CLINICAL INDICATIONS | ROUTES AND DOSAGE RANGES | |
			Adults	Children
Silver sulfadiazine (Silvadene)	• Effective against most *Pseudomonas* species, the most common pathogen in severe burn sepsis; *E. coli; Klebsiella; Proteus;* staphylococci; and streptococci • Lower incidence of pain, burning, or itching than mafenide • Does not cause electrolyte or acid–base imbalances • Significant amounts may be absorbed systemically with large burned areas and prolonged use. Monitor for adverse effects common to sulfonamides.	Same as mafenide. Usually the preferred drug	Same as mafenide	Same as mafenide

IV, intravenous; PO, oral; UTI, urinary tract infection.

fonamides. After resistance to one sulfonamide develops, cross-resistance to others is common.

Indications for Use

A **tetracycline** is the drug of choice or an alternate (sometimes as part of combination therapy) in a few infections (eg, brucellosis, chancroid, cholera, granuloma inguinale, psittacosis, Rocky Mountain spotted fever, syphilis, trachoma, typhus, gastroenteritis due to *V. cholerae* or *Helicobacter pylori*). Tetracyclines are also useful in treating some animal bites and Lyme disease. Other drugs (eg, penicillins) are usually preferred in gram-positive infections, and most gram-negative organisms are resistant to tetracyclines. However, a tetracycline may be used if bacterial susceptibility is confirmed. Specific clinical indications for tetracyclines include:

● Treatment of uncomplicated urethral, endocervical, or rectal infections caused by *Chlamydia* organisms.
● Adjunctive treatment, with other antimicrobials, in the treatment of pelvic inflammatory disease and sexually transmitted diseases.
● Postexposure prophylaxis and treatment of anthrax. Doxycycline is the tetracycline of choice as part of a single- or combination-drug regimen.

● Long-term treatment of acne. Tetracyclines interfere with the production of free fatty acids and decrease *Corynebacterium* in sebum. These actions decrease the inflammatory, pustular lesions associated with severe acne.
● As a substitute for penicillin in penicillin-allergic clients. Tetracyclines may be effective in treating syphilis when penicillin cannot be given. They should not be substituted for penicillin in treating streptococcal pharyngitis because microbial resistance is common, and tetracyclines do not prevent rheumatic fever. In addition, they should not be substituted for penicillin in any serious staphylococcal infection because microbial resistance commonly occurs.
● Doxycycline may be used to prevent traveler's diarrhea due to enterotoxic strains of *Escherichia coli*.
● Demeclocycline (Declomycin) may be used to inhibit antidiuretic hormone in the treatment of chronic inappropriate antidiuretic hormone secretion.

Sulfonamides are commonly used to treat UTI (eg, acute and chronic cystitis, asymptomatic bacteriuria) caused by *E. coli* and *Proteus* or *Klebsiella* organisms. In acute pyelonephritis, other agents are preferred. Trimethoprim-sulfamethoxazole is used in chronic bronchitis due to pneumococci, *H. influenzae*, and *Moraxella catarrhalis*. It is also the drug of choice for treatment and prophylaxis of *P. jiroveci* infection in clients with and without human immunodeficiency virus (HIV) infection. Additional uses of sulfonamides include ulcerative colitis and uncommon infections such as chancroid, lymphogranuloma venereum, nocardiosis, toxoplasmosis, and trachoma. Topical sulfonamides are used in prevention of burn wound infections and in treatment of ocular, and other soft tissue infections. For specific clinical indications of individual drugs, see Table 32-2.

Urinary antiseptics are used only for UTI. Table 32-3 summarizes information about drugs used to treat UTI.

Contraindications to Use

Both tetracyclines (except doxycycline) and sulfonamides are contraindicated in clients with renal failure. Tetracyclines are also contraindicated in pregnant women and in children up to 8 years of age. In the fetus and young child, tetracyclines are deposited in bones and teeth along with calcium. If given during active mineralization of these tissues, tetracyclines can cause permanent brown coloring (mottling) of tooth enamel and can depress bone growth. Increased photosensitivity is a common adverse effect, and clients should be warned to take precautions against sunburn while taking these drugs. Sulfonamides are also contraindicated in late pregnancy, lactation, children younger than 2 months of age (except for treatment of congenital toxoplasmosis), and people who have had hypersensitivity reactions to them or to chemically related drugs (eg, thiazide diuretics, antidiabetic sulfonylureas). Sulfasalazine (Azulfidine) is contraindicated in people who are allergic to salicylates and in people with intestinal or urinary tract obstruction.

NURSING PROCESS

General aspects of the nursing process in antimicrobial drug therapy, as described in Chapter 29, apply to the client receiving tetracyclines, sulfonamides, and urinary antiseptics. In this chapter, only those aspects related specifically to these drugs are included.

Assessment

With tetracyclines, assess for conditions in which the drugs must be used cautiously or are contraindicated, such as impaired renal or hepatic function.

With sulfonamides, assess for signs and symptoms of disorders for which the drugs are used:

● For *UTI*, assess urinalysis reports for white blood cell and bacteria counts; urine culture reports for type of bacteria; and symptoms of dysuria, frequency, and urgency of urination.

● For *burns*, assess the size of the wound, amount and type of drainage, presence of edema, and amount of eschar.
● Ask clients specifically if they have ever taken a sulfonamide and, if so, whether they had an allergic reaction.

With urinary antiseptics, assess for signs and symptoms of UTI.

Nursing Diagnoses

● Risk for Injury: Hypersensitivity reaction, kidney, liver, or blood disorders with sulfonamides
● Deficient Knowledge: Correct administration and use of tetracyclines, sulfonamides, and urinary antiseptics

Planning/Goals

The client will
● Receive or self-administer the drugs as directed
● Receive prompt and appropriate treatment if adverse effects occur

Interventions

● During tetracycline therapy for systemic infections, monitor laboratory tests of renal function for abnormal values.
● During sulfonamide therapy, encourage sufficient fluids to produce a urine output of at least 1200 to 1500 mL daily. A high fluid intake decreases the risk of crystalluria (precipitation of drug crystals in the urine).
● Avoid urinary catheterization when possible. If catheterization is necessary, use sterile technique. The urinary tract is normally sterile except for the lower third of the urethra. Introduction of any bacteria into the bladder may cause infection.
● A single catheterization may cause infection. With indwelling catheters, bacteria colonize the bladder and produce infection within 2 to 3 weeks, even with meticulous care.
● When indwelling catheters must be used, measures to decrease UTI include using a closed drainage system; keeping the perineal area clean; forcing fluids, if not contraindicated, to maintain a dilute urine; and removing the catheter as soon as possible. Do not disconnect the system and irrigate the catheter unless obstruction is suspected. *Never* raise the urinary drainage bag above bladder level.
● Force fluids in anyone with a UTI unless contraindicated. Bacteria do not multiply as rapidly in dilute urine. In addition, emptying the bladder frequently allows it to refill with uninfected urine. This decreases the bacterial population of the bladder.
● Teach women to cleanse themselves from the urethral area toward the rectum after voiding or defecating to avoid contamination of the urethral area with bacteria

Table 32-3 Drugs at a Glance: Miscellaneous Drugs for Urinary Tract Infections

GENERIC/TRADE NAME	CHARACTERISTICS	ROUTES AND DOSAGE RANGES	
		Adults	Children
Fosfomycin (Monurol)	• Approved only for treatment of uncomplicated UTI in women due to susceptible strains of *Escherichia coli* and *Enterococcus faecalis* • Most common adverse effects are diarrhea, nausea, vaginitis, and headache.	PO 3 g in a single dose, taken with or without food. Powder should be mixed with ½ cup of water and drunk immediately.	Dosage not established
Methenamine mandelate (Mandelamine)	• Antibacterial activity only at a urine pH <5.5. In acidic urine, the drug forms formaldehyde, which is the antibacterial component. Acidification of urine (eg, with ascorbic acid) is usually needed. • Formaldehyde is active against several gram-positive and gram-negative organisms, including *E. coli.* It is most useful for long-term suppression of bacteria in chronic, recurrent infections. • It is not indicated in acute infections. • Contraindicated in renal failure	PO 1 g 4 times daily after meals and at bedtime	*6–12 y:* PO 500 mg 4 times daily *<6 y:* PO 50 mg/kg/d, in 3 divided doses
Methenamine hippurate (Hiprex)	See methenamine mandelate, above	PO 1 g twice daily	*6–12 y:* PO 500 mg–1 g twice daily
Nalidixic acid (NegGram)	• Prototype of quinolones • Active against most gram-negative organisms that cause UTI, but rarely used because organisms develop resistance rapidly and other effective drugs are available	PO 4 g daily in 4 divided doses for 1–2 wk, then 2 g/d if long-term treatment is required	PO 55 mg/kg/d in 4 divided doses, reduced to 33 mg/kg/d for long-term use in children <12 y. Contraindicated in infants <3 mo. *>3 mo:* PO 5–7 mg/kg/d, in 4 divided doses
Nitrofurantoin (Furadantin, Macrodantin)	• Antibacterial activity against *E. coli* and most other organisms that cause UTI • Used for short-term treatment of UTI or long-term suppression of bacteria in chronic, recurrent UTI • Bacterial resistance develops slowly and to a limited degree. • Contraindicated in severe renal disease	PO macrocrystal capsules: 50–100 mg 4 times daily; dual-release capsules: 100 mg q12h for 7 d Prophylaxis of recurrent UTI in women, PO 50–100 mg at bedtime	*Children >12y:* Dual-release capsules: 100 mg q12h for 7 d *Children ≥1 mo:* PO macrocrystal capsules: 5–7 mg/kg/d in 4 divided doses for 7 d
Phenazopyridine (Pyridium)	• An azo dye that acts as a urinary tract analgesic and relieves symptoms of dysuria, burning, and frequency and urgency of urination, which occur with UTI • It has no anti-infective action. • It turns urine orange-red, which may be mistaken for blood. • It is contraindicated in renal insufficiency and severe hepatitis.	PO 200 mg 3 times daily after meals	*6–12 y:* PO 12 mg/kg/d, in 3 divided doses

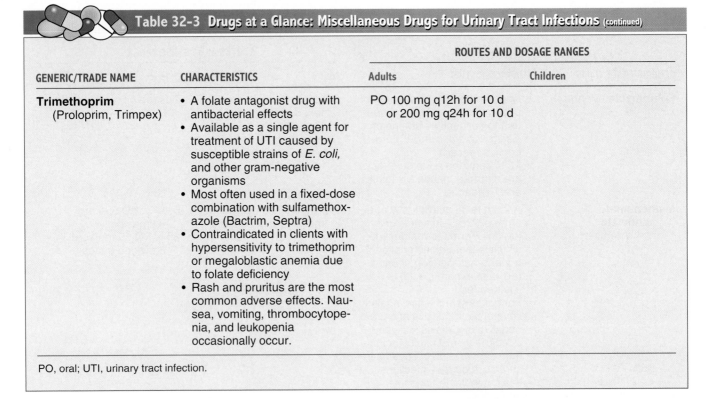

Table 32-3 Drugs at a Glance: Miscellaneous Drugs for Urinary Tract Infections (continued)

GENERIC/TRADE NAME	CHARACTERISTICS	ROUTES AND DOSAGE RANGES	
		Adults	Children
Trimethoprim (Proloprim, Trimpex)	• A folate antagonist drug with antibacterial effects • Available as a single agent for treatment of UTI caused by susceptible strains of *E. coli,* and other gram-negative organisms • Most often used in a fixed-dose combination with sulfamethoxazole (Bactrim, Septra) • Contraindicated in clients with hypersensitivity to trimethoprim or megaloblastic anemia due to folate deficiency • Rash and pruritus are the most common adverse effects. Nausea, vomiting, thrombocytopenia, and leukopenia occasionally occur.	PO 100 mg q12h for 10 d or 200 mg q24h for 10 d	

PO, oral; UTI, urinary tract infection.

from the vagina and rectum. Also, voiding after sexual intercourse helps cleanse the lower urethra and prevent UTI.
● Provide appropriate teaching related to any drug therapy (see accompanying displays).

Evaluation

● Interview and observe for improvement in the infection being treated.
● Interview and observe for adverse drug effects.

APPLYING YOUR KNOWLEDGE 32-1
Sharon will need to have adequate serum drug levels of Bactrim to treat her infection successfully. What instruction should you give Sharon in regard to fluid intake?

PRINCIPLES OF THERAPY

Tetracyclines

● Culture and susceptibility studies are needed before tetracycline therapy is started because many strains of

---

CLIENT TEACHING GUIDELINES

Oral Tetracyclines

General Considerations

✔ Because tetracyclines inhibit rather than kill bacteria, they must be taken correctly to achieve desired effects.
✔ These drugs increase sensitivity to sunlight and risks of sunburn. Avoid sunlamps, tanning beds, and intense or prolonged exposure to sunlight; if unable to avoid exposure, wear protective clothing and a sunblock preparation.
✔ Report severe nausea, vomiting, diarrhea, skin rash, or perineal itching. These symptoms may indicate a need for changing or stopping the tetracycline.

Self-Administration

✔ Take most tetracyclines on an empty stomach, at least 1 hour before or 2 hours after meals. Doxycycline and minocycline may be taken with food (except dairy products).
✔ Do not take with or within 2 hours of dairy products, antacids, or iron supplements. If an antacid must be taken, take at least 2 hours before or after tetracycline.
✔ Take each dose with at least 8 ounces of water.

CLIENT TEACHING GUIDELINES

CLIENT TEACHING GUIDELINES

Oral Sulfonamides

General Considerations

✓ Sulfonamides inhibit rather than kill bacteria. Thus, it is especially important to take them as prescribed, for the length of time prescribed.

✓ These drugs increase sensitivity to sunlight and risks of sunburn. Avoid sunlamps, tanning beds, and intense or prolonged exposure to sunlight; if unable to avoid exposure, wear protective clothing and a sunblock preparation.

✓ Notify the prescribing physician if you have blood in urine, skin rash, difficulty in breathing, fever, or sore throat. These symptoms may indicate adverse drug effects and the need to change or stop the drug.

Self-Administration

✓ Take oral sulfonamides on an empty stomach with at least 8 ounces of water.

✓ With oral suspensions, shake well, refrigerate after opening, and discard the unused portion after 14 days.

✓ Drink 2 to 3 quarts of fluid daily, if able. A good fluid intake helps the drugs to be more effective, especially in urinary tract infections, and decreases the likelihood of damaging the kidneys.

---

organisms are either drug resistant or vary greatly in drug susceptibility. Cross-sensitivity and cross-resistance are common among tetracyclines.

● The oral route of administration is usually effective and preferred. Intravenous (IV) therapy is used when oral administration is contraindicated or for initial treatment of severe infections.

● Tetracyclines decompose with age, exposure to light, and extreme heat and humidity. Because the breakdown products may be toxic, it is important to store these drugs correctly. Also, the manufacturer's expiration dates on containers should be noted and outdated drugs should be discarded.

Sulfonamides and Urinary Antiseptics

● With systemically absorbed sulfonamides, an initial loading dose may be given to produce therapeutic blood levels more rapidly. The amount is usually twice the maintenance dose.

● Urine pH is important in drug therapy with sulfonamides and urinary antiseptics.

● With sulfonamide therapy, alkaline urine increases drug solubility and helps prevent crystalluria. It also increases the rate of sulfonamide excretion and the concentration of sulfonamide in the urine. The urine can be alkalinized by giving sodium bicarbonate. Alkalinization is not needed with sulfisoxazole (because the drug is highly soluble) or sulfonamides used to treat intestinal infections or burn wounds (because there is little systemic absorption).

● With mandelamine therapy, urine pH must be acidic (<5.5) for the drug to be effective. At a higher pH, Mandelamine does not hydrolyze to formaldehyde, the antibacterial component. Urine can be acidified by concomitant administration of ascorbic acid.

● Urine cultures and susceptibility tests are indicated in suspected UTI because of wide variability in possible pathogens and their susceptibility to antibacterial drugs. The best results are obtained with drug therapy indicated by the microorganisms isolated from each client.

APPLYING YOUR KNOWLEDGE 32-2

Sharon mentions that she is going to Florida for spring break. What precaution should you teach Sharon?

Use in Special Populations

Use in Children

Tetracyclines should not be used in children younger than 8 years of age because of their effects on teeth and bones. In teeth, the drugs interfere with enamel development and may cause a permanent yellow, gray, or brown discoloration. In bone, the drugs form a stable compound in bone-forming tissue and may interfere with bone growth.

Systemic sulfonamides are contraindicated during late pregnancy, lactation, and in children younger than 2 months of age. If a fetus or young infant receives a sulfonamide by placental transfer, in breast milk, or by direct administration, the drug displaces bilirubin from binding sites on albumin. As a result, bilirubin may accumulate in the bloodstream (hyperbilirubinemia) and central nervous system (kernicterus) and cause life-threatening toxicity.

Sulfonamides are often used to treat UTI in children older than 2 months of age. Few data are available regarding the effects of long-term or recurrent use of sulfamethoxazole in children younger than 6 years with chronic renal disease. Sulfamethoxazole is often given in combination with trimethoprim (Bactrim, Septra), although trimethoprim has not been established as safe and effective in children younger than 12 years of age.

Some clinicians recommend that asymptomatic bacteriuria be treated in children younger than 5 years of age to decrease risks of long-term renal damage. Treatment is the same as for symptomatic UTI.

Use in Older Adults

A major concern with the use of tetracyclines and sulfonamides in older adults is renal impairment, which commonly occurs in this population. Sulfonamides may cause additional renal impairment. As with younger adults, a fluid intake of 2 liters daily is needed to reduce formation of crystals and stones in the urinary tract.

With the combination of trimethoprim-sulfamethoxazole, older adults are at increased risk for severe adverse effects. Severe skin reactions and bone marrow depression are most often reported. Folic acid deficiency may also occur because both of the drugs interfere with folic acid metabolism.

Use in Clients With Renal Impairment

As discussed previously, most tetracyclines are contraindicated in clients with renal impairment. High concentrations of tetracyclines inhibit protein synthesis in human cells. This antianabolic effect increases tissue breakdown (catabolism) and the amount of waste products to be excreted by the kidneys. The increased workload can be handled by normally functioning kidneys, but waste products are retained when renal function is impaired. This leads to azotemia, increased blood urea nitrogen, hyperphosphatemia, hyperkalemia, and acidosis. If a tetracycline is necessary because of an organism's sensitivity or the host's inability to take other antimicrobial drugs, doxycycline or minocycline may be given.

Systemic sulfonamides should probably be avoided in clients with renal impairment, if other effective drugs are available. Acute renal failure (ARF) has occurred when the drugs or their metabolites precipitated in renal tubules and caused obstruction. ARF is rarely associated with newer sulfonamides, which are more soluble than older ones, but has increased with the use of sulfadiazine to treat toxoplasmosis in clients with acquired immunodeficiency syndrome (AIDS). Preventive measures include an intake of 2 to 3 liters of fluid daily.

Use in Clients With Hepatic Impairment

Tetracyclines are contraindicated in pregnant women because they may cause fatal hepatic necrosis in the mother. They must be used cautiously in the presence of liver or kidney impairment. Because tetracyclines are metabolized in the liver, hepatic impairment or biliary obstruction slows drug elimination. In clients with renal impairment, high IV doses (>2 g/day) have been associated with death from liver failure. If the drug is necessary to treat clients with known or suspected renal and hepatic impairment, renal and liver function test results should be monitored. In addition, serum tetracycline levels should not exceed 15 micrograms per milliliter, and other hepatotoxic drugs should be avoided.

Sulfonamides cause cholestatic jaundice in a small percentage of clients and should be used with caution in clients with hepatic impairment.

Use in Clients With Critical Illness

Tetracyclines may be used to treat sepsis caused by rickettsial, chlamydial, or mycoplasma infection and pulmonary infection caused by *M. pneumoniae* or *Legionella pneumophila*. When necessary, doxycycline is the drug of choice because it can be given to clients with renal impairment, a common problem in critical care settings.

Sulfonamides are rarely used in critical care settings except topical silver sulfadiazine (Silvadene) used to treat burn wounds and trimethoprim-sulfamethoxazole used to treat *P. jiroveci* pneumonia. Although often given IV in critical care settings, oral or nasogastric tube administration of trimethoprim-sulfamethoxazole may be used in selected clients.

APPLYING YOUR KNOWLEDGE 32-3

While Sharon is in the clinic it would be prudent to review what she knows about her other medication. What dietary concerns should Sharon be aware of with regard to tetracycline's food–drug and drug–drug interactions?

N U R S I N G   A C T I O N S

Tetracyclines, Sulfonamides, and Urinary Agents

NURSING ACTIONS	RATIONALE/EXPLANATION
1. Administer accurately	
a. With tetracyclines:	
(1) Give oral drugs with food that does not contain dairy products; do not give with or within 2 hours of dairy products, antacids, or iron supplements. Doxycycline and minocycline may be given with food.	To decrease nausea and other gastrointestinal (GI) symptoms. Tetracyclines combine with metallic ions (eg, aluminum, calcium, iron, magnesium) and are not absorbed.

NURSING ACTIONS	RATIONALE/EXPLANATION
(2) For intravenous (IV) administration, dilute with an appropriate type and amount of IV solution, and infuse over 1–4 hours.	Rapid administration should be avoided. IV doses are usually mixed in hospital pharmacies.
b. With sulfonamides:	
(1) Give oral drugs before or after meals, with a full glass of water.	Absorption is better when taken on an empty stomach; however, taking with food decreases GI upset.
(2) Infuse IV trimethoprim-sulfamethoxazole (diluted in 125 mL of 5% dextrose in water) over 60–90 minutes. Do not mix with other drugs or solutions and flush IV lines to remove any residual drug.	Manufacturer's recommendations
(3) For topical sulfonamides to burn wounds, apply a thin layer with a sterile gloved hand after the surface has been cleansed of previously applied medication.	Burn wounds may be cleansed by whirlpool, shower, or spot cleansing with sterile saline, gauze pads, and gloves.
c. Give nitrofurantoin with or after meals.	Food decreases nausea, vomiting, and diarrhea.
2. Observe for therapeutic effects	Therapeutic effects depend on the reason for use.
a. With tetracyclines, observe for decreased signs and symptoms of the infection for which the drug is being given.	
b. With sulfonamides, observe for decreased symptoms of urinary tract infection (UTI); decreased diarrhea when given for ulcerative colitis or bacillary dysentery; lack of fever and wound drainage, and evidence of healing in burn wounds.	Topical sulfonamides for burns are used to prevent rather than treat infection.
c. With urinary antiseptics, observe for decreased symptoms of UTI.	
3. Observe for adverse effects	
a. Nausea, vomiting, diarrhea	Commonly occur with tetracyclines, sulfonamides, and urinary antiseptics, probably from local irritation of GI mucosa. After several days of an oral tetracycline, diarrhea may be caused by superinfection.
b. Hematologic disorders—anemia, neutropenia, thrombocytopenia	
c. Hypersensitivity—anaphylaxis, skin rash, urticaria, serum sickness	
d. Photosensitivity—sunburn reaction	This can be prevented or minimized by avoiding exposure to sunlight or other sources of ultraviolet light, wearing protective clothing, and using sunscreen lotions.
e. Thrombophlebitis at IV infusion sites	These drugs are irritating to tissues. Irritation can be decreased by diluting the drugs and infusing them at the recommended rates.
f. Nephrotoxicity—increased blood urea nitrogen and serum creatinine; hematuria; proteinuria; crystalluria	Nephrotoxicity is more likely to occur in people who already have impaired renal function. Keeping clients well hydrated may help prevent renal damage.
g. Hepatotoxicity—elevated aspartate aminotransferase and other enzymes	Hepatitis, cholestasis, and other serious liver disorders rarely occur with these drugs.
h. Superinfection—sore mouth; white patches on oral mucosa; black, furry tongue; diarrhea; skin rash; itching in the perineal area; pseudomembranous colitis	Superinfection may occur with tetracyclines because of their broad spectrum of antimicrobial activity. Signs and symptoms usually indicate monilial infection. Meticulous oral and perineal hygiene helps prevent these problems. The drug should be stopped if severe diarrhea occurs, with blood, mucus, or pus in stools.
i. Vertigo and dizziness	Occurs only with minocycline

(continued)

NURSING ACTIONS	RATIONALE/EXPLANATION
j. Adverse effects of sulfonamides in human immunodeficiency virus (HIV)-infected clients—rash, fever, leukopenia, elevated transaminases, thrombocytopenia	Occurs in 20%–85% of HIV-infected clients
4. Observe for drug interactions	
a. Drugs that *decrease* effects of tetracyclines:	
(1) Aluminum, calcium, iron, or magnesium preparations (eg, antacids, ferrous sulfate)	These metals combine with oral tetracyclines to produce insoluble, nonabsorbable compounds that are excreted in feces.
(2) Cathartics, didanosine	Decrease absorption
(3) Barbiturates, carbamazepine, phenytoin, rifampin	These drugs induce drug-metabolizing enzymes in the liver and may speed up metabolism of doxycycline.
b. Drugs that *increase* effects of sulfonamides:	
(1) Alkalinizing agents (eg, sodium bicarbonate)	Increase rate of urinary excretion, thereby raising levels of sulfonamides in the urinary tract and increasing effectiveness in UTIs
(2) Methenamine compounds, urinary acidifiers (eg, ascorbic acid)	These drugs increase the risk of nephrotoxicity and should not be used with sulfonamides. They may cause precipitation of sulfonamide with resultant blockage of renal tubules.
(3) Salicylates (eg, aspirin), nonsteroidal anti-inflammatory drugs (eg, ibuprofen), oral anticoagulants, phenytoin, methotrexate	Increase toxicity by displacing sulfonamides from plasma protein-binding sites, thereby increasing plasma levels of free drug
c. Drugs that *alter* effects of nitrofurantoin:	
(1) Antacids	May decrease absorption
(2) Acidifying agents	Increase antibacterial activity of nitrofurantoin by decreasing renal excretion. Nitrofurantoin is most active against organisms causing UTI when urine pH is 5.5 or less.

APPLYING YOUR KNOWLEDGE: ANSWERS

32-1 Sharon needs fluid intake of at least 2 to 3 liters daily. The fluid will keep her urine dilute and reduce the multiplication of bacteria.

32-2 The Bactrim will increase the skin's sensitivity to sunlight and sunburn. Sharon is already at risk due to the tetracycline. Advise her to wear sunscreen and protective clothing.

32-3 Tetracyclines should not be taken with food that contains dairy products; antacids; or iron supplements. The combination of a tetracycline with calcium, iron, aluminum, or magnesium results in an insoluble compound that prevents the absorption of tetracycline.

Review and Application Exercises

Short Answer Exercises

1. What foods and drugs interfere with absorption of oral tetracyclines? How can interference be prevented or minimized?

2. What are potentially serious adverse effects of tetracyclines?

3. What is the rationale for long-term, low-dose administration of a tetracycline for acne?

4. Which tetracyclines may be given to clients with renal impairment?

5. Why are sulfonamides often effective in UTI?

6. What are major adverse effects of sulfonamides, and how may they be prevented or minimized?

7. What is the rationale for combining sulfamethoxazole and trimethoprim?

8. What are important characteristics of urinary antiseptics?

NCLEX-Style Questions

9. A 6-year-old child with bronchitis is being seen in the pediatrician's office. During the nurse's assessment, the mother expresses concern about the expense of treatment. She asks if it will be all right

for her to use the leftover tetracycline prescribed for her 15-year-old son during his last bout of bronchitis. The appropriate response would not include

a. counseling the mother about the need to complete the full prescribed regimen of any antibiotic
b. instructing the mother to use her son's old prescription, but at half the dose
c. informing the mother of the adverse effects on tooth enamel for young children
d. instructing the mother to discard her son's old tetracycline medication

10. An HIV-positive client is being seen for routine follow-up care in the physician's office. His chief complaints are fever and a severe rash. The medication regimen includes trimethoprim-sulfamethoxazole for prophylaxis of *P. jiroveci* infection. The client asks if his symptoms could be due to any of his medications. The nurse's best response is

a. The likelihood of the client's fever and rash being drug-related is very low.
b. A high percentage of clients with HIV receiving trimethoprim-sulfamethoxazole develop adverse reactions such as these.
c. Adverse effects of trimethoprim-sulfamethoxazole in HIV-infected clients are rarely serious and usually self-limiting.
d. The presence of fever and rash probably indicates that the trimethoprim-sulfamethoxazole regimen is ineffective.

11. Client teaching about phenazopyridine should not include

a. Instruction that the drug is not an antibiotic and only relieves the symptoms of a UTI.
b. A warning that the drug causes a harmless orange-red discoloration of the urine.
c. Counseling to take the drug after meals.
d. Instruction that phenazopyridine will eradicate the UTI in 3 days.

12. The nurse prepares to administer the 2:00 P.M. medications to a hospitalized client. Scheduled for that time are doxycycline PO, Maalox PO, and ferrous sulfate PO. The nurse should

a. Change the doxycycline to IV to avoid drug interactions.
b. Co-administer the doxycycline and ferrous sulfate, but hold the Maalox until 4:00 P.M.
c. Reschedule the Maalox and ferrous sulfate to 4:00 P.M.
d. Give the medications with a glass of milk to decrease stomach irritation.

13. Which of the following instructions should be given to clients prescribed either tetracyclines or sulfonamides?

a. Take with at least 8 ounces of water.
b. Direct exposure to the sun should be avoided, but use of tanning beds is acceptable during therapy.
c. Take the antibiotic until no longer febrile.
d. Stop didanosine therapy during treatment with the antibiotic.

Selected References

Chambers, H. F. (2001). Antimicrobial agents: Protein synthesis inhibitors and miscellaneous antibacterial agents. In J. G. Hardman & L. E. Limbird (Eds.), *Goodman & Gilman's The pharmacological basis of therapeutics* (10th ed., pp. 1239–1271). New York: McGraw-Hill.

Drug facts and comparisons. (Updated monthly). St. Louis: Facts and Comparisons.

Marchiondo, K. (1998). A new look at urinary tract infection. *American Journal of Nursing, 98*(3), 34–38.

Petri, W. A., Jr. (2001). Antimicrobial agents: Sulfonamides, trimethoprim-sulfamethoxazole, quinolones, and agents for urinary tract infections. In J. G. Hardman & L. E. Limbird (Eds.), *Goodman & Gilman's The pharmacological basis of therapeutics* (10th ed., pp. 1171–1188). New York: McGraw-Hill.

Macrolides, Ketolides, and Miscellaneous Antibacterials

OBJECTIVES

After studying this chapter, you will be able to:

1. Discuss characteristics and specific uses of macrolide and ketolide antibacterials.
2. Compare and contrast macrolides and ketolides with other commonly used antibacterial drugs.
3. Apply principles of using macrolides and ketolides in selected client situations.
4. Discuss characteristics and clinical indications for using chloramphenicol, clindamycin, daptomycin, linezolid, metronidazole, quinupristin-dalfopristin, rifaximin, spectinomycin, and vancomycin.
5. Discuss the roles of metronidazole and oral vancomycin in the treatment of pseudomembranous colitis.

APPLYING YOUR KNOWLEDGE

Arthur Shone is a 65-year-old male who has had chronic obstructive pulmonary disease for a number of years. He presents to the doctor's office with a respiratory tract infection. He is started on azithromycin 500 mg for one dose, then 250 mg PO daily for 4 days.

INTRODUCTION

The drugs described in this chapter are heterogeneous in their antimicrobial spectra, characteristics, and clinical uses. Some are used often; some are used only in specific circumstances. The macrolides, ketolides, and selected miscellaneous drugs are described in the following sections; names, routes, and dosage ranges of individual drugs are listed in the Drugs at a Glance tables.

MACROLIDES AND KETOLIDES

Table 33-1 presents routes and dosage ranges for macrolides and ketolides.

The **macrolides,** which include erythromycin, azithromycin (Zithromax), and clarithromycin (Biaxin), have similar antibacterial spectra and mechanisms of action. Macrolides are widely distributed into body tissues and fluids and may be bacteriostatic or bactericidal, depending on drug concentration in in-

fected tissues. They are effective against gram-positive cocci, including group A streptococci, pneumococci, and most staphylococci. They are also effective against species of *Corynebacterium, Treponema, Legionella, Chlamydia, Neisseria,* and *Mycoplasma* and against some anaerobic species of organisms such as *Bacteroides* and *Clostridia.* Azithromycin and clarithromycin also are active against the atypical mycobacteria that cause *Mycobacterium avium* complex (MAC) disease. MAC disease (see Chap. 34) is an opportunistic infection that occurs mainly in people with advanced human immunodeficiency virus (HIV) infection. *Helicobacter pylori,* a pathogen implicated in peptic ulcer disease, is also treated by azithromycin or clarithromycin as part of a combination regimen.

P **Erythromycin,** the prototype, is now used less often because of microbial resistance, numerous drug interactions, and the development of newer macrolides. Erythromycin is metabolized in the liver and excreted mainly in bile; approximately 20% is excreted in urine. Depending on the specific salt formulation used, food can have a variable effect on the

Table 33-1 Drugs at a Glance: Macrolides and Ketolides

GENERIC/TRADE NAME	USUAL ROUTES AND DOSAGE RANGES	
	Adults	Children
Azithromycin (Zithromax)	Respiratory and skin infections, PO 500 mg as a single dose on the first d, then 250 mg once daily for 4 d Nongonococcal urethritis and cervicitis caused by *Chlamydia trachomatis,* 1 g as a single dose Prevention of MAC, PO 1200 mg once per wk Treatment of MAC, PO 600 mg once daily	*2 y and older:* Pharyngitis/tonsillitis, PO 12 mg/kg (not to exceed 500 mg) once daily for 5 d *6 mo and older:* Acute otitis media, PO 10 mg/kg as a single dose (not to exceed 500 mg) on the first d, then 5 mg/kg (not to exceed 250 mg) once daily for 4 d
Clarithromycin (Biaxin, Biaxin XL)	PO 250–500 mg q12h for 7–14 d Prevention of MAC, PO 500 mg q12h or 1000 mg XL daily Extended-release: bronchitis and community-acquired pneumonia, PO 1000 mg (two 500-mg tablets) once daily for 7 d Acute maxillary sinusitis, PO 1000 mg once daily for 14 d	PO 7.5 mg/kg q12h, not to exceed 500 mg q12h Prevention or treatment of MAC, same as above
Erythromycin base (E-mycin)	PO 250–500 mg q6h; severe infections, up to 4 g or more daily in divided doses	PO 30–50 mg/kg/d in divided doses q6–12h; severe infections, 100 mg/kg/d in divided doses
Erythromycin estolate	PO 250 mg q6h; maximal daily dose, 4 g	*Weight >25 kg,* PO same as adults *Weight 10–25 kg,* PO 30–50 mg/kg/d in divided doses *Weight <10 kg,* PO 10 mg/kg/d in divided doses q6–12h Dosages may be doubled in severe infections.
Erythromycin ethylsuccinate (E.E.S.)	PO 400 mg 4 times daily; severe infections, up to 4 g or more daily in divided doses	PO 30–50 mg/kg/d in 4 divided doses q6h. Severe infections, 60–100 mg/kg/d in divided doses
Erythromycin lactobionate	IV 15–20 mg/kg/d in divided doses; severe infections, up to 4 g daily	IV same as adults
Erythromycin stearate (Erythrocin stearate)	PO 250 mg q6h or 500 mg q12h; severe infections, up to 4 g daily	PO 30–50 mg/kg/d in 4 divided doses q6h; severe infections, 60–100 mg/kg/d
Telithromycin (Ketek)	Acute bacterial exacerbation of chronic bronchitis, acute bacterial sinusitis, PO 800 mg once daily for 5 d Community-acquired pneumonia, PO 800 mg once daily for 7–10 d	Not established

IV, intravenous; MAC, *Mycobacterium avium* complex; PO, oral.

absorption of oral erythromycin. Compared with erythromycin, the newer drugs have enhanced antibacterial activity; require less frequent administration; and cause less nausea, vomiting, and diarrhea. Azithromycin is excreted mainly in bile, and clarithromycin is metabolized to an active metabolite in the liver, which is then excreted in urine.

Erythromycin is available in several preparations. Ophthalmic and topical preparations are discussed in Chapters 63 and 64, respectively.

A relative of the macrolides, telithromycin (Ketek) is the first member of the **ketolide** class. In addition to sharing the general spectrum of activity of the newer macrolides, it offers better activity against macrolide-resistant strains of *Streptococcus pneumoniae,* an increasingly common cause of infections in children and adults. Telithromycin is excreted by the liver and kidneys. Food does not affect the absorption of telithromycin.

Mechanism of Action

The macrolides and ketolides enter microbial cells and reversibly bind to the 50S subunits of ribosomes, thereby inhibiting microbial protein synthesis. Ketolides have a greater affinity for ribosomal RNA, expanding their antimicrobial spectrum compared to macrolides.

Indications for Use

The macrolides are widely used for treatment of respiratory tract and skin/soft tissue infections caused by streptococci and staphylococci. Erythromycin is also used as a penicillin substitute in clients who are allergic to penicillin; for prevention of rheumatic fever, gonorrhea, syphilis, pertussis, and chlamydial conjunctivitis in newborns (ophthalmic ointment); and to treat other infections (eg, Legionnaire's disease, genitourinary infections caused by *Chlamydia trachomatis,* intestinal amebiasis caused by *Entamoeba histolytica*).

In addition, azithromycin is approved for treatment of urethritis and cervicitis caused by *C. trachomatis* organisms, and is being used for the prevention and treatment of MAC disease. For acute bacterial sinusitis, azithromycin is approved for an abbreviated 3-day treatment duration.

Clarithromycin is approved for prevention and treatment of MAC disease. Clarithromycin is also approved to treat *H. pylori* infections associated with peptic ulcer disease.

The ketolide telithromycin is approved for acute bacterial exacerbations of chronic bronchitis, acute bacterial sinusitis, and community-acquired pneumonia (including multidrug-resistant *S. pneumoniae.*)

Contraindications to Use

Macrolides and ketolides are contraindicated in people who have had hypersensitivity reactions. Telithromycin is contraindicated in people who have had hypersensitivity reactions to macrolides. Use of the estolate form of erythromycin is contraindicated in clients with pre-existing liver disease. All macrolides and telithromycin must be used with caution in clients with pre-existing liver disease. Use of erythromycin and telithromycin concurrently with drugs highly dependent on CYP3A4 liver enzymes for metabolism (eg., pimozide) is contraindicated.

MISCELLANEOUS ANTIBACTERIAL DRUGS

Table 33-2 summarizes pertinent information about miscellaneous antibacterial drugs.

Chloramphenicol (Chloromycetin) is a broad-spectrum, bacteriostatic antibiotic that is active against most gram-positive and gram-negative bacteria, rickettsiae, chlamydiae, and treponemes. It acts by interfering with microbial protein synthesis. It is well absorbed and diffuses well into body tissues and fluids, including cerebrospinal fluid (CSF), but low drug levels are obtained in urine. It is metabolized in the liver and excreted in the urine.

Chloramphenicol is rarely used now to treat infections because of the effectiveness and low toxicity of alternative drugs. It is used in serious infections for which no adequate substitute drug is available. Specific infections include meningococcal, pneumococcal, or *Haemophilus* meningitis in penicillin-allergic clients; anaerobic brain abscess; *Bacteroides fragilis* infections; and rickettsial infections and brucellosis when tetracyclines are contraindicated. In infections due to vancomycin-resistant enterococci (VRE), chloramphenicol is effective against some strains.

Clindamycin (Cleocin) is similar to the macrolides in its mechanism of action and antimicrobial spectrum. Bacteriostatic in usual doses, it is effective against gram-positive cocci, including group A streptococci, pneumococci, most staphylococci, and some anaerobes such as *Bacteroides* and *Clostridia.* Clindamycin enters microbial cells and attaches to 50S subunits of ribosomes, thereby inhibiting microbial protein synthesis.

Clindamycin is often used to treat infections caused by *B. fragilis.* Because these bacteria are usually mixed with gram-negative organisms from the gynecologic or gastrointestinal (GI) tracts, clindamycin is usually given with another drug, such as an aminoglycoside or a fluoroquinolone, to treat mixed infections. The drug may be useful as a penicillin substitute in clients who are allergic to penicillin and who have serious streptococcal (including prevention of perinatal group B streptococcal disease), staphylococcal, or pneumococcal infections in which the causative organism is susceptible to clindamycin. A topical solution is used in the treatment of acne, and a vaginal cream is available. Clindamycin does not reach therapeutic concentrations in the central nervous system (CNS) and cannot be used for treating meningitis.

Clindamycin is well absorbed with oral administration and reaches peak plasma levels within 1 hour after a dose. It is widely distributed in body tissues and fluids, except CSF, and crosses the placenta. It is highly bound (90%) to plasma proteins. It is metabolized in the liver, and the metabolites are excreted in bile and urine. Dosage may need to be reduced in clients with severe hepatic failure to prevent accumulation and toxic effects.

Daptomycin (Cubicin) belongs to the lipopeptide class, a new class of antibiotics. It is a bactericidal agent effective only for gram-positive infections due to *Staphylococcus aureus* (including oxacillin-resistant strains), *Streptococcus pyogenes,* group B streptococci, and *Enterococcus faecalis* (vancomycin-susceptible strains only). In combination with gentamicin, daptomycin is synergistic in killing staphylococci and enterococci. Its mechanism of action is unique. The drug kills bacteria by inhibiting synthesis of bacterial proteins, DNA, and RNA. Indications are limited to the treatment of complicated skin and skin structure infections caused by the above organisms.

Available only for intravenous (IV) administration, the drug reaches target concentrations by the third daily dose. Daptomycin is excreted primarily by the kidneys. Information on use in children or during pregnancy and lactation is not known. Adverse musculoskeletal effects have been seen, primarily as increased serum creatine kinase (CK) levels. These effects are usually asymptomatic but the drug should

Table 33-2 Drugs at a Glance: Miscellaneous Antibacterials

GENERIC/TRADE NAME	ROUTES AND DOSAGE RANGES	
	Adults	Children
Chloramphenicol (Chloromycetin)	IV 50–100 mg/kg/d in 4 divided doses, q6h	*Children and full-term infants >2 wk:* IV 50 mg/kg/d in 4 divided doses, q6h *Neonates <2 wk:* 25 mg/kg/d in 4 divided doses, q6h
Clindamycin hydrochloride (Cleocin)	PO 150–300 mg q6h; up to 450 mg q6h for severe infections	PO 8–16 mg/kg/d in 3 or 4 divided doses q6–8h; up to 20 mg/kg/d in severe infections
Clindamycin phosphate (Cleocin phosphate)	IV, IM 600 mg–2.7 g/d in 2–4 divided doses, q6–12h (IV up to 4.8 g/d in life-threatening infections)	*Children ≥ 1 mo:* IM, IV 20–40 mg/kg/d in 3 or 4 divided doses q6–8h; up to 40 mg/kg/d in severe infections *Neonates:* 15–20 mg/kg/d in 3 or 4 divided doses q6–8h
Clindamycin palmitate (Cleocin Pediatric– 75 mg/mL)		PO 8–12 mg/kg/d in 3 or 4 divided doses; up to 25 mg/kg/d in very severe infections. For children weighing ≤10 kg, the minimum dose is 37.5 mg, 3 times per day.
Daptomycin (Cubicin)	IV, 4 mg/kg every 24 h for 7–14 d	Dosage not established
Linezolid (Zyvox)	PO, IV 400–600 mg q12h for 10–28 d	*Children ≥12 y:* PO, IV 600 mg every 12 h *Children 7 d–11 y:* PO, IV 10 mg/kg every 8 h *Neonates <7 d:* PO, IV 10 mg/kg every 12 h
Metronidazole (Flagyl)	Anaerobic bacterial infection, IV 15 mg/kg (about 1 g for a 70-kg adult) as a loading dose, infused over 1 h, followed by 7.5 mg/kg (about 500 mg for a 70-kg adult) q6h as a maintenance dose, infused over 1 h. Duration usually 7–10 d; maximum dose 4 g/d Surgical prophylaxis, colorectal surgery, IV 500 mg infused over 30–60 min (within 0.5–1 h prior to incision) *C. difficile* colitis, PO 750 mg–2 g daily in 3 or 4 divided doses for 7–14 d; IV 500–750 mg every 6–8 h	*Children ≥1 mo:* 15–35 mg/kg daily in 3 divided doses *Neonates 1–4 wk:* 7.5 mg/kg every 24–48 h (for weight <1.2 kg), 7.5 mg/kg every 12 h (for weight 1.2–2 kg), 15 mg/kg every 12 h (for weight >2 kg) *Neonates <1 wk:* 7.5 mg/kg every 24–48 h (for weight <1.2 kg), 7.5 mg/kg every 24 h (for weight 1.2–2 kg), 7.5 mg/kg every 12 h (for weight >2 kg)
Quinupristin-dalfopristin (Synercid)	IV 7.5 mg/kg over 60 min q12h for skin and skin-structure infections, and q8h for VREF bacteremia	Same as adult
Rifaximin (Xifaxan)	PO 200 mg 3 times daily for 3 d	Dosage not established
Spectinomycin (Trobicin)	IM 2 g in a single dose	*Children ≥45 kg:* Same as adult *Children <45 kg:* IM 40 mg/kg single dose, maximum dose 2 g
Vancomycin (Vancocin)	PO, IV 500 mg q6h or 1 g q12h; maximum dose, 4 g/d PO not for treatment of systemic infections	PO 40 mg/kg/d in 3 or 4 divided doses for treating antibiotic-associated pseudomembranous colitis *Children ≥1 mo:* 40–60 mg/kg/d in 4 divided doses *Infants and neonates:* IV 15 mg/kg initially, then 10 mg/kg q12h for neonates up to 7 d of age, then q8h up to 1 mo of age PO not for treatment of systemic infections

IM, intramuscular; IV, intravenous; PO, oral; VREF, vancomycin-resistant *Enterococcus faecium.*

be discontinued in clients who develop muscle pain or weakness. The most common adverse effects are constipation, nausea, diarrhea, and vomiting.

Linezolid (Zyvox) is a member of the oxalodinone class, a newer class of antibiotics. It is active against aerobic gram-positive bacteria, in which it acts by inhibiting protein synthesis by a unique mechanism. Linezolid binds to the bacterial 23S ribosomal RNA of the 50S subunit, thus preventing an essential component of the bacterial translation process. The drug exhibits bactericidal activity against most staphylococci, enterococci, and streptococci. It is well absorbed orally, distributes widely, and undergoes hepatic elimination. Its effects in pregnancy and in children are largely unknown.

Linezolid is indicated for pneumonia (both community acquired and nosocomial); complicated and uncomplicated skin and skin structure infections; and vancomycin-resistant *Enterococcus faecium* (VREF) infections. The drug is bacteriostatic against enterococci (including *E. faecalis* and *E. faecium*) and staphylococci (including methicillin-resistant strains), and bactericidal for most streptococci.

Myelosuppression (eg, anemia, leukopenia, pancytopenia, thrombocytopenia) is a serious adverse effect that may occur with prolonged therapy over 2 weeks. The client's complete blood count should be monitored; if myelosuppression occurs, linezolid should be discontinued. Myelosuppression usually improves with drug discontinuation. Pseudomembranous colitis may also occur. Mild cases usually resolve with drug discontinuation; moderate or severe cases may require fluid and electrolyte replacement and an antibacterial drug that is effective against *Clostridium difficile* organisms. Hypertension may occur with the concomitant ingestion of linezolid and adrenergic drugs (eg, dopamine, epinephrine). Clients receiving linezolid and selective serotonin reuptake inhibitors (SSRIs) may be at risk for serotonin syndrome, characterized by fever and cognitive dysfunction. Because linezolid is a weak monoamine oxidase (MAO) inhibitor, clients should avoid food high in tyramine content (aged cheeses, fermented or air-dried meats, sauerkraut, soy sauce, tap beers, red wine) while taking the drug.

Metronidazole (Flagyl) is effective against anaerobic bacteria, including gram-negative bacilli such as *Bacteroides,* gram-positive bacilli such as *Clostridia,* and some gram-positive cocci. It is also effective against protozoa that cause amebiasis, giardiasis, and trichomoniasis (see Chap. 37). Metronidazole achieves therapeutic concentrations in body fluids and tissues and can be used to treat anaerobic brain abscesses. It is eliminated by the liver and kidneys.

Clinical indications for use include prevention or treatment of anaerobic bacterial infections (eg, in colorectal surgery, intra-abdominal infections) and treatment of *C. difficile* infections associated with pseudomembranous colitis. As part of a combination regimen, it is also useful in treatment of infections due to *H. pylori*. It is contraindicated during the first trimester of pregnancy and must be used with caution in clients with CNS or blood disorders.

Quinupristin-dalfopristin (Synercid) belongs to a class of antimicrobials referred to as *streptogramins.* Both components are active antimicrobials that affect bacterial ribosomes to decrease protein synthesis. The combination is bacteriostatic against *E. faecium* (including vancomycin-resistant strains) and bactericidal against both methicillin-susceptible and methicillin-resistant strains of staphylococci. It is not active against *E. faecalis.* The combination undergoes biliary excretion and fecal elimination.

Quinupristin-dalfopristin is indicated for skin and skin structure infections caused by *S. aureus* or group A streptococcus. It is also used for treatment of clients with serious or life-threatening infections associated with VREF bacteremia.

Quinupristin-dalfopristin is a strong inhibitor of cytochrome P450 3A4 enzymes and therefore interferes with the metabolism of drugs such as cyclosporine, antiretrovirals, carbamazepine, and many others. Toxicity may occur with the inhibited drugs.

Rifaximin (Xifaxan) is a structural analog of rifampin. It is used in infectious (travelers') diarrhea due to *Escherichia coli,* but is not effective in diarrhea due to *Campylobacter jejuni.* It is not known whether rifaximin is effective to treat diarrhea due to *Shigella* or *Salmonella* species. Because of its very limited systemic absorption (97% eliminated in feces), rifaximin cannot be used to treat systemic infections, including infections due to invasive strains of *E. coli.* Therefore, diarrhea occurring with fever or bloody stools should be treated with alternative agents. After treatment with rifaximin is started, clients reporting worsening or persistent diarrhea for longer than 24 to 48 hours; fever; or blood in the stool should be treated with an alternative agent.

Spectinomycin (Trobicin) is used for treatment of gonococcal exposure or infection in people who are allergic to or unable to take the preferred regimen (cephalosporins or fluoroquinolones). It may be used during pregnancy when clients cannot tolerate cephalosporins and when fluoroquinolones are contraindicated. Spectinomycin has no activity against infections caused by *Chlamydia* organisms, which often accompany gonorrhea.

Vancomycin (Vancocin) is active only against gram-positive microorganisms. It acts by inhibiting cell wall synthesis. Parenteral vancomycin has been used extensively to treat infections caused by methicillin-resistant *Staphylococcus aureus* (MRSA) and methicillin-resistant staphylococcal species non-aureus (SSNA, including *Staphylococcus epidermidis*), and endocarditis caused by *Streptococcus viridans* (in clients allergic to or with infections resistant to penicillins and cephalosporins) or *E. faecalis* (with an aminoglycoside). *S. pneumoniae* remain susceptible to vancomycin, although vancomycin-tolerant strains have been identified. The drug has also been widely used for prophylaxis of gram-positive infections in clients who are at high risk of developing MRSA infections (eg, those with diabetes, previous hospitalization, or MRSA in their nasal passages) and who require placement of long-term intravascular catheters and other invasive treatment or monitoring devices. Oral vancomycin is used only to treat staphylococcal enterocolitis and pseudomembranous colitis caused by *C. difficile*.

Partly because of this widespread use, VRE are being encountered more often, especially in critical care units, and treatment options for infections caused by these organisms are limited. To decrease the spread of VRE, the Centers for Disease Control and Prevention recommend limiting the use of vancomycin. Specific recommendations include avoiding or minimizing use in empiric treatment of febrile clients with neutropenia (unless the prevalence of MRSA or SSNA is high); in initial treatment for *C. difficile* colitis (metronidazole is preferred); and as prophylaxis for surgery, low birth weight infants, intravascular catheter colonization or infection, and peritoneal dialysis.

For systemic infections, vancomycin is given IV and reaches therapeutic plasma levels within 1 hour after infusion. It is very important to give IV infusions slowly, over 1 to 2 hours, to avoid an adverse reaction characterized by hypotension, flushing, and skin rash. This reaction, sometimes called "red man syndrome," is attributed to histamine release. Vancomycin is excreted through the kidneys; dosage should be reduced in the presence of renal impairment. For bacterial colitis, vancomycin is given orally because it is not absorbed from the GI tract and acts within the bowel lumen. Large amounts of vancomycin are excreted in the feces after oral administration.

NURSING PROCESS

Assessment

- Assess for infections that macrolides, ketolides, and the designated miscellaneous drugs are used to prevent or treat.
- Assess each client for signs and symptoms of the specific current infection.
- Assess culture and susceptibility reports when available.
- Assess each client for risk factors that increase risks of infection (eg, immunosuppression) or risks of adverse drug reactions (eg, impaired renal or hepatic function).

Nursing Diagnoses

- Deficient Knowledge related to type of infection and appropriate use of prescribed antimicrobial drugs
- Risk for Injury related to adverse drug effects
- Risk for Injury related to infection with antibiotic-resistant microorganisms

Planning/Goals

The client will

- Take or receive macrolides, ketolides, and miscellaneous antimicrobials accurately, for the prescribed length of time

- Experience decreased signs and symptoms of the infection being treated
- Be monitored regularly for therapeutic and adverse drug effects
- Verbalize and practice measures to prevent recurrent infection

Interventions

- Use measures to prevent and minimize the spread of infection (see Chap. 29).
- Monitor for fever and other signs and symptoms of infection.
- Monitor laboratory reports for indications of the client's response to drug therapy (eg, white blood cell count [WBC], tests of renal function).
- Encourage fluid intake to decrease fever and maintain good urinary tract function.
- Provide foods and fluids with adequate nutrients to maintain or improve nutritional status, especially if febrile and hypermetabolic.
- Assist clients to prevent or minimize infections with streptococci, staphylococci, and other gram-positive organisms.
- Provide appropriate client teaching for any drug therapy (see accompanying display).

Evaluation

- Interview and observe for improvement in the infection being treated.
- Interview and observe for adverse drug effects.

APPLYING YOUR KNOWLEDGE 33-1

What instructions should be given to Mr. Shone with regard to drug–food or drug–drug interactions, for him to accurately self-administer the azithromycin?

PRINCIPLES OF THERAPY

Culture and Susceptibility Studies

Culture and susceptibility reports and local susceptibility patterns should be reviewed to determine if an antibiotic-resistant pathogen is present in the client. This is particularly important before starting vancomycin, quinupristin-dalfopristin, daptomycin, or linezolid. These drugs have relatively narrow spectra of activity and appropriate indications for their use should be observed to decrease the likelihood of resistance.

Effects of Macrolides on Other Drugs

Erythromycin is metabolized by the cytochrome P450 3A4 isoenzymes in the liver. It interacts with other drugs metabo-

CLIENT TEACHING GUIDELINES

Macrolides and Ketolides

General Considerations

☑ Complete the full course of drug therapy. The fastest and most complete relief of infections occurs with accurate usage of antibiotics. Moreover, inaccurate use may cause other, potentially more severe, infections.

☑ These drugs are often given for infections of the respiratory tract or skin (eg, bronchitis, pneumonia, cellulitis). Good hand hygiene can help prevent the development and spread of these infections.

☑ Report symptoms of infection that recur or develop during antibiotic therapy. Such symptoms can indicate recurrence of the original infection (ie, the antibiotic is not effective because it is the wrong drug or wrong dosage for the infection or it is not being taken accurately) or a new infection with antibiotic-resistant bacteria or fungi.

☑ Report nausea, vomiting, diarrhea, abdominal cramping or pain, yellow discoloration of the skin or eyes (jaundice), dark urine, pale stools, or unusual tiredness. These symptoms may indicate liver damage, which sometimes occurs with these drugs.

☑ Telithromycin (Ketek) may interfere with accommodation, resulting in visual disturbances such as blurred vision, difficulty focusing, and diplopia. This often occurs with the first or second dose. Cau-

tion should be used while driving, operating machinery, or engaging in other potentially hazardous activities. The client should report visual disturbances that interfere with daily activities.

Self-Administration

☑ Take each dose with 6 to 8 ounces of water, at evenly spaced time intervals, preferably around the clock.

☑ With erythromycin, ask a health care provider if not instructed when to take the drug in relation to food. Erythromycin is available in several preparations. Some should be taken on an empty stomach (at least 1 hour before or 2 hours after meals) or may be taken with a small amount of food if gastrointestinal upset occurs. Some preparations may be taken without regard to meals.

☑ Take azithromycin (Zithromax) tablets and oral suspension without regard to meals. Do not take with an antacid.

☑ Take clarithromycin (Biaxin) regular tablets and the oral suspension without regard to meals. Take extended-release tablets (Biaxin XL) with food. With the oral suspension, do not refrigerate and shake well before measuring the dose.

☑ Take telithromycin (Ketek) without regard to meals.

---

lized by the same isoenzyme and interferes with the elimination of several drugs. As a result, the affected drugs are eliminated more slowly, their serum levels are increased, and they are more likely to cause adverse effects and toxicity unless dosage is reduced. Erythromycin in combination with potent inhibitors of CYP3A4 (eg, fluconazole, diltiazem) increases the risk of sudden cardiac death. A partial list of other interacting drugs includes carbamazepine (Tegretol), cyclosporine (Sandimmune), digoxin (Lanoxin), disopyramide (Norpace), lopinavir-ritonavir (Kaletra), lovastatin (Mevacor), nevirapine (Viramune), pimozide (Orap), quinidine, rifampin (Rifadin), ritonavir (Norvir), simvastatin (Zocor), theophylline (Theo-Dur), triazolam (Halcion), and warfarin (Coumadin). These drugs represent a variety of drug classes.

Although they are less potent inhibitors of CYP3A than erythromycin, clarithromycin and telithromycin also interact with many of these drugs. Azithromycin is not a potent inhibitor of the CYP3A4 isoenzyme and is less prone to drug–drug interactions. However, caution should be used with all these agents.

Preventing Toxicity

Chloramphenicol

Blood dyscrasias (potentially serious and life-threatening) have occurred in clients taking chloramphenicol. Irreversible bone marrow depression, which may lead to aplastic anemia, may appear weeks or months after therapy. A dose-related reversible bone marrow depression usually responds to discontinuation of the drug. Clients should be monitored with a

complete blood count, platelet count, reticulocyte count, and serum iron test every 2 days. In addition, periodic measurements of serum drug levels are recommended when possible. Therapeutic levels are 5 to 20 micrograms per milliliter. Therapy should be discontinued as soon as possible and the drug should not be used for trivial infections or for prophylaxis of infections. During therapy, it is recommended that the client be hospitalized to facilitate close monitoring.

Clindamycin

If diarrhea develops in a client receiving clindamycin, the drug should be stopped. If the diarrhea is severe and persistent, stools should be checked for WBCs, blood, mucus, and the presence of *C. difficile* toxin. Sigmidoscopy can be done to more definitively determine whether the client has pseudomembranous colitis, a potentially fatal adverse reaction. If lesions are seen on sigmoidoscopy, the drug should be stopped immediately. Although pseudomembranous colitis may occur with any antibiotic, it has often been associated with clindamycin therapy.

APPLYING YOUR KNOWLEDGE 33-2

Arthur Shone returns to the office with severe diarrhea and a fever. He is diagnosed with pseudomembranous colitis. His stool is positive for *C. difficile* secondary to antibiotic therapy. He is prescribed metronidazole 500 mg PO three times a day for 7 days. What adverse effects should you assess for, in a client receiving metronidazole?

Daptomycin

Unexplained increases in serum CK levels associated with symptoms of myopathy should prompt discontinuation of daptomycin. Concurrent use of daptomycin with other drugs that might produce rhabdomyolysis (eg, statin cholesterol-lowering drug) may increase the risk of musculoskeletal toxicity. If possible, these drugs should not be used concomitantly.

Use in Special Populations

Use in Children

Erythromycin is usually considered safe for treatment of infections caused by susceptible organisms. Azithromycin and clarithromycin are used in young children for some infections (eg, pharyngitis/tonsillitis, acute otitis media). Safety and effectiveness of telithromycin have not been established for children.

Dosage of chloramphenicol must be reduced in premature infants and in full-term infants less than 2 weeks of age because immature metabolism may lead to accumulation and adverse effects, including fatalities ("gray syndrome").

Clindamycin should be given to neonates and infants only if clearly indicated, and then liver and kidney function must be monitored. Diarrhea and pseudomembranous colitis may occur with topical clindamycin for treatment of acne. The safety and efficacy of metronidazole have been established in children only for the treatment of amebiasis, although the drug is used for other infections in pediatric clients without reported unusual adverse effects. Linezolid and vancomycin are used in children, including premature and full-term neonates, for the same indications as in adults. Monitoring serum drug levels is recommended with IV vancomycin.

With the newer drugs, daptomycin, quinupristin-dalfopristin and rifaximin, there has been little or no experience with their use in children, and pediatric dosages have not been identified.

Use in Older Adults

Erythromycin is generally considered safe. Because it is metabolized in the liver and excreted in bile, it may be an alternative in clients with impaired renal function. Dosage reductions are not indicated with azithromycin and telithromycin, but may be needed if clarithromycin is given to older adults with severe renal impairment. Dosage of vancomycin should be adjusted for impaired renal function in older adults as in other age groups.

Daptomycin, quinupristin-dalfopristin, and linezolid do not require dosage adjustment in older adults. The miscellaneous antibacterial drugs are used in older adults for the same indications as in younger adults.

Use in Clients With Renal Impairment

With the macrolides, dosage of erythromycin and azithromycin do not require reduction in renal impairment. However, clarithromycin dosage should be halved or the dosing interval doubled in clients with severe renal impairment (creatinine clearance [CrCl] <30 mL/minute). The dose of telithromycin for clients with severe renal impairment or those on dialysis has not been established.

Chloramphenicol concentrations may increase in clients with impaired renal function. Doses should be adjusted and serum levels monitored during therapy.

Dosage of clindamycin does not need reduction in renal impairment because it is excreted primarily by the liver. Daptomycin dosage should be reduced to every 48 hours in clients with CrCl of less than 30 milliliters per minute and in those undergoing dialysis. Dosage of vancomycin should be reduced because it is excreted mainly by the kidneys and accumulates in renal impairment. In addition, vancomycin may be nephrotoxic with IV administration, high serum concentrations, prolonged therapy, use in older adults or neonates, and concomitant use of other nephrotoxic drugs. Thus, in addition to reduced dosage, renal function and serum drug levels should be monitored (therapeutic levels are 10–25 mcg/mL). Dosage of metronidazole, quinupristin-dalfopristin, and linezolid does not need to be reduced in clients with renal failure. The use of rifaximin in renal failure has not been studied.

Use in Clients With Hepatic Impairment

Erythromycin should be used cautiously, if at all, in clients with hepatic impairment. It is metabolized in the liver to an active metabolite that is excreted in the bile. Avoiding the drug or dosage reduction may be needed in liver failure. It has also been associated with cholestatic hepatitis, most often with the estolate formulation. Symptoms, which may include nausea, vomiting, fever, and jaundice, usually occur after 1 to 2 weeks of drug administration and subside when the drug is stopped.

Other macrolides vary in their hepatic effects. Azithromycin is mainly eliminated unchanged in bile and could accumulate with impaired liver function, but dosage recommendations have not been established. It should be used with caution. Clarithromycin is metabolized in the liver to an active metabolite that is then excreted through the kidneys. Dosage reduction is not recommended for clients with hepatic impairment. The ketolide, telithromycin, does not need dosage adjustment in liver disease.

Clindamycin, chloramphenicol, and metronidazole should be used cautiously, if at all, in the presence of liver disease. Because these drugs are eliminated through the liver, they may accumulate and cause toxic effects. When feasible, other drugs should be substituted. If no effective substitutes are available, dosage should be reduced. With daptomycin, quinupristin-dalfopristin, rifaximin, and linezolid, there are currently no recommendations to alter dosage in hepatic impairment.

A common adverse reaction to many drugs is hepatotoxicity. This may occur with the administration of macrolides. What signs and symptoms should you teach the client to monitor for and report to his primary care provider?

Use in Clients With Critical Illness

Erythromycin is seldom used in critical care settings, partly because broader spectrum bactericidal drugs are usually needed in critically ill clients, and partly because it inhibits liver metabolism and slows elimination of several other drugs. For a critically ill client who needs a macrolide antibiotic, one of the newer macrolides or the ketolide, telithromycin, is preferred because they have broader spectra of antibacterial activity and fewer effects on the metabolism of other drugs.

Clindamycin should be used only when necessary (ie, for serious infections caused by susceptible anaerobes) because critically ill clients may develop hepatic impairment and pseudomembranous colitis (also called *antibiotic-associated colitis*). These clients are at high risk for development of pseudomembranous colitis because they often receive aggressive antibiotic therapy with multiple or broad-spectrum antibacterial drugs that destroy normal bowel microorganisms.

Metronidazole is often used in critically ill clients with mixed infections. These clients are at risk for drug toxicity from accumulation of active metabolites. Vancomycin penetrates tissues well in critically ill clients and achieves therapeutic levels well above the minimum inhibitory concentration (MIC) for most staphylococci and enterococci. Plasma drug levels and renal function should be monitored. Although usually given by IV infusion, vancomycin is given orally to treat pseudomembranous colitis. Quinupristin-dalfopristin, daptomycin, and linezolid are often used in critically ill clients because infections with resistant pathogens commonly occur in this population.

Use in Home Care

Most of the macrolides, telithromycin, and miscellaneous antibacterial drugs may be taken in the home setting. The role of the home care nurse is generally the same as with other antibiotic therapy; that is, the nurse may need to teach clients or caregivers about drug administration and expected effects. For clients taking oral metronidazole or vancomycin for pseudomembranous colitis, stool specimens may need to be collected and tested in the laboratory for the presence of *C. difficile* organisms or toxins.

NURSING ACTIONS

Macrolides, Ketolides, and Miscellaneous Antibacterials

NURSING ACTIONS	RATIONALE/EXPLANATION
1. Administer accurately	
a. Give oral erythromycin preparations according to manufacturers' instructions, with 6–8 ounces of water, at evenly spaced intervals, around the clock.	Some should be taken on an empty stomach; some can be taken without regard to meals. Adequate water aids absorption; regular intervals help to maintain therapeutic blood levels.
b. With azithromycin, give the tablets or oral suspension without regard to meals. Do not give oral azithromycin with aluminum- or magnesium-containing antacids.	Antacids decrease absorption of tablets and the suspension.
c. With clarithromycin, give regular tablets and the oral suspension with or without food. Give the extended-release tablets (Biaxin XL) with food. Shake the suspension well before measuring the dose.	Manufacturer's recommendations All suspensions should be mixed well to measure accurately.
d. With telithromycin, give without regard to meals.	
e. For intravenous (IV) erythromycin, consult the manufacturer's instructions for dissolving, diluting, and administering the drug. Infuse continuously or intermittently (eg, q6h over 30–60 min).	The IV formulation has limited stability in solution, and instructions must be followed carefully to achieve therapeutic effects. Also, instructions differ for intermittent and continuous infusions. IV erythromycin is the treatment of choice for Legionnaire's disease. Otherwise, it is rarely used.

NURSING ACTIONS	RATIONALE/EXPLANATION
f. With chloramphenicol: (1) Mix IV chloramphenicol in 50–100 milliliters of 5% dextrose in water and infuse over 15–30 minutes.	Do not administer intramuscularly (IM).
g. With clindamycin: (1) Give capsules with a full glass of water.	To avoid esophageal irritation
(2) Do not refrigerate reconstituted oral solution.	Refrigeration thickens the solution, making it difficult to measure and pour accurately.
(3) Give IM injections deeply, and rotate sites. Do not give more than 600 milligrams in a single injection.	To decrease pain, induration, and abscess formation
(4) For IV administration, dilute 300–600 milligrams in 50 milliliters of IV fluid and give over 10–20 minutes, or dilute 900 milligrams in 50–100 milliliters and give over 20 minutes. *Do not* give clindamycin undiluted or by direct injection.	Dilution decreases risks of phlebitis. Cardiac arrest has been reported with bolus injections of clindamycin.
h. With daptomycin: (1) Mix with normal saline or lactated Ringer's IV solution only.	The drug is incompatible with dextrose-containing IV solutions.
(2) Infuse over 30 minutes.	
i. With linezolid: (1) Give oral tablets and suspension without regard to meals.	Manufacturer's recommendations
(2) For IV administration, the drug is compatible with 5% dextrose, 0.9% sodium chloride, and lactated Ringer's solutions.	
(3) Infuse the drug over 30–120 minutes. If other drugs are being given through the same IV line, flush the line with one of the above solutions before and after linezolid administration.	
j. With IV metronidazole, check the manufacturer's instructions.	The drug requires specific techniques for preparation and administration.
k. With quinupristin-dalfopristin: (1) Give IV, mixed in a minimum of 250 milliliters of 5% dextrose solution and infused over 60 minutes.	Dilution in at least 250 milliliters of IV solution decreases venous irritation. A central venous catheter may also be used for drug administration to decrease irritation.
(2) Do *not* mix the drug or flush the IV line with saline- or heparin-containing solutions.	The drug is incompatible with saline- and heparin-containing solutions.
l. Give rifaximin without regard to meals.	
m. With spectinomycin, administer by deep IM injection in upper outer quadrant of the gluteal muscle.	
n. With vancomycin, dilute 500-milligram doses in 100 milliliters, and 1-gram doses in 200 milliliters of 0.9% NaCl or 5% dextrose injection and infuse over at least 60 minutes.	To decrease hypotension and flushing (ie, "red man syndrome") that may occur with more rapid IV administration. This reaction is attributed to histamine release and may be prevented by prior administration of diphenhydramine, an antihistamine. Dilution also decreases pain and phlebitis at the injection site.
2. Observe for therapeutic effects	See Chapter 29.
a. Decreased local and systemic signs of infection	
b. Decreased signs and symptoms of the specific infection for which the drug is being given	

(continued)

NURSING ACTIONS	RATIONALE/EXPLANATION
3. Observe for adverse effects	
a. With macrolides and ketolides:	
(1) Nausea, vomiting, diarrhea	These are the most frequent adverse reactions, reportedly less common with azithromycin, clarithromycin, and telithromycin than with erythromycin.
(2) With IV erythromycin, phlebitis at the IV infusion site	The drug is very irritating to body tissues. Phlebitis can be minimized by diluting the drug well, infusing it slowly, and not using the same vein more than 48–72 hours, if possible.
(3) Hepatotoxicity—nausea, vomiting, abdominal cramps, fever, leukocytosis, abnormal liver function, cholestatic jaundice	More likely to occur with the estolate formulation of erythromycin; less likely to occur with the newer macrolides and ketolides than with erythromycin
(4) Allergic reactions—anaphylaxis, skin rash, urticaria	Potentially serious but infrequent
b. With chloramphenicol:	
(1) Bone marrow depression—anemia, leukopenia, thrombocytopenia	Blood dyscrasias are the most serious adverse reaction to chloramphenicol.
(2) Clinical signs of infection or bleeding	
c. With clindamycin:	
(1) Nausea, vomiting, diarrhea	These are the most frequent adverse effects and may be severe enough to require stopping the drug.
(2) Pseudomembranous colitis (also called *antibiotic-associated colitis*)—severe diarrhea, fever, stools containing neutrophils and shreds of mucous membrane	May occur with most antibiotics but is more common with oral clindamycin. It is caused by *Clostridium difficile*. The organism produces a toxin that kills mucosal cells and produces superficial ulcerations that are visible with sigmoidoscopy. Discontinuing the drug and giving oral metronidazole are curative measures.
d. With daptomycin:	
(1) Increases in serum creatine kinase, muscle pain or weakness	Daptomycin discontinuation may be warranted.
e. With linezolid:	
(1) Nausea, vomiting, diarrhea	These are common effects.
(2) Bone marrow depression—anemia, leukopenia, thrombocytopenia	Complete blood counts (CBCs) are recommended weekly to monitor for myelosuppression. If it occurs, the drug should be discontinued.
f. With metronidazole:	
(1) Central nervous system effects—convulsive seizures, peripheral paresthesias, ataxia, confusion, dizziness, headache	Convulsions and peripheral neuropathy may be serious effects.
(2) GI effects—nausea, vomiting, diarrhea, unpleasant metallic taste	GI effects are most common.
(3) Dermatologic effects—skin rash, pruritus, thrombophlebitis at infusion sites	
g. With quinupristin-dalfopristin:	
(1) IV infusion site reactions—pain, edema, inflammation	The most common adverse effects during clinical trials. Moderate to severe venous irritation can occur with administration through peripheral veins. This can be prevented by infusion through a central venous IV line.
(2) Nausea, vomiting, diarrhea	These effects occurred in 2.7%–4.6% of subjects in clinical trials. Most other adverse effects occurred in fewer than 1% of subjects.
h. With rifaximin:	
(1) Flatulence, headache, abdominal pain, nausea, constipation, vomiting	Occurred with approximately the same frequency as people receiving placebo in studies.
i. With vancomycin:	
(1) Nephrotoxicity—oliguria, increased blood urea nitrogen and serum creatinine	Uncommon. Most likely to occur with large doses, concomitant administration of an aminoglycoside antibiotic, or pre-existing renal impairment. Usually resolves when vancomycin is discontinued.

NURSING ACTIONS	RATIONALE/EXPLANATION
(2) Ototoxicity—hearing loss, tinnitus	Most likely to occur in people with renal impairment or a pre-existing hearing loss
(3) "Red man syndrome"—hypotension, skin flushing	Occurs with rapid infusion of IV vancomycin. Can be prevented by adequate dilution and infusing over 1–2 hours or premedicating with diphenhydramine (an antihistamine).
4. Observe for drug interactions	
a. Drugs that *increase* effects of erythromycin:	
(1) Chloramphenicol	The combination is effective against some strains of resistant *Staphylococcus aureus*.
(2) Streptomycin	The combination is effective against the enterococcus in bacteremia, brain abscess, endocarditis, meningitis, and urinary tract infection
b. Drugs that *increase* effects of clarithromycin:	
(1) Atazanavir, delavirdine, fluconazole, lopinavir, omeprazole, ritonavir, saquinavir	Inhibits metabolism of clarithromycin; dosage reductions of clarithromycin sometimes recommended.
c. Drugs that *decrease* effects of clarithromycin:	
(1) Efavirenz, nevirapine	Consider alternatives to clarithromycin.
d. Drugs that *decrease* effects of azithromycin:	
(1) Antacids	Antacids decrease peak serum levels.
e. Drugs that *decrease* effects of telithromycin:	
(1) Phenytoin, carbamazepine, phenobarbital, rifampin	Decrease in telithromycin levels may result, with loss of antibacterial effect.
f. Drugs that *decrease* effects of chloramphenicol:	
(1) Enzyme inducers (eg, rifampin, phenobarbital)	Reduce serum levels, probably by accelerating liver metabolism of chloramphenicol
g. Drug that *decreases* effects of clindamycin:	
(1) Erythromycin	Delays absorptiom
h. Drugs that *increase* effects of daptomycin:	
(1) HMG-CoA reductase inhibitors (eg, statin cholesterol-lowering drugs)	Potential to increase the musculoskeletal adverse effects of daptomycin
i. Drug that *increases* effects of metronidazole:	
(1) Cimetidine	Inhibits hepatic metabolism of metronidazole
j. Drugs that *decrease* effects of metronidazole:	
(1) Enzyme inducers (phenobarbital, phenytoin, prednisone, rifampin)	These drugs induce hepatic enzymes and decrease effects of metronidazole by accelerating its rate of hepatic metabolism.

APPLYING YOUR KNOWLEDGE: ANSWERS

33-1 Azithromycin should be taken on an empty stomach with 6 to 8 ounces of water. Do not take any antacid products for 2 hours before or 2 hours after a dose of azithromycin. Take the medication at the same time each day until all of the pills are gone. Adequate water intake aids absorption. Taking the drug at regular intervals helps to maintain a therapeutic blood level. Finishing the drug will help decrease the risks of inadequate treatment and drug resistance.

33-2 Assess for the occurrence of adverse GI effects such as nausea, vomiting, or continued diarrhea. Mr. Shone should be aware that he may have a metallic taste in his mouth due to the metronidazole. Also observe for CNS adverse effects, such as seizures or peripheral neuropathy.

33-3 Teach Mr. Shone to monitor himself for abdominal pain, nausea, vomiting, diarrhea, and/or yellow discoloration of the eyes or skin.

Review and Application Exercises

Short Answer Exercises

1. Why is erythromycin called a "penicillin substitute"?

2. What are adverse effects with erythromycin, and how may they be prevented or minimized?

3. How do the newer macrolides differ from erythromycin?

4. How does the ketolide differ from the macrolides?

5. How would you recognize pseudomembranous colitis in a client? What would you do if you thought a client might have it? Why?

6. Why is metronidazole preferred over vancomycin for initial treatment of pseudomembranous colitis?

7. Which antibacterial drug is considered the drug of choice for MRSA and SSNA?

8. What is "red man syndrome" and how can it be prevented or minimized?

9. What is the main clinical importance of the newer drugs, linezolid, daptomycin, rifaximin, and quinupristin-dalfopristin?

NCLEX-Style Questions

10. A 35-year-old man with HIV is being seen for routine follow-up care. He is receiving highly active antiretroviral therapy (HAART). The client was recently hospitalized with an infection due to MAC disease, and the physician now decides to place the client on a preventive regimen. The best choice of drug would be
    a. erythromycin
    b. clarithromycin
    c. azithromycin
    d. telithromycin

11. A 19-year-old college student was seen in the physician's office for severe diarrhea. The physician diagnosed travelers' diarrhea because the student had recently returned from Mexico. Rifaximin 200 mg orally three times daily for 3 days was prescribed. The student calls the office 3 days later and reports to the nurse that she has a fever and that the diarrhea has not resolved. The nurse should
    a. Advise the student to return to the physician's office for further tests and a different antibiotic.
    b. Call the pharmacy and authorize one refill of rifaximin.
    c. Advise the student that it takes up to 48 to 72 hours after the completion of treatment for the diarrhea to completely resolve.
    d. Tell the student to continue to drink plenty of fluids and report back in 24 hours.

12. An 89-year-old man is admitted to the hospital from a nursing home with the diagnosis of pneumonia. The most likely pathogen is *Staphylococcus aureus*. He is also in acute renal failure with an estimated CrCl of 20 mL/min. Which of the following regimens would not require dosage adjustment because of the renal failure?
    a. vancomycin + azithromycin
    b. quinupristin-dalfopristin + azithromycin
    c. daptomycin + telithromycin
    d. linezolid + clarithromycin

13. A recent nurse graduate is preparing to administer vancomycin IV to a client. She states the client reported that he experienced flushing with his last dose of vancomycin. The nurse should
    a. Infuse the vancomycin over 30 minutes to decrease the chance of a reaction.
    b. Hold the vancomycin dose until the physician's rounds the following morning.
    c. Dilute the vancomycin in 50 mL of normal saline solution and infuse over 60 minutes.
    d. Contact the physician, report the reaction, and request an order for diphenhydramine pretreatment.

14. A client is started on clarithromycin extended-release tablets (Biaxin XL) 500 mg every 24 hours for 7 days. The teaching plan for this client should not include
    a. Complete the full 7 days of treatment.
    b. Perform thorough hand hygiene to decrease spread of infection.
    c. Contact the physician if a rash, jaundice, or diarrhea develops.
    d. Take on an empty stomach.

Selected References

Chambers, H. F. (2001). Antimicrobial agents: Protein synthesis inhibitors and miscellaneous antibacterial agents. In J. G. Hardman & L. E. Limbird (Eds.), *Goodman & Gilman's The pharmacological basis of therapeutics* (10th ed., pp. 1239–1271). New York: McGraw-Hill.

de Roux, A., & Lode, H. (2003). Recent developments in antibiotic treatment. *Infectious Disease Clinics of North America, 17*(4), 739–751.

Drug facts and comparisons. (Updated monthly). St. Louis: Facts and Comparisons.

Hospital Infection Control Practices Advisory Committee. (1995). Recommendations for preventing the spread of vancomycin resistance: Recommendations of the Hospital Infection Control Practices Advisory Committee (HICPAC). *Morbidity and Mortality Weekly Report: Recommendations and Reports, 44*(RR-12), 1–13.

Karakousis, P. C., Moore, R. D., & Chaisson, R. E. (2004). *Mycobacterium avium* complex in patients with HIV infection in the era of highly active antiretroviral therapy. *Lancet Infectious Diseases, 4*(9), 557–565.

Klein, N. C., & Cunha, B. A. (2001). New uses of older antibiotics. *Medical Clinics of North America, 85*(1), 125–132.

Lundstrom, T. S., & Sobel, J. D. (2004). Antibiotics for gram-positive bacterial infections: Vancomycin, quinupristin-dalfopristin, linezolid, and daptomycin. *Infectious Disease Clinics of North America, 18*(3), 651–668.

Zuckerman, J. M. (2004). Macrolides and ketolides: Azithromycin, clarithromycin, telithromycin. *Infectious Disease Clinics of North America, 18*(3), 621–649.

Drugs for Tuberculosis and *Mycobacterium avium* Complex (MAC) Disease

OBJECTIVES

After studying this chapter, you will be able to:

1. Describe characteristics of latent, active, and drug-resistant tuberculosis infections.
2. Identify populations at high risk for developing tuberculosis.
3. List characteristics, uses, effects, and nursing implications of using primary antitubercular drugs.
4. Describe the rationale for multiple-drug therapy in treatment of tuberculosis.
5. Discuss ways to increase adherence to antitubercular drug therapy regimens.
6. Differentiate the advantages and disadvantages of directly observed therapy (DOT).
7. Describe factors affecting the use of primary, secondary, and other drugs in the treatment of multidrug-resistant tuberculosis (MDR-TB).
8. Describe *Mycobacterium avium* complex disease and the drugs used to prevent or treat it.

APPLYING YOUR KNOWLEDGE

Fred Guth is a 58-year-old homeless man. He is spending the night at a shelter where one of your coworkers volunteers one evening a month. Fred has a productive cough. Your coworker notes that he has visibly lost weight since he was in the shelter 1 month ago. When she asks him how he feels, Fred says he sweats a lot at night and thinks he has a fever. He is sent to the free clinic the next day, where his sputum test is positive for *Mycobacterium tuberculosis.* From the clinic, Fred is sent to the county jail, where he will stay until his sputum test is negative. He is started on the following regimen:

> Isoniazid (INH) 300 mg PO daily for 6 months
> Rifampin 600 mg PO daily for 6 months
> Pyrazinamide 2000 mg PO daily for 2 months

The health department supplies his medication and is responsible for overseeing his course of therapy. You are a nurse working for the health department.

INTRODUCTION

Tuberculosis (TB) is an infectious disease that usually affects the lungs (>80% of cases) but may involve most parts of the body, including lymph nodes, pleurae, bones, joints, kidneys, and the gastrointestinal (GI) tract. It is caused by *Mycobacterium tuberculosis,* the tubercle bacillus. In general, these bacilli multiply slowly; they may lie dormant in the body for many years; they resist phagocytosis and survive in phagocytic cells; and they develop resistance to antitubercular drugs.

Tuberculosis commonly occurs in many parts of the world and causes many deaths annually. In the United States, active disease has decreased to a low level overall, but has increased in certain states (eg, California, New York, Texas) and in foreign-born members of racial/ethnic groups from Mexico, the Philippines, Vietnam, India, and China. There are also large numbers of people with inactive or latent TB infection. Contributing factors include increased exposure during a resurgence of active disease between 1985 and 1992; immigration from countries where the disease is common; and

increasing numbers of people with conditions or medications that depress the immune system.

Epidemiology of Tuberculosis

There are four phases in the initiation and progression of tuberculosis (Fig. 34-1):

1. **Transmission.** This occurs when an uninfected person inhales infected airborne particles that are exhaled by an infected person. Major factors affecting transmission are the number of bacteria expelled by the infected person and the closeness and duration of the contact between the infected and the uninfected person.
2. **Primary infection.** It is estimated that 30% of persons exposed to tuberculosis bacilli become infected and develop a mild, pneumonia-like illness that is often undiagnosed. About 6 to 8 weeks after exposure, those infected have positive reactions to tuberculin skin tests. Within approximately 6 months of exposure, spontaneous healing occurs as the bacilli are encapsulated in calcified tubercles.

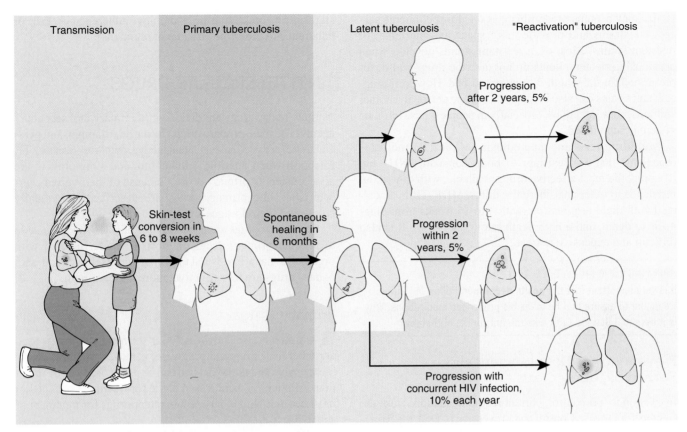

FIGURE 34-1 Transmission of tuberculosis and progression from latent infection to reactivated disease. Among persons who are seronegative for the human immunodeficiency virus (HIV), approximately 30% of heavily exposed persons will become infected. In 5% of persons with latent infection, active disease will develop within 2 years, and in an additional 5%, progression to active disease will occur later. The rate of progression to active disease is dramatically increased among persons who are coinfected with HIV. (Adapted from Small, P. M., & Fujiwara, P. I. [2001]. Management of tuberculosis in the United States. *New England Journal of Medicine, 345*[3], 189–200.)

3. **Latent tuberculosis infection (LTBI)**. The immune system is able to stop bacterial growth in most people who become infected with TB bacteria. The bacteria become inactive, although they remain alive in the body and can become active later. People with inactive or latent TB infection have no symptoms; do not feel sick; do not spread TB to others; usually have a positive skin-test reaction; and can develop active TB disease years later if the latent infection is not effectively treated. In many people with LTBI, the infection remains inactive throughout their lives. In others, the TB bacteria become active and cause tuberculosis, usually when a person's immune system becomes weak as a result of disease, immunosuppressive drugs, or aging.

4. **Active tuberculosis** usually results from reactivation of latent infection, although new infection can also occur. Both reactivated and new infections are more likely to occur in people whose immune system is depressed by disease (eg, human immunodeficiency virus [HIV] infection, diabetes mellitus, cancer) or drug therapy (eg, for cancer or organ transplantation). Among people with

LTBI, signs and symptoms of active disease (eg, cough that is persistent and often productive of sputum, chest pain, chills, fever, hemoptysis, night sweats, weight loss, weakness, lack of appetite, positive skin test, abnormal chest radiograph, positive sputum smear or culture) are estimated to develop in 5% within 2 years and in another 5% after 2 years. Among people with both LTBI and HIV infection, LTBI progresses to active disease more rapidly (approximately 10% each year), is more severe, and often involves extrapulmonary sites.

Drug-Resistant Tuberculosis

In addition to LTBI, a major concern among public health and infectious-disease authorities is an increase in drug-resistant infections. A major factor in drug-resistant infections is poor client adherence to prescribed antitubercular drug therapy.

Drug-resistant mutants of *M. tuberculosis* microorganisms are present in any infected person. When infected people receive antitubercular drugs, drug-resistant mutants continue to appear and reproduce in the presence of the drugs. These strains may become predominant as the drugs eliminate susceptible strains and provide more space and nutrients for resistant strains. Most drug-resistant strains develop when previously infected clients do not take the drugs and doses prescribed for the length of time prescribed. However, drug-resistant strains can also be spread from one person to another and cause new infections, especially in people whose immune system is suppressed.

Multidrug-resistant tuberculosis (MDR-TB) indicates organisms that are resistant to both isoniazid (INH) and rifampin, the most effective drugs available, with or without resistance to other antitubercular drugs. MDR-TB is associated with rapid progression, with 4 to 16 weeks from diagnosis to death, and a high death rate (50%–80%). It is also difficult and expensive to treat.

APPLYING YOUR KNOWLEDGE 34-1

It is very important that the health department follow Mr. Guth's treatment to assure that he takes his prescribed medications. Why is it essential that Mr. Guth take the full course of therapy?

Preventing the Development and Spread of Tuberculosis

In relation to TB control, current recommendations from the Centers for Disease Control and Prevention (CDC), the American Thoracic Society (ATS), and the Infectious Diseases Society of America (IDSA) emphasize continued treatment of active disease and expanded efforts to identify and treat latent infection (LTBI). For identification, tuberculin skin testing is recommended only for high-risk groups (Box 34-1). When LTBI is found in these groups, it should be treated to eradicate this reservoir of infection (Box 34-2).

Recommendations for treatment change as authorities strive to design more effective regimens and overcome barriers to their effective implementation. One change is the increasing use of short-course regimens. Numerous studies indicate that these regimens are effective for many people. In addition, clients are more likely to complete a shorter course of therapy, which reduces the occurrence of drug-resistant TB.

Although local health departments are largely responsible for TB control programs, some authorities urge increased testing and treatment in primary-care settings and in settings where high-risk groups are found (eg, homeless shelters). In addition, authorities urge recognition and effective management of language, social, economic, transportation, and other barriers that limit access to health care and inhibit diagnosis and treatment.

Nurses have important roles to play in TB control. Some of the roles include performing and reading tuberculin skin tests; managing TB clinics; tracking contacts of clients with active disease; assessing clients, homes, and other settings for risk factors; educating clients and families about TB infection and its treatment; administering or directing the administration of antitubercular drugs (eg, directly observed therapy [DOT]); and maintaining records (eg, skin-test results, clients starting or completing drug therapy, adherence or lack of adherence to prescribed treatment regimens).

ANTITUBERCULAR DRUGS

Antitubercular drugs are divided into primary and secondary agents. The main primary drugs (isoniazid, rifampin, and pyrazinamide) are used to treat latent, active, and drug-resistant TB infection when possible. Ethambutol and streptomycin are also considered primary drugs. Because of their varied characteristics, the primary drugs are described individually below and their dosages are listed in Table 34-1.

Secondary drugs are used only for clients who are unable to tolerate primary drugs or those who are infected with organisms that are resistant to primary drugs. In general, secondary drugs are less effective, more toxic, or both.

Primary Drugs

P **Isoniazid** (also known as **INH**), the most commonly used antitubercular drug and prototype, is bactericidal, relatively inexpensive and nontoxic, and can be given orally or by injection. Although it can be used alone for treatment of LTBI, it must be used with other antitubercular drugs for treatment of active disease.

INH penetrates body cells and mycobacteria, kills actively growing intracellular and extracellular organisms, and inhibits the growth of dormant organisms in macrophages and tuberculous lesions. Its mechanism of action is to inhibit formation of cell walls in mycobacteria.

INH is well absorbed from the GI tract, with peak serum concentrations occurring 1 to 2 hours after a 300-milligram dose. It penetrates and reaches therapeutic concentrations in essentially all body fluids and cavities. Its half-life is 1 to 4 hours. It is acetylated in the liver to acetylisoniazid, which is excreted by the kidneys. Metabolism of INH is genetically determined; some people are "slow acetylators" and others are "rapid acetylators." A person's rate of acetylation may be significant in determining response to INH. Slow acetylators have less N-acetyltransferase, the acetylating enzyme, in the liver. In these clients, INH is more likely to accumulate to toxic concentrations, and the development of peripheral neuropathy is more likely. However, there is no significant difference in the clinical effectiveness of INH. Rapid acetylators may require unusually high doses of INH. They also may be more susceptible to serious liver injury because of rapid formation of hepatotoxic metabolites. The drug is excreted in urine.

Potentially serious adverse effects include hepatotoxicity and peripheral neuropathy. Hepatotoxicity may be manifested by symptoms of hepatitis (eg, anorexia, nausea, fatigue, malaise, jaundice) or elevated liver enzymes. The drug should be stopped if hepatitis develops or liver enzymes (eg, alanine and aspartate aminotransferases [ALT and AST]) are more than five times the normal values. Hepatitis is more likely to

Box 34-1 Targeted Tuberculin Testing for Latent Tuberculosis Infection (LTBI)

Purpose
To identify people with latent tuberculosis infection (LTBI) who are at high risk of developing active tuberculosis and who would benefit from treatment of LTBI, if detected.

Who Should Be Tested?
Numerous high-risk groups have been identified, including persons with the following circumstances or conditions:

- Having recent infection with *Mycobacterium tuberculosis* organisms
- Having close contact with someone diagnosed with infectious pulmonary TB
- Immigrating from areas of the world with high rates of TB. For about 5 years, immigrants have incidence rates similar to those of their country of origin and are thought to have become infected in their native country. After 5 years, rates become similar to those of the general U.S. population.
- Belonging to younger age groups. Young children (eg, <5 years) with a positive skin test are at high risk for progression to active disease. The risk is also increased in adolescents and young adults.
- Belonging to older age groups, especially if also living or working in institutions with high-risk populations (eg, hospitals, homeless shelters, correctional facilities, nursing homes, residential homes for patients with acquired immune deficiency syndrome (AIDS)
- Being homeless
- Being an injection drug user
- Having HIV infection or AIDS. HIV infection greatly increases the risk for progression of LTBI to active TB.
- Having chest radiographs that show fibrotic lesions in the lungs. Such lesions are likely to stem from prior, untreated, healed TB.
- Being underweight, especially if more than 10%–15% under ideal weight.
- Having silicosis (a pulmonary disorder caused by inhalation of dust particles from mining or stonecutting). People with silicosis and a positive tuberculin test are about 30 times more likely to develop active disease than the general population.
- Having chronic renal failure and being on hemodialysis. These people are 10 to 25 times more likely to develop active disease than the general population.
- Having diabetes mellitus. These people are 2 to 4 times more likely to develop active TB than those without diabetes, and the risk is probably greater in those with insulin-dependent or poorly controlled diabetes.
- Having a history of gastrectomy (which is often accompanied by weight loss and malabsorption), jejunoileal bypass, renal or cardiac transplantation, carcinoma of the head or neck, lung cancer, lymphoma, or leukemia.
- Receiving high-dose corticosteroid therapy (eg, prednisone >15 mg/d or equivalent amounts of other drugs for several weeks). These people may be at risk for reactivation of TB, but the exact risk is unknown. Lower doses and intermittent administration of corticosteroids are not associated with TB.

Where Should Testing Be Done?
Traditionally, local health departments have been responsible for testing, interpreting, and providing follow-up care; some institutions have tested residents and employees, and some large businesses have tested employees. More recently, the Centers for Disease Control and Prevention (CDC) and other authorities have recommended that more testing be done in primary care settings and any other locations where high-risk individuals are. Such testing sites include neighborhood health centers, jails, homeless shelters, inner-city sites, methadone clinics, syringe and needle-exchange programs, and other community-based social service organizations. In the latter situations, local health departments are urged to assist local providers in developing, implementing, and evaluating TB screening programs appropriate for their communities.

Test Interpretation
Positive reactions differ according to the amount of induration (a nodule or area of hardened tissue, not to be confused with the area of redness, which may be larger than the area of induration) and characteristics of the group being tested, as follows:

- **Induration of 5 mm or more**. Persons at highest risk (eg, close contacts of someone with active, infectious TB; those with HIV infection or risk factors for HIV infection; and those with chest radiographs that are consistent with previous TB)
- **Induration of 10 mm or more**. Persons at high risk (eg, those with conditions or characteristics such as diabetes mellitus; silicosis; immunosuppressive drug therapy; leukemia; lymphoma; head or neck cancer; chronic renal failure; gastrectomy; jejunoileal bypass; low body weight; injecting drug users known to be seronegative for HIV infection; recent immigrants from countries that have high TB rates; residents and employees of prisons, long-term care institutions, and other congregate settings for high-risk populations; low-income groups; high-risk racial and ethnic groups; migrant farm workers; and infants, children, and adolescents exposed to adults in high-risk categories)
- **Induration of 15 mm or more**. Persons who are at low risk for developing TB and do not meet the criteria listed for the above groups. Routine testing is not recommended for low-risk groups.
- **False-positive reactions**. These may occur with infections caused by nontuberculous strains of mycobacteria or a previous intradermal injection of bacillus Calmette-Guérin (BCG), a live attenuated strain derived from *Mycobacterium bovis*. In many parts of the world, BCG is used as a vaccine against tuberculosis, especially in children. There is currently no reliable way to differentiate tuberculin reactions caused by vaccination with BCG from those caused by infection with *M. tuberculosis*. However, large areas of induration (>20 mm) are unlikely to result from BCG.
- **False-negative reactions**. These may occur with HIV infection or other conditions that suppress the immune system and inhibit the ability to react to the tuberculin antigen. Thus, a negative skin test may occur in the presence of tuberculosis infection.

Box 34–2 Treatment of Latent Tuberculosis Infection (LTBI)

Recommended Regimens for Adults

Isoniazid (INH) daily or twice weekly for 9 months is the preferred regimen, including persons with human immunodeficiency virus (HIV) infection or radiographic evidence of prior TB.

Isoniazid daily or twice weekly for 6 months. The main advantage of this regimen over the 9-month schedule is greater adherence because of the shorter length. It is also less costly. This regimen may be used for HIV-negative adults with normal chest radiographs; it is *not* recommended for HIV-positive persons, those <18 years of age, or those with fibrotic lesions as shown on chest radiographs.

Rifampin and pyrazinamide (RIF-PZA) daily or twice weekly for 2 months. This regimen may be used for contacts of clients with INH-resistant TB and for those who are unlikely to complete a longer course of treatment. Rifampin is contraindicated in HIV-positive clients who are receiving protease inhibitors or non-nucleoside reverse transcriptase inhibitors (NNRTIs), because rifampin greatly stimulates metabolism and decreases the effectiveness of the antiviral drugs. Rifabutin, which causes less enzyme induction than rifampin, may be substituted in some cases. Pyrazinamide is contraindicated during pregnancy.

This regimen was revised in 2001 because of several reports of liver failure and death. To reduce the risks of liver injury, the American Thoracic Society and the Centers for Disease Control and Prevention (CDC), with the endorsement of the Infectious Diseases Society of America, issued new recommendations for choosing clients and for more intensive clinical and laboratory monitoring, as follows:

1. The RIF-PZA regimen is not recommended for persons who have underlying liver disease or who have had INH-associated liver injury. It should be used with caution in clients who take other hepatotoxic medications or use alcohol, even if alcohol use is stopped during treatment. Persons being considered for treatment with this regimen should be informed about potential hepatotoxicity and asked whether they have had liver disease or adverse effects from INH.
2. The RIF-PZA regimen is recommended mainly for clients who are unlikely to complete longer courses of treatment and who can be monitored closely. (For other adults not infected with HIV, the 9-month daily regimen of INH is preferred, with 4 months of daily RIF as an acceptable alternative.)
3. The RIF-PZA regimen does increase risks of hepatotoxicity in clients with HIV infection. Still, INH daily for 9 months is the treatment of choice for HIV-infected persons with LTBI when completion of treatment can be assured.
4. Increase safety by limiting the pyrazinamide dose to <20 mg/kg/d and a maximum of 2 g/d; giving no more than a 2-week supply of rifampin and pyrazinamide at a time; and assessing clients at 2, 4, and 6 weeks of treatment for adherence, tolerance, and adverse effects, and at 8 weeks to document treatment completion. For non–

English-speaking clients, health care providers who speak the clients' language should instruct them to stop taking the drugs immediately and seek medical care if abdominal pain, emesis, jaundice, or other symptoms of hepatitis develop. Provider continuity is recommended for monitoring.
5. Perform liver function tests (eg, serum aspartate and alanine aminotransferases [AST and ALT] and bilirubin) at baseline and at 2, 4, and 6 weeks. RIF-PZA treatment should be stopped and not resumed if enzyme levels are higher than five times the upper limit of normal in an asymptomatic person, are higher than normal range if symptoms of hepatitis are present, or if a serum bilirubin level is above normal range.

Rifampin daily for 4 months. This regimen is used mainly for clients who cannot tolerate INH or pyrazinamide.

Special Populations

1. Pregnant women. The preferred regimen for treatment of LTBI is INH, administered daily or twice weekly for 9 or 6 months. Pregnant women taking INH should also take pyridoxine supplementation. For HIV-positive women with higher risks of progression to active TB, treatment should not be delayed; for those with lower risks, some experts recommend waiting until after delivery to start treatment. In general, INH, rifampin, and ethambutol have good safety records in pregnancy. Pyrazinamide and streptomycin are contraindicated during pregnancy.
2. Children and adolescents. INH daily or twice weekly for 9 months is recommended. Infants and children under 5 years of age with LTBI are at high risk for progression to disease. They are also more likely than older children and adults to develop life-threatening forms of TB, including meningeal and disseminated disease. INH therapy appears to be more effective for children than adults, and the risk for INH-related hepatitis is minimal in infants, children, and adolescents, who generally tolerate the drug better than adults. Routine administration of pyridoxine is not recommended for children taking INH, but should be given to breast-feeding infants, children and adolescents with pyridoxine-deficient diets, and children who experience paresthesias when taking INH.

Although few studies have been done in infants, children, and adolescents, rifampin alone, rifampin with INH, and rifampin with pyrazinamide have been used to treat LTBI with effectiveness. Although the optimal length of rifampin therapy in children with LTBI is unknown, the American Academy of Pediatrics (AAP) recommends 6 months.

There have been no reported studies of any regimen for treatment for LTBI in HIV-infected children. The AAP recommends INH for 9 months; most experts recommend routine monitoring of serum liver enzyme concentrations and pyridoxine administration.

3. Contacts of clients with drug-susceptible TB and positive skin-test reactions (>5 mm) should be treated with one of the recommended regimens described above, regardless of age.
4. Contacts of clients with INH-resistant, rifampin-susceptible TB should generally be given rifampin and pyrazinamide

Box 34-2 Treatment of Latent Tuberculosis Infection (LTBI) (continued)

for 2 months. For clients with intolerance to pyrazinamide, rifampin alone for 4 months is recommended. If rifampin cannot be used, rifabutin can be substituted.

5. Contacts of clients with multidrug-resistant (MDR)-TB who are at high risk for developing active TB are generally given pyrazinamide and ethambutol or pyrazinamide and a fluoroquinolone (levofloxacin or ofloxacin) for 6 to 12 months. Immunocompetent contacts may be observed without treatment or treated for 6 months; immuno-compromised contacts (eg, HIV-infected persons) should be treated for 12 months.

   For children exposed to MDR-TB, pyrazinamide and ethambutol are recommended for 9 to 12 months if the isolate is susceptible to both drugs. If these drugs cannot be used, two other drugs to which the infecting organism is likely susceptible should be given. Fluoroquinolones are contraindicated in children.

6. HIV-infected persons. With INH, the 9-month regimen is recommended. With rifampin, the drug is contraindicated or should be used with caution in persons who are taking protease inhibitors or NNRTIs. Rifabutin can be substituted for rifampin in some circumstances, but it should not be used with hard-gel saquinavir or delavirdine and must be used cautiously with soft-gel saquinavir and nevirapine because data are limited. Dosage of rifabutin needs to be reduced to one half the usual daily dose (ie, from 300 mg/d to 150 mg/d) with indinavir, nelfinavir, or amprenavir and to one fourth the usual dose (ie, 150 mg every other day or 3 times a week) with ritonavir. Usual dosage (300 mg/d) can be given with nevirapine and 450 or 600 mg/d are needed with efavirenz. Rifapentine is not recommended as a substitute for rifampin because its safety, effectiveness, and interactions with anti-HIV medication have not been established.

7. Bacillus Calmette-Guérin (BCG)-vaccinated persons. A history of BCG vaccination should not influence the decision to treat LTBI.

Additional Recommendations

1. Before beginning treatment for LTBI, active TB should be ruled out by history, physical examination, chest radiography, and bacteriologic studies, if indicated.

2. Allow clients to participate in choosing a treatment regimen, when feasible, by discussing options and characteristics of each (eg, the length and complexity, possible adverse effects, potential drug interactions).

3. Directly observed therapy (DOT) should be used consistently with intermittent regimens (eg, twice weekly) and when possible with 2-month regimens and in certain settings (eg, institutional settings, community outreach programs, and for persons living in households with clients who are receiving home-based DOT for active TB).

4. Try to ensure completion of treatment. This is determined by the total number of doses administered as well as the duration of therapy. For daily INH, the 9-month regimen should include at least 270 doses in 12 months and the 6-month regimen should include at least 180 doses in 9 months. For twice-weekly INH, the 9-month regimen should include at least 76 doses in 12 months and the 6-month regimen should include at least 52 doses in 9 months. For the 2-month regimen of daily rifampin (or rifabutin) and pyrazinamide, at least 60 doses should be given in 3 months. For the 4-month regimen of daily rifampin alone, at least 120 doses should be given in 6 months.

   These schedules allow minor interruptions in therapy although, ideally, clients should receive medication on a regular schedule until the course of therapy is completed. When doses are missed, the duration of therapy should be lengthened. When restarting therapy after interruptions, the original regimen may be continued as long as needed to complete the recommended duration of the particular regimen or a new regimen may be needed if interruptions were frequent or prolonged. If treatment is interrupted for longer than 2 months, the client should be reassessed for active TB before restarting drug therapy.

---

occur during the first 8 weeks of INH therapy and in people who use alcohol. Clients receiving INH should be monitored monthly for signs and symptoms of hepatitis. Because of the risk of hepatotoxicity, INH should be used cautiously in clients with pre-existing liver disease. Peripheral neuropathy may be manifested by numbness and tingling in the hands and feet. It is most likely to occur in clients who are malnourished or older, or who have alcoholism, diabetes mellitus, or uremia. Pyridoxine 25 to 50 milligrams daily is usually given with INH to minimize peripheral neuropathy.

APPLYING YOUR KNOWLEDGE 34-2

You will have multiple opportunities to assess Mr. Guth when he receives his medication. For what adverse effects of INH do you plan to monitor Mr. Guth?

Rifampin (Rifadin) is a rifamycin drug that is bactericidal for both intracellular and extracellular tuberculosis organisms. It kills mycobacteria by inhibiting synthesis of RNA and thereby causing defective, nonfunctional proteins to be produced. Its ability to penetrate intact cells contributes to its effectiveness in TB because mycobacteria are harbored in host cells. Rifampin and INH are synergistic in combination, eliminating tuberculosis bacilli from sputum and producing clinical improvement faster than any other drug regimen, unless organisms resistant to one or both drugs are causing the disease.

Rifampin is well absorbed with oral administration and diffuses well into body tissues and fluids, with highest concentrations occurring in the liver, lungs, gallbladder, and kidneys. Peak serum concentration occurs in 1 to 3 hours with oral administration and immediately with IV administration.

Table 34-1 Drugs at a Glance: Primary Antitubercular Drugs

NAME/ROUTE	DOSAGE RANGES (Maximum dose)				COMMENTS
	Adults		Children		
	DAILY	TWICE/WK	DAILY	TWICE/WK	
Isoniazid (INH) PO or IM	5 mg/kg (300 mg)	15 mg/kg (900)	10–20 mg/kg (300)	20–40 mg/kg (900)	*LTBI:* Given at least 6 mo; 9 mo preferred *Active TB:* Given at least 6 mo, with other drugs
Rifampin (Rifadin) PO or IV infusion	10 mg/kg (600 mg)	10 mg/kg (600 mg)	10–20 mg/kg (600 mg)	10–20 mg/kg (600 mg)	*LTBI:* Given 4 mo alone or 2 mo with pyrazinamide *Active TB:* Given for 6 mo, with other drugs
Pyrazinamide PO	15–30 mg/kg (2 g)	50–70 mg/kg (4 g)	15–30 mg/kg (2 g)	50–70 mg/kg (4 g)	*LTBI:* Given for 2 mo, with rifampin *Active TB:* Given for 2 mo, with INH and rifampin
Streptomycin IM	15 mg/kg (1 g)	25–30 mg/kg (1.5 g)	20–40 mg/kg (1 g)	25–30 mg/kg (1.5 g)	Used for active TB, with other drugs
Ethambutol (Myambutol) PO	15–25 mg/kg (2.5 g)	50 mg/kg (2.5 g)	15–25 mg/kg (2.5 g)	50 mg/kg (2.5 g)	Used for active TB, with other drugs, and MAC disease
Rifabutin (Mycobutin) PO	300 mg		Not established		Used to treat MAC disease and to substitute for rifampin in clients taking certain anti-HIV medications
Rifapentine (Priftin) PO		150 mg twice a wk for 2 mo, then once a wk for 4 mo	Not established		May be used instead of rifampin, with other drugs

HIV, human immunodeficiency virus; IM, intramuscular; IV, intravenous; LTBI, latent tuberculosis infection; MAC, *Mycobacterium avium* complex; PO, oral; TB, tuberculosis.

The drug is metabolized in the liver and excreted primarily in bile; a small amount is excreted in urine. Its elimination half-life is approximately 3 hours with a 300-milligram dose, and approximately 5 hours with a 600-milligram dose. Because it is a strong inducer of drug-metabolizing enzymes, its half-life becomes shorter with continued use.

Adverse effects include GI upset, skin rashes, hepatitis, and a harmless red-orange discoloration of urine, tears, sweat, and other body fluids. Soft contact lenses may be permanently stained.

Rifampin has many interactions with other drugs. It induces hepatic cytochrome P450 3A4 enzymes and accelerates the metabolism of numerous other drugs, thereby decreasing their serum concentrations, half-lives, and therapeutic effects. Affected drugs include anti–acquired immunodeficiency syndrome (AIDS) drugs (protease inhibitors [PIs] and non-nucleoside reverse transcriptase inhibitors [NNRTIs]; see Chap. 35), benzodiazepines, corticosteroids, cyclosporine, estrogens, fluconazole, methadone, metoprolol, phenytoin, propranolol, oral contraceptives, oral sulfonylureas, theophylline, verapamil, and warfarin. With warfarin, decreased anticoagulant effect occurs approximately 5 to 8 days after rifampin is started, and lasts for 5 to 7 days after rifampin is stopped. With methadone, concurrent administration with rifampin may precipitate signs and symptoms of opiate withdrawal unless methadone dosage is increased.

APPLYING YOUR KNOWLEDGE 34-3

You are teaching Mr. Guth about his medication. What adverse effect of rifampin should you include in your teaching so that Mr. Guth does not become alarmed and stop taking his medication?

Rifabutin (Mycobutin) is another rifamycin that is active against mycobacteria. However, most rifampin-resistant strains are also resistant to rifabutin. The drug's two main uses are in clients with HIV infection, to treat *Mycobacterium avium* complex (MAC) disease; and to substitute for rifampin in clients who need both antitubercular and certain antiviral drugs. The major advantages of rifabutin over rifampin are a longer serum half-life (45 hours, on average) and reduced induction of hepatic drug-metabolizing enzymes. Rifabutin has no advantage over rifampin in treatment of TB, but may be given concurrently with INH to clients who need prophylaxis against both *M. tuberculosis* and *M. avium.*

Rifabutin is well absorbed from the GI tract; a dose of 300 milligrams produces peak serum concentration in 23 hours. It is extensively metabolized in the liver (and to a lesser extent in the intestinal wall); it is excreted in urine and bile.

Like rifampin, rifabutin and its metabolites may cause a harmless red-orange discoloration of body fluids and permanent staining of soft contact lenses. Adverse effects include GI upset (nausea, vomiting, diarrhea), hepatitis, muscular aches, neutropenia, skin rash, and uveitis (an eye disorder characterized by inflammation, pain, and impaired vision). Hepatotoxicity is rare. Adverse effects increase when rifabutin is administered with a drug that inhibits cytochrome P450 3A4 enzymes (eg, clarithromycin) and inhibits rifabutin metabolism. Safety and effectiveness in children have not been established

Also similarly to rifampin, but to a lesser extent, rifabutin induces drug-metabolizing enzymes in the liver and accelerates the metabolism of numerous drugs. This action decreases concentration and clinical efficacy of beta blockers, corticosteroids, cyclosporine, digoxin, hormonal contraceptives, itraconazole, methadone, NNRTIs, oral hypoglycemic agents, phenytoin, PIs, theophylline, warfarin, and zidovudine. If these drugs are administered with rifabutin, their dosage may need to be increased.

Rifapentine (Priftin) is similar to rifampin in effectiveness, adverse effects, and enzyme induction activity. It is indicated for use in the treatment of pulmonary TB and must be used with at least one other drug to which the causative organisms are susceptible. The main advantage over rifampin is less frequent administration (once or twice weekly). Its action has a slow onset and peaks in 5 to 6 hours. It is metabolized in the liver and excreted in urine and feces. It has a half-life of 14 hours.

Ethambutol (Myambutol) is a tuberculostatic drug that inhibits synthesis of RNA and thus interferes with mycobacterial protein metabolism. It may be a component in a four-drug regimen for initial treatment of active TB that may be caused by drug-resistant organisms. When culture and susceptibility reports become available (usually after several weeks), ethambutol may be stopped if the causative organisms are susceptible to INH and rifampin, or continued if the organisms are resistant to INH or rifampin and susceptible to ethambutol. Ethambutol is not recommended for young children (eg, <5 years of age) whose visual acuity cannot be monitored, but may be considered for children of any age when organisms are susceptible to ethambutol and resistant to other drugs. Mycobacterial resistance to ethambutol develops slowly.

Ethambutol is well absorbed from the GI tract, even when given with food. Dosage is determined by body weight and should be changed during treatment if significant changes in weight occur. To obtain therapeutic serum levels, the total daily dose is given at one time. Drug action has a rapid onset, peaks in 2 to 4 hours, and lasts 20 to 24 hours. The drug has a half-life of 3 to 4 hours; is metabolized in the liver; and is excreted primarily by the kidneys, either unchanged or as metabolites. Dosage must be reduced with impaired renal function.

A major adverse effect is optic neuritis, an inflammatory, demyelinating disorder of the optic nerve that decreases visual acuity and ability to differentiate red from green. Tests of visual acuity and red–green discrimination are recommended before starting ethambutol and periodically during therapy. If optic neuritis develops, the drug should be promptly stopped. Recovery usually occurs when ethambutol is discontinued.

Pyrazinamide is used with INH and rifampin for the first 2 months of treating active TB. It is bactericidal against actively growing mycobacteria in macrophages, but its exact mechanism of action is unknown. It is well absorbed from the GI tract and penetrates most body fluids and tissues, including macrophages containing TB organisms. Its action has a rapid onset and it peaks in 2 hours. It is metabolized in the liver and excreted mainly through the kidneys. Its half-life is 9 to 10 hours.

The most common adverse effect is GI upset; the most severe adverse effect is hepatotoxicity, and the drug should not be given to a client with pre-existing liver impairment unless it is considered essential. Clients without liver impairment should be assessed for symptoms of liver dysfunction every 2 weeks during the usual 8 weeks of therapy. If symptoms occur, liver enzymes (ALT and AST) should be measured. If significant liver damage is indicated, pyrazinamide should be stopped.

Pyrazinamide inhibits urate excretion. This characteristic causes hyperuricemia in most clients and may cause acute attacks of gout.

Streptomycin, an aminoglycoside antibiotic (see Chap. 31), acts only against extracellular organisms; it does not penetrate macrophages and tuberculous lesions. It may be used in a regimen of four drugs to treat active TB when the susceptibility of the causative organism is unknown, or in a regimen of four to six drugs in the treatment of TB suspected or known to be resistant to INH, rifampin, or both. It may be discontinued when cultures become negative or after a few months of therapy.

Combination Primary Drugs

Rifamate and Rifater are combination products developed to increase convenience to clients and promote adherence to the prescribed drug-therapy regimen (for drug-susceptible TB). Each Rifamate tablet contains INH 150 milligrams and rifampin 300 milligrams, and 2 tablets daily provide the recommended doses for a 6-month, short-course treatment regimen. Rifater contains INH 50 milligrams, rifampin 120 milligrams, and pyrazinamide 300 milligrams and is approved for the first 2 months of a 6-month, short-course treatment regimen. Dosage depends on weight, with 4 tablets daily for clients weighing 44 kilograms or less; 5 tablets daily for those weighing 45 to 54 kilograms; and 6 tablets daily for those weighing 55 kilograms or more.

Secondary Drugs

Para-aminosalicylic acid (PAS), capreomycin (Capastat), cycloserine (Seromycin), and ethionamide (Trecator SC) are diverse drugs that share tuberculostatic properties. They are indicated for use only when other agents are contraindicated or in disease caused by organisms resistant to primary drugs. They must be given concurrently with other drugs to inhibit emergence of resistant mycobacteria.

Other Drugs Used in Multidrug-Resistant Tuberculosis

Amikacin and kanamycin are aminoglycoside antibiotics with activity against mycobacteria. Although they are not usually considered antitubercular drugs, one may be a component of a four- to six-drug regimen to treat suspected or known MDR-TB. Similarly, the fluoroquinolones (eg, ciprofloxacin, levofloxacin, ofloxacin) have antimycobacterial activity and may be used to treat MDR-TB.

TREATMENT OF ACTIVE TUBERCULOSIS

Adequate drug therapy of clients with active disease usually produces improvement within 2 to 3 weeks, with decreased fever and cough; weight gain; improved well-being; and improved chest radiographs. Treatment should generally be continued for at least 6 months, or 3 months after cultures become negative. Most clients have negative sputum cultures within 3 to 6 months. If the client is symptomatic or if the culture is positive after 3 months, noncompliance or drug resistance must be considered. Cultures that are positive after 6 months often include drug-resistant organisms, and an alternative drug-therapy regimen is needed. With the increasing prevalence of MDR-TB, guidelines for treatment have changed and continue to evolve in the attempt to promote client adherence to treatment and to manage MDR-TB: two of the major problems in drug therapy of tuberculosis.

- The most commonly used regimen consists of INH, rifampin, and pyrazinamide daily for 2 months, followed by INH and rifampin (daily, 2 times weekly, or 3 times weekly) for 4 additional months. If 4% or more of the tuberculosis isolates in the community are INH-resistant organisms, ethambutol or streptomycin should also be given until susceptibility reports become available. If the causative strain of *M. tuberculosis* is susceptible to INH, rifampin, and pyrazinamide, the regimen is continued as with the 3-drug regimen described and the fourth drug (ethambutol or streptomycin) is discontinued. If rifampin is not used, an 18-month course of therapy is considered the minimum. In the absence of drug resistance, INH and rifampin in a 9-month regimen are effective; adding pyrazinamide for the initial 2 months of therapy allows the regimen to be shortened to 6 months.

- For INH-resistant TB, the recommended regimen is rifampin, pyrazinamide, and ethambutol for 6 months. For rifampin-resistant TB, recommended regimens are INH and ethambutol for 18 months or INH, pyrazinamide, and streptomycin for 9 months. For MDR-TB, a five- or six-drug regimen, individualized according to susceptibility reports and containing at least three drugs to which the organism is susceptible, should be instituted. Such regimens include primary and secondary antitubercular drugs as well as other drugs with activity against *M. tuberculosis,* such as an aminoglycoside or a fluoroquinolone. Some clinicians include at least one injectable agent. The drugs should be given for 1 to 2 years after cultures become negative. Intermittent administration is not recommended for MDR-TB.

- In the intermittent schedules, health care providers (or other responsible adults) either administer the drugs or observe the client taking them (directly observed therapy [DOT]). This method was initially developed for clients unable or unwilling to self-administer the drugs independently, in an effort to increase adherence to and completion of prescribed courses of treatment. Now, DOT is recommended for all treatment regimens and is considered mandatory for intermittent regimens (eg, two or three times weekly) and regimens for MDR-TB.

- During pregnancy, a 3-drug regimen of INH, rifampin, and ethambutol is usually used, with close monitoring of liver function tests. Pyrazinamide and streptomycin should not be used during pregnancy.

MYCOBACTERIUM AVIUM COMPLEX DISEASE

Mycobacterium avium and *Mycobacterium intracellulare* are different types of mycobacteria that resemble each other so closely that they are usually grouped together as *Mycobacterium avium* complex (MAC). These atypical mycobacteria are found in water and soil throughout the United States. The organisms are thought to be transmitted by inhalation of droplets of contaminated water; there is no evidence of spread to humans from animals or other humans.

MAC rarely causes significant disease in immunocompetent people, but causes an opportunistic pulmonary infection in approximately 50% of clients with advanced HIV infection. Symptoms include a productive cough, weight loss, hemoptysis, and fever. As the disease becomes disseminated through the body, chronic lung disease develops and the organism is found in the blood, bone marrow, liver, lymph nodes, and other body tissues.

The main drugs used in prevention of MAC disease are the macrolide drugs azithromycin and clarithromycin (see Chap. 33) and rifabutin (described earlier in this chapter). Prophylactic drug therapy is recommended to be lifelong. For treatment, a three-drug regimen of azithromycin 250 milligrams daily or clarithromycin 1000 milligrams daily, rifabutin (300 mg daily), and ethambutol (25 mg/kg/d for 2 months, then 15 mg/kg/d) is often used. The drugs may also be given two or three times weekly. Drug dosages are the same for intermittent regimens except that the larger dose of ethambutol is continued throughout. Streptomycin 500 to 1000 milligrams twice weekly is usually added for the initial 3 months of treatment when extensive MAC disease is present.

NURSING PROCESS

Assessment

Assess for latent or active tuberculosis infection.

- For latent infection, identify high-risk clients (ie, people who are close contacts of someone with active TB; are elderly or undernourished; have diabetes mellitus, silicosis, Hodgkin's disease, leukemia, or AIDS; are alcoholics; are receiving immunosuppressive drugs; or are immigrants from Southeast Asia and other parts of the world where the disease is endemic).
- For active disease, clinical manifestations include fatigue, weight loss, anorexia, malaise, fever, and a productive cough. In early phases, however, there may be no symptoms. If available, check diagnostic test reports for indications of TB (chest radiograph, tuberculin skin test, sputum smear and culture).
- In children, initial signs and symptoms may occur within a few weeks after exposure, before skin tests become positive, and resemble those of bacterial pneumonia. In addition, indications of disease in lymph nodes, GI and urinary tracts, bone marrow, and meninges may be present.
- In older adults, signs and symptoms of TB are often less prominent than in younger adults, or are similar to those in other respiratory disorders. Thus, an older adult is less likely to have fever, a positive skin test, significant sputum production, hemoptysis, or night sweats. However, mental status changes and mortality rates are higher in older than in younger adults.

- In clients with HIV infection, skin tests showing 5 mm of induration are considered positive. In addition, disease manifestations in clients with AIDS differ from those in people with undamaged immune systems. For example, malaise, weight loss, weakness, and fever are prominent. Other symptoms often resemble those of bacterial pneumonia, involve multiple lobes of the lungs, and involve extrapulmonary sites of infection.
- Assess candidates for antitubercular drug therapy for previous exposure and reaction to the primary drugs and for the current use of drugs that interact with the primary drugs.
- Assess for signs and symptoms of MAC disease, especially in clients with advanced HIV infection who have a CD4+ cell count of 100/mm^3 or less.

Nursing Diagnoses

- Anxiety or Fear related to chronic illness and long-term drug therapy
- Deficient Knowledge: Disease process and need for treatment
- Noncompliance related to adverse drug effects and need for long-term treatment
- Deficient Knowledge: Consequences of noncompliance with the drug therapy regimen
- Risk for Injury: Adverse drug effects

Planning/Goals

The client will
- Take drugs as prescribed
- Keep appointments for follow-up care
- Report adverse drug effects
- Act to prevent spread of TB

Interventions

Assist clients to understand the disease process and the necessity for long-term treatment and follow-up (see accompanying client teaching display). This is extremely important for the client and the community, because lack of knowledge and failure to comply with the therapeutic regimen lead to disease progression and spread. The American Lung Association publishes many helpful pamphlets, written for the general public, that can be obtained from a local chapter and given to clients and their families. Do not use these as a substitute for personal contact, however.

Use measures to prevent the spread of tuberculosis:

- Isolate suspected or newly diagnosed hospitalized clients in a private room for 2 or 3 weeks, until drug therapy has rendered them noninfectious.
- Wear a mask with close contact, and perform thorough hand hygiene afterward.

CLIENT TEACHING GUIDELINES

Isoniazid, Rifampin, and Pyrazinamide

✔ Isoniazid (INH) is one of the most commonly used medications for tuberculosis infection. It is given to people with positive skin tests to prevent development of active disease. Vitamin B$_6$ (pyridoxine) is usually given along with the INH to prevent leg numbness and tingling. Take INH and pyridoxine in a single dose once daily. Take on an empty stomach if possible; if stomach upset occurs, the drugs may be taken with food.

✔ For treatment of active disease, INH, rifampin, and pyrazinamide are usually given daily or twice weekly for 2 months; then the pyrazinamide is stopped and the others are continued for an additional 4 months.

✔ For treatment of inactive or latent tuberculosis infection, various regimens of INH alone, rifampin and pyrazinamide, or rifampin alone may be used. Any one of these regimens can be effective in preventing active disease if the drugs are take correctly and for the time prescribed.

✔ INH, rifampin, and pyrazinamide can all cause liver damage. As a result, you should avoid alcoholic beverages and watch for signs and symptoms of hepatitis (eg, nausea, yellowing of skin or eyes, dark urine, light-colored stools). If such symptoms occur, you should stop taking the drugs and report the symptoms to the nurse or physician managing the tuberculosis infection immediately. Blood tests of liver function will also be ordered. In some cases, liver failure has occurred, most often when clients continued to take the medications for a week or longer after symptoms of liver damage occurred.

✔ Rifampin should be taken in a single dose, once daily or twice weekly, on an empty stomach, 1 hour before or 2 hours after a meal.

✔ Rifampin causes a reddish discoloration of urine, tears, saliva, and other body secretions. This is harmless, except that soft contact lenses may be permanently stained.

✔ Use all available resources to learn about tuberculosis and the medications used to prevent or treat the infection. This is extremely important because the information can help you understand the reasons long-term treatment and follow-up care are needed. In addition to personal benefit, taking medications as prescribed can help your family and community by helping to prevent spread of tuberculosis. The American Lung Association publishes many helpful pamphlets that are available from local health departments and health care providers. Additional information is available on the Internet (eg, the Centers for Disease Control and Prevention at http://www.cdc.gov).

✔ Learn how to prevent spread of tuberculosis:

  ✔ Cover mouth and nose when coughing or sneezing. This prevents expelling tuberculosis germs into the surrounding air, where they can be inhaled by and infect others.

  ✔ Cough and expectorate sputum into at least two layers of tissue. Place the used tissues in a waterproof bag, and dispose of the bag, preferably by burning.

  ✔ Wash hands after coughing or sneezing.

✔ A nourishing diet and adequate rest help healing of infection.

✔ Periodic visits to a health care provider are needed for follow-up care and to monitor medications.

✔ The importance of taking medications as prescribed cannot be overemphasized. If not taken in the doses and for the length of time needed, there is a high likelihood for development of tuberculosis infection that is resistant to the most effective antituberculosis drugs. If this happens, treatment is much longer, very expensive, and requires strong drugs that cause more adverse effects. In addition, this very serious infection can be spread to family members and other close contacts. Thus, avoiding drug-resistant tuberculosis should be a strong incentive to complete the full course of treatment.

✔ Rifampin decreases the effectiveness of oral contraceptive tablets; a different type of contraception should be used during rifampin therapy.

- Have clients wear a mask when out of the room for diagnostic tests.
- Assist clients to take antitubercular drugs as prescribed, for the length of time prescribed.

Evaluation

- Observe for improvement in signs and symptoms of TB and MAC disease.
- Interview and observe for adverse drug effects; check laboratory reports of hepatic and renal function, when available.
- Question regarding compliance with instructions for taking antitubercular and anti-MAC drugs.

PRINCIPLES OF THERAPY

Goals of Therapy

In general, the goals for treatment of TB are to cure clients with latent or active infection and to minimize transmission of the causative organism to other people. More specifically, the goal with latent TB infection is to prevent the development of active infection. The main goals with active infection are to decrease signs and symptoms; make the client noninfectious; ensure adherence to the drug therapy regimen; and cure the client (at least 6 months of treatment are usually required). Secondary goals are to identify the person from whom the client caught the infection (called the *index case*); identify other people infected by the index case or the new case of TB; and ensure that those persons are treated appropriately.

Drug-Susceptible Tuberculosis

Sputum culture and susceptibility reports require 6 to 8 weeks because the tubercle bacillus multiplies slowly. Consequently, initial drug therapy is based on other factors, such as the extent of disease; whether the client has previously received antitubercular drugs; and whether multidrug-resistant strains are being found in the particular community.

Some general guidelines for pharmacologic treatment of TB include:

- Multiple drugs are required to effectively treat the infection and inhibit emergence of drug-resistant organisms.
- Duration of drug therapy varies with the purpose, extent of disease, adherence to the drug therapy regimen, and clinical response. The trend in recent years, for treatment of both latent and active disease, is to give short courses of treatment (eg, 6 months) when possible. Such regimens are more likely to be completed, and completion decreases the prevalence of drug-resistant disease in a community. In addition to the number of months of treatment, however, the total number of medication doses is also important. For example, the usual 6-month regimen for drug-susceptible TB consists of 182 doses of INH and rifampin and 56 doses of pyrazinamide. If treatment is interrupted for any reason, it is recommended that the drugs be continued so that the total number of doses is administered within a maximum time period of 9 months.
- Fixed-dose combination tablets (eg, Rifamate, Rifater) are recommended by some authorities, because they help to prevent the emergence of drug-resistant organisms. These formulations are more expensive than separate drugs.

Multidrug-Resistant Tuberculosis

- Multidrug-resistant strains may occur anywhere. However, in the United States, they have been most evident in populations with AIDS, in closed environments (eg, hospitals, prisons, long-term care facilities, homeless shelters), and in large urban areas.
- Drug therapy regimens for people exposed to someone with MDR-TB or suspected of having MDR-TB should be designed in consultation with infectious-disease or tuberculosis specialists.
- Treatment of MDR-TB requires concurrent administration of more drugs (eg, 4 to 6), for a longer period of time (eg, 2 years or longer), than for drug-susceptible TB. The specific regimen is derived from cultures of infecting strains and susceptibility tests with primary, secondary, and other drugs with antimycobacterial

activity. It should include 2 or 3 drugs to which the isolate is sensitive and that the client has not taken before. The fluoroquinolones are not recommended for use in children.
- All drug therapy for suspected or known MDR-TB should involve daily administration and DOT.
- Treatment is extremely expensive, even in the non-HIV population, and costs many thousand dollars more than the treatment of drug-susceptible TB.

Increasing Adherence to Antitubercular Drug Therapy

Failure to complete treatment regimens is a major problem in TB management because it increases the spread of the disease and the amount of drug-resistant disease in a community. There is more difficulty with getting clients to complete treatment for latent infection than for active disease. Identifying and treating LTBI requires several steps, including administering and reading skin tests; obtaining medical evaluations of infected persons; and initiating, monitoring, and completing treatment. Nonadherence is common in all of these aspects. Numerous strategies have been proposed to increase adherence, including:

- **Educating clients, family members, and contacts of clients.** This may be especially important with treatment of LTBI. Most people are more motivated to take medications and schedule follow-up care when they have symptoms, than when they feel well and have no symptoms. The importance of treatment for the future health of the individual, significant others, and the community must be emphasized. In addition, clients should be informed about common and potential adverse effects of drug therapy and what to do if they occur.
- **Providing support services and resources.** These require substantial financial resources and may include more workers to provide DOT therapy at the client's location; flexible clinic hours; reducing waiting times for clients; and assisting clients with child care, transportation, or other social service needs that encourage them to initiate and continue treatment. Lack of these services (eg, clinics far from clients' homes, with inconvenient hours, long waiting times, unsupportive staff) may deter clients from being evaluated for a positive skin test, initiating treatment, or completing the prescribed treatment and follow-up care.
- **Individualizing treatment regimens,** when possible, to increase client convenience and minimize disruption of usual activities of daily living. Short-course regimens, intermittent dosing (eg, 2 or 3 times weekly rather than daily), and fixed-dose combinations of drugs (eg, Rifater, Rifamate) reduce the number of pills and the duration of therapy.

● **Promoting communication and continuity of care.** With clients for whom English is not their primary language, it is desirable to have a health care worker who speaks their language or who belongs to their ethnic group. This worker may be able to more effectively teach clients and others, elicit cooperation with treatment, administer DOT, and be a consistent support person.

Monitoring Antitubercular Drug Therapy

There are two main methods of monitoring client responses to treatment: clinical and laboratory. The current trend is toward increasing clinical monitoring and decreasing laboratory monitoring.

1. *Clinical monitoring* is indicated for all clients. It includes teaching clients about signs and symptoms of adverse drug effects and which effects require stopping drug therapy and obtaining medical care (eg, hepatotoxicity). It also includes regular assessment by a health care provider. Clinical monitoring should be repeated at each monthly visit. Clients should be assessed for signs of liver disease (eg, loss of appetite, nausea, vomiting, dark urine, jaundice, fatigue, abdominal tenderness, easy bruising or bleeding) at least monthly if receiving INH alone or rifampin alone and at 2, 4, and 8 weeks if receiving rifampin and pyrazinamide. In addition to detecting adverse effects, these ongoing contacts are opportunities to reinforce teaching, assess adherence with therapy since the last visit, and observe for drug interactions. A standardized interview form may be helpful in eliciting appropriate information.

2. *Laboratory monitoring* mainly involves liver function tests (ALT, AST, bilirubin). Baseline measurements are indicated for clients with possible liver disorders; those infected with HIV; women who are pregnant or early postpartum (within 3 months of delivery); those with a history of liver disease (eg, hepatitis B or C, alcoholic hepatitis or cirrhosis); those who use alcohol regularly; and those with risk factors for liver disease. Monitoring during therapy is indicated for clients who have abnormal baseline values or other risk factors for liver disease and those who develop symptoms of liver damage. Some clinicians recommend that INH be stopped for transaminase levels over three times the upper limit of normal if associated with symptoms and five times the upper limit of normal if the client is asymptomatic.

Effects of Antitubercular Drugs on Other Drugs

Isoniazid (INH) increases risks of toxicity with several drugs by inhibiting their metabolism and increasing their blood levels. These include carbamazepine, haloperidol, fluconazole, phenytoin (effects of rifampin are opposite to those of INH and tend to predominate if both drugs are given with phenytoin), and vincristine. INH increases the risk of hepatotoxicity with most of these drugs; concurrent use should be avoided when possible or blood levels of the inhibited drug should be monitored. With vincristine, INH may increase peripheral neuropathy.

The rifamycins (rifampin, rifabutin, rifapentine) induce cytochrome P450 drug-metabolizing enzymes and therefore accelerate the metabolism and decrease the effectiveness of many drugs. Rifampin is the strongest inducer and may decrease the effects of angiotensin-converting enzyme (ACE) inhibitors, anticoagulants, antidysrhythmics, some antifungals (eg, fluconazole), anti-HIV protease inhibitors (eg, amprenavir, indinavir), anti-HIV NNRTIs (eg, efavirenz, nevirapine), benzodiazepines, beta blockers, corticosteroids, cyclosporine, digoxin, diltiazem, estrogens and oral contraceptives, fexofenadine, fluoroquinolones, fluvastatin, haloperidol, lamotrigine, losartan, macrolide antibiotics, narcotic analgesics (eg, methadone, morphine), nifedipine, ondansetron, phenytoin, propafenone, sertraline, sirolimus, sulfonylureas (eg, glyburide), tacrolimus, tamoxifen, theophylline, thyroid hormones, toremifene, tricyclic antidepressants, verapamil, zaleplon, zidovudine, and zolpidem.

Rifabutin is reportedly a weaker enzyme inducer and may be substituted for rifampin in some cases. It is probably substituted most often for clients who require anti-HIV medications.

Pyrazinamide may decrease effects of allopurinol and cyclosporine.

Use in Special Populations

Use in Clients With Human Immunodeficiency Virus (HIV) Infection

Tuberculosis is a common opportunistic infection in people with advanced HIV infection and may develop from an initial infection or reactivation of an old infection. For treatment of latent infection (LTBI) in clients with positive skin tests, INH daily or twice weekly for 9 months is effective.

Treatment of active disease is similar to that in persons who do not have HIV infection. Those with HIV infection who adhere to standard treatment regimens do not have an increased risk of treatment failure. Thus, these clients are usually treated with antitubercular drugs for 6 months like HIV-seronegative clients. The regimen may be longer if the bacteriologic (eg, negative cultures) or clinical response (eg, improvement in symptoms) is slow or inadequate.

A major difficulty with treatment of TB in clients with HIV infection is that rifampin interacts with many PIs and NNRTIs. If the drugs are given concurrently, rifampin decreases blood levels and therapeutic effects of the anti-HIV drugs. Rifabutin has fewer interactions and may be substituted for rifampin. The PIs indinavir and nelfinavir and most of the NNRTIs can be used with rifabutin. Ritonavir (PI) and delavirdine (NNRTI) should not be used with rifabutin. Also, amprenavir and indinavir increase risks of rifabutin toxicity. Dosage of rifabutin should be decreased if given with one of these drugs.

Use in Children

Tuberculosis occurs in children of all ages. Infants and pre-school children need early recognition and treatment because the disease can rapidly progress from primary infection to active pulmonary disease and perhaps to extrapulmonary involvement. TB is usually discovered during examination of a sick child or investigation of the contacts of someone with newly diagnosed active TB. Most children are infected in their home. Children in close contact with a client with TB should receive skin testing, a physical examination, and a chest x-ray examination.

For treatment of latent infection, only one of the four reg-imens currently recommended for adults (INH for 9 months) is recommended for those under 18 years of age. For treat-ment of active disease, the prescribed regimens are similar to those used for adults. That is, the same primary drugs are used and may be given daily, twice weekly, or three times weekly with child-appropriate reductions in dosage. If the drug-susceptibility patterns of the *M. tuberculosis* strain causing the index case are known, the child is treated with those drugs; if this information is not available, the pattern of drug resistance in the community where the child likely became infected should be the guide for selecting the drug therapy regimen. As in adults, drug-susceptible TB is treated with INH, rifampin, and pyrazinamide for 2 months. Then, pyrazinamide is stopped and the INH and rifampin are con-tinued for 4 more months. If drug-resistant organisms have been identified in the community, a fourth drug, ethambutol or streptomycin, should be given until the client's culture and susceptibility reports become available. If pyrazinamide is not given, INH and rifampin are recommended for 9 months. When INH or rifampin cannot be used, therapy should con-tinue for 12 to 24 months.

Drug-resistant TB in children is usually acquired from an adult family member or other close contact with active, drug-resistant disease. For children exposed to MDR-TB, there is no proven preventive therapy. Several regimens are used empirically, including ethambutol and pyrazinamide or ethionamide and cycloserine. When INH and rifampin cannot be given because of MDR-TB, drug therapy should continue for 24 months after sputum smears or cultures become nega-tive. Fluoroquinolones (eg, levofloxacin, others) are used for treatment of MDR-TB in adults, but are not recommended for use in children. Clients with MDR-TB may require months of treatment before sputum smears become negative, and they are infectious during this period. To guide dosage and mini-mize adverse drug effects, serum drug levels should be mea-sured periodically, especially in clients with GI, renal, or hepatic disease, or in those with advanced HIV infection.

In children with HIV infection, the American Academy of Pediatrics recommends three drugs for at least 12 months. If drug-resistant or extrapulmonary disease is suspected, four drugs are indicated.

Overall, as with adults, drug therapy regimens vary with particular circumstances and continue to evolve. Health care providers must follow current recommendations of pediatric infectious-disease specialists.

Use in Older Adults

Although INH is the drug of choice for treatment of latent infec-tion, its use is controversial in older adults. Because risks of drug-induced hepatotoxicity are higher in this population, some clinicians believe those clients with positive skin tests should have additional risk factors (eg, recent skin-test conversion, immunosuppression, previous gastrectomy) before receiving INH. When INH is given, people who drink alcoholic bever-ages daily are most likely to sustain serious liver impairment.

For treatment of active disease caused by drug-susceptible organisms, INH, rifampin, and pyrazinamide are given, as in younger adults. Because all three drugs may cause hepato-toxicity, liver function tests should be monitored and the drugs discontinued if signs and symptoms of hepatotoxicity occur. For treatment of suspected or known MDR-TB, four to six drugs are used.

Use in Clients With Renal Impairment

Rifampin is mainly eliminated by the liver. However, up to 30% of a dose is excreted by the kidneys and dose reduction may be needed in clients with renal impairment. In addition, dosage of amikacin, capreomycin, cycloserine, ethambutol, fluoroquinolones, and streptomycin should be reduced in clients with impaired renal function. Cycloserine is con-traindicated in severe renal impairment.

Use in Clients With Hepatic Impairment

Most antitubercular drugs are metabolized in the liver and sev-eral (eg, INH, rifampin, pyrazinamide) are hepatotoxic. More-over, they are often used concomitantly, which increases risks of hepatotoxicity. To detect hepatotoxicity as early as possible, clients should be thoroughly instructed to report any signs of liver damage and health care providers who administer DOT or have any client contact should observe for and ask about symp-toms. For clients at risk of developing hepatotoxicity, serum ALT and AST should be measured before starting and period-ically during drug therapy. If hepatitis occurs, these enzyme lev-els usually increase before other signs and symptoms develop.

With INH, mild increases in AST and ALT occur in ap-proximately 10% to 20% of clients but are not considered sig-nificant and usually resolve without stopping the drug. Hepatitis and liver damage are more likely to occur during the first 8 weeks of INH therapy and in middle-aged and older adults. Clients should be assessed monthly for symptoms of hepatitis (anorexia, nausea, fatigue, malaise, jaundice). If symptoms occur or if AST and ALT increase significantly (more than five times the normal values), INH should be discontinued. INH should be used cautiously in clients with pre-existing liver disease.

With rifampin, liver damage is most likely to occur with pre-existing liver disease or concurrent use of other hepatotoxic drugs. Clients should be monitored at least monthly for symptoms of hepatotoxicity. AST and ALT may be measured before starting and periodically during rifampin therapy. If signs of liver damage occur, the drug should be stopped, serum AST and ALT should be measured, and medical evaluation should be done.

With pyrazinamide, the drug should not be given to a client with pre-existing liver impairment unless it is considered absolutely essential. For clients without liver impairment, clinical monitoring for signs and symptoms of hepatotoxicity are recommended every 2 weeks. Serum ALT and AST may also be measured periodically. If significant symptoms or elevations of serum ALT and AST levels occur, the drug must be stopped.

Use in Home Care

The home care nurse has major roles to play in the health care of clients, families, and communities. With individual clients receiving antitubercular drugs for latent or active infection, the home care nurse needs to assist in taking the drugs as directed. Specific interventions vary widely and may include administering the drugs (DOT); teaching about the importance of taking the drugs and the possible consequences of not taking them (ie, more severe disease, longer treatment regimens with more toxic drugs, spreading the disease to others); monitoring for adverse drug effects and assisting the client to manage them or reporting them to the drug prescriber; assisting in obtaining the drugs and keeping follow-up appointments for blood tests and chest x-ray examinations; and others. Family members may also need teaching related to preventing spread of the disease and assisting the client to obtain adequate treatment. In relation to community needs, the nurse needs to be active in identifying cases, investigating contacts of newly diagnosed cases, and promoting efforts to manage tuberculosis effectively.

N   U   R   S   I   N   G   A   C   T   I   O   N   S

Antitubercular Drugs

NURSING ACTIONS	RATIONALE/EXPLANATION
1. Administer accurately	
a. Give isoniazid (INH), ethambutol, and rifampin in a single dose once daily, twice a week, or 3 times a week.	A single dose with the resulting higher blood levels is more effective. Also, less-frequent administration is more convenient for clients and more likely to be completed.
b. Give INH and rifampin on an empty stomach, 1 hour before or 2 hours after a meal, with a full glass of water. INH may be given with food if gastrointestinal (GI) upset occurs.	Food delays absorption.
c. Give parenteral INH by deep intramuscular (IM) injection into a large muscle mass, and rotate injection sites.	To decrease local pain and tissue irritation. Used only when clients are unable to take the medication orally.
d. Give IV rifampin by infusion, over 1–3 hours, depending on dose and volume of IV solution.	For a 600-mg dose, reconstitute with 10 milliliters of sterile water for injection; withdraw the entire amount and add it to 500 milliliters 5% dextrose or 0.9% sodium chloride solution; infuse over 3 hours.
e. Give rifabutin 300 milligrams once daily; if GI upset occurs, may give 150 milligrams twice daily.	Manufacturer's recommendation
f. Give rifapentine on an empty stomach when possible; may give with food if GI upset occurs.	Usually given twice weekly for 2 months, with 72 hours between doses, then once weekly for 4 months, along with other antitubercular drugs, for treatment of active TB.
g. Give secondary anti-TB drugs daily. See drug literature for specific instructions.	These drugs are used only to treat TB infection caused by organisms that are resistant to the primary anti-TB drugs.
2. Observe for therapeutic effects	Therapeutic effects are usually apparent within the first 2 or 3 weeks of drug therapy for active disease.
a. With latent infection, observe for the absence of signs and symptoms.	

NURSING ACTIONS	RATIONALE/EXPLANATION
b. With active disease, observe for clinical improvement (eg, decreased cough, sputum, fever, night sweats, and fatigue; increased appetite, weight, and feeling of well-being; negative sputum smear and culture results; improvement in chest radiographs).	
3. Observe for adverse effects	
a. Nausea, vomiting, diarrhea	These symptoms are likely to occur with any of the oral antitubercular drugs.
b. Neurotoxicity:	
(1) Eighth cranial nerve damage—vertigo, tinnitus, hearing loss	A major adverse reaction to aminoglycoside antibiotics
(2) Optic nerve damage—decreased vision and color discrimination	The major adverse reaction to ethambutol
(3) Peripheral neuritis—tingling, numbness, paresthesias	Often occurs with INH but can be prevented by administering pyridoxine (vitamin B_6). Also may occur with ethambutol.
(4) Central nervous system changes—confusion, convulsions, depression	More often associated with INH, but similar changes may occur with ethambutol
c. Hepatotoxicity—increased serum alanine and aspartate aminotransferases (ALT and AST), and bilirubin; jaundice; other symptoms of hepatitis (eg, anorexia, nausea, vomiting, abdominal pain)	May occur with INH, rifampin, and pyrazinamide, especially if the client already has liver damage. Report these symptoms to the prescribing prescriber immediately, to prevent possible liver failure and death.
d. Nephrotoxicity—increased blood urea nitrogen and serum creatinine; cells in urine; oliguria	A major adverse reaction to aminoglycosides
e. Hypersensitivity—fever, tachycardia, anorexia, and malaise are early symptoms. If the drug is not discontinued, exfoliative dermatitis, hepatitis, renal abnormalities, and blood dyscrasias may occur.	Hypersensitivity reactions are more likely to occur between the third and eighth weeks of drug therapy. Early detection and drug discontinuation are necessary to prevent progressive worsening of the client's condition. Severe reactions can be fatal.
f. Miscellaneous—rifampin, rifabutin, and rifapentine can cause:	The color change is harmless, but clients should avoid wearing soft contact lenses during therapy.
(1) a red-orange discoloration of body fluids, including urine and tears	
(2) permanent staining of soft contact lenses	
(3) increased sensitivity to sunlight	
(4) unplanned pregnancy, most often associated with rifampin, which makes hormonal birth control pills and implants less effective	Women who take rifampin should use a different form of birth control.
4. Observe for drug interactions	
a. Drugs that *increase* effects of antitubercular drugs:	
(1) Other antitubercular drugs	Potentiate antitubercular effects and risks of hepatotoxicity. These drugs are always used in combinations of two or more for treatment of active tuberculosis.
b. Drugs that *increase* effects of INH:	
(1) Alcohol	Increases risk of hepatotoxicity, even if use is stopped during INH therapy

(continued)

NURSING ACTIONS	RATIONALE/EXPLANATION
(2) Carbamazepine	Accelerates metabolism of INH to hepatotoxic metabolites and increases risk of hepatotoxicity
(3) Stavudine	Increases risk of peripheral neuropathy; avoid the combination if possible.
c. Drug that *decreases* effects of INH:	
(1) Pyridoxine (vitamin B$_6$)	Decreases risk of peripheral neuritis
d. Drug that *decreases* effects of rifampin:	
(1) Ketoconazole	May decrease absorption

APPLYING YOUR KNOWLEDGE: ANSWERS

34-1 The primary reason for MDR-TB is a failure to take the medication as prescribed.

34-2 Assess for the occurrence of hepatotoxicity. The signs and symptoms might include anorexia, nausea, fatigue, malaise, and/or jaundice. You would also want to monitor the liver enzymes ALT and AST for an increase.

34-3 Rifampin may cause a red-orange coloration to the urine and other body fluids. Although it will permanently stain clothing and other objects, it is not harmful to the client.

Review and Application Exercises

Short Answer Exercises

1. How do tuberculosis infections differ from other bacterial infections?

2. Why are clients with AIDS at high risk for developing tuberculosis?

3. What are the main risk factors for development of drug-resistant tuberculosis?

4. Who should receive INH to prevent tuberculosis? Who should not be given INH? Why?

5. When INH is given alone for treatment of latent infection (LTBI), how long should it be taken?

6. If you worked in a health department with clients taking INH for treatment of LTBI, what are some interventions to promote client adherence to the drug regimen?

7. Why is active, symptomatic tuberculosis always treated with multiple drugs?

8. In a client with tuberculosis newly started on drug therapy, how could you explain the emergence of drug-resistant organisms and the importance of preventing this problem?

9. What are advantages and disadvantages of short-course (6–9 months) treatment programs?

10. What adverse effects are associated with INH, rifampin, pyrazinamide, and ethambutol, and how may they be prevented or minimized?

NCLEX-Style Questions

11. Which of the following vitamin supplements is usually given with isoniazid (INH)?
    a. niacin
    b. pyridoxine
    c. vitamin D
    d. folate

12. Which of the following adverse effects may occur in clients receiving INH and rifampin?
    a. neurotoxicity
    b. hepatotoxicity
    c. nephrotoxicity
    d. ototoxicity

13. Clients taking INH should be taught to avoid alcohol because of increased risks of
    a. severe central nervous system depression
    b. hepatitis
    c. drug-resistant *M. tuberculosis* organisms
    d. rapid drug metabolism

14. Therapeutic effects of antitubercular drugs are usually evident in
    a. 3–5 days
    b. 7–10 days
    c. 2–3 weeks
    d. 6 weeks or longer

15. A fluoroquinolone drug (eg, ciprofloxacin) may be used to treat
  a. inactive or latent tuberculosis
  b. active drug-susceptible tuberculosis
  c. MDR-TB
  d. nontuberculous mycobacterial infection

Selected References

Al-Dossary, F. S., Ong, L. T., Correa, A. G., & Starke, J. R. (2002). Treatment of childhood tuberculosis with a six month directly observed regimen of only two weeks of daily therapy. *The Pediatric Infectious Diseases Journal, 21*(2), 91–96.

American Thoracic Society, Centers for Disease Control and Prevention. (2000). Diagnostic standards and classification of tuberculosis in adults and children. *American Journal of Respiratory and Critical Care Medicine, 161,* 1376–1395.

American Thoracic Society, Centers for Disease Control and Prevention. (2000). Targeted tuberculin testing and treatment of latent tuberculosis infection. *American Journal of Respiratory and Critical Care Medicine, 161*(4), S221–S247.

American Thoracic Society, Centers for Disease Control and Prevention, Infectious Diseases Society of America. (2003). Treatment of tuberculosis. *American Journal of Respiratory and Critical Care Medicine, 167,* 603–662.

Centers for Disease Control and Prevention. (2001, August 31). Fatal and severe liver injuries associated with rifampin and pyrazinamide for latent tuberculosis infection and revisions in American Thoracic Society/CDC recommendations. *Morbidity and Mortality Weekly Report, 50*(34), 733–735.

Centers for Disease Control and Prevention. (2003). *Reported tuberculosis in the United States, 2002.* Retrieved September 26, 2005, from http://www.cdc.gov/nchstp/tb/surv/surv2002/default.htm

Iseman, M. D. (2004). Tuberculosis. In L. Goldman & D. Ausiello (Eds.), *Cecil textbook of medicine* (22nd ed., pp. 1894–1902). Philadelphia: W. B. Saunders.

Kamholz, S. L. (2001, November 4). *Current trends in multidrug-resistant tuberculosis.* Paper presented at the 67th Annual Scientific Assembly of the American College of Chest Physicians, Philadelphia.

Kim, R. B. (Ed.). (2001). *Handbook of adverse drug interactions.* New Rochelle, NY: Medical Letter.

Lacy, C. F., Armstrong, L. L., Goldman, M. P., Lance, L. L. (2004). *Lexi-Comp's drug information handbook* (12th ed.). Hudson, OH: Lexi-Comp.

Peloquin, C. A. (2002). Tuberculosis. In J. T. DiPiro, R. L. Talbert, G. C. Yee, G. R. Matzke, B. G. Wells, & L. M. Posey (Eds.), *Pharmacotherapy: A pathophysiologic approach* (5th ed., pp. 1917–1937). New York: McGraw-Hill.

Porth, C. M. (2005). Tuberculosis. In C. M. Porth, *Pathophysiology: Concepts of altered health states* (7th ed., pp. 669–673). Philadelphia: Lippincott Williams & Wilkins.

Preheim, L. C. (2004). Other mycobacterioses. In L. Goldman & D. Ausiello (Eds.), *Cecil textbook of medicine* (22nd ed., pp. 1902–1904). Philadelphia: W. B. Saunders.

Shakya, R., Rao, B. S., & Shrestha, B. (2004). Incidence of hepatotoxicity due to antitubercular medicines and assessment of risk factors. *The Annals of Pharmacotherapy, 38,* 1074–1079.

Small, P. M., & Fujiwara, P. I. (2001). Management of tuberculosis in the United States. *New England Journal of Medicine, 345*(3), 189–200.

Starke, J. R. (2002). Tuberculosis. In H. B. Jenson & R. S. Baltimore (Eds.), *Pediatric infectious diseases: Principles and practice* (2nd ed., pp. 396–419). Philadelphia: W. B. Saunders.

Antiviral Drugs

OBJECTIVES

After studying this chapter, you will be able to:

1. Describe characteristics of viruses and common viral infections.
2. Discuss difficulties in developing and using antiviral drugs.
3. Identify clients at risk for development of systemic viral infections.
4. Differentiate types of antiviral drugs used for herpesvirus, human immunodeficiency virus (HIV), influenza A virus, and respiratory syncytial virus infections.
5. Describe commonly used antiviral drugs in terms of indications for use, adverse effects, and nursing process implications.
6. Discuss the rationale for using combinations of drugs in treating HIV infection.
7. Discuss guidelines for using antiviral drugs in special populations.
8. Teach clients techniques to prevent viral infections.

APPLYING YOUR KNOWLEDGE

Tony Bronowicz is a 32-year-old man who is HIV positive. He is following a drug regimen that consists of Combivir one capsule PO twice a day and ritonavir 600 mg PO twice a day. Mr. Bronowicz is currently hospitalized and you are his nurse.

INTRODUCTION

Viruses cause many diseases, including acquired immuno-deficiency syndrome (AIDS), hepatitis, pneumonia, and other disorders that affect almost every body system. Many potentially pathogenic viral strains exist. For example, more than 150 viruses infect the human respiratory tract, including approximately 100 types of rhinovirus that cause the common cold. Viruses can be spread by secretions from infected people; ingestion of contaminated food or water; breaks in skin or mucous membrane; blood transfusions; sexual contact; pregnancy; breastfeeding; and organ transplantation. Viral infections vary from mild, localized disease with few symptoms to severe systemic illness and death. Severe infections are more common when host defense mechanisms are impaired by disease or drugs. Additional characteristics of viruses and viral infections are described in the following paragraphs; selected infections are described in Box 35-1.

- Viruses are intracellular parasites that can live and reproduce only while inside other living cells. They gain entry to human host cells by binding to receptors on cell membranes. All human cells do not have receptors for all viruses; cells that lack receptors for a particular virus are resistant to infection by that virus. Thus, the locations and numbers of the receptors determine which host cells can be infected by a virus. For example, the mucous membranes lining the tracheobronchial tree have receptors for the influenza A virus, and certain white blood cells (eg, helper T lymphocytes) have CD4 molecules, which are the receptors for the human immunodeficiency virus (HIV).

- Inside host cells, viruses use cellular metabolic activities for their own survival and replication. Viral replication involves dissolution of the protein coating and exposure of the genetic material (deoxyribonucleic acid [DNA] or ribonucleic acid [RNA]). With DNA viruses, the viral DNA enters the host cell's nucleus, where it becomes incorporated into the host cell's chromosomal DNA. Then, host cell genes are coded to produce new viruses. In addition, the viral DNA incorporated with host DNA is transmitted to the host's daughter cells

Box 35-1   Selected Viral Infections

Herpesvirus Infections
Cytomegalovirus Disease and Retinitis
Cytomegalovirus (CMV) infection is extremely common, and most people become infected by adulthood. Infection is usually asymptomatic in healthy, immunocompetent adults. Like other herpesviruses, CMV can cause a primary infection, then remain latent in body tissues, probably for life. This means the virus can be shed in secretions of an asymptomatic host and spread to others by contact with infected saliva, blood, urine, semen, breast milk, and cervical secretions. It also means the virus may lead to an opportunistic infection when the host becomes immunosuppressed. During pregnancy, CMV is transmitted to the fetus across the placenta and may cause infection in the brain, inner ears, eyes, liver, and bone marrow. Learning disabilities and mental retardation can result from congenital CMV infection. Children spread the virus to each other in saliva or urine, whereas adolescents and adults transmit the virus mainly through sexual contact.

Major populations at risk for development of active CMV infection are patients with cancer who receive immunosuppressant drugs; organ transplant recipients, who must receive immunosuppressant drugs to prevent their body's rejection of the transplanted organ; and those with advanced human immunodeficiency virus (HIV) infection. Systemic CMV infection occurs mainly from reactivation of endogenous virus, although it may occur from an exogenous source. Active CMV infection may cause cellular necrosis and inflammation in various body tissues. Common manifestations of disease include pneumonitis, hepatitis, encephalitis, adrenal insufficiency, gastrointestinal inflammation, and gastric ulcerations.

In the eye, CMV infection produces retinitis, usually characterized by blurred vision and decreased visual acuity. Visual impairment is progressive and irreversible and, if untreated, may result in blindness. CMV retinitis may also indicate systemic CMV infection or may be entirely asymptomatic.

Genital Herpes Infection
Genital herpes infection is caused by the herpes simplex virus (HSV) and produces recurrent, painful, blister-like eruptions of the skin and mucous membranes. The virus is usually transmitted from person to person by direct contact with open lesions or secretions, including genital secretions. Primary infection occurs at a site of viral entry, where the virus infects epithelial cells, produces progeny viruses, and eventually causes cell death. After primary infection, latent virus may become dormant within sensory nerve cells. In response to various stimuli, such as intense sunlight, emotional stress, febrile illness, or menstruation, this latent virus may become reactivated and lead to viral reproduction and shedding.

In the fetus, HSV may be transmitted from an infected birth canal, and neonatal herpes is a serious complication of maternal genital herpes. Neonatal herpes usually becomes evident within the first week of life and may be manifested by the typical clusters of blister-like lesions on skin or mucous membranes. Irritability, lethargy, jaundice, altered blood clotting, respiratory distress, seizures, or coma may also occur. The lesions may heal in 1 to 2 weeks, but clinicians should be aware that neonatal her-

pes carries a high mortality rate. In immunosuppressed patients, HSV infection may result in severe, systemic disease.

Herpes Zoster
Herpes zoster is caused by the varicella-zoster virus, which is highly contagious and present worldwide. Most children in the United States are infected by early school age. The virus produces chickenpox on first exposure and is spread from person to person by the respiratory route or by contact with secretions from skin lesions. Recovery from the primary infection leaves latent infection in nerve cells. Reactivation of the latent infection (usually later in life) causes herpes zoster (more commonly known as "shingles"), a localized cluster of painful, blister-like skin eruptions. The skin lesions have the same appearance as those of chickenpox and genital herpes. Over several days, the vesicles become pustules, then rupture and heal. Because the virus remains in sensory nerve cells, pain can persist for months after the skin lesions heal. Most cases of herpes zoster infection occur among the elderly and the immunocompromised.

Human Immunodeficiency Virus Infection
HIV infection is caused by a retrovirus that infects the immune system. Two types of HIV virus have been identified, HIV-1 and HIV-2. Most infections in the United States are caused by HIV-1; HIV-2 infections occur mainly in Africa. HIV binds to a receptor protein located on the surface of CD4+ cells (also called T lymphocytes or helper T cells). The binding of HIV to CD4+ cells and its impending replication eventually results in cell death. CD4+ cells play pivotal roles in controlling and regulating immune function. The destruction of CD4+ cells eventually results in impairment of the immune system and acquisition of opportunistic infections.

Progression of HIV-1 infection to acquired immunodeficiency syndrome (AIDS) occurs in phases. The initial phase of infection is characterized by influenza-like symptoms (eg, fever, chills, muscle aches) that may last several weeks. During this time, the virus undergoes rapid and significant replication. The next phase is characterized by a dramatic decline in the rate of viral replication, attributed to a partially effective immune response. During this phase, no visible manifestations of HIV infection may be present. Despite the lack of symptoms, replication of HIV continues, and antibodies may be detected in the serum (seroconversion). During this period, which may last 10 years, the person is seropositive (HIV+) and infectious but asymptomatic. Eventually, the immune system is substantially damaged and the rate of viral reproduction accelerates. When viral load and immunodeficiency reach significant levels, the illness is termed *AIDS*. This phase is characterized by decreased CD4+ cell counts, loss of immune responses, and onset of opportunistic infections such as *Pneumocystis jiroveci* pneumonia.

HIV can spread to a new host during any phase of infection. The virus is most commonly spread by sexual intercourse; injection of intravenous drugs with contaminated needles; mucous membrane contact with infected blood or body fluids; and perinatally from mother to fetus. Although the virus is

(continued)

Box 35-1 Selected Viral Infections (continued)

found in most body fluids, infection has primarily been associated with exposure to blood, semen, or vaginal secretions. The virus is not spread through casual contact. Health care workers may be infected by needle-stick injuries. They should be aware that postexposure prophylaxis is available and may significantly reduce the risk of transmission.

Respiratory Syncytial Virus Infection
The respiratory syncytial virus (RSV) is a highly contagious virus that is present worldwide and infects most children by school age. Epidemics of RSV infection often occur in nurseries, daycare centers, and pediatric hospital units during winter months. RSV infects and destroys respiratory epithelium in the bronchi, bronchioles, and alveoli. It is spread by respiratory droplets and secretions, direct contact with an infected person, and contact with fomites, including the hands of caregivers.

RSV is the most common cause of bronchiolitis and pneumonia in infants and causes severe illness in those

younger than 6 months of age. These infants usually have wheezing, cough, respiratory distress, and fever. The infection is usually self-limited and resolves in 1 to 2 weeks. Antiviral therapy with ribavirin is used in some cases. The mortality rate from RSV infection is low in children who are generally healthy but increases substantially in those with congenital heart disease or immunosuppression. Recurrent infection occurs but is usually less severe than primary infection. In older children, RSV infection produces much milder disease but may be associated with acute exacerbations of asthma.

In adults, RSV infection causes colds and bronchitis, with symptoms of fever, cough, and nasal congestion. Infection occurs most often in those with household or other close contact with children, including pediatric health care workers. In elderly adults, RSV infection may cause pneumonia requiring hospitalization. In immunocompromised patients, RSV infection may cause severe and potentially fatal pneumonia.

---

during host cell mitosis and becomes part of the inherited genetic information of the host cell and its progeny. With RNA viruses (eg, HIV), viral RNA must be converted to DNA by an enzyme called *reverse transcriptase* before replication can occur.

After new viruses are formed, they are released from the infected cell either by budding out and breaking off from the cell membrane (leaving the host cell intact) or by causing lysis of the cell. When the cell is destroyed, the viruses are released into the blood and surrounding tissues, from which they can transmit the viral infection to other host cells.

● Viruses induce antibodies and immunity. Antibodies are proteins that defend against microbial or viral invasion. They are very specific (ie, an antibody protects only against a specific virus or other antigen). For example, in a person who has had measles, antibody protection (immunity) develops against future infection by the measles virus, but immunity does not develop against other viral infections, such as chickenpox or hepatitis.

The protein coat of the virus allows the immune system of the host to recognize the virus as a "foreign invader" and to produce antibodies against it. This system works well for most viruses but does not work for the influenza A virus, which can alter its protein covering so much and so often that the immune system does not recognize it as foreign to the body. Thus, last year's antibody cannot recognize and neutralize this year's virus.

Antibodies against infecting viruses can prevent the viruses from reaching the bloodstream, or if they are already in the bloodstream, prevent their invasion of host cells. After the virus has penetrated the cell, it is pro-

tected from antibody action, and the host depends on cell-mediated immunity (lymphocytes and macrophages) to eradicate the virus along with the cell harboring it.

● Viral infection may occur without signs and symptoms of illness. If illness does occur, the clinical course is usually short and self-limited. Recovery occurs as the virus is eliminated from the body. Some viruses (eg, herpesviruses) can survive in host cells for many years and cause a chronic, latent infection that periodically becomes reactivated. Also, autoimmune diseases may be caused by viral alteration of host cells so that lymphocytes recognize the host's own tissues as being foreign.

● Symptoms usually associated with acute viral infections include fever, headache, cough, malaise, muscle pain, nausea and vomiting, diarrhea, insomnia, and photophobia. White blood cell counts usually remain normal. Other signs and symptoms vary with the type of virus and body organs involved.

ANTIVIRAL DRUGS

Numerous drugs have been developed to treat HIV infection and opportunistic viral infections that occur in hosts whose immune system is suppressed by AIDS or immunosuppressant drugs given to organ transplant recipients. Drug therapy for viral infections is still limited, however, because viruses use the metabolic and reproductive mechanisms of host cells for their own vital functions, and few drugs inhibit viruses without being excessively toxic to host tissues. Most antiviral agents inhibit viral reproduction but do not eliminate viruses from tissues. Available drugs are expensive, relatively toxic, and effective in a limited number of infections. Some may be useful in treating an established infection if given promptly and in chemoprophylaxis if given before or soon after exposure. Protection conferred by chemoprophylaxis is immediate but lasts only while the drug is being taken. Subgroups of antiviral drugs are described in the following sections; additional characteristics and dosage ranges are listed in the Drugs at a Glance tables.

Drugs for Herpesvirus Infections

Acyclovir, famciclovir, and **valacyclovir** penetrate virus-infected cells, become activated by an enzyme, and inhibit viral DNA reproduction. They are used in the treatment of herpes simplex and herpes zoster infections. Acyclovir is used to treat genital herpes, in which it decreases viral shedding and the duration of skin lesions and pain. It does not eliminate inactive virus in the body and thus does not prevent recurrence of the disease unless oral drug therapy is continued. Acyclovir is also used for treatment of herpes simplex infections in immunocompromised clients. Prolonged or repeated courses of acyclovir therapy may result in the emergence of acyclovir-resistant viral strains, especially in immunocompromised clients. Acyclovir can be given orally, intravenously (IV), or applied topically to lesions. IV use is recommended for severe genital herpes in nonimmunocompromised clients and any herpes infections in immunocompromised clients. Oral and IV acyclovir are excreted mainly in urine, and dosage should be decreased in clients who are older or who have renal impairment.

Famciclovir and valacyclovir are oral drugs for herpes zoster and recurrent genital herpes. Famciclovir is metabolized to penciclovir, its active form, and excreted mainly in the urine. Valacyclovir is metabolized to acyclovir by enzymes in the liver and/or intestine and is eventually excreted in the urine. As with acyclovir, dosage of these drugs must be reduced in the presence of renal impairment.

Cidofovir, foscarnet, ganciclovir, and **valganciclovir** also inhibit viral reproduction after the drugs are activated by a viral enzyme found in virus-infected cells. The drugs are used to treat cytomegalovirus (CMV) retinitis, which most often occurs in clients with AIDS. In addition, foscarnet is used to treat acyclovir-resistant mucocutaneous herpes simplex infections in people with impaired immune function. Valganciclovir and ganciclovir are used to prevent CMV disease, mainly in clients with organ transplants or HIV infection. Dosage of these drugs must be reduced with renal impairment. Ganciclovir causes granulocytopenia and thrombocytopenia in approximately 20% to 40% of recipients. These hematologic effects often occur during the first 2 weeks of therapy but may occur at any time. If severe bone marrow depression occurs, ganciclovir should be discontinued; recovery usually occurs within a week of stopping the drug. Foscarnet and cidofovir should be used cautiously in clients with renal disease.

Trifluridine and **vidarabine** are applied topically to treat keratoconjunctivitis and corneal ulcers caused by the herpes simplex virus (herpetic keratitis). Trifluridine should not be used longer than 21 days because of possible ocular toxicity. Vidarabine also is given IV to treat herpes zoster infections in clients whose immune system is impaired and encephalitis caused by herpes simplex viruses. IV dosage must be reduced with impaired renal function.

Table 35-1 provides indications and dosage ranges for selected drugs for herpes.

Drugs for HIV Infection and AIDS (Antiretrovirals)

Five classes of drugs currently exist for the management of HIV infection: nucleoside reverse transcriptase inhibitors (NRTIs), nucleotide reverse transcriptase inhibitors, non-nucleoside reverse transcriptase inhibitors (NNRTIs), protease inhibitors, and fusion inhibitors (see Table 35-2). The first four groups inhibit enzymes required for viral replication in human host cells. The fusion inhibitor enfuvirtide (Fuzeon), which represents a new class of antiretroviral drugs, blocks the initial attachment of the virus to the CD4+ receptor on human cells (see Fig. 35-1). To increase effectiveness and decrease viral mutations and emergence of drug-resistant viral strains, the drugs are used in combination. All of the drugs can cause serious adverse effects and require intensive monitoring.

Nucleoside Reverse Transcriptase Inhibitors (NRTIs)

The NRTIs are structurally similar to specific DNA components (adenosine, cytosine, guanosine, or thymidine) and thus easily enter human cells and viruses in human cells. For example, **P** **zidovudine,** the prototype, is able to substitute for thymidine. In infected cells, these drugs inhibit reverse transcriptase, an enzyme required by retroviruses to convert RNA to DNA and allow replication. The drugs are more active in slowing the progression of acute infection than in treating chronically infected cells. Thus, they do not cure HIV infection or prevent transmission of the virus through sexual contact or blood contamination.

Zidovudine, the first NRTI to be developed, is still widely used. However, zidovudine-resistant viral strains are common. Other NRTIs are usually given in combination with zidovudine or as a substitute for zidovudine in clients who are unable to take or do not respond to zidovudine.

Nucleotide Reverse Transcriptase Inhibitor

The nucleotide group includes one agent, tenofovir (Viread). This group, similar to the NRTIs, inhibits the reverse transcriptase enzyme. However, tenofovir differs structurally from the NRTIs, and this difference helps to circumvent acquired drug resistance. The drug is partially activated and begins inhibiting HIV replication soon after ingestion. Tenofovir can be given once daily and has also demonstrated efficacy in the treatment of hepatitis B.

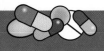

Table 35-1   Drugs at a Glance: Drugs for Prevention or Treatment of Selected Viral Infections

GENERIC/TRADE NAME	INDICATIONS FOR USE	ROUTES AND DOSAGE RANGES	
		Adults	Children
Herpesvirus Infections			
Acyclovir (Zovirax)	Oral mucocutaneous lesions (eg, cold sores, fever blisters) Genital herpes Herpes simplex encephalitis Varicella (chickenpox) in immunocompromised hosts Herpes zoster (shingles) in normal and immuno-compromised hosts	Genital herpes, PO 200 mg q4h, 5 times daily for 10 d for initial infection; 400 mg 2 times daily to prevent recurrence of chronic infection; 200 mg q4h 5 times daily for 5 d to treat recurrence Herpes zoster, PO 800 mg q4h 5 times daily for 7–10 d Chickenpox, PO 20 mg/kg (maximum dose 800 mg) 4 times daily for 5 d Mucosal and cutaneous HSV infections in ICH, IV 5 mg/kg infused at constant rate over 1 h, q8h for 7 d Varicella-zoster infections in ICH, IV 10 mg/kg, infused as above, q8h for 7 d HSV encephalitis, IV 10 mg/kg, infused as above, q8h for 10 d Topically to lesions q3h, 6 times daily for 7 d	*<12 y:* IV 250 mg/m² q8h for 7 d
Adefovir (Hepsera)	Treatment of chronic hepatitis B	PO 10 mg once daily	Dosage not established
Cidofovir (Vistide)	Treatment of CMV retinitis in persons with AIDS	IV infusion, 5 mg/kg over 1 h, every 2 wk	Dosage not established
Famciclovir (Famvir)	Acute herpes zoster Genital herpes, recurrent episodes	Herpes zoster, PO 500 mg q8h for 7 d Genital herpes, PO 125 mg twice daily for 5 d	Dosage not established
Foscarnet (Foscavir)	Treatment of CMV retinitis in persons with AIDS Treatment of acyclovir-resistant mucocutaneous HSV infections in immunocompromised clients	CMV retinitis, IV 60 mg/kg q8h for 2–3 wk, depending on clinical response, then 90–120 mg/kg/d for maintenance HSV infections, IV 40 mg/kg q8–12h for 2–3 wk or until lesions are healed Reduce dosage with impaired renal function.	
Ganciclovir (Cytovene)	CMV retinitis in immuno-compromised clients Prevention of CMV disease in clients with organ transplants or advanced HIV infection	CMV retinitis, IV 5 mg/kg q12h for 14–21 d, then 5 mg/kg once daily for 7 d/wk or 6 mg/kg once daily for 5 d/wk or PO 1000 mg 3 times daily for maintenance Prevention in transplant recipients, IV 5 mg/kg once daily 7 d/wk or 6 mg/kg once daily 5 d/wk Prevention in clients with HIV infection, PO 1000 mg 3 times daily	
Trifluridine (Viroptic)	Keratoconjunctivitis caused by herpes viruses	Topically to eye, 1% ophthalmic solution, 1 drop q2h while awake (maximum 9 drops/d) until re-epithelialization of corneal ulcer occurs; then 1 drop q4h (maximum 5 drops/d) for 7 d	
Valacyclovir (Valtrex)	Herpes zoster and recurrent genital herpes in immunocompetent clients	Herpes zoster, PO 1 g q8h for 7 d Recurrent genital herpes, PO 500 mg q12h daily for 5 d Reduce dosage with renal impairment (creatinine clearance <50 mL/min)	

Table 35-1 Drugs at a Glance: Drugs for Prevention or Treatment of Selected Viral Infections (continued)

GENERIC/TRADE NAME	INDICATIONS FOR USE	ROUTES AND DOSAGE RANGES	
		Adults	Children
Vidarabine (Vira-A)	Keratoconjunctivitis caused by herpes viruses	IV 15 mg/kg/d dissolved in 2500 mL of fluid and given over 12–24 h daily for 10 d Topically to eye, 3% ophthalmic ointment, applied q3h until re-epithelialization, then twice daily for 7 d	
Influenza Virus Infection **Amantadine** (Symmetrel)	Prevention or treatment of influenza A infection	PO 200 mg once daily or 100 mg twice daily Reduce dosage with renal impairment (creatinine clearance <50 mL/min).	*9 to 12 y:* PO 100 mg twice daily *1 to 9 y:* PO 4.4 to 8.8 mg/kg/d given in 1 single dose or 2 divided doses, not to exceed 150 mg/d
Oseltamivir (Tamiflu)	Treatment of influenza	PO 75 mg twice daily for 5 d	≥ *1 y:* Oral suspension, 30–35 mg twice daily, depending on weight, for 5d ≥ *13 y:* Same as adults
Rimantadine (Flumadine)	Prevention or treatment of influenza A infection in adults Prophylaxis of influenza A in children	PO 100 mg twice daily	*>10 y:* Same as adults *<10 y:* 5 mg/kg once daily, not exceeding 150 mg
Zanamivir (Relenza)	Treatment of influenza A or B infection	Oral inhalation, 2 inhalations twice daily for 5 d	≥ *7 y:* Same as adults
Respiratory Syncytial Virus Infection **Ribavirin** (Virazole)	Treatment of hospitalized infants and young children with severe lower respiratory tract infections Treatment of chronic hepatitis C infection (with interferon)	PO 800–1200 mg twice daily for 24–48 wk	Inhalation; diluted to a concentration of 20 mg/mL for 12–18 h/d for 3–7 d

AIDS, acquired immunodeficiency syndrome; CMV, cytomegalovirus; HSV, herpes simplex virus; ICH, immunocompromised host; IV, intravenous; PO, oral.

Non-Nucleoside Reverse Transcriptase Inhibitors (NNRTIs)

The NNRTIs inhibit viral replication in infected cells by directly binding to reverse transcriptase and preventing its function. They are used in combination with NRTIs to treat clients with advanced HIV infection. Because the two types of drugs inhibit reverse transcriptase by different mechanisms, they may have synergistic antiviral effects. NNRTIs are also used with other antiretroviral drugs because drug-resistant strains emerge rapidly when the drugs are used alone.

Protease Inhibitors

Protease inhibitors exert their effects against HIV at a different phase of its life cycle than reverse transcriptase inhibitors. Protease is an HIV enzyme required to process viral protein

(text continues on page 569)

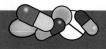

Table 35-2 Drugs at a Glance: Drugs for Human Immunodeficiency Virus Infection and Acquired Immunodeficiency Syndrome

		ROUTES AND DOSAGE RANGES	
GENERIC/TRADE NAME	CHARACTERISTICS	Adults	Children
Nucleoside Reverse Transcriptase Inhibitors (NRTIs)			
Zidovudine (AZT, ZVD, Retrovir)	Prototype NRTI Well absorbed with oral administration Metabolized in the liver to an inactive metabolite, which is excreted in urine Often causes severe anemia and granulocytopenia, which may require stopping the drug, giving blood transfusions, or giving filgrastim or sargramostim to hasten bone-marrow recovery May also cause peripheral neuropathy and pancreatitis	PO 300 mg twice daily	*3 mo to 12 y:* 180 mg/m² q6h (not to exceed 200 mg q6h) *Neonate born of HIV-infected mother who took the drug during pregnancy, labor, and delivery;* PO 2 mg/kg q6h starting within 12 h of birth and continuing until 6 wk of age. If unable to take oral drug, give 1.5 mg/kg IV q6h, infused over 30 min.
Abacavir (Ziagen)	Well absorbed with oral administration Approximately 50% bound to plasma proteins Metabolized to inactive metabolites that are excreted in urine and feces May cause serious hypersensitivity reactions	PO 300 mg twice daily	*>3 mo:* PO 8 mg/kg twice daily (maximum dose, 300 mg twice daily)
Didanosine (ddl, Videx, Videx EC)	Used for clients who do not respond to or cannot tolerate zidovudine	PO 200 mg twice daily or 400 mg (enteric-coated) once daily	*<0.4 m² BSA:* PO 25 mg q12h *0.5–0.7 m² BSA:* PO 50 mg q12h *0.8–1 m² BSA:* PO 75 mg q12h *1.1–1.4 m² BSA:* PO 100 mg q12h
Emtricitabine (Emtriva)	Well absorbed with oral administration Metabolized in the liver and excreted mainly in urine	PO 200 mg once daily	Dosage not established
Lamivudine (Epivir)	Used to treat advanced HIV infection and chronic hepatitis B Well absorbed with oral administration and mainly eliminated unchanged in urine Dosage should be reduced with renal impairment.	PO 150 mg twice daily Weight <50 kg (110 lb): PO 2 mg/kg twice daily	*12–16 y:* PO same as adults *3 mo to 12 y:* PO 4 mg/kg twice daily
Stavudine (Zerit)	Used to treat adults who do not improve with or do not tolerate other anti-HIV medications May be useful against zidovudine-resistant strains of HIV Approximately 40% is eliminated through the kidneys, and dosage should be reduced with renal impairment. May cause peripheral neuropathy	Weight ≥60 kg, PO 40 mg q12h Weight <60 kg, PO 30 mg q12h	Dosage not established

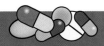

Table 35-2 Drugs at a Glance: Drugs for Human Immunodeficiency Virus Infection and Acquired Immunodeficiency Syndrome (continued)

		ROUTES AND DOSAGE RANGES	
GENERIC/TRADE NAME	CHARACTERISTICS	Adults	Children
Zalcitabine (Hivid)	Used with zidovudine to treat advanced HIV infection in adults whose condition continues to deteriorate while receiving zidovudine May cause peripheral neuropathy	PO 0.75 mg q8h (2.25 mg/d) with zidovudine 200 mg q8h (600 mg/d)	Dosage not established
Zidovudine and lamivudine (Combivir)	Combination product to reduce pill burden	One capsule twice daily	Dosage not established
Zidovudine, lamivudine, and abacavir (Trizivir)	Combination product to reduce pill burden	One capsule twice daily	Dosage not established
Nucleotide Reverse Transcriptase Inhibitor			
Tenofovir DF (Viread)	Used for salvage therapy after multiple drug failures Efficacious against hepatitis B	300 mg once daily	Dosage not established
Non-Nucleoside Reverse Transcriptase Inhibitors (NNRTIs)			
Delavirdine (Rescriptor)	Used with NRTIs and protease inhibitors Well absorbed with oral administration and metabolized in the liver Induces drug-metabolizing enzymes in the liver and increases metabolism of itself and other drugs Common adverse effects are nausea and skin rash.	PO 400 mg (four 100-mg tablets) 3 times daily	Dosage not established
Efavirenz (Sustiva)	May cause central nervous system side effects	PO 600 mg at bedtime	*Weight >40 kg:* PO same as adults *≥ 3 y and weight 10–40 kg (22–88 lb):* PO 200–400 mg, depending on weight
Nevirapine (Viramune)	Well absorbed with oral administration and metabolized in the liver Induces drug-metabolizing enzymes in the liver and increases metabolism of itself and other drugs Adverse effects include severe skin reactions and hepatotoxicity.	PO 200 mg once daily for 2 wk, then 200 mg twice daily	Dosage not established

(continued)

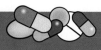

GENERIC/TRADE NAME	CHARACTERISTICS	ROUTES AND DOSAGE RANGES	
		Adults	Children
Protease Inhibitors			
Amprenavir (Agenerase)	Well absorbed after oral administration Oral solution less bioavailable than capsules, thus the two dosage forms are not equivalent on a milligram basis Highly bound to plasma proteins Metabolized in liver; small amount of unchanged drug excreted in urine and feces May cause serious skin reactions	PO 1200 mg (eight 150-mg capsules) twice daily	*13–16 y and weight ≥50 kg:* PO same as adults *4–12 y, or 13–16 y and weight <50 kg:* PO 20/mg/kg twice daily or 15 mg/kg 3 times daily (maximum daily dose, 2400 mg); oral solution, 22.5 mg/kg twice daily or 17 mg/kg 3 times daily (maximum daily dose, 2800 mg)
Atazanavir (Reyataz)	Well absorbed with few adverse effects May cause hyperbilirubinemia	PO 400 mg daily	Dosage not established
Fosamprenavir (Lexiva)	Prodrug formulation of amprenavir that allows for a reduced pill burden	Treatment-naïve: PO 1400 mg twice daily Treatment-experienced: PO 700 mg twice daily (with ritonavir 100 mg twice daily)	Dosage not established
Indinavir (Crixivan)	Well absorbed and approximately 60% bound to plasma proteins Metabolized in the liver and excreted mainly in feces May cause GI upset and kidney stones	PO 800 mg (two 400-mg capsules) q8h	Dosage not established
Nelfinavir (Viracept)	Metabolized in the liver Most common adverse effect is diarrhea, which can be controlled with over-the-counter drugs such as loperamide	1250 mg twice daily	*2–13 y:* PO 20–30 mg/kg/dose, 3 times daily
Ritonavir (Norvir)	Metabolized in the liver May cause GI upset	PO 600 mg twice daily	PO 400 mg/m² daily
Saquinavir (Fortovase)	Not well absorbed, undergoes first-pass metabolism in the liver, and is highly bound to plasma proteins Metabolized in the liver and excreted mainly in feces May cause GI upset May produce fewer drug interactions than indinavir and ritonavir	PO 1200 mg (six 200-mg tablets) 3 times daily	Dosage not established
Kaletra (Lopinavir and ritonavir)	Combination product composed of two protease inhibitors Ritonavir boosts lopinavir levels manyfold	3 capsules twice daily	*7–15 kg:* 12/3 mg/kg twice daily *15–40 kg:* 10/2.5 mg/kg twice daily

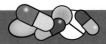

Table 35-2 Drugs at a Glance: Drugs for Human Immunodeficiency Virus Infection and Acquired Immunodeficiency Syndrome (continued)

GENERIC/TRADE NAME	CHARACTERISTICS	ROUTES AND DOSAGE RANGES	
		Adults	Children
Fusion Inhibitor			
Enfuvirtide (Fuzeon)	Highly protein bound (92%) Adverse effects include injection site reactions, nausea, and diarrhea.	Sub-Q 90 mg (1 mL) twice daily into upper arm, anterior thigh, or abdomen	*6–16 y:* Sub-Q 2 mg/kg up to a maximum of 90 mg twice daily, into upper arm, anterior thigh, or abdomen

BSA, body surface area; GI, gastrointestinal; PO, oral.

precursors into mature particles that are capable of infecting other cells. The drugs inhibit the enzyme by binding to its protease-active site. This inhibition causes the production of immature, noninfectious viral particles. These drugs are active in both acutely and chronically infected cells because they block viral maturation.

Most protease inhibitors are metabolized in the liver by the cytochrome P450 enzyme system and should be used cautiously in clients with impaired liver function. They should also be used cautiously in pregnant women because few data exist and it is unknown whether the drugs are excreted in breast milk. However, this may be irrelevant because the Centers for Disease Control and Prevention (CDC) advise women with HIV infection to avoid breastfeeding because HIV may be transmitted to an uninfected infant.

Indinavir, ritonavir, and **saquinavir** are the oldest and best known protease inhibitors. Two major concerns with

this group are viral resistance and drug interactions. Viral resistance develops fairly rapidly, with resistant strains developing in approximately half of the recipients within a year of drug therapy. In relation to drug interactions, protease inhibitors interfere with metabolism, increase plasma concentrations, and increase risks of toxicity of numerous other drugs metabolized by the cytochrome P450 enzymes in the liver.

Ritonavir is the most potent cytochrome P450 inhibitor among the protease inhibitor class. It may increase plasma concentrations of amiodarone, bupropion, clozapine, flecainide, meperidine, piroxicam, propafenone, propoxyphene, quinidine, and rifabutin. None of these drugs should be given concomitantly with ritonavir because high plasma concentrations may cause cardiac dysrhythmias, hematologic abnormalities, seizures, and other potentially serious adverse effects. In addition, ritonavir may increase sedation and respiratory

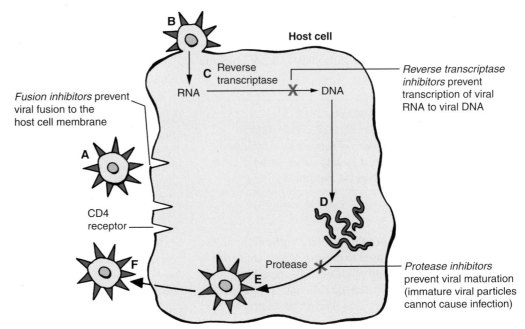

FIGURE 35-1 Human immunodeficiency virus (HIV) replication and actions of anti-HIV drugs. **(A)** The virus attaches to and fuses with receptors (eg, CD4 molecules) on the host cell membrane. **(B)** The virus becomes uncoated and releases its RNA into the host cell. **(C)** The enzyme *reverse transcriptase* converts RNA to DNA, which is necessary for viral replication. **(D)** The DNA codes for protein synthesis, which produces immature viral particles. **(E)** The enzyme *protease* assembles the immature viral particles into mature viruses. **(F)** Mature viruses are released from the host cell.

depression when used concurrently with benzodiazepines (eg, alprazolam, diazepam) and zolpidem.

Indinavir increases plasma concentrations of several of the same drugs listed previously and should not be given concomitantly with them because of potential cardiac dysrhythmias or prolonged sedation. Saquinavir may produce fewer interactions because it inhibits the cytochrome P450 enzyme system to a lesser extent than indinavir and ritonavir. However, if saquinavir is given with clindamycin, quinidine, triazolam, or a calcium channel blocker, clients should be monitored closely for increased plasma levels and adverse drug effects.

Amprenavir is a sulfonamide and should be used with caution in clients known to be allergic to sulfonamides. The likelihood of cross-sensitivity reactions between amprenavir and other sulfonamides is unknown. The drug formulation contains high concentrations of vitamin E and clients using this drug should be cautioned against taking any additional vitamin E supplements.

Fusion Inhibitor

The HIV contains a glycoprotein on its surface that allows it to bind to CD4 receptors on human cells and fuse with the cell membrane. This binding and fusion, which is the initial step of viral penetration and infection of the cell, is blocked by fusion inhibitor drugs such as **enfuvirtide** (Fuzeon).

Combination Drugs

Antiretroviral drug regimens are complex and involve the ingestion of many pills daily. Adherence to a regimen is difficult, but critical in producing therapeutic effects and preventing the development of drug resistance. Combination products decrease the "pill burden" and promote adherence. **Combivir** (lamivudine and zidovudine), **Trizivir** (abacavir, lamivudine, and zidovudine), and **Kaletra** (lopinavir and ritonavir) are currently available. Kaletra is a combination of two protease inhibitors in which ritonavir is added to increase serum concentrations of lopinavir. Lopinavir is not available as a single agent.

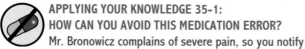 **APPLYING YOUR KNOWLEDGE 35-1:**
HOW CAN YOU AVOID THIS MEDICATION ERROR?
Mr. Bronowicz complains of severe pain, so you notify the resident and receive an order for meperidine 50 mg IM for one dose. You prepare and administer the medication.

Drugs for Influenza A

Amantadine and **rimantadine** inhibit replication of the influenza A virus and are used to prevent or treat influenza A infections. Postexposure prophylaxis with these drugs may protect persons who have had direct contact with people infected with influenza A. Seasonal prophylaxis may be used in high-risk clients if the influenza vaccine cannot be given or

may be ineffective. In epidemics, use of one of the drugs is recommended for clients at high risk who have not been vaccinated. The high-risk population includes older adults, those who have chronic lung disease, and those who have immunodeficiency disorders. During an epidemic, amantadine or rimantadine may be given for approximately 2 weeks if the client is vaccinated at the beginning of drug therapy or approximately 4 to 8 weeks if the client is un-vaccinated. Protection is lost within a few days after drug therapy is stopped. For treatment of influenza A infection, either drug may shorten the illness if started soon after onset and continued for 5 days. The drugs may also decrease viral shedding and spread.

Amantadine and rimantadine are well absorbed after oral administration. Amantadine is excreted in the urine unchanged. It accumulates in the body of older adults and others with impaired renal function, and dosage therefore should be reduced in these groups. Rimantadine is extensively metabolized, with small amounts excreted in the urine. The most common adverse effects of the drugs are gastrointestinal (anorexia, nausea) and central nervous system (CNS) (nervousness, lightheadedness, difficulty concentrating) symptoms. CNS effects are more likely to occur with amantadine than rimantadine, and high plasma levels of amantadine have been associated with delirium, hallucinations, seizures, coma, and cardiac dysrhythmias. Amantadine has also been associated with exacerbations of pre-existing seizure disorders and psychiatric symptoms. Amantadine is teratogenic in animals, and neither drug has been established as safe for pregnant women.

Amantadine is also used in the treatment of Parkinson's disease and for extrapyramidal symptoms associated with the use of certain antipsychotic drugs (see Chap. 12).

Oseltamivir (Tamiflu) and **zanamivir** (Relenza) are approved for treatment of influenza A or B in clients with symptoms for 2 days or less. Therapy should last for 5 days. Oseltamivir is an oral drug; zanamivir is a powder form for oral inhalation with a device called a Diskhaler. Zanamivir may cause bronchospasm in clients with asthma or chronic obstructive pulmonary disease.

Drug for Respiratory Syncytial Virus Respiratory Tract Infections

Ribavirin is used mainly for the treatment of bronchiolitis or pneumonia caused by the respiratory syncytial virus (RSV). It is used in hospitalized infants and young children and given by inhalation with the Viratek Small Particle Aerosol Generator. The drug is not recommended for clients on ventilators because it precipitates and may block breathing tubes, including endotracheal tubes. Deterioration of pulmonary function is a common adverse effect. The drug is absorbed systemically after administration by aerosol. Most infants and children with RSV infections have mild, self-limited disease that does not involve the lower respiratory tract and therefore does not require hospitalization or ribavirin therapy. Oral ribavirin is also being used in combination with interferon for treatment of some hepatitis C infections.

NURSING PROCESS

Assessment

- Assessment varies with the type of viral infection and may include signs and symptoms of influenza or other viral infections of the respiratory tract; genital herpes; viral infections of the eye; or other conditions.
- Assess renal function and adequacy of fluid intake.
- With HIV infection, assess baseline data to assist in monitoring response to drug therapy. Baseline data may include vital signs; weight and nutritional status; signs and symptoms of the disease; signs and symptoms of opportunistic infections associated with the disease and immunosuppression; and available reports of laboratory tests (eg, complete blood count; CD4+ lymphocyte counts; plasma levels of viral RNA, blood urea nitrogen, and serum creatinine; liver function tests.

Nursing Diagnoses

- Anxiety related to a medical diagnosis of HIV infection, genital herpes, or CMV retinitis
- Altered Sexuality Patterns related to sexually transmitted viral infections (HIV infection, genital herpes)
- Disturbed Body Image related to sexually transmitted infection
- Social Isolation related to a medical diagnosis of HIV infection or genital herpes
- Deficient Knowledge: Disease process and methods of spread; availability of vaccines and other prophylactic interventions
- Risk for Injury: Recurrent infection; adverse drug effects or interactions; infections and other problems associated with a compromised immune system in HIV infection

Planning/Goals

The client will

- Receive or take antiviral drugs as prescribed
- Be safeguarded against new or recurrent infection
- Act to prevent spread of viral infection to others and recurrence in self
- Avoid preventable adverse drug effects
- Receive emotional support and counseling to assist in coping with HIV infection or genital herpes

Interventions

- Follow recommended policies and procedures for preventing spread of viral infections.
- Assist clients in learning ways to control spread and recurrence of viral infection.
- Assist clients to maintain immunizations against viral infections.

- For clients receiving systemic antiviral drugs, monitor serum creatinine and other tests of renal function, complete blood count, and fluid balance.
- Spend time with the client when indicated to reduce anxiety and support usual coping mechanisms.
- For clients with HIV infection, monitor for changes in baseline data during each contact; prevent opportunistic infections (eg, CMV retinitis, herpes infections) when possible; and manage signs and symptoms, disease complications, and adverse effects of drug therapy to promote quality of life.

In addition, client teaching guidelines for selected antiviral and antiretroviral drugs are presented in the accompanying displays.

Evaluation

- Observe for improvement in signs and symptoms of the viral infection for which a drug is given.
- Interview outpatients regarding their compliance with instructions for taking antiviral drugs.
- Interview and observe for use of infection control measures.
- Interview and observe for adverse drug effects.
- Observe the extent and severity of any symptoms in clients with HIV infection.

APPLYING YOUR KNOWLEDGE 35-2

Mr. Bronowicz has been having a hard time with his drug regimen. He has difficulty with the proper timing of his medications. He also has complained about an upset stomach. What client education should you provide to Mr. Bronowicz?

PRINCIPLES OF THERAPY

Prevention of Viral Infections

General preventive measures include vaccination; hand hygiene; teaching infected clients to cover their mouth and nose when coughing or sneezing; treatment of symptoms; and recognition and treatment of complications. Of the sexually transmitted viral infections, spread of genital herpes can be prevented by avoiding sex when skin lesions are present and using condoms; and HIV infection can be prevented by the consistent use of condoms and use of clean needles by IV drug abusers.

Viral Vaccines

Viral vaccines are used to produce active immunity in clients before exposure or to control epidemics of viral disease in a community. Vaccines for prevention of poliomyelitis, measles, rubella, mumps, smallpox, chickenpox, and yellow fever, and

General Considerations

✔ Prevention is better than treatment, partly because medications used to treat viral infections may cause serious adverse effects. Thus, whenever possible, techniques to prevent viral infections should be employed.
  ✔ Wash hands frequently and thoroughly; this helps prevent most infections.
  ✔ Maintain immunizations against viral infections as indicated.
  ✔ With genital herpes, avoid sexual intercourse when visible lesions are present and always wash hands after touching any lesion.
✔ Drugs may relieve symptoms but do not cure viral infections. For example, treatment of genital herpes does not prevent transmis-

sion to others, and treatment of cytomegalovirus (CMV) retinitis may not prevent disease progression.
✔ Ask a health care provider for information about managing adverse drug effects.
✔ If taking foscarnet or ganciclovir for CMV retinitis, have eye examinations approximately every 6 weeks.

Self-Administration

✔ With acyclovir, famciclovir, and valacyclovir for genital herpes, start oral drugs for recurrent lesions as soon as signs and symptoms begin.
✔ Use gloves to apply acyclovir ointment to lesions.

for protection against influenza and rabies, are available (see Chap. 39). Live attenuated viral vaccines are generally safe and nontoxic. However, they should not be used in clients who are pregnant, immunodeficient, receiving high-dose, long-term corticosteroids; or receiving antineoplastic or immunosuppressive drugs or radiation. Influenza vaccines prevent infection in most clients. If infection does occur, less virus is shed in respiratory secretions. Thus, vaccination reduces transmission of influenza by decreasing the number of susceptible people and by decreasing transmission by immunized people who still become infected. The multiplicity of rhinoviruses (common cold), enteroviruses, and respiratory viruses hinders development of practical, specific vaccines for these common diseases.

Use of Antibacterial Drugs in Viral Infections

Antibacterial drugs (eg, antibiotics) should not be used to treat viral infections. They do have a role, however, in treating bacterial complications of viral infections. For example, bacterial pneumonia may develop as a complication of influenza.

Use of Antiretroviral Drugs in HIV Infection

- The goals of drug therapy include prolonging and improving quality of life, decreasing viral load to undetectable levels (<400 copies/mL) as long as possible, halting disease progression, and restoring immune function.
- Treatment of HIV infection is complex, and recommendations change often as new drugs and research reports become available. Thus, when possible, clinicians with expertise in the care of HIV-infected clients should prescribe, supervise, and monitor drug therapy. Clinicians caring for HIV-seropositive clients should always consult current treatment guidelines before initiating therapy.

- Drug therapy requires substantial commitment of time and energy by clinicians and their clients. Clinicians must keep abreast of new developments and monitor clients' responses; clients must be willing to adhere to complex regimens and manage or tolerate adverse drug effects. Nonadherence may lead to a lack of effectiveness or emergence of drug-resistant viral strains. Thus, the benefits and risks of drug therapy must be clear to all clients initiating therapy.
- Drug therapy is usually initiated early in the course of infection. The initial infection is manifested by an illness similar to influenza, with fever, chills, and muscle aches that may last for several weeks. This period is usually followed by a quiescent phase, which may last up to 10 years, during which there may be no clinical manifestations. This phase was previously thought to indicate viral latency and inactivity. However, research has shown that the initial infection is characterized by explosive viral growth and spread to body tissues, especially the lymphoid system. The period after the initial infection is characterized by a partially effective immune-system response, which decreases viral replication. However, some viral replication and destruction of lymphoid tissue continue during this period. Early treatment reduces viral load and may delay progression of the disease and development of acute clinical signs and symptoms.
- Guidelines for drug therapy in adults and adolescents, as developed by the Panel on Clinical Practices for Treatment of HIV Infection (convened by the Department of Health and Human Services and the Henry J. Kaiser Family Foundation), include the following:
  - Treatment is recommended for symptomatic clients, clients with CD4+ cell counts <350 cells/mm^3, or clients with viral loads >30–55,000 copies/mL.

General Considerations

☑ Prevention is better than treatment, partly because medications used to treat viral infections may cause serious adverse effects. Thus, whenever possible, techniques to prevent viral infections should be employed.

    ☑ Wash hands frequently and thoroughly; this helps prevent most infections.

    ☑ Maintain immunizations against viral infections as indicated.

    ☑ Always practice safer sex by using a condom.

    ☑ In cases of intravenous drug use, use and promote the use of clean needles.

☑ Drugs may relieve symptoms but do not cure human immuno-deficiency virus (HIV) infection, prevent transmission of the virus, or prevent other illnesses associated with advanced HIV infection.

☑ Effective treatment of HIV infection requires close adherence to drug therapy regimens involving several drugs and daily doses. Missing as few as one or two doses can decrease blood levels of antiretroviral drugs and result in increased HIV replication and development of drug-resistant viral strains.

☑ It is generally recommended that herbal products not be used with antiretroviral medications. The protease inhibitors are particularly sensitive to the effects of herbal remedies, and the use of these products may result in decreased serum levels. In controlled clinical trials, St. John's wort and garlic reduced serum levels of specific protease inhibitors. Echinacea should also be avoided because it may stimulate viral replication.

☑ Request information about adverse effects associated with the specific drugs you are taking and what you should do if they occur. Adverse effects vary among the drugs; some are potentially serious.

☑ Have regular blood tests including viral load, CD4+ cell count, complete blood count, and others as indicated (eg, tests of kidney and liver function).

☑ Keep your health care providers informed about all medications being taken; do not take any other drugs (including drugs of abuse, herbal preparations, vitamin/mineral supplements, non-prescription drugs) without consulting a health care provider. These preparations may make anti-HIV medications less effective or more toxic.

☑ If amprenavir is prescribed:

    ☑ Tell the prescriber if you are allergic to sulfa drugs. Amprenavir is a sulfonamide; it is unknown whether people allergic to sulfa drugs are allergic to amprenavir.

☑ Women who take hormonal contraceptives may need to use a second form of contraception.

☑ Do not take vitamin E supplements because amprenavir capsules and oral solution contain more than the recommended daily amount of vitamin E.

☑ With nelfinavir, women using oral contraceptives may need to use a second form of contraception.

Self-Administration

☑ Take the medications exactly as prescribed. Do not change doses or stop the medications without consulting a health care provider. If a dose is missed, do not double the next dose. The drugs must be taken consistently to suppress HIV infection and minimize adverse drug effects.

☑ These medications vary in their interactions with food and should be taken appropriately for optimal benefit. Unless otherwise instructed, take the drugs as follows:

    ☑ **Abacavir, amprenavir, Combivir, delavirdine, efavirenz, famciclovir, fosamprenavir, lamivudine, nevirapine, stavudine, tenofovir, Trizivir,** and **valacyclovir** may be taken with or without food. However, do not take **abacavir, amprenavir,** or **efavirenz** with a high-fat meal. Also, if taking an antacid or didanosine, take **amprenavir** at least 1 hour before or after a dose of antacid or didanosine.

    ☑ Take **didanosine** and **indinavir** on an empty stomach. This usually means 1 hour before or 2 hours after a meal. Although indinavir is best absorbed if taken on an empty stomach, with water, it may also be taken with skim milk, juice, coffee, tea, or a light meal (eg, toast, cereal). If you are taking indinavir and didanosine, the drugs should be taken at least 1 hour apart on an empty stomach.

    ☑ Take **atazanavir, ganciclovir, Kaletra, nelfinavir,** and **ritonavir** with food. The oral solution of ritonavir may be mixed with chocolate milk to improve the taste.

    ☑ Take **saquinavir** within 2 hours after a meal.

☑ **Delavirdine** tablets may be mixed in water by adding four tablets to at least 3 ounces of water, waiting a few minutes, and then stirring. Drink the mixture promptly, rinse the glass, and swallow the rinse to be sure the entire dose is taken.

☑ To give **nelfinavir** to infants and young children, the oral powder can be mixed with a small amount of water, milk, or formula. After it is mixed, the entire amount must be taken to obtain the full dose. Acidic foods or juices (eg, applesauce, orange juice, apple juice) should not be used because they produce a bitter taste.

● Combination antiretroviral therapy is the standard of care. A commonly used three-drug regimen includes two NRTIs and a protease inhibitor. Other options include two NRTIs and one NNRTI (most commonly efavirenz) or three NRTIs. The choice of specific drugs must be accomplished with consider-

ation of the client's health status, adverse drug effects, and potential drug interactions. For example, anorexia may prevent clients from following dietary recommendations to promote absorption of some protease inhibitors; bone marrow suppression induced by zidovudine may make the drug intolerable; specific combinations of NRTIs may increase the likelihood of neuropathy; and multiple drug interactions may occur, especially between protease inhibitors and many other drugs. Because of the high risk of drug interactions, clients considering initiating new drugs (including over-the-counter, herbal, or other preparations) should discuss the potential effects on their anti-HIV drug regimen with a health care provider.

Therapy with a single anti-HIV medication should never be used except during pregnancy, to reduce perinatal transmission.

- When initiating drug therapy, medications should be started concurrently and in full therapeutic doses.
- Potentially serious drug interactions, especially between protease inhibitors and other agents, are extensive and often require drug substitution or dose reduction to avoid toxicity. Clients should be assessed for signs and symptoms of adverse drug effects at least twice during the first month of treatment, and approximately every 3 months during therapy.
- Effective drug therapy usually produces significantly reduced plasma HIV RNA levels by 2 months and undetectable levels (<400 copies/mL) by 4 to 6 months. Failure to obtain an undetectable viral load may result from nonadherence to the medication regimen, inadequate drugs or doses, drug-resistant viral strains, and a number of other factors.
- Laboratory tests are used to determine when to initiate drug therapy and to assess adherence and response to therapy. Viral load is a measure of the number of HIV RNA particles within the blood; it does not measure viral levels in tissues, where viral reproduction may be continuing. Measurement is recommended at the time of diagnosis and subsequently every 3 to 4 months in untreated clients. In treated clients, HIV RNA levels should be assessed before and 2 to 8 weeks after starting drug therapy, then every 3 to 4 months. Serial measurements should be done in the same laboratory because slight variations may occur among different assay tests and techniques.

CD4+ cell counts are also assessed and used to monitor effective drug therapy. CD4+ cell counts should be measured at the time of diagnosis and approximately every 3 to 6 months thereafter. Complete blood counts, electrolyte panels, and tests of renal and hepatic function are also recommended.

- Clients receiving drug therapy for advanced HIV infection should continue medications during an opportunistic infection or malignancy, unless there are significant drug intolerances, toxicities, or interactions.
- Reasons for temporary interruption of therapy include intolerable adverse effects, drug interac-

tions, and unavailability of drug. Although interruptions increase the risk of drug resistance, the time interval between stopping drug therapy and the development of drug resistance is unknown. If one antiretroviral drug must be stopped for a prolonged period, then all medications should be discontinued. Continuing one or two drugs may select for drug-resistant strains.

- Updated treatment guidelines are readily available via the Internet at www.aidsinfo.nih.gov.

APPLYING YOUR KNOWLEDGE 35-3

During the course of therapy for Mr. Bronowicz, periodic laboratory tests will be done to monitor the effectiveness of drug therapy. What cell count is assessed and how often should it be monitored?

Use in Special Populations

Use in Children

The use of systemic antiviral drugs may be difficult in children because several of the available agents have not been tested in this group, are not available in pediatric formulations, and/or do not have pediatric dosages.

Amantadine may be given to prevent or treat influenza A in children 1 year of age or older, and rimantadine is given only for prevention in children. Oseltamivir may be used in children 1 year and older, zaramivir in children 7 years and older.

Cidofovir is highly nephrotoxic and should probably not be used in children because of long-term risks of carcinogenicity and reproductive toxicity.

Consistent with most other viral infections, few guidelines exist regarding the use of anti-HIV drugs in children. Most HIV infections in children result from perinatal transmission and HIV testing of pregnant women should be a part of routine perinatal care. HIV-seropositive females should receive zidovudine to prevent perinatal transmission. At 14 to 34 weeks of gestation, zidovudine should be administered at a dose of 100 milligrams PO five times a day until delivery. At delivery, a loading dose of 2 milligrams per kilogram of body weight should be administered, followed by 1 milligram per kilogram of body weight per hour until birth. The infant is then given zidovudine 2 milligrams per kilogram of body weight every 6 hours for the first 6 weeks of life. If perinatal infection occurs, the infant usually develops symptoms (eg, an opportunistic infection, failure to thrive) within the first 3 to 8 months of life. Zidovudine, which is approved for treatment of HIV infection in children, is usually the drug of choice. As in adults, anemia and neutropenia are common adverse effects of zidovudine.

Abacavir can be used in clients 3 months to 13 years of age; amprenavir can be used in children 4 to 16 years of age; didanosine is an alternative for children who do not respond to zidovudine; nelfinavir may be used in children 2 years of age and older; and delavirdine and zalcitabine may be used in adolescents. Kaletra can be used for children 6 months or older.

Safety and effectiveness of several antiretroviral drugs have not been established (eg, indinavir, fosamprenavir, atazanavir, and stavudine for any age group; ritonavir for those younger than 12 years of age; saquinavir for those younger than 16 years of age).

Use in Older Adults

Antiviral drug selection and dosing should proceed cautiously with older adults, who often have impaired organ function, concomitant diseases, and/or other drug therapy. Most systemic antiviral drugs are excreted by the kidneys and renal impairment is common in older adults. Therefore, greater risks of toxicity exist. These risks may be minimized by dose reduction when indicated by decreased creatinine clearance (CrCl). When amantadine is given to prevent or treat influenza A, dosage should be reduced with renal impairment, and older adults should be closely monitored for CNS (eg, hallucinations, depression, confusion) and cardiovascular (eg, congestive heart failure, orthostatic hypotension) effects.

There is little information regarding the effects of anti-HIV medications in older adults. As potent antiretroviral therapy continues to extend the lifespan of HIV-seropositive clients, clinicians can expect to encounter greater numbers of older adults who take these medications. As a general rule, renal impairment may necessitate adjustment of NRTI and NNRTI doses, and hepatic impairment will affect dosing of protease inhibitors.

Use in Clients With Renal Impairment

Antiviral drugs should be used cautiously in clients with impaired renal function because some of these drugs are nephrotoxic, most are eliminated by the kidneys, and many require dosage reductions because their elimination may be decreased. All clients with renal impairment should be monitored closely for abnormal renal function tests and drug-related toxicity. Renal effects and guidelines for usage of selected drugs are described in the following sections.

Nephrotoxic Drugs
- **Acyclovir** may precipitate in renal tubules and cause renal impairment with high doses of oral drug or IV administration (eg, to treat acute herpes zoster). This is most likely to occur in clients who are dehydrated and may be minimized by maintaining a high urine output. Although clients on hemodialysis usually need reduced doses, an additional dose is needed after dialysis because treatment removes up to 51% of serum acyclovir.
- **Cidofovir** is nephrotoxic in approximately 50% of clients. It is contraindicated in clients who are taking other nephrotoxic drugs or who have abnormal renal function tests (eg, baseline serum creatinine >1.5 mg/dL,

CrCl ≤55 mL/minute, or proteinuria ≥ 2+). Acute renal failure can occur and renal function may not return to baseline after drug discontinuation. Guidelines to minimize nephrotoxicity include avoiding higher-than-recommended doses, rates of infusion, and frequencies of administration; pre-hydration with IV 0.9% sodium chloride injection; administration of probenecid with each infusion; monitoring serum creatinine and urine protein levels 48 hours prior to each dose; and dose adjustment when indicated.
- **Foscarnet** may cause or worsen renal impairment and should be used with caution in all clients. Manifestations of renal impairment are most likely to occur during the second week of induction therapy, but may occur any time during treatment. Renal impairment may be minimized by monitoring renal function (eg, at baseline; 2 or 3 times weekly during induction; at least every 1 or 2 weeks during maintenance therapy) and reducing dosage accordingly. The drug should be stopped if CrCl drops below 0.4 mL/minute/kg. Adequate hydration should also be maintained throughout the course of drug therapy.
- **Indinavir** may cause nephrolithiasis, flank pain, and hematuria. Symptoms usually subside with increased hydration and drug discontinuation. To avoid nephrolithiasis, clients on indinavir should consume six to eight full 8-ounce glasses of water or other appropriate fluid per day.

Drugs That Require Dosage Reduction
- **Amantadine, emtricitabine, famciclovir, ganciclovir, lamivudine, stavudine, valacyclovir,** and **zalcitabine** are eliminated mainly through the kidneys. In clients with renal impairment, they may accumulate, produce higher blood levels, have longer half-lives, and cause toxicity. For all of these drugs except famciclovir and emtricitabine, dosage should be reduced with CrCl levels below 50 mL/minute. With famciclovir, dosage should be decreased with CrCl below 60 mL/minute. For clients receiving hemodialysis, dosages should be calculated according to CrCl, with daily doses given after dialysis. With emtricitabine, dosage is reduced by extending the dosage interval. Prescribers should consult manufacturers' recommendations.
- **Zidovudine** dosage should be decreased in cases of severe renal impairment. Zidovudine is mainly metabolized in the liver to an inactive metabolite that is then eliminated renally (approximately 60%–75% of a dose); another 20% is excreted as unchanged drug in the urine. Thus, mild to moderate renal impairment does not lead to drug accumulation or a need for reduced dosage. With severe impairment, however, drug half-life is prolonged, possibly because some metabolism occurs in the kidneys as well as the liver. Also, clients with renal impairment may be more likely to experience zidovudine-induced

hematologic adverse effects because of decreased production of erythropoietin. Because of these factors, it is recommended that the daily dosage be reduced by approximately 50% in clients with severe renal impairment (CrCl <25 mL/minute) and clients on hemodialysis.

● **Didanosine** doses are approximately 60% excreted in the urine as unchanged drug. The remainder is metabolized in the liver to several metabolites, including one with antiviral activity. In clients with severe renal impairment, didanosine is eliminated slowly and has a longer half-life. Thus, dosage reduction is indicated to prevent drug accumulation and toxic effects in clients with renal impairment. Also, standard didanosine tablets—unlike the enteric-coated formulation (didanosine EC)—contain sodium and magnesium, which may accumulate in clients with reduced renal function.

Use in Clients With Hepatic Impairment

The antiviral drugs of most concern in hepatic impairment are the anti-HIV agents, especially the protease inhibitors. Although most antiretroviral drugs have not been studied in clients with hepatic impairment, several are primarily metabolized in the liver and may produce high blood levels and cause adverse effects in the presence of liver dysfunction. In addition, clients with HIV infection may have concomitant liver disease that further impairs hepatic metabolism and elimination of the drugs. Although few guidelines are available, dosages should be individualized according to the severity of hepatic impairment and HIV infection; other drug therapies (for HIV infection, opportunistic infections, or other conditions); additional risk factors for drug toxicity; and the potential for drug interactions. In addition, all clients with hepatic impairment should be monitored closely for abnormal liver function tests (LFTs) and drug-related toxicity. Hepatic effects and considerations for usage of selected drugs are as follows:

● **Amprenavir, atazanavir, delavirdine, didanosine, fosamprenavir, nelfinavir, nevirapine, ritonavir, saquinavir,** and **tenofovir** may need dosage reductions in clients with impaired hepatic function.
● **Nevirapine** may cause abnormal LFTs, and a few cases of fatal hepatitis have been reported. If moderate or severe LFT abnormalities occur, nevirapine administration should be discontinued until LFTs return to baseline. If liver dysfunction recurs when the drug is resumed, nevirapine should be discontinued permanently.
● **Zidovudine** is eliminated slowly and has a longer half-life in clients with moderate to severe liver disease. Thus, daily doses should be reduced by 50% in clients with hepatic impairment.

Use in Home Care

Most antiviral drugs are self-administered or dosed by caregivers in the home setting. Precautions to prevent viral infections from occurring or spreading are important because of the close contact among members of a household. The home care nurse may be required to teach infection-control precautions and to assess the immunization status of all household members. If immunizations are indicated, the nurse may need to teach about, encourage, provide, or facilitate their administration.

Home care of clients with HIV infection may include a variety of activities, such as teaching clients and caregivers about the disease and its treatment; assisting with drug therapy for HIV or opportunistic infections; coordinating medical and social services; managing symptoms of infection or adverse drug effects; and preventing or minimizing opportunistic infections.

NURSING ACTIONS

Antiviral Drugs

NURSING ACTIONS	RATIONALE/EXPLANATION
1. Administer accurately	
a. Give oral drugs as recommended in relation to meals:	Manufacturers' recommendations to promote absorption and bioavailability
(1) Give abacavir, amprenavir, fosamprenavir, delavirdine, efavirenz, famciclovir, lamivudine, nevirapine, stavudine, tenofovir, and valacyclovir with or without food. However, do not give abacavir, amprenavir, or efavirenz with a high-fat meal. Also, if the client is taking an antacid or didanosine, give amprenavir at least 1 hour before or after a dose of antacid or didanosine. Avoid antacids in combination with atazanavir.	

NURSING ACTIONS	RATIONALE/EXPLANATION
(2) Give didanosine and indinavir on an empty stomach, 1 hour before or 2 hours after a meal. Although indinavir is best absorbed if taken on an empty stomach, with water, it may also be taken with skim milk, juice, coffee, tea, or a light meal (eg, toast, cereal). If the patient is taking indinavir and didanosine, the drugs should be given at least 1 hour apart on an empty stomach.	
(3) Give ganciclovir, nelfinavir, Kaletra, and ritonavir with food. The oral solution of ritonavir may be mixed with chocolate milk to improve the taste.	
(4) Give saquinavir within 2 hours after a meal.	
b. Delavirdine tablets may be mixed in water by adding four tablets to at least 3 ounces of water, waiting a few minutes, and then stirring. Have the client drink the mixture promptly, rinse the glass, and swallow the rinse to be sure the entire dose is taken.	
c. To give nelfinavir to infants and young children, the oral powder can be mixed with a small amount of water, milk, or formula. After it is mixed, the entire amount must be taken to obtain the full dose.	Acidic foods or juices (eg, orange juice, apple juice, applesauce) should not be used because they produce a bitter taste.
d. Give intravenous (IV) acyclovir, cidofovir, foscarnet, and ganciclovir over 1 hour.	To decrease tissue irritation and increased toxicity from high plasma levels
e. With cidofovir therapy, give probenecid 2 grams 3 hours before cidofovir, 1 gram 2 hours before cidofovir, and 1 gram 8 hours after completion of the cidofovir infusion.	To slow renal excretion of cidofovir and decrease nephrotoxic effects
f. When applying topical acyclovir, wear a glove.	
g. With administering ribavirin by inhalation, follow the manufacturer's instructions.	
2. Observe for therapeutic effects	
a. With acyclovir for genital herpes, observe for fewer recurrences when given for prophylaxis; observe for healing of lesions and decreased pain and itching when given for treatment.	
b. With amantadine, observe for absence of symptoms when given for prophylaxis of influenza A, and decreased fever, cough, muscle aches, and malaise when given for treatment.	
c. With cidofovir, ganciclovir, or foscarnet for cytomegalovirus retinitis, observe for improved vision.	
d. With ophthalmic drugs, observe for decreased signs of eye infection.	
e. With antiretroviral drugs, observe for improved clinical status and improved laboratory markers (eg, decreased viral load, increased CD4+ cell count)	
3. Observe for adverse effects	
a. General effects—anorexia, nausea, vomiting, diarrhea, fever, headache	These effects occur with most systemic antiviral drugs and may range from mild to severe.
b. With IV acyclovir—phlebitis at injection site; skin rash; urticaria; increased blood urea nitrogen or serum creatinine; encephalopathy manifested by confusion, coma, lethargy, seizures, tremors	Encephalopathy is rare but potentially serious; other effects commonly occur.

(continued)

NURSING ACTIONS	RATIONALE/EXPLANATION
c. With topical acyclovir—burning or stinging and pruritus	These effects are usually transient.
d. With amantadine and rimantadine—central nervous system (CNS) effects with anxiety, ataxia, dizziness, hyperexcitability, insomnia, mental confusion, hallucinations, slurred speech	CNS symptoms are reportedly more likely with amantadine than with rimantadine and may be similar to those caused by atropine and CNS stimulants. Adverse reactions are more likely to occur in older adults and those with renal impairment.
e. With didanosine, stavudine, and zidovudine—peripheral neuropathy (numbness, burning, pain in hands and feet), pancreatitis (abdominal pain, severe nausea and vomiting, elevated serum amylase)	Peripheral neuropathy is more likely with stavudine, and the drug should be discontinued if symptoms occur. Pancreatitis may be more likely with didanosine, especially in clients with previous episodes, alcohol consumption, elevated serum triglycerides, or advanced human immunodeficiency virus (HIV) infection. Didanosine should be stopped promptly if symptoms of pancreatitis occur.
f. With ganciclovir and foscarnet—bone marrow depression (anemia, leukopenia, neutropenia, thrombocytopenia), renal impairment (increased serum creatinine and decreased creatinine clearance), neuropathy	Renal impairment may be more likely to occur with foscarnet.
g. With indinavir, ritonavir, and saquinavir—circumoral and peripheral paresthesias, debilitation, fatigue	The most frequent adverse effects are the general ones listed above. Most are relatively mild.
h. With stavudine—peripheral neuropathy, flu-like syndrome (fever, malaise, muscle and joint aches or pain), dizziness, insomnia, depression	
i. With ophthalmic antiviral drugs—pain, itching, edema, or inflammation of the eyelids	These symptoms result from tissue irritation or hypersensitivity reactions.
j. With inhaled ribavirin—increased respiratory distress	Pulmonary function may deteriorate.
k. With zidovudine—bone marrow depression (anemia, leukopenia, granulocytopenia, thrombocytopenia); anemia and neutropenia in newborn infants	Anemia may occur within 2–4 weeks of starting the drug; granulocytopenia is more likely after 6–8 weeks. A complete blood count should be performed every 2 weeks. Colony-stimulating factors have been used to aid recovery of bone marrow function. Blood transfusions may be given for anemia. Hematologic effects may occur in newborn infants when the mothers received zidovudine during pregnancy.
4. Observe for drug interactions	Antiviral drugs are often given concomitantly with each other and with many other drugs, especially those used to treat opportunistic infections and other illnesses associated with HIV infection and organ transplantation. In general, combinations of drugs that cause similar, potentially serious adverse effects (eg, bone marrow depression, peripheral neuropathy) should be avoided, when possible.
a. Drugs that *increase* effects of acyclovir:	
(1) Probenecid	May increase blood levels of acyclovir by slowing its renal excretion
(2) Zidovudine	Severe drowsiness and lethargy may occur.
b. Drugs that *increase* effects of amantadine and rimantadine:	
(1) Anticholinergics—atropine, first-generation antihistamines, antipsychotics, tricyclic antidepressants	These drugs add to the anticholinergic effects (eg, blurred vision, mouth dryness, urine retention, constipation, tachycardia) of the antiviral agents.
(2) CNS stimulants	These drugs add to the CNS-stimulating effects (eg, confusion, insomnia, nervousness, hyperexcitability) of the antiviral agents.
c. Drugs that *increase* effects of cidofovir and foscarnet:	
(1) Aminoglycoside antibiotics, amphotericin B, didanosine, IV pentamidine	These drugs are nephrotoxic themselves and increase risks of nephrotoxicity.

NURSING ACTIONS	RATIONALE/EXPLANATION
d. Drugs that *increase* effects of ganciclovir:	
(1) Imipenem-cilastatin	Increased risk of seizures; avoid the combination if possible.
(2) Nephrotoxic drugs (eg, amphotericin B, cyclosporine)	Increased serum creatinine and potential nephrotoxicity
(3) Probenecid	May increase blood levels of ganciclovir by decreasing its renal excretion
e. Drugs that *increase* effects of indinavir:	
(1) Clarithromycin, ketoconazole, quinidine, zidovudine.	Increase blood levels of indinavir, probably by decreasing its metabolism and elimination
f. Drugs that *decrease* effects of indinavir:	
(1) Didanosine	Didanosine increases gastric pH and decreases absorption of indinavir. If the two drugs are given concurrently, give at least 1 hour apart, on an empty stomach.
(2) Fluconazole	Decreases blood levels of indinavir
(3) Rifampin, rifabutin	These drugs speed up metabolism of indinavir by inducing hepatic drug-metabolizing enzymes.
g. Drug that *increases* the effects of lamivudine:	
(1) Trimethoprim-sulfamethoxazole	Decreases elimination of lamivudine
h. Drugs that *increase* the effects of ritonavir:	
(1) Clarithromycin, fluconazole, fluoxetine	Increase blood levels, probably by slowing metabolism of ritonavir
i. Drug that *decreases* the effects of ritonavir:	
(1) Rifampin	Accelerates metabolism of ritonavir by inducing drug-metabolizing enzymes in the liver
j. Drug that *increases* the effects of saquinavir:	
(1) Ketoconazole	Increases blood levels of saquinavir
k. Drugs that *decrease* the effects of saquinavir:	
(1) Rifampin, rifabutin	Accelerate metabolism of ritonavir by inducing drug-metabolizing enzymes in the liver
l. Drugs that *increase* the effects of zalcitabine:	
(1) Chloramphenicol, cisplatin, didanosine, ethionamide, isoniazid, metronidazole, nitrofurantoin, phenytoin, ribavirin, vincristine	Zalcitabine and these drugs are associated with peripheral neuropathy; concomitant use increases risks of this adverse effect.
(2) Cimetidine, probenecid	Increase blood levels of zalcitabine by decreasing its elimination
(3) Pentamidine (IV)	Increased risk of pancreatitis. If IV pentamidine is used to treat *Pneumocystis jiroveci* pneumonia, zalcitabine should be interrupted.
m. Drugs that *decrease* effects of zalcitabine:	
(1) Antacids, metoclopramide	Decrease absorption. Do not give antacids at the same time as zalcitabine.
n. Drugs that *increase* effects of zidovudine:	
(1) Doxorubicin, vincristine, vinblastine	Increased bone marrow depression, including neutropenia
(2) Amphotericin B, flucytosine	Increased nephrotoxicity
(3) Ganciclovir, pentamidine	Increased neutropenia
(4) Probenecid, trimethoprim	May increase blood levels of zidovudine, probably by decreasing renal excretion

(continued)

NURSING ACTIONS	RATIONALE/EXPLANATION
o. Drugs that *decrease* effects of zidovudine:	
(1) Rifampin, rifabutin	Accelerate metabolism of zidovudine
p. Drugs that *decrease* effects of Kaletra:	
(1) Efavirenz	Dosage of Kaletra may need to be increased if it is given concomitantly
(2) Nevirapine	with one of these drugs.
q. Drugs that *decrease* effects of atazanavir:	Decreased stomach acidity results in reduced absorption of atazanavir.
(1) Antacids	
(2) Histamine H$_2$ antagonists, proton pump inhibitors	

APPLYING YOUR KNOWLEDGE: ANSWERS

35-1 Ritonavir may increase the plasma concentration of meperidine to dangerous levels with potentially serious adverse effects. Meperidine is contraindicated with ritonavir and should not be administered.

35-2 Both of Mr. Bronowicz's current antiretroviral medications may be taken with food, so he may take them with meals. This will also help with his stomach irritation. Encourage Mr. Bronowicz to continue the drug regimen.

35-3 In an effective drug regimen, the CD4+ cell count should be greater than 350 cells/mm^3. The cell count should be performed approximately every 3 to 6 months during treatment.

Review and Application Exercises

Short Answer Exercises

1. What are the predominant effects of antiviral drugs on susceptible viruses?

2. Which viral infections may be prevented by administration of antiviral drugs?

3. What are the major adverse effects associated with commonly used antiviral drugs? How would you assess for each of these adverse effects?

4. Why is it important to monitor renal function in any client receiving a systemic antiviral drug?

5. What is the advantage of combination drug therapy for HIV infection?

6. List nursing interventions to prevent or minimize adverse effects of anti-HIV drugs.

NCLEX-Style Questions

7. Which of the following drugs is used to treat influenza A infection?
   a. ganciclovir (Cytovene)
   b. amantadine (Symmetrel)
   c. nevirapine (Viramune)
   d. ritonavir (Norvir)

8. For a client receiving acyclovir (Zovirax) for genital herpes, an expected outcome is
   a. decreased fever
   b. decreased pain
   c. prevention of recurrence
   d. fewer and smaller lesions

9. Which of the following antiviral drugs is given to pregnant women to prevent transmission of HIV infection to an infant?
   a. zidovudine (AZT)
   b. vidarabine (Vira-A)
   c. zalcitabine (Hivid)
   d. ribavirin (Virazole)

10. A 21-year-old man is being started on a combination of drugs for treatment of AIDS. Which of the following statements indicates understanding of client teaching?
    a. "The medicines inactivate the virus and prevent recurrence of the disease."
    b. "The medicines do not promote the development of drug-resistant viral strains."
    c. "The medicines slow the progression of the disease but do not cure it."
    d. "The medicines prevent the occurrence of opportunistic infections."

11. Enfuvirtide (Fuzeon) exerts its anti-HIV viral effects by
    a. inhibiting reverse transcriptase enzymes
    b. inhibiting protease enzymes
    c. having direct toxic effects on the virus in the bloodstream
    d. preventing the virus from attaching to human cells

Selected References

Albo, T., & Terriff, C. M. 2004. Enfuvirtide: An HIV fusion inhibitor. *Advances in Pharmacy, 2*(1), 12–18.

Drug facts and comparisons. (Updated monthly). St. Louis: Facts and Comparisons.

Fletcher, C. V., Kakuda, T. N., & Collier, A. C. (2002). Human immunodeficiency virus infection. In J. T. DiPiro, R. L. Talbert, G. C. Yee, G. R. Matzke, B. G. Wells, & L. M. Posey (Eds.), *Pharmacotherapy: A pathophysiologic approach* (5th ed., pp. 2151–2174). New York: McGraw-Hill.

Masur, H. (2004). Treatment of HIV infection and AIDS. In L. Goldman & D. Ausiello (Eds.), *Cecil textbook of medicine* (22nd ed., pp. 2183–2191). Philadelphia: W. B. Saunders.

Modrzejewski, K. A., & Herman, R. A. (2004). Emtricitabine: A once-daily nucleoside reverse transcriptase inhibitor. *The Annals of Pharmacotherapy, 38,* 1006–1014.

Rivkin, A. M. (2004). Adefovir dipivoxil in the treatment of chronic hepatitis B. *The Annals of Pharmacotherapy, 38,* 625–633.

Sweeney, K. A. (2005). Acquired immunodeficiency syndrome. In C. M. Porth, *Pathophysiology: Concepts of altered health states* (7th ed., pp. 427–445). Philadelphia: Lippincott Williams & Wilkins.

Taylor, K. H., & Chung, A. M. (2004). Metabolic complications of antiretroviral therapy. *Advances in Pharmacy, 2*(1), 29–40.

Terriff, C. M. (2004). Atazanavir (Reyataz): A new HIV protease inhibitor. *Advances in Pharmacy, 2*(1), 5–11.

U.S. Department of Health and Human Services. (2004). *Public Health Service Task Force Recommendations for Use of Antiretroviral Drugs in Pregnant HIV-1-Infected Women for Maternal Health and Interventions to Reduce Perinatal HIV-1 Transmission in the United States, December 17, 2004.* Retrieved September 27, 2005, from http://www.aidsinfo.nih.gov/

Whitley, R. J. (2004). Antiviral therapy (non-AIDS). In L. Goldman & D. Ausiello (Eds.), *Cecil textbook of medicine* (22nd ed., pp. 1960–1967). Philadelphia: W. B. Saunders.

Yeni, P. G., Hammer, S. M., Hirsch, M. S., et al. (2004). Treatment for adult HIV infection: 2004 Recommendations of the International AIDS Society–USA Panel. *Journal of the American Medical Association, 292*(2), 251–265.

Antifungal Drugs

OBJECTIVES

After studying this chapter, you will be able to:

1. Describe characteristics of fungi and fungal infections.
2. Discuss antibacterial drug therapy and immunosuppression as risk factors for development of fungal infections.
3. Describe commonly used antifungal drugs in terms of indications for use, adverse effects, and nursing process implications.
4. Differentiate between adverse effects associated with systemic and topical antifungal drugs.
5. Teach clients about prevention and treatment of fungal infections.

APPLYING YOUR KNOWLEDGE

Charlotte Angelo, age 21, is on antibiotic therapy for a urinary tract infection. During the course of her therapy she develops vaginal discharge and is diagnosed with a *Candida albicans* vaginal infection. The primary care provider prescribes fluconazole (Diflucan) 150 mg PO, one dose.

INTRODUCTION

Fungi

Fungi are molds and yeasts that are widely dispersed in the environment and are either saprophytic (ie, obtain food from dead organic matter) or parasitic (ie, obtain nourishment from living organisms). *Molds* are multicellular organisms comprised of colonies of tangled strands. They form a fuzzy coating on various surfaces (eg, the mold that forms on spoiled food, the mildew that forms on clothing in damp environments). *Yeasts* are unicellular organisms. Some fungi, called *dermatophytes,* can grow only at the cooler temperatures of body surfaces. Other fungi, called *dimorphic,* can grow as molds outside the body and as yeasts in the warm temperatures of the body. As molds, these fungi produce spores that can persist indefinitely in the environment and be carried by the wind to distant locations. When these mold spores enter the body, most often by inhalation, they rapidly become yeasts that can invade body tissues. Dimorphic fungi include a number of human pathogens such as those that cause blastomycosis, histoplasmosis, and coccidioidomycosis.

Fungi that are pathogenic in humans exist in soil, decaying plants, and other environmental habitats or as part of the endoge-nous human flora. For example, *Candida albicans* organisms are part of the normal microbial flora of the skin, mouth, gastrointestinal (GI) tract, and vagina. Growth of *Candida* organisms is normally restrained by intact immune mechanisms and bacterial competition for nutrients. When these restraining forces are altered (eg, by suppression of the immune system, antibacterial drug therapy), fungal overgrowth and opportunistic infection can occur. In addition, some fungi have characteristics that enhance their ability to cause disease. *Cryptococcus neoformans* organisms, for example, can become encapsulated, which allows them to evade the normal immune defense mechanism of phagocytosis. *Aspergillus* organisms produce protease, an enzyme that allows them to destroy structural proteins and penetrate body tissues.

Structurally, fungi are larger and more complex than bacteria. They have a thick, rigid cell wall, of which glucan is one of the components. Glucan is formed by the fungal enzyme, glucan synthetase. Fungi also have a cell membrane composed mainly of ergosterol, a lipid that is similar to cholesterol in human cell membranes. Within the cell membrane, structures are mostly the same as those in human cells (eg, a nucleus, mitochondria, Golgi apparatus, ribosomes attached to endoplasmic reticulum, a cytoskeleton with microtubules and filaments).

Fungal Infections (Mycoses)

Fungal infections (mycoses) may be mild and superficial or life-threatening and systemic. Dermatophytes cause superficial infections of the skin, hair, and nails. They obtain nourishment from keratin, a protein in skin, hair, and nails. Dermatophytic infections include tinea pedis (athlete's foot) and tinea capitis (ringworm of the scalp) (see Chap. 64).

Systemic or invasive mycoses include the endemic mycoses that can cause disease (eg, blastomycosis, coccidioidomycosis, histoplasmosis, sporotrichosis) in healthy hosts who are exposed to them in the environment and the opportunistic mycoses (eg, aspergillosis, candidiasis, cryptococcosis) that cause serious infection mainly in immunosuppressed hosts. The fungi that cause endemic mycoses exist as molds in the environment; they grow in soil and decaying organic matter. Infection is acquired by inhalation of airborne spores from contaminated soil. Histoplasmosis, coccidioidomycosis, and blastomycosis usually occur as pulmonary disease but may be systemic. These infections often mimic common bacterial infections and their severity is determined both by the extent of the exposure to the organism and by the immune status of the host. The fungi that cause opportunistic mycoses may be part of the normal body flora (eg, *Candida* species) or exist in the environment (*Aspergillus, Cryptococcus*). Infection occurs after inhalation or injection of the fungus into body tissues.

The most common opportunistic infection is candidiasis. *Candida* species are part of the normal human flora and *C. albicans* is a common cause of infection. However, other candidal species also colonize clients, especially with hospitalization and the use of antifungal drugs.

Most fungal infections occur in healthy people but are more severe and invasive in immunocompromised hosts. For example, *C. albicans* organisms often cause superficial mucosal infections (eg, oral, intestinal, or vaginal candidiasis) with antibacterial drug therapy. In immunocompromised hosts, candidal infections are more likely to be deep, widespread, and caused by non-*albicans* species. Serious fungal infections continue to increase in incidence, largely because of human immunodeficiency virus (HIV) infections; the use of immunosuppressant drugs to treat clients with cancer or organ transplants; the use of indwelling intravenous (IV) catheters for prolonged drug therapy or parenteral nutrition; implantation of prosthetic devices; and widespread use of broad-spectrum antibacterial drugs. Characteristics of selected fungal infections are described in Box 36-1.

ANTIFUNGAL DRUGS

Development of drugs that are effective against fungal cells without being excessively toxic to human cells has been limited because fungal cells are similar to human cells. Most of the available drugs target the fungal cell membrane and produce potentially serious toxicities and drug interactions. In general, antifungal drugs produce their therapeutic effects by disrupting the structure and function of fungal cell components (Fig. 36-1).

Polyenes (eg, amphotericin B), azoles (eg, fluconazole), and terbinafine act on ergosterol to disrupt fungal cell membranes. Amphotericin B (and nystatin) binds to ergosterol and forms holes in the membrane, causing leakage of fungal cell contents and lysis of the cell. The azole drugs bind to an enzyme that is required for synthesis of ergosterol. This action causes production of a defective cell membrane, which also allows leakage of intracellular contents and destruction of the cell. Both types of drugs also affect cholesterol in human cell membranes, and this characteristic is considered primarily responsible for the drugs' toxicities.

Echinocandins (eg, caspofungin) are a new class of antifungal drugs that disrupt fungal cell walls rather than fungal cell membranes. They act by inhibiting glucan synthetase, an enzyme required for synthesis of glucan. Glucan is a component of the fungal cell wall; its depletion leads to leakage of cellular contents and cell death. Because human cells do not contain cell walls, these drugs are less toxic than the polyene and azole antifungals.

Drugs for superficial fungal infections of skin and mucous membranes are usually applied topically. Numerous preparations are available, many without a prescription. Drugs for systemic infections are given IV or orally. Clients with HIV infection need aggressive treatment of primary fungal infections and prolonged or lifelong secondary prophylaxis. Clients with prolonged or severe neutropenia secondary to treatment with cytotoxic cancer drugs also require aggressive treatment of fungal infections, because they are at high risk for acute, life-threatening, systemic mycoses such as candidiasis and aspergillosis. Selected antifungal drugs are further described in the following sections. In addition, pharmacokinetic characteristics of selected drugs are listed in Table 36-1; clinical indications for use and dosage ranges are listed in Table 36-2.

Polyenes

Amphotericin B is active against most types of pathogenic fungi and is fungicidal or fungistatic, depending on the concentration in body fluids and the susceptibility of the causative fungus. Because of its toxicity, the drug is used only for serious fungal infections. It is usually given for 4 to 12 weeks.

Lipid formulations (Abelcet, AmBisome, Amphotec) were developed to decrease adverse effects. Compared with the original deoxycholate formulation of amphotericin B (Fungizone), lipid formulations reach higher concentrations in diseased tissues and increase therapeutic effects. At the same time, they produce lower concentrations in normal tissues, which decreases adverse effects and also allows higher doses to be given. These products are much more expensive than

(text continues on page 586)

Box 36-1 Selected Fungal Infections

Aspergillosis occurs in debilitated and immunocompromised people, including those with leukemia, lymphoma, or acquired immunodeficiency syndrome (AIDS), and those with neutropenia from a disease process or drug therapy. Invasive aspergillosis is a serious illness characterized by inflammatory granulomatous lesions, which may develop in the bronchi, lungs, ear canal, skin, or mucous membranes of the eye, nose, or urethra. It may extend into blood vessels, which leads to infection of the brain, heart, kidneys, and other organs. It is associated with thrombosis, ischemic infarction of involved tissues, and progressive disease. It is often fatal.

Allergic bronchopulmonary aspergillosis, an allergic reaction to inhaled aspergillus spores, may develop in people with asthma and cause bronchoconstriction, wheezing, dyspnea, cough, muscle aches, and fever. The condition is aggravated if the spores germinate and grow in the airways, thereby producing chronic exposure to the antigen and permanent fibrotic damage.

Aspergillus mold is widespread in the environment; large numbers of spores are released into the air during soil excavations (eg, for construction or renovation of buildings) or handling of decaying plant matter and are carried into most human environments. Spores have been found in water (eg, hot water faucets, saunas, showerheads, swimming pools, public buildings and private homes (eg, basements, crawl spaces, bedding, humidifiers, ventilation ducts, potted plants, wicker or straw material, house dust); and foods (eg, peppers and spices, pasta, peanuts, cashews, coffee beans). In hospitals, probable sources of infections have included contaminated air from building renovations and new construction; hospital water, which may become aerosolized during activities such as client showering; and cereals, powdered milk, tea, and soy sauce ingested by neutropenic clients. As *Aspergillus* molds grow, they produce toxins (eg, aflatoxin, one of the strongest carcinogens known) that contaminate the food chain.

There are several species that cause invasive disease in humans, but *Aspergillus fumigatus* is the most common (about 90% of cases). *A. fumigatus* reproduces by releasing spores, which are small enough to reach the alveoli when inhaled. Most aspergillus organisms (80%–90%) enter the body through the respiratory system, and pulmonary aspergillosis is acquired by inhalation of the spores. Other potential entry sites include damaged skin (eg, burn wounds, intravenous [IV] catheter insertion sites), operative wounds, the cornea, and the ear. One study investigated invasive aspergillosis in an intensive care unit for liver transplant clients. The first client developed a wound infection 11 days after liver transplantation. Two other clients in the unit developed invasive pulmonary aspergillosis. The researchers concluded that *Aspergillus* organisms can form spores in infected wounds and that debriding and dressing those wounds may result in aerosolization of spores and airborne person-to-person transmission.

Blastomycosis is initiated by inhalation of spores from a fungus that grows in soil and decaying organic matter. The organism is widespread in the southeastern United States, Min-

nesota, Wisconsin, Michigan, and New York. Sporadic cases most often occur in adult males who have extensive exposure to woods and streams with vocational or recreational activities. The infection may be asymptomatic or produce pulmonary symptoms resembling pneumonia, tuberculosis, or lung cancer. It may also be systemic and involve other organs, especially the skin and bone. Skin lesions (eg, pustules, ulcerations, abscesses) may progress over a period of years and eventually involve large areas of the body. Bone invasion, with arthritis and bone destruction, occurs in 25% to 50% of clients.

Blastomycosis can occur in healthy people with sufficient exposure, but is usually more severe and more likely to involve multiple organs and central nervous system (CNS) disease in immunocompromised clients. However, it infrequently occurs in clients with human immunodeficiency virus (HIV) infection.

Candidiasis is a yeast infection that often occurs in clients with malignant lymphomas, diabetes mellitus, or AIDS and in clients receiving antibiotic, antineoplastic, corticosteroid, and immunosuppressant drug therapy. *Candida* organisms are found in soil, on inanimate objects, in hospital environments, and in food. In the human body, they are found on skin and in the gastrointestinal (GI) and genitourinary tracts, including the urine of clients with indwelling bladder catheters. Most infections arise from the normal endogenous organisms of the GI tract and are caused by *Candida albicans*. Oral, intestinal, vaginal, and systemic candidiasis can occur. Early recognition and treatment of local infections may prevent systemic candidiasis.

- **Oral candidiasis** (thrush) is characterized by painless white plaques on oral and pharyngeal mucosa. It often occurs in newborn infants who become infected during passage through an infected or colonized vagina. In older children and adults, thrush may occur as a complication of diabetes mellitus, as a result of poor oral hygiene, or after taking antibiotics or corticosteroids. It may also occur as an early manifestation of AIDS.

- **Gastrointestinal candidiasis** most often occurs after prolonged broad-spectrum antibacterial therapy, which destroys a large part of the normal flora of the intestine. The main symptom is diarrhea.

- **Vaginal candidiasis** commonly occurs in women who are pregnant, have diabetes mellitus, or take oral contraceptives or antibacterial drugs. The main symptom is a yellowish vaginal discharge. The infection may produce inflammation of the perineal area and spread to the buttocks and thighs. The organism is difficult to eradicate, and many women have recurrent infections.

- **Skin candidiasis** usually occurs in people with continuously moist skinfolds or moist surgical dressings. The organism also may cause diaper rash and perineal rashes. Skin lesions are red and macerated.

- **Systemic** or **invasive candidiasis** occurs when the organism gets into the bloodstream and is circulated throughout the body, with the brain, heart, kidneys, and eyes as the most common sites of infection. It often occurs as a nosocomial infection in clients with serious illness or who are undergoing drug therapy that suppresses the immune sys-

Box 36-1 **Selected Fungal Infections** (continued)

tem, and may be fatal. Invasive infections may be present in any organ and may produce such disorders as urinary tract infection, endocarditis, and meningitis. It is usually diagnosed by positive cultures of blood or tissue. Signs and symptoms depend on the severity of the infection and the organs affected, and are indistinguishable from those occurring with bacterial infections. The mortality rate of disseminated candidiasis approaches 40%.

The incidence of severe candidal infections has increased in recent years, in part because of increased numbers of neutropenic and immunodeficient clients. In addition, the frequent use of strong, broad-spectrum antibiotics leads to extensive candidal colonization in debilitated clients, and the widespread use of medical devices (eg, intravascular catheters, monitoring equipment, endotracheal tubes, urinary catheters) allows the organisms to reach sites that are normally sterile. People who use IV drugs also develop invasive candidiasis because the injections inoculate the fungi directly into the bloodstream.

The incidence of invasive infections caused by non-*albicans Candida* species also seems to be increasing. These infections are probably related to the widespread use of antifungal drugs such as fluconazole. In general, non-*albicans* candidal infections are less susceptible to azole antifungal drugs (eg, fluconazole, itraconazole) and are more difficult to treat effectively with the currently available agents.

Coccidioidomycosis is caused by an organism that grows as a mold in soil and decaying organic matter and is commonly found in the southwestern United States and northern Mexico. Infection results from inhalation of spores that convert to yeasts in the warm environment of the body and often cause asymptomatic or mild respiratory infection. However, the organism may cause acute pulmonary infection with fever, chest pain, cough, headache, and loss of appetite. Radiographs may show small nodules in the lung like those seen in tuberculosis. In some cases, chronic disease develops in which the organisms remain localized and cause large, organism-filled cavities in the lung. These cavities may become fibrotic and eventually require surgical excision. In a few cases, severe, disseminated disease occurs, either soon after the primary infection or after years of chronic pulmonary disease. Disseminated coccidioidomycosis may produce an acute or chronic meningitis or a generalized disease with lesions in many internal organs. Skin lesions appear as granulomas that may eventually heal or become ulcerations. Most clients with primary infection recover without treatment; clients with disseminated disease require prolonged chemotherapy.

Coccidioidomycosis may occur in healthy or immunocompromised people but is more severe and more likely to become systemic in immunocompromised clients. For example, clients with AIDS who live in endemic areas are highly susceptible to this infection. The severity of the disease also increases with intensity of exposure.

Cryptococcosis is caused by inhalation of spores of *Cryptococcus neoformans*, an organism found worldwide. *C. neoformans* organisms grow most abundantly in bird

excreta, especially pigeon droppings. They have also been isolated from non-avian sources such as fruits, vegetables, and dairy products.

When cryptococcosis occurs in healthy people, the primary infection is localized in the lungs; is asymptomatic or produces mild symptoms; and heals without treatment. However, pneumonia may occur and lead to spread of the organisms by the bloodstream. When cryptococcosis occurs in immunocompromised people, it is likely to be more severe and to become disseminated to the CNS, skin, and other body organs. People with AIDS are highly susceptible and cryptococcosis is the fourth most frequent opportunistic infection in this population. Infection most often affects the lungs and CNS. Cryptococcal pneumonia in clients with AIDS has a mortality rate of 40% or more. Cryptococcal meningitis, the most common manifestation of disseminated disease, often produces abscesses in the brain. Clinical manifestations include headache, dizziness, and neck stiffness, and the condition is often mistaken for brain tumor. Later symptoms include coma, respiratory failure, and death if the meningitis is not treated effectively.

Histoplasmosis is a common fungal infection that occurs worldwide, especially in the central and mideastern United States. The causative fungus is found in soil and organic debris around chicken houses, bird roosts, and caves inhabited by bats. Exposure to spores may result from activities such as demolishing or remodeling old buildings, clearing brush from urban parks, or cleaning chicken coops. Spores can be picked up by the wind and spread over large areas. Histoplasmosis develops when the spores are inhaled into the lungs, where they rapidly develop into the tissue-invasive yeast cells that reach the bloodstream and become distributed throughout the body. In most cases, the organisms are destroyed or encapsulated by the host's immune system. The lung lesions heal by fibrosis and calcification and resemble the lesions of tuberculosis.

Clinical manifestations may vary widely. In people with a normal immune response, manifestations can be correlated with the extent of exposure. Most infections are asymptomatic or produce minimal symptoms for which treatment is not sought. When symptoms occur, they usually resemble an acute, influenza-like respiratory infection and improve within a few weeks. However, people exposed to large amounts of spores may have a high fever and severe pneumonia, which usually resolves with a low mortality rate. Some people, most often adult men with underlying emphysema or other lung disease, develop chronic pulmonary histoplasmosis with recurrent episodes of cough, fever, and weakness. Some people (10% or fewer) also develop inflammatory complications such as arthritis, arthralgia, or pericarditis. These disorders are usually managed with anti-inflammatory drugs rather than antifungal drug therapy. Some people also develop histoplasmosis years after the primary infection, probably from reactivation of a latent infection. This is likely to occur in clients with AIDS. Histoplasmosis is the most frequent endemic fungal infection occurring in clients with HIV infection and has been recognized as an AIDS-defining illness since 1987.

(continued)

In addition, histoplasmosis occasionally infects the liver, spleen, and other organs and is rapidly fatal if not treated effectively. As with many other infections, the severe, disseminated form usually occurs in clients whose immune system is suppressed by diseases or drugs.

Sporotrichosis occurs when contaminated soil or plant material is inoculated into the skin through small wounds (eg, thorn pricks) on the fingers, hands, or arms. It is most likely to occur among people who handle sphagnum moss, roses, or baled hay. Thus, infection is a hazard for gardeners and greenhouse workers. It can occur in both healthy and immunocompromised people, but is usually more severe and disseminated in the immunocompromised host.

Initial lesions, which are usually small, painless bumps resembling insect bites, occur 1 week to 6 months after inoculation. The subcutaneous nodule develops into a necrotic ulcer, which heals slowly as new ulcers appear in adjacent areas. Local lymphatic channels and lymph nodes also develop abscesses, nodules, and ulcers that may persist for years if the disease is not treated effectively. In immunocompromised people, sporotrichosis may spread to various tissues, including the meninges.

the deoxycholate formulation. They are most likely to be used for clients with pre-existing renal impairment or conditions in which other nephrotoxic drugs are routinely given (eg, bone marrow transplant recipients) and when high doses are needed for difficult-to-treat infections. The various lipid preparations differ in their characteristics and cannot be used interchangeably.

Amphotericin B must be given IV for systemic infections. After infusion, the drug is rapidly taken up by the liver and other organs. It is then slowly released back into the bloodstream. Despite its long-term use, little is known about its distribution and metabolic pathways. Drug concentrations in most body fluids are higher in the presence of inflammation; concentrations in cerebrospinal fluid (CSF) are low with or without inflammation. The drug has an initial serum half-life of 24 hours, which represents redistribution from the bloodstream to tissues. This is followed by a second elimination phase, with a half-life of approximately 15 days, which represents elimination from tissue storage sites. Most of the drug is thought to be metabolized in the tissues; about 5% of the active drug is excreted daily in the urine. After administration is stopped, amphotericin B can be detected in the urine for several weeks.

(text continues on page 590)

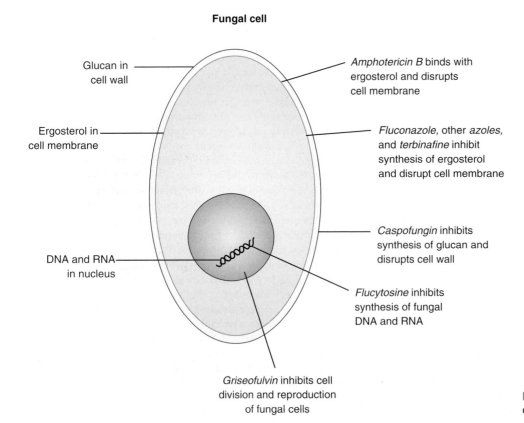

Fungal cell

Glucan in cell wall

Ergosterol in cell membrane

DNA and RNA in nucleus

Amphotericin B binds with ergosterol and disrupts cell membrane

Fluconazole, other *azoles,* and *terbinafine* inhibit synthesis of ergosterol and disrupt cell membrane

Caspofungin inhibits synthesis of glucan and disrupts cell wall

Flucytosine inhibits synthesis of fungal DNA and RNA

Griseofulvin inhibits cell division and reproduction of fungal cells

FIGURE 36-1 Actions of antifungal drugs on fungal cells.

TABLE 36-1 Pharmacokinetics of Systemic Antifungal Drugs

GENERIC/TRADE NAME	PROTEIN BINDING (%)	HALF-LIFE	METABOLISM/EXCRETION	ACTION		
				Onset	Peak	Duration
Amphotericin B deoxycholate (Fungizone)	>90	24 h, then 15 d	Tissues/urine	IV 20–30 min	1–2 h	20–24 h
Fluconazole (Diflucan)	11–12	30 h	80% eliminated in urine as unchanged drug	PO slow IV rapid	1–2 h 1 h	2–4 d 2–4 d
Flucytosine (Ancobon)	Minimal	2–4 h	Mainly eliminated in urine as unchanged drug	PO varies	2 h	10–12 h
Itraconazole (Sporanox)	99	21 h, then 64 h	Hepatic/urine	PO slow IV rapid	4 h	4–6 d
Ketoconazole (Nizoral)	99	8 h	Hepatic/bile	Varies	1–4 h	End of infusion
Terbinafine (Lamisil)	99	36 h	Hepatic/urine		2 h	
Voriconazole (Vfend)	58	6 h	Hepatic/urine	Rapid	<2 h	

IV, intravenous; PO, oral.

Table 36-2 Drugs at a Glance: Selected Antifungal Drugs

GENERIC/TRADE NAME	CLINICAL INDICATIONS	ROUTES AND DOSAGE RANGES	
		Adults	Children
Amphotericin B deoxycholate (Fungizone)	Serious, systemic fungal infections (eg, candidiasis, histoplasmosis) Cutaneous candidiasis Oral candidiasis	IV, individualized according to disease severity and client tolerance. Initial dose often 0.25 mg/kg/d, gradually increased to 0.5–1 mg/kg/d, infused over 2–6 h Topically to skin lesions 2–4 times daily for 1–4 wk Oral suspension (100 mg/mL), 1 mL "swish and swallow" 4 times daily	Same as for adults for IV, skin preparations, and oral suspension
Amphotericin B lipid complex (Abelcet)	Systemic infections in clients who do not tolerate Fungizone	IV 5 mg/kg/d	Same as adults
Liposomal amphotericin B (AmBisome)	Systemic infections in clients who do not tolerate Fungizone Empiric treatment of presumed fungal infections in febrile, neutropenic clients	IV 3–5 mg/kg/d	Same as adults
Amphotericin B cholesteryl (Amphotec)	Systemic infections in clients who do not tolerate Fungizone	IV 3–4 mg/kg/d	Same as adults

(continued)

Table 36-2 Drugs at a Glance: Selected Antifungal Drugs (continued)

GENERIC/TRADE NAME	CLINICAL INDICATIONS	ROUTES AND DOSAGE RANGES	
		Adults	Children
Butenafine (Mentax)	Tinea infections	Topically to skin lesions 1–2 times daily for 1–4 wk	Safety and efficacy not established for children <12 y
Butoconazole (Femstat, Gynazole)	Vaginal candidiasis	Intravaginally, once daily for 3 d	
Caspofungin (Cancidas)	Invasive aspergillosis Candidiasis	IV infusion over 1 h, 70 mg initially, then 50 mg daily Hepatic impairment, 70 mg initially, then 35 mg daily	Safety and efficacy not established
Ciclopirox (Loprox)	Tinea infections, cutaneous candidiasis	Topically to skin lesions, twice daily for 2–4 wk	
Clotrimazole (Lotrimin, Mycelex, Gyne-Lotrimin)	Cutaneous dermatophytosis; oral, cutaneous, and vaginal candidiasis	Orally, 1 troche dissolved in mouth 5 times daily Topically to skin daily for 2–4 wk Intravaginally, once daily for 3–7 d	Same as adults
Econazole (Spectazole)	Tinea infections, cutaneous candidiasis	Topically to skin lesions, once or twice daily for 2–4 wk	Dosage not established
Fluconazole (Diflucan)	Oropharyngeal, esophageal, vaginal, and systemic candidiasis Prevention of candidiasis after bone marrow transplantation Cryptococcal meningitis	Oropharyngeal candidiasis, PO, IV 200 mg first day, then 100 mg daily for 2 wk Esophageal candidiasis, PO, IV, 200 mg first day, then 100 mg daily for at least 3 wk Vaginal candidiasis, PO 150 mg as a single dose Systemic candidiasis, PO, IV 400 mg first day, then 200 mg daily for at least 4 wk Prophylaxis, PO, IV 400 mg once daily Cryptococcal meningitis, PO, IV, 400 mg first day, then 200–400 mg/d for 10–12 wk	Oropharyngeal candidiasis, PO, IV 6 mg/kg first day, then 3 mg/kg/d for at least 2 wk Esophageal candidiasis, PO, IV, 6 mg/kg first day, then 3 mg/kg/d for at least 3 wk Systemic candidiasis, PO, IV 6–12 mg/kg/d Cryptococcal meningitis, PO, IV 12 mg/kg first day, then 6 mg/kg/d for 10–12 wk
Flucytosine (Ancobon)	Systemic mycoses due to *Candida* species or *Cryptococcus neoformans*	PO 50–150 mg/kg/d in divided doses q6h Dosage must be decreased with impaired liver function.	Safety and efficacy not established
Griseofulvin	Dermatophytosis (skin, hair, nails)	PO 250–500 mg daily	PO 5–10 mg/kg/d (micro-size discontinued)
Haloprogin (Halotex)	Dermatophytosis, mainly tinea pedis (athlete's foot), cutaneous candidiasis	Topically to skin, 1% cream or solution twice daily for 2–4 wk	Dosage not established

Table 36-2 Drugs at a Glance: Selected Antifungal Drugs (continued)

		ROUTES AND DOSAGE RANGES	
GENERIC/TRADE NAME	CLINICAL INDICATIONS	Adults	Children
Itraconazole (Sporanox)	Systemic fungal infections, including aspergillosis, in neutropenic and immuno-compromised hosts Onychomycosis Tinea infections	Systemic infection, PO 200 mg once or twice daily for 3 mo Blastomycosis, histoplasmosis, aspergillosis, IV 200 mg twice daily for 4 doses, then 200 mg/d Fingernail onychomycosis, PO 200 mg twice daily for 1 wk, no drug for 3 wk, then repeat dosage for 1 wk Oral solution, 100–200 mg daily (10–20 mL), swish and swallow 3 times daily for 3–5 d Tinea infections, PO 100–200 mg daily for 1–4 wk	Safety and efficacy not established. *3–16-y-old* patients have been treated with 100 mg daily for systemic infections and clients *6 mo–12 y* have been treated with 5 mg/kg once daily for 2 wk without serious or unusual adverse effects.
Ketoconazole (Nizoral)	Candidiasis, histoplasmosis, coccidioidomycosis Cutaneous candidiasis Tinea infections	PO 200 mg once daily, increased to 400 mg once daily if necessary in severe infections Topically, once daily for 2–6 wk	*2 y and older:* PO 3.3–6.6 mg/kg/d as a single dose
Miconazole (Monistat)	Dermatophytosis, cutaneous and vulvovaginal candidiasis	Topically, twice daily for 2–4 wk Intravaginally, vaginal cream, once daily at bedtime for 3–7 d; vaginal suppository, once daily at bedtime (1 d for 1200 mg; 3 d for 200 mg; 7 d for 100 mg)	
Naftifine (Naftin)	Tinea infections (athlete's foot, jock itch, ringworm)	Topically, once daily (cream) or twice daily (gel)	Safety and efficacy not established
Natamycin (Natacyn)	Fungal infections of the eye	Topically, 1 drop q1–2h for 3–4 d, then 1 drop 6–8 times daily for 14–24 d	Safety and efficacy not established
Nystatin (Mycostatin)	Candidiasis of skin, mucous membrane, and intestinal tract	Oral or intestinal infection, PO tablets 1–2 (500,000–1,000,000 units) 3 times daily; oral suspension, 4–6 mL (400,000–600,000 units) 4 times daily; oral troches 1–2 (200,000–400,000 units) 4–5 times daily Topically to skin lesions, 2–3 times daily Intravaginally, 1 vaginal tablet once daily for 14 d	*>1 y:* PO oral suspension, same as adults; *infants,* 2 mL (200,000 units) 4 times daily Oral troches, same as adults for children old enough to suck on the lozenge until it dissolves

(continued)

Table 36–2 Drugs at a Glance: Selected Antifungal Drugs (continued)

GENERIC/TRADE NAME	CLINICAL INDICATIONS	ROUTES AND DOSAGE RANGES	
		Adults	Children
Oxiconazole (Oxistat)	Tinea infections	Topically to skin lesions, once or twice daily for 2–4 wk	Safety and efficacy not established
Sulconazole (Exelderm)	Tinea infections	Topically to skin lesions, once or twice daily for 3–4 wk	Safety and efficacy not established for children <12 y
Terbinafine (Lamisil)	Tinea infections Onychomycosis of fingernails or toenails	Tinea infections, topically to skin, once or twice daily for at least 1 wk and no longer than 4 wk Fingernail infections, PO 250 mg daily for 6 wk Toenail infections, PO 250 mg daily for 12 wk	
Terconazole (Terazol)	Vaginal candidiasis	Intravaginally, 1 applicator once daily at bedtime for 7 doses (0.4% cream) or 3 doses (0.8% cream) Vaginal suppository, 1 daily at bedtime for 3 d	
Tioconazole (Vagistat)	Vaginal candidiasis	Intravaginally, 1 applicator at bedtime	
Tolnaftate (Tinactin)	Cutaneous mycoses (dermatophytosis)	Topically to skin lesions, twice daily for 2–6 wk	
Triacetin (Fungoid)	Dermatophytosis (eg, athlete's foot), cutaneous candidiasis	Topically to skin lesions, 3 times daily	
Voriconazole (Vfend)	Esophageal candidiasis Invasive aspergillosis Other serious fungal infections	Esophageal candidiasis, PO 200 mg q12h for weight of ≥40 kg; 100 mg q12h for weight <40 kg. Give at least 14 d or 7 d after symptoms resolve. Aspergillosis and other serious infections, IV 6 mg/kg q12h for 2 doses (loading dose), then 4 mg/kg q12h (maintenance dose)	Safety and efficacy not established for children <12 y
Zinc undecylenate (Desenex)	Dermatophytosis	Topically to skin twice daily for 2–4 wk	Same as for adults

IV, intravenous; PO, oral.

Adverse effects include an infusion reaction characterized by fever, chills, and tachypnea. Nephrotoxicity is the most common and the most serious long-term adverse effect. The drug apparently damages the kidneys by constricting afferent renal arterioles and reducing blood flow to the kidneys. Several measures may decrease nephrotoxicity, such as keeping the client well hydrated, giving 0.9% sodium chloride IV prior to drug administration, and avoiding the concomitant administration of other nephrotoxic drugs (eg, aminoglycoside antibiotics) or diuretics. Hypokalemia and hypomagnesemia also occur and may require oral or IV mineral replacement. Additional adverse effects include anorexia, nausea, vomiting, anemia, and phlebitis at peripheral infusion sites. A central vein is preferred for administration.

Nystatin has the same mechanism of action as amphotericin B. However, it is used only for topical therapy of oral, intestinal, and vaginal candidiasis because it is too toxic for systemic use. Although given orally for oral or intestinal infections, the drug is not absorbed systemically and it is excreted in the feces after oral use. With oral use, adverse effects include nausea, vomiting, and diarrhea; with vaginal application, adverse effects include local irritation and burning.

Azoles

The azoles are the largest group of commonly used antifungal agents. Many are used topically and some are available without a prescription for dermatologic (see Chap. 64) or vaginal use (eg, butoconazole, clotrimazole, miconazole, terconazole, tioconazole). The main drugs discussed in this chapter are used systemically or both topically and systemically. In serious, invasive fungal infections, these drugs are often used long term following initial treatment with amphotericin B. However, their use as initial treatment for systemic infections is increasing.

There are currently four azoles available for systemic use: ketoconazole, fluconazole, itraconazole, and voriconazole. Compared with ketoconazole, the first azole, the other drugs have a broader spectrum of antifungal activity, better absorption with oral administration, better drug distribution in body tissues, fewer adverse effects, and fewer drug interactions. The most common adverse effects are nausea, diarrhea, and skin rash. In addition, all azoles may cause hepatotoxicity (eg, hepatitis). Therapy must be monitored closely with impaired liver function and with chronic use. Azoles are contraindicated during pregnancy. The drugs also interact with cytochrome P450 enzymes to produce significant interactions with many other drugs (in which they usually decrease the metabolism and increase the risks of toxicity with affected drugs).

APPLYING YOUR KNOWLEDGE 36-1

What assessment should be made before Charlotte takes fluconazole (Diflucan)?

Ketoconazole (Nizoral) has largely been replaced by the newer drugs. It may still be used for some clients who require long-term therapy, because it is much less expensive than other azoles. It may also be used with cyclosporine and tacrolimus because it increases blood levels of these immunosuppressant drugs and allows smaller dosages in clients with organ transplants.

Fluconazole (Diflucan) is a broad-spectrum agent that is effective for candidiasis, cryptococcosis, and coccidioidomycosis and may be used as first-line or second-line (after amphotericin B) therapy. It is often the drug of choice for localized candidal infections (eg, urinary tract infections, thrush, esophagitis, peritonitis) and is useful for severe disseminated candidiasis. In vaginal candidiasis, a single oral dose of 150 milligrams is usually effective. However, more infections with resistant strains of *Candida* organisms are being seen with the extensive use of fluconazole during recent years. Fluconazole is also used for long-term suppression of cryptococcal meningitis in clients with acquired immunodeficiency syndrome (AIDS) after initial use of amphotericin B. Aspergillosis does not respond to fluconazole therapy, and fluconazole has less activity against blastomycosis and histoplasmosis than itraconazole.

Fluconazole can be given orally or IV and, except for a more rapid onset with IV use, pharmacokinetics and dosage are similar with the two routes. Oral drug is well absorbed and the drug reaches therapeutic levels in most body fluids and tissues, including normal and inflamed meninges. With a one-time loading dose of twice the usual daily dose, steady-state blood levels are reached in about 2 days; without a loading dose, 5 to 10 days are required. Once-daily dosing may be effective in some clients with normal renal function. Most of the drug is excreted as unchanged drug in urine; dosage may need to be reduced in clients with impaired renal function.

Fluconazole is usually well tolerated. Adverse effects, including nausea, vomiting, diarrhea, abdominal pain, headache, and skin rash, have been reported in fewer than 3% of clients. In addition, elevation of liver enzymes and hepatic necrosis have been reported, and alopecia often occurs in clients receiving prolonged, high-dose treatment.

Fluconazole increases the effects of several drugs, including cyclosporine, phenytoin, oral sulfonylureas, and warfarin, but apparently has fewer interactions than ketoconazole and itraconazole.

Itraconazole (Sporanox) is a broad-spectrum agent similar to fluconazole. It is a drug of choice for many fungal infections, including blastomycosis, histoplasmosis, and sporotrichosis. It is also useful in treating aspergillosis and many superficial fungal infections of the skin and mucous membranes (eg, vaginal candidiasis, tinea infections, dermatophytic infections, onychomycosis [fungal infection of nails]). It is contraindicated for the treatment of dermatophytic infections and onychomycosis in clients with heart failure.

Itraconazole can be given orally or IV. The capsules require adequate gastric acidity for absorption and therefore should be taken with food; the oral suspension is better absorbed than the capsule and should be taken on an empty stomach. Drug absorption may be decreased in clients with HIV infection who have achlorhydria and in those receiving a concurrent antacid, histamine H_2 antagonist, or proton pump inhibitor. Serum levels should be measured to ensure adequate absorption. Drug concentrations are higher in visceral organs than in serum; little drug appears in urine or CSF.

The drug is well tolerated in usual doses but may cause nausea and gastric distress. Higher doses may cause impotence, hypokalemia, hypertension, edema, and heart failure. Itraconazole has significant interactions with several commonly prescribed drugs. Drugs that increase the pH of gastric acid (eg, antacids, histamine H_2 blockers, proton pump inhibitors) decrease absorption of itraconazole and should be given at least 2 hours after itraconazole. Drugs that induce drug-metabolizing enzymes (eg, carbamazepine, phenytoin, rifampin) decrease serum levels and therapeutic effectiveness of itraconazole. Itraconazole increases serum levels of cyclosporine, digoxin, oral sulfonylureas, and warfarin. It decreases serum levels of carbamazepine, phenytoin, and rifampin.

Voriconazole (Vfend) has a broad spectrum of antifungal activity, including activity against clinically important species of *Candida* and *Aspergillus*. The drug is indicated for treatment of esophageal candidiasis and invasive aspergillosis.

Voriconazole is well absorbed with oral administration and reaches peak serum levels in less than 2 hours. It is widely distributed in body tissues; metabolized in the liver by cytochrome P450 enzymes 2C9, 2C19, and 3A4; and the metabolites are excreted renally. Transient visual disturbance is a common adverse effect, occurring in approximately 30% of recipients.

Clinically significant drug interactions include reduced voriconazole levels with enzyme inducers (eg, rifampin, rifabutin, carbamazepine) and increased sirolimus levels with voriconazole administration, possibly to toxic levels. These drugs are contraindicated during voriconazole therapy and concomitant cyclosporine, tacrolimus, or warfarin administration requires vigilant monitoring. Dosage of voriconazole should be reduced with impaired liver function.

APPLYING YOUR KNOWLEDGE 36-2

The dose of Diflucan is not effective and Charlotte returns to the office 2 weeks later with an active *C. albicans* infection. The primary care provider prescribes Diflucan 200 mg PO for one dose, then 100 mg PO daily for 14 days. What adverse effects should you monitor for in the client taking Diflucan?

Miscellaneous Antifungal Drugs

Caspofungin (Cancidas), an echinocandin, inhibits glucan synthase, the enzyme that forms the glucan component of fungal cells walls. Depletion of glucan leads to leakage of cellular contents and cell death. Because human cells do not have cell walls or contain glucan, echinocandin drugs are less toxic than other systemic antifungal drugs.

Caspofungin has fungicidal activity against most *Aspergillus* and *Candida* species, including azole-resistant *Candida* strains; some activity against the organisms that cause blastomycosis and histoplasmosis; and little to no activity against *Cryptococcus* organisms. At present, caspofungin is indicated for treatment of invasive aspergillosis and a few studies indicate a synergistic effect with itraconazole, voriconazole, or amphotericin B in *Aspergillus* infections. It is also being used to treat esophageal candidiasis, candidemia, and invasive candidiasis; in these conditions, it is reportedly as effective as, and better tolerated than, amphotericin B.

Caspofungin is given IV and is highly bound to plasma albumin. After a single 1-hour infusion, plasma levels decline in three main phases. A short phase occurs soon after infusion; an intermediate phase has a half-life of 8 to 11 hours; and a longer phase has a half-life of 40 to 50 hours. There is minimal biotransformation or excretion during the first 30 hours after infusion, then the drug is metabolized slowly and excreted in feces and urine.

Caspofungin is usually well tolerated with doses of 50 milligrams per day. Adverse effects include fever, headache, nausea, skin rash, vomiting, and phlebitis at injection sites. Abnormal laboratory reports (eg, decreased white blood cells, hemoglobin and hematocrit; increased serum potassium and liver alanine and aspartate aminotransferase [ALT and AST] enzymes) may also occur. Dosage must be reduced with moderate hepatic impairment (eg, after a 70-mg loading dose, a 35-mg daily dose is recommended rather than the 50 mg daily recommended for clients with normal liver function). No dosage reduction is needed for renal impairment.

Cyclosporine increases the effects of caspofungin, including potential liver damage, and concomitant use is not recommended. Drugs that decrease effects include anti-HIV drugs (eg, efavirenz, nelfinavir, nevirapine), anticonvulsants (eg, carbamazepine, phenytoin), dexamethasone, and rifampin. Concurrent administration may significantly reduce caspofungin blood levels and therapeutic effectiveness unless dosage is increased (eg, from the usual 50 mg to 70 mg daily).

Flucytosine is converted to 5-fluorouracil (5-FU) inside the fungal cell. The 5-FU is then metabolized to products that interfere with the synthesis of fungal RNA and DNA. Flucytosine has little activity against molds or dimorphic fungi and is mainly used for yeast infections. It has significant activity against *Candida* and *C. neoformans* organisms. Flucytosine is not used alone because drug resistance develops. It is most often used in combination with amphotericin B to treat systemic candidiasis and cryptococcal meningitis. The combination allows smaller doses of amphotericin B and prevents emergence of flucytosine resistance.

Flucytosine is well absorbed with oral use and widely distributed into most body fluids, including CSF. Most is excreted unchanged in urine. Dosage must be reduced and serum drug levels monitored in the presence of impaired renal function.

Flucytosine causes fewer adverse effects than amphotericin B and the azole antifungals, but may be associated with GI upset (nausea, vomiting, diarrhea) and bone marrow depression (eg, leukopenia, thrombocytopenia), especially when given concurrently with amphotericin B. AIDS clients with systemic fungal infections do not tolerate flucytosine well because of their baseline leukopenia. Adverse effects are attributed to conversion of flucytosine to toxic metabolites in human cells.

Griseofulvin has long been used orally for dermatophyte infections of the scalp and nails and for skin eruptions that were too extensive to be treated with topical agents alone. The drug acts by interfering with cell division and reproduction in actively growing fungal cells. In infections of keratinized tissues, the drug binds to keratin (a protein in hair, nails, and the epidermis of the skin). Over time, the infected tissues are shed and replaced by uninfected tissues. Dermatophytic infections (eg, ringworm) of skin usually improve in 3 to 8 weeks. A year or more may be needed to eliminate onychomycosis of toenails. As a result, griseofulvin is being used less often and itraconazole, which is effective with shorter courses of therapy, is being used more often. Griseofulvin is contraindicated for clients with liver disease.

Oral griseofulvin is poorly absorbed; absorption is improved by reducing the particle size and by taking the drug with fatty meals. The drug is usually well tolerated. Common adverse effects include GI upset (eg, nausea, vomiting, diarrhea), fatigue, headache, insomnia, and skin rash. Hepatotoxicity may also occur. Griseofulvin may decrease the effects of cyclosporine, oral contraceptives, salicylates, and warfarin. Warfarin doses may need to be increased and an alternative method of contraception may be needed during griseofulvin therapy.

Terbinafine (Lamisil) is a synthetic allylamine with a broad spectrum of antifungal activity. It inhibits an enzyme needed for synthesis of ergosterol, a structural component of fungal cell membranes. Terbinafine has fungicidal activity against dermatophytes and has been used primarily for topical treatment of ringworm infections and oral treatment of onychomycosis. Therapeutic effects may not be evident until months after drug therapy is stopped, because of the time required for growth of healthy nail. Because of its activity against *Candida, Aspergillus,* and possibly other organisms, terbinafine may be used in combination with other antifungal drugs in serious infections.

Oral terbinafine is about 70% absorbed, but first-pass metabolism reduces bioavailability to approximately 40%. The drug is extensively metabolized to inactive metabolites and excreted in the urine.

Adverse effects with topical terbinafine are minimal. Common effects with oral use are headache, diarrhea, and abdominal discomfort. Oral drug may also cause skin reactions and liver failure with long-term therapy of onychomycosis. Hepatotoxicity is uncommon, but has occurred in people with and without pre-existing liver disease and has led to liver transplant or death. Terbinafine is not recommended for clients with chronic or active liver disease, and serum ALT and AST should be checked before starting the drug.

NURSING PROCESS

Assessment

Assess for fungal infections. Specific signs and symptoms vary with location and type of infection as well as the immune state of the client.

- Superficial lesions of skin, hair, and nails are usually characterized by pain, burning, and itching. Some lesions are moist; others are dry and scaling. They also may appear inflamed or discolored.
- Candidiasis occurs in warm, moist areas of the body. Skin lesions are likely to occur in perineal and intertriginous areas. They are usually moist, inflamed, pruritic areas with papules, vesicles, and pustules. Oral lesions are white patches that adhere to the buccal mucosa. Vaginal infection causes a cheesy vaginal discharge, burning, and itching. Intestinal infection causes diarrhea. Systemic infection causes chills and fever, myalgia, arthralgia, and prostration.

- Blastomycosis, coccidioidomycosis, and histoplasmosis may be asymptomatic or mimic influenza, pneumonia, or tuberculosis, with cough, fever, malaise, and other pulmonary manifestations. Severe histoplasmosis may also cause fever, anemia, enlarged spleen and liver, leukopenia, and GI tract ulcers.
- Cryptococcosis may involve the lungs, skin, and other body organs. In clients with AIDS or other immunosuppressant disorders, it often involves the central nervous system (CNS) and produces mental status changes, headache, dizziness, and neck stiffness.
- Sporotrichosis involves the skin and lymph nodes. It usually produces small nodules that look like insect bites initially and ulcerations later. Nodules and ulcers also may develop in local lymphatic channels and nodes. The infection can spread to other parts of the body in immunocompromised clients.
- Systemic mycoses produce severe symptoms and may be life-threatening. They are confirmed by recovery of organisms from specimens of body tissues or fluids.

Nursing Diagnoses

- Risk for Injury related to fungal infection
- Deficient Knowledge: Prevention of fungal infection; accurate drug usage
- Noncompliance related to the need for long-term therapy
- Risk for Injury: Adverse drug effects with systemic antifungal drugs

Planning/Goals

The client will

- Take or receive systemic antifungal drugs as prescribed
- Apply topical drugs accurately
- Act to prevent recurrence of fungal infection
- Avoid preventable adverse effects from systemic drugs

Interventions

Use measures to prevent spread of fungal infections.

- Observe Standard Precautions while assessing or providing care to clients with skin lesions. Superficial infections (eg, ringworm) are highly contagious and can be spread by sharing towels and hairbrushes. Systemic mycoses are not usually considered contagious.
- Decrease client exposure to environmental fungi. For inpatients who are neutropenic or otherwise immunocompromised, do not allow soil-containing plants in the room and request regular cleaning and inspection of air-conditioning systems. Aspergillosis has occurred after

inhalation of airborne mold spores from air-conditioning units and hospital water supplies. For outpatients, assist to identify and avoid areas of potential exposure (eg, soil contaminated by chicken, bird, or bat droppings; areas where buildings are being razed, constructed, or renovated). If exposure is unavoidable, instruct to spray areas with water to minimize airborne spores and to wear disposable clothing and a face mask. For clients at risk of exposure to sporotrichosis (eg, those who garden or work in plant nurseries), assist to identify risk factors and preventive measures (eg, wearing gloves and long sleeves).

● For obese clients with skin candidiasis, apply dry padding to intertriginous areas to help prevent irritation and candidal growth.

● For clients with oropharyngeal ulcerations, provide soothing oral hygiene, nonacidic fluids, and soft, bland foods.

● For clients with systemic fungal infections, monitor respiratory, cardiovascular, and neurologic status at least every 8 hours. Provide comfort measures and medications (eg, analgesics, antihistamines, antipyretics, antiemetics) for clients receiving IV amphotericin B.

In addition, client teaching guidelines for oral and topical antifungals are presented in the accompanying display.

Evaluation

● Observe for relief of symptoms for which an antifungal drug was prescribed.
● Interview outpatients regarding their compliance with instructions for using antifungal drugs.
● Interview and observe for adverse drug effects with systemic antifungal agents.

CLIENT TEACHING GUIDELINES

Oral and Topical Antifungal Drugs

General Considerations

☑ If you have a condition or take a medicine that suppresses your immune system (eg, bone marrow or organ transplant, leukemia, lymphoma, diabetes mellitus, human immunodeficiency virus (HIV) infection, cancer chemotherapy, corticosteroid therapy), avoid exposure to molds and fungi when possible. For example, aspergillus organisms, which can be in the air, dust, soil, and other environments, can cause serious illness and death. To minimize exposure, avoid areas of building construction or renovation, avoid cleaning carpets or potentially moldy areas, and avoid potted plants and live flowers.

☑ With skin lesions, wash hands often and do not share towels, hairbrushes, or other personal items.

☑ With vaginal yeast infections, do not use over-the-counter medications repeatedly without consulting a physician or other health care provider. Recurrent infections may indicate inadequate treatment, reinfection, or a bacterial infection (for which an antifungal drug is not effective), and a different treatment may be needed.

☑ With histoplasmosis and other potentially serious fungal infections, avoid or minimize future exposure to chicken, pigeon, and bat excreta.

☑ If you work with plants (eg, roses, sphagnum moss) or baled hay, prevent sporotrichosis by wearing gloves and long sleeves and avoiding injuries that cause breaks in the skin.

Self-Administration

☑ Use antifungal drugs as prescribed.
☑ With topical skin preparations, wash and dry the area before each application of medication.
☑ With vaginal antifungal preparations:
  ☑ Read instructions carefully, with prescribed and over-the-counter drugs.

☑ Insert high into the vagina (except during pregnancy).
☑ Continue use through menstruation.
☑ Wear a minipad to avoid staining clothing; do not use a tampon.
☑ Wash applicator with mild soap and rinse thoroughly after each use.
☑ Avoid sexual intercourse while using the drug.

☑ With flucytosine, take capsules a few at a time over 15 minutes to decrease nausea and vomiting.

☑ With oral ketoconazole, take with food to decrease gastrointestinal upset. However, do not take with antacids or drugs such as ranitidine (Zantac) or omeprazole (Prilosec). If one of these drugs is required, take it approximately 2 hours after a dose of ketoconazole.

☑ With itraconazole capsules, take after a full meal for best absorption. With the oral suspension, take on an empty stomach, usually by swishing in the mouth and then swallowing it.

☑ With oral voriconazole, take 1 hour before or after a meal.

☑ With nystatin suspension for mouth lesions (thrush), swish the medication around in the mouth for a few minutes (to increase drug contact with the lesions), then swallow the medication.

☑ With oral fluconazole (Diflucan), itraconazole (Sporanox), ketoconazole (Nizoral), or terbinafine (Lamisil), notify a health care provider of unusual fatigue, loss of appetite, nausea, vomiting, jaundice, dark urine, pale stools, fever, abdominal pain, or diarrhea. These may be signs of liver damage or other adverse drug effects. Drug therapy may need to be discontinued.

☑ With griseofulvin, avoid prolonged exposure to sunlight or sunlamps; the drug may cause photosensitivity.

☑ With voriconazole, do not drive at night because vision may be blurred.

PRINCIPLES OF THERAPY

Nonpharmacologic Treatment

Some fungal infections are asymptomatic or resolve spontaneously without treatment. In addition, some candidal infections respond to the removal of predisposing factors such as antibacterial drugs; corticosteroids or other immunosuppressive drugs; and indwelling IV or bladder catheters.

Drug Selection

Drug therapy for potentially serious fungal infections should be planned in consultation with an infectious-disease specialist when possible. Drug selection is determined mainly by the type of fungal infection. For example, drugs that are effective in candidiasis are not usually effective in dermatophytic infections, and vice versa. For serious infections, amphotericin B has long been the drug of choice, especially for invasive aspergillosis and systemic infections in immunocompromised hosts. However, fluconazole, itraconazole, voriconazole, and caspofungin are increasingly being used for first-line treatment of some infections. The systemic azoles are also used for initial therapy in less acutely ill clients, and as long-term treatment after a brief initial course of amphotericin B. However, all azoles are contraindicated during pregnancy.

Drug Dosage and Administration

Dosages depend on illness severity, with large amounts required for systemic infections, especially in immunocompromised hosts. Routes are determined mainly by location and severity of infection. For example, local infections can often be treated by topical applications, whereas more serious or systemic infections require oral or IV routes.

Duration of Therapy

When antifungal drug therapy is required, it is usually long term, over weeks to months. In some cases, it may be continued for years or lifelong. If drug therapy is stopped too soon, relapse of the infection commonly occurs. However, in clients with AIDS, who often require long-term antifungal drug therapy, drug-resistant infections may develop. Fluconazole-resistant candidiasis is becoming increasingly recognized in this population. Clients with an impaired immune response often become reinfected after effective antifungal drug therapy and may require repeated courses.

Drug Treatment of Specific Infections

- **Aspergillosis.** Itraconazole for approximately 1 year may be effective in mild to moderate infection. Amphotericin B is indicated for serious invasive disease, and large doses are required. Voriconazole or caspofungin may also be used.

- **Blastomycosis.** Clients with skin, pulmonary, or other manifestations of systemic disease should receive systemic antifungal drug therapy to prevent further progression. Mild to moderate disease may be treated with itraconazole for 6 to 12 months. For severe disease and clients with CNS infection or immunosuppression, amphotericin B is the drug of first choice. After initial amphotericin B therapy and clinical improvement, itraconazole may be given for 6 to 12 months.

- **Candidiasis.** Most mucocutaneous infections may be initially treated with local applications of drug. For **oral candidiasis,** clotrimazole troches are preferred; oral fluconazole, itraconazole, or nystatin suspension may also be used. **Vaginal candidiasis** may be treated with a single oral dose of fluconazole or multiple doses of vaginal tablets, creams, or suppositories containing butoconazole, clotrimazole, miconazole, nystatin, terconazole, or tioconazole. Some of these preparations are available over-the-counter. One concern about self-treatment with nonprescription products is an incorrect diagnosis. Antifungal preparations do not help a bacterial vaginal infection. Pregnant clients should consult their obstetrician before using these drugs. **Esophageal candidiasis** should be treated with a systemically absorbed agent such as fluconazole or itraconazole. **Systemic candidiasis** may be treated with amphotericin B, fluconazole, itraconazole, voriconazole, or caspofungin. Fluconazole is usually preferred; amphotericin B is preferred if the client has previously received fluconazole or if the infection is caused by non-*albicans Candida*. If the CNS is involved, flucytosine is used in conjunction with amphotericin B, although some strains of *C. albicans* are resistant to flucytosine. Chronic systemic candidiasis usually requires months of drug therapy.

- **Coccidioidomycosis.** Many coccidioidal infections are chronic in nature and require long-term drug therapy to control disease activity. Mild infections are usually treated with an oral azole (eg, fluconazole, itraconazole) for 6 to 12 months. Amphotericin B is preferred for severe or disseminated disease and is usually given for 1 to 3 months. Clients with meningitis may require lifelong therapy with an azole drug to prevent recurrence.

- **Cryptococcosis.** A combination of IV amphotericin B and oral flucytosine for 2 to 6 weeks is the initial treatment of first choice, including clients with CNS infections and/or AIDS. This may be followed by 6 to 12 months of oral fluconazole for treatment of meningitis. Clients with AIDS are usually given fluconazole long term to suppress recurrence.

- **Histoplasmosis.** Itraconazole is the drug of choice for mild to moderate histoplasmosis, and amphotericin B is the drug of choice for severe disease. Clients who also have AIDS may be given itraconazole twice daily for 12 weeks, then maintained on daily itraconazole to suppress recurrence. Flucytosine and ketoconazole are second-line agents.

- **Sporotrichosis.** Itraconazole, for 3 to 6 months, is probably the drug of choice for localized lymphocutaneous infection. Amphotericin B is used to treat pulmonary, disseminated, and relapsing infections.

Characteristics and Usage of Amphotericin B

Amphotericin B has long been the gold standard of drug therapy for serious fungal infections. However, its use is problematic because of different preparations, special requirements for administration, and toxicity. These aspects are summarized as follows:

- **Preparations.** The deoxycholate preparation (Fungizone), often called "conventional amphotericin B," is the oldest, most widely used form. Lipid preparations were developed to decrease the toxicity of the deoxycholate form, and three are currently available. These preparations have similar antifungal spectra, but they differ from the deoxycholate formulation and from each other in other respects. The cholesteryl form (Amphotec) and the lipid-complex form (Abelcet) have longer half-lives than the liposomal form (AmBisome). Because they are less toxic to normal tissues, these formulations can be given in higher doses than Fungizone.

- **Administration.** These drugs should be reconstituted and prepared for IV administration in a pharmacy. If not prepared in a pharmacy, the manufacturer's instructions should be followed for each preparation. Additional factors include the following:

    - A test dose is usually recommended to assess the client's tolerance of the drug. Some authorities question the need for a test dose.
    - Maintenance doses can be doubled and infused on alternate days. However, a single daily dose of Fungizone should not exceed 1.5 mg/kg; overdoses can result in cardiorespiratory arrest.
    - Small initial doses (eg, 5–10 mg/day) are recommended for clients with impaired cardiovascular or renal function or a severe reaction to the test dose.
    - Larger doses of lipid preparations are needed to achieve therapeutic effects similar to those of the deoxycholate preparation.
    - Administer through a separate IV line when possible. If injecting into an existing IV line, the line should be flushed with 5% dextrose solution before and after drug administration (both deoxycholate and lipid formulations).
    - An in-line filter may be used with Fungizone and AmBisome but should not be used with Abelcet or Amphotec.
    - Prepared solutions should be infused within 8 hours of reconstitution.

- **Decreasing adverse effects.** Several recommendations for reducing toxicity of IV amphotericin B have evolved, but most of them have not been tested in controlled studies. Recommendations to decrease nephrotoxicity are listed at "Use in Clients With Renal Impairment"; those to decrease fever and chills include premedication with acetaminophen, diphenhydramine, and a corticosteroid; and those to decrease phlebitis at injection sites include administering on alternate days, adding 500 to 2000 units of heparin to the infusion, rotating infusion sites, administering through a large central vein, removing the needle after infusion, and using a pediatric scalp vein needle. A test dose is often given, but this does not reliably predict or rule out anaphylaxis, which is a rare adverse effect of both conventional and lipid formulations.

    Supplemental potassium may be used to treat hypokalemia, and recombinant erythropoietin may be used to treat anemia if the client has a low plasma level of erythropoietin.

APPLYING YOUR KNOWLEDGE 36-3

A fungal infection that is severe or systemic may need to be treated with amphotericin B. Proper administration and assessment for adverse effects are part of the nurse's role. What adverse effects do you assess for in Charlotte while her amphotericin B is infusing?

Effects of Antifungals on Other Drugs

Amphotericin B increases effects of cyclosporine (nephrotoxicity); digoxin (risk of hypokalemia and resultant cardiac dysrhythmias); nephrotoxic drugs (eg, aminoglycoside antibiotics); skeletal muscle relaxants (amphotericin B–induced hypokalemia may enhance muscle relaxation); and thiazide and loop diuretics (risk of hypokalemia). Serum potassium levels should be monitored.

Azoles inhibit the metabolism of many drugs (by inhibiting cytochrome P450 drug-metabolizing enzymes in the liver and small intestine, especially 3A4 enzymes) and therefore increase their effects and risks of toxicity. These drugs include benzodiazepines (alprazolam, midazolam, triazolam); calcium channel blockers (felodipine, nifedipine); cyclosporine; phenytoin; statin cholesterol-lowering drugs (lovastatin, simvastatin); sulfonylureas; tacrolimus; theophylline; warfarin; vincristine; and zidovudine.

Although the main concern about azole drug interactions is increased toxicity of inhibited drugs, ketoconazole is being given concurrently with cyclosporine and tacrolimus to decrease dosages and costs of the immunosuppressant drugs. There may also be a reduced risk of fungal infections, which commonly occur in people with an impaired immune system.

Fluconazole is apparently a less potent inhibitor of cytochrome P450 3A4 enzymes than ketoconazole and itraconazole. As a result, drug interactions with fluconazole are of lesser magnitude and usually occur only with dosages of 200 milligrams per day or more. However, fluconazole is a strong inhibitor of cytochrome P450 2C9 enzymes, and concurrent administration of losartan, phenytoin, sulfamethoxazole, or warfarin results in greater risks of toxicity with the inhibited drugs.

Caspofungin decreases serum levels of tacrolimus; serum levels of tacrolimus should be monitored with concurrent use of the two drugs. **Griseofulvin** decreases the effects of cyclosporine, oral contraceptives, salicylates, and warfarin, probably by inducing hepatic drug-metabolizing enzymes and accelerating their metabolism.

Terbinafine is a strong inhibitor of cytochrome P450 2D6 enzymes and may increase the effects of propafenone (an antidysrhythmic); metoprolol (a beta blocker); and desipramine and nortriptyline (tricyclic antidepressants).

Use in Special Populations

Use in Children

Guidelines for the use of topical antifungal drugs in children are generally the same as those for adults. With most oral and parenteral agents, safety, effectiveness, and guidelines for use have not been established. In addition, some agents have no established pediatric dosages and others have age restrictions. Despite these limitations, most oral and parenteral drugs have been used successfully to treat children with serious fungal infections, without unusual or severe adverse effects. These include conventional and lipid formulations of amphotericin B; fluconazole; and itraconazole. As in other populations receiving these drugs, children should receive the lowest effective dosage and be monitored closely for adverse effects. The safety and efficacy of caspofungin in children have not been established.

Use in Older Adults

Specific guidelines for the use of antifungal drugs have not been established. The main concern is with oral or parenteral drugs because topical agents produce few adverse effects.

Virtually all adults receiving IV amphotericin B experience adverse effects. With the impaired renal and cardiovascular functions that usually accompany aging, older adults are especially vulnerable to serious adverse effects. They must be monitored closely to reduce the incidence and severity of nephrotoxicity, hypokalemia, and other adverse drug reactions. Lipid formulations of amphotericin B are less nephrotoxic than the conventional deoxycholate formulation and may be preferred for older adults. Azole drugs should probably be stopped if hypertension, edema, or hypokalemia occur. In addition, itraconazole has been associated with heart failure, a common condition in older adults.

Use in Clients With Cancer

Clients with cancer are at high risk for development of serious, systemic fungal infections. In clients receiving cytotoxic anticancer drugs, antifungal therapy is often used to prevent or treat infections caused by *Candida* and *Aspergillus* organisms. For prophylaxis, topical, oral, or IV agents are given before and during periods of drug-induced neutropenia, often to prevent recurrence of infection that occurred during previous neutropenic episodes. For treatment, oral or IV drugs may be given at the onset of fever and neutropenia; when fever persists or recurs in a neutropenic client despite appropriate antimicrobial therapy; or when maintenance therapy is needed after initial treatment of coccidioidomycosis, cryptococcosis, or histoplasmosis. These infections often relapse if antifungal drugs are discontinued. Clients must be closely monitored for adverse effects of antifungal drugs.

Use in Clients With Renal Impairment

Amphotericin B deoxycholate (Fungizone), the conventional formulation, is nephrotoxic. Renal impairment occurs in most clients (up to 80%) within the first 2 weeks of therapy but usually subsides with dosage reduction or drug discontinuation. Permanent impairment occurs in a few clients. Recommendations to decrease nephrotoxicity include hydrating clients with a liter of 0.9% sodium chloride solution IV and monitoring serum creatinine and blood urea nitrogen (BUN) at least weekly. If BUN exceeds 40 milligrams per deciliter, or serum creatinine exceeds 3 milligrams per deciliter, the drug should be stopped or dosage should be reduced until renal function recovers. Another strategy is to give a lipid formulation (eg, Abelcet, AmBisome, Amphotec), which is less nephrotoxic. For clients who already have renal impairment or other risk factors for development of renal impairment, a lipid formulation is indicated. Renal function should still be monitored frequently.

Caspofungin does not require dosage reduction for renal impairment and is not removed by hemodialysis. **Fluconazole** is mainly excreted in the urine as unchanged drug. For clients with a creatinine clearance (CrCl) above 50 milliliters per minute, full dosage may be given. For those with a CrCl of 50 milliliters per minute or less, dosage should be reduced by one half. However, for clients receiving hemodialysis, an extra dose may be needed because 3 hours of hemodialysis lowers plasma drug levels by approximately 50%. **Itraconazole** can be given to clients with mild to moderate renal impairment but is contraindicated in those with a CrCl of 30 milliliters per minute or less. It is not removed by hemodialysis. **Voriconazole** has been associated with acute renal failure; renal function should be closely monitored during use.

Flucytosine is excreted renally and may accumulate in renal impairment. Accumulation may increase BUN and serum creatinine and lead to renal failure unless dosage is reduced. Plasma drug levels should be monitored, and dosage should be adjusted to maintain blood levels below 100 micrograms per milliliter. **Terbinafine** clearance is reduced by 50% in clients with significant renal impairment (CrCl of 50 mL/minute or less). Its use is not recommended.

Use in Clients With Hepatic Impairment

Although the main concern with **amphotericin B** is nephrotoxicity, it is recommended that liver function tests be monitored during use. **Caspofungin** dosage must be reduced with moderate hepatic impairment; the drug has not been studied in clients with severe hepatic impairment.

The azole antifungals may cause hepatotoxicity, ranging from mild elevations in ALT and AST to clinical hepatitis, cholestasis, hepatic failure, and death. Fatal hepatic damage has occurred primarily in clients with serious underlying conditions, such as AIDS or malignancy, and with multiple concomitant medications. The drugs are relatively contraindicated in clients with increased liver enzymes, active liver disease, or a history of liver damage with other drugs. They should be given only if expected benefits outweigh risks of liver injury. ALT, AST, and serum bilirubin should be checked before drug use, after several weeks of drug use, and every 1 to 2 months during long-term therapy. If ALT and AST increase to more than three times the normal range, the azole should be discontinued. Hepatotoxicity may be reversible if drug therapy is stopped.

Griseofulvin may cause hepatotoxicity, especially if given in large doses for prolonged periods. **Terbinafine** has been associated with liver failure, and its clearance is reduced by 50% in clients with hepatic cirrhosis. Its use is not recommended for clients with chronic or active liver disease, and liver function tests should be done in all clients before starting therapy. Hepatotoxicity has been reported in clients with and without pre-existing liver disease.

Use in Clients With Critical Illness

Amphotericin B, caspofungin, and the azoles are often used for serious fungal infections. **Amphotericin B** penetrates tissues well, except for CSF, and only small amounts are excreted in urine. With prolonged administration, the half-life increases from 1 to 15 days. Hemodialysis does not remove the drug. Lipid formulations may be preferred in critically ill clients because of less nephrotoxicity. **Fluconazole** penetrates tissues well, including CSF. Although IV administration may be necessary in many critically ill clients, the drug is well absorbed when administered orally or by nasogastric tube. Significantly impaired renal function may require reduced dosage, and impaired hepatic function may require discontinuation. When **itraconazole** is used in critically ill clients, a loading dose of 200 milligrams three times daily (600 mg/day) may be given for the first 3 days. Treatment should be continued for at least 3 months; inadequate treatment may lead to recurrent infection.

Use in Home Care

Antifungal drugs may be taken at home by various routes. For topical and oral routes, the role of the home care nurse may be teaching correct usage and encouraging clients to persist with the long-term treatment usually required. With IV antifungal drugs for serious infections, the home care nurse may need to assist in managing the environment, administering the drug, and monitoring for adverse effects. Because the immune function of these clients is often severely suppressed, protective interventions are needed. These may include teaching about frequent and thorough hand hygiene by clients, all members of the household, and visitors; safe food preparation and storage; removing potted plants and fresh flowers; and avoiding activities that generate dust in the client's environment. In addition, air conditioning and air filtering systems should be kept meticulously clean and any plans for renovations should be postponed or canceled.

N U R S I N G   A C T I O N S

Antifungal Drugs

NURSING ACTIONS	RATIONALE/EXPLANATION
1. Administer accurately	
a. Give intravenous (IV) amphotericin B according to manufacturers' recommendations for each product:	Test doses and all other solutions should be prepared in the pharmacy.
(1) Follow recommendations for administration of test doses.	Preparation, concentration, and recommended infusion times vary among formulations.
(2) Use an infusion pump.	To regulate flow accurately
(3) Use a separate IV line if possible; if necessary to use an existing line, flush with 5% dextrose in water before and after each infusion.	
(4) Fungizone IV—give in 5% dextrose in water, over 2–6 hours; use an in-line filter; do not mix with other IV medications.	Administration times can vary according to client tolerance.

NURSING ACTIONS	RATIONALE/EXPLANATION
(5) Abelcet—give IV over approximately 2 hours; if infusion time exceeds 2 hours, shake the container every 2 hours to mix contents; do not use an in-line filter.	
(6) AmBisome—infuse over 2 hours or longer; may use an in-line filter.	
(7) Amphotec—refrigerate after reconstitution and use within 24 hours; infuse over at least 2 hours; do not use an in-line filter.	
(8) Apply cream or lotion liberally to skin lesions and rub in gently.	
b. Give azoles according to manufacturers' recommendations:	
(1) With IV fluconazole and voriconazole, follow instructions for preparation carefully. Give fluconazole as a continuous infusion at a maximum rate of 200 mg/h. Give voriconazole over 1 to 2 hours.	
(2) Shake the oral suspension of fluconazole thoroughly before measuring the dose.	To resuspend medication in the liquid vehicle and ensure accurate dosage
(3) Give itraconazole capsules after a full meal; give the oral solution on an empty stomach and ask the client to swish the medication around in the mouth, then swallow the medication.	To decrease gastrointestinal (GI) upset and increase absorption. The oral solution is used to treat oropharyngeal and esophageal candidiasis, and correct administration enhances contact with mucosal lesions.
(4) Give ketoconazole tablets with food. However, do not give with antacids or other gastric-acid suppressants. If such drugs are required, give them 2 hours after a dose of ketoconazole.	Food decreases GI upset. Antacids and other drugs that suppress gastric acid decrease absorption because the drug is dissolved and absorbed only in an acidic environment.
c. With IV caspofungin, infuse over approximately 1 hour. Be sure it is added to 0.9% sodium chloride solutions only (dextrose solutions should be avoided). Do not mix or co-infuse with any other medications.	Caspofungin should be prepared in a pharmacy according to manufacturer's instructions. The drug is available in single-dose vials of 50 or 70 milligrams. It must be reconstituted with 0.9% sodium chloride solution, then added to 250 milliliters of 0.9% sodium chloride solution.
d. With flucytosine, have the client take 1 or 2 capsules at a time over 15 minutes.	To decrease nausea and vomiting
2. Observe for therapeutic effects	Most antifungal drug therapy is long term, over weeks, months, or years. With skin infections, optimal therapeutic effects may occur 2–4 weeks after drug therapy is stopped. With nail infections, optimal effects may occur 6–9 months after drug therapy is stopped.
a. Decreased fever and malaise with systemic mycoses	
b. Healing of lesions on skin and mucous membranes	
c. Diminished diarrhea with intestinal candidiasis	
d. Decreased vaginal discharge and discomfort with vaginal candidiasis	
3. Observe for adverse effects	
a. With IV amphotericin B, observe for fever, chills, anorexia, nausea, vomiting, renal damage (elevated blood urea nitrogen and serum creatinine), hypokalemia, hypomagnesemia, headache, stupor, coma, convulsions, anemia from bone marrow depression, phlebitis at venipuncture sites, and anaphylaxis.	Amphotericin B is a highly toxic drug and most recipients develop adverse reactions, including some degree of renal damage. Antipyretic and antiemetic drugs may be given to help minimize adverse reactions and promote client comfort. Adequate hydration and lipid formulations may decrease renal damage. Anaphylaxis is uncommon; however, appropriate treatment medications and supplies should be available during infusions. If severe respiratory distress occurs, the drug infusion should be stopped immediately and no additional doses should be given.
b. With fluconazole, itraconazole, or ketoconazole, observe for unusual fatigue, loss of appetite, nausea, vomiting, jaundice, dark urine, pale stools, fever, abdominal pain, or diarrhea. With ketoconazole, observe for nausea, vomiting, pruritus, and abdominal pain.	These may be signs of liver damage or other adverse effects. Drug therapy may need to be discontinued. With ketoconazole, GI upset occurs in about 20% of clients taking 200 milligrams daily and in 50% or more of clients taking 400 milligrams daily.

(continued)

NURSING ACTIONS	RATIONALE/EXPLANATION
c. With caspofungin 50 milligrams daily, observe for nausea, vomiting, and phlebitis at infusion sites. With larger doses (50–70 mg daily), observe for the above plus fever, headache, and abnormal laboratory reports (eg, decreased white blood cells, hemoglobin, and hematocrit; increased serum potassium and liver aminotransferase enzymes).	The drug is usually well tolerated.
d. With flucytosine, observe for nausea, vomiting, and diarrhea.	These are common effects. Hepatic, renal, and hematologic functions also may be affected.
e. With griseofulvin, observe for GI symptoms, hypersensitivity (urticaria, photosensitivity, skin rashes, angioedema), headache, mental confusion, fatigue, dizziness, peripheral neuritis, and blood dyscrasias (leukopenia, neutropenia, granulocytopenia).	The incidence of serious reactions is very low.
f. With oral terbinafine, observe for diarrhea, dyspepsia, headache, skin rash or itching, and liver enzyme abnormalities.	Elevated liver enzymes (alanine and aspartate aminotransferases [ALT and AST]) may indicate liver damage and may occur in clients with or without pre-existing liver disease.
g. With topical drugs, observe for skin rash and irritation.	Adverse reactions are usually minimal with topical drugs, although hypersensitivity may occur.
4. Observe for drug interactions	
a. Drugs that *increase* effects of amphotericin B:	
(1) Antineoplastic drugs	May increase risks of nephrotoxicity, hypotension, and bronchospasm
(2) Corticosteroids	May potentiate hypokalemia and precipitate cardiac dysfunction
(3) Zidovudine	Increases renal and hematologic adverse effects of the liposomal formulation of amphotericin B. Renal and hematologic functions should be monitored closely.
(4) Nephrotoxic drugs (eg, aminoglycoside antibiotics, cyclosporine)	Increase nephrotoxicity
b. Drug that *increases* effects of fluconazole:	
(1) Hydrochlorothiazide	Increases serum levels of fluconazole, attributed to decreased renal excretion
c. Drugs that *decrease* effects of fluconazole:	
(1) Cimetidine	Decreased absorption
(2) Rifampin	Accelerated metabolism from enzyme induction
d. Drugs that *decrease* effects of itraconazole and ketoconazole:	
(1) Antacids, histamine H₂ antagonists, proton pump inhibitors	These drugs decrease gastric acid, which inhibits absorption of itraconazole and ketoconazole. If one of these drugs is required, it should be given at least 2 hours after the azole drug.
(2) Phenytoin, rifampin	Decrease serum levels, probably from accelerated metabolism
e. Drug that *increases* effects of caspofungin:	
(1) Cyclosporine	Increases serum levels
f. Drugs that *decrease* effects of caspofungin:	
(1) Enzyme inducers (efavirenz, nelfinavir, nevirapine, dexamethasone, carbamazepine, phenytoin, rifampin)	Decrease serum levels by accelerating caspofungin metabolism. The daily dose of caspofungin may need to be increased to 70 mg/d (instead of 50 mg/d) if given with one of these drugs.

NURSING ACTIONS	RATIONALE/EXPLANATION
g. Drugs that *decrease* effects of griseofulvin:	
(1) Enzyme inducers (eg, rifampin)	Enzyme inducers inhibit effects of griseofulvin by increasing its rate of metabolism.
h. Drug that *increases* effects of terbinafine:	
(1) Cimetidine	Slows metabolism and elimination of terbinafine so that serum levels are increased
i. Drug that *decreases* effects of terbinafine:	
(1) Rifampin	Causes rapid clearance of terbinafine

APPLYING YOUR KNOWLEDGE: ANSWERS

36-1 Charlotte should be assessed for pregnancy before taking fluconazole. Azole drugs are contraindicated in pregnancy.

36-2 Assess for nausea, vomiting, diarrhea, abdominal pain, headache, or skin rash, although these symptoms only occur in about 3% of clients. You should also be aware of the risk of liver dysfunction.

36-3 Clients who receive IV amphotericin B should be assessed for fever, chills, and tachypnea. Infusion reactions from IV amphotericin B should be reported. Charlotte should be premedicated with acetaminophen, diphenhydramine, and a corticosteroid.

Review and Application Exercises

Short Answer Exercises

1. What environmental factors predispose clients to development of fungal infections?

2. What signs and symptoms occur with candidiasis, and how would you assess for these?

3. Which fungal infections often mimic other respiratory infections?

4. What are the clinical indications for use of IV amphotericin B?

5. What are nursing interventions to decrease adverse effects of IV amphotericin B?

6. What are the differences between amphotericin B deoxycholate and the lipid formulations?

7. What are the clinical indications for use of oral antifungal drugs?

8. What are some early indications that a client is developing nephrotoxicity or hepatotoxicity?

9. Which population groups are at high risk of developing serious fungal infections and what can be done to protect them?

NCLEX-Style Questions

10. A major risk factor for serious fungal infections is
    a. immunosuppression
    b. mild exposure to a causative organism
    c. poor hand hygiene technique
    d. taking an antibacterial drug for 5 days

11. Which of the following drugs may be used to treat oral candidiasis (thrush)?
    a. terbinafine (Lamisil)
    b. flucytosine (Ancobon)
    c. fluconazole (Diflucan)
    d. butoconazole (Gynazole)

12. Which of the following is a major adverse effect of IV amphotericin B?
    a. bone marrow depression
    b. nephrotoxicity
    c. hepatotoxicity
    d. neurotoxicity

13. What is a major adverse effect of the azole antifungal drugs?
    a. bone marrow depression
    b. nephrotoxicity
    c. hepatotoxicity
    d. neurotoxicity

14. Which of the following medications is given with IV amphotericin B to decrease infusion reactions?
    a. an antihistamine
    b. an antibacterial
    c. a diuretic
    d. a local anesthetic

Selected References

Anaissie, E. J., Stratton, S. L, Dignani, M. C., et al. (2002). Pathogenic *Aspergillus* species recovered from a hospital water system: A 3-year prospective study. *Clinical Infectious Diseases, 34*(6), 780–789.

Brown, T. E. R., & Chin, T. W. F. (2002). Superficial fungal infections. In J. T. DiPiro, R. L. Talbert, G. C. Yee, G. R. Matzke, B. G. Wells, & L. M. Posey (Eds.), *Pharmacotherapy: A pathophysiologic approach* (5th ed., pp. 2043–2058). New York: McGraw-Hill.

Carver, P. L. (2002). Invasive fungal infections. In J. T. DiPiro, R. L. Talbert, G. C. Yee, G. R. Matzke, B. G. Wells, & L. M. Posey (Eds.), *Pharmacotherapy: A pathophysiologic approach* (5th ed., pp. 2059–2088). New York: McGraw-Hill.

Drug facts and comparisons. (Updated monthly.) St. Louis: Facts and Comparisons.

Ernst, E. J. (2001). Investigational antifungal agents. *Pharmacotherapy, 21*(8, Pt. 2), 165S–174S.

Goldman, L., & Ausiello, D. (Eds.). (2004). *Cecil textbook of medicine* (22nd ed., pp. 2043–2067). Philadelphia: W. B. Saunders.

Kauffman, C. A. (2004). Introduction to the mycoses. In L. Goldman & D. Ausiello (Eds.), *Cecil textbook of medicine* (22nd ed., pp. 2042–2043). Philadelphia: W. B. Saunders.

Kontoyiannis, D. P. (2001). A clinical perspective for the management of invasive fungal infections: Focus on IDSA guidelines. *Pharmacotherapy, 21*(8, Suppl.), 175S–187S.

Lewis, R. E., & Kontoyiannis, D. P. (2001). Rationale for combination antifungal therapy. *Pharmacotherapy, 21*(8, Pt. 2), 149S–164S.

Morrison, C., & Lew, E. (2001). Aspergillosis. *American Journal of Nursing, 101*(8), 40–48.

Pegues, D. A., Lasker, B. A., McNeil, M. M., et al. (2002). Cluster of cases of invasive aspergillosis in a transplant intensive care unit: Evidence of person-to-person airborne transmission. *Clinical Infectious Diseases, 34*(3), 412–416.

Reed, M. D., & Blumer, J. L. (2002). Anti-infective therapy. In H. B. Jenson & R. S. Baltimore (Eds.), *Pediatric infectious diseases: Principles and practice* (2nd ed., pp. 147–215). Philadelphia: W. B. Saunders.

Sidbury, R., & Schwarzenberger, K. (2002). Superficial cutaneous infections. In H. B. Jenson & R. S. Baltimore (Eds.), *Pediatric infectious diseases: Principles and practice* (2nd ed., pp. 544–577). Philadelphia: W. B. Saunders.

Wingard, J. R. (2002). Antifungal chemoprophylaxis after blood and marrow transplantation. *Clinical Infectious Diseases, 34*(10), 1386–1390.

Antiparasitics

OBJECTIVES

After studying this chapter, you will be able to:

1. Describe environmental and other major factors in prevention and recognition of selected parasitic diseases.
2. Discuss assessment and treatment of pinworm infestations and pediculosis in school-age children.
3. Discuss the drugs used to treat *Pneumocystis jiroveci* pneumonia in clients with acquired immunodeficiency syndrome.
4. Teach preventive interventions to clients planning travel to a malarious area.

APPLYING YOUR KNOWLEDGE

Lacy Michelsen is a 35-year-old woman who is a missionary. She has just returned from a 2-year stay in a developing country. Ms. Michelsen comes to the clinic today with severe diarrhea, fever, chills, headache, and myalgia. She is diagnosed with giardiasis and malaria and is prescribed chloroquine 500 mg daily for 3 weeks, and metronidazole 250 mg PO three times a day for 7 days.

INTRODUCTION

A *parasite* is a living organism that survives at the expense of another organism, called the *host*. Parasitic infestations are common human ailments worldwide. The effects of parasitic diseases on human hosts vary from minor to major and life threatening. Parasitic diseases discussed in this chapter are those caused by protozoa, helminths (worms), scabies, and pediculi (lice). Protozoa and helminths can infect the digestive tract and other body tissues; scabies and pediculi affect the skin.

Protozoal Infections

Amebiasis

Amebiasis is a common disease in Africa, Asia, and Latin America, but it can occur in any geographic region. In the United States, it is most likely to occur in residents of institutions for the mentally challenged; men who have sex with men; and residents or travelers in countries with poor sanitation.

Amebiasis is caused by the pathogenic protozoan *Entamoeba histolytica,* which exists in two forms. The cystic form is inactive and resistant to a number of factors, including drugs, heat, cold, and drying. The cystic form can survive outside the body for long periods. Amebiasis is transmitted by the fecal–oral route, such as by ingesting food or water contaminated with human feces containing amebic cysts. After they are ingested, some cysts open in the ileum to release amebae, which produce trophozoites. Other cysts remain intact, to be expelled in feces and continue the chain of infection. Trophozoites are active amebae that feed, multiply, move about, and produce clinical manifestations of amebiasis. Trophozoites produce an enzyme that allows them to invade body tissues. They may form erosions and ulcerations in the intestinal wall with resultant diarrhea (this form of the disease is called *intestinal amebiasis* or *amebic dysentery*), or they may penetrate blood vessels and be carried to other organs, where they form abscesses. These abscesses are usually found in the liver (hepatic amebiasis), but also may occur in the lungs or brain.

Drugs used to treat amebiasis (amebicides) are classified according to their site of action. For example, iodoquinol is an intestinal amebicide because it acts within the lumen of the bowel; and chloroquine is a tissue or extraintestinal amebicide because it acts in the bowel wall, liver, and other tissues. Metronidazole (Flagyl) is effective in both intestinal and extraintestinal amebiasis. No amebicides are currently recommended for prophylaxis of amebiasis.

Giardiasis

Giardiasis is caused by *Giardia lamblia,* a common intestinal parasite. It is spread by food or water contaminated with human feces containing encysted forms of the organism or by contact with infected people or animals. Person-to-person spread often occurs among children in daycare centers, institutionalized people, and men who have sex with men. The organism is also found in people who camp or hike in wilderness areas or who drink untreated well water in areas where sanitation is poor. Giardiasis may affect children more than adults and may cause community outbreaks of diarrhea.

Giardial infections occur 1 to 2 weeks after ingestion of the cysts and may be asymptomatic or produce diarrhea, abdominal cramping, and distention. If untreated, giardiasis may resolve spontaneously or progress to a chronic disease with anorexia, nausea, malaise, weight loss, and continued diarrhea with large, foul-smelling, light-colored, fatty stools. Deficiencies of vitamin B_{12} and fat-soluble vitamins may occur. Adults and children older than 8 years of age with symptomatic giardiasis are usually treated with oral metronidazole.

Malaria

Malaria is a common cause of morbidity and mortality in many parts of the world, especially in tropical regions. In the United States, malaria is rare and affects travelers or immigrants from malarious areas.

Malaria is caused by four species of protozoa of the genus *Plasmodium.* The human being is the only natural reservoir of these parasites. All types of malaria are transmitted only by *Anopheles* mosquitoes. *Plasmodium vivax, Plasmodium malariae,* and *Plasmodium ovale* cause recurrent malaria by forming reservoirs in the human host. In these types of malaria, signs and symptoms may occur months or years after the initial attack. *Plasmodium falciparum* causes the most life-threatening type of malaria but does not form a reservoir. This type of malaria may be cured and prevented from recurring.

Plasmodia have a life cycle in which one stage of development occurs within the human body. When a mosquito bites a person with malaria, it ingests blood that contains gametocytes (male and female forms of the protozoan parasite). From these forms, sporozoites are produced and transported to the mosquito's salivary glands. When the mosquito bites the next person, the sporozoites are injected into that person's bloodstream. From the bloodstream, the organisms lodge in the liver and other tissues, where they reproduce and form merozoites. The liver cells containing the parasite eventually rupture and release the merozoites into the bloodstream, where they invade red blood cells. After a period of growth and reproduction, merozoites rupture red blood cells, invade other erythrocytes, form gametocytes, and continue the cycle. After several cycles, clinical symptoms of malaria occur because of the large parasite burden. The characteristic cycles of chills and fever correspond to the release of merozoites from erythrocytes.

Antimalarial drugs act at different stages in the life cycle of plasmodial parasites. Some drugs (eg, chloroquine) are effective against erythrocytic forms and are therefore useful in preventing or treating acute attacks of malaria. These drugs do not prevent infection with the parasite, but they do prevent clinical manifestations. Other drugs (eg, primaquine) act against exoerythrocytic or tissue forms of the parasite to prevent initial infection and recurrent attacks or to cure some types of malaria. Combination drug therapy, administered concomitantly or consecutively, is common with antimalarial drugs.

Pneumocystosis

Pneumocystosis is caused by *Pneumocystis jiroveci* (formerly *Pneumocystis carinii*), a parasitic organism once considered a protozoan but now considered a fungus. Sources and routes of spread have not been clearly delineated. It is apparently widespread in the environment, and most people are exposed at an early age. Infections are mild or asymptomatic in immunocompetent people. However, the organism can form cysts in the lungs, persist for long periods, and become activated in immunocompromised hosts. Activation produces an acute, life-threatening pneumonia characterized by cough, fever, dyspnea, and presence of the organism in sputum. Groups at risk include human immunodeficiency virus (HIV) seropositive persons; those receiving corticosteroids or antineoplastics and other immunosuppressive drugs; and caregivers of infected people.

Toxoplasmosis

Toxoplasmosis is caused by *Toxoplasma gondii,* a parasite spread by ingesting undercooked meat or other food containing encysted forms of the organism; by contact with feces from infected cats; and by congenital spread from mothers with acute infection. After infection, the organism may persist in tissue cysts for the life of the host. However, symptoms rarely occur unless the immune system is impaired or becomes impaired at a later time. Although symptomatic infection may occur in anyone with immunosuppression (eg, people with cancer or organ transplantation), it is especially common and serious in people with AIDS, in whom it often causes encephalitis and death.

Trichomoniasis

The most common form of trichomoniasis is a vaginal infection caused by *Trichomonas vaginalis.* The disease is usually spread by sexual intercourse. Antitrichomonal drugs may be administered systemically (ie, metronidazole) or applied locally as douche solutions or vaginal creams. Because trichomoniasis is transmitted by sexual intercourse, partners should be treated simultaneously to prevent reinfection.

Helminthiasis

Helminthiasis, or infestation with parasitic worms, is a common finding in many parts of the world. Helminths are most often found in the gastrointestinal (GI) tract. However, several types of parasitic worms penetrate body tissues or produce larvae that migrate to the blood, lymph channels, lungs, liver, and other body tissues. Helminthic infections are described in Box 37-1.

Drugs used for treatment of helminthiasis are called *anthelmintics*. Most anthelmintics act locally to kill or cause expulsion of parasitic worms from the intestines; some anthelmintics act systemically against parasites that have penetrated various body tissues. The goal of anthelmintic therapy may be to eradicate the parasite completely or to decrease the magnitude of infestation ("worm burden").

Scabies and Pediculosis

Scabies and pediculosis are parasitic infestations of the skin. Scabies is caused by the "itch mite" (*Sarcoptes scabiei*), which burrows into the skin and lays eggs that hatch in 4 to 8 days. The burrows may produce visible skin lesions, most often between the fingers and on the wrists.

Pediculosis may be caused by one of three types of lice. Pediculosis capitis (head lice) is the most common type of pediculosis in the United States. It is diagnosed by finding louse eggs (nits) attached to hair shafts close to the scalp. Pediculosis corporis (body lice) is diagnosed by finding lice in clothing, especially in seams. Body lice can transmit typhus and other diseases. Pediculosis pubis (pubic or crab lice) is diagnosed by the presence of nits in the pubic and genital areas. Although scabies and pediculosis are caused by different parasites, the conditions have several common characteristics, as follows:

- They are more likely to occur in areas of poverty, overcrowding, and poor sanitation. However, they may occur in any geographic area and socioeconomic group.
- They are highly communicable and transmitted by direct contact with an infected person or the person's personal effects (eg, clothing, combs and hairbrushes, bed linens).

Box 37-1 Helminthic Infections

Hookworm infections are caused by *Necator americanus*, a species found in the United States, and *Ancylostoma duodenale*, a species found in Europe, the Middle East, and North Africa. Hookworm is spread by ova-containing feces from infected people. Ova develop into larvae when deposited on the soil. Larvae burrow through the skin (eg, if the person walks on the soil with bare feet), enter blood vessels, and migrate through the lungs to the pharynx, where they are swallowed. Larvae develop into adult hookworms in the small intestine and attach themselves to the intestinal mucosa.

Pinworm infections (enterobiasis), caused by *Enterobius vermicularis*, are the most common parasitic worm infections in the United States. They are highly communicable and often involve schoolchildren and household contacts. Infection occurs from contact with ova in food or water or on bed linens. The female pinworm migrates from the bowel to the perianal area to deposit eggs, especially at night. Touching or scratching the perianal area deposits ova on hands and any objects touched by the contaminated hands.

Roundworm infections (ascariasis), caused by *Ascaris lumbricoides*, are the most common parasitic worm infections in the world. They occur most often in tropical regions but may occur wherever sanitation is poor. The infection is transmitted by ingesting food or water contaminated with feces from infected people. Ova are swallowed and hatch into larvae in the intestine. The larvae penetrate blood vessels and migrate through the lungs before returning to the intestines, where they develop into adult worms.

Tapeworms attach themselves to the intestinal wall and may grow as long as several yards. Segments called *proglottids*, which contain tapeworm eggs, are expelled in feces. Tapeworms are transmitted by ingestion of contaminated, raw, or improperly cooked beef, pork, or fish. Beef and fish tapeworm infections are not usually considered serious illnesses. Pork tapeworm, which is uncommon in the United States, is more serious because it produces larvae that enter the bloodstream and migrate to other body tissues (ie, muscles, liver, lungs, and brain).

Threadworm infections (strongyloidiasis), caused by *Strongyloides stercoralis*, are potentially serious infections. This worm burrows into the mucosa of the small intestine, where the female lays eggs. The eggs hatch into larvae that can penetrate all body tissues.

Trichinosis, a parasitic worm infection caused by *Trichinella spiralis*, occurs worldwide. It is caused by ingestion of inadequately cooked meat, especially pork. Encysted larvae are ingested in infected pork. In the intestine, the larvae excyst, mature, and produce eggs that hatch into new larvae. The larvae enter blood and lymphatic vessels and are transported throughout the body. They penetrate various body tissues (eg, muscles and brain) and evoke inflammatory reactions. Eventually, the larvae are re-encysted or walled off in the tissues and may remain for 10 years or longer.

Whipworm infections (trichuriasis) are caused by *Trichuris trichiura*. Whipworms attach themselves to the wall of the colon.

- Pruritus is usually the major symptom. It results from an allergic reaction to parasite secretions and excrement. In addition to the intense discomfort associated with pruritus, scratching is likely to cause skin excoriation with secondary bacterial infection and formation of vesicles, pustules, and crusts.
- They are treated with many of the same topical medications.

ANTIPARASITIC DRUGS

Antiparasitic drugs include amebicides, antimalarials, other antiprotozoal agents, anthelmintics, scabicides, and pediculicides. Their descriptions are in the following text and are also listed in Table 37-1.

Antiprotozoal Agents

Amebicides

Chloroquine (Aralen) is used primarily for its antimalarial effects. When used as an amebicide, the drug is effective in extraintestinal amebiasis (ie, hepatic amebiasis) but usually ineffective in intestinal amebiasis. The phosphate salt is given orally. When the oral route is contraindicated; severe nausea and vomiting occur; or the infection is severe, the hydrochloride salt can be given intramuscularly. Treatment is usually combined with an intestinal amebicide.

Iodoquinol (Yodoxin) is an iodine compound that acts against active amebae (trophozoites) in the intestinal lumen. It may be used alone in asymptomatic intestinal amebiasis to decrease the number of amebic cysts passed in the feces. When given for symptomatic intestinal amebiasis (eg, amebic dysentery), it is usually given with other amebicides in concurrent or alternating courses. Iodoquinol is ineffective in amebic hepatitis and abscess formation. Its use is contraindicated with iodine allergy and liver disease.

Metronidazole (Flagyl) is effective against protozoa that cause amebiasis, giardiasis, and trichomoniasis and against anaerobic bacilli, such as *Bacteroides* and *Clostridia* (see Chap. 33). In amebiasis, metronidazole is amebicidal at intestinal and extraintestinal sites of infection. It is a drug of choice for all forms of amebiasis except asymptomatic intestinal amebiasis (in which amebic cysts are expelled in the feces). In trichomoniasis, metronidazole is more effective than any locally active agent.

Metronidazole is usually contraindicated during the first trimester of pregnancy and must be used with caution in clients with central nervous system (CNS) or blood disorders. Clients should also avoid all forms of ethanol while on this medication.

Tetracycline and **doxycycline** are antibacterial drugs (see Chap. 32) that act against amebae in the intestinal lumen by altering the bacterial flora required for amebic viability. One of these drugs may be used with other amebicides in the treatment of all forms of amebiasis except asymptomatic intestinal amebiasis.

Tinidazole (Tindamax) is a newer drug approved for the treatment of amebiasis, giardiasis, and trichomoniasis. It is chemically related to metronidazole. It is metabolized in the liver by cytochrome P450 3A4 enzymes and should be used cautiously in people with impaired liver function. The most common adverse effects are a metallic/bitter taste and nausea.

APPLYING YOUR KNOWLEDGE 37-1
What important information about contraindications to metronidazole should you teach to Ms. Michelsen?

Antimalarial Agents

Chloroquine is a widely used antimalarial agent. It acts against erythrocytic forms of plasmodial parasites to prevent or treat malarial attacks. When used for prophylaxis, it is given before, during, and after travel or residence in endemic areas. When used for treatment of malaria caused by *P. vivax, P. malariae,* or *P. ovale,* chloroquine relieves symptoms of the acute attack. However, the drug does not prevent recurrence of malarial attacks because it does not act against the tissue (exoerythrocytic) forms of the parasite. When used for treatment of malaria caused by *P. falciparum,* chloroquine relieves symptoms of the acute attack and eliminates the parasite from the body because *P. falciparum* does not form tissue reservoirs. Concern about chloroquine-resistant strains of *P. falciparum* has developed in many areas.

Chloroquine is also used in protozoal infections other than malaria, including extraintestinal amebiasis and giardiasis. It should be used with caution in clients with hepatic disease or severe neurologic, GI, ocular, or blood disorders.

Hydroxychloroquine (Plaquenil) is a derivative of chloroquine with essentially the same actions and uses with fewer adverse effects. It has also been used to treat rheumatoid arthritis and lupus erythematosus.

Chloroquine with **primaquine** is a mixture available in tablets containing chloroquine phosphate 500 milligrams (equivalent to 300 mg of chloroquine base) and primaquine phosphate 79 milligrams (equivalent to 45 mg of primaquine base). This combination is effective for prophylaxis of malaria and may be more acceptable to clients. It also may be more convenient for use in children because no pediatric formulation of primaquine is available.

Malarone is a newer combination product containing atovaquone and proguanil. The drugs inhibit different pathways in plasmodial synthesis of nucleic acids. Malarone may be used for both the prevention and treatment of malarial infections, particularly those caused by *P. falciparum.* It also seems to be effective in chloroquine-resistant areas and has fewer adverse effects than mefloquine. The drug should be taken daily with food or milk starting 1 to 2 days before entering an endemic area and for 7 days upon return.

(text continues on page 611)

Table 37-1 Drugs at a Glance: Antiparasitic Drugs

GENERIC/TRADE NAME	INDICATIONS FOR USE	ROUTES AND DOSAGE RANGES	
		Adults	Children
Amebicides **Chloroquine** (Aralen)	Extraintestinal amebiasis	Phosphate, PO 1 g/d for 2 d, then 500 mg/d for 2–3 wk Hydrochloride, IM 200 to 250 mg/d for 10–12 d	Phosphate, PO 20 mg/kg/d, in 2 divided doses, for 2 d, then 10 mg/kg/d for 2–3 wk Hydrochloride, IM 15 mg/kg/d for 2 d, then 7.5 mg/kg/d for 2–3 wk
Iodoquinol (Yodoxin)	Intestinal amebiasis	Asymptomatic carriers, PO 650 mg/d Symptomatic intestinal amebiasis, PO 650 mg 3 times daily after meals for 20 d; repeat after 2–3 wk if necessary	PO 40 mg/kg/d in 3 divided doses for 20 d (maximum dose, 2 g/d); repeat after 2–3 wk if necessary
Metronidazole (Flagyl)	Intestinal and extraintestinal amebiasis Giardiasis Trichomoniasis	Amebiasis, PO 500–750 mg 3 times daily for 5–10 d Giardiasis, PO 250 mg 3 times daily for 7 d Trichomoniasis, PO 250 mg 3 times daily for 7 d, 1 g twice daily for 1 d, or 2 g in a single dose. Repeat after 4–6 wk, if necessary. *Gardnerella vaginalis* vaginitis, PO 500 mg twice daily for 7 d	Amebiasis, PO 35–50 mg/kg/d in 3 divided doses, for 10 d Giardiasis, PO 15 mg/kg/d in 3 divided doses, for 7 d
Tetracycline (Sumycin) and **doxycycline** (Vibramycin)	Intestinal amebiasis	PO 250–500 mg q6h, up to 14 d	PO 25–50 mg/kg/d in 4 divided doses, for 7–10 d
Tinidazole (Tindamax)	Amebiasis Giardiasis Trichomoniasis	Amebiasis, PO 2 g daily for 3–5 d Giardiasis and trichomoniasis, PO 2 g as a single dose	Amebiasis, *3 y and older,* PO 50 mg/kg, up to 2 g, daily for 3–5 d Giardiasis and trichomoniasis, PO 50 mg/kg, up to 2 g, as a single dose
Antimalarial Agents **Chloroquine phosphate** and **chloroquine hydrochloride** (Aralen)	Prevention and treatment of malaria	Prophylaxis, PO 5 mg/kg (chloroquine base) weekly (maximum of 300 mg weekly), starting 2 wk before entering a malarious area and continuing for 8 wk after return Treatment, PO 1 g (600 mg of base) initially, then 500 mg (300 mg of base) after 6–8 h, then 500 mg daily for 2 d (total of 2.5 g in 4 doses) Treatment of malarial attacks, (hydrochloride) IM 250 mg (equivalent to 200 mg of chloroquine base) initially, repeated q6h if necessary, to a maximal dose of 800 mg of chloroquine base in 24 h	Treatment, PO 10 mg/kg (chloroquine base) initially, then 5 mg/kg after 6 h, then 5 mg/kg/d for 2 d (total of 4 doses) Treatment of malarial attacks, (hydrochloride) IM 5 mg/kg (chloroquine base) initially, repeated after 6 h if necessary; maximal dose, 10 mg/kg/24 h

(continued)

Table 37-1 Drugs at a Glance: Antiparasitic Drugs (continued)

		ROUTES AND DOSAGE RANGES	
GENERIC/TRADE NAME	**INDICATIONS FOR USE**	Adults	Children
Hydroxychloroquine (Plaquenil)	Erythrocytic malaria	Prophylaxis, PO 5 mg/kg, not to exceed 310 mg (of hydroxychloroquine base), once weekly for 2 wk before entry to and 8 wk after return from malarious areas Treatment of acute malarial attacks, PO 620 mg initially, then 310 mg 6 h later, and 310 mg/d for 2 d (total of 4 doses)	Prophylaxis, PO 5 mg/kg (of hydroxychloroquine base) once weekly for 2 wk before entry to and 8 wk after return from malarious areas Treatment of acute malarial attacks, PO 10 mg/kg initially, then 5 mg/kg 6 h later, and 5 mg/kg/d for 2 doses (total of 4 doses)
Chloroquine with **primaquine**	Prophylaxis of malaria	PO 1 tablet weekly for 2 wk before entering and 8 wk after leaving malarious areas	PO same as adults for children weighing >45 kg; ½ tablet for children weighing 25–45 kg. For younger children, a suspension is prepared (eg, 40 mg of chloroquine and 6 mg of primaquine in 5 mL). Dosages are then 2.5 mL for children weighing 5–7 kg, 5 mL for 8–11 kg, 7.5 mL for 12–15 kg, 10 mL for 16–20 kg, and 12.5 mL for 21–24 kg. Dosages are given weekly for 2 wk before entering and 8 wk after leaving malarious areas.
Atovaquone/proguanil (Malarone)	Prevention and treatment of malaria	Prophylaxis, one adult tablet daily 1–2 d before and 7 d after travel. Treatment, 4 adult tablets daily for 3 d	*11–40 kg:* Prophylaxis, 1–3 pediatric tablets 1–2 d before and 7 d after travel Treatment, 1–4 adult tablets daily for 3 d *<40 kg:* PO 8 mg/kg according to the schedule for adults
Mefloquine (Lariam)	Prevention and treatment of malaria	Prophylaxis, PO 250 mg 1 wk before travel, then 250 mg weekly during travel and for 4 wk after leaving a malarious area Treatment, 1250 mg (5 tablets) as a single dose	Prophylaxis, PO ¼ tablet for 15–19 kg weight; ½ tablet for 20–30 kg; ¾ tablet for 31–45 kg; and 1 tablet for >45 kg, according to the schedule for adults
Primaquine	Prevention of malaria	PO 26.3 mg (equivalent to 15 mg of primaquine base) daily for 14 d, beginning immediately after leaving a malarious area, or 79 mg (45 mg of base) once weekly for 8 wk. To prevent relapse, the same dose is given with chloroquine or a related drug daily for 14 d.	PO 0.3 mg of base/kg/d for 14 d, according to the schedule for adults, or 0.9 mg of base/kg/wk for 8 wk

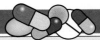

Table 37-1 Drugs at a Glance: Antiparasitic Drugs (continued)

GENERIC/TRADE NAME	INDICATIONS FOR USE	ROUTES AND DOSAGE RANGES	
		Adults	**Children**
Pyrimethamine (Daraprim)	Prevention of malaria	PO 25 mg once weekly, starting 2 wk before entering and continuing for 8 wk after returning from malarious areas	*>10 y:* PO 25 mg once weekly, as for adults *<10 y:* 6.25–12.5 mg once weekly
Quinine	Treatment of malaria	PO 650 mg q8h for 10–14 d	PO 25 mg/kg/d in divided doses q8h for 10–14 d
Other Antiprotozoal Agent			
Nitazoxanide (Alinia)	Diarrhea caused by giardiasis or cryptosporidiosis in children 1–11 y		*≥ 12y,* 1 tab (500 mg) or 25 ml oral suspension q12h for 3d *4–11 y,* 10 mL q12h for 3 d *12–47 mo,* 5 mL q12h for 3 d
Anti–Pneumocystis _jiroveci_ Agents			
Trimethoprim–sulfamethoxazole or **TMP-SMZ** (Bactrim, others)	Prevention and treatment of pneumocystis pneumonia	Prophylaxis, PO 1 double-strength tablet (160 mg TMP and 800 mg SMZ) q24h. Treatment, IV 15–20 mg/kg/d (based on trimethoprim) q6–8h, for up to 14 d; PO 15–20 mg/kg TMP/100 mg/kg SMZ per day, in divided doses, q6h, for 14–21 d	Prophylaxis, PO 150 mg/m^2 TMP/750 mg/m^2 SMZ per d, in divided doses q12h, on 3 consecutive d per wk. Maximum daily dose, 320 mg TMP/1600 mg SMZ. Treatment, IV 15–20 mg/kg/d (based on trimethoprim) q6–8h, for up to 14 d; PO 15–20 mg/kg TMP/100 mg/kg SMZ per d, in divided doses, q6h, for 14–21 d
Atovaquone (Mepron)	Prevention and treatment of pneumocystis pneumonia in people who are unable to take TMP-SMZ	Prevention, PO 1500 mg once daily with a meal. Treatment, PO 750 mg twice daily with food for 21 d	*13–16 y:* Same as adults *<13 y:* Dosage not established
Dapsone (Avlosulfon)	Prevention of pneumocystis pneumonia	PO 100 mg daily	*>1 mo:* 2 mg/kg/d, maximum dose, 100 mg daily
Pentamidine (Pentam 300, NebuPent)	Prevention and treatment of pneumocystis pneumonia	Treatment, IM, IV 4 mg/kg once daily for 14 d. Prophylaxis, inhalation, 300 mg every 4 wk	IM, IV same as adults. Inhalation, dosage not established
Trimetrexate (Neutrexin)	Treatment of pneumocystis pneumonia in immunocompromised clients who are unable to take TMP-SMZ	IV infusion 45 mg/m^2 daily, over 60–90 min, for 21 d (with leucovorin, PO, IV 20 mg/m^2 q6h for 24 d; give IV doses over 5–10 min)	Dosage not established
Anthelmintics **Mebendazole** (Vermox)	Treatment of hookworm, pinworm, roundworm, whipworm, and tapeworm infections	Most infections, PO 100 mg morning and evening for 3 consecutive d. For pinworms, a single 100-mg dose may be sufficient. A second course may be given in 3 wk, if necessary.	Same as adults

(continued)

Table 37-1 Drugs at a Glance: Antiparasitic Drugs (continued)

		ROUTES AND DOSAGE RANGES	
GENERIC/TRADE NAME	INDICATIONS FOR USE	Adults	Children
Pyrantel (Pin-Rid)	Treatment of roundworm, pinworm, and hook-worm infections	Roundworms and pinworms, PO 11 mg/kg (maximal dose, 1 g) as a single dose; for hookworms, the same dose is given daily for 3 consecutive d. The course of therapy may be repeated in 1 mo, if necessary.	Same as adults
Thiabendazole (Mintezol)	Treatment of threadworm, pinworm, hookworm, roundworm, and whip-worm infections	PO 22 mg/kg (maximal single dose, 3 g) twice daily after meals: 1 d for pinworms, repeated after 1–2 wk; 2 d for other infections, except trichinosis, which requires approximately 5 d	Same as adults
Ivermectin (Stromectol)	Treatment of strongy-loidiasis	200 mcg/kg as a single dose	≥5 y: 150 mcg/kg as a single dose
Scabicides and Pediculicides **Permethrin** (Nix, Elimite)	Pediculosis Scabies	Scabies, massage Elimite into the skin over the entire body except the face, leave on for 8–14 h, wash off. Pediculosis, apply Nix after shampooing, rinsing, and towel-drying hair. Saturate hair and scalp, leave on for 10 min, rinse off with water.	Same as adults
Gamma benzene hexachloride (Lindane)	Pediculosis Scabies	Scabies, apply topically to entire skin except the face, neck, and scalp; leave in place for 24 h; then remove by shower. Pediculosis, rub cream or lotion into affected area, leave in place for 12 h, then wash or shampoo (rub into the affected area for 4 min and rinse thoroughly).	Same as adults
Malathion (Ovide)	Pediculosis (head lice)	Apply to hair, rub in well to wet hair, then dry hair with-out covering or using a hair dryer. After 8–12 h, shampoo, rinse, and comb hair with a fine-toothed comb to remove dead lice and eggs. If nec-essary, treatment can be repeated in 7–9 d.	>2 y: Same as adults <2 y: Safety and effectiveness not established

IM, intramuscular; IV, intravenous; PO, oral.

Mefloquine (Lariam) is used to prevent *P. falciparum* malaria, including chloroquine-resistant strains, and to treat acute malaria caused by *P. falciparum* or *P. vivax.*

Primaquine is used to prevent the initial occurrence of malaria; to prevent recurrent attacks of malaria caused by *P. vivax, P. malariae,* and *P. ovale;* and to achieve "radical cure" (ie, eradicating the exoerythrocytic forms of the plasmodium and preventing survival of the blood forms) of these three types of malaria. The clinical usefulness of primaquine stems primarily from its ability to destroy tissue (exoerythrocytic) forms of the malarial parasite. Primaquine is especially effective in *P. vivax* malaria. Thus far, plasmodial strains causing the three relapsing types of malaria have not developed resistance to primaquine. When used to prevent initial occurrence of malaria (causal prophylaxis), primaquine is given concurrently with a suppressive agent (eg, chloroquine, hydroxychloroquine) after the client has returned from a malarious area. Primaquine is not effective for treatment of acute attacks of malaria.

Pyrimethamine (Daraprim) is a folic acid antagonist used to prevent malaria caused by susceptible strains of plasmodia. It is sometimes used with a sulfonamide and quinine to treat chloroquine-resistant strains of *P. falciparum.* Folic acid antagonists and sulfonamides act synergistically against plasmodia because they block different steps in the synthesis of folic acid, a nutrient required by the parasites.

Quinine is derived from the bark of the cinchona tree. Quinine was the primary antimalarial drug for many years but has been largely replaced by synthetic agents that cause fewer adverse reactions. However, it may still be used in the treatment of chloroquine-resistant *P. falciparum* malaria, usually in conjunction with pyrimethamine and a sulfonamide. Quinine also relaxes skeletal muscles and has been used for prevention and treatment of nocturnal leg cramps.

Other Antiprotozoal Agent

Nitazoxanide (Alinia) is approved for treatment of diarrhea caused by giardiasis or cryptosporidiosis in children. It is the first drug approved for treatment of cryptosporidiosis, which may be life-threatening in immunocompromised hosts.

Anti-*Pneumocystis jiroveci* Agents

Trimethoprim-sulfamethoxazole or **TMP-SMZ** (Bactrim, others) (see Chap. 32) is the drug of choice for prevention and treatment of *Pneumocystis* pneumonia (also called PCP). Prophylaxis may be indicated for adults and adolescents with HIV and CD4+ cell counts of less than 200; organ transplant recipients; clients with leukemia or lymphoma who are receiving cytotoxic chemotherapy; and clients receiving high doses of corticosteroids (equivalent to 20 mg or more daily of prednisone) for prolonged periods of time (>2 weeks).

Common adverse effects include nausea, vomiting, and skin rash. These effects are more common in clients who are HIV seropositive.

Atovaquone (Mepron) is used for both prophylaxis and treatment of *Pneumocystis* pneumonia in people who are unable to take TMP-SMZ. Adverse effects include nausea, vomiting, diarrhea, fever, insomnia, and elevated hepatic enzymes.

Dapsone may be used for the prophylaxis of *Pneumocystis* infection in HIV-seropositive clients who are unable to tolerate TMP-SMZ. Clients who are glucose-6-phosphate dehydrogenase (G6PD) deficient develop hemolytic anemia with dapsone therapy and should be assessed for this condition before and during therapy. Common adverse effects include nausea, vomiting, and rash.

Pentamidine (Pentam 300, NebuPent) may be used both for prophylaxis and treatment of *Pneumocystis* infection. Pentamidine interferes with production of ribonucleic acid (RNA) and deoxyribonucleic acid (DNA) by the organism. The drug may be given parenterally for treatment of *Pneumocystis* pneumonia and by inhalation for prophylaxis. It is excreted by the kidneys and accumulates in the presence of renal failure, so dosage should be reduced in clients with renal impairment. In addition, the intravenous form of pentamidine is highly pancreotoxic and appropriate tests (eg, complete blood count, platelet count, serum creatinine, blood urea nitrogen, blood glucose, serum calcium, electrocardiogram) should be performed before, during, and after treatment.

Trimetrexate (Neutrexin) is a folate antagonist (which must be used with leucovorin rescue) approved only for treatment of moderate to severe *Pneumocystis* pneumonia in immunocompromised clients, including those with advanced HIV infection who are unable to take TMP-SMZ. Hematologic toxicity is the main dose-limiting adverse effect. To minimize hematologic effects, leucovorin should be given daily during trimetrexate therapy and for 72 hours after the last trimetrexate dose. Dosage of trimetrexate must be reduced, and dosage of leucovorin must be increased with significant neutropenia or thrombocytopenia.

Anthelmintics

Ivermectin (Stromectol) is used for numerous parasitic infections and is most active against strongyloidiasis. Ivermectin has also been used for the oral treatment of resistant lice infestations. The drug has relatively few adverse effects but may cause some nausea and vomiting.

Mebendazole (Vermox) is a broad-spectrum anthelmintic used in the treatment of parasitic infections by hookworms, pinworms, roundworms, and whipworms. It is also useful but less effective in tapeworm infection. Mebendazole kills helminths by preventing uptake of the glucose necessary for parasitic metabolism. The helminths become immobilized and die slowly, so they may be expelled from the GI tract up to 3 days after drug therapy is completed. Mebendazole acts locally in the GI tract, and little drug is absorbed systemically.

Mebendazole is usually the drug of choice for single or mixed infections caused by the aforementioned parasitic worms. The drug is contraindicated during pregnancy because of teratogenic effects in rats; it is relatively contraindicated in children younger than 2 years of age.

Pyrantel (Pin-Rid) is effective in infestations of roundworms, pinworms, and hookworms. The drug acts locally to paralyze worms in the intestinal tract. Pyrantel is poorly absorbed from the GI tract, and most of an administered dose may be recovered in feces. Pyrantel is contraindicated in pregnancy and is not recommended for children younger than 1 year of age.

Thiabendazole (Mintezol) is most effective against threadworms and pinworms. It is useful but less effective against hookworms, roundworms, and whipworms. Because of the broad spectrum of anthelmintic activity, thiabendazole may be especially useful in mixed parasitic infestations. In trichinosis, thiabendazole decreases symptoms and eosinophilia but does not eliminate larvae from muscle tissues. The mechanism of anthelmintic action is uncertain but probably involves interference with parasitic metabolism. The drug is relatively toxic compared with other anthelmintic agents.

Thiabendazole is a drug of choice for threadworm infestations. For other types of helminthiasis, it is usually considered an alternative drug. It is rapidly absorbed after oral administration and most of the drug is excreted in urine within 24 hours. It should be used with caution in clients with liver or kidney disease.

Scabicides and Pediculicides

Permethrin is the drug of choice for both pediculosis and scabies. Although a single application eliminates parasites and ova, two applications are generally recommended. For pediculosis, permethrin is available as a 1% over-the-counter liquid (Nix). For scabies, a 5% permethrin cream (Elimite) is available by prescription and a single application is considered curative. Permethrin is safer than other scabicides and pediculicides, especially for infants and children.

Permethrin is derived from a chrysanthemum plant, and people with a history of allergy to ragweed or chrysanthemum flowers should use it cautiously. The most frequent adverse effect is pruritus.

To avoid reinfection, close contacts should be treated simultaneously. With pediculosis, clothing and bedding should be sterilized by boiling or steaming, and seams of clothes should be examined to verify that all lice are eliminated.

Gamma benzene hexachloride (Lindane) is a second-line drug for scabies and pediculosis. It may be used for people who have hypersensitivity reactions or resistance to treatment with permethrin. It is applied topically, and substantial amounts are absorbed through intact skin. CNS toxicity has been reported with excessive use, especially in infants and children. The drug is available in a 1% concentration in a cream, lotion, and shampoo.

Malathion (Ovide) is a pediculicide used in the treatment of resistant head lice infestations, and **Pyrethrin** preparations (eg, Barc, RID) are available over-the-counter as gels, shampoos, and liquid suspensions for treatment of pediculosis. These preparations require two applications approximately 10 days apart.

NURSING PROCESS

Assessment

Assess for conditions in which antiparasitic drugs are used.

- Assess for exposure to parasites. Although exposure is influenced by many variables (eg, geographic location, personal hygiene, environmental sanitation), some useful questions may include the following:
  - Does the person live in an institution, an area of poor sanitation, an underdeveloped country, a tropical region, or an area of overcrowded housing? These conditions predispose to parasitic infestations with lice, scabies, protozoa, and worms.
  - Are parasitic diseases present in the person's environment? For example, head lice, scabies, and pinworm infestations often affect school-age children and their families.
  - Has the person recently traveled (within the previous 1–3 weeks) in malarious regions? If so, were prophylactic measures used appropriately?
  - With vaginal trichomoniasis, assess in relation to sexual activity. The disease is spread by sexual intercourse, and sexual partners need simultaneous treatment to prevent reinfection.
  - With pubic (crab) lice, assess sexual activity. Lice may be transmitted by sexual and other close contact and by contact with infested bed linens.
- Assess for signs and symptoms. These vary greatly, depending on the type and extent of parasitic infestation.
  - **Amebiasis.** The person may be asymptomatic; have nausea, vomiting, diarrhea, abdominal cramping, and weakness; or experience symptoms from ulcerations of the colon or abscesses of the liver (amebic hepatitis) if the disease is severe, prolonged, and untreated. Amebiasis is diagnosed by identifying cysts or trophozoites of *E. histolytica* in stool specimens.
  - **Malaria.** Initial symptoms may resemble those produced by influenza (eg, headache, myalgia). Characteristic paroxysms of chills, fever, and copious perspiration may not be present in early malaria. During acute malarial attacks, the cycles occur every 36 to 72 hours. Additional manifestations include nausea and vomiting, splenomegaly, hepatomegaly, anemia, leukopenia, thrombocytopenia, and hyperbilirubinemia. Malaria is diagnosed by identifying

the plasmodial parasite in peripheral blood smears (by microscopic examination).

- **Trichomoniasis.** Women usually have vaginal burning, itching, and yellowish discharge; men may be asymptomatic or have symptoms of urethritis. The condition is diagnosed by finding *T. vaginalis* organisms in a wet smear of vaginal exudate, semen, prostatic fluid, or urinary sediment (by microscopic examination). Cultures may be necessary.

- **Helminthiasis.** Light infestations may be asymptomatic. Heavy infestations produce symptoms according to the particular parasitic worm. Hookworm, roundworm, and threadworm larvae migrate through the lungs and may cause symptoms of pulmonary congestion. The hookworm may cause anemia by feeding on blood from the intestinal mucosa; the fish tapeworm may cause megaloblastic or pernicious anemia by absorbing folic acid and vitamin B_{12}. Large masses of roundworms or tapeworms may cause intestinal obstruction. The major symptom usually associated with pinworms is intense itching in the perianal area (pruritus ani). Helminthiasis is diagnosed by microscopic identification of parasites or ova in stool specimens. Pinworm infestation is diagnosed by identifying ova on anal swabs, obtained by touching the sticky side of cellophane tape to the anal area. (Early-morning swabs are best because the female pinworm deposits eggs during sleeping hours.)

- **Scabies and pediculosis.** Pruritus is usually the primary symptom. Secondary symptoms result from scratching and often include skin excoriation and infection (ie, vesicles, pustules, and crusts). Pediculosis is diagnosed by visual identification of lice or ova (nits) on the client's body or clothing.

Nursing Diagnoses

- Deficient Knowledge: Management of disease process and prevention of recurrence
- Deficient Knowledge: Accurate drug administration
- Imbalanced Nutrition: Less Than Body Requirements related to parasitic disease or drug therapy
- Self-Esteem Disturbance related to a medical diagnosis of parasitic infestation
- Noncompliance related to need for hygienic and other measures to prevent and treat parasitic infestations

Planning/Goals

The client will

- Experience relief of symptoms for which antiparasitic drugs were taken
- Self-administer drugs accurately
- Avoid preventable adverse effects

- Act to prevent recurrent infestation
- Keep appointments for follow-up care

Interventions

Use measures to avoid exposure to or prevent transmission of parasitic diseases.

- Environmental health measures include the following:
  - Sanitary sewers to prevent deposition of feces on surface soil and the resultant exposure to helminths
  - Monitoring of community water supplies, food-handling establishments, and food-handling personnel
  - Follow-up examination and possibly treatment of household and other close contacts of people with helminthiasis, amebiasis, trichomoniasis, scabies, and pediculosis
  - Mosquito control in malarious areas and prophylactic drug therapy for travelers to malarious areas. In addition, teach travelers to decrease exposure to mosquito bites (eg, wear long-sleeved, dark clothing; use an effective insect repellent such as DEET; sleep in well-screened rooms or under mosquito netting). These measures are especially needed at dusk and dawn, the maximal feeding times for mosquitoes.
- Personal and other health measures include the following:
  - Maintain personal hygiene (ie, regular bathing and shampooing, performing hand hygiene before eating or handling food and after defecation or urination).
  - Avoid raw fish and undercooked meat. This is especially important for anyone with immunosuppression.
  - Avoid contaminating streams or other water sources with feces.
  - Control flies and avoid foods exposed to flies.
  - With scabies and pediculosis infestations, drug therapy must be accompanied by adjunctive measures to avoid reinfection or transmission to others. For example, close contacts should be examined carefully and treated if indicated. Clothes, bed linens, and towels should be washed and dried on hot cycles. Clothes that cannot be washed should be dry cleaned. With head lice, combs and brushes should be cleaned and disinfected; carpets and upholstered furniture should be vacuumed.
  - With pinworms, clothing, bed linens, and towels should be washed daily on hot cycles. Toilet seats should be disinfected daily.
  - Ensure follow-up measures, such as testing of stool specimens; vaginal examinations; anal swabs; smears; and cultures.
  - With vaginal infections, avoid sexual intercourse, or have the male partner use a condom.

- Provide client teaching for any drug therapy (see accompanying display).

Evaluation

- Interview and observe for relief of symptoms.
- Interview outpatients regarding compliance with instructions for taking antiparasitic drugs and measures to prevent recurrence of infestation.
- Interview and observe for adverse drug effects.
- Interview and observe regarding food intake or changes in weight.

APPLYING YOUR KNOWLEDGE 37-2

Ms. Michelsen should be taught measures to prevent parasitic infection or reinfection. What would you include in this teaching plan?

PRINCIPLES OF THERAPY

Antiparasitic drugs should be used along with personal and public health control measures to prevent the spread of parasitic infestations. Specific measures vary according to the type of organism, the environment, and the host.

Many of the drugs described in this chapter are quite toxic; they should be used only when clearly indicated (ie, laboratory documentation of parasitic infection).

Use in Special Populations

Use in Children

Children often receive an antiparasitic drug for head lice or worm infestations. These products should be used exactly as directed and with appropriate precautions to prevent reinfection. Malaria is usually more severe in children than in adults, and children should be protected from exposure when possible. When chemoprophylaxis or treatment for malaria is indicated, the same drugs are used for children as for adults, with appropriate dosage adjustments. The tetracyclines are an exception and should not be given to children younger than 8 years of age.

Use in Older Adults

Older adults are more likely to experience adverse effects of antiparasitic drugs because they often have impaired renal and hepatic function.

Use in Home Care

Most antiparasitic drugs are given primarily in the home setting. The home care nurse may need to examine close contacts

---

CLIENT TEACHING GUIDELINES

Antiparasitic Drugs

General Considerations

- ✔ Use measures to prevent parasitic infection or reinfection:
  - ✔ Support public health measures to maintain a clean environment (ie, sanitary sewers, clean water, regulation of food-handling establishments and food-handling personnel).
  - ✔ When traveling to wilderness areas or to tropical or underdeveloped countries, check with the local health department about precautions needed to avoid parasitic infections.
  - ✔ Practice good hand hygiene and other personal hygienic practices.
  - ✔ When a family member or other close contact contracts a parasitic infection, be sure appropriate treatment and follow-up care are completed.
  - ✔ Avoid raw fish and undercooked meat.
  - ✔ With vaginal infections, avoid sexual intercourse, or use a condom.

Self- or Caregiver Administration

- ✔ Use antiparasitic drugs as prescribed; their effectiveness depends on accurate use.

- ✔ Take atovaquone, chloroquine and related drugs, iodoquinol, oral metronidazole, and tinidazole with or after meals. Food increases absorption of atovaquone and decreases gastrointestinal irritation with the other drugs.
- ✔ To use pentamidine by inhalation, dissolve the contents of one vial in 6 milliliters of sterile water, place the solution in the nebulizer chamber of a Respirgard II device, and deliver by way of oxygen or compressed air flow until the nebulizer chamber is empty (approximately 30–45 minutes).
- ✔ Take or give most anthelmintics without regard to mealtimes or food ingestion. Mebendazole tablets should be chewed or crushed and mixed with food; thiabendazole should be taken with food to decrease stomach upset. Chew chewable tablets thoroughly before swallowing.
- ✔ Use pediculicides and scabicides as directed on the label or product insert. Instructions vary among preparations.

of the infected person and assess their need for treatment; assist parents and clients so that drugs are used appropriately; and teach personal and environmental hygiene measures to prevent reinfection. When children have parasitic infestations, the home care nurse may need to collaborate with daycare centers and schools to prevent or control outbreaks.

N U R S I N G   A C T I O N S

Antiparasitics

NURSING ACTIONS	RATIONALE/EXPLANATION
1. Administer accurately	
a. Give atovaquone, chloroquine and related drugs, iodoquinol, oral metronidazole, and tinidazole with or after meals.	Food improves absorption of atovaquone and decreases gastrointestinal (GI) irritation with the other drugs.
b. With pentamidine:	
(1) For intravenous administration, dissolve the calculated dose in 3–5 milliliters of sterile water or 5% dextrose in water. Dilute further with 50–250 milliliters of 5% dextrose solution and infuse over 60 minutes.	
c. Give anthelmintics without regard to mealtimes or food ingestion. Mebendazole tablets may be chewed, swallowed, or crushed and mixed with food.	Food in the GI tract does not decrease effectiveness of most anthelmintics.
d. For pediculicides and scabicides, follow the label or manufacturer's instructions.	Instructions vary among preparations.
2. Observe for therapeutic effects	
a. With chloroquine for acute malaria, observe for relief of symptoms and negative blood smears.	Fever and chills usually subside within 24–48 hours, and blood smears are negative for plasmodia within 24–72 hours.
b. With amebicides, observe for relief of symptoms and negative stool examinations.	Relief of symptoms does not indicate cure of amebiasis; laboratory evidence is required. Stool specimens should be examined for amebic cysts and trophozoites periodically for approximately 6 months.
c. With anti–*Pneumocystis jiroveci* agents for prophylaxis, observe for absence of symptoms; when used for treatment, observe for decreased fever, cough, and respiratory distress.	
d. With anthelmintics, observe for relief of symptoms, absence of the parasite in blood or stool for three consecutive examinations, or a reduction in the number of parasitic ova in the feces.	The goal of anthelmintic drug therapy may be complete eradication of the parasite or reduction of the "worm burden."
e. With pediculicides, inspect affected areas for lice or nits.	For most clients, one treatment is effective. For others, a second treatment may be necessary.
3. Observe for adverse effects	
a. With amebicides, observe for anorexia, nausea, vomiting, epigastric burning, diarrhea.	GI effects may occur with all amebicides.
(1) With iodoquinol, observe for agitation, amnesia, peripheral neuropathy, optic neuropathy.	These effects are most likely to occur with large doses or long-term drug administration.
b. With antimalarial agents, observe for nausea, vomiting, diarrhea, pruritus, skin rash, headache, central nervous system (CNS) stimulation.	These effects may occur with most antimalarial agents. However, adverse effects are usually mild because small doses are used for prophylaxis, and the larger doses required for treatment of acute malarial attacks are given only for short periods.

(continued)

NURSING ACTIONS	RATIONALE/EXPLANATION
(1) With pyrimethamine, observe for anemia, thrombocytopenia, leukopenia.	This drug interferes with folic acid metabolism.
(2) With quinine, observe for signs of cinchonism (headache, tinnitus, decreased auditory acuity, blurred vision).	These effects occur with usual therapeutic doses of quinine. They do not usually necessitate discontinuance of quinine therapy.
c. With metronidazole, observe for convulsions, peripheral paresthesias, nausea, diarrhea, unpleasant taste, vertigo, headache, and vaginal and urethral burning sensation.	CNS effects are most serious; GI effects are most common.
d. With parenteral pentamidine, observe for leukopenia, thrombocytopenia, hypoglycemia, hyperglycemia, hypocalcemia, hypokalemia, hypotension, acute renal failure.	Severe hypotension may occur after a single parenteral dose. Deaths from hypotension, hypoglycemia, and cardiac dysrhythmias have been reported.
e. With aerosolized pentamidine, observe for fatigue, shortness of breath, bronchospasm, cough, dizziness, rash, anorexia, nausea, vomiting, chest pain.	These are the most common adverse effects.
f. With atovaquone, observe for nausea, vomiting, diarrhea, fever, headache, skin rash.	
g. With trimetrexate, observe for anemia, neutropenia, thrombocytopenia, increased bilirubin and liver enzymes (aspartate and alanine aminotransferase [AST and ALT], alkaline phosphatase), fever, skin rash, pruritus, nausea, vomiting, hyponatremia, hypocalcemia.	
h. With topical antitrichomonal agents, observe for hypersensitivity reactions (eg, rash, inflammation), burning, and pruritus.	Hypersensitivity reactions are the major adverse effects. Other effects are minor and rarely require that drug therapy be discontinued.
i. With permethrin, observe for pruritus, burning, or tingling; with Lindane, observe for CNS stimulation (nervousness, tremors, insomnia, convulsions).	Antihistamines or topical corticosteroids may be used to decrease itching. CNS toxicity is more likely to occur with excessive use of Lindane (ie, increased amounts, leaving in place longer than prescribed, or applying more frequently than prescribed).
4. Observe for drug interactions	Few clinically significant drug interactions occur because many antiparasitic agents are administered for local effects in the GI tract or on the skin. Most of the drugs also are given for short periods.
a. Drugs that *alter* effects of chloroquine:	
(1) Acidifying agents (eg, ascorbic acid)	Inhibit chloroquine by increasing the rate of urinary excretion
(2) Alkalinizing agents (eg, sodium bicarbonate)	Potentiate chloroquine by decreasing the rate of urinary excretion
(3) Monoamine oxidase (MAO) inhibitors	Increase risk of toxicity and retinal damage by inhibiting metabolism
b. Drugs that *alter* effects of metronidazole:	
(1) Phenobarbital, phenytoin	These drugs induce hepatic enzymes and decrease effects of metronidazole by accelerating its rate of hepatic metabolism.
(2) Cimetidine	May increase effects by inhibiting hepatic metabolism of metronidazole
c. Drugs that *decrease* effects of atovaquone and trimetrexate:	Although few interactions have been reported, any enzyme-inducing drug can potentially decrease effects of atovaquone and trimetrexate by accelerating their metabolism in the liver.
(1) Rifampin and other drugs that induce cytochrome P450 drug-metabolizing enzymes in the liver	

APPLYING YOUR KNOWLEDGE: ANSWERS

37-1 Metronidazole is contraindicated in the first trimester of pregnancy. Also, the client should avoid all forms of alcohol while taking this medication.

37-2 Teach Ms. Michelsen to use proper hand and other personal hygiene techniques. She should avoid raw fish and undercooked meat. Encourage Ms. Michelsen to take all of her medication and to have follow-up care.

37-3 Chloroquine should be taken with meals to decrease GI irritation.

Review and Application Exercises

Short Answer Exercises

1. What groups are at risk for development of parasitic infections (eg, amebiasis, giardiasis, malaria, pediculosis, helminthiasis)?

2. What interventions are needed to prevent parasitic infections?

3. How would you assess for a parasitic infection in a client who has been in an environment associated with a particular infestation?

4. How can you assess a client's personal hygiene practices and environmental sanitation facilities?

5. How would you instruct a child's mother regarding treatment and prevention of reinfection with head lice or pinworms?

6. What are adverse effects of commonly used antiparasitic drugs, and how might they be prevented or minimized?

NCLEX-Style Questions

7. A client being treated for amebiasis should be informed that which of the following adverse drug effects may occur?
   a. dizziness and numbness of extremities
   b. weight gain and reduced urine output
   c. nausea, vomiting, and diarrhea
   d. low blood pressure and a fast pulse

8. For a client taking metronidazole (Flagyl) for trichomoniasis, which of the following statements indicates understanding of a precaution needed for safe drug usage?
   a. "I will limit my intake of caffeine."
   b. "I will eat a low-sodium diet for a week."
   c. "I will increase my daily intake of potassium."
   d. "I will not drink any alcoholic beverages."

9. The drug of choice for prevention or treatment of *Pneumocystis* pneumonia is
   a. trimethoprim-sulfamethoxazole (Bactrim)
   b. trimetrexate (Neutrexin)
   c. mebendazole (Vermox)
   d. permethrin (Nix, Elimite)

10. The usual drug of choice for prevention or treatment of malaria is
    a. chloroquine (Aralen)
    b. metronidazole (Flagyl)
    c. pentamidine (Pentam 300)
    d. pyrantel (Pin-Rid)

11. Clients taking antiparasitic drugs should be taught
    a. to watch for all potential adverse drug effects
    b. to have blood tests weekly
    c. ways to prevent reinfection
    d. ways to maintain pre-infection activities of daily living

Selected References

Anandan, J. V. (2002). Parasitic diseases. In J. T. DiPiro, R. L. Talbert, G. C. Yee, G. R. Matzke, B. G. Wells, & L. M. Posey (Eds.), *Pharmacotherapy: A pathophysiologic approach* (5th ed., pp. 1967–1980). New York: McGraw-Hill.

Bailey, J. M., & Erramouspe, J. (2004). Nitazoxanide treatment for giardiasis and cryptosporidiosis in children. *The Annals of Pharmacotherapy, 38*, 634–640.

Bartels, C. L., Peterson, K. E., & Taylor, K. L. (2001). Head lice resistance: Itching that just won't stop. *The Annals of Pharmacotherapy, 35*, 109–112.

Drug facts and comparisons. (Updated monthly). St. Louis: Facts and Comparisons.

Goldman, L., & Ausiello, D. (Eds.). (2004). *Cecil textbook of medicine* (22nd ed.). Philadelphia: W. B. Saunders.

Greenwood, B., & Mutabingwa, T. (2002). Malaria in 2002. *Nature, 415*, 670–672.

Grover, J. K., Vats, V., & Yadav, S. (2001) Anthelmintics: A review. *Tropical Gastroenterology, 22*, 180–189.

Kain, C. K., Shanks, D., & Keystone, J. S. (2001) Malaria chemoprophylaxis in the age of drug resistance: Currently recommended drug regimens. *Clinical Infectious Diseases, 33*, 226–234.

Sepkowitz, K. A. (2002). Opportunistic infections in clients with and clients without acquired immunodeficiency syndrome. *Clinical Infectious Disease, 34*, 1098–1107.

Winstanley, P. (2001). Modern chemotherapeutic options for malaria. *Lancet Infectious Diseases, 1*, 242–250.

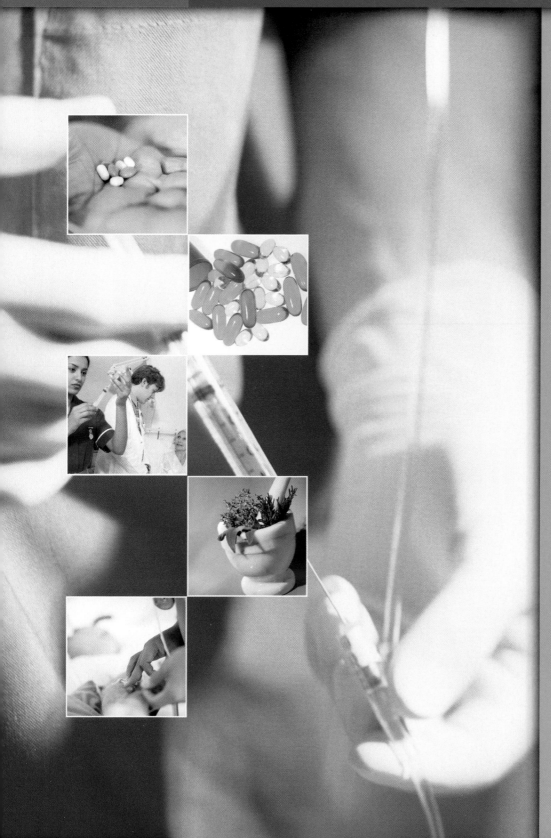

CHAPTER OUTLINE

38 Physiology of the Hematopoietic and Immune Systems

39 Immunizing Agents

40 Hematopoietic and Immunostimulant Drugs

41 Immunosuppressants

42 Drugs Used in Oncologic Disorders

Physiology of the Hematopoietic and Immune Systems

INTRODUCTION

Hematopoietic and immune blood cells originate in bone marrow in stem cells, which are often called *pluripotent* stem cells because they are capable of becoming different types of cells. As these stem cells reproduce, some cells are exactly like the original cells and are retained in bone marrow to maintain a continuing supply. However, most reproduced stem cells differentiate to form other types of cells. The early offspring are committed to become a particular type of cell, and a committed stem cell that will produce a cell type is called a *colony-forming unit* (CFU), such as CFU-erythrocyte or CFU-granulocyte. Hematopoietic growth factors or cytokines control the reproduction, growth, and differentiation of stem cells and CFUs. They also initiate the processes required to produce fully mature cells. Overall, cytokines are involved in numerous physiologic responses, including hematopoiesis, cellular proliferation and differentiation, inflammation, wound healing, and cellular and humoral immunity.

HEMATOPOIETIC CYTOKINES

Cytokines (Table 38-1) are substances produced by bone marrow cells, activated helper T cells, activated macrophages, and other cells. They regulate many cellular activities by acting as chemical messengers among cells. Some of these structurally and functionally diverse cytokines are growth factors that induce proliferation and differentiation of blood cells.

Cytokines act by binding to receptors on the same cells that secreted them, on target cells near the cells that produced them, or on target cells in distant parts of the body. After binding, the cytokine–receptor complexes trigger signal-transduction pathways that alter gene expression in the target cells. Cytokine actions and functions are affected by several factors. First, although the immune response to an antigen may include the production of cytokines, cytokines do not act in response to specific antigens. Instead, they affect whatever cells they encounter that have cytokine receptors and are able to respond. Cytokine receptors are often expressed on a cell only after that cell has

TABLE 38-1 Hematopoietic and Immune Cytokines

TYPE/NAME	MAIN SOURCE	MAIN FUNCTIONS
Colony-Stimulating Factors (CSFs)		
G-CSF	Leukocytes	Stimulates growth of bone marrow
		Generates neutrophils
M-CSF		Generates and stimulates growth of macrophages
GM-CSF		Stimulates growth of granulocyte–macrophages
Erythropoietin	Kidneys	Stimulates production of red blood cells by bone marrow
Thrombopoietin	Liver and kidneys	Stimulates production of platelets by bone marrow
Interferons		
Interferon alfa	Leukocytes	Inhibits viral replication in uninfected cells (antiviral effects)
		Has antiproliferative and immunomodulating effects
Interferon beta	Fibroblasts	Inhibits viral replication in uninfected cells
		Helps to regulate immune-cell functions
Interferon gamma	Circulating T and NK cells	Inhibits viral replication
		Induces cell-membrane antigens (eg, MHC)
		Acts on B cells to alter antibody production
		Influences functions of basophils and mast cells by increasing their ability to release histamine and decreasing their capacity for growth
		Helps regulate delayed-type hypersensitivity
		May have greater antitumor, cytolytic, and immunomodulatory effects than interferon alfa or beta
Interleukins (IL)		
IL-1	Monocytes	Stimulates growth of blood cells, especially B and T lymphocytes
	Monocyte–macrophages	Enhances interactions between monocytes and lymphocytes
	B cells, vascular endothelial cells, other cell types	Interacts with tumor necrosis factor to induce other growth factors
		Promotes chemotaxis and inflammation
		Acts on hypothalamus to cause fever
IL-2	T lymphocytes	Activates and promotes growth of T cells, B cells, and NK cells
	Helper T cells	Augments production of other cytokines, such as interferon gamma
		Influences the expression of histocompatibility antigens
		May inhibit granulocyte–macrophage colony formation and erythropoiesis
IL-3 (multi-CSF)	T lymphocytes	Stimulates bone marrow; growth factor for all blood cells
		Stimulates growth and histamine secretion of mast cells
IL-4	Helper T cells	Stimulates growth of T and B cells, mast cells, and NK cells
		Stimulates activation and differentiation of B cells; promotes production of immunoglobulins
		Increases phagocytic activity of macrophages
IL-5	Helper T cells	Stimulates B-cell growth, differentiation, and antibody secretion
		Stimulates eosinophils
IL-6	Fibroblasts and others	Acts on myeloid stem cells to stimulate growth and differentiation of B and T cells, megakaryocytes, and granulocyte–macrophages
		Promotes differentiation of B cells into plasma cells; then stimulates plasma cells to produce antibodies
		Interacts with other growth factors to stimulate growth and differentiation of T cells
		Enhances inflammatory responses
IL-7	Stromal cells of bone marrow	Acts on lymphoid stem cells to generate pre–B and pre–T cells, stimulate lymphocyte growth, and activate B and T cells
		Acts on resting T cells to increase expression of IL-2 and its receptor
IL-8	Macrophages and others	Regulates growth and movement of neutrophils and lymphocytes
		Induces immediate inflammatory responses (eg, acts on neutrophils to attract them to sites of cell injury, promote their adherence to vascular endothelium, and promote their movement from the bloodstream into tissues)
IL-9	T lymphocytes	Stimulates production of red blood cells, platelets, and helper T cells
IL-10	T and B lymphocytes, macrophages	Acts on macrophages to inhibit cytokine production and on antigen-presenting cells to reduce expression of class II MHC genes

TABLE 38-1 Hematopoietic and Immune Cytokines (continued)

TYPE/NAME	MAIN SOURCE	MAIN FUNCTIONS
IL-11	Stromal cells of bone marrow	Stimulates growth and differentiation of megakaryocytes, B cells, and blast cells Stimulates hepatocytes to produce acute-phase proteins (eg, fibrinogen and C-reactive protein, as part of the inflammatory response)
IL-12	Lymphocytes Macrophages and B cells	Stimulates activation and proliferation of T lymphocytes and NK cells Acts synergistically with IL-2 to stimulate cytotoxic T cells
IL-13	Activated lymphocytes Helper T cells	Similar to IL-4 Promotes proliferation of B lymphocytes Helps to regulate inflammatory process by inhibiting activation and release of inflammatory cytokines from macrophages
IL-14	T cells and malignant B cells	Promotes proliferation of B cells Inhibits B-cell production of immunoglobulins May stimulate growth of non-Hodgkin's lymphoma
IL-15	T lymphocytes	Stimulates growth of T cells, NK cells, and activated B cells
IL-16	T lymphocytes (mainly cytotoxic) and eosinophils	Acts on helper T cells to induce chemotaxis, synthesis of cytokines, and other functions
IL-17	T lymphocytes	Promotes T-cell chemotaxis and function Acts on macrophages to initiate and maintain inflammation Stimulates bone marrow stem cells to differentiate into neutrophils
IL-18	Activated macrophages	Acts on T cells to stimulate production of interferon gamma and on NK cells to enhance cytotoxicity
Tumor Necrosis Factors (TNFs) TNF-alpha	T lymphocytes, macrophages, mast cells	Cytotoxic effects on tumor cells Enhances inflammatory and immune responses (eg, stimulates production of cytokines)
TNF-beta	T lymphocytes	Cytotoxic and other effects on tumor cells, similar to TNF-alpha Enhances phagocytic activity of macrophages and neutrophils

MHC, major histocompatibility complex; NK, natural killer.

interacted with an antigen, so that cytokine activation is limited to antigen-activated lymphocytes. Second, the actions of most cytokines have been determined in laboratories by analysis of the effects of recombinant cytokines, often at nonphysiologic concentrations, and added individually to in vitro systems. Within the human body, however, cytokines rarely, if ever, act alone. Instead, a target cell is exposed to an environment containing a mixture of cytokines, which may have synergistic or antagonistic effects on each other. Third, cytokines often induce the synthesis of other cytokines. The resulting actions and interactions among cytokines may profoundly alter physiologic responses. Fourth, proteins that act as cytokine antagonists are found in the bloodstream and other extracellular fluids. These proteins may bind directly to a cytokine and inhibit its activity or bind to a cytokine receptor but fail to activate the cell. The main groups of cytokines are categorized as colony-stimulating factors (CSFs), interferons, and interleukins.

Colony-Stimulating Factors

As their name indicates, CSFs stimulate the production of red blood cells (erythropoietin), platelets (thrombopoietin), gran-

ulocytes (G-CSF), granulocyte–macrophages (GM-CSF), and monocyte–macrophages (M-CSF). In addition to granulocytes (neutrophils, basophils, and eosinophils), G-CSF also affects other blood cells (eg, erythrocytes, platelet precursors, macrophages). Interleukin-3 (IL-3) is sometimes called *multi-CSF* because it stimulates the production of all types of blood cells.

Interferons

Interferons "interfere" with the ability of viruses in infected cells to replicate and spread to uninfected cells. They also inhibit reproduction and growth of other cells, including tumor cells, and activate natural killer (NK) cells. These antiproliferative and immunomodulatory activities play important roles in normal host defense mechanisms.

Interleukins

Interleukins (ILs) were initially named because they were thought to be produced by and to act only on leukocytes. However, they can be produced by body cells other than leukocytes and they can act on nonhematopoietic cells. Interleukins 1 through 18 have been identified. Especially important ILs include IL-3 (stimulates growth of stem-cell precursors of all blood cells), IL-2 (stimulates T and B lymphocytes), IL-12 (stimulates hematopoietic cells and lymphocytes), and IL-11 (stimulates platelets and other cells). Interleukin action may occur only when combined with another factor; may be suppressive rather than stimulatory (eg, IL-10); or may involve a specific function (eg, IL-8 mainly promotes movement of leukocytes into injured tissues as part of the inflammatory response).

OVERVIEW OF BODY DEFENSE MECHANISMS

The immune system is one of several mechanisms that protect the body from potentially harmful substances, including pathogenic microorganisms. The body's primary external defense mechanism is intact skin, which prevents entry of foreign substances and produces secretions that inhibit microbial growth. The mucous membranes lining the gastrointestinal (GI) and respiratory tracts are internal defense mechanisms that act as physical barriers and produce mucus that traps foreign substances so they may be expelled from the body. Mucous membranes also produce other secretions (eg, gastric acid) that kill ingested microorganisms. Additional internal mechanisms include the normal microbial population, which is usually nonpathogenic and controls potential pathogens; and secretions (eg, perspiration, tears, saliva) that contain lysozyme, an enzyme that destroys the cell walls of gram-positive bacteria.

If a foreign substance gets through the aforementioned defenses to penetrate body tissues and cause cellular injury, an inflammatory response begins immediately. Cellular injury may be caused by chemicals, hypoxia, ischemia, microorganisms, excessive heat or cold, radiation, and nutritional deficiencies or excesses. The cellular response to injury involves inflammation, a generalized reaction to any tissue damage, which attempts to remove the damaging agent and repair the damaged tissue. The hemodynamic aspect of inflammation includes vasodilation, which increases blood supply to the injured area; and increased capillary permeability, which allows fluid to leak into tissue spaces. The cellular aspect involves the movement of white blood cells (WBCs) into the area of injury. WBCs are attracted to the injured area by bacteria, tissue debris, plasma protein fractions (complement), and other substances, in a process called *chemotaxis.* After they reach the area, they phagocytize causative agents and tissue debris.

The final defense mechanism is the immune response, and an effective response involves lymphoid cells, inflammatory cells, and hematopoietic cells. The immune response stimulates production of antibodies and activated lymphocytes to destroy foreign invaders and mutant body cells (eg, abnormal cells, cancer cells).

Inflammatory and immune responses interact in complex ways and share a number of processes, including phagocytosis. They produce their effects indirectly, through interactions among cytokines and other chemical mediators. Cytokines induce WBC replication, phagocytosis, antibody production, fever, inflammation, and tissue repair. Other chemical mediators (eg, histamine, prostaglandins) are synthesized or released by mast cells and other cells. After they are activated, mediators may exert their effects on tissues locally or at distant target sites. They also may induce or enhance other mediators. Little information is available about the chemical mediators of chronic inflammation, but immunologic mechanisms are thought to play an important role.

IMMUNITY

Immunity indicates protection from a disease, and the main function of the immune system is host protection. To this end, the immune system detects and eliminates foreign substances that may cause tissue injury or disease. It also regulates tissue homeostasis and repair as cells of the immune system identify and remove injured, damaged, dead, or malignant cells.

To perform these functions, the immune system must be able to differentiate body tissues (self) from foreign substances (non-self). Self tissues are recognized by distinctive protein molecules on the surface membranes of body cells. These molecules or markers are encoded by a group of genes called the major histocompatibility complex (MHC). MHC markers are essential to immune system function because they regulate the antigens to which a person responds and allow immune cells (eg, lymphocytes, macrophages) to recognize and communicate with each other. Non-self or foreign antigens are also recognized by distinctive molecules, called *epitopes,* on their surfaces. Epitopes vary widely in type, number, and ability to elicit an immune response.

A normally functioning immune system does not attack body tissues labeled as self, but attacks non-self substances. An abnormally functioning immune system causes numerous diseases. When the system is hypoactive, immunodeficiency disorders develop because the person is highly susceptible to infectious and neoplastic diseases. When the system is hyperactive, it perceives ordinarily harmless environmental substances (eg, foods, plant pollens) as harmful and induces allergic reactions. When the system is inappropriately activated (it loses its ability to distinguish between self and non-self, so an immune response is aroused against the host's own body tissues), the result is autoimmune disorders such as rheumatoid arthritis and systemic lupus erythematosus (SLE). Many other disorders, including diabetes mellitus, myasthenia gravis, and inflammatory bowel diseases, are thought to involve autoimmune mechanisms. To aid understanding of the immune response and drugs used to alter immune response, more specific characteristics, processes, and functions of the immune system are described.

Types of Immunity

Innate immunity, which is not produced by the immune system, includes the general protective mechanisms described.

Adaptive or **acquired immunity** develops during gestation or after birth and may be active or passive. *Active immunity* is produced by the person's own immune system in response to a disease caused by a specific antigen or administration of an antigen (eg, a vaccine) from a source outside the body, usually by injection. The immune response stimulated by the antigen produces activated lymphocytes and antibodies against the antigen. When an antigen is present for the first time, production of antibodies requires several days. As a result, the serum concentration of antibodies does not reach protective levels for 7 to 10 days, and the disease develops in the host. When the antigen is eliminated, the antibody concentration gradually decreases over several weeks.

The duration of active immunity may be brief (eg, to influenza viruses), or it may last for years or a lifetime. Long-term active immunity has a unique characteristic called *memory*. When the host is re-exposed to the antigen, lymphocytes are activated and antibodies are produced rapidly, and the host does not contract the disease. This characteristic allows "booster" doses of antigen to increase antibody levels and maintain active immunity against some diseases.

Passive immunity occurs when antibodies are formed by the immune system of another person or animal and transferred to the host. For example, an infant is normally protected for several months by maternal antibodies received through the placenta during gestation. Also, antibodies previously formed by a donor can be transferred to the host by an injection of immune serum. These antibodies act against antigens immediately. Passive immunity is short-term, lasting only a few weeks or months.

Cellular and Humoral Immunity

Types of adaptive immunity have traditionally been separated into cellular immunity (mainly involving activated T lymphocytes in body tissues) and humoral immunity (mainly involving B lymphocytes and antibodies in the blood). However, it is now known that the two types are closely connected; that virtually all antigens elicit both cellular and humoral responses; and that most humoral (B cell) responses require cellular (T cell) stimulation.

Although most humoral immune responses occur when antibodies or B cells encounter antigens in blood, some occur when antibodies or B cells encounter antigens in other body fluids (eg, tears, sweat, saliva, mucus, breast milk). The antibodies in body fluids other than blood are produced by a part of humoral immunity sometimes called the *secretory* or *mucosal immune system*. The B cells of the mucosal system migrate through lymphoid tissues of tear ducts, salivary glands, breasts, bronchi, intestines, and genitourinary structures. The antibodies (mostly immunoglobulin A [IgA]; some IgM and IgG) secreted at these sites act locally rather than systemically.

This local protection combats foreign substances, especially pathogenic microorganisms, that are inhaled, swallowed, or otherwise come in contact with external body surfaces. When the foreign substances bind to local antibodies, they are unable to attach to and invade mucosal tissue.

Antigens

Antigens are the foreign (non-self) substances (eg, microorganisms, other proteins, polysaccharides) that initiate immune responses. Antigens have specific sites that interact with immune cells to induce the immune response. The number of antigenic sites on a molecule depends largely on its molecular weight. Large protein and polysaccharide molecules are complete antigens because of their complex chemical structure and multiple antigenic sites. Smaller molecules (eg, animal danders, plant pollens, most drugs) are incomplete antigens (called *haptens*) and cannot act as antigens by themselves. However, they have antigenic sites and can combine with carrier substances to become antigenic. In discussions of hypersensitivity (allergic) conditions, antigens are often called *allergens*.

Immune Responses to Antigens

The immune response involves antigens that induce the formation of antibodies or activated T lymphocytes. The initial response occurs when an antigen is first introduced into the body. B lymphocytes recognize the antigen as foreign and develop antibodies against it. Antibodies are proteins called *immunoglobulins* (Ig) that interact with specific antigens.

Antigen–antibody interactions may result in formation of antigen–antibody complexes; agglutination or clumping of cells; neutralization of bacterial toxins; destruction of pathogens or cells; attachment of antigen to immune cells; coating of the antigen so that it is more readily recognized by phagocytic cells (opsonization); or activation of complement (a group of plasma proteins activated by recognition of an antigen–antibody complex, bacteria, or viruses and essential to normal inflammatory and immunologic responses). Activated complement stimulates *chemotaxis* (movement of monocytes, neutrophils, basophils, and eosinophils toward the antigen) and the release of hydrolytic enzymes, actions that result in the destruction or inactivation of the invading antigen. With a later exposure to the antigen, antibody is rapidly produced. The number of exposures required to produce enough antibodies to bind a significant amount of antigen is unknown. Thus, an allergic reaction may occur with the second exposure or after several exposures, when sufficient antibodies have been produced.

Antigen–T lymphocyte interactions stimulate production and function of other T lymphocytes and help to regulate antibody production by B lymphocytes. T cells are involved in delayed hypersensitivity reactions, rejection of tissue or organ transplants, and responses to neoplasms and some infections.

IMMUNE CELLS

Immune cells (Fig. 38-1) are WBCs that circulate in the blood and lymphatic vessels or reside in lymphoid tissues. These cells (neutrophils, eosinophils, basophils, monocyte–macrophages, dendritic cells, NK cells, and lymphocytes) are present in virtually every body tissue and their ability to circulate throughout the body and to migrate between blood and lymphoid tissues are major components of host defenses. The cells are activated by exposure to an antigen. Although all WBCs play a role, neutrophils, monocytes, and lymphocytes are especially important in phagocytic and immune processes.

Neutrophils

Neutrophils are the major WBCs in the bloodstream and the body's main defense against pathogenic bacteria. They usually arrive at sites of tissue injury within 90 minutes. They localize the area of injury and phagocytize organisms or particles by releasing digestive enzymes and oxidative metabolites that kill engulfed pathogens or destroy other types of foreign particles. The number of neutrophils increases greatly during the inflammatory process. These cells circulate in the bloodstream for approximately 10 hours, then move into tissues, where they live for 1 to 3 days.

Eosinophils and Basophils

Eosinophils increase in number and activity during allergic reactions and parasitic infections. In parasitic infections, they bind to and kill the parasites. In hypersensitivity reactions, they produce enzymes that inactivate histamine and leukotrienes and may produce other enzymes that destroy antigen–antibody complexes. Despite these generally beneficial effects, eosinophils also may aggravate tissue damage by releasing cytotoxic substances. Basophils release histamine, a major chemical mediator in inflammatory and immediate hypersensitivity reactions. However, the function of basophils in normal immune responses is not well understood.

Monocytes

Monocytes arrive several hours after injury and usually replace neutrophils as the predominant WBC within 48 hours. They are the largest WBCs, and their lifespan is much longer than that of the neutrophils. Monocytes can phagocytize larger sizes and amounts of foreign material than neutrophils. In addition to their activity in the bloodstream, monocytes can leave blood vessels and enter tissue spaces (and then are called *tissue macrophages*). Tissue macrophages are widely distributed in connective tissue and in other areas (eg, Kupffer's cells in the liver, alveolar macrophages in the lungs, others in the lymph nodes and spleen) and form the mononuclear phagocyte system. Both mobile and fixed monocyte–macrophages are important in inflammatory processes and both can initiate the immune response by activating lymphocytes. They perform this function as part of phagocytosis, in which they engulf a circulating antigen (eg, foreign material, cellular debris), break it into fragments, combine the fragments with MHC molecules, and return the antigenic fragments to the cell surface. The antigenic fragments are recognized as foreign material by circulating T and B lymphocytes, and an immune response is initiated. Because the monocytes prepare the antigen to interact with T and B lymphocytes, they are called *antigen-presenting cells* (APCs). In addition to phagocytosis, activated macrophages also secrete many products (eg, enzymes, cytokines); remove antigen–antibody complexes; remove dying and dead host cells; and can destroy virus-infected cells or tumor cells.

Dendritic Cells

Dendritic cells are surface macrophages found in peripheral lymphoid tissues and peripheral tissues through which microorganisms and other foreign antigens enter the body (eg, skin, mucosa, bronchial airways). They are star-shaped, with a large surface area through which they can recognize, capture, and ingest antigens. Their main function is the presentation of antigen to T lymphocytes, which activates the T cells and initiates the adaptive immune response.

Dendritic cells become active APCs when stimulated by injury or cytokines such as tumor necrosis factor–alpha (TNF-alpha) or interferon alfa. Activation also causes the antigen-containing cells to enter lymph vessels and migrate to regional lymph nodes, where the T cells are located.

Lymphocytes

Lymphocytes are the main immune cells, and those in tissues are in dynamic equilibrium with those in circulating blood. These cells continuously travel through blood and lymph vessels from one lymphoid organ to another. The three types of lymphocytes are NK cells, T cells, and B cells.

Natural Killer Cells

Natural killer cells, so called because they do not need to interact with a specific antigen to become activated, destroy infectious microorganisms and malignant cells by releasing powerful chemicals. These cells are thought to provide the first line of defense against viral infections and other intracellular pathogens while adaptive immune responses are being generated. NK cells are sensitized by cytokines released from macrophages and dendritic cells. They function mainly by secreting interferon gamma, which activates macrophages and other cells. In addition to their ability to kill virus-infected cells, they are thought to kill certain tumor cells.

T Lymphocytes

T lymphocytes, the main regulators of the immune response, are involved in both cell-mediated and humoral immunity

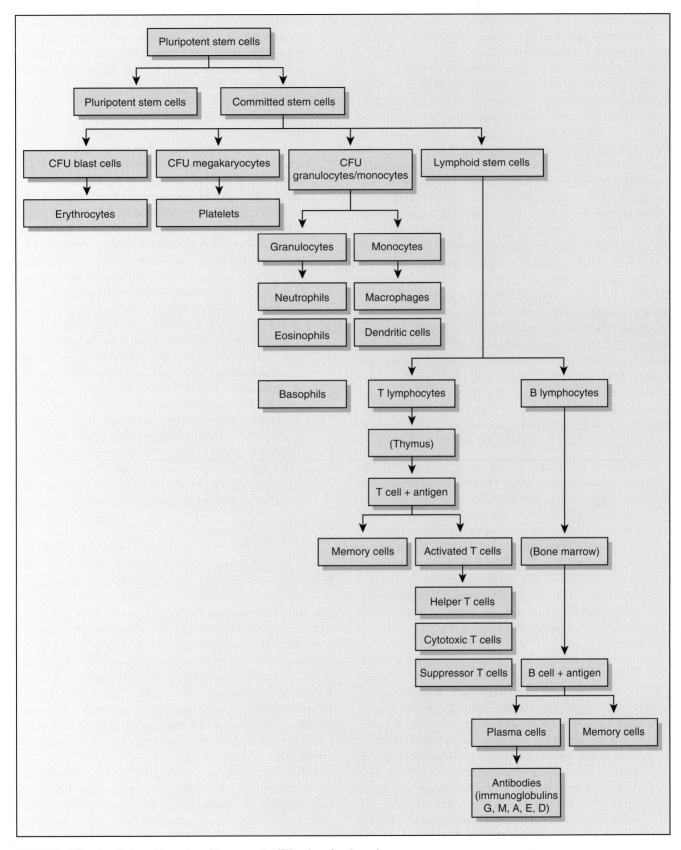

FIGURE 38-1 Hematopoiesis and formation of immune cells. CFU, colony-forming unit.

because they direct the activities of B cells and macrophages. T cells must be activated by antigens before they can fulfill their immune functions, and they have proteins on their cell-membrane surfaces that act as receptors for antigens.

Each T cell reacts only with a specific type of antigen and is capable of forming only one type of T cell. When a specific antigen attaches to cell-membrane receptors to form an antigen–antibody complex, the complex activates the T cell to form tremendous numbers of duplicate T cells (clones) that are exactly like the parent cell. T-cell clones are sensitized or activated T cells that are released into lymphatic ducts, carried to the blood, circulated through all tissue fluids, then returned to lymphatic ducts and recirculated. Additional participants in the activation process are phagocytic macrophages and helper T cells, which secrete cytokines that regulate the growth, reproduction, and function of lymphocytes.

T lymphocytes originate in stem cells in the bone marrow and differentiate into immune cells in the thymus gland. The thymus produces a substance called *thymosin,* which is necessary for T-cell maturation. When T cells bind with an antigen, specific genes are activated to produce substances that direct T-cell proliferation and differentiation. One such substance is IL-2, which stimulates T-cell DNA replication and mitosis. Cell division is necessary for production of large numbers of antigen-reactive cells and for cellular changes associated with the different subgroups of T cells. Specific types and functions of T cells include the following:

- *Helper T cells* (also called T_H or *CD4+* cells), the largest subgroup, regulate virtually all immune functions by producing protein substances called *cytokines.* The cytokines stimulate the growth of bone marrow and other cells of the immune system (eg, cytotoxic T and B cells). They also activate macrophages and facilitate phagocytosis. Important cytokines include IL-2, -3, -4, -5, and -6; GM-CSF; and interferon gamma. The devastating effects of acquired immunodeficiency syndrome (AIDS) result primarily from the ability of the human immunodeficiency virus (HIV) to destroy helper T cells.

  Subsets of helper T cells have recently been identified as T_H1, T_H2, and suppressor T cells. Both T_h1 and T_h2 cells secrete IL-3 and GM-CSF, but differ in the other cytokines they secrete. The T_H1 subset is responsible for many cell-mediated functions (eg, delayed-type hypersensitivity reactions, activation of cytotoxic T cells) and for the production of IgG antibodies that promote recognition of antigens. These cells are also associated with excessive inflammation and tissue injury. The T_H2 subset stimulates the activation and differentiation of eosinophils, and stimulates B cells (eg, to produce immunoglobulins such as IgM and IgE). These cells are also associated with hypersensitivity reactions. Suppressor T cells are thought to stop the immune response (ie, decrease the activities of B

cells and other T cells) when an antigen has been destroyed. This activity is considered important in preventing further tissue damage. For example, in autoimmune disorders, suppressor T cell function is impaired and extensive tissue damage may result.

- *Cytotoxic T cells* (also called T_C or *CD8+* cells) are recruited and activated by helper T cells. More specifically, helper T cells secrete IL-2, which is necessary for activation and proliferation (clonal expansion) of cytotoxic T cells. When activated by antigen and IL-2, cytotoxic T cells bind to antigens on the surfaces of target cells. After binding to antigen, the T cells are thought to destroy target cells by one or more of three mechanisms. One mechanism involves the formation of holes in the target cell membrane that allow fluids to enter and swell the cell until it bursts. Another is the insertion of enzymes that break down or digest the cell. A third mechanism is to induce apoptosis (programmed cell death). After these cytotoxic cells have damaged the target cells, they can detach themselves and attack other target cells.

  Cytotoxic T cells are especially lethal to virus-infected cells because virus particles become entrapped in the membranes of the cells and act as strong antigens that attract the T cells. These cells persist in tissues for months, even after destruction of all the invaders that elicited the original cytotoxic activity. Thus, cytotoxic T cells are especially important in killing body cells that have been invaded by foreign microorganisms or cells that have become malignant. Cytotoxic T cells also play a role in the destruction of transplanted organs and delayed hypersensitivity reactions.

B Lymphocytes

B cells are involved in humoral immunity; they secrete antibodies that can neutralize pathogens before their entry into host cells. B cells must be activated by antigens before they can fulfill their immune functions, and they have proteins on their cell-membrane surfaces that act as receptors for antigens. Each B lymphocyte reacts only with a specific type of antigen, and is capable of forming only one type of antibody. When a specific antigen attaches to cell-membrane receptors to form an antigen–antibody complex, the complex activates the lymphocyte to form tremendous numbers of duplicate lymphocytes (clones) that are exactly like the parent cell. Clones of a B lymphocyte eventually secrete antibodies that circulate throughout the body.

B lymphocytes originate in stem cells in the bone marrow, differentiate into cells capable of forming antibodies (also in the bone marrow), and migrate to the spleen, lymph nodes, or other lymphoid tissue. In lymphoid tissue, the cells may be dormant until exposed to an antigen. In response to an antigen and IL-2 from helper T cells, B cells multiply rapidly, enlarge, and differentiate into plasma cells, which then produce antibodies (immunoglobulins [Ig]) to oppose the antigen. Immunoglobulins are secreted into lymph and transported to the bloodstream for circulation throughout the body. There are five main classes of immunoglobulins:

1. *IgG* is the most abundant immunoglobulin, constituting approximately 80% of the antibodies in human serum. It protects against bacteria, toxins, and viruses as it circulates in the bloodstream. Molecules of IgG combine with molecules of antigen, and the antigen–antibody complex activates complement. Activated complement causes an inflammatory reaction, promotes phagocytosis, and inactivates or destroys the antigen. IgG also crosses the placenta to provide maternally acquired antibodies (passive immunity) to the infant.

2. *IgA* is the main immunoglobulin in mucous membranes and body secretions. It is found in saliva, breast milk, and nasal, respiratory, prostatic, and vaginal secretions. It protects against pathogens and other antigens that gain access to these areas. For example, it prevents attachment of viruses and bacteria to mucous membranes.

3. *IgM* constitutes approximately 10% of serum antibodies. It protects against bacteria, toxins, and viruses that gain access to the bloodstream and is important in early immune responses. It acts only in the bloodstream, because its large molecular size prevents its movement or transport through capillary walls. It activates complement to destroy microorganisms.

4. *IgE* binds to mast cells and basophils. It is present in body fluids and readily enters body tissues. It is involved in parasitic infections and hypersensitivity reactions, including anaphylaxis. IgE sensitizes mast cells, which then release histamine and other chemical mediators that cause bronchoconstriction, edema, urticaria, and other manifestations of allergic reactions. IgE does not activate complement. The production of IgE is stimulated by T lymphocytes and IL-4, -5, and -6 and is inhibited by the interferons. Small amounts of IgE are present in the serum of nonallergic people; larger amounts are produced by people with allergies.

5. *IgD* is found on the cell membranes of B lymphocytes. It functions as an antigen receptor for initiating the differentiation and maturation of B lymphocytes.

IMMUNE SYSTEM CYTOKINES

Cytokines (Fig. 38-2) are the primary means of communication between immune cells and other tissues and organs of the body. They also regulate the intensity and duration of the immune response by stimulating or inhibiting the activation, proliferation, and/or differentiation of various cells and by regulating the secretion of antibodies or other cytokines. Although the hematopoietic cytokines described include the immune system cytokines, the emphasis here is on those that affect immune cells. It is thought that cytokines formed by

activated macrophages enter the bone marrow, where they induce the synthesis and release of other cytokines that activate resting stem cells to produce more granulocytes and monocytes–macrophages. Newly formed granulocytes and monocytes leave the bone marrow and enter the circulating blood in approximately 3 days.

Cytokine binding to target cells elicits wide-ranging effects, including increased expression of cytokine receptors and increased production of other cytokines. In general, the cytokines secreted by antigen-activated lymphocytes can affect the activity of most cells involved in the immune response. For example, cytokines produced by activated helper T cells influence the activity of B cells, cytotoxic T cells, NK cells, macrophages, granulocytes, and hematopoietic stem cells. As a result, a network of interacting cells is activated.

Some cytokines enhance macrophage activity by two main mechanisms. First, they cause macrophages to accumulate in damaged tissues by delaying or stopping macrophage migration from the area. Second, they increase the capacity and effectiveness of phagocytosis. Some cytokines, especially IL-2, directly stimulate helper T cells and enhance their antiantigenic activity. They also enhance the antiantigenic activity of the entire immune system. IL-4, -5, and -6 are especially important in B-cell activities.

Tumor necrosis factors (TNF) are produced by activated macrophages and other cells and act on many immune and nonimmune target cells. They participate in the inflammatory response and cause hemorrhagic necrosis in several types of tumor cells. TNF-alpha is structurally the same as cachectin, a substance associated with debilitation and weight loss in clients with cancer. TNF-beta is also called *lymphotoxin*.

CLIENT-RELATED FACTORS THAT INFLUENCE IMMUNE FUNCTION

Age

Fetuses and Neonates

During the first few months of gestation, the fetal immune system is deficient in antibody production and phagocytic activity. During the last trimester, the fetal immune system may be able to respond to infectious antigens, such as cytomegalovirus, rubella virus, and *Toxoplasma*. However, most fetal protection against infectious microorganisms is by maternal antibodies that reach the fetal circulation through the placenta.

At birth, the neonatal immune system is still immature, but IgG levels (from maternal blood) are near adult levels in umbilical cord blood. However, the source of maternal antibodies is severed at birth. Antibody titers in infants decrease over approximately 6 months as maternal antibodies are catabolized. Although the infant does start producing IgG, the rate of production is lower than the rate of breakdown of

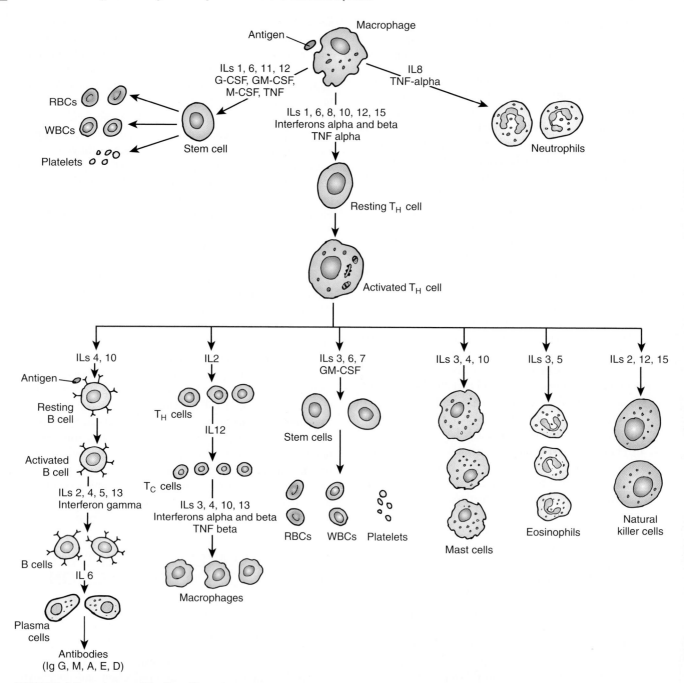

FIGURE 38-2 Macrophage and T-cell cytokines, their target cells, and the products of target cells. These elements overlap and interact to regulate the immune response. CSF, colony-stimulating factor; G-CSF, granulocyte–colony-stimulating factor; GM-CSF, granulocyte macrophage colony-stimulating factor; Ig, immunoglobulin; IL, interleukin; M-CSF, monocyte–macrophage colony-stimulating factor; RBCs, red blood cells; T$_C$, cytotoxic T cell; T$_H$, helper T cell; TNF, tumor necrosis factor; WBCs, white blood cells.

maternal antibodies. Cell-mediated immunity is probably completely functional at birth.

Older Adults

Both humoral and cell-mediated immune functions decline with aging, and this decline is probably a major factor in the older adult's increased susceptibility to infections and neoplasms. Lymphocytes are less able to proliferate in response to antigenic stimulation, and a relative state of immunodeficiency prevails. With T lymphocytes, function is impaired, and the numbers in peripheral blood may be decreased. The functional impairment includes decreased activity of helper T cells. With B lymphocytes, the cells are less able to form antibodies in response to antigens. Abnormal antibody production results from impaired function of B cells and helper T cells. Other aspects of immune system function also decline with age. For example, older adults have increased blood levels of antibodies against their own tissues (autoantibodies), which may account for the greater frequency of autoimmune diseases in this age group.

Impaired immune mechanisms have several implications for clinicians who care for older clients, including the following:

- Older adults are more likely to develop infections (including reactivation of infections such as tuberculosis and herpes zoster) and less able to recover from them. Therefore, older adults need protective measures, such as rigorous personal hygiene; good nutrition; adequate exercise, rest, and sleep; minimal exposure to potential pathogens, when possible; and appropriate immunizations (eg, influenza, pneumonia, tetanus). When an infection develops in older adults, signs and symptoms (eg, fever, drainage) may be absent or less pronounced than in younger adults.
- Older adults have impaired immune responses to antigens. Thus, achieving protective antibody titers may require higher doses of immunizing antigens in older adults than in younger adults.
- Older adults often exhibit a less intense positive reaction in skin tests for tuberculosis (indicating a decreased delayed hypersensitivity response).

Nutritional Status

Nutritional status can have profound effects on immune function. Adequate nutrient intake contributes to immunocompetence (ability of the immune system to function effectively). Malnutrition contributes to immunodeficiency. A severe lack of calories or protein decreases numbers and functions of T cells; complement activity; neutrophil chemotaxis; and phagocytosis. An inadequate zinc intake can depress the functions of T and B cells. Zinc is a cofactor for many enzymes, some of which are found in lymphocytes and are required for lymphocyte function. Zinc deficiency also may result from inadequate absorption in the GI tract or excessive losses in urine, feces, or through the skin with such disorders as chronic renal disease, chronic diarrhea, burns, or severe psoriasis. Vitamin deficiencies may also depress T- and B-cell function because several (eg, A, E, folic acid, pantothenic acid, pyridoxine) also are enzyme cofactors in lymphocytes.

Stress

There is evidence that stress depresses immune function and therefore increases risks for development of infection and cancer. The connection between the stress response and the immune response is thought to involve neuroendocrine mechanisms. The stress response is characterized by increased activity of catecholamine neurotransmitters in the central and autonomic nervous systems (eg, norepinephrine, epinephrine) and increased secretion of cortisol from the adrenal cortex. Cortisol and other corticosteroids are well known to suppress immune function and are used therapeutically for that purpose. The immune response is affected by these neuroendocrine influences on lymphoid organs and lymphocyte functions because lymphocytes have receptors for many neurotransmitters and hormones.

IMMUNE DISORDERS

Dysfunction of the immune system is related to many different disease processes, including allergic, autoimmune, immunodeficiency, and neoplastic disorders. These disorders are described below to assist in understanding the use of drugs to alter immune functions.

Allergies

In allergic disorders, the body erroneously perceives normally harmless substances (eg, foods, pollens) as antigens and mounts an immune response. More specifically, IgE binds to antigen on the surface of mast cells and causes the release of chemical mediators (eg, histamine) that produce the allergic manifestations. These reactions may cause tissue damage ranging from mild skin rashes to life-threatening anaphylaxis.

Autoimmune Disorders

In autoimmune disorders, the body erroneously perceives its own tissues as antigens and elicits an immune response, usually chronic and inflammatory in nature. Hashimoto's thyroiditis, multiple sclerosis, myasthenia gravis, rheumatoid arthritis, SLE, and type 1 diabetes mellitus are considered autoimmune disorders. Autoimmune processes, which are similar to the processes elicited by pathogenic microorganisms and environmental antigens, may damage virtually every body tissue.

Immunodeficiency Disorders

Defects in any immune system components can compromise host protection and greatly increase susceptibility to infections and malignant neoplasms. Immunodeficiency disorders can be inherited or acquired. Common causes of acquired disorders include infection with HIV, advanced age, cytotoxic anticancer chemotherapy, and immunosuppressive drugs used to treat transplant rejection or autoimmune disorders. The HIV paralyzes the immune system by targeting helper T cells, macrophages, and dendritic cells. More specifically, it decreases the numbers and almost all functions of T lymphocytes and several functions of B lymphocytes and monocytes. Advanced age is associated with reduced ability to produce T cells, and chemotherapy is often associated with permanent deficits in the numbers and functions of T cells.

Neoplastic Disorders

In neoplastic disease, immune cells lose their ability to recognize and destroy mutant cells or early malignant cells. This effect could result from immunodeficiency states or from cancer cells that are overwhelming in number or highly malignant. Mutant cells constantly occur during cell division, but few survive or lead to cancer. Most mutant cells simply die; some survive but retain the normal controls that prevent excessive growth; and some are destroyed by immune processes activated by the abnormal proteins found in most mutant cells.

DRUGS THAT ALTER HEMATOPOIETIC AND IMMUNE RESPONSES

Drugs that modify the immune system (often called *biologic response modifiers* or *immunomodulators*) can enhance or restrict immune responses to various disease processes. Thus, they may be immunostimulants or immunosuppressants. Specific drug groups include hematopoietic growth factors, interferons, interleukins, and monoclonal antibodies. Interferons have antiviral and antiproliferative actions as well as immuno-modulatory functions.

These drugs are heterogenous in their uses and characteristics. They are used to prevent or treat symptoms (eg, anemia, neutropenia) caused by disease processes or their treatments; prevent or treat infections; prevent or treat rejection of transplanted tissues or organs; treat autoimmune disorders; and treat immunodeficiency disorders and cancer. In cancer, the drugs are used to modify host responses; to destroy tumor cells by suppressing their growth or killing the cells; or to modify tumor cell biology. Vaccines for melanoma and prostate cancer are being investigated.

Methods of modifying immune functions include administering exogenous antigens (eg, immunizations, desensitization procedures) or strengthening antigens (eg, an antigen that is too weak to elicit an immune response), or suppressing the normal response to an antigen. In desensitization procedures, weak extracts of antigenic substances (eg, foods, plant pollens, penicillin) are prepared as drugs and administered in small, increasing amounts so the client develops a tolerance for the substances and avoids serious allergic reactions.

Overall, drugs can be given to stimulate immune responses (see Chap. 39); stimulate hematopoiesis and immune responses

(see Chap. 40); suppress normal immune responses (see Chap. 41); and manage various aspects of oncologic disorders (see Chap. 42).

Review and Application Exercises

Short Answer Exercises

1. What is the difference between innate and acquired immunity?

2. What are methods of producing active acquired immunity?

3. Which WBCs are phagocytes?

4. Describe phagocytosis.

5. Where are T lymphocytes formed, and what are their functions?

6. Where are B lymphocytes formed, and what are their functions?

7. What are antigens, and how do they elicit an immune response?

8. What are cytokines, and how do they function in the immune response?

9. What is complement, and how does it function in the immune response?

10. What are the main consequences of immunodeficiency states?

Selected References

English, D. (2003). Blood components, immunity, and hemostasis. In R. A. Rhoades & G. A. Tanner, *Medical physiology* (2nd ed., pp. 191–209). Philadelphia: Lippincott Williams & Wilkins.

Goldman, L., & Ausiello, D. (Eds.). (2004). *Cecil textbook of medicine* (22nd ed.). Philadelphia: W. B. Saunders.

Goronzy, J. J., & Weyand, C. M. (2004). The innate and adaptive immune systems. In L. Goldman & D. Ausiello (Eds.), *Cecil textbook of medicine* (22nd ed., pp. 208–217). Philadelphia: W. B. Saunders.

Hall, P. D., & Karlix, J. L. (2002). Function and evaluation of the immune system. In J. T. DiPiro, R. L. Talbert, G. C. Yee, G. R. Matzke, B. G. Wells, & L. M. Posey (Eds.), *Pharmacotherapy: A pathophysiologic approach* (5th ed., pp. 1557–1568). New York: McGraw-Hill.

Quesenberry, P. J. (2004). Hematopoiesis and hematopoietic growth factors. In L. Goldman & D. Ausiello (Eds.), *Cecil textbook of medicine* (22nd ed., pp. 958–963). Philadelphia: W. B. Saunders.

Rhoades, R. A., & Tanner, G. A. (2003). *Medical physiology* (2nd ed.). Philadelphia: Lippincott Williams & Wilkins.

Sommer, C. (2005). The immune response. In C. M. Porth, *Pathophysiology: Concepts of altered health states* (7th ed., pp. 365–385). Philadelphia: Lippincott Williams & Wilkins.

Immunizing Agents

OBJECTIVES

After studying this chapter, you will be able to:

1. Discuss common characteristics of immunizations.
2. Discuss the importance of immunizations in promoting health and preventing disease.
3. Identify authoritative sources for immunization information.
4. Identify immunizations recommended for children.
5. Identify immunizations recommended for adults.
6. Discuss ways to promote immunization of all age groups.
7. Teach parents about recommended immunizations and record keeping.

APPLYING YOUR KNOWLEDGE

Deborah Stein is a 29-year-old woman who is planning a trip abroad this year. She is visiting her health care provider to plan for the necessary immunizations for her trip. She is unsure about her immunization history, and she is new to this medical practice.

INTRODUCTION

Immune responses and types of immunity are described in Chapter 38. Many antigens that activate the immune response are microorganisms that cause infectious diseases. Early scientists observed that people who contracted certain diseases were thereafter protected despite repeated exposure to the disease. As knowledge evolved, it was discovered that protection stemmed from body substances called *antibodies,* and that antibodies could also be induced by deliberate, controlled exposure to the antigen. Subsequently, immunization techniques were developed.

Although immunizations against some diseases have long been used, the development of immunizing agents and recommendations for their use continue. Some recommendations and changes of recent years are summarized as follows:

- The American Academy of Pediatrics (AAP; www.aap.org) recommends that only the inactivated poliomyelitis vaccine (IPV) be used in the United States. The oral vaccine used for many years contained live virus and caused viral shedding and a few cases of polio. The main disadvantages of IPV are that it must be injected and it is more expensive.

- Hepatitis B virus (HBV) infection can cause serious liver diseases such as acute and chronic hepatitis, cirrhosis, and hepatocellular carcinoma. Chronic carriers of HBV may be asymptomatic reservoirs for viral transmission. Children who become infected are at high risk of becoming chronically infected. Because of these circumstances, hepatitis B vaccine is now recommended for all newborns and for unimmunized children before starting school, as well as other at-risk groups. Overall, the goal is to achieve universal immunization, decrease transmission, and eradicate the disease.

- Everyone should be immunized against diphtheria and tetanus every 7 to 10 years for life.

- Strategies to promote immunization continue to evolve. One strategy is to combine vaccines so that only one injection is required when the need and time for multiple vaccines coincide. In addition to the long-used measles-mumps-rubella (MMR) and diphtheria-tetanus-pertussis (DTaP) combinations, available combinations include *Haemophilus influenzae* b (Hib) with hepatitis B (eg, Comvax); DTaP with *H. influenzae* b (DTaP-HIB) (eg, TriHIBit); and hepatitis A and hepatitis B (eg, Twinrix). Another strategy is to give multiple vaccines (in separate syringes, at different sites) at one visit to a health care provider when feasible. For example, several vaccines can be given at the same time for routine immunization of infants and young children. In addition, influenza and pneumococcal vaccines can be administered concurrently, and at least one study indicates that varicella and MMR vaccines can be given at the same office visit.

Immunization

Immunization or *vaccination* involves administration of an antigen to induce antibody formation (for active immunity) or administration of serum from immune people (for passive immunity). Preparations used for immunization are biologic products prepared by pharmaceutical companies and regulated by the United States Food and Drug Administration (FDA).

GENERAL CHARACTERISTICS OF IMMUNIZING AGENTS

Agents for Active Immunity

The biologic products used for active immunity are vaccines and toxoids. **Vaccines** are suspensions of microorganisms or their antigenic products that have been killed or attenuated (weakened or reduced in virulence) so that they can induce antibody formation while preventing or causing very mild forms of the disease. Many vaccines produce long-lasting immunity. Attenuated live vaccines produce immunity, usually lifelong, that is similar to that produced by natural infection. However, there is a small risk of producing disease with live vaccines, especially in people with impaired immune function. Vaccines developed with recombinant DNA technology have a low risk for causing active disease.

Toxoids are bacterial toxins or products that have been modified to destroy toxicity while retaining antigenic properties (ie, ability to induce antibody formation). Immunization with toxoids is not permanent; scheduled repeat doses (boosters) are required to maintain immunity.

Additional components of vaccines and toxoids may include aluminum phosphate, aluminum hydroxide, or calcium phosphate. Products containing aluminum should be given intramuscularly only, because they cannot be given intravenously and greater tissue irritation occurs with subcutaneous injections. These additives are used to delay absorption and increase antigenicity.

For maximum effectiveness, vaccines and toxoids must be given before exposure to the pathogenic microorganism. They should also be given by the recommended route to ensure the desired immunologic response.

Indications for Use

Clinical indications for use of vaccines and toxoids include the following:

- Routine immunization of all children against diphtheria, *H. influenzae* b infection, hepatitis B, mumps, pertussis,

pneumococcal infection, poliomyelitis, rubella (German measles), rubeola (red measles), tetanus, and varicella
- Immunization of adolescents and adults against diphtheria and tetanus
- Immunization of prepubertal girls or women of childbearing age against rubella. Rubella during the first trimester of pregnancy is associated with a high incidence of birth defects in the newborn.
- Immunization of people at high risk of serious morbidity or mortality from a particular disease. For example, influenza and pneumococcal vaccines are recommended for selected groups of people.
- Immunization of adults and children at high risk of exposure to a particular disease. For example, some diseases (eg, yellow fever) rarely occur in most parts of the world. Thus, immunization is recommended only for people who live in or travel to geographic areas where the disease can be contracted.

Contraindications to Use

Vaccines and toxoids are usually contraindicated during febrile illnesses; immunosuppressive drug therapy (see Chap. 41); immunodeficiency states; leukemia, lymphoma, or generalized malignancy; and pregnancy.

APPLYING YOUR KNOWLEDGE 39-1
What nursing assessments will you perform to evaluate Ms. Stein for possible contraindications for immunization?

Agents for Passive Immunity

Immune serums are the biologic products used for passive immunity. They are used to provide temporary immunity in people exposed to or experiencing a particular disease. The goal of therapy is to prevent or modify the disease process (ie, decrease the incidence and severity of symptoms).

Immune globulin products are made from the serum of individuals with high concentrations of the specific antibody or immunoglobulin (Ig) required. These products may consist of whole serum or of the immunoglobulin portion of serum in which the specific antibodies are concentrated. Immunoglobulin fractions are preferred over whole serum because they are more likely to be effective. Plasma used to prepare these products is negative for hepatitis B surface antigen (HbsAg). Hyperimmune serums are available for cytomegalovirus, hepatitis B, rabies, rubella, tetanus, varicella zoster (shingles), and respiratory syncytial virus infections.

INDIVIDUAL IMMUNIZING AGENTS

Vaccines, toxoids, and immune serums are listed in Tables 39-1 and 39-2.

(*text continues on page 643*)

Table 39-1 Drugs at a Glance: Vaccines and Toxoids for Active Immunity

NAME/CHARACTERISTICS	CLINICAL INDICATIONS	ROUTES AND DOSAGE RANGES	
		Adults	Children
Vaccines			
***Haemophilus influenzae* b (Hib) conjugate vaccine** (ActHIB, HibTITER, PedvaxHIB) Formed by conjugating a derivative of the organism with a protein. The protein increases antigenicity.	To prevent infection with Hib, a common cause of serious bacterial infections, including meningitis, in children younger than 5 y		**ActHIB, HibTITER,** age 2–6 mo, IM 0.5 mL every 2 mo for 3 doses; age 15 mo, 0.5 mL as a single booster dose Age 7–11 mo, IM 0.5 mL every 2 mo for 2 doses; age 15 mo, 0.5 mL as a single booster dose Age 12–14 mo, IM 0.5 mL as single dose; age 15 mo, 0.5 mL as a single booster dose, at least 2 mo after the first dose Age 15–71 mo, IM 0.5 mL as a single dose (no booster dose) **Pedvax HIB,** age 2–14 mo, IM 0.5 mL every 2 mo for 2 doses; age 12–15 mo, 0.5 mL as a booster dose Age 15–71 mo, IM 0.5 mL as a single dose (no booster dose)
***Haemophilus influenzae* b (Hib) conjugate vaccine with hepatitis B vaccine** (Comvax) May be given at the same time as DTaP; measles, mumps, rubella (MMR); injected polio vaccine (IPV), but with separate syringes and in separate sites	Routine immunization of children 6 wk–15 mo of age born to HBsAg-negative mothers		IM, 0.5 mL at 2, 4, and 12–15 months of age
Hepatitis A vaccine (Havrix, Vaqta) Inactivated whole virus More than 90% effective Contraindicated during febrile illness, immunosuppression With Havrix, the adult form contains 1440 units in 1 mL; the pediatric form contains 360 or 720 units in 0.5 mL With Vaqta, the adult form contains 50 units/mL; the pediatric form contains 25 units/0.5 mL	Workers in daycare centers, laboratories, food-handling establishments; men who have sex with men; IV drug users; military personnel; travelers to areas where hepatitis A is endemic; community residents during an outbreak; people with chronic liver disease (eg, hepatitis B or C, cirrhosis)	Havrix, IM in deltoid, 1440 units initially and 6–12 mo later (total of 2 doses) Vaqta, IM in deltoid, 50 units initially and 6–12 mo later (total of 2 doses)	Havrix, 2–18 y, IM, 360 units initially, 1 mo later, and 6–12 mo later (total of 3 doses) or 720 units initially and 6–12 mo later (total of 2 doses) Vaqta, IM, 25 units initially and 6–18 mo later (total of 2 doses)

(continued)

Table 39-1 Drugs at a Glance: Vaccines and Toxoids for Active Immunity (continued)

NAME/CHARACTERISTICS	CLINICAL INDICATIONS	ROUTES AND DOSAGE RANGES	
		Adults	Children
Hepatitis B vaccine (recombinant) (Recombivax HB, Engerix-B) Prepared by inserting the gene coding for production of HBsAg into yeast cells Contains no blood or blood products Approximately 96% effective in children and young adults; approximately 88% effective in adults >40 y Duration of protection unknown; can measure serum antibody levels periodically (protective levels approximately 10 million units/mL)	Pre-exposure immunization of high-risk groups, such as health care providers (nurses, physicians, dentists, laboratory workers); clients with cancer, organ transplants, hemodialysis, immunosuppressant drug therapy, or multiple infusions of blood or blood products; men who have sex with men; IV drug abusers; household contacts of hepatitis B virus carriers; residents and staff of institutions for mentally challenged people Persons requiring postexposure vaccine include infants born to carrier mothers, people with accidental exposure of skin or mucous membrane to infected blood (eg, needlestick injuries), and household contacts or sexual partners of persons with acute hepatitis B infection	*20 y and older:* **Engerix-B,** IM, 20 mcg (1 mL) initially and 1 mo and 6 mo later (3 doses) Predialysis and dialysis clients, IM, 40 mcg (2 mL) initially and 1, 2, and 6 mo later (4 doses) **Recombivax HB,** IM, 10 mcg (1 mL) initially and 1 mo and 6 mo later (3 doses) Predialysis and dialysis clients, IM, 40 mcg (1 mL) initially and 1 mo and 6 mo later (3 doses)	*Neonates to 19 y:* **Engerix-B**, IM, 10 mcg (0.5 mL) initially and 1 mo and 6 mo later (3 doses) *Neonates to 19 y:* **Recombivax**, IM, 5 mcg (0.5 mL) initially and 1 mo and 6 mo later (3 doses)
Hepatitis A, inactivated, and hepatitis B, recombinant (Twinrix) Contains 720 units of hepatitis A and 20 mcg of hepatitis B antigens per mL	Adults exposed to hepatitis A or B (eg, medical personnel, staff in institutional settings such as daycare centers, prisons) Adults at risk of exposure, including travelers to areas of high incidence; people with chronic liver disease; laboratory workers, police, emergency medical personnel, sanitation workers	IM 1 mL initially and 1 mo and 6 mo later (total of 3 doses)	
Influenza vaccine (Fluzone, Fluvirin, FluMist) Inactivated strains of A and B influenza viruses, formulated annually to include current strains Provides protective antibody concentrations for about 6 mo **Note: Fluvirin** is indicated only in children 4 y and older. **FluMist** is indicated in healthy children and adolescents 5–17 y of age, and in healthy adults 18–49 y of age (except during pregnancy).	Children between 6 mo and 2 y of age, their household contacts, out-of-home caregivers, and health care providers Recommended annually for all adults older than 50 y of age; health care providers; and people chronically ill with pulmonary, cardiovascular, or renal disorders, diabetes mellitus, or adrenocortical insufficiency Injected vaccine recommended for pregnant women in their second or third trimester during "flu" season	*All adults:* IM 0.5 mL in a single dose *Healthy adults 18–49 y:* Intranasal spray 0.5 mL per season	**Injectable form** *6–35 mo:* IM, 0.25 mL, 1 dose if previously vaccinated; 2 doses at least 1 mo apart if first vaccination *3–8 y:* IM, 0.5 mL, 1 dose if previously vaccinated; 2 doses at least 1 mo apart if first vaccination *9 y and older:* IM, 0.5 mL in a single dose **Intranasal spray** *5–8 y* (not previously vaccinated with FluMist): 0.5 mL per dose, 60 d apart for a total of 2 doses *5–8 y* (previously vaccinated with FluMist): 0.5 mL in a single dose per season *9 y and older:* 0.6 mL in a single dose per season

Table 39-1 Drugs at a Glance: Vaccines and Toxoids for Active Immunity (continued)

NAME/CHARACTERISTICS	CLINICAL INDICATIONS	ROUTES AND DOSAGE RANGES	
		Adults	Children
Measles vaccine (Attenuvax) Preparation of live, attenuated measles (rubeola) virus Protects approximately 95% of recipients for several years or lifetime Measles vaccine should not be given for 3 mo after administration of immune serum globulin, plasma, or whole blood	Routine immunization of children up to 1 y of age Immunization of adults not previously immunized	Sub-Q 0.5 mL in a single dose	Same as adults
Measles, mumps, and rubella vaccine (M-M-R II) Mixture of rubeola, rubella, and mumps vaccines Preferred over single immunizing agents	Immunization at 15 mo, entry to kindergarten or first grade, and again at entry to middle or junior high school		Sub-Q 0.5 mL per dose
Meningitis vaccine (Menomune-A/C/Y/W-135) Suspension prepared from *Neisseria meningitidis* Protective levels of antibody usually achieved 7–10 d after immunization	Immunization of people at risk in epidemic or endemic areas	Sub-Q 0.5 mL	Sub-Q 0.5 mL
Mumps vaccine (Mumpsvax) Suspension of live, attenuated mumps virus Provides immunity in about 97% of children and 93% of adults for at least 10 y Most often given in combination with measles and rubella vaccines	Routine immunization of children up to 1 y old and adults	Sub-Q 0.5 mL in a single dose (Reconstituted vaccine retains potency for 8 h if refrigerated. Discard if not used within 8 h.)	*>1 y:* Same as adults (Vaccination not indicated in children <1 y.)
Pneumococcal vaccine, polyvalent (Pneumovax 23, Pnu-Imune 23) Consists of 23 strains of pneumococci, which cause approximately 85%–90% of the serious pneumococcal infections in the United States	Adults with chronic disorders associated with increased risk of pneumococcal infection (eg, cardiovascular or pulmonary disease, diabetes mellitus, Hodgkin's disease, multiple myeloma, cirrhosis, alcohol dependence, renal failure, immunosuppression)	Sub-Q, IM 0.5 mL as a single dose–may be repeated after 5 y	Same as adults–may be repeated after 3 y

(continued)

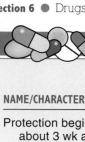

Table 39-1 Drugs at a Glance: Vaccines and Toxoids for Active Immunity (continued)

NAME/CHARACTERISTICS	CLINICAL INDICATIONS	ROUTES AND DOSAGE RANGES	
		Adults	Children
Protection begins about 3 wk after vaccination and lasts years. Not recommended for children <2 y because they may be unable to produce adequate antibody levels.	Adults 65 y and older who are otherwise healthy. Children 2 y and older with chronic disease associated with increased risk of pneumococcal infection (eg, asplenia, nephrotic syndrome, immunosuppression)		
Pneumococcal 7-valent conjugate vaccine (Prevnar) Contains 7 *Streptococcus pneumoniae* antigens conjugated to a protein to increase antigenicity	Active immunization to prevent invasive pneumococcal infections in young children		*Birth–6 mo:* IM 0.5 mL at 2, 4, and 6 mo and at 12–15 mo (4 doses) *7–11 mo:* IM 0.5 mL initially, at least 4 wk later, and after 1 y birthday (3 doses) *12–23 mo:* IM 0.5 ml initially and at least 2 mo later (2 doses) *24 mo–9 y:* IM 0.5 mL in a single dose
Poliomyelitis vaccine, inactivated (IPV) (IPOL) A suspension of inactivated poliovirus types I, II, and III	Routine immunization of infants. Immunization of adults not previously immunized and at risk of exposure (eg, health care or laboratory workers)	Sub-Q, 0.5 mL monthly for 2 doses, then a third dose 6–12 mo later	Sub-Q, 0.5 mL at 2, 4, and 6–18 mo, and 4–6 y of age (4 doses) or at 2 and 4 mo (2 doses)
Rabies vaccine (human diploid cell rabies vaccine [HDCV]) (Imovax) An inactivated virus vaccine. Immunity develops in 7–10 d and lasts 1 y or longer	Pre-exposure immunization in people at high risk of exposure (veterinarians, animal handlers, laboratory personnel who work with rabies virus). Postexposure prophylaxis in people who have been bitten by potentially rabid animals or who have skin scratches or abrasions exposed to animal saliva (eg, animal licking of wound), urine, or blood	Pre-exposure prophylaxis, IM, 1.0 mL for 3 doses. The second dose is given 1 wk after the first; the third dose is given 3–4 wk after the first. Then, booster doses (1 mL) every 2–5 y based on antibody titers. Postexposure, IM, 1 mL for 5 doses. After the initial dose, other doses are given 3, 7, 14, and 28 d later. Rabies immunoglobulin is administered at the same time as the initial dose of HDCV vaccine.	Same as adults
Rubella vaccine (Meruvax II) Sterile suspension of live, attenuated rubella virus. Protects about 95% of recipients at least 15 y, probably for lifetime	Routine immunization of children 1 y and older. Initial or repeat immunization of adolescent girls or women of childbearing age *if* serum antibody levels are low	Sub-Q 0.5 mL in a single dose	Same as adults

Table 39-1 Drugs at a Glance: Vaccines and Toxoids for Active Immunity (continued)

NAME/CHARACTERISTICS	CLINICAL INDICATIONS	ROUTES AND DOSAGE RANGES	
		Adults	Children
Should not be given for 3 mo after receiving immune serum globulin, plasma, or whole blood Usually given with measles and mumps vaccines			
Rubella and mumps vaccine (Biavax II) A mixture of mumps and rubella virus strains Less frequently used than measles, mumps, and rubella vaccine	Immunization of children		*Up to 1 y:* Sub-Q, total volume of reconstituted vial
Tuberculosis vaccine (bacillus Calmette-Guérin) (TICE BCG) Suspension of attenuated tubercle bacilli Converts negative tuberculin reactors to positive reactors; therefore, precludes use of the tuberculin skin test for screening or early diagnosis of tuberculosis Contraindicated in clients with impaired immune responses	People at high risk for exposure, including newborns of women with tuberculosis	Percutaneous, by multiple puncture disk, 0.2–0.3 mL	*Newborns:* Percutaneous, by multiple puncture disk, 0.1 mL *>1 mo:* Same as adults
Typhoid vaccine (Vivotif Berna, Typhim Vi) Suspension of attenuated or killed typhoid bacilli Protects 50%–77% of recipients Not recommended for routine use in United States	High-risk people (household contacts of typhoid carriers or people whose occupation or travel predisposes to exposure)	Sub-Q, 0.5 mL for 2 doses at least 4 wk apart, then a booster dose of 0.5 mL (or 0.1 mL intradermal) at least every 3 y for repeated or continued exposure PO 1 capsule every other day for 4 doses; repeat every 5 y as a booster dose with repeated or continued exposure	**Sub-Q form** *6 mo–10 y:* Sub-Q 0.25 mL for 2 doses at least 4 wk apart, then a booster dose of 0.25 mL (or 0.1 mL intradermal) every 3 y if indicated *>10 y:* Sub-Q 0.5 mL for 2 doses at least 4 wk apart, then a booster dose of 0.5 mL at least every 3 y for repeated or continued exposure **PO form** *>6 y:* PO same as adults
Varicella virus vaccine (Varivax) Contains live, attenuated varicella virus	Immunization of children 12 mo and older Immunization of adults	Sub-Q 0.5 mL, followed by a second dose of 0.5 mL 4–8 wk after the first dose	*1–12 y:* Sub-Q 0.5 mL in a single dose *Adolescents, 13 y and older:* Same as adults

(continued)

Table 39-1 Drugs at a Glance: Vaccines and Toxoids for Active Immunity (continued)

NAME/CHARACTERISTICS	CLINICAL INDICATIONS	ROUTES AND DOSAGE RANGES	
		Adults	Children
Contraindicated in people with hematologic or lymphatic malignancy, immunosuppression, febrile illness, or pregnancy			
Yellow-fever vaccine (YF-Vax) Suspension of live, attenuated yellow-fever virus Protects about 95% of recipients for 10 y or longer	Laboratory personnel at risk of exposure Travel to endemic areas (Africa, South America)	Sub-Q 0.5 mL; booster dose of 0.5 mL every 10 y if in endemic areas	*>6 mo:* Same as adults
Toxoids			
Diphtheria and tetanus toxoids and acellular pertussis vaccine (DTaP) (Tripedia, Infanrix) The pertussis component is acellular bacterial particles, which decrease the adverse effects associated with the whole-cell vaccine used formerly.	Active immunization of children aged 6 wk–7 y		IM 0.5 mL at approximately 2, 4, 6, and 18 mo of age and at 4–6 y
Diphtheria and tetanus toxoids and acellular pertussis and *Haemophilus influenzae* type B conjugate vaccines (DTaP-HIB) (TriHIBit) A combination product, to decrease the number of injections and increase compliance	Active immunization of children 15–18 mo of age who have been previously immunized against diphtheria, tetanus, and pertussis		IM 0.5 mL within 30 min or less after reconstitution
Diphtheria and tetanus toxoids, adsorbed (pediatric type) (DT) Contains a larger amount of diphtheria antigen than "tetanus and diphtheria toxoids, adult type (Td)"	Routine immunization of infants and children 6 y and younger in whom pertussis vaccine is contraindicated (ie, those who have adverse reactions to initial doses of diphtheria-tetanus-pertussis [DTP] vaccine)		*Infants and children 6 y and younger:* IM 0.5 mL for 2 doses at least 4 wk apart, followed by a reinforcing dose 1 y later and at the time the child starts school

Table 39-1 Drugs at a Glance: Vaccines and Toxoids for Active Immunity (continued)

NAME/CHARACTERISTICS	CLINICAL INDICATIONS	ROUTES AND DOSAGE RANGES	
		Adults	Children
Tetanus toxoid, adsorbed Protects about 100% of recipients for 10 y or more Usually given in combination (eg, DTaP or DT) for primary immunization of infants and children 6 y of age or older Usually given alone or combined with diphtheria toxoid (eg, Td adult type) for primary immunization of adults	Routine immunization of infants and young children Primary immunization of adults Prevention of tetanus in previously immunized people who sustain a potentially contaminated wound	Primary immunization in adults not previously immunized, IM 0.5 mL for 3 doses: initially, 4–8 wk later, then at 6–12 mo. Then, 0.5 mL booster dose every 10 y. Prophylaxis, IM 0.5 mL if wound severely contaminated and no booster dose was received for 5 y; 0.5 mL if wound is clean and no booster dose was received for 10 y	Primary immunization and prophylaxis, same as adults
Tetanus and diphtheria toxoids, adsorbed (adult type) (Td) Contains a smaller amount of diphtheria antigen than "diphtheria and tetanus toxoids, pediatric type (DT)"	Primary immunization or booster doses in adults and children >6 y of age	IM 0.5 mL for 2 doses, at least 4 wk apart, followed by a reinforcing dose 6–12 mo later and every 10 y thereafter	*>6 y:* Same as adults

HBsAg, hepatitis B surface antigen; IM, intramuscular; IV, intravenous; PO, oral; Sub-Q, subcutaneous.

Table 39-2 Drugs at a Glance: Immune Serums for Passive Immunity

NAME/CHARACTERISTICS	CLINICAL INDICATIONS	ROUTES AND DOSAGE RANGES
Cytomegalovirus immune globulin, intravenous, human (CMV-IGIV) (CytoGam) Contains antibodies against CMV Dosage varies with type of transplant	Prevention of CMV infection in heart, kidney, liver, lung, and pancreas transplant recipients	Post-transplantation, IV infusion, 150 mg/kg within 72 h, then 100–150 mg/kg at 2, 4, 6, and 8 wk, then 50–100 mg/kg at 12 and 16 wk
Hepatitis B immune globulin, human (HBIG) (BayHep B, Nabi-HB) A solution of immunoglobulins that contains antibodies to HBsAg	To prevent hepatitis after exposure. Neonates born to HBsAg-positive or unknown-status mothers are given HBIG and the first dose of hepatitis B vaccine within 12 h of birth.	*Adults and children:* IM, 0.06 mL/kg (usual adult dose is 3–5 mL) as soon as possible after exposure, preferably within 7 d. Repeat dose in 1 mo.
Immune globulin (human) (IG; IGIM) (BayGam) Given IM only Commonly called "gamma globulin" Obtained from pooled plasma of normal donors Consists primarily of IgG, which contains concentrated antibodies Produces adequate serum levels of IgG in 2–5 d	To decrease the severity of hepatitis A, measles, and varicella after exposure To treat immunoglobulin deficiency Adjunct to antibiotics in severe bacterial infections and burns To lessen possibility of fetal damage in pregnant women exposed to rubella virus (however, routine use in early pregnancy is not recommended)	*Adults and children:* Exposure to hepatitis A, IM, 0.02 mL/kg Exposure to measles, IM, 0.25 mL/kg given within 6 d of exposure Exposure to varicella, IM, 0.6–1.2 mL/kg Exposure to rubella (pregnant women only), IM, 0.55 mL/kg Immunoglobulin deficiency, IM, 1.3 mL/kg initially, then 0.6 mL/kg every 3–4 wk Bacterial infections, IM, 0.5–3.5 mL/kg

(continued)

Table 39-2 Drugs at a Glance: Immune Serums for Passive Immunity (continued)

NAME/CHARACTERISTICS	CLINICAL INDICATIONS	ROUTES AND DOSAGE RANGES
Immune globulin intravenous (IGIV) (Gammagard, Iveegam, Polygam S/D, Panglobulin, Sandoglobulin, Venoglobulin-S) Given IV only Provides immediate antibodies Half-life about 3 wk Mechanism of action in ITP unknown **Warning:** IGIV products have been associated with renal dysfunction and failure and death. They should be used cautiously in clients with or at risk of developing renal impairment.	Immunodeficiency syndrome ITP	*Sandoglobulin:* IV infusion, 200 mg/kg once a mo. May be given more often or increased to 300 mg/kg if clinical response or serum level of IgG is inadequate. ITP, IV infusion, 400 mg/kg daily for 2–5 consecutive d Other products, see manufacturers' literature
Rabies immune globulin (human) RIG (BayRab, Imogam) Gamma globulin obtained from plasma of people hyper-immunized with rabies vaccine Not useful in treatment of clinical rabies infection	Postexposure prevention of rabies, in conjunction with rabies vaccine	*Adults and children:* IM, 20 units/kg (half the dose may be injected around the wound) as soon as possible after possible exposure (eg, animal bite)
Respiratory syncytial virus immune globulin intravenous (human) (RSV-IGIV) (RespiGam) Reduces severity of RSV illness and the incidence and duration of hospitalization in high-risk infants May cause fluid overload Not established as safe and effective in children with congenital heart disease	Prevention of serious RSV infections in high-risk children <2 y (ie, those with bronchopulmonary dysplasia or history of premature birth [gestation of 35 wk or less]) Treatment of RSV lower respiratory tract infections in hospitalized infants and young children	*Children:* IV infusion via infusion pump, 1.5 mL/kg/h for 15 min, then 3 mL/kg/h for 15 min, then 6 mL/kg/h until the infusion is completed, then once monthly, if tolerated. Maximum monthly dose, 750 mg/kg
Rh₀(D) immune globulin (human) (RhoGAM) Prepared from fractionated human plasma A sterile concentrated solution of specific immunoglobulin (IgG) containing anti-Rh₀(D)	To prevent sensitization in a subsequent pregnancy to the Rho(D) factor in an Rh-negative mother who has given birth to an Rh-positive infant by an Rh-positive father Also available in microdose form (MICRhoGAM) for the prevention of maternal Rh immunization after abortion or miscarriage up to 12 wk gestation	*Obstetric use:* Inject contents of 1 vial IM for every 15 mL fetal packed red cell volume within 72 h after delivery, miscarriage, or abortion. Consult package instructions for blood typing and drug administration procedures.
Tetanus immune globulin (human) (BayTet) Solution of globulins from plasma of people hyperimmunized with tetanus toxoid Tetanus toxoid (Td) should also be given to initiate active immunization if minor wound and >10 y since Td, if major wound and >5 y since Td, or if Td primary immunization series was incomplete.	To prevent tetanus in clients with wounds possibly contaminated with *Clostridium tetani* and whose immunization history is uncertain or incomplete Treatment of tetanus infection	*Adults and children:* Prophylaxis, IM, 250 units as a single dose Treatment of clinical disease, IM 3000–6000 units in a single dose

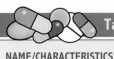

Table 39-2 Drugs at a Glance: Immune Serums for Passive Immunity (continued)

NAME/CHARACTERISTICS	CLINICAL INDICATIONS	ROUTES AND DOSAGE RANGES
Varicella-zoster immune globulin (human) (VZIG) (Varicella-zoster immune globulin) The globulin fraction of human plasma Antibodies last 1 mo or longer.	Postexposure to chickenpox or shingles, to prevent or decrease severity of infections in children <15 y of age who have not been immunized or who are immunodeficient because of illness or drug therapy Infants born to mothers who develop varicella 5 d before or 2 d after delivery and premature infants <28 wk gestation	IM 125 units/10 kg up to a maximum of 625 units within 48 h after exposure if possible; may be given up to 96 h after exposure. Minimal dose, 125 units

CMV, cytomegalovirus; IgG, immunoglobulin G; IM, intramuscular; ITP, idiopathic thrombocytopenic purpura; IV, intravenous; RSV, respiratory syncytial virus; HBsAg, hepatitis B surface antigen.

NURSING PROCESS

Assessment

Assess the client's immunization status by obtaining the following information:

- Determine the client's previous history of diseases for which immunizing agents are available (eg, measles, influenza).
- Ask if the client has had previous immunizations.
  - For which diseases were immunizations received?
  - Which immunizing agent was received?
  - Were any adverse effects experienced? If so, what symptoms occurred, and how long did they last?
  - Was tetanus toxoid given for any cuts or wounds?
  - Did any foreign travel require immunizations?
- Determine whether the client has any conditions that contraindicate administration of immunizing agents (eg, malignancy, pregnancy, immunosuppressive drug therapy).
- For pregnant women not known to be immunized against rubella, serum antibody titer should be measured to determine resistance or susceptibility to the disease.
- For clients with wounds, assess the type of wound and determine how, when, and where it was sustained. Such information may reveal whether tetanus immunization is needed.
- For clients exposed to infectious diseases, try to determine the extent of exposure (eg, household or brief, casual contact) and when it occurred.

Nursing Diagnoses

- Deficient Knowledge: Importance of maintaining immunizations for both children and adults
- Risk for Fluid Volume Deficit related to inadequate intake and febrile reactions to immunizing agent
- Noncompliance in obtaining recommended immunizations related to fear of adverse effects
- Risk for Injury related to hypersensitivity, fever, and other adverse drug effects

Planning/Goals

The client will

- Avoid diseases for which immunizations are available and recommended
- Obtain recommended immunizations for children and self
- Keep appointments for immunizations

Interventions

Use measures to prevent infectious diseases, and provide information about the availability of immunizing agents. General measures include those to promote health and resistance to disease (eg, nutrition, rest, exercise). Additional measures include the following:

- Education of the public, especially parents of young children, regarding the importance of immunizations to personal and public health. Include information about the diseases that can be prevented and where immunizations can be obtained (see accompanying Client Teaching Guidelines).
- Assisting clients in developing a system to maintain immunization records for themselves and their children. This is important because immunizations are often obtained at different places and over a period of years. Written, accurate, up-to-date records help to prevent diseases and unnecessary immunizations.
- Prevention of disease transmission. The following are helpful measures:
  - Hand hygiene (probably the most effective method)

CLIENT TEACHING GUIDELINES

Vaccinations

☑ Appropriate vaccinations should be maintained for adults as well as for children. Consult a health care provider periodically because recommendations and personal needs change fairly often.

☑ Maintain immunization records for yourself and your children. This is important because immunizations are often obtained at different places and over a period of years. Written, accurate, up-to-date records help to prevent diseases and unnecessary immunizations.

☑ If a physician recommends an immunization and you do not know whether you have had the immunization or the disease, it is probably safer to take the immunization than to risk having the disease. Immunization after a previous immunization or after having the disease usually is not harmful.

☑ To avoid rubella-induced abnormalities in fetal development, women of childbearing age who receive a rubella immunization must avoid becoming pregnant (ie, must use effective contraceptive methods) for 3 months.

☑ Women of childbearing age who receive a varicella immunization must avoid becoming pregnant (ie, must use effective contraceptive methods) for 3 months.

☑ Most vaccines cause fever and soreness at the site of injection. Acetaminophen (Tylenol) can be taken two to three times daily for 24 to 48 hours (by adults and children) to decrease fever and discomfort.

☑ After receiving varicella vaccine (to prevent chickenpox), avoid close contact with newborns, pregnant women, and anyone whose immune system is impaired. Also, use effective methods of contraception to avoid pregnancy for at least 3 months after immunization. Vaccinated people may transmit the vaccine virus to susceptible close contacts. Effects of the vaccine on the fetus are unknown, but fetal harm has occurred with natural varicella infection during pregnancy.

☑ After receiving a vaccine, stay in the area for approximately 30 minutes. If an allergic reaction is going to occur, it will usually do so within that time.

● Avoiding contact with people who have known or suspected infectious diseases, when possible

● Using isolation techniques when appropriate

● Using medical and surgical aseptic techniques

● For someone exposed to rubeola, administration of measles vaccine within 48 hours to prevent the disease

● For someone with a puncture wound or a dirty wound, administration of tetanus immune globulin to prevent tetanus, a life-threatening disease

● For someone with an animal bite, washing the wound immediately with large amounts of soap and water. Health care should then be sought. Administration of rabies vaccine may be needed to prevent rabies, a life-threatening disease.

● Explaining to the client that contracting rubella or undergoing rubella immunization during pregnancy, especially during the first trimester, may cause severe birth defects in the infant. The goal of immunization is to prevent congenital rubella syndrome. Current recommendations are to immunize children against rubella at 12 to 15 months of age. It is recommended that previously unimmunized girls 11 to 13 years of age be immunized against rubella. Furthermore, nonpregnant women of childbearing age should have rubella antibody tests. If antibody concentrations are low, the woman should be immunized. Pregnancy should be avoided for 3 months after immunization.

Evaluation

● Interview and observe for symptoms.

● Interview and observe for adverse drug effects.

● Check immunization records when indicated.

PRINCIPLES OF THERAPY

Keeping Up-to-Date With Immunization Recommendations

Recommendations regarding immunizations change periodically as additional information and new immunizing agents become available. Consequently, health care providers should update their knowledge at least annually. The best source of information regarding current recommendations is the Centers for Disease Control and Prevention (CDC), whose headquarters are in Atlanta, Georgia (Internet address: www.cdc.gov).

The main source of CDC recommendations is the Advisory Committee on Immunization Practices (ACIP; www.cdc.gov/nip/acip), which consists of 15 experts appointed by the Secretary of the United States Department of Health and Human Services to advise the Secretary, the Assistant Secretary for Health, and the CDC on strategies to prevent vaccine-preventable diseases. Other sources of information include the American Academy of Pediatrics (AAP; www.aap.org) and the American Academy of Family Physicians (AAFP; www.aafp.org). Local health departments can also be consulted about routine immunizations and those required for foreign travel. These sources can also provide information on new vaccine releases and vaccine supply, and statements on usage of specific vaccines.

APPLYING YOUR KNOWLEDGE 39-2
You are unaccustomed to providing immunizations other than the usual childhood ones. How should you obtain current information from Ms. Stein, and how often should this information be obtained?

Storage of Vaccines

To maintain effectiveness of vaccines and other biologic preparations, the products must be stored properly. Most products require refrigeration at 2°C to 8°C (35.6°–46.4°F); some (eg, MMR) require protection from light. Manufacturers' instructions for storage should be strictly followed.

Vaccine Shortages

From 2000 to 2002, approximately, shortages of several vaccines occurred. Some shortages were localized, and some were widespread. These shortages interrupted the recommended schedules for many immunizations, especially those for routine immunizations of children. Long-term consequences of altered immunization schedules are largely unknown.

During the shortages, public health officials regularly issued updates on availability and priorities for usage among at-risk populations. One postulated reason for the shortages was the withdrawal of some manufacturers from vaccine production, probably because of relatively low profits and difficulties in complying with FDA regulations for manufacturing vaccines. For example, a regulation requiring removal of thiomerosal, a mercury-based preservative, resulted in the need for single-dose vials rather than multiple-dose vials and a smaller amount of marketable product from the same amount of vaccine. Mercury is toxic to humans, especially to infants.

APPLYING YOUR KNOWLEDGE 39-3:
HOW CAN YOU AVOID THIS MEDICATION ERROR?
You look in the supply area for the vaccines to be provided to Ms. Stein at this visit. You find the MMR on the shelf above the sink and prepare the injection.

Use in Special Populations

Use in Children

Routine immunization of children has greatly reduced the prevalence of many common childhood diseases. However, many children are not being immunized appropriately, and diseases for which vaccines are available still occur. Children's health care providers should follow standards of practice and the annual "Recommended Childhood Immunization Schedule" (American Academy of Pediatrics Committee on Infectious Diseases, 2002) of the AAP, the ACIP, and the AAFP, issued in January of each year. Guidelines for children whose immunizations begin in early infancy are listed below; different schedules are recommended for children 1 to 5 years of age and for those older than 6 years of age who are being immunized for the first time.

- Hepatitis B vaccine to all newborns, with a second dose 4 weeks after the first dose, and a third dose at least 8 weeks after the third dose or 16 weeks after the first dose. The last dose in the series (third or fourth dose) should not be given before 6 months of age. This schedule is for monovalent vaccine (hepatitis B vaccine only) and infants whose mothers were negative for HbsAg. If a combined hepatitis B, *H. influenzae* b vaccine is used (the combination can be used for all but the first dose in newborns), the second dose should not be given before 6 weeks of age. Also, if the mother's HbsAg status is positive or unknown, newborns should be given hepatitis B vaccine within 12 hours of birth, along with a dose of hepatitis B immune globulin (HBIG).
- DTaP (diphtheria and tetanus toxoids and acellular pertussis vaccine) at 2 months, 4 months, 6 months, 15 to 18 months, and 4 to 6 years of age
- *H. influenzae* b vaccine (Hib) at 2, 4, 6, and 12 to 15 months of age. There are three Hib conjugate vaccines approved for use in infants. If PedvaxHIB or ComVax is given at 2 and 4 months of age, a dose at 6 months is not needed. DTaP/Hib combination products should not be used for primary immunization at 2, 4, or 6 months of age but can be used as boosters after any Hib vaccine.
- Inactivated poliomyelitis vaccine (IPV) injection at 2 and 4 months of age, at 6 to 18 months, and at 4 to 6 years of age
- MMR at 15 months of age, as a combined vaccine. These vaccines are given later than DTaP and IPV because sufficient antibodies may not be produced until passive immunity acquired from the mother dissipates (at about 15 months of age).
- Pneumococcal 7-valent conjugate vaccine (Prevnar) to all children at 2 to 23 months of age and pneumococcal polyvalent vaccine (Pneumovax 23, Pnu-Imune 23) to children 2 years and older with chronic illnesses that increase their risk for developing serious pneumococcal infections
- Varicella at 12 to 18 months and again at approximately 12 years of age
- For children with chronic illnesses such as asthma, heart disease, diabetes, and others, influenza vaccine is recommended annually after 6 months of age. In 2004, the American Academy of Pediatrics (AAp; updated its guidelines to recommend influenza vaccine for all healthy children between 6 months and 2 years of age, as well as their household contacts, out-of-home caregivers, and health care providers.

- For children with human immunodeficiency virus (HIV) infection, live viral and bacterial vaccines (MMR, varicella, bacillus Calmette-Guérin [BCG]) are contraindicated because they may cause the disease rather than prevent it. However, immunizations with DTaP, IPV, and Hib are recommended even though they may be less effective than in children with a competent immune system. Also recommended are annual administration of influenza vaccine for children older than 6 months of age and one-time administration of pneumococcal vaccine for children older than 2 years of age.

Use in Healthy Adolescents, Young Adults, and Middle-Aged Adults

Adolescents who received all primary immunizations as infants and young children should have hepatitis B vaccine (if not received earlier) and a tetanus-diphtheria booster (adult type) at 14 to 16 years of age and every 10 years thereafter. Young adults who are health care workers, are sexually active, or belong to high-risk groups should have hepatitis B vaccine if not previously received; a tetanus-diphtheria booster every 10 years; MMR if not pregnant and rubella titer is inadequate or proof of immunization is unavailable; and varicella vaccine. In addition, young adults who are health care providers should have influenza vaccine annually. Middle-aged adults should maintain immunizations against tetanus; high-risk groups (eg, those with chronic illness) and health care providers should receive hepatitis B vaccine once (if not previously taken) and influenza vaccine annually at 50 years of age and older.

Use in Older Adults

Annual influenza vaccine and one-time administration of pneumococcal vaccine at 65 years of age are recommended for healthy older adults and those with chronic respiratory, cardiovascular, and other diseases. A second dose of pneumococcal vaccine may be given at 65 years if the first dose was given 5 years previously. As with younger adults, immunization for most other diseases is recommended for older adults at high risk of exposure.

Use in Clients With Immunosuppression

Compared with healthy, immunocompetent individuals, the antibody response to immunization is usually adequate but reduced in immunosuppressed people. Immunizations should be individualized. In general, those with diabetes mellitus or chronic pulmonary, renal, or hepatic disorders who are not receiving immunosuppressant drugs may be given both live attenuated and killed vaccines and toxoids to induce active immunity. However, they may need higher doses or more frequent administration to induce adequate immunity. With

hepatitis B vaccine, for example, larger doses may be required initially and booster doses may be needed later if antibody concentrations fall.

Clients with active malignant disease may be given killed vaccines or toxoids but should not be given live vaccines (an exception is persons with leukemia who have not received chemotherapy for at least 3 months). When vaccines are used, they should be given at least 2 weeks before the start of chemotherapy or 3 months after chemotherapy is completed. Passive immunity with immunoglobulins may be used in place of active immunity.

Clients receiving a systemic corticosteroid in high doses (eg, prednisone 20 mg or equivalent daily) or for longer than 2 weeks should wait at least 3 months before being given a live-virus vaccine. Immunizations are not contraindicated with short-term use (less than 2 weeks) or low to moderate doses (less than 20 mg of prednisone daily). In addition, long-term alternate-day therapy with short-acting agents; maintenance physiologic doses; and the use of topical, aerosol, or intra-articular injections are not contraindications to immunization.

Clients with HIV infection have less-than-optimal responses to immunizing agents because the disease produces major defects in cell-mediated and humoral immunity. Live bacterial (BCG, oral typhoid) or viral (MMR, varicella, yellow fever) vaccines should not be given because the bacteria or viruses may be able to reproduce and cause active infection. Persons with asymptomatic HIV infection should receive inactivated vaccines; those exposed to measles or varicella may be given immune globulin or varicella-zoster immune globulin for passive immunization.

For children with HIV infection, the AAP and ACIP recommend administration of most routine immunizations (DTaP, IPV, MMR, Hib, influenza). MMR is not recommended in children with severe immunosuppression and varicella vaccine is recommended only for children with no evidence of immunosuppression. Pneumococcal vaccine is recommended for HIV-infected persons over 2 years of age.

Use in Clients With Cancer

For clients with active malignant disease, live vaccines should not be given. Although killed vaccines and toxoids may be given, antibody production may be inadequate to provide immunity. When possible, clients should receive needed immunizations 2 weeks before or 3 months after immunosuppressive radiation or chemotherapy treatments. For example, clients with Hodgkin's lymphoma who are more than 2 years old should be immunized with pneumococcal and Hib vaccines 10 to 14 days before therapy is started. In addition, clients who have not received chemotherapy for 3 to 4 weeks may have an adequate antibody response to influenza vaccine.

N U R S I N G   A C T I O N S

Immunizing Agents

NURSING ACTIONS	RATIONALE/EXPLANATION
1. Administer accurately	
a. Read the package insert and check the expiration date on all biologic products (eg, vaccines, toxoids, human immune serums).	Concentration, dosage, and administration of biologic products often vary with the products. Fresh products are preferred; avoid administration of expired products. Also, use reconstituted products within designated time limits because they are usually stable for only a few hours.
b. Check the child's temperature before giving diphtheria, tetanus, and pertussis (DTaP) vaccine.	If the child's temperature is elevated, do not give the vaccine.
c. Give DTaP in the lateral thigh muscle of the infant.	The vastus lateralis is the largest skeletal muscle mass in the infant and the preferred site for all intramuscular (IM) injections.
d. With measles, mumps, rubella (MMR) vaccine, use only the diluent provided by the manufacturer, and administer the vaccine subcutaneously (Sub-Q) within 8 hours after reconstitution.	The reconstituted preparation is stable for approximately 8 hours. If not used within 8 hours, discard the solution.
e. Give hepatitis B vaccine IM in the anterolateral thigh of infants and young children and in the deltoid of older children and adults. Although the IM route is preferred, the drug can be given Sub-Q in people at high risk of bleeding from IM injections (eg, clients with hemophilia).	Higher blood levels of protective antibodies are produced when the vaccine is given in the thigh or deltoid than when it is given in the buttocks, probably because of injection into fatty tissue rather than gluteal muscles.
f. Give IM human immune serum globulin with an 18- to 20-gauge needle, preferably in gluteal muscles. If the dose is 5 milliliters or more, divide it and inject it into two or more IM sites. Follow manufacturer's instructions for preparation and administration of intravenous (IV) formulations.	To promote absorption and minimize tissue irritation and other adverse reactions
g. Aspirate carefully before IM or Sub-Q injection of any immunizing agent.	To avoid inadvertent IV administration and greatly increased risks of severe adverse effects
h. Have aqueous epinephrine 1:1000 readily available before administering any vaccine.	For immediate treatment of allergic reactions
i. After administration of an immunizing agent in a clinic or office setting, have the client stay in the area for at least 30 minutes.	To observe for allergic reactions, which usually occur within 30 minutes
2. Observe for therapeutic effects	
a. Absence of diseases for which immunized	
b. Decreased incidence and severity of symptoms when given to modify disease processes	
3. Observe for adverse effects	Most adverse effects are mild and transient. However, serious reactions occasionally occur. The risk of serious adverse effects from immunization is usually much smaller than the risk of the disease immunized against.
	Adverse effects may be caused by the immunizing agent or by foreign protein incorporated with the immunizing agent (eg, egg protein in viral vaccines grown in chick embryos).
a. General reactions:	
(1) Pain, tenderness, redness at injection sites	Local tissue irritation may occur with injected immunizing agents.
(2) Fever, malaise, muscle aches	These adverse effects commonly occur with vaccines and toxoids. They rarely occur with human immune serums given for passive immunity.
(3) Anaphylaxis—cardiovascular collapse, shock, laryngeal edema, urticaria, angioneurotic edema, severe respiratory distress	Anaphylaxis occasionally occurs with immunizing agents. It is a medical emergency that requires immediate treatment with Sub-Q epinephrine (0.5 mL for adults; 0.01 mL/kg for children). Anaphylaxis is most likely to occur within 30 minutes after immunizing agents are injected.

(continued)

NURSING ACTIONS	RATIONALE/EXPLANATION
(4) Serum sickness—urticaria, fever, arthralgia, enlarged lymph nodes	Serum sickness is a delayed hypersensitivity reaction that occurs several days or weeks after an injection of serum. Treatment is symptomatic. Symptoms are usually relieved by acetaminophen, antihistamines, and corticosteroids.
b. With DTaP:	
(1) Soreness, erythema, edema at injection sites	These effects are common.
(2) Anorexia, nausea	
(3) Severe fever, encephalopathy, seizures	These are rare adverse reactions and are less likely to occur with the acellular pertussis component now used. If they occur, they are thought to be caused by the pertussis antigen, and further administration of pertussis vaccine or DTaP may be contraindicated.
c. With *Haemophilus influenzae* b vaccine—pain and erythema at injection sites	These effects occur in about 25% of recipients but are usually mild and resolve within 24 hours.
d. With hepatitis B vaccine:	
(1) Injection site soreness, erythema, induration	Soreness and fever commonly occur and can be relieved by acetaminophen or ibuprofen. Anaphylaxis and other severe reactions rarely occur.
(2) Fever	
(3) Anaphylaxis	
e. With influenza vaccine:	
(1) Via injection—pain, induration, and erythema at injection sites; flu-like symptoms such as chills, fever, malaise, muscle aches	Adverse effects can be minimized by giving acetaminophen at the time of immunization and at 4, 8, and 12 hours later. Injection site reactions and flu-like symptoms may start within 12 hours after vaccination.
(2) Via intranasal spray—runny nose; headache; cough; sore throat; irritability in children	
f. With MMR vaccine:	
(1) Mild symptoms of measles—cough, fever up to 39.4°C (102°F), headache, malaise, photophobia, skin rash, sore throat	These symptoms may occur 6–11 days after immunization.
(2) Febrile seizures	These are rare, but are more likely to occur in children <2 years of age.
(3) Arthralgia (joint pain)	Joint pain has been reported in as many as 25% of adult females 2–6 weeks after receiving rubella vaccine.
(4) Anaphylaxis in recipients who are allergic to eggs	The measles and mumps viruses used in MMR vaccine are grown in chick-embryo cell cultures. Recipients who are allergic to eggs should be observed for 90 minutes after the vaccine is injected. MMR vaccine should be given only in a setting where personnel and equipment are available to treat anaphylaxis.
g. With pneumococcal vaccine:	
(1) Local effects—soreness, induration, and erythema at injection sites	Local effects occur in 40%–90% of recipients; systemic effects occur less frequently.
(2) Systemic effects—chills, fever, headache, muscle aches, nausea, photophobia, weakness	
h. With polio vaccine:	
(1) Soreness at injection sites	Adverse effects are usually mild. Anaphylaxis rarely occurs. However, if it occurs within 24 hours after administration of polio vaccine, no additional doses of the vaccine should be given.
(2) Fever	
(3) Anaphylaxis	
i. With varicella vaccine:	
(1) Early effects—transient soreness or erythema at injection sites	Injection site reactions occur in 20%–35% of recipients; a skin rash develops in a few (about 8%) recipients within a month. Those who develop a rash from the vaccine have milder symptoms of shorter duration than those who develop varicella naturally.
(2) Late effect—a mild, maculopapular skin rash with a few lesions	

NURSING ACTIONS	RATIONALE/EXPLANATION
j. With immune globulin intravenous (IGIV):	
(1) Chills; dizziness; dyspnea; fever; flushing; headache; nausea; urticaria; vomiting; tightness in chest; pain in chest, hip, or back	These effects are related to the rate of infusion. If they occur, the infusion should be stopped until the symptoms subside, then be restarted at a slower rate. The symptoms can also be prevented or minimized by pre-infusion administration of acetaminophen and diphenhydramine or a corticosteroid.
(2) Renal dysfunction, acute renal failure, death	Acute renal failure is most likely to occur in clients older than 65 years of age; in those with pre-existing renal insufficiency, diabetes mellitus, volume depletion, or sepsis; or in those taking known nephrotoxic drugs.
4. Observe for drug interactions	
a. Drugs that *decrease* effects of vaccines in general:	
(1) Immunosuppressants (eg, corticosteroids, antineoplastic drugs, phenytoin [Dilantin])	Vaccines may be contraindicated in clients receiving immunosuppressive drugs. These clients cannot produce sufficient amounts of antibodies for immunity and may develop the illness produced by the particular organism contained in the vaccine. The disease is most likely to occur with the live-virus vaccines (measles, mumps, rubella). Similar effects occur when the client is receiving radiation and phenytoin, an anticonvulsant drug that suppresses both cellular and humoral immune responses.
b. Drugs that *decrease* effects of measles and MMR vaccines:	
(1) Immunosuppressants	May decrease effectiveness of immunization; clients may remain susceptible to measles despite immunization.
(2) Immune globulins (eg, RIG, RSV-IGIV, VZIG, IGIV)	To avoid inactivation of the attenuated virus, give measles or MMR vaccine at least 14–30 days before or 6–8 weeks after the immune globulin. Alternatively, may check antibody titers or repeat the measles vaccine dose 3 months after immune globulin administration
(3) Interferon	May inhibit antibody response to the vaccine
c. Drugs that *decrease* effects of meningococcal vaccine:	
(1) Measles vaccine	These vaccines should be given at least 1 month apart.
d. With varicella vaccine, salicylates may *increase* risk of Reye's syndrome.	Aspirin and other salicylates should be avoided for 6 weeks after vaccine administration because of potential for Reye's syndrome, which has been reported with salicylate use after natural varicella infection.

APPLYING YOUR KNOWLEDGE: ANSWERS

39-1 Assess for the presence of fever, immunosuppressive drug therapy, immunodeficiency states, and pregnancy. Vaccines and toxoids are usually contraindicated with these conditions.

39-2 The best source for current immunization information is the CDC Web site (www.cdc.gov). Health care providers should update their knowledge at least annually.

39-3 Do not use any vaccine that has been stored at room temperature. To maintain effectiveness of the vaccine, MMR requires refrigeration and protection from light.

Review and Application Exercises

Short Answer Exercises

1. What is the difference between active immunity and passive immunity?

2. How do vaccines act to produce active immunity?

3. What are the sources and functions of immune serums?

4. List common childhood diseases for which immunizing agents are available.

5. Which immunizations are recommended for adults?

6. What are advantages of administering a combination of immunizing agents rather than single agents?

7. What are common adverse reactions to immunizing agents, and how may they be prevented or minimized?

8. Why should live vaccines not be given to people whose immune system is suppressed by drugs or diseases?

NCLEX-Style Questions

9. Vaccines provide
   a. active immunity
   b. passive immunity
   c. innate immunity
   d. nonspecific immunity

10. Severe immunosuppression is a contraindication to
    a. all injectable immunizations
    b. the use of live bacterial or viral vaccines
    c. the use of immune globulins for passive immunity
    d. the use of most immunizing agents in children

11. To decrease fever and discomfort after an immunization, adults and children can take
    a. an opioid analgesic every 6 to 8 hours for 48 hours
    b. acetaminophen every 4 to 6 hours for at least 24 hours
    c. an antihistamine for 2 days before and 2 days after vaccine administration
    d. a sedative at bedtime to aid sleep

12. For a child receiving an immunization, parents should be informed that common aftereffects include

    a. skin rash and swelling
    b. redness and soreness at the injection site
    c. muscle weakness and difficulty in walking
    d. nausea, vomiting, and diarrhea

13. Adults should be given tetanus toxoid vaccine every
    a. year
    b. 2 years
    c. 5 years
    d. 10 years

Selected References

American Academy of Pediatrics Committee on Infectious Diseases. (2002). Recommended childhood immunization schedule: United States, 2002. *Pediatrics, 109*(1), 162.

Association for Professionals in Infection Control and Epidemiology (APIC) Guidelines Committee. (1999). APIC position paper: Immunization. *American Journal of Infection Control, 27,* 52–53.

Bertino, J. S., Jr., & Hayney, M. S. (2002). Vaccines, toxoids, and other immunobiologics. In J. T. DiPiro, R. L. Talbert, G. C. Yee, G. R. Matzke, B. G. Wells, & L. M. Posey (Eds.), *Pharmacotherapy: A pathophysiologic approach* (5th ed., pp. 2123–2149). New York: McGraw-Hill.

Drug facts and comparisons. (Updated monthly). St. Louis: Facts and Comparisons.

Orenstein, W. A. (2004). Immunization. In L. Goldman & D. Ausiello (Eds.), *Cecil textbook of medicine* (22nd ed., pp. 64–74). Philadelphia: W. B. Saunders.

Porth, C. M. (2005). *Pathophysiology: Concepts of altered health states* (7th ed.). Philadelphia: Lippincott Williams & Wilkins.

Shinefield, H. R., Black, S. B., Staehle, B. O., et al. (2002). Vaccination with measles, mumps and rubella vaccine and varicella vaccine: Safety, tolerability, immunogenicity, persistence of antibody and duration of protection against varicella in healthy children. *Pediatric Infectious Diseases Journal, 21*(6), 555–561.

Smeltzer, S. C., & Bare, B. G. (2004). *Brunner & Suddarth's textbook of medical-surgical nursing* (10th ed., pp. 2114–2146). Philadelphia: Lippincott Williams & Wilkins.

Hematopoietic and Immunostimulant Drugs

OBJECTIVES

After studying this chapter, you will be able to:

1. Describe the goals and methods of enhancing hematopoietic and immune functions.
2. Discuss the use of hematopoietic agents in the treatment of anemia and thrombocytopenia.
3. Discuss the use of filgrastim and sargramostim in neutropenia and bone marrow transplantation.
4. Describe the adverse effects and nursing process implications of administering filgrastim and sargramostim.
5. Discuss interferons in terms of clinical uses, adverse effects, and nursing process implications.

APPLYING YOUR KNOWLEDGE

Alice Miller is a 76-year-old woman undergoing chemotherapy for inoperable liver cancer. She receives a combination chemotherapy regimen every 6 weeks. She is in the oncologist's office for her routine laboratory work 10 days after chemotherapy and complains of severe fatigue. The results of her blood work are:

    Hemoglobin 11.2 g
    Hematocrit 32%
    WBC 2000
    ANC 800
    Platelet count 120,000

INTRODUCTION

Enhancing a person's own body systems to fight infection and cancer is a concept that continues to evolve. Hematopoietic and immunostimulant drugs (also called *biologic response modifiers* and *immunomodulators*) are given to restore normal function or increase the ability of the immune system to eliminate potentially harmful invaders. Drugs available for therapeutic use include hematopoietic colony-stimulating factors (CSF; eg, darbepoetin alfa, epoetin alfa, filgrastim, sargramostim), several interferons, and two interleukins. These drugs, which are the primary focus of this chapter, are described in the following sections and in Table 40-1.

Bacillus Calmette-Guérin (BCG) vaccine, used in the treatment of bladder cancer, is also discussed. Other drugs with immunostimulant properties are discussed in other chapters. These include traditional immunizing agents (see Chap. 39); levamisole (Ergamisol), which restores functions of macrophages and T cells and is used with fluorouracil in the treatment of intestinal cancer (see Chap. 42); and antiviral drugs used in the treatment of acquired immunodeficiency syndrome (AIDS) (see Chap. 35). Levamisole and antiviral drugs

are more accurately called *immunorestoratives* because they help a compromised immune system regain normal function rather than stimulating "supranormal" function. In AIDS, the human immunodeficiency virus (HIV) causes severe immune system dysfunction, so the antiviral drugs indirectly improve immunologic function.

GENERAL CHARACTERISTICS OF HEMATOPOIETIC AND IMMUNOSTIMULANT DRUGS

- Most hematopoietic and immunostimulant drugs are synthetic versions of natural endogenous protein substances called *cytokines* (see Chap. 38). Techniques of molecular biology are used to delineate the type and sequence of amino acids and to identify the genes responsible for producing the substances. These genes are then inserted into bacteria (usually *Escherichia coli*) or yeasts capable of producing the substances exogenously. Cloning of the genes that encode interferons, for

(text continues on page 655)

Table 40-1 Drugs at a Glance: Hematopoietic and Immunostimulant Agents

GENERIC/TRADE NAME	INDICATIONS FOR USE	ROUTES AND DOSAGE RANGES	COMMENTS
Hematopoietic Agents **Darbepoetin alfa** (Aranesp)	Anemia associated with chronic renal failure (CRF)	Sub-Q, IV 0.45 mcg/kg once weekly, adjusted to achieve and maintain hemoglobin level no greater than 12 g/dL	Main advantage over epoetin alfa is that it is given less often
Epoetin alfa (Epogen, Procrit)	Prevention and treatment of anemia associated with CRF, zidovudine therapy, or anticancer chemotherapy Reduction of blood transfusions in anemic clients undergoing elective noncardiac, nonvascular surgery	*CRF:* IV, Sub-Q 50–100 units/kg 3 times weekly to achieve or maintain a hematocrit of 30%–36% *Zidovudine therapy:* IV, Sub-Q 100 units/kg 3 times weekly, increased if necessary *Cancer chemotherapy:* Sub-Q 150–300 units/kg 3 times weekly *Surgery:* Sub-Q 300 units/kg/d for 10 d before surgery, on the day of surgery and for 4 d after surgery	Most patients need an iron supplement during epoetin alfa therapy.
Colony-Stimulating Factors (CSF) **Filgrastim (G-CSF)** (Neupogen)	To prevent infection in patients with neutropenia induced by cancer chemotherapy or bone marrow transplantation To mobilize stem cells from bone marrow to peripheral blood, where they can be collected and reinfused after chemotherapy that depresses bone marrow function To treat severe chronic neutropenia	*Myelosuppressive chemotherapy:* Sub-Q injection, IV infusion over 15–30 min, or continuous Sub-Q or IV infusion 5 mg/kg/d, up to 2 wk until ANC reaches 10,000/mm³ *Bone marrow transplantation:* IV or Sub-Q infusion, 10 mcg/kg/d initially, then titrated according to neutrophil count (5 mcg/kg/d if ANC >1000/mm³ for 3 consecutive days; stop drug if >1000/mm³ for 6 d. If ANC drops below 1000/mm³, restart filgrastim at 5 mcg/kg/d). *Collection of peripheral stem cells:* Sub-Q 10 mcg/kg/d for 6–7 d, with collection on the last 3 d of drug administration *Severe, chronic neutropenia:* Sub-Q 5 or 6 mcg/kg, once or twice daily, depending on clinical response and ANC	Do not give 24 h before or after a dose of cytotoxic chemotherapy. Dosage may be increased if indicated by neutrophil count. Stop the drug if ANC exceeds 10,000/mm³.
Pegfilgrastim (Neulasta)	To prevent infection in patients with neutropenia induced by cancer chemotherapy	Sub-Q 6 mg once per chemotherapy cycle. Do not give between 14 d before and 24 h after cytotoxic chemotherapy.	
Sargramostim (GM-CSF) (Leukine)	After bone marrow transplantation to promote bone marrow function or to treat graft failure or delayed function	*Bone marrow reconstitution:* IV infusion over 2 h, 250 mcg/m²/d, starting 2–4 h after bone marrow infusion, and continuing for 21 d	

Table 40-1 Drugs at a Glance: Hematopoietic and Immunostimulant Agents (continued)

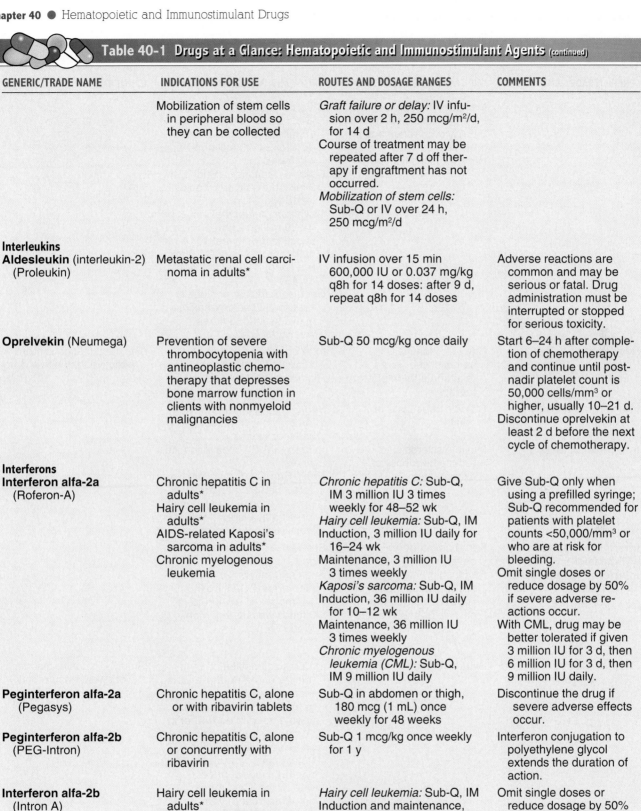

GENERIC/TRADE NAME	INDICATIONS FOR USE	ROUTES AND DOSAGE RANGES	COMMENTS
	Mobilization of stem cells in peripheral blood so they can be collected	*Graft failure or delay:* IV infusion over 2 h, 250 mcg/m²/d, for 14 d Course of treatment may be repeated after 7 d off therapy if engraftment has not occurred. *Mobilization of stem cells:* Sub-Q or IV over 24 h, 250 mcg/m²/d	
Interleukins **Aldesleukin** (interleukin-2) (Proleukin)	Metastatic renal cell carcinoma in adults*	IV infusion over 15 min 600,000 IU or 0.037 mg/kg q8h for 14 doses: after 9 d, repeat q8h for 14 doses	Adverse reactions are common and may be serious or fatal. Drug administration must be interrupted or stopped for serious toxicity.
Oprelvekin (Neumega)	Prevention of severe thrombocytopenia with antineoplastic chemotherapy that depresses bone marrow function in clients with nonmyeloid malignancies	Sub-Q 50 mcg/kg once daily	Start 6–24 h after completion of chemotherapy and continue until post-nadir platelet count is 50,000 cells/mm³ or higher, usually 10–21 d. Discontinue oprelvekin at least 2 d before the next cycle of chemotherapy.
Interferons **Interferon alfa-2a** (Roferon-A)	Chronic hepatitis C in adults* Hairy cell leukemia in adults* AIDS-related Kaposi's sarcoma in adults* Chronic myelogenous leukemia	*Chronic hepatitis C:* Sub-Q, IM 3 million IU 3 times weekly for 48–52 wk *Hairy cell leukemia:* Sub-Q, IM Induction, 3 million IU daily for 16–24 wk Maintenance, 3 million IU 3 times weekly *Kaposi's sarcoma:* Sub-Q, IM Induction, 36 million IU daily for 10–12 wk Maintenance, 36 million IU 3 times weekly *Chronic myelogenous leukemia (CML):* Sub-Q, IM 9 million IU daily	Give Sub-Q only when using a prefilled syringe; Sub-Q recommended for patients with platelet counts <50,000/mm³ or who are at risk for bleeding. Omit single doses or reduce dosage by 50% if severe adverse reactions occur. With CML, drug may be better tolerated if given 3 million IU for 3 d, then 6 million IU for 3 d, then 9 million IU daily.
Peginterferon alfa-2a (Pegasys)	Chronic hepatitis C, alone or with ribavirin tablets	Sub-Q in abdomen or thigh, 180 mcg (1 mL) once weekly for 48 weeks	Discontinue the drug if severe adverse effects occur.
Peginterferon alfa-2b (PEG-Intron)	Chronic hepatitis C, alone or concurrently with ribavirin	Sub-Q 1 mcg/kg once weekly for 1 y	Interferon conjugation to polyethylene glycol extends the duration of action.
Interferon alfa-2b (Intron A)	Hairy cell leukemia in adults* AIDS-related Kaposi's sarcoma in adults* Condylomata (genital warts) Chronic hepatitis (B and C)	*Hairy cell leukemia:* Sub-Q, IM Induction and maintenance, 2 million IU/m² 3 times weekly up to 6 mo *Kaposi's sarcoma:* Sub-Q, IM Induction and maintenance, 30 million IU/m² 3 times weekly	Omit single doses or reduce dosage by 50% if severe adverse reactions occur.

(continued)

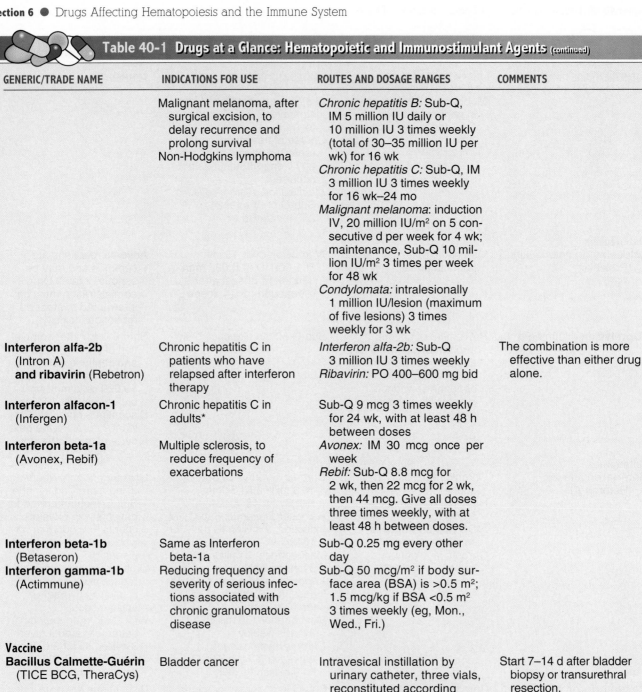

Table 40-1 Drugs at a Glance: Hematopoietic and Immunostimulant Agents (continued)

GENERIC/TRADE NAME	INDICATIONS FOR USE	ROUTES AND DOSAGE RANGES	COMMENTS
	Malignant melanoma, after surgical excision, to delay recurrence and prolong survival Non-Hodgkins lymphoma	*Chronic hepatitis B:* Sub-Q, IM 5 million IU daily or 10 million IU 3 times weekly (total of 30–35 million IU per wk) for 16 wk *Chronic hepatitis C:* Sub-Q, IM 3 million IU 3 times weekly for 16 wk–24 mo *Malignant melanoma:* induction IV, 20 million IU/m² on 5 consecutive d per week for 4 wk; maintenance, Sub-Q 10 million IU/m² 3 times per week for 48 wk *Condylomata:* intralesionally 1 million IU/lesion (maximum of five lesions) 3 times weekly for 3 wk	
Interferon alfa-2b (Intron A) **and ribavirin** (Rebetron)	Chronic hepatitis C in patients who have relapsed after interferon therapy	*Interferon alfa-2b:* Sub-Q 3 million IU 3 times weekly *Ribavirin:* PO 400–600 mg bid	The combination is more effective than either drug alone.
Interferon alfacon-1 (Infergen)	Chronic hepatitis C in adults*	Sub-Q 9 mcg 3 times weekly for 24 wk, with at least 48 h between doses	
Interferon beta-1a (Avonex, Rebif)	Multiple sclerosis, to reduce frequency of exacerbations	*Avonex:* IM 30 mcg once per week *Rebif:* Sub-Q 8.8 mcg for 2 wk, then 22 mcg for 2 wk, then 44 mcg. Give all doses three times weekly, with at least 48 h between doses.	
Interferon beta-1b (Betaseron)	Same as Interferon beta-1a	Sub-Q 0.25 mg every other day	
Interferon gamma-1b (Actimmune)	Reducing frequency and severity of serious infections associated with chronic granulomatous disease	Sub-Q 50 mcg/m² if body surface area (BSA) is >0.5 m²; 1.5 mcg/kg if BSA <0.5 m² 3 times weekly (eg, Mon., Wed., Fri.)	
Vaccine **Bacillus Calmette-Guérin** (TICE BCG, TheraCys)	Bladder cancer	Intravesical instillation by urinary catheter, three vials, reconstituted according to manufacturer's instructions, then diluted further in 50 mL of sterile, preservative-free saline solution (total volume per dose, 53 mL). Repeat once weekly for 6 wk, then give one dose monthly for 6–12 mo (TICE BCG) or one dose at 3, 6, 12, 18, and 24 mo (TheraCys).	Start 7–14 d after bladder biopsy or transurethral resection.

*18 y of age and older.

AIDS, acquired immunodeficiency syndrome; ANC, absolute neutrophil count; IM, intramuscular; IV, intravenous; PO, oral; Sub-Q, Subcutaneous.

example, has made it possible to produce large amounts of these substances for research and clinical use.

● Despite extensive research efforts, relatively few cytokine-like drugs are available for clinical use. One of the difficulties in using cytokines is maintaining effective dose levels over treatment periods of weeks or months. During a "natural" immune response, interacting body cells produce adequate concentrations of cytokines around target cells. However, achieving adequate local concentrations from injected, exogenous cytokines is difficult.

A second difficulty is that some of the drugs have a short half-life and require frequent administration. Some newer formulations (eg, darbepoetin alfa, pegfilgrastim, peginterferon alfa 2b) can be given less often. With peginterferon, pegylation (conjugation with polyethylene glycol [PEG]) increases half-life and allows once-weekly administration.

A third difficulty is that the substances are powerful biologic response modifiers and they can cause unanticipated adverse effects.

● Exogenous drug preparations have the same mechanisms of action as the endogenous products. Thus, CSF bind to receptors on the cell surfaces of immature blood cells in the bone marrow and increase the number, maturity, and functional ability of the cells. Interferons, called *alfa, beta,* or *gamma* according to specific characteristics, also bind to specific cell-surface receptors and alter intracellular activities. In viral infections, they induce enzymes that inhibit protein synthesis and degrade viral ribonucleic acid. As a result, viruses are less able to enter uninfected cells, reproduce, and release new viruses.

In addition to their antiviral effects, interferons also have antiproliferative and immunoregulatory activities. They can increase expression of major histocompatibility complex (MHC) molecules; augment the activity of natural killer (NK) cells; increase the effectiveness of antigen-presenting cells in inducing the proliferation of cytotoxic T cells; aid the attachment of cytotoxic T cells to target cells; and inhibit angiogenesis. Because of these characteristics, the interferons are used mainly to treat viral infections and cancers. In chronic hepatitis C, interferon improves liver function in approximately 50% of clients, but relapse often occurs when drug therapy is stopped. In multiple sclerosis, the action of interferon beta is unknown. The drugs are being investigated for additional uses. Systemic interferons are usually well absorbed, widely distributed, and eliminated primarily by the kidneys.

● In cancer, the exact mechanisms by which interferons and interleukins exert antineoplastic effects are unknown. However, their immunostimulant effects are thought to enhance activities of immune cells (ie, NK cells, T cells,

B cells, and macrophages); induce tumor-cell antigens (which make tumor cells more easily recognized by immune cells); or alter the expression of oncogenes (genes that can cause a normal cell to change to a cancer cell). BCG vaccine is thought to act against cancer of the urinary bladder by stimulating the immune system and eliciting a local inflammatory response, but its exact mechanism of action is unknown.

● They are given by subcutaneous (Sub-Q) or intravenous (IV) injection because they are proteins that would be destroyed by digestive enzymes if given orally. Darbepoetin alfa (Aranesp), epoetin alfa (Epogen, Procrit), filgrastim (Neupogen, Neulasta), oprelvekin (Neumega), and the interferons are often self- or caregiver-administered to ambulatory clients.

● They may produce adverse effects so that clients do not feel better when taking one of these drugs.

● The combination of injections and adverse effects may lead to noncompliance in taking the drugs as prescribed.

● All of the drugs are contraindicated for use in clients who have previously experienced hypersensitivity reactions to any component of the pharmaceutical preparations.

CLASSIFICATIONS AND INDIVIDUAL DRUGS

Hematopoietic Agents

Darbepoetin alfa and **epoetin alfa** are drug formulations of erythropoietin, a hormone from the kidney that stimulates bone marrow production of red blood cells (RBCs). They are used to prevent or treat anemia. In chronic renal failure, epoetin has a serum half-life of 4 to 13 hours and produces detectable blood levels of erythropoietin within 24 hours with IV administration. With Sub-Q administration, peak serum levels occur within 5 to 24 hours and then decline slowly. Darbepoetin has a much longer half-life (about 49 hours) in clients with chronic renal failure, and peak plasma levels occur in about 34 hours.

Colony-Stimulating Factors

Filgrastim and **sargramostim** are drug formulations of granulocyte colony-stimulating factor (G-CSF) and granulocyte macrophage colony-stimulating factor (GM-CSF), respectively, produced by recombinant DNA technology. They are used to stimulate blood cell production by the bone marrow in clients with bone marrow transplantation or chemotherapy-induced neutropenia. They can greatly reduce the incidence and severity of infections. GM-CSF is also being used to promote growth of blood vessels (angiogenesis) in clients with ischemic heart disease. The drug apparently promotes growth of arterioles around blocked areas in coronary arteries. It may be more effective than drugs that stimulate capillary growth, because arterioles are larger and can carry more blood.

Interleukins

Aldesleukin (Proleukin) is a recombinant DNA version of interleukin-2 (IL-2). It differs from native IL-2 but has the same biologic activity (eg, activates cellular immunity; produces tumor necrosis factor, interkeukin-1 [IL-1], and interferon gamma; inhibits tumor growth). It is used to treat metastatic renal cell carcinoma and melanoma and is being investigated for use in other types of cancer. The drug is given by IV infusion, after which it is rapidly distributed to extravascular, extracellular spaces and eliminated by metabolism in the kidneys.

Aldesleukin is contraindicated for initial use in clients who have had organ transplantation or those with serious cardiovascular disease (eg, an abnormal thallium stress test, which reflects coronary artery disease) or serious pulmonary disease (eg, abnormal pulmonary function tests). It is contraindicated for repeated courses of therapy in clients who had serious toxicity during earlier courses, including the following:

- Cardiac—dysrhythmias unresponsive to treatment or ventricular tachycardia lasting for five beats or more; recurrent episodes of chest pain with electrocardiographic evidence of angina or myocardial infarction; pericardial tamponade
- Gastrointestinal—bleeding requiring surgery; bowel ischemia or perforation
- Respiratory—intubation required longer than 72 hours
- Central nervous system—coma or toxic psychosis lasting longer than 72 hours; repetitive or hard-to-control seizures

Oprelvekin (Neumega) is recombinant IL-11, which stimulates platelet production. It is used to prevent severe thrombocytopenia and reduce the need for platelet transfusions in clients with cancer who are receiving chemotherapy that depresses the bone marrow.

Interferons

Interferons alfa-2a and **alfa-2b,** structurally the same except for one amino acid, are used to treat hairy-cell leukemia (a type of B-cell leukemia in which the cells are covered with fine, hairlike structures), Kaposi's sarcoma associated with AIDS, and chronic hepatitis. Interferon alfa-2b is also approved for the treatment of condylomata acuminata (genital warts associated with infection by human papillomavirus), non-Hodgkins lymphoma, and malignant melanoma. In chronic hepatitis C, interferon alfa-2b may be combined with ribavirin, another antiviral drug, to increase effectiveness. In condylomata, interferon alfa-2b is injected directly into the lesions for several weeks, and most of the lesions disappear completely.

Interferon alfa-n1 and **alfacon-1** are approved for treatment of chronic hepatitis C, a condition that can lead to liver failure. **Interferon gamma** is used to treat chronic granulomatous disease, which involves impaired phagocytosis of ingested microbes and frequent infections. Drug therapy reduces the incidence and severity of infections. **Interferon beta** is used for multiple sclerosis, an autoimmune neurologic disorder in which the drug reduces progression of neurologic dysfunction, prolongs remissions, and reduces the severity of relapses.

Interferons are being investigated for additional uses, especially in cancer and viral infections, including AIDS. In cancer, for example, interferon alfa has demonstrated antitumor effects in multiple myeloma, renal cell carcinoma, and others. In chronic myelogenous leukemia (CML), 70% response rates have been reported and some clients undergo complete remission. Common solid tumors of the breast, lung, and colon are unresponsive.

Although the main adverse effects are flulike symptoms, alfa interferons may also cause or aggravate serious, life-threatening neuropsychiatric (including depression and some reports of suicide), autoimmune, ischemic, and infectious disorders. Clients receiving the drugs should be closely monitored with clinical and laboratory examinations and the drugs should be discontinued if persistently severe or worsening signs or symptoms of these disorders occur. In many but not all cases, these disorders resolve after stopping interferon alfa.

Bacillus Calmette-Guérin

Bacillus Calmette-Guérin vaccine is a suspension of attenuated *Mycobacterium bovis,* long used as an immunizing agent against tuberculosis. The drug's immunostimulant properties stem from its ability to stimulate cell-mediated immunity. It is used as a topical agent to treat superficial cancers of the urinary bladder, in which approximately 80% of clients achieve a therapeutic response. BCG is contraindicated in immunosuppressed clients because the live tubercular organisms may cause tuberculosis in this high-risk population.

NURSING PROCESS

Assessment

- Assess the client's status in relation to conditions for which hematopoietic and immunostimulant drugs are used (eg, infection, neutropenia, cancer).
- Assess nutritional status, including appetite and weight.
- Assess functional abilities in relation to activities of daily living (ADLs).
- Assess adequacy of support systems for outpatients (eg, transportation for clinic visits).

● Assess ability and attitude toward planned drug therapy and associated monitoring and follow-up.

● Assess coping mechanisms of client and significant others in stressful situations.

● Assess client for factors predisposing to infection (eg, skin lesions, invasive devices, cigarette smoking).

● Assess environment for factors predisposing to infection (eg, family or health care providers with infections).

● Assess baseline values of laboratory and other diagnostic test reports to aid monitoring of responses to hematopoietic and immunostimulant drug therapy.

Nursing Diagnoses

● Risk for Injury: Infection related to drug-induced neutropenia, immunosuppression, malnutrition, chronic disease; bleeding related to anemia or thrombocytopenia

● Risk for Injury: Adverse drug effects

● Activity Intolerance related to weakness, fatigue from debilitating disease, or drug therapy

● Anxiety related to the diagnosis of cancer, hepatitis, multiple sclerosis, or HIV infection

● Deficient Knowledge: Disease process; hematopoietic and immunostimulant drug therapy

Planning/Goals

The client will

● Participate in interventions to prevent or decrease infection

● Remain afebrile during immunostimulant therapy

● Experience increased immunocompetence as indicated by increased white blood cell (WBC) count (if initially leukopenic) or tumor regression

● Avoid preventable infections

● Experience relief or reduction of disease symptoms

● Maintain independence in ADLs when able; be assisted appropriately when unable

● Maintain adequate levels of nutrition and fluids, rest and sleep, and exercise

● Maintain or increase appetite and weight if initially anorexic and underweight

● Learn to self-administer medications accurately when indicated

Interventions

● Practice and promote good hand hygiene techniques by clients and all others in contact with the client.

● Use sterile technique for all injections, IV site care, wound dressing changes, and any other invasive diagnostic or therapeutic measures.

● Screen staff and visitors for signs and symptoms of infection; if infection is noted, do not allow contact with the client.

● Allow clients to participate in self-care and decision making when possible and appropriate.

● Use isolation procedures when indicated, usually when the neutrophil count is less than 500/mm³.

● Promote adequate nutrition, with nutritious fluids, supplements, and snacks when indicated.

● Promote adequate rest, sleep, and exercise (eg, schedule frequent rest periods, avoid interrupting sleep when possible, individualize exercise or activity according to the client's condition).

● Inform clients about diagnostic test results, planned changes in therapeutic regimens, and evidence of progress.

● Allow family members or significant others to visit clients when feasible.

● Monitor complete blood count (CBC) and other diagnostic test reports for normal or abnormal values.

● Schedule and coordinate drug administration, diagnostic tests, and other elements of care to conserve clients' energy and decrease stress.

● Consult other health care providers (eg, physician, dietitian, social worker) on the client's behalf when indicated.

● Assist clients to learn ways to prevent or reduce the incidence of infections (eg, meticulous personal hygiene, avoiding contact with infected people).

● Assist clients to learn ways to enhance immune mechanisms and other body defenses by healthy lifestyle habits, such as a nutritious diet, adequate rest and sleep, and avoidance of tobacco and alcohol (see accompanying Client Teaching Guidelines).

● Assist clients or caregivers in learning how to prepare and inject darbepoetin alfa, epoetin alfa, filgrastim, an interferon, or oprelvekin, when indicated.

Evaluation

● Determine the number and type of infections that have occurred in neutropenic clients.

● Compare current CBC reports with baseline values for changes toward normal levels (eg, WBC count 5000–10,000/mm³).

● Compare weight and nutritional status with baseline values for maintenance or improvement.

● Observe and interview for decreased numbers or severity of disease symptoms.

● Observe for increased energy and ability to participate in ADLs.

● Observe and interview outpatients regarding compliance with follow-up care.

● Observe and interview regarding the mental and emotional status of the client and family members.

CLIENT TEACHING GUIDELINES

Blood Cell and Immune System Stimulants

General Considerations

- Help your body maintain immune mechanisms and other defenses by healthy lifestyle habits, such as a nutritious diet, adequate rest and sleep, and avoidance of tobacco and alcohol.
- Practice meticulous personal hygiene and avoid people and circumstances in which you are exposed to infection.
- Keep appointments with health care providers for follow-up care, blood tests, and so forth.
- Inform any other physician, dentist, or health care provider about your condition and the medications you are taking.
- Several of these medications can be taken at home, even though they are taken by injection. If you are going to self-inject a medication at home, allow sufficient time to learn and practice the techniques under the supervision of a health care provider. Correct preparation and injection are necessary to increase beneficial effects and decrease adverse effects.
- With oprelvekin, report the occurrence of ankle edema, shortness of breath, or dizzy spells. Edema and breathing difficulty may be caused by fluid retention, a common adverse effect, and dizziness may result from an irregular heartbeat, which is most likely to occur in older adults.
- With interferons, report the occurrence of depression or thoughts of suicide, dizziness, hives, itching, chest tightness, cough, diffi-

culty breathing or wheezing, or visual problems. These symptoms may require that the drug be stopped or the dosage reduced. In addition, avoid pregnancy (use effective contraceptive methods) and avoid prolonged exposure to sunlight, wear protective clothing, and use sunscreens.

Self- or Caregiver Administration

- Take the drugs as prescribed. Although this is important with all medications, it is especially important with these. Obtaining beneficial effects and decreasing adverse effects depend to a great extent on how the drugs are taken.
- Use correct techniques to prepare and inject the medications. Instructions for mixing the drugs should be followed exactly.
- With interferons:
  - Store in the refrigerator.
  - Do not freeze or shake the drug vial.
  - Do not change brands (changes in dosage may result).
  - Take at bedtime to reduce some common adverse effects (eg, flu-like symptoms such as fever, headache, fatigue, anorexia, nausea, and vomiting).
  - Take acetaminophen (eg, Tylenol, others), if desired, to prevent or decrease fever and headache.
  - Maintain a good fluid intake (eg, 2 to 3 quarts daily).

APPLYING YOUR KNOWLEDGE 40-1

With her low WBC count and ANC (Absolute Neutrophil Count), Mrs. Miller is at great risk for infection. What should you teach her regarding infection prevention?

PRINCIPLES OF THERAPY

Drug Administration: Inpatient Versus Outpatient Settings

Choosing inpatient or outpatient administration of hematopoietic and immunostimulant therapy depends on many factors, including the condition of the client, route of drug administration, expected duration of therapy, and potential severity of adverse drug reactions. Most of these drugs are proteins, and anaphylactic or other allergic reactions may occur, especially with parenteral administration. Thus, initial doses should be given where appropriate supplies and personnel are available to treat allergic reactions.

Darbepoetin alfa, epoetin alfa, filgrastim, interferons, and oprelvekin may be taken at home if the client or a caregiver can prepare and inject the medication. Because severe, life-threatening adverse effects may occur with high-dose aldesleukin, this drug should be given only in a hospital with

intensive care facilities, under the supervision of health care providers experienced in critical care.

Drug Dosage

With darbepoetin alfa and epoetin alfa, dosage is adjusted according to response. With darbepoetin, dosage is adjusted to achieve and maintain a hemoglobin value of approximately 12 grams per deciliter. With epoetin, dosage is adjusted to achieve and maintain a hematocrit value of 30% to 36%. Dosage should be reduced when the hematocrit approaches 36% or increases by more than 4 points in any 2-week period. Dosage should be increased if hematocrit does not increase by 5 to 6 points after 8 weeks of drug therapy and is below the recommended range. When doses are changed, measurable differences in hematocrit do not occur for 2 to 6 weeks because of the time required for maturation of RBCs and their release into the circulation. Thus, the hematocrit should be checked twice weekly for at least 2 to 6 weeks after any dosage change. In general, dose adjustments should not be made more often than once monthly.

Optimal dosages for interferons and aldesleukin have not been established. For clients who experience severe adverse reactions with interferon alfa, dosage should be reduced by 50% or administration stopped until the reaction subsides.

For clients who experience severe reactions to aldesleukin, dosage reduction is not recommended. Instead, one or more doses should be withheld, or the drug should be discontinued. Withhold the dose for cardiac dysrhythmias, hypotension, chest pain, agitation or confusion, sepsis, renal impairment (oliguria, increased serum creatinine), hepatic impairment (encephalopathy, increasing ascites), positive stool guaiac test, or severe dermatitis, until the condition is resolved. The drug should be discontinued for the occurrence of any of the conditions listed as contraindications for repeat courses of aldesleukin therapy (eg, sustained ventricular tachycardia, angina, myocardial infarction, pulmonary intubation, renal dialysis, coma, GI bleeding).

Laboratory Monitoring

With darbepoetin and epoetin, iron stores (transferrin saturation and serum ferritin) should be measured before and periodically during treatment. Clients usually require supplemental iron. Check hemoglobin (with darbepoetin) once weekly or hematocrit (with epoetin) twice weekly until stabilized and maintenance drug doses are established.

With most of the hematopoietic and immunostimulant drugs, a CBC with WBC differential and platelet count should be done before and during treatment to monitor response and prevent avoidable adverse reactions. With CSF, these tests are recommended twice weekly during drug administration. With aldesleukin, these tests plus electrolytes and renal and liver function tests are recommended daily during drug administration. With interferons alfacon-1 and alfan1, tests of platelet and neutrophil counts, hemoglobin, serum creatinine or creatinine clearance, serum albumin, and thyroid-stimulating hormone are recommended for all clients before starting therapy, 2 weeks later, and periodically thereafter during the 24 weeks of therapy.

Use in Special Populations

Use in Clients With Cancer

Colony-Stimulating Factors

Filgrastim and sargramostim are used to restore, promote, or accelerate bone marrow function in clients with cancer who are undergoing chemotherapy or bone marrow transplantation. In cancer chemotherapy, many therapeutic drugs cause bone marrow depression and result in anemia and neutropenia. Neutropenic clients are at high risk for development of infections, often from the normal microbial flora of the client's body or environmental microorganisms, and they may involve bacteria, fungi, and viruses. The client is most vulnerable to infection when the neutrophil count falls below 500/mm³. Filgrastim helps to prevent infection by reducing the incidence, severity, and duration of neutropenia associated with several chemotherapy regimens. Most clients

taking filgrastim have fewer days of fever, infection, and antimicrobial drug therapy. In addition, by promoting bone marrow recovery after a course of cytotoxic antineoplastic drugs, filgrastim also may allow higher doses or more timely administration of subsequent antitumor drugs.

When filgrastim is given to prevent infection in neutropenic clients with cancer, the drug should be started at least 24 hours after the last dose of the antineoplastic agent (it must also not be given 24 hours before a dose of cytotoxic chemotherapy). It should then be continued during the period of maximum bone marrow suppression and the lowest neutrophil count (nadir) and during bone marrow recovery. CBC and platelet counts should be performed twice weekly during therapy, and the drug should be stopped if the neutrophil count exceeds 10,000/mm³. When sargramostim is given to clients with cancer who have had bone marrow transplantation, the drug should be started 2 to 4 hours after the bone marrow infusion and at least 24 hours after the last dose of antineoplastic chemotherapy or 12 hours after the last radiotherapy treatment. CBC should be done twice weekly during therapy, and the neutrophil count should not exceed approximately 20,000/mm³.

Epoetin alfa may be used to prevent or treat anemia in clients with cancer. An adequate intake of iron is required for drug effectiveness. In addition to dietary sources, a supplement is usually necessary.

 APPLYING YOUR KNOWLEDGE 40-2:
HOW CAN YOU AVOID THIS MEDICATION ERROR?
Mrs. Miller is having her blood work done the day prior to her next chemotherapy treatment. Her WBC count is still low, and you administer filgrastim according to the standing orders for a WBC count of less than 2000. What should you have taken into consideration before giving the injection?

Interleukins

Aldesleukin is a highly toxic drug and contraindicated in clients with pre-existing serious cardiovascular or pulmonary impairment. Therefore, when it is used to treat metastatic renal cell carcinoma, clients must be carefully selected, evaluated, and monitored. The drug is most effective in clients with prior nephrectomy and low tumor burden. Still, only approximately 15% to 25% of clients experience therapeutic responses.

Measures to decrease toxicity are also needed. One strategy is to give the drug by continuous infusion rather than bolus injection. Another is to use cancer-fighting T cells found within tumors. These T cells, called *tumor-infiltrating lymphocytes,* can be removed from the tumors, incubated in vitro with aldesleukin, and reinjected into the client. Tumor-infiltrating lymphocytes return to the tumor and are more active in killing malignant cells than untreated T cells. This technique allows lower and therefore less toxic doses of aldesleukin. Corticosteroids can also decrease toxicity, but their use is not recommended because they also decrease the antineoplastic effects of aldesleukin.

In addition, any pre-existing infection should be treated and resolved before initiating aldesleukin therapy because the drug may impair neutrophil function and increase the risk of infections, including septicemia and bacterial endocarditis. Clients with indwelling central IV devices should be given prophylactic antibacterials that are effective against *Staphylococcus aureus* (eg, nafcillin, vancomycin).

Oprelvekin may be used to prevent or treat thrombocytopenia and risks of bleeding in clients with cancer.

Interferons

In hairy-cell leukemia, interferons normalize WBC counts in 70% to 90% of clients, with or without prior splenectomy. Drug therapy must be continued indefinitely to avoid relapse, which usually develops rapidly after the drug is discontinued. In AIDS-related Kaposi's sarcoma, larger doses are required than in other clinical uses, with resultant increases in toxicity. Interferon alfa is recommended for clients with CD4 cell counts higher than 200 per milliliter (CD4 cells are the helper T cells attacked by the AIDS virus), who have no systemic symptoms, and who have had no opportunistic infections. Approximately 40% of these clients achieve a therapeutic response that lasts 1 to 2 years. In addition to antineoplastic effects, data indicate that viral replication is suppressed in responding clients. Research studies suggest that a combination of interferon alfa and zidovudine, an antiviral drug used in the treatment of AIDS, may have synergistic antineoplastic and antiviral effects. Lower doses of interferon must be used when the drug is combined with zidovudine, to minimize neutropenia.

Bacillus Calmette-Guérin

Bacillus Calmette-Guérin, when instilled into the urinary bladder of clients with superficial bladder cancer, causes remission in up to 82% of clients for an average of 4 years. Early, successful treatment of carcinoma in situ also prevents development of invasive bladder cancer. A specific protocol has been developed for administration of BCG solution, and it should be followed accurately.

APPLYING YOUR KNOWLEDGE 40-3
Epoetin alfa is prescribed for Mrs. Miller's anemia. What dietary considerations should you be aware of?

Use in Clients Undergoing Bone Marrow and Stem Cell Transplantation

Filgrastim and sargramostim are used to treat clients who undergo bone marrow transplantation for Hodgkin's disease, non-Hodgkin's lymphoma, or acute lymphoblastic leukemia. Before receiving a bone marrow transplant, the client's immune system is suppressed by anticancer drugs or irradiation. After transplantation, it takes 2 to 4 weeks for the engrafted bone mar-

row cells to mature and begin producing blood cells. During this time, the client has virtually no functioning granulocytes and is at high risk for infection. Sargramostim promotes engraftment and function of the transplanted bone marrow, thereby decreasing risks of infection. If the graft is successful, the granulocyte count starts to rise in approximately 2 weeks. Sargramostim also is used to treat graft failure.

In stem cell transplantation, filgrastim or sargramostim is used to stimulate the movement of hematopoietic stem cells from the bone marrow to circulating blood, where they can be readily collected (in a process called *peripheral blood progenitor cell collection*). Transplantation of large numbers of stem cells can lead to more rapid engraftment and recovery, with less risk of transplant failure and complications.

Use in Children

There has been limited experience with hematopoietic and immunostimulant drugs in children (younger than 18 years of age), and the drugs' safety and effectiveness have not been established. Filgrastim and sargramostim have been used in children with therapeutic and adverse effects similar to those in adults. In clinical trials, filgrastim produced a greater incidence of subclinical spleen enlargement in children than in adults, but whether this affects growth and development or has other long-term consequences is unknown.

Oprelvekin has been given to a few children with adverse effects similar to those observed in adults. Reports indicate that tachycardia occurs more often in children and that larger doses are needed (eg, a dose of 75–100 mcg/kg in children produces similar plasma levels to a dose of 50 mcg/kg in adults). Long-term effects on growth and development are unknown.

Little information is available about the use of interferons in children and most are not recommended. Interferon alfa-2b may be used to treat chronic hepatitis B in children. It is given Sub-Q in doses of 3 million units/m² three times per week for the first week, then 6 million units/m² three times per week for 16 to 24 weeks. Dosage should be reduced by 50% or the drug discontinued if serious adverse effects or laboratory abnormalities develop.

Use in Older Adults

In general, hematopoietic and immunostimulant agents have the same uses and responses in older adults as in younger adults. Older adults may be at greater risk of adverse effects, especially if large doses are used. Oprelvekin should be used with caution in clients with a history of or risk factors for atrial fibrillation or flutter; these dysrhythmias occurred in approximately 10% of clients during clinical trials. In addition, older adults are more likely to have fluid retention with oprelvekin, with resultant symptoms of peripheral edema, dyspnea on exertion, and dilutional anemia.

Use in Clients With Renal Impairment

Except for darbepoetin alfa and epoetin alfa, which are used to treat anemia in clients with chronic renal failure, little information is available about the use of hematopoietic and immunostimulant drugs in clients with renal impairment. In some clients with pre-existing renal impairment, sargramostim increased serum creatinine. Values declined to baseline levels when the drug was stopped or its dosage reduced. Renal function tests are recommended every 2 weeks in clients with pre-existing impairment.

With aldesleukin, renal impairment occurs during therapy. This impairment may be increased if other nephrotoxic drugs are taken concomitantly. In addition, drug-induced renal impairment may delay elimination of other medications and increase risks of adverse effects.

Use in Clients With Hepatic Impairment

In some clients with pre-existing hepatic impairment, sargramostim increased serum bilirubin and liver enzymes. Values declined to baseline levels when the drug was stopped or its dosage reduced. Hepatic function tests are recommended every 2 weeks in clients with pre-existing impairment.

With aldesleukin, hepatic impairment occurs during therapy. This impairment may be increased if other hepatotoxic drugs are taken concomitantly. In addition, drug-induced hepatic impairment may delay metabolism and elimination of other medications and increase risks of adverse effects.

Interferons may aggravate hepatic impairment. Interferons alfa-2b, alfacon-1, and alfa-n1 are contraindicated in clients with decompensated liver disease (ie, signs and symptoms such as jaundice, ascites, bleeding disorders, or decreased serum albumin), autoimmune hepatitis, a history of autoimmune disease, or posttransplantation immunosuppression. Worsening of liver disease, with jaundice, hepatic encephalopathy, hepatic failure, and death, has occurred in these clients. The drugs should be discontinued in clients with signs and symptoms of liver failure.

Use in Home Care

Darbepoetin alfa (Aranesp), epoetin alfa (Epogen, Procrit), filgrastim (Neupogen, Neulasta), oprelvekin (Neumega), and the interferons are often self-administered or given by a caregiver to chronically ill clients. The home care nurse may need to teach clients or caregivers accurate drug preparation and injection techniques, as well as proper disposal of needles and syringes. Assistance may also be needed in obtaining appropriate laboratory tests (eg, CBC, platelet count, tests of renal or hepatic function) to monitor clients' responses to the medications. Other interventions depend on the drug being taken. For example, epoetin alfa is not effective unless sufficient iron is present, and most clients need an iron supplement. When an iron preparation is prescribed, the home care nurse may need to emphasize the importance of taking it. With filgrastim, the nurse may need to help the client and family with techniques to reduce exposure to infection.

N U R S I N G   A C T I O N S

Hematopoietic and Immunostimulant Agents

NURSING ACTIONS	RATIONALE/EXPLANATION
1. Administer accurately	For hospitalized clients, the drugs may be prepared for administration in a pharmacy. When nurses prepare the drugs, they should consult the manufacturer's instructions.
a. Give darbepoetin alfa intravenously (IV) or subcutaneously (Sub-Q) once weekly.	Outpatients may be taught self-administration techniques. Omit the dose if the hemoglobin level is >12g/dL.
b. Give epoetin alfa IV or Sub-Q; do not shake the vial; and discard any remainder of multidose vials 21 days after opening.	For clients with chronic renal failure on hemodialysis, epoetin alfa can be given by bolus injection at the end of dialysis. For other patients with an IV line, the drug can be given IV. For patients without an IV line or who are ambulatory, the drug is injected Sub-Q.
	Shaking can inactivate the medication; the manufacturer does not ensure sterility or stability of multidose vials after 21 days.
c. Give filgrastim (Neupogen) according to indication for use: (1) With cancer chemotherapy, give by Sub-Q bolus injection, IV infusion over 15–30 minutes, or continuous Sub-Q or IV infusion. (2) For bone marrow transplantation, give by IV infusion over 4 hours or by continuous IV or Sub-Q infusion.	Manufacturer's recommendations

NURSING ACTIONS	RATIONALE/EXPLANATION
(3) For collection of stem cells, give as a bolus or a continuous infusion.	
(4) For chronic neutropenia, give Sub-Q.	
d. Give pegfilgrastim (Neulasta) Sub-Q only.	
e. Give sargramostim by IV infusion over 2 hours, after reconstitution with 1 mL sterile water for injection and addition to 0.9% sodium chloride.	Manufacturer's recommendation
f. With aldesleukin, review institutional protocols or the manufacturer's instructions for administration.	This drug has limited uses and is rarely given. Thus, most nurses will need to review instructions each time.
g. With interferons:	
(1) Read drug labels carefully to ensure having the correct drug preparation.	Available drugs have similar names but often differ in indications for use, dosages, and routes of administration.
(2) Give most interferons Sub-Q, 3 times weekly, on a regular schedule (eg, Mon., Wed., and Fri.), at about the same time of day, at least 48 hours apart.	Manufacturer's recommendation
(3) Inject interferon for condylomata intralesionally into the base of each wart with a small-gauge needle. For large warts, inject at several points.	Manufacturer's recommendation
h. With intravesical *Bacillus Calmette-Guérin (BCG)*:	
(1) Reconstitute solution (see Table 40-1).	Reconstituted solution should be used immediately or refrigerated. Discard if not used within 2 hours.
(2) Wear gown and gloves.	
(3) Insert a sterile urethral catheter and drain bladder.	
(4) Instill medication slowly by gravity.	
(5) Remove catheter.	
(6) Have the patient lie on abdomen, back, and alternate sides for 15 min in each position. Then, allow to ambulate but ask to retain solution for a total of 2 hours before urinating, if able.	
(7) Dispose of all equipment in contact with BCG solution appropriately.	BCG contains live mycobacterial organisms and is therefore infectious material.
(8) Do not give if catheterization causes trauma (eg, bleeding), and wait 1 week before a repeat attempt.	
2. Observe for therapeutic effects	
a. With darbepoetin alfa and epoetin alfa, observe for increased red blood cells, hemoglobin, and hematocrit.	Therapeutic effects depend on the dose and the client's underlying condition. The goal is usually to achieve and maintain a hematocrit between 30% and 36% (with epoetin) or hemoglobin of no more than 12 g/dL (with darbepoetin). With epoetin, it takes 2–6 weeks for the hematocrit to change after a dosage change.
b. With oprelvekin, observe for maintenance of a normal or near-normal platelet count when used to prevent thrombocytopenia and an increased platelet count or fewer platelet transfusions when used to treat thrombocytopenia.	Platelet counts usually increase in approximately 1 week and continue to increase for approximately 1 week after the drug is stopped. Then, counts decrease toward baseline during the next 2 weeks.
c. With aldesleukin, observe for tumor regression (improvement in signs and symptoms).	Tumor regression may occur as early as 4 weeks after the first course of therapy and may continue up to 12 months.
d. With parenteral interferons, observe for improvement in signs and symptoms.	With hairy-cell leukemia, hematologic tests may improve within 2 months, but optimal effects may require 6 months of drug therapy. With Kaposi's sarcoma, skin lesions may resolve or stabilize over several weeks. With chronic hepatitis, liver function tests may improve within a few weeks.

NURSING ACTIONS	RATIONALE/EXPLANATION
e. With intralesional interferon, observe for disappearance of genital warts.	Lesions usually disappear after several weeks of treatment.
3. Observe for adverse effects	
a. With darbepoetin alfa and epoetin alfa, observe for nausea, vomiting, diarrhea, arthralgias, and hypertension.	The drugs are usually well tolerated, with adverse effects similar to those of placebo and which may result from the underlying disease processes.
b. With oprelvekin, observe for atrial fibrillation or flutter, dyspnea, edema, fever, mucositis, nausea, neutropenia, tachycardia, vomiting.	In clinical trials, most adverse events were mild or moderate in severity and reversible after stopping drug administration. Atrial dysrhythmias are more likely to occur in older adults. Dyspnea and edema are attributed to fluid retention.
c. With filgrastim, observe for bone pain, erythema at Sub-Q injection sites, and increased serum lactate dehydrogenase, alkaline phosphatase, and uric acid levels.	Bone pain reportedly occurs in 20%–25% of patients and can be treated with acetaminophen or a nonsteroidal anti-inflammatory drug (NSAID).
d. With sargramostim, observe for bone pain, fever, headache, muscle aches, generalized maculopapular skin rash, and fluid retention (peripheral edema, pleural effusion, pericardial effusion).	Pleural and pericardial effusions are more likely at doses greater than 20 mcg/kg/d. Adverse effects occur more often with sargramostim than filgrastim.
e. With interferons, observe for acute flu-like symptoms (eg, fever, chills, fatigue, muscle aches, headache), chronic fatigue, depression, leukopenia, and increased liver enzymes. Anemia and depressed platelet and WBC counts may also occur but are infrequent.	Acute effects occur in most patients, increasing with higher doses and decreasing with continued drug administration. Most symptoms can be relieved by acetaminophen. Fatigue and depression occur with long-term administration and are dose-limiting effects.
f. With aldesleukin, observe for capillary leak syndrome (hypotension, shock, angina, myocardial infarction, dysrhythmias, edema, respiratory distress, gastrointestinal bleeding, renal insufficiency, mental status changes). Other effects may involve most body systems, such as chills and fever, blood (anemia, thrombocytopenia, eosinophilia), central nervous system (CNS) (seizures, psychiatric symptoms), skin (erythema, burning, pruritus), hepatic (cholestasis), endocrine (hypothyroidism), and bacterial infections. In addition, drug-induced tumor breakdown may cause hypocalcemia, hyperkalemia, hyperphosphatemia, hyperuricemia, renal failure, and electrocardiogram changes.	Adverse effects are frequent, often serious, and sometimes fatal. Most subside within 2 to 3 days after stopping the drug. Capillary leak syndrome, which may begin soon after treatment starts, is characterized by a loss of plasma proteins and fluids into extravascular space. Signs and symptoms result from decreased organ perfusion, and most patients can be treated with vasopressor drugs, cautious fluid replacement, diuretics, and supplemental oxygen.
g. With intravesical BCG, assess for symptoms of bladder irritation (eg, frequency, urgency, dysuria, hematuria) and systemic symptoms of fever, chills, and malaise.	These effects occur in more than 50% of patients, usually starting a few hours after administration and lasting 2 to 3 days. They can be decreased by phenazopyridine (Pyridium), a urinary tract analgesic; propantheline (Pro-Banthine) or oxybutynin (Ditropan), antispasmodics; and acetaminophen (Tylenol) or ibuprofen (Motrin), analgesic–antipyretic agents.
4. Observe for drug interactions	
a. Drugs that *increase* effects of sargramostim:	
(1) Corticosteroids, lithium	These drugs have myeloproliferative (bone-marrow stimulating) effects of their own, which may add to those of sargramostim.
b. Drugs that *increase* effects of aldesleukin:	All of the listed drug groups may potentiate adverse effects of aldesleukin.
(1) Aminoglycoside antibiotics (eg, gentamicin, others)	Increased nephrotoxicity
(2) Antihypertensives	Increased hypotension
(3) Antineoplastics (eg, asparaginase, doxorubicin, methotrexate)	Increased toxic effects on bone marrow, heart, and liver. Aldesleukin is usually given as a single antineoplastic agent; its use in combination with other antineoplastic drugs is being evaluated.

(continued)

NURSING ACTIONS	RATIONALE/EXPLANATION
(4) Opioid analgesics	Increased CNS adverse effects
(5) NSAIDs (eg, ibuprofen)	Increased nephrotoxicity
(6) Sedative-hypnotics	Increased CNS adverse effects
c. Drugs that *decrease* effects of aldesleukin:	
(1) Corticosteroids	These drugs should not be given concurrently with aldesleukin, because they decrease the drug's therapeutic anticancer effects.

APPLYING YOUR KNOWLEDGE: ANSWERS

40-1 Teach Mrs. Miller to get adequate rest and sleep, to eat a nutritious diet, and to practice meticulous personal hygiene.

40-2 Filgrastim should not be given for 24 hours before or after a dose of chemotherapy.

40-3 An adequate intake of iron is needed for the drug to be effective. A nutritional supplement is usually necessary, in addition to dietary sources.

Review and Application Exercises

Short Answer Exercises

1. What are the hematopoietic, colony-stimulating cytokines, and how do they function in the body?

2. What are adverse effects of filgrastim and sargramostim, and how may they be prevented or minimized?

3. What are the clinical uses of pharmaceutical interleukins and interferons?

4. What are the adverse effects of interleukins and interferons, and how can they be prevented or minimized?

5. Describe the clinical uses of hematopoietic and immunostimulant drugs in the treatment of anemia, neutropenia, thrombocytopenia, cancer, and bone marrow transplantation.

NCLEX-Style Questions

6. The expected outcome of administering epoetin alfa (Epogen) or darbepoetin alfa (Aranesp) to a client with chronic renal failure is
   a. decreased bleeding
   b. increased WBC production
   c. increased RBC production
   d. improved renal function

7. Most clients who take epoetin or darbopoetin also need to take
   a. iron
   b. potassium
   c. antacids
   d. analgesics

8. An expected outcome after the administration of filgrastim (Neupogen) is
   a. fewer infections
   b. decreased anemia
   c. longer life expectancy
   d. less nausea and vomiting

9. An interferon may be used to treat
   a. most types of cancer
   b. chronic hepatitis C
   c. flulike symptoms
   d. mental depression

10. BCG for bladder cancer would be contraindicated for clients with a history of
    a. heart disease
    b. diabetes mellitus
    c. pulmonary fibrosis
    d. organ transplantation

Selected References

Darbepoetin (Aranesp)—A long-acting erythropoietin. (2001, December 10). *The Medical Letter on Drugs and Therapeutics, 43*(1120), 109–110.

DiPiro, J. T., Talbert, R. L., Yee, G. C., Matzke, G. R., Wells, B. G., & Posey, L. M. (Eds.). (2002). *Pharmacotherapy: A pathophysiologic approach* (5th ed.). New York: McGraw-Hill.

Drug facts and comparisons. (Updated monthly). St. Louis: Facts and Comparisons.

Goldman, L., & Ausiello, D. (Eds.). (2004). *Cecil textbook of medicine* (22nd ed.). Philadelphia: W. B. Saunders.

Porth, C. M. (2005). *Pathophysiology: Concepts of altered health states* (7th ed.). Philadelphia: Lippincott Williams & Wilkins.

Rhoades, R. A., & Tanner, G. A. (2003). *Medical physiology* (2nd ed.). Philadelphia: Lippincott Williams & Wilkins.

Smeltzer, S. C., & Bare, B. G. (2004). *Brunner & Suddarth's textbook of medical-surgical nursing* (10th ed.). Philadelphia: Lippincott Williams & Wilkins.

Immunosuppressants

OBJECTIVES

After studying this chapter, you will be able to:

1. Describe characteristics and consequences of immunosuppression.
2. Discuss characteristics and uses of major immunosuppressant drugs in autoimmune disorders and organ transplantation.
3. Identify adverse effects of immunosuppressant drugs.
4. Discuss nursing interventions to decrease adverse effects of immunosuppressant drugs.
5. Teach clients, family members, and caregivers about safe and effective immunosuppressant drug therapy.
6. Assist clients and family members to identify potential sources of infection in the home care environment.

APPLYING YOUR KNOWLEDGE

Edward Kinney is a 48-year-old salesman who has had long-standing hypertension. He had severe kidney damage and required a renal transplant. His transplant was successful and was completed 2 years ago. He is receiving prednisone 10 mg PO daily, cyclosporine, sirolimus, and mycophenolate.

INTRODUCTION

Immunosuppressant drugs interfere with the production or function of immune cells and cytokines. The drugs are used to decrease an undesirable immune response.

The immune response is normally a protective mechanism (see Chap. 38) that helps the body defend itself against potentially harmful agents. However, numerous disease processes develop when the immune system perceives the person's own body tissues as harmful invaders and tries to eliminate them. This inappropriate activation of the immune response is a major factor in diseases believed to involve autoimmune processes, including rheumatoid arthritis (RA), Crohn's disease, psoriasis, psoriatic arthritis, and others.

An appropriate but undesirable immune response is elicited when foreign tissue is transplanted into the body. If the immune response is not sufficiently suppressed, the body reacts as with other antigens and attempts to destroy (reject) the foreign organ or tissue. Although numerous advances have been made in transplantation technology, the immune response remains a major factor in determining the success or failure of transplantation.

Many of the available immunosuppressant drugs inhibit the immune response in a general or nonspecific manner. However, the number of drugs that suppress the immune response to specific antigens is increasing. Drugs used therapeutically as immunosuppressants comprise a diverse group, several of which also are used for other purposes. These include corticosteroids (see Chap. 23) and certain cytotoxic antineoplastic drugs (see Chap. 42). These drugs are discussed here in relation to their effects on the immune response. The drugs used to treat inflammatory autoimmune disorders or to prevent or treat transplant rejection reactions are the main focus of this chapter (Fig. 41-1). These drugs are described in the following sections and in Table 41-1. To aid understanding of immunosuppressive drug therapy, selected inflammatory autoimmune disorders, tissue and organ transplantation, and rejection reactions are described.

Autoimmune Disorders

Autoimmune disorders occur when a person's immune system loses its ability to differentiate between antigens on its own cells (called *self-antigens* or *autoantigens*) and antigens on foreign cells. As a result, an immune response is aroused

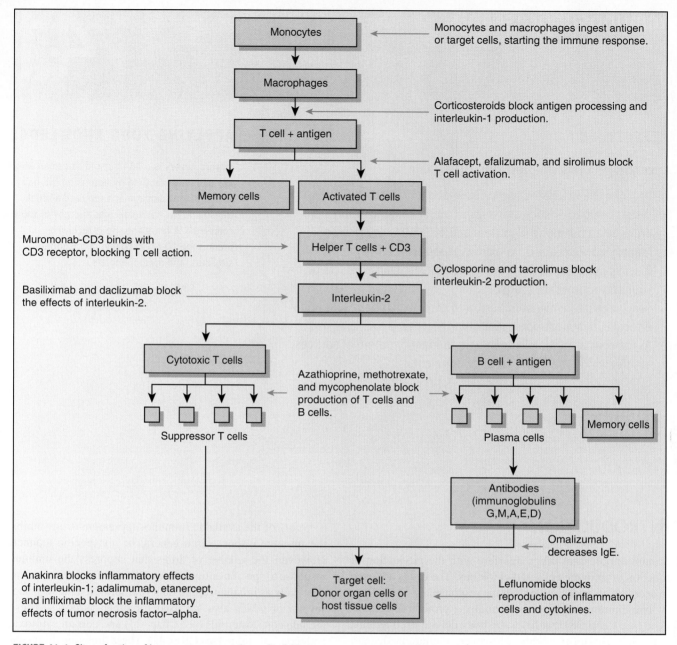

FIGURE 41-1 Sites of action of immunosuppressant drugs. Available immunosuppressants inhibit the immune response by blocking that response at various sites.

against host tissues. Autoantigens for some disorders have been identified as specific proteins and are found in affected tissues; in other disorders, the autoantigen is unknown. Even when the autoantigen is known, the mechanism by which it is altered to elicit an immune response is unclear. Potential mechanisms include genetic susceptibility and possible "triggering" events (eg, tissue damage by microorganisms or trauma, similarities between autoantigens and foreign antigens). After an autoantigen is changed so that it is perceived as foreign or "nonself," the immune response may involve T lymphocytes in direct destruction of tissue, production of

proinflammatory cytokines that attract and activate phagocytes, and stimulation of B lymphocytes to produce autoantibodies that lead to inflammation and tissue damage.

In recent years, much progress has been made in delineating the roles of inflammatory cells and cytokines in the immunologic response to tissue injury. One example involves tumor necrosis factor (TNF)–alpha, a cytokine synthesized and released mainly by macrophages, that plays a major role in the response to infection. Specific functions of TNF include activation of monocytes, macrophages, and cytotoxic T cells; enhancement of natural killer (NK) cell functions;

increased leukocyte movement into areas of tissue injury; increased phagocytosis by neutrophils; stimulation of B cells; and expansion of T-cell clones. Despite beneficial effects of a "normal" amount of TNF, however, an excessive TNF response has been associated with the pathogenesis of autoimmune disorders such as RA and Crohn's disease.

In addition to the factors that activate an immune response, there are also factors that prevent the immune system from "turning off" the abnormal immune or inflammatory process. One of these factors may be a deficient number of suppressor T cells, which are thought to be a subpopulation of helper or cytotoxic T cells. Another factor may be inadequate amounts of anti-inflammatory cytokines (eg, interleukin [IL]-10).

In general, autoimmune disorders share inflammation as a major mechanism of tissue damage. Allergic asthma, Crohn's disease, psoriasis, psoriatic arthritis, and RA are inflammatory disorders that may be treated with immunosuppressant drugs.

Tissue and Organ Transplantation

Tissue and organ transplantation involves replacing diseased host tissue with healthy donor tissue. The goal of such treatment is to save or enhance the quality of the host's life. Skin and renal grafts are commonly and successfully performed; heart, liver, lung, pancreas, and bone marrow transplantations are increasing. Although numerous factors affect graft survival, including the degree of matching between donor tissues and recipient tissues, drug-induced immunosuppression is a major part of transplantation technology. The goal is to provide adequate, but not excessive, immunosuppression. If immunosuppression is inadequate, graft-rejection reactions occur with solid organ transplantation, and graft-versus-host disease (GVHD) occurs with bone marrow transplantation. If immunosuppression is excessive, the client develops serious infections and other adverse effects because the drug actions that slow the proliferation of activated lymphocytes also affect any rapidly dividing nonimmune cells (eg, epithelial cells of the gastrointestinal [GI] tract, hematopoietic stem cells of the bone marrow). Serious complications can occur.

Rejection Reactions With Solid Organ Transplantation

A rejection reaction occurs when the host's immune system is stimulated to destroy the transplanted organ. The immune cells of the transplant recipient attach to the donor cells of the transplanted organ and react against the antigens of the donor organ. The rejection process involves T and B lymphocytes, antibodies, multiple cytokines, and inflammatory mediators. In general, T-cell activation and proliferation are more important in the rejection reaction than B-cell activation and formation of antibodies. Cytotoxic and helper T cells are activated; activated helper T cells stimulate B cells to produce antibodies and lead to a delayed hypersensitivity reaction.

The initial target of the recipient antibodies is the blood vessels of the transplanted organ. The antibodies can injure the transplanted organ by activating complement, producing antigen–antibody complexes, or causing antibody-mediated tissue breakdown. This reaction can destroy the solid organ graft within 2 weeks, unless the recipient's immune system is adequately suppressed by immunosuppressant drugs.

Rejection reactions are designated as hyperacute, acute, or chronic, depending on the time elapsed between transplantation and rejection. *Hyperacute* reactions occur within 24 hours. This rare type of reaction occurs in recipients who have previously formed antibodies against antigens in the graft. The antibodies bind to the graft and induce intense inflammation with extensive infiltration of neutrophils into the grafted tissue. The inflammatory reaction causes massive blood clots within the capillaries and prevents vascularization and function of the graft. *Acute* reactions, which may occur from 10 days to a few months after transplantation, mainly involve a cellular response with the proliferation of T lymphocytes. Characteristics include signs of organ failure and vasculitis lesions that often lead to arterial narrowing or obliteration. Treatment with immunosuppressant drugs is usually effective in ensuring short-term survival of the transplant, but does not prevent chronic rejection. *Chronic* reactions, which may occur after months or years of normal function, are caused by both cellular and humoral immunity and do not respond to increased immunosuppressive drug therapy. Characteristics include fibrosis of blood vessels and progressive failure of the transplanted organ.

Rejection reactions produce general manifestations of inflammation and specific manifestations depending on the organ involved. With renal transplantation, for example, acute rejection reactions produce fever, flank tenderness over the graft organ site, and symptoms of renal failure (eg, increased serum creatinine; decreased urine output; edema; weight gain; hypertension). Chronic rejection reactions are characterized by a gradual increase in serum creatinine levels over approximately 4 to 6 months.

Bone Marrow Transplantation and Graft-Versus-Host Disease

With bone marrow transplantation, the donor bone marrow mounts an immune response (mainly by stimulating T lymphocytes) against antigens on the host's tissues, producing GVHD. Tissue damage is produced directly by the action of cytotoxic T cells or indirectly through the release of inflammatory mediators such as complement and cytokines such as TNF–alpha and interleukins.

Acute GVHD occurs in 30% to 50% of clients, usually within 6 weeks. Signs and symptoms include delayed recovery of blood cell production in the bone marrow, skin rash, liver dysfunction (indicated by increased alkaline phosphatase, aminotransferases, and bilirubin), and diarrhea. The skin reaction is usually a pruritic maculopapular rash that begins on the palms and soles and may extend over the entire body. Liver involvement can lead to bleeding disorders and coma.

Chronic GVHD occurs when symptoms persist or occur 100 days or more after transplantation. It is characterized by abnormal humoral and cellular immunity, severe skin disorders, and liver disease. Chronic GVHD appears to be an autoimmune disorder in which activated T cells perceive self-antigens as foreign antigens.

CLASSIFICATIONS AND INDIVIDUAL DRUGS

Drug therapy to suppress the immune system began with the corticosteroids in the 1950s. Since then, many other agents have been developed. Drugs used as immunosuppressants are diverse agents with often overlapping mechanisms of actions and effects. Older drugs generally depress the immune system (ie, are nonspecific and suppress the immune response to all antigens). This greatly increases risks of serious infections with bacteria, viruses, fungi, or protozoa, at any time during the immunosuppressed state. In addition, many immunosuppressant drugs slow the proliferation of activated lymphocytes and damage rapidly dividing nonimmune cells (eg, mucosal cells, intestinal cells, bone marrow hematopoietic stem cells). As a result, serious, life-threatening complications can occur. For example, clients on long-term immunosuppressant drug therapy (eg, with autoimmune disorders, organ transplantation) are at increased risk of serious infections, cancer (especially lymphoma), hypertension, and metabolic bone disease.

For many reasons, including adverse effects of older drugs and the efforts to develop more effective agents, extensive research has been done to develop drugs that *modify* the immune response (often called *immunomodulators* or *biologic response modifiers*). As a result, several drugs with more specific immunosuppressive actions have been approved in recent years. Most are used in combination with older immunosuppressants for synergistic effects.

Immunosuppressants are discussed here as corticosteroids, cytotoxic antiproliferative agents, conventional antirejection agents, antibody preparations, cytokine inhibitors, and miscellaneous drugs. Table 41-1 provides pertinent information for the drugs. Most of the drugs could also fit in one or more other categories (eg, the cytotoxic drugs and most of the antibody preparations are also antirejection drugs).

APPLYING YOUR KNOWLEDGE 41-1

Mr. Kinney has a depressed immune system secondary to the medications necessary to prevent organ rejection. What is Mr. Kinney at risk to develop?

Corticosteroids

Corticosteroids are potent anti-inflammatory drugs that act to suppress the immune response at many levels. In many disorders, they relieve signs and symptoms by decreasing the accumulation of lymphocytes and macrophages and the production of cell-damaging cytokines at sites of inflammatory reactions. Because inflammation is a common response to chemical mediators or antigens that cause tissue injury, the anti-inflammatory and immunosuppressive actions of corticosteroids often overlap and are indistinguishable. However, corticosteroid effects on the immune response are emphasized here. In general, the drugs suppress growth of all lymphoid tissue and therefore decrease formation and function of antibodies and T cells. For clients with autoimmune disorders, corticosteroids decrease inflammation but do not prevent tissue damage. For clients with transplanted tissues, a corticosteroid is usually given with other agents (eg, azathioprine) to prevent acute episodes of graft rejection. Specific effects include the following:

- Increased numbers of circulating neutrophils (more are released from bone marrow and fewer leave the circulation to enter inflammatory exudates). In terms of neutrophil functions, corticosteroids increase chemotaxis and release of lysosomal enzymes.
- Decreased numbers of circulating basophils, eosinophils, and monocytes. The reduced availability of monocytes is considered a major factor in the anti-inflammatory activity of corticosteroids. Functions of monocyte–macrophages are also impaired. Corticosteroids suppress phagocytosis and initial antigen processing (necessary to initiate an immune response), impair migration to areas of tissue injury, and block the differentiation of monocytes to macrophages.
- Decreased numbers of circulating lymphocytes (immune cells), resulting from impaired production (ie, inhibition of deoxyribonucleic acid [DNA], ribonucleic acid [RNA], and protein synthesis), sequestration in lymphoid tissues, or lysis of the cells. T cells are markedly reduced; B cells are moderately reduced.
- Impaired function of cellular (T-cell) and humoral (B-cell) immunity. Corticosteroids inhibit the production of immunostimulant cytokines (eg, IL-1, IL-2) required for activation and clonal expansion of lymphocytes and cytotoxic cytokines, such as TNF and interferons. When administered for 2 to 3 weeks, the drugs also inhibit immune reactions to antigenic skin tests and reduce serum concentrations of some antibodies (immunoglobulins [Ig] G and A, but not IgM).

Cytotoxic, Antiproliferative Agents

Cytotoxic, antiproliferative drugs damage or kill cells that are able to reproduce, such as immunologically competent lymphocytes. These drugs are used primarily in cancer chemother-

Table 41-1 Drugs at a Glance: Immunosuppressants

GENERIC/TRADE NAME	INDICATIONS FOR USE	CONTRAINDICATIONS	ROUTES AND DOSAGE RANGES
Adalizumab (Humira)	Rheumatoid arthritis	Hypersensitivity to any component of the drug formulation	Sub-Q 40 mg every other week
Alefacept (Amevive)	Psoriasis	Hypersensitivity to any component of the drug formulation Infection History of malignancy	IM 15 mg once weekly for 12 wk IV 7.5 mg once weekly for 12 wk
Anakinra (Kineret)	Rheumatoid arthritis	Active infection Hypersensitivity to *Escherichia coli*–derived proteins or any component of the drug formulation	Sub-Q 100 mg once daily
Azathioprine (Imuran)	Prevent renal transplant rejection Severe rheumatoid arthritis unresponsive to other treatment	Pregnancy Allergy to azathioprine	*Renal transplant:* PO, IV 3–5 mg/kg/d initially, decreased (1–3 mg/kg/d) for maintenance and in presence of renal impairment *Rheumatoid arthritis:* PO 1 mg/kg/d (50–100 mg), increased by 0.5 mg/kg/d after 8 wk, then every 5 wk to a maximum dose of 2.5 mg/kg/d. Decrease dosage for maintenance.
Basiliximab (Simulect)	Prevent renal transplant rejection	Hypersensitivity to any component of the drug formulation	*Adults:* IV 20 mg within 2 h before transplantation and 20 mg 4 d after transplantation (total of two doses) *Children (2–15 y):* IV 12 mg/m² up to a maximum of 20 mg for two doses as for adults
Cyclosporine (Sandimmune, Neoral)	Prevent rejection of solid organ (eg, heart, kidney, liver) transplant Prevent and treat graft-versus-host disease in bone marrow transplantation Psoriasis Rheumatoid arthritis	Allergy to cyclosporine or polyoxyethylated castor oil (in IV preparation only) Cautious use during pregnancy or lactation	*Sandimmune:* PO 15 mg/kg 4–12 h before transplant surgery, then 15 mg/kg once daily for 1–2 wk, then decrease by 5% per week to a maintenance dose of 5–10 mg/kg/d *IV* 5–6 mg/kg infused over 2–6 h *Neoral:* PO, the first dose in clients with new transplants is the same as the first oral dose of Sandimmune; later doses are titrated according to the desired cyclosporine blood level
Daclizumab (Zenapax)	Prevent renal transplant rejection	Hypersensitivity to any component of the drug formulation	IV 1 mg/kg over 15 min. First dose within 24 h before transplantation, then a dose every 14 d for four doses (total of five doses)

(continued)

Table 41-1 Drugs at a Glance: Immunosuppressants (continued)

GENERIC/TRADE NAME	INDICATIONS FOR USE	CONTRAINDICATIONS	ROUTES AND DOSAGE RANGES
Efalizumab (Raptiva)	Psoriasis	Should not be given with any other immunosuppressant drug Hypersensitivity to any component of the drug formulation	Sub-Q 0.7 mg/kg initially, then 1 mg/kg once weekly
Etanercept (Enbrel)	Rheumatoid arthritis Psoriatic arthritis Ankylosing spondylitis Juvenile chronic arthritis	Sepsis Hypersensitivity to any component of the drug formulation	*Adults:* Sub-Q 25 mg twice weekly, 72–96 h apart *Children (4–17 y):* Sub-Q 0.4 mg/kg up to a maximum of 25 mg per dose, twice weekly, 72–96 h apart
Infliximab (Remicade)	Crohn's disease, moderate to severe or fistulizing Rheumatoid arthritis	Hypersensitivity to mouse proteins or any other component of the formulation	*Crohn's disease, moderate to severe:* IV infusion 5 mg/kg as a single dose *Crohn's disease, fistulizing:* IV infusion 5 mg/kg initially and 2 and 6 wk later (total of three doses)
Leflunomide (Arava)	Rheumatoid arthritis	Hypersensitivity to any component of the drug formulation Pregnancy	PO 100 mg once daily for 3 d, then 20 mg once daily
Lymphocyte immune globulin, antithymocyte globulin (Equine) (Atgam)	Prevent or treat renal transplant rejection Treat aplastic anemia	Allergy to horse serum or prior allergic reaction to Atgam	IV 15 mg/kg/d for 14 d, then every other day for 14 d (21 doses)
Methotrexate (MTX) (Rheumatrex)	Severe rheumatoid arthritis unresponsive to other therapy Psoriasis	Allergy to methotrexate Pregnancy, lactation Liver disease Blood dyscrasias	PO 7.5 mg/wk as single dose, or 2.5 mg q12h for three doses once weekly
Muromonab-CD3 (Orthoclone OKT3)	Treatment of renal, cardiac, and hepatic transplant rejection	Allergy to muromonab-CD3 Signs of fluid overload (eg, heart failure, weight gain during week before starting drug therapy) Cautious use during pregnancy	IV 5 mg bolus injection once daily for 10–14 d
Mycophenolate mefetil (CellCept, Myfortic)	Prevent renal, cardiac, and hepatic transplant rejection	Hypersensitivity to the drug or any component of the product	*Renal transplantation:* PO, IV 1 g twice daily *Cardiac and hepatic transplantation:* PO, IV 1.5 g twice daily *Extended-release tablets (Myfortic):* PO 720 mg twice daily
Omalizumab (Xolair)	Allergic asthma	Hypersensitivity to any component of the drug formulation Acute bronchospasm Status asthmaticus	Sub-Q variable according to weight and serum IgE levels. See manufacturer's instructions.
Sirolimus (Rapamune)	Prevent renal transplant rejection	Hypersensitivity to any component of the drug formulation	*Adults:* PO 6 mg as soon after transplantation as possible, then 2 mg daily *Children >13 y:* PO 3 mg/m² as loading dose, then 1 mg/m² daily

Table 41-1 Drugs at a Glance: Immunosuppressants (continued)			
GENERIC/TRADE NAME	**INDICATIONS FOR USE**	**CONTRAINDICATIONS**	**ROUTES AND DOSAGE RANGES**
Tacrolimus (Prograf)	Prevent liver, kidney, and heart transplant rejection	Hypersensitivity to the drug or the castor oil used in the IV formulation	*Adults:* IV infusion, 25–50 mcg/kg/d, starting no sooner than 6 h after transplantation, until the patient can tolerate oral administration, usually 2–3 d PO 150–200 mcg/kg/d, in two divided doses q12h, with the first dose 8–12 h after stopping the IV infusion *Children:* IV 50–100 mcg/kg/d PO 200–300 mcg/kg/d

IgE, immunoglobulin E; IM, intramuscular; IV, intravenous; PO, oral; Sub-Q, subcutaneous.

apy. However, in small doses, some also exhibit immunosuppressive activities and are used to treat autoimmune disorders (eg, methotrexate) and to prevent rejection reactions in organ transplantation (ie, azathioprine). These drugs cause generalized suppression of the immune system and can kill lymphocytes and nonlymphoid proliferating cells (eg, bone marrow blood cells, GI mucosal cells, germ cells in gonads).

Azathioprine is an antimetabolite that interferes with production of DNA and RNA and thus blocks cellular reproduction, growth, and development. After it is ingested, azathioprine is metabolized by the liver to 6-mercaptopurine, a purine analog. The purine analog is then incorporated into the DNA of proliferating cells in place of the natural purine bases, leading to the production of abnormal DNA. Rapidly proliferating cells are most affected, including T and B lymphocytes, which normally reproduce rapidly in response to stimulation by an antigen. The drug acts especially on T cells to block cell division, clonal proliferation, and differentiation.

Azathioprine is well absorbed after oral administration, with peak serum concentrations in 1 to 2 hours and a half-life of less than 5 hours. The mercaptopurine resulting from initial biotransformation is inactivated mainly by the enzyme xanthine oxidase. Impaired liver function may decrease metabolism of azathioprine to its active metabolite and therefore decrease pharmacologic effects.

The drug is used mainly to prevent organ graft rejection and has little effect on acute rejection reactions. It is also used to treat severe RA. When used to prevent graft rejection, azathioprine is used lifelong. Dosage varies among transplantation centers and types of transplants, but depends largely on white blood cell (WBC) and platelet counts.

Methotrexate is a folate antagonist. It inhibits dihydrofolate reductase, the enzyme that converts dihydrofolate to the tetrahydrofolate required for biosynthesis of DNA and cell reproduction. The resultant DNA impairment inhibits production and function of immune cells, especially T cells. Methotrexate has long been used in the treatment of cancer. Other uses have evolved from its immunosuppressive effects, including treatment of autoimmune or inflammatory disorders, such as severe arthritis and psoriasis, that do not respond to other treatment measures. It is also used (with cyclosporine) to prevent GVHD associated with bone marrow transplantation. Lower doses are given for these conditions than for cancers, and adverse drug effects are fewer and less severe.

Mycophenolate is similar to azathioprine. It is used for prevention and treatment of rejection reactions with renal, cardiac, and hepatic transplantation. It inhibits proliferation and function of T and B lymphocytes. It has synergistic effects with corticosteroids and cyclosporine and is used in combination with these drugs.

After oral or intravenous (IV) administration, the drug is rapidly broken down to mycophenolic acid, the active component. Mycophenolic acid is further metabolized to inactive metabolites that are eliminated in bile and urine. Neutropenia and thrombocytopenia may occur but are less common and less severe than with azathioprine. Infections with mycophenolate occur at approximately the same rate as with other immunosuppressant drugs. Because of its lesser toxicity, mycophenolate may be preferred over azathioprine, at least in clients who are unable to tolerate azathioprine.

APPLYING YOUR KNOWLEDGE 41-2

Mr. Kinney is prescribed mycophenolate. Related to the administration of mycophenolate, you should assess Mr. Kinney for what adverse effects?

Conventional Antirejection Agents

Cyclosporine, tacrolimus, and sirolimus are fungal metabolites with strong immunosuppressive effects. Cyclosporine and tacrolimus are chemically unrelated but have a similar action. They inhibit the synthesis of a cytokine, IL-2, which is required for activation of T cells and B cells. Sirolimus is structurally similar to tacrolimus. It inhibits T-cell activation and proliferation in response to several interleukins (eg, IL-2, IL-4, IL-15). It also inhibits antibody production. Sirolimus and tacrolimus may have stronger immunosuppressant activity than cyclosporine.

By inhibiting helper–T-cell proliferation and cytokine expression, these three drugs reduce the activation of various cells involved in graft rejection, including cytotoxic T cells, NK cells, macrophages, and B cells. Consequently, they are widely used in heart, liver, kidney, and bone marrow transplantation.

Cyclosporine is used to prevent rejection reactions and prolong graft survival after solid organ transplantation (eg, kidney, liver, heart, lung), or to treat chronic rejection in clients previously treated with other immunosuppressive agents. The drug inhibits both cellular and humoral immunity but affects T lymphocytes more than B lymphocytes. With T cells, cyclosporine reduces proliferation of helper and cytotoxic T cells and synthesis of several cytokines (eg, IL-2, interferons). With B cells, cyclosporine reduces production and function to some extent, but considerable activity is retained.

Transplant rejection reactions mainly involve cellular immunity or T cells. With cyclosporine-induced deprivation of IL-2, T cells stimulated by the graft antigen do not undergo clonal expansion and differentiation, and graft destruction is inhibited. In addition to its use in solid organ transplantation, cyclosporine is used to prevent and treat GVHD, a complication of bone marrow transplantation. In GVHD, T lymphocytes from the transplanted marrow of the donor mount an immune response against the tissues of the recipient.

Absorption of cyclosporine is slow and incomplete with oral administration. The drug is highly bound to plasma proteins (90%), and approximately 50% is distributed in erythrocytes, so drug levels in whole blood are significantly higher than those in plasma. Peak plasma levels occur 4 to 5 hours after a dose, and the elimination half-life is 10 to 27 hours. Cyclosporine is metabolized in the liver and excreted in bile; less than 10% is excreted unchanged in urine.

Because the drug is insoluble in water, other solvents are used in commercial formulations. Thus, it is prepared in alcohol and olive oil for oral administration and in alcohol and castor oil for IV administration. Anaphylactic reactions, attributed to the castor oil, have occurred with the IV formulation. Neoral is a microemulsion formulation of cyclosporine that is better absorbed than oral Sandimmune. The two formulations are not equivalent and cannot be used interchangeably. Neoral is available in capsules and an oral solution; Sandimmune is available in capsules, oral solution, and an IV solution.

Nephrotoxicity is a major adverse effect. Acute nephrotoxicity may occur and progress to chronic nephrotoxicity and kidney failure.

Sirolimus is used to prevent renal transplant rejection. It acts by inhibiting T-cell activation. It is given concomitantly with a corticosteroid and cyclosporine. It may have synergistic effects with cyclosporine because it has a different mechanism of action. However, the two drugs are metabolized by the same cytochrome P450 3A4 enzymes and cyclosporine increases blood levels of sirolimus, possibly to toxic levels. Consequently, the drugs should not be given at the same time; sirolimus should be taken 4 hours after a dose of cyclosporine. Sirolimus is contraindicated in clients who are allergic to the drug or who are pregnant or breast-feeding.

Sirolimus is well absorbed with oral administration. Its action has a rapid onset and peaks within 1 hour. It has a long half-life of 62 hours. It is metabolized in the liver and excreted mainly in feces (>90%), with a small amount eliminated in urine.

Reported adverse effects include abdominal pain, acne, anemia, constipation, diarrhea, edema, headache, hepatotoxicity, hypercholesterolemia, hypertension, insomnia, leukopenia, nausea, nephrotoxicity, skin rash, thrombocytopenia, and tremor. Because of the high risk of infection with sirolimus, as with other immunosuppressant drugs, antimicrobial prophylaxis is recommended for cytomegalovirus (CMV) infection for 3 months and *Pneumocystis* pneumonia for 1 year after transplantation.

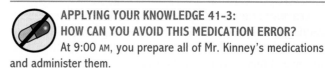

APPLYING YOUR KNOWLEDGE 41-3:
HOW CAN YOU AVOID THIS MEDICATION ERROR?
At 9:00 AM, you prepare all of Mr. Kinney's medications and administer them.

Tacrolimus is similar to cyclosporine in its mechanisms of action, pharmacokinetic characteristics, and adverse effects. It prevents rejection of transplanted organs by inhibiting growth and proliferation of T lymphocytes. Although survival of clients and grafts is approximately the same as with cyclosporine, the use of tacrolimus allows less corticosteroid therapy and shorter hospitalizations.

Tacrolimus is not well absorbed orally, so higher oral doses than IV doses must be given to obtain similar blood levels. With IV administration, action onset is rapid and peak action occurs in 1 to 2 hours; with oral administration, onset varies and peak action occurs in 1.5 to 3.5 hours. The drug is well distributed through the body and reaches higher concentrations in erythrocytes than in plasma. It is metabolized in the liver and intestine to several metabolites, which are excreted in bile and urine. It has a half-life of 6 hours. Impaired liver function may slow its metabolism and elimination.

Dosage ranges of tacrolimus vary according to clinical response, adverse effects, and blood concentrations. Serum drug levels are routinely monitored, with therapeutic ranges approximately 10 to 20 nanograms per milliliter for 6 months after transplantation, then 5 to 15 nanograms per milliliter. Children with transplants metabolize tacrolimus more rapidly than adults with transplants, on a body-weight basis. Thus, children require higher doses, based on milligrams of drug per kilogram of body weight, to maintain similar plasma drug levels. Dosage does not need to be reduced in clients with renal insufficiency because there is little renal elimination of the drug.

There are numerous potential drug interactions that increase or decrease blood levels and effects of tacrolimus. Because tacrolimus is metabolized mainly by the cytochrome P450 enzymes that metabolize cyclosporine, drug interactions known to alter cyclosporine effects are likely to alter tacrolimus effects. For example, antacids and enzyme inducers (eg, rifampin, carbamazepine, phenytoin) may reduce therapeutic effects; nephrotoxic drugs (eg, amphotericin B, aminoglycoside antibiotics) may increase nephrotoxic effects; and enzyme inhibitors (eg, erythromycin, fluconazole and related antifungals) may increase plasma levels and toxic effects.

The use of tacrolimus in transplantation has expanded in recent years, mainly because cyclosporine is given with corticosteroids. Using tacrolimus rather than cyclosporine may allow corticosteroids to be reduced or stopped, thereby decreasing the adverse effects of long-term corticosteroid therapy. Nephrotoxicity occurs at an approximately equal rate with the two drugs.

Antibody Preparations

Antibody preparations are produced in the laboratory or derived from animals injected with human lymphoid tissue to stimulate an immune response. Such preparations are being extensively used in inflammatory autoimmune disorders, transplantation rejection reactions, and cancer. They are also being used in diagnostic imaging technology.

The antibodies may be polyclonal or monoclonal. *Polyclonal* preparations are a mixture of antibodies (IgA, IgD, IgE, IgG, IgM) produced by several clones of B lymphocytes. Each clone produces a structurally and functionally different antibody, even though the humoral immune response was induced by a single antigen. *Monoclonal antibodies* are produced in the laboratory by procedures that isolate and clone individual B lymphocytes, resulting in the production of identical antibody molecules. The antigen to which the desired antibody will respond is first injected into a mouse. The mouse mounts an immune response in which its B lymphocytes are stimulated to produce a specific antibody against that antigen. The B lymphocytes are then recovered from the spleen of the mouse and mixed with myeloma cells (a cell line that can live forever in culture) in polyethylene glycol. This treatment results in fusion of the cells and produces an antibody-secreting hybridoma, which can be cloned to produce large amounts of the desired antibody. The antibodies can be isolated from the culture and prepared for clinical use. Because the antibodies are proteins and would be destroyed if taken orally, they must be given by injection.

Older animal-derived antibodies (eg, LIG, ATG; muromonab-CD3) are themselves antigenic; they usually elicit human antibodies against the animal cells within 2 weeks. Newer murine (mouse-derived) antibodies (eg, basiliximab) have had human antibodies added by recombinant DNA technology and are less likely to elicit an immune response. However, because the products are proteins, there is some risk of hypersensitivity reactions.

Because they are derived from one cell line or clone, monoclonal antibodies can be designed to suppress the specific components of the immune system that are causing tissue damage in particular disorders. They cause cell destruction by eliciting an antigen–antibody reaction, activating complement, targeting molecules on the cell surface that are necessary for growth or differentiation of that cell, or inhibiting proinflammatory cytokines.

Note that the generic names of monoclonal antibodies used as drugs end in *mab* and thus identify their origin.

Polyclonal Antibody

Lymphocyte immune globulin, antithymocyte globulin (LIG, ATG [Atgam]) is a nonspecific antibody with activity against all blood cells, although it acts mainly against T lymphocytes. LIG, ATG is obtained from the serum of horses immunized with human thymus tissue or T lymphocytes. It contains antibodies that destroy lymphoid tissues and decrease the number of circulating T cells, thereby suppressing cellular and humoral immune responses. In addition to its high concentration of antibodies against T lymphocytes, the preparation contains low concentrations of antibodies against other blood cells. A skin test is recommended before administration to determine whether the client is allergic to horse serum. Because there is a high risk of anaphylactic reactions in recipients previously sensitized to horse serum, clients with positive skin tests should be desensitized before drug therapy is begun. LIG, ATG may be given for a few weeks to treat rejection reactions after solid organ transplantation, and it may be used to treat aplastic anemia.

Monoclonal Antibodies

Alefacept (Amevive) and **efalizumab** (Raptiva) are monoclonal antibodies used to treat moderate to severe psoriasis. Psoriasis involves activated T lymphocytes that secrete inflammatory mediators. The drugs bind to receptors on the surface of T lymphocytes, inhibit the receptors from interacting with particular antigens, and thereby inhibit activation of T lymphocytes.

Alefacept is given intramuscularly (IM) or IV, usually once weekly for 12 weeks. Its half-life after IV administration is about 10 days. Common adverse effects include lymphopenia and injection-site reactions (eg, edema, inflammation, pain). Efalizumab is given subcutaneously (Sub-Q) once weekly for 12 weeks. It reaches steady-state concentration in

4 weeks and is excreted over 3 weeks. Common adverse effects include headache, infection, lymphocytosis, and a first-dose reaction characterized by chills, fever, muscle aches, and nausea.

Basiliximab (Simulect) and **daclizumab** (Zenapax) are similar drugs. They are humanized IgE (ie, a combination of human and murine antibodies). They are called IL-2 receptor antagonists because they bind to IL-2 receptors on the surface of activated lymphocytes. This action inhibits the ability of IL-2 to stimulate proliferation and cytokine production of lymphocytes, a critical component of the cellular immune response involved in allograft rejection. The drugs are used to prevent organ rejection in clients receiving renal transplants and are given in combination with cyclosporine and a corticosteroid.

Basiliximab is given IV and its effects last an average of 36 days. Its elimination half-life is about 7 days in adults, 9 days in children. Daclizumab is also given IV and its elimination half-life is about 20 days in adults, 13 days in children. Common adverse effects include constipation, diarrhea, edema, fever, headache, hypertension, infection, nausea, and vomiting.

Muromonab-CD3 (Orthoclone OKT3) is a monoclonal antibody that acts against an antigenic receptor called CD3, which is found on the surface membrane of most T cells in blood and body tissues. CD indicates *clusters of differentiation,* or groups of cells with the same surface markers (antigenic receptors). The CD3 molecule is associated with the antigen recognition structure of T cells and is essential for T-cell activation. Muromonab-CD3 binds with its antigen (CD3) and therefore blocks all known functions of T cells containing the CD3 molecule. Because rejection reactions are mainly T-cell–mediated immune responses against antigenic (nonself) tissues, the drug's ability to suppress such reactions accounts for its therapeutic effects in treating renal, cardiac, and hepatic transplant rejection. It is usually given for 10 to 14 days. After treatment, CD3-positive T cells reappear rapidly and reach pretreatment levels within 1 week. The drug's name is derived from its source (murine or mouse cells) and its action (monoclonal antibody against the CD3 antigen). Because the drug is a protein and induces antibodies in most clients, decreased effectiveness and serious allergic reactions may occur if it is readministered later. Second courses of treatment must be undertaken cautiously.

Omalizumab (Xolair) is a humanized monoclonal antibody approved for treatment of moderate to severe allergic asthma that is not relieved by inhaled corticosteroids. An additional benefit is that dosage of corticosteroids can usually be reduced, thereby reducing the adverse effects of long-term corticosteroid therapy.

IgE is a major factor in the pathogenesis of allergic reactions and asthma. When stimulated by an allergen, it combines with a receptor on mast cells and basophils and causes the release of allergic and proinflammatory mediators. Omalizumab binds with the IgE and reduces the amount of IgE free to bind to the receptors on mast cells and basophils. This action inhibits IgE-induced tissue injury.

Omalizumab is given Sub-Q and slowly absorbed. Peak concentration is reached in about 1 week and it has a half-life of 3 to 4 weeks. It is metabolized in the liver. Dosage and frequency of administration are determined by body weight and total serum IgE level, which should be measured before the start of treatment and periodically during treatment. The drug is generally well tolerated in adults and children. Common adverse effects include injection-site reactions and infections (eg, viral, upper respiratory tract, pharyngitis, sinusitis).

Cytokine Inhibitors

Two major cytokines in chronic, inflammatory autoimmune disorders are IL-1 and TNF–alpha. This knowledge led to the development and clinical use of biologic agents directed against these cytokines. The cytokine inhibitors used as drugs (some of which are monoclonal antibodies) inhibit one of these cytokines to suppress inflammation and promote tissue repair in disorders such as RA, Crohn's disease, psoriasis, and psoriatic arthritis. (Two additional cytokine inhibitors are basiliximab and daclizumab, which inhibit IL-2 to prevent rejection reactions in transplantation immunology. They are previously described with monoclonal antibodies.)

Cytokine inhibitors can greatly improve signs and symptoms of arthritis, Crohn's disease, and psoriasis. Despite their substantial therapeutic effects, however, cytokine inhibitors also increase the risks of serious infections, especially the TNF–alpha inhibitors. A wide range of infections has occurred, including tuberculosis characterized by increased extrapulmonary and/or disseminated disease. Other serious infections include pneumococcal infections, necrotizing fasciitis, *Pneumocystis* pneumonia, and systemic infections such as aspergillosis, cryptococcosis, and others.

Interleukin Blocking Agents

Anakinra (Kineret) is a recombinant interleukin-receptor antagonist. It binds to the IL-1 receptor and thereby blocks the inflammatory effects of IL-1. It is used to treat moderate to severe RA in adults. It may be used alone or in combination with other disease-modifying antirheumatic drugs (except TNF blocking agents).

Anakinra is well absorbed with Sub-Q injection and reaches its peak concentration in 3 to 7 hours. Its elimination half-life is 4 to 6 hours. Common adverse effects include headache, injection-site reactions (redness, bruising, inflammation, pain), infection, nausea, diarrhea, decreased WBCs, sinusitis, and flu-like symptoms.

Tumor Necrosis Factor–Alpha (TNF–Alpha) Blocking Agents

Adalimumab (Humira) is a recombinant monoclonal antibody that binds to TNF–alpha receptor sites and prevents endogenous TNF–alpha from binding to the sites and exerting its injurious effects. The drug is used to treat moderate to severe RA. In RA, the drug reduces the elevated levels of TNF–alpha in synovial fluid that are thought responsible for pain and joint destruction.

Adalimumab is given Sub-Q, peak serum concentration occurs within 2 to 5 days, and its elimination half-life is about 2 weeks. Excretion is decreased in clients over 40 years of age. Common adverse effects include injection-site reactions, upper respiratory tract infections, headache, nausea, and skin rash.

Etanercept (Enbrel) is a manufactured TNF receptor that binds with TNF and prevents it from binding with its "normal" receptors on cell surfaces. This action inhibits TNF activity in inflammatory and immune responses. The drug is used to treat moderate to severe RA in adults and children. In this condition, TNF is increased in joint synovial fluid and considered important in joint inflammation and destruction. Etanercept can be used in combination with methotrexate in clients who do not respond adequately to methotrexate alone.

Etanercept is given Sub-Q and reaches its peak concentration in about 3 days. Onset of action occurs within 2 to 3 weeks and its elimination half-life is about 5 days. Common adverse effects include headache, injection-site reactions, and respiratory tract and other infections.

Infliximab (Remicade) is a humanized IgG monoclonal antibody used to treat RA and Crohn's disease. It inhibits TNF–alpha from binding to its receptors and thus neutralizes its actions. Infliximab's ability to neutralize TNF–alpha accounts for its anti-inflammatory effects.

Infliximab is given IV. Its half-life elimination is about 8 days and its onset of action in Crohn's disease is about 2 weeks. Adverse effects include formation of autoimmune antibodies and hypersensitivity reactions. Dyspnea, hypotension, and urticaria have occurred. The drug should be administered in settings in which personnel and supplies (eg, epinephrine, antihistamines, corticosteroids) are available for treatment of hypersensitivity reactions, and should be discontinued if severe reactions occur. In addition, infections developed in approximately 21% of clients in clinical trials and the drug may aggravate congestive heart failure.

Miscellaneous Immunosuppressant

Leflunomide (Arava) has antiproliferative and anti-inflammatory activities that are attributed to its effects on the immune system. The drug inhibits the synthesis of pyrimidines, which are components of DNA and RNA, and therefore blocks the expansion of T cells. Leflunomide is used to treat RA in adults and its efficacy is similar to that of methotrexate. In addition to relieving signs and symptoms, the drug also slows the destruction of joint tissues.

After oral administration, leflunomide is metabolized to an active metabolite (called *M1*) that exerts most of the drug's effects. M1 has a half-life of about 2 weeks, and a loading dose of leflunomide is usually given for 3 days to achieve therapeutic blood levels more rapidly. The metabolite is highly bound to serum albumin and eventually eliminated by further metabolism and renal or biliary excretion. Some of the M1 excreted in bile is reabsorbed, and this contributes to its long half-life. Most adverse effects in clinical trials were similar to those of placebos.

NURSING PROCESS

Assessment

- Assess clients receiving or anticipating immunosuppressant drug therapy for signs and symptoms of current infection or factors predisposing them to potential infection (eg, impaired skin integrity, invasive devices, cigarette smoking).
- Assess the environment for factors predisposing to infection (eg, family or health care providers with infections, contact with young children, potential exposure to childhood infectious diseases).
- Assess nutritional status, including appetite and weight.
- Assess baseline values of laboratory and other diagnostic test results to aid monitoring of responses to immunosuppressant drug therapy. With pretransplantation clients, this includes assessing for impaired function of the diseased organ and for abnormalities that need treatment before surgery.
- Assess adequacy of support systems for transplant recipients.
- Assess posttransplantation clients for surgical wound healing, manifestations of organ rejection, and adverse effects of immunosuppressant drugs.
- Assess clients with autoimmune disorders (eg, RA, Crohn's disease) for manifestations of the disease process and responses to drug therapy.

Nursing Diagnoses

- Risk for Injury: Adverse drug effects
- Risk for Injury: Infection and cancer related to immunosuppression and increased susceptibility
- Deficient Knowledge: Disease process and immunosuppressant drug therapy
- Anxiety related to the diagnosis of serious disease or need for organ transplantation
- Social Isolation related to activities to reduce exposure to infection

Planning/Goals

The client will
- Participate in decision making about the treatment plan
- Receive or take immunosuppressant drugs correctly
- Verbalize or demonstrate essential drug information

- Participate in interventions to prevent infection (eg, maintain good hygiene, avoid known sources of infection) while immunosuppressed
- Experience relief or reduction of disease symptoms
- Maintain adequate levels of nutrition and fluids, rest and sleep, and exercise
- Be assisted to cope with anxiety related to the disease process and drug therapy
- Keep appointments for follow-up care
- Have adverse drug effects prevented or recognized and treated promptly
- Maintain diagnostic test values within acceptable limits
- Maintain family and other emotional or social support systems
- Receive optimal instructions and information about the treatment plan, self-care in activities of daily living, reporting adverse drug effects, and other concerns
- Before and after tissue or organ transplantation, receive appropriate care, including prevention or early recognition and treatment of rejection reactions

Interventions

- Practice and emphasize good personal and hand hygiene techniques by clients and all others in contact with clients.
- Use sterile technique for all injections, IV site care, wound dressing changes, and any other invasive diagnostic or therapeutic measures.
- Screen staff and visitors for signs and symptoms of infection; if infection is noted, do not allow contact with the client.
- Report fever and other manifestations of infection *immediately*.
- Allow clients to participate in decision making when possible and appropriate.
- Use isolation techniques according to institutional policies, usually after transplantation or when the neutrophil count is less than 500/mm³.
- Assist clients to maintain adequate nutrition, rest and sleep, and exercise.
- Inform clients about diagnostic test results, planned changes in therapeutic regimens, and evidence of progress.
- Allow family members or significant others to visit clients when feasible.
- Monitor complete blood count (CBC) and other diagnostic test results related to blood, liver, and kidney function throughout drug therapy. Specific tests vary with the client's health or illness status and the immunosuppressant drugs being taken.
- Schedule and coordinate drug administration to maximize therapeutic effects and minimize adverse effects.
- Consult other health care providers (eg, physician,

dietitian, social worker) on the client's behalf when indicated. Multidisciplinary consultation is essential for transplantation clients and desirable for clients with autoimmune disorders.
- Assist clients in learning strategies to manage day-to-day activities during long-term immunosuppression (see accompanying Client Teaching Guidelines).

Evaluation

- Interview and observe for accurate drug administration.
- Interview and observe for personal hygiene practices and infection-avoiding maneuvers.
- Interview and observe for therapeutic and adverse drug effects with each client contact.
- Interview regarding knowledge and attitude toward the drug therapy regimen, including follow-up care and symptoms to report to health care providers.
- Determine the number and types of infections that have occurred in the neutropenic client.
- Compare current CBC and other reports with baseline values for acceptable levels, according to the client's condition.
- Observe and interview outpatients regarding compliance with follow-up care.
- Interview and observe for organ function and absence of rejection reactions in posttransplantation clients.

APPLYING YOUR KNOWLEDGE 41-4
What are the specific teaching points to be covered with Mr. Kinney regarding proper self-administration of his medication?

PRINCIPLES OF THERAPY

Risk–Benefit Factors

Immunosuppression is a serious, life-threatening condition that may result from disease or drug therapy. At the same time, immunosuppressant drugs are used to treat serious illnesses, and their use may be required. Rational use of these drugs requires thorough assessment of a client's health or illness status, clear-cut indications for use, a lack of more effective and safer alternative treatments, cautious administration, and vigilant monitoring of the client's response. If a decision is then made that immunosuppressant drug therapy is indicated and benefits outweigh risks, the therapeutic plan must be discussed with the client (ie, reasons, expected benefits, consequences for the client's health and lifestyle).

In addition to the specific risks of individual immunosuppressant drugs, general risks of immunosuppression include *infection* and *cancer*. Infection is a major cause

CLIENT TEACHING GUIDELINES

Immunosuppressant Drugs

General Considerations

☑ People taking medications that suppress the immune system are at high risk for development of infections. As a result, clients, caregivers, and others in the client's environment need to wash their hands often and thoroughly, practice meticulous personal hygiene, avoid contact with infected people, and practice other methods of preventing infection.

☑ Report adverse drug effects (eg, signs or symptoms of infection such as sore throat or fever, decreased urine output if taking cyclosporine, easy bruising or bleeding if taking azathioprine or methotrexate) to a health care provider.

☑ Try to maintain healthy lifestyle habits, such as a nutritious diet, adequate rest and sleep, and avoiding tobacco and alcohol. These measures enhance immune mechanisms and other body defenses.

☑ Carry identification that lists the drugs being taken; the dosage; the physician's name, address, and telephone number; and instructions for emergency treatment. This information is needed if an accident or emergency situation occurs.

☑ Inform all health care providers that you are taking these drugs.

☑ Maintain regular medical supervision. This is extremely important for detecting adverse drug reactions, evaluating disease status, evaluating drug responses and indications for dosage change, and having blood tests or other monitoring tests when needed.

☑ Take no other drugs, prescription or nonprescription, without notifying the physician who is managing immunosuppressant therapy. Immunosuppressant drugs may influence reactions to other drugs, and other drugs may influence reactions to the immunosuppressants. Thus, taking other drugs may decrease therapeutic effects or increase adverse effects. In addition, vaccinations may be less effective, and some should be avoided while taking immunosuppressant drugs.

☑ People of reproductive capability who are sexually active should practice effective contraceptive techniques during immunosuppressive drug therapy. With methotrexate, use contraception during and for at least 3 months (men) or one ovulatory cycle (women) after stopping the drug. With mycophenolate, effective contraception should be continued for 6 weeks after the drug is stopped. With sirolimus, effective contraception must be used before, during, and for 12 weeks after drug therapy. The drug was toxic to embryos and fetuses in animal studies.

☑ Wear protective clothing and use sunscreens to decrease exposure of skin to sunlight and risks of skin cancers. Also, methotrexate and sirolimus increase sensitivity to sunlight and may increase sunburn.

Self-Administration

☑ Follow instructions about taking the drugs. This is vital to achieving beneficial effects and decreasing adverse effects. If unable to take a medication, report to the prescribing physician or other health care provider; do not stop unless advised to do so. For transplant recipients, missed doses may lead to transplant rejection; for clients with autoimmune diseases, missed doses may lead to acute flareups of symptoms. In addition, take at approximately the same time each day to maintain consistent drug levels in the blood.

☑ Take oral azathioprine in divided doses, after meals, to decrease stomach upset.

☑ With cyclosporine oral solution, use the same solution consistently. The two available solutions (Neoral and Sandimmune) are not equivalent and cannot be used interchangeably. If a change in formulation is necessary, it should be made cautiously and only under supervision of the prescribing physician.

Measure oral cyclosporine solution with the dosing syringe provided; add to orange or apple juice that is at room temperature (avoid grapefruit juice); stir well and drink at once (do not allow diluted solution to stand before drinking). Use a glass container, not plastic. Rinse the glass with more diluent to ensure the total dose is taken. Do not rinse the dosing syringe with water or other cleaning agents. Take on a consistent schedule with regard to time of day and meals.

These are the manufacturer's recommendations. Mixing with orange or apple juice improves taste; grapefruit juice should not be used because it affects metabolism of cyclosporine. The amount of fluid should be large enough to increase palatability, especially for children, but small enough to be consumed quickly. Rinsing ensures the entire dose is taken.

☑ Take mycophenolate on an empty stomach; food decreases the amount of active drug by 40%. Do not crush mycophenolate tablets and do not open or crush the capsules.

☑ Take sirolimus consistently with or without food; do *not* mix or take the drug with grapefruit juice. Grapefruit juice inhibits metabolism and increases adverse effects. If also taking cyclosporine, take the sirolimus 4 hours after a dose of cyclosporine.

If taking the oral solution, use the syringe that comes with the medication to measure and withdraw the dose from the bottle. Empty the dose into a glass or plastic container with at least 2 oz (¼ cup or 60 mL) of water or orange juice. *Do not use any other liquid to dilute the drug.* Stir the mixture vigorously, and drink it immediately. Refill the container with at least 4 oz (½ cup or 120 mL) of water or orange juice, stir vigorously, and drink at once.

☑ Take tacrolimus with food to decrease stomach upset.

☑ If giving or taking an injected drug (eg, etanercept), be sure you understand how to mix and inject the medication correctly. For example, with etanercept, rotate injection sites, give a new injection at least 1 inch from a previous injection site, and do not inject the medication into areas where the skin is tender, bruised, red, or hard. When possible, practice the required techniques and perform at least the first injection under supervision of a qualified health care professional.

of morbidity and mortality, especially in clients who are neutropenic (neutrophil count <1000/mm³) from cytotoxic immunosuppressant drugs, who take TNF inhibitors, or who have had bone marrow or solid organ transplantation. For those with solid organ transplantation, who must continue lifelong immunosuppression to avoid graft rejection, serious infection is a constant hazard. Extensive efforts are made to prevent infections; if these efforts are unsuccessful, infections may be fatal unless recognized promptly and treated aggressively. Common infections are bacterial (gram-positive, such as *Staphylococcus aureus* or *S. epidermidis;* and gram-negative, such as *Escherichia coli, Klebsiella,* and *Pseudomonas* species), fungal (candidiasis, aspergillosis), or viral (CMV, herpes simplex, or herpes zoster). In addition, severe, disseminated tuberculosis is associated with the use of TNF inhibitors.

Cancer may result from immunosuppression. When T lymphocytes and NK cells are suppressed and unable to recognize and eliminate abnormal cells, the abnormal cells may undergo spontaneous malignant transformation and result in widespread and often aggressive malignancies. Most of the available information is related to posttransplant cancer development.

With early transplantations, major causes of death were graft rejection and infection. Now, improvements in transplantation technology and drug therapy are leading to more transplants, older transplant recipients, and longer survival rates among recipients. One consequence of long-term survival and chronic immunosuppression is increased risk of developing a posttransplant malignancy. The incidence in the United States is unknown, but often estimated at 20% or more after 10 years of immunosuppression. As a result, cancer has become the second most common cause of mortality in transplant recipients and its incidence is expected to increase.

The most common malignancies among transplant recipients are skin cancers (including squamous cell, basal cell, and melanoma) and lymphomas. Other malignancies include solid organ tumors, some of which occur at similar rates in the general and posttransplant populations (eg, brain, breast, lung, prostate) and some of which occur more often in the posttransplant population (eg, renal cell cancer in renal transplant recipients; colon cancers; cervical, perineal/anal, and vulvar cancers in women). When breast cancer occurs posttransplantation, it often occurs at a younger age and grows more aggressively than in the general population. In addition, men with transplants are more likely to develop breast cancer than men in the general population.

Immunosuppressant drugs often associated with posttransplantation cancer include azathioprine and cyclosporine. Azathioprine has a strong link with carcinogenesis. Tacrolimus is considered safer than formerly and cyclosporine because smaller doses are being given and serum drug levels are being monitored. Other immunosuppressants considered less likely to promote carcinogenesis include mycophenolate, polyclonal antibodies, and sirolimus. Few data exist regarding the cancer-causing potential of newer immunosuppressants. However, some may be safer because they suppress specific immune cells and cytokines and have more limited effects than the older drugs that suppress multiple immune components and cause general immunosuppression.

When cancer develops, treatment includes reduced immunosuppressant drug therapy as well as treatment of the malignancy. Reducing dosages of immunosuppressant drugs increases risks of rejection reactions and the need for retransplantation.

Use in Autoimmune Disorders

Allergic Asthma

Allergic asthma is characterized by increased production of IgE in response to inhaled allergens. IgE molecules then interact with allergen molecules to form IgE–allergen complexes that damage tissues and produce signs and symptoms. Omalizumab (Xolair), the only noncorticosteroid immunosuppressant used in the treatment of asthma, combines with free IgE so that there is less IgE available to combine with allergens. It is considered second-line therapy for clients with allergic asthma whose symptoms are not adequately controlled with inhaled corticosteroids.

Crohn's Disease

Crohn's disease is a chronic, recurrent, inflammatory bowel disorder that can affect any area of the GI tract. The inflammation is attributed to a strong mixture of inflammatory mediators (eg, IL-1 and -6, TNF–alpha) produced by activated macrophages. The focus of treatment is to decrease inflammation and promote healing of bowel lesions. Several medications are effective, including corticosteroids, cyclosporine, 6-mercaptopurine, metronidazole, and sulfasalazine. Because elevated concentrations of TNF–alpha are found in clients' stools and correlate with episodes of increased disease activity, infliximab (Remicade) is also used. Infliximab reduces infiltration of inflammatory cells, production of TNF–alpha in inflamed areas of the intestine, and the number of cells that can produce TNF–alpha. It is indicated for clients with moderate to severe disease who do not respond adequately to other treatment measures.

Psoriasis and Psoriatic Arthritis

Psoriasis is a skin disorder of unknown cause. It is thought that activated T lymphocytes produce cytokines that stimulate abnormal growth of affected skin cells and blood vessels. The accompanying inflammation results from infiltration of neutrophils and monocytes. Several medications (eg, beta blockers, lithium) may precipitate or aggravate psoriasis. Corticosteroids and other immunosuppressants (eg, cyclosporine, methotrexate) have long been used to treat psoriasis because they suppress inflammation and proliferation of T cells. Newer biologic immunosuppressants (eg, alefacept, efalizumab) also reduce the activity of T lymphocytes and the inflammation of skin lesions.

Psoriatic arthritis is a type of arthritis associated with psoriasis that is also similar to RA. It may be characterized by extensive and disabling joint damage, especially in hand and finger joints. Etanercept (Enbrel) is a TNF–alpha inhibitor approved for treatment.

Rheumatoid Arthritis

Rheumatoid arthritis is an abnormal immune response that leads to inflammation and damage of joint cartilage and bone. It is thought to involve the activation of T lymphocytes, release of inflammatory cytokines, and formation of antibodies. Research in recent years has increased understanding of the major role that TNF–alpha and IL-1 play in the pathophysiology of RA. This understanding led to the development of drugs directed against TNF–alpha (eg, adalimumab, etanercept, infliximab) and IL-1 (eg, anakinra).

These drugs are highly effective in relieving joint pain and inflammation and they also slow progression of RA, as measured by serial radiographs. Because of their ability to slow disease progression, they are called *disease-modifying anti-rheumatic drugs* (DMARDs). They act more rapidly than older DMARDs (eg, methotrexate) and greatly improve the quality of life for clients with RA. However, their use is also associated with significant risks of serious infections, especially with the TNF–alpha antagonists. To decrease the adverse effects of the TNF inhibitors, the following guidelines have been developed for clients receiving these drugs:

● Tuberculin testing before starting a TNF inhibitor and antitubercular prophylaxis for clients with positive skin-test results
● Administration of pneumococcal and perhaps meningococcal vaccine
● Administration of trimethoprim-sulfamethoxazole (TMP-SMX) to prevent infection
● Consideration of fluconazole administration to clients at high risk of developing coccidioidomycosis and cryptococcosis
● Education of clients and caregivers to avoid potential exposures to infection in the community
● Provision of antibiotics for immediate initiation at home with the onset of fever or upper respiratory infection, followed by seeking emergency care

Use in Transplantation

The use of immunosuppressant drugs in transplantation continues to evolve. Although specific protocols vary among transplantation centers and types of transplants, newer immunosuppressant regimens and effective treatment of infections have shifted the focus from client and organ survival to the complications of transplantation. Many transplant clients have preexisting conditions that are aggravated by immunosuppressant drug therapy (eg, diabetes mellitus, hypertension, dyslipidemia). Nephrotoxicity, osteoporosis, and malignancies also occur. Thus, when immunosuppressant drug therapy is started, measures to prevent the development of new diseases or the worsening of pre-existing conditions are needed.

One strategy to decrease posttransplantation complications is to decrease the use or dosage of immunosuppressant drugs, especially corticosteroids and cyclosporine. This strategy must be used with vigilant monitoring to catch possible rejection reactions early, when restarting immunosuppressant drugs or increasing their dosage can still save the transplant.

Another strategy is to increase and improve cancer surveillance. Most monitoring is the same as for the nontransplant population (eg, annual chest radiograph; annual Pap smear in women over 18 years of age; regular mammograms for middle-aged and older women; colonoscopy at age 50, then every 5 years unless clinical symptoms or guaiac-positive stools occur; annual digital prostate examination and serum prostate-specific antigen [PSA] test). In addition, because of increased risks of skin cancer, transplant recipients should undergo complete skin inspection at least annually, especially if they live in geographic areas of high sun exposure.

Posttransplant Combinations of Immunosuppressant Drugs

In transplantation, immunosuppressants are used to prevent rejection of transplanted tissues. The rejection reaction involves T and B lymphocytes and multiple inflammatory cytokines. Thus, drug combinations are rational because they act on different components of the immune response and often have overlapping and synergistic effects. They may also allow lower doses of individual drugs, which usually cause fewer or less severe adverse effects. For example, most organ transplantation centers use a combination regimen (eg, azathioprine, a corticosteroid, and either cyclosporine, sirolimus, or tacrolimus) for prevention and treatment of rejection reactions. After the transplanted tissue is functioning and rejection has been successfully prevented or treated, it often is possible to maintain the graft with fewer drugs or lower drug dosages. Some recommendations to increase safety or effectiveness of drug combinations include the following:

● *Lymphocyte immune globulin, antithymocyte globulin* is usually given with azathioprine and a corticosteroid.
● *Azathioprine* is usually given with cyclosporine and prednisone.
● *Basiliximab* and *daclizumab* are given with cyclosporine and a corticosteroid.

- *Corticosteroids* may be given alone or included in multidrug regimens with cyclosporine and muromonab-CD3. A corticosteroid should always accompany cyclosporine administration to enhance immunosuppression. In prophylaxis of organ transplant rejection, the combination seems more effective than azathioprine alone or azathioprine and a corticosteroid. A corticosteroid may not be required, at least long-term, with tacrolimus.
- *Cyclosporine* should be used cautiously with immunosuppressants other than corticosteroids to decrease risks of excessive immunosuppression and its complications.
- *Methotrexate* may be used alone or with cyclosporine for prophylaxis of GVHD after bone marrow transplantation.
- *Muromonab-CD3* may be given cautiously with reduced numbers or dosages of other immunosuppressants. When co-administered with prednisone and azathioprine, the maximum daily dose of prednisone is 0.5 mg/kg, and the maximum for azathioprine is 25 mg. When muromonab-CD3 is co-administered with cyclosporine, cyclosporine dosage should be reduced or the drug temporarily discontinued. If discontinued, cyclosporine is restarted 3 days before completing the course of muromonab-CD3 therapy, to resume a maintenance level of immunosuppression.
- *Mycophenolate* is used with cyclosporine and a corticosteroid. It may be used instead of azathioprine.
- *Sirolimus* is used with cyclosporine and a corticosteroid.
- *Tacrolimus* is substituted for cyclosporine in some long-term immunosuppressant regimens. An advantage of tacrolimus is that corticosteroid therapy can often be discontinued.

Drug Dosage

Immunosuppressant drugs are relatively toxic, and adverse effects occur more often and are more severe with higher doses. Thus, the general principle of using the smallest effective dose for the shortest period of time is especially important with immunosuppressant drug therapy. Dosage must be individualized according to the client's serum drug levels and clinical response (ie, improvement in signs and symptoms or occurrence of adverse effects). Factors to be considered in drug dosage decisions include the following:

- *Azathioprine* dosage should be reduced or the drug discontinued if severe bone marrow depression occurs (eg, reduced red blood cells, WBCs, and platelets on complete blood count [CBC]). If it is necessary to stop the drug, administration may be resumed at a smaller dosage after the bone marrow has recovered. With renal transplant recipients, the dosage required to prevent rejection and minimize toxicity varies. When given long-term for maintenance of immunosuppression, the lowest effective dose is recommended. If given concomitantly with muromonab-CD3, the dosage is reduced to 25 mg/day.

- *Corticosteroid* dosages vary among transplantation centers. The highest doses are usually given immediately after transplantation and during treatment of acute graft-rejection reactions. Doses are usually tapered by 6 months after the transplantation, and long-term maintenance doses of prednisone are usually under 10 mg/day. Doses of corticosteroids may also be reduced when the drugs are given in combination with other immunosuppressants. For some clients, the drugs may be discontinued.
- *Cyclosporine* dosage should be individualized according to drug concentration in blood, serum creatinine levels, and the client's clinical status. Higher doses are given for approximately 3 months posttransplantation and may be given IV for a few days after surgery (at one third the oral dosage). Higher doses are also given when cyclosporine is used with one other drug than when it is used with two other drugs. After a few months, the dose is reduced for long-term maintenance of immunosuppression after solid organ transplantation. When a client receiving cyclosporine is given muromonab-CD3, cyclosporine is stopped temporarily or given in reduced doses.
- Dosage of *mycophenolate, muromonab-CD3, sirolimus,* and *tacrolimus* should follow established recommendations.

Drug Administration

The effectiveness of immunosuppressant therapy may be enhanced by appropriate timing of drug administration. For example, corticosteroids are most effective when given just before exposure to the antigen, whereas the cytotoxic agents (eg, azathioprine, methotrexate) are most effective when given soon after exposure (ie, during the interval between exposure to the antigen and the production of sensitized T cells or antibodies). The newer drugs, basiliximab and daclizumab, are started a few hours before transplantation and continued for a few doses afterward.

Drug Selection and Type of Transplant

Cardiac transplant recipients are usually given azathioprine, cyclosporine, and prednisone. Tacrolimus may be used instead of cyclosporine. Because rejection reactions are more likely to occur during the first 6 months after transplantation, transvenous endomyocardial biopsies are performed at regular intervals up to a year, then as needed according to the client's clinical status.

Renal transplant recipients receive variable immunosuppressive drug therapy, depending on the time interval since the transplant surgery. For several days posttransplantation, high doses of IV methylprednisolone are usually given. The dose is tapered and discontinued as oral prednisone is initiated. Cyclosporine may not be used because of its unpredictable absorption and its nephrotoxicity. If used, it is given in low doses. If not used, adequate immunosuppression must be maintained with other agents. Whichever drugs are used in the immediate postoperative period and up to 3 months posttransplantation, high doses are required to prevent organ rejection. These high doses may result in serious complications, such as infection and corticosteroid-induced diabetes. Doses are usually reduced if clients have serious adverse effects (eg, infection, nephrotoxicity, hepatotoxicity).

After approximately 3 months, maintenance immunosuppressant therapy usually consists of azathioprine and prednisone alone or with cyclosporine or tacrolimus. Doses are gradually decreased over 6 to 12 months, and some drugs may be discontinued (eg, prednisone, when tacrolimus is given). In addition, cyclosporine may be discontinued if chronic nephrotoxicity or severe hypertension occurs.

Liver transplant recipients may be given various drugs, and there are several effective regimens. Most regimens use methylprednisolone initially, with cyclosporine or tacrolimus; some include azathioprine or mycophenolate. At some centers, corticosteroids are eventually discontinued and clients are maintained on tacrolimus alone. Treatment of rejection reactions also varies among liver transplantation centers and may include the addition of high-dose corticosteroids and muromonab-CD3 or LIG, ATG for 7 to 14 days. In addition, clients on tacrolimus may be given higher doses. Those on cyclosporine usually do not receive higher doses because of nephrotoxicity.

An additional consideration is that liver and biliary tract functions vary among clients. As a result, the pharmacokinetics of some immunosuppressant drugs are altered. Cyclosporine has been studied most in this setting. When liver function is impaired, for example, oral cyclosporine is poorly absorbed and higher oral doses or IV administration are required to maintain adequate blood levels. When liver function and bile flow are restored, absorption of oral cyclosporine is greatly improved and dosage must be substantially reduced to maintain stable blood concentrations. Absorption of other lipid-soluble drugs is also improved. In addition, serum albumin levels are usually decreased for months after transplantation, producing higher blood levels of drugs that normally bind to albumin.

Still another consideration is that neurologic adverse effects (eg, ataxia, psychosis, seizures) occur in almost half of liver transplant recipients. These effects have been associated with corticosteroids, cyclosporine, muromonab-CD3, and tacrolimus.

Bone marrow transplant recipients are usually given cyclosporine and a corticosteroid.

Laboratory Monitoring

With *azathioprine*, bone marrow depression (eg, severe leukopenia or thrombocytopenia) may occur. To monitor bone marrow function, CBC and platelet counts should be checked weekly during the first month, every 2 weeks during the second and third months, then monthly. If dosage is changed or a client's health status worsens at any time during therapy, more frequent blood tests are needed.

With oral *cyclosporine,* blood levels are monitored periodically for low or high values. Subtherapeutic levels may lead to organ transplant rejection. They are more likely to occur with the Sandimmune formulation than with Neoral because Sandimmune is poorly absorbed. High levels increase adverse effects. The blood levels are used to regulate dosage. In addition, renal (serum creatinine, blood urea nitrogen) and liver (bilirubin, aminotransferase enzymes) function tests should be performed regularly to monitor for nephrotoxicity and hepatotoxicity.

With *leflunomide,* renal and liver function tests should be done periodically.

With *methotrexate,* CBC and platelet counts and renal and liver function tests should be done periodically.

With *muromonab-CD3,* WBC and differential counts should be performed periodically.

With *mycophenolate,* a CBC is recommended weekly during the first month, twice monthly during the second and third months, and monthly during the first year.

With *sirolimus,* serum drug levels should be monitored in clients who are likely to have altered drug metabolism (eg, those 13 years and older who weigh less than 40 kg, those with impaired hepatic function, those who also are receiving enzyme-inducing or inhibiting drugs). Trough concentrations of 15 nanograms per milliliter or more are associated with increased frequency of adverse effects. In addition, tests related to hyperlipidemia and renal function should also be performed periodically.

With *tacrolimus,* periodic measurements of serum creatinine, potassium, and glucose are recommended to monitor for the adverse effects of nephrotoxicity, hyperkalemia, and hyperglycemia.

Use in Special Populations

Use in Children

Most immunosuppressants are used in children for the same disorders and with similar effects as in adults. *Corticosteroids* impair growth in children. As a result, some transplantation centers avoid prednisone therapy until a rejection episode occurs. When prednisone is used, administering it every other day may improve growth rates. *Cyclosporine* has been safely and effectively given to children as young as 6 months of age and *muromonab-CD3* has been used successfully in children as young as 2 years of age. *Mycophenolate* has been used in a few children undergoing renal transplantation. In children with impaired renal function, recommended doses of mycophenolate cause a high incidence of adverse effects. Thus, dosage should be adjusted for the level of renal function. *Tacrolimus* has been used in children younger than 12 years of age who were undergoing liver transplantation. This usage indicates that children require higher doses to maintain therapeutic blood levels than adults because they metabolize the drug more rapidly.

Little information is available about the use of newer immunosuppressants in children. Safety and effectiveness have not been established for *basiliximab, daclizumab, inflix-imab,* or *leflunomide.* Leflunomide is not recommended for children under 18 years of age. *Etanercept* is approved for clients 4 to 17 years of age with juvenile RA. In clinical trials, effects in children were similar to those in adults. Most children in a 3-month study had an infection while receiving etanercept, but the infections were usually mild. Children reported abdominal pain, nausea, vomiting, and headache with etanercept more often than adults. Other medications (eg, a corticosteroid, methotrexate, a nonsteroidal anti-inflammatory drug, an analgesic) may be continued during treatment.

For children age 12 and older with allergic asthma, *omalizumab* is the only immunosuppressant drug approved for use. Dosages and frequency of administration are determined by body weight and serum levels of IgE. The drug is generally well tolerated in children.

Use in Older Adults

Immunosuppressants are used for the same purposes and produce similar therapeutic and adverse effects in older adults as in younger adults. Because older adults often have multiple disorders and organ impairments, it is especially important that drug choices, dosages, and monitoring tests are individualized. In addition, infections occur more commonly in older adults, and this tendency is increased with immunosuppressant therapy.

Use in Clients With Renal Impairment

- *Azathioprine* metabolites are excreted in urine but they are inactive, and the dose does not need to be reduced in clients with renal impairment.
- *Cyclosporine* is nephrotoxic but commonly used in clients with renal and other transplants. Nephrotoxicity has been noted in 25% of renal, 38% of cardiac, and 37% of liver transplant recipients, especially with high doses. It usually subsides with decreased dosage or stopping the drug.

  In renal transplant recipients, when serum creatinine and blood urea nitrogen levels remain elevated, a complete evaluation of the client must be done to differentiate cyclosporine-induced nephrotoxicity from a transplant rejection reaction (although up to 20% of clients may have simultaneous nephrotoxicity and rejection). If renal function is deteriorating from cyclosporine, dosage reduction may be needed. If dosage reduction does not improve renal function, another immunosuppressant is preferred.

  If renal function is deteriorating from a rejection reaction, decreasing cyclosporine dosage would increase the severity of the reaction. With severe rejection that does not respond to treatment with corticosteroids and monoclonal antibodies, it is preferable to allow the kidney transplant to be rejected and removed

rather than increase cyclosporine dosage to high levels in an attempt to reverse the rejection.

To decrease risks of nephrotoxicity, dosage is adjusted according to cyclosporine blood levels and renal function test results, and other nephrotoxic drugs should be avoided. An additional factor is the potential for significant drug interactions with microsomal enzyme inhibitors and inducers. Drugs that inhibit hepatic metabolism (eg, cimetidine) raise cyclosporine blood levels, whereas those that stimulate metabolism decrease levels.

- *Methotrexate* is mainly excreted in urine, so its half-life is prolonged in clients with renal impairment, with risks of accumulation to toxic levels and additional renal damage. However, the risks are less with the small doses used for treatment of RA than for the high doses used in cancer chemotherapy. To decrease these risks, adequate renal function should be documented before the drug is given and clients should be well hydrated.
- *Muromonab-CD3* has caused increased serum creatinine and decreased urine output in a few clients during the first 1 to 3 days of use. This was attributed to the release of cytokines with resultant renal function impairment or delayed renal allograft function. The renal function impairment was reversible.
- *Mycophenolate* produces higher plasma levels in renal transplant recipients with severe, chronic renal impairment than in clients with less severe renal impairment and healthy volunteers. Doses higher than 1 g twice a day should be avoided in these clients. There is no information about mycophenolate use in cardiac transplant recipients with severe, chronic renal impairment.
- *Sirolimus* is eliminated mainly in feces; dosage does not need to be reduced with renal impairment.
- *Tacrolimus* is often associated with high rates of nephrotoxicity when given IV, so oral dosing is preferred. Renal impairment does not increase drug half-life.

Little information is available about the use of *basiliximab, etanercept, infliximab,* or *leflunomide* in clients with renal impairment. However, leflunomide metabolites are partly excreted renally and the drug should be used cautiously. *Daclizumab* dosage does not need to be adjusted with renal impairment.

Use in Clients With Hepatic Impairment

- *Azathioprine* is normally metabolized to its active metabolite in the liver. As a result, pharmacologic action is decreased in clients with hepatic impairment. When azathioprine is used in liver transplantation, clients sometimes experience hepatotoxicity. Liver function usually improves within a week if azathioprine is discontinued.

- *Cyclosporine* reportedly causes hepatotoxicity (eg, elevated serum aminotransferases and bilirubin) in approximately 4% of renal and liver transplant recipients and 7% of cardiac transplant recipients. This is most likely to occur during the first month of therapy, when high doses of cyclosporine are usually given, and usually subsides with reduced dosage.
- *Methotrexate* is metabolized in the liver and may cause hepatotoxicity, even in the low doses used in RA and psoriasis. Several studies indicate that these clients eventually sustain liver changes that may include fatty deposits, lobular necrosis, fibrosis, and cirrhosis. Progression to cirrhosis may be related to the deposition of methotrexate and its metabolites in the liver. Many clinicians recommend serial liver biopsies for clients on long-term, low-dose methotrexate (eg, after each cumulative dose of 1–1.5 g) because fibrosis and cirrhosis may not produce clinical manifestations.

  In addition, in clients with or without initial liver impairment, liver function tests should be performed to monitor clients for hepatotoxicity and to guide drug dosage. In general, methotrexate dosage should be decreased by 25% if bilirubin (normal = 0.1–1.0 mg/dL) is between 3 and 5 mg/dL or aspartate aminotransferase (AST) (normal = 10–40 IU/L) is above 180 IU/L, and the drug should be omitted if bilirubin is above 5 mg/dL.

- *Muromonab-CD3* may cause a transient increase in liver aminotransferase enzymes (eg, AST, alanine aminotransferase [ALT]) with the first few doses.
- *Mycophenolate* is metabolized in the liver to an active metabolite that is further metabolized to inactive metabolites. Liver impairment presumably could interfere with these processes and affect both action and elimination.
- *Sirolimus* is extensively metabolized in the liver and may accumulate in the presence of hepatic impairment. The maintenance dose should be reduced by 35%; it is not necessary to reduce the loading dose.
- *Tacrolimus* is metabolized in the liver by the microsomal P450 enzyme system. Impaired liver function may decrease presystemic (first-pass) metabolism of oral tacrolimus and produce higher blood levels. Also, the elimination half-life is significantly longer for IV or oral drug. As a result, dosage must be decreased in clients with impaired liver function.

  An additional factor is the potential for significant drug interactions with microsomal enzyme inhibitors and inducers. Drugs that inhibit hepatic metabolism (eg, cimetidine) raise tacrolimus blood levels, whereas those that stimulate metabolism decrease levels.

There is little or no information about the use of *basiliximab, daclizumab, etanercept,* or *infliximab* in clients with liver impairment. *Leflunomide* may be hepatotoxic in clients with normal liver function and is not recommended for use in clients with liver impairment or positive serology tests for hepatitis B or C. Considerations and guidelines include the following:

- Leflunomide is metabolized to an active metabolite. The site of metabolism is unknown but thought to be the liver and the wall of the intestine. With liver impairment, less formation of the active metabolite may result in reduced therapeutic effect.
- The active metabolite is further metabolized and excreted through the kidneys and biliary tract. Some of the drug excreted in bile is reabsorbed. Leflunomide's long half-life is attributed to this biliary recycling.
- The role of the liver in drug metabolism and excretion in bile increases risks of hepatotoxicity. The drug increased liver enzymes (mainly AST and ALT) in clinical trials. Most elevations were mild and usually subsided with continued therapy. Higher elevations were infrequent and subsided if dosage was reduced or the drug was discontinued. It is recommended that liver enzymes, especially ALT, be measured before starting leflunomide, every month during therapy until stable, then as needed.
- When ALT elevation is more than twice the upper limits of normal (ULN), leflunomide dosage should be reduced to 10 mg/day (half the usual daily maintenance dose). If ALT levels are more than twice but not more than three times the ULN and persist despite dosage reduction, liver biopsy is recommended if continued drug use is desired. If elevations are more than three times the ULN and persist despite dosage reduction and cholestyramine (see below), leflunomide should be discontinued. ALT levels should be monitored and cholestyramine readministered as indicated.
- When leflunomide is stopped, a special procedure is recommended to eliminate the drug (otherwise it could take as long as 2 years). The procedure involves administration of cholestyramine (see Chap. 55) 8 g three times daily for 11 days (the 11 days do not need to be consecutive unless blood levels need to be lowered rapidly). If plasma levels are still above the goal level of less than 0.02 mcg/mL, additional cholestyramine may be needed.

Use in Home Care

With clients who are taking immunosuppressant drugs, a major role of the home care nurse is to assess the environment for potential sources of infection, assist clients and other members of the household to understand the client's susceptibility to infection, and teach ways to decrease risks of infection. Although infections often develop from the client's own body flora, other potential sources include people with infections, caregivers, water or soil around live plants, and raw fruits and vegetables. Meticulous environmental cleansing as well as personal and hand hygiene are required. In addition, the nurse may need to assist with clinic visits for monitoring and follow-up care.

Immunosuppressants

NURSING ACTIONS	RATIONALE/EXPLANATION

1. Administer accurately

a. For prepared intravenous (IV) solutions, check for appropriate dilution, discoloration, particulate matter, and expiration time. If okay, give by infusion pump, for the recommended time.

IV drugs should be reconstituted and diluted in a pharmacy, and the manufacturers' instructions should be followed exactly. After they are mixed, most of these drugs are stable only for a few hours and some do not contain preservatives.

b. Give oral **azathioprine** in divided doses, after meals; give IV drug by infusion, usually over 30 to 60 minutes.

To decrease nausea and vomiting with oral drug

c. With **basiliximab,** infuse through a peripheral or central vein over 20–30 minutes. Use the reconstituted solution within 4 hours at room temperature or 24 hours if refrigerated.

The first dose is given within 2 hours before transplantation surgery and the second dose 4 days after transplantation.

d. With **IV cyclosporine,** infuse over 2–6 hours.

IV drug is given to patients who are unable to take it orally; resume oral administration when feasible.

e. With **oral cyclosporine** solutions, measure doses with the provided syringe; add to room-temperature orange or apple juice (avoid grapefruit juice); stir well and have the patient drink at once (do not allow diluted solution to stand before drinking). Use a glass container, not plastic. Rinse the glass with more juice to ensure the total dose is taken. Do not rinse the dosing syringe with water or other cleaning agents. Give on a consistent schedule in relation to time of day and meals.

These are the manufacturers' recommendations. Mixing with orange or apple juice improves taste; grapefruit juice should not be used because it affects metabolism of cyclosporine.

The amount of fluid should be large enough to increase palatability, especially for children, but small enough to be consumed quickly. Rinsing ensures the entire dose is taken.

Oral cyclosporine may be given to clients who have had an anaphylactic reaction to the IV preparation, because the reaction is attributed to the oil diluent rather than the drug.

f. Infuse reconstituted and diluted **daclizumab** through a peripheral or central vein over 15 minutes. After it is mixed, use within 4 hours or refrigerate up to 24 hours.

The first dose is given approximately 24 hours before transplantation, followed by a dose every 2 weeks for four doses (total of five doses).

g. With **etanercept,** slowly inject 1 mL of the supplied Sterile Bacteriostatic Water for Injection into the vial, without shaking (to avoid excessive foaming). Give subcutaneously, rotating sites so that a new dose is injected at least 1 inch from an old site and never into areas where the skin is tender, bruised, red, or hard.

This drug may be administered at home, by a client or a caregiver, with appropriate instructions and supervised practice in mixing and injecting the drug.

h. Infuse reconstituted and diluted **infliximab** over approximately 2 hours, starting within 3 hours of preparation (contains no antibacterial preservatives).

Infliximab should be prepared in a pharmacy because special equipment is required for administration.

i. Give **lymphocyte immune globulin, antithymocyte globulin** (diluted to a concentration of 1 mg/mL) into a large or central vein, using an in-line filter and infusion pump, over at least 4 hours. After it is diluted, use within 24 hours.

Manufacturer's recommendations. Using a high-flow vein decreases phlebitis and thrombosis at the IV site. The filter is used to remove any insoluble particles.

j. Give **muromonab-CD3** in an IV bolus injection once daily. Do not give by IV infusion or mix with other drug solutions.

Manufacturer's recommendations

k. Infuse **IV mycophenolate** over approximately 2 hours, within 4 hours of solution preparation (contains no antibacterial preservatives).

The IV drug must be reconstituted and diluted with 5% dextrose to a concentration of 6 mg/mL (1 g reconstituted drug in 140 mL or 1.5 g in 210 mL).

Handle the drug cautiously to avoid contact with skin and mucous membranes. If such contact occurs, wash thoroughly with soap and water; rinse eyes with plain water.

l. Give **oral mycophenolate** on an empty stomach. Do not crush the tablets; do not open or crush the capsules; and ask clients to swallow the capsules whole, without biting or chewing.

Food decreases absorption. Avoid inhaling the powder from the capsules or getting on skin or mucous membranes. Such contacts produced teratogenic effects in animals.

NURSING ACTIONS	RATIONALE/EXPLANATION
m. With **sirolimus,** give 4 hours after a dose of cyclosporine; give consistently with or without food; and do not give with grapefruit juice.	Serum drug levels of sirolimus are increased if the two drugs are taken at the same time; consistent timing in relation to food provides more consistent absorption and blood levels; grapefruit juice inhibits the enzymes that metabolize sirolimus, thereby increasing blood levels of drug and increasing risks of toxicity.
With oral sirolimus solution, use the amber oral-dose syringe to withdraw a dose from the bottle; empty the dose into a glass or plastic container with at least 60 mL of water or orange juice (do not use any other diluent); stir the mixture vigorously and ask the patient to drink it immediately; refill the container with at least 120 mL of water or orange juice; stir vigorously and ask the patient to drink all of the fluid.	Manufacturer's recommendations
n. Give **IV tacrolimus** as a continuous infusion by infusion pump.	
o. Give the first dose of **oral tacrolimus** 8–12 hours after stopping the IV infusion.	Oral tacrolimus can usually be substituted for IV drug 2–3 days after transplantation.
2. Observe for therapeutic effects	
a. When a drug is given to suppress the immune response to organ transplants, therapeutic effect is the absence of signs and symptoms indicating rejection of the transplanted tissue.	
b. When azathioprine or methotrexate is given for rheumatoid arthritis, observe for decreased pain.	With azathioprine, therapeutic effects usually occur after 6–8 weeks. If no response occurs within 12 weeks, other treatment measures are indicated. With methotrexate, therapeutic effects usually occur within 3–6 weeks.
c. When adalimumab, etanercept, or infliximab is given for rheumatoid arthritis, observe for decreased symptoms and less joint destruction on x-ray examination reports.	
d. When infliximab is given for Crohn's disease, observe for decreased symptoms.	
e. When alafacept or efalizumab is given for psoriasis, observe for improvement in skin lesions.	
3. Observe for adverse effects	
a. Observe for infection (fever, sore throat, wound drainage, productive cough, dysuria, and so forth).	Frequency and severity increase with higher drug dosages. Risks are high in immunosuppressed clients. Infections may be caused by almost any microorganism and may affect any part of the body, although respiratory and urinary tract infections may occur more often.
b. With azathioprine, observe for:	
(1) Bone marrow depression (anemia, leukopenia, thrombocytopenia, abnormal bleeding)	The incidence of adverse effects is high in transplant recipients. Dosage reduction or stopping azathioprine may be indicated.
(2) Nausea and vomiting	Can be reduced by dividing the daily dosage and giving after meals
c. With basiliximab and daclizumab, observe for gastrointestinal (GI) disorders (nausea, vomiting, diarrhea, heartburn, abdominal distention).	GI symptoms were often reported in clinical trials. Although adverse effects involving all body systems were reported, the number and type were similar for basiliximab, daclizumab, and placebo groups. All patients were also receiving cyclosporine and a corticosteroid.
d. With cyclosporine, observe for:	
(1) Nephrotoxicity (increased serum creatinine and blood urea nitrogen [BUN], decreased urine output, edema, hyperkalemia)	This is a major adverse effect, and it may produce signs and symptoms that are difficult to distinguish from those caused by renal graft rejection. Rejection usually occurs within the first month after surgery. If it occurs, dosage must be reduced and the patient observed for improved renal function.
	Also, note that graft rejection and drug-induced nephrotoxicity may be present simultaneously. The latter may be decreased by reducing dosage. Nephrotoxicity often occurs 2–3 months after transplantation and results in a stable but decreased level of renal function (BUN of 35–45 mg/dL and serum creatinine of 2.0–2.5 mg/dL).

(continued)

NURSING ACTIONS	RATIONALE/EXPLANATION
(2) Hepatotoxicity (increased serum enzymes and bilirubin)	The reported incidence is less than 8% after kidney, heart, or liver transplantation. It usually occurs during the first month, when high doses are used, and decreases with dosage reduction.
(3) Hypertension	This is especially likely to occur in clients with heart transplants and may require antihypertensive drug therapy. Do not give a potassium-sparing diuretic as part of the antihypertensive regimen because of increased risk of hyperkalemia.
(4) Anaphylaxis (with IV cyclosporine) (urticaria, hypotension or shock, respiratory distress)	This is rare but may occur. The allergen is thought to be the polyoxyethylated castor oil because people who had allergic reactions with the IV drug have later taken oral doses without allergic reactions. During IV administration, observe the client continuously for the first 30 minutes and often thereafter. Stop the infusion if a reaction occurs, and give emergency care (eg, epinephrine 1:1000).
(5) Central nervous system (CNS) toxicity (confusion, depression, hallucinations, seizures, tremor)	These effects are relatively uncommon and may be caused by factors other than cyclosporine (eg, nephrotoxicity).
(6) Other (gingival hyperplasia, hirsutism)	Gingival hyperplasia can be minimized by thorough oral hygiene.
e. With infliximab, observe for:	
(1) Infusion reactions (fever, chills, pruritus, urticaria, chest pain)	
(2) GI upset (nausea, vomiting, abdominal pain)	
(3) Respiratory symptoms (bronchitis, chest pain, coughing, dyspnea)	
f. With leflunomide, observe for:	The drug was, in general, well tolerated in clinical trials, with the number and type of most adverse effects similar to those occurring with placebo.
(1) GI upset (nausea, diarrhea)	
(2) Hepatotoxicity (elevation of transaminases)	
(3) Skin disorders (alopecia, rash)	
g. With lymphocyte immune globulin, antithymocyte globulin, observe for:	
(1) Anaphylaxis (chest pain, respiratory distress, hypotension, or shock)	An uncommon but serious allergic reaction to the animal protein in the drug that may occur anytime during therapy. If it occurs, stop the drug infusion, inject 0.3 mL epinephrine 1:1000 Sub-Q or IM, and provide other supportive emergency care as indicated.
(2) Chills and fever	Fever occurs in approximately 50% of clients; it may be decreased by premedicating with acetaminophen, an antihistamine, or a corticosteroid.
h. With methotrexate, observe for:	
(1) GI disorders (nausea, vomiting, diarrhea, ulcerations, bleeding)	
(2) Bone marrow depression (anemia, neutropenia, thrombocytopenia)	Monitor complete blood count (CBC) regularly. Bone marrow depression is less likely to occur with the small doses used for inflammatory disorders than with doses used in cancer chemotherapy.
(3) Hepatotoxicity (yellow discoloration of skin or eyes, dark urine, elevated liver aminotransferases)	Long-term, low-dose methotrexate may produce fatty changes, fibrosis, necrosis, and cirrhosis in the liver.
i. With muromonab-CD3, observe for:	
(1) An acute reaction called the cytokine release syndrome (high fever, chills, chest pain, dyspnea, hypertension, nausea, vomiting, diarrhea)	This reaction is attributed to the release of cytokines by activated lymphocytes or monocytes. Symptoms may range from "flu-like" to a less frequent but severe, shock-like reaction that may include serious cardiovascular and CNS disorders.
(2) Hypersensitivity (edema, difficulty in swallowing or breathing, skin rash, urticaria, rapid heart beat)	Symptoms usually occur within 30–60 minutes after administration of a dose, especially the first dose, and may last several hours. The reaction usually subsides with later doses, but may recur with dosage increases or restarting after a period without the drug. Patients experiencing a hypersensitivity reaction should receive immediate treatment.

NURSING ACTIONS	RATIONALE/EXPLANATION
(3) Nausea, vomiting, diarrhea	
j. With mycophenolate, observe for:	
(1) GI effects (nausea, vomiting, diarrhea)	GI effects are more likely when mycophenolate is started and may subside if dosage is reduced.
(2) Hematologic effects (anemia, neutropenia)	Monitor CBC reports regularly. Up to 2% of renal and 2.8% of cardiac transplant recipients taking mycophenolate have severe neutropenia (absolute neutrophil count <500/mm^3). The neutropenia may be related to mycophenolate, concomitant medications, viral infections, or a combination of these causes. If a client has neutropenia, interrupt drug administration or reduce the dose and initiate appropriate treatment as soon as possible.
(3) CNS effects (dizziness, headache, insomnia)	
k. With sirolimus, observe for:	Most reactions were common (ie, occurred in >10% of recipients). However, patients were also receiving cyclosporine and a corticosteroid.
(1) GI effects (abdominal pain, nausea, vomiting, constipation, diarrhea, hepatotoxicity)	
(2) Hematologic effects (anemia, leukopenia, thrombocytopenia, hypercholesterolemia)	
(3) Cardiovascular effects (edema, hypertension)	
(4) CNS effects (insomnia, headache, tremor)	
l. With tacrolimus, observe for:	
(1) Nephrotoxicity (increased serum creatinine, decreased urine output)	Nephrotoxicity has occurred in one third or more of liver transplant recipients who received tacrolimus. The risk is greater with higher doses.
(2) Neurotoxicity (minor effects include insomnia, mild tremors, headaches, photophobia, nightmares; major effects include confusion, seizures, coma, expressive aphasia, psychosis, and encephalopathy)	Neurologic symptoms are common and occur in approximately 10%–20% of clients receiving tacrolimus.
(3) Infection (cytomegalovirus (CMV) infection and others)	CMV infection commonly occurs.
(4) Hyperglycemia	Glucose intolerance may require insulin therapy.
4. Observe for drug interactions	Drug interactions have not been reported with the newer biologic immunosuppressants (adalimumab, alefacept, anakinra, basiliximab, daclizumab, etanercept, infliximab, omalizumab).
a. Drugs that *increase* effects of azathioprine:	
(1) Allopurinol	Inhibits hepatic metabolism, thereby increasing pharmacologic effects. If the two drugs are given concomitantly, the dose of azathioprine should be reduced drastically to 25%–35% of the usual dose.
(2) Corticosteroids	Increased immunosuppression and risk of infection
b. Drugs that *increase* effects of cyclosporine:	
(1) Aminoglycoside antibiotics (eg, gentamicin), antifungals (eg, amphotericin B)	Increased risk of nephrotoxicity. Avoid other nephrotoxic drugs when possible.
(2) Antifungals (fluconazole, itraconazole), calcium channel blockers (diltiazem, nicardipine, verapamil), macrolide antibiotics (erythromycin, clarithromycin), cimetidine	Decreased hepatic metabolism, increased serum drug levels, and increased risk of toxicity
c. Drugs that *decrease* effects of cyclosporine:	
(1) Enzyme inducers, including anticonvulsants (carbamazepine, phenytoin), rifampin	Enzyme-inducing drugs stimulate hepatic metabolism of cyclosporine, thereby reducing blood levels. If concurrent administration is necessary, monitor cyclosporine blood levels to avoid subtherapeutic levels and decreased effectiveness.

(continued)

NURSING ACTIONS	RATIONALE/EXPLANATION
d. Drugs that *increase* effects of leflunomide:	
(1) Rifampin	Rifampin induces liver enzymes and accelerates metabolism of leflunomide to its active metabolite.
(2) Hepatotoxic drugs (eg, methotrexate)	Additive hepatotoxicity
e. Drugs that *decrease* effects of leflunomide:	
(1) Charcoal	These drugs may be used to lower blood levels of leflunomide.
(2) Cholestyramine	
f. Drugs that *increase* effects of methotrexate:	
(1) Probenecid	Probenecid, salicylates, and sulfonamides may increase both therapeutic and toxic effects. The mechanism is unknown, but may involve slowing of methotrexate elimination through the kidneys or displacement of methotrexate from plasma protein-binding sites.
(2) Salicylates	
(3) Sulfonamides	
(4) Non-steroidal anti-inflammatory drugs (NSAIDs)	NSAIDs are often used concomitantly with methotrexate by clients with rheumatoid arthritis. There may be an increased risk of GI ulceration and bleeding.
(5) Procarbazine	Procarbazine may increase nephrotoxicity.
(6) Alcohol and other hepatotoxic drugs	Hepatotoxic drugs increase hepatotoxicity.
g. Drug that *decreases* effects of methotrexate:	
(1) Folic acid	Methotrexate acts by blocking folic acid. Its effectiveness is decreased by folic acid supplementation, alone or in multivitamin preparations.
h. Drugs that *increase* effects of mycophenolate:	
(1) Acyclovir, ganciclovir	Increase blood levels of mycophenolate, probably by decreasing renal excretion
(2) Probenecid, salicylates	Increase blood levels
i. Drug that *decreases* effects of mycophenolate:	
(1) Cholestyramine	Decreases absorption
j. Drugs that *increase* effects of sirolimus:	
(1) Cyclosporine	Increases blood levels of sirolimus and should not be given at same time (give sirolimus 4 hours after a dose of cyclosporine)
(2) CYP3A4 enzyme inhibitors—azole antifungal drugs (eg, fluconazole, itraconazole), calcium channel blockers (eg, diltiazem, nicardipine, verapamil), macrolide antibiotics (eg, erythromycin, clarithromycin), protease inhibitors (eg, ritonavir, indinavir), cimetidine	These drugs inhibit metabolism of sirolimus, which increases blood levels and risks of toxicity.
k. Drugs that *decrease* effects of sirolimus:	
(1) Enzyme inducers—anticonvulsants (eg, carbamazepine, phenytoin), rifamycins (eg, rifampin, rifabutin, rifapentine), St. John's wort	These drugs speed up the metabolism and elimination of sirolimus.
l. Drugs that *increase* effects of tacrolimus:	
(1) Nephrotoxic drugs (eg, aminoglycoside antibiotics, amphotericin B, cisplatin, NSAIDs)	Increased risk of nephrotoxicity
(2) Antifungals (clotrimazole, fluconazole, itraconazole); erythromycin and other macrolides; calcium channel blockers (diltiazem, verapamil); cimetidine; danazol; methylprednisolone; metoclopramide	These drugs may increase blood levels of tacrolimus, probably by inhibiting or competing for hepatic drug-metabolizing enzymes.
(3) Angiotensin-converting enzyme inhibitors, potassium supplements	Increased risk of hyperkalemia. Serum potassium levels should be monitored closely.

NURSING ACTIONS	RATIONALE/EXPLANATION
m. Drugs that *decrease* effects of tacrolimus:	
(1) Antacids	With oral tacrolimus, antacids adsorb the drug or raise the pH of gastric fluids and increase its degradation. If ordered conco-mitantly, an antacid should be given at least 2 hours before or after tacrolimus.
(2) Enzyme inducers—carbamazepine, phenytoin, rifampin, rifabutin	Induction of drug-metabolizing enzymes in the liver may accelerate metabolism of tacrolimus and decrease its blood levels.

APPLYING YOUR KNOWLEDGE: ANSWERS

41-1 Mr. Kinney is at a greatly increased risk of a serious infection and perhaps a life-threatening complication. In addition to the immunosuppressed state putting Mr. Kinney at risk for infection, the immunosuppressant drugs slow the proliferation of lymphocytes and damage rapidly dividing nonimmune cells.

41-2 Monitor Mr. Kinney's WBC and platelet counts. The adverse reactions to mycophenolate are neutropenia and thrombocytopenia.

41-3 Cyclosporine and sirolimus should not be given at the same time. The drugs should be taken 4 hours apart. The concomitant administration of cyclosporine and sirolimus can increase the blood level of sirolimus to possible toxic levels.

41-4 The following teaching points are appropriate: Do not substitute brands of cyclosporine, and report to the primary care provider if a decreased urinary output is observed. Take mycophenolate on an empty stomach. Take sirolimus 4 hours after the dose of cyclosporine and do not take it with grapefruit juice. All of these drugs should be taken at the same time each day and you should report to the primary care provider if you cannot take the medication as ordered for any reason. Take no other drugs without medical supervision. Take precautions to prevent infection.

Review and Application Exercises

Short Answer Exercises

1. List clinical indications for use of immunosuppressant drug therapy.

2. How do the different types of drugs exert their immunosuppressant effects?

3. What are major adverse effects of immunosuppressant drugs?

4. When assessing a client receiving one or more immunosuppressant drugs, what specific signs and symptoms indicate adverse drug effects?

5. For a client taking one or more immunosuppressant drugs, prepare a teaching plan related to safe and effective drug therapy.

NCLEX-Style Questions

6. In addition to organ transplantation, immunosuppressant drugs are used to treat
   a. serious infections
   b. Crohn's disease and rheumatoid arthritis
   c. gastroesophageal reflux disease
   d. seizure disorders

7. After organ transplantation, immunosuppressants are given to prevent
   a. nephrotoxicity
   b. hepatotoxicity
   c. rejection reactions
   d. bleeding disorders

8. The most common malignancies that occur with immunosuppression include
   a. skin cancers and lymphomas
   b. cancers of the GI tract
   c. renal and liver cancers
   d. brain and spinal cord cancers

9. Clients taking immunosuppressant drugs should be taught
   a. ways to decrease infections
   b. to avoid weight gain
   c. to maintain a good fluid intake
   d. to increase rest and decrease exercise

Selected References

Anderson, D. L. (2004). TNF inhibitors: A new age in rheumatoid arthritis treatment. *American Journal of Nursing, 104*(2), 60–68.

Davis, L. A. (2004). Omalizumab: A novel therapy for allergic asthma. *Annals of Pharmacotherapy, 38,* 1236–1242.

Imperato, A. K., Smiles, S., & Abramson, S. B. (2004). Long-term risks associated with biologic response modifiers used in rheumatic diseases. *Current Opinions in Rheumatology, 16*(3), 199–205.

Johnson, H. J., & Heim-Duthoy, K. L. (2002). Renal transplantation. In J. T. DiPiro, R. L. Talbert, G. C. Yee, G. R. Matzke, B. G. Wells, & L. M. Posey (Eds.), *Pharmacotherapy: A pathophysiologic approach* (5th ed., pp. 843–866). New York: McGraw-Hill.

Olsen, N. J., & Stein, C. M. (2004). New drugs for rheumatoid arthritis. *New England Journal of Medicine, 350,* 2167–2179.

Panaccione, R., & Sandborn, W. J. (2004). Medical therapy of Crohn disease. *Current Opinions in Gastroenterology, 20*(4), 351–359.

Porth, C. M. (2005). *Pathophysiology: Concepts of altered health states* (7th ed.). Philadelphia: Lippincott Williams & Wilkins.

Ruffin, C. G., & Busch, B. E. (2004). Omalizumab: A recombinant humanized anti-IgE antibody for allergic asthma. *American Journal of Health-System Pharmacy, 61*(14), 1449–1459.

Stoffel, J. A., & Somani, A. Z. (2002). Liver transplantation. In J. T. DiPiro, R. L. Talbert, G. C. Yee, G. R. Matzke, B. G. Wells, & L. M. Posey (Eds.), *Pharmacotherapy: A pathophysiologic approach* (5th ed., pp. 743–752). New York: McGraw-Hill.

Suissa, S., Ernst, P., Hudson, M., et al. (2004). Newer disease-modifying antirheumatic drugs and the risk of serious hepatic adverse events in clients with rheumatoid arthritis. *American Journal of Medicine, 117,* 87–92.

Tolkoff-Rubin, N. E., & Rubin, R. H. (2004). The compromised host. In L. Goldman & D. Ausiello (Eds.), *Cecil textbook of medicine* (22nd ed., pp. 1735–1744). Philadelphia: W. B. Saunders.

Wallis, R. S., Broder, M. S., Wong, J. Y., et al. (2004). Granulomatous infectious diseases associated with tumor necrosis factor antagonists. *Clinical Infectious Diseases, 38,* 1261–1265.

Drugs Used in Oncologic Disorders

OBJECTIVES

After studying this chapter, you will be able to:

1. Contrast normal and malignant cells.
2. Describe major types of antineoplastic drugs in terms of mechanism of action, indications for use, administration, and nursing process implications.
3. Discuss the rationales for using antineoplastic drugs in combination with each other, with surgical treatment, and with radiation therapy.
4. Discuss adverse drug effects and their prevention or management.
5. Assist clients/caregivers in preventing or managing symptoms associated with chemotherapy regimens.
6. Teach, promote, and practice reduction of risk factors for development of cancer; early recognition of cancer signs and symptoms; and early implementation of effective treatment measures.

APPLYING YOUR KNOWLEDGE

Julia Gardner is a 60-year-old retired teacher. She has been diagnosed with cancer in her right breast. Prior to her mastectomy, Julia is receiving neoadjuvant chemotherapy. Julia receives trastuzumab (Herceptin), doxorubicin, and paclitaxel (Taxol) IV every 3 weeks. She takes methotrexate PO 2 times a week.

INTRODUCTION

Oncology is the study of malignant neoplasms and their treatment. Drugs used in oncologic disorders include those used to kill, damage, or slow the growth of cancer cells, and those used to prevent or treat adverse drug effects. Antineoplastic drug therapy is a major treatment modality for cancer, along with surgery and radiation therapy.

Major groups of anticancer drugs are the traditional cytotoxic agents (eg, alkylating agents, antimetabolites, antitumor antibiotics, plant alkaloids), newer cytotoxic "biologic targeted therapies" (eg, monoclonal antibodies, growth-factor inhibitors), and hormone inhibitors, which are not cytotoxic. In addition, several drugs are used to ameliorate the adverse effects of cytotoxic drugs (eg, cytoprotectants, including some immunostimulants discussed in Chap. 40). To aid understanding of the drugs used in oncologic disorders, selected characteristics of cancer and the drugs are described below.

Cancer

The term *cancer* is used to describe many disease processes with the common characteristics of uncontrolled cell growth, invasiveness, and metastasis, as well as numerous etiologies, clinical manifestations, and treatments.

Normal Versus Malignant Cells

Normal cells reproduce in response to a need for tissue growth or repair and stop reproduction when the need has been met. The normal cell cycle is the interval between the "birth" of a cell and its division into two daughter cells (Fig. 42-1). The daughter cells may then enter the resting phase (G_0) or proceed through the reproductive cycle to form more new cells. Normal cells are also well differentiated in appearance and function and have a characteristic lifespan.

Malignant cells occupy space, take blood and nutrients away from normal tissues, and serve no useful purpose. They

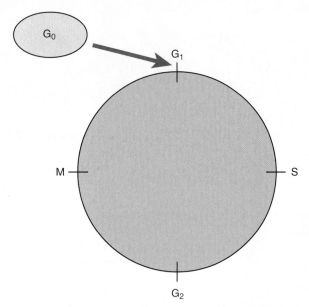

FIGURE 42-1 Normal cell cycle. The normal cell cycle (the interval between the birth of a cell and its division into two daughter cells) involves several phases. During the resting phase (G_0), cells perform all usual functions except replication; that is, they are not dividing but are capable of doing so when stimulated. Different types of cells spend different lengths of time in this phase, after which they either reenter the cell cycle and differentiate or die. During the first active phase (G_1), ribonucleic acid (RNA) and enzymes required for production of deoxyribonucleic acid (DNA) are developed. During the next phase (S), DNA is synthesized for chromosomes. During G_2, RNA is synthesized, and the mitotic spindle is formed. Mitosis occurs in the final phase (M). The resulting two daughter cells may then enter the resting phase (G_0) or proceed through the reproductive cycle.

grow in an uncontrolled fashion and avoid the restraints (eg, contact with other cells) that stop the growth of normal cells. They are undifferentiated, which means they have lost the structural and functional characteristics of the cells from which they originated. They are loosely connected, so that cells break off from the primary tumor and invade adjacent tissues. Loose cells also enter blood and lymph vessels, circulate through the body, and produce additional neoplasms at sites distant from the primary tumor.

A malignant cell develops from a transformed normal cell. The transformation may begin with a random mutation (abnormal structural change in the genetic material of a cell). A mutated cell may be destroyed by body defenses (eg, an immune response), or it may replicate. When the mutated cell eludes destruction by the immune system and begins to reproduce, additional changes that occur during succeeding cell divisions may produce cells with progressively fewer normal and more malignant characteristics. It usually takes years for malignant cells to produce a clinically detectable neoplasm.

Development of Cancer

The cause of cancer is unknown. One theory is that it is caused by mutation of genes, abnormal activation of genes that regu-

late cell growth and mitosis, or lack of tumor-suppressor genes. The abnormal genes, called *oncogenes,* are mutations of normal growth-regulating genes called *proto-oncogenes,* which are present in all body cells. When proto-oncogenes are exposed to carcinogens and genetically altered to oncogenes, they may operate continuously and cause abnormal, disordered, and unregulated cell growth. Unregulated cell growth and proliferation increases the probability of neoplastic transformation of the cell. Tumors of the breast, colon, lung, and bone have been linked to activation of oncogenes.

Tumor-suppressor genes (anti-oncogenes) normally function to inhibit inappropriate cellular growth and proliferation. Abnormal tumor-suppressor genes (ie, absent, damaged, mutated, or inactivated) may be inherited or result from exposure to carcinogens. When these genes are inactivated, a block to proliferation is removed and the cells begin unregulated growth. One tumor suppressor gene, p53, is present in virtually all normal tissues. When cellular deoxyribonucleic acid (DNA) is damaged, the p53 gene allows time for DNA repair and restricts proliferation of cells with abnormal DNA. Mutations of the p53 gene, a common genetic change in cancer, are associated with more than 90% of small cell lung cancers and more than 50% of breast and colon cancers. Mutant p53 proteins can also form complexes with normal p53 proteins and inactivate the function of the normal suppressor gene.

Thus, activation of oncogenes and inactivation of anti-oncogenes probably both play roles in cancer development. Multiple genetic abnormalities are characteristic of cancer cells and may occur concurrently or sequentially.

Overall, evidence indicates that neoplastic transformation is a progressive process involving several generations of cells, with each new generation becoming more like malignant cells. Thus, malignancy probably results from a combination of factors experienced over a person's lifetime, including random cell mutations, exposure to carcinogens, and host characteristics or lifestyle habits that increase susceptibility to cancer development. Some known carcinogens and risk factors are listed in Box 42-1.

After a cancer develops, factors influencing its growth include blood and nutrient supply, immune response, and hormonal stimulation (eg, in tumors of the breast, uterus, ovary, and prostate). Malignant tumors are able to form new blood vessels (a process called *angiogenesis*) to support their growth.

Classification of Malignant Neoplasms

Malignant neoplasms are classified according to the type of tissue involved and other characteristics. With the exception of the acute leukemias, they are considered chronic diseases.

Hematologic malignancies involve the bone marrow and lymphoid tissues; they include leukemias, lymphomas, and multiple myeloma. *Leukemias* are cancers of the bone marrow characterized by overproduction of abnormal white blood cells. The four main types are acute lymphocytic; acute myelogenous; chronic lymphocytic; and chronic myelogenous. *Lymphomas* are tumors of lymphoid tissue characterized by

Box 42-1 Carcinogens and Risk Factors

Environmental Carcinogens

Biologic carcinogens. Viruses linked to cancer include Epstein-Barr (Burkitt's lymphoma, Hodgkin's disease); hepatitis B and C (liver); herpes simplex II (cervix and vulva); human papilloma (cervix, penis, oral cavity, esophagus, larynx); human immunodeficiency (Kaposi's sarcoma); and human T-cell lymphotropic (T-cell leukemia or lymphoma). In addition, *Helicobacter pylori* bacteria are associated with gastric cancer and gastric lymphoma.

Radiation (eg, from sunlight) can damage DNA and cause cell mutations.

Chemicals include many substances that can damage cellular structures and interfere with cell regulation. *Industrial carcinogens* include benzene (bladder cancer), hydrocarbons (lung and skin cancer), polyvinyl chloride (liver cancer), and other substances used in the production of various products. Workers who manufacture the products and people who live in the plant vicinity are most likely to be affected. *Tobacco products,* including cigarettes and smokeless products, contain numerous carcinogens and are associated with cancers of the lungs, mouth, pharynx, larynx, esophagus, and bladder.

Therapeutic drugs are associated with both hematologic and solid neoplasms. The *alkylating antineoplastic drugs* are associated with leukemia, lymphoma, and other cancers. The drugs damage DNA and interfere with growth or replication of tumor cells. At the same time, they may damage the DNA of normal cells and transform some of them into malignant cells. *Immunosuppressants* (eg, azathioprine, cyclosporine, tacrolimus, corticosteroids) are associated with an increased risk of non-Hodgkin's lymphoma and skin cancer in renal transplant patients. Other clients taking immunosuppressant drugs (eg, for rheumatoid arthritis) are at risk for lymphomas, squamous cell carcinoma of skin, and soft tissue sarcomas, but at lower rates than transplant recipients.

Sex hormones are growth factors for certain cells. In women, *estrogens* are associated with breast and endometrial cancer. The antiestrogen tamoxifen is associated with endometrial cancer. In men, *androgens* are associated with prostate cancer; and *anabolic steroids,* especially in high doses and with prolonged use, are associated with hepatic neoplasms.

Host Factors

Age. Except for a few early-childhood cancers, the risks of cancer increase with age.

Alcohol use is associated with cancers of the breast, head and neck, and liver.

Diet. A high-fat diet is associated with breast, colon, and prostate cancer; a low-fiber diet may increase risks of colon cancer.

Gender. Men are more likely to have leukemia and cancer of the urinary bladder, stomach, and pancreas; women are at risk of cancer of the breast, cervix, and endometrium. Lung and colon cancer occur equally in both sexes.

Geography and **ethnicity** are more environmental than hereditary or racial. Immigrants who adopt dietary and lifestyle habits of natives have similar risks and people who live in cities have greater risks because of greater exposure to air pollutants and other carcinogens. In the United States, African Americans have higher rates of multiple myeloma and cancers of the lung, prostate, esophagus, and pancreas than white people.

Heredity. In some families, there is a tendency toward development of cancer (eg, close relatives of premenopausal women with breast cancer are at high risk for breast cancer).

Immunosuppression, whether caused by disease or drug therapy, is associated with an increased risk of lymphomas, skin cancers, and other malignancies.

Obesity is associated with increased risks of developing cancer of the breast, colon, endometrium, esophagus, liver, pancreas, and prostate gland.

Previous cancer is associated with a higher risk of other cancers in those who are treated with chemotherapy or radiation and survive. Secondary cancers are usually attributed to treatments that damage DNA and eventually transform normal cells into malignant cells.

Tobacco use is a major risk factor for cancers of the lung, esophagus, and head and neck. Chemicals in cigarette smoke cause most lung cancer, in smokers and other people exposed to cigarette smoke. Children whose parents smoke have an increased risk of brain cancer, lymphomas, and acute lymphocytic leukemia.

---

abnormal proliferation of the white blood cells normally found in lymphoid tissue. They usually develop within lymph nodes and may occur anywhere, because virtually all body tissues contain lymphoid structures. The two main types are Hodgkin's disease and non-Hodgkin's lymphoma. *Multiple myeloma* is a tumor of the bone marrow in which abnormal plasma cells proliferate. Because normal plasma cells produce antibodies and abnormal plasma cells cannot fulfill this function, the body's immune system is impaired. As the malignant cells expand, they crowd out normal cells, interfere with other bone marrow functions, infiltrate and destroy bone, and eventually metastasize to other tissues, such as the spleen, liver, and lymph nodes.

Solid neoplasms are composed of a mass of malignant cells (parenchyma) and a supporting structure of connective tissue, blood vessels, and lymphatics (stroma). The two major classifications are carcinomas and sarcomas. *Carcinomas* are derived from epithelial tissues (skin, mucous membrane, linings and coverings of viscera) and are the most common type of malignant tumors. They are further classified by cell type, such as adenocarcinoma or basal cell carcinoma. *Sarcomas* are derived from connective tissue (muscle, bone, cartilage, fibrous tissue, fat, blood vessels). They are subclassified by cell type (eg, osteogenic sarcoma, angiosarcoma).

Grading and Staging of Malignant Neoplasms

When a malignant neoplasm is identified, it is further "graded" according to the degree of malignancy and "staged" according to tissue involvement. Grades 1 and 2 are similar to the normal tissue of origin and show cellular differentiation; grades 3 and 4 are unlike the normal tissue of origin, less differentiated, and more malignant. Staging indicates whether the neoplasm is localized or metastasized and which organs are involved. These characteristics assist in treatment (eg, localized tumors are usually amenable to surgical or radiation therapy; metastatic disease requires systemic chemotherapy).

Effects of Cancer on the Host

Effects vary according to the location and extent of the disease process. There are few effects initially. As the neoplasm grows, effects occur when the tumor becomes large enough to cause pressure, distortion, or deficient blood supply in surrounding tissues; interfere with organ function; obstruct ducts and organs; and impair nutrition of normal tissues. More specific effects include anemia, malnutrition, pain, immunosuppression, infection, hemorrhagic tendencies, thromboembolism, hypercalcemia, cachexia, and various symptoms related to impaired function of affected organs and tissues.

Overview of Antineoplastic Drug Therapy

One definition of *chemotherapy* is the use of medications to treat cancer (rather than surgical or radiation therapy). However, the term is most often used to indicate the use of traditional cytotoxic antineoplastic drugs (as differentiated from biologic or hormonal therapy). Actually, except for hormone inhibitors that slow the growth of cancer cells stimulated by hormones, the purpose of all antineoplastic drugs is to damage or kill cancer cells (ie, be cytotoxic). Most chemotherapy regimens involve a combination of drugs that work together to kill cancer cells. Combining drugs with different actions at the cellular level is thought to destroy a greater number of cancer cells and reduce the risk of the cancer developing drug resistance. Chemotherapy is usually administered in cycles, depending on the type of cancer and which drugs are used. Cycles involve taking the drugs daily, weekly, or monthly for a few months or several months, with a recovery period following each treatment cycle. Recovery periods allow time for the client's body to rest and produce new, healthy cells.

Because the consequences of inappropriate or erroneous drug therapy may be fatal for clients (from the disease or the treatment), chemotherapy regimens should be managed by medical oncologists experienced in use of the drugs. Because of the drugs' toxicity, nurses who administer intravenous (IV) cytotoxic chemotherapy should be specially trained and certified in handling and administering the drugs safely and accurately.

TRADITIONAL CYTOTOXIC ANTINEOPLASTIC DRUGS

These drugs comprise the largest, oldest, and most diverse group of antineoplastic drugs. They are described below and in Table 42-1.

General Characteristics

● Most drugs kill malignant cells by interfering with cell replication, with the supply and use of nutrients (eg, amino acids, purines, pyrimidines), or with the genetic materials in the cell nucleus (DNA or RNA).

● The drugs act during the cell's reproductive cycle (Fig. 42-2). Some, called *cell cycle–specific,* act mainly during specific phases such as DNA synthesis or formation of the mitotic spindle. Others act during any phase of the cell cycle and are called *cell cycle–nonspecific.*

● Cytotoxic drugs are most active against rapidly dividing cells, both normal and malignant. Commonly damaged normal cells are those of the bone marrow, the lining of the gastrointestinal (GI) tract, and the hair follicles. Healthy cells usually recover fairly soon.

● Each drug dose kills a specific percentage of cells. To achieve a cure, all malignant cells must be killed or reduced to a small number that can be killed by the person's immune system.

● Antineoplastic drugs may induce drug-resistant malignant cells. Mechanisms may include inhibiting drug uptake or activation, increasing the rate of drug inactivation, pumping the drug out of the cell before it can act, increasing cellular repair of DNA damaged by the drugs, or altering metabolic pathways and target enzymes of the drugs. Mutant cells also may emerge.

● Most cytotoxic antineoplastic drugs are potential teratogens.

● Most antineoplastic drugs are given orally or IV; some are given topically, intrathecally, or by instillation into a body cavity.

● A few drugs are available in liposomal preparations. These preparations increase drug concentration in malignant tissues and decrease concentration in normal tissues, thereby increasing effectiveness while decreasing toxicity. For example, liposomal doxorubicin and daunorubicin reduce the drugs' cardiotoxic effects.

● Common adverse effects include alopecia, anemia, bleeding, fatigue, mucositis, nausea and vomiting, neutropenia, and thrombocytopenia. Less common problems may include damage to the heart, liver, lungs, kidneys, or nerves. In general, adverse effects depend on the specific drugs used and the client's health status.

● With treatment of leukemias and lymphomas, a serious, life-threatening adverse effect called *tumor lysis syndrome* may occur. This syndrome occurs when large numbers of cancer cells are killed or damaged and release their contents into the bloodstream. As a result, hyper-

(text continues on page 698)

Table 42-1 Drugs at a Glance: Cytotoxic Antineoplastic Drugs

GENERIC/TRADE NAME	ROUTES AND DOSAGE RANGES*	CLINICAL USES	ADVERSE EFFECTS
Alkylating Drugs			
NITROGEN MUSTARD DERIVATIVES			
Chlorambucil (Leukeran)	PO 0.1–0.2 mg/kg/d for 3–6 wk. Maintenance therapy, 0.03–0.1 mg/kg/d	Chronic lymphocytic leukemia, Hodgkin's and non-Hodgkin's lymphomas	Bone marrow depression, hepatotoxicity, secondary leukemia
Cyclophosphamide (Cytoxan)	Induction therapy, PO 1–5 mg/kg/d; IV 20–40 mg/kg in divided doses over 2–5 days. Maintenance therapy, PO 1–5 mg/kg daily	Hodgkin's disease; non-Hodgkin's lymphomas; leukemias; cancer of breast, lung, or ovary; multiple myeloma; neuroblastoma	Bone marrow depression, nausea, vomiting, alopecia, hemorrhagic cystitis, hypersensitivity reactions, secondary leukemia or bladder cancer
Ifosfamide (Ifex)	IV 1.2 g/m^2/d for 5 consecutive d. Repeat every 3 wk or after white blood cell and platelet counts return to normal after a dose.	Germ cell testicular cancer	Bone marrow depression, hemorrhagic cystitis, nausea and vomiting, alopecia, CNS depression, seizures
Melphalan (Alkeran)	PO 6 mg/d for 2–3 wk, then 28 drug-free days, then 2 mg daily IV 16 mg/m^2 every 2 wk for 4 doses, then every 4 wk	Multiple myeloma, ovarian cancer	Bone marrow depression, nausea and vomiting, hypersensitivity reactions
NITROSOUREAS			
Carmustine (BiCNU, Gliadel)	IV 150–200 mg/m^2 every 6 wk Wafer, implanted in brain after tumor resection	Hodgkin's disease, non-Hodgkin's lymphomas, multiple myeloma, brain tumors	Bone marrow depression, nausea, vomiting
Lomustine (CCNU)	PO 130 mg/m^2 every 6 wk	Hodgkin's disease, brain tumors	Nausea and vomiting, bone marrow depression
PLATINUM COMPOUNDS			
Carboplatin (Paraplatin)	IV infusion 360 mg/m^2 on day 1 every 4 wk	Palliation of ovarian cancer	Bone marrow depression, nausea and vomiting, nephrotoxicity
Cisplatin (Platinol)	IV 100 mg/m^2 once every 4 wk	Advanced carcinomas of testes, bladder, ovary	Nausea, vomiting, anaphylaxis, nephrotoxicity, bone marrow depression, ototoxicity
Oxaliplatin (Eloxatin)	IV infusion 85 mg/m^2 every 2 wk	Advanced colon cancer	Anaphylaxis, anemia, increased risk of bleeding or infection
Antimetabolites			
Capecitabine (Xeloda)	PO 1250 mg/m^2 q12h for 2 wk, then a rest period of 1 wk, then repeat cycle	Metastatic breast cancer, colorectal cancer	Bone marrow depression, nausea, vomiting, diarrhea, mucositis
Cladribine (Leustatin)	IV infusion 0.09 mg/kg/d for 7 consecutive d	Hairy cell leukemia	Bone marrow depression, nausea, vomiting
Cytarabine (Cytosar-U)	IV infusion 100 mg/m^2/d for 7 d	Leukemias of adults and children	Bone marrow depression, nausea, vomiting, anaphylaxis, mucositis, diarrhea
Fludarabine (Fludara)	IV 25 mg/m^2/d for 5 consecutive d; repeat every 28 d	Chronic lymphocytic leukemia	Bone marrow depression, nausea, vomiting, diarrhea
Fluorouracil (5-FU) (Adrucil, Efudex, Fluoroplex)	IV 12 mg/kg/d for 4 d, then 6 mg/kg every other day for 4 doses	Carcinomas of the breast, colon, stomach, and pancreas	Bone marrow depression, nausea, vomiting, mucositis

(continued)

Table 42-1 Drugs at a Glance: Cytotoxic Antineoplastic Drugs (continued)

GENERIC/TRADE NAME	ROUTES AND DOSAGE RANGES*	CLINICAL USES	ADVERSE EFFECTS
	Topical, apply to skin cancer lesion twice daily for several weeks	Solar keratoses, basal cell carcinoma	Pain, pruritus, burning at site of application
Gemcitabine (Gemzar)	IV 1000 mg/m² once weekly up to 7 wk or toxicity, withhold for 1 wk, then once weekly for 3 wk and withhold for 1 wk	Lung and pancreatic cancer	Bone marrow depression, nausea, vomiting, flu-like symptoms, skin rash
Mercaptopurine (Purinethol)	PO 2.5 mg/kg/d (100–200 mg for average adult)	Acute and chronic leukemias	Bone marrow depression, nausea, vomiting, mucositis
P Methotrexate (MTX) (Rheumatrex)	Acute leukemia in children, induction, PO, IV 3 mg/m²/d; maintenance, PO 30 mg/m² twice weekly Choriocarcinoma, PO, IM 15 mg/m² daily for 5 d	Leukemias; non-Hodgkin's lymphomas; osteosarcoma; choriocarcinoma of testes; cancers of breast, lung, head and neck	Bone marrow depression, nausea, vomiting, mucositis, diarrhea, fever, alopecia
Pemetrexed (Alimta)	IV infusion 500 mg/m² over 10 min, every 21 d	Non–small cell lung cancer	Mucositis, skin rash
Antitumor Antibiotics **Bleomycin** (Blenoxane)	IV, IM, Sub-Q 0.25–0.5 units/kg once or twice weekly	Squamous cell carcinoma, Hodgkin's and non-Hodgkin's lymphomas, testicular carcinoma	Pulmonary toxicity, mucositis, alopecia, nausea, vomiting, hypersensitivity reactions
Dactinomycin (Actinomycin D, Cosmegen)	IV 15 mcg/kg/d for 5 d and repeated every 2–4 wk	Rhabdomyosarcoma, Wilms' tumor, choriocarcinoma, testicular carcinoma, Ewing's sarcoma	Bone marrow depression, nausea, vomiting. Extravasation may lead to tissue necrosis.
Daunorubicin conventional	IV 25–45 mg/m² daily for 3 d every 3–4 wk	Acute leukemias, lymphomas	Same as doxorubicin, below
Daunorubicin liposomal (DaunoXome)	IV infusion, 40 mg/m² every 2 wk	AIDS-related Kaposi's sarcoma	Bone marrow depression, nausea, vomiting
Doxorubicin conventional (Adriamycin)	Adults, IV 60–75 mg/m² every 21 d Children, IV 30 mg/m² daily for 3 d, repeated every 4 wk	Acute leukemias; lymphomas; carcinomas of breast, lung, and ovary	Bone marrow depression, alopecia, mucositis, GI upset, cardiomyopathy. Extravasation may lead to tissue necrosis.
Doxorubicin liposomal (Doxil)	IV infusion, 20 mg/m², once every 3 wk	AIDS-related Kaposi's sarcoma	Bone marrow depression, nausea, vomiting, fever, alopecia
Epirubicin (Ellence)	IV infusion 120 mg/m² every 3–4 wk	Breast cancer	Cardiotoxicity
Idarubicin (Idamycin)	IV injection 12 mg/m²/d for 3 d, with cytarabine	Acute myeloid leukemia	Same as doxorubicin, above
Mitomycin (Mutamycin)	IV 20 mg/m² every 6–8 wk	Metastatic carcinomas of stomach and pancreas	Bone marrow depression, nausea, vomiting. Extravasation may lead to tissue necrosis.
Mitoxantrone (Novantrone)	IV infusion 12 mg/m² on days 1–3, for induction of remission in leukemia	Acute nonlymphocytic leukemia, prostate cancer	Bone marrow depression, congestive heart failure, nausea
Pentostatin (Nipent)	IV 4 mg/m² every other week	Hairy cell leukemia unresponsive to interferon alfa	Bone marrow depression, hepatotoxicity, nausea, vomiting
Valrubicin (Valstar)	Intravesically, 800 mg once weekly for 6 wk	Bladder cancer	Dysuria, urgency, frequency, bladder spasms, hematuria

Table 42-1 Drugs at a Glance: Cytotoxic Antineoplastic Drugs (continued)

GENERIC/TRADE NAME	ROUTES AND DOSAGE RANGES*	CLINICAL USES	ADVERSE EFFECTS
Plant Alkaloids			
CAMPTOTHECINS			
Irinotecan (Camptosar)	IV infusion, 125 mg/m² once weekly for 4 wk, then a 2-wk rest period; repeat regimen	Metastatic cancer of colon or rectum	Bone marrow depression, diarrhea
Topetecan (Hycamtin)	IV infusion 1.5 mg/m² daily for 5 consecutive days every 21 d	Advanced ovarian cancer, small-cell lung cancer	Bone marrow depression, nausea, vomiting, diarrhea
PODOPHYLLOTOXINS			
Etoposide (VePesid)	IV 50–100 mg/m²/d on days 1–5, or 100 mg/m²/d on days 1, 3, and 5, every 3–4 wk PO 2 times the IV dose	Testicular cancer, small-cell lung cancer	Bone marrow depression, allergic reactions, nausea, vomiting, alopecia
Teniposide (Vumon)	IV infusion 165 mg/m² twice weekly for 8–9 doses	Acute lymphocytic leukemia in children	Same as etoposide, above
TAXANES			
Docetaxel (Taxotere)	IV infusion 60–100 mg/m², every 3 wk	Advanced breast cancer, non–small cell lung cancer	Bone marrow depression, nausea, vomiting, hypersensitivity reactions,
Paclitaxel (Taxol)	IV infusion 135 mg/m² every 3 wk	Advanced ovarian cancer, advanced breast cancer, non–small cell lung cancer, AIDS-related Kaposi's sarcoma	Bone marrow depression, allergic reactions, hypotension, bradycardia, nausea, vomiting
VINCA ALKALOIDS			
Vinblastine (Velban)	Adults, IV 3.7–11.1 mg/m² (average 5.5–7.4 mg/m²) weekly Children, IV 2.5–7.5 mg/m² weekly	Metastatic testicular carcinoma, Hodgkin's disease	Bone marrow depression, nausea, vomiting. Extravasation may lead to tissue necrosis.
Vincristine (Oncovin)	Adults, IV 1.4 mg/m² weekly Children, IV 2 mg/m² weekly	Hodgkin's and other lymphomas, acute leukemia, neuroblastoma, Wilms' tumor	Peripheral neuropathy. Extravasation may lead to tissue necrosis.
Vinorelbine (Navelbine)	IV injection 30 mg/m² once weekly	Non–small cell lung cancer	Bone marrow depression, peripheral neuropathy. Extravasation may lead to tissue necrosis.
Miscellaneous Agents			
L-Asparaginase (Elspar)	IV 1000 IU/kg/d for 10 d	Acute lymphocytic leukemia	Hypersensitivity reactions, including anaphylaxis
Hydroxyurea (Hydrea)	PO 80 mg/kg as a single dose every third day or 20–30 mg/kg as a single dose daily	Chronic myelocytic leukemia, melanoma, ovarian cancer, head and neck cancer	Bone marrow depression, nausea, vomiting, peripheral neuritis
Levamisole (Ergamisol)	PO 50 mg q8h for 3 d every 2 wk	Colon cancer, with fluorouracil	Nausea, vomiting, diarrhea
Procarbazine (Matulane)	PO 2–4 mg/kg/d for 1 wk, then 4–6 mg/kg/d	Hodgkin's disease	Bone marrow depression, mucositis, CNS depression
Temozolomide (Temodar)	PO 150 mg/m² once daily for 5 d, then 200 mg/m² every 28 d	Brain tumors	Bone marrow depression

*Dosages may vary significantly or change often, according to use in different types of cancer and in different combinations.

AIDS, acquired immunodeficiency syndrome; IM, intramuscular; IV, intravenous; PO, oral; Sub-Q, subcutaneous.

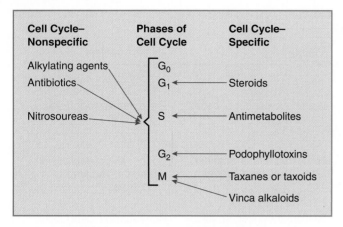

Cell Cycle– Nonspecific	Phases of Cell Cycle	Cell Cycle– Specific
Alkylating agents	G_0	
Antibiotics	G_1 ←	Steroids
Nitrosoureas	S ←	Antimetabolites
	G_2 ←	Podophyllotoxins
	M ←	Taxanes or taxoids
		Vinca alkaloids

FIGURE 42–2 Cell cycle effects of cytotoxic antineoplastic drugs.

kalemia, hyperphosphatemia, hyperuricemia, hypomagnesemia, hypocalcemia, and acidosis develop. Signs and symptoms depend on the severity of the metabolic imbalances, but may include GI upset, fatigue, altered mental status, hypertension, muscle cramps, paresthesias (numbness and tingling), tetany, seizures, electrocardiographic changes (eg, wide QRS waves, dysrhythmias), cardiac arrest, reduced urine output, and acute renal failure. The condition can be prevented or minimized by aggressive hydration with IV normal saline, alkalinization with IV sodium bicarbonate, and administration of allopurinol (eg, 300 mg daily for adults and 10 mg/kg/d for children) to reduce uric acid levels. Maintaining a urine pH of 7 or more prevents renal failure from precipitation of uric acid crystals in the kidneys. Treatment of hyperkalemia may include IV dextrose and regular insulin (to drive potassium into cells) or Kayexalate to eliminate potassium in feces. Treatment of hyperphosphatemia may include administration of aluminum hydroxide or another phosphate-binding agent. Hemodialysis may be used if the other measures are ineffective.

Indications for Use

Cytotoxic antineoplastic drugs are used to cure the disease, relieve symptoms, or induce or maintain remissions (symptom-free periods). In hematologic neoplasms, drug therapy is the treatment of choice because the disease is systemic rather than localized. In solid tumors, drug therapy may be used before or after surgery or radiation therapy and when metastasis occurs.

Antineoplastic drugs are sometimes used in the treatment of nonmalignant conditions. For example, small doses of methotrexate (MTX) are used for rheumatoid arthritis and psoriasis.

Classifications and Mechanisms of Action

Cytotoxic antineoplastic drugs are usually classified in terms of their mechanisms of action (alkylating agents and antimetabolites) or their sources (plant alkaloids, antibiotics).

Alkylating Agents

Alkylating agents include nitrogen mustard derivatives, nitrosoureas, and platinum compounds. *Nitrogen mustard derivatives* (eg, cyclophosphamide) interfere with cell division and the structure of DNA during all phases of the malignant cell cycle. As a result, they have a broad spectrum of activity. They are most effective in hematologic malignancies but also are used to treat breast, lung, and ovarian tumors. All of these drugs cause significant bone marrow depression (myelosuppression) and frequent complete blood counts (CBCs) are required.

Nitrosoureas also interfere with DNA replication and RNA synthesis and may inhibit essential enzymatic reactions of cancer cells. They are cell cycle–nonspecific and have been used in clients with GI, lung, and brain tumors. They are highly lipid soluble and therefore enter the brain and cerebrospinal fluid more readily than other antineoplastic drugs. They cause delayed bone marrow depression, with maximum leukopenia and thrombocytopenia occurring 5 to 6 weeks after drug administration. As a result, the drugs are given less often than other drugs, and CBCs are needed weekly for at least 6 weeks after a dose.

Platinum compounds are cell cycle–nonspecific agents that inhibit DNA, RNA, and protein synthesis. Cisplatin is used to treat both hematologic and solid cancers. Adverse effects include severe nausea and vomiting and nephrotoxicity. Carboplatin is used to treat endometrial and ovarian carcinomas and it produces bone marrow depression as a major adverse effect. Oxaliplatin (Eloxatin) is used to treat colorectal cancer, with 5-fluorouracil and leucovorin. Adverse effects include peripheral neuropathy, vomiting, diarrhea, and anemia.

Antimetabolites

Antimetabolites are diverse drugs that are allowed to enter cancer cells because they are similar to metabolites or nutrients needed by the cells for reproduction. Inside the cell, the drugs may replace normal metabolites or inhibit essential enzymes. These actions deprive the cell of substances needed for formation of DNA or cause formation of abnormal DNA. The drugs are cell cycle–specific because they exert their cytotoxic effects only during the S phase of the cell's reproductive cycle, when DNA is being synthesized.

This group includes folic acid antagonists (eg, 🅟 methotrexate, pemetrexed), purine antagonists (eg, mercaptopurine), and pyrimidine antagonists (eg, fluorouracil). These drugs have been used to treat many types of cancers, but they are most effective against rapidly growing tumors, and individual drugs vary in their effectiveness with different kinds of cancer. Toxic effects include bone marrow depression, mucositis and ulceration of the GI tract, and hair loss (alopecia). Pemetrexed (Alimta), a newer antimetabolite which blocks folate and enzymes essential for cancer cell reproduction, may also increase blood levels of homocysteine. Homocysteine is produced when proteins are broken down in the blood and elevated blood levels are considered a risk factor for coronary artery disease and stroke. Treatment with folic acid and vitamin B$_{12}$ supplements, which can reduce homocysteine blood levels, is required for all clients taking the drug.

APPLYING YOUR KNOWLEDGE 42-1
Because Julia is being treated as an outpatient, it is extremely important that an appropriate plan of care be made to allow her to care for the adverse effects of these medications at home. What are the most common adverse effects of the methotrexate and what nursing interventions should be anticipated?

Antitumor Antibiotics

These drugs (eg, **doxorubicin**) bind to DNA so that DNA and RNA transcription is blocked. They are active in all phases of the cell cycle and their cytotoxic effects are similar to those of the alkylating agents. Major toxicities are bone marrow depression and GI upset. Doxorubicin and related drugs also cause cardiotoxicity and tissue necrosis if extravasation (leaking of medication into soft tissues around the venipuncture site) occurs. Bleomycin may cause significant pulmonary toxicity.

Plant Alkaloids

Plant alkaloids include derivatives of camptothecin (eg, topotecan), podophyllotoxin (eg, etoposide), taxanes (eg, paclitaxel), and plants of the *Vinca* genus (eg, **vincristine**). These drugs vary in their characteristics and clinical uses.

Camptothecins (also called *DNA topoisomerase inhibitors*) inhibit an enzyme required for DNA replication and repair. They have activity in several types of cancers, including colorectal, lung, and ovarian cancers. Dose-limiting toxicity is myelosuppression.

Podophyllotoxins act mainly in the G$_2$ phase of the cell cycle and prevent mitosis. Etoposide is used mainly to treat testicular and small cell lung cancer; teniposide is used mainly for childhood acute lymphocytic leukemia. Dose-limiting toxicity is myelosuppression.

Taxanes inhibit cell division (antimitotic effects). They are used mainly for advanced breast and ovarian cancers. Dose-limiting toxicity is neutropenia.

Vinca alkaloids are cell cycle–specific agents that stop mitosis. These drugs have similar structures but different antineoplastic activities and adverse effects. Vincristine is used to treat Hodgkin's disease, acute lymphoblastic leukemia, and non-Hodgkin's lymphomas. Vinblastine is used to treat Hodgkin's disease and choriocarcinoma; vinorelbine is used to treat non–small cell lung cancer. The drugs can cause severe tissue damage with extravasation. In addition, vinblastine and vinorelbine are more likely to cause bone marrow depression, and vincristine is more likely to cause peripheral nerve toxicity.

Miscellaneous Cytotoxic Agents

Miscellaneous agents vary in their sources, mechanisms of action, indications for use, and toxic effects. *L-Asparaginase* (Elspar) is an enzyme that inhibits protein synthesis and reproduction by depriving cells of required amino acids. It is used to treat acute lymphocytic leukemia and can cause allergic reactions, including anaphylaxis. *Pegaspargase* (Oncaspar) is a modified formulation for people who are hypersensitive to Elspar. *Hydroxyurea* acts in the S phase of the cell cycle to impair DNA synthesis. It is used to treat leukemia, melanoma, and advanced ovarian cancer. A major adverse effect is myelosuppression. *Procarbazine* inhibits DNA, RNA, and protein synthesis. It is used to treat Hodgkin's disease. It is a monoamine oxidase inhibitor and may cause hypertension if given with adrenergic drugs, tricyclic antidepressants, or foods with high tyramine content (see Chap. 10). Common adverse effects include leukopenia and thrombocytopenia.

BIOLOGIC TARGETED ANTINEOPLASTIC DRUGS

Two major mechanisms in cancer development are thought to be failure of the immune system to eliminate mutant, premalignant, and malignant cells and failure of the growth-regulating mechanisms to control the proliferation of mutant, premalignant, and malignant cells. As increased understanding of cancer-cell biology has evolved during recent years, much research has focused on biologic agents to stimulate the immune system to fight cancer cells or to inhibit biologic processes that allow cancer cells to grow and proliferate.

Treatment of cancer with biologic agents is a growing modality as researchers try to increase anticancer effectiveness and decrease the adverse effects of traditional cytotoxic chemotherapy. Biologic antineoplastic drugs include immunotherapy drugs and some newer drugs that "target" biologic processes of malignant cells. Some immunologic anticancer drugs are discussed in Chapter 40 (eg, bacillus Calmette-Guérin vaccine for bladder cancer; interferon alfa for AIDS-related Kaposi's sarcoma, selected leukemias, malignant melanoma, and non-Hodgkin's lymphoma; and interleukin-2 for renal cell carcinoma). Other available drugs are monoclonal antibodies, tyrosine kinase inhibitors, and a proteasome inhibitor. These drugs are described below and in Table 42-2.

Monoclonal Antibodies

Monoclonal antibodies (see Chap. 41) are produced from one cell line. Early murine (mouse-derived) antibodies produced problems as hosts' immune systems reacted against the foreign protein. Most currently available drugs are partially or wholly humanized and were developed to target specific cellular components. In cancer, these drugs act by one of three main mechanisms. **Alemtuzumab** (Campath) and **rituximab** (Rituxan) bind to an antigen on normal T and B lymphocytes and malignant lymphoid cells to activate antibody- and complement-mediated cytotoxicity. **Bevacizumab** (Avastin), **cetuximab**

Table 42–2 Drugs at a Glance: Biologic Antineoplastic Drugs

GENERIC/TRADE NAMES	ROUTES AND DOSAGE RANGES	CLINICAL USES	ADVERSE EFFECTS
Monoclonal Antibodies			
Alemtuzumab (Campath IH)	IV infusion, initially, 3 mg/d as a 2-hour infusion; increase to 10 mg/d, then to 30 mg/d as tolerated. Maintenance, 30 mg/d 3 times weekly on alternate days for up to 12 wk	Treat B-cell chronic lymphocytic leukemia in patients who have been previously treated with alkylating agents and fludarabine	Allergic infusion reactions (dyspnea, fever, chills, skin rash), immunosuppression, hypotension, hypertension, peripheral edema, nausea, vomiting, diarrhea, mucositis
Bevacizumab (Avastin)	IV infusion, 5 mg/kg once every 14 d until disease progression is detected	Colorectal cancer	Heart failure, hemorrhage, hypertension, diarrhea, leukopenia, pain, dyspnea, dermatitis, stomatitis, vomiting
Cetuximab (Erbitux)	IV infusion, initially, 400 mg/m^2 over 2 h; maintenance, 250 mg/m^2 over 1 h once weekly	Metastatic colorectal cancer	Anemia, leukopenia, infusion reaction, nausea, sepsis, skin rash, diarrhea, stomatitis, vomiting, dyspnea, fever
Gemtuzumab ozogamicin (Mylotarg)	IV infusion, 9 mg/m^2, for 2 doses, 14 d apart	Acute myeloid leukemia	Chills, fever, nausea, vomiting, diarrhea
Ibritumomab tiuxetan (Zevalin)	See literature	Non-Hodgkin's lymphoma, with rituximab	Severe or fatal infusion reaction, severe bone marrow depression
Rituximab (Rituxan)	IV infusion, 375 mg/m^2 once weekly for 4 doses	Non-Hodgkin's lymphoma	Hypersensitivity reactions, cardiac dysrhythmias
Tositumomab and Iodine 131-Itositumomab (Bexxar)	See literature	Non-Hodgkin's lymphoma	Fever, chills, nausea, vomiting, skin rash, headache, cough, infection, pain
Trastuzumab (Herceptin)	IV infusion, 4 mg/kg initially, then 2 mg/kg once weekly	Metastatic breast cancer	Cardiotoxicity (dyspnea, edema, heart failure)
Tyrosine Kinase Inhibitors			
Gefitinib (Iressa)	PO 250 mg daily	Non–small cell lung cancer	Nausea, vomiting, diarrhea, skin rash
			Nausea, vomiting, diarrhea, skin rash
Erlotinib (Tarceva)	PO 150 mg daily	Non-small cell lung cancer; brain glioma	Dyspnea, edema, fever, nausea, vomiting, diarrhea, hemorrhage, neutropenia, thrombocytopenia, musculoskeletal pain
Imatinib (Gleevec)	Adults, PO 400–800 mg daily. Children 3 y and older, 260–340 mg/m^2/d	Chronic myeloid leukemia, gastrointestinal stromal tumors	
Proteasome Inhibitor			
Bortezomib (Velcade)	IV injection, 1.3 mg/m^2, twice weekly for 2 wk (eg, days 1, 4, 8, 11) followed by 10-d rest period	Multiple myeloma	Edema, hypotension, nausea, vomiting, diarrhea, dyspnea, anemia, neutropenia, thrombocytopenia.

IV, intravenous; PO, oral.

(Erbitux), and **trastuzumab** (Herceptin) bind to growth factors or growth factor receptors found on blood vessels, colorectal cancer cells, and breast cancer cells, respectively, to prevent the growth factors from becoming activated and stimulating cell growth. For example, bevacizumab was developed to bind with vascular endothelial growth factor (VEGF) and inhibit the formation of the new blood vessels required for tumor growth. In addition, trastuzumab was developed to bind with human epidermal growth factor receptor 2 (HER2), of which 25% to 30% of women with breast cancer have an excessive number. **Gemtuzumab ozogamicin** (Mylotarg), **ibritumomab tiuxetan** (Zevalin), and **tositumomab and iodine I 131 tositumomab** (Bexxar) are conjugated with a radioisotope or toxin to increase anticancer effectiveness.

Serious adverse effects of these drugs include a potentially fatal hypersensitivity-type infusion reaction (eg, chills, fever, bronchospasm, dyspnea, skin rash or urticaria) and bone marrow depression (eg, anemia, leukopenia, thrombocytopenia). To prevent or decrease infusion reactions, premedication with diphenhydramine (Benadryl) and acetaminophen is recommended. With alemtuzumab, a very high risk of infection results because the drug depletes normal B and T lymphocytes. As a result, prophylactic antimicrobial drugs are recommended during and for 3 months after alemtuzumab administration. Severe cardiotoxicity, including heart failure, has also been reported, more often with bevacizumab and trastuzumab. With trastuzumab, clients at higher risk of cardiotoxicity include those 60 years and older and those who have received doxorubicin (or a related drug) or cyclophosphamide. Left ventricular function should be evaluated in all clients before and during treatment and trastuzumab should be discontinued in those who develop significant decreases.

Monoclonal antibodies may be used alone or in combination with traditional cytotoxic antineoplastic drugs and other treatment modalities. Most of the drugs are relatively new and their roles in clinical oncology continue to be investigated. Most are also being investigated for use in additional types of cancer and some other conditions.

APPLYING YOUR KNOWLEDGE 42-2
Julia asks why she must take the Herceptin because there are such serious concerns about an allergic reaction to the monoclonal antibodies. How would you respond?

Growth Factor and Tyrosine Kinase Inhibitors

Growth factors such as epidermal growth factor (EGF, which stimulates the growth of epithelial cells in the skin and other organs) and platelet-derived growth factor (PDGF, which stimulates the proliferation of vascular smooth muscle and endothelial cells) bind to receptors on cell membrane surfaces or within cells and initiate intracellular events that result in cell growth. EGF is normally produced in the kidneys and salivary glands and is found in almost all body fluids. When EGF binds to the external portion of the EGF receptor, it stimulates gene expression, cell proliferation, programmed cell death (apoptosis), and angiogenesis.

The EGF receptor (EGFR; also called the erbB1 and tyrosine kinase receptor), which is found in normal body cells and some malignant cells, has three distinctive areas (see Fig. 42-3). One area is on the cell membrane surface and available to combine with EGF. A second area crosses the cell membrane. A third, an intracellular area, contains tyrosine kinase enzymes. Tyrosine kinase enzymes play an important role in the proliferation and differentiation of cells.

Gefitinib (Iressa) and **erlotinib** (Tarceva) inhibit the tyrosine kinase enzyme portion of the EGFR. This action inhibits cell proliferation and induces cell death. Both drugs are used to treat advanced non-small cell lung cancer, the most common type of lung cancer, which is known to overexpress the EGFR. Erlotinib is also used to treat malignant glioma, a type of brain tumor. Adverse effects of these drugs include skin rash, diarrhea, nausea, and vomiting. In addition, interstitial lung disease has been reported in some clients, with a few deaths. Clients should be monitored for acute onset of dyspnea, shortness of breath, or pneumonitis. If interstitial lung disease is confirmed, gefitinib or erlotinib should be discontinued. These drugs are pregnancy risk category D and women of childbearing potential should avoid pregnancy during drug use and for at least 2 weeks afterward.

Gefitinib is slowly absorbed with oral administration, reaches peak plasma levels in 3 to 7 hours, and has a half-life of about 48 hours. It is metabolized in the liver and excreted mainly in feces (86%). Erlotinib is approximately 60% absorbed after an oral dose; peak plasma levels occur 4 hours after dosing and food increases bioavailability. The drug is highly protein bound (93%), has a half-life of 36 hours, is metabolized in the liver, and is excreted mainly (83%) in feces. Both of these drugs are metabolized mainly by cytochrome P450 3A4 enzymes and interact with drugs that induce (eg, rifampin, phenytoin) or inhibit (eg, clarithromycin, itraconazole) these enzymes. Dosage may need to be increased with concurrent administration of inducers or decreased with concurrent use of inhibitors.

Imatinib (Gleevec) inhibits several tyrosine kinase enzymes that are essential to the growth of some cancer cells, including an abnormal type of tyrosine kinase thought to be the main cause of chronic myelogenous leukemia (CML) and the tyrosine kinases activated by PDGF and stem cell factor (SCF). This action inhibits cell proliferation and induces cell death. The drug is used to treat CML and a rare type of cancer called gastrointestinal stromal tumor. It is well absorbed with oral administration, and peak serum levels are reached in 2 to 4 hours. It is highly protein bound (95%), its elimination half-life is 18 hours, it is metabolized in the liver, and it is excreted mainly as metabolites in feces (66%) and as unchanged drug (20%). Adverse effects include edema, musculoskeletal pain, nausea, and anemia. Imatinib is pregnancy risk category D and women of childbearing potential should avoid pregnancy while taking the drug.

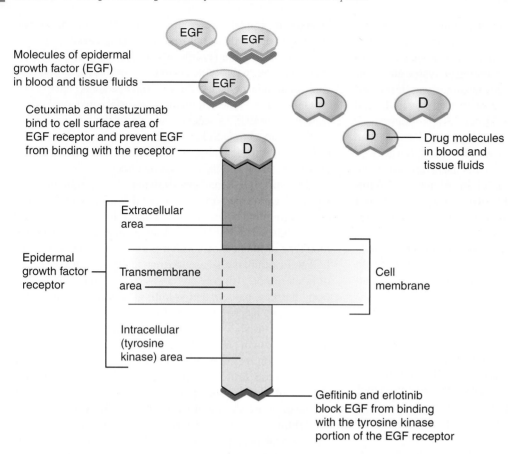

FIGURE 42-3 Actions of selected biologic targeted drugs. These drugs prevent epidermal growth factor (EGF) from combining with its receptors and thereby prevent or decrease cell growth. Cetuximab and trastuzumab bind with the extracellular portion of the EGF receptor; gefitinib and erlotinib block the intracellular (tyrosine kinase) portion of the EGF receptor.

Imatinib is metabolized mainly by cytochrome P450 3A4 enzymes and interacts with drugs that induce (eg, rifampin, phenytoin) or inhibit (eg, clarithromycin, itraconazole) these enzymes. Dosage may need to be increased with concurrent administration of inducers or decreased with concurrent use of inhibitors.

Proteasome Inhibitor

Proteasomes are enzyme complexes in the cytoplasm and nucleus of all body cells, both normal and malignant. These enzymes regulate intracellular proteins. **Bortezomib** (Velcade) inhibits proteasomes, affects multiple proteins within cells, and is thought to have multiple mechanisms of cytotoxicity (eg, preventing formation of new blood vessels in tumors and accelerating death of malignant cells). In general, the drug leads to cell cycle arrest, delayed tumor growth, and cell death. It is indicated for treatment of multiple myeloma in clients who have received two prior therapies and had disease progression during the previous treatment.

Bortezomib is moderately protein bound (83%) and metabolized by several cytochrome P450 enzymes in the liver. The drug should be used with caution in clients with impaired hepatic or renal function.

Adverse effects include dehydration, edema, fever, hypotension, nausea, skin rash, and peripheral neuropathy. The risk of neuropathy may be increased with previous use of neurotoxic agents or pre-existing peripheral neuropathy and dosage adjustment may be required.

ANTINEOPLASTIC HORMONE INHIBITOR DRUGS

The main hormonal agents used in the treatment of cancer are the corticosteroids (see Chap. 23) and drugs that block the production or activity of estrogens and androgens. Corticosteroids suppress or kill malignant lymphocytes and are most useful in the treatment of leukemias, lymphomas, and multiple myeloma. They are also used to treat complications of cancer (eg, brain metastases, hypercalcemia). Prednisone and dexamethasone are commonly used. Sex-hormone blocking drugs are used mainly to control tumor growth and relieve symptoms. They are not cytotoxic and adverse effects are usually mild.

Sex hormones are growth factors in some malignancies (eg, estrogens in breast and uterine cancer; androgens in prostate cancer). The hormones may be normally produced within the body or administered as drugs. For example, oral contraceptives and long-term estrogen replacement therapy are associated with breast cancer.

Surgery or antihormonal drugs may be used to decrease hormonal stimulation of cancer growth. Estrogens and androgens are normally produced from cholesterol through a series of chemical conversions involving the hypothalamus, anterior pituitary, adrenal glands, and ovaries in females and testes in males. Preventing production anywhere along this path or blocking estrogens and androgens from combining with their receptors in target tissues can decrease the growth of cells stimulated by the hormones. Historically, several methods have been used, including surgical excision of the anterior pituitary,

adrenal glands, and ovaries or testes, and pharmacologic doses of estrogens or androgens (which decreased the number of receptors in target tissues) and opposing hormones (eg, estrogens were used to oppose androgens in prostate cancer and androgens were used to oppose estrogens in metastatic breast cancer). Now, excision of the ovaries or testes (surgical castration) and antihormonal drugs (medical or chemical castration) are commonly used. The ovaries are most likely to be removed in premenopausal women with breast cancer and the testes may be removed in men with prostate cancer. In general, currently used drugs interfere with hormone production or hormone action at the cellular level (see Fig. 42-4).

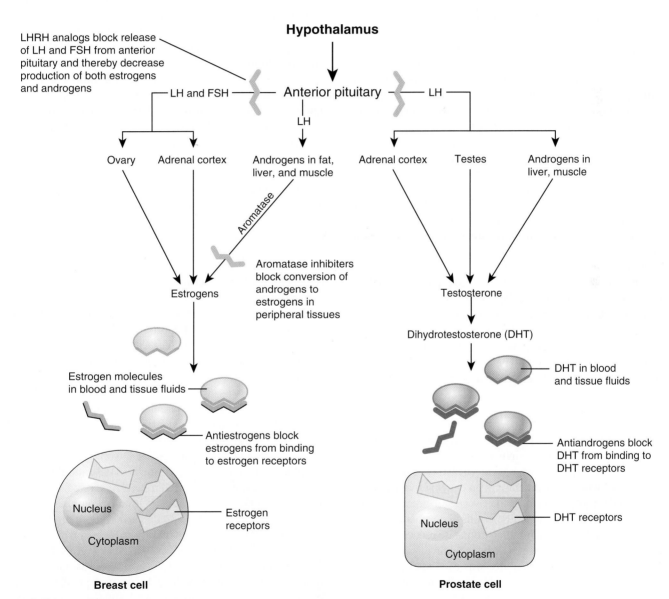

FIGURE 42-4 Actions of hormone inhibitor drugs. Drugs used to treat breast cancer block the production of estrogens (eg, LHRH analogs, aromatase inhibitors) or prevent estrogens from binding to receptors in breast cancer cells (antiestrogens). Drugs used to treat prostate cancer block the production of androgens (eg, LHRH analogs) or prevent DHT, the active form of testosterone, from binding to receptors in prostate cancer cells (antiandrogens).

The main hormone inhibitor drugs are the antiestrogens, aromatase inhibitors, antiandrogens, and luteinizing hormone releasing hormone (LHRH; also known as gonadotropin-releasing hormone [GnRH]) analogs. These are described as follows and in Table 42-3.

Antiestrogens

Antiestrogens (also called *estrogen receptor modulators*) used in the treatment of cancer include **fulvestrant** (Faslodex), **tamoxifen** (Nolvadex), and **toremifene** (Fareston). These drugs bind to estrogen receptors in normal and malignant cells. In breast cancer, the drugs compete with estrogen for receptor binding sites and thereby decrease the estrogen growth-stimulating action on malignant cells. Tamoxifen has been widely used to prevent recurrence of breast cancer after surgical excision and to treat metastatic breast cancer in postmenopausal women with receptor-positive disease. Tamoxifen plus traditional cytotoxic chemotherapy improves survival in both premenopausal and postmenopausal women with estrogen or progesterone receptor–positive disease. For prevention, the drug is usually taken for 2 to 5 years.

Tamoxifen becomes ineffective after about 5 years and several studies indicate greater effectiveness when an aromatase inhibitor is given instead of tamoxifen after 2 to 5 years. Although antiestrogens and aromatase inhibitors both block the growth of breast tumors that respond to estrogen, their mechanisms of action are different. For example, tamoxifen inhibits the ability of breast cancer cells to use estrogen for growth, whereas an aromatase inhibitor inhibits the production of estrogen in fat, muscle, and other tissues. Adverse effects of antiestrogens include increased risk of blood clots or stroke, vaginal bleeding, and muscle cramps.

Sexually active premenopausal women who take tamoxifen should use effective nonhormonal contraception during and for 2 months after tamoxifen is discontinued. (Premenopausal women may also be treated with an LHRH analog, which may be as effective as antiestrogen therapy.)

Aromatase Inhibitors

Anastrazole (Arimidex), **exemestane** (Aromasin), and **letrozole** (Femara) are aromatase inhibitors used to treat or prevent recurrence of estrogen-responsive breast cancer in postmenopausal women. Aromatase is an enzyme that catalyzes the production of estrogen in the ovaries of premenopausal women and in fat, liver, and muscle cells of postmenopausal or castrated women. Thus, inhibiting aromatase reduces estrogen levels in the blood and target tissues, including the breast.

Earlier, an aromatase inhibitor was used after 5 years of tamoxifen therapy. More recently, numerous studies have indicated that changing to an aromatase inhibitor after 2 or 3 years of tamoxifen therapy is more effective in decreasing recurrent breast cancer. Most studies were done with letrozole or exemestane. Letrozole therapy after 5 years of tamoxifen is considered the current standard of care and exemestane is being considered as first-line therapy (instead of tamoxifen) for metastatic breast cancer in postmenopausal women.

Adverse effects include nausea, diarrhea, headache, hot flashes, joint pain, bone loss and fractures, and vision disturbances. Because aromatase inhibitors promote bone loss, these drugs may not be appropriate for women at high risk of bone fractures.

Antiandrogens

Bicalutamide (Casodex), **flutamide** (Eulexin), and **nilutamide** (Nilandron) are used to treat prostate cancer, usually with an LHRH analog (see below). The drugs bind to androgen receptors in cells of the prostate gland and thereby block dihydrotestosterone (DHT) stimulation of malignant cell growth.

In the prostate gland, normal cell growth and differentiation depends on the presence of androgens, specifically DHT, the active form of testosterone. These androgens are produced mainly by the testes and the adrenal glands through a series of chemical conversions also involving the hypothalamus and anterior pituitary. In prostate cancer, androgenic stimulation of tumor growth can be reduced by surgical excision of the organs involved in androgen production (usually the testes) or administering drugs that inhibit the production or action of androgens (eg, antiandrogens, LHRH analogs). Adverse drug effects include hot flashes, breast enlargement and tenderness, nausea, vomiting, constipation, diarrhea, and pain.

Luteinizing Hormone Releasing Hormone (LHRH) Analogs

Goserelin (Zoladex), **leuprolide** (Eligard, Lupron, Viadur), and **triptorelin** (Trelstar) are synthetic versions of the hypothalamic LHRH (also known as GnRH) that initiates production of both estrogens and androgens. Therapeutic doses of LHRH analogs initially increase the release of luteinizing hormone (LH) and follicle-stimulating hormone (FSH) from the anterior pituitary, then decrease their release by downregulating receptors. Inhibiting the release of LH and FSH reduces the production of ovarian estrogen in women to postmenopausal levels and testicular testosterone in men to castration levels. These effects occur within 2 to 4 weeks after drug therapy is begun. In premenopausal women with estrogen receptor–positive breast cancer, medical castration with these drugs is increasingly being used instead of surgical excision of the ovaries. One of these drugs is usually combined with an antiestrogen. In men with prostate cancer, these drugs reduce androgens to the levels seen with surgical excision of the testes. In metastatic prostate cancer, an LHRH analog is often given with an antiandrogen, to increase effectiveness. Goserelin is approved for treatment of both breast and prostate cancer; leuprolide and triptorelin are approved only for prostate cancer.

Adverse effects are basically those of estrogen or testosterone deficiency and may include nausea and hot flashes. The drugs may also cause or aggravate depression. Impotence occurs in men, but may be reversible when the drug is

Table 42-3 Drugs at a Glance: Antineoplastic Hormone Inhibitors

GENERIC/TRADE NAMES	ROUTES AND DOSAGE RANGES	CLINICAL USES	ADVERSE EFFECTS
Antiestrogens			
Fulvestrant (Faslodex)	IM 250 mg once monthly (one 5-mL or two 2.5-mL injections)	Advanced breast cancer in postmenopausal women	GI upset, hot flashes, injection site reactions
Tamoxifen (Nolvadex)	PO 20 mg once or twice daily	Breast cancer, after surgery or radiation; prophylaxis in high-risk women; and treatment of metastatic disease	Hot flashes, nausea, vomiting, vaginal discharge, risk of endometrial cancer in nonhysterectomized women
Toremifene (Fareston)	PO 60 mg once daily	Metastatic breast cancer in postmenopausal women	Hot flashes, nausea, hypercalcemia, tumor flare
Aromatase Inhibitors			
Anastrazole (Arimidex)	PO 1 mg once daily	Breast cancer in postmenopausal women	Nausea, hot flashes, edema
Exemestane (Aromasin)	PO 25 mg once daily	Breast cancer in postmenopausal women	Hot flashes, nausea, depression, insomnia, anxiety, dyspnea, pain
Letrozole (Femara)	PO 2.5 mg once daily	Breast cancer in postmenopausal women	Nausea, hot flashes
Antiandrogens			
Bicalutamide (Casodex)	PO 500 mg once daily (with goserelin or leuprolide)	Advanced prostatic cancer	Nausea, vomiting, diarrhea, hot flashes, pain, breast enlargement
Flutamide (Eulexin)	PO 250 mg every 8 h	Advanced prostatic cancer	Nausea, vomiting, diarrhea, hot flashes, hepatotoxicity
LHRH Analogs			
Nilutamide (Nilandron)	PO 300 mg daily for 30 d, then 150 mg daily	Advanced breast cancer in postmenopausal women	Diarrhea, GI bleeding, heart failure, hyperglycemia
Goserelin (Zoladex)	Sub-Q implant, 3.6 mg every 28 d or 10.8 mg every 12 wk	Advanced prostatic or breast cancer, endometriosis	Hot flashes, transient increase in bone pain
Leuprolide (Eligard, Lupron, Viadur)	Sub-Q 7.5 mg/mo IM 7.5 mg/mo, 22.5 mg/ 3 mo, or 30 mg/4 mo	Advanced prostatic cancer	Same as for goserelin, above
Triptorelin (Trelstar LA, Trelstar Depot)	IM implant 65 mg/12 mo IM 3.75 mg/28 d or 11.25 mg/3 mo	Advanced prostatic cancer	Same as for goserelin and leuprolide, above

GI, gastrointestinal; IM, intramuscular; PO, oral; Sub-Q, subcutaneous.

discontinued. When given for prostate cancer, the drugs may cause increased bone pain and increased difficulty in urinating during the first few weeks of use.

CYTOPROTECTANT DRUGS

Cytoprotectants reduce the adverse effects of cytotoxic drugs, which may be severe, debilitating, and life threatening (Box 42-2). Severe adverse effects may also limit drug dosage or fre-

quency of administration, thereby limiting the effectiveness of chemotherapy. Several cytoprotectants are available to protect certain body tissues from one or more adverse effects and allow a more optimal dose and schedule of cytotoxic agents. To be effective, administration and scheduling must be precise in relation to administration of the cytotoxic agent. A cytoprotective agent does not prevent or treat all adverse effects of a particular cytotoxic agent and it may have adverse effects of its own.

Amifostine produces a metabolite that combines with cisplatin and decreases cisplatin-induced renal damage.

Box 42-2 Management of Chemotherapy Complications

Complications of cytotoxic chemotherapy range from minor to life threatening. Vigilant efforts toward prevention or early detection and treatment are needed.

- **Nausea** and **vomiting** commonly occur and are treated with antiemetics (see Chap. 62), which are most effective when started before chemotherapy and continued on a regular schedule for 24 to 48 hours afterward. An effective regimen is a serotonin receptor antagonist (eg, ondansetron) and a corticosteroid (eg, dexamethasone), given orally or IV. Other measures include a benzodiazepine (eg, lorazepam) for anticipatory nausea and vomiting and limiting oral intake for a few hours.

- **Anorexia** interferes with nutrition. Well-balanced meals, with foods the client is able and willing to eat, and nutritional supplements, to increase intake of protein and calories, are helpful.

- **Fatigue** is often caused or aggravated by anemia and can be prevented or treated with administration of erythropoietin. An adequate diet and light-to-moderate exercise, as tolerated, may also be helpful.

- **Alopecia** occurs with cyclophosphamide, doxorubicin, MTX, and vincristine. Counsel clients taking these drugs that hair loss is temporary and that hair may grow back a different color and texture; suggest the purchase of wigs, hats, and scarves before hair loss is expected to occur; and instruct women to use a mild shampoo and avoid rollers, permanent waves, hair coloring, and other treatments that damage the hair.

- **Mucositis** (also called *stomatitis*) often occurs with the antimetabolites, antibiotics, and plant alkaloids and usually lasts 7 to 10 days. It may interfere with nutrition; lead to oral ulcerations, infections, and bleeding; and cause pain. Nurse or client interventions to minimize or treat mucositis include the following:
  - Brush the teeth after meals and at bedtime with a soft toothbrush and floss once daily. Stop brushing and flossing if the platelet count drops below 20,000/mm³ because gingival bleeding is likely. Teeth may then be cleaned with soft, sponge-tipped or cotton-tipped applicators.
  - Rinse the mouth several times daily, especially before meals (to decrease unpleasant taste and increase appetite) and after meals (to remove food particles that promote growth of microorganisms). One suggested solution is 1 teaspoon of table salt and 1 teaspoon of baking soda in 1 quart of water. Commercial mouthwashes are not recommended, because their alcohol content causes drying of oral mucous membranes.
  - Encourage the client to drink fluids. Systemic dehydration and local dryness of the oral mucosa contribute to the development and progression of mucositis. Pain and soreness contribute to dehydration. Fluids usually tolerated include tea, carbonated beverages, ices (eg, popsicles), and plain gelatin desserts. Fruit juices may be diluted with water, ginger ale, Sprite, or 7-Up to decrease pain, burning, and further tissue irritation. Drinking fluids through a straw may be more comfortable, because this decreases contact of fluids with painful ulcerations.
  - Encourage the client to eat soft, bland, cold, nonacidic foods. Although individual tolerances vary, it is usually better to avoid highly spiced or rough foods.
  - Remove dentures entirely or for at least 8 hours daily because they may irritate oral mucosa.
  - Inspect the mouth daily for signs of inflammation and lesions.
  - Give medications for pain. Local anesthetic solutions, such as viscous lidocaine, can be taken a few minutes before meals. Because the mouth and throat are anesthetized, swallowing and detecting the temperature of hot foods may be difficult, and aspiration or burns may occur. Doses should not exceed 15 mL every 3 hours or 120 mL in 24 hours. If systemic analgesics are used, they should be taken 30 to 60 minutes before eating.
  - For oral infections resulting from mucositis, local or systemic antimicrobial drugs are used. Fungal infections with *Candida albicans* can be treated with antifungal tablets, suspensions, or lozenges. Severe infections may require systemic antibiotics, depending on the causative organism as identified by cultures of mouth lesions.

- **Infection** is common because the disease and its treatment lower host resistance to infection.
  - If fever occurs, especially in a neutropenic client, possible sources of infection are usually cultured and antibiotics are started immediately.
  - Severe neutropenia can be prevented or its extent and duration minimized by administering filgrastim or sargramostim to stimulate the bone marrow to produce leukocytes. A protective environment may be needed to decrease exposure to pathogens.
  - Instruct the client to avoid exposure to infection by avoiding crowds, anyone with a known infection, and contact with fresh flowers, soil, animals, or animal excrement.
  - Frequent and thorough hand hygiene by the client and everyone involved in his or her care is necessary to reduce exposure to pathogenic microorganisms.
  - The client should take a bath daily and put on clean clothes. In addition, the perineal area should be washed with soap and water after each urination or defecation.
  - When venous access devices are used, take care to prevent them from becoming sources of infection. For implanted catheters, inspect and cleanse around exit sites according to agency policies and procedures. Use strict sterile technique when changing dressings or flushing the catheters. For peripheral venous lines, the same principles of care apply, except that sites should be changed every 3 days or if signs of phlebitis occur.
  - Avoid indwelling urinary catheters when possible. When they are necessary, cleanse the perineal area with soap and water at least once daily and provide sufficient fluids to ensure an adequate urine output.
  - Help the client maintain a well-balanced diet. Oral hygiene and analgesics before meals may increase food intake. High-protein, high-calorie foods and fluids can be given between meals. Nutritional supplements can be taken with or between

Box 42-2 Management of Chemotherapy Complications (continued)

meals. Provide fluids with high nutritional value (eg, milk-shakes or nutritional supplements) if the client can tolerate them and has an adequate intake of water and other fluids.

- **Bleeding** may be caused by thrombocytopenia and may occur spontaneously or with minor trauma. Precautions should be instituted if the platelet count drops to 50,000/mm³ or below. Measures to avoid bleeding include giving oprelvekin to stimulate platelet production and prevent thrombocytopenia; avoiding trauma, including venipuncture and injections, when possible; using an electric razor for shaving; checking skin, urine, and stool for blood; and for platelet counts less than 20,000/mm³, stop brushing and flossing the teeth.

- **Extravasation.** Several drugs (called *vesicants*) cause severe inflammation, pain, ulceration, and tissue necrosis if they leak into soft tissues around veins. Thus, efforts are needed to prevent extravasation or to minimize tissue damage if it occurs.
  - Identify clients at risk for extravasation, including those who are unable to communicate (eg, sedated clients, infants), have vascular impairment (eg, from multiple attempts at venipuncture), or have obstructed venous drainage after axillary node surgery.
  - Be especially cautious with the anthracyclines (eg, doxorubicin) and the vinca alkaloids (eg, vincristine). Choose peripheral IV sites carefully, avoiding veins that are small

or located in an edematous extremity or near a joint. Inject the drugs slowly (1–2 mL at a time) into the tubing of a rapidly flowing IV infusion, for rapid dilution and detection of extravasation. Observe the venipuncture site for swelling and ask the client about pain or burning. After a drug has been injected, continue the rapid flow rate of the IV fluid for 2 to 5 minutes to flush the vein.

- If using a central IV line, do not give the drug unless patency is indicated by a blood return. Using a central line does not eliminate the risk of extravasation.
- When extravasation occurs, the drug should be stopped immediately. Techniques to decrease tissue damage include aspirating the drug (about 5 mL of blood, if able) through the IV catheter before it is removed, elevating the involved extremity, and applying warm (with dacarbazine, etoposide, vinblastine, and vincristine) or cold (with daunorubicin and doxorubicin) compresses. Nurses involved in cytotoxic chemotherapy must know the procedure to be followed if extravasation occurs so that it can be instituted immediately.

- **Hyperuricemia** from rapid breakdown of malignant cells can lead to kidney damage. Risks of nephropathy can be decreased by high fluid intake, high urine output, alkalinizing the urine with sodium bicarbonate, and giving allopurinol to inhibit uric acid formation.

Dexrazoxane decreases cardiac toxicity of doxorubicin. **Erythropoietin, filgrastim, oprelvekin,** and **sargramostim** are colony-stimulating factors (see Chap. 40) that stimulate the bone marrow to produce blood cells. Erythropoietin stimulates production of red blood cells and is used for anemia; oprelvekin stimulates production of platelets and is used to prevent thrombocytopenia; filgrastim and sargramostim stimulate production of white blood cells and are used to reduce neutropenia and infection. **Leucovorin** is used with high-dose MTX. **Mesna** is used with ifosfamide, which produces a metabolite that causes hemorrhagic cystitis. Mesna combines with and inactivates the metabolite and thereby decreases cystitis. Dosages and routes of administration for these medications are listed in Table 42-4.

NURSING PROCESS

Assessment

- Assess all clients for risk factors, screening behaviors, and/or manifestations of cancer, in order to prevent cancer, if possible, or recognize and seek treatment for cancer as early as possible. Risk factors include use of tobacco products (including inhalation of secondhand cigarette smoke in home or work environments); drink-

ing more than one drink a day (for women) or two drinks a day (for men); being overweight; damage to skin unprotected by sunscreen; and unsafe sexual behaviors. Screening behaviors include the use of breast self-examinations, regular mammograms, colonoscopy when indicated, measurement of prostate-specific antigen (PSA), and so forth.

- Assess the client's condition before chemotherapy is started and often during treatment. Useful information includes the type, grade, and stage of the tumor as well as the signs and symptoms of cancer. General manifestations include anemia, malnutrition, weight loss, pain, and infection; specific manifestations depend on the organs affected.

- Assess for other diseases and organ dysfunctions (eg, cardiac, renal, hepatic) that influence response to chemotherapy.

- Assess emotional status, coping mechanisms, family relationships, financial resources, and social support mechanisms. Anxiety and depression are common features during cancer diagnosis and treatment.

- Assess laboratory test results before chemotherapy to establish baseline data and during chemotherapy to monitor drug effects.
  - **Blood tests for tumor markers** (tumor-specific antigens on cell surfaces). *Alpha-fetoprotein* is a fetal

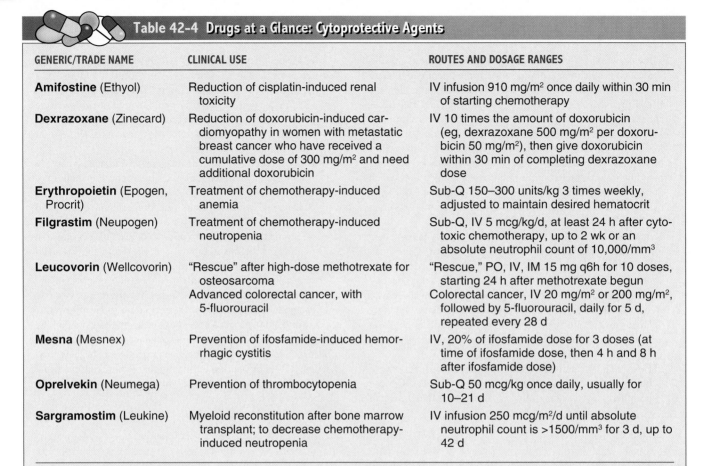

Table 42-4 Drugs at a Glance: Cytoprotective Agents

GENERIC/TRADE NAME	CLINICAL USE	ROUTES AND DOSAGE RANGES
Amifostine (Ethyol)	Reduction of cisplatin-induced renal toxicity	IV infusion 910 mg/m^2 once daily within 30 min of starting chemotherapy
Dexrazoxane (Zinecard)	Reduction of doxorubicin-induced cardiomyopathy in women with metastatic breast cancer who have received a cumulative dose of 300 mg/m^2 and need additional doxorubicin	IV 10 times the amount of doxorubicin (eg, dexrazoxane 500 mg/m^2 per doxorubicin 50 mg/m^2), then give doxorubicin within 30 min of completing dexrazoxane dose
Erythropoietin (Epogen, Procrit)	Treatment of chemotherapy-induced anemia	Sub-Q 150–300 units/kg 3 times weekly, adjusted to maintain desired hematocrit
Filgrastim (Neupogen)	Treatment of chemotherapy-induced neutropenia	Sub-Q, IV 5 mcg/kg/d, at least 24 h after cytotoxic chemotherapy, up to 2 wk or an absolute neutrophil count of 10,000/mm^3
Leucovorin (Wellcovorin)	"Rescue" after high-dose methotrexate for osteosarcoma Advanced colorectal cancer, with 5-fluorouracil	"Rescue," PO, IV, IM 15 mg q6h for 10 doses, starting 24 h after methotrexate begun Colorectal cancer, IV 20 mg/m^2 or 200 mg/m^2, followed by 5-fluorouracil, daily for 5 d, repeated every 28 d
Mesna (Mesnex)	Prevention of ifosfamide-induced hemorrhagic cystitis	IV, 20% of ifosfamide dose for 3 doses (at time of ifosfamide dose, then 4 h and 8 h after ifosfamide dose)
Oprelvekin (Neumega)	Prevention of thrombocytopenia	Sub-Q 50 mcg/kg once daily, usually for 10–21 d
Sargramostim (Leukine)	Myeloid reconstitution after bone marrow transplant; to decrease chemotherapy-induced neutropenia	IV infusion 250 mcg/m^2/d until absolute neutrophil count is >1500/mm^3 for 3 d, up to 42 d

IM, intramuscular; IV, intravenous; PO, oral; Sub-Q, subcutaneous.

antigen normally present during intrauterine and early postnatal life but absent in adulthood. Increased amounts may indicate hepatic or testicular cancer. *Carcinoembryonic antigen* (CEA) is secreted by several types of malignant cells (eg, CEA is present in approximately 75% of people with colorectal cancer). A rising level may indicate tumor progression and levels that are elevated before surgery and disappear after surgery indicate adequate tumor excision. If CEA levels rise later, it probably indicates tumor recurrence. With chemotherapy, falling CEA levels indicate effectiveness. Other tumor markers are *immunoglobulins* (elevated levels may indicate multiple myeloma) and *PSA* (elevated levels may indicate prostatic cancer).

● **CBC** to check for anemia, leukopenia, and thrombocytopenia because most cytotoxic antineoplastic drugs cause bone marrow depression. A CBC and white blood cell differential are done before each cycle of chemotherapy to determine dosage and frequency of drug administration, to monitor bone mar-

row function so fatal bone marrow depression does not occur, and to assist the nurse in planning care. For example, the client is very susceptible to infection when the leukocyte count is low, and bleeding is likely when the platelet count is low.

● **Other tests.** These include tests of kidney and liver function, serum calcium, uric acid, and others, depending on the organs affected by the cancer or its treatment.

Nursing Diagnoses

● Pain, nausea and vomiting, weakness, and activity intolerance related to disease process or chemotherapy
● Imbalanced Nutrition: Less Than Body Requirements related to disease process or chemotherapy
● Anxiety related to the disease, its possible progression, and its treatment
● Ineffective Family Coping related to illness and treatment of a family member
● Deficient Fluid Volume related to chemotherapy-induced nausea, vomiting, and diarrhea

- Risk for Injury: Infection related to drug-induced neutropenia; bleeding related to drug-induced thrombocytopenia; stomatitis related to damage of GI mucosal cells
- Deficient Knowledge about cancer chemotherapy and managing adverse drug effects

Planning/Goals

The client will
- Receive assistance in coping with the diagnosis of cancer
- Experience reduced anxiety and fear
- Receive chemotherapy accurately and safely
- Experience reduction of tumor size, change of laboratory values toward normal, or other therapeutic effects of chemotherapy
- Experience minimal bleeding, infection, nausea and vomiting, and other consequences of chemotherapy
- Maintain adequate food and fluid intake and body weight
- Receive assistance in activities of daily living when needed
- Be informed about community resources for cancer care (eg, hospice, Reach to Recovery, other support groups)

Interventions

- Participate in and promote efforts to prevent cancer.
  - Follow and promote the diet recommended by the American Cancer Society (ie, decrease fat; eat at least five servings of fruits and vegetables daily; increase intake of dietary fiber; minimize intake of salt-cured or smoked foods).
  - Promote weight control. Obesity may contribute to the development of several cancers, including breast and endometrial cancer in women.
  - Identify cancer-causing agents in homes and workplaces and strategies to reduce exposure to them when possible.
  - Strengthen host defenses by promoting a healthful lifestyle (eg, good nutrition, adequate rest and exercise, stress management techniques, avoiding or minimizing alcohol and tobacco use).
  - Avoid smoking cigarettes and being around smokers. Passive smoking increases risk of lung cancer in spouses of smokers and risks of brain cancer, lymphomas, and acute lymphogenous leukemia in children of smokers.
  - Minimize exposure to sunlight, use sunscreens liberally, and wear protective clothing to prevent skin cancer.
- Participate in and promote cancer screening tests in nonsymptomatic people, especially those at high risk, to detect cancer before signs and symptoms occur. These tests include regular examination of breasts, cervix (Pap test), testicles, and skin, and tests for colon cancer such as hemoccult tests on stool and colonoscopy. Early recognition of risk factors, premalignant tissue changes (dysplasia), biochemical tumor markers, and beginning malignancies may be life saving; early treatment can greatly reduce the suffering and problems associated with advanced cancer.
- For clients receiving cytotoxic anticancer drugs, try to prevent or minimize the incidence and severity of adverse reactions (see Box 42-2 and accompanying teaching guidelines).
- Provide supportive care to clients and families. Physiologic care includes pain management, comfort measures, and assistance with nutrition, hygiene, ambulation, and other activities of daily living as needed. Psychological care includes allowing family members or significant others to be with the client and participate in care when desired, and keeping clients and families informed.

Evaluation

- Monitor drug administration for accuracy.
- Observe and interview for therapeutic effects of chemotherapy.
- Compare current laboratory reports with baseline values for changes toward normal values.
- Compare weight and nutritional status with baseline values for maintenance or improvement.
- Observe and interview for adverse drug effects and interventions to prevent or manage them.
- Observe and interview for adequate pain management and other symptom control.

PRINCIPLES OF THERAPY

Overview of Cancer Treatment

For many clients, cancer treatment involves surgery, radiation, and chemotherapy during the course of their disease. *Surgery* is used to excise localized tumors, which may be curative, and to treat complications of cancer, such as bowel obstruction. *Radiation therapy* is used to treat most types of cancer. It may be used alone for some malignancies, such as Hodgkin's disease or cervical cancer. It may be used with surgery to reduce the need for radical surgery; to eliminate malignant cells (eg, positive lymph nodes) that remain after surgery; with chemotherapy to control growth of tumors; and to relieve symptoms in clients with metastatic bone or brain involvement.

Chemotherapy may be used to eliminate or control the growth of malignant cells or to relieve symptoms and improve the client's quality of life. It is most effective when started before extensive tumor growth or when the tumor burden has been reduced by surgical excision or radiation therapy. After they metastasize, solid tumors become systemic diseases and

CLIENT TEACHING GUIDELINES

Managing Chemotherapy

Most chemotherapy is given intravenously, in outpatient clinics, by nurses who are specially trained to administer the medications and monitor your condition. The medications are usually given in cycles such as every few weeks. There are many different chemotherapy drugs, and the ones used for a particular client depend on the type of malignancy, its location, and other factors.

The goal of chemotherapy is to be as effective as possible with tolerable side effects. Particular side effects vary with the medications used; some increase risks of infection, and some cause anemia, nausea, or hair loss. All of these can be managed effectively, and several medications can help prevent or minimize side effects. In addition, some helpful activities are listed below.

✔ Keep all appointments for chemotherapy, blood tests, and check-ups. This is extremely important. Chemotherapy effectiveness depends on its being given on time; blood tests help to determine when the drugs should be given and how the drugs affect your body tissues.

✔ Do everything you can to avoid infection, such as avoiding other people who have infections and washing your hands frequently and thoroughly. If you have a fever, chills, sore throat, or cough, notify your oncologist.

✔ Try to maintain or improve your intake of nutritious food and fluids; this will help you feel better. A dietitian can be helpful in designing a diet to meet your needs.

✔ If your chemotherapy may cause bleeding, you can decrease the likelihood by shaving with an electric razor, avoiding aspirin and other non-steroidal anti-inflammatory drugs (including over-the-counter Advil, Aleve, and others), and avoiding injections, cuts, and other injuries when possible. If you notice excessive bruising; bleeding gums when you brush your teeth; or blood in your urine or bowel movement, notify your oncologist immediately.

✔ If hair loss is expected with the medications you take, you can use wigs, scarves, and hats. These should be purchased before starting chemotherapy, if possible. Hair loss is temporary; your hair will grow back!

✔ Inform any other physician, dentist, or health care provider that you are taking chemotherapy before any diagnostic test or treatment is begun. Some procedures may be contraindicated or require special precautions.

✔ If you are of childbearing age, effective contraceptive measures should be carried out during and a few months after chemotherapy.

✔ A few chemotherapy medications and medications to prevent or treat side effects are taken at home. Instructions for taking the drugs should be followed exactly for the most beneficial effects.

✔ Although specific instructions vary with the drugs you are taking, the following are a few precautions with some commonly used drugs:

   ✔ With **cyclophosphamide,** take the tablets on an empty stomach. If severe stomach upset occurs, take with food. Also, drink 2 or 3 quarts of fluid daily, if possible, and urinate often, especially at bedtime. If blood is seen in the urine or signs of cystitis occur (eg, burning with urination), report to a health care provider. The drug is irritating to the bladder lining and may cause cystitis. High fluid intake and frequent emptying of the bladder help to decrease bladder damage.

   ✔ With **doxorubicin,** the urine may turn red for 1 to 2 days after drug administration. This discoloration is harmless; it does not indicate bleeding. Also, report to a health care provider if you have edema, shortness of breath, and excessive fatigue. Doxorubicin may need to be stopped if these symptoms occur.

   ✔ With **fluorouracil,** drink plenty of liquids while taking.

   ✔ With **methotrexate,** avoid alcohol, aspirin, and prolonged exposure to sunlight.

   ✔ With **vincristine,** eat high-fiber foods, such as raw fruits and vegetables and whole cereal grains, if you are able, to prevent constipation. Also try to maintain a high fluid intake. A stool softener or bulk laxative may be prescribed for daily use.

---

are not accessible to surgical excision or radiation therapy. *Neoadjuvant chemotherapy* is used before surgery or radiation, to reduce the size of tumors; *adjuvant chemotherapy* is used after surgery or radiation to destroy or reduce microscopic metastases (eg, in the treatment of clients with carcinomas of the breast, colon, lung, ovaries, or testes). *Palliative chemotherapy* is used in advanced cancer to relieve symptoms and treat or prevent complications.

Drug Selection

Drug therapy for a particular client depends on the type and stage of cancer, the effectiveness of particular drugs in that type and stage of cancer, and the client's age and health status, including liver and kidney function. Most regimens use combinations of drugs because they are more effective, less toxic, and less likely to cause drug resistance than single agents. Numerous combinations have been developed for use in specific types of cancer. Effective combinations include drugs that act by different mechanisms, act at different times in the reproductive cycle of malignant cells, and differ in their adverse effects. Bleomycin is often combined with myelosuppressive drugs because it rarely causes myelosuppression. However, it can cause severe allergic reactions with hypotension and pulmonary toxicity (eg, interstitial pneumonitis, pulmonary fibrosis). Increasingly, biologic drugs are being added to traditional cytotoxic drug regimens.

Drug Dosage

Dosage must be calculated and regulated carefully to minimize toxicity. The client's age, nutritional status, blood count, kidney and liver function, and previous chemotherapy or radiation therapy must be considered. Additional guidelines include the following:

- High doses, to the limits of tolerance of normal tissues (eg, bone marrow), are usually most effective.
- Doses are usually calculated according to body surface area, which includes both weight and height, and are expressed as milligrams of drug per square meter of body surface area (mg/m^2). Doses also can be expressed as milligrams per kilogram of body weight (mg/kg). Because dosages based on body surface area consider the client's size, they are especially important for children. If the client's weight changes more than a few pounds during treatment, dosages should be recalculated.
- Dosage may be reduced for neutropenia, thrombocytopenia, stomatitis, diarrhea, and renal or hepatic impairment that reduces the client's ability to eliminate the drugs.
- Total dose limits for doxorubicin (550 mg/m^2) and bleomycin (450 units) should not be exceeded.

Drug Administration

- Dosage schedules are largely determined by clinical trials and should be followed as exactly as possible.
- Antineoplastic drugs are usually given in relatively high doses, on an intermittent or cyclic schedule. This regimen seems more effective than low doses given continuously or massive doses given once. It also produces less immunosuppression and provides drug-free periods during which normal tissues can repair themselves from damage inflicted by the drugs. Succeeding doses are given when tissue repair occurs, usually when leukocyte and platelet counts return to acceptable levels.
- Each antineoplastic drug should be used in the schedule, route, and dosage judged to be most effective for a particular type of cancer. With combinations of drugs, the recommended schedule should be followed precisely because safety and effectiveness may be schedule dependent. When chemotherapy is used as an adjuvant to surgery, it usually should be started as soon as possible after surgery; given in maximal tolerated doses just as if advanced disease were present; and continued for several months.
- IV drugs should be given by experienced personnel who ensure free flow of fluid to the vein and verify adequate blood return. Infusion should be through a large, upper-extremity vein. When possible, veins of the antecubital fossa, wrist, dorsum of the hand, and the arm where an axillary lymph node dissection has been done should be avoided. An indwelling central venous catheter is often inserted for clients with poor peripheral venous access or who require many doses of chemotherapy.
- With bleomycin, a test dose of 1 to 2 mg should be given subcutaneously before starting full doses. Severe allergic reactions with hypotension may occur.
- With paclitaxel and docetaxel, premedication is needed to decrease severe hypersensitivity reactions with dys-

pnea, hypotension, angioedema, and urticaria. A few deaths have occurred despite premedication. With paclitaxel, one regimen is oral dexamethasone 20 mg at 12 and 6 hours before, with IV diphenhydramine (Benadryl) 50 mg and cimetidine 300 mg, famotidine 20 mg, or ranitidine 50 mg at 30 to 60 minutes before. Additional paclitaxel is contraindicated for clients who experience severe hypersensitivity reactions. With docetaxel, an oral corticosteroid (eg, dexamethasone 8 mg twice daily) is recommended for 3 days, starting 1 day before docetaxel administration. This reduces risk and severity of hypersensitivity reactions and fluid retention.
- Premedication with diphenhydramine and acetaminophen is recommended prior to administration of several antineoplastic monoclonal antibodies, to decrease potentially serious allergic reactions to drug infusions.

Hormone Inhibitor Therapy

Sex hormone inhibitors (eg, antiestrogens, aromatase inhibitors, antiandrogens, LHRH analogs) are often used to treat breast or prostate cancer. Decreasing the hormones that stimulate tumor growth in these tissues can decrease symptoms and prolong survival.

In some clients with breast cancer, the presence of receptors for estrogen indicates a likely response to drugs that decrease estrogen availability. After initial surgery and/or radiation therapy, tamoxifen or a related drug is often used to treat breast cancers in clients with estrogen receptors because it inhibits estrogen binding to estrogen receptors. However, tumors may become resistant to tamoxifen because of mutations in receptors that alter receptor functions. An aromatase inhibitor drug (eg, letrozole, exemestane) is increasingly being used after 2 to 5 years of tamoxifen therapy and is being investigated for use as first-line therapy instead of tamoxifen. In clients with prostate cancer, antiandrogens (eg, bicalutamide) and LHRH analogs decrease androgen availability.

When both hormone inhibitor and cytotoxic drug therapies are needed, they are not given concurrently because hormone antagonists decrease malignant cell growth and cytotoxic agents are most effective when the cells are actively dividing. In clients with breast cancer, a hormone-inhibiting drug is usually given before cytotoxic chemotherapy in metastatic disease and after chemotherapy when used for adjuvant treatment.

Planning With Client and Family

Clients with cancer and their families should be provided with information about their disease, their treatment options, and the preferred treatment. When cytotoxic chemotherapy is recommended, discussions should include expected benefits; adverse drug effects and their prevention or management; specific information about when and how the drugs will be administered; and the importance of regular blood tests to monitor drug effects. For those with Internet access, helpful information can be obtained at:

CancerNet: http://www.cancer.gov/cancer_information
Cancer News on the Net:
   http://www.cancernews.com/default2.asp
OncoLink: http://cancer.med.upenn.edu

APPLYING YOUR KNOWLEDGE 42-3

Julia still appears concerned about a possible adverse reaction to the Herceptin. What should you tell Julia about the precautions taken when administering this drug?

Safety Precautions With Cytotoxic Antineoplastic Drugs

Most cytotoxic antineoplastic drugs are carcinogenic, mutagenic, and teratogenic. Exposure during pregnancy increases risks of fetal abnormalities, ectopic pregnancy, and spontaneous abortion. In addition, parenteral solutions are irritating to the skin and mucous membranes and may cause contact dermatitis, cough, nausea, vomiting, and diarrhea. As a result, guidelines have been established for nurses who administer these drugs, to increase the safety of both clients and nurses. These guidelines include the following:

- Ensure appropriate orders (eg, be sure the prescriber is qualified to write chemotherapy orders; do not accept verbal or telephone orders).
- Do not give injectable drugs unless certified to administer chemotherapy.
- Check all IV drug preparations for appropriate dilution, dosage that corresponds to the prescriber's order, absence of precipitates, expiration dates, and so forth.
- Avoid direct contact with solutions for injection by wearing gloves, face shields, and protective clothing (eg, disposable, liquid-impermeable gowns).
- If handling a powder form of a drug, avoid inhaling the powder.
- Do not prepare the drugs in eating areas (to decrease risks of oral ingestion).
- Dispose of contaminated materials (eg, needles, syringes, ampules, vials, IV tubing and bags) in puncture-proof containers labeled "Warning: Hazardous Material."
- Wear gloves when handling clients' clothing, bed linens, or excreta. Blood and body fluids are contaminated with drugs or metabolites for about 48 hours after a dose.
- Wash hands thoroughly after exposure or potential exposure.
- Wear a respiratory mask and follow recommended procedures for cleaning up spills.

Use in Special Populations

Use in Children

Children are at risk for a wide range of malignancies, including acute leukemias, lymphomas, brain tumors, Wilms' tumor, and sarcomas of muscle and bone. Children whose parents smoke have an increased risk of brain cancer, lymphomas, and acute lymphocytic leukemia. Smokeless tobacco products are also carcinogens. Although traditional cytotoxic chemotherapy drugs are widely used in children, few studies have been done and their safety and effectiveness are not established. As with adults, chemotherapy is often used with surgery or radiation therapy.

Chemotherapy should be designed, ordered, and supervised by pediatric oncologists. Dosage of cytotoxic drugs should be based on body surface area because this takes size into account. Long-term effects on growth and development of survivors are not clear and special efforts are needed to maintain nutrition, organ function, psychological support, and other aspects of growth and development.

After successful chemotherapy, children should be closely monitored because they are at increased risk for development of cancers in adulthood (eg, leukemia). After radiation therapy, they are at increased risk of developing breast, thyroid, or brain cancer. Children treated for Hodgkin's disease seem to have the highest risk of developing a new cancer later. In addition, children who are given an anthracycline drug (eg, doxorubicin) are at increased risk of developing cardiotoxic effects (eg, heart failure) during treatment or after receiving the drug. Efforts to reduce cardiotoxicity include using alternative drugs when effective, giving smaller cumulative doses of anthracycline drug, and observing clients closely so that early manifestations can be recognized and treated before heart failure occurs.

Most of the newer anticancer drugs (eg, biologic or hormone inhibiting) are used to treat malignancies that do not commonly occur in children and little is known about their effects in children.

Use in Older Adults

Older adults are at risk for a wide range of cancers. Although they also are likely to have chronic cardiovascular, renal, and other disorders that increase their risks of serious adverse effects, they should not be denied the potential benefits of traditional cytotoxic chemotherapy on the basis of age alone (see Research Brief). Instead, greater vigilance is needed to maximize benefits and minimize hazards of chemotherapy. For example, older adults are more sensitive to the neurotoxic effects of vincristine and need reduced dosages of some drugs (eg, cyclophosphamide, MTX) if renal function is impaired. Creatinine clearance (CrCl) should be monitored; serum creatinine level is not a reliable indicator of renal function in older adults because of their decreased muscle mass.

Estrogen- and androgen-inhibiting drugs are often used in older adults to treat breast or prostate cancer. The drugs may be used with or instead of other treatment modalities and are usually well tolerated. Newer biologic drugs (eg, for colorectal or lung cancer) will probably be widely used in older adults, but guidelines for their use have not been established.

RESEARCH BRIEF

Adjuvant Chemotherapy in Treatment of Breast Cancer

SOURCE:

Muss, H. B., Woolf, S., Berry, D., et al. (2005). Adjuvant chemotherapy in older and younger women with lymph node–positive breast cancer. *Journal of the American Medical Association, 293*(9), 1073–1081.

SUMMARY:

The incidence of breast cancer increases with age, and almost half of all new breast cancers in the United States occur in women 65 years of age or older. Studies indicate that adjuvant chemotherapy significantly improves time-to-relapse and survival in women with early-stage breast cancer. The researchers were concerned that many older women are not receiving optimal chemotherapy, at least partly because some medical oncologists do not believe older women can tolerate the adverse effects of cytotoxic chemotherapy. To compare the benefits and toxic effects of adjuvant chemotherapy in women 50 years and younger, 51 to 64 years, and 65 years and older, the researchers reviewed four randomized clinical trials that enrolled 6487 women with lymph node–positive breast cancer between 1975 and 1999. The median follow-up period was 9.6 years. Of these women, 542 were 65 years or older and 159 were 70 years or older. The results indicated that older women and younger women obtained similar reductions in breast cancer mortality and recurrence from treatment regimens containing more chemotherapy, although older women had a slight increase in chemotherapy-associated toxic effects and treatment-related mortality. The researchers concluded that age alone should not bar the use of optimal chemotherapy regimens in older women who are in good general health.

NURSING IMPLICATIONS:

The main role for most nurses may be helping women reach informed decisions about participating in adjuvant chemotherapy when offered or suggested by oncologists or initiating discussion about the topic when not offered or suggested by oncologists.

Use in Clients With Renal Impairment

Some antineoplastic drugs are nephrotoxic (eg, cisplatin, MTX) and many are excreted through the kidneys. In the presence of impaired renal function, risks of further impair-ment or accumulation of toxic drug levels are increased. Thus, renal function should be monitored carefully during therapy and drug dosages are often reduced according to CrCl levels. In cases of advanced cancer, CrCl may not be reliable because these clients are often in catabolic states characterized by increased production of creatinine from breakdown of skeletal muscle and other proteins. Renal effects of selected cytotoxic chemotherapy drugs are as follows:

- **Carmustine** and **lomustine** are associated with azotemia and renal failure, usually with long-term IV administration and large cumulative doses.
- **Cisplatin** is nephrotoxic, and acute overdosage can cause renal failure. Because nephrotoxicity is increased with repeated doses, cisplatin is given at 3- or 4-week intervals and renal function tests (eg, serum creatinine, blood urea nitrogen [BUN]), serum electrolytes [eg, sodium, potassium, calcium]) are measured before each course of therapy. Renal function is usually allowed to return to normal before another dose is given. Nephrotoxicity may be reduced by the use of amifostine or IV hydration and mannitol.
- **Cyclophosphamide** may cause hemorrhagic ureteritis and renal tubular necrosis with IV doses above 50 mg/kg. These effects usually subside when the drug is stopped.
- **Ifosfamide** may increase BUN and serum creatinine, but its major effect on the urinary tract is hemorrhagic cystitis, manifested by hematuria. Cystitis can be reduced by the use of mesna, vigorous hydration, and delaying drug administration if a predose urinalysis shows hematuria.
- **Irinotecan** dosage should be reduced (eg, 0.75 mg/m^2) in clients with moderate impairment (CrCl 20–39 mL/minute). No dosage reduction is recommended with mild impairment (CrCl 40–60 mL/minute), and there are inadequate data for recommendations with severe impairment.
- **Melphalan** should be reduced in dosage when given IV, to reduce accumulation and increased bone marrow toxicity. It is unknown whether dosage reduction is needed with oral drug.
- **Mercaptopurine** should be given in smaller doses because the drug may be eliminated more slowly.
- **MTX** is excreted mainly by the kidneys and its use in clients with impaired renal function may lead to accumulation of toxic amounts or additional renal damage. The client's renal status should be evaluated before and during MTX therapy. If significant renal impairment occurs, the drug should be discontinued or reduced in dosage until renal function improves.

In clients who receive high doses for treatment of osteosarcoma, MTX may cause renal damage leading to acute renal failure. Nephrotoxicity is attributed to precipitation of MTX and a metabolite in renal tubules. Renal impairment may be reduced by monitoring renal function closely, ensuring adequate hydration, alkalinizing the urine, and measuring serum drug levels.

- **Procarbazine** may cause more severe adverse effects if given to clients with impaired renal function. Hospitalization is recommended for the first course of treatment.

Many other drugs should be used with caution in clients with renal impairment. **L-Asparaginase** often causes azotemia (eg, increased BUN); acute renal failure and fatal renal insufficiency have been reported. **Bleomycin** is rarely associated with nephrotoxicity but its elimination half-life is prolonged in clients with a CrCl of less than 35 milliliters per minute. **Cytarabine** is detoxified mainly by the liver. However, clients with renal impairment may have more central nervous system (CNS)-related adverse effects, and dosage reduction may be needed. **Gemcitabine** should be used with caution, although it has not been studied in clients with pre-existing renal impairment. Mild proteinuria and hematuria were commonly reported during clinical trials, and hemolytic-uremic syndrome (HUS) was reported in a few clients. HUS may be manifested by anemia, indications of blood-cell breakdown (eg, elevated bilirubin and reticulocyte counts), and renal failure. The drug should be stopped immediately if HUS occurs; hemodialysis may be required.

With the newer biologic drugs, bortezomib should be used with caution; no dosage adjustment is needed for gefitinib or imatinib.

Use in Clients With Hepatic Impairment

Some antineoplastic drugs are hepatotoxic and many are metabolized in the liver. With impaired hepatic function, risks of further impairment or accumulation of toxic drug levels are increased. Hepatic function should be monitored with most drugs and dosage reduction is needed with some. However, abnormal values for the usual liver function tests (eg, serum aspartate aminotransferase [AST] and alanine aminotransferase [ALT], bilirubin, alkaline phosphatase) may indicate liver injury but do not indicate decreased ability to metabolize drugs. Clients with metastatic cancer often have impaired liver function.

Hepatotoxic drugs include the anthracyclines (eg, doxorubicin), mercaptopurine, MTX, paclitaxel, and vincristine. Hepatic effects of these and selected other drugs are as follows:

- **L-Asparaginase** is hepatotoxic in most clients and may increase pre-existing hepatic impairment. It may also increase hepatotoxicity of other medications. Signs of liver impairment, which usually subside when the drug is discontinued, include increased AST, ALT, alkaline phosphatase, and bilirubin and decreased serum albumin, cholesterol, and plasma fibrinogen.
- **Capecitabine** blood levels are significantly increased with hepatic impairment, and clients with mild to moderate impairment caused by liver metastases should be

monitored closely. The effects of severe impairment have not been studied.

- **Carmustine** may increase AST, ALT, alkaline phosphatase, and bilirubin when given IV.
- **Cisplatin** may cause a transient increase in liver enzymes and bilirubin that should be measured periodically during cisplatin therapy.
- **Cytarabine** is metabolized in the liver and clients with impaired liver function are more likely to have CNS-related adverse effects. The drug should be used with caution and dosage may need to be reduced.
- **Dacarbazine,** an alkylating agent, is hepatotoxic, and a few cases of hepatic-vein thrombosis and fatal liver necrosis have been reported.
- **Daunorubicin,** liposomal formulation, should be reduced in dosage according to serum bilirubin (eg, bilirubin 1.2–3 mg/dL, give three fourths the normal dose; bilirubin >3 mg/dL, give one half the normal dose).
- **Doxorubicin** is excreted primarily in bile and toxicity is increased with impaired hepatic function. Liver function tests should be done before drug administration, and dosage of both regular and liposomal formulations should be reduced according to the serum bilirubin (eg, bilirubin 1.2 to 3 mg/dL, give one half the normal dose; bilirubin >3 mg/dL, give one fourth the normal dose).
- **Gemcitabine** should be used with caution; transient increases in serum aminotransferases occurred in most clients during clinical trials.
- **Idarubicin** should not be given to clients with a serum bilirubin above 5 mg/dL.
- **Irinotecan** has been associated with abnormal liver function tests in clients with liver metastases.
- **Mercaptopurine** causes hepatotoxicity, especially with higher doses (>2.5 mg/kg/day) and in combination with doxorubicin. Encephalopathy and fatal liver necrosis have occurred. The drug should be stopped if signs of hepatotoxicity (eg, jaundice, hepatomegaly, liver function tests indicating toxic hepatitis or biliary stasis) occur. Serum aminotransferases, alkaline phosphatase, and bilirubin should be monitored weekly initially, then monthly. Liver function tests may be needed more often in clients who have pre-existing liver impairment or are receiving other hepatotoxic drugs.
- **MTX** may cause acute (increased serum aminotransferases, hepatitis) and chronic (fibrosis and cirrhosis) hepatotoxicity. Chronic toxicity is potentially fatal. It is more likely to occur after prolonged use (eg, 2 years or longer) and after a total dose of at least 1.5 g. Cautious use of MTX is especially indicated in clients with pre-existing liver damage or impaired hepatic function. Liver function tests should be closely monitored.
- **Paclitaxel** is mainly metabolized by the liver and may cause more toxicity in clients with impaired hepatic function.

- **Procarbazine** causes more toxic effects in clients with hepatic impairment. Hospitalization is recommended for the first course of therapy.
- **Topotecan** is cleared from plasma more slowly in clients with hepatic impairment, but dosage reductions are not recommended.
- **Vinblastine** and **vincristine** may cause more toxicity with hepatic impairment and dosage should be reduced 50% for clients with a direct serum bilirubin value above 3 mg/dL.

Other drugs that should be used with caution include the antineoplastic hormone inhibitors. The antiandrogens include bicalutamide, flutamide, and nilutamide. **Bicalutamide** has a long serum half-life in clients with severe hepatic impairment. Excretion may be delayed and the drug may accumulate. The drug should be used with caution in clients with moderate to severe hepatic impairment, and liver function tests are needed periodically during long-term therapy. **Flutamide** is associated with serum aminotransferase abnormalities, cholestatic jaundice, hepatic encephalopathy, hepatic necrosis, and a few deaths. Liver function tests should be performed periodically and at the first sign or symptom of liver dysfunction (eg, pruritus, dark urine, jaundice). Flutamide should be discontinued if jaundice develops in clients who do not have liver metastases or if serum aminotransferase levels increase more than 2 to 3 times the upper limit of normal. Liver damage usually subsides if flutamide is discontinued or if dosage is reduced. **Nilutamide** may cause hepatitis or increases in liver enzymes. Liver enzymes should be checked at baseline and every 3 months. If symptoms of liver injury occur or if aminotransferases increase over 2 to 3 times the upper limits of normal, nilutamide should be discontinued.

Medroxyprogesterone should be stopped if any manifestations of impaired liver function develop. Tamoxifen and toremifene are antiestrogens. **Tamoxifen** is associated with changes in liver enzyme levels and occasionally more severe liver damage, including fatty liver, cholestasis, hepatitis, and hepatic necrosis. **Toremifene**'s elimination half-life is prolonged in clients with hepatic cirrhosis or fibrosis.

With the newer biologic drugs, **bortezomib** should be used with caution in clients with impaired hepatic function. With **gefitinib**, no dosage adjustments are necessary in clients with moderate to severe hepatic impairment.

Use in Home Care

Clients may receive parenteral cytotoxic drugs as outpatients and return home, or these and other antineoplastic drugs may be administered at home by the client or a caregiver. The home care nurse may be involved in a wide range of activities associated with antineoplastic drug therapy, including administering the drugs; administering other drugs to prevent or manage adverse effects; and assessing client and family responses to therapy. In addition, a major role involves teaching about the disease process, management of pain and other symptoms, the anticancer drugs, prevention or management of adverse drug effects, preventing infection, maintaining food and fluid intake, and other aspects of care. If a client is receiving erythropoietin or oprelvekin subcutaneously, the client or a caregiver may need to be taught injection technique.

The home care nurse also needs to teach clients and caregivers about safe handling of the traditional cytotoxic agents, including items contaminated with the drugs and client body fluids or excreta. Precautions need to be similar to those used in health care agencies.

APPLYING YOUR KNOWLEDGE 42-4

Julia has a long drive to the clinic to receive her chemotherapy and has to arrange with a friend or relative to bring her. Julia arrives at the clinic and you look for her orders. You are unable to locate any written orders so you call the physician, who gives you the orders over the telephone.

N U R S I N G   A C T I O N S

Antineoplastic Drugs

NURSING ACTIONS	RATIONALE/EXPLANATION
1. **Administer accurately**	
a. With oral cytotoxic drugs, follow specific instructions for individual drugs. For most drugs, the total daily dose can be given at one time.	These drugs are usually taken at home by clients or administered by a caregiver.
b. With **intravenous (IV) cytotoxic drugs,** general instructions include the following:	These drugs should be prepared in a pharmacy and given only by nurses who are certified to do so, who administer the drugs regularly, and who maintain their knowledge base about use of the drugs in oncology.

(continued)

NURSING ACTIONS	RATIONALE/EXPLANATION
(1) Compare labels on prepared solutions to medication orders in terms of the drug, concentration, expiration date, and instructions for administration.	Many of the drugs must be reconstituted from a powder and further diluted in an IV solution. Drug solutions should be prepared in the pharmacy.
(2) Follow instructions for administering each drug. Common methods include injecting the drug into the tubing of a rapidly flowing IV or infusing the drug over a specified period of minutes to hours.	Because the drugs are highly toxic, every precaution must be taken to ensure accurate and safe administration.
(3) For clients with a long-term venous access device (eg, Hickman or Groshong catheter), follow agency protocols for drug administration and catheter care.	Long-term devices decrease the number of venipunctures a client must undergo, but require special care to maintain patency and prevent infection.
(4) Follow agency protocols for skin exposure or spills of cytotoxic drug solutions.	These solutions are hazardous materials that require special handling.
c. With **monoclonal antibodies,** general instructions include the following:	The drugs should be prepared in a pharmacy. They may be given in an outpatient setting but patients receiving them must be closely monitored.
(1) Compare labels on prepared solutions to medication orders in terms of the drug, concentration, expiration date, and instructions for administration.	To ensure accurate administration of these diverse products.
(2) Administer by IV infusion; do *not* give as an IV push or bolus injection; do *not* mix with any other drugs.	Manufacturers' recommendations
(3) Follow instructions *exactly* re: rates of infusion.	Recommended rates vary according to the individual drugs and whether the first or later doses are being given.
(4) Pre-medicate with diphenhydramine and acetaminophen when ordered.	To prevent allergic-type infusion reactions, which are associated with alemtuzumab, cetuximab, gemtuzumab, rituximab
d. Give **gefitinib** without regard to food intake. Give **imatinib** with a meal and large glass of water; give doses of 400 or 600 mg once daily and doses of 800 mg as 400 mg twice daily. For patients unable to swallow the tablets, dissolve the tablets in water or apple juice (50 mL for 200-mg tablet and 100 mL for 400-mg tablet). Stir and have the patient drink the suspension when the tablet is completely dissolved.	Manufacturers' recommendations
e. Give reconstituted **bortezomib** as a bolus IV injection.	The drug is reconstituted with 3.5 mL of 0.9% sodium chloride injection, preferably in a pharmacy.
f. Give **goserelin** and **leuprolide** according to the manufacturers' instructions.	These drugs require specific techniques.
g. Give **letrozole**, **tamoxifen**, and **toremifene** without regard to meals; give exemestane after a meal.	Manufacturers' recommendations
h. Give **fulvestrant** intramuscularly (IM), into buttock, as a single 5 mL injection or as two 2.5 mL injections.	
2. **Observe for therapeutic effects** a. Increased appetite b. Increased feelings of well-being c. Improved mobility d. Decreased pain e. Laboratory and diagnostic tests that indicate improvement	Therapeutic effects depend to a large extent on the type of malignancy being treated. They may not become evident for several weeks after drug therapy is begun. With traditional cytotoxic drugs, some clients experience anorexia, nausea, and vomiting for 2 to 3 weeks after each cycle of drug therapy.

NURSING ACTIONS	RATIONALE/EXPLANATION
3. Observe for adverse effects	
a. With traditional cytotoxic drugs:	Cytotoxic drugs may have adverse effects on virtually any body tissue. These effects range from common to rare, from relatively mild to life threatening, and occur with usual dosage ranges. Myelosuppressive effects are used to guide drug therapy.
(1) Hematologic effects: bone marrow depression with anemia, leukopenia, and thrombocytopenia; decreased antibodies and lymphocytes	For most drugs, white blood cell (WBC) and platelet counts reach their lowest points (nadirs) 7 to 14 days after drug administration and return toward normal after 21 days. Normal leukocyte and platelet counts indicate recovery of bone marrow function. Anemia may occur later because the red blood cell lives longer than WBCs and platelets. Most of these drugs have immunosuppressant effects, which impair body defenses against infection.
(2) Gastrointestinal (GI) effects—anorexia, nausea, vomiting, diarrhea, constipation, oral and intestinal mucositis and mucosal ulcerations, oral candidiasis	Nausea and vomiting are common, usually occur within a few hours of drug administration, and often subside within 12 to 24 hours. Constipation is most likely to occur with vincristine. Mucositis may occur anywhere in the GI tract; may interfere with nutrition and cause significant discomfort; may lead to infection, hemorrhage, or perforation; and may require that drug therapy be stopped.
(3) Dermatologic effects—alopecia, dermatitis, tissue irritation at injection sites	Complete hair loss may take several weeks to occur. Some drugs may cause phlebitis and sclerosis of veins used for injections, as well as pain and tissue necrosis if allowed to leak into tissues around the injection site.
(4) Renal effects:	
(a) Hyperuricemia and uric acid nephropathy	When malignant cells are destroyed, they release uric acid into the bloodstream. Uric acid crystals may precipitate in the kidneys and cause impaired function or failure. Adverse effects on the kidneys are especially associated with methotrexate and cisplatin.
(b) With cisplatin, nephrotoxicity (increased blood urea nitrogen [BUN] and serum creatinine; decreased creatinine clearance)	Nephrotoxicity is a major adverse effect. Decreasing the dose or frequency of administration; vigorous hydration; and amifostine administration can reduce the incidence.
(c) With cyclophosphamide or ifosfamide, hemorrhagic cystitis (blood in urine, dysuria, burning on urination)	Hemorrhagic cystitis occurs in about 10% of clients. It is attributed to irritating effects of drug metabolites on the bladder mucosa. The drug is stopped if this occurs. Cystitis can be decreased by an ample fluid intake. In addition, mesna is given with ifosfamide.
(d) Pulmonary effects—cough, dyspnea, chest x-ray examination changes	Adverse effects on the lungs are associated mainly with bleomycin and methotrexate. With bleomycin, pulmonary toxicity may be severe and progress to pulmonary fibrosis.
(e) Cardiovascular effects—heart failure (dyspnea, edema, fatigue), dysrhythmias, electrocardiographic changes	Cardiomyopathy is associated mainly with doxorubicin and related drugs. This is a life-threatening adverse reaction. The heart failure may be unresponsive to digoxin.
(f) Central nervous system effects—peripheral neuropathy with vincristine, manifested by muscle weakness, numbness and tingling of extremities, foot drop, and decreased ability to walk	This common effect of vincristine may worsen for several weeks after drug administration. There is usually some recovery of function eventually.
(g) Endocrine effects—menstrual irregularities, sterility in men and women	
b. With monoclonal antibodies:	Although these drugs act more specifically than the traditional cytotoxic drugs, they may still affect normal cells and produce serious adverse effects.

(continued)

NURSING ACTIONS	RATIONALE/EXPLANATION
(1) Hypersensitivity-type infusion reaction—chills, fever, bronchospasm, dyspnea, skin rash or urticaria	These products are proteins and may contain other components capable of arousing an allergic reaction. Premedication with diphenhydramine (Benadryl) and acetaminophen is recommended with most of the drugs (eg, alemtuzumab, cetuximab, gemtuzumab, rituximab) to prevent or decrease infusion reactions.
(2) Hematologic effects—bone marrow depression (anemia, leukopenia, thrombocytopenia); high risk of infection, with chills, fever, respiratory and other symptoms	These effects occur with most of the drugs and leukopenia may be especially severe with alemtuzumab, for which prophylactic antimicrobial drugs are recommended during and for 2 to 3 months after drug administration.
(3) GI effects—anorexia, nausea, vomiting, stomatitis, diarrhea	These effects commonly occur.
(4) Cardiovascular effects—hypertension, hypotension, peripheral edema, heart failure, especially with alemtuzumab, bevacizumab, gemtuzumab, and trastuzumab	Severe cardiotoxicity leading to heart failure may be more likely to occur with bevacizumab and trastuzumab. With trastuzumab, cardiotoxicity is most likely to develop in patients who are 60 years or older and those who have received doxorubicin or cyclophosphamide. Left ventricular function should be evaluated in all patients before and during treatment and trastuzumab should be discontinued in those who develop significant decreases in left ventricular function (ie, ejection fraction).
(5) Miscellaneous effects with most of the drugs—joint and muscle pain, weakness, dyspnea, headache, dizziness	
c. With gefitinib and imatinib—anorexia, bleeding, edema, fatigue, fever, nausea, vomiting, diarrhea, neutropenia and infection, joint and muscle pain, skin rash, weakness	In addition, interstitial lung disease has been reported in 1% of patients taking gefitinib, with a few deaths. Patients should be monitored for acute onset of respiratory distress. If interstitial lung disease is confirmed, gefitinib should be discontinued.
d. With bortezomib—dehydration, edema, fever, hypotension, nausea, vomiting, skin rash, peripheral neuropathy	The risk of neuropathy may be increased with previous use of neurotoxic agents or pre-existing peripheral neuropathy.
e. With hormone inhibitors:	Hot flashes and nausea are the most common adverse effect of drugs that decrease estrogen.
(1) Aromatase inhibitors—hot flashes, fatigue, headache, nausea, musculoskeletal pain	
(2) Antiestrogens—hot flashes, nausea, fluid retention, weight loss, musculoskeletal pain, vaginal discharge and menstrual irregularities in premenopausal women	
(3) LHRH analogs—headache, depression, hot flashes, sexual dysfunction in males and females, infections in females	Hot flashes were the most commonly reported effect in both males and females; headache and depression were reported much more often in females than in males.
(4) Antiandrogens—hot flashes, breast tenderness and enlargement, chest pain, heart failure, weight gain, muscle pain, neuropathy	
4. Observe for drug interactions	
a. Drugs that *increase* effects of cytotoxic antineoplastic drugs:	
(1) Anticoagulants, oral	Increased risk of bleeding
(2) Bone marrow depressants	Increased bone marrow depression
(3) Other antineoplastic drugs	Additive cytotoxic effects, both therapeutic and adverse
b. Drugs that *increase* effects of cyclophosphamide:	
(1) Anesthetics, inhalation	Lethal combination. Discontinue cyclophosphamide at least 12 hours before general inhalation anesthesia is to be given.
(2) Carbamazepine, phenytoin, rifampin	Potentiate cyclophosphamide by induction of liver enzymes, which accelerate transformation of the drug into its active metabolites
(3) Other myelosuppressive antineoplastic drugs	Increased bone marrow depression

NURSING ACTIONS	RATIONALE/EXPLANATION
c. Drug that *increases* the effect of mercaptopurine:	
(1) Allopurinol	Allopurinol increases formation of the active mercaptopurine metabolite; doses of mercaptopurine must be reduced to one third to one fourth the usual dose.
d. Drugs that *increase* effects of methotrexate (MTX):	
(1) Alcohol	Additive liver toxicity. Avoid concomitant use.
(2) Aspirin, nonsteroidal anti-inflammatory drugs (NSAIDs), phenytoin, procarbazine, sulfonamides	Potentiate MTX by displacing it from protein-binding sites in plasma. Salicylates also block renal excretion of methotrexate. This may cause pancytopenia and liver toxicity.
(3) Other hepatotoxic drugs	Additive liver toxicity
(4) Other antineoplastic drugs	Additive cytotoxic effects, both therapeutic and adverse. Cisplatin may induce renal damage that impairs MTX excretion, increases blood levels, and increases toxicity.
(5) Trimethoprim-sulfamethoxazole (TMP-SMX, Bactrim)	Increased MTX toxicity; avoid concurrent administration if possible.
e. Drug that *decreases* effects of methotrexate (MTX):	
(1) Leucovorin (folinic acid)	Leucovorin antagonizes the toxic effects of MTX and is used as an antidote for high-dose MTX regimens or for overdose. It must be given exactly at the specified time, before affected cells become too damaged to respond.
f. Drugs that *increase* effects of vinca alkaloids:	
(1) Erythromycin increases vinblastine toxicity; itraconazole increases vincristine toxicity.	These drugs probably inhibit metabolism of vinblastine and vincristine.
g. Drugs that *alter* effects of monoclonal antibodies:	
(1) Paclitaxel may increase blood levels and effects of trastuzumab.	Interactions have not been studied with these drugs.
h. Drugs that *alter* effects of biologic targeted drugs:	
(1) Enzyme inhibitors (eg, cimetidine, clarithromycin, erythromycin, itraconazole, others) *increase* effects; enzyme inducers (eg, carbamazepine, phenytoin, rifampin, others) *decrease* effects.	Most interactions are thought to occur with drugs metabolized by CYP3A4 enzymes. If imatinib is given concurrently with an enzyme inducer, dosage must be increased by approximately 50% for therapeutic effects and patients must be carefully monitored.
(2) With gefitinib, drugs that cause sustained elevations in gastric pH (eg, cimetidine, ranitidine, sodium bicarbonate) may *decrease* effects.	
(3) With imatinib, chronic use of acetaminophen may *increase* risks of hepatotoxicity.	
i. Drugs that *alter* effects of hormone inhibitors:	
(1) With tamoxifen and toremifene, enzyme inhibitors *increase* effects and enzyme inducers *decrease* effects (see **h.** (1), above).	
(2) With flutamide, amiodarone, fluoroquinolones, and fluvoxamine may *increase* effects; carbamazepine and rifampin may *decrease* effects.	
(3) With nilutamide, delavirdine, fluconazole, fluvoxamine, gemfibrozil, isoniazid, and omeprazole may *increase* effects; carbamazepine and rifampin may *decrease* effects.	

APPLYING YOUR KNOWLEDGE: ANSWERS

42-1 The most common adverse effects are bone marrow depression, mucositis, alopecia, and GI ulceration. Julia will need periodic blood tests to determine the degree of bone marrow depression. Nutrition will be important. Julia should have a plan for the alopecia (perhaps including purchasing a wig prior to her hair loss). Be sure to review medications to prevent and treat the adverse effects with Julia.

42-2 Although there is some risk, the benefit is that Herceptin will bind with a substance called *human epidermal growth factor receptor 2,* which is present in excess in 25%–30% of women with breast cancer.

42-3 Tell Julia that every precaution is taken when administering this medication and that she will be medicated before the infusion with diphenhydramine and acetaminophen to reduce the occurrence of a serious allergic reaction.

42-4 Ensure that the orders are appropriate; do not accept verbal or telephone orders.

Review and Application Exercises

Short Answer Exercises

1. List major characteristics of malignant cells.

2. Which common cancers are attributed mainly to environmental factors? Which are attributed to genetic factors?

3. Which cytotoxic antineoplastic drugs are associated with serious adverse effects (eg, bone marrow suppression, cardiotoxicity, hepatotoxicity, nephrotoxicity, neurotoxicity)?

4. Which drugs are associated with second malignancies?

5. How do the newer biologic agents differ from traditional cytotoxic drugs?

6. What is the basis for the anticancer effects of hormone inhibiting drugs?

7. For which cytotoxic drugs are cytoprotective drugs available?

8. List at least one intervention to prevent or minimize each of the following adverse effects of traditional cytotoxic chemotherapy: anemia, bleeding, infection, nausea and vomiting, neutropenia, stomatitis.

9. What measures are used to prevent or decrease the allergic infusion reactions associated with several antineoplastic monoclonal antibodies?

NCLEX-Style Questions

10. A priority nursing diagnosis for a client receiving cytotoxic chemotherapy is
   a. Risk for Impaired Skin Integrity
   b. Risk for Injury: Infection
   c. Body Image Disturbance related to alopecia
   d. Ineffective Family Coping

11. For a client receiving a drug that causes bone marrow depression, which of the following should be especially emphasized with the client and family members or caregivers?
   a. Wash hands often and avoid people with colds, flu, or other infections.
   b. Fatigue and weakness are uncommon.
   c. More nausea and vomiting may occur when the blood-cell counts are low.
   d. Take acetaminophen for fever.

12. An important characteristic of cytotoxic chemotherapy is that it
   a. damages both malignant and nonmalignant cells
   b. causes few adverse effects
   c. stimulates growth of cancer cells
   d. must be given daily

13. Biologic drugs used in the treatment of cancer
   a. are highly cytotoxic to both cancer cells and normal cells
   b. target specific antigens or vital processes of cancer cells
   c. change the hormonal environment of cancer cells
   d. protect normal cells from cytotoxic drugs

14. A *vesicant* antineoplastic drug can
   a. cause skin irritation
   b. cause extensive tissue damage
   c. only be given through a central IV line
   d. be given by deep intramuscular injection if diluted with normal saline

Selected References

Aberle, M. F., & McLeskey, S. W. (2003). Biology of lung cancer with implications for new therapies. *Oncology Nursing Forum, 30*(2), 273–280.

Agraharkar, M. L., Cinclair, R. D., Kuo, Y. F., et al. (2004). Risk of malignancy with long-term immunosuppression in renal transplant recipients. *Kidney International, 66,* 383–389.

Balmer, C. M., & Valley, A. W. (2002). Cancer treatment and chemotherapy. In J. T. DiPiro, R. L. Talbert, G. C. Yee, G. R. Matzke, B. G. Wells, & L. M. Posey (Eds.), *Pharmacotherapy: A pathophysiologic approach* (5th ed., pp. 2175–2222). New York: McGraw-Hill.

Berlin, J. D. (2002). Targeting vascular endothelial growth factor in colorectal cancer. *Oncology, 16*(8, Suppl. 7), 13–15.

Bertino, J. R., & Hait, W. (2004). Principles of cancer therapy. In L. Goldman & D. Ausiello (Eds.), *Cecil textbook of medicine* (22nd ed., pp. 1137–1150). Philadelphia: W. B. Saunders.

Coyle, B., & Polovich, M. (2004). Handling hazardous drugs. *American Journal of Nursing, 104*(2), 104.

Davidson, M. B., Thakkar, S., Hix, J. K., et al. (2004). Pathophysiology, clinical consequences, and treatment of tumor lysis syndrome. *American Journal of Medicine, 116,* 546–554.

Drug facts and comparisons. (Updated monthly). St. Louis: Facts and Comparisons.

Duffy, K. M. (2003). Innovations in the management of leukemia: Role of biologic therapies. *Cancer Nursing, 26*(6, Suppl.), 26S–31S.

Eilers, J. (2004). Nursing interventions and supportive care for the prevention and treatment of oral mucositis associated with cancer treatment. *Oncology Nursing Forum, 31*(Suppl. 4), 13–23.

Gillespie, T. W. (2003). Anemia in cancer: Therapeutic implications and interventions. *Cancer Nursing, 26*(2), 119–123.

Hansten, P. D., & Horn, J. R. (2004). *The top 100 drug interactions: A guide to patient management.* Edmonds, WA: H & H.

Kremer, L., & Caron, H. N. (2004). Anthracycline cardiotoxicity in children. *New England Journal of Medicine, 351*(2), 120–121.

Lacy, C. F., Armstrong, L. L., Goldman, M. P., et al. (2004). *Lexi-Comp's drug information handbook* (12th ed.). Hudson, OH: Lexi-Comp.

Naughton, M. (2004). Medical management of malignant disease. In G. B. Green, I. S. Harris, G. A. Lin, et al. (Eds.), *The Washington manual of medical therapeutics* (31st ed., pp. 440–479). Philadelphia: Lippincott Williams & Wilkins.

Nirenberg, A. (2003). Managing hematologic toxicities. *Cancer Nursing, 26*(6, Suppl.), 32S–37S.

Pitot, H. C. (2002). *Fundamentals of oncology* (4th ed.). New York: Marcel Dekker.

Porth, C. M. (2004). *Pathophysiology: Concepts of altered health states* (7th ed.). Philadelphia: Lippincott Williams & Wilkins.

Rokita, S. A. (2004). Oncology: Nursing management in cancer care. In S. C. Smeltzer & B. G. Bare (Eds.), *Brunner & Suddarth's textbook of medical-surgical nursing* (10th ed., pp. 315–368). Philadelphia: Lippincott Williams & Wilkins.

Rosen, R. H. (2002). Management of chemotherapy-induced nausea and vomiting. *Journal of Pharmacy Practice, 15*(1), 32–41.

Twite, K. (2004). Neoplasia. In C. M. Porth, *Pathophysiology: Concepts of altered health states* (7th ed., pp. 155–184). Philadelphia: Lippincott Williams & Wilkins.

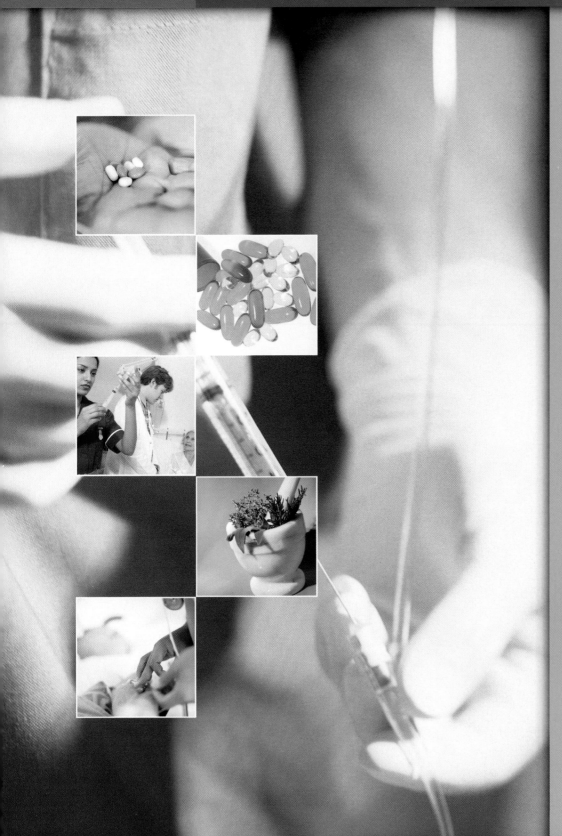

Drugs Affecting the Respiratory System

CHAPTER OUTLINE

43 Physiology of the Respiratory System

44 Drugs for Asthma and Other Broncho-constrictive Disorders

45 Antihistamines and Allergic Disorders

46 Nasal Decongestants, Antitussives, and Cold Remedies

Physiology of the Respiratory System

OBJECTIVES

After studying this chapter, you will be able to:

1. Review roles and functions of the main respiratory tract structures in oxygenation of body tissues.
2. Describe the role of carbon dioxide in respiration.
3. List common signs and symptoms affecting respiratory function.
4. Identify general categories of drugs used to treat respiratory disorders.

OVERVIEW OF THE RESPIRATORY SYSTEM

The respiratory system helps meet the basic human need for oxygen (O_2). Oxygen is necessary for the oxidation of foodstuffs, by which energy for cellular metabolism is produced. When the oxygen supply is inadequate, cell function is impaired; when oxygen is absent, cells die. Permanent brain damage occurs within 4 to 6 minutes of anoxia. In addition to providing oxygen to all body cells, the respiratory system also removes carbon dioxide (CO_2), a major waste product of cell metabolism. Excessive accumulation of CO_2 damages or kills body cells.

The efficiency of the respiratory system depends on the quality and quantity of air inhaled, the patency of air passageways, the ability of the lungs to expand and contract, and the ability of O_2 and CO_2 to cross the alveolar–capillary membrane. In addition to the respiratory system, the circulatory, nervous, and musculoskeletal systems have important functions in respiration. Additional characteristics of the respiratory system and the process of respiration are described in the following sections.

Respiration

Respiration is the process of gas exchange by which O_2 is obtained and CO_2 is eliminated. This gas exchange occurs between the lung and the blood across the alveolar–capillary membrane and between the blood and body cells. More specifically, the four parts of respiration are:

- *Ventilation*—the movement of air between the atmosphere and the alveoli of the lungs
- *Perfusion*—blood flow through the lungs
- *Diffusion*—the process by which O_2 and CO_2 are transferred between alveoli and blood and between blood and body cells
- *Regulation* of breathing by the respiratory muscles and nervous system

Respiratory Tract

The respiratory tract is a series of branching tubes with progressively smaller diameters. These tubes (nose, pharynx, larynx, trachea, bronchi, and bronchioles) function as air passageways and air "conditioners" that filter, warm, and humidify incoming air. Most of the conditioning is done by the ciliated mucous membrane that lines the entire respiratory tract, except the pharynx and alveoli. *Cilia* are tiny, hair-like projections that sweep mucus toward the pharynx to be expectorated or swallowed. The mucous membrane secretes mucus, which forms a protective blanket and traps foreign particles, such as bacteria and dust.

When air is inhaled through the nose, it is conditioned by the nasal mucosa. When the nasal passages are blocked, the mouth serves as an alternate airway. The oral mucosa may warm and humidify air but cannot filter it.

Pharynx, Larynx, and Trachea

Air passes from the nasal cavities to the pharynx (throat). Pharyngeal walls are composed of skeletal muscle, and their lining is composed of mucous membrane. The pharynx contains the palatine tonsils, which are large masses of lymphatic tissue. The pharynx is a passageway for food, fluids, and air. Food and fluids go from the pharynx to the esophagus, and air passes from the pharynx into the trachea.

The larynx is composed of nine cartilages joined by ligaments and controlled by skeletal muscles. It contains the vocal cords and forms the upper end of the trachea. It closes on swallowing to prevent aspiration of food and fluids into the lungs.

The trachea is the passageway between the larynx and the main stem bronchi. It is a cartilaginous tube lined with ciliated epithelium and mucus-secreting cells. Cilia and mucus help to protect and defend the lungs.

Lungs

The lungs begin where the trachea divides into the right and left mainstem *bronchi* and contain the remaining respiratory structures. They are divided into five lobes, each with a secondary bronchus. The lobes are further subdivided into bronchopulmonary segments supplied by smaller bronchi. The bronchopulmonary segments contain lobules, which are the functional units of the lung (the site where gas exchange takes place). Each lobule is supplied by a bronchiole, an arteriole, a venule, and a lymphatic vessel. Blood enters the lobules through a pulmonary artery and exits through a pulmonary vein. Lymphatic structures surround the lobule and aid in the removal of plasma proteins and other particles from interstitial spaces.

The mainstem bronchi branch into smaller bronchi, then into bronchioles. *Bronchioles* are approximately the size of a pencil lead and do not contain cartilage or mucus-secreting glands. The walls of the bronchioles contain smooth muscle, which is controlled by the autonomic nervous system. Stimulation of parasympathetic nerves causes constriction; stimulation of sympathetic nerves causes relaxation or dilation.

The epithelial lining of the bronchioles becomes thinner with progressive branchings until only one cell layer is apparent. The bronchioles give rise to the *alveoli,* which are grape-like clusters of air sacs surrounded by capillaries.

The alveoli are composed of two types of cells. Type I cells are flat, thin epithelial cells that fuse with capillaries to form the alveolar–capillary membrane across which gas exchange occurs. Oxygen enters the bloodstream to be transported to body cells; CO_2 enters the alveoli to be exhaled from the lungs. Type II cells produce surfactant, a lipoprotein substance that decreases the surface tension in the alveoli and aids lung inflation. The alveoli also contain macrophages that help to protect and defend the lungs.

The lungs are encased in a membrane called the *pleura,* which is composed of two layers. The inner layer, which adheres to the surface of the lung, is called the *visceral pleura.* The outer layer, which lines the thoracic cavity, is called the *parietal pleura.* The potential space between the layers is called the *pleural cavity.* It contains fluid that allows the layers to glide over each other and minimizes friction.

The lungs expand and relax in response to changes in pressure relationships (intrapulmonic and intrapleural pressures). Elastic tissue in the bronchioles and alveoli allows the lungs to stretch or expand to accommodate incoming air. This ability is called *compliance.* The lungs also recoil (like a stretched rubber band) to expel air. Some air remains in the lungs after expiration, which allows gas exchange to continue between respirations.

In addition to exchanging O_2 and CO_2, the lungs synthesize, store, release, remove, metabolize, or inactivate a variety of biologically active substances. These substances, which may be locally released or carried in blood or tissue fluids, participate in both physiologic and pathologic processes. Specific substances that may be released from the lungs include biogenic amines (eg, catecholamines, histamine, serotonin), arachidonic acid metabolites (eg, prostaglandins, leukotrienes), angiotensin-converting enzyme, and heparin. The amines are important in regulating smooth muscle tone (ie, constriction or dilation) in the airways and blood vessels. Prostaglandins and leukotrienes are important in inflammatory processes. Angiotensin-converting enzyme converts angiotensin I to angiotensin II, which is important in regulating blood pressure. Heparin helps to dissolve blood clots, especially in the capillaries, where small clots are trapped. The lungs also process peptides, lipids, hormones, and drugs and inactivate bradykinin.

Lung Circulation

The pulmonary circulatory system transports O_2 and CO_2. After oxygen enters the bloodstream across the alveolar–capillary membrane, it combines with hemoglobin in red blood cells for transport to body cells, where it is released. Carbon dioxide combines with hemoglobin in the cells for return to the lungs and elimination from the body.

The lungs receive the total cardiac output of blood and are supplied with blood from two sources, the pulmonary and bronchial circulations. The pulmonary circulation provides for gas exchange because the pulmonary arteries carry deoxygenated blood to the lungs and the pulmonary veins return oxygenated blood to the heart. The bronchial arteries arise from the thoracic aorta and supply the air passages and supporting structures. The bronchial circulation also warms and humidifies incoming air and can form new vessels and develop collateral circulation when normal vessels are blocked (eg, in pulmonary embolism). The latter ability helps to keep lung tissue alive until circulation can be restored.

Capillaries in the lungs are lined by a single layer of epithelial cells called *endothelium*. Once thought to be a passive conduit for blood, it is now known that the endothelium performs several important functions. First, it forms a barrier that prevents leakage of water and other substances into lung tissue. Second, it participates in the transport of respiratory gases, water, and solutes. Third, it secretes vasodilating substances such as nitric oxide and prostacyclin. Nitric oxide also regulates smooth muscle tone in the bronchi, and prostacyclin also inhibits platelet aggregation. When pulmonary endothelium is injured (eg, by endotoxins or drugs such as bleomycin, an anticancer drug), these functions are impaired.

The Nervous System's Role in Respiration

The nervous system regulates the rate and depth of respiration by the respiratory center in the medulla oblongata, the pneumotaxic center in the pons, and the apneustic center in the reticular formation. The respiratory center is stimulated primarily by increased CO_2 in the fluids of the center. (However, excessive CO_2 depresses the respiratory center.) When the center is stimulated, the rate and depth of breathing are increased, and excessive CO_2 is exhaled. A lesser stimulus to the respiratory center is decreased oxygen in arterial blood.

The nervous system also operates several reflexes important to respiration. The cough reflex is especially important because it helps protect the lungs from foreign particles, air pollutants, bacteria, and other potentially harmful substances. A cough occurs when nerve endings in the respiratory tract mucosa are stimulated by dryness, pressure, cold, irritant fumes, or excessive secretions.

The Musculoskeletal System's Role in Respiration

The musculoskeletal system participates in chest expansion and contraction. Normally, the diaphragm and external intercostal muscles expand the chest cavity and are called *muscles of inspiration*. The abdominal and internal intercostal muscles are the *muscles of expiration*.

Summary of Respiratory Function

Overall, normal respiration requires:

1. Atmospheric air containing at least 21% O_2.
2. Adequate ventilation. Ventilation, in turn, requires patent airways, expansion and contraction of the chest, expan-

sion and contraction of the lungs, and maintenance of a normal range of intrapulmonic and intrapleural pressures.
3. Adequate diffusion of O_2 and CO_2 through the alveolar–capillary membrane. Factors influencing diffusion include the thickness and surface area of the membrane and pressure differences between gases on each side of the membrane.
4. Adequate perfusion or circulation of blood and sufficient hemoglobin to carry needed O_2.

In addition, normal breathing occurs 16 to 20 times per minute and is quiet, rhythmic, and effortless. Approximately 500 mL of air is inspired and expired with a normal breath (tidal volume); deep breaths or "sighs" occur 6 to 10 times per hour to ventilate more alveoli. Fever, exercise, pain, and emotions such as anger increase respirations. Sleep or rest and various medications, such as antianxiety drugs, sedatives, and opioid analgesics, slow respiration.

DISORDERS OF THE RESPIRATORY SYSTEM

The respiratory system is subject to many disorders that interfere with respiration and other lung functions. These disorders may be caused by agents that reach the system through inhaled air or through the bloodstream and include respiratory tract infections, allergic disorders, inflammatory disorders, and conditions that obstruct airflow (eg, excessive respiratory tract secretions, asthma, other chronic obstructive pulmonary diseases). Injury to the lungs by various disorders (eg, anaphylaxis, asthma, mechanical stimulation such as hyperventilation, pulmonary thromboembolism, pulmonary edema, acute respiratory distress syndrome) is associated with the release of histamine and other biologically active chemical mediators from the lungs. These mediators often cause inflammation and constriction of the airways.

The ciliated epithelial cells of the larger airways, the type I epithelial cells of the alveoli, and the capillary endothelial cells of the alveolar area are especially susceptible to injury. When they are injured, cellular functions are impaired (eg, decreased mucociliary clearance). Common signs and symptoms of respiratory disorders include cough, increased secretions, mucosal congestion, and bronchospasm. Severe disorders or inadequate treatment may lead to cell necrosis or respiratory failure.

DRUG THERAPY

In general, drug therapy is more effective in relieving respiratory symptoms than in curing the underlying disorders that cause the symptoms. Major drug groups used to treat respiratory symptoms are bronchodilating and anti-inflammatory agents (see Chap. 44), antihistamines (see Chap. 45), and nasal decongestants, antitussives, and cold remedies (see Chap. 46).

Review and Application Exercises

Short Answer Exercises

1. What is the main function of the respiratory system?

2. Where does the exchange of oxygen and carbon dioxide occur?

3. List factors that stimulate rate and depth of respiration.

4. List factors that depress rate and depth of respiration.

5. What are common signs and symptoms of respiratory disorders for which drug therapy is often used?

Selected References

Guyton, A. C., & Hall, J. E. (2000). *Textbook of medical physiology* (10th ed.). Philadelphia: W. B. Saunders.

Porth, C. M. (2005). *Pathophysiology: Concepts of altered health states* (7th ed.). Philadelphia: Lippincott Williams & Wilkins.

Drugs for Asthma and Other Bronchoconstrictive Disorders

OBJECTIVES

After studying this chapter, you will be able to:

1. Describe the main pathophysiologic characteristics of asthma and other bronchoconstrictive disorders.
2. Discuss the uses and effects of bronchodilating drugs, including adrenergics, anticholinergics, and xanthines.
3. Differentiate between short-acting and long-acting inhaled beta$_2$-adrenergic agonists in terms of uses and nursing process implications.
4. Discuss the uses of anti-inflammatory drugs, including corticosteroids, leukotriene modifiers, and mast cell stabilizers.
5. Discuss reasons for using inhaled drugs when possible.
6. Differentiate between "quick relief" and long-term control of asthma symptoms.
7. Discuss the use of antiasthmatic drugs in special populations.
8. Teach clients self-care and long-term control measures.

APPLYING YOUR KNOWLEDGE

Kenneth Cuff is a 56-year-old male who has adult-onset asthma. His medications include salmeterol and fluticasone (Advair); zafirlukast; and albuterol when needed. Mr. Cuff works as a sales manager at a large corporation. You are the on-site nurse for the office.

INTRODUCTION

The drugs described in this chapter are used to treat respiratory disorders characterized by bronchoconstriction, inflammation, mucosal edema, and excessive mucus production (asthma, bronchitis, and emphysema). Asthma is emphasized because of its widespread prevalence, especially in urban populations. Compared with Caucasians, African Americans and Hispanics have a higher prevalence and African Americans have a higher death rate from asthma. However, the differences are usually attributed to urban living and lesser access to health care rather than race or ethnic group. Occupational asthma (ie, asthma resulting from repeated and prolonged exposure to industrial inhalants) is also a major health problem. Persons with occupational asthma often have symptoms while in the work environment, with improvement on days off and during vacations. Symptoms sometime persist after termination of exposure. Asthma may occur at any age but is especially common in children and older adults. Children who are exposed to allergens and airway irritants such as tobacco smoke during infancy are at high risk for development of asthma.

Asthma

Symptoms

Asthma is an airway disorder characterized by bronchoconstriction, inflammation, and hyperreactivity to various stimuli. Resultant symptoms include dyspnea, wheezing, chest tightness, cough, and sputum production. Wheezing is a high-pitched, whistling sound caused by turbulent airflow through an obstructed airway. Thus, any condition that produces significant airway occlusion can cause wheezing. However, a chronic cough may be the only symptom for some people. Symptoms vary in incidence and severity from occasional episodes of mild respiratory distress, with normal functioning between "attacks," to persistent, daily, or continual respiratory distress if not adequately controlled. Inflammation and damaged airway mucosa are chronically present, even when clients appear symptom free.

Acute symptoms of asthma may be precipitated by numerous stimuli, and hyperreactivity to such stimuli may initiate both inflammation and bronchoconstriction. Viral infections of the respiratory tract are often the causative agents, especially in infants and young children whose airways are small and easily obstructed. Asthma symptoms may persist for days or weeks after the viral infection resolves. In about 25% of clients with asthma, aspirin and other nonsteroidal anti-inflammatory drugs (NSAIDs) can precipitate an attack. Some clients are allergic to sulfites and may experience life-threatening asthma attacks if they ingest foods processed with these preservatives (eg, beer, wine, dried fruit). The Food and Drug Administration (FDA) has banned the use of sulfites on foods meant to be served raw, such as open salad bars. Clients with severe asthma should be cautioned against ingesting food and drug products containing sulfites or metabisulfites.

Gastroesophageal reflux disease (GERD), a common disorder characterized by heartburn and esophagitis, is also associated with asthma. Asthma that worsens at night may be associated with nighttime acid reflux. The reflux of acidic gastric contents into the esophagus is thought to initiate a vagally mediated, reflex type of bronchoconstriction. (Asthma may also aggravate GERD, because antiasthma medications that dilate the airways also relax muscle tone in the gastroesophageal sphincter and may increase acid reflux.) Additional precipitants may include allergens (eg, pollens, molds), airway irritants and pollutants (eg, chemical fumes, cigarette smoke, automobile exhaust), cold air, and exercise. Acute episodes of asthma may last minutes to hours.

Pathophysiology

Bronchoconstriction (also called *bronchospasm*) involves strong muscle contractions that narrow the airways. Airway smooth muscle extends from the trachea through the bronchioles. It is wrapped around the airways in a spiral pattern, and contraction causes a sphincter type of action that can completely occlude the airway lumen. Bronchoconstriction is aggravated by inflammation, mucosal edema, and excessive mucus and may be precipitated by the numerous stimuli described above.

When lung tissues are exposed to causative stimuli, mast cells release substances that cause bronchoconstriction and inflammation. Mast cells are found throughout the body in connective tissues and are abundant in tissues surrounding capillaries in the lungs. When sensitized mast cells in the lungs or eosinophils in the blood are exposed to allergens or irritants, multiple cytokines and other chemical mediators (eg, acetylcholine, cyclic guanosine monophosphate [GMP], histamine, interleukins, leukotrienes, prostaglandins, serotonin) are synthesized and released. These chemicals act directly on target tissues of the airways, causing smooth muscle constriction, increased capillary permeability and fluid leakage, and changes in the mucus-secreting properties of the airway epithelium.

Bronchoconstrictive substances are antagonized by cyclic adenosine monophosphate (cyclic AMP). Cyclic AMP is an intracellular substance that initiates various intracellular activities, depending on the type of cell. In lung cells, cyclic AMP inhibits release of bronchoconstrictive substances and thus indirectly promotes bronchodilation. In mild to moderate asthma, bronchoconstriction is usually recurrent and reversible, either spontaneously or with drug therapy. In advanced or severe asthma, airway obstruction becomes less reversible and worsens because chronically inflamed airways undergo structural changes (eg, fibrosis, enlarged smooth muscle cells, enlarged mucous glands), called "airway remodeling," that inhibit their function.

National Asthma Education and Prevention Program (NAEPP)

Because of asthma's significance as a public health problem, the National Heart, Lung, and Blood Institute (NHLBI) of the National Institutes of Health (NIH) established the NAEPP. The NAEPP assembled a group of experts who established "Guidelines for the Diagnosis and Management of Asthma." These guidelines (Box 44-1) were updated in 1997; selected aspects, mainly related to children, were updated in 2002. The guidelines are the current "standard of care" for adults and children with asthma. Additional information can be obtained from:

NHLBI Health Information Network
P.O. Box 30105
Bethesda, MD 20824-0105
Phone: (301) 592-8573
Fax: (301) 592-8563
Web: http://www.nhlbi.nih.gov

Chronic Bronchitis and Emphysema

Chronic bronchitis and *emphysema,* commonly called *chronic obstructive pulmonary disease* (COPD), usually develop after long-standing exposure to airway irritants such as cigarette smoke. In these conditions, bronchoconstriction and inflammation are more constant and less reversible than with asthma. Anatomic and physiologic changes occur over several years and lead to increasing dyspnea and activity intolerance. These conditions usually affect middle-aged or older adults.

Drug Therapy

Two major groups of drugs used to treat asthma, acute and chronic bronchitis, and emphysema are bronchodilators and anti-inflammatory drugs. Bronchodilators are used to prevent and treat bronchoconstriction; anti-inflammatory drugs are used to prevent and treat inflammation of the airways. Reducing inflammation also reduces bronchoconstriction by decreasing mucosal edema and mucus secretions that narrow airways and by decreasing airway hyperreactivity to various stimuli.

Box 44-1 National Asthma Education and Prevention Program (NAEPP) Expert Panel Guidelines*

Definition

Asthma is "a chronic inflammatory disorder of the airways in which many cells and cellular elements play a role, in particular, mast cells, eosinophils, T lymphocytes, macrophages, neutrophils, and epithelial cells."

Goals of Therapy

1. Minimal or no chronic symptoms day or night
2. Minimal or no exacerbations
3. No limitations on activities; for children, no school/parent's work missed
4. Minimal use of short-acting inhaled beta$_2$ agonist (<1 time per day, <1 canister/month)
5. Minimal or no adverse effects from medications

General Recommendations

- Establish and teach patients/parents/caregivers about quick relief measures and long-term control measures. Assist to identify and control environmental factors that aggravate asthma.
- For acute attacks, gain control as quickly as possible (a short course of systemic corticosteroids may be needed); then step down to the least medication necessary to maintain control.
- Review the treatment regimen every 1 to 6 months. If control is adequate and goals are being met, a gradual stepwise reduction in medication may be possible. If control is inadequate, the treatment regimen may need to be changed. For example, frequent or increasing use of a short-acting beta$_2$ agonist (>2 times a week with intermittent asthma; daily or increasing use with persistent asthma) may indicate the need to initiate or increase long-term control therapy. However, first reassess patients' medication techniques (eg, correct use of inhalers), adherence, and environmental control measures.

Quick Relief for Acute Exacerbations

- **Adults and children > 5 years:** Short-acting, inhaled, beta$_2$ agonist, 2–4 puffs as needed. If symptoms are severe, patients may need up to 3 treatments at 20-minute intervals or a nebulizer treatment. A short course of a systemic corticosteroid may also be needed.
- **Children 5 years and younger:** Short-acting beta$_2$ agonist by nebulizer or face mask and spacer or holding chamber. Alternative: oral beta$_2$ agonist. With viral respiratory infections, the beta$_2$ agonist may be needed q4–6h up to 24 hours or longer and a systemic corticosteroid may be needed.

Long-Term Control

- **Step 1 Mild Intermittent** (symptoms 2 days/week or less or 2 nights/month or less): No daily medication needed; treat acute exacerbations with an inhaled beta$_2$ agonist and possibly a short course of a systemic corticosteroid.
- **Step 2 Mild Persistent** (symptoms >2/week but <1×/day or >2 nights/month):
  - **Adults and children > 5 years:** Low-dose inhaled corticosteroid. Alternatives: cromolyn or nedocromil, a leukotriene

modifier, or sustained-release theophylline to maintain a serum theophylline drug level of 5–15 mcg/mL.
- **Children 5 years and younger:** Administer the inhaled corticosteroid by a nebulizer or metered-dose inhaler (MDI) with a holding chamber. Alternatives: cromolyn (via nebulizer or MDI with holding chamber) or a leukotriene modifier.
- **Step 3 Moderate Persistent** (symptoms daily and >1 night/ week):
  - **Adults and children > 5 years:** Low- to medium-dose inhaled corticosteroid and a long-acting beta$_2$ agonist. Alternatives: increase corticosteroid dose or continue low to medium dose of corticosteroid and add a leukotriene modifier or theophylline.
  - **Children < 5 years:** Low-dose inhaled corticosteroid and a long-acting beta$_2$ agonist or medium-dose inhaled corticosteroid.
- **Step 4 Severe Persistent** (symptoms continual during daytime hours and frequent at night):
  - **Adults and children > 5 years:** High-dose inhaled corticosteroid and long-acting beta$_2$ agonist and, if necessary, a systemic corticosteroid (2 mg/kg/d, not to exceed 60 mg/d). Reduce systemic corticosteroid when possible.
  - **Children < 5 years:** Same as for adults and older children.

Low (L), Medium (M), and High (H) Doses of Inhaled Corticosteroids:

	Adults (mcg)	Children (12 y and younger) (mcg)
Beclomethasone (42 or 84 mcg/puff)	L: 168–504 M: 504–840 H: >840	L: 84–336 M: 336–672 H: >672
Beclomethasone (40–80 mcg/puff)	L: 80–240 M: 240–480 H: >480	L: 80–160 M: 160–320 H: >320
Budesonide (200 mcg/ inhalation)	L: 200–600 M: 600–1200 H: >1200	L: 200–400 M: 400–800 H: >800
Budesonide inhalation suspension for nebulization (child dose only)		L: 0.5 mg M: 1.0 mg H: 2.0 mg
Flunisolide (250 mcg/puff)	L: 500–1000 M: 1000–2000 H: >2000	L: 500–750 M: 1000–1250 H: >1250
Fluticasone aerosol (44, 110, or 220 mcg/puff)	L: 88–264 M: 264–660 H: >660	L: 88–176 M: 176–440 H: >440
Fluticasone powder (50, 100, or 250 mcg/puff)	L: 100–300 M: 300–600 H: >600	L: 100–200 M: 200–400 H: >400
Triamcinolone acetonide (100 mcg/puff)	L: 400–1000 M: 1000–2000 H: >2000	L: 400–800 M: 800–1200 H: >1200

*Adapted from NAEPP Expert Panel Report 2 (NIH Publication No. 97-4051, 1997) and the Update on Selected Topics 2002 (NIH Publication No. 02-5075).

The drugs are described in the following sections; pharmacokinetic characteristics of inhaled drugs are listed in Table 44-1.

BRONCHODILATORS

Table 44-2 lists routes and dosage ranges of the bronchodilators.

Adrenergics

Adrenergic drugs (see Chap. 17) stimulate beta$_2$-adrenergic receptors in the smooth muscle of bronchi and bronchioles. The receptors, in turn, stimulate the enzyme adenyl cyclase to increase production of cyclic AMP. The increased cyclic AMP produces bronchodilation. Some beta-adrenergic drugs (eg, epinephrine) also stimulate beta$_1$-adrenergic receptors in the heart to increase the rate and force of contraction. Cardiac stimulation is an adverse effect when the drugs are given for bronchodilation. These drugs are contraindicated in clients with cardiac tachydysrhythmias and severe coronary artery disease; they should be used cautiously in clients with hypertension, hyperthyroidism, diabetes mellitus, and seizure disorders.

Epinephrine may be injected subcutaneously in an acute attack of bronchoconstriction, with therapeutic effects in approximately 5 minutes and lasting for approximately 4 hours. However, an inhaled selective beta$_2$ agonist is the drug of choice in this situation. Epinephrine is also available without prescription in a pressurized aerosol form (eg, Primatene). Almost all over-the-counter aerosol products promoted for use in asthma contain epinephrine. These products are often abused and may delay the client from seeking medical attention. Clients should be cautioned that excessive use may produce hazardous cardiac stimulation and other adverse effects.

Albuterol, levalbuterol, and **pirbuterol** are short-acting beta$_2$-adrenergic agonists used for prevention and treatment of bronchoconstriction. These drugs act more selectively on beta$_2$ receptors and cause less cardiac stimulation than epinephrine. Most often taken by inhalation, they are also the most effective bronchodilators and the treatment of first choice to relieve acute asthma. Because the drugs can be effectively delivered by aerosol or nebulization, even to young children and to clients on mechanical ventilation, there is seldom a need to give epinephrine or other nonselective adrenergic drugs by injection.

The beta$_2$ agonists are usually self-administered by metered-dose inhalers (MDIs). Although most drug references still list a regular dosing schedule (eg, every 4 to 6 hours), asthma experts recommend that the drugs be used when needed (eg, to treat acute dyspnea or prevent dyspnea during exercise). If these drugs are overused, they lose their bronchodilating effects because the beta$_2$-adrenergic receptors become unresponsive to stimulation. This tolerance does not occur with the long-acting beta$_2$ agonists.

Formoterol and **salmeterol** are long-acting beta$_2$-adrenergic agonists used only for *prophylaxis* of acute bronchoconstriction. They are not effective in acute attacks because they have a slower onset of action than the short-acting drugs (up to 20 minutes for salmeterol). Effects last 12 hours and the drugs should *not* be taken more frequently. If additional bronchodilating medication is needed, a short-acting agent (eg, albuterol) should be used.

Metaproterenol is a relatively selective, intermediate-acting beta$_2$-adrenergic agonist that may be given orally or by

TABLE 44-1 Pharmacokinetics of Selected Inhaled Antiasthma Medications

| GENERIC NAME | ACTION | | | METABOLISM/EXCRETION | HALF-LIFE (HOURS) |
	Onset (min)	Peak (hours)	Duration (hours)		
Adrenergics					
Albuterol	5	1.5–2	3–6	Liver/urine	2–4
Levalbuterol	5	1	6–8	Liver/urine	4–6
Pirbuterol	5		5	Liver, tissue/urine	ND
Salmeterol	13–20	3–4	7.5–17	Liver/feces	ND
Anticholinergic					
Ipratropium	15	1–2	3–4		1.6
Corticosteroids					
Beclomethasone	Rapid	1–2 wk		Liver/feces	3–15
Budesonide	Immediate	Rapid	8–12	Liver/urine (60%) & feces	2.8
Flunisolide	Slow	10–30	4–6	Liver/renal (50%), feces (40%)	1–2
Fluticasone	Slow		24	Liver/feces & urine	3.1

ND, not determined.

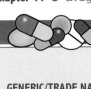

Table 44-2 Drugs at a Glance: Bronchodilating Drugs

GENERIC/TRADE NAME	ROUTES AND DOSAGE RANGES	
	Adults	**Children**
Bronchodilators		
ADRENERGICS		
Albuterol (Proventil, Ventolin, AccuNeb, Proventil, Repetab)	Inhalation* aerosol (90 mcg/actuation): 1–2 oral inhalations q4–6h; prevention of exercise-induced bronchospasm, 2 inhalations 1 min before exercise Inhalation solution via nebulizer, 2.5 mg 3–4 times daily (in 2.5 mL sterile saline, over 5–15 min) Regular tablets: PO 2–4 mg 3–4 times daily Extended-release tablets: Proventil Repetabs PO 4–8 mg q12h, initially. Increase if necessary to a maximum of 32 mg/d, in divided doses, q12h.	*Inhalation aerosol:* 4 y and older (12 y and older for Proventil), same as adults Nebulizer solution, 12 y and older, same as adults; 2–12 y (AccuNeb), 1.25 mg 3–4 times daily, as needed, over 5–15 min *Regular tablets:* 12 y and older, same as adults; 6–12 y, 2 mg 3–4 times daily *Extended-release tablets:* 12 y and older, same as adults: 6–12 y: PO 4 mg q12h initially; increase if necessary to a maximum of 24 mg/d, in divided doses, q12h (both Volmax and Proventil Repetab).
Epinephrine (Adrenalin, Bronkaid)	Aqueous solution (epinephrine 1:1000), Sub-Q 0.2–0.5 mL; dose may be repeated after 20 min if necessary Inhalation by inhaler, one or two inhalations 4–6 times per day Inhalation by nebulizer, 0.25–0.5 mL of 2.25% racemic epinephrine in 2.5 mL normal saline	Aqueous solution (epinephrine 1:1000), Sub-Q 0.01 mL/kg q4h as needed. A single dose should not exceed 0.5 mL. Inhalation, same as adults for both inhaler and nebulizer
Formoterol (Foradil)	Oral inhalation by special inhaler (Aerolizer), 12 mcg (contents of 1 capsule) twice daily, q12h	5 y and older, same as adults
Levalbuterol (Xopenex)	Nebulizer, 0.63–1.25 mg 3 times daily, q6–8h	12 y and older, same as adults *6–11 y:* Nebulizer, 0.31 mg 3 times daily, q6–8h
Metaproterenol (Alupent)	Inhalation,* 1–3 puffs (0.65 mg/dose), 4 times per day; maximum dose, 12 inhalations/d	Inhalation, not recommended for use in children <12 y
Pirbuterol (Maxair)	Inhalation,* two puffs (0.4 mg/dose), 4–6 times per day; maximum dose, 12 inhalations/d	*>12 y:* Same as adults; not recommended for use in children <12 y
Salmeterol (Serevent)	Inhalation powder: 1 inhalation (50 mcg) q12h	<12 y, dosage not established Inhalation powder: 4 y and older, same as adults
Terbutaline (Brethine)	PO 2.5–5 mg q6–8h; maximum dose, 15 mg/d Sub-Q 0.25 mg, repeated in 15–30 min if necessary, q4–6h Inhalation,* two inhalations (400 mcg/dose) q4–6h	PO 2.5 mg 3 times per day for children 12 y and older; maximum dose, 7.5 mg/d Sub-Q dosage not established Inhalation, same as adults for children 12 y and older
ANTICHOLINERGICS		
Ipratropium bromide (Atrovent)	Two inhalations (36 mcg) from the metered-dose inhaler 4 times per day	Dosage not established
Tiotropium (Spiriva)	One tablet (18 mcg) in HandiHaler once daily	Dosage not established
Xanthines **Short-acting theophylline** (Aminophylline)	PO, 500 mg initially, then 200–300 mg q6–8h; IV infusion, 6 mg/kg over 30 min, then 0.1–1.2 mg/kg/h	PO, 7.5 mg/kg initially, then 5–6 mg/kg q6–8h; IV infusion, 6 mg/kg over 30 min, then 0.6–0.9 mg/kg/h

(continued)

Table 44-2 Drugs at a Glance: Bronchodilating Drugs (continued)

	ROUTES AND DOSAGE RANGES	
GENERIC/TRADE NAME	**Adults**	**Children**
ANTICHOLINERGICS **Xanthines**		
Long-acting theophylline (Theochron, others)	PO, 150–300 mg q8–12h; maximal dose 13 mg/kg or 900 mg daily, whichever is less	PO, 100–200 mg q8–12h; maximal dose, 24 mg/kg/d
Combination Drugs **Fluticasone/Salmeterol** (Advair)	Oral inhalation, one inhalation, twice daily	*12 y and older:* same as adults
Ipratropium/Albuterol (Combivent, DuoNeb)	Aerosol: two inhalations 4 times daily Nebulizing solution: 1 vial 4 times daily, increased to 6 times daily if necessary	Dosage not established

*Short-acting adrenergic bronchodilators are used mainly by inhalation, as needed, rather than on a regular schedule.
IV, intravenous; PO, oral; Sub-Q, subcutaneous.

MDI. It is used to treat acute bronchospasm and to prevent exercise-induced asthma. In high doses, metaproterenol loses some of its selectivity and may cause cardiac and central nervous system (CNS) stimulation.

Terbutaline is a relatively selective beta$_2$-adrenergic agonist that is a long-acting bronchodilator. When given subcutaneously, terbutaline loses its selectivity and has little advantage over epinephrine. Muscle tremor is the most frequent side effect with this agent.

Anticholinergics

Anticholinergics (see Chap. 20) block the action of acetylcholine in bronchial smooth muscle when given by inhalation. This action reduces intracellular GMP, a bronchoconstrictive substance.

Ipratropium was formulated to be taken by inhalation for maintenance therapy of bronchoconstriction associated with chronic bronchitis and emphysema. Improved pulmonary function usually occurs in a few minutes. Ipratropium acts synergistically with adrenergic bronchodilators and may be used concomitantly. It improves lung function about 10% to 15% over an inhaled beta$_2$ agonist alone. Ipratropium may also be used to treat rhinorrhea associated with allergic rhinitis and the common cold. It is available as a nasal spray for such usage. Ipratropium is poorly absorbed and produces few systemic effects. However, cautious use is recommended in clients with narrow-angle glaucoma and prostatic hypertrophy. The most common adverse effects are cough, nervousness, nausea, gastrointestinal upset, headache, and dizziness.

Tiotropium (Spiriva) was approved to be taken once daily by inhalation for maintenance therapy of bronchoconstriction

associated with chronic bronchitis and emphysema. Tiotropium has differences in its pharmacokinetic and pharmacologic properties that may make it superior to ipratropium as an anticholinergic agent. The primary adverse effect of tiotropium is dry mouth, though other effects include headache, dizziness, abdominal pain, constipation, diarrhea, flulike symptoms, and chest pain. Cautious use is recommended in clients with narrow-angle glaucoma.

Xanthines

The main xanthine used clinically is **theophylline.** Despite many years of use, the drug's mechanism of action is unknown. Various mechanisms have been proposed, such as inhibiting phosphodiesterase enzymes that metabolize cyclic AMP, increasing endogenous catecholamines, inhibiting calcium ion movement into smooth muscle, inhibiting prostaglandin synthesis and release, or inhibiting the release of bronchoconstrictive substances from mast cells and leukocytes. In addition to bronchodilation, other effects that may be beneficial in asthma and COPD include inhibiting pulmonary edema by decreasing vascular permeability; increasing the ability of cilia to clear mucus from the airways; strengthening contractions of the diaphragm; and decreasing inflammation. Theophylline also increases cardiac output, causes peripheral vasodilation, exerts a mild diuretic effect, and stimulates the CNS. The cardiovascular and CNS effects are adverse effects. Serum drug levels should be monitored to help regulate dosage and avoid adverse effects. Theophylline preparations are contraindicated in clients with acute gastritis and peptic ulcer disease; they should be used cautiously in those with cardiovascular disorders that could be aggravated by drug-induced cardiac stimulation.

Theophylline was formerly used extensively in the prevention and treatment of bronchoconstriction associated with asthma, bronchitis, and emphysema. Now, it is considered a second-line agent that may be added in severe disease inadequately controlled by first-line drugs. Numerous dosage forms of theophylline are available. Theophylline ethylenediamine (aminophylline) contains approximately 85% theophylline and is the only formulation that can be given intravenously (IV). However, IV aminophylline is not recommended for emergency treatment of acute asthma because studies indicate little, if any, added benefit in adults or children. Oral theophylline preparations may be used for long-term treatment. Most formulations contain anhydrous theophylline (100% theophylline) as the active ingredient, and sustained-action tablets (eg, Theochron) are more commonly used than other formulations. Theophylline is metabolized in the liver; metabolites and some unchanged drug are excreted through the kidneys.

APPLYING YOUR KNOWLEDGE 44-1:
HOW CAN YOU AVOID THIS MEDICATION ERROR?
Mr. Cuff is having difficulty breathing and visits the on-site clinic. You administer an inhaled bronchodilator, the Advair.

ANTI-INFLAMMATORY AGENTS

Table 44-3 provides routes and dosage ranges of anti-inflammatory antiasthmatic drugs.

Corticosteroids

Corticosteroids (see Chap. 23) are used in the treatment of acute and chronic asthma and other bronchoconstrictive disorders, in which they have two major actions. First, they suppress inflammation in the airways by inhibiting the following processes: movement of fluid and protein into tissues; migration and function of neutrophils and eosinophils; synthesis of histamine in mast cells; and production of proinflammatory substances (eg, prostaglandins, leukotrienes, several interleukins). Beneficial effects of suppressing airway inflammation include decreased mucus secretion, decreased edema of airway mucosa, and repair of damaged epithelium, with subsequent reduction of airway reactivity. A second action is to increase the number and sensitivity of beta$_2$-adrenergic receptors, which restores or increases the effectiveness of beta$_2$-adrenergic bronchodilators. The number of beta$_2$ receptors increases within approximately 4 hours, and improved responsiveness to beta$_2$ agonists occurs within approximately 2 hours.

In acute, severe asthma, a systemic corticosteroid in relatively high doses is indicated in clients whose respiratory distress is not relieved by multiple doses of an inhaled beta$_2$ agonist (eg, every 20 minutes for 3 to 4 doses). The corticosteroid may be given IV or orally, and IV administration offers no therapeutic advantage over oral administration. After the drug is started, pulmonary function usually improves in 6 to 8 hours. Most clients achieve substantial benefit within 48 to 72 hours and the drug is usually continued for 7 to 10 days. Multiple doses are usually given because studies indicate that maintaining the drug concentration at steroid receptor sites in the lung is more effective than high single doses. High single or pulse doses do not increase therapeutic effects; they may increase risks of developing myopathy and other adverse effects, however. In some infants and young children with acute, severe asthma, oral prednisone for 3 to 10 days has relieved symptoms and prevented hospitalization.

In chronic asthma, a corticosteroid is usually taken by inhalation, on a daily schedule. It is often given concomitantly with one or more bronchodilators and may be given with another anti-inflammatory drug such as a leukotriene modifier or a mast cell stabilizer. In some instances, the other drugs allow smaller doses of the corticosteroid. For acute flare-ups of symptoms during treatment of chronic asthma, a systemic corticosteroid may be needed temporarily to regain control.

In early stages of the progressive disease, clients with COPD are unlikely to need corticosteroid therapy. In later stages, however, they usually need periodic short-course therapy for episodes of respiratory distress. When needed, the corticosteroid is given orally or parenterally because effectiveness of inhaled corticosteroids has not been established in COPD. In end-stage COPD, clients often become "steroid-dependent" and require daily doses because any attempt to reduce dosage or stop the drug results in respiratory distress. Such clients experience numerous serious adverse effects of prolonged systemic corticosteroid therapy.

Corticosteroids should be used with caution in clients with peptic ulcer disease, inflammatory bowel disease, hypertension, congestive heart failure, and thromboembolic disorders. However, they cause fewer and less severe adverse effects when taken in short courses or by inhalation than when taken systemically for long periods of time.

Beclomethasone, budesonide, flunisolide, fluticasone, mometasone, and **triamcinolone** are topical corticosteroids for inhalation. Topical administration minimizes systemic absorption and adverse effects. These preparations may substitute for or allow reduced dosage of systemic corticosteroids. In people with asthma who are taking an oral corticosteroid, the oral dosage is reduced slowly (over weeks to months) when an inhaled corticosteroid is added. The goal is to give the lowest oral dose necessary to control symptoms. Beclomethasone, flunisolide, and fluticasone also are available in nasal solutions for treatment of allergic rhinitis, which may play a role in bronchoconstriction. Because systemic absorption occurs in clients using inhaled corticosteroids (about 20% of a dose), high doses should be reserved for those otherwise requiring oral corticosteroids.

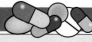

Table 44-3 Drugs at a Glance: Anti-Inflammatory Antiasthmatic Drugs

GENERIC/TRADE NAME	ROUTES AND DOSAGE RANGES	
	Adults	Children
Corticosteroids		
Beclomethasone (QVAR)	Oral inhalation, two inhalations (0.84 mg/dose) three or four times daily; maximum, 20 inhalations/24 h	*6–12 y:* Oral inhalation, one or two inhalations three or four times per day; maximum dose, 10 inhalations/24 h
Beclomethasone (Beconase AQ)	1 spray in each nostril 2–4 times/day or 2 sprays in each nostril twice daily (total dose 168–336 mcg/day)	
Budesonide (Pulmocort Turbuhaler)	Oral inhalation, 200–400 mcg twice daily	*6 y:* Oral inhalation 200 mcg twice daily
Flunisolide (AeroBid)	Oral inhalation, two inhalations (0.50 mg/dose) twice daily, morning and evening; maximum dose, four inhalations twice daily (2 mg)	*6–15 y:* Oral inhalation, two inhalations twice daily
Fluticasone (Flonase)	4 sprays in each nostril once daily (265 mcg/day)	*12 y and older:* Same as adults *4–11 y:* 1 spray in each nostril once daily; may increase to 2 sprays in each nostril for desired effect
Fluticasone aerosol (Flovent)	Aerosol, 88–440 mcg twice daily	Dosage not established
Fluticasone powder (Flovent Rotadisk)	Powder, 100–500 mcg twice daily	*12 y and older:* Same as adults *4–11 y:* Powder, 50–100 mcg twice daily
Hydrocortisone sodium phosphate and sodium succinate	IV 100–200 mg q4–6h initially, then decreased or switched to an oral dosage form	IV 1–5 mg/kg q4–6h
Methylprednisolone sodium succinate	IV 10–40 mg q4–6h for 48–72 h	IV 0.5 mg/kg q4–6h
Mometasone (Asmanex Twisthaler, Nasonex)	Nasal inhalation two sprays (50 mcg/spray) in each nostril once daily	*12 y and older:* Same as adults *2–11 y:* 1 spray (50 mcg) in each nostril once daily
Prednisone	PO 20–60 mg/d	PO 2 mg/kg/d initially
Triamcinolone (Azmacort)	Oral inhalation, two inhalations 3 or 4 times per day; maximum dose, 16 inhalations/24 h	*6–12 y:* one or two inhalations 3 or 4 times per day; maximum dose, 12 inhalations/24 h
Leukotriene Modifiers		
Montelukast (Singulair)	PO 10 mg once daily in the evening or at bedtime	*15 y and older:* Same as adults *6–14 y:* PO 5 mg once daily in the evening *2–5 y:* 4 mg once daily
Zafirlukast (Accolate)	PO 20 mg twice daily, 1 h before or 2 h after a meal	*12 y and older:* Same as adults *5–11 y:* PO 10 mg twice daily
Zileuton (Zyflo)	PO 600 mg 4 times daily	*12 y and older:* Same as adults *<12 y:* Dosage not established
Mast Cell Stabilizers		
Cromolyn (Intal)	Nebulizer solution, oral inhalation, 20 mg 4 times daily	*2 y and older:* Same as adults
	Aerosol spray, oral inhalation, two sprays 4 times daily	*5 y and older:* Same as adults
Nedocromil (Tilade)	Inhalation, 4 mg q6–12h	*>12 y:* Same as adults

IV, intravenous; PO, oral.

Hydrocortisone, prednisone, and **methylprednisolone** are given to clients who require systemic corticosteroids. Prednisone is given orally; hydrocortisone and methylprednisolone may be given IV to clients who are unable to take an oral medication.

APPLYING YOUR KNOWLEDGE 44-2
Mr. Cuff has a friend who takes prednisone for his breathing problems. Mr. Cuff asks why he isn't taking the same medication. How would you respond?

Leukotriene Modifiers

Leukotrienes are strong chemical mediators of bronchoconstriction and inflammation, the major pathologic features of asthma. They can cause sustained constriction of bronchioles and immediate hypersensitivity reactions. They also increase mucus secretion and mucosal edema in the respiratory tract. Leukotrienes are formed by the lipoxygenase pathway of arachidonic acid metabolism (Fig. 44-1) in response to cellular injury. They are designated by LT, the letter B, C, D, or E, and the number of chemical bonds in their structure (eg, LTB4, LTC4, and LTE4, also called *slow releasing substances of anaphylaxis* or *SRS-A,* because they are released more slowly than histamine).

Leukotriene modifier drugs were developed to counteract the effects of leukotrienes and are indicated for long-term treatment of asthma in adults and children. The drugs help to prevent acute asthma attacks induced by allergens, exercise, cold air, hyperventilation, irritants, and aspirin or NSAIDs. They are not effective in relieving acute attacks. However, they may be continued concurrently with other drugs during acute episodes.

The leukotriene modifiers include three agents with two different mechanisms of action. **Zileuton** inhibits lipoxygenase and thereby reduces formation of leukotrienes; **montelukast** and **zafirlukast** are leukotriene receptor antagonists. Zileuton is used infrequently because it requires multiple daily dosing, may cause hepatotoxicity, and may inhibit the metabolism of drugs metabolized by the cytochrome P450 3A4 enzymes. Zafirlukast and montelukast improve symptoms and pulmonary function tests (PFTs), decrease nighttime symptoms, and decrease the use of beta$_2$ agonist drugs. They are effective with oral administration, can be taken once or twice a day, can be used with bronchodilators and corticosteroids, and elicit a high degree of client adherence and satisfaction. However, they are less effective than low doses of inhaled corticosteroids.

Montelukast and zafirlukast are well absorbed with oral administration. They are metabolized in the liver by the

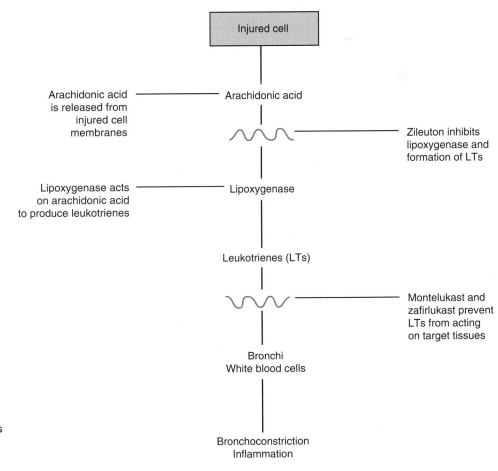

FIGURE 44-1 Formation of leukotrienes and actions of leukotriene-modifying drugs.

cytochrome P450 enzyme system and may interact with other drugs metabolized by this system. Most metabolites are excreted in the feces. Zafirlukast is excreted in breast milk and should not be taken during lactation. The most common adverse effects reported in clinical trials were headache, nausea, diarrhea, and infection.

Zileuton is well absorbed, highly bound to serum albumin (93%), and metabolized by the cytochrome P450 liver enzymes; metabolites are excreted mainly in urine. It is contraindicated in clients with active liver disease or substantially elevated liver enzymes (three times the upper limit of normal values). When used, hepatic aminotransferase enzymes should be monitored during therapy and the drug should be discontinued if enzyme levels reach five times the normal values or if symptoms of liver dysfunction develop. Elevation of liver enzymes was the most serious adverse effect during clinical trials; other adverse effects include headache, pain, and nausea. In addition, zileuton increases serum concentrations of propranolol, theophylline, and warfarin.

Mast Cell Stabilizers

Cromolyn and **nedocromil** stabilize mast cells and prevent the release of bronchoconstrictive and inflammatory substances when mast cells are confronted with allergens and other stimuli. The drugs are indicated only for prophylaxis of acute asthma attacks in clients with chronic asthma; they are not effective in acute bronchospasm or status asthmaticus and should not be used in these conditions. Use of one of these drugs may allow reduced dosage of bronchodilators and corticosteroids.

The drugs are taken by inhalation. Cromolyn is available in a metered-dose aerosol and a solution for use with a power-operated nebulizer. A nasal solution is also available for prevention and treatment of allergic rhinitis. Nedocromil is available in a metered-dose aerosol.

Mast cell stabilizers are contraindicated in clients who are hypersensitive to the drugs. They should be used with caution in clients with impaired renal or hepatic function. Also, the propellants in the aerosols may aggravate coronary artery disease or dysrhythmias.

Immunosuppressant Monoclonal Antibody

Omalizumab (Xolair) works by binding to immunoglobulin E (IgE), blocking receptors on the surfaces of mast cells and basophils. This prevents IgE from attaching to the cells, thus preventing the release of substances in the body that can trigger an allergic reaction and preventing the development of inflammation. Omalizumab is indicated in clients with allergic asthma whose symptoms do not respond adequately to inhaled steroids. Further discussion of this drug is found in Chapter 41.

Herbal and Dietary Supplements

Numerous preparations are promoted to relieve symptoms of asthma and clients with asthma are increasingly using alternative and complementary therapies. Some herbs have a pharmacologic basis for effect. However, most are less potent or more toxic than traditional asthma medications. For example, caffeine is a xanthine and therefore has bronchodilating effects similar to, but weaker than, those of theophylline. Caffeine-containing products, including coffee and tea, may slightly enhance bronchodilation. However, they also increase the adverse effects associated with adrenergic bronchodilators or theophylline (eg, symptoms of excessive cardiac and CNS stimulation such as tachycardia, dysrhythmias, insomnia, nervousness).

In general, herbal and dietary therapies in asthma, as in other disorders, have not been studied in controlled clinical trials and should be avoided. Because asthma can result in death in a matter of minutes, clients should be counseled *not* to use dietary or herbal supplements in place of prescribed bronchodilating and anti-inflammatory medications. Delays in appropriate treatment can have serious, even fatal, consequences.

NURSING PROCESS

Assessment

Assess the client's pulmonary function.

- General assessment factors include rate and character of respiration, skin color, arterial blood gas analysis, and pulmonary function tests. Abnormal breathing patterns (eg, rate below 12 or above 24 per minute, dyspnea, cough, orthopnea, wheezing, "noisy" respirations) may indicate respiratory distress. Severe respiratory distress is characterized by tachypnea, dyspnea, use of accessory muscles of respiration, and hypoxia. Early signs of hypoxia include mental confusion, restlessness, anxiety, and increased blood pressure and pulse rate. Late signs include cyanosis and decreased blood pressure and pulse. Hypoxemia is confirmed if arterial blood gas analysis shows decreased partial pressure of oxygen (Po_2).
- In acute bronchospasm, a medical emergency, the client is in obvious and severe respiratory distress. A characteristic feature of bronchospasm is forceful expiration or wheezing.
- If the client has chronic asthma, try to determine the frequency and severity of acute attacks; factors that precipitate or relieve acute attacks; antiasthmatic medications taken occasionally or regularly; allergies; and condition between acute attacks, such as restrictions in activities of daily living due to asthma.

● If the client has chronic bronchitis or emphysema, assess for signs of respiratory distress, hypoxia, cough, amount and character of sputum, exercise tolerance (eg, dyspnea on exertion, dyspnea at rest), medications, and nondrug treatment measures (eg, breathing exercises, chest physiotherapy).

Nursing Diagnoses

● Impaired Gas Exchange related to bronchoconstriction and excessive mucus production
● Activity Intolerance related to impaired gas exchange and fatigue
● Risk for Injury: Severe bronchospasm with asthma and adverse effects with antiasthmatic drugs
● Noncompliance: Overuse of adrenergic bronchodilators
● Deficient Knowledge: Factors precipitating bronchoconstriction and strategies to avoid precipitating factors
● Deficient Knowledge: Accurate self-administration of drugs, including use of inhalers

Planning/Goals

The client will
● Self-administer bronchodilating and other drugs accurately
● Experience relief of symptoms
● Avoid preventable adverse drug effects
● Avoid overusing bronchodilating drugs
● Avoid exposure to stimuli that cause bronchospasm when possible
● Avoid respiratory infections when possible

Interventions

Use measures to prevent or relieve bronchoconstriction when possible. General measures include those to prevent respiratory disease or promote an adequate airway. Some specific measures include the following:

● Use mechanical measures for removing excessive respiratory tract secretions and preventing their retention. Effective measures include coughing, deep breathing, percussion, and postural drainage.
● Help the client identify and avoid exposure to conditions that precipitate bronchoconstriction. For example, allergens may be removed from the home, school, or work environment; cigarette smoke should be avoided when possible. When bronchospasm is precipitated by exercise, prophylaxis by prior inhalation of bronchodilating agents is better than avoiding exercise, especially in children.
● Assist clients with asthma to identify early signs of difficulty, including increased need for beta-adrenergic

agonists, activity limitations, and waking at night with asthma symptoms.
● Monitor peak expiratory flow rate (PEFR) when indicated. Portable meters are available for use in clinics, physicians' offices, and clients' homes. This is an objective measure of airflow/airway obstruction and helps to evaluate the client's treatment regimen.
● Assist clients with moderate to severe asthma in obtaining meters and learning to measure PEFR. Clients with a decreased PEFR may need treatment to prevent acute, severe respiratory distress.
● Assist clients and at least one family member in managing acute attacks of bronchoconstriction, including when to seek emergency care.
● Try to prevent or reduce anxiety, which may aggravate bronchospasm. Stay with the client during an acute asthma attack if feasible. Clients experiencing severe and prolonged bronchospasm (status asthmaticus) should be admitted or transferred to a hospital intensive care unit.
● With any clients who smoke cigarettes, encourage cessation of smoking and provide information, resources, and assistance in doing so. Emphasize the health benefits of improved respiratory function.
● In addition, provide appropriate client teaching related to drug therapy (see accompanying display).

Evaluation

● Observe for relief of symptoms and improved arterial blood gas values.
● Interview and observe for correct drug administration, including use of inhalers.
● Interview and observe for tachydysrhythmias, nervousness, insomnia, and other adverse drug effects.
● Interview about and observe behaviors to avoid stimuli that cause bronchoconstriction and respiratory infections.

APPLYING YOUR KNOWLEDGE 44-3
Mr. Cuff comes into the clinic and you suspect he is experiencing respiratory distress. You focus your assessment on what signs/symptoms?

PRINCIPLES OF THERAPY

Drug Selection and Administration

Choice of drug and route of administration are determined largely by the severity of the disease process and the client's response to therapy. Some guidelines include the following:

● A selective, short-acting, inhaled beta$_2$-adrenergic agonist (eg, albuterol) is the initial drug of choice for acute bronchospasm.

General Considerations

☑ Asthma and other chronic lung diseases are characterized by constant inflammation of the airways and periodic or persistent labored breathing from constriction or narrowing of the airways. Antiasthmatic drugs are often given in combination to combat these problems. Thus, it is extremely important to know the type and purpose of each drug.

☑ Except for the short-acting, inhaled bronchodilators (eg, albuterol), antiasthmatic medications are used long term to control symptoms and prevent acute asthma attacks. This means they must be taken on a regular schedule and continued when symptom free.

☑ When an asthma attack (ie, acute bronchospasm with shortness of breath, wheezing respirations, cough) occurs, the only fast-acting, commonly used medication to relieve these symptoms is an inhaled, short-acting bronchodilator (eg, albuterol). Other inhaled and oral drugs are not effective and should not be used.

☑ Try to prevent symptoms. For example, respiratory infections can precipitate difficulty in breathing. Avoiding infections (eg, by good hand hygiene, avoiding people with infections, annual influenza vaccinations, and other measures) can prevent acute asthma attacks. If you are allergic to tobacco smoke, perfume, or flowers, try to avoid or minimize exposure.

☑ A common cause of acute asthma attacks is not taking medications correctly. Some studies indicate that one third to two thirds of clients with asthma do not comply with instructions for using their medications. Factors that contribute to noncompliance with drug therapy include long-term use, expense, and adverse effects. If you have difficulty taking medications as prescribed, discuss the situation with a health care provider. Cheaper medications or lower doses may be effective alternatives. Just stopping the medications may precipitate acute breathing problems.

☑ If unable to prevent symptoms, early recognition and treatment may help prevent severe distress and hospitalizations. Signs of impending difficulty include increased needs for bronchodilator inhalers, activity limitations, waking at night because of asthma symptoms, and variability in the peak expiratory flow rate (PEFR), if you use a PEFR meter at home. The first treatment is to use a short-acting, inhaled bronchodilator. If this does not improve breathing, seek emergency care.

☑ Keep adequate supplies of medications on hand. Missing a few doses of long-term control or "preventive" medications may precipitate an acute asthma attack; not using an inhaled bronchodilator for early breathing difficulty may lead to more severe problems and the need for emergency treatment or hospitalization.

☑ Be sure you can use your metered-dose inhalers correctly. According to several research studies, many patients do not.

☑ Drinking 2 to 3 quarts of fluids daily helps thin secretions in the throat and lungs and makes them easier to remove.

☑ Avoid tobacco smoke and other substances that irritate breathing passages (eg, aerosol hair spray, antiperspirants, cleaning products, and automobile exhaust) when possible.

☑ Avoid excessive intake of caffeine-containing fluids such as coffee, tea, and cola drinks. These beverages may increase bronchodilation but also may increase heart rate and cause palpitations, nervousness, and insomnia with bronchodilating drugs.

☑ Take influenza vaccine annually and pneumococcal vaccine at least once if you have chronic lung disease.

☑ Inform all health care providers about the medications you are taking and do not take over-the-counter drugs or herbal supplements without consulting a health care provider. Some drugs can decrease beneficial effects or increase adverse effects of antiasthmatic medications. For example, over-the-counter nasal decongestants, asthma remedies, cold remedies, and antisleep medications can increase the rapid heartbeat, palpitations, and nervousness often associated with bronchodilators. With herbal remedies, none are as effective as standard antiasthmatic medication, and they may cause serious or life-threatening adverse effects.

Self-Administration

☑ Follow instructions carefully. Better breathing with minimal adverse effects depends on accurate use of prescribed medications. If help is needed with metered-dose inhalers, consult a health care provider.

☑ Use short-acting bronchodilator inhalers as needed, not on a regular schedule. If desired effects are not achieved or if symptoms worsen, inform the prescribing physician. Do not increase dosage or frequency of taking medication. Overuse increases adverse drug effects and decreases drug effectiveness.

☑ If taking formoterol or salmeterol, which are long-acting, inhaled bronchodilators, do not use more often than every 12 hours. If constricted breathing occurs, use a short-acting bronchodilator inhaler between doses of a long-acting drug. Salmeterol does not relieve acute shortness of breath because it takes approximately 20 minutes to start acting and 1 to 4 hours to achieve maximal bronchodilating effects.

☑ If taking an oral or inhaled corticosteroid, take on a regular schedule, at approximately the same time each day. The purpose of these drugs is to relieve inflammation in the airways and prevent acute respiratory distress. They are not effective unless taken regularly.

☑ If taking oral theophylline, take fast-acting preparations before meals with a full glass of water, at regular intervals around the clock. If gastrointestinal upset occurs, take with food. Take long-acting preparations every 8 to 12 hours; do not chew or crush.

☑ Take zafirlukast 1 hour before or 2 hours after a meal; montelukast and zileuton may be taken with or without food. Take montelukast in the evening or at bedtime. This schedule provides maximum beneficial effects during the night and early morning, when asthma symptoms often occur or worsen.

☑ Use inhalers correctly:
1. Shake well immediately before each use.
2. Remove the cap from the mouthpiece.
3. Exhale to the end of a normal breath.

C L I E N T   T E A C H I N G   G U I D E L I N E S

Antiasthmatic Drugs (continued)

4. With the inhaler in the upright position, place the mouthpiece just inside the mouth, and use the lips to form a tight seal or hold the mouthpiece approximately two finger-widths from the open mouth.

5. While pressing down on the inhaler, take a slow, deep breath for 3 to 5 seconds, hold the breath for approximately 10 seconds, and exhale slowly.

6. Wait 3 to 5 minutes before taking a second inhalation of the drug.

7. Rinse the mouth with water after each use.

8. Rinse the mouthpiece and store the inhaler away from heat.

9. If you have difficulty using an inhaler, ask your physician about a spacer device (a tube attached to the inhaler that makes it easier to use).

- Because aerosol products act directly on the airways, drugs given by inhalation can usually be given in smaller doses and produce fewer adverse effects than oral or parenteral drugs.

- Ipratropium and tiotropium, the anticholinergic bronchodilators, are most useful in the long-term management of COPD. They are ineffective in relieving acute bronchospasm by themselves, but they add to the bronchodilating effects of adrenergic drugs.

- Theophylline is used less often than formerly and is now considered a second-line drug. When used, it is usually given orally in an extended-release formulation for chronic disorders, such as COPD. IV aminophylline is no longer used to treat acute asthma attacks.

- Cromolyn and nedocromil are used prophylactically; they are ineffective in acute bronchospasm.

- Because inflammation has been established as a major component of asthma, an inhaled corticosteroid is being used early in the disease process, often with a bronchodilator or mast cell stabilizer. In acute episodes of bronchoconstriction, a corticosteroid is often given orally or IV for several days.

- In chronic disorders, inhaled corticosteroids should be taken on a regular schedule. These drugs may be effective when used alone or with relatively small doses of an oral corticosteroid. Optimal schedules of administration are not clearly established, but more frequent dosing (eg, every 6 hours) may be more effective than less frequent dosing (eg, every 12 hours), even if the total amount is the same. As with systemic glucocorticoid therapy, the recommended inhaled corticosteroid dose is the lowest amount required to control symptoms. High doses suppress adrenocortical function, but much less than systemic drugs. Small doses may impair bone metabolism and predispose adults to osteoporosis by decreasing calcium deposition and increasing calcium resorption from bone. In children, chronic administration of corticosteroids may retard growth. Local adverse effects (oropharyngeal candidiasis, hoarseness) can be decreased by reducing the dose, administering less often, rinsing the mouth after use, or using a spacer device. These measures decrease the amount of drug deposited in the oral cavity. The inhaled drugs are well tolerated with chronic use.

- A common regimen for treatment of moderate asthma is an inhaled corticosteroid on a regular schedule, two to four times daily, and a short-acting, inhaled beta$_2$-adrenergic agonist as needed for prevention or treatment of bronchoconstriction. For more severe asthma, an inhaled corticosteroid is continued and both a short-acting and a long-acting beta$_2$ agonist may be given. A leukotriene modifier may also be added to the regimen to further control symptoms and reduce the need for corticosteroids and inhaled bronchodilators.

- Multidrug regimens are commonly used and one advantage is that smaller doses of each agent can usually be given. This may decrease adverse effects and allow dosages to be increased when exacerbation of symptoms occurs. Available combination inhalation products include Combivent (albuterol and ipratropium) and Advair (salmeterol and fluticasone). Advair, which was developed to treat both inflammation and bronchoconstriction, was more effective than the individual components at the same doses and as effective as concurrent use of the same drugs at the same doses. In addition, the combination reduced the corticosteroid dose by 50% and was more effective than higher doses of fluticasone alone in reducing asthma exacerbations. The combination improved symptoms within 1 week. Additional combination products are likely to be marketed and may improve client compliance with prescribed drug therapy.

Drug Dosage

Dosage of antiasthmatic drugs must be individualized to attain the most therapeutic effects and the fewest adverse effects. Larger doses of bronchodilators and corticosteroids (inhaled, systemic, or both) are usually required to relieve the symptoms of acute, severe bronchoconstriction or status asthmaticus. Then, doses should be reduced to the smallest effective amounts for long-term control.

Dosage of theophylline preparations should be based mainly on serum theophylline levels (therapeutic range is 5–15 mcg/mL; toxic levels are 20 mcg/mL or above). Blood for serum levels should be drawn 1 to 2 hours after immediate-release dosage forms and about 4 hours after sustained-release forms are taken. In addition, children and cigarette smokers usually need higher doses to maintain therapeutic blood levels because they metabolize theophylline rapidly, and clients with liver disease, congestive heart failure, chronic pulmonary disease, or acute viral infections usually need smaller doses because these conditions impair theophylline metabolism. For obese clients, theophylline dosage should be calculated on the basis of lean or ideal body weight because theophylline is not highly distributed in fatty tissue.

Toxicity: Recognition and Management

With antiasthmatic drugs, signs and symptoms of overdose and toxicity are probably most likely to occur when clients with acute or chronic bronchoconstrictive disorders overuse bronchodilators in their efforts to relieve dyspnea. General management of acute poisoning includes early recognition of signs and symptoms, stopping the causative drug, and instituting other treatment measures as indicated. Specific measures include the following:

- **Bronchodilator overdose.** With inhaled or systemic adrenergic bronchodilators, major adverse effects are excessive cardiac and CNS stimulation. Symptoms of cardiac stimulation include angina, tachycardia, and palpitations; serious dysrhythmias and cardiac arrest have also been reported. Symptoms of CNS stimulation include agitation, anxiety, insomnia, seizures, and tremors. Severe overdoses may cause delirium, collapse, and coma. In addition, hypokalemia, hyperglycemia, and hypotension or hypertension may occur. Management includes discontinuing the causative medications and using general supportive measures. Emesis, gastric lavage, or activated charcoal may be useful with oral drugs if benefit exceeds risk. For cardiac symptoms, monitor blood pressure, pulse, and electrocardiogram. Cautious use of a beta-adrenergic blocking drug (eg, propranolol) may be indicated. However, a nonselective beta blocker may induce bronchoconstriction.
- **Theophylline overdose.** Signs and symptoms include anorexia, nausea, vomiting, agitation, nervousness, insomnia, tachycardia and other dysrhythmias, and tonic-clonic convulsions. Ventricular dysrhythmias or convulsions may be the first sign of toxicity. Serious adverse effects rarely occur at serum drug levels below 20 mcg/mL. Overdoses with sustained-release preparations may cause a dramatic increase in serum drug concentrations much later (12 hours or longer) than the immediate-release preparations. Early treatment helps

but does not prevent these delayed increases in serum drug levels.

In clients without seizures, induce vomiting unless the level of consciousness is impaired. In these clients, precautions to prevent aspiration are needed, especially in children. If overdose is identified within an hour of drug ingestion, gastric lavage may be helpful if unable to induce vomiting or vomiting is contraindicated. Administration of activated charcoal and a cathartic is also recommended, especially for overdoses of sustained-release formulations if benefit exceeds risk.

In clients with seizures, treatment includes securing the airway, giving oxygen, injecting IV diazepam (0.1–0.3 mg/kg, up to 10 mg), monitoring vital signs, maintaining blood pressure, providing adequate hydration, and monitoring serum theophylline levels until below 20 mcg/mL. Also, symptomatic treatment of dysrhythmias may be needed.

- **Leukotriene modifiers and mast cell stabilizers.** These drugs seem relatively devoid of serious toxicity. There have been few reports of toxicity in humans and little clinical experience in managing it. If toxicity occurs, general supportive and symptomatic treatment is indicated.

Use in Special Populations

Use in Children

The American Academy of Pediatrics endorses the clinical practice guidelines established by the NAEPP (see Box 44-1). In general, antiasthmatic medications are used in children and adolescents for the same indications as for adults. With adrenergic bronchodilators, recommendations for use vary according to route of administration, age of the child, and specific drug formulations. However, even infants and young children can be treated effectively with aerosolized or nebulized drugs. In addition, some oral drugs can be given to children as young as 2 years and most can be given to children 6 to 12 years of age.

With theophylline, use in children should be closely monitored because dosage needs and rates of metabolism vary widely. In children younger than 6 months, especially premature infants and neonates, drug elimination may be prolonged because of immature liver function. Except for preterm infants with apnea, theophylline preparations are not recommended for use in this age group. Children 6 months to 16 years of age, approximately, metabolize theophylline more rapidly than younger or older clients. Thus, they may need higher doses than adults in proportion to size and weight. If the child is obese, the dosage should be calculated on the basis of lean or ideal body weight because the drug is not highly distributed in fatty tissue. Long-acting dosage forms are not recommended for children younger than 6 years of age. Children may become hyperactive and disruptive from the CNS-stimulating effects of theophylline. Tolerance to these effects usually develops with continued use of the drug.

Corticosteroids are being used earlier in children as in adults and inhaled corticosteroids are first-line drugs for treatment of persistent bronchoconstrictive disorders. The effectiveness and safety of inhaled corticosteroids in children older than 3 years of age is well established; few data are available on the use of inhaled drugs in those younger than 3 years. Major concerns about long-term use in children include decreased adrenal function, growth, and bone mass. Most corticosteroids are given by inhalation, and dosage, type of inhaler device, and characteristics of individual drugs influence the extent and severity of these systemic effects.

Adrenal insufficiency is most likely to occur with systemic or high doses of inhaled corticosteroids. Dose-related inhibition of growth has been reported in short and intermediate studies but long-term studies have found few, if any, decreases in expected adult height. Inhaled corticosteroids have not been associated with significant decreases in bone mass but more studies of high doses and of drug therapy in adolescents are needed. Bone growth should be monitored closely in children taking corticosteroids. Although inhaled corticosteroids are the most effective anti-inflammatory medications available for asthma, high doses in children are still of concern. The risk of high doses is especially great in children with other allergic conditions that require topical corticosteroid drugs. The risk can be decreased by using the lowest effective dose, administration techniques that minimize swallowed drug, and other antiasthmatic drugs to reduce corticosteroid dose.

Leukotriene modifiers have not been extensively studied in children and adolescents. With montelukast, the 10-milligram film-coated tablet is recommended for adolescents 15 years of age and older and a 4-milligram chewable tablet is recommended for children 2 to 5 years of age. Safety and effectiveness of zafirlukast in children younger than 12 years have not been established.

Cromolyn aerosol solution may be used in children 5 years of age and older, and nebulizer solution is used with children 2 years and older. Nedocromil is not established as safe and effective in children younger than 12 years of age.

Use in Older Adults

Older adults often have chronic pulmonary disorders for which bronchodilators and antiasthmatic medications are used. As with other populations, administering the medications by inhalation and giving the lowest effective dose decrease adverse effects. The main risks with adrenergic bronchodilators are excessive cardiac and CNS stimulation.

Theophylline use must be carefully monitored because drug effects are unpredictable. On the one hand, cigarette smoking and drugs that stimulate drug-metabolizing enzymes in the liver (eg, phenobarbital, phenytoin) increase the rate of metabolism and therefore dosage requirements. On the other hand, impaired liver function, decreased blood flow to the liver, and some drugs (eg, cimetidine, erythromycin) impair metabolism and therefore decrease dosage requirements. Adverse effects include cardiac and CNS stimulation. Safety can be increased by measuring serum drug levels and adjusting dosage to maintain therapeutic levels of 5 to 15 micrograms per milliliter. If the client is obese, dosage should be based on lean or ideal body weight because theophylline is not highly distributed in fatty tissue.

Corticosteroids increase the risks of osteoporosis and cataracts in older adults. Leukotriene modifiers usually are well tolerated by older adults, with pharmacokinetics and effects similar to those in younger adults. With zafirlukast, however, blood levels are higher and elimination is slower than in younger adults. Zileuton is contraindicated in older adults with underlying hepatic dysfunction.

Use in Clients With Renal Impairment

Bronchodilating and anti-inflammatory drugs can usually be given without dosage adjustments in clients with impaired renal function. Beta agonists may be given by inhalation or parenteral routes. Theophylline can be given in usual doses, but serum drug levels should be monitored. Most corticosteroids are eliminated by hepatic metabolism, and dosage reductions are not needed in clients with renal impairment. No data are available about the use of montelukast, and no dosage adjustments are recommended for zafirlukast or zileuton.

Cromolyn is eliminated by renal and biliary excretion; the drug should be given in reduced doses, if at all, in clients with renal impairment.

Use in Clients With Hepatic Impairment

Montelukast and zafirlukast produce higher blood levels and are eliminated more slowly in clients with hepatic impairment. However, no dosage adjustment is recommended for clients with mild to moderate hepatic impairment. Zileuton is associated with hepatotoxicity and contraindicated in clients with active liver disease or aminotransferase elevations of three times the upper limit of normal or higher. Recommendations to avoid hepatotoxicity include measuring hepatic aminotransferases (eg, alanine aminotransferase) before starting zileuton, once a month for the first 3 months of therapy; every 2 to 3 months for the remainder of the first year; and periodically thereafter. The drug should be discontinued if symptoms of liver dysfunction develop (eg, right upper quadrant pain, nausea, fatigue, pruritus, jaundice, flulike symptoms) or aminotransferase levels increase to more than five times the upper limit of normal.

Cromolyn is eliminated by renal and biliary excretion; the drug should be given in reduced doses, if at all, in clients with hepatic impairment.

Use in Clients With Critical Illness

Acute, severe asthma (status asthmaticus) is characterized by severe respiratory distress and requires emergency treatment. Beta$_2$ agonists should be given in high doses and as often as every 20 minutes for 1 to 2 hours (by MDIs with spacer devices or by compressed-air nebulization). However, high doses of nebulized albuterol have been associated with tachycardia, hypokalemia, and hyperglycemia. After symptoms are controlled, dosage can usually be reduced and dosing intervals extended. High doses of systemic corticosteroids are also given for several days, IV or orally. If the client is able to take an oral drug, there is no therapeutic advantage to IV administration.

When respiratory function improves, efforts to prevent future episodes are needed. These efforts may include identifying and avoiding suspected triggers; evaluation and possible adjustment of the client's treatment regimen; and assessment of the client's adherence to the prescribed regimen.

Use in Home Care

All of the drugs discussed in this chapter are used in the home setting. A major role of the home care nurse is to assist clients in using the drugs safely and effectively. Several studies have indicated that many people do not use MDIs and other inhalation devices correctly. The home care nurse needs to observe a client using an inhalation device when possible. If errors in technique are assessed, teaching or reteaching may be needed. With inhaled medications, a spacer device may be useful, especially for children and older adults, because less muscle coordination is required to administer a dose. Adverse effects may be minimized as well.

For clients with asthma, especially children, assess the environment for potential triggers of acute bronchospasm, such as cigarette smoking. In addition, assist clients to recognize and treat (or get help for) exacerbations before respiratory distress becomes severe.

With theophylline, the home care nurse needs to assess the client and the environment for substances that may affect metabolism of theophylline and decrease therapeutic effects or increase adverse effects. In addition, the nurse needs to reinforce the importance of not exceeding the prescribed dose, not crushing long-acting formulations, reporting adverse effects, and keeping appointments for follow-up care.

N U R S I N G   A C T I O N S

Drugs for Asthma and Other Bronchoconstrictive Disorders

NURSING ACTIONS	RATIONALE/EXPLANATION
1. Administer accurately	
a. Be sure clients have adequate supplies of inhaled bronchodilators and corticosteroids available for self-administration. Observe technique of self-administration for accuracy and assist if needed.	
b. Give immediate-release oral theophylline before meals with a full glass of water, at regular intervals around the clock. If gastrointestinal upset occurs, give with food.	To promote dissolution and absorption. Taking with food may decrease nausea and vomiting.
c. Give sustained-release theophylline q8–12h, with instructions not to chew or crush.	Sustained-release drug formulations should never be chewed or crushed because doing so causes immediate release of potentially toxic doses.
d. Give zafirlukast 1 hour before or 2 hours after a meal; montelukast and zileuton may be given with or without food.	The bioavailability of zafirlukast is reduced approximately 40% if taken with food. Food does not significantly affect the bioavailability of montelukast and zileuton.
e. Give montelukast in the evening or at bedtime.	This schedule provides high drug concentrations during the night and early morning, when asthma symptoms tend to occur or worsen.
2. Observe for therapeutic effects	
a. Decreased dyspnea, wheezing, and respiratory secretions	Relief of bronchospasm and wheezing should be evident within a few minutes after giving subcutaneous epinephrine, or aerosolized adrenergic bronchodilators.
b. Reduced rate and improved quality of respirations	
c. Reduced anxiety and restlessness	
d. Therapeutic serum levels of theophylline (5–15 mcg/mL)	
e. Improved arterial blood gas levels (normal values: Po$_2$, 80 to 100 mm Hg; Pco$_2$, 35 to 45 mm Hg; pH, 7.35 to 7.45)	

NURSING ACTIONS	RATIONALE/EXPLANATION
f. Improved exercise tolerance	
g. Decreased incidence and severity of acute attacks of bronchospasm with chronic administration of drugs	
3. Observe for adverse effects	
a. With adrenergic bronchodilators, observe for tachycardia, dysrhythmias, palpitations, restlessness, agitation, insomnia.	These signs and symptoms result from cardiac and central nervous system (CNS) stimulation.
b. With ipratropium and tiotropium, observe for cough or exacerbation of symptoms.	Ipratropium and tiotropium produces few adverse effects because it is not absorbed systemically.
c. With xanthine bronchodilators, observe for tachycardia, dysrhythmias, palpitations, restlessness, agitation, insomnia, nausea, vomiting, convulsions.	Theophylline causes cardiac and CNS stimulation. Convulsions occur at toxic serum concentrations (>20 mcg/mL). They may occur without preceding symptoms of toxicity and may result in death. IV diazepam (Valium) may be used to control seizures. Theophylline also stimulates the chemoreceptor trigger zone in the medulla oblongata to cause nausea and vomiting.
d. With inhaled corticosteroids, observe for hoarseness, cough, throat irritation, and fungal infection of mouth and throat.	Inhaled corticosteroids are unlikely to produce the serious adverse effects of long-term systemic therapy (see Chap. 23).
e. With leukotriene inhibitors, observe for headache, infection, nausea, pain, elevated liver enzymes (eg, alanine aminotransferase [ALT]), and liver dysfunction.	These drugs are usually well tolerated. A highly elevated ALT and liver dysfunction are more likely to occur with zileuton.
f. With cromolyn, observe for dysrhythmias, hypotension, chest pain, restlessness, dizziness, convulsions, CNS depression, anorexia, nausea and vomiting. Sedation and coma may occur with overdosage.	Some of the cardiovascular effects are thought to be caused by the propellants used in the aerosol preparation.
4. Observe for drug interactions	
a. Drugs that *increase* effects of bronchodilators:	
(1) Monoamine oxidase inhibitors	These drugs inhibit the metabolism of catecholamines. The subsequent administration of bronchodilators may increase blood pressure.
(2) Erythromycin, clindamycin, cimetidine	These drugs may decrease theophylline clearance and thereby increase plasma levels.
b. Drugs that *decrease* effects of bronchodilators:	
(1) Lithium	Lithium may increase excretion of theophylline and therefore decrease therapeutic effectiveness.
(2) Phenobarbital	This drug may increase the metabolism of theophylline by way of enzyme induction.
(3) Propranolol, other nonselective beta blockers	These drugs may cause bronchoconstriction and oppose effects of bronchodilators.
c. Drugs that *alter* effects of zafirlukast:	
(1) Aspirin	Increases blood levels
(2) Erythromycin, theophylline	Decrease blood levels

APPLYING YOUR KNOWLEDGE: ANSWERS

44-1 The salmeterol in the Advair is only for prophylaxis of acute bronchoconstriction. The appropriate medication for acute attacks is the albuterol.

44-2 Explain to Mr. Cuff that he is receiving the same type of medication in his inhaled Advair (with contains fluticasone). An inhaled corticosteroid will minimize systemic absorption and the adverse effects. Topical application will reduce the inflammation.

44-3 Respiratory assessment should consist of observation of the client's breathing pattern. Observe for a rate less than 12 or above 24 breaths per minute, dyspnea, cough, or wheezing respirations. Indications of severe respiratory distress include tachypnea, the use of accessory muscles, and hypoxia.

Review and Application Exercises

Short Answer Exercises

1. What are some causes of bronchoconstriction, and how can they be prevented or minimized?

2. How do beta-adrenergic agonists act as bronchodilators?

3. What adverse effects are associated with bronchodilators, and how can they be prevented or minimized?

4. For what effects are corticosteroids used in the treatment of bronchoconstrictive respiratory disorders?

5. How do cromolyn and nedocromil act to prevent acute asthma attacks?

6. What are the main elements of treating respiratory distress from acute bronchospasm?

NCLEX-Style Questions

7. The nurse notes that a client's serum theophylline level is 25 mcg/mL and that a scheduled dose of the medication is due. The nurse should
   a. Hold the scheduled dose, contact the health care provider, and assess the client for signs of theophylline toxicity.
   b. Administer the dose as scheduled.
   c. Administer only half of the dose and repeat the theophylline level in 4 hours.
   d. Hold the dose until the next meal and administer at that time.

8. A client, taking a short-acting inhaled bronchodilator and a steroid inhaler at the same scheduled time, asks the nurse if the order of administration of the inhalers matters. The best response by the nurse is
   a. "You should not take both inhalers at the same time."
   b. "The short-acting inhaled bronchodilator should be used first, followed by the steroid inhaler."
   c. "Either medication can effectively be used first."
   d. "The steroid inhaler should be used first, followed by the short-acting inhaled bronchodilator."

9. A client on a steroid inhaler complains of anorexia and discomfort when he eats. The nurse noted that the client has oropharyngeal candidiasis. This adverse affect can be decreased by all of the following except
   a. reducing the dose
   b. administering the drug more frequently
   c. rinsing the mouth after use
   d. using a spacer device

10. Montelukast is effective in relieving the inflammation and bronchoconstriction associated with acute asthmatic attacks through which principal action?
    a. stabilizing mast cells
    b. blocking leukotriene receptors
    c. binding to immunoglobulin E (IgE)
    d. decreasing prostaglandin synthesis

Selected References

Allen, D. B. (2002). Inhaled corticosteroid therapy for asthma in preschool children: Growth issues. *Pediatrics, 109*(2), 373–380.

Allen, D. B. (2002). Safety of inhaled corticosteroids in children. *Pediatric Pulmonology, 33,* 208–220.

American Academy of Pediatrics. (2002). *Practice guideline endorsement. Guidelines for the diagnosis and management of asthma: Update on selected topics.* Retrieved August 6, 2002, from http://www.aap.org/policy/astmaref.html

Blake, K. (2000). Asthma. In E. T. Herfindal & D. R. Gourley (Eds.), *Textbook of therapeutics: Drug and disease management* (7th ed., pp. 727–764). Philadelphia: Lippincott Williams & Wilkins.

Drazen, J. M. (2004). Asthma. In L. Goldman & D. Ausiello (Eds.), *Cecil textbook of medicine* (22nd ed., pp. 502–509). Philadelphia: W. B. Saunders.

Drug facts and comparisons. (Updated monthly). St. Louis: Facts and Comparisons.

Fulco, P. P., Lone, A. A., & Pugh, C. B. (2002). Intravenous versus oral corticosteroids for treatment of acute asthma exacerbations. *The Annals of Pharmacotherapy, 36,* 565–570.

Gallagher, C. (2002). Childhood asthma: Tools that help parents manage it. *American Journal of Nursing, 102*(8), 71–83.

Kelly, H. W., & Sorkness, C. A. (2002). Asthma. In J. T. DiPiro, R. L. Talbert, G. C. Yee, G. R. Matzke, B. G. Wells, & L. M. Posey (Eds.), *Pharmacotherapy: A pathophysiologic approach* (5th ed., pp. 475–510). New York: McGraw-Hill.

Lacy, C. F., Armstrong, L. L., Goldman, M. P., et al. (2004). *Lexi-Comp's drug information handbook* (12th ed.). Hudson, OH: Lexi-Comp.

Lazarus, S. C., Boushey, H. A., Fahy, J. V., et al. (2001). Long-acting beta₂-agonist monotherapy vs. continued therapy with inhaled corticosteroids in clients with persistent asthma: A randomized controlled trial. *Journal of the American Medical Association, 285*(20), 2583–2593.

Lemanske, R. F., Jr. (2002). Inflammation in childhood asthma and other wheezing disorders. *Pediatrics, 109*(2), 368–372.

National Asthma Education and Prevention Program. (1997, February). *Expert panel report 2: Guidelines for the diagnosis and management of asthma* (NIH Publication No. 97-4051). Retrieved July 27, 2005, from http://www.nhlbi.nih.gov/guidelines/asthma/asthgdln.pdf. Bethesda, MD: National Institutes of Health, National Heart, Lung, and Blood Institute.

National Asthma Education and Prevention Program. (2002, June). *Expert panel report: Guidelines for the diagnosis and management of asthma—Update on selected topics 2002* (NIH Publication No. 02-5075). Retrieved July 27, 2005, from http://www.nhlbi.nih.gov/guidelines/asthma/asthma-fullrpt.pdf. Bethesda, MD: National Institutes of Health, National Heart, Lung, and Blood Institute.

Pope, B. B. (2002). Client education series: Asthma. *Nursing 2002, 32*(5), 44–45.

Porth, C. M. (2005). *Pathophysiology: Concepts of altered health states* (7th ed.). Philadelphia: Lippincott Williams & Wilkins.

Sin, D. D., Man, J., Sharpe, H., Gan, Q. W., & Man, S. F. M. (2004). Pharmacological management to reduce exacerbations in adults with asthma: A systematic review and meta-analysis. *JAMA, 292*(3), 367–376.

Sorkness, C. A. (2001). Leukotriene receptor antagonists in the treatment of asthma. *Pharmacotherapy, 21*(2, Pt. 3), 34S–37S.

Togger, D. A., & Brenner, P. S. (2001). Metered dose inhalers. *American Journal of Nursing, 101*(10), 26–32.

Williams, D. M. (2001). Clinical considerations in the use of inhaled corticosteroids for asthma. *Pharmacotherapy, 21*(3, Pt. 2), 38S–48S.

Wood, R. A. (2002). Pediatric asthma. *JAMA, 288*(6), 745–747.

Antihistamines and Allergic Disorders

OBJECTIVES

After studying this chapter, you will be able to:

1. Delineate effects of histamine on selected body tissues.
2. Differentiate histamine receptors.
3. Describe the types of hypersensitivity or allergic reactions.
4. Discuss allergic rhinitis, allergic contact dermatitis, and drug allergies as conditions for which antihistamines are commonly used.
5. Identify the effects of histamine that are blocked by histamine$_1$ (H$_1$) receptor antagonist drugs.
6. Differentiate first- and second-generation antihistamines.
7. Describe antihistamines in terms of indications for use, adverse effects, and nursing process implications.
8. Discuss the use of antihistamines in special populations.

APPLYING YOUR KNOWLEDGE

Linda Fisher, age 32, suffers from seasonal allergies. You work at a community health clinic. Ms. Fisher comes to the clinic seeking your advice about what medication might provide relief of her symptoms of runny nose and eyes, nasal congestion, and productive cough.

INTRODUCTION

Antihistamines are drugs that antagonize the action of histamine. Thus, to understand the use of these drugs, it is necessary to understand histamine and its effects on body tissues; characteristics of allergic reactions; and selected conditions for which antihistamines are used.

Histamine and Its Receptors

Histamine is the first chemical mediator to be released in immune and inflammatory responses. It is synthesized and stored in most body tissues, with high concentrations in tissues exposed to environmental substances (eg, the skin and mucosal surfaces of the eye, nose, lungs, and gastrointestinal [GI] tract). It is also found in the central nervous system (CNS). In these tissues, histamine is located mainly in secretory granules of mast cells (tissue cells surrounding capillaries) and basophils (circulating blood cells).

Histamine is discharged from mast cells and basophils in response to certain stimuli (eg, allergic reactions, cellular injury, extreme cold). After it is released, it diffuses rapidly into other tissues, where it interacts with histamine receptors

on target organs, called H_1 and H_2. H$_1$ receptors are located mainly on smooth muscle cells in blood vessels and the respiratory and GI tracts. When histamine binds with these receptors and stimulates them, effects include:

- Contraction of smooth muscle in the bronchi and bronchioles (producing bronchoconstriction and respiratory distress)
- Stimulation of vagus nerve endings to produce reflex bronchoconstriction and cough
- Increased permeability of veins and capillaries, which allows fluid to flow into subcutaneous tissues and form edema
- Increased secretion of mucous glands. Mucosal edema and increased nasal mucus produce the nasal congestion characteristic of allergic rhinitis and the common cold.
- Stimulation of sensory peripheral nerve endings to cause pain and pruritus. Pruritus is especially prominent with allergic skin disorders.
- Dilation of capillaries in the skin, to cause flushing

When H$_2$ receptors are stimulated, the main effects are increased secretion of gastric acid and pepsin, increased rate and force of myocardial contraction, and decreased immunologic and proinflammatory reactions (eg, decreased release of histamine from basophils, decreased movement of neutrophils and basophils into areas of injury, inhibited T- and B-lymphocyte function). Stimulation of both H_1 and H_2 receptors causes peripheral vasodilation (with hypotension, headache, and skin flushing) and increases bronchial, intestinal, and salivary secretion of mucus.

Hypersensitivity (Allergic) Reactions

Hypersensitivity or allergic reactions are immune responses (see Chap. 38) in which a person's body overreacts to an environmental or ingested substance that does not cause a reaction in most people. That is, the person is hypersensitive or allergic to the substance (called an *antigen* or *allergen*). Allergic reactions may result from specific antibodies, sensitized T lymphocytes, or both, formed during exposure to an antigen.

Types of Allergic Reactions

- *Type I* (also called *immediate hypersensitivity* because it occurs within minutes of exposure to the antigen) is an immunoglobulin E (IgE)-induced response that causes release of histamine and other mediators. For example, *anaphylaxis* is a type I response that may be mild (characterized mainly by urticaria, other dermatologic manifestations, or rhinitis) or severe and life threatening (characterized by respiratory distress and cardiovascular collapse). It is uncommon and does not occur on first exposure to an antigen; it occurs with a second or later exposure, after antibody formation was induced by an earlier exposure. Severe anaphylaxis (sometimes called anaphylactic shock; see Chap. 51) is characterized by cardiovascular collapse from profound vasodilation and pooling of blood in the splanchnic system so that the client has severe hypotension and functional hypovolemia. Respiratory distress often occurs from laryngeal edema and bronchoconstriction. Urticaria often occurs because the skin has many mast cells to release histamine. Anaphylaxis is a systemic reaction that usually involves the respiratory, cardiovascular, and dermatologic systems. Severe anaphylaxis may be fatal if not treated promptly and effectively.
- *Type II* responses are mediated by IgG or IgM. They produce direct damage to the cell surface. These cytotoxic reactions include blood transfusion reactions, hemolytic disease of newborns, autoimmune hemolytic anemia, and some drug reactions.
- *Type III* is an IgG- or IgM-mediated reaction characterized by formation of antigen–antibody complexes that induce an acute inflammatory reaction in the tissues. *Serum sickness,* the prototype of these reactions, occurs when excess antigen combines with antibodies to form immune complexes. The complexes then diffuse into affected tissues, where they cause tissue damage by activating the complement system and

initiating the immune response. If small amounts of immune complexes are deposited locally, the antigenic material can be phagocytized and digested by white blood cells and macrophages without tissue destruction. If large amounts are deposited locally or reach the bloodstream and become deposited in blood vessel walls, the lysosomal enzymes released during phagocytosis may cause permanent tissue destruction.
- *Type IV* hypersensitivity (also called *delayed hypersensitivity* because it usually occurs several hours or days after exposure to the antigen) is a cell-mediated response in which sensitized T lymphocytes react with an antigen to cause inflammation mediated by release of lymphokines, direct cytotoxicity, or both.

Allergic Rhinitis

Allergic rhinitis is inflammation of nasal mucosa caused by a type I hypersensitivity reaction to inhaled allergens. It is a very common disorder characterized by nasal congestion, itching, sneezing, and watery drainage. Itching of the throat, eyes, and ears often occurs as well.

There are two types of allergic rhinitis. Seasonal disease (often called *hay fever*) produces acute symptoms in response to the protein components of airborne pollens from trees, grasses and weeds, mainly in spring or fall. Perennial disease produces chronic symptoms in response to nonseasonal allergens such as dust mites, animal dander, and molds. Actually, mold spores can cause both seasonal and perennial allergies because they are present year round, with seasonal increases. Some people have both types, with chronic symptoms plus acute seasonal symptoms.

People with a personal or family history of other allergic disorders are likely to have allergic rhinitis. When nasal mucosa is inflamed, symptoms can be worsened by nonallergenic irritants such as tobacco smoke, strong odors, air pollution, and climatic changes.

Allergic rhinitis is an immune response in which normal nasal breathing and filtering of air brings inhaled antigens into contact with mast cells and basophils in nasal mucosa, blood vessels, and submucosal tissues. With initial exposure, the inhaled antigens are processed by lymphocytes that produce IgE, an antigen-specific antibody that binds to mast cells. With later exposures, the IgE interacts with inhaled antigens and triggers the breakdown of the mast cell. This breakdown causes the release of histamine and other inflammatory mediators such as prostaglandins and leukotrienes (Fig. 45-1). These mediators, of which histamine may be the most important, dilate and engorge blood vessels to produce nasal congestion, stimulate secretion of mucus, and attract inflammatory cells (eg, eosinophils, lymphocytes, monocytes, macrophages). In people with allergies, mast cells and basophils are increased in both number and reactivity. Thus, these cells may be capable of releasing large amounts of histamine and other mediators.

Allergic rhinitis that is not effectively treated may lead to chronic fatigue, impaired ability to perform usual activities

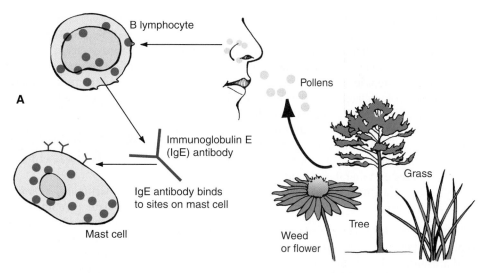

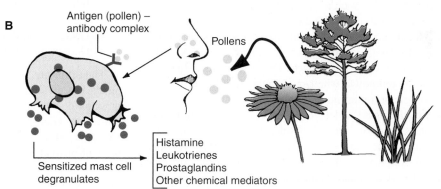

FIGURE 45-1 Type I hypersensitivity reaction: allergic rhinitis. **(A)** The first exposure of mast cells in nasal mucosa to inhaled antigens (eg, pollens from weeds, grasses, trees) leads to the formation of immunoglobulin E (IgE) antibody molecules. These molecules then bind to the surface membranes of mast cells. This process sensitizes mast cells to the effects of inhaled antigens (allergens). **(B)** When sensitized mast cells are re-exposed to inhaled pollens or other antigens, they release histamine and other chemical mediators which then act on nasal mucosa to produce characteristic symptoms of allergic rhinitis.

of daily living, difficulty sleeping, sinus infections, postnasal drip, cough, and headache. In addition, this condition is a strong risk factor for asthma.

Allergic Contact Dermatitis

Allergic contact dermatitis is a type IV hypersensitivity reaction resulting from direct contact with antigens to which a person has previously become sensitized (eg, poison ivy or poison oak, cosmetics, hair dyes, metals, drugs applied topically to the skin). This reaction, which may be acute or chronic, usually occurs more than 24 hours after re-exposure to an antigen and may last from days to weeks.

Affected areas of the skin are usually inflamed, warm, edematous, intensely pruritic, and tender to touch. Skin lesions are usually erythematous macules, papules, and vesicles (blisters) that may drain, develop crusts, and become infected. Lesion location may indicate the causative antigen.

Allergic Drug Reactions

Virtually any drug may induce an immunologic response in susceptible people, and any body tissues may be affected. Allergic drug reactions are complex and diverse and may include any of the types of hypersensitivity described previ-

ously. A single drug may induce one or more of these states and multiple symptoms. There are no specific characteristics that identify drug-related reactions, although some reactions commonly attributed to drugs (eg, skin rashes, drug fever, hematologic reactions, hepatic reactions) rarely occur with plant pollens and other naturally occurring antigens. Usually, however, the body responds to a drug as it does to other foreign materials (antigens). In addition, some reactions may be caused by coloring agents, preservatives, and other additives rather than the drug itself.

Allergic drug reactions should be considered when new signs and symptoms develop or when they differ from the usual manifestations of the illness being treated, especially if a reaction

- Follows ingestion of a drug, especially one known to produce allergic reactions
- Is unpredictable and occurs in only a few clients when many clients receive the suspected drug
- Occurs approximately 7 to 10 days after initial exposure to the suspected drug (to allow antibody production)
- Follows a previous exposure to the same or similar drug (sensitizing exposure)
- Occurs minutes or hours after a second or subsequent exposure

- Occurs after small doses (reduces the likelihood that the reaction is due to dose-related drug toxicity)
- Occurs with other drugs that are chemically or immunologically similar to the suspected drug
- Produces signs and symptoms that differ from the usual pharmacologic actions of the suspected drug
- Produces signs and symptoms usually considered allergic in nature (eg, anaphylaxis, urticaria, serum sickness)
- Produces similar signs and symptoms to previous allergic reactions to the same or a similar drug
- Increases eosinophils in blood or tissue
- Resolves within a few days of discontinuing the suspected drug

Virtually all drugs have been implicated in **anaphylactic reactions.** Penicillins and other antimicrobials, radiocontrast media, aspirin and other nonsteroidal anti-inflammatory drugs, and antineoplastics such as L-asparaginase and cisplatin are more common offenders. Less common causes include anesthetics (local and general), opioid analgesics, skeletal muscle relaxants used with general anesthetics, and vaccines. Approximately 10% of severe anaphylactic reactions are fatal. In many cases, it is unknown whether clinical manifestations are immunologic or nonimmunologic in origin.

Serum sickness is a delayed hypersensitivity reaction most often caused by drugs, such as antimicrobials. In addition, many drugs that produce anaphylaxis also produce serum sickness. With initial exposure to the antigen, symptoms usually develop within 7 to 10 days and include urticaria, lymphadenopathy, myalgia, arthralgia, and fever. The reaction usually resolves within a few days but may be severe or even fatal. With repeated exposure to the antigen, after prior sensitization of the host, accelerated serum sickness may develop within 2 to 4 days, with similar but often more severe signs and symptoms.

Systemic lupus erythematosus (SLE) is an autoimmune disorder that may be idiopathic from nondrug causes or induced by hydralazine, procainamide, isoniazid, and other drugs. Clinical manifestations vary greatly, depending on the location and severity of the inflammatory and immune processes, and may include skin lesions, fever, pneumonia, anemia, arthralgia, arthritis, nephritis, and others. Drug-induced lupus produces less renal and CNS involvement than idiopathic SLE.

Fever often occurs with allergic drug reactions. It may occur alone, with a skin rash and eosinophilia, or with other drug-induced allergic reactions such as serum sickness, SLE, vasculitis, and hepatitis.

Dermatologic conditions (eg, skin rash, urticaria, inflammation) commonly occur with allergic drug reactions and may be the first and most visible manifestations.

Pseudoallergic Drug Reactions

Pseudoallergic drug reactions resemble immune responses (because histamine and other chemical mediators are released) but they do not produce antibodies or sensitized T lymphocytes. **Anaphylactoid reactions** are like anaphylaxis in terms of immediate occurrence, symptoms, and life-threatening severity. The main difference is that they are not antigen–antibody reactions and therefore may occur on first exposure to the causative agent. The drugs bind directly to mast cells, activate the cells, and cause the release of histamine and other vasoactive chemical mediators. Contrast media for radiologic diagnostic tests are often implicated.

GENERAL CHARACTERISTICS OF ANTIHISTAMINES

The term *antihistamines* generally indicates classic or traditional drugs. With increased knowledge about histamine receptors, these drugs are often called H_1 *receptor antagonists*. These drugs prevent or reduce most of the physiologic effects that histamine normally induces at H_1 receptor sites. Thus, they

- Inhibit smooth muscle constriction in blood vessels and the respiratory and GI tracts
- Decrease capillary permeability
- Decrease salivation and tear formation

The drugs are similar in effectiveness as histamine antagonists but differ in adverse effects. These are the antihistamines discussed in this chapter. Cimetidine (Tagamet), ranitidine (Zantac), famotidine (Pepcid), and nizatidine (Axid) are H_2 receptor antagonists or blocking agents used to prevent or treat peptic ulcer disease. These are discussed in Chapter 59. Selected H_1 antagonists are described in the following sections and in Table 45-1.

Mechanism of Action

Antihistamines are structurally related to histamine and occupy the same receptor sites as histamine, which prevents histamine from acting on target tissues (Fig. 45-2). Thus, the drugs are effective in inhibiting vascular permeability, edema formation, bronchoconstriction, and pruritus associated with histamine release. They do not prevent histamine release or reduce the amount released.

Indications for Use

Antihistamines are used for a variety of allergic and nonallergic disorders to prevent or reverse target organ inflammation and its effects on organ function. The drugs can relieve symptoms but do not relieve the hypersensitivity.

- **Allergic rhinitis.** Of people with seasonal allergic rhinitis, 75% to 95% experience some relief of sneezing, rhinorrhea, nasal congestion, and conjunctivitis with the use of antihistamines. People with perennial allergic rhinitis usually experience decreased nasal congestion and drying of nasal mucosa. However, many people require an additional drug to relieve symptoms. Cromolyn, ipratropium, and several corticosteroids are available in intranasal preparations for this purpose. These drugs, with dosage ranges for adults and children, are listed in Table 45-2.

Table 45-1 Drugs at a Glance: Commonly Used Antihistamines

GENERIC/TRADE NAME	INDICATIONS FOR USE	ROUTES AND DOSAGE RANGES	
		Adults	Children
First Generation **Brompheniramine** (LoHist)	Allergic rhinitis	1–2 tablets (6–12 mg) q12h	≥ 12 y and older: Same as adults. 6–12 1 tablet (6 mg) q12h
Chlorpheniramine (Chlor-Trimeton)	Allergic rhinitis	PO 4 mg q4–6h; maximal dose, 24 mg in 24h Timed-release forms, PO 8 mg q8–12h or 12 mg q12h; maximal dose, 24 mg in 24h	≥ 12 y: Same as adults 6–12 y: PO 2 mg q4–6h; maximal dose, 12 mg in 24h 2–6 y: PO 1 mg q4–6h Timed-release forms, ≥ 12 y: PO 8 mg q8–12h or 12 mg q12h; maximal dose, 24 mg in 24h
Clemastine (Tavist)	Allergic rhinitis Urticaria/angioedema	Allergic rhinitis, PO 1.34 mg twice daily, increased up to a maximum of 8.04 mg daily, if necessary Urticaria/angioedema, PO 2.68 mg one to three times daily	Allergic rhinitis, 6–12 y (syrup only): PO 0.67 mg twice daily, increased up to a maximum of 4.02 mg daily, if necessary Urticaria/angioedema, 6–12 y (syrup only): PO 1.34 mg twice daily
Cyproheptadine	Hypersensitivity reactions (allergic rhinitis, conjunctivitis, dermatitis)	PO 4 mg q8h initially, increase if necessary. Maximal dose 0.5 mg/kg/d	(Calculate total daily dosage as 0.25 mg/kg or 8 mg/m^2) 7–14 y: PO 4 mg q8–12h; maximal dose, 16 mg/d 2–6 y: 2 mg q8–12h; maximal dose, 12 mg/d
Dexchlorpheniramine	Hypersensitivity reactions (allergic rhinitis, conjunctivitis, dermatitis)	Regular tablets and syrup, PO 2 mg q4–6h Timed-release tablets, PO 4–6 mg at bedtime or q8–12h	≥ 12 y: Same as adults 6–11 y: PO 1 mg q4–6h 2–5 y: PO 0.5 mg q4–6h Timed-release tablets, ≥ 12 y: Same as adults; 6–12 y: 4 mg once daily, at bedtime
P Diphenhydramine (Benadryl)	Hypersensitivity reactions (allergic rhinitis, conjunctivitis, dermatitis) Motion sickness Parkinsonism Insomnia Antitussive (syrup only)	Hypersensitivity reaction, motion sickness, parkinsonism, PO 25–50 mg q4–8h; IV or deep IM 10–50 mg, increased if necessary to a maximal daily dose of 400 mg Insomnia, PO 50 mg at bedtime Syrup for cough, PO 25 mg (10 mL) q4h, not to exceed 100 mg (40 mL) in 24 h	Weight >10 kg (22 lbs): PO 12.5–25 mg q6–8h, 5 mg/kg/d, or 150 mg/m^2/d; IV 5 mg/kg/d, or 150 mg/m^2/d. Maximum oral or parenteral dosage, 300 mg daily Insomnia, ≥ 12 y: Same as adults Syrup for cough, 6–12 y: PO 12.5 mg (5 mL) q4h, not to exceed 50 mg (20 mL) in 24 h; 2–6 y: PO 6.25 mg (2.5 mL) q4h, not to exceed 25 mg (10 mL) in 24 h
Hydroxyzine (Vistaril)	Pruritus Sedation Antiemetic	PO 25 mg q6–8h; IM 25–100 mg as needed	>6 y: PO 50–100 mg daily in divided doses <6 y: PO 50 mg daily in divided doses

(continued)

Table 45-1 Drugs at a Glance: Commonly Used Antihistamines (continued)

GENERIC/TRADE NAME	INDICATIONS FOR USE	ROUTES AND DOSAGE RANGES	
		Adults	Children
Phenindamine (Nolahist)	Allergic rhinitis	PO 25 mg q4–6h; maximal dose 150 mg in 24 h	≥12 y: Same as adults 6–11 y: PO 12.5 mg q4–6h; maximal dose 75 mg in 24 h
Promethazine (Phenergan)	Hypersensitivity reactions (allergic rhinitis, conjunctivitis, dermatitis) Sedation Antiemetic Motion sickness	PO, IM, rectally, 25 mg q4–6h as needed	≥2 y: 12.5 mg q4–6h as needed
Triprolidine (Zymine)	Allergic rhinitis	PO 10 mL (1.2 mg/5 mL) q4–6h, not to exceed 40 mL/24h	≥12y: Same as adults 6–12 y: 5 mL q4–6h, not to exceed 20 mL/24h 4–6 y: 3.75 mL q4–6h, not to exceed 15 mL/24h 2–4 y: 2.5 mL q4–6h, not to exceed 10 mL/24h 4 m–2 y: 1.25 mL q4–6h, not to exceed 5 mL/24h
Second Generation **Azelastine** (Astelin)	Allergic rhinitis	Nasal inhalation, two sprays per nostrils q12h	≥12 y: Same as adults
Cetirizine (Zyrtec)	Allergic rhinitis Chronic idiopathic urticaria	PO 5–10 mg once daily Renal or hepatic impairment, PO 5 mg once daily	≥6 y: Same as adults 6 mo–5y: PO 2.5 mg (one-half tsp) once daily
Desloratadine (Clarinex)	Allergic rhinitis Chronic idiopathic urticaria	5 mg once daily	≥12 y: Same as adults <12 y: Dosage not established
Fexofenadine (Allegra)	Allergic rhinitis	PO 60 mg twice daily Renal impairment, PO 60 mg once daily	≥12 y: Same as adults 6–11 y: PO 30 mg twice daily
Loratadine (Claritin)	Allergic rhinitis Chronic idiopathic urticaria	PO 10 mg once daily Renal or hepatic impairment, PO 10 mg every other day	≥6 y: Same as adults 2–5 y: PO 5 mg daily

IM, intramuscular; IV, intravenous; PO, oral.

● **Anaphylaxis.** Antihistamines are helpful in treating urticaria and pruritus but are not effective in treating bronchoconstriction and hypotension. Epinephrine, rather than an antihistamine, is the drug of choice for treating severe anaphylaxis.

● **Allergic conjunctivitis.** This condition, which is characterized by redness, itching, and tearing of the eyes, is often associated with allergic rhinitis. Antihistamine eye medications may be given (see Chap. 63).

● **Drug allergies and pseudoallergies.** Antihistamines may be given to prevent or treat reactions to drugs. When used for prevention, they should be given before exposure (eg, before a diagnostic test that uses an iodine preparation as a contrast medium; before an intravenous infusion of amphotericin B). When antihistamines are used for treatment, giving the antihistamine and stopping the causative drug usually relieve signs and symptoms within a few days.

● **Transfusions of blood and blood products.** Premedication with an antihistamine is often used to prevent allergic reactions.

● **Dermatologic conditions.** Antihistamines are the drugs of choice for treatment of allergic contact dermatitis and acute urticaria (a vascular reaction of the skin characterized by papules or wheals and severe itching, often called *hives*). Urticaria often occurs because the skin has many mast cells to release histamine. Other indications for use include drug-induced skin reactions, pruritus ani, and pruritus vulvae. Systemic drugs are used; topical preparations are not recommended because they often induce skin rashes themselves. With pruritus, oral cyproheptadine and hydroxyzine (Vistaril) are especially effective.

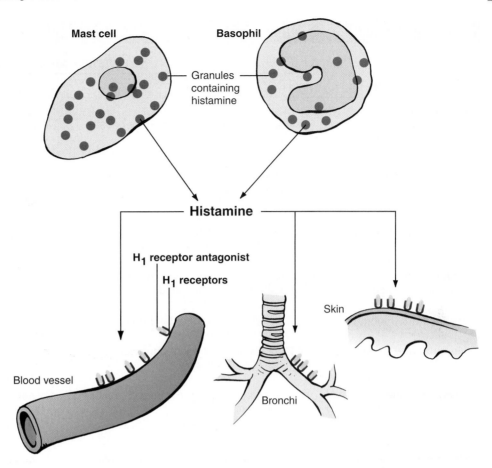

FIGURE 45-2 Action of antihistamine drugs. Histamine$_1$ (H$_1$) receptor antagonists bind to H$_1$ receptors. This prevents histamine from binding to its receptors and acting on target tissues.

● **Miscellaneous.** Some antihistamines are commonly used for nonallergic disorders, such as motion sickness, nausea and vomiting (eg, promethazine, hydroxyzine; see Chap. 62), and sleep (eg, diphenhydramine). The active ingredient in over-the-counter (OTC) sleep aids (eg, Compoz, Sominex) is a sedating antihistamine. Antihistamines are also common ingredients in OTC cold remedies (see Chap. 46).

Contraindications to Use

Antihistamines are contraindicated or must be used with caution in pregnant clients and clients with hypersensitivity to the drugs, narrow-angle glaucoma, prostatic hypertrophy, stenosing peptic ulcer, and bladder neck obstruction.

CLASSIFICATIONS AND INDIVIDUAL DRUGS

First-Generation H$_1$ Receptor Antagonists

These chemically diverse antihistamines (also called *non-selective* or *sedating agents*) bind to both central and peripheral H$_1$ receptors and can cause CNS depression or stimulation. They usually cause CNS depression (drowsiness, sedation) with therapeutic doses and may cause CNS stimulation (anxiety, agitation) with excessive doses, especially in children. They also have substantial anticholinergic effects (eg, cause dry mouth, urinary retention, constipation, blurred vision).

Brompheniramine, chlorpheniramine (Chlor-Trimeton), and **dexchlorpheniramine** cause minimal drowsiness. P **Diphenhydramine** (Benadryl), the prototype of first-generation antihistamines, causes a high incidence of drowsiness and anticholinergic effects. **Hydroxyzine** (Vistaril) and **promethazine** (Phenergan) are strong CNS depressants and cause extensive drowsiness.

First-generation antihistamines are usually well absorbed after oral administration. Immediate-release oral forms act within 15 to 60 minutes and last 4 to 6 hours. Enteric-coated or sustained-release preparations last 8 to 12 hours. Most drugs are given orally; a few may be given parenterally. These drugs are primarily metabolized by the liver, with metabolites and small amounts of unchanged drug excreted in urine within 24 hours. Several of these drugs are available without prescription. Brompheniramine, chlorpheniramine, and diphenhydramine are available alone and in combination with adrenergic nasal decongestants, analgesics, and allergy, cold, and sinus remedies.

Table 45-2 Drugs at a Glance: Intranasal Drugs for Allergic Rhinitis

GENERIC/TRADE NAME	ROUTES AND DOSAGE RANGES	
	Adults	Children
Anticholinergic		
Ipratropium (Atrovent nasal spray)	2 sprays (42 mcg or 84 mcg) per nostril 2–4 times daily	*12 y and older:* Same as adults
Corticosteroids		
Beclomethasone (Beconase)	1 inhalation (42 mcg) in each nostril 2–4 times daily	*12 y and older:* Same as adults 6–12 y: 1 inhalation in each nostril 3 times daily
Budesonide (Rhinocort)	256 mcg daily as 2 sprays per nostril twice daily or 4 sprays per nostril once daily	6 y and older: Same as adults
Flunisolide (Nasalide, Nasarel)	2 sprays (50 mcg) in each nostril 2 times daily, increase to 3 times daily if necessary	*6–14 y:* 1 spray (25 mcg) in each nostril 3 times daily or 2 sprays per nostril (50 mcg) 2 times daily
Fluticasone (Flonase)	2 sprays (50 mcg each) per nostril once daily (200 mcg daily)	*4 y and older:* 1 spray per nostril per day (100 mcg daily)
Mometasone (Nasonex)	2 sprays (50 mcg each) per nostril once daily (200 mcg daily)	*12 y and older:* Same as adults *3–11 y:* 1 spray per nostril once daily (100 mcg daily)
Triamcinolone (Nasacort, Nasacort AQ)	2 sprays (55 mcg/spray) in each nostril once daily	*6 y and older:* Same as adults initially, then reduce to 1 spray per nostril per day
Mast Cell Stabilizer		
Cromolyn (Nasalcrom)	1 spray in each nostril 3–6 times daily, q4–6h	*6 y and older:* Same as adults

Second-Generation H₁ Receptor Antagonists

Second-generation H$_1$ antagonists (also called *selective* or *nonsedating agents*) were developed mainly to produce less sedation than the first-generation drugs. They cause less CNS depression because they are selective for peripheral H$_1$ receptors and do not cross the blood–brain barrier. These drugs have been available only by prescription. Loratadine (Claritin) is available for OTC sales. Proponents of OTC availability usually argue that the drugs are safer than the first-generation drugs that have been available OTC for many years.

Azelastine (Astelin) is the only antihistamine formulated as a nasal spray for topical use. When applied to nasal mucosa, it produces peak levels in 2 to 3 hours and lasts 12 to 24 hours. It is metabolized in the liver to an active metabolite and is excreted mainly in feces. The other drugs are well absorbed with oral administration and have a rapid onset of action. **Cetirizine** (Zyrtec) is an active metabolite of hydroxyzine that causes less drowsiness than hydroxyzine. It reaches maximal serum concentration in 1 hour and is about 93% protein bound. About half of a dose is metabolized in the liver; the other half is excreted unchanged in the urine. **Fexofenadine** (Allegra) reaches peak serum con-

centrations in about 2.5 hours, is 60% to 70% protein bound, and 95% is excreted unchanged in bile and urine. **Loratadine** (Claritin) effects occur within 1 to 3 hours, reach a maximum in 8 to 12 hours, and last 24 hours or longer. Loratadine is metabolized in the liver and its long duration of action is due, in part, to an active metabolite. The patent for loratadine expired in December, 2002, clearing the way for generic formulations. **Desloratadine** (Clarinex), an active metabolite of loratadine and marketed by the manufacturer of Claritin, seems to offer no advantage over loratadine or other second-generation drugs.

NURSING PROCESS

Assessment

● Assess the client's condition in relation to disorders for which antihistamines are used. For the client with known allergies, try to determine the factors that precipitate or relieve allergic reactions and specific signs and symptoms experienced during a reaction.

- Assess every client for a potential hypersensitivity reaction. For example, it is standard practice on first contact to ask a client if he or she has any food, drug, or other allergies. The health care provider is likely to get more complete information by asking clients about allergic reactions to specific drugs (eg, antibiotics such as penicillin, local anesthetics) rather than asking if they are allergic to or cannot take any drugs.

    If a drug allergy is identified, ask about specific signs and symptoms as well as any drugs currently being taken. With previous exposure and sensitization to the same or a similar drug, immediate allergic reactions may occur. With a new drug, antibody formation and allergic reactions usually require a week or longer. Most reactions appear within a month of starting a drug.

    When a suspected allergic reaction occurs (eg, skin rash, fever, edema, dyspnea), interview the client or consult medical records about the drug, dose, route, and time of administration. In addition, evaluate all the drugs a client is taking as a potential cause of the reaction. This assessment may involve searching drug literature to see if the suspected drug is associated with allergic reactions, and discussion with physicians and pharmacists.

Nursing Diagnoses

- Risk for Injury related to drowsiness with first-generation antihistamines
- Deficient Knowledge: Safe and accurate drug use
- Deficient Knowledge: Strategies for minimizing exposure to allergens and irritants

Planning/Goals

The client will

- Experience relief of symptoms
- Take antihistamines accurately
- Avoid hazardous activities if sedated from antihistamines
- Avoid preventable adverse drug effects
- Avoid taking sedative-type antihistamines with alcohol or other sedative drugs

Interventions

- For clients with known allergies, assist in identifying and avoiding precipitating factors when possible. If it is a drug allergy, encourage the client to carry a medical alert device that identifies the drug.
- Monitor the client closely for excessive drowsiness during the first few days of therapy with antihistamines known to cause sedation.
- Encourage a fluid intake of 2000 to 3000 mL daily, if not contraindicated.

- Because antihistamines are most effective before exposure to the stimulus that causes histamine release, assist clients in learning when to take the drugs (eg, during seasons of high pollen and mold counts).
- When indicated, obtain an order and administer an antihistamine before situations known to elicit allergic reactions (eg, blood transfusions, diagnostic tests that involve contrast media).
- For clients who have experienced an allergic or pseudo-allergic drug reaction, assist them in learning about the drug thought responsible (including the generic and commonly used trade names), suitable alternatives for future drug therapy, and potential sources of the drug.
- Provide appropriate client teaching regarding any drug therapy (see accompanying display).

Evaluation

- Observe for relief of symptoms.
- Interview and observe for correct drug usage.
- Interview and observe for excessive drowsiness.

APPLYING YOUR KNOWLEDGE 45-1

Ms. Fisher starts taking OTC loratadine. What client teaching points are appropriate?

PRINCIPLES OF THERAPY

Prevention of Histamine-Releasing Reactions

When possible, avoiding exposure to known allergens can prevent allergic reactions. If antihistamine therapy is required, it is more effective if started before exposure to allergens because the drugs can then occupy receptor sites before histamine is released.

Drug Selection

- Choosing an antihistamine is based on the desired effect, duration of action, adverse effects, and other characteristics of available drugs. For most people, a second-generation drug is the first drug of choice. However, they are quite expensive. If costs are prohibitive for a client, a first-generation drug may be used with minimal daytime sedation if taken at bedtime or in low initial doses, with gradual increases over a week or two. Azelastine nasal spray also causes little sedation, but it leaves an unpleasant taste. Overall, safety should be the determining factor. Some studies have shown cognitive and performance impairment with the first-generation drugs even when the person does not feel drowsy or impaired.
- For treatment of acute allergic reactions, a rapid-acting agent of short duration is preferred.

CLIENT TEACHING GUIDELINES

Antihistamines

General Considerations

✔ Some antihistamines should not be taken by people with glaucoma, peptic ulcer, urinary retention, or pregnancy. Inform your physician if you have any of these conditions or, for over-the-counter (OTC) antihistamines, read the label to see if you should avoid a particular drug.

✔ Antihistamines may dry and thicken respiratory tract secretions and make them more difficult to remove. Thus, do not take diphenhydramine (Benadryl), which is available OTC, if you have active asthma, bronchitis, or pneumonia.

✔ Some antihistamines cause drowsiness or dizziness and impair mental alertness, judgment, and physical coordination, especially during the first few days. Do not smoke, drive a car, operate machinery, or perform other tasks requiring alertness and physical dexterity until drowsiness has worn off, to avoid injury.

✔ Avoid using sedating antihistamines with other sedative-type drugs (eg, alcohol, medications to relieve nervousness or produce sleep), to avoid adverse effects and dangerous drug interactions. Alcohol and other drugs that depress brain function may cause excessive sedation, respiratory depression, and death.

✔ Do not take more than one antihistamine at a time (eg, two prescription drugs, two OTC drugs, or a combination of prescription and OTC drugs) because adverse effects are likely. If you do not know whether a particular medication is an antihistamine, consult a health care provider. For example, many OTC cold remedies and "nighttime" or "PM" allergy or sinus preparations contain an antihistamine. In addition, the active ingredient in OTC sleep aids is a sedating antihistamine, usually diphenhydramine (Benadryl).

✔ Avoid prolonged exposure to sunlight and use sunscreens and protective clothing; some antihistamines may increase sensitivity to sunlight and risks of skin damage from sunburn.

✔ Report adverse effects, such as excessive drowsiness. The physician may be able to change drugs or dosages to decrease adverse effects.

✔ Store antihistamines out of reach of children to avoid accidental ingestion.

✔ If you experience an allergic reaction to a medication, obtain information about the drug thought responsible (including its various names), acceptable alternatives for future drug therapy, and potential sources of the drug. In addition, read the list of ingredients on labels of OTC drug preparations, inform all health care providers about the drug reaction before taking any newly prescribed drug, and wear a medical alert device that lists drugs to be avoided. Note that people may be allergic to additives (eg, dyes, binders, others) rather than the active drug.

Self-Administration

✔ Take antihistamines only as prescribed or as instructed on packages of OTC preparations to increase beneficial effects and decrease adverse effects. If you miss a dose, do not take a double dose.

✔ Take most antihistamines with meals to decrease stomach upset. Take loratadine (Claritin) on an empty stomach for better absorption; cetirizine (Zyrtec) and desloratadine (Clarinex) may be taken with or without food.

✔ Do not chew or crush sustained-release tablets and do not open sustained-release capsules. Such actions can cause rapid drug absorption, high blood levels, and serious adverse effects, rather than the slow absorption and prolonged action intended with these products.

● For chronic allergic symptoms (eg, allergic rhinitis), long-acting preparations provide more consistent relief. A client may respond better to one antihistamine than to another. Thus, if one does not relieve symptoms or produces excessive sedation, another may be effective.

● For treatment of the common cold, studies have demonstrated that antihistamines do not relieve symptoms and are not recommended. However, an antihistamine is often included in prescription and OTC combination products for the common cold.

APPLYING YOUR KNOWLEDGE 45-2

Ms. Fisher returns to the clinic. She states, "The medication makes me feel better, but it is so expensive. I have a hard time affording it." What advice can you offer?

Use in Special Populations

Use in Children

First-generation antihistamines (eg, diphenhydramine) may cause drowsiness and decreased mental alertness in children as in adults. Young children may experience paradoxical excitement. These reactions may occur with therapeutic dosages. In overdosage, hallucinations, convulsions, and death may occur. Close supervision and appropriate dosages are required for safe drug usage in children.

Diphenhydramine is not recommended for use in newborn infants (premature or full-term) or children with chickenpox or a flulike infection. When used in young children, doses should be small because of drug effects on the brain and nervous system. *Promethazine* should not be used in children with hepatic disease, Reye's syndrome, a history of sleep apnea, or a family history of sudden infant death syndrome.

The second-generation drugs vary in recommendations for use according to age groups. *Cetirizine* and *loratadine* may be used in children 2 years and older. Syrup formulations are available for use in younger children. *Azelastine* may be used in children 5 years and older; *fexofenadine* may be used in children 6 years of age and older; and *desloratadine* may be used in children 12 years and older.

APPLYING YOUR KNOWLEDGE 45-3:
HOW CAN YOU AVOID THIS MEDICATION ERROR?
During her visit, Ms. Fisher tells you that her 18-month-old daughter has a cold. Last night, she gave her daughter a dose of the loratadine to relieve her symptoms and help the child get some rest.

Use in Older Adults

First-generation antihistamines (eg, *diphenhydramine*) may cause confusion (with impaired thinking, judgment, and memory), dizziness, hypotension, sedation, syncope, unsteady gait, and paradoxical CNS stimulation in older adults. These effects, especially sedation, may be misinterpreted as senility or mental depression. Older men with prostatic hypertrophy may have difficulty voiding while taking these drugs. Some of these adverse reactions derive from anticholinergic effects of the drugs and are likely to be more severe if the client is also taking other drugs with anticholinergic effects (eg, tricyclic antidepressants, older antipsychotic drugs, some antiparkinson drugs). Despite the increased risk of adverse effects, however, diphenhydramine is sometimes prescribed as a sleep aid for occasional use in older adults. As with many other drugs, smaller-than-usual dosages are indicated.

In general, second-generation antihistamines should be used for older adults. They are much safer because they do not impair consciousness, thinking, or ability to perform activities of daily living (eg, driving a car or operating various machines).

Use in Clients With Renal Impairment

Little information is available about using antihistamines in clients with impaired renal function. With *diphenhydramine,* the dosing interval should be extended to 12 to 18 hours in clients with severe kidney failure. With *cetirizine* (5 mg once daily), *desloratadine* (5 mg every other day), *fexofenadine* (60 mg once daily), and *loratadine* (10 mg every other day), recommended doses for initial use are approximately one half of those used for young and middle-aged adults. No data are available regarding use of *azelastine.* However, because the drug is metabolized in the liver and excreted mainly in feces, it is unlikely that a dosage reduction is needed in clients with renal impairment.

Use in Clients With Hepatic Impairment

Little information is available about using antihistamines in clients with impaired hepatic function. With *diphenhydramine,* single doses are probably safe but the effects of multiple doses have not been studied in this population. With *promethazine,* cholestatic jaundice has been reported and the drug should be used with caution. With *cetirizine* (5 mg once daily) and *loratadine* (10 mg every other day), smaller-than-usual doses are recommended. No data are available regarding use of *azelastine.* However, because the drug is metabolized in the liver and excreted mainly in feces, cautious use and a possible dosage reduction may be needed in clients with hepatic impairment.

Use in Clients With Critical Illness

Antihistamines are not often used in the treatment of clients with critical illness. Most are given orally, and many critically ill clients are unable to take oral drugs. *Diphenhydramine* may be given by injection, usually as a single dose, to a client who is having a blood transfusion or a diagnostic test, to prevent allergic reactions. *Hydroxyzine* or *promethazine* may be given by injection for nausea and vomiting or to provide sedation, but are not usually the first drugs of choice for these indications.

Use in Home Care

Antihistamines are often taken in the home setting, especially for allergic rhinitis and other allergic disorders. Most people are familiar with the uses and side effects of antihistamines. The home care nurse is unlikely to be involved in antihistamine drug therapy unless visiting a client for other care and purposes. If a first-generation drug is being used, the home care nurse needs to assess for drowsiness and safety hazards in the environment (eg, operating a car or other potentially hazardous machinery). In most people, tolerance develops to the sedative effects within a few days if they are not taking other sedative-type drugs or alcoholic beverages.

If a client has an allergic disorder, the home care nurse may need to assist in identifying and alleviating environmental allergens (eg, cigarette smoke, animal dander, dust mites).

Antihistamines

NURSING ACTIONS	RATIONALE/EXPLANATION
1. Administer accurately	
a. Give most oral antihistamines with food; give loratadine on an empty stomach; give cetirizine or desloratadine with or without food.	To decrease gastrointestinal (GI) effects of the drugs
b. Give intramuscular antihistamines deeply into a large muscle mass.	To decrease tissue irritation
c. Inject intravenous (IV) antihistamines slowly, over a few minutes.	Severe hypotension may result from rapid IV injection.
d. When a drug is used to prevent motion sickness, give it 30–60 minutes before travel.	
2. Observe for therapeutic effects	Therapeutic effects depend on the reason for use.
a. A verbal statement of therapeutic effect (relief of symptoms)	
b. Decreased nausea and vomiting when given for antiemetic effects	
c. Decreased dizziness and nausea when taken for motion sickness	
d. Drowsiness or sleep when given for sedation	
3. Observe for adverse effects	
a. First-generation drugs	
(1) Sedation	Drowsiness due to central nervous system (CNS) depression is the most common adverse effect.
(2) Paradoxical excitation—restlessness, insomnia, tremors, nervousness, palpitations	This reaction is more likely to occur in children. It may result from the anticholinergic effects of antihistamines.
(3) Convulsive seizures	Antihistamines, particularly the phenothiazines, may lower the seizure threshold.
(4) Dryness of mouth, nose, and throat; blurred vision; urinary retention; constipation	Due to anticholinergic effects
(5) GI distress—anorexia, nausea, vomiting	
b. Second-generation drugs	Adverse effects are few and mild.
(1) Drowsiness	Drowsiness and dry mouth are more likely to occur with cetirizine; headache is more likely to occur with loratadine; desloratadine and fexofenadine reportedly produce minimal adverse effects.
(2) Dry mouth	
(3) Fatigue	
(4) Headache	
(5) GI upset	
4. Observe for drug interactions	Note: No documented drug interactions have been reported with intranasal azelastine or oral cetirizine or desloratadine.
a. Drugs that *increase* effects of first-generation antihistamines:	
(1) Alcohol and other CNS depressants (eg, antianxiety and antipsychotic agents, opioid analgesics, sedative-hypnotics)	Additive CNS depression. Concomitant use may lead to drowsiness, lethargy, stupor, respiratory depression, coma, and death.
(2) Monoamine oxidase inhibitors	Inhibit metabolism of antihistamines, leading to an increased duration of action; increased incidence and severity of sedative and anticholinergic adverse effects.
(3) Tricyclic antidepressants	Additive anticholinergic side effects
b. Drugs that *increase* effects of loratadine:	All of these drugs increase plasma levels of loratadine by decreasing its metabolism.
(1) Macrolide antibacterials (azithromycin, clarithromycin, erythromycin)	
(2) Azole antifungals (fluconazole, itraconazole, ketoconazole, miconazole)	
(3) Cimetidine	
c. Drugs that may *decrease* effects of fexofenadine:	
(1) Rifampin	Rifampin may induce enzymes that accelerate metabolism of fexofenadine.

APPLYING YOUR KNOWLEDGE: ANSWERS

45-1 Loratadine should be taken on an empty stomach. Do not take both loratadine and diphenhydramine. Wear sunscreen if exposed to sunlight. Inform your physician if you become pregnant, and do not consume alcohol.

45-2 First-generation antihistamines such as diphenhydramine are less costly and may provide an alternative to the higher cost of the second-generation antihistamines. Caution Ms. Fisher that if she switches drugs, the first-generation drugs cause more drowsiness.

45-3 Since the nurse is unlikely to have an opportunity to teach about individual OTC medications, it is important to advise. Ms. Fisher to read the medication label on all OTC medication. She needs to be especially careful when medicating a small child. Loratadine is only approved for use in children 2 years and older.

Review and Application Exercises

Short Answer Exercises

1. Describe several factors that cause histamine release from cells.

2. What signs and symptoms are produced by the release of histamine?

3. How do antihistamines act to block the effects of histamine?

4. Differentiate between H_1 and H_2 receptor antagonists in terms of pharmacologic effects and clinical indications for use.

5. In general, when should an antihistamine be taken to prevent or treat allergic disorders?

6. Compare and contrast the first- and second-generation antihistamines.

NCLEX-Style Questions

7. Second-generation H_1 antagonists differ from first-generation antagonists in that they
   a. cause greater CNS sedation
   b. are available only by prescription
   c. are less expensive
   d. do not cross the blood–brain barrier

8. Studies have demonstrated that for treatment of the common cold, antihistamines
   a. are effective in relieving cold symptoms
   b. do not relieve symptoms and are not recommended
   c. should be compounded with other products to be effective
   d. relieve nonallergenic symptoms only

9. The drug of choice for severe allergic reactions is
   a. atropine
   b. cimetidine (Tagamet)
   c. epinephrine
   d. loratadine (Claritin)

10. Diphenhydramine (Benadryl) is recommended for use in
    a. premature or full-term infants
    b. adults to prevent allergic reactions
    c. children with chickenpox
    d. children with a flulike infection

11. Due to the action of antihistamines on target tissues, these drugs are effective in producing all of the following actions except
    a. inhibiting vascular permeability
    b. reducing bronchoconstriction
    c. minimizing edema formation
    d. preventing histamine release

Selected References

Desloratadine (Clarinex). (2002, March 18). *The Medical Letter on Drugs and Therapeutics, 44*(1126).
Drug facts and comparisons. (Updated monthly). St. Louis: Facts and Comparisons.
Guyton, A. C., & Hall, J. E. (2000). *Textbook of medical physiology* (10th ed.). Philadelphia: W. B. Saunders.
Hussex, T. C. (2002). Allergic rhinitis: a focus on nonprescription therapy. *Pharmacy Times, 68*(5), 63–67.
Karch, A. M. (2005). *2006 Lippincott's nursing drug guide.* Philadelphia: Lippincott Williams & Wilkins.
Kim, R. B. (Ed.). (2001). *Handbook of adverse drug interactions.* New Rochelle, NY: Medical Letter.
Lacy, C. F., Armstrong, L. L., Goldman, M. P., et al. (2004). *Lexi-Comp's drug information handbook* (12th ed.). Hudson, OH: Lexi-Comp.
Porth, C. M. (2005). *Pathophysiology: Concepts of altered health states* (7th ed.). Philadelphia: Lippincott Williams & Wilkins.
Sampey, C. S., & Follin, S. L. (2001). Second generation antihistamines: The OTC debate. *Journal of the American Pharmaceutical Association, 43*(3), 454–457.
Terr, A. I. (2000). Approach to the patient with allergies. In H. D. Humes (Ed.), *Kelley's Textbook of internal medicine* (4th ed., pp. 1340–1346). Philadelphia: Lippincott Williams & Wilkins.

Nasal Decongestants, Antitussives, and Cold Remedies

OBJECTIVES

After studying this chapter, you will be able to:

1. Describe characteristics of selected upper respiratory disorders and symptoms.
2. Review decongestant and adverse effects of adrenergic drugs.
3. Describe general characteristics and effects of antitussive agents.
4. Discuss the advantages and disadvantages of using combination products to treat the common cold.
5. Evaluate over-the-counter allergy, cold, cough, and sinus remedies for personal or clients' use.

APPLYING YOUR KNOWLEDGE

Archie Hobbs is a 45-year-old welder at an industrial plant. As the occupational nurse for the facility, you observe a high rate of people with colds. Archie comes to the health office complaining about his nasal congestion and cough.

INTRODUCTION

The drugs discussed in this chapter are used to treat upper respiratory disorders and symptoms such as the common cold, sinusitis, nasal congestion, cough, and excessive secretions. Some of these diverse drugs are discussed more extensively in other chapters; they are discussed here in relation to their use in upper respiratory conditions.

Common Respiratory Disorders

The Common Cold

The common cold, a viral infection of the upper respiratory tract, is the most common respiratory tract infection. Adults usually have two to four colds per year; schoolchildren may have as many as 10 per year. A cold often begins with dry, stuffy feelings in the nose and throat, an increased amount of clear nasal secretions, and tearing of the eyes. As the mucous membranes of the nose and throat become more inflamed, other common symptoms include cough, increased nasal congestion and drainage, sore throat, hoarseness, headache, and general malaise. Colds can be caused by many types of virus, most often the rhinovirus. Shedding of these viruses by infected people, mainly from nasal mucosa, can result in rapid spread to other people.

The major mode of transmission is contamination of skin or environmental surfaces. The infected person, with viruses on the hands from contact with nasal secretions (eg, sneezing, coughing), touches various objects (eg, doorknobs, faucet handles, telephones). The uninfected person touches these contaminated surfaces with the fingers and then transfers the viruses by touching nasal or eye mucosal membranes. The viruses can enter the body through mucous membranes. Cold viruses can survive for several hours on the skin and hard surfaces, such as wood and plastic. There may also be airborne spread from sneezing and coughing, but this source is considered secondary. After the viruses gain entry, the incubation period is about 5 days, the most contagious period is about 3 days after symptoms begin, and the cold usually lasts about 7 days. Because of the way cold viruses are spread, frequent and thorough hand hygiene (by both infected and uninfected people) is the most important protective and preventive measure.

Sinusitis

Sinusitis is inflammation of the paranasal sinuses, air cells that connect with the nasal cavity and are lined by similar mucosa. As in other parts of the respiratory tract, ciliated mucous membranes help move fluid and microorganisms out of the sinuses and into the nasal cavity. This movement becomes impaired when sinus openings are blocked by nasal swelling, and the impairment is considered a major cause of sinus infections. Another contributing factor is a lower oxygen content in the sinuses, which aids the growth of microorganisms and impairs local defense mechanisms. Rhinitis (inflammation and congestion of nasal mucosa) and upper respiratory tract infections are the most common causes of sinusitis. Symptoms may include moderate to severe headache, tenderness or pain in the affected sinus area, and fever.

APPLYING YOUR KNOWLEDGE 46-1

Mr. Hobbs works in an area with many other people. What should you emphasize to help prevent the further spread of infection throughout the plant?

Common Signs and Symptoms of Respiratory Disorders

Nasal Congestion

Nasal congestion is manifested by obstructed nasal passages ("stuffy nose") and nasal drainage ("runny nose"). It is a prominent symptom of the common cold and rhinitis (including allergic rhinitis; see Chap. 45). Nasal congestion results from dilation of the blood vessels in the nasal mucosa and engorgement of the mucous membranes with blood. At the same time, nasal membranes are stimulated to increase mucus secretion. Related symptomatic terms are *rhinorrhea* (secretions discharged from the nose) and *rhinitis* (inflammation of nasal mucosa, usually accompanied by nasal congestion, rhinorrhea, and sneezing).

Cough

Cough is a forceful expulsion of air from the lungs. It is normally a protective reflex for removing foreign bodies, environmental irritants, or accumulated secretions from the respiratory tract. The cough reflex involves central and peripheral mechanisms. Centrally, the cough center in the medulla oblongata receives stimuli and initiates the reflex response (deep inspiration, closed glottis, buildup of pressure within the lungs, and forceful exhalation). Peripherally, cough receptors in the pharynx, larynx, trachea, or lungs may be stimulated by air, dryness of mucous membranes, or excessive secretions. A cough is productive when secretions are expectorated; it is nonproductive when it is dry and no sputum is expectorated.

Cough is a prominent symptom of respiratory tract infections (eg, the common cold, influenza, bronchitis, pharyngitis)

and chronic obstructive pulmonary diseases (eg, emphysema, chronic bronchitis).

Increased Secretions

Increased secretions may result from excessive production or decreased ability to cough or otherwise remove secretions from the respiratory tract. Secretions may seriously impair respiration by obstructing airways and preventing air flow to and from alveoli, where gas exchange occurs. Secretions also may cause atelectasis (a condition in which part of the lung is airless and collapses) by blocking air flow, and they may cause or aggravate infections by supporting bacterial growth.

Respiratory disorders characterized by retention of secretions include influenza, pneumonia, upper respiratory infections, acute and chronic bronchitis, emphysema, and acute attacks of asthma. Nonrespiratory conditions that predispose to secretion retention include immobility, debilitation, cigarette smoking, and postoperative status. Surgical procedures involving the chest or abdomen are most likely to be associated with retention of secretions because pain may decrease the client's ability to cough, breathe deeply, and ambulate.

GENERAL CHARACTERISTICS OF DRUGS USED IN/FOR RESPIRATORY DISORDERS

Numerous drugs are available and widely used to treat the symptoms of respiratory disorders. Many are nonprescription drugs and can be obtained alone or in combination products. Available products include nasal decongestants, antitussives, and expectorants.

Nasal Decongestants

Nasal decongestants are used to relieve nasal obstruction and discharge. Adrenergic (sympathomimetic) drugs are most often used for this purpose (see Chap. 17). These agents relieve nasal congestion and swelling by constricting arterioles and reducing blood flow to nasal mucosa. Oxymetazoline (Afrin) is a commonly used nasal spray; pseudoephedrine (Sudafed) is taken orally. Rebound nasal swelling can occur with excessive or extended use of nasal sprays (eg, >7 days, perhaps sooner).

Nasal decongestants are most often used to relieve rhinitis associated with respiratory infections or allergies. They also may be used to reduce local blood flow before nasal surgery and to aid visualization of the nasal mucosa during diagnostic examinations.

These drugs are contraindicated in clients with severe hypertension or coronary artery disease because of their cardiac stimulating and vasoconstricting effects. They also are contraindicated for clients with narrow-angle glaucoma and those taking tricyclic or monoamine oxidase inhibitor antidepressants. They must be used with caution in the presence of cardiac dysrhythmias, hyperthyroidism, diabetes mellitus, glaucoma, and prostatic hypertrophy.

APPLYING YOUR KNOWLEDGE 46-2:
HOW CAN YOU AVOID THIS MEDICATION ERROR?
Mr. Hobbs has been sick for more than 7 days. He feels that he is getting worse. When you ask him what medication he is taking, he reports that he is using a nasal spray that you had recommended the last time he was congested. He feels that he is getting worse.

Antitussives

Antitussive agents suppress cough by depressing the cough center in the medulla oblongata or the cough receptors in the throat, trachea, or lungs. Centrally acting antitussives include narcotics (eg, codeine, hydrocodone) and non-narcotics (eg, dextromethorphan). Locally acting agents (eg, throat lozenges, cough drops) may suppress cough by increasing the flow of saliva and by containing demulcents or local anesthetics to decrease irritation of pharyngeal mucosa. Flavored syrups are often used as vehicles for other drugs.

The major clinical indication for use of antitussives is a dry, hacking, nonproductive cough that interferes with rest and sleep. It is not desirable to suppress a productive cough because the secretions need to be removed. Although antitussives continue to be used and some people report beneficial effects, some research studies indicate that cough medicines are no more effective than placebos in children or adults. The American Academy of Pediatrics and several other groups advise against the use of antitussives.

Expectorants

Expectorants are agents given orally to liquefy respiratory secretions and allow for their easier removal. Guaifenesin is the most commonly used expectorant. It is available alone and as an ingredient in many combination cough and cold remedies, although research studies do not support its effectiveness and many authorities do not recommend its use.

Mucolytics

Mucolytics are administered by inhalation to liquefy mucus in the respiratory tract. Solutions of mucolytic drugs may be nebulized into a face mask or mouthpiece or instilled directly into the respiratory tract through a tracheostomy. Sodium chloride solution and acetylcysteine (Mucomyst) are the only agents recommended for use as mucolytics. Acetylcysteine is effective within 1 minute after inhalation, and maximal effects occur within 5 to 10 minutes. It is effective immediately after direct instillation. Oral acetylcysteine is widely used in the treatment of acetaminophen overdosage (see Chap. 7).

Cold Remedies

Many combination products are available for treating symptoms of the common cold. Many of the products contain an antihistamine, a nasal decongestant, and an analgesic. Some contain antitussives, expectorants, and other agents as well. Many cold remedies are over-the-counter (OTC) formulations. Commonly used ingredients include chlorpheniramine (antihistamine), pseudoephedrine (adrenergic nasal decongestant), acetaminophen (analgesic and antipyretic), dextromethorphan (antitussive), and guaifenesin (expectorant). Although antihistamines are popular OTC drugs because they dry nasal secretions, they are not recommended because they can also dry lower respiratory secretions and worsen secretion retention and cough. The use of OTC products containing ephedrine and pseudoephedrine to manufacture methamphetamine has increased at an alarming rate. Some states have passed laws placing these products behind pharmacy counters to restrict sales.

Many products come in several formulations, with different ingredients, and are advertised for different purposes (eg, allergy, sinus disorders, multisymptom cold and flu remedies). For example, allergy remedies contain an antihistamine; "nondrowsy" or "daytime" formulas contain a nasal decongestant, but do not contain an antihistamine; "PM" or "night" formulas contain a sedating antihistamine to promote sleep; pain, fever, and multisymptom formulas usually contain acetaminophen; and "maximum strength" preparations usually refer only to the amount of acetaminophen per dose, usually 1000 milligrams for adults. In addition, labels on OTC combination products list ingredients by generic name, without identifying the type of drug. As a result of these bewildering products, consumers, including nurses and other health care providers, may not know what medications they are taking or whether some drugs increase or block the effects of other drugs.

APPLYING YOUR KNOWLEDGE 46-3
Mr. Hobbs also complains of a productive cough. He has been taking chlorpheniramine to treat it. What advice should you give to Mr. Hobbs with regard to the appropriate treatment of a productive cough?

INDIVIDUAL DRUGS

Individual decongestants, antitussives, expectorants, and mucolytics are listed in Table 46-1; selected combination products are listed in Table 46-2.

Herbal and Dietary Supplements

Several supplements are commonly used to prevent or treat symptoms of the common cold. In general, there is minimal or no support for such use.

Echinacea preparations differ in chemical composition depending on which of the nine species or parts of the plant (eg, leaves, roots, whole plant) are used, as well as the season

Table 46-1 Drugs at a Glance: Nasal Decongestants, Antitussives, Expectorants and Mucolytics

GENERIC/TRADE NAME	ROUTES AND DOSAGE RANGES	
	Adults	Children
Nasal Decongestants		
Ephedrine sulfate 0.25% solution	Topically, 2–3 sprays in each nostril no more often than q4h. Maximum, 6 doses/24 h	*12 y and older:* Same as adults *6–11 y:* 1–2 sprays in each nostril no more often than q4h. Maximum, 6 doses/24 h *<6 y:* Not recommended
Naphazoline (Privine) 0.05% spray or drops	Topically, 1–2 sprays or drops no more often than q6h. Maximum, 4 doses/24 h	*12 y and older:* Same as adults *<12 y:* Not recommended
Oxymetazoline (Afrin) 0.05% spray	Topically, 2–3 sprays in each nostril, q10–12h. Maximum, 2 doses/24 h	*6 y and older:* Same as adults *<6 y:* Not recommended
Phenylephrine (Neo-Synephrine)	PO 10–20 mg q4h. Maximum 120 mg/24 h Topically, 2–3 sprays or drops of 0.25%, 0.5%, or 1% solution in each nostril no more often than q4h. Maximum, 6 doses/24 h	*12 y and older:* Same as adults *6–11 y:* PO 10 mg q4h. Maximum 60 mg/24 h Topically, 2–3 sprays of 0.25% solution in each nostril no more often than q4h. Maximum, 6 doses/24 h *2–5 y:* Topically, 2–3 drops of 0.125% solution no more often than q4h. Maximum 6 doses/24 h
Pseudoephedrine (Sudafed, Dimetapp)	Regular tablets, PO 60 mg q4–6 h Extended-release tablets, PO 120 mg q12h or 240 mg q24h. Maximum, 240 mg in 24 h	*12 y and older:* Same as adults for regular and extended-release tablets *6–12 y:* 30 mg q4–6h. Maximum, 120 mg/24 h *2–5 y:* PO 15 mg q4–6h. Maximum, 60 mg/24 h *<2 y:* Consult pediatrician
Tetrahydrozoline (Tyzine) 0.1% solution	Topically, 2–4 drops or 3–4 sprays in each nostril, no more often than q3h. Maximum, 8 doses/24 h	*6 y and older:* Same as adults *2–5 y:* Spray not recommended. 2–3 drops of 0.05% solution in each nostril no more often than q3h. Maximum, 8 doses/24 h
Xylometazoline (Otrivin)	Topically, 0.1% solution, 1–3 sprays or 2–3 drops in each nostril q8–10h. Maximum, 3 doses/24 h	*12 y and older:* Same as adult *2–11 y:* Topically, 0.05%, 1 spray or 2–3 drops in each nostril q8–10h. Maximum, 3 doses/24 h
Narcotic Antitussive **Codeine**	PO 10–20 mg q4–6h. Maximum, 120 mg/24 h	*6–12 y:* PO 5–10 mg q4–6h. Maximum, 60 mg/24 h *2–6 y:* PO 2.5–5 mg q4–6h. Maximum, 30 mg/24 h
Hydrocodone bitrartate (Hycodan)	PO 1 (5 mg) tablet q4–6h up to 6 daily	Not recommended
Non-Narcotic Antitussive **Dextromethorphan** (Benylin DM, others)	Liquid, lozenges, and syrup, 10–30 mg q4–8h. Maximum, 120 mg/24 h Sustained-action liquid (Delsym), PO 60 mg q12h	*>12 y:* Same as adults *6–12 y:* 5–10 mg q4h or 15 mg q6–8h; Maximum, 60 mg/24 h *2–6 y:* 2.5–7.5 mg q4–8h. Maximum, 30 mg/24 h Sustained-action liquid, *6–12 y:* 30 mg q12h *2–5 y:* 15 mg q12h
Expectorant **Guaifenesin** (glyceryl guaiacolate) (Robitussin, others)	PO 100–400 mg q4h. Maximum, 2400 mg/24 h	*12 y and older:* Same as adults *6–12 y:* PO 100–200 mg q4h. Maximum, 1200 mg/24 h *2–6 y:* PO 50–100 mg q4h. Maximum, 600 mg/24 h

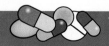

Table 46-1 Drugs at a Glance: Nasal Decongestants, Antitussives, Expectorants and Mucolytics (continued)

	ROUTES AND DOSAGE RANGES	
GENERIC/TRADE NAME	**Adults**	**Children**
Mucolytic **Acetylcysteine** (Mucomyst)	Nebulization, 1–10 mL of a 20% solution or 2–20 mL of a 10% solution q2–6h Instillation, 1–2 mL of a 10% or 20% solution q1–4h Acetaminophen overdosage, PO 140 mg/kg initially, then 70 mg/kg q4h for 17 doses; dilute a 10% or 20% solution to a 5% solution with cola, fruit juice, or water	Acetaminophen overdosage, see literature

PO, oral.

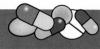

Table 46-2 Drugs at a Glance: Representative Multi-Ingredient Nonprescription Cold, Cough, and Sinus Remedies

	INGREDIENTS				
TRADE NAME	**Antihistamine**	**Nasal Decongestant**	**Analgesic**	**Antitussive**	**Expoectorant**
Actifed Cold & Allergy	Triprolidine 2.5 mg/tablet	Pseudoephedrine 60 mg/tablet			
Advil Cold and Sinus Tablets		Pseudoephedrine 30 mg/tablet	Ibuprofen 200 mg/tablet		
Cheracol D Cough Liquid				Dextromethorphan 10 mg/5 mL	Guaifenesin 100 mg/5 mL
Comtrex Cold & Sinus Tablets	Brompheniramine 2 mg/tablet	Pseudoephedrine 30 mg/tablet	Acetaminophen 500 mg/tablet		
Contac Day & Night Cold & Flu Tablets	(Night) Diphen-hydramine 50 mg/tablet	Pseudoephedrine 60 mg/tablet Pseudoephedrine 60 mg/tablet	Acetaminophen 650 mg/tablet Acetaminophen 650 mg/tablet	(Day) Dextrometh-orphan 30 mg/tablet	
Coricidin D Cold, Flu & Sinus Tablets	Chlorpheniramine 2 mg/tablet	Pseudoephedrine 30 mg/tablet	Acetaminophen 325 mg/tablet		
Dimetapp Cold and Allergy Elixir	Brompheniramine 1 mg/5 mL	Pseudoephedrine 15 mg/5 mL			
Dristan Cold Formula	Chlorpheniramine 2 mg/tablet	Phenylephrine 5 mg/tablet	Acetaminophen 325 mg/tablet		
Motrin Sinus Tablets		Pseudoephedrine 30 mg/tablet	Ibuprofen 200 mg/tablet		
Robitussin Cold and Flu Tablets		Pseudoephedrine 10 mg/tablet	Acetaminophen 325 mg/tablet	Dextromethorphan 30 mg/tablet	Guaifenesin 200 mg/tablet
Sinutab Sinus Allergy Maxi-mum Strength Tablets	Chlorpheniramine 2 mg/tablet	Pseudoephedrine 30 mg/tablet	Acetaminophen 500 mg/tablet	Dextromethorphan 10 mg/tablet	
TheraFlu Flu, Cold, and Cough Powder	Chlorpheniramine 4 mg/pack	Pseudoephedrine 60 mg/pack	Acetaminophen 650 mg/pack	Dextromethorphan 20 mg/pack	
Vicks NyQuil Cold & Flu Capsules	Doxylamine 6.25 mg/capsule	Pseudoephedrine 30 mg/capsule	Acetaminophen 250 mg/capsule	Dextromethorphan 10 mg/capsule	

of harvesting. Also, which constituents of the plants are pharmacologically active is unclear.

Some studies indicating effectiveness of echinacea in preventing or treating colds are considered flawed in methodology, but may indicate the use of different products with different chemical components. A double-blind, placebo-controlled study showed no benefit of using echinacea for preventing respiratory infection or the common cold. However, after a cold occurred, the symptoms did not last quite as long in the echinacea group. In general, randomized, placebo-controlled research studies indicate no significant differences between echinacea groups and placebo groups in the incidence, duration, or severity of upper respiratory infections. Thus, there is no convincing evidence that echinacea is effective. Moreover, the purity and potency of echinacea products are unknown or variable among products. Although generally considered safe, allergic reactions, including anaphylaxis, have been reported.

Vitamin C, usually in large doses of more than 1000 milligrams daily, is used to reduce the incidence and severity of colds and influenza. However, such usage is not recommended or justified by clinical data. In general, high doses of vitamin C demonstrate little or no benefit in shortening the duration of symptoms or reducing viral shedding. In addition, they may cause adverse effects and about 90% of large doses is excreted in the urine. Very little is absorbed and blood levels of vitamin C are raised only slightly.

Zinc gluconate lozenges are marketed as a cold remedy. However, some studies indicate beneficial effects and others do not. Most of the studies suggesting benefit are considered flawed in methodology. For example, although some studies were supposed to be blind, the lozenges' distinctive taste likely allowed the drug to be distinguished from placebo.

NURSING PROCESS

Assessment

Assess the client's condition in relation to disorders for which the drugs are used.

- With nasal congestion, observe for decreased ability to breathe through the nose. If nasal discharge is present, note the amount, color, and thickness. Question the client about the duration and extent of nasal congestion and factors that precipitate or relieve the symptom.
- With coughing, a major assessment factor is whether the cough is productive of sputum or dry and hacking. If the cough is productive, note the color, odor, viscosity, and amount of sputum. In addition, assess factors that stimulate or relieve cough and the client's ability and willingness to cough effectively.
- Assess fluid intake and hydration status.

Nursing Diagnoses

- Risk for Injury related to cardiac dysrhythmias, hypertension, and other adverse effects of nasal decongestants
- Noncompliance: Overuse of nasal decongestants
- Deficient Knowledge: Appropriate use of single- and multi-ingredient drug formulations

Planning/Goals

The client will
- Experience relief of symptoms
- Take drugs accurately and safely
- Avoid overuse of decongestants
- Avoid preventable adverse drug effects
- Act to avoid recurrence of symptoms

Interventions

- Encourage clients to use measures to prevent or minimize the incidence and severity of symptoms:
  - Avoid smoking cigarettes or breathing secondhand smoke, when possible. Cigarette smoke irritates respiratory tract mucosa, and this irritation causes cough, increased secretions, and decreased effectiveness of cilia in cleaning the respiratory tract.
  - Avoid or limit exposure to crowds, especially during winter when the incidence of colds and influenza is high.
  - Avoid contact with people who have colds or other respiratory infections. This is especially important for clients with chronic lung disease, because upper respiratory infections may precipitate acute attacks of asthma or bronchitis.
  - Maintain a fluid intake of 2000 to 3000 mL daily unless contraindicated by cardiovascular or renal disease.
  - Maintain nutrition, rest, activity, and other general health measures.
  - Practice good hand hygiene techniques.
  - Annual vaccination for influenza is recommended for clients who are elderly or have chronic respiratory, cardiovascular, or renal disorders.
- Provide appropriate teaching related to drug therapy (see accompanying display).

Evaluation

- Interview and observe for relief of symptoms.
- Interview and observe for tachycardia, hypertension, drowsiness, and other adverse drug effects.
- Interview and observe for compliance with instructions about drug use.

CLIENT TEACHING GUIDELINES

Nasal Decongestants, Anticough Medications, and Multi-Ingredient Cold Remedies

General Considerations

☑ These drugs may relieve symptoms but do not cure the disorder causing the symptoms.

☑ An adequate fluid intake, humidification of the environment, and sucking on hard candy or throat lozenges can help relieve mouth dryness and cough.

☑ Over-the-counter (OTC) cold remedies should not be used longer than 1 week. Do not use nose drops or sprays more often or longer than recommended. Excessive or prolonged use may damage nasal mucosa and produce chronic nasal congestion.

☑ Do not increase dosage if symptoms are not relieved by recommended amounts.

☑ See a health care provider if symptoms persist longer than 1 week.

☑ Read the labels of OTC allergy, cold, and sinus remedies for information about ingredients, dosages, conditions or other medications with which the drugs should not be taken, and adverse effects.

☑ Do not combine two drug preparations containing the same or similar active ingredients. For example, pseudoephedrine is the nasal decongestant component of most prescription and OTC sinus and multi-ingredient cold remedies. The recommended dose for immediate-release preparations is usually 30 to 60 mg of pseudoephedrine; doses in extended-release preparations are usually 120 mg. Taking more than one preparation containing pseudoephedrine (or phenylephrine, a similar drug) may increase dosage to toxic levels and cause irregular heartbeats and extreme nervousness.

☑ Note that many combination products contain acetaminophen or ibuprofen as pain relievers. If you are taking another form of one of these drugs (eg, Tylenol or Advil), there is a risk of overdosage and adverse effects. Acetaminophen can cause liver damage; ibuprofen is a relative of aspirin that can cause gastrointestinal upset and bleeding. Thus, you need to be sure your total daily dosage is not excessive (with Tylenol, above four doses of 1000 mg each; with ibuprofen, above 2400 mg).

☑ Individuals with diabetes mellitus should read OTC labels for sugar content because many decongestants and cough medicines may contain sucrose, glucose, or corn syrup as a base.

Self-Administration

☑ Take medications as prescribed or as directed on the labels of OTC preparations. Taking excessive amounts or taking recommended amounts too often can lead to serious adverse effects.

☑ Do not chew or crush long-acting tablets or capsules (eg, those taken once or twice daily). Such actions can cause rapid drug absorption, high blood levels, and serious adverse effects, rather than the slow absorption and prolonged action intended with these products.

☑ For OTC drugs available in different dosage strengths, start with lower recommended doses rather than "maximum strength" formulations or the highest recommended doses. It is safer to see how the drugs affect you, then increase doses if necessary and not contraindicated.

☑ With topical nasal decongestants:
1. Use only preparations labeled for intranasal use. For example, phenylephrine (Neo-Synephrine) is available in both nasal and eye formulations. The two types of solutions cannot be used interchangeably. In addition, phenylephrine preparations may contain 0.125%, 0.25%, 0.5%, or 1% of drug. Be sure the concentration is appropriate for the person to receive it (eg, an infant, young child, or older adult).
2. Blow the nose gently before instilling nasal solutions or sprays. This clears nasal passages and increases effectiveness of medications.
3. To instill nose drops, lie down or sit with the neck hyperextended and instill medication without touching the dropper to the nostrils (to avoid contamination of the dropper and medication). Rinse the medication dropper after each use.
4. For nasal sprays, sit or stand, squeeze the container once to instill medication, and rinse the spray tip after each use. Most nasal sprays are designed to deliver one dose when used correctly.
5. If decongestant nose drops are ordered for nursing infants, give a dose 20 to 30 minutes before feeding. Nasal congestion interferes with an infant's ability to suck.

☑ Take or give cough syrups undiluted and avoid eating and drinking for approximately 30 minutes. Part of the beneficial effect of cough syrups stems from soothing effects on pharyngeal mucosa. Food or fluid removes the medication from the throat.

☑ Report palpitations, dizziness, drowsiness, or rapid pulse. These effects may occur with nasal decongestants and cold remedies and may indicate excessive dosage.

PRINCIPLES OF THERAPY

Drug Selection and Administration

Choice of drugs and routes of administration are influenced by several client- and drug-related variables. Some guidelines include the following:

● Single-drug formulations allow flexibility and individualization of dosage, whereas combination products may contain unneeded ingredients and are more expensive. However, many people find combination products more convenient to use.

● With nasal decongestants, topical preparations (ie, nasal solutions or sprays) are often preferred for short-term use. They are rapidly effective because they come into direct contact with nasal mucosa. If used longer than 7 consecutive days or in excessive amounts, however, these products may produce rebound nasal congestion. Oral drugs are preferred for long-term use (>7 days). For clients with cardiovascular disease, topical nasal decongestants are usually preferred. Oral agents are usually contraindicated because of cardiovascular effects (eg, increased force of myocardial contraction, increased heart rate, increased blood pressure).

- Antihistamines are clearly useful in allergic conditions (eg, allergic rhinitis; see Chap. 45), but their use to relieve cold symptoms is controversial. First-generation antihistamines (eg, chlorpheniramine, diphenhydramine) have anticholinergic effects that may reduce sneezing, rhinorrhea, and cough. Also, their sedative effects may aid sleep. Many multi-ingredient cold remedies contain an antihistamine.

- Cough associated with the common cold usually stems from postnasal drainage and throat irritation. Most antitussives are given orally as tablets or cough syrups. Syrups serve as vehicles for antitussive drugs and may exert antitussive effects of their own by soothing irritated pharyngeal mucosa. Dextromethorphan is the antitussive drug of choice in most circumstances and is the antitussive ingredient in almost all OTC cough remedies (often designated by "DM" on the product label). However, as discussed previously, some authorities question the effectiveness of antitussives and do not recommend them for use in children or adults.

- Ipratropium (Atrovent), an anticholinergic drug, in a 0.06% nasal spray, is Food and Drug Administration (FDA) approved for treatment of rhinorrhea associated with the common cold.

- Cromolyn, a mast cell stabilizer, used by oral or intranasal inhalation, seems effective in reducing the symptoms and duration of the common cold but it is not FDA approved for this purpose. In one study, it was used every 2 hours for the first 2 days, then 4 times daily. The nasal solution (Nasalcrom) is available OTC.

- For treatment of excessive respiratory tract secretions, mechanical measures (eg, coughing, deep breathing, ambulation, chest physiotherapy, forcing fluids) are more likely to be effective than expectorant drug therapy.

Use in Special Populations

Use in Children

Upper respiratory infections with nasal congestion, sore throat, cough, and increased secretions are common in children, and the drugs described in this chapter are often used. However, there are differences of opinion regarding use of the drugs and most authorities agree that more research is needed regarding dosage, safety, and effectiveness of cough and cold mixtures in children. Some considerations include the following:

- Most infections are viral in origin and antibiotics are not generally recommended. For sore throat, a throat culture for streptococcus organisms should be performed and the results obtained before an antibiotic is prescribed. For bronchitis, which is almost always viral, antibiotics are not usually indicated unless pneumonia is suspected or the cough lasts 10 to 14 days without improvement.

- Cough medicines are not considered effective by some authorities.

- With nasal decongestants, pseudoephedrine is considered effective in children older than 5 years of age, but research studies are inconclusive about its effectiveness in younger children. One consideration is that the low doses found in children's preparations may be insufficient to produce therapeutic effects. As a result, some pediatricians do not recommend usage while others say the drug may be useful in some children.

- Nasal congestion may interfere with an infant's ability to nurse. Phenylephrine nasal solution, applied just before feeding time, is usually effective. However, excessive amounts or too-frequent administration of topical agents may result in rebound nasal congestion and systemic effects of cardiac and central nervous system stimulation. Therefore, the drug should be given to infants only when recommended by a pediatric specialist.

- Parents often administer a medication (eg, acetaminophen, ibuprofen) for pain and fever when a child has cold symptoms, whether the child has pain and fever or not. Some pediatricians suggest treating fevers above 101 degrees if the child seems uncomfortable but not to treat them otherwise. Parents may need to be counseled that fever is part of the body's defense mechanism and may help the child recover from an infection.

Use in Older Adults

A major consideration is that older adults are at high risk of adverse effects from oral nasal decongestants (eg, hypertension, cardiac dysrhythmias, nervousness, insomnia). Adverse effects from topical agents are less likely, but rebound nasal congestion and systemic effects may occur with overuse. Older adults with significant cardiovascular disease should avoid the drugs. Also, as in other populations, antitussives and expectorants have questionable effectiveness.

Use in Home Care

These drugs are used primarily in home settings and household members may ask the home care nurse for advice about OTC

N U R S I N G   A C T I O N S

Nasal Decongestants, Antitussives, and Cold Remedies

NURSING ACTIONS

RATIONALE/EXPLANATION

1. **Administer accurately**

   a. With topical nasal decongestants:

   (1) Use only preparations labeled for intranasal use.

   Intranasal preparations are usually dilute, aqueous solutions prepared specifically for intranasal use. Some agents (eg, phenylephrine) are available in ophthalmic solutions as well. The two types of solutions *cannot* be used interchangeably.

   (2) Use the drug concentration ordered.

   Some drug preparations are available in several concentrations. For example, phenylephrine preparations may contain 0.125%, 0.25%, 0.5%, or 1% of drug.

   (3) For instillation of nose drops, have the client lie down or sit with the neck hyperextended. Instill medication without touching the dropper to the nares. Rinse the medication dropper after each use.

   To avoid contamination of the dropper and medication

   (4) For nasal sprays, have the client sit, squeeze the container once to instill medication, avoid touching the spray tip to the nares, and rinse the spray tip after each use.

   Most nasal sprays are designed to deliver one dose when used correctly. If necessary, secretions may be cleared and a second spray used. Correct usage and cleansing prevents contamination and infection.

   (5) Give nasal decongestants to infants 20–30 minutes before feeding.

   Nasal congestion interferes with an infant's ability to suck.

   b. Administer cough syrups undiluted and instruct the client to avoid eating and drinking for approximately 30 minutes.

   Part of the therapeutic benefit of cough syrups stems from soothing effects on pharyngeal mucosa. Food or fluid removes the medication from the pharynx.

2. **Observe for therapeutic effects**

   Therapeutic effects depend on the reason for use.

   a. When nasal decongestants are given, observe for decreased nasal obstruction and drainage.

   b. With antitussives, observe for decreased coughing.

   The goal of antitussive therapy is to suppress nonpurposeful coughing, not productive coughing.

   c. With cold and allergy remedies, observe for decreased nasal congestion, rhinitis, muscle aches, and other symptoms.

3. **Observe for adverse effects**

   a. With nasal decongestants, observe for:

   (1) Tachycardia, cardiac dysrhythmias, hypertension

   These effects may occur with any of the adrenergic drugs (see Chap. 17). When adrenergic drugs are used as nasal decongestants, cardiovascular effects are more likely to occur with oral agents. However, topically applied drugs also may be systemically absorbed through the nasal mucosa or by being swallowed and absorbed through the gastrointestinal tract.

   (2) Rebound nasal congestion, chronic rhinitis, and possible ulceration of nasal mucosa

   Adverse effects on nasal mucosa are more likely to occur with excessive or long-term (>10 d) use.

   b. With antitussives, observe for:

   (1) Excessive suppression of the cough reflex (inability to cough effectively when secretions are present)

   This is a potentially serious adverse effect because retained secretions may lead to atelectasis, pneumonia, hypoxia, hypercarbia, and respiratory failure.

   (2) Nausea, vomiting, constipation, dizziness, drowsiness, pruritus, and drug dependence

   These are adverse effects associated with narcotic agents (see Chap. 6). When narcotics are given for antitussive effects, however, they are given in relatively small doses and are unlikely to cause adverse reactions.

NURSING ACTIONS	RATIONALE/EXPLANATION
(3) Nausea, drowsiness, and dizziness with non-narcotic antitussives	Adverse effects are infrequent and mild with these agents.
c. With combination products (eg, cold remedies), observe for adverse effects of individual ingredients (ie, antihistamines, adrenergics, analgesics, and others).	Adverse effects are rarely significant when the products are used as prescribed. There may be subtherapeutic doses of one or more component drugs, especially in over-the-counter formulations. Also, the drowsiness associated with antihistamines may be offset by stimulating effects of adrenergics. Ephedrine, for example, has central nervous system (CNS)–stimulating effects.
4. Observe for drug interactions	
a. Drugs that *increase* effects of nasal decongestants:	These interactions are more likely to occur with oral decongestants than topically applied drugs.
(1) Cocaine, digoxin, general anesthetics, monoamine oxidase (MAO) inhibitors, other adrenergic drugs, thyroid preparations, and xanthines	Increased risks of cardiac dysrhythmias
(2) Antihistamines, epinephrine, ergot alkaloids, MAO inhibitors, methylphenidate	Increased risks of hypertension due to vasoconstriction
b. Drugs that *increase* antitussive effects of codeine:	
(1) CNS depressants (alcohol, antianxiety agents, barbiturates, and other sedative-hypnotics)	Additive CNS depression. Codeine is given in small doses for antitussive effects, and risks of significant interactions are minimal.
c. Drugs that *alter* effects of dextromethorphan:	
(1) MAO inhibitors	This combination is contraindicated. Apnea, muscular rigidity, hyperpyrexia, laryngospasm, and death may occur.
d. Drugs that may *alter* effects of combination products for coughs, colds, and allergies:	Interactions depend on the individual drug components of each formulation. Risks of clinically significant drug interactions are increased with use of combination products.
(1) Adrenergic (sympathomimetic) agents (see Chap. 17)	
(2) Antihistamines (see Chap. 45)	
(3) CNS depressants (see Chaps. 6, 8, and 13)	
(4) CNS stimulants (see Chap. 15)	

remedies for conditions such as allergies, colds, coughs, and sinus headaches. Before recommending a particular product, the nurse needs to assess the intended recipient for conditions or other medications that contraindicate the product's use. For example, the nasal decongestant component may cause or aggravate cardiovascular disorders (eg, hypertension). In addition, other medications the client is taking need to be evaluated in terms of potential drug interactions with the remedy.

The home care nurse also must emphasize the need to read the label of any OTC medication for ingredients, precautions, contraindications, drug interactions, administration instructions, and so forth.

APPLYING YOUR KNOWLEDGE: ANSWERS

46-1 Remind everyone of the need for frequent and thorough hand hygiene. Infected people with viruses on their hands touch objects that uninfected people will touch, thereby transferring the viruses.

46-2 Appropriate client teaching with regard to nasal sprays should include not using a nasal spray for more than 7 days. Rebound nasal swelling can occur with excessive or extended use.

46-3 Nonpharmacologic measures would be most appropriate to consider. Intake of adequate fluids, frequent and thorough hand hygiene, and proper disposal of soiled tissues should be reinforced. Chlorpheniramine is an antihistamine. Mr. Hobbs should avoid using an antihistamine; it will dry nasal secretions but it will also dry lower respiratory secretions and may worsen secretion retention and cough. The use of expectorants, such as guaifenesin, has not clearly been supported by research, and many authories do not support its use.

Review and Application Exercises

Short Answer Exercises

1. How do adrenergic drugs relieve nasal congestion?

2. Who should usually avoid OTC nasal decongestants and cold remedies?

3. What are advantages and disadvantages of multi-ingredient cold remedies?

4. Given a client with a productive cough, what are nondrug interventions to promote removal of secretions?

5. Given a client who uses echinacea, vitamin C, or zinc lozenges and asks you what you think about the products as cold remedies, how would you reply?

NCLEX-Style Questions

6. A common mucolytic used to liquefy mucus in the respiratory tract is
   a. acetylcysteine (Mucomyst)
   b. ipratropium (Atrovent)
   c. dextromethorphan
   d. pseudoephedrine (Sudafed)

7. Adrenergic drugs are used as nasal decongestants to relieve symptoms by
   a. constricting arterioles and reducing blood flow to nasal mucosa
   b. stimulating air movement in the lungs
   c. stabilizing mast cells
   d. initiating the cough reflex

8. A nasal decongestant, such as oxymetazoline (Afrin), is often preferred for short-term use because excessive use may produce
   a. copious lower respiratory tract secretions
   b. ringing in the ears
   c. rebound nasal congestion
   d. a suppressed cough reflex

9. Cold remedies listed as "nondrowsy" or "daytime" formulas do not contain
   a. a nasal decongestant
   b. an antihistamine
   c. a pain reliever
   d. any of the above

Selected References

Drug facts and comparisons. (Updated monthly). St. Louis: Facts and Comparisons.

Echinacea for prevention and treatment of upper respiratory infections. (2002, April 1). *The Medical Letter on Drugs and Therapeutics, 44*(1127).

Guyton, A. C., & Hall, J. E. (2000). *Textbook of medical physiology* (10th ed.). Philadelphia: W. B. Saunders.

Kim, R. B. (Ed.). (2001). *Handbook of adverse drug interactions.* New Rochelle, NY: Medical Letter.

Lacy, C. F., Armstrong, L. L., Goldman, M. P., et al. (2004). *Lexi-Comp's drug information handbook* (12th ed.). Hudson, OH: Lexi-Comp.

Nix, D. E. (2000). Upper respiratory infections. In E. T. Herfindal & D. R. Gourley (Eds.), *Textbook of therapeutics: Drug and disease management* (7th ed., pp. 1385–1401). Philadelphia: Lippincott Williams & Wilkins.

Porth, C. M. (2005). *Pathophysiology: Concepts of altered health states* (7th ed.). Philadelphia: Lippincott Williams & Wilkins.

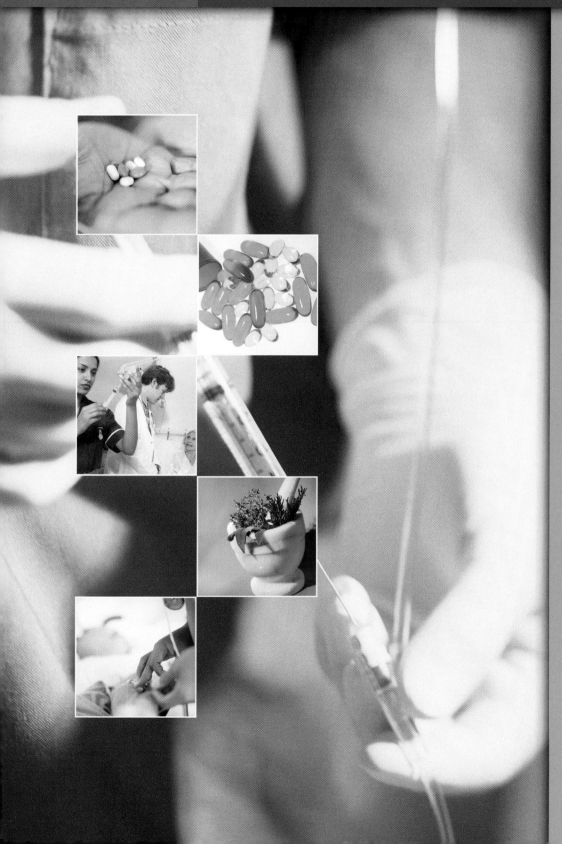

CHAPTER OUTLINE

47 Physiology of the Cardiovascular System

48 Drug Therapy for Heart Failure

49 Antidysrhythmic Drugs

50 Antianginal Drugs

51 Drugs Used in Hypotension and Shock

52 Antihypertensive Drugs

53 Diuretics

54 Drugs That Affect Blood Coagulation

55 Drugs for Dyslipedemia

Physiology of the Cardiovascular System

INTRODUCTION

The cardiovascular or circulatory system is composed of the heart, blood vessels, and blood. The general functions of the system are to carry oxygen, nutrients, hormones, antibodies, and other substances to all body cells and to remove waste products of cell metabolism (carbon dioxide and others). The efficiency of the system depends on the heart's ability to pump blood, the patency and functions of blood vessels, and the quality and quantity of blood.

HEART

The heart is a hollow, muscular organ that functions as a two-sided pump to circulate five to six liters of blood through the body every minute. Major components and characteristics are described in the following sections.

Chambers of the Heart

The heart has four chambers: two atria and two ventricles. The *atria* are receiving chambers. The right atrium receives deoxygenated blood from the upper part of the body by way of the superior vena cava; from the lower part of the body by way of the inferior vena cava; and from veins and sinuses within the heart itself. The left atrium receives oxygenated blood from the lungs through the pulmonary veins. The *ventricles* are distributing chambers. The right ventricle sends deoxygenated blood through the pulmonary circulation. It is small and thin walled because it contracts against minimal pressure. The left ventricle pumps oxygenated blood through the systemic circuit. It is much more muscular and thick walled because it contracts against relatively high pressure. The right atrium and right ventricle form one pump, and the left atrium and left ventricle form another. A muscular wall called the *septum* separates the right and left sides of the heart.

Layers of the Heart

The layers of the heart are the endocardium, myocardium, and epicardium. The *endocardium* is the membrane lining the heart chambers. It is continuous with the endothelial lining of blood vessels entering and leaving the heart, and it covers the heart valves. The *myocardium* is the strong muscular layer of the heart that provides the pumping power for circulation of blood. The *epicardium* is the outer, serous layer of the heart. The heart is enclosed in a fibroserous sac called the *pericardium*.

Heart Valves

Heart valves function to maintain the one-way flow of blood and prevent backflow. The *mitral* valve separates the left atrium and left ventricle. The *tricuspid* valve separates the right atrium and right ventricle. The *pulmonic* valve separates the right ventricle and pulmonary artery. The *aortic* valve separates the left ventricle and aorta.

Conduction System

The heart contains special cells that can carry electrical impulses much more rapidly than ordinary muscle fibers. This special conduction system consists of the sinoatrial (SA) node, the atrioventricular node, bundle of His, right and left bundle branches, and Purkinje fibers. The SA node, the normal pacemaker of the heart, generates a burst of electrical energy approximately 60 to 100 times each minute under normal circumstances. The electrical current flows over the heart in an orderly way to produce contraction of both atria, then both ventricles.

A unique characteristic of the heart is that any cell in any chamber can generate its own electrical impulse to contract. For example, the ventricles can beat independently, but at a rate of less than 40 beats per minute. This provides a backup mechanism should the SA node fail to fire, with an inherent rate that does not compete with SA node firing. In addition, the heart does not require nervous stimulation to contract. However, the autonomic nervous system does influence heart rate. Sympathetic nerves increase heart rate (through the release of epinephrine and norepinephrine); parasympathetic nerves (by way of the vagus nerve) decrease heart rate.

Blood Supply

The heart receives its blood supply from the coronary arteries. Coronary arteries originate at the base of the aorta in the aortic cusps and fill during *diastole,* the resting or filling phase of the cardiac cycle. Coronary arteries branch into smaller arteries that supply specific parts of the myocardium, without an overlapping supply from other arterial branches. However, artery-to-artery anastomoses occur between many adjacent vessels. These anastomotic arteries may not supply sufficient blood to the heart if a major artery is suddenly occluded, but they may dilate to considerable size when disease (usually coronary atherosclerosis) develops slowly. The resultant *collateral circulation* may provide a sufficient blood supply for myocardial function, at least during rest.

BLOOD VESSELS

There are three types of blood vessels: arteries, veins, and capillaries. Arteries and veins are similar in that they have three layers. The *intima,* the inner lining, is composed of a layer of endothelial cells next to the blood (to provide a smooth surface for blood circulation) and an elastic layer that joins the media. The *media* is the middle layer of muscle and elastic tissue. The *adventitia* is the outer layer of connective tissue.

Blood vessel walls are composed of two types of cells, *smooth muscle cells* and *endothelial cells.* Vascular smooth muscle functions to maintain blood pressure and blood flow. It contracts and relaxes in response to numerous stimuli, including local and circulating mediators. Contractile properties also vary among blood vessels, with some being more responsive to stimuli than others. Overall, regulation of tone in vascular smooth muscle depends on the intracellular concentration of calcium ions. Increased intracellular calcium leads to increased vascular tone. There are several mechanisms by which calcium ions can enter the cell.

Endothelial cells, once thought to be passive conduits for blood flow, are now known to perform two extremely important functions in maintaining homeostatic processes. One function is structural, in which the cells act as a permeability barrier and regulate passage of molecules and cells across the blood vessel wall. The second function is metabolic, in which the cells secrete opposing mediators that maintain a balance between bleeding and clotting of blood (including activation and inhibition of platelet functions and fibrinolysis), constriction and dilation of blood vessels, and promotion and inhibition of vascular cell growth and inflammation. Selected mediators are listed in Table 47-1; some are discussed in more detail in later chapters.

Arteries

Arteries and arterioles contain a well-developed layer of smooth muscle (the media) and are sometimes called *resistance* vessels. Their efficiency depends on their patency and ability to constrict or dilate in response to various stimuli. The degree of constriction or dilation (vasomotor tone) determines peripheral vascular resistance, which is a major determinant of blood pressure.

Veins

Veins and venules have a thin media and valves that assist blood flow against gravity. They are sometimes called *capacitance* vessels, because blood may accumulate in various parts of the venous system. Their efficiency depends on patency, competency of valves, and the contraction and relaxation action of muscles around veins.

Capillaries

Capillaries, the smallest blood vessels, connect the arterial and venous segments of the circulation. They consist of a single layer of connected endothelial cells and a few smooth muscle cells. Gases, nutrients, cells, and waste prod-

TABLE 47-1 Endothelial Mediators That Regulate Cardiovascular Function

PROMOTING FACTORS	INHIBITING FACTORS
Vasomotor Tone	
Vasodilators	**Vasoconstrictors**
Endothelial-derived hyper-polarizing factor (EDHF)	Angiotensin II
	Endothelin
Nitric oxide (also called endothelial-derived relaxing factor, or EDRF)	Endothelium-derived constricting factor
	Platelet-derived growth factor
Prostacyclin (prostaglandin I₂)	Thromboxane A₂
Blood Coagulation	
Procoagulants	**Anticoagulants**
Tissue factor	Heparin sulfate
Von Willebrand factor	Thrombomodulin
Platelet activators	**Platelet inhibitors**
Platelet-activating factor	Nitric oxide
Von Willebrand factor	Prostacyclin
Profibrinolytic factors	**Antifibrinolytic factor**
Tissue plasminogen activator (t-PA)	Plasminogen activator inhibitor-1
Urokinase-type plasminogen activator	
Cell Growth	
Angiotensin II	Heparin
Endothelin	Nitric oxide
Platelet-derived growth factor	Prostacyclin
Inflammation	
Proinflammatory factors	**Anti-inflammatory factors**
Cellular and intercellular adhesion molecules	Nitric oxide
Monocyte chemotactic protein-1	
Interleukin-8	

BLOOD

Blood functions to nourish and oxygenate body cells, protect the body from invading microorganisms, and initiate hemostasis when a blood vessel is injured. Specific functions and components are listed in the following sections.

Functions

- Transports oxygen to cells and carbon dioxide from cells to lungs for removal from the body
- Transports absorbed food products from the gastrointestinal tract to tissues; at the same time, carries metabolic wastes from tissues to the kidneys, skin, and lungs for excretion
- Transports hormones from endocrine glands to other parts of the body
- Transports leukocytes and antibodies to sites of injury, infection, and inflammation
- Assists in regulation of body temperature by transferring heat produced by cell metabolism to the skin, where it can be released
- Transports platelets to injured areas for hemostasis

Components

- *Plasma* comprises approximately 55% of the total blood volume, and it is more than 90% water. Other components are
  - Serum albumin, which helps maintain blood volume by exerting colloid osmotic pressure
  - Fibrinogen, which is necessary for hemostasis
  - Gamma globulin, which is necessary for defense against microorganisms
  - Less than 1% antibodies, nutrients, metabolic wastes, respiratory gases, enzymes, and inorganic salts
- *Solid particles* or cells comprise approximately 45% of total blood volume. Cells include erythrocytes (red blood cells or RBCs); leukocytes (white blood cells or WBCs); and thrombocytes (platelets). The bone marrow produces all RBCs, 60% to 70% of WBCs, and all platelets. Lymphatic tissues (spleen and lymph nodes) produce 20% to 30% of WBCs, and reticuloendothelial tissues (spleen, liver, lymph nodes) produce 4% to 8% of WBCs. Cell characteristics include the following:
  - Erythrocytes function primarily to transport oxygen. Almost all oxygen (95%–97%) is transported in combination with hemoglobin; very little is dissolved in blood. The lifespan of a normal RBC is approximately 120 days.
  - Leukocytes function primarily as a defense mechanism against microorganisms. They leave the bloodstream to enter injured tissues and phagocytize the

ucts are exchanged between blood and extracellular fluid across capillary walls. The endothelial lining acts as a semipermeable membrane to regulate the exchange of plasma solutes with extracellular fluid. Lipid-soluble materials diffuse directly through the capillary cell membrane; water and water-soluble materials enter and leave the capillary through the junctions or gaps between endothelial cells.

Lymphatics

Lymphatic vessels, which are composed mainly of endothelium, parallel the veins and empty into the venous system. They drain tissue fluid that has filtered through the endothelium of capillaries and venules from the plasma. They then carry lymphocytes, large molecules of protein and fat, microorganisms, and other materials to regional lymph nodes.

injurious agent. They also produce antibodies. The lifespan of a normal WBC is a few hours.

● Platelets are fragments of large cells, called *megakaryocytes,* found in the bone marrow. Platelets are essential for blood coagulation. For example, when a blood vessel is injured, platelets adhere to each other and the edges of the injury to form a cluster of activated platelets (ie, a platelet thrombus or "plug") that adheres to the vessel wall and prevents leakage of blood. In addition, the clustered platelets release substances (eg, adenosine diphosphate, thromboxane A_2, von Willebrand factor) that promote recruitment and aggregation of new platelets.

Platelets have no nucleus and cannot replicate. If not used, they circulate for approximately a week before being removed by phagocytic cells of the spleen.

CARDIOVASCULAR DISORDERS

Cardiovascular disorders, which are common causes of morbidity and mortality, often stem from blood vessel abnormalities. In turn, most vascular diseases result from the malfunction of endothelial cells or smooth muscle cells. Dysfunctional endothelium is considered a major factor in atherosclerosis, acute coronary syndromes (symptomatic myocardial ischemia, asymptomatic myocardial infarction [MI], and MI with or without ST-segment elevation), hypertension, and thromboembolic disorders. The main cause of endothelial dysfunction is injury to the blood vessel wall from trauma or disease processes. The injury alters the normal regulatory forces and leads to vasospasm, thrombosis, growth of the intimal layer of the blood vessel, rupture of atherosclerotic plaque, tissue ischemia and infarction, and dysrhythmias. Pathologic changes in the structure of the capillary and venular endothelium also result in the accumulation of excess fluid in interstitial space (edema), a common symptom of cardiovascular and other disorders.

Overall, cardiovascular disorders may involve any structure or function of the cardiovascular system. Because the circulatory system is a closed system, a disorder in one part of the system eventually disturbs the function of all other parts.

DRUG THERAPY USED FOR CARDIOVASCULAR DISORDERS

Cardiovascular disorders usually managed with drug therapy include atherosclerosis, heart failure, cardiac dysrhythmias,

ischemia, myocardial infarction, hypertension, hypotension, and shock. Peripheral vascular disease and valvular disease are usually managed surgically. Blood disorders that respond to drug therapy include certain types of anemia and coagulation disorders.

The goal of drug therapy in cardiovascular disorders is to restore homeostasis or physiologic balance between opposing factors (eg, coagulant vs. anticoagulant, vasoconstriction vs. vasodilation). Cardiovascular drugs may be given to increase or decrease cardiac output, blood pressure, and heart rate; to alter heart rhythm; to increase or decrease blood clotting; to alter the quality of blood; and to decrease chest pain of cardiac origin. In addition, these drugs may be given for palliation of symptoms without alteration of the underlying disease process.

Review and Application Exercises

Short Answer Exercises

1. How does the heart muscle differ from skeletal muscle?

2. What is the normal pacemaker of the heart?

3. In what circumstances do other parts of the heart take over as pacemaker?

4. What is the effect of parasympathetic (vagal) stimulation on the heart?

5. What is the effect of sympathetic stimulation on the heart and blood vessels?

6. List five chemical mediators produced by endothelial cells and their roles in maintaining cardiovascular function.

7. How does endothelial cell dysfunction contribute to cardiovascular disorders?

Selected References

Gokce, N., & Vita, J. A. (2003). Clinical manifestations of endothelial dysfunction. In J. Loscalzo & A. I. Schafer (Eds.), *Thrombosis and hemorrhage* (3rd ed., pp. 685–706). Baltimore: Williams & Wilkins.

Guyton, A. C., & Hall, J. E. (2000). *Textbook of medical physiology* (10th ed.). Philadelphia: W. B. Saunders.

Porth, C. M. (2005). *Pathophysiology: Concepts of altered health states* (7th ed.). Philadelphia: Lippincott Williams & Wilkins.

Smeltzer, S. C., & Bare, B. G. (2004). *Brunner & Suddarth's textbook of medical-surgical nursing* (10th ed.). Philadelphia: Lippincott Williams & Wilkins.

Drug Therapy for Heart Failure

OBJECTIVES

After studying this chapter, you will be able to:

1. Describe major manifestations of heart failure (HF).
2. Discuss the role of endothelial dysfunction in HF.
3. Differentiate the types of drugs used to treat HF.
4. List characteristics of digoxin in terms of effects on myocardial contractility and cardiac conduction, indications for use, principles of therapy, and nursing process implications.
5. Differentiate therapeutic effects of digoxin in HF and atrial fibrillation.
6. Differentiate digitalizing and maintenance doses of digoxin.
7. Identify therapeutic and excessive serum digoxin levels.
8. Identify clients at risk for development of digoxin toxicity.
9. Discuss interventions to prevent or minimize digoxin toxicity.
10. Explain the roles of potassium chloride, lidocaine, atropine, and digoxin immune fab in the management of digoxin toxicity.
11. Teach clients ways to increase safety and effectiveness of digoxin.
12. Discuss important elements of using digoxin in special populations.

APPLYING YOUR KNOWLEDGE

Clara Motsinger is a 70-year-old woman who has HF. She has been treated with an ACE inhibitor and a diuretic for several years but this drug regimen has now failed to control her HF. Her cardiologist has added digoxin 0.125 mg daily (tablets) to her treatment regimen.

INTRODUCTION

Heart failure (HF) is a common condition that occurs when the heart cannot pump enough blood to meet tissue needs for oxygen and nutrients. It may result from impaired myocardial contraction during systole (systolic dysfunction), impaired relaxation and filling of ventricles during diastole (diastolic dysfunction), or a combination of systolic and diastolic dysfunction. HF has also been referred to as congestive heart failure (CHF) because frequently there is congestion (fluid accumulation) in the lungs and peripheral tissues. Many clients, however, do not have congestive symptoms; therefore, *heart failure* is the preferred term.

Causes of Heart Failure

At the cellular level, HF stems from dysfunction of contractile myocardial cells and the endothelial cells that line the heart and blood vessels (see Chap. 47). Vital functions of the endothelium include maintaining equilibrium between vasodilation and vasoconstriction, coagulation and anticoagulation, and cellular growth promotion and inhibition. Endothelial dysfunction allows processes that narrow the blood vessel lumen (eg, buildup of atherosclerotic plaque, growth of cells, inflammation, activation of platelets) and lead to blood-clot formation and vasoconstriction that further narrow the blood vessel lumen. These are major factors in coronary artery disease and hypertension, the most common conditions leading to HF.

Other causative factors include hyperthyroidism, excessive intravenous (IV) fluids or blood transfusions, and drugs that decrease the force of myocardial contraction (eg, antidysrhythmic drugs) or cause retention of sodium and water (eg, corticosteroids, estrogens, nonsteroidal anti-inflammatory agents). These factors impair the pumping ability or increase the workload of the heart so an adequate cardiac output cannot be maintained.

Compensatory Mechanisms of Heart Failure

As the heart fails, the low cardiac output and inadequately filled arteries activate the neurohormonal system by several feedback mechanisms. One mechanism is increased sympathetic activity and circulating catecholamines (neurohormones), which increases the force of myocardial contraction, increases heart rate, and causes vasoconstriction. The effects of the baroreceptors in the aortic arch and carotid sinus that normally inhibit undue sympathetic stimulation are blunted in clients with HF, and the effects of the high levels of circulating catecholamines are intensified. Endothelin, a neurohormone secreted primarily by endothelial cells, is the most potent endogenous vasoconstrictor and may exert direct toxic effects on the heart and result in myocardial cell proliferation.

Another mechanism is activation of the renin–angiotensin–aldosterone system. Renin is an enzyme produced in the kidneys in response to impaired blood flow and tissue perfusion. When released into the bloodstream, renin stimulates the production of angiotensin II, a powerful vasoconstrictor. Arterial vasoconstriction impairs cardiac function by increasing the resistance (afterload) against which the ventricle ejects blood. This raises filling pressures inside the heart, increases stretch and stress on the myocardial wall, and predisposes to subendocardial ischemia. In addition, clients with severe HF have constricted arterioles in cerebral, myocardial, renal, hepatic, and mesenteric vascular beds. This results in increased organ hypoperfusion and dysfunction. Venous vasoconstriction limits venous capacitance, resulting in venous congestion and increased diastolic ventricular filling pressures (preload). Angiotensin II also promotes sodium and water retention by stimulating aldosterone release from the adrenal cortex and the release of vasopressin (antidiuretic hormone) from the posterior pituitary gland.

All of these mechanisms combine to increase blood volume and pressure in the heart chambers, stretch muscle fibers, and produce dilation, hypertrophy, and changes in the shape of the heart (a process called *cardiac* or *ventricular remodeling*) that make it contract less efficiently. Overall, the compensatory mechanisms increase preload (amount of venous blood returning to the heart), workload of the heart, afterload (amount of resistance in the aorta and peripheral blood vessels that the heart must overcome to pump effectively), and blood pressure. These compensatory mechanisms that initially preserve cardiac function result in progressive deterioration of myocardial function over time.

Signs and Symptoms of Heart Failure

Clients with compensated (asymptomatic) HF usually have no symptoms at rest and no edema; dyspnea and fatigue occur only with activities involving moderate or higher levels of exertion. Symptoms that occur with minimal exertion or at rest and are accompanied by ankle edema and distention of the jugular vein (from congestion of veins and leakage of fluid into tissues) reflect decompensation (symptomatic HF). Acute, severe cardiac decompensation is manifested by pulmonary edema, a medical emergency that requires immedi-

ate treatment. Two models currently exist for classification of HF. The New York Heart Association (NYHA) classifies HF based on functional limitations. A newer system of staging HF, proposed by the American College of Cardiology (ACC) and the American Heart Association (AHA), is based on the progression of HF. These classifications complement each other and are often used together to determine and evaluate therapy (Table 48-1).

Drug Therapy for Heart Failure

Several drugs are used to treat acute HF. A diuretic, in combination with an angiotensin-converting enzyme (ACE) inhibitor or angiotensin II receptor blocker (ARB), is first-line therapy for chronic failure. Digoxin, a beta-adrenergic blocking agent, or an aldosterone inhibitor may be added to the ACE inhibitor or ARB and diuretic regimen.

Drug therapy for HF continues to evolve as the pathophysiologic mechanisms are better understood and research studies indicate more effective regimens. Combinations of drugs are commonly used in efforts to improve circulation, alter the compensatory mechanisms, and reverse heart damage. Most of the drugs used to treat HF are also used in other disorders and are discussed in other chapters; their effects in HF are described in Box 48-1. The primary focus of this chapter is inotropic agents, which include digoxin (a cardiac glycoside) and the phosphodiesterase inhibitors inamrinone and milrinone. Two additional classifications of drugs, human B-type natriuretic peptides and endothelin receptor antagonists, are also presented. These drugs are discussed in the following sections and in Table 48-2.

INOTROPES

Cardiac Glycosides (Digoxin)

Digoxin (Lanoxin) is the only commonly used digitalis glycoside. In the following discussion, the terms *digitalization* and *digitalis toxicity* refer to digoxin.

General Characteristics

When digoxin is given orally, absorption varies among available preparations. Lanoxicaps, which are liquid-filled capsules, and the elixir used for children are better absorbed than tablets. With tablets, the most frequently used formulation, differences in bioavailability are important because a person who is stabilized on one formulation may be underdosed or overdosed if another formulation is taken. Differences are attributed to the rate and extent of tablet dissolution rather than amounts of digoxin. In addition to drug dosage forms, other factors that may decrease digoxin absorption include the presence of food in the GI tract, delayed gastric emptying, malabsorption syndromes, and concurrent administration of some drugs (eg, antacids, cholestyramine).

TABLE 48-1 Classifying Signs and Symptoms of Heart Failure to Determine Treatment

NEW YORK HEART ASSOCIATION (NYHA) CLASSIFICATION	AMERICAN COLLEGE OF CARDIOLOGY (ACC)/AMERICAN HEART ASSOCIATION (AHA) GUIDELINES	RECOMMENDATIONS
	Stage A. Patient at high risk for developing heart failure (HF) but without structural heart disease or signs and symptoms of HF.	• Treat hypertension, lipid disorders, diabetes. • Encourage patient to stop smoking and to exercise regularly. • Discourage use of alcohol, illicit drugs. • ACE inhibitor if indicated
Class I. Ordinary physical activity does not cause undue fatigue, palpitations, dyspnea, or angina.	*Stage B.* Structural heart disease, but without signs and symptoms of HF.	• All stage A therapies • ACE inhibitor unless contraindicated • Beta-blocker unless contraindicated
Class II. Slight limitation of physical activity but asymptomatic at rest. Ordinary physical activity causes fatigue, palpitations, dyspnea, or anginal pain. *Class III.* Marked limitation of physical activity, but typically asymptomatic at rest. Less-than-ordinary physical activity causes fatigue, palpitations, dyspnea, or angina.	*Stage C.* Structural heart disease with prior or current signs and symptoms of HF.	• All stage A and B therapies • Sodium-restricted diet • Diuretics • Digoxin • Avoid or withdraw antiarrhythmic agents, most calcium channel blockers, and nonsteroidal anti-inflammatory drugs. • Consider aldosterone antagonists, angiotensin receptor blockers, hydralazine, and nitrates.
Class IV. Unable to perform any physical activity without discomfort; symptoms may be present at rest. Discomfort increases with physical activity.	*Stage D.* End-stage disease requiring specialized treatment strategies, such as mechanical circulatory support, continuous inotropic infusion, or heart transplant.	• All therapies for stages A, B, and C • Mechanical assist device, such as biventricular pacemaker or left ventricular assist device • Continuous inotropic therapy • Hospice care

Source: Naylor, L., Howe, L., Eggert, J., & Heifferon, B. (2004). CHF in the elderly: Using ACEIs appropriately. *Nurse Practitioner, 29*(7), 46–53.

Digoxin is distributed to most body tissues and high concentrations are found in the myocardium, brain, liver, and skeletal muscle. It also crosses the placenta, and serum levels in neonates are similar to those in the mother. Digoxin circulates mainly in a free state, with only 20% to 30% bound to serum proteins. Therapeutic serum levels of digoxin are 0.5 to 2 nanograms per milliliter; toxic serum levels are above 2. In the elderly and in the presence of renal failure, therapeutic serum levels are 0.5 to 1.3 nanograms per milliliter. Research in the past decade has suggested that serum levels of 1.0 nanograms per milliliter or less are more appropriate in those with HF (see Research Brief). However, toxicity may occur at virtually any serum level. Dosage must be reduced in the presence of renal failure because most of the digoxin (60%–70%) is excreted unchanged by the kidneys to prevent drug accumulation and toxicity. The remainder is metabolized or excreted by nonrenal routes.

Mechanisms of Action

In HF, digoxin exerts a cardiotonic or positive inotropic effect that improves the pumping ability of the heart. The mechanism by which digoxin increases the force of myocardial contraction is thought to be inhibition of Na,K-adenosine triphosphatase (Na,K-ATPase), an enzyme in cardiac cell membranes that decreases the movement of sodium out of myocardial cells after contraction. As a result, calcium enters the cell in exchange for sodium, causing additional calcium to be released from intracellular binding sites. With the increased intracellular concentration of free calcium ions, more calcium is available

Box 48-1 Drugs Used to Treat Heart Failure

Adrenergics

Dopamine or dobutamine (see Chaps. 17 and 51) may be used in acute, severe heart failure (HF) when circulatory support is required, usually in a critical care unit. Given by intravenous (IV) infusion, these drugs strengthen myocardial contraction (inotropic or cardiotonic effects) and increase cardiac output. Dosage or flow rate is titrated to hemodynamic effects; minimal effective doses are recommended because of vasoconstrictive effects. The drugs also cause tachycardia and hypertension and increase cardiac workload and oxygen consumption.

Angiotensin-Converting Enzyme (ACE) Inhibitors

Captopril and other ACE inhibitors (see Chap. 52) are drugs of first choice in treating clients with chronic HF. ACE inhibitors are usually given in combination with a diuretic. All of the drugs have similar effects, but captopril, enalapril, lisinopril, quinapril, and ramipril are Food and Drug Administration (FDA)-approved for treatment of HF. Some clinicians use captopril initially because it has a short half-life and is rapidly eliminated when stopped, then switch to a long-acting drug if captopril is tolerated by the client. Digoxin, a beta-adrenergic blocking agent, or an aldosterone inhibitor may be added to the ACE-inhibitor/diuretic regimen.

These drugs improve cardiac function and decrease mortality. They also relieve symptoms, increase exercise tolerance, and delay further impairment of myocardial function and progression of HF (ie, ventricular dilatation and enlargement [ventricular remodeling]). They act mainly to decrease activation of the renin–angiotensin–aldosterone system, a major pathophysiologic mechanism in HF. More specifically, the drugs prevent inactive angiotensin I from being converted to angiotensin II. Angiotensin II produces vasoconstriction and retention of sodium and water; inhibition of angiotensin II decreases vasoconstriction and retention of sodium and water. Thus, major effects of the drugs are dilation of both veins and arteries, decreased preload and afterload, decreased workload of the heart, and increased perfusion of body organs and tissues.

During ACE-inhibitor therapy, clients usually need to see a health care provider frequently for dosage titration and monitoring of serum creatinine and potassium levels for increases. Elevated creatinine levels may indicate impaired renal function, in which case dosage needs to be reduced; elevated potassium levels indicate hyperkalemia, an adverse effect of the drugs.

Angiotensin II Receptor Blockers (ARBs)

Losartan and other angiotensin receptor blockers (see Chap. 52) are similar to ACE inhibitors in their effects on cardiac function, although the mechanism of action is at the angiotensin II receptor site rather than inhibiting the conversion of angiotensin I to angiotensin II. All ARBs are approved for treatment of hypertension; however, only valsartan has received FDA approval for treatment of clients with moderate to severe HF and those unable to tolerate an ACE inhibitor due to adverse effects such as cough. Studies indicate that the addition of an ARB to a regimen that includes ACE inhibitors may result in a decrease in hospitalizations, but does not reduce the mortality rate.

Beta-Adrenergic Blocking Agents

Although beta blockers (see Chaps. 18, 49, and 52) were formerly considered contraindicated, numerous research studies indicate they decrease morbidity (ie, symptoms and hospitalizations) and mortality in clients with chronic HF. The change evolved from a better understanding of the mechanisms causing chronic HF.

Beta blockers suppress activation of the sympathetic nervous system and the resulting catecholamine excess that eventually damages myocardial cells, reduces myocardial beta receptors, and reduces cardiac output. As a result, over time, ventricular remodeling regresses, the heart returns toward a more normal shape and function, and cardiac output increases.

Beta blockers are not recommended for clients in acute HF because of the potential for an initial decrease in myocardial contractility. A beta blocking agent is started after normal blood volume is restored and edema and other symptoms are relieved. The goal of beta blocker therapy is to shrink the ventricle back to its normal size (reverse remodeling). The beta blocker is added to the ACE-inhibitor/diuretic regimen, usually near the end of a hospital stay or as outpatient therapy. Most studies have been done with bisoprolol, carvedilol, or metoprolol; it is not yet known whether some beta blockers are more effective than others. When used in clients with chronic HF, recommendations include starting with a low dose (because symptoms may initially worsen in some clients), titrating the dose upward at approximately 2-week intervals, and monitoring closely. Significant hemodynamic improvement usually requires 2 to 3 months of therapy, but effects are long lasting. Beneficial effects can be measured by increases in the left ventricular ejection fraction (ie, cardiac output).

Diuretics

Diuretics (see Chap. 53) are used in treating both acute and chronic HF. Thiazides (eg, hydrochlorothiazide) can be used for mild diuresis in clients with normal renal function; loop diuretics (eg, furosemide) should be used in clients who have impaired renal function or who need strong diuresis.

For clients in acute HF, which is characterized by fluid accumulation, a diuretic is the initial treatment. It acts to decrease plasma volume (extracellular fluid volume) and increase excretion of sodium and water, thereby decreasing preload. With early or mild HF, starting or increasing the dose of an oral thiazide may be effective. With moderate to severe HF (pulmonary edema), an IV loop diuretic is indicated. IV furosemide also has a vasodilator effect that helps relieve vasoconstriction (afterload). Although diuretic therapy relieves symptoms, it does not improve left ventricular function and decrease mortality rates. Some clients may also need drugs to increase myocardial contractility and vasodilators to decrease preload, afterload, or both.

In clients with chronic HF, an oral diuretic is a common component of treatment regimens. Depending on the severity of symptoms or degree of HF, the regimen may also include an ACE inhibitor or ARB, a beta blocker, and digoxin.

Potassium-sparing diuretics (eg, amiloride, triamterene) are often given concurrently with potassium-losing diuretics

Box 48-1 Drugs Used to Treat Heart Failure (continued)

(eg, thiazides or loop diuretics) to help maintain normal serum potassium levels. Concomitant use of ACE inhibitors and non-steroidal anti-inflammatory drugs and the presence of diabetes mellitus increase risks of hyperkalemia.

With all diuretic therapy, serum potassium levels must be measured periodically to monitor for hypokalemia and hyperkalemia. Both hypokalemia and hyperkalemia are cardiotoxic and impair heart function.

Aldosterone Antagonist

Increasingly, spironolactone is also being added to the drug regimen for clients with moderate to severe HF. Increased aldosterone, a major factor in the pathophysiology of HF, results in increased interstitial fibrosis that may decrease systolic function and increase the risk of ventricular dysrhythmias. Spironolactone is an aldosterone antagonist that reduces the aldosterone-induced retention of sodium and water and impaired vascular function. Although ACE inhibitors also decrease aldosterone initially, this effect is transient. Spironolactone is given in a daily dose of 12.5 to 25 mg, along with standard doses of an ACE inhibitor, a loop diuretic, and usually digoxin. In clients with adequate renal function (ie, serum creatinine 2.5 mg/dL or less), the addition of spironolactone usually allows smaller doses of loop diuretics and potassium

supplements. Overall, studies indicate that the addition of spironolactone improves cardiac function and reduces symptoms, hospitalizations, and mortality. In 2003, a second drug, eplerenone, was given approval to be used in the management of HF after a myocardial infarction to improve survival.

Vasodilators

Vasodilators are essential components of treatment regimens for HF, and the beneficial effects of ACE inhibitors and angiotensin II receptor antagonists stem significantly from their vasodilating effects (ie, preventing or decreasing angiotensin-induced vasoconstriction). Other vasodilators may also be used. Venous dilators (eg, nitrates) decrease preload; arterial dilators (eg, hydralazine) decrease afterload. Isosorbide dinitrate and hydralazine may be combined to decrease both preload and afterload. The combination has similar effects to those of an ACE inhibitor or an ARB, but may not be as well tolerated by clients. Nitrates are discussed in Chapter 50; hydralazine and other vasodilators are discussed in Chapter 52.

Oral vasodilators usually are used in clients with chronic HF and parenteral agents are reserved for those who have severe HF or are unable to take oral medications. Vasodilators should be started at low doses, titrated to desired hemodynamic effects, and discontinued slowly to avoid rebound vasoconstriction.

---

to activate the contractile proteins actin and myosin, and increase myocardial contractility. Overall, digoxin helps to relieve symptoms and decrease hospitalizations, but does not prolong survival. In HF, it is given concomitantly with a diuretic and an ACE inhibitor or ARB.

In clients with atrial dysrhythmias, digoxin slows the rate of ventricular contraction (negative chronotropic effect). Negative chronotropic effects are probably caused by several factors. First, digoxin has a direct depressant effect on cardiac conduction tissues, especially the atrioventricular node. This action decreases the number of electrical impulses allowed to reach the ventricles from supraventricular sources. Second, digoxin indirectly stimulates the vagus nerve. Third, increased efficiency of myocardial contraction and vagal stimulation decrease compensatory tachycardia that results from the sympathetic nervous system response to inadequate circulation.

Indications for Use

The clinical uses of digoxin include management of HF, atrial fibrillation, and atrial flutter. Digoxin may be used in clients with acute or chronic conditions, for digitalization, or for maintenance therapy. Although the use of digoxin in clients with normal sinus rhythm has been questioned, studies indicate improved ejection fraction and exercise tolerance in clients who receive digoxin. In addition, in clients with HF who are stabilized on digoxin, a diuretic, and an ACE inhibitor or ARB, symptoms worsen if digoxin is discontinued.

Contraindications to Use

Digoxin is contraindicated in clients with severe myocarditis, ventricular tachycardia, or ventricular fibrillation and must be used cautiously in those with acute myocardial infarction, heart block, Adams-Stokes syndrome, Wolff-Parkinson-White syndrome (risk of fatal dysrhythmias), electrolyte imbalances (hypokalemia, hypomagnesemia, hypercalcemia), and renal impairment.

Administration and Digitalization

Digoxin is given orally or IV. Although it can be given intramuscularly, this route is not recommended because pain and muscle necrosis may occur at injection sites. When given orally, onset of action occurs in 30 minutes to 2 hours, and peak effects occur in approximately 6 hours. When given IV, the onset of action occurs within 10 to 30 minutes, and peak effects occur in 1 to 5 hours.

In the heart, maximum drug effect occurs when a steady-state tissue concentration has been achieved. This occurs in approximately 1 week (five half-lives) unless loading doses are given for more rapid effects. Traditionally, a loading dose is called a *digitalizing dose*. Digitalization (administration of an amount sufficient to produce therapeutic effects) may be accomplished rapidly by giving a total dose of 0.75 to 1.5 milligrams of digoxin in divided doses, 6 to 8 hours apart, over a 24-hour period. Because rapid digitalization engenders higher risks of toxicity, it is usually done for atrial tachydys-

Table 48-2 Drugs at a Glance: Drugs for Heart Failure

GENERIC/TRADE NAME	ROUTES AND DOSAGE RANGES	
	Adults	Children
Inotropic Agents CARDIAC GLYCOSIDE **Digoxin** (Lanoxin)	Digitalizing dose, PO 0.75–1 mg in 3 or 4 divided doses over 24 h; IV 0.5–0.75 mg in divided doses over 24 h. Maintenance dose, PO, IV 0.125–0.5 mg/d (average, 0.25 mg)	*>10 y:* Same as adult. *2–10 y:* Digitalizing dose, PO 0.02–0.04 mg/kg in 4 divided doses over 24 h. Maintenance dose, PO, IV approximately 20%–35% of the digitalizing dose or a maximum dose of 100–150 mcg/d *1 mo–2 y:* Digitalizing dose, PO 0.035–0.06 mg/kg in 4 divided doses over 24 h; IV, 0.035–0.05 mg/kg in 4 divided doses over 24 h. Maintenance dose, PO, IV, approximately 20%–35% of the digitalizing dose *Newborns:* Digitalizing dose, PO 0.025–0.035 mg/kg in 4 divided doses over 24 h. Maintenance dose, PO, IV, approximately 20%–35% of the digitalizing dose.
PHOSPHODIESTERASE INHIBITORS **Inamrinone**	IV injection (loading dose), 0.75 mg/kg slowly, over 2–3 min IV infusion (maintenance dose), 5–10 mcg/kg/min, diluted in 0.9% or 0.45% NaCl solution to a concentration of 1–3 mg/mL. May give another bolus dose 30 min after start of therapy. Maximum dose 10 mg/kg/d	*1y and older:* Same as adult. *Infant:* IV injection (loading dose), 3–4.5 mcg/kg, in divided doses. IV infusion (maintenance dose), 10 mcg/kg/min *Neonate:* IV injection (loading dose), 3–4.5 mcg/kg, in divided doses. IV infusion (maintenance dose), 3–5 mcg/kg/min
Milrinone (Primacor)	IV bolus infusion (loading dose), 50 mcg/kg over 10 min IV continuous infusion (maintenance dose), 0.375–0.75 mcg/kg/min, diluted in 0.9% or 0.45% NaCl or 5% dextrose solution	Not established
HUMAN B-TYPE NATRIURETIC PEPTIDE **Nesiritide** (Natrecor)	IV bolus infusion (loading dose), 2 mcg/kg followed by continuous infusion of 0.01 mcg/kg/min. Use for >48 hours not studied.	Safety not established
ENDOTHELIN RECEPTOR ANTAGONISTS **Bosentan** (Tracleer)	PO 62.5 mg twice daily for 4 wks and then increased to a maintenance dosage of 125 mg twice daily	

IM, intramuscular; IV, intravenous; PO, oral.

rhythmias, with continuous cardiac monitoring, rather than for HF. Slow digitalization may be accomplished by initiating therapy with a maintenance dose of digoxin. When digoxin is discontinued, elimination of the drug requires approximately 1 week.

APPLYING YOUR KNOWLEDGE 48-1

Ms. Motsinger is due for her first dose of digoxin. Her physician has decided to digitalize the client. What does digitalization involve and why would this be desirable in Ms. Motsinger's case?

RESEARCH BRIEF

Use of Digoxin in Men and Women

SOURCES:

Digitalis Investigation Group. (1997). The effect of digoxin on mortality and morbidity in patients with heart failure. *New England Journal of Medicine, 336:* 525–533.

Rathore, S. S., Wang, Y., & Krumholz, H. (2002). Sex-based differences in the effect of digoxin for the treatment of heart failure. *New England Journal of Medicine, 347:* 1403–1411.

SUMMARY:

In 2002, Rathore, Wang, and Krumholz performed a retrospective analysis of data collected in 1997 to assess the impact of digoxin on morbidity and mortality in an attempt to determine if digoxin had different effects on men and women. The death rate was 33.1% for women taking digoxin and 28.9% for those taking a placebo. Cause of the increase is unknown; however, possibilities include differences in myocardial cell growth and function, autonomic function, signal transduction, or muscle metabolism between the sexes. It is also likely that plasma digoxin levels may have been excessively high in women who died. Unfortunately, drug levels were not measured regularly in all subjects. These findings do suggest that digoxin doses and serum levels must be keep as low as possible (0.5 to 1 ng/mL) and that the benefits of a small decrease in risk of hospitalization (4%) may not justify the risk of possible drug-induced death.

NURSING IMPLICATIONS:

Typically digoxin should be reserved for clients who do not respond well to the first line medicines of ACE inhibitors, diuretics, and beta blockers. Until further research is done, caution should be used with digoxin, which should not be withheld from those likely to benefit, especially those with atrial fibrillation and heart failure, nor should it be discontinued indiscriminately.

Digoxin Toxicity

Digoxin has a low therapeutic index (ie, a dose adequate for therapeutic effects may be accompanied by signs of toxicity). Digoxin toxicity may result from many contributing factors:

- Accumulation of larger-than-necessary maintenance doses
- Rapid loading or digitalization, whether by one or more large doses or frequent administration of small doses
- Impaired renal function, which delays excretion of digoxin
- Age extremes (young or old)
- Electrolyte imbalance (eg, hypokalemia, hypomagnesemia, hypercalcemia)

- Hypoxia due to heart or lung disease, which increases myocardial sensitivity to digoxin
- Hypothyroidism, which slows digoxin metabolism and may cause accumulation
- Concurrent treatment with other drugs affecting the heart, such as quinidine, verapamil, or nifedipine

APPLYING YOUR KNOWLEDGE 48-2

Ms. Motsinger has been taking digoxin for 2 days. You must assess her drug level before administration of digoxin; blood for the test was drawn this morning. What should her drug level be to be in the therapeutic range?

Phosphodiesterase Inhibitors

Inamrinone (Inocor), formerly amrinone, and **milrinone IV** (Primacor) are cardiotonic–inotropic agents used in short-term management of acute, severe HF that is not controlled by digoxin, diuretics, and vasodilators. The drugs increase levels of cyclic adenosine monophosphate (cAMP) in myocardial cells by inhibiting phosphodiesterase, the enzyme that normally metabolizes cAMP. They also relax vascular smooth muscle to produce vasodilation and decrease preload and afterload. In HF, inotropic and vasodilator effects increase cardiac output. The effects of these drugs are additive to those of digoxin and may be synergistic with those of adrenergic drugs (eg, dobutamine). There is a time delay before the drugs reach therapeutic serum levels as well as inter-individual variability in therapeutic doses.

Compared with inamrinone, milrinone is more potent as an inotropic agent and causes fewer adverse effects. Both drugs are given IV by bolus injection followed by continuous infusion. Flow rate is titrated to maintain adequate circulation. Milrinone can be used alone or with other drugs such as dobutamine and nitroprusside. Its dosage should be reduced in the presence of renal impairment. Dose-limiting adverse effects of the drugs include tachycardia, atrial or ventricular dysrhythmias, and hypotension. Hypotension is more likely to occur in clients who are hypovolemic. Milrinone has a long half-life of approximately 80 hours and may accumulate with prolonged infusions.

HUMAN B-TYPE NATRIURETIC PEPTIDE (NESIRITIDE)

Nesiritide (Natrecor) is the first in this class of drugs to be used in the management of acute HF. Produced by recombinant DNA technology, nesiritide is identical to endogenous human B-type natriuretic peptide (BNP), which is secreted primarily by the ventricles in response to fluid and pressure overload. This drug acts to compensate for deteriorating cardiac function by reducing preload and afterload, increasing diuresis and secretion of sodium, suppressing the renin–angiotensin–aldosterone system, and decreasing secretion of the neurohormones endothelin and norepinephrine. Onset of action is immediate with peak effects attained in 15 minutes with a bolus dose followed by continuous IV infusion. Administration should be by a separate IV line because nesiritide is incompatible with many other drugs. Hemodynamic monitoring of pulmonary artery pressure is indicated to determine drug effectiveness. Clearance of the drug is proportional to body weight and partially by the kidneys; however, no adjustment in dosing is required for age, gender, race/ethnicity, or renal function impairment. Clinical studies have not been conducted on the use of nesiritide for more than 48 hours.

ENDOTHELIN RECEPTOR ANTAGONISTS (BOSENTAN)

This class of drugs relaxes blood vessels and improves blood flow by targeting endothelin-1 (a neurohormone) that is produced in excess in HF. Endothelin-1 causes blood vessels to constrict, forcing the ailing heart to work harder to pump blood through the narrowed vessels. Studies indicate that endothelin antagonist drugs improve heart function, as measured by cardiac index; animal studies indicate that structural changes of HF (eg, hypertrophy) may be reversed by the drugs. Currently, one endothelin receptor antagonist, **bosentan** (Tracleer), a dual-receptor antagonist, is approved by the Food and Drug Administration (FDA), but only for treatment of pulmonary hypertension. The selective endothelin receptor-A antagonists sitaxsentan and ambrisentan are currently undergoing investigation. Additional data are being collected to support specific indications for these drugs in the management of HF.

NURSING PROCESS

Assessment

Assess clients for current or potential HF.
- Identify risk factors for HF.
  - **Cardiovascular disorders:** atherosclerosis, hypertension, coronary artery disease, myocardial infarction, cardiac dysrhythmias, and cardiac valvular disease
  - **Noncardiovascular disorders:** severe infections, hyperthyroidism, pulmonary disease (eg, cor pulmonale—right-sided HF resulting from lung disease)
  - **Other factors:** excessive amounts of IV fluids, rapid infusion of IV fluids or blood transfusions, advanced age
- Interview and observe for signs and symptoms of **chronic** HF. Within the clinical syndrome of HF, clinical manifestations vary from few and mild to many and severe, including the following:
  - **Mild HF:** Common signs and symptoms of mild HF are ankle edema, dyspnea on exertion, and fatigue

with ordinary physical activity. Edema results from increased venous pressure, which allows fluids to leak into tissues; dyspnea and fatigue result from tissue hypoxia.
  - **Moderate or severe HF:** More extensive edema, dyspnea, and fatigue at rest are likely to occur. Additional signs and symptoms include orthopnea, postnocturnal dyspnea, and cough (from congestion of the respiratory tract with venous blood); mental confusion (from cerebral hypoxia); oliguria and decreased renal function (from decreased blood flow to the kidneys); and anxiety.
- Observe for signs and symptoms of **acute** HF. Acute pulmonary edema indicates acute HF and is a medical emergency. Pulmonary edema occurs when left ventricular failure results in accumulation of blood and fluid in pulmonary veins and tissues. Causes include acute myocardial infarction, cardiac dysrhythmias, severe hypertension, acute fluid or salt overload, and certain drugs (eg, quinidine and other cardiac depressants; propranolol and other antiadrenergics; phenylephrine, norepinephrine, and other alpha-adrenergic stimulants). As a result, the person experiences severe dyspnea, hypoxia, hypertension, tachycardia, hemoptysis, frothy respiratory tract secretions, and anxiety.

Assess clients for signs and symptoms of atrial tachydysrhythmias.
- Record the rate and rhythm of apical and radial pulses. Atrial fibrillation, the most common atrial dysrhythmia, is characterized by tachycardia, pulse deficit (faster apical rate than radial rate), and a very irregular rhythm. Fatigue, dizziness, and fainting may occur.
- Check the electrocardiogram (ECG) for abnormal P waves, rapid rate of ventricular contraction, and QRS complexes of normal configuration but irregular intervals.

Assess baseline vital signs; weight; edema; laboratory results for potassium, magnesium, and calcium levels; and other tests of cardiovascular function when available.

Assess a baseline ECG before digoxin therapy when possible. If a client is in normal sinus rhythm, later ECGs may aid recognition of digitalis toxicity (ie, drug-induced dysrhythmias). If a client has an atrial tachydysrhythmia and is receiving digoxin to slow the ventricular rate, later ECGs may aid recognition of therapeutic and adverse effects. For clients who are already receiving digoxin at the initial contact, a baseline ECG can still be valuable because changes in later ECGs may promote earlier recognition and management of drug-induced dysrhythmias.

Nursing Diagnoses

- Ineffective Tissue Perfusion related to decreased cardiac output
- Anxiety related to chronic illness and lifestyle changes
- Impaired Gas Exchange related to venous congestion and fluid accumulation in lungs
- Imbalanced Nutrition: Less Than Body Requirements related to digoxin-induced anorexia, nausea, and vomiting
- Noncompliance related to the need for long-term drug therapy and regular medical supervision
- Deficient Knowledge: Managing drug therapy regimen safely and effectively

Planning/Goals

The client will
- Take digoxin and other medications safely and accurately
- Experience improved breathing and less fatigue and edema
- Maintain serum digoxin levels within therapeutic ranges
- Be closely monitored for therapeutic and adverse effects, especially during digitalization; when dosage is being changed; and when other drugs are added to or removed from the management regimen
- Keep appointments for follow-up monitoring of vital signs, serum potassium levels, serum digoxin levels, and renal function

Interventions

- Use measures to prevent or minimize HF and atrial dysrhythmias. In the broadest sense, preventive measures include sensible eating habits (a balanced diet; avoiding excess saturated fat and salt; weight control), avoiding cigarette smoking, and regular exercise. In the client at risk for development of HF and dysrhythmias, preventive measures include the following:
  - Treatment of hypertension
  - Avoidance of hypoxia
  - Weight control
  - Avoidance of excess sodium in the diet
  - Avoidance of fluid overload, especially in elderly clients
  - Maintenance of management programs for HF, atrial dysrhythmias, and other cardiovascular or noncardiovascular disorders
- Monitor vital signs, weight, urine output, and serum potassium level regularly, and compare with baseline values.
- Monitor ECGs when available, and compare with baseline or previous tracings.
- Provide appropriate teaching related to drug therapy (see accompanying display).

Evaluation

- Interview and observe for relief of symptoms (weight loss, increased urine output, less extremity edema, easier breathing, improved activity tolerance and self-care ability, slower heart rate).
- Observe serum drug levels for normal or abnormal values, when available.
- Interview regarding compliance with instructions for taking the drug.
- Interview and observe for adverse drug effects, especially cardiac dysrhythmias.

 APPLYING YOUR KNOWLEDGE 48-3: HOW CAN YOU AVOID THIS MEDICATION ERROR?
You are giving Ms. Motsinger her morning medication. The pharmacy has sent Lanoxicaps for today's dose of digoxin. You administer the 0.125-mg capsule.

PRINCIPLES OF THERAPY

Goals of Therapy

The goals for clients with compensated HF are to maintain function as nearly normal as possible and to prevent symptomatic (acute, congestive, or decompensated) HF, hospitalizations, and death. When symptoms (decompensation) occur, the goals are to relieve symptoms, restore function, and prevent progressive cardiac deterioration.

Nonpharmacologic Management Measures

- Prevent or treat conditions that precipitate cardiac decompensation and failure (eg, fluid and sodium retention, factors that impair myocardial contractility or increase cardiac workload).
- Restrict dietary sodium intake to reduce edema and other symptoms and allow a decrease in diuretic dosage. For most clients, sodium restriction need not be severe. A common order, "no added salt," may be accomplished by avoiding obviously salty foods (eg, ham, potato chips, snack foods) and by not adding salt during cooking or eating. For clients with more severe HF, dietary intake may be more restricted (eg, no more than 2 g daily). A major source of sodium intake is table salt: a level teaspoonful contains 2300 mg of sodium.
- If hyponatremia (serum sodium <130 mEq/L) develops from sodium restrictions and diuretic therapy, fluids may need to be restricted (eg, 1.5 L/day or less) until the serum sodium level increases. Severe hyponatremia (<125 mEq/L) may lead to dysrhythmias.

CLIENT TEACHING GUIDELINES

Digoxin

General Considerations

✔ This drug is prescribed for two types of heart disease. One type is heart failure, in which digoxin strengthens your heartbeat and helps to relieve such symptoms as ankle swelling, shortness of breath, and fatigue. The other type is a fast heartbeat called *atrial fibrillation,* in which digoxin slows the heartbeat and decreases symptoms such as fatigue. Because these are chronic conditions, digoxin therapy is usually long term. Ask your health care provider why you are being given digoxin and what effects you can expect, both beneficial and adverse.

✔ It is extremely important to take digoxin (and other cardiovascular medications) as prescribed, usually once daily. The drug must be taken regularly to maintain therapeutic blood levels, but overuse can cause serious adverse effects.

✔ Precautions to increase the drug's safety and effectiveness include the following:

　✔ As a general rule, *do not* miss a dose. It is helpful to develop a routine of taking the medication at approximately the same time each day and maintaining a written record, such as a dated checklist. If you forget a dose at the usual time and remember it within a few hours (approximately 6), go ahead and take the daily dose.

　✔ *Do not* take an extra dose. For example, do not take a double dose to make up for a missed dose.

　✔ *Do not* take other prescription or nonprescription (eg, antacids, cold remedies, diet pills) drugs without consulting the health care provider who prescribed digoxin. Many drugs interact with digoxin to increase or decrease its effects.

　✔ You will need periodic physical examinations, electrocardiograms, and blood tests to check digoxin and electrolyte (sodium, potassium, magnesium) levels to monitor your response to digoxin and see whether changes in dosage are needed.

✔ Digoxin is often one drug in a management regimen of several drugs for heart disease. The drugs are all needed to help the heart and blood vessels work better. Together, the drugs help maintain a balance in the cardiovascular system. As a result, changing any aspect of one of the drugs can upset the balance and lead to symptoms. For example, stopping one drug because of adverse effects can lead to problems. If you think a drug needs to be stopped or its dosage reduced, talk with a health care provider. *Do not* make changes on your own; serious illness or even death could result.

✔ Small doses (eg, 0.125 milligrams [125 micrograms] daily or every other day) are usually given to older adults, and other people with impaired kidney function. Digoxin is eliminated through the kidneys; it can accumulate and cause adverse effects if dosage is not reduced in clients with kidney impairment.

✔ You may need to limit your salt (sodium chloride) intake and get an adequate supply of potassium. Follow your health care provider's recommendations about any diet changes. People taking digoxin are often taking a diuretic, a drug that increases urine production and loss of sodium and potassium from the body. If potassium levels get too low, adverse effects of digoxin are more likely to occur. However, too much potassium can also be harmful. Do not use salt substitutes (potassium chloride) without consulting a health care provider.

✔ Report adverse drug effects (eg, undesirable changes in heart rate or rhythm, nausea and vomiting, or visual problems) to a health care provider. These symptoms may indicate that digoxin dosage needs to be reduced.

✔ Use the same brand and type of digoxin all the time. For example, whether using generic digoxin or trade-name Lanoxin tablets, get the same one each time a prescription is refilled. In addition, there is a capsule form and a liquid form. These forms and concentrations are different and cannot be used interchangeably. Underdoses and overdoses may occur. Lanoxin tablets are the most commonly used formulation.

Self- or Caregiver Administration

✔ If instructed to do so by your health care provider, count your pulse before each dose. In some circumstances, you may be advised to skip that scheduled dose. *Do not* skip doses unless specifically instructed to do so.

✔ Take or give digoxin tablets approximately the same time each day to maintain more even blood levels and help in remembering to take the drug. The tablets may be crushed and can be taken with or after food, if desired, although milk and dairy products may delay absorption.

✔ Digoxin capsules should be swallowed whole.

✔ If taking or giving a liquid form of digoxin, it is extremely important to measure it accurately. A few drops more could produce overdosage, with serious adverse effects; a few drops less could produce underdosage, with a loss or decrease of therapeutic effects.

● For clients who are obese, weight loss is desirable to decrease systemic vascular resistance and myocardial oxygen demand.

● Reduce physical activity in clients with symptomatic HF. This decreases the workload and oxygen consumption of the myocardium. If bed rest is instituted, antithrombotic measures such as compression stockings/devices or heparin therapy should be prescribed to prevent deep vein thrombosis.

● Administer oxygen, if needed, to relieve dyspnea, improve oxygen delivery, reduce the work of breathing, and decrease constriction of pulmonary blood vessels (which is a compensatory measure in clients with hypoxemia).

Pharmacologic Management

Drug Selection

A combination of drugs is the standard of care for both acute and chronic HF. Specific drug components depend on the client's symptoms and hemodynamic status.

Acute Heart Failure

For acute HF, the first drugs of choice may include an IV loop diuretic, a cardiotonic–inotropic agent (eg, digoxin, dobutamine, milrinone), and vasodilators (eg, nitroglycerin and hydralazine or nitroprusside). For clients with decompensated acute HF, nesiritide may be used for initial treatment (<48 hours) or may be given in combination with diuretics, inotropes, or vasodilators. These combinations reduce preload and afterload and increase myocardial contractility.

In acute HF, there is a high risk of hypokalemia because large doses of potassium-losing diuretics are often given. Serum potassium levels should be monitored regularly and supplemental potassium may be needed.

Chronic Heart Failure

For **chronic HF,** an ACE inhibitor or ARB and a diuretic are the basic standard of care. Digoxin, a beta-adrenergic blocking agent, and spironolactone may also be added. Although the use of digoxin in clients with normal sinus rhythm has been questioned, studies indicate improved ejection fraction and exercise tolerance in clients who receive digoxin. In addition, in clients stabilized on digoxin, a diuretic, and an ACE inhibitor or ARB, symptoms worsen if digoxin is discontinued.

In chronic HF, hypokalemia may be less likely to occur because lower doses of potassium-losing diuretics are usually being given. In addition, there may be more extensive use of potassium-sparing diuretics (eg, amiloride, triamterene) and the aldosterone antagonist, spironolactone. Note, however, that hyperkalemia must also be prevented because it is cardiotoxic. Overall, these drugs improve clients' quality of life by decreasing their symptoms and increasing their ability to function in activities of daily living. They also decrease hospitalizations and deaths from HF.

Digoxin Dosage and Administration

- Digoxin dosages are usually stated as the average amounts needed for digitalization and maintenance therapy. These dosages must be interpreted with consideration of specific client characteristics. Digitalizing or loading doses are safe *only* for a short period, usually 24 hours. In addition, loading doses should be used cautiously in clients who have taken digoxin within the previous 2 or 3 weeks. Maintenance doses, which are much smaller than digitalizing doses, may be safely used to initiate digoxin therapy and are always used for long-term therapy.
- In general, larger doses are needed to slow the heart rate in atrial tachydysrhythmias than to increase myocardial contractility in HF. Larger doses may also be needed to

reach therapeutic serum levels of digoxin in a small group of clients (about 10%) who have digoxin-metabolizing bacteria in their colons. Members of this group are at risk for development of digoxin toxicity if they are given antibacterial drugs that destroy colonic bacteria.

- Smaller doses (loading and maintenance) should be given to clients who are elderly or have hypothyroidism. Because metabolism and excretion of digoxin are delayed in such people, the drug may accumulate and cause toxicity if dosage is not reduced. Dosage also should be reduced in clients with hypokalemia, extensive myocardial damage, or cardiac conduction disorders. These conditions increase risks of digoxin-induced dysrhythmias.
- Dosage can be titrated according to client response. In HF, severity of symptoms, ECGs, and serum drug concentrations are useful. In atrial fibrillation, dosage can be altered to produce the desired decrease in the ventricular rate of contraction. Optimal dosage is the lowest amount that relieves signs and symptoms of HF or alters heart rate and rhythm toward normal without producing toxicity.
- IV dosage of digoxin should be 20% to 30% less than oral dosage.
- Digoxin dosage must be reduced by approximately half in clients with renal failure, to avoid drug accumulation and toxicity. Dosage should be based on signs and symptoms of toxicity, creatinine clearance, and serum drug levels.
- Dosage of digoxin must be reduced by approximately half when certain drugs are given concurrently, to avoid drug accumulation and toxicity. For example, amiodarone, quinidine, nifedipine, and verapamil slow digoxin excretion and increase serum digoxin levels.
- When a hospitalized client is unable to take a daily maintenance dose of digoxin at the scheduled time because of diagnostic tests, treatment measures, or other reasons, the dose should usually be given later rather than omitted. If the client is having surgery, the nurse often must ask the surgeon whether the drug should be given on the day of surgery (ie, orally with a small amount of water or parenterally) and if the drug should be reordered after surgery. Many clients require continued digoxin therapy. However, if a dose is missed, probably no ill effects will occur because the pharmacologic actions of digoxin persist longer than 24 hours.
- **Electrolyte balance** must be monitored and maintained during digoxin therapy, particularly normal serum levels of potassium (3.5–5 mEq/L), magnesium (1.5–2.5 mg/100 mL), and calcium (8.5–10 mg/100 mL). Hypokalemia and hypomagnesemia increase cardiac excitability and ectopic pacemaker activity, leading to dysrhythmias; hypercalcemia enhances the effects of digoxin. These electrolyte abnormalities increase the risk of digoxin toxicity. Hypocalcemia increases excitability of nerve and muscle cell membranes and

causes myocardial contraction to be weak (leading to a decrease in digoxin effect).

Digoxin Toxicity: Recognition and Management

Recognition of digoxin toxicity may be difficult because of nonspecific early manifestations (eg, anorexia, nausea, confusion) and the similarity between the signs and symptoms of heart disease for which digoxin is given and the signs and symptoms of digoxin intoxication. Continued atrial fibrillation with a rapid ventricular response may indicate inadequate dosage. However, other dysrhythmias may indicate toxicity. Premature ventricular contractions commonly occur. Serum drug levels and ECGs may be helpful in verifying suspected toxicity. Blood for serum digoxin testing should be drawn just before a dose. Drug distribution to tissues requires about 6 hours after a dose is given; if the blood is drawn before 6 hours, the level may be high.

When signs and symptoms of digoxin toxicity occur, management may include any or all of the following interventions, depending on the client's condition:

- Digoxin should be discontinued, not just reduced in dosage. Most clients with mild or early toxicity recover completely within a few days after the drug is stopped.
- If serious cardiac dysrhythmias are present, several drugs may be used, including
  - **Potassium chloride,** if serum potassium level is low. It is a myocardial depressant that acts to decrease myocardial excitability. The dose depends on the severity of toxicity, serum potassium level, and client response. Potassium is contraindicated in renal failure and should be used with caution in the presence of cardiac conduction defects.
  - **Lidocaine,** an antidysrhythmic local anesthetic agent used to decrease myocardial irritability
  - **Atropine** or **isoproterenol,** used in the management of bradycardia or conduction defects
  - **Other antidysrhythmic drugs** may be used, but are in general less effective in digoxin-induced dysrhythmias than in dysrhythmias due to other causes.
  - **Digoxin immune fab** (Digibind) is a digoxin-binding antidote derived from antidigoxin antibodies produced in sheep. It is recommended only for serious toxicity. It combines with digoxin and pulls digoxin out of tissues and into the bloodstream. This causes serum digoxin levels to be high, but the drug is bound to the antibody and therefore inactive. Digoxin immune fab is given IV, as a bolus injection if the client is in danger of immediate cardiac arrest, but preferably over 15 to 30 minutes. Dosage varies and is calculated according to the amount of digoxin ingested or serum digoxin levels (see manufacturer's instructions).

Use in Special Populations

Use in Children

Digoxin is commonly used in children for the same indications as for adults and should be prescribed or supervised by a pediatric cardiologist when possible. The response to a given dose varies with age, size, and renal and hepatic function. There may be little difference between a therapeutic dose and a toxic dose. Very small amounts are often given to children. These factors increase the risks of dosage errors in children. In a hospital setting, institutional policies may require that each dose be verified with another nurse before it is administered. ECG monitoring is desirable when digoxin therapy is started.

As in adults, dosage of digoxin should be individualized and carefully titrated. Digoxin is primarily excreted by the kidneys, and dosage must be reduced with impaired renal function. In general, divided daily doses should be given to infants and children younger than 10 years, and adult dosages adjusted to their weight should be given to children older than 10 years of age. Larger doses are usually needed to slow a too-rapid ventricular rate in children with atrial fibrillation or flutter. Differences in bioavailability of different preparations (parenterals, capsules, elixirs, and tablets) must be considered when switching from one preparation to another.

Neonates vary in tolerance of digoxin depending on their degree of maturity. Premature infants are especially sensitive to drug effects. Dosage must be reduced, and digitalization should be even more individualized and cautiously approached than in more mature infants and children. Early signs of toxicity in newborns are undue slowing of sinus rate, sinoatrial arrest, and prolongation of the P–R interval.

Use in Older Adults

Digoxin is widely used and a frequent cause of adverse effects in older adults. Reduced dosages are usually required because of decreased liver or kidney function, decreased lean body weight, and advanced cardiovascular disease. All of these characteristics are common in older adults. Impaired renal function leads to slower drug excretion and increased risk of accumulation. Dosage must be reduced by approximately 50% with renal failure or concurrent administration of amiodarone, quinidine, nifedipine, or verapamil. These drugs increase serum digoxin levels and increase risks of toxicity if dosage is not reduced. The most commonly recommended dose is 0.125 milligrams daily. Antacids decrease absorption of oral digoxin and should not be given at the same time.

Use in Clients With Renal Impairment

Digoxin should be used cautiously, in reduced dosages, because renal impairment delays its excretion. Both loading and maintenance doses should be reduced. Clients with advanced renal impairment can achieve therapeutic serum concentrations with a dosage of 0.125 milligrams three to five times per week.

In addition, in clients with reduced blood flow to the kidneys (eg, fluid volume depletion, acute HF), digoxin may be reabsorbed in renal tubules. As a result, less digoxin is excreted through the kidneys and maintenance doses may need even greater decreases than those calculated according to creatinine clearance. Thus, digoxin toxicity develops more often and lasts longer in renal impairment. Clients with renal impairment who are receiving digoxin, even in small doses, should be monitored closely for adverse effects, and serum digoxin levels should be monitored periodically.

There is no information available about the use of inamrinone in renal impairment. However, pharmacokinetic data indicate higher plasma levels with HF-induced reductions in renal perfusion. Also, the drug and its metabolites are excreted primarily by the kidneys.

With milrinone, which is also excreted primarily by the kidneys, renal impairment significantly increases elimination half-life, drug accumulation, and adverse effects. Dosage should be reduced according to creatinine clearance (see manufacturer's instructions).

Use in Clients With Hepatic Impairment

Hepatic impairment has little effect on digoxin clearance, and no dosage adjustments are needed. Inamrinone is extensively metabolized in the liver and may be hepatotoxic. If significant increases in liver enzymes and clinical symptoms occur, inamrinone should be discontinued. If smaller increases in liver enzymes occur without clinical symptoms, inamrinone may be continued with reduced dosage or discontinued, depending on the client's need for the drug.

Use in Clients With Critical Illness

Critically ill clients often have multiple cardiovascular and other disorders that require drug therapy. Acute HF may be the primary critical illness. It may also be precipitated by other illnesses or treatments that alter fluid balance, impair myocardial contractility, or increase the workload of the heart beyond its capacity to accommodate. Management is often symptomatic, with choice of drug and dosage requiring careful titration and frequent monitoring of the client's response. Cardiotonic, diuretic, and vasodilator drugs are often required. All of the drugs should be used with caution in critically ill clients.

Use in Home Care

Most digoxin is taken at home, and the home care nurse shares responsibility for teaching clients how to use the drug effectively and circumstances to be reported to a health care provider. Accurate dosing is vitally important because under-use may cause recurrence of symptoms and overuse may cause toxicity. Either condition may be life threatening and require emergency care. The home care nurse also needs to monitor clients' responses to the drug and changes in conditions or drug therapy that increase risks of toxicity.

When clients are receiving a combination of drugs for management of HF, the nurse needs to assist them in understanding that the different types of drugs have different actions and produce different responses. As a result, they work together to be more effective and maintain a more balanced state of cardiovascular function. Changing drugs or dosages can upset the balance and lead to acute and severe symptoms that require hospitalization and may even cause death from HF. Thus, it is extremely important that they take all the medications as prescribed. If unable to take the medications for any reason, clients or caregivers should notify the prescribing health care provider. They should be instructed not to wait until symptoms become severe before seeking care.

Use in Clients Taking Herbal and Dietary Supplements

Use of nonprescription herbal and dietary supplements is frequently not reported by the client even though one third of the adults in the United States use these agents. Significant interactions can occur between supplements and prescribed drugs. Natural licorice blocks the effects of spironolactone and causes sodium retention and potassium loss, effects that may worsen HF and potentiate the effects of digoxin. Hawthorn should be used cautiously as it may increase the effects of ACE inhibitors and digoxin. Use of ginseng can result in digoxin toxicity. Clients may utilize herbs such as dandelion root and juniper berries for their diuretic effect. Herbal and dietary supplements should not be taken instead of prescribed drug therapies.

N U R S I N G A C T I O N S

Cardiotonic-Inotropic Drugs

NURSING ACTIONS	RATIONALE/EXPLANATION
1. Administer accurately	
a. With digoxin:	
(1) Read the drug label and the health care provider's order carefully when preparing a dose.	For accurate administration

(continued)

NURSING ACTIONS	RATIONALE/EXPLANATION
(2) Give only the ordered dosage form (eg, tablet, Lanoxicap, or elixir).	Digoxin formulations vary in concentration and bioavailability and *cannot* be used interchangeably.
(3) Check the apical pulse before each dose. If the rate is less than 60 in adults, 70 in older children, or 100 in younger children and infants, omit the dose, and notify the health care provider.	Bradycardia is an adverse effect.
(4) Have the same nurse give digoxin to the same clients when possible because it is important to detect changes in rate and rhythm (see *Observe for therapeutic effects* and *Observe for adverse effects,* later).	
(5) Give oral digoxin with food or after meals.	This may minimize gastric irritation and symptoms of anorexia, nausea, and vomiting. However, these symptoms probably arise from drug stimulation of chemoreceptors in the medulla rather than as a direct irritant effect of the drug on the gastrointestinal (GI) tract.
(6) Inject intravenous (IV) digoxin slowly (over at least 5 min).	Digoxin should be given slowly because the diluent, propylene glycol, has toxic effects on the cardiac conduction system if given too rapidly. Digoxin may be given undiluted or diluted with a fourfold or greater volume of sterile water for injection, 0.9% sodium chloride injection, or 5% dextrose injection. If diluted, use the solution immediately.
b. With inamrinone:	
(1) Give undiluted or diluted to a concentration of 1 to 3 mg/mL.	Manufacturer's recommendations
(2) Dilute with 0.9% or 0.45% sodium chloride solution; use the diluted solution within 24 hours. Do not dilute with solutions containing dextrose.	Inamrinone may be injected into IV tubing containing a dextrose solution because contact is brief. However, a chemical interaction occurs with prolonged contact.
(3) Give bolus injections into the tubing of an IV infusion, over 2 to 3 minutes.	
(4) Administer maintenance infusions at a rate of 5–10 mcg/kg/min.	
c. With milrinone:	
(1) Dilute with 0.9% or 0.45% sodium chloride or 5% dextrose solution; use the diluted solution within 24 hours.	Manufacturer's recommendations
(2) Give the loading dose by bolus infusion over 10 minutes.	
(3) Give maintenance infusions at a standard rate of 0.5 mcg/kg/min; this rate may be increased or decreased according to response.	Manufacturer's recommendations
d. With nesiritide:	
(1) Dilute with 5 mL of 0.9% or 0.45% sodium chloride or 5% dextrose solution from a 250 mL IV container; add mixed drug to the container and use diluted solution within 24 hours.	Manufacturer's recommendations
(2) Prime infusion tubing with 25 mL prior to connecting to the patient; withdraw a bolus loading dose from infusion solution.	Manufacturer's recommendations
(3) Give a bolus injection of 2 mcg/kg over 1 minute.	
(4) Give the maintenance infusion at a rate of 0.01 mcg/kg/min.	
(5) Do not mix with any other drug solution; administer through a separate line.	Incompatible with most drugs

NURSING ACTIONS	RATIONALE/EXPLANATION

2. Observe for therapeutic effects

a. When the drugs are given in heart failure (HF), observe for:

(1) Fewer signs and symptoms of pulmonary congestion (dyspnea, orthopnea, cyanosis, cough, hemoptysis, crackles, anxiety, restlessness)

> The pulmonary symptoms that develop with HF are a direct result of events initiated by inadequate cardiac output. The left side of the heart is unable to accommodate incoming blood flow from the lungs. The resulting back pressure in pulmonary veins and capillaries causes leakage of fluid from blood vessels into tissue spaces and alveoli. Fluid accumulation may result in severe respiratory difficulty and pulmonary edema, a life-threatening development. The improved strength of myocardial contraction resulting from cardiotonic-inotropic drugs reverses this potentially fatal chain of events.

(2) Decreased edema—absence of pitting, decreased size of ankles or abdominal girth, decreased weight

> Diuresis and decreased edema result from improved circulation and increased renal blood flow.

(3) Increased tolerance of activity

> Indicates a more adequate supply of blood to tissues

b. When digoxin is given in atrial dysrhythmias, observe for:

(1) Gradual slowing of the heart rate to 70 to 80 beats/min

(2) Elimination of the pulse deficit

(3) Change in rhythm from irregular to regular

> In clients with atrial fibrillation, slowing of the heart rate and elimination of the pulse deficit are clinical indicators that digitalization has been achieved.

3. Observe for adverse effects

a. With digoxin observe for:

> There is a high incidence of adverse effects with digoxin therapy. Therefore, every client receiving digoxin requires close observation. Severity of adverse effects can be minimized with early detection and treatment.

(1) Cardiac dysrhythmias:

> Digoxin toxicity may cause any type of cardiac dysrhythmia. These are the most serious adverse effects associated with digoxin therapy. They are detected as abnormalities in electrocardiograms and in pulse rate or rhythm.

(a) Premature ventricular contractions (PVCs)

> PVCs are among the most common digoxin-induced dysrhythmias. They are not specific for digoxin toxicity because there are many possible causes. They are usually perceived as "skipped" heartbeats.

(b) Bradycardia

> Excessive slowing of the heart rate is an extension of the drug's therapeutic action of slowing conduction through the atrioventricular (AV) node and probably depressing the sinoatrial node as well.

(c) Paroxysmal atrial tachycardia with heart block

(d) AV nodal tachycardia

(e) AV block (second- or third-degree heart block)

> Electrocardiogram study is necessary for identification of nodal rhythms and heart block.

(2) Anorexia, nausea, vomiting

> These GI effects commonly occur with digoxin therapy. Because they are caused at least in part by stimulation of the vomiting center in the brain, they occur with parenteral and oral administration. The presence of these symptoms raises suspicion of digitalis toxicity, but they are not specific because many other conditions may cause anorexia, nausea, and vomiting. Also, clients receiving digoxin are often taking other medications that cause these side effects, such as diuretics and potassium supplements.

(3) Headache, drowsiness, confusion

> These central nervous system effects are most common in older adults.

(4) Visual disturbances (eg, blurred vision, photophobia, altered perception of colors, flickering dots)

> These are due mainly to drug effects on the retina and may indicate acute toxicity.

(continued)

NURSING ACTIONS	RATIONALE/EXPLANATION
b. With inamrinone, observe for:	
(1) Thrombocytopenia	Thrombocytopenia is more likely to occur with prolonged therapy and is usually reversible if dosage is reduced or the drug is discontinued.
(2) Anorexia, nausea, vomiting, abdominal pain	GI symptoms can be decreased by reducing drug dosage.
(3) Hypotension	Hypotension probably results from vasodilatory effects of inamrinone.
(4) Hepatotoxicity	If marked changes in liver enzymes occur in conjunction with clinical symptoms, the drug should be discontinued.
c. With milrinone, observe for ventricular dysrhythmias, hypotension, and headache.	Ventricular dysrhythmias reportedly occur in 12% of clients, hypotension and headache in approximately 3% of clients.
d. With nesiritide, observe for hypotension, headache, nausea, back pain, ventricular tachycardia, dizziness, anxiety, insomnia, bradycardia, and vomiting.	Hypotension occurs in approximately 11% of clients; headache in 8%; nausea and back pain in 4%; and other adverse effects in 1%–3%.
4. Observe for drug interactions	Most significant drug interactions increase risks of toxicity. Some alter absorption or metabolism to produce under-digitalization and decreased therapeutic effect.
a. Drugs that *increase* effects of digoxin:	
(1) Adrenergic drugs (eg, ephedrine, epinephrine, isoproterenol)	Increase risks of cardiac dysrhythmias
(2) Antidysrhythmics (eg, amiodarone, propafenone, quinidine)	Decrease clearance of digoxin, thereby increasing serum digoxin levels and risks of toxicity. Dosage of digoxin should be reduced if one of these drugs is given concurrently (25% with propafenone and 50% with amiodarone and quinidine).
(3) Anticholinergics	Increase absorption of oral digoxin by slowing transit time through the GI tract
(4) Calcium preparations	Increase risks of cardiac dysrhythmias. IV calcium salts are contraindicated in digitalized clients.
(5) Calcium channel blockers (eg, diltiazem, felodipine, nifedipine, verapamil)	Decrease clearance of digoxin, thereby increasing serum digoxin levels and risks of toxicity. Dosage of digoxin should be reduced 25% if verapamil is given concurrently.
b. Drugs that *decrease* effects of digoxin:	
(1) Antacids, cholestyramine, colestipol, laxatives, oral aminoglycosides (eg, neomycin)	Decrease absorption of oral digoxin

APPLYING YOUR KNOWLEDGE: ANSWERS

48-1 Digitalization in adults is accomplished by the administration of a total dose of 0.75 to 1.0 mg of digoxin in divided doses over a 24-hour period. Although digitalization engenders a higher risk of toxicity, the maximum drug effect will be reached more rapidly.

48-2 The normal digoxin level is 0.5 to 2.0 ng/mL. Toxic serum levels are greater than 2 ng/mL; however, toxicity may occur at any serum level.

48-3 When taken orally, the absorption of digoxin depends on the preparation. Capsules have better absorption than the tablets and should not be substituted equally.

Review and Application Exercises

Short Answer Exercises

1. What signs and symptoms usually occur with HF? How would you assess for these?

2. What are the physiologic effects of digoxin on the heart?

3. How does digoxin produce or assist diuresis?

4. Differentiate between a digitalizing dose of digoxin and a daily maintenance dose.

5. Why do nurses need to check heart rate and rhythm before giving digoxin?

6. When is it appropriate to withhold a dose of digoxin?

7. What are adverse effects associated with digoxin, and how may they be prevented or minimized?

8. Why is it important to maintain a therapeutic serum potassium level during digoxin therapy?

9. What is the specific antidote for severe digoxin toxicity?

NCLEX-Style Questions

10. A 65-year-old client develops digoxin toxicity 1 month after beginning 0.25 mg of digoxin PO daily. Which factor affects the duration of such an adverse reaction?
   a. daily drug dosage
   b. half-life of the drug
   c. form of the drug prescribed
   d. duration of therapy

11. A 5-year-old child is placed on digoxin. Which electrolyte imbalance will place her at a greater risk for digoxin toxicity?
   a. hyponatremia
   b. hyperkalemia
   c. hypocalcemia
   d. hypokalemia

12. When administering the daily dose of digoxin 0.125 mg PO to a client with a history of type 1 diabetes mellitus who is now in heart failure, the nurse should
   a. Give it with orange juice.
   b. Monitor for dysrhythmias.
   c. Administer it 1 hour before the morning insulin.
   d. Withhold it if the apical pulse rate is less than 80 beats per minute.

13. A 44-year-old client develops blurring of vision with yellow spots in his visual fields while taking digoxin. The nurse recognizes that the visual changes may indicate
   a. a need for a vision exam
   b. adjustment of the retina to the drug
   c. acute toxicity
   d. therapeutic effects

14. As the nurse prepares to administer a scheduled dose of digoxin to an adult client, she reviews lab results from earlier in the day and notes that the plasma level of digoxin is 1.5 ng/mL. Based on this report, the nurse should
   a. Withhold the drug and notify the health care provider during rounds.
   b. Withhold the drug and notify the health care provider immediately.
   c. Administer Digibind to counteract the toxicity.
   d. Check the client's pulse and if it is greater than 60 beats per minute, administer the dose of digoxin.

Selected References

Carelock, J., & Clark, A. P. (2001). Heart failure: Pathophysiologic mechanisms. *American Journal of Nursing, 101*(12), 26–33.

Channick, R. N., Sitbon, O., Barst, R. J., Manes, A., & Rubin, L. J. (2004). Endothelin receptor antagonists in pulmonary arterial hypertension. *Journal of American College of Cardiology, 43*(12, Suppl. 1), S62–S66.

Cohen, H., Chahine, C., Hui, A., & Mukherji, R. (2004). Bosentan therapy for arterial hypertension. *American Journal of Health System Pharmacists, 61,* 1107–1119.

Drug facts and comparisons. (Updated monthly). St. Louis: Facts and Comparisons.

Hockenberry, M. J., Wilson, D., Winkelstein, M. L., & Kline, N. E. (2003). *Wong's Nursing care of infants and children* (7th ed., pp. 1476–1484). St. Louis: Mosby.

Hunt, S. A., Baker, D. W., Chin, M. H., Cinquegrani, M. P., Feldman, A. M., Francis, G. S., et al. (2001). *ACC/AHA guidelines for the evaluation and management of chronic heart failure in the adult: A report of the American College of Cardiology/American Heart Association Task Force on Practice Guidelines (Committee to Revise the 1995 Guidelines for the Evaluation and Management of Heart Failure).* Retrieved July 30, 2005, from http://www.org/clinical/guidelines/failure/hf_index.htm

Johnson, J. A., Parker, R. B., & Patterson, J. H. (2002). Heart failure. In J. T. DiPiro, R. L. Talbert, G. C. Yee, G. R. Matzke, B. G. Wells, & L. M. Posey (Eds.), *Pharmacotherapy: A pathophysiologic approach* (5th ed., pp. 185–218). New York: McGraw-Hill.

Karch, A. M. (2005). *2006 Lippincott's nursing drug guide.* Philadelphia: Lippincott Williams & Wilkins.

Naylor, L., Howe, L., Eggert, J., & Heifferon, B. (2004). CHF in the elderly: Using ACEIs appropriately. *Nurse Practitioner, 29*(7), 46–53.

North American Nursing Diagnosis Association. (2003). *Nursing diagnoses: Definitions & classification 2003–2004.* Philadelphia: Author.

Porth, C. M. (2005). *Pathophysiology: Concepts of altered health states* (7th ed., pp. 603–630). Philadelphia: Lippincott Williams & Wilkins.

Scow, D. T., Smith, E. G., & Shaughnessy, A. E. (2002). Combination therapy with ACE inhibitors and angiotensin-receptor blockers in heart failure. *American Family Physician, 68,* 1795–1798.

Skidmore-Roth, L. (2004). *Mosby's handbook of herbs & natural supplements* (2nd ed.). St. Louis: Mosby.

Smeltzer, S. C., & Bare, B. G. (2004). *Brunner & Suddarth's textbook of medical-surgical nursing* (10th ed., pp. 787–806). Philadelphia: Lippincott Williams & Wilkins.

Antidysrhythmic Drugs

OBJECTIVES

After studying this chapter, you will be able to:

1. Differentiate between supraventricular and ventricular dysrhythmias in terms of etiology and hemodynamic effects.
2. Describe nonpharmacologic measures to prevent or minimize tachydysrhythmias.
3. Discuss the roles of beta-adrenergic blocking agents, calcium channel blockers, digoxin, and quinidine in the management of supraventricular tachydysrhythmias.
4. Discuss the effects of lidocaine in the management of ventricular tachycardia.
5. Describe adverse effects and nursing process implications related to the use of selected antidysrhythmic drugs.

APPLYING YOUR KNOWLEDGE

Butch Brown is a 74-year-old male who recently had coronary artery bypass surgery with three vessel grafts. During his postoperative period, he developed premature ventricular complexes (PVCs) and atrial fibrillation (AF).

INTRODUCTION

Antidysrhythmic agents are diverse drugs used for prevention and management of cardiac dysrhythmias. Dysrhythmias, also called *arrhythmias,* are abnormalities in heart rate or rhythm. They become significant when they interfere with cardiac function and ability to perfuse body tissues. To aid in understanding of dysrhythmias and antidysrhythmic drug therapy, the physiology of cardiac conduction and contractility is reviewed.

Cardiac Electrophysiology

The heart is an electrical pump. The "electrical" activity resides primarily in the specialized tissues that can generate and conduct an electrical impulse. Although impulses are conducted through muscle cells, the rate is much slower. The mechanical or "pump" activity resides in contractile tissue. Normally, these activities result in effective cardiac contraction and distribution of blood throughout the body. Each heartbeat or cardiac cycle occurs at regular intervals and consists of four events. These are *stimulation* from an electrical impulse, *transmission* of the electrical impulse to adjacent conductive or contractile tissue, *contraction* of atria and ventricles, and *relaxation* of atria and ventricles, during which they refill with blood in preparation for the next contraction.

Automaticity

Automaticity is the heart's ability to generate an electrical impulse. Any part of the conduction system can spontaneously start an impulse, but the sinoatrial (SA) node normally has the highest degree of automaticity and therefore the highest rate of spontaneous impulse formation. With its faster rate of electrical discharge or depolarization than other parts of the conduction system, the SA node serves as pacemaker and controls heart rate and rhythm.

Initiation of an electrical impulse depends on the movement of sodium and calcium ions into a myocardial cell and movement of potassium ions out of the cell. Normally, the cell membrane becomes more permeable to sodium and opens pores or channels to allow its rapid movement into the cell. Calcium ions follow sodium ions into the cell at a slower rate. As sodium and calcium ions move into cells, potassium ions move out of cells. The movement of the ions changes the membrane from its resting state of electrical neutrality to an activated state of electrical energy buildup. When the electrical energy is discharged (depolarization), muscle contraction occurs.

Some cells in the cardiac conduction system depolarize in response to the entry of calcium ions rather than entry of sodium ions. In these calcium-respondent cells, which are found mainly in the SA and atrioventricular (AV) nodes, the electrical impulse is conducted more slowly and recovery of excitability takes longer than in sodium-respondent cells. Overall, activation of the SA and AV nodes depends on a slow depolarizing current through calcium channels, and activation of the atria and ventricles depends on a rapid depolarizing current through sodium channels. These two types of conduction tissues are often called *slow* and *fast channels*, respectively, and they differ markedly in their responses to drugs that affect conduction of electrical impulses.

The ability of a cardiac muscle cell to respond to an electrical stimulus is called *excitability* or *irritability*. The stimulus must reach a certain intensity or threshold to cause contraction. After contraction, sodium and calcium ions return to the extracellular space, potassium ions return to the intracellular space, muscle relaxation occurs, and the cell prepares for the next electrical stimulus and contraction.

Following contraction there is also a period of decreased excitability (called the *absolute refractory period*) during which the cell cannot respond to a new stimulus. Before the resting membrane potential is reached, a stimulus greater than normal can evoke a response in the cell. This period is called the *relative refractory period.*

Conductivity

Conductivity is the ability of cardiac tissue to transmit electrical impulses. Although the electrophysiology of a single myocardial cell can assist understanding of the process, the orderly, rhythmic transmission of impulses to all cells is needed for effective myocardial contraction.

Normally, electrical impulses originate in the SA node and are transmitted to atrial muscle, where they cause atrial contraction, and then to the AV node, bundle of His, bundle branches, Purkinje fibers, and ventricular muscle, where they cause ventricular contraction. The cardiac conduction system is shown in Figure 49-1.

Cardiac Dysrhythmias

Cardiac dysrhythmias can originate in any part of the conduction system or from atrial or ventricular muscle. They result from disturbances in electrical impulse formation (automaticity), conduction (conductivity), or both. The characteristic of automaticity allows myocardial cells other than the SA node to depolarize and initiate the electrical impulse that culminates in atrial and ventricular contraction. This

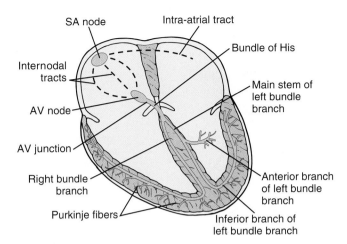

FIGURE 49-1 The conducting system of the heart. Impulses originating in the SA node are transmitted through the atria, into the AV node to the bundle of His, and by way of Purkinje fibers through the ventricles.

may occur when the SA node fails to initiate an impulse or does so too slowly. When the electrical impulse arises anywhere other than the SA node, it is an abnormal or ectopic focus. If the ectopic focus depolarizes at a rate faster than the SA node, the ectopic focus becomes the dominant pacemaker. Ectopic pacemakers may arise in the atria, AV node, Purkinje fibers, or ventricular muscle. They may be activated by hypoxia, ischemia, or hypokalemia. Ectopic foci indicate myocardial irritability (increased responsiveness to stimuli) and potentially serious impairment of cardiac function.

A common mechanism by which abnormal conduction causes dysrhythmias is called *reentry excitation*. During normal conduction, the electrical impulse moves freely down the conduction system until it reaches recently excited tissue that is refractory to stimulation. This causes the impulse to be extinguished. The SA node then recovers, fires spontaneously, and the conduction process starts over again. Reentry excitation means that an impulse continues to reenter an area of the heart rather than becoming extinguished. For this to occur, the impulse must encounter an obstacle in the normal conducting pathway. The obstacle is usually an area of damage, such as myocardial infarction. The damaged area allows conduction in only one direction and causes a circular movement of the impulse (Fig. 49-2).

Dysrhythmias may be mild or severe, acute or chronic, episodic or relatively continuous. They are clinically significant if they interfere with cardiac function (ie, the heart's ability to pump sufficient blood to body tissues). The normal heart can maintain an adequate cardiac output with ventricular rates ranging from 40 to 180 beats per minute. The diseased heart, however, may not be able to maintain an adequate cardiac output with heart rates below 60 or above 120. Dysrhythmias are usually categorized by rate, location, or patterns of conduction. Common types of dysrhythmias are described in Box 49-1.

Normal conduction

Nerve impulse

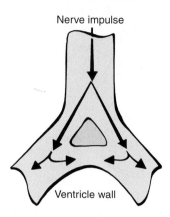

Ventricle wall

**Unidirectional
blockage of conduction**

Impulse
blocked by
injured
myocardial cells —

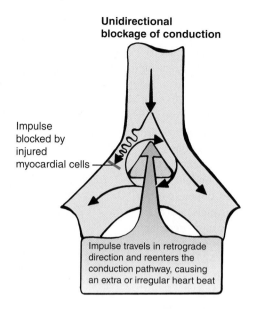

Impulse travels in retrograde
direction and reenters the
conduction pathway, causing
an extra or irregular heart beat

FIGURE 49-2 Reentry excitation of
dysrhythmias.

GENERAL CHARACTERISTICS OF ANTIDYSRHYTHMIC DRUGS

Antidysrhythmic drugs alter the heart's electrical conduction system. Atropine for bradydysrhythmias is discussed in Chapter 20; digoxin and its use in treating atrial fibrillation (AF) are discussed in Chapter 48. The focus of this chapter is the drugs used for tachydysrhythmias. These drugs are described in the following sections and listed in Table 49-1.

Clinical use of antidysrhythmic drugs for tachydysrhythmias has undergone significant changes. One change is that the goal of drug therapy is to prevent or relieve symptoms or prolong survival, not just suppress dysrhythmias. This change resulted from studies in which clients treated for some dysrhythmias had a higher mortality rate than clients who did not receive antidysrhythmic drug therapy. The higher mortality rate was attributed to prodysrhythmic effects (ie, worsening existing dysrhythmias or causing new dysrhythmias). Overall, there is decreasing use of class I drugs (eg, quinidine) and increasing use of class II (beta blockers) and class III (eg, amiodarone) drugs.

Another change is the greater use of nonpharmacologic management of dysrhythmias. These methods include destroying dysrhythmogenic foci in the heart with radio waves (radiofrequency catheter ablation) or surgical procedures and implanting devices for sensing, cardioverting, defibrillating, or pacing (eg, the implantable cardioverter–defibrillator [ICD]).

Indications for Use

Antidysrhythmic drug therapy commonly is indicated in the following conditions:

- To convert AF or atrial flutter to normal sinus rhythm (NSR)
- To maintain NSR after conversion from AF or flutter

- When the ventricular rate is so fast or irregular that cardiac output is impaired. Decreased cardiac output leads to symptoms of decreased systemic, cerebral, and coronary circulation.
- When dangerous dysrhythmias occur and may be fatal if not quickly terminated. For example, ventricular tachycardia may cause cardiac arrest.

Mechanisms of Action

Drugs used for rapid dysrhythmias mainly *reduce automaticity* (spontaneous depolarization of myocardial cells, including ectopic pacemakers), *slow conduction* of electrical impulses through the heart, and *prolong the refractory period* of myocardial cells (so they are less likely to be prematurely activated by adjacent cells). Several different groups of drugs perform one or more of these actions. They are classified according to their mechanisms of action and effects on the conduction system, even though they differ in other respects. Additionally, some drugs have characteristics of more than one classification.

CLASSIFICATIONS AND INDIVIDUAL DRUGS

Class I Sodium Channel Blockers

Class I drugs block the movement of sodium into cells of the cardiac conducting system. This results in a membrane-stabilizing effect and decreased formation and conduction of electrical impulses. This group of drugs is declining in clinical use, mainly because of prodysrhythmic effects and resultant increased mortality rates. The higher mortality rates occur most often in clients with significant structural heart disease.

(text continues on page 802)

Box 49-1 Types of Dysrhythmias

Sinus dysrhythmias are usually significant only if they are severe or prolonged. Tachycardia increases the workload of the heart and may lead to heart failure or angina pectoris. Sinus tachycardia may cause anginal pain (myocardial ischemia) by two related mechanisms. One mechanism involves increased myocardial oxygen consumption. The other mechanism involves a shortened diastole so that coronary arteries may not have adequate filling time between heartbeats. Thus, additional blood flow to the myocardium is required at the same time that a decreased blood supply is delivered.

Sinus tachycardia (Fig. A) may be caused by numerous conditions such as fever, hypotension, heart failure, thyrotoxicosis, stimulation of the sympathetic nervous system (eg, stress or drugs, including asthma remedies and nasal decongestants), and lifestyle drugs such as alcohol, caffeine, and nicotine. Thus, the initial assessment of a client with sinus tachycardia should include a search for underlying causes. The rate usually may be slowed by treating the underlying cause or by stimulating the vagus nerve (eg, by carotid sinus massage or Valsalva maneuver).

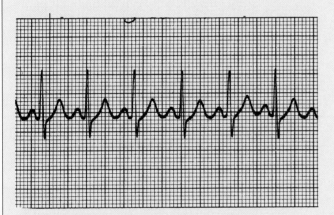

FIGURE A Sinus tachycardia.

Sinus bradycardia (Fig. B) may occur with excessive vagal stimulation, deficient sympathetic tone, and sinus node dysfunction. It often occurs in healthy young adults, especially in athletes and during sleep. Other conditions associated with sinus bradycardia include hypothyroidism, hypothermia, vasovagal reactions, and with the use of drugs such as beta-adrenergic blocking agents, amiodarone, diltiazem, lithium, and verapamil. Thus, as with sinus tachycardia, efforts to identify the underlying cause are needed. Asymptomatic sinus bradycardia does not require treatment. Acute, symptomatic sinus bradycardia can be treated with atropine or a temporary pacemaker (eg, an external transthoracic, a transvenous, or an external pacemaker). Chronic symptomatic sinus bradycardia requires insertion of a permanent pacemaker.

Atrial dysrhythmias are most significant in the presence of underlying heart disease. Atrial fibrillation and atrial flutter commonly occur, especially in older adults. Numerous conditions may lead to these dysrhythmias, including myocardial ischemia or infarction, hypertension, cardiomyopathy, valvular disorders, pulmonary embolus, pulmonary hypertension, thyrotoxicosis, alcohol withdrawal, sepsis, or excessive physical

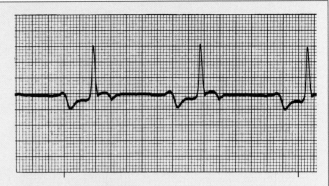

FIGURE B Sinus bradycardia.

exertion. One characteristic of *atrial fibrillation* (Fig. C) is disorganized, tremor-like movement of the atria. This lack of effective atrial contraction impairs ventricular filling, decreases cardiac output, and may lead to the formation of atrial thrombi, with a high potential for embolization. Another characteristic is a very rapid atrial rate (400–600 beats/minute). Some of the atrial impulses penetrate the atrioventricular (AV) conduction system to reach the ventricles, and some do not. This results in irregular activation of the ventricles and a slower ventricular rate (120–180 beats/minute) than atrial rate.

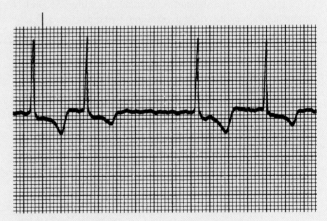

FIGURE C Atrial fibrillation.

Atrial flutter (Fig. D) occurs less often than atrial fibrillation but causes similar symptoms. Atrial flutter is characterized by a rapid (270–330 atrial beats/minute) but regular atrial activation and a regular ventricular pulse rate.

For some clients, the main goal of management for atrial fibrillation or flutter is restoration of sinus rhythm by pharmacologic or electrical cardioversion. Then, long-term drug therapy is usually given to prevent recurrence. For clients who do not successfully convert to normal sinus rhythm with drug therapy or who are not considered candidates for cardioversion, the goals are to slow the ventricular response rate (with antidysrhythmic medication) and to prevent stroke or other thromboembolic complications (eg, with aspirin, warfarin, or both).

(continued)

Box 49-1 Types of Dysrhythmias (continued)

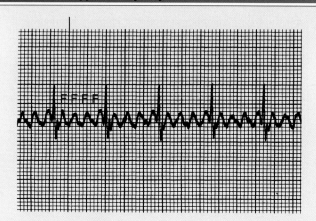

FIGURE D Atrial flutter.

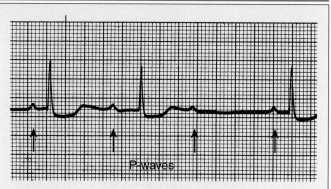

FIGURE F Mobitz Type I (second-degree) heart block.

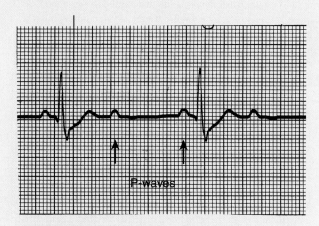

FIGURE G Mobitz Type II (second-degree) heart block.

Nodal dysrhythmias may involve tachycardia and increased workload of the heart or bradycardia from heart block. Either tachycardia or bradycardia may decrease cardiac output. Heart block involves impaired conduction of the electrical impulse through the AV node. With first-degree heart block(Fig. E), conduction is slowed, but not significantly. With second-degree heart block, every second, third, or fourth atrial impulse is blocked and does not reach the ventricles (2:1, 3:1, or 4:1 block). Thus, atrial and ventricular rates differ. Second-degree heart block has been divided into two types (Mobitz type I [or Wenckebach's phenomenon] and Mobitz type II) and may interfere with cardiac output. Mobitz type I (Fig. F) has been associated with individuals with inferior wall myocardial infarction (MI) or digoxin toxicity and usually does not require temporary pacing because it is transient in nature. Mobitz type II (Fig. G) occurs in clients with anterior wall MI, may progress to third-degree block, and often requires cardiac pacing because it is associated with a high mortality rate. Third-degree (Fig. H) is the most serious type of heart block because no impulses reach the ventricles. As a result, AV dissociation occurs and the ventricles beat independently at a rate less than 40 beats/minute. This slow ventricular rate severely reduces cardiac output and hemodynamic stability.

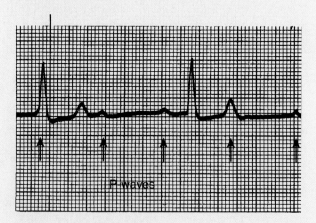

FIGURE H Third-degree heart block.

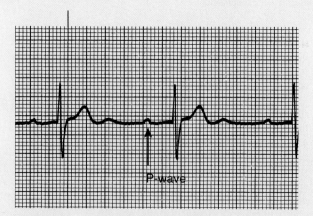

FIGURE E First-degree heart block.

Ventricular dysrhythmias include premature ventricular contractions (PVCs), ventricular tachycardia, and ventricular fibrillation. PVCs (Fig. I) occur in healthy individuals as well as those with heart disease and may cause no symptoms or only mild palpitations. Serious PVCs often occur with ischemic heart disease, especially after acute MI. PVCs are considered serious

Box 49-1 Types of Dysrhythmias (continued)

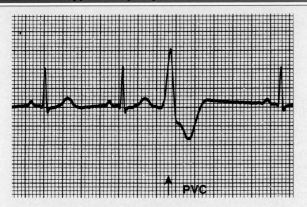

FIGURE I Premature ventricular contractions.

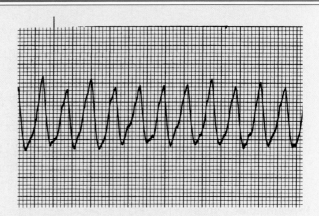

FIGURE J Ventricular tachycardia.

if they produce significant symptoms (eg, anginal pain, dyspnea, or syncope), occur more than five times per minute, are coupled or grouped, are multifocal, or occur during the resting phase of the cardiac cycle (*R on T phenomenon*). Serious PVCs indicate a high degree of myocardial irritability and may lead to life-threatening ventricular tachycardia, ventricular fibrillation, or asystole. The goal of treatment is to decrease myocardial irritability, relieve symptoms, and prevent progression to more serious dysrhythmias.

Ventricular tachycardia (VT) (Fig. J) is characterized by a ventricular rate of 160 to 250 beats/minute. It is diagnosed when three or more PVCs occur in a row at a rate greater than 100 beats/minute. VT may be sustained (lasts longer than 30 seconds or requires termination because of hemodynamic collapse) or nonsustained (stops spontaneously in less than 30 seconds). Occasional brief episodes of VT may be asymptomatic; frequent or relatively long episodes may result in hemodynamic collapse, a life-threatening situation. An acute episode most often occurs during an acute MI. Other precipitating factors include severe electrolyte imbalances (eg, hypokalemia), hypoxemia, or digoxin toxicity. Correction of these precipitating factors usually prevents recurrences of VT. Clients with organic heart disease may have a chronic recurrent form of VT. Torsades de pointes is an especially serious type of VT that may deteriorate into ventricular fibrillation. Predisposing factors include severe bradycardia, electrolyte deficiencies (eg, hypokalemia, hypomagnesemia), and several drug groups (eg, class IA antidysrhythmics, phenothiazine antipsychotics, and tricyclic antidepressants). VT can be treated with intravenous lidocaine (a loading dose and continuous infusion), direct-current countershock, external pacing, or insertion of a transvenous pacing wire for overdrive pacing.

Ventricular fibrillation (VF), Figure K, produces no myocardial contraction so that there is no cardiac output and sudden cardiac death (SCD) occurs. Death results unless effective cardiopulmonary resuscitation or defibrillation is instituted within approximately 4 to 6 minutes. VF most often occurs in clients with ischemic heart disease, especially acute MI. Direct-current countershock and antidysrhythmic drug therapy may be used to restore a functional heart rhythm. For primary VF that occurs during the first 72 hours following an MI, antidysrhythmic drug therapy is not indicated because the VF is unlikely to recur. For VF without an identifiable or a reversible cause, successful resuscitation should be followed by long-term antidysrhythmic drug therapy or a transvenous implantable cardioverter-defibrillator (ICD). ICDs improve survival rates in sudden cardiac death (SCD) better than antidysrhythmic drug therapy. However, beta blocker therapy for the first year after an MI significantly improves survival and reduces the occurrence of SCD. Other effective treatments for VT/VF include myocardial revascularization surgery or radiofrequency catheter ablation of the dysrhythmogenic focus.

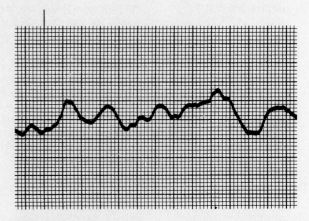

FIGURE K Ventricular fibrillation.

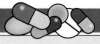

Table 49-1 Drugs at a Glance: Antidysrhythmic Drugs

DRUGS FOR TACHYDYSRHYTHMIAS	ROUTES AND DOSAGE RANGES	
	Adults	Children

Class I Sodium Channel Blockers

CLASS 1A

Treatment of symptomatic premature ventricular contractions, supraventricular tachycardia, and ventricular tachycardia; prevention of ventricular fibrillation

P Quinidine	PO 200–600 mg q6h; maximum dose, 3–4 g/d; maintenance dose, PO 200–600 mg q6h, or 1 or 2 extended-action tablets, 2 or 3 times per day IM (quinidine gluconate) 600 mg initially, then 400 mg q4–6h	PO 6 mg/kg q4–6h
Procainamide (Pronestyl, Procanbid)	PO 1 g loading dose initially, then 250–500 mg q3–4h (q6h for sustained-release tablets) IM loading dose, 500–1000 mg followed by oral maintenance doses IV 25–50 mg/min; maximum dose, 1000 mg	PO 50 mg/kg/d in 4–6 divided doses
Disopyramide (Norpace)	PO loading dose, 300 mg, followed by 150 mg q6h; usual dose, PO 400–800 mg/d in 4 divided doses	*12–18 y:* 6–15 mg/kg/d in 4 divided doses *4–12 y:* 10–15 mg/kg/d in 4 divided doses *1–4 y:* 10–20 mg/kg/d in 4 divided doses *<1 y:* 10–30 mg/kg/d in 4 divided doses

CLASS 1B

Treatment of symptomatic premature ventricular contractions and ventricular tachycardia; prevention of ventricular fibrillation

P Lidocaine (Xylocaine)	IV 1–2 mg/kg, not to exceed 50–100 mg, as a single bolus injection over 2 min, followed by a continuous infusion (1 g of lidocaine in 500 mL of 5% dextrose in water) at a rate to deliver 1–4 mg/min; maximum dose, 300 mg/h IM 4–5 mg/kg as a single dose; may repeat in 60–90 min	IV injection 1 mg/kg, followed by IV infusion of 20–50 mcg/kg/min
Mexiletine (Mexitil)	PO 200 mg q8h initially, increased by 50–100 mg every 2–3 d if necessary to a maximum of 1200 mg/d	1.4–5 mg/kg per dose, given every 8 h
Phenytoin (Dilantin)	PO, loading dose 13 mg/kg (approximately 1000 mg) first day, 7.5 mg/kg second and third days; maintenance dose 4–6 mg/kg/d (average 400 mg) in 1 or 2 doses starting on the fourth day IV 100 mg every 5 min until the dysrhythmia is reversed or toxic effects occur; maximum dose, 1 g/24 h	1.25 mg/kg every 5 min, may repeat up to total loading dose of 15 mg/kg

CLASS 1C

Treatment of life-threatening ventricular tachycardia or fibrillation and supraventricular tachycardia unresponsive to other drugs

Flecainide (Tambocor)	PO 100 mg q12h initially, increased by 50 mg q12h every 4 d until effective; maximum dose, 400 mg/d	Initial 1–3 mg/kg/d in 3 divided doses; usual 3–6 mg/kg/d in 3 divided doses up to 8 mg/kg/d
Propafenone (Rythmol)	PO 150 mg q8h initially, increased to a maximum dose of 1200 mg/d if necessary; usual maintenance dose 150–300 mg q8h	Safety and efficacy not established

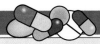

Table 49-1 Drugs at a Glance: Antidysrhythmic Drugs (continued)

DRUGS FOR TACHYDYSRHYTHMIAS	ROUTES AND DOSAGE RANGES	
	Adults	**Children**
CLASS 1 MISCELLANEOUS Treatment of life-threatening ventricular dysrhythmias		
Moricizine (Ethmozine)	PO 200–300 mg q8h	Safety and efficacy not established
Class II Beta Blockers Treatment of supraventricular tachycardia		
Acebutolol (Sectral)	PO 200 mg twice daily, increased gradually until optimal response is obtained (usually 600–1200 mg/d in divided doses)	Safety and efficacy not established
Esmolol (Brevibloc)	IV infusion 500 mcg/kg/min initially as a loading dose, followed by a maintenance dose of 50 mcg/kg/min over 4 min. Repeat the same loading dose, and increase maintenance doses in 50 mcg/kg increments every 5–10 min until therapeutic effects are obtained. Average maintenance dose, 100 mcg/kg/min	IV infusion 500 mcg/kg/min initially as a loading dose over 1 min, with a maximum dose of 50–250 mcg/kg/min
Ⓟ **Propranolol** (Inderal)	IV injection 1–3 mg at a rate of 1 mg/min PO 10–30 mg 3 or 4 times per day	IV injection 0.01–0.1 mg/kg slow IVP over 10 min, with a maximum dose of 1 mg Initial PO dose of 0.5–1.0 mg/kg/d in divided doses every 6–8 h. May adjust every 3–7 d to a maximum of 16 mg/kg/d or 60 mg/d
Class III Potassium Channel Blockers Treatment of ventricular tachycardia and fibrillation; conversion of atrial fibrillation or flutter to sinus rhythm; maintenance of sinus rhythm (amiodarone)		
Amiodarone (Cordarone)	Loading dose, IV 150 mg over 10 min (15 mg/min), then 360 mg over the next 6 h (1 mg/min), then 540 mg over the next 18 h (0.5 mg/min); maintenance dose, IV 720 mg/24 h (0.5 mg/min) Loading dose, PO 800–1600 mg/d for 1–3 wk, with a gradual decrease to 600–800 mg/d for 1 mo; maintenance dose, PO 400 mg/d	IV safety and efficacy not established Loading dose, PO 10–15 mg/kg/d in 1–2 divided doses for up to 14 d or until dysrhythmia controlled. Dose should then be reduced to 5 mg/kg/d once daily for several weeks. Minimal maintenance dose, PO 2.5 mg/kg/d for 5–7 d/wk
Bretylium (Bretylol)	IM 5 mg/kg, repeated in 1–2 h then q6–8h IV 5–10 mg/kg (diluted in at least 50 mL of IV fluid and infused over 10–20 min) During cardiopulmonary resuscitation, IV 5 mg/kg given by direct injection (undiluted); may be repeated every 15–30 min to a maximum total dose of 30 mg/kg	Dosage not well established; following dosages suggested: IM 2–5 mg/kg in one dose IV 5 mg/kg over 1 min (undiluted); may be repeated with 10 mg/kg over 1 min (undiluted); may be repeated every 15–30 min to a maximum total dose of 30 mg/kg
Dofetilide (Tikosyn)	IV 500 mcg twice daily with creatinine clearance > 60 mL/min, adjusted to manage adverse effects	Safety and efficacy not established
Ibutilide (Corvert)	Weight ≥60 kg: IV infusion over 10 min, 1 mg Weight <60 kg: IV infusion over 10 min, 0.01 mg/kg The dose can be repeated once, after 10 min, if necessary.	Safety and efficacy not established

(continued)

Table 49-1 Drugs at a Glance: Antidysrhythmic Drugs (continued)

	ROUTES AND DOSAGE RANGES	
DRUGS FOR TACHYDYSRHYTHMIAS	**Adults**	**Children**
Sotalol (Betapace)	PO 80 mg q12h initially, titrated to response; average dose, 160–320 mg daily. See manufacturer's recommendations for dosing in renal failure.	Safety and efficacy not established
Class IV Calcium Channel Blockers Treatment of supraventricular tachycardia		
Diltiazem (Cardizem)	IV injection 0.25 mg/kg (average dose 20 mg) over 2 min. A second dose of 0.35 mg/kg (average, 25 mg) may be given in 15 min, and an IV infusion of 5–15 mg/h may be given up to 24 h, if necessary.	Safety and efficacy not established
Verapamil (Calan, Isoptin)	PO 40–120 mg q6–8h IV 5–10 mg initially, then 10 mg 30 min later, if necessary	*1–15 y:* IV injection 0.1–0.3 mg/kg (usual range 2–5 mg for a single dose) over 2 min with continuous ECG monitoring; repeat in 30 min if necessary *<1 y:* IV injection 0.1–0.2 mg/kg (usual range, 0.75–2.0 mg for a single dose) over 2 min with continuous ECG monitoring
Unclassified Adenosine is used to treat supraventricular tachycardia; magnesium sulfate is used to treat torsades de pointes		
Adenosine (Adenocard)	IV 6 mg given rapidly over 1–2 sec. If first dose does not slow the supraventricular tachycardia within 1–2 min, give 12 mg rapidly, and repeat one time, if necessary.	*Neonates:* Initial IV dose 0.05 mg/kg. If first dose does not slow the supraventricular tachycardia within 1–2 min, increase dose by 0.25 mg/kg. *Infants and children:* 0.1 mg/kg. If first dose does not slow the supraventricular tachycardia, give 0.2 mg/kg.
Magnesium sulfate	IV 1–2 g (2–4 mL of 50% solution), diluted in 10 mL of 5% dextrose solution	Safety and efficacy not established for treatment of torsades de pointes

ECG, electrocardiogram; IM, intramuscular; IV, intravenous; IVP, intravenous push; PO, oral.

Class IA

Class IA drugs have a broad spectrum of antidysrhythmic effects and are used for both supraventricular and ventricular dysrhythmias. P **Quinidine**, the prototype, reduces automaticity, slows conduction, and prolongs the refractory period. It has long been used to maintain NSR in clients with AF or flutter who have been converted to NSR with digoxin or electrical cardioversion. However, such use is declining because clients may have recurrent AF and have higher mortality rates with long-term quinidine therapy.

Quinidine is well absorbed after oral administration. Therapeutic serum levels (2–6 mcg/mL) are attained within 1 hour and persist for 6 to 8 hours. Quinidine is highly bound to serum albumin and has a half-life of about 6 hours. It is metabolized by the liver (about 80%) and excreted in the urine (about 20%). In alkaline urine (ie, pH > 7), renal excretion of quinidine decreases, and serum levels may rise. Serum levels greater than 8 micrograms per milliliter are toxic.

Quinidine's low therapeutic ratio and high incidence of adverse effects limit its clinical usefulness. The drug is usually contraindicated in clients with severe, uncompensated heart failure or with heart block because it depresses myocardial contractility and conduction through the AV node.

Quinidine salts used clinically include the generic forms of quinidine sulfate and quinidine gluconate. These salts differ in the amount of active drug (quinidine base) they contain and the rate of absorption with oral administration. The sulfate salt contains 83% quinidine base, and peak effects occur in 0.5 to 1.5 hours (4 hours for sustained-release forms). The gluconate salt contains 62% active drug, and peak effects occur in 3 to 4 hours. Quinidine preparations are usually given orally. The gluconate salt reportedly causes less gastrointestinal (GI) irritation than quinidine sulfate; this is probably related to its lower quinidine content.

Disopyramide is similar to quinidine in pharmacologic actions and may be given orally to adults with ventricular tachydysrhythmias. It is well absorbed after oral administration and reaches peak serum levels (2–8 mcg/mL) within 30 to 60 minutes. Drug half-life is 5 to 8 hours. Disopyramide is excreted by the kidneys and the liver in almost equal proportions. Dosage must be reduced in renal insufficiency.

Procainamide is related to the local anesthetic procaine and is similar to quinidine in actions and uses. Quinidine may be preferred for long-term use because procainamide produces a high incidence of adverse effects, including a syndrome resembling lupus erythematosus. Procainamide has a short duration of action (3–4 hours); sustained-release tablets (Procanbid) prolong action to about 6 hours. Therapeutic serum levels are 4 to 8 micrograms per milliliter.

Class IB

P **Lidocaine**, a local anesthetic (see Appendix F), is the prototype of class IB. It is the drug of choice for treating serious ventricular dysrhythmias associated with acute myocardial infarction, cardiac surgery, cardiac catheterization, and electrical cardioversion. Lidocaine decreases myocardial irritability (automaticity) in the ventricles. It has little effect on atrial tissue and is not useful in treating atrial dysrhythmias. It differs from quinidine in that

- It must be given by injection.
- It does not decrease AV conduction or myocardial contractility with usual therapeutic doses.
- It has a rapid onset and short duration of action. After intravenous (IV) administration of a bolus dose, therapeutic effects occur within 1 to 2 minutes and last approximately 20 minutes. This characteristic is advantageous in emergency management but limits lidocaine use to acute care settings.
- It is metabolized in the liver. Dosage must be reduced in clients with hepatic insufficiency or heart failure to avoid drug accumulation and toxicity.
- It is less likely to cause heart block, cardiac asystole, ventricular dysrhythmias, and heart failure.

Therapeutic serum levels of lidocaine are 2 to 5 micrograms per milliliter. Lidocaine may be given intramuscularly (IM) in emergencies when IV administration is impossible. When given IM, therapeutic effects occur in about 15 minutes and last about 90 minutes. Lidocaine is contraindicated in clients allergic to related local anesthetics (eg, procaine). Anaphylactic reactions may occur in sensitized individuals.

Mexiletine is an oral analog of lidocaine with similar pharmacologic actions. The drug is used to suppress ventricular fibrillation or ventricular tachycardia. It is well absorbed from the GI tract, and peak serum levels are obtained within

3 hours. Taking the drug with food delays but does not decrease absorption.

Phenytoin, an anticonvulsant (see Chap. 11), may be used to treat dysrhythmias produced by digoxin intoxication. Phenytoin decreases automaticity and improves conduction through the AV node. Decreased automaticity helps control dysrhythmias, whereas enhanced conduction may improve cardiac function. Further, because heart block may result from digoxin, quinidine, or procainamide, phenytoin may relieve dysrhythmias without intensifying heart block. Phenytoin is not a cardiac depressant. Its only quinidine-like action is to suppress automaticity; otherwise, it counteracts the effects of quinidine and procainamide largely by increasing the rate of conduction. Phenytoin also has a longer half-life (22–36 hours) than other antidysrhythmic drugs. Given IV, a therapeutic plasma level (10–20 mcg/mL) can be obtained rapidly. Given orally, however, the drug may not reach a steady-state concentration for approximately 1 week unless loading doses are given initially.

APPLYING YOUR KNOWLEDGE 49-1

You are assigned to care for Mr. Brown. He is prescribed lidocaine and started on IV lidocaine to control his PVCs. What therapeutic level should you monitor for?

Class IC

Flecainide and **propafenone** are oral agents that greatly decrease conduction in the ventricles. They may initiate new dysrhythmias or aggravate pre-existing dysrhythmias, sometimes causing sustained ventricular tachycardia or ventricular fibrillation. These effects are more likely to occur with high doses and rapid dose increases. The drugs are recommended for use only in life-threatening ventricular dysrhythmias.

Miscellaneous Class I Drug

Moricizine is a class I agent with properties of the other subclasses (ie, IA, IB, and IC). It is indicated for management of life-threatening ventricular dysrhythmias, such as sustained ventricular tachycardia, and contraindicated in clients with heart block, cardiogenic shock, and hypersensitivity reactions to the drug. After oral administration, onset of action occurs within 2 hours, and duration of action is 10 to 24 hours. The drug is 95% protein bound, extensively metabolized in the liver, and excreted in the urine. Because moricizine may cause new dysrhythmias or aggravate pre-existing dysrhythmias, therapy should be initiated in hospitalized clients with continuous electrocardiographic (ECG) monitoring.

Class II Beta-Adrenergic Blockers

These agents (see Chap. 18) exert antidysrhythmic effects by blocking sympathetic nervous system stimulation of beta receptors in the heart and decreasing risks of ventricular fibrillation.

Blockage of receptors in the SA node and ectopic pacemakers decreases automaticity, and blockage of receptors in the AV node increases the refractory period. The drugs are effective for management of supraventricular dysrhythmias and those resulting from excessive sympathetic activity. Thus, they are most often used to slow the ventricular rate of contraction in supraventricular tachydysrhythmias (eg, AF, atrial flutter, paroxysmal supraventricular tachycardia [PSVT]).

As a class, beta blockers are being used more extensively because of their effectiveness and their ability to reduce mortality in a variety of clinical settings, including post–myocardial infarction and heart failure. Reduced mortality may result from the drugs' ability to prevent ventricular fibrillation. Only four of the beta blockers marketed in the United States are approved by the Food and Drug Administration (FDA) for management of dysrhythmias.

Acebutolol may be given orally for chronic therapy to prevent ventricular dysrhythmias, especially those precipitated by exercise. **Esmolol** has a rapid onset and short duration of action. It is given IV for supraventricular tachydysrhythmias, especially during anesthesia, surgery, or other emergency situations when the ventricular rate must be reduced rapidly. It is not used for chronic therapy. **Propranolol** may be given orally for chronic therapy to prevent ventricular dysrhythmias, especially those precipitated by exercise. It may be given IV for life-threatening dysrhythmias or those occurring during anesthesia. **Sotalol** is a noncardioselective beta blocker (class II) that also has properties of class III antidysrhythmic drugs. Because its class III characteristics are considered more important in its antidysrhythmic effects, it is a class III drug (see next section).

Class III Potassium Channel Blockers

These drugs act to prolong duration of the action potential, slow repolarization, and prolong the refractory period in both atria and ventricles. Although the drugs share a common mechanism of action, they are very different drugs. As with beta blockers, clinical use of class III agents is increasing because they are associated with less ventricular fibrillation and decreased mortality compared with class I drugs.

Although classified as a potassium channel blocker, **amiodarone** also has electrophysiologic characteristics of sodium channel blockers, beta blockers, and calcium channel blockers. Thus, it has vasodilating effects and decreases systemic vascular resistance; it prolongs conduction in all cardiac tissues and decreases heart rate; and it decreases contractility of the left ventricle.

Intravenous and oral amiodarone differ in their electrophysiologic effects. When given IV, the major effect is slowing conduction through the AV node and prolonging the effective refractory period. Thus, it is given IV mainly for acute suppression of refractory, hemodynamically destabilizing ventricular tachycardia and ventricular fibrillation. The drug has assumed an increasing role as a preferred agent in the American Heart Association Advanced Cardiac Life Support (ACLS) algorithm for this purpose. It is given orally to treat recurrent ventricular tachycardia or ventricular fibrillation and to maintain an NSR after conversion of AF and flutter. Low doses (100–200 mg/day) may prevent recurrence of AF with less toxicity than higher doses of amiodarone or usual doses of other agents, including quinidine.

Amiodarone is extensively metabolized in the liver and produces active metabolites. The drug and its metabolites accumulate in the liver, lung, fat, skin, and other tissues. With IV administration, the onset of action usually occurs within several hours. With oral administration, the action may be delayed from a few days up to a week or longer. Because of its long serum half-life, loading doses are usually given and larger loading doses reduce the time required for therapeutic effects. Also, effects may persist for several weeks after the drug is discontinued.

Amiodarone is an iodine-rich drug that has been associated with thyroid dysfunction, with hypothyroidism occurring more frequently than hyperthyroidism. Other adverse effects include pulmonary fibrosis, myocardial depression, hypotension, bradycardia, hepatic dysfunction, central nervous system (CNS) disturbances (depression, insomnia, nightmares, hallucinations), peripheral neuropathy and muscle weakness, bluish discoloration of skin and corneal deposits that may cause photosensitivity, appearance of colored halos around lights, and reduced visual acuity. Most adverse effects are considered dose dependent and reversible.

When oral amiodarone is used long term, it also increases the effects of numerous drugs, including anticoagulants, beta blockers, calcium channel blockers, class I antidysrhythmics (quinidine, flecainide, lidocaine, procainamide), cyclosporine, digoxin, methotrexate, phenytoin, and theophylline.

Bretylium initially increases release of catecholamines and therefore increases heart rate, blood pressure, and myocardial contractility. This is followed in a few minutes by a decrease in vascular resistance, blood pressure, and heart rate. Bretylium previously has been used primarily in critical care settings for acute control of recurrent ventricular fibrillation, especially in clients with recent myocardial infarction. It is given by IV infusion, with a loading dose followed by a maintenance dose, or in repeated IV injections. However, bretylium has been eliminated from the ACLS protocol because of a lack of proven efficacy.

Because it is excreted almost entirely by the kidney, drug half-life is prolonged with renal impairment and dosage must be reduced. Adverse effects include hypotension and dysrhythmias.

Dofetilide is indicated for the maintenance of NSR in symptomatic clients who are in AF of more than 1 week's duration. Adverse effects increase with decreasing creatinine clearance levels so renal function must be assessed and initial dosage is dependent on creatinine clearance levels. High dosages in clients with renal dysfunction result in drug accumulation and prodysrhythmia (torsades de pointes). The drug has an elimination half-life of approximately 8 hours with the kidneys being the major route of elimination. The drug should initially be administered in a setting with personnel and equipment available for emergency use.

Ibutilide is indicated for management of recent onset of AF or atrial flutter, in which the goal is conversion to NSR. The drug enhances the efficacy of cardioversion. Ibutilide is structurally similar to sotalol but lacks clinically significant beta-blocking activity. Ibutilide is widely distributed and has an elimination half-life of about 6 hours. Most of a dose is metabolized, and the metabolites are excreted in urine and feces. Adverse effects include supraventricular and ventricular dysrhythmias (particularly torsades de pointes) and hypotension. Ibutilide should be administered in a setting with personnel and equipment available for emergency use.

Sotalol has both beta-adrenergic–blocking and potassium channel–blocking activity. Beta-blocking effects predominate at lower doses and class III effects predominate at higher doses. The drug is well absorbed after oral administration, and peak serum level is reached in 2 to 4 hours. It has an elimination half-life of approximately 12 hours, and 80% to 90% is excreted unchanged by the kidneys. Sotalol is approved for prevention or management of ventricular tachycardia and fibrillation. It has also been used, usually in smaller doses, to prevent or treat AF. However, it is less effective than amiodarone in the prophylaxis of AF. It is contraindicated in clients with asthma, sinus bradycardia, heart block, cardiogenic shock, heart failure, and previous hypersensitivity to sotalol. Dosage should be individualized, reduced with renal impairment, and increased slowly (eg, every 2 to 3 days with normal renal function, at longer intervals with impaired renal function). Dysrhythmogenic effects are most likely to occur when therapy is started or when dosage is increased. Heart failure may occur in clients with markedly depressed left ventricular systolic function. Most adverse effects are attributed to beta-blocking activity.

Like amiodarone, sotalol may be preferred over a class I agent because it is more effective in reducing recurrent ventricular tachycardia, ventricular fibrillation, and death.

APPLYING YOUR KNOWLEDGE 49-2

Mr. Brown's AF is converted to NSR pharmacologically. The physician prescribes amiodarone at 200 mg PO daily. Why is Mr. Brown given this drug and what adverse effects should you monitor?

Class IV Calcium Channel Blockers

Calcium channel blockers (see Chap. 50) block the movement of calcium into conductile and contractile myocardial cells. As antidysrhythmic agents, they act primarily against tachycardias at SA and AV nodes because the cardiac cells and slow channels that depend on calcium influx are found mainly at these sites. Thus, they reduce automaticity of the SA and AV nodes, slow conduction, and prolong the refractory period

in the AV node. They are effective only in supraventricular tachycardias.

Diltiazem and **verapamil** are the only calcium channel blockers approved for management of dysrhythmias. Both drugs may be given IV to terminate acute PSVT, usually within 2 minutes, and in AF and flutter. They are also effective in exercise-related tachycardias. When given IV, the drugs act within 15 minutes and last up to 6 hours. Oral verapamil may be used in the chronic management of the aforementioned dysrhythmias. Diltiazem and verapamil are metabolized by the liver, and metabolites are primarily excreted by the kidneys. The drugs are contraindicated in digoxin toxicity because they may worsen heart block. If used with propranolol or digoxin, caution must be exercised to avoid further impairment of myocardial contractility. *Do not* use IV verapamil with IV propranolol; potentially fatal bradycardia and hypotension may occur.

Unclassified Drugs

Adenosine, a naturally occurring component of all body cells, differs chemically from other antidysrhythmic drugs but acts like the calcium channel blockers. It depresses conduction at the AV node and is used to restore NSR in clients with PSVT; it is ineffective in other dysrhythmias. The drug has a very short duration of action (serum half-life is less than 10 seconds) and a high degree of effectiveness. It must be given by a rapid bolus injection, preferably through a central venous line. If given slowly, it is eliminated before it can reach cardiac tissues and exert its action.

Magnesium sulfate is given IV in the management of several dysrhythmias, including prevention of recurrent episodes of torsades de pointes and management of digitalis-induced dysrhythmias. Its antidysrhythmic effects may derive from imbalances of magnesium, potassium, and calcium.

Hypomagnesemia increases myocardial irritability and is a risk factor for both atrial and ventricular dysrhythmias. Thus, serum magnesium levels should be monitored in clients at risk and replacement therapy instituted when indicated. However, in some instances, the drug seems to have antidysrhythmic effects even when serum magnesium levels are normal.

NURSING PROCESS

Assessment

Assess the client's condition in relation to cardiac dysrhythmias.

- Identify conditions or risk factors that may precipitate dysrhythmias. These include the following:
  - Hypoxia
  - Electrolyte imbalances (eg, hypokalemia, hypomagnesemia)
  - Acid–base imbalances

- Ischemic heart disease (angina pectoris, myocardial infarction)
- Cardiac valvular disease
- Febrile illness
- Respiratory disorders (eg, chronic lung disease)
- Exercise
- Emotional upset
- Excessive ingestion of caffeine-containing beverages (eg, coffee, tea, colas)
- Cigarette smoking
- Drug therapy with digoxin, antidysrhythmic drugs, CNS stimulants, anorexiants, and tricyclic antidepressants
- Hyperthyroidism
- Observe for clinical signs and symptoms of dysrhythmias. Mild or infrequent dysrhythmias may be perceived by the client as palpitations or skipped heartbeats. More severe dysrhythmias may produce manifestations that reflect decreased cardiac output and other hemodynamic changes, as follows:
  - Hypotension, bradycardia or tachycardia, and irregular pulse
  - Shortness of breath, dyspnea, and cough from impaired respiration
  - Syncope or mental confusion from reduced cerebral blood flow
  - Chest pain from decreased coronary artery blood flow. Angina pectoris or myocardial infarction may occur.
  - Oliguria from decreased renal blood flow
- When ECG monitoring is available (eg, 12-lead ECG or continuous ECG monitoring), assess for indications of dysrhythmias.

Nursing Diagnoses

- Decreased Cardiac Output related to ineffective pumping action of the heart
- Ineffective Tissue Perfusion, cerebral and peripheral, related to compromised cardiac output or drug-induced hypotension
- Activity Intolerance related to weakness and fatigue
- Impaired Gas Exchange related to decreased tissue perfusion
- Anxiety related to potentially serious illness
- Deficient Knowledge: Pharmacologic and nonpharmacologic management of dysrhythmias
- Excess Fluid Volume: Peripheral edema and pulmonary congestion related to decreased cardiac output

Planning/Goals

The client will

- Receive or take antidysrhythmic drugs accurately
- Avoid conditions that precipitate dysrhythmias, when feasible

- Experience improved heart rate, circulation, and activity tolerance
- Be closely monitored for therapeutic and adverse drug effects
- Avoid preventable adverse drug effects
- Have adverse drug effects promptly recognized and treated if they occur
- Keep follow-up appointments for monitoring responses to treatment measures

Interventions

Use measures to prevent or minimize dysrhythmias.

- Treat underlying disease processes that contribute to dysrhythmia development. These include cardiovascular (eg, acute myocardial infarction) and noncardiovascular (eg, chronic lung disease) disorders.
- Prevent or treat other conditions that predispose to dysrhythmias (eg, hypoxia, electrolyte imbalance).
- Help the client avoid cigarette smoking, overeating, excessive coffee drinking, and other habits that may cause or aggravate dysrhythmias. Long-term supervision and counseling may be needed.
- For the client receiving antidysrhythmic drugs, implement the preceding measures to minimize the incidence and severity of acute dysrhythmias, and help the client comply with drug therapy.
- Monitor heart rate and rhythm and blood pressure every 4 to 6 hours.
- Check laboratory reports of serum electrolytes and serum drug levels when available. Report abnormal values.

Provide appropriate client teaching related to drug therapy (see accompanying display).

Evaluation

- Check vital signs for improved heart rate and rhythm.
- Interview and observe for relief of symptoms and improved functioning in activities of daily living.
- Interview and observe for hypotension and other adverse drug effects.
- Interview and observe for compliance with instructions for taking antidysrhythmic drugs and other aspects of care.

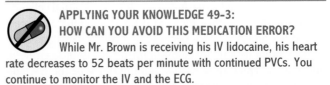

APPLYING YOUR KNOWLEDGE 49-3:
HOW CAN YOU AVOID THIS MEDICATION ERROR?
While Mr. Brown is receiving his IV lidocaine, his heart rate decreases to 52 beats per minute with continued PVCs. You continue to monitor the IV and the ECG.

General Considerations

☑ A fast heartbeat normally occurs in response to exercise, fever, and other conditions so that more blood can be pumped and carried to body tissues. An irregular heartbeat occurs occasionally in most individuals. However, when you are prescribed a long-term medication to slow or regularize your heartbeat, this means that you have a potentially serious condition. In addition, the medications can cause potentially serious adverse effects. Thus, it is extremely important that you take the medications exactly as prescribed. Taking extra doses is dangerous; skipping doses or waiting longer between doses may lead to loss of control of the heart problem.

☑ You may be given a drug classified as an antidysrhythmic or a drug from another group that has antidysrhythmic effects (eg, a beta blocker such as propranolol, a calcium channel blocker such as verapamil or diltiazem, or digoxin). Instructions should be provided for the specific drug ordered.

☑ Be sure you know the names (generic and brand) of the medication, why you are receiving it, and what effects you can expect (therapeutic and adverse).

☑ You will need continued medical supervision, along with periodic measurements of heart rate and blood pressure, blood tests, and electrocardiograms.

☑ Try to learn the triggers for your irregular heartbeats and avoid them when possible (eg, excessive caffeinated beverages, strenuous or excessive exercise).

☑ Avoid over-the-counter cold and asthma remedies, appetite suppressants, and antisleep preparations. These drugs are stimulants that can cause or aggravate irregular heartbeats.

Self- or Caregiver Administration

☑ Take or give medications at evenly spaced intervals to maintain adequate blood levels.

☑ Take or give amiodarone, mexiletine, and quinidine with food to decrease gastrointestinal symptoms.

☑ Do not crush or chew sustained-release tablets or capsules.

☑ Report dizziness or fainting spells. This may mean the medication is decreasing your blood pressure, which is more likely to occur when starting or increasing the dose of an antidysrhythmic drug. Drug dosage may need to be adjusted.

PRINCIPLES OF THERAPY

Nonpharmacologic Management of Dysrhythmias

Nonpharmacologic management is preferred, at least initially, for several dysrhythmias. For example, sinus tachycardia usually results from such disorders as infection, dehydration, or hypotension and management should attempt to relieve the underlying cause. For PSVT with mild or moderate symptoms, Valsalva's maneuver, carotid sinus massage, or other measures to increase vagal tone are preferred. For ventricular fibrillation, immediate defibrillation by electrical countershock is the initial management of choice.

In addition to these strategies, others are being increasingly used. The impetus for nonpharmacologic management developed mainly from studies demonstrating that antidysrhythmic drugs could worsen existing dysrhythmias, cause new dysrhythmias, and cause higher mortality rates in clients receiving the drugs than clients not receiving the drugs. Current technology allows clinicians to insert pacemakers and defibrillators (eg, ICD) to control bradydysrhythmias or tachydysrhythmias and to use radio waves (radiofrequency catheter ablation) or surgery to deactivate ectopic foci.

Pharmacologic Management of Dysrhythmias

Rational drug therapy for cardiac dysrhythmias requires accurate identification of the dysrhythmia, understanding of the basic mechanisms causing the dysrhythmia, observation of the hemodynamic and ECG effects of the dysrhythmia, knowledge of the pharmacologic actions of specific antidysrhythmic drugs, and the expectation that therapeutic effects will outweigh potential adverse effects. Even when these criteria are met, antidysrhythmic drug therapy is somewhat empiric. Although some dysrhythmias usually respond to particular drugs, different drugs or combinations of drugs are often required. General trends and guidelines for drug therapy of supraventricular and ventricular dysrhythmias are described in the following sections. General trends include:

● There is a relative consensus of opinion among clinicians about appropriate management for acute, symptomatic dysrhythmias, in which the goals are to abolish the abnormal rhythm, restore NSR, and prevent recurrence of the dysrhythmia. There is less agreement about long-term use of the drugs, which is probably indicated only for clients who experience recurrent symptomatic episodes.

● Class I agents do not prolong survival in any group of clients and their use is declining. For example, quinidine is no longer recommended to slow heart rate or prevent recurrence of AF. Some clinicians recommend restricting this class to clients without structural heart disease, who are less likely to experience increased mortality than others.

- Class II and class III drugs are being used increasingly, because of demonstrated benefits in relieving symptoms and decreasing mortality rates in clients with heart disease.

Treatment of Supraventricular Tachydysrhythmias

- **Propranolol** and other beta blockers are being increasingly used for tachydysrhythmias, especially in clients with myocardial infarction, heart failure, or exercise-induced dysrhythmias. In addition to controlling dysrhythmias, the drugs decrease the mortality rate in these clients. Also, a beta blocker is the management of choice if a rapid heart rate is causing angina or other symptoms in a client with known coronary artery disease.

- **Atrial fibrillation** is the most common dysrhythmia. Management may involve conversion to NSR by electrical or pharmacologic means or long-term drug therapy to slow the rate of ventricular response. Advantages of conversion to NSR include improvement of symptoms and decreased risks of heart failure or thromboembolic problems. If pharmacologic conversion is chosen, IV **adenosine, dofetilide, ibutilide, verapamil,** or **diltiazem** may be used. After being converted to NSR, clients usually require long-term drug therapy. Low-dose **amiodarone** seems to be emerging as the drug of choice for preventing recurrent AF after electrical or pharmacologic conversion. The low doses cause fewer adverse effects than the higher ones used for life-threatening ventricular dysrhythmias.

  When clients are not converted to NSR, drugs are given to slow the heart rate. This strategy is used for clients who
  - Have chronic AF but are asymptomatic
  - Have had AF for longer than 1 year
  - Are elderly
  - Have not responded to multiple drugs

  In addition to amiodarone, other drugs used to slow the heart rate include a **beta blocker, digoxin, verapamil,** or **diltiazem.** In most clients, a beta blocker, verapamil, or diltiazem may be preferred. In clients with heart failure, digoxin may be preferred. In addition, the class IC agents **flecainide** or **propafenone** may be used to suppress paroxysmal atrial flutter and fibrillation in clients with minimal or no heart disease.

- IV **adenosine, ibutilide, verapamil,** or **diltiazem** may be used to convert PSVT to an NSR. These drugs block conduction across the AV node.

Treatment of Ventricular Dysrhythmias

- Treatment of asymptomatic PVCs and nonsustained ventricular tachycardia (formerly standard practice with lidocaine in clients who are post–myocardial infarction) is not recommended.

- A **beta blocker** may be preferred as a first-line drug for symptomatic ventricular dysrhythmias. **Amiodarone, flecainide, propafenone,** and **sotalol** are also used in the management of life-threatening ventricular dysrhythmias, such as sustained ventricular tachycardia. The use of **bretylium** for the management of ventricular dysrhythmias is on the decline. Class I agents (eg, **lidocaine, mexiletine**) may be used in clients with structurally normal hearts. Lidocaine may also be used for treating digoxin-induced ventricular dysrhythmias.

- **Amiodarone, sotalol,** or a **beta blocker** may be used to prevent recurrence of ventricular tachycardia or fibrillation in clients resuscitated from cardiac arrest.

- **Moricizine** is infrequently used in the United States because of its potential for causing undesirable cardiac events. It may be used to treat life-threatening ventricular dysrhythmias (eg, sustained ventricular tachycardia) that have not responded to safer drugs.

Use in Special Populations

Use in Children

Antidysrhythmic drugs are less often needed in children than in adults, and their use has decreased with increased use of catheter ablative techniques. Catheter ablation uses radio waves to destroy dysrhythmia-producing foci in cardiac tissue and reportedly causes fewer adverse effects and complications than long-term antidysrhythmic drug therapy.

Antidysrhythmic drug therapy is also less clear-cut in children. The only antidysrhythmic drug that is FDA approved for use in children is digoxin. However, pediatric cardiologists have used various drugs and developed guidelines for their use, especially dosages. As with adults, the drugs should be used only when clearly indicated, and children should be monitored closely because all of the drugs can cause adverse effects, including hypotension and new or worsened dysrhythmias.

Supraventricular tachydysrhythmias are the most common sustained dysrhythmias in children. IV **adenosine, digoxin, procainamide,** or **propranolol** can be used acutely to terminate supraventricular tachydysrhythmias. IV verapamil, which is often used in adults to terminate supraventricular tachydysrhythmias, is contraindicated in infants and small children. Although it can be used cautiously in older children, some clinicians recommend that IV verapamil be avoided in the pediatric population. **Digoxin** or a beta blocker may be used for long-term management of supraventricular tachydysrhythmias.

Propranolol is the beta blocker most commonly used in children. It is one of the few antidysrhythmic drugs available in a liquid solution. Propranolol has a shorter half-life (3–4 hours) in infants than in children older than 1 to 2 years of age and adults (6 hours). When given IV, antidysrhythmic effects are rapid, and clients require careful monitoring for bradycardia and hypotension. **Esmolol** is being used more frequently to treat tachydysrhythmias in children, especially those occurring after surgery.

Lidocaine may be used to treat ventricular dysrhythmias precipitated by cardiac surgery or digitalis toxicity. Class I or III drugs are usually started in a hospital setting, at lower dosage ranges, because of prodysrhythmic effects. Prodysrhythmia is more common in children with structural heart disease or significant dysrhythmias. In general, serum levels should be monitored with class IA and IC drugs and IV lidocaine. Flecainide is the class IC drug most commonly used in children. Class III drugs are used in pediatrics mainly to treat life-threatening refractory tachydysrhythmias.

As in adults, most antidysrhythmic drugs and their metabolites are excreted through the kidneys and may accumulate in children with impaired renal function.

Use in Older Adults

Cardiac dysrhythmias are common in older adults, but in general only those causing symptoms of circulatory impairment should be treated with antidysrhythmic drugs. Compared with younger adults, older adults are more likely to experience serious adverse drug effects, including aggravation of existing dysrhythmias, production of new dysrhythmias, hypotension, and heart failure. Cautious use is required, and dosage usually needs to be reduced to compensate for heart disease or impaired drug-elimination processes.

Use in Clients With Renal Impairment

Antidysrhythmic drug therapy in clients with renal impairment should be very cautious, with close monitoring of drug effects (eg, plasma drug levels, ECG changes, symptoms that may indicate drug toxicity). The kidneys excrete most antidysrhythmic drugs and their metabolites. As a result, decreased renal perfusion or other renal impairment can reduce drug elimination and lead to accumulation and adverse effects if dosage is not reduced. As a general rule, dosage of bretylium, digoxin, disopyramide, flecainide, lidocaine, moricizine, procainamide, propafenone, quinidine, and sotalol should be reduced in clients with significant impairment of renal function. Dosage of adenosine, amiodarone, ibutilide, and mexiletine does not require reduction.

Use in Clients With Hepatic Impairment

As with renal impairment, antidysrhythmic drug therapy in clients with hepatic impairment should be very cautious, with close monitoring of drug effects (eg, plasma drug levels, ECG changes, symptoms that may indicate drug toxicity).

Amiodarone may be hepatotoxic and cause serious, sometimes fatal, liver disease. Hepatic enzyme levels are often elevated without accompanying symptoms of liver impairment. However, liver enzymes should be monitored regularly, especially in clients receiving relatively high maintenance doses. If enzyme levels are above three times the normal range or double in a client whose baseline levels were elevated, dosage reduction or drug discontinuation should be considered.

Hepatic impairment increases plasma half-life of several antidysrhythmic drugs, and dosage usually should be reduced. These drugs include disopyramide, flecainide, lidocaine, mexiletine, moricizine, procainamide, propafenone, quinidine, and tocainide.

Dosages of adenosine and ibutilide are unlikely to need reductions in clients with hepatic impairment.

Use in Clients With Critical Illness

Critically ill clients often have multiple cardiovascular and other disorders that increase their risks for development of acute, serious, and potentially life-threatening dysrhythmias. They may also have refractory dysrhythmias that require strong, potentially toxic antidysrhythmic drugs. Thus, antidysrhythmic drugs are often given IV in critical care settings for rapid reversal of a fast rhythm. After reversal, IV or oral drugs may be given to prevent recurrence of the dysrhythmia.

Because serious problems may stem from either dysrhythmias or their treatment, health care providers should be adept in preventing, recognizing, and treating conditions that predispose to the development of serious dysrhythmias (eg, electrolyte imbalances, hypoxia). If dysrhythmias cannot be prevented, early recognition and treatment are needed.

Overall, any antidysrhythmic drug therapy in critically ill clients is preferably performed or at least initiated in critical care units or other facilities with appropriate equipment and personnel. For example, nurses who work in emergency departments or critical care units must be certified in cardiopulmonary resuscitation and ACLS. With ACLS, the American Heart Association and others have developed algorithms to guide drug therapy of dysrhythmias.

Use in Home Care

Clients receiving chronic antidysrhythmic drug therapy are likely to have significant cardiovascular disease. With each visit, the home care nurse needs to assess the client's physical, mental, and functional status and evaluate pulse and blood pressure. In addition, clients and caregivers should be taught to report symptoms (eg, dizziness or fainting, chest pain) and avoid over-the-counter drugs unless discussed with a health care provider.

N U R S I N G   A C T I O N S

Antidysrhythmic Drugs

NURSING ACTIONS	RATIONALE/EXPLANATION
1. Administer accurately	
a. Check apical and radial pulses before each dose. Withhold the dose and report to the physician if marked changes are noted in rate, rhythm, or quality of pulses.	Bradycardia may indicate impending heart block or cardiovascular collapse.
b. Check blood pressure at least once daily in hospitalized clients.	To detect hypotension, which is most likely to occur when antidysrhythmic drug therapy is being initiated or altered
c. During intravenous (IV) administration of antidysrhythmic drugs, maintain continuous cardiac monitoring and check blood pressure about every 5 minutes.	For early detection of hypotension and impending cardiac collapse. These drug side effects are more likely to occur with IV use.
d. Give oral drugs at evenly spaced intervals.	To maintain adequate blood levels
e. With oral amiodarone, give once daily or in two divided doses if stomach upset occurs.	
f. With IV amiodarone, mix and give loading and maintenance infusions according to the manufacturer's instructions.	Specific instructions are required for accurate mixing and administration, partly because concentrations and infusion rates vary. The drug should be given in a critical care setting, by experienced personnel, preferably through a central venous catheter.
g. Give mexiletine and quinidine with food.	To decrease gastrointestinal (GI) symptoms
h. Give lidocaine parenterally only, as a bolus injection or a continuous drip. Use only solutions labeled "For cardiac dysrhythmias," and do not use solutions containing epinephrine. Give an IV bolus over 2 minutes.	Lidocaine solutions that contain epinephrine are used for local anesthesia only. They should never be given intravenously to clients with cardiac dysrhythmias because the epinephrine can cause or aggravate dysrhythmias. Rapid injection (within approximately 30 sec) produces transient blood levels several times greater than therapeutic range limits. Therefore, there is increased risk of toxicity without a concomitant increase in therapeutic effectiveness.
2. Observe for therapeutic effects	
a. Conversion to normal sinus rhythm	After a single oral dose, peak plasma levels are reached in approximately 1–4 hours with quinidine, procainamide, and propranolol and in 6–12 hours with phenytoin. Equilibrium between plasma and tissue levels is reached in 1 or 2 days with quinidine, procainamide, and propranolol; in approximately 1 week with phenytoin; in 1–3 weeks with amiodarone; and in just a few minutes with IV lidocaine.
b. Improvement in rate, rhythm, and quality of apical and radial pulses and the electrocardiogram (ECG)	
c. Signs of increased cardiac output—blood pressure near normal range, urine output more adequate, no complaints of dizziness	
d. Serum drug levels (mcg/mL) within therapeutic ranges (Table 49-2)	Serum drug levels must be interpreted in light of the client's clinical status.
3. Observe for adverse effects	
a. Heart block—may be indicated on the ECG by a prolonged PR interval, prolonged QRS complex, or absence of P waves	Owing to depressant effects on the cardiac conduction system
b. Dysrhythmias—aggravation of existing dysrhythmia, tachycardia, bradycardia, premature ventricular contractions, ventricular tachycardia or fibrillation	Because they affect the cardiac conduction system, antidysrhythmic drugs may worsen existing dysrhythmias or cause new dysrhythmias.
c. Hypotension	Owing to decreased cardiac output
d. Additional adverse effects with specific drugs:	
(1) Disopyramide—mouth dryness, blurred vision, urinary retention, other anticholinergic effects	These effects commonly occur.

NURSING ACTIONS	RATIONALE/EXPLANATION

TABLE 49-2 Therapeutic Serum Drug Level Ranges of Common Antidysrhythmics

DRUG	THERAPEUTIC RANGE (mcg/mL)
Class IA	
Disopyramide	2–8
Procainamide	4–8
Quinidine	2–6
Class IB	
Lidocaine	1.5–6
Mexiletine	0.5–2
Phenytoin	10–20
Tocainide	4–10
Class IC	
Flecainide	0.2–1
Propafenone	0.06–1
Class II	
Propranolol	0.05–0.1
Class III	
Amiodarone	0.5–2.5
Bretylium	0.5–1.5
Class IV	
Verapamil	0.08–0.3

(2) Lidocaine—drowsiness, paresthesias, muscle twitching, convulsions, changes in mental status (eg, confusion), hypersensitivity reactions (eg, urticaria, edema, anaphylaxis)

Most adverse reactions result from drug effects on the central nervous system (CNS). Convulsions are most likely to occur with high doses. Hypersensitivity reactions may occur in individuals who are allergic to related local anesthetic agents.

(3) Phenytoin—nystagmus, ataxia, slurring of speech, tremors, drowsiness, confusion, gingival hyperplasia

CNS changes are caused by depressant effects.

(4) Propranolol—weakness or dizziness, especially with activity or exercise

The beta-adrenergic blocking action of propranolol blocks the normal sympathetic nervous system response to activity and exercise. Clients may have symptoms caused by deficient blood supply to body tissues.

(5) Quinidine—hypersensitivity, cinchonism (tinnitus, vomiting, severe diarrhea, vertigo, headache), and torsades de pointes

These are the most frequent adverse effects.

(6) Tocainide—lightheadedness, dizziness, nausea, paresthesia, tremor

4. **Observe for drug interactions**

a. Drugs that *increase* effects of antidysrhythmics:

These drugs may potentiate therapeutic effects or increase risk of toxicity.

(1) Antidysrhythmic agents

When antidysrhythmic drugs are combined, there are additive cardiac depressant effects.

(continued)

NURSING ACTIONS	RATIONALE/EXPLANATION
(2) Antihypertensives, diuretics, phenothiazine antipsychotic agents	Additive hypotension
(3) Cimetidine	Increases effects by inhibiting hepatic metabolism of quinidine, procainamide, lidocaine, tocainide, flecainide, and phenytoin
b. Drugs that *decrease* effects of antidysrhythmic agents:	
(1) Atropine sulfate	Atropine is used to reverse propranolol-induced bradycardia.
(2) Phenytoin, rifampin	Decrease effects by inducing drug-metabolizing enzymes in the liver and accelerating the metabolism of quinidine, disopyramide, and mexiletine

APPLYING YOUR KNOWLEDGE: ANSWERS

49-1 The normal therapeutic serum level of lidocaine is 2 to 5 mcg/mL. The risk of adverse effects is reduced when the drug is administered within the therapeutic range. Lidocaine will also not decrease AV conduction or myocardial contractility with therapeutic doses.

49-2 The amiodarone is given to prevent the recurrence of AF and at this low dose it has less toxicity. You should monitor for thyroid dysfunction, pulmonary fibrosis, myocardial depression, hypotension, bradycardia, hepatic dysfunction, CNS disturbances, peripheral neuropathy, bluish discoloration of the skin, and reduced visual acuity.

49-3 Bradycardia may indicate impending heart block or cardiovascular collapse. You should stop the IV infusion and report to the physician if there are marked changes in the rate, rhythm, or quality of the pulse.

Review and Application Exercises

Short Answer Exercises

1. Which tissues in the heart are able to generate an electrical impulse and therefore serve as a pacemaker?

2. What risk factors predispose a client to development of dysrhythmias?

3. Name interventions that clients or health care providers can perform to decrease risks of dysrhythmias.

4. Differentiate the hemodynamic effects of common dysrhythmias.

5. What are the classes of antidysrhythmic drugs?

6. How do beta-adrenergic blocking agents act on the conduction system to slow heart rate?

7. What are common and potentially serious adverse effects of antidysrhythmic drugs?

NCLEX-Style Questions

8. The clinical use of class III agents is increasing because they are associated with
   a. less ventricular fibrillation
   b. increased mortality
   c. more sustained effects
   d. mild adverse effects

9. A patient being monitored in the critical care unit has been receiving quinidine. The nurse notes that the patient's serum quinidine level is 8 mcg/mL, and the patient has developed diarrhea. The most appropriate action by the nurse is to
   a. Hold the medication and report the findings to the health care prescriber immediately.
   b. Administer the medication as ordered.
   c. Anticipate that the dosage of the medication will be increased.
   d. Anticipate that the dosage of the medication will be decreased.

10. Mr. Conley, age 53, is about to be discharged from the hospital after treatment for recurrent ventricular fibrillation unresponsive to other agents. To prevent further ventricular ectopy, the health care provider prescribes amiodarone (Cordarone), 1000 mg PO daily as a loading dose for 2 weeks. Why is such a large loading dose required?
   a. Most of the drug is destroyed in the GI tract.
   b. Males require larger dosages because of their faster metabolisms.
   c. A history of ventricular dysrhythmia necessitates a higher dose.
   d. The drug has a long serum half-life.

11. Phenytoin, an anticonvulsant, may be used to treat dysrhythmias produced by
  a. digoxin toxicity
  b. quinidine intoxication
  c. lidocaine overdose
  d. procainamide toxicity

12. Ms. Ferguson, age 58, is admitted to the coronary care unit for treatment of an acute anterior myocardial infarction. That evening, she experiences frequent runs of ventricular tachycardia. The health care provider tells the nurse to prepare an IV bolus dose of lidocaine. Why is lidocaine administered IV instead of orally?
  a. Lidocaine absorption is too erratic when administered orally.
  b. Lidocaine is inactivated by hydrochloric acid.
  c. Most of an absorbed oral dose undergoes first-pass metabolism in the liver.
  d. Onset of action for oral lidocaine is over 8 hours.

Selected References

Bauman, J. L., & Schoen, M. D. (2002). The arrhythmias. In J. T. DiPiro, R. L. Talbert, G. C. Yee, G. R. Matzke, B. G. Wells, & L. M. Posey (Eds.), *Pharmacotherapy: A pathophysiologic approach* (5th ed., pp. 273–304). New York: McGraw-Hill.

Brater, D. C. (2000). Clinical pharmacology of cardiovascular drugs. In H. D. Humes (Ed.), *Kelley's Textbook of internal medicine* (4th ed., pp. 651–672). Philadelphia: Lippincott Williams & Wilkins.

Drug facts and comparisons. (Updated monthly). St. Louis: Facts and Comparisons.

Faddis, M. N. (2001). Cardiac arrhythmias. In S. N. Ahya, K. Flood, & S. Paranjothi (Eds.), *The Washington manual of medical therapeutics* (30th ed., pp. 96–130). Philadelphia: Lippincott Williams & Wilkins.

Feller, D. B., & Grauer, K. (2002). Atrial fibrillation: How best to use rate control and anticoagulation. *Consultant, 42*(4), 526–531.

Guyton, A. C., & Hall, J. E. (2000). *Textbook of medical physiology* (10th ed.). Philadelphia: W. B. Saunders.

Haugh, K. H. (2002). Antidysrhythmic agents at the turn of the twenty-first century: A current review. *Critical Care Nursing Clinics of North America, 14*(1), 53–69.

Kern, K. B., Halperin, H. R., & Field, J. (2001). New guidelines for cardio-pulmonary resuscitation and emergency cardiac care: Changes in the management of cardiac arrest. *Journal of the American Medical Association, 285*(10):1267–1269.

Winters, J. M. (2005). Cardiac conduction and rhythm disorders. In C. M. Porth, *Pathophysiology: Concepts of altered health states* (7th ed., pp. 581–601). Philadelphia: Lippincott Williams & Wilkins.

Antianginal Drugs

OBJECTIVES

After studying this chapter, you will be able to:

1. Describe the types, causes, and effects of angina pectoris.
2. Describe general characteristics and types of antianginal drugs.
3. Discuss nitrate antianginals in terms of indications for use, routes of administration, adverse effects, nursing process implications, and drug tolerance.
4. Differentiate between short-acting and long-acting dosage forms of nitrate antianginal drugs.
5. Discuss calcium channel blockers in terms of their effects on body tissues, clinical indications for use, common adverse effects, and nursing process implications.
6. Teach clients ways to prevent, minimize, or manage acute anginal attacks.

APPLYING YOUR KNOWLEDGE

Richard Gerald is a 72-year-old man with a history of hypertension, coronary artery disease (CAD), and a myocardial infarction (MI). He stopped smoking and began a regular exercise program after his MI.

INTRODUCTION

Angina pectoris is a clinical syndrome characterized by episodes of chest pain. It occurs when there is a deficit in myocardial oxygen supply (myocardial ischemia) in relation to myocardial oxygen demand. It is most often caused by atherosclerotic plaque in the coronary arteries but may also be caused by coronary vasospasm. The development and progression of atherosclerotic plaque is called *coronary artery disease* (CAD). Atherosclerotic plaque narrows the lumen, decreases elasticity, and impairs dilation of coronary arteries. The result is impaired blood flow to the myocardium, especially with exercise or other factors that increase the cardiac workload and need for oxygen.

The continuum of CAD progresses from angina to myocardial infarction (MI). There are three main types of angina: classic angina, variant angina, and unstable angina (Box 50-1). The Canadian Cardiovascular Society classifies clients with angina according to the amount of physical activity they can tolerate before anginal pain occurs (Box 50-2). These categories can assist in clinical assessment and evaluation of therapy.

Classic anginal pain is usually described as substernal chest pain of a constricting, squeezing, or suffocating nature. It may radiate to the jaw, neck, or shoulder; down the left or both arms; or to the back. The discomfort is sometimes mistaken for arthritis, or for indigestion, because the pain may be associated with nausea, vomiting, dizziness, diaphoresis, shortness of breath, or fear of impending doom. The discomfort is usually brief, typically lasting 5 minutes or less until the balance of oxygen supply and demand is restored.

Current research indicates that gender differences exist in the type and quality of cardiac symptoms, with women reporting epigastric or back discomfort. Additionally, older adults may have atypical symptoms of CAD and may experience "silent" ischemia that may delay them from seeking professional help. Individuals with diabetes mellitus may present without classic angina, although they may experience related symptoms. The American Heart Association has released guidelines for the management of angina.

Box 50-1 Types of Angina Pectoris

Classic

Classic angina (also called *stable, typical,* or *exertional angina*) occurs when atherosclerotic plaque obstructs coronary arteries and the heart requires more oxygenated blood than the blocked arteries can deliver. Chest pain is usually precipitated by situations that increase the workload of the heart, such as physical exertion, exposure to cold, and emotional upset. Recurrent episodes of classic angina usually have the same pattern of onset, duration, and intensity of symptoms. Pain is usually relieved by rest, a fast-acting preparation of nitroglycerin, or both.

Variant

Variant angina (also called *atypical, Prinzmetal's,* or *vasospastic angina*) is caused by spasms of the coronary artery that decrease blood flow to the myocardium. The spasms occur most often in coronary arteries that are already partly blocked by atherosclerotic plaque. Variant angina usually occurs during rest or with minimal exercise and often occurs at night. It often occurs at the same time each day. Pain is usually relieved by nitroglycerin. Long-term management includes avoidance of conditions that precipitate vasospasm, when possible (eg, exposure to cold, smoking, and emotional stress), as well as antianginal drugs.

Unstable

Unstable angina (also called *rest, preinfarction,* and *crescendo angina*) is a type of myocardial ischemia that falls between classic angina and myocardial infarction. It usually occurs in clients with advanced coronary atherosclerosis and produces increased frequency, intensity, and duration of symptoms. It often leads to myocardial infarction.

Unstable angina usually develops when a minor injury ruptures atherosclerotic plaque. The resulting injury to the endothelium causes platelets to aggregate at the site of injury, form a thrombus, and release chemical mediators that cause vasoconstriction (eg, thromboxane, serotonin, platelet-derived growth factor). The disrupted plaque, thrombus, and vasoconstriction combine to obstruct blood flow further in the affected coronary artery. When the plaque injury is mild, blockage of the coronary artery may be intermittent and cause silent myocardial ischemia or episodes of anginal pain at rest. Thrombus formation and vasoconstriction may progress until the coronary artery is completely occluded, producing myocardial infarction. Endothelial injury, with subsequent thrombus formation and vasoconstriction, may also result from therapeutic procedures (eg, angioplasty, atherectomy).

The Agency for Healthcare Research and Quality, in its clinical practice guidelines for the management of angina, defines unstable angina as meeting one or more of the following criteria:

- Anginal pain at rest that usually lasts longer than 20 minutes
- Recent onset (<2 months) of exertional angina of at least Canadian Cardiovascular Society Classification (CCSC) class III severity
- Recent (<2 months) increase in severity as indicated by progression to at least CCSC class III

However, myocardial ischemia may also be painless or silent in a substantial number of clients. Overall, the diagnosis is usually based on chest pain history, electrocardiographic evidence of ischemia, and other signs of impaired cardiac function (eg, heart failure).

Because unstable angina often occurs hours or days before acute myocardial infarction, early recognition and effective management are extremely important in preventing progression to infarction, heart failure, or sudden cardiac death.

Numerous overlapping factors contribute to the development and progression of CAD. To aid understanding of drug therapy for angina, these factors are described in the following sections.

Coronary Atherosclerosis

Atherosclerosis (see Chap. 47) begins with accumulation of lipid-filled macrophages (ie, foam cells) on the inner lining of coronary arteries. Foam cells, which promote growth of atherosclerotic plaque, develop in response to elevated blood cholesterol levels. Initially, white blood cells (monocytes) become attached to the endothelium and move through the endothelial layer into subendothelial spaces, where they ingest lipid and become foam cells. These early lesions progress to fibrous plaques containing foam cells covered by smooth muscle cells and connective tissue. Advanced lesions also contain hemorrhages, ulcerations, and scar tissue. Factors contributing

Box 50-2 Canadian Cardiovascular Society Classification of Patients with Angina Pectoris

Class I: Ordinary physical activity (eg, walking, climbing stairs) does not cause angina. Angina occurs with strenuous, rapid, or prolonged exertion at work or recreation.

Class II: Slight limitation of ordinary activity. Angina occurs on walking or climbing stairs rapidly, walking uphill, walking or stair climbing after meals, or in cold, in wind, or under emotional stress. Walking more than two blocks on the level and climbing more than one flight of ordinary stairs at a normal pace and in normal conditions can elicit angina.

Class III: Marked limitations of ordinary physical activity. Angina occurs on walking one or two blocks on the level and climbing one flight of stairs in normal conditions and at a normal pace.

Class IV: Inability to carry on any physical activity without discomfort—anginal symptoms may be present at rest.

to plaque development and growth include endothelial injury, lipid infiltration (ie, cholesterol), recruitment of inflammatory cells (mainly monocytes and T lymphocytes), and smooth muscle cell proliferation. Endothelial injury may be the initiating factor in plaque formation because it allows monocytes, platelets, cholesterol, and other blood components to come in contact with and stimulate abnormal growth of smooth muscle cells and connective tissue in the arterial wall.

Atherosclerosis commonly develops in the coronary arteries. As the plaque lesions develop over time, they become larger and extend farther into the lumen of the artery. The lesions may develop for decades before they produce symptoms of reduced blood flow. Eventually, events such as plaque rupture, mural hemorrhage, formation of a thrombus that partly or completely occludes an artery, and vasoconstriction precipitate myocardial ischemia. Thus, serious impairment of blood flow may occur with a large atherosclerotic plaque or a relatively small plaque with superimposed vasospasm and thrombosis. If stenosis blocks approximately 80% of the artery, blood flow cannot increase in response to increased need; if stenosis blocks 90% or more of the artery, blood flow is impaired when the client is at rest.

When coronary atherosclerosis develops slowly, collateral circulation develops to increase blood supply to the heart. Collateral circulation develops from anastomotic channels that connect the coronary arteries and allow perfusion of an area by more than one artery. When one artery becomes blocked, the anastomotic channels become larger and allow blood from an unblocked artery to perfuse the area typically supplied by the occluded artery. Endothelium-derived relaxing factors such as nitric oxide (NO) can dilate collateral vessels and facilitate regional myocardial blood flow. Although collateral circulation may prevent myocardial ischemia in the client at rest, it has limited ability to increase myocardial perfusion with increased cardiac workload.

Myocardial ischemia impairs blood flow to the myocardium, especially with exercise, mental stress, exposure to cold, or other factors that increase the cardiac workload. Most individuals with myocardial ischemia have advanced coronary atherosclerosis. Hypertension is also a major risk factor for myocardial ischemia.

Myocardial Ischemia

Myocardial ischemia occurs when the coronary arteries are unable to provide sufficient blood and oxygen for normal cardiac functions. Also known as *ischemic heart disease, CAD,* and *coronary heart disease,* myocardial ischemia may present as an acute coronary syndrome with three main consequences. One consequence is unstable angina, with the occurrence of pain (symptomatic myocardial ischemia). A second is MI that is silent or asymptomatic and diagnosed by biochemical markers only. A third is MI, with or without ST-segment elevation, which occurs when the ischemia is persistent or severe.

Resultant Cardiovascular Impairments

With normal cardiac function, coronary blood flow can increase to meet needs for an increased oxygen supply with exercise or other conditions that increase cardiac workload. When coronary arteries are partly blocked by atherosclerotic plaque, vasospasm, or thrombi, blood flow may not be able to increase sufficiently.

The endothelium of normal coronary arteries synthesizes numerous substances (see Chap. 47) that protect against vasoconstriction and vasospasm, bleeding and clotting, inflammation, and excessive cell growth. Impaired endothelium (eg, by rupture of atherosclerotic plaque or the shear force of hypertension) leads to vasoconstriction, vasospasm, clot formation, formation of atherosclerotic plaque, and growth of smooth muscle cells in blood vessel walls.

One important substance produced by the endothelium of coronary arteries is NO (also called endothelium-derived relaxing factor). NO, which is synthesized from the amino acid arginine, is released by shear stress on the endothelium, sympathetic stimulation of exercise, and interactions with acetylcholine, histamine, prostacyclin, serotonin, thrombin, and other chemical mediators. NO relaxes vascular smooth muscle and inhibits adhesion and aggregation of platelets. When the endothelium is damaged, these vasodilating and antithrombotic effects are lost. At the same time, production of strong vasoconstrictors (eg, angiotensin II, endothelin-1, thromboxane A_2) is increased. In addition, inflammatory cells enter the injured area and growth factors stimulate growth of smooth muscle cells. All of these factors participate in blocking coronary arteries.

Sympathetic nervous system stimulation normally produces dilation of coronary arteries, tachycardia, and increased myocardial contractility to handle an increased need for oxygenated blood. Atherosclerosis of coronary arteries, especially if severe, may cause vasoconstriction as well as decrease blood flow by obstruction.

Nonpharmacologic Management of Angina

For clients at any stage of CAD development, irrespective of symptoms of myocardial ischemia, optimal management involves lifestyle changes and medications, if necessary, to control or reverse risk factors for disease progression. Risk factors are frequently additive in nature and are classified as nonmodifiable and modifiable. Nonmodifiable risk factors include age, race, gender, and family history. The risk factors that can be altered include smoking, hypertension, hyperlipidemia, obesity, sedentary lifestyle, stress, and the use of drugs that increase cardiac workload (eg, adrenergics, corticosteroids). Thus, efforts are needed to assist clients in reducing blood pressure, weight, and serum cholesterol levels, when indicated, and developing an exercise program. For clients with diabetes mellitus, glucose and blood pressure control can reduce the microvascular changes associated with the condition.

In addition, clients should avoid circumstances known to precipitate acute attacks, and those who smoke should stop. Smoking is harmful to clients because

- Nicotine increases catecholamines which, in turn, increase heart rate and blood pressure.
- Carboxyhemoglobin, formed from the inhalation of carbon monoxide in smoke, decreases delivery of blood and oxygen to the heart, decreases myocardial contractility, and increases the risks of life-threatening cardiac dysrhythmias (eg, ventricular fibrillation) during ischemic episodes.
- Both nicotine and carbon monoxide increase platelet adhesiveness and aggregation, thereby promoting thrombosis.
- Smoking increases the risks for MI, sudden cardiac death, cerebrovascular disease (eg, stroke), peripheral vascular disease (eg, arterial insufficiency), and hypertension. It also reduces high-density lipoprotein, the "good" cholesterol.

Additional nonpharmacologic management strategies include surgical revascularization (eg, coronary artery bypass graft) and interventional procedures that reduce blockages (eg, percutaneous transluminal coronary angioplasty [PTCA], intracoronary stents, laser therapy, rotational atherectomy). However, most clients still require antianginal and other cardiovascular medications to manage their disease.

Drug Management

Drugs used for myocardial ischemia are the organic nitrates, the beta-adrenergic blocking agents, and the calcium channel blocking agents. These drugs relieve anginal pain by reducing myocardial oxygen demand or increasing blood supply to the myocardium. Nitrates and beta blockers are described in the following sections; dosage ranges for these drugs are listed in Table 50-1. Calcium channel blockers are described in a following section; indications for use and dosage ranges are listed in Table 50-2.

ANTIANGINAL DRUGS: CLASSIFICATIONS AND INDIVIDUAL DRUGS

Organic Nitrates

General Characteristics

Organic nitrates relax smooth muscle in blood vessel walls. This action produces vasodilation, which relieves anginal pain by several mechanisms. First, dilation of veins reduces venous pressure and venous return to the heart. This decreases blood volume and pressure within the heart (preload), which in turn decreases cardiac workload and oxygen demand. Second,

nitrates dilate coronary arteries at higher doses and can increase blood flow to ischemic areas of the myocardium. Third, nitrates dilate arterioles, which lowers peripheral vascular resistance (afterload). This results in lower systolic blood pressure and, consequently, reduced cardiac workload. The prototype and most widely used nitrate is **nitroglycerin.**

Nitrates are converted to NO in vascular smooth muscle. NO activates guanylate cyclase, an enzyme that catalyzes formation of cyclic guanine monophosphate, which decreases calcium levels in vascular smooth muscle cells. Because intracellular calcium is required for contraction of vascular smooth muscle, the result of decreased calcium is vasodilation. The NO derived from nitrate medications can be considered a replacement or substitute for the NO that a damaged endothelium can no longer produce.

Clinical indications for nitroglycerin and other nitrates are management and prevention of acute chest pain caused by myocardial ischemia. For acute angina and prophylaxis before a situation deemed likely to precipitate acute angina, fast-acting preparations (sublingual or chewable tablets, transmucosal spray or tablet) are used. For management of recurrent angina, long-acting preparations (oral and sustained-release tablets or transdermal ointment and discs) are used. However, they may not be effective long-term because tolerance develops to their hemodynamic effects. Intravenous (IV) nitroglycerin is used to manage angina that is unresponsive to organic nitrates via other routes or beta-adrenergic blocking agents. It also may be used to control blood pressure in perioperative or emergency situations and to reduce preload and afterload in severe heart failure.

Contraindications include hypersensitivity reactions, severe anemia, hypotension, and hypovolemia. The drugs should be used cautiously in the presence of head injury or cerebral hemorrhage because they may increase intracranial pressure. Additionally, males taking nitroglycerin or any other nitrate should not take phosphodiesterase enzyme type 5 inhibitors such as sildenafil (Viagra) and vardenafil (Levitra) for erectile dysfunction. Nitrates and phosphodiesterase enzyme type 5 inhibitors decrease blood pressure and the combined effect can produce profound, life-threatening hypotension.

Individual Nitrates

P **Nitroglycerin** (Nitro-Bid, others), the prototype drug, is used to relieve acute angina pectoris, prevent exercise-induced angina, and decrease the frequency and severity of acute anginal episodes. Oral dosage forms are rapidly metabolized in the liver, and relatively small proportions of doses reach the systemic circulation. In addition, oral doses act slowly and do not help relieve acute chest pain.

For these reasons, several alternative dosage forms have been developed, including transmucosal tablets and sprays administered sublingually or buccally; transdermal ointments and adhesive discs applied to the skin; and an IV preparation. When given sublingually, nitroglycerin is absorbed directly into the systemic circulation. It acts within 1 to 3 minutes and

Table 50-1 Drugs at a Glance: Nitrate and Beta-Blocker Antianginal Drugs

GENERIC/TRADE NAME	INDICATIONS FOR USE	ROUTES AND DOSAGE RANGES
Nitrates		
P Nitroglycerin (Nitro-Bid, others)	Relieve acute angina Prevent exercise-induced angina Long-term prophylaxis to decrease the frequency and severity of acute anginal episodes	PO immediate-release tablets, 2.5–9 mg 2 or 3 times per day PO sustained-release tablets or capsules, 2.5 mg 3 or 4 times per day SL 0.15–0.6 mg PRN for chest pain Translingual spray, one or two metered doses (0.4 mg/dose) sprayed onto oral mucosa at onset of anginal pain, to a maximum of 3 doses in 15 min Transmucosal tablet, 1 mg q3–5h while awake, placed between upper lip and gum or cheek and gum Topical ointment, 1/2–2 inches q4–8h; do not rub in Topical transdermal disc, applied once daily IV 5–10 mcg/min initially, increased in 10- to 20-mcg/min increments up to 100 mcg/min or more if necessary to relieve pain
Isosorbide dinitrate (Isordil)	Treatment and prevention of angina	SL 2.5–10 mg PRN or q2–4h PO regular tablets, 10–60 mg q4–6h PO chewable tablets, 5–10 mg q2–3h PO sustained-release capsules, 40 mg q6–12h
Isosorbide mononitrate (Ismo, Imdur)	Treatment and prevention of angina	PO 20 mg twice daily, with first dose on arising and the second dose 7 h later PO extended-release tablets (Imdur), 30–60 mg once daily in the morning, increased after several days to 120 mg once daily if necessary
Beta Blockers		
P Propranolol (Inderal)	Long-term management of angina, to reduce frequency and severity of anginal episodes	PO 10–80 mg 2 to 4 times per day IV 0.5–3 mg q4h until desired response is obtained
Atenolol (Tenormin)	Long-term management of angina, to reduce frequency and severity of anginal episodes	PO 50 mg once daily, initially, increased to 100 mg/d after 1 wk if necessary
Metoprolol (Lopressor)	Long-term management of angina, to reduce frequency and severity of anginal episodes	PO 50 mg twice daily initially, increased up to 400 mg daily if necessary
Nadolol (Corgard)	Long-term management of angina, to reduce frequency and severity of anginal episodes	PO 40–240 mg/d in a single dose

IV, intravenous; PO, oral; SL, sublingual.

lasts 30 to 60 minutes. When applied topically to the skin, nitroglycerin is also absorbed directly into the systemic circulation. However, absorption occurs at a slower rate, and topical nitroglycerin has a longer duration of action than other forms. It is available in an ointment, which is effective for 4 to 8 hours, and in a transdermal disc, which is effective for about 12 hours. An IV form of nitroglycerin is used to relieve acute anginal pain that does not respond to other agents. Regardless of the route, nitroglycerin has a half-life of 1 to 5 minutes, supporting the beneficial use of transdermal patches and sustained-release tablets.

Isosorbide dinitrate (Isordil) is used to reduce the frequency and severity of acute anginal episodes. When given sublingually or in chewable tablets, it acts in about 2 min-

Table 50-2 Drugs at a Glance: Calcium Channel Blockers

GENERIC/TRADE NAME	INDICATIONS FOR USE	ROUTES AND DOSAGE RANGES
Amlodipine (Norvasc)	Angina Hypertension	PO 5–10 mg once daily
Diltiazem (Cardizem)	Angina Hypertension Atrial fibrillation and flutter PSVT	Angina or hypertension, immediate-release, PO 60–90 mg 4 times daily before meals and at bedtime Hypertension, sustained-release only, PO 120–180 mg twice daily Dysrhythmias (Cardizem IV only), IV injection 0.25 mg/kg (average dose 20 mg) over 2 min with a second dose of 0.35 mg/kg (average dose 25 mg) in 15 min if necessary, followed by IV infusion of 5–15 mg/h up to 24 h
Felodipine (Plendil)	Hypertension	PO 5–10 mg once daily
Isradipine (DynaCirc)	Hypertension	PO 2.5–5 mg twice daily
Nicardipine (Cardene)	Angina Hypertension	Angina, immediate-release only, PO 20–40 mg 3 times daily Hypertension, immediate-release, same as for angina, above; sustained-release, PO 30–60 mg twice daily
Nifedipine (Adalat, Procardia)	Angina Hypertension	Angina, immediate-release, PO 10–30 mg 3 times daily; sustained-release, PO 30–60 mg once daily Hypertension, sustained-release only, 30–60 mg once daily
Nimodipine (Nimotop)	Subarachnoid hemorrhage	PO 60 mg q4h for 21 consecutive days. If patient unable to swallow, aspirate contents of capsule into a syringe with an 18-gauge needle, administer by nasogastric tube, and follow with 30 mL normal saline.
Nisoldipine (Sular)	Hypertension	PO, initially 20 mg once daily, increased by 10 mg/wk or longer intervals to a maximum of 60 mg daily. Average maintenance dose, 20–40 mg daily. Adults with liver impairment or >65 y, PO, initially 10 mg once daily
Verapamil (Calan, Isoptin)	Angina Atrial fibrillation or flutter PSVT Hypertension	Angina, PO 80–120 mg 3 times daily Dysrhythmias, PO 80–120 mg 3 to 4 times daily; IV injection, 5–10 mg over 2 min or longer, with continuous monitoring of electrocardiogram and blood pressure Hypertension, PO 80 mg 3 times daily or 240 mg (sustained-release) once daily

IV, intravenous; PO, oral; PSVT, paroxysmal supraventricular tachycardia.

utes, and its effects last 2 to 3 hours. When higher doses are given orally, more drug escapes metabolism in the liver and produces systemic effects in approximately 30 minutes. Therapeutic effects last about 4 hours after oral administration. The effective oral dose is usually determined by increasing the dose until headache occurs, indicating the maximum tolerable dose. Sustained-release capsules also are available.

Isosorbide mononitrate (Ismo, Imdur) is the metabolite and active component of isosorbide dinitrate. It is well absorbed after oral administration and almost 100% bioavailable. Unlike other oral nitrates, this drug is not subject to first-pass hepatic metabolism. Onset of action occurs within 1 hour, peak effects occur between 1 and 4 hours, and the elimination half-life is approximately 5 hours. It is used only for prophylaxis of angina; it does not act rapidly enough to relieve acute attacks.

APPLYING YOUR KNOWLEDGE 50-1:
HOW CAN YOU AVOID THIS MEDICATION ERROR?
Mr. Gerald is prescribed nitroglycerin in both sublingual form and as a transdermal patch. He has had a history of erectile dysfunction and has some medication in the medicine cabinet that was prescribed for him before his MI.

Beta-Adrenergic Blocking Agents

General Characteristics

Beta-adrenergic blocking agents are often prescribed in a variety of clinical conditions. Their actions, uses, and adverse effects are discussed in Chapter 18. In this chapter, the drugs are discussed only in relation to their use in angina pectoris.

Sympathetic stimulation of beta$_1$ receptors in the heart increases heart rate and force of myocardial contraction, both of which increase myocardial oxygen demand and may precipitate acute anginal attacks. Beta-blocking drugs prevent or inhibit sympathetic stimulation. Thus, the drugs reduce heart rate and myocardial contractility, particularly when sympathetic output is increased during exercise. A slower heart rate may improve coronary blood flow to the ischemic area. Beta blockers also reduce blood pressure, which in turn decreases myocardial workload and oxygen demand. Studies indicate that beta blockers are more effective than nitrates or calcium channel blockers in decreasing the likelihood of silent ischemia and improving the mortality rate after transmural MI. In angina pectoris, beta-adrenergic blocking agents are used in long-term management to decrease the frequency and severity of anginal attacks, decrease the need for sublingual nitroglycerin, and increase exercise tolerance. When a beta blocker is being discontinued after prolonged use, it should be tapered in dosage and gradually discontinued or rebound angina can occur.

These drugs should not be given to clients with known or suspected coronary artery spasms because they may intensify the frequency and severity of vasospasm. This probably results from unopposed stimulation of alpha-adrenergic receptors, which causes vasoconstriction, when beta-adrenergic receptors are blocked by the drugs. Clients who continue to smoke may have reduced efficacy with the use of beta blockers. Clients with asthma should be observed for bronchospasm from blockage of beta$_2$ receptors in the lung. Beta blockers should be used with caution in clients with diabetes mellitus because they can conceal signs of hypoglycemia (except for sweating).

Individual Drugs

P **Propranolol**, the prototype beta blocker, is used to reduce the frequency and severity of acute attacks of angina. It is usually added to the antianginal drug regimen when nitrates do not prevent anginal episodes. It is especially useful in preventing exercise-induced tachycardia, which can precipitate anginal attacks.

Propranolol is well absorbed after oral administration. It is then metabolized extensively in the liver; a relatively small proportion of an oral dose (approximately 30%) reaches the systemic circulation. For this reason, oral doses of propranolol are much higher than IV doses. Onset of action is 30 minutes after oral administration and 1 to 2 minutes after IV injection. Because of variations in the degree of hepatic metabolism, clients vary widely in the dosages required to maintain a therapeutic response.

Atenolol, metoprolol, and **nadolol** have the same actions, uses, and adverse effects as propranolol, but they have long half-lives and can be given once daily. They are excreted by the kidneys, and dosage must be reduced in clients with renal impairment.

APPLYING YOUR KNOWLEDGE 50-2

APPLYING YOUR KNOWLEDGE 50-2

In addition to nitroglycerin, the physician prescribes metoprolol. Mr. Gerald understands why nitroglycerin is beneficial to his condition. He asks about the metoprolol and why he needs to take this medication. How should you respond?

Calcium Channel Blocking Agents

Calcium channel blockers act on contractile and conductive tissues of the heart and on vascular smooth muscle. For these cells to function normally, the concentration of intracellular calcium must be increased. This is usually accomplished by movement of extracellular calcium ions into the cell (through calcium channels in the cell membrane) and release of bound calcium from the sarcoplasmic reticulum in the cell. Thus, calcium plays an important role in maintaining vasomotor tone, myocardial contractility, and conduction. Calcium channel blocking agents prevent the movement of extracellular calcium into the cell. As a result, coronary and peripheral arteries are dilated, myocardial contractility is decreased, and the conduction system is depressed in relation to impulse formation (automaticity) and conduction velocity (Fig. 50-1).

In angina pectoris, the drugs improve the blood supply to the myocardium by dilating coronary arteries and decrease the workload of the heart by dilating peripheral arteries. In variant angina, calcium channel blockers reduce coronary artery vasospasm. In atrial fibrillation or flutter and other supraventricular tachydysrhythmias, diltiazem and verapamil slow the rate of ventricular response. In hypertension, the drugs lower blood pressure primarily by dilating peripheral arteries.

Calcium channel blockers are well absorbed after oral administration but undergo extensive first-pass metabolism in the liver. Most of the drugs are more than 90% protein bound and reach peak plasma levels within 1 to 2 hours (6 hours or longer for sustained-release forms). Most also have short elimination half-lives (<5 hours), so doses must be given three or four times daily unless sustained-release formulations are used. Amlodipine (30–50 hours), and felodipine (11–16 hours) have long elimination half-lives and therefore can be given once daily. The drugs are metabolized in the liver, and dosage should be reduced in clients with severe liver disease. Dosage reductions are not required with renal disease.

The calcium channel blockers approved for use in the United States vary in their chemical structures and effects on body tissues. Seven of these are chemically dihydropyridines, of which nifedipine is the prototype. Diltiazem and verapamil differ chemically from the dihydropyridines and each other. Nifedipine and related drugs act mainly on vascular smooth muscle to produce vasodilation, whereas verapamil and diltiazem have greater effects on the cardiac conduction system.

The drugs also vary in clinical indications for use; most are used for angina or hypertension, and only diltiazem and

Muscle relaxation

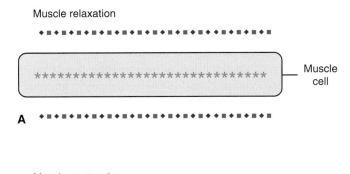

A

Muscle contraction

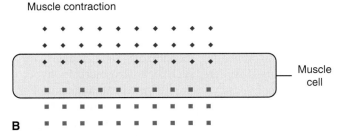

Calcium-blocking drugs

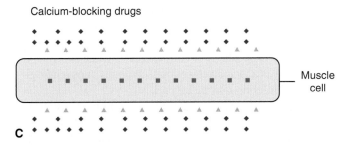

C

FIGURE 50-1 Calcium channel blockers: mechanism of action. **(A)** During muscle relaxation, potassium ions are inside the muscle cell and calcium and sodium ions are outside the muscle cell. **(B)** For muscle contraction to occur, potassium ions leave the cell and sodium and calcium ions enter the cell through open channels in the cell membrane. **(C)** When calcium channels are blocked by drug molecules, muscle contraction is decreased because calcium ions cannot move through the cell membrane into the muscle cell. (Calcium ions = ◆; sodium ions = ■; potassium ions = *; calcium channel blocking drugs = ▲.)

verapamil are used to manage supraventricular tachydysrhythmias. In clients with CAD, the drugs are effective as monotherapy but are commonly prescribed in combination with beta blockers. In addition, nimodipine is approved for use only in subarachnoid hemorrhage, in which it decreases spasm in cerebral blood vessels and limits the extent of brain damage. In animal studies, nimodipine exerted greater effects on cerebral arteries than on other arteries, probably because it is highly lipid soluble and penetrates the blood–brain barrier.

Contraindications include second- or third-degree heart block, cardiogenic shock, and severe bradycardia, heart failure, or hypotension. The drugs should be used cautiously with milder bradycardia, heart failure, or hypotension and with renal or hepatic impairment.

Adjunctive Antianginal Drugs

In addition to antianginal drugs, several other drugs may be used to control risk factors and prevent progression of myocardial ischemia to MI and sudden cardiac death. These may include:

- **Aspirin.** This drug has become the standard of care because of its antiplatelet (ie, antithrombotic) effects. Recommended doses vary from 81 mg daily to 325 mg daily or every other day; apparently all doses are beneficial in reducing the possibility of myocardial reinfarction, stroke, and death. Clopidogrel (see Chap. 54), 75 mg/day, is an acceptable alternative for individuals with aspirin allergy.
- **Antilipemics.** These drugs (see Chap. 55) may be needed by clients who are unable to lower serum cholesterol levels sufficiently with a low-fat diet. Lovastatin or a related "statin" is often used. The goal is usually to reduce the serum cholesterol level below 200 mg/dL and low-density lipoprotein cholesterol to below 130 mg/dL.
- **Antihypertensives.** These drugs (see Chap. 52) may be needed for clients with hypertension. Because beta blockers and calcium channel blockers are used to manage hypertension as well as angina, one of these drugs may be effective for both disorders.

NURSING PROCESS

Assessment

Assess the client's condition in relation to angina pectoris. Specific assessment data vary with each client but usually should include the following:

- During the initial nursing history interview, try to answer the following questions:
  - How long has the client been taking antianginal drugs? For what purpose are they being taken (prophylaxis, treatment of acute attacks, or both)?
  - What is the frequency and duration of acute anginal attacks? Has either increased recently? (An increase could indicate worsening coronary atherosclerosis and increased risk of MI.)
  - Do symptoms other than chest pain occur during acute attacks (eg, sweating, nausea)?
  - Are there particular activities or circumstances that provoke acute attacks? Do attacks ever occur when the client is at rest? Where does the client fit in the

Canadian Cardiovascular Society classification system?

- What measures relieve symptoms of acute angina?
- If the client takes nitroglycerin, ask how often it is required, how many tablets are needed for relief of pain, how often the supply is replaced, and where the client stores or carries the drug.

- Assess blood pressure and pulse, electrocardiogram (ECG) reports, serum cholesterol, and cardiac enzyme reports. Elevated cholesterol is a significant risk factor for coronary atherosclerosis and angina, and the risk is directly related to the degree of elevation. Cardiac enzyme levels, such as troponin, creatine kinase (CK), lactate dehydrogenase (LDH), and aspartate amino-transferase (AST), should all be normal in clients with angina.

- During an acute attack, assess the following:
  - Location and quality of the pain. Chest pain is non-specific. It may be a symptom of numerous disorders, such as pulmonary embolism, esophageal spasm or inflammation (heartburn), costochondritis, or anxiety. Chest pain of cardiac origin is caused by myocardial ischemia and may indicate angina pectoris or MI.
  - Precipitating factors. For example, what was the client doing, thinking, or feeling just before the onset of chest pain?
  - Has the client had invasive procedures to diagnose or treat his or her CAD (eg, cardiac catheterization, angioplasty, revascularization surgery)?

Nursing Diagnoses

- Decreased Cardiac Output related to altered stroke volume or drug therapy
- Acute pain in chest related to inadequate perfusion of the myocardium
- Activity Intolerance related to chest pain
- Deficient Knowledge related to management of disease process and drug therapy
- Ineffective Individual Coping related to chronic disease process
- Sexual Dysfunction related to fear of precipitating chest pain

Planning/Goals

The client will

- Receive or take antianginal drugs accurately
- Experience relief of acute chest pain
- Have fewer episodes of acute chest pain
- Have increased activity tolerance
- Identify and manage situations that precipitate anginal attacks

- Be closely monitored for therapeutic and adverse effects, especially when drug therapy is started
- Avoid preventable adverse effects
- Verbalize essential information about the disease process, needed dietary and lifestyle changes to improve health status, and drug therapy
- Recognize signs and symptoms that necessitate professional intervention
- Keep appointments for follow-up care and monitoring

Interventions

Use the following measures to prevent acute anginal attacks.

- Assist in preventing, recognizing, and managing contributory disorders, such as atherosclerosis, hypertension, hyperthyroidism, hypoxia, and anemia. For example, hypertension is a common risk factor for CAD and morbidity and mortality increase progressively with the degree of either systolic or diastolic elevation. Management of hypertension reduces morbidity and mortality rates. However, most studies indicate that the reductions stem more from fewer strokes, less renal failure, and less heart failure, than from less CAD.
- Help the client recognize and avoid precipitating factors (eg, heavy meals, strenuous exercise) when possible. If anxiety is a factor, relaxation techniques or psychological counseling may be helpful.
- Help the client develop a more healthful lifestyle in terms of diet and weight control, adequate rest and sleep, regular exercise, and not smoking. Ideally, these self-help interventions are practiced before illness occurs; they can help prevent or delay illness. However, most individuals are unmotivated until illness develops, and perhaps after it develops as well. These interventions are beneficial at any stage of CAD. For example, for a client who already has angina, a supervised exercise program helps develop collateral circulation. Smoking has numerous ill effects on the client with angina and decreases effectiveness of antianginal drugs.

During an acute anginal attack in a client known to have angina or CAD, take the following actions.

- Assume that any chest pain may be of cardiac origin.
- Have the client lie down or sit down to reduce cardiac workload and provide rest.
- Check vital signs and compare them with baseline values.
- Record the characteristics of chest pain and the presence of other signs and symptoms.
- Have the client take a fast-acting nitroglycerin preparation (previously prescribed), up to three sublingual tablets or three oral sprays, each 5 minutes apart, as necessary.
- If chest pain is not relieved with rest and nitroglycerin, assume that an MI has occurred until proven otherwise.

In a health care setting, keep the client at rest and notify the client's physician immediately. Outside of a health care setting, call 911 for immediate assistance.

- Leave sublingual nitroglycerin at the bedside of hospitalized clients (per hospital policy). The tablets or spray should be within reach so that they can be used immediately. Record the number of tablets used daily, and ensure that an adequate supply is available.

Provide appropriate client teaching related to drug therapy (see accompanying display).

Evaluation

- Observe and interview for relief of acute chest pain.
- Observe and interview regarding the number of episodes of acute chest pain.
- Identify CAD lifestyle factors that are being successfully modified or require modification (eg, diet, weight, activity, smoking cessation).
- Interview regarding success and compliance with drug therapy.

PRINCIPLES OF THERAPY

Goals of Therapy

The goals of drug therapy are to relieve acute anginal pain; reduce the number and severity of acute anginal attacks; improve exercise tolerance and quality of life; delay progression of CAD; prevent MI; and prevent sudden cardiac death.

Drug Selection and Dosage

For relief of acute angina and prophylaxis before events that cause acute angina, nitroglycerin (sublingual tablets or translingual spray) is usually the primary drug of choice. Sublingual or chewable tablets of isosorbide dinitrate also may be used. For long-term prevention or management of recurrent angina, oral or topical nitrates, beta-adrenergic blocking agents, or calcium channel blocking agents are used. Combination drug therapy with a nitrate and one of the other drugs is common and effective. Clients taking one or more long-acting antianginal drugs should carry a short-acting drug as well, to be used for acute attacks.

Dosage of all antianginal drugs should be individualized to achieve optimal benefit and minimal adverse effects. This is usually accomplished by starting with relatively small doses and increasing them at appropriate intervals as necessary. Doses may vary widely among individuals.

Tolerance to Long-Acting Nitrates

Clients who take long-acting dosage forms of nitrates on a regular schedule develop tolerance to the vasodilating (antianginal) effects of the drug. The clients more likely to develop tolerance are those on high-dose, uninterrupted therapy. Although tolerance decreases the adverse effects of hypotension, dizziness, and headache, therapeutic effects also may be decreased. As a result, episodes of chest pain may occur more often or be more severe than expected. In addition, short-acting nitrates may be less effective in relieving acute pain.

Opinions seem divided about the best way to prevent or manage nitrate tolerance. Some authorities recommend using short-acting nitrates when needed and avoiding the long-acting forms. Others recommend using the long-acting forms for 12 to 16 hours daily during active periods and omitting them during inactive periods or sleep. Thus, a dose of an oral nitrate or topical ointment would be given every 6 hours for three doses daily, allowing a rest period of 6 hours without a dose. Transdermal discs should be removed at bedtime. If anginal symptoms occur during sleeping hours, short-acting nitrates may be beneficial in relieving the symptoms. All nitrates should be administered at the lowest effective dosage.

Use in Special Populations

Use in Children

The safety and effectiveness of antianginal drugs have not been established for children. Nitroglycerin has been given IV for heart failure and intraoperative control of blood pressure, with the initial dose adjusted for weight and later doses titrated to response.

Use in Older Adults

Antianginal drugs are often used because cardiovascular disease and myocardial ischemia are common problems in older adults. Adverse drug effects, such as hypotension and syncope, are likely to occur, and they may be more severe than in younger adults. Blood pressure and ability to ambulate safely should be closely monitored, especially when drug therapy is started or dosages are increased. Ambulatory clients also should be monitored for their ability to take the drugs correctly.

With calcium channel blockers, older adults may have higher plasma concentrations of verapamil, diltiazem, nifedipine, and amlodipine. This is attributed to decreased hepatic metabolism of the drugs, probably because of decreased hepatic blood flow. In addition, older adults may experience more hypotension with verapamil, nifedipine, and felodipine than younger clients. Blood pressure should be monitored with these drugs.

Use in Clients With Renal Impairment

Little information is available about the use of antianginal drugs in clients with impaired renal function. A few studies indicate that advanced renal failure may alter the pharmacokinetics of calcium channel blockers. Although the pharmacokinetics of diltiazem and verapamil are quite similar in clients with normal and impaired renal function, caution is

General Considerations

☑ Angina is chest pain that occurs because your heart is not getting enough blood and oxygen. The most common causes are hypertension and atherosclerosis of the coronary arteries. The chest pain usually lasts less than 5 minutes and episodes can be managed for years without causing permanent heart damage. However, if the pain is severe or prolonged, a heart attack and heart damage may develop. You need to seek information about your heart condition to prevent or decrease episodes of angina and prevent a heart attack.

☑ Several types of drugs are used in angina, and you may need a combination of drugs for the best effects. Most clients take one or more long-acting drugs to prevent anginal attacks and a fast, short-acting drug (usually nitroglycerin tablets that you dissolve under your tongue, or a nitroglycerin solution that you spray into your mouth) to relieve acute attacks. You should seek emergency care immediately if rest and three sublingual tablets or oral sprays 5 minutes apart do not relieve your chest pain. The long-acting medications are not effective in relieving sudden anginal pain.

☑ As with any medications for serious or potentially serious conditions, it is extremely important to take antianginal medications as prescribed. Do not increase dosage or discontinue the drugs without specific instructions from your health care provider.

☑ With sublingual nitroglycerin tablets, keep them in the original container; carry them so that they are always within reach but not where they are exposed to body heat; and replace them approximately every 6 months because they become ineffective.

☑ It may be helpful to record the number and severity of anginal episodes, the number of nitroglycerin tablets required to relieve the attack, and the total number of tablets taken daily. Such a record can help your health care provider know when to change your medications or your dosages.

☑ Headache and dizziness may occur with nitrate antianginal drugs, especially sublingual nitroglycerin. These effects are usually temporary and dissipate with continued therapy. If dizziness occurs, avoid strenuous activity and stand up slowly for approximately an hour after taking the drugs. If headache is severe, you may take aspirin or acetaminophen with the nitrate drug. Do not reduce drug dosage or take the drug less often to avoid headache; loss of effectiveness may occur.

☑ Keep family members or support individuals informed about the location and use of antianginal medications in case help is needed.

☑ Avoid over-the-counter decongestants, cold remedies, and diet pills, which stimulate the heart and constrict blood vessels and thus may cause angina.

☑ With nitrate antianginal drugs, avoid alcohol. Both the drugs and alcohol dilate blood vessels and an excessive reduction in blood pressure (with dizziness and fainting) may occur with the combination.

☑ Several calcium channel blockers are available in both immediate-acting and long-acting (sustained-release) forms. The brand names often differ very little (eg, Procardia is a brand name of immediate-release nifedipine; Procardia XL is a long-acting formulation). It is extremely important that the correct formulation is used consistently.

Self- or Caregiver Administration

☑ Take or give as instructed; specific instructions differ with the type of antianginal drug being taken.

☑ Take or give antianginal drugs on a regular schedule, at evenly spaced intervals. This increases drug effectiveness in preventing acute attacks of angina.

☑ With nitroglycerin and other nitrate preparations:

　☑ Use according to instructions for the particular dosage form. The dosage forms were developed for specific routes of administration and are not interchangeable.

　☑ For sublingual nitroglycerin tablets, place them under the tongue until they dissolve. Take at the first sign of an anginal attack, before severe pain develops. If chest pain is not relieved in 5 minutes, dissolve a second tablet under the tongue. If pain is not relieved within another 5 minutes, dissolve a third tablet. If pain continues or becomes more severe, notify your health care provider immediately or report to the nearest hospital emergency room. Sit down when you take the medications. This may help to relieve your pain and prevent dizziness from the drug.

　☑ For the translingual solution of nitroglycerin, spray onto or under the tongue; do not inhale the spray.

　☑ For transmucosal tablets of nitroglycerin, place them under the upper lip or between the cheek and gum and allow them to dissolve slowly over 3 to 5 hours. Do not chew or swallow the tablets.

　☑ Take oral nitrates on an empty stomach with a glass of water. Oral isosorbide dinitrate is available in regular and chewable tablets; be sure each type is taken appropriately. Do not crush or chew sustained-release nitroglycerin tablets.

　☑ For sublingual isosorbide dinitrate tablets, place them under the tongue until they dissolve.

　☑ If an oral nitrate and topical nitroglycerin are being used concurrently, stagger the times of administration. This minimizes dizziness from low blood pressure and headache, which are common adverse effects of nitrate drugs.

　☑ For nitroglycerin ointment, use the special paper to measure the dose. Place the ointment on a nonhairy part of the upper body and apply with the applicator paper. Cover the area with plastic wrap or tape. Rotate application sites (because the ointment can irritate the skin) and wipe off the previous dose before applying a new dose. Wash hands after applying the ointment.

　　The measured paper must be used for accurate dosage. The paper is used to apply the ointment because the drug is readily absorbed through the skin. Skin contact should be avoided except on the designated area of the body. Plastic wrap or tape aids absorption and prevents removal of the drug. It also prevents soiling of clothes and linens.

C L I E N T   T E A C H I N G   G U I D E L I N E S

Antianginal Drugs (Continued)

✔ For nitroglycerin patches, apply at the same time each day to clean, dry, hairless areas on the upper body or arms. Rotate sites. Avoid applying below the knee or elbow or in areas of skin irritation or scar tissue. Correct application is necessary to promote effective and consistent drug absorption. The drug is not as well absorbed from distal portions of the extremities because of decreased blood flow. Rota-

tion of sites decreases skin irritation. Also, used patches must be disposed of properly because there is enough residual nitroglycerin to be harmful, especially to children and pets.

✔ With sustained-release forms of calcium channel blockers, which are usually taken once daily, do not take more often than prescribed and do not crush or chew.

---

still advised. With verapamil, about 70% of a dose is excreted as metabolites in urine.

Dosage reductions are considered unnecessary with verapamil and diltiazem but may be needed with nifedipine and several other dihydropyridine derivatives. With nifedipine, protein binding is decreased and the elimination half-life is prolonged with renal impairment. In a few clients, reversible elevations in blood urea nitrogen and serum creatinine have occurred. With nicardipine, plasma concentrations are higher in clients with renal impairment, and dosage should be reduced.

Use in Clients With Hepatic Impairment

Nitrates, beta blockers (see Chap. 18), and calcium channel blockers are metabolized in the liver, and all should be used with caution in clients with significant impairment of hepatic function from reduced blood flow or disease processes.

With oral nitrates, it is difficult to predict effects. On the one hand, first-pass metabolism is reduced, which increases the bioavailability (amount of active drug) of a given dose. On the other hand, the nitrate reductase enzymes that normally deactivate the drug may increase if large doses are given. In this case, more enzymes are available and the drug is metabolized more rapidly, possibly reducing therapeutic effects of a given dose. Relatively large doses of oral nitrates are sometimes given to counteract the drug tolerance (reduced hemodynamic effects) associated with chronic use. In addition, metabolism of nitroglycerin and isosorbide dinitrate normally produces active metabolites. Thus, if metabolism is reduced by liver impairment, drug effects may be decreased and shorter in duration.

With calcium channel blockers, impairment of liver function has profound effects on the pharmacokinetics and pharmacodynamics of most of these drugs. Thus, the drugs should be used with caution, dosages should be substantially reduced, and clients should be closely monitored for drug effects (including periodic measurements of liver enzymes). These recommendations stem from the following effects.

- An impaired liver produces fewer drug-binding plasma proteins such as albumin. This means that a greater proportion of a given dose is unbound and therefore active.
- In clients with cirrhosis, bioavailability of oral drugs is greatly increased and metabolism (of both oral and parenteral drugs) is greatly decreased. Both of these effects increase plasma levels of drug from a given dose (essentially an overdose). The effects result from shunting of blood around the liver so that drug molecules circulating in the bloodstream do not come in contact with drug-metabolizing enzymes and therefore are not metabolized. For example, the bioavailability of verapamil, nifedipine, felodipine, and nisoldipine is approximately double and their clearance is approximately one third that of clients without cirrhosis.
- Although hepatotoxicity is uncommon, clinical symptoms of hepatitis, cholestasis, or jaundice and elevated liver enzymes (eg, alkaline phosphatase, creatine kinase [CK], lactate dehydrogenase [LDH], aspartate aminotransferase [AST], alanine aminotransferase [ALT]) have occurred, mainly with diltiazem, nifedipine, and verapamil. These changes resolve if the causative drug is stopped.

Use in Clients With Critical Illness

Antianginal drugs have multiple cardiovascular effects and may be used alone or in combination with other cardiovascular drugs in clients with critical illness. They are probably used most often to manage severe angina, severe hypertension, or serious cardiac dysrhythmias. For example, IV nitroglycerin may be used for angina and hypertension; an IV beta blocker or calcium channel blocker may be used to improve cardiovascular function with angina, hypertension, or supraventricular tachydysrhythmias. With any of these drugs, dosage must be carefully titrated and clients must be closely monitored for hypotension and other drug effects.

In addition, absorption of oral drugs or topical forms of nitroglycerin may be impaired in clients with extensive edema, heart failure, hypotension, or other conditions that impair blood flow to the gastrointestinal tract or skin.

Use in Home Care

The role of the home care nurse may vary, depending largely on the severity of the client's illness. Initially, the nurse should assess the frequency and severity of anginal attacks and how the attacks are managed. In addition, the nurse can assess the home setting for lifestyle and environmental factors that may precipitate myocardial ischemia. When causative factors are identified, plans can be developed to avoid or minimize them. Other aspects of home care may include monitoring the client's response to antianginal medications; teaching clients and caregivers how to use, store, and replace medications to ensure a constant supply; and discussing circumstances for which the client should seek emergency care.

NURSING ACTIONS

Antianginal Drugs

NURSING ACTIONS	RATIONALE/EXPLANATION
1. Administer accurately	
a. Check blood pressure and heart rate before each dose of an antianginal drug. Withhold the drug if systolic blood pressure is below 90 mm Hg. If the dose is omitted, record and report to the health care provider.	Hypotension is an adverse effect of antianginal drugs. Bradycardia is an adverse effect of propranolol and nadolol. Dosage adjustments may be necessary if these effects occur.
b. Give antianginal drugs on a regular schedule, at evenly spaced intervals.	To increase effectiveness in preventing acute attacks of angina
c. If oral nitrates and topical nitroglycerin are being used concurrently, stagger times of administration.	To minimize risks of additive hypotension and headache
d. For sublingual nitroglycerin and isosorbide dinitrate, instruct the client to place the tablets under the tongue until they dissolve.	
e. For oral isosorbide dinitrate, regular and chewable tablets are available. Be sure each type of tablet is taken appropriately.	
f. For sublingual nitroglycerin, check the expiration date on the container.	Sublingual tablets of nitroglycerin are volatile. After the bottle has been opened, they become ineffective after approximately 6 months and should be replaced.
g. To apply nitroglycerin ointment, use the special paper to measure the dose. Place the ointment on a nonhairy part of the body, and apply with the applicator paper. Cover the area with plastic wrap or tape. Rotate application sites and wipe off previous ointment before applying a new dose.	The measured paper must be used for accurate dosage. The paper is used to apply the ointment because the drug is readily absorbed through the skin. Skin contact should be avoided except on the designated area of the body. Plastic wrap or tape aids absorption and prevents removal of the drug. It also prevents soiling of clothes and linens. Application sites should be rotated because the ointment can irritate the skin.
h. For nitroglycerin patches, apply at the same time each day to clean, dry, hairless areas on the upper body or arms. Rotate sites. Avoid applying below the knee or elbow or in areas of skin irritation or scar tissue.	To promote effective and consistent drug absorption. The drug is not as well absorbed from distal portions of the extremities because of decreased blood flow. Rotation of sites decreases skin irritation.
i. For intravenous (IV) nitroglycerin, dilute the drug and give by continuous infusion, with frequent monitoring of blood pressure and heart rate. Use only with the special administration set supplied by the manufacturer to avoid drug adsorption onto tubing.	The drug should not be given by direct IV injection. The drug is potent and may cause hypotension. Dosage (flow rate) is adjusted according to response (pain relief or drop in systolic blood pressure of 20 mm Hg).
j. With IV verapamil, inject slowly, over 2–3 minutes.	To decrease hypotension and other adverse effects
2. Observe for therapeutic effects	
a. Relief of chest pain with acute attacks	Sublingual nitroglycerin usually relieves pain within 5 minutes. If pain is not relieved, two additional tablets may be given, 5 minutes apart. If pain is not relieved after three tablets, report to the health care provider or seek emergency care.

NURSING ACTIONS	RATIONALE/EXPLANATION
b. Reduced incidence and severity of acute attacks with prophylactic antianginal drugs	
c. Increased exercise tolerance	
3. Observe for adverse effects	
a. With nitrates, observe for hypotension, dizziness, lightheadedness, tachycardia, palpitations, and headache.	Adverse effects are extensions of pharmacologic action. Vasodilation causes hypotension, which in turn causes dizziness from cerebral hypoxia and tachycardia from compensatory sympathetic nervous system stimulation. Hypotension can decrease blood flow to coronary arteries and precipitate angina pectoris or myocardial infarction. Hypotension is most likely to occur within an hour after drug administration. Vasodilation also causes headache, the most common adverse effect of nitrates.
b. With beta-adrenergic blocking agents, observe for hypotension, bradycardia, bronchospasm, and heart failure.	Beta blockers lower blood pressure by decreasing myocardial contractility and cardiac output. Excessive bradycardia may contribute to hypotension and cardiac dysrhythmias. Bronchospasm is more likely to occur in clients with asthma or other chronic respiratory problems.
c. With calcium channel blockers, observe for hypotension, dizziness, lightheadedness, weakness, peripheral edema, headache, heart failure, pulmonary edema, nausea, and constipation. Bradycardia may occur with verapamil and diltiazem; tachycardia may occur with nifedipine and nicardipine.	Adverse effects result primarily from reduced smooth muscle contractility. These effects, except constipation, are much more likely to occur with nifedipine and other dihydropyridines. Nifedipine may cause profound hypotension, which activates the compensatory mechanisms of the sympathetic nervous system and the renin–angiotensin–aldosterone system. Peripheral edema may require the administration of a diuretic. Constipation is more likely to occur with verapamil. Diltiazem reportedly causes few adverse effects.
4. Observe for drug interactions	
a. Drugs that *increase* effects of antianginal drugs:	
(1) Antidysrhythmics, antihypertensive drugs, diuretics, phenothiazine antipsychotic agents	Additive hypotension
(2) Cimetidine	May increase beta-blocking effects of propranolol by slowing its hepatic clearance and elimination. Increases effects of all calcium channel blockers by inhibiting hepatic metabolism and increasing serum drug levels.
(3) Digoxin	Additive bradycardia when given with beta-blocking agents
b. Drugs that *decrease* effects of antianginal drugs:	
(1) Adrenergic drugs (eg, epinephrine, isoproterenol)	Adrenergic drugs, which stimulate beta receptors, can reverse bradycardia induced by beta blockers.
(2) Anticholinergic drugs	Drugs with anticholinergic effects can increase heart rate, offsetting slower heart rates produced by beta blockers.
(3) Calcium salts	May decrease therapeutic effectiveness of calcium channel blockers
(4) Carbamazepine, phenytoin, rifampin	May decrease effects of calcium channel blockers by inducing hepatic enzymes and thereby increasing their rate of metabolism

APPLYING YOUR KNOWLEDGE: ANSWERS

50-1 Mr. Gerald should be taught to never take sildenafil or other drugs in this class while on nitroglycerin. The combination can produce life-threatening hypotension.

50-2 Beta blockers are used in the treatment of CAD for a number of reasons. They reduce the frequency and severity of anginal attacks. Beta blockers also decrease exercise-induced tachycardia. They additionally are more effective at decreasing the likelihood of silent ischemia and improve the mortality rate after an MI.

50-3 Diltiazem is a calcium channel blocker. The drug will improve blood supply to the myocardium and decrease the workload on the heart. In addition, the diltiazem will reduce coronary artery vasospasm, which is most likely the cause of the pain that Mr. Gerald experiences at rest.

Review and Application Exercises

Short Answer Exercises

1. What is angina pectoris?

2. What is the role of endothelial dysfunction in the development of coronary artery atherosclerosis and myocardial ischemia?

3. How do nitrates relieve angina?

4. Develop a teaching plan for a client who is beginning nitrate therapy.

5. How do beta blockers relieve angina?

6. Why should beta blockers be tapered and discontinued slowly in clients with angina?

7. How do calcium channel blockers relieve angina?

8. Develop a teaching plan for a client taking a calcium channel blocker.

NCLEX-Style Questions

9. The nurse removes a client's transdermal nitroglycerin disc at bedtime as ordered to minimize nitrate tolerance. The client awakens during the night and complains of anginal symptoms. The nurse's first action is to
   a. Notify the health care provider.
   b. Apply a new transdermal disc.
   c. Obtain further history of complaints.
   d. Administer a short-acting nitrate as ordered.

10. The health care provider prescribes nitroglycerin 2% ointment, 1.5-inch dose every 4 hours. To accurately apply the ointment, the client should be instructed to
    a. Rub the ointment into the skin to enhance absorption.
    b. Leave previous ointment on for 4 hours after applying a new dose.
    c. Rotate application sites to decrease skin irritation.
    d. Place the ointment on a distal part of the lower body to increase absorption.

11. Concurrent use of nitrates in any form or route of administration with phosphodiesterase enzyme inhibitors produces
    a. enhanced erectile potential
    b. significant tachycardia
    c. severe hypotensive effects
    d. mild bronchodilation

12. A client who is taking metoprolol (Lopressor) is seen in the cardiac clinic following an MI and reports that he continues to smoke. The nurse recognizes that smoking may contribute to what effect on beta-blocking activity?
    a. reduce the efficacy
    b. potentiate an increase in intracranial pressure
    c. precipitate ventricular fibrillation
    d. increase the incidence of side effects

13. A client with angina pectoris, being discontinued from his beta blockers, asks the nurse, "Why can't I just stop taking the drug today if it's not working anyway?" The nurse instructs the client that failure to taper the drug slowly may lead to
    a. worsening of his angina symptoms
    b. significant bronchoconstriction
    c. development of congestive heart failure
    d. drug fever

Selected References

Brater, D. C. (2000). Clinical pharmacology of cardiovascular drugs. In H. D. Humes (Ed.), *Kelley's Textbook of internal medicine* (4th ed., pp. 651–672). Philadelphia: Lippincott Williams & Wilkins.

Braunwald, E., Antman, E. M., Beasley, J. W., et al. (2002). ACC/AHA guidelines for the management of patients with unstable angina and non–ST-segment elevation myocardial infarction: Executive summary and recommendations. A report of the American College of Cardiology/American Heart Association Task Force on Practice Guidelines (Committee on the Management of Patients with Unstable Angina). *Circulation, 106,* 1893–1900.

Drug facts and comparisons. (Updated monthly). St. Louis: Facts and Comparisons.

Jones, S. (2001). Oral or intravenous beta blockers in acute myocardial infarction. *Emergency Medicine Journal, 18*(4), 270–271.

Lacy, C. F., Armstrong, L. L., Goldman, M. P., et al. (2004). *Lexi-Comp's drug information handbook* (12th ed.). Hudson, OH: Lexi-Comp.

Porth, C. M. (2004). *Pathophysiology: Concepts of altered health states* (7th ed.). Philadelphia: Lippincott Williams & Wilkins.

Schwartz, D., & Goldberg, A. C. (2004). Ischemic heart disease. In G. B. Green, S. Harris, G. A. Lin, & K. C. Moylan (Eds.), *The Washington manual of medical therapeutics* (31st ed., pp. 92–125). Philadelphia: Lippincott Williams & Wilkins.

Talbert, R. L. (2002). Ischemic heart disease. In J. T. DiPiro, R. L. Talbert, G. C. Yee, G. R. Matzke, B. G. Wells, & L. M. Posey (Eds.), *Pharmacotherapy: A pathophysiologic approach* (5th ed., pp. 219–250). New York: McGraw-Hill.

Drugs Used in Hypotension and Shock

OBJECTIVES

After studying this chapter, you will be able to:

1. Identify clients at risk for development of hypovolemia and shock.
2. Identify common causes of hypotension and shock.
3. Discuss assessment of a client in shock.
4. Describe therapeutic and adverse effects of vasopressor drugs used in the management of hypotension and shock.

APPLYING YOUR KNOWLEDGE

Karl Savage is an 80-year-old man who has been admitted to the ICU suffering from hypovolemic shock. He has had aggressive fluid resuscitation; however, his BP remains low. His physician orders an IV dopamine drip to be started at 3 mcg/kg/min.

INTRODUCTION

Shock is a clinical syndrome characterized by decreased blood supply to body tissues. Clinical symptoms depend on the degree of impaired perfusion of vital organs (eg, brain, heart, kidneys). Common signs and symptoms include oliguria, heart failure, mental confusion, cool extremities, and coma. Most, but not all, people in shock are hypotensive. In a previously hypertensive person, shock may be present if a drop in blood pressure of greater than 50 mm Hg has occurred, even if current blood pressure readings are "normal."

An additional consequence of inadequate blood flow to tissues is that cells change from aerobic (oxygen-based) to anaerobic metabolism. Lactic acid produced by anaerobic metabolism leads to generalized metabolic acidosis and eventually to organ failure and death if blood flow is not promptly restored.

Types of Shock

There are three general categories of shock that are based on the circulatory mechanisms involved. These mechanisms are intravascular volume, the ability of the heart to pump, and vascular tone.

Hypovolemic shock involves a loss of intravascular fluid volume that may be due to actual blood loss or relative loss from fluid shifts within the body.

Cardiogenic shock, also called *pump failure,* occurs when the myocardium has lost its ability to contract efficiently and maintain an adequate cardiac output.

Distributive or *vasogenic shock* is characterized by severe, generalized vasodilation, which results in severe hypotension and impairment of blood flow. Distributive shock is further divided into anaphylactic, neurogenic, and septic shock.

- *Anaphylactic shock* results from a hypersensitivity (allergic) reaction to drugs or other substances (see Chap. 17).
- *Neurogenic shock* results from inadequate sympathetic nervous system (SNS) stimulation. The SNS normally maintains sufficient vascular tone (ie, a small amount of vasoconstriction) to support adequate blood circulation. Neurogenic shock may occur with depression of the vasomotor center in the brain or decreased sympathetic outflow to blood vessels.
- *Septic shock* can result from almost any organism that gains access to the bloodstream but is most often associated with gram-negative and gram-positive bacterial infections and fungi.

It is important to know the etiology of shock because management varies among the types. The types of shock, with their causes and symptoms, are summarized in Table 51-1.

GENERAL CHARACTERISTICS OF ANTISHOCK DRUGS

Drugs used in the management of shock are primarily the adrenergic drugs, which are discussed more extensively in Chapter 17. In this chapter, the drugs are discussed only in relation to their use in hypotension and shock. In these conditions, drugs with alpha-adrenergic activity (eg, norepinephrine, phenylephrine) are used to increase peripheral vascular resistance and raise blood pressure. Drugs with beta-adrenergic activity (eg, dobutamine, isoproterenol) are used to increase myocardial contractility and heart rate, which in turn raises blood pressure. Some drugs have both alpha- and beta-adrenergic activity (eg, dopamine, epinephrine). In many cases, a combination of drugs is used, depending on the type

of shock and the client's response to treatment. In an emergency, the drugs may be used to maintain adequate perfusion of vital organs until sufficient fluid volume is replaced and circulation is restored.

Adrenergic drugs with beta activity may be relatively contraindicated in shock states precipitated or complicated by cardiac dysrhythmias. Beta-stimulating drugs also should be used cautiously in cardiogenic shock after myocardial infarction because increased contractility and heart rate will increase myocardial oxygen consumption and extend the area of infarction. Individual drugs are described in the following section; indications for use and dosage ranges are listed in Table 51-2.

INDIVIDUAL DRUGS

Dopamine is a naturally occurring catecholamine that functions as a neurotransmitter. Dopamine exerts its actions by stimulating alpha, beta, or dopaminergic receptors, depending on the dose being used. In addition, dopamine acts indirectly by releasing norepinephrine from sympathetic nerve endings and the adrenal glands. Peripheral dopamine receptors are located in splanchnic and renal vascular beds. At low doses (0.5–10 mcg/kg/min), dopamine selectively stimulates dopaminergic receptors that may increase renal blood flow and glomerular filtration rate (GFR). It has long been accepted that stimulation of dopamine receptors by low doses of exogenous dopamine produces vasodilation in the renal circulation and increases urine output. More recent studies indicate that low-dose dopamine enhances renal function only when cardiac function is improved. At doses greater than 3 micrograms per kilogram per minute, dopamine binds to beta and alpha receptors; the selectivity of dopaminergic receptors is lost beyond 10 micrograms per kilogram per minute. At doses that stimulate beta receptors (3–20 mcg/kg/min), there is an increase in heart rate, myocardial contractility, and blood pressure. At the highest doses (20–50 mcg/kg/min), beta activity remains, but increasing alpha stimulation (vasoconstriction) may overcome its actions.

Dopamine is useful in hypovolemic and cardiogenic shock. Adequate fluid therapy is necessary for the maximal pressor effect of dopamine. Acidosis decreases the effectiveness of dopamine.

APPLYING YOUR KNOWLEDGE 51-1

Think back to Mr. Savage's case. Why has this dosage of dopamine been prescribed? What is the advantage of administration at this dosage?

APPLYING YOUR KNOWLEDGE 51-2

Mr. Savage's BP remains low even after the dopamine drip is initiated. The dose is ordered to be increased to keep his systolic BP above 90 mm Hg. What is the physiologic effect of dopamine at dosages greater than 20 mcg/kg/min?

TABLE 51-1 Types of Shock

TYPE OF SHOCK	POSSIBLE CAUSES	CLINICAL MANIFESTATIONS
Hypovolemic	Trauma Gastrointestinal bleed Ruptured aneurysms Third spacing Dehydration	Hypotension Tachycardia Cool, clammy skin Diaphoresis Pallor Oliguria
Cardiogenic	Acute myocardial infarction Cardiac surgery Dysrhythmias Cardiomyopathy	Signs and symptoms of heart failure Signs and symptoms of decreased cardiac output
Distributive Neurogenic	Spinal cord damage Spinal anesthesia Severe pain Drugs	Hypotension Bradycardia Warm, dry skin Hypotension
Septic	Infection (eg, urinary tract, upper respiratory infections) Invasive procedures	Cool or warm, dry skin Hypothermia or hyperthermia Hypotension
Anaphylactic	Contrast dyes Drugs Insect bites Foods	Hives Bronchospasm

Table 51-2 Drugs at a Glance: Drugs Used for Hypotension and Shock

GENERIC/TRADE NAME	INDICATIONS FOR USE	ROUTES AND DOSAGE RANGES	
		Adults	**Children**
Dopamine (Intropin)	Increase cardiac output Treat hypotension Increase urine output	IV 2–5 mcg/kg/min initially, gradually increasing to 20–50 mcg/kg/min if necessary Prepare by adding 200 mg of dopamine to 250 mL of IV fluid for a final concentration of 800 mcg/mL or to 500 mL IV fluid for a final concentration of 400 mcg/mL.	Same as adults
Dobutamine (Dobutrex)	Increase cardiac output	IV 2.5–15 mcg/kg/min, increased to 40 mcg/kg/min if necessary Reconstitute the 250-mg vial with 10 mL of sterile water or 5% dextrose injection. The resulting solution should be diluted to at least 50 mL with IV solution before administering (5000 mcg/mL). Add 250 mg of drug to 500 mL of diluent for a concentration of 500 mcg/mL.	
Epinephrine (Adrenalin)	Treat anaphylactic shock Reverse bronchoconstriction Increase cardiac output Treat cardiac arrest	IV 1–4 mcg/min. Prepare the solution by adding 2 mg (2 mL) of epinephrine injection 1:1000 to 250 or 500 mL of IV fluid. The final concentration is 8 or 4 mcg/mL, respectively. IV direct injection, 100–1000 mcg of 1:10,000 injection, every 5–15 min, injected slowly. Prepare the solution by adding 1 mL epinephrine 1:1000 to 9 mL sodium chloride injection. The final concentration is 100 mcg/mL. Cardiac arrest, IV injection, 0.5–1.0 mg of 1:10,000 solution, repeated every 5 min as needed	IV infusion, 0.025–0.3 mcg/kg/min IV direct injection, 5 to 10 mcg/kg, slowly Sub-Q, 0.01 mg/kg of 1:1000 solution
Isoproterenol (Isuprel)	Treat atropine-refractory bradycardias	IV infusion, 0.5–10 mcg/min Prepare solution by adding 2 mg to 250 mL of IV fluid. Final concentration is 8 mcg/mL.	IV infusion, 0.05–0.3 mcg/kg/min
Metaraminol (Aramine)	Treat hypotension due to spinal anesthesia	IM 2–10 mg IV injection, 0.5–5 mg IV infusion, add 15–500 mg of metaraminol to 250 or 500 mL of IV fluid. Adjust flow rate (dosage) to maintain the desired blood pressure.	IM 0.1 mg/kg IV injection, 0.01 mg/kg IV infusion, 1 mg/25 mL of diluent. Adjust flow rate to maintain the desired blood pressure.
Milrinone (Primacor)	Increase cardiac output in cardiogenic shock	IV injection (loading dose), 50 mcg/kg over 10 min IV infusion (maintenance dose), 0.375–0.75 mcg/kg/min diluted in 0.9% or 0.45% sodium chloride or 5% dextrose solution. Maximum dose, 1.13 mg/kg/d	
Norepinephrine (Levophed)	Treat hypotension Increase cardiac output	IV infusion, 2–4 mcg/min, to a maximum of 20 mcg/min. Prepare solution by adding 2 mg to 500 mL of IV fluid. Final concentration is 4 mcg/mL.	IV infusion, 0.03–0.1 mcg/kg/min
Phenylephrine (Neo-Synephrine)	Treat hypotension	IV infusion, 100–180 mcg/min initially, then 40–60 mcg/min Prepare solution by adding 10 mg of phenylephrine to 250 or 500 mL of IV fluid. Final concentration is 20 or 40 mcg/mL, respectively. IV injection, 0.1–0.5 mg every 10–15 min	Sub-Q, IM 0.5–1 mg/11 kg

IM, intramuscular; IV, intravenous; Sub-Q, subcutaneous.

Dobutamine is a synthetic catecholamine developed to provide less vascular activity than dopamine. It acts mainly on beta$_1$ receptors in the heart to increase the force of myocardial contraction with a minimal increase in heart rate. Dobutamine also may increase blood pressure with large doses. It is less likely to cause tachycardia, dysrhythmias, and increased myocardial oxygen demand than dopamine and isoproterenol. It is most useful in cases of shock that require increased cardiac output without the need for blood pressure support. It is recommended for short-term use only. It may be used with dopamine to augment the beta$_1$ activity that is sometimes overridden by alpha effects when dopamine is used alone at doses greater than 10 micrograms per kilogram per minute.

Dobutamine has a short plasma half-life and therefore must be administered by continuous intravenous (IV) infusion. A loading dose is not required because the drug has a rapid onset of action and reaches steady state within approximately 10 minutes after the infusion is begun. It is rapidly metabolized to inactive metabolites.

Epinephrine is a naturally occurring catecholamine produced by the adrenal glands. At low doses, epinephrine stimulates beta receptors, which increases cardiac output by increasing the rate and force of myocardial contractility. It also causes bronchodilation. Larger doses act on alpha receptors to increase blood pressure.

Epinephrine is the drug of choice for management of anaphylactic shock because of its rapid onset of action and anti-allergic effects. It prevents the release of histamine and other mediators that cause symptoms of anaphylaxis, thereby reversing vasodilation and bronchoconstriction. In early management of anaphylaxis, it may be given subcutaneously to produce therapeutic effects within 5 to 10 minutes, with peak activity in approximately 20 minutes.

Epinephrine is also used to manage other kinds of shock and is usually given by continuous IV infusion. However, bolus doses may be given in emergencies, such as cardiac arrest. Epinephrine may produce excessive cardiac stimulation, ventricular dysrhythmias, and reduced renal blood flow. Epinephrine has an elimination half-life of about 2 minutes and is rapidly inactivated to metabolites, which are then excreted by the kidneys.

Isoproterenol is a synthetic catecholamine that acts exclusively on beta receptors to increase heart rate, myocardial contractility, and systolic blood pressure. However, it also stimulates vascular beta$_2$ receptors, which causes vasodilation, and may decrease diastolic blood pressure. For this reason, isoproterenol has limited usefulness as a pressor agent. It also may increase myocardial oxygen consumption and decrease coronary artery blood flow, which in turn causes myocardial ischemia. Cardiac dysrhythmias may result from excessive beta stimulation. Because of these limitations, use of isoproterenol is limited to shock associated with slow heart rates and myocardial depression.

Metaraminol is used mainly for hypotension associated with spinal anesthesia. It acts indirectly by releasing norepi-

nephrine from sympathetic nerve endings. Thus, its vasoconstrictive actions are similar to those of norepinephrine, except that metaraminol is less potent and has a longer duration of action.

Milrinone is discussed in Chapter 48 as a treatment for heart failure. It is also used to manage cardiogenic shock in combination with other inotropic agents or vasopressors. It increases cardiac output and decreases systemic vascular resistance without significantly increasing heart rate or myocardial oxygen consumption. The increased cardiac output improves renal blood flow, which then leads to increased urine output, decreased circulating blood volume, and decreased cardiac workload.

Norepinephrine (Levophed) is a pharmaceutical preparation of the naturally occurring catecholamine norepinephrine. It stimulates alpha-adrenergic receptors and thus increases blood pressure primarily by vasoconstriction. It also stimulates beta$_1$ receptors and therefore increases heart rate, force of myocardial contraction, and coronary artery blood flow. It is useful in cardiogenic and septic shock, but reduced renal blood flow limits its prolonged use. Norepinephrine is used mainly with clients who are unresponsive to dopamine or dobutamine. As with all drugs used to manage shock, blood pressure should be monitored frequently during infusion.

Phenylephrine (Neo-Synephrine) is an adrenergic drug that stimulates alpha-adrenergic receptors. As a result, it constricts arterioles and raises systolic and diastolic blood pressures. Phenylephrine resembles epinephrine but has fewer cardiac effects and a longer duration of action. Reduction of renal and mesenteric blood flow limits prolonged use.

APPLYING YOUR KNOWLEDGE 51-3

Mr. Savage continues to have a BP that is less than 90 mm Hg. The physician orders the dopamine drip to be discontinued and to start a Levophed drip to keep the BP above 90 mm Hg. Why has this change in medication been made?

NURSING PROCESS

Assessment

Assess the client's condition in relation to hypotension and shock.

● Check blood pressure; heart rate; urine output; skin temperature and color of extremities; level of consciousness; orientation to person, place, and time; and adequacy of respiration. Abnormal values are not specific indicators of hypotension and shock, but they may indicate a need for further evaluation. In general, report blood pressure less than 90/60 mm Hg, heart rate greater than 100 beats/minute, and urine output less than 30 mL/hour.

● Assess electrocardiogram and cardiac and hemodynamic status for indications of impaired cardiac function.

● Monitor available laboratory reports for abnormal values (eg, decreased oxygen saturation levels indicate decreased oxygenation of tissues; abnormal arterial blood gases may indicate metabolic acidosis; an increased hematocrit may indicate hypovolemia; an increased eosinophil count may indicate anaphylaxis; the presence of bacteria in blood cultures may indicate sepsis; increased serum creatinine and blood urea nitrogen may indicate impending renal failure).

Nursing Diagnoses

● Decreased Cardiac Output related to altered stroke volume
● Ineffective Tissue Perfusion: Decreased related to compromised cardiac output
● Deficient Fluid Volume related to fluid loss or vasodilation
● Anxiety related to potentially life-threatening illness
● Risk for Injury: Myocardial infarction, stroke, or renal damage related to decreased blood flow to vital organs

Planning/Goals

● Have improved tissue perfusion and relief of symptoms
● Have improved vital signs
● Be guarded against recurrence of hypotension and shock if possible
● Be assessed for therapeutic and adverse effects of adrenergic drugs
● Avoid preventable adverse effects of adrenergic drugs

Interventions

Use measures to prevent or minimize hypotension and shock.
● General measures include those to maintain the airway, maintain fluid balance, control hemorrhage, manage infections, prevent hypoxia, and control other causative factors.
● Learn to recognize impending shock so management can be initiated early. Do not wait until symptoms are severe. The earlier the management, the greater the likelihood of reversing shock and preventing end-stage organ damage.
● Assist in recognizing and managing the underlying cause of shock in a particular client (eg, replacing fluids; preventing further loss of blood or other body fluids).

Monitor clients during shock and vasopressor drug therapy.

● Titrate adrenergic drug infusions to maintain blood pressure and tissue perfusion without causing hypertension.

● Check blood pressure and pulse constantly or at least every 5 to 15 minutes during acute shock and vasopressor drug therapy. Intra-arterial monitoring may be more reliable than cuff blood-pressure measurements in shock conditions.
● Monitor mental status, distal pulses, urine output, and skin temperature and color closely to assess tissue perfusion.
● Assess venipuncture sites frequently for signs of infiltration or extravasation. Have phentolamine (Regitine), an alpha-adrenergic blocking agent that reverses vasoconstriction, readily available in any setting where IV adrenergic drugs are used. If infiltration occurs, instill phentolamine through the IV catheter prior to removal.
● Keep family members informed about client status and management measures, including drug therapy, monitoring equipment, and the need for close observation of vital signs, IV infusion site, urine output, and so forth.

Provide client teaching regarding drug therapy (see accompanying display).

Evaluation

Observe for improved vital signs, color and temperature of skin, urine output, and mental responsiveness.

PRINCIPLES OF THERAPY

Goal of Therapy

The goal of adrenergic drug therapy in hypotension and shock is to restore and maintain adequate tissue perfusion, especially to vital organs.

Drug Selection

The choice of drug depends primarily on the pathophysiology involved. For cardiogenic shock and decreased cardiac output, dopamine or dobutamine is given. With severe heart failure characterized by decreased cardiac output and high peripheral vascular resistance, vasodilator drugs (eg, nitroprusside, nitroglycerin) may be given along with the cardiotonic drug. The combination increases cardiac output and decreases cardiac workload by decreasing preload and afterload. However, vasodilators should not be used alone because of the risk of severe hypotension and further compromising tissue perfusion. Milrinone may be given when other drugs fail.

For distributive shock characterized by severe vasodilation and decreased peripheral vascular resistance, a vasoconstrictor or vasopressor drug, such as norepinephrine, is the drug of first choice. Drug dosage must be carefully titrated to avoid excessive vasoconstriction and hypertension, which causes impairment rather than improvement in tissue perfusion.

Guidelines for Management of Hypotension and Shock

- Vasopressor drugs are less effective in the presence of inadequate blood volume, electrolyte abnormalities, and acidosis. These conditions also must be treated if present. In addition, normalizing the blood pH and body temperature facilitates the release of oxygen from hemoglobin to the cells.
- Minimal effective doses of adrenergic drugs are recommended because of their extreme vasoconstrictive effects that can produce lactic acidosis at the cell level and create metabolic acidosis. Because catecholamine drugs have short half-lives, varying the flow rate of IV infusions can easily control dosage. Dosage and flow rate usually are titrated to maintain a low-normal blood pressure. Such titration depends on frequent and accurate blood pressure measurements.
- Septic shock due to bacterial infection requires appropriate antibiotic therapy in addition to other management measures (see Section 5). If an abscess is the source of infection, it must be surgically drained.
- Hypovolemic shock is most effectively managed by IV fluids that replace the type of fluid lost; that is, blood loss should be replaced with whole blood; gastrointestinal losses should be replaced with solutions containing electrolytes (eg, Ringer's lactate or sodium chloride solutions with added potassium chloride).
- Cardiogenic shock may be complicated by pulmonary congestion, for which diuretic drugs are indicated and IV fluids are contraindicated (except to maintain a patent IV line).
- Anaphylactic shock is often managed by nonadrenergic drugs as well as epinephrine. For example, the histamine-induced cardiovascular symptoms (eg, vasodilation and increased capillary permeability) are thought to be mediated through both types of histamine receptors. Thus, management may include a histamine$_1$ receptor blocker (eg, diphenhydramine 1 mg/kg IV) and a histamine$_2$ receptor blocker (eg, cimetidine 4 mg/kg IV), given over at least 5 minutes. In addition, IV corticosteroids are often given, such as methylprednisolone (20–100 mg) or hydrocortisone (100–500 mg). Doses may need to be repeated every 2 to 4 hours. Corticosteroids increase tissue responsiveness to adrenergic drugs in approximately 2 hours but do not produce anti-inflammatory effects for several hours.

Use in Special Populations

Use in Children

Little information is available about adrenergic drugs for the management of hypotension and shock in children. Children who lose up to one fourth of their circulating blood volume may produce minimal changes in arterial blood pressure and a relatively low heart rate. In general, management is the same as for adults, with drug dosages adjusted for weight.

Use in Older Adults

Older adults often have disorders such as atherosclerosis, peripheral vascular disease, and diabetes mellitus and may not demonstrate common symptoms of volume depletion (eg, thirst, skin turgor changes). Also, when adrenergic drugs are given, their vasoconstricting effects may decrease blood flow and increase risks of tissue ischemia and thrombosis. Careful monitoring of vital signs, skin color and temperature, urine output, and mental status is essential.

Use in Clients With Renal Impairment

Although adrenergic drugs may be life saving, they can reduce renal blood flow and cause renal failure because of their vasoconstrictive effects. Renal impairment may occur in clients with previously normal renal function and may be worsened in clients whose renal function is already impaired. Low-dose dopamine is commonly used to increase renal perfusion in oliguric clients, but the effectiveness of this practice is being questioned.

In men with benign prostatic hypertrophy, oliguric renal failure may need to be differentiated from post–renal failure (urinary retention) because some adrenergic drugs (eg, epinephrine, norepinephrine, phenylephrine) cause urinary retention.

Most adrenergic drugs are metabolized in the liver and the metabolites are excreted in the urine. However, little accumulation of the drugs or metabolites is likely because the drugs have short half-lives.

Use in Clients With Hepatic Impairment

Catecholamine drugs are metabolized by monoamine oxidase (MAO) and catechol-*O*-methyl transferase (COMT). MAO is widely distributed in most body tissues, whereas COMT is located mainly in the liver. Thus, the drugs are eliminated mainly by liver metabolism and must be used cautiously in clients with impaired liver function. Clients should be monitored closely and drug dosage should be adjusted as symptoms warrant. However, the half-life of most adrenergic drugs is very brief, and this decreases the chances of drug accumulation in hepatically impaired clients.

Use in Clients With Critical Illness

The adrenergic catecholamines (eg, dopamine, dobutamine, epinephrine, norepinephrine) are widely used in clients with a low cardiac output that persists despite adequate fluid replacement and correction of electrolyte imbalance. By improving circulation, the drugs also help to prevent tissue injury from ischemia (eg, renal failure).

Although the drugs may be used initially in almost any setting, most clients with hypotension and shock are managed in critical care units. Dobutamine and dopamine are usually the cardiotonic agents of choice in critically ill clients. Dopamine varies in clearance rate in adult and pediatric clients. However, this variance may result from the use of non–steady-state plasma concentrations in calculating the clearance rate. When a dopamine IV infusion is started, it may take 1 to 2 hours to achieve a steady-state plasma level. Relatively large doses of dopamine are given for cardiotonic and vasoconstrictive effects.

Epinephrine and norepinephrine are also widely used in critically ill clients. Recommended infusion rates in critically ill clients vary from 0.01 to 0.15 micrograms per kilogram per minute for epinephrine and from 0.06 to 0.15 for norepinephrine. All clients receiving drugs for management of hypotension and shock should be closely monitored regarding drug dosage, vital signs, relevant laboratory test results, and other indicators of clinical status. Continuous invasive hemodynamic monitoring with an arterial catheter and a pulmonary artery catheter may be indicated to titrate drug dosage and monitor the response to drug therapy. Close monitoring of the critically ill is essential because these clients often have multiple organ impairments and are clinically unstable.

APPLYING YOUR KNOWLEDGE 51-4:
HOW CAN YOU AVOID THIS MEDICATION ERROR?
Jason, a nurse on your floor, is monitoring the dopamine drip for his patient and does not observe an increase in BP after the infusion has been running for about 30 minutes. He calls the physician to obtain orders to change the dopamine to some other vasopressor.

N U R S I N G   A C T I O N S

Drugs Used in Hypotension and Shock

NURSING ACTIONS	RATIONALE/EXPLANATION
1. Administer accurately	
a. Use a large vein for the venipuncture site.	To decrease risks of extravasation
b. Dilute drugs for continuous infusion in 250 or 500 mL of intravenous (IV) fluid. A 5% dextrose injection is compatible with all of the drugs and is most often used. For use of other IV fluids, consult drug manufacturers' literature. Dilute drugs for bolus injections to at least 10 mL with sodium chloride or water for injection.	To avoid adverse effects, which are more likely to occur with concentrated drug solutions
c. Use a separate IV line or a "piggyback" IV setup.	This allows the adrenergic drug solution to be regulated or discontinued without disruption of other IV lines.
d. Use an infusion pump.	To administer the drug at a consistent rate and prevent wide fluctuations in blood pressure and other cardiovascular functions
e. Discard any solution with a brownish color or precipitate.	Most of the solutions are stable for 24–48 hours. Epinephrine and isoproterenol decompose on exposure to light, producing a brownish discoloration.
f. Start the adrenergic drug slowly, and increase as necessary to obtain desired responses in blood pressure and other parameters of cardiovascular function.	Flow rate (dosage) is titrated according to client response.
g. Stop the drug gradually.	Abrupt discontinuance of pressor drugs may cause rebound hypotension.
h. Manage the client, not the monitor.	Abnormal monitor readings (ie, blood pressure monitors) should be confirmed with a manual reading before adjusting medication dosage.
2. Observe for therapeutic effects	
a. Systolic blood pressure of 80–100 mm Hg	These levels are adequate for tissue perfusion. Higher levels may increase cardiac workload, resulting in reflex bradycardia and decreased cardiac output. However, higher levels may be necessary to maintain cerebral blood flow in older adults.

(continued)

NURSING ACTIONS	RATIONALE/EXPLANATION
b. Heart rate of 60–100, improved quality of peripheral pulses	These indicate improved tissue perfusion and cardiovascular function.
c. Improved urine output	Increased urine output indicates improved blood flow to the kidneys.
d. Improved skin color and temperature	These indicate improved peripheral tissue perfusion.
e. Pulmonary capillary wedge pressure between 15 and 20 mm Hg in cardiogenic shock	Normal pulmonary capillary wedge pressure is 6–12 mm Hg. Higher levels are required to maintain cardiac output in cardiogenic shock.
3. Observe for adverse effects	
a. Bradycardia	Reflex bradycardia may occur with norepinephrine, metaraminol, and phenylephrine.
b. Tachycardia	This is most likely to occur with isoproterenol, but may occur with dopamine and epinephrine.
c. Dysrhythmias	Serious dysrhythmias may occur with any of the agents used in hypotension and shock. Causes may include high doses that result in excessive adrenergic stimulation of the heart, low doses that result in inadequate perfusion of the myocardium, or the production of lactic acid by ischemic tissue.
d. Hypertension	This is most likely to occur with high doses of norepinephrine, metaraminol, and phenylephrine.
e. Hypotension	This is most likely to occur with low doses of dopamine and isoproterenol, owing to vasodilation.
f. Angina pectoris—chest pain, dyspnea, palpitations	All pressor agents may increase myocardial oxygen consumption and induce myocardial ischemia.
g. Tissue necrosis if extravasation occurs	This may occur with solutions containing dopamine, norepinephrine, metaraminol, and phenylephrine, owing to local vasoconstriction and impaired blood supply. Tissue necrosis may be prevented by injecting 5–10 mg of phentolamine (Regitine) through the catheter or subcutaneously, around the area of extravasation. Phentolamine is most effective if injected within 12 hours after extravasation.
4. Observe for drug interactions	
a. Drugs that *increase* effects of pressor agents:	
(1) General anesthetics (eg, halothane)	Halothane and other halogenated anesthetics increase cardiac sensitivity to sympathomimetic drugs and increase the risks of cardiac dysrhythmias.
(2) Anticholinergic drugs (eg, atropine)	Atropine and other drugs with anticholinergic activity may potentiate the tachycardia that often occurs with pressor agents, especially isoproterenol.
(3) Monoamine oxidase (MAO) inhibitors (eg, tranylcypromine)	All effects of exogenously administered adrenergic drugs are magnified in clients taking MAO inhibitors because MAO is the circulating enzyme responsible for metabolism of adrenergic agents.
(4) Oxytocics (eg, oxytocin)	The risk of severe hypertension is increased.
b. Drugs that *decrease* effects of pressor agents:	
(1) Beta-blocking agents (eg, propranolol)	Beta-blocking agents antagonize the cardiac stimulation of some pressor agents (eg, dobutamine, isoproterenol). Decreased heart rate, myocardial contractility, and blood pressure may result.

APPLYING YOUR KNOWLEDGE: ANSWERS

51-1 Dopamine at a dosage this low may provide the BP support to raise Mr. Savage's BP to a clinically satisfactory level. At this dosage, the dopamine may also increase renal blood flow and GFR.

51-2 Dopamine at dosages from 20 to 50 mcg/kg/min will have an increased vasoconstrictive effect due to the increasing alpha adrenergic stimulation.

51-3 Levophed has a primary alpha-adrenergic effect that will raise the BP by vasoconstriction. It will also increase heart rate, the force of myocardial contraction, and coronary artery blood flow with beta$_1$ receptor stimulation. Levophed is used for patients like Mr. Savage who have been unresponsive to dopamine.

51-4 Dopamine can take up to 1 to 2 hours to reach a steady-state plasma level. The first measure to increase BP would normally be to increase dosage.

Review and Application Exercises

Short Answer Exercises

1. How do adrenergic drugs improve circulation in hypotension and shock?

2. Which adrenergic drug should be readily available for management of anaphylactic shock?

3. What are major adverse effects of adrenergic drugs?

4. How would you assess the client for therapeutic or adverse effects of an adrenergic drug being given by continuous IV infusion?

5. Why is it important to prevent extravasation of adrenergic drug infusions into tissues surrounding the vein?

6. In hypovolemic shock, should fluid volume be replaced before or after an adrenergic drug is given? Why?

NCLEX-Style Questions

7. During administration of dopamine, a client complains of pain at the infusion site. The nurse should recognize that the
   a. client is hypersensitive to the drug
   b. infusion rate is too fast
   c. infusion site should be immediately changed
   d. medication is not effective

8. A client in cardiogenic shock is started on dobutamine (Dobutrex). The health care provider's order reads: dobutamine 10 mcg/kg/min IV. What effect should the nurse expect after beginning drug therapy?
   a. enhanced cardiac contraction and contractility via stimulation of alpha$_1$, beta$_1$, and beta$_2$ receptors
   b. dilated blood vessels via stimulation of dopamine receptors
   c. increased cardiac output through stimulation of beta$_1$ receptors
   d. constricted blood vessels and increased cardiac output through stimulation of alpha$_1$ receptors

9. A client receiving norepinephrine (Levophed) for shock has an arterial line in place. The client's blood pressure has been near 90/42 mm Hg for most of the morning. The blood pressure reading on the monitor suddenly shows a blood pressure of 130/80. The nurse should:
   a. Decrease the rate of the norepinephrine.
   b. Call the health care provider.
   c. Stop the norepinephrine infusion.
   d. Confirm the blood pressure with a manual reading.

10. A client who is in anaphylactic shock presents to the emergency department. The nurse should anticipate that the drug of choice for this type of shock would be
    a. dobutamine
    b. dopamine
    c. isoproterenol
    d. epinephrine

Selected References

Dax, J. M., & Hermey, C. L. (2000). Shock and multiple organ dysfunction syndrome. In S. M. Lewis, M. M. Heitkemper, & S. R. Dirksen (Eds.), *Medical-surgical nursing: Assessment and management of clinical problems* (5th ed., pp. 1865–1894). St. Louis: Mosby.

Erstad, B. L. (2002). Hypovolemic shock. In J. T. DiPiro, R. L. Talbert, G. C. Yee, G. R. Matzke, B. G. Wells, & L. M. Posey (Eds.), *Pharmacotherapy: A pathophysiologic approach* (5th ed., pp. 453–466). New York: McGraw-Hill.

Karch, A. M. (2003). *2004 Lippincott's nursing drug guide.* Philadelphia: Lippincott Williams & Wilkins.

Lacy, C. F., Armstrong, L. L., Goldman, M. P., et al. (2004). *Lexi-Comp's drug information handbook* (12th ed.). Hudson, OH: Lexi-Comp.

Porth, C. M. (2005). *Pathophysiology: Concepts of altered health states* (7th ed.). Philadelphia: Lippincott Williams & Wilkins.

Rudis, M. I., & Dasta, J. F. (2002). Vasopressors and inotropes in shock. In J. T. DiPiro, R. L. Talbert, G. C. Yee, G. R. Matzke, B. G. Wells, & L. M. Posey (Eds.), *Pharmacotherapy: A pathophysiologic approach* (5th ed., pp. 435–451). New York: McGraw-Hill.

Antihypertensive Drugs

OBJECTIVES

After studying this chapter, you will be able to:

1. Describe factors that control blood pressure.
2. Define/describe hypertension.
3. Identify clients at risk for development of hypertension and its sequelae.
4. Discuss nonpharmacologic measures to control hypertension.
5. Review the effects of alpha-adrenergic blockers, beta-adrenergic blockers, calcium channel blockers, and diuretics in hypertension.
6. Discuss angiotensin-converting enzyme inhibitors and angiotensin II receptor blockers in terms of mechanisms of action, indications for use, adverse effects, and nursing process implications.
7. Describe the rationale for using combination drugs in the management of hypertension.
8. Discuss interventions to increase therapeutic effects and minimize adverse effects of antihypertensive drugs.
9. Discuss the use of antihypertensive drugs in special populations.

APPLYING YOUR KNOWLEDGE

Harold Olms is a 55-year-old, African-American male. He is married, has four children, and works as an automobile salesman. Mr. Olms has experienced hypertension for the past 15 years. His current drug regimen to keep his blood pressure at less than 140/90 mm Hg consists of:
  Valsartan 80 mg PO daily
  Amlodipine 10 mg PO daily
  Hydrochlorothiazide 12.5 mg PO daily

INTRODUCTION

Antihypertensive drugs are used to treat hypertension, a common, chronic disorder affecting an estimated 50 to 60 million adults and an unknown number of children and adolescents in the United States. Hypertension increases risks of myocardial infarction, heart failure, cerebral infarction and hemorrhage, and renal disease. To understand hypertension and antihypertensive drug therapy, it is necessary first to understand the physiologic mechanisms that normally control blood pressure; characteristics of hypertension; and characteristics of antihypertensive drugs.

Regulation of Blood Pressure

Arterial blood pressure reflects the force exerted on arterial walls by blood flow. Blood pressure normally remains constant because of homeostatic mechanisms that adjust blood flow to meet tissue needs. The two major determinants of arterial blood pressure are cardiac output (systolic pressure) and peripheral vascular resistance (diastolic pressure).

Cardiac output equals the product of the heart rate and stroke volume ($CO = HR \times SV$). Stroke volume is the amount of blood ejected with each heartbeat (approximately 60–90 mL). Thus, cardiac output depends on the force of myocardial contraction, blood volume, and other factors. Peripheral vascular resistance is determined by local blood flow and the degree of constriction or dilation in arterioles and arteries (vascular tone).

Autoregulation of Blood Flow

Autoregulation is the ability of body tissues to regulate their own blood flow. Local blood flow is regulated primarily by nutritional needs of the tissue, such as lack of oxygen or accumulation of products of cellular metabolism (eg, carbon dioxide, lactic acid). Local tissues produce vasodilating and vasoconstricting substances to regulate local blood flow. Important tissue factors include histamine, bradykinin, serotonin, and prostaglandins.

Histamine is found mainly in mast cells surrounding blood vessels and is released when these tissues are injured.

In some tissues, such as skeletal muscle, mast cell activity is mediated by the sympathetic nervous system (SNS) and histamine is released when SNS stimulation is blocked or withdrawn. In this case, vasodilation results from increased histamine release and the withdrawal of SNS vasoconstrictor activity. *Bradykinin* is released from a protein in body fluids. Kinins dilate arterioles, increase capillary permeability, and constrict venules. *Serotonin* is released from aggregating platelets during the blood clotting process. It causes vasoconstriction and plays a major role in control of bleeding. *Prostaglandins* are formed in response to tissue injury and include vasodilators (eg, prostacyclin) and vasoconstrictors (eg, thromboxane A_2).

An important component of regulating local blood flow is the production of several vasoactive substances by the endothelial cells that line blood vessels. Vasoconstricting substances, which increase vascular tone and blood pressure, include angiotensin II, endothelin-1, and thromboxane A_2. Vasodilating substances, which decrease vascular tone and blood pressure, include nitric oxide and prostacyclin. Excessive vasoconstrictors or deficient vasodilators may contribute to the development of atherosclerosis, hypertension, and other diseases. Injury to the endothelial lining of blood vessels (eg, by the shear force of blood flow with hypertension, by rupture of atherosclerotic plaque) leads to vasoconstriction, vasospasm, thrombus formation, and thickening of the blood vessel wall. All of these factors narrow the blood vessel lumen and increase peripheral vascular resistance.

Overall, regulation of blood pressure involves a complex, interacting, overlapping network of hormonal, neural, and vascular mechanisms, and any condition that affects heart rate, stroke volume, or peripheral vascular resistance affects arterial blood pressure. Many of these mechanisms are compensatory effects that attempt to restore balance when hypotension or hypertension occurs. The mechanisms are further described in Box 52-1 and are referred to in the following discussion of antihypertensive drugs and their actions in lowering high blood pressure.

Response to Hypotension

When hypotension (and decreased tissue perfusion) occurs, the SNS is stimulated, the hormones epinephrine and norepinephrine are secreted by the adrenal medulla, angiotensin II and aldosterone are formed, and the kidneys retain fluid. These compensatory mechanisms raise the blood pressure. Specific effects include the following:

- Constriction of arterioles, which increases peripheral vascular resistance
- Constriction of veins and increased venous tone
- Stimulation of cardiac beta-adrenergic receptors, which increases heart rate and force of myocardial contraction
- Activation of the renin–angiotensin–aldosterone mechanism

Response to Hypertension

When arterial blood pressure is elevated, the following sequence of events occurs.

- Kidneys excrete more fluid (increase urine output).
- Fluid loss reduces both extracellular fluid volume and blood volume.
- Decreased blood volume reduces venous blood flow to the heart and therefore decreases cardiac output.
- Decreased cardiac output reduces arterial blood pressure.
- The vascular endothelium produces vasodilating substances (eg, nitric oxide, prostacyclin), which reduce blood pressure.

Hypertension

Hypertension is persistently high blood pressure that results from abnormalities in regulatory mechanisms. It is usually defined as a systolic pressure above 140 mm Hg or a diastolic pressure above 90 mm Hg on multiple blood pressure measurements.

Primary or essential hypertension (that for which no cause can be found) makes up 90% to 95% of known cases. Secondary hypertension may result from renal, endocrine, or central nervous system disorders and from drugs that stimulate the SNS or cause retention of sodium and water. Primary hypertension can be controlled with appropriate therapy; secondary hypertension can sometimes be cured by surgical therapy.

The Seventh Report of the Joint National Committee on Prevention, Detection, Evaluation, and Treatment of High Blood Pressure (JNC 7), guidelines published in 2003, classified blood pressures in adults (in mm of Hg) as follows:

- Normal = systolic <120 <u>and</u> diastolic <80
- Prehypertension = systolic 120–139 <u>or</u> diastolic 80–89
- Stage 1 hypertension = systolic 140–159 <u>or</u> diastolic 90–99
- Stage 2 hypertension = systolic >160 <u>or</u> diastolic 100 or more

This classification is markedly different from the four stages previously defined. The addition of a prehypertension stage targets individuals who are twice as likely to progress to hypertension as those with lower pressure values. Stages 3 and 4 have been eliminated. These newer guidelines also recommend a goal blood pressure for those with diabetes or renal disease of less than 130/80 mmHg. A systolic pressure of 140 or above, with a diastolic pressure below 90, is called *isolated systolic hypertension* and is more common in the elderly.

Hypertension profoundly alters cardiovascular function by increasing the workload of the heart and causing thickening and sclerosis of arterial walls. As a result of increased cardiac workload, the myocardium hypertrophies as a compensatory mechanism and heart failure eventually occurs. As a result of

Box 52-1   Mechanisms That Regulate Blood Pressure

Neural

Neural regulation of blood pressure mainly involves the sympathetic nervous system (SNS). In the heart, SNS neurons control heart rate and force of contraction. In blood vessels, SNS neurons control muscle tone by maintaining a state of partial contraction, with additional constriction or dilation accomplished by altering this basal state. When hypotension and inadequate tissue perfusion occur, the SNS is activated and produces secretion of epinephrine and norepinephrine by the adrenal medulla; constriction of blood vessels in the skin, gastrointestinal tract, and kidneys; and stimulation of beta-adrenergic receptors in the heart, which increases heart rate and force of myocardial contraction. All of these mechanisms act to increase blood pressure and tissue perfusion, especially of the brain and heart.

The SNS is activated by the vasomotor center in the brain, which constantly receives messages from baroreceptors and chemoreceptors located in the circulatory system. Adequate function of these receptors is essential for rapid and short-term regulation of blood pressure. The vasomotor center interprets the messages from these receptors and modifies cardiovascular functions to maintain adequate blood flow.

More specifically, baroreceptors detect changes in pressure or stretch. For example, when a person moves from a lying to a standing position, blood pressure falls and decreases stretch in the aorta and arteries. This elicits increased heart rate and vasoconstriction to restore adequate circulation. The increased heart rate occurs rapidly and blood pressure is adjusted within 1 to 2 minutes. This quick response prevents orthostatic hypotension with dizziness and possible syncope. (Antihypertensive medications may blunt this response and cause orthostatic hypotension.)

Chemoreceptors, which are located in the aorta and carotid arteries, are in close contact with arterial blood and respond to changes in the oxygen, carbon dioxide, and hydrogen ion content of blood. Although their main function is to regulate ventilation, they also communicate with the vasomotor center and can induce vasoconstriction. Chemoreceptors are stimulated when blood pressure drops to a certain point because oxygen is decreased and carbon dioxide and hydrogen ions are increased in arterial blood.

The central nervous system (CNS) also regulates vasomotor tone and blood pressure. Inadequate blood flow to the brain results in ischemia of the vasomotor center. When this occurs, neurons in the vasomotor center stimulate widespread vasoconstriction in an attempt to raise blood pressure and restore blood flow. This reaction, the CNS ischemic response, is an emergency measure to preserve blood flow to vital brain centers. If blood flow is not restored within 3 to 10 minutes, the neurons of the vasomotor center are unable to function, the impulses that maintain vascular muscle tone stop, and blood pressure drops to a fatal level.

Hormonal

The renin–angiotensin–aldosterone (RAA) system and vasopressin are important hormonal mechanisms in blood pressure regulation.

The *RAA system* is activated in response to hypotension and acts as a compensatory mechanism to restore adequate blood flow to body tissues. Renin is an enzyme that is synthesized,

stored, and released from the kidneys in response to decreased blood pressure, SNS stimulation, or decreased sodium concentration in extracellular fluid. When released into the bloodstream, where its action lasts 30 to 60 minutes, renin converts angiotensinogen (a plasma protein) to angiotensin I. Angiotensin-converting enzyme (ACE) in the endothelium of pulmonary blood vessels then acts on angiotensin I to produce angiotensin II. Angiotensin II strongly constricts arterioles (and weakly constricts veins), increases peripheral resistance, and increases blood pressure by direct vasoconstriction, stimulation of the SNS, and stimulation of catecholamine release from the adrenal medulla. It also stimulates secretion of aldosterone from the adrenal cortex, which then causes the kidneys to retain sodium and water. Retention of sodium and water increases blood volume, cardiac output, and blood pressure.

Vasopressin, also called antidiuretic hormone or ADH, is a hormone secreted by the posterior pituitary gland that regulates reabsorption of water by the kidneys. It is released in response to decreased blood volume and decreased blood pressure. It causes retention of body fluids and vasoconstriction, both of which act to raise blood pressure.

Vascular

The endothelial cells that line blood vessels synthesize and secrete several substances that play important roles in regulating cardiovascular functions, including blood pressure. These substances normally maintain a balance between vasoconstriction and vasodilation. When the endothelium is damaged (eg, by trauma, hypertension, hypercholesterolemia, or atherosclerosis), the resulting imbalance promotes production of vasoconstricting substances and also causes blood vessels to lose their ability to relax in response to dilator substances. In addition, changes in structure of endothelial and vascular smooth muscle cells (vascular remodeling) further impair vascular functions.

Vasoconstrictors increase vascular tone (ie, constrict or narrow blood vessels so that higher blood pressure is required to pump blood to body tissues). Vasoconstricting substances produced by the endothelium include angiotensin II, endothelin-1, platelet-derived growth factor (PDGF), and thromboxane A_2. Endothelin-1 is the strongest endogenous vasoconstrictor known. Angiotensin II and thromboxane A_2 can also be produced by other types of cells, but endothelial cells can produce both. Thromboxane A_2, a product of arachidonic acid metabolism, also promotes platelet aggregation and thrombosis.

Vasodilators decrease vascular tone and blood pressure. Major vasodilating substances produced by the endothelium include nitric oxide and prostacyclin (prostaglandin I_2)

Nitric oxide (NO) is a gas that can diffuse through cell membranes, trigger biochemical reactions, and then dissipate rapidly. It is formed by the action of the enzyme NO synthase on the amino acid L-arginine and continually released by normal endothelium. Its production is tightly regulated and depends on the amount of ionized calcium in the fluid portion of endothelial cells. Several substances (eg, acetylcholine, bradykinin, catecholamines, substance P, and products of aggregating platelets such as adenosine diphosphate and serotonin) act on receptors in endothelial cell membranes to

(continued)

Box 52-1 Mechanisms That Regulate Blood Pressure (continued)

increase the cytosolic concentration of ionized calcium, activate NO synthase, and increase NO production. In addition, increased blood flow or blood pressure increases shear stress at the endothelial surface and stimulates production of NO.

Once produced, endothelium-derived NO produces vasodilation primarily by activating guanylyl cyclase in vascular smooth muscle cells and increasing intracellular cyclic 3,5′-guanosine monophosphate as a second messenger. NO also inhibits platelet aggregation and production of platelet-derived vasoconstricting substances. Because NO is released into the vessel wall (to relax smooth muscle) and into the vessel lumen (to inactivate platelets), it is thought to have protective effects against vasoconstriction and thrombosis.

NO is also produced in leukocytes, fibroblasts, and vascular smooth muscle cells and may have pathologic effects when large amounts are produced. In these tissues, NO seems to have other functions, such as modifying nerve activity in the nervous system.

Prostacyclin is synthesized and released from endothelium in response to stimulation by several factors (eg, bradykinin, interleukin-1, serotonin, thrombin, PDGF). It produces vasodilation by activating adenylyl cyclase and increasing levels of cyclic adenosine monophosphate in smooth muscle cells. In addition, like NO, prostacyclin also inhibits platelet aggregation and production of platelet-derived vasoconstricting substances. The vasodilating effects of prostacyclin may occur independently or in conjunction with NO.

Overall, excessive vasoconstrictors or deficient vasodilators may contribute to the development of atherosclerosis, hypertension, and other diseases. Injury to the endothelial lining of blood vessels (eg, by the shear force of blood flow with hypertension or by rupture of atherosclerotic plaque) decreases vasodilators and leads to vasoconstriction, vasospasm, thrombus formation, and thickening of the blood vessel wall. All of these factors require the blood to flow through a narrowed lumen and increase blood pressure.

Vascular Remodeling

Vascular remodeling is similar to the left ventricular remodeling that occurs in heart failure (see Chap. 48). It results from

endothelial dysfunction and produces a thickening of the blood vessel wall and a narrowing of the blood vessel lumen. Thickening of the wall makes blood vessels less flexible and less able to respond to vasodilating substances. There are also changes in endothelial cell structure (ie, the connections between endothelial cells become looser) that lead to increased permeability. The mechanisms of these vascular changes, which promote and aggravate hypertension, are described below.

As discussed in previous chapters, normal endothelium helps maintain a balance between vasoconstriction and vasodilation, procoagulation and anticoagulation, proinflammation and antiinflammation, and progrowth and antigrowth. In the inflammatory process, normal endothelium acts as a physical barrier against the movement of leukocytes into the subendothelial space. Endothelial products such as nitric oxide may also inhibit leukocyte activity. However, inflammatory cytokines such as tumor necrosis factor–alpha and interleukin-1 activate endothelial cells to produce adhesion molecules (which allow leukocytes to adhere to the endothelium), interleukin-8 (which attracts leukocytes to the endothelium and allows them to accumulate in subendothelial cells), and foam cells (lipid-filled monocyte/macrophages that form fatty streaks, the beginning lesions of atherosclerotic plaque). Although activation of endothelial cells may be a helpful component of the normal immune response, the resulting inflammation may contribute to disease development.

In terms of cell growth, normal endothelium limits the growth of vascular smooth muscle that underlies the endothelium and forms the vessel wall. Growth-inhibiting products of the endothelium include nitric oxide, which also inhibits platelet activation and production of growth-promoting substances. When the endothelium is damaged, endothelial cells become activated and also produce growth-promoting products. Other endothelial products (eg, angiotensin II and endothelin-1) may also stimulate growth of vascular smooth muscle cells. Thus, damage or loss of endothelial cells stimulates growth of smooth muscle cells in the intimal layer of the blood vessel wall.

---

endothelial dysfunction and arterial changes (vascular remodeling), the arterial lumen is narrowed, blood supply to tissues is decreased, and risks of thrombosis are increased. In addition, necrotic areas may develop in arteries, and these may rupture with sustained high blood pressure. The areas of most serious damage are the heart, brain, kidneys, and eyes. These are often called *target organs.*

Initially and perhaps for years, primary hypertension may produce no symptoms. If symptoms occur, they are usually vague and nonspecific. Hypertension may go undetected, or it may be incidentally discovered when blood pressure measurements are taken as part of a routine physical examination, screening test, or assessment of other disorders. Eventually, symptoms reflect target organ damage. Hypertension is often

discovered after a person experiences angina pectoris, myocardial infarction, heart failure, stroke, or renal disease.

Hypertensive emergencies are episodes of severely elevated blood pressure that may be an extension of malignant (rapidly progressive) hypertension or caused by cerebral hemorrhage, dissecting aortic aneurysm, renal disease, pheochromocytoma, or eclampsia. These require immediate management, usually with intravenous (IV) antihypertensive drugs, to lower blood pressure. Symptoms include severe headache, nausea, vomiting, visual disturbances, neurologic disturbances, disorientation, and decreased level of consciousness (drowsiness, stupor, coma). Hypertensive emergencies require immediate blood pressure reduction with parenteral antihypertensive drugs to limit damage to target organs. Hypertensive urgencies are episodes of marked elevation in blood pressure without target organ damage and are often managed with oral drugs. The goal of management is to lower blood pressure within 24 hours. In most instances, it is better to lower blood pressure gradually and to avoid wide fluctuations in blood pressure.

ANTIHYPERTENSIVES: CLASSIFICATIONS AND INDIVIDUAL DRUGS

Drugs used in the management of primary hypertension belong to several different groups, including angiotensin-converting enzyme (ACE) inhibitors; angiotensin II receptor blockers (ARBs), also called *angiotensin II receptor antagonists* (AIIRAs); antiadrenergics; calcium channel blockers; diuretics; and direct vasodilators. In general, these drugs act to decrease blood pressure by decreasing cardiac output or peripheral vascular resistance.

Antihypertensive agents are shown in Table 52-1; antihypertensive–diuretic combination products are listed in Table 52-2. Adult dosages are based on product labeling and JNC 7 recommendations. Pediatric dosages are based on product labeling and recommendations from the National High Blood Pressure Education Program Working Group on High Blood Pressure in Children and Adolescents (2004).

Angiotensin-Converting Enzyme Inhibitors

Angiotensin-converting enzyme (also called *kininase*) is mainly located in the endothelial lining of blood vessels, which is the site of production of most angiotensin II. This same enzyme also metabolizes bradykinin, an endogenous substance with strong vasodilating properties.

ACE inhibitors block the enzyme that normally converts angiotensin I to the potent vasoconstrictor angiotensin II. By blocking production of angiotensin II, the drugs decrease vasoconstriction (having a vasodilating effect) and decrease aldosterone production (reducing retention of sodium and water). In addition to inhibiting formation of angiotensin II, the drugs also inhibit the breakdown of bradykinin, prolonging its vasodilating effects. These effects and possibly others help to prevent or reverse the remodeling of heart muscle and blood vessel walls that impairs cardiovascular function and exacerbates cardiovascular disease processes. Because of their effectiveness in hypertension and beneficial effects on the heart, blood vessels, and kidneys, these drugs are increasing in importance and use. Widely used to treat heart failure and hypertension, the drugs may also decrease morbidity and mortality in other cardiovascular disorders. They improve post–myocardial infarction survival when added to the standard therapy of aspirin, a beta blocker, and a thrombolytic.

ACE inhibitors may be used alone or in combination with other antihypertensive agents, such as thiazide diuretics. Although the drugs can cause or aggravate proteinuria and renal damage in nondiabetic people, they decrease proteinuria and slow the development of nephropathy in diabetic clients.

Most ACE inhibitors (captopril, enalapril, fosinopril, lisinopril, ramipril, and quinapril) also are used in the management of heart failure because they decrease peripheral vascular resistance, cardiac workload, and ventricular remodeling. **P Captopril** and other ACE inhibitors are recommended as first-line agents for treating hypertension in diabetic clients, particularly those with type 1 diabetes and/or diabetic nephropathy, because they reduce proteinuria and slow progression of renal impairment.

ACE inhibitors are well absorbed with oral administration; produce effects within 1 hour that last approximately 24 hours; have prolonged serum half-lives with impaired renal function; and most are metabolized to active metabolites that are excreted in urine and feces. These drugs are well tolerated, with a low incidence of serious adverse effects (eg, neutropenia, agranulocytosis, proteinuria, glomerulonephritis, angioedema). However, a persistent cough develops in approximately 10% to 20% of clients and may lead to stopping the drug. Also, acute hypotension may occur when an ACE inhibitor is started, especially in clients with fluid volume deficit. This reaction may be prevented by starting with a low dose taken at bedtime, or by stopping diuretics and reducing dosage of other antihypertensive drugs temporarily. Hyperkalemia may develop in clients who have diabetes mellitus or renal impairment or who are taking nonsteroidal anti-inflammatory drugs, potassium supplements, or potassium-sparing diuretics.

These drugs are contraindicated during pregnancy because serious illnesses, including renal failure, have occurred in neonates whose mothers took an ACE inhibitor during the second and third trimesters.

Angiotensin II Receptor Blockers

Angiotensin II receptor blockers (ARBs) were developed to block the strong blood pressure–raising effects of angiotensin II. Instead of decreasing production of angiotensin II, as the ACE inhibitors do, these drugs compete with angiotensin II for tissue binding sites and prevent angiotensin II from combining with its receptors in body tissues. Although multiple types of receptors have been identified, the AT1 receptors located in brain, renal, myocardial, vascular, and adrenal tissue determine most of the effects of angiotensin II on cardiovascular and renal functions. ARBs block the angiotensin II AT1 receptors and decrease arterial blood pressure by decreasing systemic vascular resistance (Fig. 52-1).

These drugs are similar to ACE inhibitors in their effects on blood pressure and hemodynamics and are as effective as ACE inhibitors in the management of hypertension and probably

(text continues on page 846)

Table 52-1 Drugs at a Glance: Antihypertensive Drugs

	ROUTES AND DOSAGE RANGES	
GENERIC/TRADE NAME	Adults	Children 1–17 Years of Age (unless otherwise stated)
Angiotensin-Converting Enzyme (ACE) Inhibitors		
Benazepril (Lotensin)	PO 10 mg once daily initially, increased to 40 mg daily if necessary, in 1 or 2 doses	
P **Captopril** (Capoten)	PO 25 mg, 2 to 3 times daily initially, gradually increased to 50, 100, or 150 mg 2 to 3 times daily, if necessary; maximum dose, 450 mg/d	PO 1.5 mg/kg/d in divided doses, q8h; maximum dose, 6 mg/kg/d Neonates: PO 0.03–0.15 mg/kg/d, q8–24h; maximum dose, 2 mg/kg/d
Enalapril (Vasotec)	PO 5 mg once daily, increased to 10–40 mg daily, in 1 or 2 doses, if necessary	PO 0.15 mg q12–24h
Fosinopril (Monopril)	Same as benazepril, above	
Lisinopril (Prinivil, Zestril)	PO 10 mg once daily, increased to 40 mg if necessary	
Moexipril (Univasc)	PO initial dose 7.5 mg (3.75 mg for those who have renal impairment or are taking a diuretic). Maintenance dose, 7.5–30 mg daily, in 1 or 2 doses, adjusted according to blood-pressure control	
Perindopril (Aceon)	PO 4–16 mg daily, in 1 or 2 doses	
Quinapril (Accupril)	PO 10 mg once daily initially, increased to 20, 40, or 80 mg daily if necessary, in 1 or 2 doses. Wait at least 2 wk between dose increments.	
Ramipril (Altace)	PO 2.5 mg once daily, increased to 20 mg daily if necessary, in 1 or 2 doses	
Trandolapril (Mavik)	PO initial dose 1 mg once daily (0.5 mg for those who have hepatic or renal impairment or are taking a diuretic; 2 mg for African Americans). Maintenance dose, 2–4 mg daily, in a single dose, adjusted according to blood-pressure control	
Angiotensin II Receptor Blockers		
Candesartan (Atacand)	PO 16 mg once daily initially, increased if necessary to a maximum of 32 mg daily, in 1 or 2 doses	
Eprosartan (Teveten)	PO 600 mg once daily initially; may be increased to 800 mg daily, in 1 or 2 doses	
Irbesartan (Avapro)	PO 150 mg once daily initially, increased up to 300 mg once daily, if necessary	
Losartan (Cozaar)	PO 50 mg once daily initially (25 mg for those who have hepatic impairment or are taking a diuretic). Maintenance dose, 35–100 mg daily, in 1 or 2 doses, adjusted according to blood-pressure control	
Olmesartan (Benicar)	PO 20 mg once daily initially, increased to 40 mg after 2 wk	
Telmisartan (Micardis)	PO 40 mg once daily initially, increased to a maximum of 80 mg daily if necessary	
Valsartan (Diovan)	PO 80 mg once daily initially, when used as monotherapy in clients who are not volume depleted. Maintenance dose may be increased. However, adding a diuretic is more effective than increasing dose beyond 80 mg.	

Table 52-1 Drugs at a Glance: Antihypertensive Drugs (continued)

	ROUTES AND DOSAGE RANGES	
GENERIC/TRADE NAME	Adults	Children 1–17 Years of Age (unless otherwise stated)
Antiadrenergic Agents		
ALPHA₁-ADRENERGIC BLOCKING AGENTS		
Doxazosin (Cardura)	PO 1 mg once daily initially, increased to 2 mg, then to 4, 8, and 16 mg daily if necessary	
Prazosin (Minipress)	PO 1 mg 2 to 3 times daily initially, increased if necessary to 20 mg in divided doses. Average maintenance dose, 6–15 mg daily	
Terazosin (Hytrin)	PO 1 mg at bedtime initially, may be increased gradually. Usual maintenance dose, 1–5 mg once daily	
ALPHA₂ AGONISTS		
Clonidine (Catapres)	PO 0.1 mg 2 times daily initially, gradually increased up to 2.4 mg daily, if necessary. Average maintenance dose, 0.2–0.8 mg daily	PO 5–25 mcg/kg/d, in divided doses, q6h; increase at 5- to 7-day intervals, if needed
Guanabenz (Wytensin)	PO 4 mg twice daily, increased by 4–8 mg daily every 1–2 wk if necessary to a maximum of 32 mg twice daily	
Guanfacine (Tenex)	PO 1 mg daily at bedtime, increased to 2 mg after 3–4 wk, then to 3 mg if necessary	
Methyldopa	PO 250 mg 2 or 3 times daily initially, increased gradually until blood pressure is controlled or a daily dose of 3 g is reached	PO 10 mg/kg/d in 2 to 4 divided doses initially, increased or decreased according to response. Maximum dose, 65 mg/kg/d or 3 g daily, whichever is less
POSTGANGLIONIC-ACTIVE DRUG		
Guanadrel (Hylorel)	PO 10 mg daily initially. Usual dosage range, 20–75 mg daily in divided doses	
BETA-ADRENERGIC BLOCKING AGENTS		
Acebutolol (Sectral)	PO 400 mg once daily initially, increased to 800 mg daily if necessary	
Atenolol (Tenormin)	PO 50 mg once daily initially, increased in 1–2 wk to 100 mg once daily, if necessary	
Betaxolol (Kerlone)	PO 10–20 mg once daily	
Bisoprolol (Zebeta)	PO 5 mg once daily, increased to a maximum of 20 mg daily if necessary	
Carteolol (Cartrol)	PO 2.5 mg once daily initially, gradually increased to a maximum of 10 mg daily if necessary. Usual maintenance dose, 2.5–5 mg once daily. Extend dosage interval to 48 h for a creatinine clearance of 20–60 mL/min and to 72 h for a creatinine clearance below 20 mL/min.	
Metoprolol (Lopressor)	PO 50 mg twice daily, gradually increased in weekly or longer intervals if necessary. Maximum dose, 450 mg daily	
Nadolol (Corgard)	PO 40 mg once daily initially, gradually increased if necessary. Average dose, 80–320 mg daily	
Penbutolol (Levatol)	PO 20 mg once daily	
Pindolol (Visken)	PO 5 mg 2 or 3 times daily initially, increased by 10 mg/d at 3- to 4-wk intervals to a maximum of 60 mg daily	

(continued)

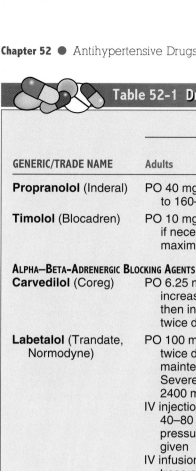

Table 52-1 Drugs at a Glance: Antihypertensive Drugs (continued)

	ROUTES AND DOSAGE RANGES	
GENERIC/TRADE NAME	Adults	Children 1–17 Years of Age (unless otherwise stated)
Propranolol (Inderal)	PO 40 mg twice daily initially, gradually increased to 160–640 mg daily	PO 1 mg/kg/d initially, gradually increased to a maximum of 10 mg/kg/d
Timolol (Blocadren)	PO 10 mg twice daily initially, increased gradually if necessary. Average daily dose, 20–40 mg; maximal daily dose, 60 mg	
ALPHA–BETA-ADRENERGIC BLOCKING AGENTS		
Carvedilol (Coreg)	PO 6.25 mg twice daily for 7–14 days, then increase to 12.5 mg twice daily for 7–14 days, then increase to a maximal dose of 25 mg twice daily if tolerated and needed	
Labetalol (Trandate, Normodyne)	PO 100 mg twice daily, increased by 100 mg twice daily every 2–3 days if necessary. Usual maintenance dose, 200–400 mg twice daily. Severe hypertension may require 1200–2400 mg daily. IV injection, 20 mg slowly over 2 min, followed by 40–80 mg every 10 min until the desired blood pressure is achieved or 300 mg has been given IV infusion, add 200 mg to 250 mL of 5% dextrose or 0.9% sodium chloride solution and infuse at a rate of 2 mg/min. Adjust flow rate according to blood pressure, and substitute oral labetalol when blood pressure is controlled.	
Calcium Channel Blocking Agents		
Amlodipine (Norvasc)	PO 5–10 mg once daily	
Diltiazem (sustained release) (Cardizem SR)	PO 60–120 mg twice daily. Extended-release tablets; swallow whole, do not crush or chew.	
Felodipine (Plendil)	PO 5–10 mg once daily. Extended-release tablets; swallow whole, do not crush or chew.	
Isradipine (DynaCirc)	PO 2.5–5 mg twice daily	
Nicardipine (Cardene, Cardene SR, Cardene IV)	PO 20–40 mg three times daily Sustained-release, PO 30–60 mg twice daily; IV infusion 5–15 mg/h	
Nifedipine (Adalat, Procardia, Procardia XL)	Sustained-release only, PO 30–60 mg once daily, increased over 1–2 wk if necessary	
Nisoldipine (Sular)	PO, 20 mg once daily initially, increased by 10 mg/wk or longer intervals to a maximum of 60 mg daily. Average maintenance dose, 20–40 mg daily Adults with liver impairment or >65 y, PO, 10 mg once daily initially	
Verapamil (Calan, Calan SR, Isoptin SR)	Immediate-release, PO 80 mg 3 times daily Sustained-release, PO 240 mg once daily IV, see manufacturer's instructions	IV, see manufacturer's instructions

Table 52-1   Drugs at a Glance: Antihypertensive Drugs (continued)

	ROUTES AND DOSAGE RANGES	
GENERIC/TRADE NAME	Adults	Children 1–17 Years of Age (unless otherwise stated)
Other Vasodilators **Fenoldopam** (Corlopam)	IV infusion, initial dose based on body weight, then flow rate titrated to achieve desired response. Mix with 0.9% sodium chloride or 5% dextrose to a concentration of 40 mcg/mL (eg, 40 mg of drug [4 mL of concentrate] in 1000 mL of IV fluid).	
Hydralazine (Apresoline)	Chronic hypertension, PO 10 mg 4 times daily for 2–4 d, gradually increased up to 300 mg/d, if necessary Hypertensive crisis, IM, IV 10–20 mg, increased to 40 mg if necessary. Repeat dose as needed.	Chronic hypertension, 0.75 mg/kg/d initially in 4 divided doses. Gradually increase over 3–4 wk to a maximal dose of 7.5 mg/kg/d if necessary. Hypertensive crisis, IM, IV 0.1–0.2 mg/kg every 4–6 h as needed
Minoxidil (Loniten)	PO 5 mg once daily initially, increased gradually until blood pressure is controlled. Average daily dose, 10–40 mg; maximal daily dose, 100 mg in single or divided doses	<12 y, PO 0.2 mg/kg/d initially as a single dose, increased gradually until blood pressure is controlled. Average daily dose, 0.25–1.0 mg/kg; maximal dose, 50 mg/d
Sodium nitroprusside (Nipress)	IV infusion 0.5–10 mcg/kg/min; average dose, 3 mcg/kg/min. Prepare solution by adding 50 mg of sodium nitroprusside to 250–1000 mL of 5% dextrose in water, and cover promptly to protect from light.	Same as for adults

IV, intravenous; PO, oral.

heart failure. They are less likely to cause hyperkalemia than ACE inhibitors, and the occurrence of a persistent cough is rare. Overall, the drugs are well tolerated, and the incidence of most adverse effects is similar to that of placebo.

P **Losartan**, the first ARB, is readily absorbed and rapidly metabolized by the cytochrome P450 liver enzymes to an active metabolite. Both losartan and the metabolite are highly bound to plasma albumin, and losartan has a shorter duration of action than its metabolite. When losartan therapy is started, maximal effects on blood pressure usually occur within 3 to 6 weeks. If losartan alone does not control blood pressure, a low dose of a diuretic may be added. A combination product of losartan and hydrochlorothiazide is available.

Antiadrenergics

Antiadrenergic (sympatholytic) drugs inhibit activity of the SNS. When the SNS is stimulated (see Chap. 16), the nerve impulse travels from the brain and spinal cord to the ganglia. From the ganglia, the impulse travels along postganglionic fibers to effector organs (eg, heart, blood vessels). Although SNS stimulation produces widespread effects in the body, the effects relevant to this discussion are the increases in heart rate, force of myocardial contraction, cardiac output, and blood pressure that occur. When the nerve impulse is inhibited or blocked at any location along its pathway, the result is decreased blood pressure (see Chap. 18).

Alpha$_1$-adrenergic receptor blocking agents (eg, prazosin) dilate blood vessels and decrease peripheral vascular resistance. These drugs can be used alone or in multidrug regimens. One adverse effect, called the *first-dose phenomenon*, results in orthostatic hypotension with palpitations, dizziness, and perhaps syncope 1 to 3 hours after the first dose or an increased dose. To prevent this effect, first doses and first increased doses are taken at bedtime. Another effect, associated with long-term use or higher doses, leads to sodium and fluid retention and a need for concurrent diuretic therapy. Centrally acting sympatholytics (eg, clonidine) stimulate presynaptic alpha$_2$ receptors in the brain and are classified as alpha$_2$ receptor agonists. When these drugs are taken, less norepinephrine is released and sympathetic outflow from the vasomotor center is reduced. Stimulation of presynaptic alpha$_2$ receptors peripherally may also contribute to the decreased sympathetic activity. Reduced sympathetic activity leads to decreased cardiac output, heart rate,

(text continues on page 849)

Table 52-2 Drugs at a Glance: Oral Antihypertensive Combination Products*

			COMPONENTS			
TRADE NAME	Angiotensin II Receptor Blocker	Angiotensin-Converting Enzyme Inhibitor	Beta Blocker	Calcium Channel Blocker	Diuretic	Non–Beta-Blocker Antiadrenergic	DOSAGE RANGES
Aldoril					HCTZ 15, 25, 30, or 50 mg	Methyldopa 250 or 500 mg	1 tablet 2 to 3 times daily for 48 h, then adjusted according to response
Avalide	Irbesartan 150 or 300 mg				HCTZ 12.5 mg		1 tablet once daily
Capozide		Captopril 25 or 50 mg			HCTZ 15 or 25 mg		1 tablet 2 to 3 times daily
Corzide			Nadolol 40 or 80 mg		Bendroflumethi-azide 5 mg		1 tablet daily
Diovan HCT	Valsartan 80 or 160 mg				HCTZ 12.5 mg		1 tablet daily
Hyzaar	Losartan 50 mg				HCTZ 12.5 mg		1 tablet once daily
Inderide			Propranolol 40 or 80 mg		HCTZ 25 mg		1–2 tablets twice daily
Lexxel		Enalapril 5 mg		Felodipine 5 mg			1–2 tablets once daily
Lopressor HCT			Metoprolol 50 or		HCTZ 25 or 50 mg		1–2 tablets daily

(continued)

Table 52-2 Drugs at a Glance: Oral Antihypertensive Combination Products* (continued)

TRADE NAME	Angiotensin II Receptor Blocker	Angiotensin-Converting Enzyme Inhibitor	Beta Blocker	Calcium Channel Blocker	Diuretic	Non–Beta-Blocker Antiadrenergic	DOSAGE RANGES
				COMPONENTS			
Lotensin HCT		Benazepril 5, 10, or 20 mg			HCTZ 12.5 or 25 mg		1 tablet daily
Lotrel		Benazepril 10 or 20 mg		Amlodipine 2.5 or 5 mg			1 capsule daily
Minizide					Polythiazide 0.5 mg	Prazosin 1, 2, or 5 mg	1 capsule 2 to 3 times daily
Prinzide		Lisinopril 20 mg			HCTZ 12.5 or 25 mg		1 tablet daily
Tarka		Trandolapril 1, 2, or 4 mg		Verapamil 180 or 240 mg			1 tablet daily
Teczem		Enalapril 5 mg		Diltiazem 180 mg			1 tablet daily
Tenoretic			Atenolol 50 or 100 mg		Chlorthalidone 25 mg		1 tablet daily
Timolide			Timolol 10 mg		HCTZ 12.5 mg		1–2 tablets 1 or 2 times daily
Vaseretic		Enalapril 5 mg			HCTZ 12.5 mg		1–2 tablets daily
Zestoretic		Lisinopril 10 or 20 mg			HCTZ 12.5 or 25 mg		1 tablet daily
Ziac		Bisoprolol 2.5, 5, or 10 mg			HCTZ 6.25 mg		1 tablet daily

*Note that one trade-name product may be available in multiple formulations, with variable amounts of antihypertensive, diuretic, or both components.
HCTZ, hydrochlorothiazide.

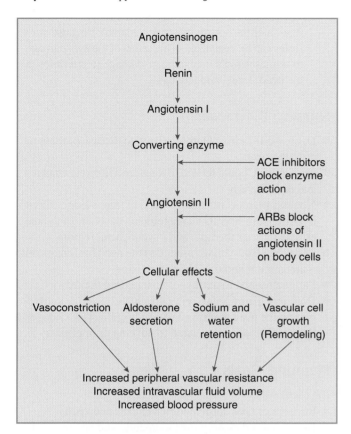

Angiotensinogen

↓

Renin

↓

Angiotensin I

↓

Converting enzyme ←— ACE inhibitors block enzyme action

↓

Angiotensin II ←— ARBs block actions of angiotensin II on body cells

↓

Cellular effects

↙ ↓ ↓ ↘

Vasoconstriction | Aldosterone secretion | Sodium and water retention | Vascular cell growth (Remodeling)

Increased peripheral vascular resistance
Increased intravascular fluid volume
Increased blood pressure

FIGURE 52-1 Angiotensin-converting enzyme (ACE) inhibitors inhibit angiotensin-converting enzyme and thereby prevent formation of angiotensin II; angiotensin II receptor blockers (ARBs) prevent angiotensin II from connecting with its receptors and thereby prevent it from acting on body tissues containing those receptors (eg, blood vessels, adrenal cortex).

peripheral vascular resistance, and blood pressure. Chronic use of clonidine and related drugs may result in sodium and fluid retention, especially with higher doses.

Beta-adrenergic blocking agents (eg, propranolol) decrease heart rate, force of myocardial contraction, cardiac output, and renin release from the kidneys. Other antiadrenergics include guanadrel and related drugs, which act at postganglionic nerve endings; and two other alpha blockers (phentolamine and phenoxybenzamine), which occasionally are used in hypertension resulting from catecholamine excess. Individual antiadrenergic drugs are discussed in Chapter 18 and listed in Tables 18-1 and 18-2.

Calcium Channel Blocking Agents

Calcium channel blockers (eg, verapamil) are used for several cardiovascular disorders. The mechanism of action and use in the management of tachydysrhythmias and angina pectoris are discussed in Chapters 49 and 50. In hypertension, the drugs mainly dilate peripheral arteries and decrease peripheral vascular resistance by relaxing vascular smooth muscle.

Most of the available drugs are approved for use in hypertension. Nifedipine, a short-acting calcium channel blocker,

has been used to treat hypertensive emergencies or urgencies, often by puncturing the capsule and squeezing the contents under the tongue or having the client bite and swallow the capsule. Such use is no longer recommended, because this practice is associated with an increased risk of adverse cardiovascular events precipitated by a rapid and severe decrease in blood pressure.

As a group, the calcium channel blockers are well absorbed from the gastrointestinal tract following oral administration and are highly bound to protein. The drugs are metabolized in the liver and excreted in urine.

Diuretics

Antihypertensive effects of diuretics are usually attributed to sodium and water depletion. In fact, diuretics usually produce the same effects as severe dietary sodium restriction. In many cases of hypertension, diuretic therapy alone may lower blood pressure. When diuretic therapy is begun, blood volume and cardiac output decrease. With long-term administration of a diuretic, cardiac output returns to normal, but there is a persistent decrease in peripheral vascular resistance. This has been attributed to a persistent small reduction in extracellular water and plasma volume; decreased receptor sensitivity to vasopressor substances such as angiotensin; direct arteriolar vasodilation; and arteriolar vasodilation secondary to electrolyte depletion in the vessel wall. In moderate or severe hypertension that does not respond to a diuretic alone, the diuretic may be continued and another antihypertensive drug added, or monotherapy with a different type of antihypertensive drug may be tried.

Thiazide diuretics (eg, hydrochlorothiazide) are most commonly used in the management of hypertension. Loop diuretics (eg, furosemide) or potassium-sparing diuretics (eg, spironolactone) may be useful in some circumstances. Diuretics are discussed in Chapter 53 and listed in Table 53-1.

Vasodilators (Direct Acting)

Vasodilator antihypertensive drugs directly relax smooth muscle in blood vessels, resulting in dilation and decreased peripheral vascular resistance. They also reduce afterload and may be used in management of heart failure. Hydralazine and minoxidil act mainly on arterioles; nitroprusside acts on arterioles and venules. These drugs have a limited effect on hypertension when used alone because the vasodilating action that lowers blood pressure also stimulates the SNS and triggers reflexive compensatory mechanisms (vasoconstriction, tachycardia, and increased cardiac output), which raise blood pressure. This effect can be prevented during long-term therapy by also giving a drug that prevents excessive sympathetic stimulation (eg, propranolol, an adrenergic blocker). These drugs also cause sodium and water retention, which may be minimized by concomitant diuretic therapy.

NURSING PROCESS

Assessment

Assess the client's condition in relation to hypertension.
- Identify conditions and risk factors that may lead to hypertension. These include
  - Obesity
  - Elevated serum cholesterol (total and low-density lipoprotein) and triglycerides
  - Cigarette smoking
  - Sedentary lifestyle
  - Family history of hypertension or other cardiovascular disease
  - African-American race
  - Renal disease (eg, renal artery stenosis)
  - Adrenal disease (eg, hypersecretion of aldosterone, pheochromocytoma)
  - Other cardiovascular disorders (eg, atherosclerosis, left ventricular hypertrophy)
  - Diabetes mellitus
  - Use of oral contraceptives, corticosteroids, appetite suppressants, nasal decongestants, nonsteroidal anti-inflammatory agents
  - Neurologic disorders (eg, brain damage)
- Observe for signs and symptoms of hypertension.
  - Check blood pressure accurately and repeatedly. As a rule, multiple measurements in which systolic pressure is greater than 140 mm Hg, and/or diastolic pressure is greater than 90 mm Hg, are necessary to establish a diagnosis of hypertension.

    The importance of accurate blood pressure measurements cannot be overemphasized because there are many possibilities for errors. Some ways to improve accuracy and validity include using correct equipment (eg, proper cuff size), having the client rested and in the same position each time blood pressure is measured (eg, sitting or supine with arm at heart level), and using the same arm for repeated measurements.
  - In most cases of early hypertension, elevated blood pressure is the only clinical manifestation. If symptoms do occur, they are usually nonspecific (eg, headache, weakness, fatigue, tachycardia, dizziness, palpitations, epistaxis).
  - Eventually, signs and symptoms occur as target organs are damaged. Heart damage is often evidenced as angina pectoris, myocardial infarction, or heart failure. Chest pain, tachycardia, dyspnea, fatigue, and edema may occur. Brain damage may be indicated by transient ischemic attacks or strokes of varying severity with symptoms ranging from syncope to hemiparesis. Renal damage may be reflected by proteinuria, increased blood urea nitrogen (BUN), and increased serum creatinine. Ophthalmoscopic examination may reveal hemorrhages, sclerosis of arterioles, and inflammation of the optic nerve (papilledema). Because arterioles can be visualized in the retina of the eye, damage to retinal vessels may indicate damage to arterioles in the heart, brain, and kidneys.

Nursing Diagnoses

- Decreased Cardiac Output related to disease process or drug therapy
- Ineffective Coping related to long-term lifestyle changes and drug therapy
- Noncompliance related to lack of knowledge about hypertension and its management, costs and adverse effects of drug therapy, and psychosocial factors
- Disturbed Body Image related to the need for long-term management and medical supervision
- Fatigue related to antihypertensive drug therapy
- Deficient Knowledge related to hypertension, antihypertensive drug therapy, and nondrug lifestyle changes
- Sexual Dysfunction related to adverse drug effects

Planning/Goals

The client will
- Receive or take antihypertensive drugs correctly
- Be monitored closely for therapeutic and adverse drug effects, especially when drug therapy is started, when changes are made in choice of drugs, and when dosages are increased or decreased
- Use nondrug measures to assist in blood pressure control
- Avoid, manage, or report adverse drug reactions
- Verbalize or demonstrate knowledge of prescribed drugs and recommended lifestyle changes
- Keep follow-up appointments

Interventions

Implement measures to prevent or minimize hypertension. Preventive measures are mainly lifestyle changes to reduce risk factors. These measures should be started in childhood and continued throughout life. After hypertension is diagnosed, lifetime adherence to a therapeutic regimen may be necessary to control the disease and prevent complications. The nurse's role is important in the prevention, early detection, and management of hypertension. Some guidelines for intervention at community, family, and personal levels include the following:
- Participate in programs to promote healthful lifestyles (eg, improving eating habits, increasing exercise, managing stress more effectively, avoiding cigarette smoking).
- Participate in community screening programs, and make appropriate referrals when abnormal blood pressures are detected. If hypertension develops in women taking

oral contraceptives, the drug should be discontinued for 3 to 6 months to see whether blood pressure decreases without antihypertensive drugs.

- Help the hypertensive client comply with prescribed therapy (see accompanying client teaching display). Noncompliance is high among clients with hypertension. Reasons given for noncompliance include lack of symptoms; lack of motivation and self-discipline to make needed lifestyle changes (eg, lose weight, stop smoking, restrict salt intake); perhaps experiencing more symptoms from medications than from hypertension; the cost of therapy; and the client's failure to realize the importance of effective management, especially as related to prevention of major cardiovascular diseases (myocardial infarction, stroke, and death). In addition, several studies have shown that compliance decreases as the number of drugs and number of doses increase.

  The nurse can help increase compliance by teaching the client about hypertension, helping the client make necessary lifestyle changes, and maintaining supportive interpersonal relationships. Losing weight, stopping smoking, and other changes are most likely to be effective if attempted one at a time.

- Use recommended techniques for measuring blood pressure. Poor techniques are too often used (eg, the client's arm up or down rather than at heart level; cuff applied over clothing, too loosely, deflated too rapidly, or reinflated before completely deflated; a regular-sized cuff used on large arms that need a large cuff; using the stethoscope diaphragm rather than the bell). It is disturbing to think that antihypertensive drugs may be prescribed and dosages changed on the basis of inaccurate blood pressures.

Evaluation

- Observe for blood pressure measurements within goal or more nearly normal ranges.
- Observe and interview regarding compliance with instructions about drug therapy and lifestyle changes.
- Observe and interview regarding adverse drug effects.

APPLYING YOUR KNOWLEDGE 52-1
Mr. Olms is noncompliant with his drug regimen. How should you react?

PRINCIPLES OF THERAPY

Therapeutic Regimens

After the diagnosis of hypertension is established, a therapeutic regimen must be designed and implemented. The goal of management for most clients is to achieve and maintain blood pressure below 140/90 mm Hg. The target blood pressure for

diabetic clients is 130/80 mm Hg. If the goal cannot be achieved, lowering blood pressure to any extent is still considered beneficial in decreasing the incidence of coronary artery disease and stroke.

The Joint National Committee on Prevention, Detection, Evaluation, and Treatment of High Blood Pressure (JNC 7) recommends management guidelines in which initial interventions are lifestyle modifications (ie, reduction of weight and sodium intake, regular physical activity, moderate alcohol intake, and no smoking) to maintain normal blood pressure or for those in the prehypertension group. If these modifications do not produce goal blood pressure or substantial progress toward goal blood pressure, antihypertensive drug therapy should be initiated and the lifestyle modifications should be continued. The JNC 7 guidelines suggest thiazide diuretics be used as first-line therapy, either alone (monotherapy) or with a beta blocker, ACE inhibitor, ARB, or calcium channel blocker. If the initial drug (and dose) does not produce the desired blood pressure, options for further management include increasing the drug dose, substituting another drug, or adding a second drug from a different group. If the response is still inadequate, a second or third drug may be added, including a diuretic if not previously prescribed. When current management is ineffective, reassess the client's compliance with lifestyle modifications and drug therapy. In addition, review other factors that may decrease the therapeutic response, such as the use of over-the-counter appetite suppressants, dietary or herbal supplements, or nasal decongestants, which raise blood pressure.

The World Health Organization and the International Society of Hypertension guidelines for management of hypertension include considering age, ethnicity, and concomitant cardiovascular disorders when choosing an antihypertensive drug; starting with a single drug, in the lowest available dose; changing to a drug from a different group, rather than increasing dosage of the first drug or adding a second drug, if the initial drug is ineffective or not well tolerated; and using long-acting drugs (ie, a single dose effective for 24 hours). The guidelines also note that many clients require two or more drugs to achieve adequate blood pressure control. When this is the case, fixed-dose combinations or long-acting agents may be preferred, as they decrease the number of drugs and doses that are required and may increase compliance.

APPLYING YOUR KNOWLEDGE 52-2
The JNC 7 has identified specific management guidelines for the client with hypertension. What should you teach a client with hypertension relative to the guidelines?

Drug Selection

Because many effective antihypertensive drugs are available, choices depend primarily on client characteristics and responses. Some general guidelines include:

- **ACE inhibitors** may be effective alone in Caucasian hypertensive clients or in combination with a diuretic in

CLIENT TEACHING GUIDELINES

Antihypertensive Drugs

General Considerations

☑ Hypertension is a major risk factor for heart attack, stroke (sometimes called brain attack), and kidney failure. Although it rarely causes symptoms unless complications occur, it can be controlled by appropriate management. Consequently, you need to learn all you can about the disease process, the factors that cause or aggravate it, and its management. In few other conditions is your knowledge and understanding about your condition as important as with hypertension.

☑ For many people, lifestyle changes (ie, a diet to avoid excessive salt and control weight and fat intake; regular exercise; and avoiding smoking) may be sufficient to control blood pressure. If drug therapy is prescribed, these measures should be continued.

☑ When drug therapy is needed, your physician will try to choose a drug and develop a regimen that works for you. There are numerous antihypertensive drugs and many can be taken once a day, which makes their use more convenient and less disruptive of your usual activities of daily living. You may need several office visits to find the right drug or combination of drugs and the right dosage. Changes in drugs or dosages may also be needed later, especially if you develop other conditions or take other drugs that alter your response to the antihypertensive drugs.

☑ Antihypertensive drug therapy is usually long term, may require more than one drug, and may produce side effects. You need to know the brand and generic names of any prescribed drugs and how to take each drug for optimal benefit and minimal adverse effects.

☑ Antihypertensive drugs must be taken as prescribed for optimal benefits, even if you do not feel well when a medication is started or when dosage is increased. *No antihypertensive drug should be stopped abruptly.* If problems develop, they should be discussed with the health care provider who is treating the hypertension. If treatment is stopped, blood pressure usually increases gradually as the medications are eliminated from the body. However, sometimes blood pressure rapidly increases to pretreatment levels or even higher. With any of these situations, you are at risk of a heart attack or stroke. In addition, stopping one drug of a multidrug regimen may lead to increased adverse effects as well as decreased antihypertensive effectiveness. To avoid these problems, antihypertensive drugs should be tapered in dosage and discontinued gradually, as directed by your health care provider.

☑ Blood pressure measurements are the only way you can tell if your medication is working. Thus, you may want to monitor your blood pressure at home, especially when starting drug therapy, changing medications, or changing dosages. If so, a blood pressure machine may be purchased at a medical supply store. Follow instructions regarding use, take your blood pressure approximately the same time(s) each day (eg, before morning and evening meals), and keep a record to show to your health care provider.

☑ People sometimes feel dizzy or faint while taking antihypertensive medications. This usually means your blood pressure drops momentarily and is most likely to occur when you start a medication, increase dosage, or stand up suddenly from a sitting or lying position. This can be prevented or decreased by moving to a standing position slowly, sleeping with the head of the bed elevated, wearing elastic stockings, exercising legs, avoiding prolonged standing, and avoiding hot baths. If episodes still occur, you should sit or lie down to avoid a fall and possible injury.

☑ It is very important to keep appointments for follow-up care.

Self- or Caregiver Administration

☑ Take or give antihypertensive drugs at prescribed time intervals, about the same time each day. For example, take once-daily drugs as close to every 24 hours as you can manage; twice-a-day drugs should be taken every 12 hours. If ordered four times daily, take approximately every 6 hours. Taking doses too close together can increase dizziness, weakness, and other adverse effects. Taking doses too far apart may not control blood pressure adequately and may increase risks of heart attack or stroke.

☑ Take oral captopril on an empty stomach. Food decreases drug absorption.

☑ Take most oral antihypertensive agents with or after food intake to decrease gastric irritation. Candesartan (Atacand), irbesartan (Avapro), losartan (Cozaar), telmisartan (Micardis), and valsartan (Diovan) may be taken with or without food.

☑ With prazosin, doxazosin, or terazosin, take the first dose and the first increased dose at bedtime to prevent dizziness and possible fainting.

☑ With the clonidine skin patch, apply to a hairless area on the upper arm or torso once every 7 days. Rotate sites.

African-American hypertensive clients. They are also recommended for hypertensive adults with diabetes mellitus and kidney damage because they slow the progression of albuminuria. Based on research studies that indicate reduced morbidity and mortality from cardiovascular diseases, these drugs are increasingly being prescribed as a component of a multidrug regimen.

● **ARBs** have therapeutic effects similar to those of ACE inhibitors, with fewer adverse effects. They may be used in most clients with hypertension.

● **Antiadrenergics** may be effective in any hypertensive population. **Alpha agonists** and **antagonists** are most often used in multidrug regimens in stage 2 hypertension, because they may cause postural hypotension and syncope. Clonidine is available in a skin patch that is applied once a week and reportedly reduces adverse effects and increases compliance. An additional advantage of transdermal clonidine is that clients who cannot take oral medications can use it. A disadvantage of this system is a delayed onset of effect (2–3 days), so other antihypertensive medications must also be given during the first 2 to 3 days of clonidine transdermal therapy. Other disadvantages include cost, a 20% incidence of local skin rash or irritation, and a 2- to 3-day delay in "offset" of action when transdermal therapy is discontinued.

Beta adrenergic blockers are the drugs of first choice for clients younger than 50 years of age with high-renin hypertension, tachycardia, angina pectoris, myocardial infarction, or left ventricular hypertrophy. Most beta blockers are approved for use in hypertension and are probably equally effective. However, the cardioselective drugs (see Chap. 18) are preferred for hypertensive clients who also have asthma, peripheral vascular disease, or diabetes mellitus. Research studies demonstrate reduced morbidity and mortality with diuretics and beta blockers used in combination, especially after a myocardial infarction.

- **Calcium channel blockers** may be used for monotherapy or in combination with other drugs. They may be especially useful for hypertensive clients who also have angina pectoris or other cardiovascular disorders. The JNC 7 recommends that calcium channel blockers be considered the drug of first choice in African Americans with stage 2 hypertension. Note that sustained-release forms of nifedipine, diltiazem, verapamil and other long-acting drugs (eg, amlodipine, felodipine) are recommended rather than the short-acting forms because they do not cause precipitous lowering of pressure.

- **Diuretics** are preferred for initial therapy in all clients, but specifically in older and African-American hypertensive clients. They should be included in any multidrug regimen for these and other populations. Thiazide and related diuretics are equally effective. Hydrochlorothiazide is most commonly used. Diazoxide, usually in parenteral form, is indicated for short-term treatment of malignant hypertension. Loop diuretics are indicated in those with renal insufficiency. Potassium-sparing diuretics may precipitate hyperkalemia. Recently, the selective aldosterone blocker, eplerenone, has demonstrated efficacy in African Americans.

- **Vasodilators** are used in combination with a beta blocker and a diuretic to prevent hypotension-induced compensatory mechanisms (stimulation of the SNS and fluid retention) that raise blood pressure.

- **Combination products** usually combine two drugs with different mechanisms of action (eg, a thiazide or related diuretic plus a beta blocker or other antiadrenergic, an ACE inhibitor, an ARB, or a calcium channel blocker). Most are available in various formulations (see Table 52-2). Potential advantages of fixed-dose combination products include comparable or improved effectiveness, smaller doses of individual components, fewer adverse effects, improved compliance, and possibly decreased costs.

Drug Dosage

Dosage of antihypertensive drugs must be titrated according to individual response. Dosage should be started at minimal levels and increased if necessary. Lower doses decrease the incidence and severity of adverse effects.

For many clients, it may be more beneficial to change drugs or add another drug rather than increase dosage. Two or three drugs in small doses may be more effective and cause fewer adverse effects than a single drug in large doses. When two or more drugs are given, the dose of each drug may need to be reduced.

Clients who maintain control of their blood pressure for 1 year or so may be candidates for reduced dosages or reduced numbers of drugs. Any such adjustments must be gradual and carefully supervised by a health care provider. Expected benefits include fewer adverse effects and greater compliance.

Sodium Restriction

Therapeutic regimens for hypertension include sodium restriction. Severe restrictions usually are not acceptable to clients; however, moderate restrictions (4–6 g of salt a day) are beneficial and more easily implemented. Avoiding heavily salted foods (eg, cured meats, sandwich meats, pretzels, potato chips) and not adding salt to food at the table can achieve this. Research and clinical observations indicate the following:

- Sodium restriction alone reduces blood pressure.
- Sodium restriction potentiates the antihypertensive actions of diuretics and other antihypertensive drugs. Conversely, excessive sodium intake decreases the antihypertensive actions of all antihypertensive drugs. Clients with unrestricted salt intake who are taking thiazides may lose excessive potassium and become hypokalemic.
- Sodium restriction may decrease dosage requirements of antihypertensive drugs, thereby decreasing the incidence and severity of adverse effects.

Use in Special Populations

Use in Various Ethnic Groups

For most antihypertensive drugs, there have been few research studies comparing their effects in different genetic or ethnic groups. However, several studies indicate that beta blockers have greater effects in people of Asian heritage compared with their effects in Caucasians. For hypertension, Asians in general need much smaller doses because they metabolize and excrete beta blockers slowly. Other populations known to metabolize beta blockers slowly include Arab and Egyptian Americans, and possibly German Americans. In African Americans, diuretics are effective and recommended as initial drug therapy; calcium channel blockers, alpha$_1$ receptor blockers, and the alpha–beta blocker labetalol are reportedly equally effective in African Americans and Caucasians. ACE inhibitors, some ARBs (eg, losartan, telmisartan), and beta blockers are less effective as monotherapy in African Americans. When beta blockers are used, they are usually one component of a multidrug regimen, and higher doses may be required. Overall, African Americans are more likely to have severe hypertension and require multiple drugs as a result of having low circulating renin, increased salt sensitivity, and a higher incidence of obesity.

Use in Children

Most principles of managing adult hypertension apply to managing childhood and adolescent hypertension; some additional elements include the following:

- Children may have primary or secondary hypertension, but the incidence is unknown and treatment is not well defined. In recent years, increased blood pressure measurements during routine pediatric examinations have led to the discovery of significant asymptomatic hypertension and the realization that mild elevations in blood pressure are more common during childhood, especially in adolescents, than previously thought. Hypertension in children and adolescents may indicate underlying disease processes (eg, cardiac, endocrine, renovascular, renal parenchymal disorders) or the early onset of primary hypertension. Routine blood pressure measurement is especially important for children who are overweight or who have a hypertensive parent. Increased blood pressure in children often correlates with hypertension in young adults.

- The National High Blood Pressure Education Program Working Group on High Blood Pressure in Children and Adolescents produced the fourth report on the diagnosis, evaluation, and treatment of high blood pressure in children and adolescents in 2004. These guidelines established parameters for blood pressure in children and adolescents of comparable age, body size (height and weight), and sex. Normal blood pressure is defined as systolic and diastolic values less than the 90th percentile; prehypertension is defined as an average of systolic or diastolic pressures within the 90th to 95th percentiles; hypertension is defined as pressures beyond the 95th percentile. Blood pressure values obtained with a child or adolescent should be compared with norms and recorded in permanent health care records. Measurements are recorded on three or more occasions. Multiple accurate measurements are especially important in diagnosing hypertension because blood pressure may be more labile in children and adolescents.

- Children have a greater incidence of secondary hypertension than adults. In general, the higher the blood pressure and the younger the child, the greater the likelihood of secondary hypertension. Diagnostic tests may

be needed to rule out renovascular disease or coarctation of the aorta in those younger than 18 years of age with blood pressure above 140/90 mm Hg, and young children with blood pressures above the 95th percentile for their age group. Oral contraceptives may cause secondary hypertension in adolescents.

- The goals of management are to reduce blood pressure to below the 95th percentile and prevent the long-term effects of persistent hypertension. As in adults, prevention of obesity, avoiding excessive sodium intake, and exercise are important nonpharmacologic measures. Obese adolescents who lose weight may lower their blood pressure, especially when they also increase physical activity.

- Most children with secondary hypertension require drug therapy, which should be directed at the cause of hypertension if known. Drug therapy should be cautious and conservative because few studies have been done in children and long-term effects are unknown. The fewest drugs and the lowest doses should be used. Thus, if an initial drug is ineffective, it may be better to give a different single drug than to add a second drug to the regimen.

- Based on the current recommendations of the National High Blood Pressure Education Program Working Group on High Blood Pressure in Children and Adolescents released in 2004, guidelines for choosing drugs include the following:
  - Beta blockers are used in children of all ages and are the preferential drug for children with hypertension and migraine headache; they should probably be avoided in children with resting pulse rates under 60.
  - Thiazide diuretics may be used, and they do not commonly produce hyperglycemia, hyperuricemia, or hypercalcemia in children as they do in adults.
  - ACE inhibitors have been used to treat hypertension in children 6 years of age and over. The safety and efficacy of these drugs is continually being documented with studies and clinical practice. ACE inhibitors are preferred for managing hypertension in children who also have coexisting diabetes, microalbuminuria, or proteinuric renal diseases. Also, because of teratogenic effects, these drugs should be used very cautiously, if at all, in adolescent girls who may be sexually active.
  - ARBs may be used in children 6 years of age or older who do not tolerate ACE inhibitors in the same way the JNC 7 recommends for adults. Further research and documentation regarding safety and efficacy are continuing.
  - Calcium channel blockers are used in treating acute and chronic childhood hypertension. With chronic hypertension, immediate-release forms have a short duration of action and require frequent administration. Amlodipine may be given once daily and has specific pediatric labeling information.

- Hydralazine seems to be less effective in childhood and adolescent hypertension than in adult disease.
- Fixed-dose combination preparations, with the exception of biosprolol and hydrocholothiazide, have not had extensive study and are not recommended for routine use.
- Although all clients with primary hypertension need regular supervision and assessment of blood pressure, this is especially important with young children and adolescents because of growth and developmental changes.

Use in Older Adults

Most principles of managing hypertension in other populations apply to older adults (>65 years). In addition, the following factors require consideration.

- There are basically two types of hypertension in older adults. One is systolic hypertension, in which systolic blood pressure is above 140 mm Hg, but diastolic pressure is below 90 mm Hg. The other type, systolic–diastolic hypertension, involves elevations of both systolic and diastolic pressures.
- Both types increase cardiovascular morbidity and mortality, especially heart failure and stroke, and should be treated.
- Nonpharmacologic management should be tried alone or with drug therapy. For example, weight reduction, limited alcohol intake, moderate sodium restriction, and smoking cessation may be the initial treatment of choice if the client is hypertensive and overweight.
- If antihypertensive drug therapy is required, drugs used for younger adults may be used alone or in combination. A diuretic is usually the drug of first choice in older adults and may be effective alone. ACE inhibitors and calcium channel blocking agents may also be effective as monotherapy; beta blockers are usually less effective as monotherapy. Some ACE inhibitors (eg, lisinopril, ramipril, quinapril, moexipril) or their active metabolites produce higher plasma concentrations in older adults than in younger ones. This is attributed to decreased renal function rather than age itself. Additional guidelines include the following:
  - The goal of drug therapy for systolic–diastolic hypertension is usually a systolic pressure below 140 mm Hg and a diastolic below 90 mm Hg in clients with no other complications. For those with diabetes or renal failure, the goal is a systolic pressure below 130 mm Hg and a diastolic below 80 mm Hg. However, the latter goal may be difficult for most clients to meet because it requires rather stringent lifestyle restrictions and may require the use of two or more antihypertensive drugs.
  - Older adults may be especially susceptible to the adverse effects of antihypertensive drugs because their homeostatic mechanisms are less efficient. For example, if hypotension occurs, the mechanisms that raise blood pressure are less efficient and syncope may occur. In addition, renal and liver function may be reduced, making accumulation of drugs more likely.
- Initial drug doses should be approximately half of the recommended doses for younger adults, and increases should be smaller and spaced at longer intervals. Lower drug dosages (eg, hydrochlorothiazide 12.5 mg daily) are often effective and reduce risks of adverse effects.
- Blood pressure should be reduced slowly to facilitate adequate blood flow through arteriosclerotic vessels. Rapid lowering of blood pressure may produce cerebral insufficiency (syncope, transient ischemic attacks, stroke).
- A further incentive for successful management of hypertension in older clients is the benefit of reducing the incidence of dementia with antihypertensives.
- If blood pressure control is achieved and maintained for approximately 6 to 12 months, drug dosage should be gradually reduced, if possible.

Use in Clients With Renal Impairment

Antihypertensive drugs are frequently required by clients with renal impairment ranging from mild insufficiency to end-stage failure. A temporary decrease in renal function may occur in these clients when blood pressure is initially lowered. Guidelines include the following:

- In hypertensive clients with primary renal disease or diabetic nephropathy, drug therapy may slow progression of renal impairment.
- Diuretics are usually required because sodium retention is an important element of hypertension in these clients. Thiazides are usually contraindicated because they are ineffective if serum creatinine is above 2 mg/dL. However, metolazone, a thiazide-related drug, may be used and relatively large doses may be required. Loop diuretics, such as furosemide, are more often used, and relatively large doses may be required.
- ACE inhibitors are usually effective in clients with renal impairment, but responses may vary and the following factors should be considered.
  - When a client with renal impairment is started on an ACE inhibitor, careful monitoring is required, especially during the first few weeks of therapy, to prevent irreversible renal failure. For some clients, it may not be possible to normalize blood pressure and maintain adequate renal perfusion.
  - In clients with severe atherosclerosis, especially those with unilateral or bilateral stenosis of renal arteries, ACE inhibitors can impair renal blood flow and worsen renal impairment (ie, increase BUN and

serum creatinine). This may require stopping the drug. In addition, some clients without renal artery stenosis have developed increased BUN and serum creatinine levels. Although these are usually minor and transient, the drug may need to be discontinued or reduced in dosage.

- Approximately 25% of clients taking an ACE inhibitor for heart failure experience an increase in BUN and serum creatinine levels. These clients usually do not require drug discontinuation unless they have severe, pre-existing renal impairment. In clients with severe heart failure, whose renal function may depend on the activity of the renin–angiotensin–aldosterone system, management with an ACE inhibitor may worsen renal impairment. However, acute renal failure rarely occurs.

- The mechanisms are unclear, but ACE inhibitors also have renal protective effects in hypertensive clients with some renal impairment and clients with diabetic nephropathy. A possible mechanism is less damage to the endothelium and less vascular remodeling (ie, less narrowing of the lumen and less thickening of the vessel wall).

- The elimination half-life of most ACE inhibitors and their active metabolites is prolonged in clients with renal impairment. Dosage may need to be reduced with benazepril, lisinopril, quinapril, and ramipril.

- ARBs also inhibit the renin–angiotensin–aldosterone system and may produce effects similar to those of the ACE inhibitors. As with ACE inhibitors, some clients with severe heart failure have had oliguria or worsened renal impairment. These drugs are also likely to increase BUN and serum creatinine in clients with stenosis of one or both renal arteries.

  Dosage reductions usually are not required for clients with renal impairment. However, fluid volume deficits (eg, from diuretic therapy) should be corrected before starting the drug, and blood pressure should be monitored closely during drug therapy. Clients on hemodialysis may have orthostatic hypotension with telmisartan and possibly other drugs of this group.

- Most beta blockers are eliminated primarily by the kidneys and serum half-life is prolonged in clients with renal impairment. Most of the drugs should be used with caution and in reduced dosages. Dosage of metoprolol does not need to be reduced. An additional consideration is that cardiac output and blood pressure should not be lowered enough to impair renal blood flow and aggravate renal impairment.

- Calcium channel blockers are often used in clients with renal impairment because, in general, they are effective and well tolerated; they maintain renal blood flow even during blood pressure reduction in most clients; and

they are mainly eliminated by hepatic metabolism. However, cautious use is still recommended because several agents produce active metabolites that are excreted by the kidneys (see "Use in Clients With Renal Impairment," Chap. 53).

Use in Clients With Hepatic Impairment

Little information is available about the use of antihypertensive drugs in clients with impaired hepatic function. However, many of the drugs are metabolized in the liver and hepatic impairment can increase and prolong plasma concentrations.

- ACE inhibitors have occasionally been associated with complex symptoms that start with cholestatic jaundice and progress to hepatic necrosis and possible death. The mechanism of liver impairment is unknown. Clients who have jaundice or marked elevations of hepatic enzymes while taking an ACE inhibitor should have the drug discontinued. In addition, therapeutic effects can be decreased with several of the drugs (eg, fosinopril, quinapril, ramipril) because less of a given dose is converted to an active metabolite. Clearance of fosinopril, quinapril, and probably other ACE inhibitors that are metabolized is reduced in clients with alcoholic or biliary cirrhosis.

- ARBs should be used cautiously in clients with biliary tract obstruction or hepatic impairment. For some of these drugs (eg, candesartan, irbesartan, valsartan), dosage reduction is unnecessary. However, a lower starting dose is recommended for losartan because plasma concentrations of the drug and its active metabolite are increased and clearance is decreased approximately 50%. With telmisartan, plasma concentrations are increased and bioavailability approaches 100%. In addition, the drug is eliminated mainly by biliary excretion and clients with biliary tract obstruction or hepatic impairment have reduced clearance. The drug should be used with caution, but dosage forms that allow dosage reduction below 40 mg are not available. Thus, an alternative drug should probably be considered for clients with hepatic impairment.

- Beta blockers that normally undergo extensive first-pass hepatic metabolism (eg, acebutolol, metoprolol, propranolol, timolol) may produce excessive blood levels in clients with cirrhosis because the blood containing the drug is shunted around the liver into the systemic circulation. Dosage should be started at a low dose and titrated carefully in these clients. Dosage of bisoprolol and pindolol should also be reduced in clients with cirrhosis or other hepatic impairment.

- Calcium channel blockers should be used with caution, dosages should be substantially reduced, liver enzymes should be monitored periodically, and clients should be closely monitored for drug effects (see "Use in Clients With Hepatic Impairment," Chap. 50).

Use in Clients Undergoing Surgery

Drug therapy should be continued until surgery and restarted as soon as possible after surgery. If clients cannot take drugs orally, parenteral diuretics, antiadrenergic agents, ACE inhibitors, calcium channel blockers, or vasodilators may be given to avoid the rebound hypertension associated with abrupt discontinuance of some antiadrenergic antihypertensive agents. Transdermal clonidine also may be used. The anesthesiologist and surgeon must be informed about the client's hypertension and medication status.

Use in Clients With Critical Illness

Antihypertensive drugs are frequently prescribed for clients with critical illness and must be used cautiously, usually with reduced dosages and careful monitoring of responses. In many cases, the drugs are continued during critical illnesses caused by both cardiovascular and noncardiovascular disorders. If the client cannot take oral drugs, drug choices are narrowed because many commonly used drugs are not available in a dosage form that can be given parenterally, by gastrointestinal tube, or topically (eg, like a clonidine skin patch). Thus, clients' drug therapy must usually be re-titrated. In one way, this may be more difficult, because critically ill clients are often unstable in their conditions and responses to drug therapy. In another way, it may be easier in a critical care unit, where hemodynamic monitoring is commonly used. The goal of management is usually to maintain adequate tissue perfusion while avoiding both hypotension and hypertension.

Antihypertensive drugs are also used to treat hypertensive urgencies and emergencies, which involve dangerously high blood pressures and actual or potential damage to target organs. Although there are risks with severe hypertension, there are also risks associated with lowering blood pressure excessively or too rapidly, including stroke, myocardial infarction, and acute renal failure. Thus, the goal of management is usually to lower blood pressure over several minutes to several hours, with careful titration of drug dosage to avoid precipitous drops.

Urgencies can be treated with oral antihypertensive agents such as **captopril** 25 to 50 milligrams every 1 to 2 hours or **clonidine** 0.2 milligram initially, then 0.1 milligram hourly until diastolic blood pressure falls below 110 mm Hg or 0.7 milligram has been given.

A hypertensive emergency, defined as a diastolic pressure of 120 mm Hg or higher and target organ damage, requires an IV drug. The goal of management is usually to lower diastolic pressure to 100 to 110 mm Hg and maintain it there for several days to allow adjustment of the physiologic mechanisms that normally regulate blood pressure. Then, the blood pressure can be lowered to normotensive levels.

Several drugs can be given to treat a hypertensive emergency. **Fenoldopam** is a fast-acting drug indicated only for short-term use (<48 hours) in hospitalized patients. Dosage is calculated according to body weight and desired effects on blood pressure. Administration is by an infusion pump, with frequent monitoring of blood pressure. **Nitroglycerin** is especially beneficial in clients with both severe hypertension and myocardial ischemia. The dose is titrated according to blood pressure response and may range from 5 to 100 micrograms per minute. Tolerance develops to IV nitroglycerin over 24 to 48 hours. **Nitroprusside,** which has a rapid onset and short duration of action, is given as a continuous infusion at a rate of 0.5 to 8 micrograms per kilogram of body weight per minute. Intra-arterial blood pressure should be monitored during the infusion. Nitroprusside is metabolized to thiocyanate, and serum thiocyanate levels should be measured if the drug is given longer than 72 hours. The infusion should be stopped after 72 hours if the serum thiocyanate level is more than 12 milligrams per deciliter; it should be stopped at 48 hours in clients with renal impairment. Symptoms of thiocyanate toxicity (eg, nausea, vomiting, muscle twitching or spasm, seizures) can be reversed with hemodialysis. Other drugs that may be used include IV **hydralazine, labetalol,** and **nicardipine;** see Table 52-1.

Use in Home Care

Antihypertensive drugs are commonly self-administered in the home setting. The home care nurse is most likely to be involved when making home visits for other reasons. Whether the client or another member of the household is taking antihypertensive medications, the home care nurse may be helpful in teaching about the drugs, monitoring for drug effects, and promoting compliance with the prescribed regimen (pharmacologic and lifestyle modifications).

Noncompliance with prescribed antihypertensive drug therapy is a major problem, and consequences may be catastrophic. The home care nurse is well situated to assess for actual or potential barriers to compliance. For example, several antihypertensive medications are quite expensive and clients may not take the drugs at all or they may take fewer than the prescribed number of doses. If the nurse's assessment reveals this sort of situation, he or she may contact the prescribing health care provider and discuss the possibility of using less expensive drugs. If the provider is unwilling to try alternative drugs, the nurse may be able to identify resources for obtaining the needed medications.

Use in Clients Taking Herbal and Dietary Supplements

Use of nonprescription herbal and dietary supplements is frequently not reported by the client even though one third of adults in the United States use these agents. Significant interactions can occur between herbs or dietary supplements and prescribed drugs. Many nonprescription medications such as antihistamines, cold/cough preparations, and weight loss products can decrease the effectiveness of antihypertensive drugs or worsen hypertension. Caffeine, by its stimulating effects, may increase blood pressure. Yohimbe, used to treat erectile dysfunction, is a central nervous system stimulant and can affect blood pressure.

APPLYING YOUR KNOWLEDGE 52-3

Mr. Olms asks you why amlodipine was chosen to control his hypertension. What is the most appropriate response?

N U R S I N G   A C T I O N S

Antihypertensive Drugs

NURSING ACTIONS	RATIONALE/EXPLANATION
1. Administer accurately	
a. Give oral captopril and moexipril on an empty stomach, 1 hour before meals.	Food decreases drug absorption.
b. Give most other oral antihypertensives with or after food intake.	To decrease gastric irritation
c. Give angiotensin II receptor blockers with or without food.	Food does not impair drug absorption.
d. For intravenous injection of propranolol or labetalol, the client should be attached to a cardiac monitor. In addition, parenteral atropine and isoproterenol (Isuprel) must be readily available.	For early detection and management of excessive myocardial depression and dysrhythmias. Atropine may be used to treat excessive bradycardia. Isoproterenol may be used to stimulate myocardial contractility and increase cardiac output.
e. Give the first dose and the first increased dose of prazosin, doxazosin, and terazosin at bedtime.	To prevent orthostatic hypotension and syncope
f. For administration of fenoldopam and nitroprusside, use the manufacturers' instructions to develop a unit protocol for preparation of infusion solutions, dosages, flow rates, durations of use, and monitoring of blood pressure during infusion.	These drugs are used to lower blood pressure rapidly in hypertensive emergencies, usually in an emergency department or critical care unit. They also have specific requirements for preparation and administration. A protocol established beforehand can save valuable time in an emergency situation.
2. Observe for therapeutic effects	The choice of drugs and drug dosages often requires adjustment to maximize beneficial effects and minimize adverse effects. Thus, optimal therapeutic effects may not occur immediately after drug therapy is begun.
a. Decreased blood pressure. The usual goal is a normal blood pressure (ie, less than 140/90 mm Hg).	
3. Observe for adverse effects	Adverse effects are most likely to occur in clients who are elderly, have impaired renal function, and are receiving multiple antihypertensive drugs or large doses of antihypertensive drugs.
a. Orthostatic hypotension, dizziness, weakness	This is an extension of the expected pharmacologic action. Orthostatic hypotension results from drug blockage of compensatory reflexes (vasoconstriction, decreased venous pooling in extremities and increased venous return to the heart) that normally maintain blood pressure in the upright position. This adverse reaction may be aggravated by other conditions that cause vasodilation (eg, exercise, heat or hot weather, and alcohol consumption).
b. Sodium and water retention; increased plasma volume; perhaps edema and weight gain	These effects result from decreased renal perfusion. This reaction can be prevented or minimized by concurrent administration of a diuretic.
c. Prolonged atrioventricular conduction, bradycardia	Due to increased vagal tone and stimulation
d. Gastrointestinal disturbances, including nausea, vomiting, and diarrhea	These effects are more likely to occur with hydralazine, methyldopa, propranolol, and captopril.
e. Mental depression (with reserpine)	Apparently caused by decreased levels of catecholamines and serotonin in the brain

NURSING ACTIONS	RATIONALE/EXPLANATION
f. Bronchospasm (with nonselective beta blockers)	The drugs may cause bronchoconstriction and are contraindicated in patients with asthma and other bronchoconstrictive lung disorders.
g. Hypertensive crisis (with abrupt withdrawal of clonidine or guanabenz).	This may be prevented by tapering dosage over several days before stopping the drug.
h. Cough and hyperkalemia with angiotensin-converting enzyme (ACE) inhibitors	A chronic, nonproductive cough is a relatively common adverse effect; hyperkalemia occurs in 1%–4% of clients.
4. Observe for drug interactions	
a. Drugs that *increase* effects of antihypertensives:	
(1) Other antihypertensive agents	Combinations of two or three drugs with different mechanisms of action are often given for their additive effects and efficacy in controlling blood pressure when a single drug is ineffective.
(2) Alcohol, other central nervous system depressants (eg, opioid analgesics, phenothiazine antipsychotics)	These drugs have hypotensive effects when used alone and increased hypotension occurs when they are combined with antihypertensive drugs.
(3) Digoxin	Additive bradycardia with beta blockers
b. Drugs that *decrease* effects of antihypertensives:	
(1) Adrenergics	These drugs stimulate the sympathetic nervous system and raise blood pressure. They include over-the-counter nasal decongestants, cold remedies, bronchodilators, and appetite suppressants.
(2) Antacids	May decrease bioavailability of ACE inhibitors, especially captopril. Give antacids 2 hours before or after ACE inhibitors.
(3) Nonsteroidal anti-inflammatory drugs, oral contraceptives	These drugs tend to increase blood pressure by causing retention of sodium and water.

APPLYING YOUR KNOWLEDGE: ANSWERS

52-1 Be aware that compliance is a common problem with clients who have hypertension. Explore the reasons for the noncompliance, such as: is the client unable to make lifestyle changes; is the client experiencing adverse effects from the medication; is the client able to afford the cost of the medication; and does the client understand this asymptomatic disorder and the many complications that hypertension can cause? As always, provide appropriate teaching.

52-2 Encourage the client to reduce weight and sodium intake, to get regular physical activity, to stop smoking, and to moderate alcohol intake. These measures can prevent prehypertension and reduce blood pressure in clients with elevated blood pressure. The client should also understand antihypertensive drug therapy. Always review other behaviors that may decrease the therapeutic response, such as taking over-the-counter medication.

52-3 Due to their efficacy, calcium channel blockers are the drugs of first choice for the treatment of hypertension in African Americans, according to the JNC 7.

Review and Application Exercises

Short Answer Exercises

1. Describe the physiologic mechanisms that control blood pressure.

2. What are common factors that raise blood pressure?

3. Why is it important to measure blood pressure accurately and repeatedly?

4. How do ACE inhibitors, ARBs, alpha- and beta-adrenergic blockers, calcium channel blockers, and direct vasodilators lower blood pressure?

5. What are adverse effects of each group of antihypertensive drugs, and how may they be prevented or minimized?

6. List at least two major considerations in using antihypertensive drugs in children, older adults, and clients who have renal or hepatic impairment.

7. How would you assess a client being treated for hypertension for compliance with the prescribed lifestyle and drug therapy regimen?

NCLEX-Style Questions

8. Which of the following is a common adverse reaction to therapy with an ACE inhibitor?
   a. tinnitus
   b. dry, nonproductive, persistent cough
   c. muscle weakness
   d. constipation

9. A client with a history of hypertension comes to the emergency department with double vision and a blood pressure of 240/120 mm Hg. The physician prescribes sodium nitroprusside (Nipress) by continuous infusion and continual blood pressure monitoring. The nurse understands that this drug's immediate action is to lower blood pressure by
   a. increasing peripheral vascular resistance
   b. increasing cardiac output
   c. dilating venous and arterial vessels
   d. decreasing heart rate

10. Which of the following is indicated for initial drug therapy in a client newly diagnosed with uncomplicated hypertension (stage 1)?
   a. calcium channel blocker
   b. potassium-sparing diuretic
   c. direct-acting vasodilator
   d. thiazide diuretic

11. Orthostatic or postural hypotension is a potential outcome that places the elderly at risk for injury.

Instructions given to the client to decrease this effect of antihypertensive therapy include
   a. Take the dose in the early afternoon.
   b. Change position slowly when rising from bed or chair.
   c. Increase fluid intake by 500 mL/day.
   d. Decrease the dose until symptoms disappear.

12. Single-drug therapy with an ACE inhibitor would be least effective in
   a. children
   b. the elderly
   c. Hispanics
   d. African Americans

Selected References

Carter, B. L., & Saseen, J. L. (2002). Hypertension. *In* J. T. DiPiro, R. L. Talbert, G. C. Yee, G. R. Matzke, B. G. Wells, & L. M. Posey (Eds.), *Pharmacotherapy: A pathophysiologic approach* (5th ed., pp. 157–183). New York: McGraw-Hill.

Drug facts and comparisons. (Updated monthly). St. Louis: Facts and Comparisons.

Ferdinand, K. C. (2003, October). Treatment guidelines for hypertension in African Americans. *The Clinical Advisor,* (CME Suppl.), 3–10.

Hockenberry, M. J., Wilson, D., Winkelstein, M. L., & Kline, N. E. (2003). *Wong's Nursing care of infants and children* (7th ed., pp. 1476–1484). St. Louis: Mosby.

Joint National Committee on Prevention, Detection, Evaluation, and Treatment of High Blood Pressure. (2003). *The seventh report of the Joint National Committee on Prevention, Detection, Evaluation, and Treatment of High Blood Pressure: The JNC 7 report.* Retrieved July 30, 2005, from http://www.nhlbi.nih.gov/guidelines/hypertension.

Karch, A. M. (2005). *2006 Lippincott's nursing drug guide.* Philadelphia: Lippincott Williams & Wilkins.

National High Blood Pressure Education Program Working Group on High Blood Pressure in Children and Adolescents. The Fourth Report on the Diagnosis, Evaluation, and Treatment of High Blood Pressure in Children and Adolescents. Retrieved September 28, 2005, from http://www.pediatrics.org/cgi/content/full/114/2/S2/555

North American Nursing Diagnosis Association. (2003). *Nursing diagnoses: Definitions & classification 2003–2004.* Philadelphia: Author.

Porth, C. M. (2005). *Pathophysiology: Concepts of altered health states* (7th ed., pp. 505–533). Philadelphia: Lippincott Williams & Wilkins.

Skidmore-Roth, L. (2004). *Mosby's handbook of herbs & natural supplements* (2nd ed.). St. Louis: Mosby.

Smeltzer, S. C., & Bare, B. G. (2004). *Brunner & Suddarth's textbook of medical-surgical nursing* (10th ed., pp. 787–806). Philadelphia: Lippincott Williams & Wilkins.

World Health Organization, International Society of Hypertension (ISH) Writing Group (2003). ISH Statement on management of hypertension. *Journal of Hyptertension, 21*(11), 1983–1992.

Diuretics

OBJECTIVES

After studying this chapter, you will be able to:

1. List characteristics of diuretics in terms of mechanism of action, indications for use, principles of therapy, and nursing process implications.
2. Discuss major adverse effects of thiazide, loop, and potassium-sparing diuretics.
3. Identify clients at risk for developing adverse reactions to diuretic administration.
4. Recognize commonly used potassium-losing and potassium-sparing diuretics.
5. Discuss the rationale for using combination products containing a potassium-losing and a potassium-sparing diuretic.
6. Discuss the rationale for concomitant use of a loop diuretic and a thiazide or related diuretic.
7. Teach clients to manage diuretic therapy effectively.
8. Discuss important elements of diuretic therapy in special populations.

APPLYING YOUR KNOWLEDGE

Agnes Bass is a 68-year-old woman who has lower-leg edema. She is being treated with furosemide 40 mg PO daily.

INTRODUCTION

Diuretics are drugs that increase renal excretion of water, sodium, and other electrolytes, thereby increasing urine formation and output. They are important therapeutic agents widely used in the management of both edematous (eg, heart failure, renal and hepatic disease) and nonedematous (eg, hypertension, ophthalmic surgery) conditions. Diuretics are also useful in preventing renal failure by their ability to sustain urine flow. To aid understanding of diuretic drug therapy, renal physiology related to drug action and characteristics of edema are reviewed.

Renal Physiology

The primary function of the kidneys is to regulate the volume, composition, and pH of body fluids. The kidneys receive approximately 25% of the cardiac output. From this large amount of blood flow, the normally functioning kidney is efficient in retaining substances needed by the body and eliminating those not needed.

The Nephron

The nephron is the functional unit of the kidney; each kidney contains approximately 1 million nephrons. Each nephron is composed of a glomerulus and a tubule (Fig. 53-1). The glomerulus is a network of capillaries that receives blood from the renal artery. Bowman's capsule is a thin-walled structure that surrounds the glomerulus, then narrows and continues as the tubule. The tubule is a thin-walled structure of epithelial cells surrounded by peritubular capillaries. The tubule is divided into three main segments, the proximal tubule, loop of Henle, and distal tubule, which differ in structure and function. The tubules are often called *convoluted tubules* because of their many twists and turns. The convolutions provide a large surface area that brings the blood flowing through the peritubular capillaries and the glomerular filtrate flowing through the tubular lumen into close proximity. Consequently, substances can be readily exchanged through the walls of the tubules.

The nephron functions by three processes: glomerular filtration, tubular reabsorption, and tubular secretion. These processes normally maintain the fluid volume, electrolyte

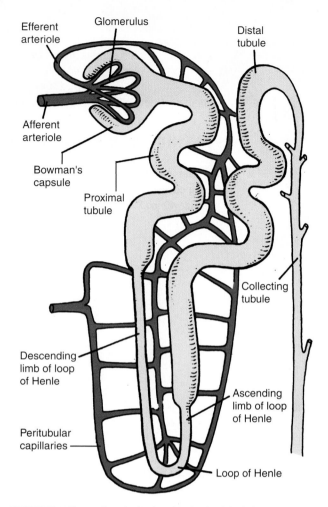

FIGURE 53-1 The nephron is the functional unit of the kidney.

concentration, and pH of body fluids within a relatively narrow range. They also remove waste products of cellular metabolism. A minimum daily urine output of approximately 400 milliliters is required to remove normal amounts of metabolic end products.

Glomerular Filtration

Arterial blood enters the glomerulus by the afferent arteriole at the relatively high pressure of approximately 70 mm Hg. This pressure pushes water, electrolytes, and other solutes out of the capillaries into Bowman's capsule and then to the proximal tubule. This fluid, called *glomerular filtrate,* contains the same components as blood except for blood cells, fats, and proteins that are too large to be filtered.

The glomerular filtration rate (GFR) is about 180 liters per day, or 125 milliliters per minute. Most of this fluid is reabsorbed as the glomerular filtrate travels through the tubules. The end product is about 2 liters of urine daily. Because filtration is a nonselective process, the reabsorption and secretion processes determine the composition of the urine. After

it is formed, urine flows into collecting tubules, which carry it to the renal pelvis, then through the ureters, bladder, and urethra for elimination from the body.

Blood that does not become part of the glomerular filtrate leaves the glomerulus through the efferent arteriole. The efferent arteriole branches into the peritubular capillaries that eventually empty into veins, which return the blood to systemic circulation.

Tubular Reabsorption

The term *reabsorption,* in relation to renal function, indicates movement of substances from the tubule (glomerular filtrate) to the blood in the peritubular capillaries. Most reabsorption occurs in the proximal tubule. Almost all glucose and amino acids are reabsorbed; about 80% of water, sodium, potassium, chloride, and most other substances is reabsorbed. As a result, about 20% of the glomerular filtrate enters the loop of Henle. In the descending limb of the loop of Henle, water is reabsorbed; in the ascending limb, sodium is reabsorbed. A large fraction of the total amount of sodium (up to 30%) filtered by the glomeruli is reabsorbed in the loop of Henle. Additional sodium is reabsorbed in the distal tubule, primarily by the exchange of sodium ions for potassium ions secreted by epithelial cells of tubular walls. Final reabsorption of water occurs in the distal tubule and small collecting tubules. The remaining water and solutes are now appropriately called *urine.*

Antidiuretic hormone from the posterior pituitary gland promotes reabsorption of water from the distal tubules and the collecting ducts of the kidneys. This conserves water needed by the body and produces more concentrated urine. Aldosterone, a hormone from the adrenal cortex, promotes sodium–potassium exchange mainly in the distal tubule and collecting ducts. Thus, aldosterone promotes sodium reabsorption and potassium loss.

Tubular Secretion

The term *secretion,* in relation to renal function, indicates movement of substances from blood in the peritubular capillaries to glomerular filtrate flowing through the renal tubules. Secretion occurs in the proximal and distal tubules, across the epithelial cells that line the tubules. In the proximal tubule, uric acid, creatinine, hydrogen ions, and ammonia are secreted; in the distal tubule, potassium ions, hydrogen ions, and ammonia are secreted. Secretion of hydrogen ions is important in maintaining acid–base balance in body fluids.

Alterations in Renal Function

Many clinical conditions alter renal function. In some conditions, excessive amounts of substances (eg, sodium, water) are retained; in others, needed substances (eg, potassium, proteins) are eliminated. These conditions include cardiovascular, renal, hepatic, and other disorders that may be managed with diuretic drugs.

Edema

Edema is the excessive accumulation of fluid in body tissues. It is a symptom of many disease processes and may occur in any part of the body. Additional characteristics include the following:

- Edema formation results from one or more of the following mechanisms that allow fluid to leave the bloodstream (intravascular compartment) and enter interstitial (third) spaces.
  - Increased capillary permeability occurs as part of the response to tissue injury. Thus, edema may occur with burns and trauma or allergic and inflammatory reactions.
  - Increased capillary hydrostatic pressure results from a sequence of events in which increased blood volume (from fluid overload or sodium and water retention) or obstruction of venous blood flow causes a high venous pressure and a high capillary pressure. This is the primary mechanism for edema formation in heart failure, pulmonary edema, and renal failure.
  - Decreased plasma oncotic pressure may occur with decreased synthesis of plasma proteins (caused by liver disease or malnutrition) or increased loss of plasma proteins (caused by burn injuries or the nephrotic syndrome). Plasma proteins are important in keeping fluids within the bloodstream. When plasma proteins are lacking, fluid seeps through the capillaries and accumulates in tissues.
- Edema interferes with blood flow to tissues. Thus, it interferes with delivery of oxygen and nutrients and removal of metabolic waste products. If severe, edema may distort body features, impair movement, and interfere with activities of daily living.

- Specific manifestations of edema are determined by its location and extent. A common type of localized edema occurs in the feet and ankles (dependent edema), especially with prolonged sitting or standing. A less common but more severe type of localized edema is pulmonary edema, a life-threatening condition that occurs with circulatory overload (eg, of intravenous [IV] fluids, blood transfusions) or acute heart failure. Generalized massive edema (anasarca) interferes with the functions of many body organs and tissues.

GENERAL CHARACTERISTICS OF DIURETIC DRUGS

Diuretic drugs act on the kidneys to decrease reabsorption of sodium, chloride, water, and other substances. Major subclasses are the thiazides and related diuretics, loop diuretics, and potassium-sparing diuretics, which act at different sites in the nephron (Fig. 53-2).

Major clinical indications for diuretics are edema, heart failure, and hypertension. In edematous states, diuretics mobilize tissue fluids by decreasing plasma volume. In hypertension, the exact mechanism by which diuretics lower blood pressure is unknown, but antihypertensive action is usually attributed to sodium depletion. Initially, diuretics decrease blood volume and cardiac output. With chronic use, cardiac output returns to normal, but there is a persistent decrease in plasma volume and peripheral vascular resistance. Sodium depletion may have a vasodilating effect on arterioles.

The use of diuretic agents in the management of heart failure and hypertension is discussed further in Chapters 48 and 52, respectively. Types of diuretics are described in the following section, and individual drugs are listed in Table 53-1.

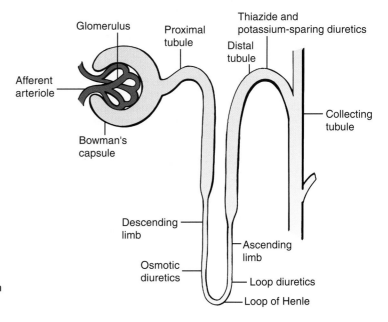

FIGURE 53-2 Diuretic sites of action in the nephron. Diuretics act at different sites in the nephron to decrease reabsorption of sodium and water and increase urine output.

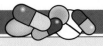

Table 53-1 Drugs at a Glance: Diuretic Agents

GENERIC (TRADE) NAME	ROUTES AND DOSAGE RANGES	
	Adults	Children
Thiazide and Related Diuretics		
Bendroflumethiazide (Naturetin)	PO 5 mg daily initially. For maintenance, 2.5–20 mg daily or intermittently	PO up to 0.4 mg/kg/d initially, in 2 divided doses. For maintenance, 0.05–0.1 mg/kg/d in a single dose
Chlorothiazide (Diuril)	PO 500–1000 mg 1 or 2 times daily IV 500 mg twice daily	PO 22 mg/kg/d in 2 divided doses Infants <6 mo, up to 33 mg/kg/d in 2 divided doses IV not recommended
Chlorthalidone (Hygroton)	PO 25–100 mg daily	PO 3 mg/kg 3 times weekly, adjusted according to response
Hydrochlorothiazide (HydroDIURIL, Esidrix, Oretic)	PO 25–100 mg 1 or 2 times daily Elderly, 12.5–25 mg daily	PO 2 mg/kg/d in two divided doses Infants <6 mo, up to 3.3 mg/kg/d in 2 divided doses
Hydroflumethiazide (Saluron)	PO 25–200 mg daily	PO 1 mg/kg/d
Indapamide (Lozol)	PO 2.5–5 mg daily	Dosage not established
Methyclothiazide (Enduron)	PO 2.5–10 mg daily	PO 0.05–0.2 mg/kg/d
Metolazone (Zaroxolyn, Mykrox)	PO 5–20 mg daily, depending on severity of condition and response	
Trichlormethiazide (Naqua)	PO 2–4 mg one or two times daily initially. For maintenance, 1–4 mg once daily	PO 0.07 mg/kg/d in single or divided doses
Loop Diuretics		
Bumetanide (Bumex)	PO 0.5–2 mg daily as a single dose. May be repeated q4–6h to a maximal dose of 10 mg, if necessary. Giving on alternate days or for 3–4 d with rest periods of 1–2 d is recommended for long-term control of edema. IV, IM 0.5–1 mg, repeated in 2–3 h if necessary, to a maximal daily dose of 10 mg. Give IV injections over 1–2 min.	Not recommended for children <18 y
Ethacrynic acid (Edecrin)	Edema, PO 50–100 mg daily, increased or decreased according to severity of condition and response. Maximal daily dose, 400 mg Rapid mobilization of edema, IV 50 mg or 0.5–1 mg/kg injected slowly to a maximum of 100 mg/dose	PO 25 mg daily No recommended parenteral dose in children
P Furosemide (Lasix)	Edema, PO 20–80 mg as a single dose initially. If an adequate diuretic response is not obtained, dosage may be gradually increased by 20- to 40-mg increments at intervals of 6–8 h. For maintenance, dosage range and frequency of administration vary widely and must be individualized. Maximal daily dose, 600 mg Hypertension, PO 40 mg twice daily, gradually increased if necessary Rapid mobilization of edema, IV 20–40 mg initially, injected slowly. This dose may be repeated in 2 h. With acute pul-	PO 2 mg/kg 1 or 2 times daily initially, gradually increased by increments of 1–2 mg/kg per dose if necessary at intervals of 6–8 h. Maximal daily dose, 6 mg/kg IV 1 mg/kg initially. If diuretic response is not adequate, increase dosage by 1 mg/kg no sooner than 2 h after previous dose. Maximal dose, 6 mg/kg

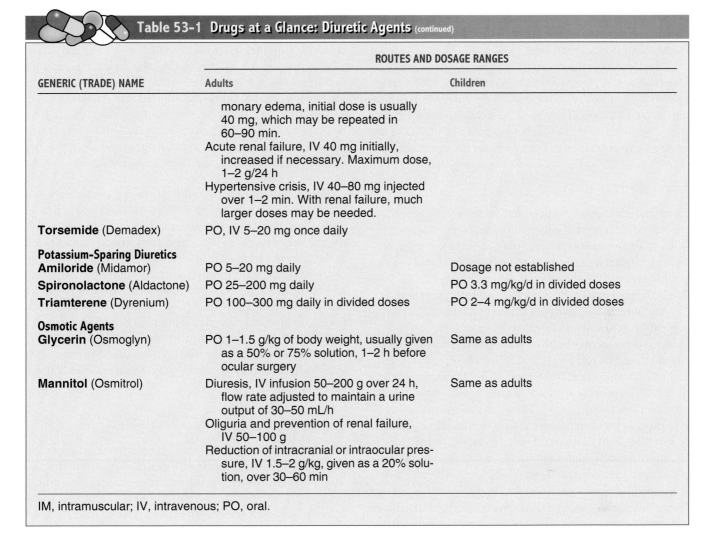

Table 53-1 Drugs at a Glance: Diuretic Agents (continued)

	ROUTES AND DOSAGE RANGES	
GENERIC (TRADE) NAME	**Adults**	**Children**
	monary edema, initial dose is usually 40 mg, which may be repeated in 60–90 min. Acute renal failure, IV 40 mg initially, increased if necessary. Maximum dose, 1–2 g/24 h Hypertensive crisis, IV 40–80 mg injected over 1–2 min. With renal failure, much larger doses may be needed.	
Torsemide (Demadex)	PO, IV 5–20 mg once daily	
Potassium-Sparing Diuretics		
Amiloride (Midamor)	PO 5–20 mg daily	Dosage not established
Spironolactone (Aldactone)	PO 25–200 mg daily	PO 3.3 mg/kg/d in divided doses
Triamterene (Dyrenium)	PO 100–300 mg daily in divided doses	PO 2–4 mg/kg/d in divided doses
Osmotic Agents		
Glycerin (Osmoglyn)	PO 1–1.5 g/kg of body weight, usually given as a 50% or 75% solution, 1–2 h before ocular surgery	Same as adults
Mannitol (Osmitrol)	Diuresis, IV infusion 50–200 g over 24 h, flow rate adjusted to maintain a urine output of 30–50 mL/h Oliguria and prevention of renal failure, IV 50–100 g Reduction of intracranial or intraocular pressure, IV 1.5–2 g/kg, given as a 20% solution, over 30–60 min	Same as adults

IM, intramuscular; IV, intravenous; PO, oral.

TYPES OF DIURETICS AND INDIVIDUAL DRUGS

Thiazide and Related Diuretics

Thiazide diuretics are synthetic drugs that are chemically related to the sulfonamides and differ mainly in their duration of action. **Hydrochlorothiazide** is the most commonly used; chlorothiazide is the only one that can be given IV. Related diuretics are nonthiazides whose pharmacologic actions are essentially the same as those of the thiazides; they include chlorthalidone, and metolazone.

Thiazides and related diuretics are frequently prescribed in the long-term management of heart failure and hypertension. They act to decrease reabsorption of sodium, water, chloride, and bicarbonate in the distal convoluted tubule. Most sodium is reabsorbed before it reaches the distal convoluted tubule and only a small amount is reabsorbed at this site. Thus, these drugs are not strong diuretics. In addition,

they are ineffective when immediate diuresis is required (because of their slow onset of action) and relatively ineffective with decreased renal function. They work efficiently only when urine flow is adequate.

A dose of diuretic that yields a near-maximum diuretic response is called the *ceiling dose* or *threshold.* The ceiling dose is dependent on the type of diuretic and the extent of an individual's disease. Thiazide diuretics have a ceiling threshold. As the maximum effect is reached, a subsequent increase in dose does not enhance efficacy. In addition, there is a direct correlation between the dosage increase and the possible onset of adverse effects. When the diuretic dose is less than at ceiling, postdiuresis fluid retention results.

These drugs are well absorbed, widely distributed in body fluids, and highly bound to plasma proteins. They accumulate only in the kidneys. Diuretic effects usually occur within 2 hours, peak at 4 to 6 hours, and last 6 to 24 hours. Antihypertensive effects usually last long enough to allow use of a single daily dose. Most of the drugs are excreted unchanged by the kidneys within 3 to 6 hours; some (eg, chlorthalidone) have longer durations of action (48–72 hours), attributed to slower excretion.

Thiazides and related drugs must be used cautiously in clients allergic to sulfonamide drugs as there is a known cross-sensitivity of some sulfonamide-allergic clients to a sulfonamide nonantibiotic. They must be used cautiously during pregnancy because they cross the placenta and may have adverse effects on the fetus by compromising placental perfusion.

Loop Diuretics

Loop diuretics inhibit sodium and chloride reabsorption in the ascending limb of the loop of Henle, where reabsorption of most filtered sodium occurs. Thus, these potent drugs produce significant diuresis, their sodium-losing effect being up to 10 times greater than that of thiazide diuretics. Dosage can be titrated upward as needed to produce greater diuretic effects. Overall, loop diuretics are the most effective and versatile diuretics available for clinical use.

Loop diuretics may be given orally or IV. After oral administration, diuretic effects occur within 30 to 60 minutes, peak in 1 to 2 hours, and last 6 to 8 hours. After IV administration, diuretic effects occur within 5 minutes, peak within 30 minutes, and last about 2 hours. Thus, the drugs produce extensive diuresis for short periods, after which the kidney tubules regain their ability to reabsorb sodium. Actually, the kidneys reabsorb more sodium than usual during this postdiuretic phase, so a high dietary intake of sodium can cause sodium retention and reduce or cancel the diuretic-induced sodium loss. Thus, dietary sodium restriction is required to achieve optimum therapeutic benefits. The drugs are metabolized and excreted by the kidneys, and drug accumulation does not occur even with repeated doses.

Loop diuretics are the diuretics of choice when rapid effects are required (eg, in pulmonary edema) and when renal function is impaired (creatinine clearance <30 mL/min). The drugs are contraindicated during pregnancy unless absolutely necessary.

P **Furosemide** is the most commonly used loop diuretic and serves as the prototype for the group. Bumetanide may be used to produce diuresis in some clients who are allergic to or no longer respond to furosemide. It is more potent than furosemide on a drug weight basis, and large doses can be given in small volumes. These drugs differ mainly in potency and produce similar effects at equivalent doses (eg, furosemide 40 mg = bumetanide 1 mg).

Potassium-Sparing Diuretics

Sodium is normally reabsorbed in the distal tubule in exchange for potassium and hydrogen ions. Potassium-sparing diuretics act at the distal tubule to decrease sodium reabsorption and potassium excretion. This group includes

three drugs. One is **spironolactone,** an aldosterone antagonist. Aldosterone is a hormone secreted by the adrenal cortex. It promotes retention of sodium and water and excretion of potassium by stimulating the sodium–potassium exchange mechanism in the distal tubule. Spironolactone blocks the sodium-retaining effects of aldosterone, and aldosterone must be present for spironolactone to be effective. The other two drugs, **amiloride** and **triamterene,** act directly on the distal tubule to decrease the exchange of sodium for potassium, and have similar diuretic activity.

Potassium-sparing diuretics are weak diuretics when used alone. Thus, they are usually given in combination with potassium-losing diuretics to increase diuretic activity and decrease potassium loss. They are contraindicated in the presence of renal insufficiency because their use may cause hyperkalemia through the inhibition of aldosterone and subsequent retention of potassium. Hyperkalemia is the major adverse effect of these drugs; clients receiving potassium-sparing diuretics should *not* be given potassium supplements and *should not be* encouraged to eat foods high in potassium or allowed to use salt substitutes. Salt substitutes contain potassium chloride rather than sodium chloride.

Osmotic Diuretics

Osmotic agents produce rapid diuresis by increasing the solute load (osmotic pressure) of the glomerular filtrate. The increased osmotic pressure causes water to be pulled from extravascular sites into the bloodstream, thereby increasing blood volume and decreasing reabsorption of water and electrolytes in the renal tubules. **Mannitol** is useful in managing oliguria or anuria, and it may prevent acute renal failure during prolonged surgery, trauma, or infusion of cisplatin, an antineoplastic agent. Mannitol is effective even when renal circulation and GFR are reduced (eg, in hypovolemic shock, trauma, dehydration). Other important clinical uses of hyperosmolar agents include reduction of intracranial pressure before or after neurosurgery, reduction of intraocular pressure before certain types of ophthalmic surgery, and urinary excretion of toxic substances. Another osmotic agent, glycerin, is listed in Table 53-1.

Combination Products

Thiazide and related diuretics are available in numerous fixed-dose combinations with nondiuretic antihypertensive agents (see Chap. 52) and with potassium-sparing diuretics (see Table 53-2 for combination diuretic products). A major purpose of the antihypertensive combinations is to increase client convenience and compliance with drug therapy regimens. A major purpose of the diuretic combinations is to prevent potassium imbalances.

| | THIAZIDE (POTASSIUM- | POTASSIUM-SPARING | |
TRADE NAME	LOSING) DIURETIC	DIURETIC	ADULT DOSAGE
Aldactazide 25/25	HCTZ 25 mg	Spironolactone 25 mg	PO 1–8 tablets daily
Aldactazide 50/50	HCTZ 50 mg	Spironolactone 50 mg	PO 1–4 tablets daily
Dyazide, Maxzide 25 mg	HCTZ 25 mg	Triamterene 37.5 mg	Hypertension, PO 1 capsule bid initially, then adjusted according to response Edema, PO 1–2 capsules bid
Maxzide	HCTZ 50 mg	Triamterene 75 mg	PO 1 tablet daily
Moduretic	HCTZ 50 mg	Amiloride 5 mg	PO 1–2 tablets daily with meals

Table 53-2 Drugs at a Glance: Combination Diuretic Products

bid, twice a day; HCTZ, hydrochlorothiazide; PO, oral.

NURSING PROCESS

Assessment

Assess the client's status in relation to baseline data and conditions in which diuretic drugs are used.

- Useful baseline data include serum electrolytes, creatinine, glucose, blood urea nitrogen (BUN), and uric acid, because diuretics may alter these values. Other data are blood pressure readings, weight, amount and appearance of urine output, and measurement of edematous areas such as ankles or abdomen.
- Observe for edema. Visible edema often occurs in the feet and legs of ambulatory clients. Rapid weight gain may indicate fluid retention.
  - With heart failure, numerous signs and symptoms result from edema of various organs and tissues. For example, congestion in the gastrointestinal (GI) tract may cause nausea and vomiting; liver congestion may cause abdominal pain and tenderness; and congestion in the lungs (pulmonary edema) causes rapid, labored breathing; hypoxemia; frothy sputum; and other manifestations of severe respiratory distress.
  - Cerebral edema may be manifested by confusion, headache, dizziness, convulsions, unconsciousness, bradycardia, or failure of the pupils to react to light.
  - Ascites, which occurs with hepatic cirrhosis, is an accumulation of fluid in the abdominal cavity. The abdomen appears much enlarged.
- With heart failure, fatigue and dyspnea, in addition to edema, are common symptoms.
- Hypertension (blood pressure greater than 140/90 mm Hg on several measurements) may be the only clinical manifestation present.

Nursing Diagnoses

- Excess Fluid Volume in edematous clients, related to retention of sodium and water

- Deficient Fluid Volume related to increased diuresis during diuretic drug therapy
- Imbalanced Nutrition: Less Than Body Requirements related to excessive loss of potassium with thiazide and loop diuretics
- Risk for Injury: Hypotension and dizziness as adverse drug effects
- Deficient Knowledge related to the need for and correct use of diuretics
- Sexual Dysfunction related to adverse drug effects

Planning/Goals

The client will

- Take or receive diuretic drugs as prescribed
- Experience reduced edema and improved control of blood pressure
- Reduce dietary intake of sodium and increase dietary intake of potassium
- Avoid preventable adverse drug effects
- Keep appointments for follow-up monitoring of blood pressure, edema, and serum electrolytes

Interventions

Promote measures to prevent or minimize conditions for which diuretic drugs are used.

- With edema, helpful measures include the following:
  - Decreasing dietary sodium intake
  - Losing weight, if obese
  - Elevating legs when sitting
  - Avoiding prolonged standing or sitting
  - Wearing support hose or elastic stockings
  - Treating the condition causing edema
- With heart failure and in older adults, administer IV fluids or blood transfusions carefully to avoid fluid overload and pulmonary edema. Fluid overload may occur with rapid administration or excessive amounts of IV fluids.

- With hypertension, helpful measures include decreasing dietary sodium intake, exercising regularly, and losing weight, if obese.
- With edematous clients, interventions to monitor fluid losses include weighing under standardized conditions, measuring urine output, and measuring edematous sites such as the ankles or the abdomen. After the client reaches "dry weight," these measurements stabilize and can be done less often.
- With clients who are taking digoxin, a potassium-losing diuretic, and a potassium supplement, help them understand that the drugs act together to increase therapeutic effectiveness and avoid adverse effects (eg, hypokalemia, digoxin toxicity). Thus, stopping or changing dosage of one of these drugs can lead to serious illness.

Provide client teaching regarding drug therapy (see accompanying display).

Evaluation

- Observe for reduced edema and body weight.
- Observe for reduced blood pressure.
- Observe for increased urine output.
- Monitor serum electrolytes for normal values.
- Interview regarding compliance with instructions for diet and drug therapy.
- Monitor compliance with follow-up appointments in outpatients.

APPLYING YOUR KNOWLEDGE 53-1
While caring for Ms. Bass, she tells you that she enjoys snacks like potato chips and pretzels. What response would you have?

APPLYING YOUR KNOWLEDGE 53-2:
HOW CAN YOU AVOID THIS MEDICATION ERROR?
The physician orders an extra dose of furosemide 20 mg IV for Ms. Bass, to be given now. You prepare the injection and administer it over 15 seconds.

PRINCIPLES OF THERAPY

Drug Selection

The choice of diuretic drug depends primarily on the client's condition.

- **Thiazides and related diuretics** are the drugs of choice for most clients who require diuretic therapy, especially for long-term management of heart failure and hypertension. All the drugs in this group have similar effects. For most clients, hydrochlorothiazide is effective.

- A **loop diuretic** (eg, furosemide) is preferred when rapid diuretic effects are required or when renal impairment is present.
- A **potassium-sparing diuretic** may be given concurrently with a potassium-losing diuretic to prevent or manage hypokalemia and to augment the diuretic effect. The two drugs can be given separately or in a fixed-dose combination product (see Table 53-2).
- Two **potassium-losing diuretics** are sometimes given concurrently when an inadequate diuretic response occurs with one of the drugs. The combination of a loop and a thiazide diuretic has synergistic effects because the drugs act in different segments of the renal tubule. The synergistic effects probably result from the increased delivery of sodium to the distal tubule (where thiazides act) because a loop diuretic blocks sodium reabsorption in the loop of Henle. A commonly used combination is furosemide and hydrochlorothiazide (chlorothiazide can be given IV in clients who are unable to take an oral drug). Furosemide and metolazone have also been used. Because a thiazide–loop diuretic combination can induce profound diuresis, with severe sodium, potassium, and volume depletion, its use should be reserved for hospitalized patients who can be closely monitored. If used for ambulatory clients, the thiazide diuretic should be given in very low doses or only occasionally, to avoid serious adverse events.

Drug Dosage and Administration

Dosage of diuretics depends largely on the client's condition and response and should be individualized to administer the minimal effective amount.

- With hydrochlorothiazide, smaller doses (eg, 12.5–25 mg daily) are effective for most people and produce fewer adverse effects (eg, hypokalemia) than larger doses. Some of the fixed-dose combinations of hydrochlorothiazide and a potassium-sparing diuretic contain 50 mg of hydrochlorothiazide. As a result, despite the convenience of a combination product, it may be better to give the drugs separately so that dosage can be titrated to the client's needs.
- Clients who do not achieve an adequate diuretic response with usual doses of an oral drug may need larger doses or an IV drug.
- With torsemide, which is highly bioavailable after oral administration, oral and IV doses are equivalent and clients may be switched from one route to the other without changing dosage.
- In liver disease, small doses of all diuretics are usually indicated because diuretic-induced electrolyte imbalances may precipitate or aggravate hepatic coma.
- In renal disease, furosemide is often given in large doses to achieve a diuretic response. Bumetanide may be a useful alternative, because it can be given in smaller dose volumes.

CLIENT TEACHING GUIDELINES

Diuretics

General Considerations

✔ Diuretics increase urine output and are commonly used to manage hypertension, heart failure, and edema (swelling) from heart, kidney, liver, and other disorders.

✔ While taking a diuretic drug, you need to maintain regular medical supervision so drug effects can be monitored and dosages adjusted when indicated.

✔ Reducing sodium intake in your diet helps diuretic drugs be more effective and allows smaller doses to be taken. Smaller doses are less likely to cause adverse effects. Thus, you need to avoid excessive table salt and obviously salty foods (eg, ham, packaged sandwich meats, potato chips, dill pickles, most canned soups). These foods may aggravate edema or hypertension by causing sodium and water retention.

✔ Diuretics may cause blood potassium imbalances, and either too little or too much damages heart function. Periodic measurements of blood potassium and other substances is one of the major reasons for regular visits to a health care provider.

Too little potassium (hypokalemia) may result from the use of potassium-losing diuretics such as hydrochlorothiazide, furosemide (Lasix), and several others. To prevent or treat hypokalemia, your doctor may prescribe a potassium chloride supplement or a combination of a potassium-losing and a potassium-saving diuretic (either separately or as a combined product such as Dyazide, Maxzide, or Aldactazide). He or she may also recommend increased dietary intake of potassium-containing foods (eg, bananas, orange juice).

Too much potassium (hyperkalemia) can result from the use of potassium-saving diuretics, the overuse of potassium supplements, or from the use of salt substitutes. Potassium-saving diuretics are not a major cause of hyperkalemia because they are usually given along with a potassium-losing diuretic. If potassium supplements are prescribed, they should be taken as directed. You should **not** use salt substitutes without consulting your primary health care provider because they contain potassium chloride instead of sodium chloride. Hyperkalemia is most likely to occur in people with decreased kidney function, which often occurs in older adults and people with diabetes.

✔ With diuretic therapy, you will have increased urination, which usually lasts only a few days or weeks if you do not have edema. If you do have edema (eg, in your ankles), you can expect weight loss and decreased swelling as well as increased urination. It is a good idea to check and record your weight 2 to 3 times per week. Rapid changes in weight often indicate gain or loss of fluid.

✔ Some commonly used diuretics may increase blood sugar levels and cause or aggravate diabetes. If you have diabetes, you may need larger doses of your antidiabetic medications.

✔ Diuretics may cause sensitivity to sunlight. Thus, you need to avoid prolonged exposure to sunlight, use sunscreens, and wear protective clothing.

✔ Do not drink alcoholic beverages or take other medications without the approval of your health care provider.

✔ If you are taking a diuretic to lower your blood pressure, especially with other antihypertensive drugs, you may feel dizzy or faint when you stand up suddenly. This can be prevented or decreased by changing positions slowly. If dizziness is severe, notify your health care provider.

Self- or Caregiver Administration

✔ Take or give a diuretic early in the day, if ordered daily, to decrease nighttime trips to the bathroom. Fewer bathroom trips means less interference with sleep and less risk of falls. Ask someone to help you to the bathroom if you are elderly, weak, dizzy, or unsteady in walking (or use a bedside commode).

✔ Take or give most diuretics with or after food to decrease stomach upset. Torsemide (Demadex) may be taken without regard to meals.

✔ If you are taking digoxin, a potassium-losing diuretic, and a potassium supplement, it is very important that you take these drugs as prescribed. This is a common combination of drugs for clients with heart failure and the drugs work together to increase beneficial effects and avoid adverse effects. Stopping or changing the dose of one of these medications while continuing the others can lead to serious illness.

● When metolazone is given concurrently with furosemide, the initial dose is usually metolazone 2.5 to 10 mg. The dose is then doubled every 24 hours until the desired response is achieved. If an adequate diuretic effect occurs with the first dose of metolazone, the dose of furosemide can be decreased. Hydrochlorothiazide 50 mg may also be used with furosemide and may be safer than metolazone because of its shorter duration of action.

Use in Edema

When diuretics are used to manage clients with edema, the underlying cause of the edema should be addressed, not just the edema itself. When treating such clients, it is preferable to aim for a weight loss of approximately 2 pounds (1 kg) per day. Rapid and excessive diuresis may cause dehydration and decreased blood volume with circulatory collapse. In some clients, giving a diuretic every other day or 3 to 5 days per week may be effective and is less likely to cause electrolyte imbalances.

Use With Digoxin

When digoxin and diuretics are given concomitantly, as is common for clients with heart failure, the risk of digoxin toxicity is increased. Digoxin toxicity is related to diuretic-induced hypokalemia. Potassium is a myocardial depressant and antidysrhythmic; it has essentially opposite cardiac effects to those of digoxin. In other words, extracellular potassium decreases the excitability of myocardial tissue, but digoxin increases excitability. The higher the serum potassium, the less effective a given dose of digoxin will be. Conversely, decreased serum potassium increases the likelihood of digoxin-induced cardiac dysrhythmias, even with small doses and therapeutic serum levels of digoxin.

Supplemental potassium chloride, a potassium-sparing diuretic, and other measures to prevent hypokalemia are often used to maintain normal serum potassium levels (3.5–5.0 mEq/L).

Prevention and Management of Potassium Imbalances

Potassium imbalances (see Chap. 57) may occur with diuretic therapy. Hypokalemia and hyperkalemia are cardiotoxic and should be prevented when possible.

- **Hypokalemia** (serum potassium level <3.5 mEq/L) may occur with potassium-losing diuretics (eg, hydrochlorothiazide, furosemide). Measures to prevent or manage hypokalemia include the following:
  - Giving low doses of the diuretic (eg, 12.5–25 mg daily of hydrochlorothiazide)
  - Giving supplemental potassium, usually potassium chloride, in an average dosage range of 20 to 60 mEq daily. Sustained-release tablets are usually better tolerated than liquid preparations.
  - Giving a potassium-sparing diuretic along with the potassium-losing drug
  - Increasing food intake of potassium. Many texts advocate this approach as preferable to supplemental potassium or combination diuretic therapy, but its effectiveness is not clearly established. Although the minimal daily requirement of potassium is unknown, usual recommendations are 40 to 50 mEq daily for the healthy adult. Potassium loss with diuretic drugs may be several times this amount.

    Some foods (eg, bananas) have undeserved reputations for having high potassium content; actually, large amounts must be ingested. To provide 50 mEq of potassium daily, estimated amounts of certain foods include 1000 milliliters of orange juice, 1600 milliliters of apple or grape juice, 1200 milliliters of pineapple juice, four to six bananas, or 30 to 40 prunes. Some of these foods are high in calories and may be contraindicated, at least in large amounts, for obese clients. Also, the amount of carbohydrate in these foods may be a concern for clients with diabetes mellitus.
  - Restricting dietary sodium intake. This reduces potassium loss by decreasing the amount of sodium available for exchange with potassium in renal tubules.
- **Hyperkalemia** (serum potassium level >5 mEq/L) may occur with potassium-sparing diuretics. The following measures help prevent hyperkalemia.

- Avoiding use of potassium-sparing diuretics and potassium supplements in clients with renal impairment
- Avoiding excessive amounts of potassium chloride supplements
- Avoiding salt substitutes
- Maintaining urine output, the major route for eliminating potassium from the body

Use in Special Populations

Use in Children

Although they have not been extensively studied in children, diuretics are commonly used to manage heart failure, which often results from congenital heart disease; hypertension, which is usually related to cardiac or renal dysfunction; bronchopulmonary dysplasia and respiratory distress syndrome, which are often associated with pulmonary edema; and edema, which may occur with cardiac or renal disorders such as the nephrotic syndrome.

With most thiazides, safety and effectiveness have not been established for use in children. **Hydrochlorothiazide** is used in doses of approximately 2.2 milligrams per kilogram of body weight per day. IV chlorothiazide usually is not recommended. Thiazides do not commonly cause hyperglycemia, hyperuricemia, or hypercalcemia in children, as they do in adults.

Although **metolazone,** a thiazide-related drug, is not usually recommended, it is sometimes used. Metolazone has some advantages over a thiazide because it is a stronger diuretic, causes less hypokalemia, and can produce diuresis in renal failure. In children, it is most often used with furosemide, in which case it is most effective when given 30 to 60 minutes before the furosemide.

Furosemide is the loop diuretic used most often in children. Oral therapy is preferred when feasible, and doses above 6 milligrams per kilogram of body weight per day are not recommended. In preterm infants, furosemide stimulates production of prostaglandin E_2 in the kidneys and may increase the incidence of patent ductus arteriosus and neonatal respiratory distress syndrome. In neonates, furosemide may be given with indomethacin to prevent nonsteroidal anti-inflammatory drug–induced nephrotoxicity during therapeutic closure of a patent ductus arteriosus. In both preterm and full-term infants, furosemide half-life is prolonged but becomes shorter as renal and hepatic functions develop.

Adverse effects of furosemide include fluid and electrolyte imbalances (eg, hyponatremia, hypokalemia, fluid volume deficit) and ototoxicity. Serum electrolytes should be closely monitored in children because of frequent changes in kidney function and fluid distribution associated with growth and development. Ototoxicity, which is associated with high plasma drug levels (>50 mcg/mL), can usually be avoided by dividing oral doses, and by slow injection or continuous infusion of IV doses.

Safety and effectiveness of bumetanide, ethacrynic acid, and torsemide have not been established. However, **bumetanide** may cause less ototoxicity and thus may be preferred for children who are taking other ototoxic drugs (eg, premature and ill neonates are often given gentamicin, an aminoglycoside antibiotic). Bumetanide may also cause less hypokalemia. The half-life of bumetanide is about 2 hours in critically ill infants and 1 hour in children.

Spironolactone is the most widely used potassium-sparing diuretic in children. It is used with other diuretics to decrease potassium loss and hypokalemia. Spironolactone accumulates in renal failure, and dosage should be reduced. It usually should not be used in severe renal failure.

Use in Older Adults

Thiazide diuretics are often prescribed for the management of hypertension and heart failure, which are common in older adults. Older adults are especially sensitive to adverse drug effects, such as hypotension and electrolyte imbalance. Thiazides may aggravate renal or hepatic impairment. With rapid or excessive diuresis, myocardial infarction, renal impairment, or cerebral thrombosis may occur from fluid volume depletion and hypotension. The smallest effective dose is recommended, usually a daily dose of 12.5 to 25 milligrams of hydrochlorothiazide or equivalent doses of other thiazides and related drugs. Risks of adverse effects may exceed benefits at doses of hydrochlorothiazide greater than 25 milligrams.

With loop diuretics, older adults are at greater risk of excessive diuresis, hypotension, fluid volume deficit, and possibly thrombosis or embolism. Rapid diuresis may cause urinary incontinence. With potassium-sparing diuretics, hyperkalemia is more likely to occur in older adults because of the renal impairment that occurs with aging.

Use in Clients With Renal Impairment

Most clients with renal impairment require diuretics as part of their drug therapy regimens. In these clients, the diuretic response may be reduced and edema of the GI tract may limit absorption of oral medications.

Thiazides may be useful in managing edema due to renal disorders such as nephrotic syndrome and acute glomerulonephritis. However, their effectiveness decreases as the GFR decreases, and the drugs become ineffective when the GFR is less than 30 milliliters per minute. The drugs may accumulate and increase adverse effects in clients with impaired renal function. Thus, renal function tests should be performed periodically. If progressive renal impairment becomes evident (eg, a rising serum creatinine or BUN), a thiazide usually should be discontinued and metolazone, indapamide, or a loop diuretic may be given. Metolazone and indapamide are thiazide-related diuretics that may be effective in clients with significantly impaired renal function.

Loop diuretics are effective in clients with renal impairment. However, in chronic renal failure, they have lower peak concentrations at their site of action, which decreases diuresis.

Renal elimination of the drugs is also prolonged. If renal dysfunction becomes more severe during treatment (eg, oliguria, increases in BUN or creatinine) the diuretic may need to be discontinued. If high doses of furosemide are used, a volume-controlled IV infusion at a rate of 4 milligrams or less per minute may be used. For continuous infusion, furosemide should be mixed with normal saline or lactated Ringer's solution because D5W may accelerate degradation of furosemide. If IV bumetanide is given to clients with chronic renal impairment, a continuous infusion (eg, 12 mg over 12 hours) produces more diuresis than equivalent-dose intermittent injections. Continuous infusion also produces lower serum drug levels and therefore may decrease adverse effects.

Potassium-sparing diuretics are contraindicated in clients with renal impairment because of the high risk of hyperkalemia. If they are used at all, frequent monitoring of serum electrolytes, creatinine, and BUN is needed.

Use in Clients With Hepatic Impairment

Diuretics are often used to manage edema and ascites in clients with hepatic impairment. These drugs must be used with caution because diuretic-induced fluid and electrolyte imbalances may precipitate or worsen hepatic encephalopathy and coma. In clients with cirrhosis, diuretic therapy should be initiated in a hospital setting, with small doses and careful monitoring. To prevent hypokalemia and metabolic alkalosis, supplemental potassium or spironolactone may be needed.

Use in Clients With Critical Illness

Fast-acting, potent diuretics such as furosemide and bumetanide are the most likely diuretics to be used in critically ill clients (eg, those with pulmonary edema). In clients with severe renal impairment, high doses are required to produce diuresis. Large doses may produce fluid volume depletion and worsen renal function. Although IV bolus doses of the drugs are often given, continuous IV infusions may be more effective and less likely to produce adverse effects in critically ill clients.

Use in Home Care

Diuretics are often taken in the home setting. The home care nurse may need to assist clients and caregivers in using the drugs safely and effectively; monitor client responses (eg, with each home visit, assess nutritional status, blood pressure, weight, use of over-the-counter medications that may aggravate edema or hypertension); and provide information as indicated. In some cases, the home care nurse may need to assist the client in obtaining medications or blood for blood tests (eg, serum potassium levels).

APPLYING YOUR KNOWLEDGE 53-3

Ms. Bass has spironolactone added to her treatment regimen to increase diuresis. Why was this added to her regimen instead of increasing her dose of furosemide?

N   U   R   S   I   N   G   A   C   T   I   O   N   S

Diuretics

NURSING ACTIONS	RATIONALE/EXPLANATION
1. Administer accurately	
a. Give in the early morning if ordered daily.	So that peak action will occur during waking hours and not interfere with sleep
b. Take safety precautions. Keep a bedpan or urinal within reach. Keep the call light within reach, and be sure the client knows how to use it. Assist to the bathroom anyone who is elderly, weak, dizzy, or unsteady in walking.	Mainly to avoid falls
c. Give amiloride and triamterene with or after food.	To decrease gastrointestinal (GI) upset
d. Give intravenous (IV) injections of furosemide and bumetanide over 1–2 minutes; give torsemide over 2 minutes.	To decrease or avoid high peak serum levels, which increase risks of adverse effects, including ototoxicity
e. Give high-dose furosemide continuous IV infusions at a rate of 4 mg/min or less.	To decrease or avoid high peak serum levels, which increase risks of adverse effects, including ototoxicity
2. Observe for therapeutic effects	
a. Decrease or absence of edema, increased urine output, decreased blood pressure	Most oral diuretics act within 2 hours; IV diuretics act within minutes. Optimal antihypertensive effects occur in approximately 2–4 weeks.
(1) Weigh the client daily while edema is present and two to three times weekly thereafter. Weigh under standard conditions: early morning before eating or drinking, after urination, with the same amount of clothing, and using the same scales.	Body weight is a very good indicator of fluid gain or loss. A weight change of 2.2 lb (1 kg) may indicate a gain or loss of 1000 mL of fluid. Also, weighing assists in dosage regulation to maintain therapeutic benefit without excessive or too rapid fluid loss.
(2) Record fluid intake and output every shift for hospitalized clients.	Normally, oral fluid intake approximates urinary output (1500 mL/24 h). With diuretic therapy, urinary output may exceed intake, depending on the amount of edema or fluid retention, renal function, and diuretic dosage. All sources of fluid gain, including IV fluids, must be included; all sources of fluid loss (perspiration, fever, wound drainage, GI tract drainage) are important. Clients with abnormal fluid losses have less urine output with diuretic therapy. Oliguria (decreased excretion of urine) may require stopping the drug. Output greater than 100 mL/h may indicate that side effects are more likely to occur.
(3) Observe and record characteristics of urine.	Dilute urine may indicate excessive fluid intake or greater likelihood of fluid and electrolyte imbalance due to rapid diuresis. Concentrated urine may mean oliguria or decreased fluid intake.
(4) Assess for edema daily or with each client contact: ankles for the ambulatory client, sacral area and posterior thighs for clients at bed rest. Also, it is often helpful to measure abdominal girth, ankles, and calves to monitor gain or loss of fluid.	Expect a decrease in visible edema and size of measured areas. If edema reappears or worsens, a thorough reassessment of the client is in order. Questions to be answered include: (1) Is the prescribed diuretic being taken correctly? (2) What type of diuretic and what dosage is ordered? (3) Is there worsening of the underlying condition(s) that led to edema formation? (4) Has other disease developed?
(5) In clients with heart failure or acute pulmonary edema, observe for decreased dyspnea, crackles, cyanosis, and cough.	Decreased fluid in the lungs leads to improved respirations as more carbon dioxide and oxygen gas exchange takes place and greater tissue oxygenation occur.
(6) Record blood pressure 2 to 4 times daily when diuretic therapy is initiated.	Although thiazide diuretics do not lower normal blood pressure, other diuretics may, especially with excessive or rapid diuresis.

NURSING ACTIONS	RATIONALE/EXPLANATION
3. Observe for adverse effects	Major adverse effects are fluid and electrolyte imbalances.
a. With potassium-losing diuretics (thiazides, bumetanide, furosemide, ethacrynic acid), observe for:	
(1) Hypokalemia	Potassium is required for normal muscle function. Thus, potassium depletion causes weakness of cardiovascular, respiratory, digestive, and skeletal muscles. Clients most likely to have hypokalemia are those who are taking large doses of diuretics, potent diuretics (eg, furosemide), or adrenal corticosteroids; those who have decreased food and fluid intake; or those who have increased potassium losses through vomiting, diarrhea, chronic laxative or enema use, or GI suction. Clinically significant symptoms are most likely to occur with a serum potassium level below 3 mEq/L.
(a) Serum potassium levels below 3.5 mEq/L	
(b) Electrocardiographic (ECG) changes (eg, low voltage, flattened T wave, depressed ST segment)	
(c) Cardiac dysrhythmias; weak, irregular pulse	
(d) Hypotension	
(e) Weak, shallow respirations	
(f) Anorexia, nausea, vomiting	
(g) Decreased peristalsis or paralytic ileus	
(h) Skeletal muscle weakness	
(i) Confusion, disorientation	
(2) Hyponatremia, hypomagnesemia, hypochloremic alkalosis, changes in serum and urinary calcium levels	In addition to potassium, sodium chloride, magnesium, and bicarbonate also are lost with diuresis. Thiazides and related diuretics cause hypercalcemia and hypocalciuria. They have been used to prevent calcium nephrolithiasis (kidney stones). Furosemide and other loop diuretics tend to cause hypocalcemia and hypercalciuria.
(3) Dehydration	Fluid volume depletion occurs with excessive or rapid diuresis. If it is prolonged or severe, hypovolemic shock may occur.
(a) Poor skin turgor, dry mucous membranes	
(b) Oliguria, urine of high specific gravity	
(c) Thirst	
(d) Tachycardia; hypotension	
(e) Decreased level of consciousness	
(f) Elevated hematocrit (above 45%)	
(4) Hyperglycemia—blood glucose above 120 mg/100 mL, polyuria, polydipsia, polyphagia, glycosuria	Hyperglycemia is more likely to occur in clients with known or latent diabetes mellitus. Larger doses of hypoglycemic agents may be required. The hyperglycemic effect may be reversible when diuretic therapy is discontinued. Long-term use of a thiazide or loop diuretic may alter glucose metabolism. One mechanism is thought to involve diuretic-induced hypokalemia and hypomagnesemia, which then leads to decreased postprandial insulin release. Another mechanism may be development or worsening of insulin resistance. Because glucose intolerance is an important risk factor for coronary artery disease, diuretics should be used with caution in prediabetic or diabetic hypertensive clients.
(5) Hyperuricemia—serum uric acid above 7.0 mg/100 mL	Hyperuricemia is usually asymptomatic except for clients with gout, a predisposition toward gout, or chronic renal failure. Apparently, decreased renal excretion of uric acid allows its accumulation in the blood.
(6) Pulmonary edema (with osmotic diuretics)	Pulmonary edema is most likely to occur in clients with heart failure who cannot tolerate the increased blood volume produced by the drugs.

(continued)

NURSING ACTIONS	RATIONALE/EXPLANATION
(7) Ototoxicity (with furosemide and ethacrynic acid)	Reversible or transient hearing impairment, tinnitus, and dizziness are more common, although irreversible deafness may occur. Ototoxicity is more likely to occur with high serum drug levels (eg, high doses or use in clients with severe renal impairment) or when other ototoxic drugs (eg, aminoglycoside antibiotics) are being taken concurrently.
b. With potassium-sparing diuretics (spironolactone, triamterene, amiloride), observe for:	
(1) Hyperkalemia	Hyperkalemia is most likely to occur in clients with impaired renal function or those who are ingesting additional potassium (eg, salt substitutes).
(a) Serum potassium levels above 5 mEq/L	
(b) ECG changes (ie, prolonged P-R interval; wide QRS complex; tall, peaked T wave; depressed ST segment)	
(c) Cardiac dysrhythmias, which may progress to ventricular fibrillation and asystole	
4. Observe for drug interactions	
a. Drugs that *increase* effects of diuretics:	
(1) Aminoglycoside antibiotics	Additive ototoxicity with ethacrynic acid
(2) Antihypertensive agents	Additive hypotensive effects. In addition, angiotensin-converting enzyme inhibitor therapy significantly increases risks of hyperkalemia with spironolactone.
(3) Corticosteroids	Additive hypokalemia
b. Drugs that *decrease* effects of diuretics:	
(1) Nonsteroidal anti-inflammatory drugs (eg, aspirin, ibuprofen, others)	These drugs cause retention of sodium and water.
(2) Oral contraceptives	Retention of sodium and water
(3) Vasopressors (eg, epinephrine, norepinephrine)	These drugs may antagonize hypotensive effects of diuretics by decreasing responsiveness of arterioles.

APPLYING YOUR KNOWLEDGE: ANSWERS

53-1 This provides an opportunity to teach Ms. Bass that avoiding foods high in sodium will help her diuretic to work more effectively. Table salt is an obvious food to avoid, but she should also read the sodium content of food containers and avoid those high in sodium, such as potato chips and other salty snacks.

53-2 IV-push furosemide should be given over 1 to 2 minutes, up to a 40-milligram dose. Too-rapid administration may lead to increased ototoxicity.

53-3 Spironolactone is a potassium-sparing diuretic. This diuretic will enhance diuresis without depleting potassium like furosemide would. You should observe for hyperkalemia with clients taking a potassium-sparing diuretic.

Review and Application Exercises

Short Answer Exercises

1. What are clinical indications for the use of diuretics?

2. What is the general mechanism by which diuretics act?

3. How can you assess a client for therapeutic effects of a diuretic?

4. Compare and contrast the main groups of diuretics in terms of adverse effects.

5. Why should serum potassium levels be monitored during diuretic therapy?

6. Which prescription and over-the-counter drugs may decrease the effects of a diuretic?

7. For a client who is starting diuretic therapy, what are important points to teach the client about safe and effective drug usage?

8. For a client who is taking a potassium-losing diuretic and a potassium chloride supplement, explain the possible consequences of discontinuing one drug while continuing the other.

NCLEX-Style Questions

9. A client receives furosemide 80 mg IV for symptoms of severe heart failure. The nurse recognizes that administering the drug slowly IV push will reduce the likelihood of which of the following adverse effects of drug therapy?
   a. hyponatremia
   b. hypokalemia
   c. fluid volume deficit
   d. ototoxicity

10. A client who is taking an oral hypoglycemic for management of his type 2 diabetes mellitus is started on hydrochlorothiazide (HydroDIURIL). The nurse should monitor for which of the following serum laboratory changes?
    a. hypocalcemia
    b. hypercalciuria
    c. hyperglycemia
    d. hypernatremia

11. A nurse is instructing a client on dietary considerations while taking spironolactone (Aldactone). Which of the following statements made by the client indicates that further teaching is necessary?
    a. "I should not eat foods high in potassium while taking this medication."
    b. "I should use a salt substitute instead of regular salt."
    c. "I should call my nurse practitioner if I have any significant adverse effects from my medications."
    d. "I should not take large amounts of potassium chloride supplements."

12. What assessment finding in a client with heart failure receiving furosemide (Lasix) would indicate an improvement in her fluid volume status?
    a. absence of crackles on auscultation of lungs
    b. complaints of proximal nocturnal dyspnea
    c. bounding radial pulse
    d. decrease in hematocrit

13. Mrs. Conley, age 53, has had hypertension for 10 years and admits that she does not comply with her prescribed antihypertensive therapy. Recently she has begun to experience shortness of breath and ankle swelling. The nurse practitioner diagnoses renal insufficiency. What classification of diuretic is the drug of choice for Mrs. Conley?
    a. thiazide
    b. loop
    c. osmotic
    d. potassium-sparing

Selected References

Applegate, W. B. (2000). Approach to the elderly client with hypertension. In H. D. Humes (Ed.), *Kelley's Textbook of internal medicine* (4th ed., pp. 3026–3031). Philadelphia: Lippincott Williams & Wilkins.

Brater, D. C. (2000). Clinical pharmacology of cardiovascular drugs. In H. D. Humes (Ed.), *Kelley's Textbook of internal medicine* (4th ed., pp. 651–672). Philadelphia: Lippincott Williams & Wilkins.

Carter, B. L., & Saseen, J. J. (2002). Hypertension. In J. T. DiPiro, R. L. Talbert, G. C. Yee, G. R. Matzke, B. G. Wells, & L. M. Posey (Eds.), *Pharmacotherapy: A pathophysiologic approach* (5th ed., pp. 157–183). New York: McGraw-Hill.

Drug facts and comparisons. (Updated monthly). St. Louis: Facts and Comparisons.

Guyton, A. C., & Hall, J. E. (2000). *Textbook of medical physiology* (10th ed.). Philadelphia: W. B. Saunders.

Johnson, J. A., Parker, R. B., & Patterson, J. H. (2002). Heart failure. In J. T. DiPiro, R. L. Talbert, G. C. Yee, G. R. Matzke, B. G. Wells, & L. M. Posey (Eds.), *Pharmacotherapy: A pathophysiologic approach* (5th ed., pp. 185–218). New York: McGraw-Hill.

Lacy, C. F., Armstrong, L. L., Goldman, M. P., et al. (2004). *Lexi-Comp's drug information handbook* (12th ed.). Hudson, OH: Lexi-Comp.

Porth, C. M. (2005). *Pathophysiology: Concepts of altered health states* (7th ed.). Philadelphia: Lippincott Williams & Wilkins.

Strom, B. L., Schinnar, R., Apter, A. J., Margolis, D. J., Lautenbach, E., Hennessy, S., et al. (2003). Absence of cross-reactivity between sulfonamide antibiotics and sulfonamide non-antibiotics. *New England Journal of Medicine 349, 17,* 1628–1635.

Drugs That Affect Blood Coagulation

OBJECTIVES

After studying this chapter, you will be able to:

1. Describe important elements in the physiology of hemostasis and thrombosis.
2. Discuss potential consequences of blood clotting disorders.
3. Discribe characteristics and uses of anticoagulant, antiplatelet, and thrombolytic agents.
4. Compare and contrast heparin and warfarin in terms of indications for use, onset and duration of action, route of administration, blood tests used to monitor effects, and nursing process implications.
5. Teach clients on long-term warfarin therapy protective measures to prevent abnormal bleeding.
6. Discuss antiplatelet agents in terms of indications for use and effects on blood coagulation.
7. With aspirin, contrast the dose and frequency of administration for antiplatelet effects with those for analgesic, antipyretic, and anti-inflammatory effects.
8. Describe thrombolytic agents in terms of indications and contraindications for use, routes of administration, and major adverse effects.
9. Discuss the use of anticoagulant, antiplatelet, and thrombolytic drugs in special populations.
10. Describe systemic hemostatic agents for treating overdoses of anticoagulant and thrombolytic drugs.

APPLYING YOUR KNOWLEDGE

Andrew Dusseau is a 45-year-old man who has suffered an acute myocardial infarction with the complication of atrial fibrillation. He is started on a IV heparin. You are the nurse providing his care.

INTRODUCTION

Anticoagulant, antiplatelet, and thrombolytic drugs are used in the prevention and management of thrombotic and thromboembolic disorders. Thrombosis involves the formation (thrombogenesis) or presence of a blood clot (thrombus) in the vascular system. Blood clotting is a normal body defense mechanism to prevent blood loss. Thus, thrombogenesis may be life saving when it occurs as a response to hemorrhage; however, it may be life threatening when it occurs at other times, because the thrombus can obstruct a blood vessel and block blood flow to tissues beyond the clot. When part of a thrombus breaks off and travels to another part of the body, it is called an *embolus*.

Atherosclerosis is the basic disease process that often leads to pathologic thrombosis. Atherosclerosis begins with accumulation of lipid-filled macrophages (ie, foam cells) on the inner lining of arteries. Foam cells develop in response to elevated blood lipid levels and eventually become fibrous plaques (ie, foam cells covered by smooth muscle cells and connective tissue). Advanced atherosclerotic lesions also contain hemorrhages, ulcerations, and scar tissue.

Atherosclerosis can affect any organ or tissue, but often involves the arteries supplying the heart, brain, and legs. Over time, plaque lesions become larger and extend farther into the lumen of the artery. Eventually, a thrombus may develop at plaque sites and partially or completely occlude an artery. In coronary arteries, a thrombus may precipitate myocardial ischemia (angina or infarction) (see Chap. 50); in carotid or cerebral arteries, a thrombus may precipitate a stroke; in peripheral arteries, a thrombus may cause intermittent claudication (pain in the legs with exercise) or acute occlusion. Thus, serious impairment of blood flow may occur with a large atherosclerotic plaque or a relatively small plaque with superimposed vasospasm and thrombosis. Consequences and clinical manifestations of thrombi and emboli depend primarily on their location and size.

Normally, thrombi are constantly being formed and dissolved (thrombolysis), but the blood stays fluid and flow is not significantly obstructed. If the balance between thrombogenesis and thrombolysis is upset, thrombotic or bleeding disorders result. Thrombotic disorders occur much more often than bleeding disorders and are emphasized in this chapter; bleeding disorders may result from excessive amounts of drugs that inhibit clotting. To aid understanding of drug therapy for thrombotic disorders, normal hemostasis; endothelial functions in relation to blood clotting; platelet functions; blood coagulation; and characteristics of arterial and venous thrombosis are described.

Hemostasis

Hemostasis is prevention or stoppage of blood loss from an injured blood vessel and is the process that maintains the integrity of the vascular compartment. It involves activation of several mechanisms, including vasoconstriction, formation of a platelet plug (a cluster of aggregated platelets), sequential activation of clotting factors (Table 54-1) in the blood, and growth of fibrous tissue (fibrin) into the blood clot to make it more stable and to repair the tear (opening) in the damaged blood vessel. Overall, normal hemostasis is a complex process involving numerous interacting activators and inhibitors, including endothelial factors, platelets, and blood coagulation factors (Box 54-1).

Clot Lysis

When a blood clot is being formed, plasminogen (an inactive protein found in many body tissues and fluids) is bound to fibrin and becomes a component of the clot. After the outward blood flow is stopped and the tear in the blood vessel is repaired, plasminogen is activated by plasminogen activator (produced by endothelial cells or the coagulation cascade) to produce plasmin. Plasmin is an enzyme that breaks down the fibrin meshwork that stabilizes the clot; this fibrinolytic or thrombolytic action dissolves the clot.

Thrombotic and Thromboembolic Disorders

Thrombosis may occur in both arteries and veins. Arterial thrombosis is usually associated with atherosclerotic plaque, hypertension, and turbulent blood flow. These conditions damage arterial endothelium and activate platelets to initiate the coagulation process. Arterial thrombi cause disease by obstructing blood flow. If the obstruction is incomplete or temporary, local tissue ischemia (deficient blood supply) occurs. If the obstruction is complete or prolonged, local tissue death (infarction) occurs.

Venous thrombosis is usually associated with venous stasis. When blood flows slowly, thrombin and other procoagulant substances present in the blood become concentrated in local areas and initiate the clotting process. With a normal rate of blood flow, these substances are rapidly removed from the blood, primarily by Kupffer's cells in the liver. A venous thrombus is less cohesive than an arterial thrombus, and an

TABLE 54-1 Blood Coagulation Factors

NUMBER	NAME	FUNCTIONS
I	Fibrinogen	Forms fibrin, the insoluble protein strands that compose the supporting framework of a blood clot. Thrombin and calcium are required for the conversion.
II	Prothrombin	Forms thrombin, which catalyzes the conversion of fibrinogen to fibrin
III	Thromboplastin	Converts prothrombin to thrombin
IV	Calcium	Catalyzes the conversion of prothrombin to thrombin
V	Labile factor	Required for formation of active thromboplastin
VI (Va)	Accelerin	This is Va, redundant to Factor V
VII	Proconvertin or stable factor	Accelerates action of tissue thromboplastin
VIII	Antihemophilic factor	Promotes breakdown of platelets and formation of active platelet thromboplastin
IX	Christmas factor	Similar to factor VIII
X	Stuart factor	Promotes action of thromboplastin
XI	Plasma thromboplastin antecedent	Promotes platelet aggregation and breakdown, with subsequent release of platelet thromboplastin
XII	Hageman factor	Similar to factor XI
XIII	Fibrin-stabilizing factor	Converts fibrin meshwork to the dense, tight mass of the completely formed clot

Box 54-1 Hemostasis and Thrombosis

The blood vessels and blood normally maintain a balance between procoagulant and anticoagulant factors that favors anticoagulation and keeps the blood fluid. Injury to blood vessels and tissues causes complex reactions and interactions among vascular endothelial cells, platelets, and blood coagulation factors that shift the balance toward procoagulation and thrombosis.

Endothelial Cells

Endothelial cells play a role in all aspects of hemostasis and thrombosis. Normal endothelium helps to prevent thrombosis by producing anticoagulant factors, inhibiting platelet reactivity, and inhibiting activation of the coagulation cascade. However, endothelium promotes thrombosis when its continuity is lost (eg, the blood vessel wall is torn by rupture of atherosclerotic plaque, hypertension, trauma), its function is altered, or when blood flow is altered or becomes static. After a blood clot is formed, the endothelium also induces its dissolution and restoration of blood flow.

Antithrombotic Functions

- Synthesizes and releases prostacyclin (prostaglandin I_2), which inhibits platelet aggregation
- Releases endothelium-derived relaxing factor (nitric oxide), which inhibits platelet adhesion and aggregation
- Blocks platelet exposure to subendothelial collagen and other stimuli for platelet aggregation
- May inhibit platelet reactivity by inactivating adenosine diphosphate (ADP), a platelet product that promotes platelet aggregation
- Produces plasminogen activators (eg, tissue-type or tPA) in response to shear stress and such agonists as histamine and thrombin. These activators convert inactive plasminogen to plasmin, which then breaks down fibrin and dissolves blood clots (fibrinolytic effects).
- Produces thrombomodulin, a protein that helps prevent formation of intravascular thrombi by inhibiting thrombin-mediated platelet aggregation. Thrombomodulin also reacts with thrombin to activate proteins C and S, which inhibit the plasma cascade of clotting factors.

Prothrombotic Functions

- Produces antifibrinolytic factors. Normally, the balance between profibrinolysis and antifibrinolysis favors fibrinolysis (clot dissolution). In pathologic conditions, including atherosclerosis, fibrinolysis may be limited and thrombosis enhanced.
- In pathologic conditions, may induce synthesis of prothrombotic factors such as von Willebrand factor. Von Willebrand factor serves as a site for subendothelial platelet adhesion and as a carrier for blood coagulation factor VIII in plasma. Several disease states are associated with increased or altered production of von Willebrand factor, including atherosclerosis.
- Produces tissue factor, which activates the extrinsic coagulation pathway after exposure to oxidized low-density lipoprotein cholesterol, homocysteine, and cytokines (eg, interleukin-1, tumor necrosis factor–alpha)

Platelets

Platelets (also called *thrombocytes*) are fragments of large cells called *megakaryocytes.* They are produced in the bone marrow and released into the bloodstream, where they circulate for approximately 7 to 10 days before they are removed by the spleen. They contain no nuclei and therefore cannot repair or replicate themselves.

The cell membrane of a platelet contains a coat of glycoproteins that prevents the platelet from adhering to normal endothelium but allows it to adhere to damaged areas of endothelium and subendothelial collagen in the blood vessel wall. It also contains receptors for ADP; collagen; blood coagulation factors such as fibrinogen; and other substances. Breakdown of the cell membrane releases arachidonic acid (which can be metabolized to produce thromboxane A_2) and allows leakage of platelet contents (eg, thromboplastin and other clotting factors), which function to stop bleeding.

The cytoplasm of a platelet contains storage granules with ADP, fibrinogen, histamine, platelet-derived growth factor, serotonin, von Willebrand factor, enzymes that produce thromboxane A_2, and other substances. The cytoplasm also contains contractile proteins that contract storage granules so they empty their contents and help a platelet plug to retract and plug a hole in a torn blood vessel.

The only known function of platelets is hemostasis. When platelets come in contact with a damaged vascular surface, they become activated and undergo changes in structure and function. They enlarge, express receptors on their surfaces, release mediators from their storage granules, become sticky so that they adhere to endothelial and collagen cells, and form a platelet thrombus (ie, a cluster or aggregate of activated platelets) within seconds. The thrombus blocks the tear in the blood vessel and prevents further leakage of blood. Platelets usually disappear from a blood clot within 24 hours and are replaced by fibrin.

Formation of a platelet thrombus proceeds through the phases of activation, adhesion, aggregation, and procoagulation.

Activation

Platelet activation occurs when agonists such as thrombin, collagen, ADP, or epinephrine bind to their specific receptors on the platelet cell membrane surface. Activated platelets release von Willebrand factor, which aids platelet adhesion to blood vessel walls. They also secrete ADP and thromboxane A_2 into the blood. The ADP and thromboxane A_2 activate and recruit nearby platelets.

Adhesion

Platelet adhesion involves changes in platelets that allow them to adhere to endothelial cells and subendothelial collagen exposed by damaged endothelium. Adhesion is mediated by interactions between platelets and substances in the subendothelial tissues. Platelets contain binding sites for several subendothelial tissue proteins, including collagen and von Willebrand factor. In capillaries, where blood shear rates are high, platelets also can bind indirectly to collagen through von Willebrand factor. Von

(continued)

Box 54-1 Hemostasis and Thrombosis (continued)

Willebrand factor is synthesized by endothelial cells and mega-karyocytes. Although it contains binding sites for platelets and collagen, it does not normally bind with platelets until they are activated.

Aggregation

Aggregation involves the accumulation of platelets at a site of injury to a blood vessel wall and is stimulated by ADP, collagen, thromboxane A_2, thrombin, and other factors. It requires the binding of extracellular fibrinogen to platelet fibrinogen receptors. The fibrinogen receptor is located on a complex of two glycoproteins (GPIIb and IIIa) in the platelet cell membrane. Although many GP IIb/IIIa com-plexes are on the surface of each platelet, they do not func-tion as fibrinogen receptors until the platelet is activated by an agonist. Each activated GP IIb/IIIa complex is capable of binding a single fibrinogen molecule. However, a fibrinogen molecule may bind to receptors on adjacent activated platelets, thus acting as a bridge to connect the platelets. Activated GP IIb/IIIa complexes can also bind von Wille-brand factor and promote platelet aggregation when fibri-nogen is lacking.

Aggregated platelets produce and release thromboxane A_2, which acts with ADP from platelet storage granules to pro-mote additional GP IIb/IIIa activation, platelet secretion, and aggregate formation. The exposure of functional GP IIb/IIIa complexes is also stimulated by thrombin, which can directly stimulate thromboxane A_2 synthesis and granule secretion without initial aggregation. Collagen stimulates additional aggregation by increasing the production of thromboxane A_2 and storage granule secretion.

Overall, aggregated platelets release substances that recruit new platelets and stimulate additional aggregation. This activ-ity helps the platelet plug become large enough to block blood flow out of a damaged blood vessel. If the opening is small, the platelet plug can stop blood loss. If the opening is large, a platelet plug and a blood clot are both required to stop the bleeding.

Procoagulant Activity

In addition to forming a platelet thrombus, platelets also acti-vate and interact with circulating blood coagulation factors to form a larger and more stable blood clot. Activation of the pre-viously inactive blood coagulation factors leads to formation of fibrin threads that attach to the platelets and form a tight meshwork of a fully developed blood clot.

More specifically, the platelet plug provides a surface on which coagulation enzymes, substrates, and cofactors interact at high local concentrations. These interactions lead to activa-tion of coagulation factor X and the conversion of prothrom-bin to thrombin.

Blood Coagulation

The blood coagulation process causes hemostasis within 1 to 2 minutes. It involves sequential activation of clotting fac-tors that are normally present in blood and tissues as inactive precursors and formation of a meshwork of fibrin strands that cements blood components together to form a stable, dense clot. Major phases include release of thromboplastin by disin-tegrating platelets and damaged tissue; conversion of pro-thrombin to thrombin, which requires thromboplastin and calcium ions; and conversion of fibrinogen to fibrin by thrombin.

Blood coagulation results from activation of the intrinsic or extrinsic coagulation pathway. Both pathways, which are acti-vated when blood passes out of a blood vessel, are needed for normal hemostasis. The intrinsic pathway occurs in the vascu-lar system; the extrinsic pathway occurs in the tissues. Although the pathways are initially separate, the terminal steps (ie, activation of factor X and thrombin-induced formation of fibrin) are the same.

The intrinsic pathway is activated when blood comes in contact with collagen in the injured vessel wall and coagula-tion factor XII interacts with biologic surfaces. The normal endothelium prevents factor XII from interacting with such surfaces. The activated form of factor XII is a protease that starts the interactions among factors involved in the intrinsic pathway (eg, prekallikrein, factor IX, factor VIII).

The extrinsic pathway is activated when blood is exposed to tissue extracts and tissue factor interacts with circulating coagulation factor VII. Activated factors VII and IX both act on factor X to produce activated factor X, which then inter-acts with factor V, calcium, and platelet factor 3. Platelet fac-tor 3, a component of the platelet cell membrane, becomes available on the platelet surface only during platelet activa-tion. The interactions among these substances lead to forma-tion of thrombin, which then activates fibrinogen to form fibrin, and the clot is complete.

---

embolus can easily become detached and travel to other parts of the body.

Venous thrombi cause disease by two mechanisms. First, thrombosis causes local congestion, edema, and perhaps inflammation by impairing normal outflow of venous blood (eg, thrombophlebitis, deep vein thrombosis [DVT]). Sec-ond, embolization obstructs the blood supply when the embo-lus becomes lodged. The pulmonary arteries are common sites of embolization.

DRUGS USED IN THROMBOTIC AND THROMBOEMBOLIC DISORDERS: CLASSIFICATIONS AND INDIVIDUAL DRUGS

Drugs given to prevent or treat thrombosis alter some aspect of the blood coagulation process. Anticoagulants are widely used in thrombotic disorders. They are more effective in preventing venous thrombosis than arterial thrombosis. Antiplatelet drugs are used to prevent arterial thrombosis. Thrombolytic agents are used to dissolve thrombi and limit tissue damage in selected thromboembolic disorders. These drugs are described in the following sections and in Table 54-2.

Anticoagulants

Anticoagulant drugs are given to prevent formation of new clots and extension of clots already present. They do not dissolve formed clots, improve blood flow in tissues around the clot, or prevent ischemic damage to tissues beyond the clot. Heparins and warfarin are commonly used anticoagulants; argatroban, lepirudin, and tinzaparin are newer agents. Clinical indications include prevention or management of thromboembolic disorders, such as thrombophlebitis, DVT, and pulmonary embolism. The main adverse effect is bleeding.

Heparin

Heparin is a pharmaceutical preparation of the natural anticoagulant produced primarily by mast cells in pericapillary connective tissue. Endogenous heparin is found in various body tissues, most abundantly in the liver and lungs. Exogenous heparin is obtained from bovine lung or porcine intestinal mucosa and standardized in units of biologic activity.

Heparin combines with antithrombin III (a natural anticoagulant in the blood) to inactivate clotting factors IX, X, XI, and XII; inhibit the conversion of prothrombin to thrombin; and prevent thrombus formation. After thrombosis has developed, heparin can inhibit additional coagulation by inactivating thrombin, preventing the conversion of fibrinogen to fibrin, and inhibiting factor XIII (the fibrin-stabilizing factor). Other effects include inhibiting factors V and VIII and platelet aggregation.

Heparin acts immediately after intravenous (IV) injection and within 20 to 30 minutes after subcutaneous (Sub-Q) injection. It is metabolized in the liver and excreted in the urine, primarily as inactive metabolites. Heparin does not cross the placental barrier and is not secreted in breast milk, making it the anticoagulant of choice for use during pregnancy and lactation.

Prophylactically, low doses of heparin are given to prevent DVT and pulmonary embolism in clients at risk for development of these disorders, such as the following:

- Clients with major illnesses (eg, acute myocardial infarction, heart failure, serious pulmonary infections, stroke)
- Clients having major abdominal or thoracic surgery
- Clients with a history of thrombophlebitis or pulmonary embolism, including pregnant women
- Clients having gynecologic surgery, especially if they have been taking estrogens or oral contraceptives or have other risk factors for DVT
- Clients expected to be on bed rest or to have limited activity for longer than 5 days

Therapeutically, heparin is used for management of acute thromboembolic disorders (eg, DVT, thrombophlebitis, pulmonary embolism). In these conditions, the aim of therapy is to prevent further thrombus formation and embolization. Heparin is also used in disseminated intravascular coagulation (DIC), a life-threatening condition characterized by widespread clotting, which depletes the blood of coagulation factors. The depletion of coagulation factors then produces widespread bleeding. The goal of heparin therapy in DIC is to prevent blood coagulation long enough for clotting factors to be replenished and thus be able to control hemorrhage.

Heparin is also used to prevent clotting during cardiac and vascular surgery, extracorporeal circulation, hemodialysis, and blood transfusions, and in blood samples to be used in laboratory tests.

Contraindications include GI ulcerations (eg, peptic ulcer disease, ulcerative colitis), intracranial bleeding, dissecting aortic aneurysm, blood dyscrasias, severe kidney or liver disease, severe hypertension, polycythemia vera, and recent surgery of the eye, spinal cord, or brain. Heparin should be used with caution in clients with hypertension, renal or hepatic disease, alcoholism, history of GI ulcerations, drainage tubes (eg, nasogastric tubes, indwelling urinary catheters), threatened abortion, endocarditis, and any occupation with high risks of traumatic injury.

Disadvantages of heparin are its short duration of action and the subsequent need for frequent administration; the necessity for parenteral injection (because it is not absorbed from the gastrointestinal [GI] tract); and local tissue reactions at injection sites.

Heparin-induced thrombocytopenia (HIT) may occur in 1% to 3% of those receiving heparin and is a very serious adverse effect of heparin. HIT is an immune-mediated process that results in development of antibodies that activate platelets. The activated platelets are rapidly consumed by the reticuloendothelial system, thereby triggering a subsequent release of procoagulant microparticles that cause platelet aggregation and a hyper-thrombotic state. All clients exposed to any heparin at therapeutic or prophylactic doses or minute amounts in heparin flushes or on heparin-coated catheters, as well as those receiving low–molecular-weight heparin, are at risk. All heparin administration must be discontinued and anticoagulation managed with a thrombin inhibitor such as argatroban.

Low–Molecular-Weight Heparins

Standard heparin is a mixture of high– and low–molecular-weight fractions, but most anticoagulant activity is attributed to the low–molecular-weight portion. **Low–molecular-weight heparins** (LMWHs) contain the low–molecular-weight fraction and are as effective as IV heparin in treating thrombotic disorders. Indications for use include prevention or management of thromboembolic complications associated with surgery or ischemic complications of unstable angina and myocardial infarction. Currently available LMWHs

Table 54-2 Drugs at a Glance: Anticoagulant, Antiplatelet, and Thrombolytic Agents

GENERIC/TRADE NAME	INDICATIONS FOR USE	ROUTES AND DOSAGE RANGES
Anticoagulants		
Heparin	Prevention and management of thrombo-embolic disorders (eg, DVT, pulmonary embolism, atrial fibrillation with embolization)	*Adults:* IV injection, 5000 units initially, followed by 5000–10,000 units q4–6h, to a maximum dose of 25,000 units/d; IV infusion, 5000 units (loading dose), then 15–25 units/kg/h DIC, IV injection, 50–100 units/kg q4h; IV infusion, 20,000–40,000 units/d at initial rate of 0.25 units/kg/min, then adjusted according to aPTT; Sub-Q 10,000–12,000 units q8h, or 14,000–20,000 units q12h Low-dose prophylaxis, Sub-Q 5000 units 2 h before surgery, then q12h until discharged from hospital or fully ambulatory *Children:* DIC, IV injection, 25–50 units/kg q4h; IV infusion, 50 units/kg initially, followed by 100 units/kg q4h or 20,000 units/m² over 24 h
Argatroban (Argatroban)	Thrombosis prophylaxis or management in heparin-induced thrombocytopenia	IV continuous infusion 2 mcg/kg/min
Bivalirudin (Angiomax)	Clients with unstable angina undergoing PTCA	IV bolus dose of 1 mg/kg followed by 4 h infusion at rate of 2.5 mg/kg/min
Dalteparin (Fragmin)	Prophylaxis of DVT in clients having hip replacement surgery; also clients at high risk of thromboembolic disorders who are having abdominal surgery	Abdominal surgery, Sub-Q 2500 IU 1–2 h before surgery and then once daily for 5–10 days after surgery Hip replacement surgery, Sub-Q 2500 IU 1–2 h before surgery and the evening of surgery (at least 6 h after first dose) and then 5000 IU once daily for 5 days
Enoxaparin (Lovenox)	Prevention and management of DVT and pulmonary embolism Management of unstable angina, to prevent myocardial infarction	DVT prophylaxis in clients having hip or knee replacement surgery, Sub-Q 30 mg twice daily, with first dose within 12–24 h after surgery and continued for 7–10 days Abdominal surgery, Sub-Q 40 mg once daily with first dose given 2 h before surgery, for 7–10 days DVT/pulmonary embolism management, outpatients, Sub-Q 1 mg/kg q12h; inpatients, 1 mg/kg q12h or 1.5 mg/kg q24h Unstable angina 1 mg/kg q12h in conjunction with oral aspirin (100–325 mg once daily)
Fondaparinux (Arixtra)	Prevention of DVT following hip fracture surgery or knee or hip replacement	Sub-Q 2.5 mg daily, with first dose 6–8 h after surgery and continuing for a maximum of 11 days
Lepirudin (Refludan)	Heparin alternative for anticoagulation in clients with heparin-induced thrombocytopenia and associated thromboembolic disorders	IV injection, 0.4 mg/kg over 15–20 sec, followed by continuous IV infusion of 0.15 mg/kg for 2–10 days or longer if needed
Tinzaparin (Innohep)	Management of DVT, with or without PE; may be given in conjunction with warfarin	Sub-Q injection 175 IU/kg daily for at least 6 days and until adequately anticoagulated with warfarin
Warfarin (Coumadin)	Long-term prevention or management of venous thromboembolic disorders, including DVT, PE, and embolization associated with atrial fibrillation and prosthetic heart valves. May also be used after myocardial infarction to decrease reinfarction, stroke, venous thromboembolism, and death	PO 2–5 mg/d for 2–3 days, then adjusted according to the international normalized ratio (INR); average maintenance daily dose, 2–5 mg

Table 54-2 Drugs at a Glance: Anticoagulant, Antiplatelet, and Thrombolytic Agents (continued)

GENERIC/TRADE NAME	INDICATIONS FOR USE	ROUTES AND DOSAGE RANGES
Antiplatelet Agents		
Aspirin	Prevention of myocardial infarction Prevention of thromboembolic disorders in clients with prosthetic heart valves or TIAs	PO 81–325 mg daily
Abciximab (ReoPro)	Used with PTCA to prevent rethrombosis of treated arteries Intended for use with aspirin and heparin	IV bolus injection, 0.25 mg/kg 10–60 min before starting PTCA, then a continuous IV infusion of 10 mcg/min for 12 h
Anagrelide (Agrylin)	Essential thrombocythemia, to reduce the elevated platelet count, the risk of thrombosis, and associated symptoms	PO 0.5 mg 4 times daily or 1 mg twice daily initially, then titrate to lowest dose effective in maintaining platelet count <600,000/mm^3
Cilostazol (Pletal)	Intermittent claudication, to increase walking distance (before leg pain occurs)	PO 100 mg twice daily, 30 min before or 2 h after breakfast and dinner; reduce to 50 mg twice daily with concurrent use of fluconazole, itraconazole, erythromycin, or diltiazem
Clopidogrel (Plavix)	Reduction of atherosclerotic events (myocardial infarction, stroke, vascular death) in clients with atherosclerosis documented by recent stroke, recent myocardial infarction, or established peripheral artery disease	PO 75 mg once daily with or without food
Dipyridamole (Persantine)	Prevention of thromboembolism after cardiac valve replacement, given with warfarin	PO 25–75 mg 3 times per day, 1 h before meals
Dipyridamole and aspirin (Aggrenox)	Reduction of stroke risk in clients with previous TIA or thrombotic event	PO 1 capsule (200 mg extended-release dipyridamole/25 mg aspirin) twice daily
Eptifibatide (Integrilin)	Acute coronary syndromes, including clients who are to be managed medically and those undergoing PTCA	IV bolus injection, 180 mcg/kg, followed by continuous infusion of 2 mcg/kg/min. See manufacturer's instructions for preparation and administration.
Ticlopidine (Ticlid)	Prevention of thrombosis in clients with coronary artery or cerebral vascular disease (eg, clients who have had stroke precursors or a completed thrombotic stroke)	PO 250 mg twice daily with food
Tirofiban (Aggrastat)	Acute coronary syndromes, with heparin, for clients who are to be managed medically or those undergoing PTCA Acute myocardial infarction Pulmonary embolism	IV infusion, 0.4 mcg/kg/min for 30 min, then 0.1 mcg/kg/min. Patients with severe renal impairment (creatinine clearance <30 mL/min) should receive half the usual rate of infusion. See manufacturer's instructions for preparation and administration.
Treprostinil (Remodulin)	Pulmonary arterial hypertension	Continuous infusion by Sub-Q catheter and infusion pump at initial dose of 1.25 mg/kg/min, increasing by no more than 1.25 mg/kg/min per week for first 4 weeks, and then by no more than 2.5 mg/kg/min per week for remaining duration of infusion
Thrombolytic Agents		
Alteplase (Activase)	Acute ischemic stroke Acute myocardial infarction Pulmonary emboli	IV infusion, 100 mg over 3 h (first hour, 60 mg with a bolus of 6–10 mg over 1–2 min initially; second hour, 20 mg; third hour, 20 mg)
Drotrecogin alfa, activated (Xigris)	Reduction of mortality in severe sepsis	IV infusion of 24 mcg/kg/h for 96 h

(continued)

GENERIC/TRADE NAME	INDICATIONS FOR USE	ROUTES AND DOSAGE RANGES
Reteplase, recombinant (Retavase)	Acute myocardial infarction	IV injection, 10 units over 2 min, repeated in 30 min. Inject into a flowing IV infusion line that contains no other medications.
Streptokinase (Streptase)	Management of acute, severe pulmonary emboli or iliofemoral thrombophlebitis Used to dissolve clots in arterial or venous cannulas or catheters May be injected into a coronary artery to dissolve a thrombus if done within 6 h of onset of symptoms	IV 250,000 units over 30 min, then 100,000 units/h for 24–72 h
Tenecteplase (TNKase)	Acute myocardial infarction	IV bolus dose based on weight, 30 mg (for <60 kg) not to exceed 50 mg (>90 kg)
Urokinase (Abbokinase)	Coronary artery thrombi Pulmonary emboli Clearance of clogged IV catheters	IV 4400 units/kg over 10 min, followed by continuous infusion of 4400 units/kg/h for 12 h For clearing IV catheters, see manufacturer's instructions.

Table 54-2 Drugs at a Glance: Anticoagulant, Antiplatelet, and Thrombolytic Agents (continued)

aPTT, activated partial thromboplastin time; DIC, disseminated intravascular coagulation; DVT, deep vein thrombosis; IV, intravenous; PE, pulmonary embolism; PO, oral; PTCA, percutaneous transluminal coronary angioplasty or atherectomy; Sub-Q, subcutaneous; TIA, transient ischemic attack.

(dalteparin, enoxaparin, tinzaparin) differ from standard heparin and each other; they cannot be used interchangeably (ie, unit for unit).

LMWHs are given Sub-Q and do not require close monitoring of blood coagulation tests. These characteristics allow outpatient anticoagulant therapy, an increasing trend. The drugs are also associated with less thrombocytopenia than standard heparin. However, platelet counts should be monitored during therapy.

APPLYING YOUR KNOWLEDGE 54-1

Before providing care for Mr. Dusseau, you review his chart (medical diagnosis and medication orders). What is the main reason for clients to receive an anticoagulant and for what adverse effect should you monitor Mr. Dusseau?

Warfarin

Warfarin is the most commonly used oral anticoagulant. It acts in the liver to prevent synthesis of vitamin K–dependent clotting factors (ie, factors II, VII, IX, and X). Warfarin is similar to vitamin K in structure and therefore acts as a competitive antagonist to hepatic use of vitamin K. Anticoagulant effects do not occur for 3 to 5 days after warfarin is started because clotting factors already in the blood follow their normal pathway of elimination. Warfarin has no effect on circulating clotting factors or on platelet function.

Warfarin is well absorbed after oral administration. It is highly bound to plasma proteins (98%), mainly albumin. It is metabolized in the liver and primarily excreted as inactive metabolites by the kidneys.

Warfarin is most useful in long-term prevention or management of venous thromboembolic disorders, including DVT, pulmonary embolism, and embolization associated with atrial fibrillation and prosthetic heart valves. In addition, warfarin therapy after myocardial infarction may decrease reinfarction, stroke, venous thromboembolism, and death. Smaller doses are being used now than formerly, with similar antithrombotic effects and decreased risks of bleeding.

Like heparin, warfarin is contraindicated in clients with GI ulcerations; blood disorders associated with bleeding; severe kidney or liver disease; severe hypertension; and recent surgery of the eye, spinal cord, or brain. It should be used cautiously in clients with mild hypertension, renal or hepatic disease, alcoholism, history of GI ulcerations, drainage tubes (eg, nasogastric tubes, indwelling urinary catheters), and occupations with high risks of traumatic injury. In addition, warfarin is contraindicated during pregnancy.

Other Anticoagulant Drugs

Fondaparinux produces anticoagulant effects by directly binding to circulating and clot-bound factor Xa, accelerating the activity of antithrombin and inhibiting thrombin production. It is used in the prevention of DVT in clients having surgery for hip fracture or joint replacement surgery of the knee or hip.

Lepirudin, bivalirudin, and **argatroban** are direct thrombin inhibitors that prevent blood coagulation by inactivating thrombin. They are used as a heparin substitute for clients who need anticoagulation but have thrombocytopenia with heparin.

Antiplatelet Drugs

Antiplatelet drugs prevent one or more steps in the prothrombotic activity of platelets. As described previously, platelet activity is very important in both physiologic hemostasis and pathologic thrombosis. Arterial thrombi, which are composed primarily of platelets, may form on top of atherosclerotic plaque and block blood flow in the artery. They may also form on heart walls and valves and embolize to other parts of the body.

Drugs used clinically for antiplatelet effects act by a variety of mechanisms to inhibit platelet activation, adhesion, aggregation, or procoagulant activity. These include drugs that block platelet receptors for thromboxane A_2, adenosine diphosphate (ADP), glycoprotein (GP) IIb/IIIa, and phosphodiesterase.

Thromboxane A_2 Inhibitors

Aspirin is a commonly used analgesic–antipyretic–anti-inflammatory drug (see Chap. 7) with potent antiplatelet effects. Aspirin exerts pharmacologic actions by inhibiting synthesis of prostaglandins. In this instance, aspirin acetylates cyclooxygenase, the enzyme in platelets that normally synthesizes thromboxane A_2, a prostaglandin product that causes platelet aggregation. Thus, aspirin prevents formation of thromboxane A_2 and thromboxane A_2–induced platelet aggregation and thrombus formation. A single dose of 300 to 600 milligrams or multiple doses of 30 milligrams (eg, daily for several days) inhibit the cyclooxygenase in circulating platelets almost completely. These antithrombotic effects persist for the life of the platelet (7–10 days). Aspirin may be used long term for prevention of myocardial infarction or stroke, and in clients with prosthetic heart valves. It is also used for the immediate treatment of suspected or actual acute myocardial infarction, for transient ischemic attacks (TIAs), and for evolving thrombotic strokes. Adverse effects are uncommon with the small doses used for antiplatelet effects. However, there is an increased risk of bleeding, including hemorrhagic stroke. Because approximately 85% of strokes are thrombotic, the benefits of aspirin or other antiplatelet agents are thought to outweigh the risks of hemorrhagic strokes (approximately 15%).

Nonsteroidal anti-inflammatory drugs (NSAIDs), including ibuprofen and many other aspirin-related drugs, inhibit cyclooxygenase reversibly. Their antiplatelet effects subside when the drugs are eliminated from the circulation and the drugs usually are not used for antiplatelet effects. However, clients who take an NSAID daily (eg, for arthritis pain) may not need to take additional aspirin for antiplatelet effects. Acetaminophen does not affect platelets in usual doses (see Chap. 7).

Adenosine Diphosphate Receptor Antagonists

Ticlopidine inhibits platelet aggregation by preventing ADP-induced binding between platelets and fibrinogen. This reaction inhibits platelet aggregation irreversibly, and effects persist for the lifespan of the platelet. The drug is indicated for prevention of thrombotic stroke in people who have had stroke precursor events (eg, TIAs) or a completed thrombotic stroke. Ticlopidine is considered a second-line drug for clients who cannot take aspirin. The adverse effects (eg, neutropenia, diarrhea, skin rashes) and greater cost make it prohibitive for use by many clients. Contraindications include active bleeding disorders (eg, GI bleeding from peptic ulcer, intracranial bleeding), neutropenia, thrombocytopenia, severe liver disease, and hypersensitivity to the drug.

Ticlopidine is rapidly absorbed after oral administration and reaches peak plasma levels about 2 hours after a dose. It is highly protein bound (98%), extensively metabolized in the liver, and excreted in urine and feces. As with other antiplatelet drugs, there is increased risk of bleeding with ticlopidine.

Clopidogrel is chemically related to ticlopidine and causes similar effects. It is indicated for reduction of myocardial infarction, stroke, and vascular death in clients with atherosclerosis and reportedly causes fewer or less severe adverse effects than ticlopidine.

Glycoprotein IIb/IIIa Receptor Antagonists

Abciximab is a monoclonal antibody that prevents the binding of fibrinogen, von Willebrand factor, and other molecules to GP IIb/IIIa receptors on activated platelets. This action inhibits platelet aggregation.

Abciximab is used with percutaneous transluminal coronary angioplasty or removal of atherosclerotic plaque to prevent rethrombosis of treated arteries. It is used with aspirin and heparin and is contraindicated in clients who have recently received an oral anticoagulant or IV dextran. Other contraindications include active bleeding, thrombocytopenia, history of a serious stroke, surgery or major trauma within the previous 6 weeks, uncontrolled hypertension, or hypersensitivity to drug components.

Eptifibatide and **tirofiban** inhibit platelet aggregation by preventing activation of GP IIb/IIIa receptors on the platelet surface and the subsequent binding of fibrinogen and von Willebrand factor to platelets. Antiplatelet effects occur during drug infusion and stop when the drug is stopped. The drugs are indicated for acute coronary syndrome (eg, unstable angina, myocardial infarction) in clients who are to be treated medically or by angioplasty or atherectomy.

Drug half-life is approximately 2.5 hours for eptifibatide and 2 hours for tirofiban; the drugs are cleared mainly by renal excretion. With tirofiban, plasma clearance is approximately 25% lower in older adults and approximately 50% lower in clients with severe renal impairment (creatinine clearance <30 mL/minute).

The drugs are contraindicated in clients with hypersensitivity to any component of the products; current or previous bleeding (within previous 30 days); a history of thrombocytopenia after previous exposure to tirofiban; a history of stroke within 30 days or any history of hemorrhagic stroke; major surgery or severe physical trauma within the previous month; severe hypertension (systolic blood pressure >180 mm Hg with tirofiban or >200 mm Hg with eptifibatide, or diastolic blood pressure >110 mm Hg with either drug); a history of intracranial hemorrhage, neoplasm, arteriovenous malformation, or aneurysm; a platelet count less than 100,000 mm³; serum creatinine 2 milligrams per deciliter or above (for the 180 mcg/kg bolus and the 2 mcg/kg/min infusion) or 4 milligrams per deciliter or above (for the 135 mcg/kg bolus and the 0.5 mcg/kg/min infusion); or dependency on dialysis (eptifibatide).

Bleeding is the most common adverse effect, with most major bleeding occurring at the arterial access site for cardiac catheterization. If bleeding occurs and cannot be controlled with pressure, the drug infusion and heparin should be discontinued.

These drugs should be used cautiously if given with other drugs that affect hemostasis (eg, warfarin, thrombolytics, other antiplatelet drugs).

Phosphodiesterase Inhibitor

Cilostazol inhibits phosphodiesterase, an enzyme that metabolizes cyclic adenosine monophosphate (cAMP). This inhibition increases intracellular cAMP, which then inhibits platelet aggregation and produces vasodilation. The drug reversibly inhibits platelet aggregation induced by various stimuli (eg, thrombin, ADP, collagen, arachidonic acid, epinephrine, shear stress). It is indicated for management of intermittent claudication. Symptoms usually improve within 2 to 4 weeks, but may take as long as 12 weeks. The drug is contraindicated in clients with heart failure.

Cilostazol is highly protein bound (95%–98%), mainly to albumin; extensively metabolized by hepatic cytochrome P450 enzymes; and excreted in urine (74%) and feces. The drug and two active metabolites accumulate with chronic administration and reach steady state within a few days. The most common adverse effects are diarrhea and headache.

Other Agents

Anagrelide inhibits platelet aggregation induced by cAMP phosphodiesterase, ADP, and collagen. However, it is indicated only to reduce platelet counts for clients with essential thrombocythemia (a disorder characterized by excessive numbers of platelets). Doses to reduce platelet production are smaller than those required to inhibit platelet aggregation.

Dipyridamole inhibits platelet adhesion, but its mechanism of action is unclear. It is used for prevention of thromboembolism after cardiac valve replacement and is given with warfarin. The combination of dipyridamole and aspirin is indicated for prevention of stroke in those who have had stroke precursors (TIAs) or a previously completed thrombotic stroke.

Thrombolytic Agents

Thrombolytic agents are given to dissolve thrombi. They stimulate conversion of plasminogen to plasmin (also called *fibrinolysin*), a proteolytic enzyme that breaks down fibrin, the framework of a thrombus. The main use of thrombolytic agents is for management of acute, severe thromboembolic disease, such as myocardial infarction, pulmonary embolism, and iliofemoral thrombosis.

The goal of thrombolytic therapy is to re-establish blood flow as quickly as possible and prevent or limit tissue damage. Drugs with shorter half lives increase the risk of rethrombosis or infarction. Anticoagulant drugs, such as heparin and warfarin, and antiplatelet agents are given following thrombolytic therapy to decrease reformation of a thrombus. Thrombolytic drugs are also used to dissolve clots in arterial or venous cannulas or catheters.

Streptokinase and **urokinase** are enzymes that break down fibrin. They are used mainly to lyse coronary artery clots in acute myocardial infarction. Streptokinase may also be used to dissolve clots in vascular catheters and to treat acute, severe pulmonary emboli or iliofemoral thrombophlebitis. Urokinase is recommended for use in clients allergic to streptokinase. As with other anticoagulants and thrombolytic agents, bleeding is the main adverse effect.

Alteplase, reteplase, and **tenecteplase** are tissue plasminogen activators used mainly in acute myocardial infarction to dissolve clots obstructing coronary arteries and re-establish perfusion of tissues beyond the thrombotic area. The drugs bind to fibrin in a clot and act locally to dissolve the clot. The most common adverse effect is bleeding, which may be internal (eg, intracranial, GI, genitourinary) or external (eg, venous or arterial puncture sites, surgical incisions). The drugs are contraindicated in the presence of bleeding, a history of stroke, central nervous system surgery or trauma within the previous 2 months, and severe hypertension.

Drotrecogin alfa is a recombinant version of human activated protein C that is approved for use in severe sepsis or septic shock. Severe sepsis is characterized by an excessive inflammatory reaction to infection, inappropriate blood clot formation, and impaired breakdown of clots. Drotrecogin alfa is given for its thrombolytic effects, along with other therapies for inflammation and infection. The major adverse effect is bleeding.

Drugs Used to Control Bleeding

Anticoagulant, antiplatelet, and thrombolytic drugs profoundly affect hemostasis, and their major adverse effect is bleeding. As a result, systemic hemostatic agents (antidotes) may be needed to prevent or treat bleeding episodes. Antidotes should be used cautiously because overuse can increase risks of recurrent thrombotic disorders. These drugs are described in this section and in Table 54-3.

Aminocaproic acid and **tranexamic acid** are used to stop bleeding caused by overdoses of thrombolytic agents. Aminocaproic acid also may be used in other bleeding disorders caused by hyperfibrinolysis (eg, in cardiac surgery, blood disorders, hepatic cirrhosis, prostatectomy, neoplastic disorders). Tranexamic acid also is used for short periods

Table 54-3 Drugs at a Glance: Systemic Hemostatic Drugs

GENERIC/TRADE NAME	INDICATIONS FOR USE	DOSAGE
Aminocaproic acid (Amicar)	Control bleeding caused by overdoses of thrombolytic agents or bleeding disorders caused by hyperfibrinolysis (eg, cardiac surgery, blood disorders, hepatic cirrhosis, prostatectomy, neoplastic disorders)	PO, IV infusion, 5 g initially, followed by 1.0 to 1.25 g/h for 8 h or until bleeding is controlled; maximum dose, 30 g/24 h
Aprotinin (Trasylol)	Used in selected clients undergoing coronary artery bypass graft surgery to decrease blood loss and blood transfusions	See manufacturer's literature for test dose, loading dose, "pump prime" dose, and constant infusion.
Protamine sulfate	Treatment of heparin overdosage	Depends on the amount of heparin given within the previous 4 h
Tranexamic acid (Cyklokapron)	Control bleeding caused by overdoses of thrombolytic agents Prevent or decrease bleeding from tooth extraction in clients with hemophilia	PO 25 mg/kg 3 to 4 times daily, starting 1 d before surgery, or IV 10 mg/kg immediately before surgery, followed by 25 mg/kg PO 3 to 4 times daily for 2–8 d
Vitamin K (Mephyton)	Antidote for warfarin overdosage	PO 10–20 mg in a single dose

IV, intravenous; PO, oral.

(2–8 days) in clients with hemophilia to prevent or decrease bleeding from tooth extraction. Dosage of tranexamic acid should be reduced in the presence of moderate or severe renal impairment.

Aprotinin is a natural protease inhibitor obtained from bovine lung that has a variety of effects on blood coagulation. It inhibits plasmin and kallikrein, thus inhibiting fibrinolysis, and inhibits breakdown of blood clotting factors. It is used to decrease bleeding in selected clients undergoing coronary artery bypass surgery.

Protamine sulfate is an antidote for standard heparin and LMWHs. Because heparin is an acid and protamine sulfate is a base, protamine neutralizes heparin activity. Protamine dosage depends on the amount of heparin administered during the previous 4 hours. Each milligram of protamine neutralizes approximately 100 units of heparin or dalteparin and 1 milligram of enoxaparin. A single dose should not exceed 50 milligrams.

The drug is given by slow IV infusion over at least 10 minutes (to prevent or minimize adverse effects of hypotension, bradycardia, and dyspnea). Protamine effects occur immediately and last for approximately 2 hours. A second dose may be required because heparin activity lasts approximately 4 hours.

Protamine sulfate can cause severe hypotensive and anaphylactoid reactions. Thus, it should be given in settings with equipment and personnel for resuscitation and management of anaphylactic shock.

Vitamin K is the antidote for warfarin overdosage. An oral dose of 10 to 20 milligrams usually stops minor bleeding and returns the international normalized ratio (INR; see "Drug Dosage and Administration: Regulation of Heparin and Warfarin Dosage") to a normal range within 24 hours.

NURSING PROCESS

Assessment

Assess the client's status in relation to thrombotic and thromboembolic disorders.

- Risk factors for thromboembolism include
  - Immobility (eg, limited activity or bed rest for more than 5 days)
  - Obesity
  - Cigarette smoking
  - History of thrombophlebitis, DVT, or pulmonary emboli
  - Congestive heart failure
  - Pedal edema
  - Lower limb trauma
  - Myocardial infarction
  - Atrial fibrillation
  - Mitral or aortic stenosis
  - Prosthetic heart valves
  - Abdominal, thoracic, pelvic, or major orthopedic surgery
  - Atherosclerotic heart disease or peripheral vascular disease
  - Use of oral contraceptives
- Signs and symptoms of thrombotic and thromboembolic disorders depend on the location and size of the thrombus.
  - DVT and thrombophlebitis usually occur in the legs. The conditions may be manifested by edema (the affected leg is often measurably larger than the other) and pain, especially in the calf when the foot

is dorsiflexed (Homans' sign). If thrombophlebitis is superficial, it may be visible as a red, warm, tender area following the path of a vein.

- Pulmonary embolism, if severe enough to produce symptoms, is manifested by chest pain, cough, hemoptysis, tachypnea, and tachycardia. Massive emboli cause hypotension, shock, cyanosis, and death.
- DIC is usually manifested by bleeding, which may range from petechiae or oozing from a venipuncture site to massive internal bleeding or bleeding from all body orifices.

Nursing Diagnoses

- Ineffective Tissue Perfusion related to thrombus or embolus or drug-induced bleeding
- Acute Pain related to tissue ischemia
- Impaired Physical Mobility related to bed rest and pain
- Ineffective Coping related to the need for long-term prophylaxis of thromboembolic disorders or fear of excessive bleeding
- Anxiety related to fear of myocardial infarction or stroke
- Deficient Knowledge related to anticoagulant or antiplatelet drug therapy
- Risk for Injury related to drug-induced impairment of blood coagulation

Planning/Goals

The client will
- Receive or take anticoagulant and antiplatelet drugs correctly
- Be monitored closely for therapeutic and adverse drug effects, especially when drug therapy is started and when changes are made in drugs or dosages
- Use nondrug measures to decrease venous stasis and prevent thromboembolic disorders
- Act to prevent trauma from falls and other injuries
- Inform any health care provider when taking an anticoagulant or antiplatelet drug
- Avoid or report adverse drug reactions
- Verbalize or demonstrate knowledge of safe management of anticoagulant drug therapy
- Keep follow-up appointments for tests of blood coagulation and drug dosage regulation
- Avoid preventable bleeding episodes

Interventions

Use measures to prevent thrombotic and thromboembolic disorders.
- Have the client ambulate and exercise legs regularly, especially after surgery.

- For clients who cannot ambulate or do leg exercises, do passive range-of-motion and other leg exercises several times daily when changing the client's position or performing other care.
- Have the client wear elastic stockings. Elastic stockings should be removed every 8 hours and replaced after inspecting the skin. Improperly applied elastic stockings can impair circulation rather than aid it. For clients on bed rest, intermittent pneumatic compression devices can also be used.
- Avoid trauma to lower extremities.
- Maintain adequate fluid intake (1500–3000 mL/day) to avoid dehydration and hemoconcentration.
- Assist clients to promote good blood circulation (eg, exercise) and avoid situations that impair circulation (eg, wearing tight clothing, crossing the legs at the knees, prolonged sitting or standing, bed rest, placing pillows under the knees when in bed).

For the client receiving anticoagulant therapy, implement safety measures to prevent trauma and bleeding.

- For clients who cannot ambulate safely because of weakness, sedation, or other conditions, keep the call light within reach, keep bed rails elevated, and assist in ambulation.
- Provide an electric razor for shaving.
- Avoid intramuscular injections, venipunctures, and arterial punctures when possible.
- Avoid intubations when possible (eg, nasogastric tubes, indwelling urinary catheters).

For the client receiving tirofiban or eptifibatide:

- Monitor the femoral artery access site closely. This is the most common site of bleeding.
- Avoid invasive procedures as much as possible (eg, arterial and venous punctures, intramuscular injections, urinary catheters, nasotracheal suction, nasogastric tubes). If venipuncture must be done, avoid sites where pressure cannot be applied (eg, subclavian or jugular veins).
- While the vascular sheath is in place, keep clients on complete bed rest with the head of the bed elevated 30 degrees and the affected limb restrained in a straight position.
- Discontinue heparin for 3 to 4 hours and be sure the activated clotting time is less than 180 seconds or the activated partial thromboplastin time (aPTT) is less than 45 seconds before removing the vascular sheath.
- After the vascular sheath is removed, apply pressure to the site and observe closely. For outpatients, be sure there is no bleeding for at least 4 hours before hospital discharge.

For the client receiving a thrombolytic drug or a revascu-larization procedure for acute myocardial infarction:

- Monitor closely for bleeding.
- Assist the client and family to understand the impor-tance of diligent efforts to reverse risk factors con-tributing to coronary artery disease (eg, diet and perhaps medication to lower serum cholesterol to less than 200 mg/dL and low-density lipoprotein choles-terol to less than 130 mg/dL; weight reduction if over-weight; control of blood pressure if hypertensive; avoidance of smoking; stress-reduction techniques; exercise program designed and supervised by a health care provider).
- Assist the client and family to understand the impor-tance of complying with medication orders to prevent reinfarction and other complications, and continued medical supervision (see accompanying Client Teach-ing Guidelines).

Evaluation

- Observe for signs and symptoms of thromboembolic disorders or bleeding.
- Check blood coagulation tests for therapeutic ranges.
- Observe and interview regarding compliance with instructions about drug therapy.
- Observe and interview regarding adverse drug effects.

PRINCIPLES OF THERAPY

Drug Selection

Choices of anticoagulant and antiplatelet drugs depend on the reason for use and other drug and client characteristics.

- Heparin is the anticoagulant of choice in acute venous thromboembolic disorders because the anticoagulant effect begins immediately with IV administration.
- Warfarin is the anticoagulant of choice for long-term maintenance therapy (ie, several weeks or months) because it can be given orally.
- Aspirin has long been the most widely used antiplatelet drug for prevention of myocardial reinfarction and arte-rial thrombosis in clients with TIAs and prosthetic heart valves. However, clopidogrel may be more effective than aspirin.
- When anticoagulation is required during pregnancy, heparin is used because it does not cross the placenta. Warfarin is contraindicated during pregnancy.
- Various combinations of antithrombotic drugs are used concomitantly or sequentially (eg, abciximab is used with aspirin and heparin; thrombolytic drugs are usually followed with heparin and warfarin).

Drug Dosage and Administration: Regulation of Heparin and Warfarin Dosage

Heparin dosage is regulated by the activated partial throm-boplastin time (aPTT), which is sensitive to changes in blood clotting factors, except factor VII. Thus, normal or control values indicate normal blood coagulation; therapeutic values indicate low levels of clotting factors and delayed blood coagulation. During heparin therapy, the aPTT should be maintained at approximately 1.5 to 2.5 times the control or baseline value. The normal control value is 25 to 35 seconds; therefore, therapeutic values are 45 to 70 seconds, approxi-mately. With continuous IV infusion, blood for the aPTT may be drawn at any time; with intermittent administration, blood for the aPTT should be drawn approximately 1 hour before a dose of heparin is scheduled. Monitoring of aPTT is not necessary with low-dose standard heparin given Sub-Q for prophylaxis of thromboembolism or with the LMWHs (eg, enoxaparin).

APPLYING YOUR KNOWLEDGE 54-2
Mr. Dusseau's aPTT is measured to regulate the amount of heparin he receives. What is the aPTT goal for a therapeutic value?

Warfarin dosage is regulated according to the INR, for which therapeutic values are 2.0 to 3.0 in most conditions. An average daily dose of 4 to 5 milligrams maintains a thera-peutic INR; stopping warfarin returns an elevated INR to nor-mal in approximately 4 days in most clients.

The INR is based on prothrombin time (PT). PT is sensi-tive to changes in three of the four vitamin K–dependent coagulation factors. Thus, normal or control values indicate normal levels of these factors; therapeutic values indicate low levels of the factors and delayed blood coagulation. A normal baseline or control PT is approximately 12 seconds; a therapeutic value is approximately 1.5 times the control, or 18 seconds.

When warfarin is started, PT and INR should be assessed daily until a stable daily dose is reached (the dose that main-tains PT and INR within therapeutic ranges and does not cause bleeding). Thereafter, PT and INR are determined every 2 to 4 weeks for the duration of oral anticoagulant drug therapy. If the warfarin dose is changed, PT and INR mea-surements are needed more often until a stable daily dose is again established.

For many years, PT was used to regulate warfarin dosage. PT is determined by adding a mixture of thromboplastin and calcium to citrated plasma and measuring the time (in seconds) it takes for the blood to clot. However, values vary among laboratories according to the type of thrombo-plastin and the instrument used to measure PT. The INR system standardizes PT by comparing a particular throm-boplastin with a standard thromboplastin designated by the World Health Organization. Advantages of the INR

CLIENT TEACHING GUIDELINES

Drugs to Prevent or Treat Blood Clots

General Considerations

✔ Antiplatelet and anticoagulant drugs are given to people who have had, or who are at risk of having, a heart attack, stroke, or other problems from blood clots. For prevention of a heart attack or stroke, you are most likely to be given an antiplatelet drug (eg, aspirin, clopidogrel) or warfarin (Coumadin). For home management of deep vein thrombosis, which usually occurs in the legs, you are likely to be given heparin injections for a few days, followed by warfarin for long-term therapy. These medications help to prevent the blood clot from getting larger, traveling to your lungs, or recurring later.

✔ All of these drugs can increase your risk of bleeding, so you need to take safety precautions to prevent injury.

✔ To help prevent blood clots from forming and decreasing blood flow through your arteries, you need to reduce risk factors that contribute to cardiovascular disease. This can be done by a low-fat, low-cholesterol diet (and medication if needed) to lower total cholesterol to below 200 mg/dL and low-density lipoprotein cholesterol to below 130 mg/dL; weight reduction if overweight; control of blood pressure if hypertensive; avoidance of smoking; stress-reduction techniques; and regular exercise.

✔ To help prevent blood clots from forming in your leg veins, avoid or minimize situations that slow blood circulation, such as wearing tight clothing; crossing the legs at the knees; prolonged sitting or standing; and bed rest. For example, on automobile trips, stop and walk around every 1 to 2 hours; on long plane trips, exercise your feet and legs at your seat and walk around when you can.

✔ Following instructions regarding these medications is extremely important. Too little medication increases your risk of problems from blood clot formation; too much medication can cause bleeding.

✔ While taking any of these medications, you need regular medical supervision and periodic blood tests. The blood tests can help your health care provider regulate drug dosage and maintain your safety.

✔ You need to take the drugs as directed; avoid taking other drugs without the health care provider's knowledge and consent; inform any health care provider (including dentists) that you are taking an antiplatelet or anticoagulant drug before any invasive diagnostic tests or treatments are begun; and keep all appointments for continuing care.

✔ With warfarin therapy, you need to avoid walking barefoot; avoid contact sports; use an electric razor; avoid injections when possible; and carry an identification card, necklace, or bracelet (eg, MedicAlert) stating the name of the drug and the health care provider's name and telephone number. Also, avoid large amounts of certain vegetables (eg, broccoli, brussels sprouts, cabbage, cauliflower, chives, collard greens, kale, lettuce, mustard greens, peppers, spinach, turnips, and watercress), tomatoes, bananas, or fish; these foods contain vitamin K and may decrease anticoagulant effects.

✔ For home management of deep vein thrombosis, both warfarin and enoxaparin (Lovenox) are given for 3 months or longer. With Lovenox, you need an injection, usually every 12 hours. You or someone close to you may be instructed in injecting the medication, or a visiting nurse may do the injections, if necessary.

Even if a nurse is not needed to give the injections, one will usually visit your home each day to perform a finger stick blood test. The results of this test determine your daily dose of warfarin. After the blood test and the warfarin dose stabilize, the blood tests are done less often (eg, every 2 weeks).

✔ Report any sign of bleeding (eg, excessive bruising of the skin; blood in urine or stool). If superficial bleeding occurs, apply direct pressure to the site for 3 to 5 minutes or longer if necessary.

Self-Administration

✔ Take aspirin with food or after meals, with 8 oz of water, to decrease stomach irritation. However, stomach upset is uncommon with the small doses used for antiplatelet effects. Do not crush or chew coated tablets (long-acting preparations).

✔ Take cilostazol (Pletal) 30 minutes before or 2 hours after morning and evening meals for better absorption and effectiveness.

✔ Take ticlopidine (Ticlid) with food or after meals to decrease GI upset. Clopidogrel (Plavix) may be taken with or without food.

✔ With Lovenox, wash hands and cleanse skin to prevent infection; inject deep under the skin, around the navel, upper thigh, or buttocks; and change the injection site daily. If excessive bruising occurs at the injection site, rubbing an ice cube over an area before the injection may be helpful.

---

include consistent values among laboratories, more consistent warfarin dosage with less risk of bleeding or thrombosis, and more consistent reports of clinical trials and other research studies. Some laboratories report both PT and INR.

Warfarin dosage may need to be reduced in clients with biliary tract disorders (eg, obstructive jaundice), liver disease (eg, hepatitis, cirrhosis), malabsorption syndromes (eg, steatorrhea), hyperthyroidism, or fever. These conditions increase anticoagulant drug effects by reducing absorption of vitamin K; decreasing hepatic synthesis of blood clotting factors; or increasing the breakdown of clotting factors. Despite these influencing factors, however, the primary determinant of dosage is the PT and INR.

Warfarin interacts with many other drugs to cause increased, decreased, or unpredictable anticoagulant effects (see Nursing Actions). Thus, warfarin dosage may need to be increased or decreased when other drugs are given concomitantly. Most drugs can be given if warfarin dosage is titrated according to the PT or INR and altered appropriately when an interacting drug is added or stopped. INR or PT measurements and vigilant observation are needed whenever a drug is added to or removed from a drug therapy regimen containing warfarin.

APPLYING YOUR KNOWLEDGE 54-3:
HOW CAN YOU AVOID THIS MEDICATION ERROR?
In anticipation of Mr. Dusseau's discharge from the hospital, the physician changes his medication from heparin to warfarin. The order is for warfarin 5 mg PO daily and for evaluation of baseline PT and INR. You administer the warfarin and order the bloodwork for the next morning.

Thrombolytic Therapy

- Thrombolytic therapy should be performed only by experienced personnel in an intensive care or diagnostic/interventional setting with cardiac and other monitoring devices in place.

- All of the available agents are effective with recommended uses. Thus, the choice of a thrombolytic agent depends mainly on risks of adverse effects and costs. All of the drugs may cause bleeding. Alteplase may act more specifically on the fibrin in a clot and cause less systemic depletion of fibrinogen, but this agent is very expensive. Streptokinase, the least expensive agent, may cause allergic reactions because it is a foreign protein. Combination therapy (eg, with alteplase and streptokinase) may also be used.

- Before a thrombolytic agent is begun, INR, aPTT, platelet count, and fibrinogen should be checked to establish baseline values and to determine if a blood coagulation disorder is present. Two or 3 hours after thrombolytic therapy is started, the fibrinogen level can be measured to determine that fibrinolysis is occurring. Alternatively, INR or aPTT can be checked for increased values because the breakdown products of fibrin exert anticoagulant effects.

- Major factors in decreasing risks of bleeding are selecting recipients carefully, avoiding invasive procedures when possible, and omitting anticoagulant or antiplatelet drugs while thrombolytics are being given. If bleeding does occur, it is most likely from a venipuncture or invasive procedure site, and local pressure may control it. If bleeding cannot be controlled or involves a vital organ, the thrombolytic drug should be stopped and fibrinogen replaced with whole blood plasma or cryoprecipitate. Aminocaproic acid or tranexamic acid may also be given.

- When the drugs are used in acute myocardial infarction, cardiac dysrhythmias may occur when blood flow is re-established. Therefore, antidysrhythmic drugs should be readily available.

Use in Special Populations

Use in Children

Little information is available about the use of anticoagulants in children. Heparin solutions containing benzyl alcohol as a preservative should not be given to premature infants because fatal reactions have been reported. When given for systemic anticoagulation, heparin dosage should be based on the child's weight (approximately 50 units/kg). Safety and effectiveness of LMWHs (eg, enoxaparin) have not been established in children.

Warfarin is given to children after cardiac surgery to prevent thromboembolism, but doses and guidelines for safe, effective use have not been developed. Accurate drug administration; close monitoring of blood coagulation tests; safety measures to prevent trauma and bleeding; avoiding interacting drugs; and informing others in the child's environment (eg, teachers, babysitters, health care providers) are necessary.

Antiplatelet and thrombolytic drugs have no established indications for use in children.

Use in Older Adults

Older adults often have atherosclerosis and thrombotic disorders, including myocardial infarction, thrombotic stroke, and peripheral arterial insufficiency, for which they receive an anticoagulant or an antiplatelet drug. They are more likely than younger adults to experience bleeding and other complications of anticoagulant and antiplatelet drugs. For example, aspirin or clopidogrel is commonly used to prevent thrombotic stroke, but both drugs increase risks of hemorrhagic stroke.

With standard heparin, general principles for safe and effective use apply. With LMWHs, elimination may be delayed in older adults with renal impairment and the drugs should be used cautiously. They should also be used with caution in clients taking a platelet inhibitor (eg, aspirin, clopidogrel) to prevent myocardial infarction or thrombotic stroke, or an NSAID for arthritis pain. NSAIDs, which are commonly used by older adults, also have antiplatelet effects. Clients who take an NSAID daily may not need low-dose aspirin for antithrombotic effects.

With warfarin, dosage should be reduced because impaired liver function and decreased plasma proteins increase the risks of bleeding. Also, many drugs interact with warfarin to increase or decrease its effect, and older adults often take multiple drugs. Starting or stopping any drug may require that warfarin dosage be adjusted.

Use in Clients With Renal Impairment

Most anticoagulant, antiplatelet, and thrombolytic drugs may be used in clients with impaired renal function. For example, heparin and warfarin can be used in usual dosages, and thrombolytic agents (eg, streptokinase, urokinase) may be used to dissolve clots in IV catheters or vascular access sites for hemodialysis. Dosage of LMWHs should be reduced in clients with severe renal impairment (creatinine clearance <30 mL/minute) because they are excreted by the kidneys and elimination is slowed. In addition, home management of DVT with LMWHs and warfarin is contraindicated in clients with severe renal impairment. Guidelines for the use of other drugs include the following:

- *Anagrelide* may be given to clients with renal impairment (eg, serum creatinine <2 mg/dL) if potential benefits outweigh risks. Clients receiving this medication should be monitored closely for signs of renal toxicity.
- *Cilostazol* is probably safe to use in clients with mild or moderate renal impairment. However, severe renal impairment alters drug protein binding and increases blood levels of metabolites.
- *Clopidogrel* does not need dosage reduction in clients with renal impairment.
- *Eptifibatide* does not need dosage reduction in clients with mild to moderate renal impairment. No data are available for clients with severe impairment or those on hemodialysis.
- *Lepirudin* is excreted by the kidneys and may accumulate in clients with impaired renal function. Dosage should be reduced.
- *Ticlopidine* may be more likely to cause bleeding in clients with renal impairment because the plasma drug concentration is increased and elimination is slower.
- *Tirofiban* clearance from plasma is decreased approximately 50% in clients with severe renal impairment (eg, creatinine clearance <30 mL/minute), including those receiving hemodialysis. Dosage must be reduced by approximately 50%.

Use in Clients With Hepatic Impairment

Little information is available about the use of most anticoagulant, antiplatelet, and thrombolytic drugs in clients with impaired liver function. However, such drugs should be used very cautiously because these clients may already be predisposed to bleeding due to decreased hepatic synthesis of clotting factors. Additional considerations include the following:

- *Warfarin* is more likely to cause bleeding in clients with liver disease, because of decreased synthesis of vitamin K. In addition, warfarin is eliminated only by hepatic metabolism and may accumulate with liver impairment.
- *LMWHs* are contraindicated for home management of DVT in clients with severe liver disease because of high risks of excessive bleeding.
- *Anagrelide* is metabolized in the liver and may accumulate with hepatic impairment. Clients with evidence of impairment (eg, bilirubin or aspartate aminotransferase more than 1.5 times the upper limit of normal)

should receive anagrelide only if potential benefits outweigh potential risks. When anagrelide is given, clients should be closely monitored for signs of hepatotoxicity.
- *Clopidogrel* is metabolized in the liver and may accumulate with hepatic impairment. It should be used cautiously.
- *Dipyridamole* is metabolized in the liver and excreted in bile.

Use in Home Care

Antiplatelet agents and warfarin are used for long-term prevention or management of thromboembolism and are often taken at home. For prevention, antiplatelet agents and warfarin are usually self-administered at home, with periodic office or clinic visits for blood tests and other follow-up care.

For home management of DVT, warfarin may be self-administered, but a nurse usually visits, performs a finger-stick INR, and notifies the prescriber, who then prescribes the appropriate dose of warfarin. Precautions are needed to decrease risks of bleeding. The risk of bleeding has lessened in recent years because of the lower doses of warfarin being used. In addition, bleeding during warfarin therapy may be caused by medical conditions other than anticoagulation.

Heparin may also be taken at home. Standard heparin may be taken Sub-Q, but use of LMWHs for home management of venous thrombosis has become standard practice. Enoxaparin is approved by the Food and Drug Administration for outpatient use. Daily visits by a home care nurse may be needed if the client or a family member is unable or unwilling to inject the medication. Platelet counts should be done before and every 2 to 3 days during heparin therapy. Heparin should be discontinued if the platelet count falls below 100,000 or to less than half the baseline value.

Most home management regimens involve a structured protocol. Clients and family members should be educated about the disorder (usually DVT), including the potential consequences of either overcoagulation or undercoagulation, and the need for blood tests.

The home care nurse needs to assess clients in relation to knowledge about prescribed drugs and ability and willingness to comply with instructions for taking the drugs, obtaining blood tests when indicated, and taking safety precautions. In addition, assess the environment for risk factors for injury. Interventions vary with clients, environments, and assessment data, but may include reinforcing instructions for safe use of the drugs, assisting clients to obtain laboratory tests, and teaching how to observe for signs and symptoms of bleeding.

Use of Herbal and Dietary Supplements

Many commonly used herbs and supplements have a profound effect on drugs used for anticoagulation. Multivitamin supplements may contain 25 to 28 micrograms of vitamin K and should be taken consistently to avoid fluctuating vitamin K levels. Doses of vitamin C in excess of 500 milligrams per day may lower INR, and vitamin E in excess of 400 international units per day may increase warfarin effects. Herbs commonly used that may increase the effects of warfarin include alfalfa, celery, clove, feverfew, garlic, ginger, ginkgo, ginseng, and licorice. Clients taking warfarin should be questioned care-fully about their use of herbs as well as vitamin or mineral supplements.

APPLYING YOUR KNOWLEDGE 54-4

After 6 months of treatment with warfarin, the physician orders Mr. Dusseau to change to aspirin therapy. What is the purpose of aspirin therapy?

N U R S I N G   A C T I O N S

Drugs That Affect Blood Coagulation

NURSING ACTIONS	RATIONALE/EXPLANATION
1. Administer accurately	
a. With standard heparin:	
(1) When handwriting a heparin dose, write out "units" rather than using the abbreviation "U."	This is a safety precaution to avoid erroneous dosage. For example, 1000 U (1000 units) may be misread as 10,000 units.
(2) Check dosage and vial label carefully.	Underdosage may cause thromboembolism, and overdosage may cause bleeding. In addition, heparin is available in several concentrations (1000, 2500, 5000, 10,000, 15,000, 20,000, and 40,000 units/mL).
(3) For subcutaneous (Sub-Q) heparin:	
(a) Use a 26-gauge, ½-inch needle.	To minimize trauma and risk of bleeding
(b) Leave a small air bubble in the syringe to follow dose.	Locks drug into subcutaneous space and minimizes trauma
(c) Grasp a skinfold and inject the heparin into it, at a 90-degree angle, without aspirating.	To give the drug in a deep subcutaneous or fat layer, with minimal trauma
(d) Do not massage site after injection.	
(4) For intermittent intravenous (IV) administration:	
(a) Give by direct injection into a heparin lock or tubing injection site.	These methods prevent repeated venipunctures.
(b) Dilute the dose in 50–100 mL of any IV fluid (usually 5% dextrose in water).	
(5) For continuous IV administration:	This is usually the preferred method because it maintains consistent serum drug levels and decreases risks of bleeding.
(a) Use a volume-control device and an infusion-control device.	To regulate dosage and flow rate accurately
(b) Add only enough heparin for a few hours. One effective method is to fill the volume-control set (eg, Volutrol) with 100 mL of 5% dextrose in water and add 5000 units of heparin to yield a concentration of 50 units/mL. Dosage is regulated by varying the flow rate. For example, administration of 1000 units/h requires a flow rate of 20 mL/h. Another method is to add 25,000 units of heparin to 500 mL of IV solution.	To avoid inadvertent administration of large amounts. Whatever method is used, it is desirable to standardize concentration of heparin solutions within an institution. Standardization is safer, because it reduces risks of errors in dosage.

NURSING ACTIONS	RATIONALE/EXPLANATION

b. With low–molecular-weight heparins:

   (1) Give by deep Sub-Q injection, into an abdominal skin fold, with the patient lying down, using the same technique as standard heparin. Do not rub the injection site.

To decrease bruising

   (2) Rotate sites.

c. After the initial dose of warfarin, check the international normalized ratio (INR) before giving a subsequent dose. Do not give the dose if the INR is above 3.0. Notify the health care provider.

The INR is measured daily until a maintenance dose is established, then periodically throughout warfarin therapy. An elevated INR indicates a high risk of bleeding.

d. Give ticlopidine with food or after meals; give cilostazol 30 minutes before or 2 hours after morning and evening meals; give clopidogrel with or without food.

e. With eptifibatide, tirofiban, and thrombolytic agents, follow manufacturers' instructions for reconstitution and administration.

These drugs require special preparation and administration techniques.

2. Observe for therapeutic effects

  a. With prophylactic heparins and warfarin, observe for the absence of signs and symptoms of thrombotic disorders.

  b. With therapeutic heparins and warfarin, observe for decrease or improvement in signs and symptoms (eg, less edema and pain with deep vein thrombosis, less chest pain and respiratory difficulty with pulmonary embolism).

  c. With prophylactic or therapeutic warfarin, observe for an INR between 2.0 and 3.0.

Frequency of INR determinations varies, but the test should be done periodically in all clients taking warfarin.

  d. With therapeutic heparin, observe for an activated partial thromboplastin time of 1.5 to 2 times the control value.

  e. With anagrelide, observe for a decrease in platelet count.

Platelet counts should be done every 2 days during the first week of management and weekly until a maintenance dose is reached. Counts usually begin to decrease within the first 2 weeks of therapy.

  f. With aspirin, clopidogrel, and other antiplatelet drugs, observe for the absence of thrombotic disorders (eg, myocardial infarction, stroke).

  g. With cilostazol, observe for ability to walk farther without leg pain (intermittent claudication).

Improvement may occur within 2–4 weeks or take as long as 12 weeks.

3. Observe for adverse effects

  a. Bleeding:

Bleeding is the major adverse effect of anticoagulant drugs. It may occur anywhere in the body, spontaneously or in response to minor trauma.

With eptifibatide and tirofiban, most major bleeding occurs at the arterial access site for cardiac catheterization.

Hypotension and tachycardia may indicate internal bleeding.

   (1) Record vital signs regularly.

   (2) Check stools for blood (melena).

Gastrointestinal (GI) bleeding is fairly common; risks are increased with intubation. Blood in stools may be bright red, tarry (blood that has been digested by GI secretions), or occult (hidden to the naked eye but present with a guaiac test). Hematemesis also may occur.

   (3) Check urine for blood (hematuria).

Genitourinary bleeding also is fairly common; risks are increased with catheterization or instrumentation. Urine may be red (indicating fresh bleeding) or brownish or smoky gray (indicating old blood). Or bleeding may be microscopic (red blood cells are visible only on microscopic examination during urinalysis).

(continued)

NURSING ACTIONS	RATIONALE/EXPLANATION
(4) Inspect the skin and mucous membranes daily.	Bleeding may occur in the skin as petechiae, purpura, or ecchymoses. Surgical wounds, skin lesions, parenteral injection sites, the nose, and gums may be bleeding sites.
(5) Assess for excessive menstrual flow.	
b. Other adverse effects:	
(1) With heparin, tissue irritation at injection sites, transient alopecia, reversible thrombocytopenia, paresthesias, and hypersensitivity	These effects are uncommon. They are more likely to occur with large doses or prolonged administration.
(2) With warfarin, dermatitis, diarrhea, and alopecia	These effects occur only occasionally. Warfarin has been given for prolonged periods without toxicity.
(3) With anagrelide, adverse cardiovascular effects (eg, tachycardia, vasodilation, heart failure)	These effects are most likely to occur in clients with known heart disease.
(4) With clopidogrel and ticlopidine, GI upset, skin rash, neutropenia, and thrombocytopenia	Neutropenia and thrombocytopenia are more likely to occur with ticlopidine than clopidogrel.
c. With thrombolytic drugs, observe for bleeding with all uses and reperfusion dysrhythmias when used for acute myocardial infarction.	Bleeding is most likely to occur at sites of venipuncture or other invasive procedures. Reperfusion dysrhythmias may occur when blood supply is restored to previously ischemic myocardium.
4. Observe for drug interactions	
a. Drugs that *increase* risks of bleeding with anticoagulant, antiplatelet, and thrombolytic agents:	These drugs are often used concurrently or sequentially to decrease risks of myocardial infarction or stroke.
(1) Any one of these drugs in combination with any other drug that affects hemostasis	
(2) A combination of these drugs	
b. Drugs that *increase* effects of heparins:	
(1) Antiplatelet drugs (eg, aspirin, clopidogrel, others)	
(2) Warfarin	Additive anticoagulant effects and increased risks of bleeding
(3) Parenteral penicillins and cephalosporins	Some may affect blood coagulation and increase risks of bleeding.
c. Drugs that *decrease* effects of heparins:	
(1) Antihistamines, digoxin, tetracyclines	These drugs antagonize the anticoagulant effects of heparin. Mechanisms are not clear.
(2) Protamine sulfate	The antidote for heparin overdose
d. Drugs that *increase* effects of warfarin:	Mechanisms by which drugs may increase effects of warfarin include inhibiting warfarin metabolism, displacing warfarin from binding sites on serum albumin, causing antiplatelet effects, inhibiting bacterial synthesis of vitamin K in the intestinal tract, and others.
(1) Analgesics (eg, acetaminophen, aspirin and other nonsteroidal anti-inflammatory drugs)	
(2) Androgens and anabolic steroids	
(3) Antibacterial drugs (eg, aminoglycosides, erythromycin, fluoroquinolones, isoniazid, metronidazole, penicillins, cephalosporins, trimethoprim-sulfamethoxazole, tetracyclines)	
(4) Antifungal drugs (eg, fluconazole, ketoconazole, miconazole), including intravaginal use	
(5) Antiseizure drugs (eg, phenytoin)	
(6) Cardiovascular drugs (eg, amiodarone, beta blockers, loop diuretics, gemfibrozil, lovastatin, propafenone, quinidine)	
(7) Gastrointestinal drugs (eg, cimetidine, omeprazole)	
(8) Thyroid preparations (eg, levothyroxine)	

NURSING ACTIONS	RATIONALE/EXPLANATION
e. Drugs that *decrease* effects of warfarin:	
(1) Antacids and griseofulvin	May decrease GI absorption
(2) Carbamazepine, disulfiram, rifampin	These drugs activate liver metabolizing enzymes, which accelerate the rate of metabolism of warfarin.
(3) Cholestyramine	Decreases absorption
(4) Diuretics	Increase synthesis and concentration of blood clotting factors
(5) Estrogens, including oral contraceptives	Increase synthesis of clotting factors and have thromboembolic effect
(6) Vitamin K	Restores prothrombin and other vitamin K–dependent clotting factors in the blood. Antidote for overdose of warfarin.
f. Drug that may *increase* or *decrease* effects of warfarin:	
(1) Alcohol	Alcohol may induce liver enzymes, which decrease effects by accelerating the rate of metabolism of the anticoagulant drug. However, with alcohol-induced liver disease (ie, cirrhosis), effects may be increased owing to impaired metabolism of warfarin.
g. Drugs that *increase* effects of cilostazol:	
(1) Diltiazem	These drugs inhibit the main cytochrome P450 enzyme (CYP3A4) that metabolizes cilostazol. Grapefruit juice also inhibits drug metabolism and should be avoided.
(2) Erythromycin	
(3) Itraconazole, ketoconazole	

APPLYING YOUR KNOWLEDGE: ANSWERS

54-1 The main reason anticoagulants are used is to prevent the formation of new clots and the extension of clots that are already present. Heparin does not dissolve a clot that is already formed. The main adverse effect is bleeding.

54-2 The goal of therapy with heparin is to maintain the aPTT at 1.5 to 2.5 times the baseline value. In most clients, the goal will be 45 to 70 seconds.

54-3 Have the bloodwork evaluated before any warfarin is given. Subsequent assessment of PT/INR should be performed before the second dose of warfarin is given.

54-4 Aspirin therapy is used in long-term therapy for the prevention of future myocardial infarction.

Review and Application Exercises

Short Answer Exercises

1. What are the major functions of the endothelium, platelets, and coagulation factors in hemostasis and thrombosis?

2. What are the indications for use of heparin and warfarin?

3. How do heparin and warfarin differ in mechanism of action, onset and duration of action, and method of administration?

4. List interventions to protect clients from anticoagulant-induced bleeding.

5. When is it appropriate to use protamine sulfate as an antidote for heparin?

6. When is it appropriate to use vitamin K as an antidote for warfarin?

7. How do antiplatelet drugs differ from heparin and warfarin?

8. For what conditions are antiplatelet drugs indicated?

9. When is it appropriate to use a thrombolytic drug?

10. How do aminocaproic acid and tranexamic acid stop bleeding induced by thrombolytics?

11. Compare and contrast nursing care needs of clients receiving anticoagulant therapy in hospital and home settings.

NCLEX-Style Questions

12. The following statements about warfarin are true except
    a. Warfarin is a vitamin K antagonist.
    b. Warfarin does not cross the placenta.
    c. Warfarin is used for long-term anticoagulation therapy.
    d. Warfarin is metabolized by the liver.

13. The nurse is reviewing the laboratory results of a patient receiving heparin therapy for pulmonary embolism. The aPTT is 50 seconds. The nurse should
    a. not give the next dose because the level is too high
    b. continue the present order because the level is appropriate
    c. notify the provider that the aPTT is low and the dose should be increased
    d. request an order for warfarin now that the patient is heparinized

14. The nurse explains to a client that aspirin suppresses blood clotting by
    a. inactivating thrombin
    b. promoting fibrin degradation
    c. decreasing synthesis of clotting factors
    d. decreasing platelet aggregation

15. A patient's Port-a-Cath has become occluded with thrombus. The nurse expects which agent will likely be used to lyse the clot?
    a. heparin
    b. tirofiban
    c. urokinase
    d. abciximab

16. Ticlopidine is indicated for
    a. prevention of thrombotic stroke in patients who have had TIAs or previous stroke
    b. adjunctive therapy to warfarin for DVT
    c. heparin-induced thrombocytopenia
    d. patients in whom bleeding is a consideration

Selected References

Activated protein C (Xigris) for severe sepsis. (2002, February 18). *The Medical Letter on Drugs and Therapeutics, 44*(1124), 17–18.

Drug facts and comparisons. (Updated monthly). St. Louis: Facts and Comparisons.

Duplaga, B. A., Rivers, C. W., & Nutescu, E. (2001). Dosing and monitoring of low-molecular-weight heparins in special populations. *Pharmacotherapy, 21*(2), 218–234.

Gaspard, K. J. (2005). Disorders of hemostasis. In C. M. Porth, *Pathophysiology: Concepts of altered health states* (7th ed., pp. 287–298). Philadelphia: Lippincott Williams & Wilkins.

Haines, S. T, Racine, E., & Zeolla, M. (2002). Venous thromboembolism. In J. T. DiPiro, R. L. Talbert, G. C. Yee, G. R. Matzke, B. G. Wells, & L. M. Posey (Eds.), *Pharmacotherapy: A pathophysiologic approach* (5th ed., pp. 337–373). New York: McGraw-Hill.

Karch, A. M. (2005). *2006 Lippincott's nursing drug guide.* Philadelphia: Lippincott Williams & Wilkins.

North American Nursing Diagnosis Association. (2003). *Nursing diagnoses: Definitions & classification 2003–2004.* Philadelphia: Author.

Skidmore-Roth, L. (2004). *Mosby's handbook of herbs & natural supplements* (2nd ed.). St. Louis: Mosby.

Smeltzer, S. C., & Bare, B. G. (2004). *Brunner & Suddarth's textbook of medical-surgical nursing* (10th ed., pp. 787–806). Philadelphia: Lippincott Williams & Wilkins.

Drugs for Dyslipidemia

OBJECTIVES

After studying this chapter, you will be able to:

1. Discuss the role of dyslipidemia in the etiology of atherosclerosis.
2. Identify sources and functions of cholesterol and triglycerides.
3. Describe dyslipidemic drugs in terms of mechanism of action, indications for use, major adverse effects, and nursing process implications.
4. Teach clients pharmacologic and nonpharmacologic measures to prevent or reduce dyslipidemia.

APPLYING YOUR KNOWLEDGE

Lewis Watkins is a 62-year-old man who has had elevated cholesterol and triglyceride levels during his two previous visits to the physician. He has tried diet modification and increasing exercise; however, his lipid levels remain elevated. His physician decides to prescribe atorvastatin 10 mg PO daily and gemfibrozil 600 mg PO bid. You are the home care nurse assigned to his care.

INTRODUCTION

Dyslipidemic drugs are used in the management of clients with elevated blood lipids, a major risk factor for atherosclerosis and vascular disorders such as coronary artery disease, strokes, and peripheral arterial insufficiency. These drugs have proven efficacy and are being used increasingly to reduce morbidity and mortality from coronary heart disease and other atherosclerosis-related cardiovascular disorders. To understand clinical use of these drugs, it is necessary to understand characteristics of blood lipids, atherosclerosis, and types of blood lipid disorders.

Blood Lipids

Blood lipids, which include cholesterol, phospholipids, and triglycerides, are derived from the diet or synthesized by the liver and intestine. Most cholesterol is found in body cells, where it is a component of cell membranes and performs other essential functions. In cells of the adrenal glands, ovaries, and testes, cholesterol is required for the synthesis of steroid hormones (eg, cortisol, estrogen, progesterone, testosterone). In liver cells, cholesterol is used to form cholic acid. The cholic acid is then conjugated with other substances to form bile salts, which promote absorption and digestion of fats. In addition, a small amount of cholesterol is found in blood serum. Serum cholesterol is the portion of total body cholesterol involved in formation of atherosclerotic plaques. Unless a person has a genetic disorder of lipid metabolism, the amount of cholesterol in the blood is strongly related to dietary intake of saturated fat. Phospholipids are essential components of cell membranes, and triglycerides provide energy for cellular metabolism.

Blood lipids are transported in plasma by specific proteins called *lipoproteins*. Each lipoprotein contains cholesterol, phospholipid, and triglyceride bound to protein. The lipoproteins vary in density and amounts of lipid and protein. Density is determined mainly by the amount of protein, which is more dense than fat. Thus, density increases as the proportion of protein increases. The lipoproteins are differentiated according to these properties, which can be measured in the laboratory. For example, high-density lipoprotein (HDL) cholesterol contains larger amounts of protein and smaller amounts of lipid; low-density lipoprotein (LDL) cholesterol contains less protein and larger amounts of lipid. Other plasma lipoproteins are chylomicrons and very–low-density lipoproteins (VLDL). Additional characteristics of lipoproteins are described in Box 55-1.

Box 55-1 Types of Lipoproteins

Chylomicrons, the largest lipoprotein molecules, are synthesized in the wall of the small intestine. They carry recently ingested dietary cholesterol and triglycerides that have been absorbed from the gastrointestinal tract. Hyperchylomicronemia normally occurs after a fatty meal, reaches peak levels in 3 to 4 hours, and subsides within 12 to 14 hours. Chylomicrons carry triglycerides to fat and muscle cells, where the enzyme lipoprotein lipase breaks down the molecule and releases fatty acids to be used for energy or stored as fat. This process leaves a remnant containing cholesterol, which is then transported to the liver. Thus, chylomicrons transport triglycerides to peripheral tissues and cholesterol to the liver.

Low-density lipoprotein (LDL) cholesterol, sometimes called "bad cholesterol," transports approximately 75% of serum cholesterol and carries it to peripheral tissues and the liver. LDL cholesterol is removed from the circulation by receptor and nonreceptor mechanisms. The receptor mechanism involves the binding of LDL cholesterol to receptors on cell surface membranes. The bound LDL molecule is then engulfed into the cell, where it is broken down by enzymes and releases free cholesterol into the cytoplasm.

Most LDL cholesterol receptors are located in the liver. However, nonhepatic tissues (eg, adrenal glands, smooth muscle cells, endothelial cells, and lymphoid cells) also have receptors by which they obtain the cholesterol needed for building cell membranes and synthesizing hormones. These cells can regulate their cholesterol intake by adding or removing LDL receptors.

Approximately two thirds of the LDL cholesterol is removed from the bloodstream by the receptor-dependent mechanism. The number of LDL receptors on cell membranes determines the amount of LDL degradation (ie, the more receptors on cells, the more LDL is broken down). Conditions that decrease the number or function of receptors (eg, high dietary intake of cholesterol, saturated fat, or calories), increase blood levels of LDL.

The remaining one third is removed by mechanisms that do not involve receptors. Nonreceptor uptake occurs in various cells, especially when levels of circulating LDL cholesterol are high. For example, macrophage cells in arterial walls can attach LDL, thereby promoting accumulation of cholesterol and the development of atherosclerosis. The amount of LDL cholesterol removed by nonreceptor mechanisms is increased with inadequate numbers of receptors or excessive amounts of LDL cholesterol.

A high serum level of LDL cholesterol is atherogenic and a strong risk factor for coronary heart disease. The body normally attempts to compensate for high serum levels by inhibiting hepatic synthesis of cholesterol and cellular synthesis of new LDL receptors.

Very–low-density lipoprotein (VLDL) contains approximately 75% triglycerides and 25% cholesterol. It transports endogenous triglycerides (those synthesized in the liver and intestine, not those derived exogenously, from food) to fat and muscle cells. There, as with chylomicrons, lipoprotein lipase breaks down the molecule and releases fatty acids to be used for energy or stored as fat. The removal of triglycerides from VLDL leaves a cholesterol-rich remnant, which returns to the liver. Then the cholesterol is secreted into the intestine, mostly as bile acids, or it is used to form more VLDL and recirculated.

High-density lipoprotein (HDL) cholesterol, often referred to as "good cholesterol," is a small but very important lipoprotein. It is synthesized in the liver and intestine and some is derived from the enzymatic breakdown of chylomicrons and VLDL. It contains moderate amounts of cholesterol. However, this cholesterol is transported from blood vessel walls to the liver for catabolism and excretion. This reverse transport of cholesterol has protective effects against coronary heart disease.

The mechanisms by which HDL cholesterol exerts protective effects are unknown. Possible mechanisms include clearing cholesterol from atheromatous plaque; increasing excretion of cholesterol so less is available for reuse in the formation of LDL cholesterol; and inhibiting cellular uptake of LDL cholesterol. Regular exercise and moderate alcohol consumption are associated with increased levels of HDL cholesterol; obesity, diabetes mellitus, genetic factors, smoking, and some medications (eg, steroids and beta blockers) are associated with decreased levels. HDL cholesterol levels are not directly affected by diet.

Atherosclerosis

Atherosclerosis is a major cause of ischemic heart disease (eg, angina pectoris, myocardial infarction), heart failure, stroke, peripheral vascular disease, and death (see Chaps. 48, 50, and 54). It is a systemic disease characterized by lesions in the endothelial lining of arteries throughout the body. These lesions (called *fatty plaques* or *atheromas*) start with injury to the endothelium and involve progressive accumulation of lipids (eg, cholesterol), vascular smooth muscle cells, macrophages, lymphocytes, and connective tissue proteins. Over time, the lesions interfere with nutrition of the blood vessel lining; the normally smooth endothelium becomes roughened; and thrombi, necrosis, scarring, and calcification occur. As the lesions develop and enlarge, they protrude into the lumen of the artery, reduce the size of the lumen, reduce blood flow, and may eventually occlude the artery. Severely impaired blood flow leads to damage or death of tissue supplied by the artery. Clinical manifestations vary according to the arteries involved and the extent of vessel obstruction.

Dyslipidemia

Dyslipidemia (also called *hyperlipidemia*) is associated with atherosclerosis and its many pathophysiologic effects (eg, myocardial ischemia and infarction, stroke, peripheral arterial occlusive disease). Ischemic heart disease has a high rate of morbidity and mortality. Elevated total cholesterol and LDL cholesterol, and reduced HDL cholesterol, are the abnormalities that are major risk factors for coronary artery disease. Elevated triglycerides also play a role in cardiovascular disease. For example, high blood levels reflect excessive caloric intake (excessive dietary fats are stored in adipose tissue; excessive proteins and carbohydrates are converted to triglycerides and also stored in adipose tissue) and obesity. High caloric intake also increases the conversion of VLDL to LDL cholesterol, and high dietary intake of triglycerides and saturated fat decreases the activity of LDL receptors and increases synthesis of cholesterol. Very high triglyceride levels are associated with acute pancreatitis.

Dyslipidemia may be primary (ie, genetic or familial) or secondary to dietary habits, other diseases (eg, diabetes mellitus, alcoholism, hypothyroidism, obesity, obstructive liver disease), and medications (eg, beta blockers, cyclosporine, oral estrogens, glucocorticoids, sertraline, thiazide diuretics, anti–human immunodeficiency virus protease inhibitors). Types of dyslipidemias (also called *hyperlipoproteinemias* because increased blood levels of lipoproteins accompany increased blood lipid levels) are described in Box 55-2. Although hypercholesterolemia is usually emphasized, hypertriglyceridemia is also associated with most types of hyperlipoproteinemia.

Initial Management of Dyslipidemia

The Third Report of The National Cholesterol Education Program Expert Panel on Detection, Evaluation, and Treatment of High Blood Cholesterol in Adults (NCEP III) classified blood lipid levels and proposed the following guidelines as treatment goals for clients with lipid abnormalities:

Total serum cholesterol (mg/dL)
Normal or desirable = less than 200
Borderline high = 200 to 239
High = 240 or above
LDL cholesterol (mg/dL)
Optimal = less than 100
Near or above optimal = 100 to 129
Borderline high = 130 to 159
High = 160 to 189
Very high = 190 or above
HDL cholesterol (mg/dL)
High = more than 60
Low = less than 40
Triglycerides (mg/dL)
Normal or desirable = less than 150
Borderline high = 150 to 199
High = 200 to 499
Very high = 500 or above

Overall, the most effective blood lipid profile for prevention or management of atherosclerosis and its sequelae is high HDL cholesterol, low LDL cholesterol, and low total choles-

Box 55-2 Types of Dyslipidemias

Type I is characterized by elevated or normal serum cholesterol, elevated triglycerides, and chylomicronemia. This rare condition may occur in infancy and childhood.

Type IIa (familial hypercholesterolemia) is characterized by a high level of low-density lipoprotein (LDL) cholesterol, a normal level of very–low-density lipoprotein (VLDL), and a normal or slightly increased level of triglycerides. It occurs in children and is a definite risk factor for development of atherosclerosis and coronary artery disease.

Type IIb (combined familial hyperlipoproteinemia) is characterized by increased levels of LDL, VLDL, cholesterol, and triglycerides and lipid deposits (xanthomas) in the feet, knees, and elbows. It occurs in adults.

Type III is characterized by elevations of cholesterol and triglycerides plus abnormal levels of LDL and VLDL. This type usually occurs in middle-aged adults (40–60 years) and is associated with accelerated coronary and peripheral vascular disease.

Type IV is characterized by normal or elevated cholesterol levels, elevated triglycerides, and increased levels of VLDL. This type usually occurs in adults and may be the most common form of hyperlipoproteinemia. Type IV is often secondary to obesity, excessive intake of alcohol, or other diseases. Ischemic heart disease may occur at 40 to 50 years of age.

Type V is characterized by elevated cholesterol and triglyceride levels with an increased level of VLDL and chylomicronemia. This uncommon type usually occurs in adults. Type V is not associated with ischemic heart disease. Instead, it is associated with fat and carbohydrate intolerance, abdominal pain, and pancreatitis, which are relieved by lowering triglyceride levels.

terol. A low triglyceride level is also desirable. For accurate interpretation of a client's lipid profile, blood samples for laboratory testing of triglycerides should be drawn after the client has fasted for 12 hours. Fasting is not required for cholesterol testing.

NCEP III recommends treatment of clients according to their blood levels of total and LDL cholesterol and their risk factors for cardiovascular disease (Table 55-1). Note that therapeutic lifestyle changes (TLC), including exercise, smoking cessation, changes in diet, and drug therapy, are recommended at lower serum cholesterol levels in clients who already have cardiovascular disease or diabetes mellitus. Also, the target LDL serum level is lower in these clients.

Guidelines include the following:

● Assess for, and treat, if present, conditions known to increase blood lipids (eg, diabetes mellitus, hypothyroidism).
● Stop medications known to increase blood lipids, if possible.

TABLE 55-1 National Cholesterol Education Program Recommendations for Treatment of Dyslipidemia

CLIENT'S CARDIOVASCULAR DISEASE STATUS	THERAPEUTIC LIFESTYLE CHANGES (TLC) LDL Cholesterol (mg/dL)	DRUG THERAPY LDL Cholesterol (mg/dL)	GOAL OF THERAPY LDL Cholesterol (mg/dL)
No or one risk factor	≥160	≥190	<160
More than two risk factors	≥130	≥160	<130
Has cardiovascular disease	≥100	≥130	<100

LDL, low-density lipoprotein.

● Start a low-fat diet. A Step I diet contains no more than 30% of calories from fat, less than 10% of calories from saturated fats (eg, meat, dairy products), and less than 300 mg of cholesterol per day. A Step II diet contains no more than 30% of calories from fat, less than 7% of calories from saturated fat, and less than 200 mg of cholesterol per day. The Step II diet is more stringent and may be used initially in clients with more severe dyslipidemia, cardiovascular disease, or diabetes mellitus. It can decrease LDL cholesterol levels by 8% to 15%. Diets with more stringent fat restrictions than the Step II diet are not recommended because they produce little additional reduction in LDL cholesterol; raise serum triglyceride levels; and lower HDL cholesterol concentrations.

● Use the "Mediterranean diet," which includes moderate amounts of monounsaturated fats (eg, canola, olive oils) and polyunsaturated fats (eg, safflower, corn, cottonseed, sesame, soybean, sunflower oils), to also decrease risks of cardiovascular disease.

● Increase dietary intake of soluble fiber (eg, psyllium preparations, oat bran, pectin, fruits and vegetables). This diet lowers serum LDL cholesterol by 5% to 10%.

● Dietary supplements (eg, Cholestin) and cholesterol-lowering margarines (eg, Benecol, Take Control) can help reduce cholesterol levels. These products are considered to be foods, not drugs, and are costly.

● Start a weight-reduction diet if the client is overweight or obese. Weight loss can increase HDL and decrease LDL.

● Emphasize regular aerobic exercise (usually 30 minutes at least three times weekly). This strategy increases blood levels of HDL.

● If the client smokes, assist to develop a cessation plan. In addition to numerous other benefits, HDL levels are higher in nonsmokers.

● If the client is postmenopausal, hormone replacement therapy can raise HDL and lower LDL.

● If the client has elevated serum triglycerides, initial management includes efforts to achieve desirable body weight; ingest low amounts of saturated fat and cho-

lesterol; exercise regularly; stop smoking; and reduce alcohol intake, if indicated. The goal is to reduce serum triglyceride levels to 200 mg/dL or less.

● Unless lipid levels are severely elevated, 6 months of intensive diet therapy and lifestyle modification may be undertaken before drug therapy is considered. It is essential that TLC continue during drug therapy because the benefits of diet, exercise, and drug therapy are additive.

Since the publication of the NCEP III in 2001, numerous clinical trials of statin therapy have been published. In 2004, more intensive treatment recommendations were established for those in the category of "very high" risk. Factors contributing to the increased risk include the presence of established cardiovascular disease or an acute coronary syndrome, with multiple major risk factors such as diabetes, obesity, hypertension (evidence of metabolic syndrome), high triglycerides, low HDL, and severe or poorly controlled risk factors such as continued cigarette smoking. These recommendations included consideration of treatment goals for LDL cholesterol to less than 70 milligrams per deciliter and earlier initiation of drug therapy in the presence of elevated triglyceride and low HDL levels. As current trials are continuing, the lower levels of LDL should be considered a therapeutic option for those at increased risk, with the goal of less than 100 milligrams per deciliter remaining as a strong recommendation for those not at high risk.

GENERAL CHARACTERISTICS OF DRUGS USED FOR MANAGEMENT OF DYSLIPIDEMIA

Dyslipidemic drugs are used to decrease blood lipids; prevent or delay the development of atherosclerotic plaque; promote the regression of existing atherosclerotic plaque; and reduce morbidity and mortality from cardiovascular disease. Clinical data suggest that drug therapy may be efficacious even for those with mild to moderate elevations of LDL cholesterol. The drugs act by altering the production, absorption, metabolism, or removal of lipids and lipoproteins. Drug therapy is initiated when 6 months of dietary and other lifestyle changes fail to decrease dyslipidemia to an acceptable level. It is also recommended for clients with signs and symptoms of coronary heart disease, a strong family history of coronary heart disease or dyslipidemia, or other risk factors for atherosclerotic vascular disease (eg, hypertension, diabetes mellitus, cigarette smoking). Although several dyslipidemic drugs are available, none is effective in all types of dyslipidemia.

DYSLIPIDEMIC DRUGS: CLASSIFICATIONS AND INDIVIDUAL DRUGS

Categories of drugs are described in this section; individual drugs are listed in Table 55-2.

HMG-CoA Reductase Inhibitors

The HMG-CoA reductase inhibitors or statins (eg, **atorvastatin**) inhibit an enzyme (hydroxymethylglutaryl-coenzyme A reductase) required for hepatic synthesis of cholesterol. By decreasing production of cholesterol, these drugs decrease total serum cholesterol, LDL cholesterol, VLDL cholesterol, and triglycerides. They reduce LDL cholesterol within 2 weeks and reach maximal effects in approximately 4 to 6 weeks. HDL cholesterol levels remain unchanged or may increase.

These drugs are useful in treating most of the major types of dyslipidemia and are the most widely used dyslipidemic drugs. Studies indicate that these drugs can reduce the blood levels of C-reactive protein, which is associated with severe arterial inflammation that leads to heart attacks and strokes. The incidence of coronary artery disease is reduced by 25% to 60% and the risk of death from any cause by approximately 30%. Statins also reduce the risk of angina pectoris and peripheral arterial disease as well as the need for angioplasty and coronary artery grafting to increase or restore blood flow to the myocardium.

APPLYING YOUR KNOWLEDGE 55-1
You are counseling Mr. Watkins about his medication. He asks when he will need to have his laboratory work completed. How do you respond?

Atorvastatin is currently the most widely used statin and one of the most widely used drugs in the United States. There is indication that pravastatin may be preferred in clients who have had a transplant or who are receiving immunosuppressants, because it interacts less with immunosuppressant agents than other statins. There is controversy regarding clinical and subclinical effects of individual agents. Several studies have suggested that atorvastatin and **rosuvastatin** may possess some benefits that other statins do not. Multiple outcomes including intimal thickness, results of imaging studies, mortality, incidence of stroke, and progression of

lesions have been studied, but there continue to be questions about the benefit profiles of individual drugs.

Absorption following oral administration varies by drug. **Lovastatin** and **pravastatin** are poorly absorbed; **fluvastatin** has the highest rate of absorption. Most of the statins undergo extensive first-past metabolism by the liver, which results in low levels of drug available for general circulation. Metabolism occurs in the liver, with 80% to 85% of drug metabolites excreted in feces and the remaining excreted in urine.

Statins are usually well tolerated; the most common adverse effects (nausea, constipation, diarrhea, abdominal cramps or pain, headache, skin rash) are usually mild and transient. More serious reactions include rare occurrences of hepatotoxicity and myopathy. Liver function studies should be monitored before onset of therapy, after 6 and 12 weeks of therapy, and intermittently during the course of therapy to detect any elevation or change. Statins can injure muscle tissue, resulting in muscle ache or weakness. Rarely is there progression to myositis and subsequent rhabdomyolysis, defined as muscle disintegration or dissociation. Factors that increase risk of myopathy include advanced age, frail or small body frame, high dosage of statins, concomitant use with fibrates, hypothyroidism, and multiple systemic diseases such as renal insufficiency secondary to diabetic nephropathy. Clients should be advised to notify their health care provider if unexplained muscle pain or tenderness occurs.

APPLYING YOUR KNOWLEDGE 55-2
When educating Mr. Watkins about his new medication, you teach him about common adverse effects. What would be included in your teaching about the adverse effects of atorvastatin? What signs and symptoms of complications would you discuss with him?

Bile Acid Sequestrants

Bile acid sequestrants (eg, **cholestyramine**) bind bile acids in the intestinal lumen. This causes the bile acids to be excreted in feces and prevents their being recirculated to the liver. Loss of bile acids stimulates hepatic synthesis of more bile acids from cholesterol. As more hepatic cholesterol is used to produce bile acids, more serum cholesterol moves into the liver to replenish the supply, thereby lowering serum cholesterol (primarily LDL). LDL cholesterol levels decrease within a week of starting these drugs and reach maximal reductions within a month. When the drugs are stopped, pretreatment LDL cholesterol levels return within a month.

These drugs are used mainly to reduce LDL cholesterol further in clients who are already taking a statin drug. The inhibition of cholesterol synthesis by a statin drug makes bile acid–binding drugs more effective. In addition, the combination increases HDL cholesterol and can further reduce the risk of cardiovascular disorders.

These drugs are not absorbed systemically and their main adverse effects are abdominal fullness, flatulence, and constipation. They may decrease absorption of many oral medications

Table 55-2 Drugs at a Glance: Dyslipidemic Agents

GENERIC/TRADE NAME	CLINICAL INDICATIONS (TYPE OF DYSLIPIDEMIA)	ROUTES AND DOSAGE RANGES	
		Adults	Children
HMG–CoA Reductase Inhibitors (Statins)			
Atorvastatin (Lipitor)	Types IIa and IIb	PO 10–80 mg daily in a single dose	
Fluvastatin (Lescol, Lescol XL)	Types IIa and IIb	PO 40–80 mg daily in 1 or 2 doses	
Lovastatin (Mevacor, Altocor)	Types IIa and IIb	PO 10–80 mg daily in 1 or 2 doses	*<10 y:* not recommended *10–17 y:* 10–40 mg once daily
Pravastatin (Pravachol)	Types IIa and IIb	PO 40–80 mg once daily Elderly, PO 10 mg once daily	
Rosuvastatin (Crestor)	Types IIa and IIb, IV	PO 10–40 mg once daily	*<18 y:* not recommended
Simvastatin (Zocor)	Types 11a, 11b, IV, V	PO 5–80 mg once daily in the evening Elderly, PO 5–20 mg once daily in the evening	
Fibrates			
Fenofibrate (Tricor)	Types IV, V (hypertriglyceridemia)	PO 67 mg once daily, increased if necessary to a maximum dose of 201 mg daily	
Gemfibrozil (Lopid)	Types IV, V (hypertriglyceridemia)	PO 900–1500 mg daily, usually 1200 mg in 2 divided doses, 30 min before morning and evening meals	
Bile Acid Sequestrants			
Cholestyramine (Questran)	Type IIa	PO tablets, 4 g once or twice daily initially, gradually increased at monthly intervals to 8–16 g daily in 2 divided doses. Maximum daily dose, 24 g PO powder, 4 g 1–6 times daily	240 mg/kg/d in 3 divided doses
Colesevelam (Welchol)	Type IIa	PO 3.75 g daily in 1 or 2 doses. Maximum daily dose, 4.375 g	
Colestipol	Type IIa	PO tablets, 2 g once or twice daily initially, gradually increased at 1- to 2-mo intervals, up to 16 g daily PO granules, 5 g daily initially, gradually increased at 1- to 2-mo intervals, up to 30 g daily in single or divided doses	
Cholesterol Absorption Inhibitor			
Ezetimibe (Zetia)	Types IIa and IIb	PO 10 mg once daily	*<10 y:* not recommended *≥10 y:* PO 10 mg once daily
Miscellaneous			
Niacin (immediate-release)	Types II, III, IV, V	PO 2–6 g daily, in 3 or 4 divided doses, with or just after meals	PO 55–87 mg/kg/d, in 3 or 4 divided doses, with or just after meals
Niacin (extended-release)	Types IIa and IIb	PO 500–2000 mg daily	

PO, oral.

(eg, digoxin, folic acid, glipizide, propranolol, tetracyclines, thiazide diuretics, thyroid hormones, fat-soluble vitamins, warfarin). Other drugs should be taken at least 1 hour before or 4 hours after bile acid sequestrants. In addition, dosage of the interactive drug may need to be changed when a bile acid sequestrant is added or withdrawn.

Fibrates

Fibrates are derivatives of fibric acid (eg, **gemfibrozil, fenofibrate**) and are similar to endogenous fatty acids. The drugs increase the oxidation of fatty acids in liver and muscle tissue and thereby decrease hepatic production of triglycerides; decrease VLDL cholesterol; and increase HDL cholesterol. These are the most effective drugs for reducing serum triglyceride levels, and their main indication for use is high serum triglyceride levels (>500 mg/dL). They are also useful for clients with low HDL cholesterol levels. In clients with coronary artery disease, management with gemfibrozil is associated with regression of atherosclerotic lesions on angiography.

These drugs are well absorbed following oral administration. Metabolism occurs in the liver and excretion is by urinary elimination. The main adverse effects are gastrointestinal discomfort and diarrhea, which may occur less often with fenofibrate than with gemfibrozil. The drugs may also increase cholesterol concentration in the biliary tract and formation of gallstones. For clients receiving warfarin, the warfarin dosage should be substantially decreased because fibrates displace warfarin from binding sites on serum albumin.

Niacin

Niacin (nicotinic acid) decreases both cholesterol and triglycerides. It inhibits mobilization of free fatty acids from peripheral tissues, thereby reducing hepatic synthesis of triglycerides and secretion of VLDL, which leads to decreased production of LDL cholesterol. Niacin is the most effective drug for increasing the concentration of HDL cholesterol. Disadvantages of niacin are the high doses required for dyslipidemic effects and the subsequent adverse effects. Niacin commonly causes skin flushing, pruritus, and gastric irritation and may cause hyperglycemia, hyperuricemia, elevated hepatic aminotransferase enzymes, and hepatitis. Flushing can be reduced by starting with small doses, gradually increasing doses, taking doses with meals, and taking 325 milligrams of aspirin about 30 minutes before niacin doses.

Niacin is rapidly absorbed from the gastrointestinal tract. Minimal metabolism occurs by the liver and the majority of the drug is excreted unchanged in the urine.

Niacin is most effective in preventing heart disease when used in combination with another dyslipidemic drug such as a bile acid sequestrant or a fibrate. Its use with a statin lowers serum LDL cholesterol more than either drug alone, but the combination has not been studied in relation to preventing cardiovascular disease.

Cholesterol Absorption Inhibitor

The cholesterol absorption inhibitor (eg, **ezetimibe**), the newest class of dyslipidemic drugs, acts in the small intestine to inhibit absorption of cholesterol and decrease the delivery of intestinal cholesterol to the liver, resulting in reduced hepatic cholesterol stores and increased clearance of cholesterol from the blood. This distinct mechanism is complementary to that of HMG-CoA reductase inhibitors.

This drug reduces total cholesterol and triglycerides, and increase HDL. The drug is indicated as an adjunctive therapy to dietary management of hyperlipidemia. Administration may be with or without food, but it should be taken 2 hours before or 4 hours after a bile acid sequestrant. Therapeutic response is achieved within 2 weeks of initiation of therapy and maintained with continued use. The most common adverse effects include hypersensitivity reactions such as rash and nausea. This drug is contraindicated in pregnancy.

NURSING PROCESS

Assessment

Assess the client's status in relation to atherosclerotic vascular disease.
● Identify risk factors:
  ● Hypertension
  ● Diabetes mellitus
  ● High intake of dietary fat and refined sugars
  ● Obesity
  ● Inadequate exercise
  ● Cigarette smoking
  ● Family history of atherosclerotic disorders
  ● Dyslipidemia
● Signs and symptoms depend on the specific problem:
  ● Dyslipidemia is manifested by elevated serum cholesterol (>200 mg/100 mL), triglycerides (>150 mg/100 mL), or both.
  ● Coronary artery atherosclerosis is manifested by myocardial ischemia (angina pectoris, myocardial infarction).
  ● Cerebrovascular insufficiency may be manifested by syncope, memory loss, transient ischemic attacks (TIAs), or strokes. Impairment of blood flow to the brain is caused primarily by atherosclerosis in the carotid, vertebral, or cerebral arteries.
  ● Peripheral arterial insufficiency is manifested by impaired blood flow in the legs (weak or absent pulses; cool, pale extremities; intermittent claudication; leg pain at rest; and development of gangrene, usually in the toes because they are most distal to blood supply). This condition results from atherosclerosis in the distal abdominal aorta, the iliac arteries, and the femoral and smaller arteries in the legs.

Nursing Diagnoses

- Ineffective Tissue Perfusion related to interruption of arterial blood flow
- Imbalanced Nutrition: More Than Body Requirements of fats and calories
- Anxiety related to risks of atherosclerotic cardiovascular disease
- Disturbed Body Image related to the need for lifestyle changes
- Noncompliance related to dietary restrictions and adverse drug reactions
- Deficient Knowledge related to drug and diet therapy of dyslipidemia

Planning/Goals

The client will
- Take lipid-lowering drugs as prescribed
- Decrease dietary intake of saturated fats and cholesterol
- Lose weight if obese and maintain the lower weight
- Have periodic measurements of blood lipids
- Avoid preventable adverse drug effects
- Receive positive reinforcement for efforts to lower blood lipid levels
- Feel less anxious and more in control as risks of atherosclerotic cardiovascular disease are decreased

Interventions

Use measures to prevent, delay, or minimize atherosclerosis.

- Help clients control risk factors. Ideally, primary prevention begins in childhood with healthful eating habits (eg, avoiding excessive fats, meat, and dairy products; obtaining adequate amounts of all nutrients, including dietary fiber; avoiding obesity), exercise, and avoiding cigarette smoking. However, changing habits to a more healthful lifestyle is helpful at any time, before or after disease manifestations appear. Weight loss often reduces blood lipids and lipoproteins to a normal range. Changing habits is difficult for most people, even those with severe symptoms.
- Use measures to increase blood flow to tissues:
  - Exercise is helpful in developing collateral circulation in the heart and legs. Collateral circulation involves use of secondary vessels in response to tissue ischemia related to obstruction of the principal vessels. Clients with angina pectoris or previous myocardial infarction require a carefully planned and supervised program of progressive exercise. Those with peripheral arterial insufficiency usually can increase exercise tolerance by walking regularly. Distances should be determined by occurrence of pain and must be individualized.
  - Posture and position may be altered to increase blood flow to the legs in clients with peripheral arterial insufficiency. Elevating the head of the bed and having the legs horizontal or dependent may help. Elevating the feet is usually contraindicated unless edema is present or likely to develop.
- Although drug therapy is being increasingly used to prevent or manage atherosclerotic disorders, a major therapeutic option for management of occlusive vascular disease is surgical removal of atherosclerotic plaque or revascularization procedures. Thus, severe angina pectoris may be relieved by a coronary artery bypass procedure that detours blood flow around occluded vessels. This procedure also may be done after a myocardial infarction. The goal is to prevent infarction or reinfarction. TIAs may be relieved by carotid endarterectomy; the goal is to prevent a stroke. Peripheral arterial insufficiency may be relieved by aortofemoral, femoropopliteal, or other bypass grafts that detour around occluded vessels. Although these procedures increase blood flow to ischemic tissues, they do not halt progression of atherosclerosis.

  The nursing role in relation to these procedures is to provide excellent preoperative and postoperative nursing care to promote healing, prevent infection, maintain patency of grafts, and help the client to achieve optimum function.

- Provide appropriate teaching related to drug therapy (see accompanying display).
- Any dyslipidemic drug therapy must be accompanied by an appropriate diet; refer clients to a nutritionist. Overeating or gaining weight may decrease or cancel the lipid-lowering effects of the drugs.
- Encourage adult clients to have their serum cholesterol level measured at least once every 5 years. Adults and children with a personal or family history of dyslipidemia or other risk factors should be tested more often.
- The most effective measures for preventing dyslipidemia and atherosclerosis are those related to a healthful lifestyle (eg, diet low in cholesterol and saturated fats, weight control, exercise).
- Help clients and family members understand the desirability of lowering high blood lipid levels before serious cardiovascular diseases develop.

Evaluation

- Observe for decreased blood levels of total and LDL cholesterol and triglycerides; observe for increased levels of HDL cholesterol.
- Observe and interview regarding compliance with instructions for drug, diet, and other therapeutic measures.
- Observe and interview regarding adverse drug effects.
- Validate the client's ability to identify foods high and low in cholesterol and saturated fats.

General Considerations

☑ Heart and blood vessel disease causes a great deal of illness and many deaths. The basic problem is usually atherosclerosis, in which the arteries are partly blocked by cholesterol deposits. Cholesterol, a waxy substance made in the liver, is necessary for normal body functioning. However, excessive amounts in the blood increase the likelihood of having a heart attack, stroke, or leg pain from inadequate blood flow. One type of cholesterol (low-density lipoprotein [LDL] or "bad") attaches to artery walls, where it can enlarge over time and block blood flow. The other type (high-density lipoprotein [HDL] or "good") carries cholesterol away from the artery and back to the liver, where it can be broken down. Thus, the healthiest blood cholesterol levels are low total cholesterol (<200 mg/dL), low LDL (<130 mg/dL), and high HDL (>35 mg/dL). High levels of blood triglycerides, another type of fat, are also unhealthy.

☑ Dyslipidemic drugs are given to lower high concentrations of fats (total cholesterol, LDL cholesterol, and triglycerides) in your blood. The goal of management is to prevent heart attack, stroke, and peripheral arterial disease. If you already have heart and blood vessel disease, the drugs can improve your symptoms, activity level, and quality of life.

☑ A low-fat diet is needed. This is often the first step in treating high cholesterol or triglyceride levels, and may be prescribed for 6 months or longer before drug therapy is begun. When drug therapy is prescribed, the diet should be continued. An important part is reducing the amount of saturated fat (from meats, dairy products). In addition, eating a bowl of oat cereal daily can help lower cholesterol by 5% to 10%. Diet counseling by a dietitian or nutritionist can be helpful in developing guidelines that fit your needs and lifestyle. Overeating or gaining weight may decrease or cancel the lipid-lowering effects of the drugs.

☑ Other lifestyle changes that can help improve cholesterol levels include regular aerobic exercise (raises HDL); losing weight (raises HDL, lowers LDL, lowers triglycerides); and not smoking (HDL levels are higher in nonsmokers).

☑ Adults should have measurements of total cholesterol and HDL cholesterol at least once every 5 years. People with a personal or family history of dyslipidemia or other risk factors for cardiovascular disease should be tested more often.

☑ Techniques for home monitoring of cholesterol levels are improving and are more available for self-use. Clients may be instructed to perform self-monitoring and report their results to their health care provider. At present, equipment and supplies can be expensive, and most are not reimbursed by insurance companies.

☑ Atorvastatin and other statin-type dyslipidemic drugs may increase sensitivity to sunlight. Avoid prolonged exposure to the sun, use sunscreens, and wear protective clothing.

☑ Gemfibrozil may cause dizziness or blurred vision and should be used cautiously while driving or performing other tasks that require alertness, coordination, or physical dexterity. It also may cause abdominal pain, diarrhea, nausea, or vomiting. Notify a health care provider if these symptoms become severe.

☑ Skin flushing may occur with niacin. If it is distressing, taking one regular aspirin tablet (325 mg) 30 to 60 minutes before the niacin dose may decrease this reaction. Flushing usually decreases in a few days, but may recur when niacin dosage is increased. Ask your health care provider if there is any reason you should not take aspirin.

☑ Cholestyramine and colestipol can cause constipation. Increasing intake of dietary fiber can help prevent this adverse effect.

Self-Administration

☑ Take lovastatin with food; take atorvastatin, fluvastatin, pravastatin, or simvastatin in the evening, with or without food. Food decreases stomach upset associated with lovastatin. All of these drugs may be more effective if taken in the evening or at bedtime, probably because more cholesterol is produced at nighttime and the drugs block cholesterol production.

☑ Take fenofibrate with food; food increases drug absorption.

☑ Take gemfibrozil on an empty stomach, 30 minutes before morning and evening meals.

☑ Take immediate-release niacin with meals to decrease stomach upset; take timed-release niacin without regard to meals.

☑ Mix cholestyramine powder and colestipol granules with water or other fluids, soups, cereals, or fruits such as applesauce and follow with more fluid. These drug forms should not be taken dry.

☑ Do not take cholestyramine, coleseveiam, or colestipol with other drugs because they may prevent absorption of the other drugs. If taking other drugs, take them 1 hour before or 4 to 6 hours after cholestyramine or colestipol.

☑ Swallow colestipol tablets whole; do not cut, crush, or chew.

☑ Take ezetimibe with or without food at the same time each day. If taken in combination with a statin, take it at the same time (usually in the evening).

APPLYING YOUR KNOWLEDGE 55-3:
HOW CAN YOU AVOID THIS MEDICATION ERROR?
You arrive at Mr. Watkins's home at 8:45AM. Mr. Watkins greets you and asks if you mind waiting a moment while he finishes his breakfast. While you are waiting, you prepare the correct doses of both his atorvastatin and gemfibrozil, which he receives routinely at 9:00AM. You then administer his medication.

PRINCIPLES OF THERAPY

Drug Selection

Drug selection is based on the type of dyslipidemia and its severity. For single-drug therapy to lower cholesterol, a statin is preferred. To lower both cholesterol and triglycerides, a statin, a cholesterol absorption inhibitor, gemfibrozil, or niacin may be used. To lower triglycerides, gemfibrozil, a cholesterol absorption inhibitor, or niacin may be used. Gemfibrozil, rather than niacin, is usually preferred for people with diabetes because niacin increases blood sugar.

When monotherapy is not effective, combination therapy is rational because the drugs act by different mechanisms. In general, a statin combined with a cholesterol absorption inhibitor or a bile acid sequestrant, or niacin combined with a bile acid sequestrant are the most effective combinations in reducing total and LDL cholesterol. A fibrate, a cholesterol absorption inhibitor, or niacin may be used when a goal of therapy is to increase the level of HDL cholesterol. However, a fibrate–statin combination should be avoided because of increased risks of severe myopathy, and a niacin–statin combination increases the risks of hepatotoxicity. Adverse reactions from combination statin and cholesterol absorption inhibitor therapy are reported to be similar to those from statins alone.

Use in Special Populations

Use in Various Ethnic Groups

Little information has been reported on racial or ethnic differences for lipid-lowering drugs. Members of minority populations (eg, African Americans, Mexican Americans) are less likely to be treated than Caucasians. Despite an increased prevalence of diabetes and obesity, American Indians appear to have lower cholesterol levels than the United States population as a whole. This suggests that diet and exercise may be more useful than lipid-lowering drugs for this group.

Use in Children

Dyslipidemia occurs in children and may lead to atherosclerotic cardiovascular disease, including myocardial infarction, in early adulthood. Dyslipidemia is diagnosed with total serum cholesterol levels of 200 milligrams per deciliter or above (desirable level, <170) and LDL cholesterol levels of 130 milligrams per deciliter or above (desirable level, <110). Early identification and management are needed. As with adults, initial management consists of diet therapy (for 6–12 months) and management of any secondary causes, especially with younger children. With additional risk factors or primary familial hypercholesterolemia (type IIa), however, these measures are not likely to be effective without drug therapy.

Dyslipidemic drugs are not recommended for children younger than 10 years of age. Lovastatin is approved for use in children 10 to 17 years old. Oral dosing recommendations are 10 to 20 milligrams daily with a meal, initially, and increasing up to 40 milligrams daily as necessary with increases made at least 4 weeks apart. Other statin drugs are not recommended in children younger than 18 years of age, and the safety and effectiveness of the fibrates have not been established. Bile acid sequestrants are considered the drugs of choice, and niacin also may be used. Despite considerable use of bile acid sequestrants, children's dosages have only

been established for cholestyramine. Recommendations for oral dosing of cholestyramine are 240 milligrams per kilogram of body weight per day, to be given in three divided doses. Niacin dosage is 55 to 87 milligrams per kilogram of body weight per day, to be given orally 3 to 4 times a day with or just after meals. The long-term consequences of dyslipidemic drug therapy in children are unknown.

Use in Older Adults

As with younger adults, diet, exercise, and weight control should be tried first. When drug therapy is required, statins are effective for lowering LDL cholesterol and usually are well tolerated by older adults. However, they are expensive. Niacin and bile acid sequestrants are effective, but older adults do not tolerate their adverse effects very well. In postmenopausal women, estrogen replacement therapy increases HDL cholesterol.

Older adults often have diabetes, impaired liver function, or other conditions that raise blood lipid levels. Thus, management of secondary causes is especially important. The older adult is also likely to have cardiovascular and other disorders that increase the adverse effects of dyslipidemic drugs. Overall, use of dyslipidemic drugs should be cautious, with close monitoring for therapeutic and adverse effects. Lower starting dosages are recommended for fenofibrate (67 mg/day), pravastatin (10 mg/day), and simvastatin (5 mg/day). *Cholesterol absorption inhibitor* as monotherapy (without statins) does not require dosage reduction in geriatric clients.

Use in Clients With Renal Impairment

Statins are metabolized by the liver and excreted partly through the kidneys (their main route of excretion is through bile). Drug plasma concentrations may be increased in clients with renal impairment and these drugs should be used cautiously; some need reduced dosage.

- With *atorvastatin,* plasma levels are not affected and dosage reductions are not needed.
- With *fluvastatin,* because it is cleared hepatically and less than 6% of the dose is excreted in urine, dosage reduction for mild to moderate renal impairment is unnecessary. Use caution with severe impairment.
- With *lovastatin,* plasma concentrations are increased in clients with severe renal impairment (creatinine clearance <30 mL/minute), and doses above 20 mg/day should be used with caution.
- With *pravastatin,* initiate therapy with 10 mg/day.
- With *simvastatin,* initiate therapy with 5 mg/day and monitor closely.

Cholesterol absorption inhibitors as monotherapy (without statins) do not require dosage reduction in renal insufficiency.

Fibrates are excreted mainly by the kidneys and therefore accumulate in the serum of clients with renal impairment. With *gemfibrozil*, there have been reports of worsening renal impairment in clients whose baseline serum creatinine levels were higher than 2 milligrams per deciliter. A different type of dyslipidemic drug may be preferred in these clients. *Fenofibrate* is contraindicated in clients with severe renal impairment, and the recommended starting dose is 67 milligrams per day in clients with a creatinine clearance of less than 50 milliliters per minute. Drug and dose effects on renal function and triglyceride levels should be evaluated before dosage is increased.

Use in Clients With Hepatic Impairment

Statins are metabolized in the liver and may accumulate in clients with impaired hepatic function. They are contraindicated in clients with active liver disease or unexplained elevations of serum aspartate or alanine aminotransferase. They should be used cautiously, in reduced dosages, for clients who ingest substantial amounts of alcohol or who have a history of liver disease.

Liver function tests are recommended before starting a statin, at 6 and 12 weeks after starting the drug or increasing the dose, then every 6 months. Monitor clients who have increased serum aminotransferases until the abnormal values resolve. If the increases are more than three times the upper limit of normal levels and persist, the dose should be reduced or the drug discontinued.

Cholesterol absorption inhibitors as monotherapy (without statins) do not require dosage reduction in mild hepatic insufficiency. *Fibrates* may cause hepatotoxicity. Abnormal elevations of serum aminotransferases have occurred with both gemfibrozil and fenofibrate, but they usually subside when the drug is discontinued. Fenofibrate is contraindicated in severe hepatic impairment, including clients with primary biliary cirrhosis, pre-existing gallbladder disease, and persistent elevations in liver function test results. In addition, hepatitis (hepatocellular, chronic active, and cholestatic) has been reported after use of fenofibrate from a few weeks to several years. Liver function tests should be monitored during the first year of drug administration. The drug should be discontinued if elevated enzyme levels persist at more than three times the normal limit.

Niacin may cause hepatotoxicity, especially with doses above 2 grams daily, with timed-release preparations, and if given in combination with a statin or a fibrate.

Use in Home Care

For a client with dyslipidemia, the home care nurse should reinforce teaching about the role of blood lipids in causing myocardial infarction, stroke, and peripheral arterial insufficiency; the prescribed management regimen and its goals; and the importance of improving dyslipidemia in preventing or improving cardiovascular disorders. In addition, the client may need assistance in obtaining blood tests (eg, lipids, liver function tests) and dietary counseling. Increasing availability of home cholesterol-monitoring devices will require additional client teaching about technique and interpretation of the results.

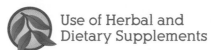 ## Use of Herbal and Dietary Supplements

Flax or flax seed is used internally as a laxative and a dyslipidemic agent. Absorption of all medications may be decreased when taken with flax, resulting in a less than therapeutic effect. Garlic is reportedly used as a dyslipidemic agent and as a possible antihypertensive, but there is little scientific support for such use. Bleeding may be increased when garlic is used with anticoagulants, and insulin doses may need to be decreased as a result of the hypoglycemic effect of garlic. Green tea is commonly used for its dyslipidemic effect and the caffeinated product can be a central nervous system stimulant. Soy is used as a food source and has been researched extensively. Use of soy to lower cholesterol (LDL and total cholesterol) has been documented. Significant interactions with other herbs or drugs have not been reported.

N U R S I N G   A C T I O N S

Drugs for Dyslipidemia

NURSING ACTIONS	RATIONALE/EXPLANATION
1. Administer accurately	
a. Give lovastatin with food; give fluvastatin on an empty stomach or at bedtime. Atorvastatin, pravastatin, or simvastatin may be given with or without food in the evening. Avoid giving with grapefruit juice.	Food decreases gastrointestinal (GI) upset associated with lovastatin. These drugs are more effective if taken in the evening or at bedtime, because more cholesterol is produced by the liver at night and the drugs block cholesterol production. Grapefruit juice increases serum drug levels.

(continued)

NURSING ACTIONS	RATIONALE/EXPLANATION
b. Give fenofibrate with food.	Food increases drug absorption.
c. Give gemfibrozil on an empty stomach, about 30 minutes before morning and evening meals.	
d. Give immediate-release niacin with meals; give timed-release niacin without regard to meals.	The immediate-release formulation may cause gastric irritation.
e. Mix cholestyramine powder and colestipol granules with water or other fluids, soups, cereals, or fruits such as applesauce and follow with more fluid.	These drug forms should not be taken dry.
f. Do not give cholestyramine or colestipol with other drugs; give them 1 hour before or 4–6 hours after cholestyramine or colestipol.	Cholestyramine and colestipol prevent absorption of many drugs.
g. Instruct clients to swallow colestipol tablets whole; do not cut, crush, or chew.	
h. Give ezetimibe with or without food at the same time each day; give at night if used in combination with a statin.	Food does not affect absorption.
i. Give ezetimibe 2 hours before or 4 hours after bile sequestrants.	Cholestyramine and colestipol prevent absorption of many drugs.

2. Observe for therapeutic effects

a. Decreased levels of total serum cholesterol, low-density lipoprotein cholesterol, and triglycerides, and increased levels of high-density lipoprotein cholesterol.	With statins, effects occur in 1–2 wk, with maximum effects in 4–6 wk. With fibrates and niacin, effects occur in approximately 1 mo. With cholestyramine and colestipol, maximum effects occur in approximately 1 mo.

3. Observe for adverse effects

a. GI problems—nausea, vomiting, flatulence, constipation or diarrhea, abdominal discomfort	GI symptoms are the most common adverse effects of dyslipidemic drugs. Constipation is especially common with cholestyramine and colestipol.
b. With lovastatin and related drugs, observe for GI upset (see 2a), skin rash, pruritus, and myopathy.	Adverse effects are usually mild and of short duration. A less common but potentially serious effect is liver dysfunction, usually manifested by increased levels of serum aminotransferases. Serum aminotransferases (aspartate and alanine aminotransferase) should be measured before starting the drug, every 4–6 weeks during the first 3 months, then every 6–12 weeks or after dosage increases for 1 year, then every 6 months.
c. With niacin, flushing of the face and neck, pruritus, and skin rash may occur, as well as tachycardia, hypotension, and dizziness.	These symptoms may be prominent when nicotinic acid is used to lower blood lipids because relatively high doses are required. Aspirin 325 mg, 30 minutes before nicotinic acid, decreases the flushing reaction.

4. Observe for drug interactions

a. Drugs that *increase* effects of lovastatin and related drugs:	
(1) Azole antifungals (eg, fluconazole, itraconazole)	Risk of myopathy is increased. It is recommended that statin therapy be interrupted temporarily if systemic azole antifungals are needed.
(2) Cyclosporine	Risk of severe myopathy or rhabdomyolysis is increased.
(3) Erythromycin	Risk of severe myopathy or rhabdomyolysis is increased.
(4) Fibrate dyslipidemics (eg, fenofibrate, gemfibrozil)	Risk of severe myopathy or rhabdomyolysis is increased.
(5) Niacin	Risk of severe myopathy or rhabdomyolysis is increased.
(6) Drugs that *increase* effects of fluvastatin:	
(a) Alcohol, cimetidine, ranitidine, omeprazole	Increased blood levels

NURSING ACTIONS	RATIONALE/EXPLANATION
(7) Drugs that *increase* effects of ezetimibe:	
(a) Cyclosporine	Increased blood levels
b. Drugs that *decrease* effects of lovastatin and related drugs:	
(1) Bile acid sequestrant dyslipidemics	Decreased blood levels unless the drugs are taken 1–4 hours apart
(2) Antacids	Decrease absorption of atorvastatin
(3) Isradipine	This calcium channel blocker may decrease blood levels of lovastatin and its metabolites by increasing their hepatic metabolism.
(4) Rifampin	Decreases blood levels of fluvastatin
c. Drugs that *decrease* effects of fibrate dyslipidemic drugs:	
(1) Bile acid sequestrant dyslipidemic drugs	Decrease absorption unless the fibrate is taken about 1 hour before or 4–6 hours after the bile acid sequestrant

APPLYING YOUR KNOWLEDGE: ANSWERS

55-1 Inform Mr. Watkins that he will need to have blood analysis performed in 4 to 6 weeks. He will need to be without food for the triglyceride level. In addition to lipid levels, the physician will check liver function.

55-2 Although this group of drugs is usually well tolerated, potential adverse effects include nausea, constipation, diarrhea, abdominal cramps or pain, headache, and skin rash. Tell Mr. Watkins to notify his health care provider if he notices **unexplained muscle pain or tenderness:** This can be a warning sign of rhabdomyolysis, a destruction of the muscle. Clients at higher risk are the elderly; those on a high dose of a statin; those with a small body frame; and those concurrently taking gemfibrozil, such as Mr. Watkins.

55-3 Gemfibrozil must be administered at least 30 minutes before food and on an empty stomach.

Review and Application Exercises

Short Answer Exercises

1. How would you describe dyslipidemia to a client?

2. What is the goal of management of dyslipidemia?

3. Differentiate lipid-lowering drugs according to their mechanisms of action.

4. What are the main nonpharmacologic measures to decrease total and LDL cholesterol and increase HDL cholesterol?

5. What are the main nonpharmacologic measures to decrease serum triglyceride levels?

NCLEX-Style Questions

6. The primary focus for decreasing lipids is which of the following?
   a. HDL
   b. triglycerides
   c. LDL
   d. total cholesterol

7. HMG-CoA reductase inhibitors (statins) are best administered
   a. with breakfast
   b. at noon
   c. with a snack in the afternoon
   d. at night or bedtime

8. Flushing, a common adverse effect of niacin therapy, can be decreased by
   a. taking half the dose in the morning and half the dose at night
   b. taking 325 mg aspirin 30 min before the niacin
   c. taking the drug on an empty stomach
   d. taking niacin as monotherapy for dyslipidemia

9. A 48-year-old man visits the health care provider for his annual checkup. Assessment findings reveal a slight increase in blood pressure and a total serum cholesterol of 240 mg/dL. What can the nurse anticipate as the preferred treatment for this client?
   a. a low-lipid diet and an exercise program
   b. a low-lipid diet and a cholesterol synthesis inhibitor
   c. an exercise program and a fibrate
   d. a low-lipid diet, an exercise program, and niacin

10. A 36-year-old female client has been taking lovastatin 40 mg PO daily for 6 months to treat dyslipidemia. At a clinic appointment, she tells the nurse she is 6 weeks' pregnant. The nurse understands that her pregnancy will require
   a. increasing the dose of prenatal vitamins
   b. reducing the dosage to 20 mg PO daily
   c. increasing the dosage to 40 mg PO twice daily
   d. discontinuing the drug immediately

Selected References

Drug facts and comparisons. (Updated monthly). St. Louis: Facts and Comparisons.

Karch, A. M. (2005). *2006 Lippincott's nursing drug guide.* Philadelphia: Lippincott Williams & Wilkins.

Matfin, G., & Porth, C. M. (2005). Alterations in cardiac function. In C. M. Porth (Ed.), *Pathophysiology: Concepts of altered health states* (7th ed., pp. 475–504). Philadelphia: Lippincott Williams & Wilkins.

National Institutes of Health Expert Panel. (2001). *Third report of the National Cholesterol Education Program (NCEP) Expert Panel on Detection, Evaluation, and Treatment of High Blood Cholesterol in Adults (Adult Treatment Panel III)* (NIH Publication No. 01-3670). Bethesda, MD: National Institutes of Health.

North American Nursing Diagnosis Association. (2003). *Nursing diagnoses: Definitions & classification 2003–2004.* Philadelphia: Author.

Ross, J. (2003). Home test measures total cholesterol. *Nurse Practitioner, 28*(7), 52–53.

Skidmore-Roth, L. (2004). *Mosby's handbook of herbs & natural supplements* (2nd ed.). St. Louis: Mosby.

Smeltzer, S. C., & Bare, B. G. (2004). *Brunner & Suddarth's textbook of medical-surgical nursing* (10th ed., pp. 712–762). Philadelphia: Lippincott Williams & Wilkins.

Talbert, R. L. (2002). Hyperlipidemia. In J. T. DiPiro, R. L. Talbert, G. C. Yee, G. R. Matzke, B. G. Wells, & L. M. Posey (Eds.), *Pharmacotherapy: A pathophysiologic approach* (5th ed., pp. 395–418). New York: McGraw-Hill.

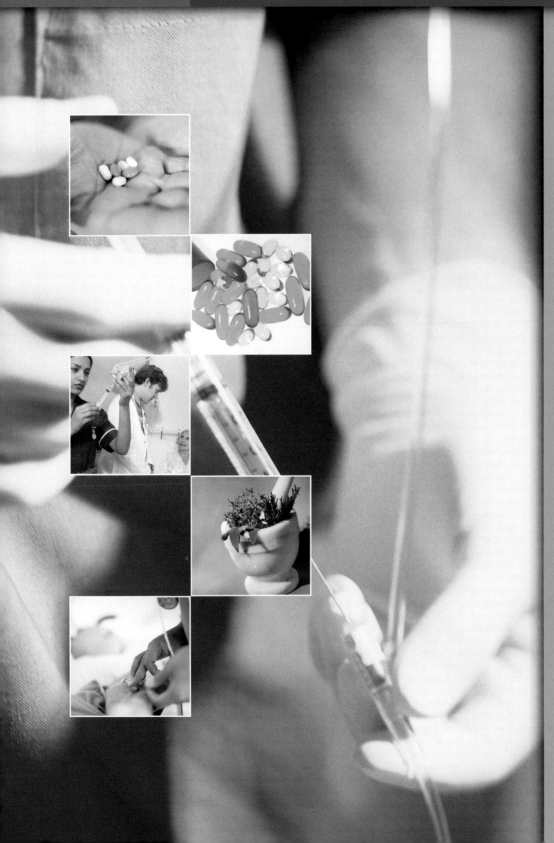

SECTION

9

Drugs Affecting the Digestive System

CHAPTER OUTLINE

56 Physiology of the Digestive System

57 Nutritional Support Products, Vitamins and Mineral—Electrolytes

58 Drugs to Aid Weight Management

59 Drugs Used for Peptic Ulcer and Acid Reflux Disorders

60 Laxatives and Cathartics

61 Antidiarrheals

62 Antiemetics

Physiology of the Digestive System

OBJECTIVES

After studying this chapter, you will be able to:

1. Review roles of the main digestive tract structures.
2. List common signs and symptoms affecting gastrointestinal functions.
3. Identify general categories of drugs used to treat gastrointestinal disorders.
4. Discuss the effects of nongastrointestinal drugs on gastrointestinal functioning.

INTRODUCTION

The digestive system (Figure 56-1) consists of the alimentary canal (a tube extending from the oral cavity to the anus, approximately 25 to 30 feet [7.5–9 m] long) and the accessory organs (salivary glands, gallbladder, liver, and pancreas). The main function of the system is to provide the body with fluids, nutrients, and electrolytes in a form that can be used at the cellular level. The system also disposes of waste products that result from the digestive process.

The alimentary canal has the same basic structure throughout. The layers of the wall are mucosa, connective tissue, and muscle. Peristalsis propels food through the tract and mixes the food bolus with digestive juices. Stimulation of the parasympathetic nervous system (by vagus nerves) increases motility and secretions. Sympathetic stimulation promotes sphincter function and inhibits motility. The tract has an abundant blood supply, which increases cell regeneration and healing. Blood flow increases during digestion and absorption. Blood flow decreases with strenuous exercise, sympathetic nervous system stimulation (ie, "fight or flight"), aging (secondary to decreased cardiac output and atherosclerosis),

and conditions that shunt blood away from the digestive tract (eg, heart failure, atherosclerosis).

STRUCTURES OF THE DIGESTIVE SYSTEM

Oral Cavity

In the oral cavity, chewing mechanically breaks food into smaller particles, which can be swallowed more easily and provide a larger surface area for enzyme action. Food is also mixed with saliva, which lubricates the food bolus for swallowing and initiates the digestion of starch.

Esophagus

The esophagus is a musculofibrous tube about 10 inches (25 cm) long; its main function is to convey food from the pharynx to the stomach. It secretes a small amount of mucus and has some peristaltic movement. Each end of the esophagus functions as a sphincter. The upper esophageal sphincter prevents air from entering the esophagus during inspiration.

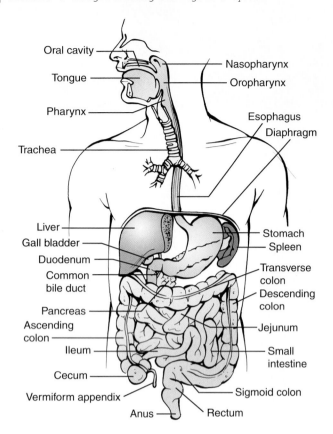

FIGURE 56-1 The digestive system.

The last 2 centimeters of the esophagus is the lower esophageal sphincter (LES). The function of the LES is to prevent reflux of acidic gastric contents into the esophagus.

Stomach

The stomach is a dilated area that serves as a reservoir. It churns and mixes the food with digestive juices; secretes mucus, hydrochloric acid, and enzymes; starts protein break-down; and secretes intrinsic factor, which is necessary for absorption of vitamin B$_{12}$ from the ileum. Although there is much diffusion of water and electrolytes through the gastric mucosa in both directions, there is little absorption of these substances. Carbohydrates and amino acids are also poorly absorbed. Only a few highly lipid-soluble substances, such as alcohol and some drugs, are absorbed in moderate quan-tities from the stomach.

The inlet of the stomach, the cardiac orifice, is at the ter-minal end of the esophagus. The stomach outlet is the pylorus, a ring-like muscle that opens into the beginning of the duo-denum. The stomach normally holds about 1000 milliliters comfortably and empties in about 4 hours. Nu3merous factors influence the rate of gastric emptying, including the size of the pylorus, gastric motility, type of food, fluidity of chyme (the material produced by gastric digestion of food), and the

state of the duodenum. Factors that cause rapid emptying include carbohydrate foods, increased motility, fluid chyme, and an empty duodenum. The stomach empties more slowly with decreased gastric tone and motility, fatty foods, chyme of excessive acidity, and a duodenum that contains fats, pro-teins, or chyme of excessive acidity. When fats are present, the duodenal mucosa produces a hormone, enterogastrone, which inhibits gastric secretion and motility. This allows a longer time for the digestion of fats in the small intestine.

Small Intestine

The small intestine consists of the duodenum, jejunum, and ileum and is approximately 20 feet (6 m) long. The duodenum makes up the first 10 to 12 inches (25–30 cm) of the small intestine. The pancreatic and bile ducts empty into the duode-num at the papilla of Vater. The small intestine contains numer-ous glands that secrete digestive enzymes, hormones, and mucus. For the most part, digestion and absorption occur in the small intestine, including absorption of most orally admin-istered drugs.

Large Intestine

The large intestine consists of the cecum, colon, rectum, and anus. The ileum opens into the cecum. The colon secretes mucus and absorbs water.

Pancreas

The pancreas secretes enzymes required for the digestion of carbohydrates, proteins, and fats. It also secretes insulin and glucagon, hormones that regulate glucose metabolism and blood sugar levels.

Gallbladder

The gallbladder is a small pouch attached to the underside of the liver that stores and concentrates bile. It has a capacity of 50 to 60 milliliters. The gallbladder releases bile when fats are present in the duodenum.

Liver

The liver is a vital organ that performs numerous functions. It receives about 1500 milliliters of blood per minute, or 25% to 30% of the total cardiac output. About three fourths of the blood flow is venous blood from the stomach, intestines, spleen, and pancreas (portal circulation); the remainder is arterial blood through the hepatic artery. The hepatic artery carries blood to the connective tissue of the liver and bile ducts, then empties into the hepatic sinuses. Arterial blood mixes with blood from the portal circulation. Venous blood from the liver flows into the inferior vena cava for return to the systemic circulation. The ample blood flow facilitates specific hepatic functions, which include the following:

- **Blood reservoir.** The liver can eject 500 to 1000 mL of blood into the general circulation in response to stress, decreased blood volume, and sympathetic nervous system stimulation (eg, hemorrhagic or hypovolemic shock).

- **Blood filter and detoxifier.** Kupffer's cells in the liver phagocytize bacteria carried from the intestines by the portal vein. They also break down worn-out erythrocytes, saving iron for reuse in hemoglobin synthesis, and form bilirubin, a waste product excreted in bile. The liver metabolizes many body secretions and most drugs to prevent accumulation and harmful effects on body tissues.

    Most drugs are active as the parent compound and are metabolized in the liver to an inactive metabolite, which is then excreted by the kidneys. However, some drugs become active only after formation of a metabolite in the liver.

    The liver detoxifies or alters substances by oxidation, hydrolysis, or conjugation. Conjugation involves combining a chemical substance with an endogenous substance to produce an inactive or harmless compound. Essentially all steroid hormones, including adrenal corticosteroids and sex hormones, are at least partially conjugated in the liver and secreted into the bile. When the liver is damaged, these hormones may accumulate in body fluids and cause symptoms of hormone excess.

- **Metabolism of carbohydrate, fat, and protein.** In carbohydrate metabolism, the liver converts glucose to glycogen for storage and reconverts glycogen to glucose when needed to maintain an adequate blood sugar concentration. Excess glucose that cannot be converted to glycogen is converted to fat. The liver also changes fructose and galactose, which cannot be used by body cells, to glucose, which provides energy for cellular metabolism. Fats are synthesized and catabolized by the liver. Amino acids from protein breakdown may be used to form glycogen, plasma proteins, and enzymes.

- **Storage of nutrients.** In addition to glycogen, the liver also stores fat-soluble vitamins (ie, vitamins A, D, E, K), vitamin B_{12}, iron, phospholipids, cholesterol, and small amounts of protein and fat.

- **Synthesis** of bile; serum albumin and globulin; prothrombin; fibrinogen; blood coagulation factors V, VII, VIII, IX, XI, and XII; and urea. Formation of urea removes ammonia from body fluids. Large amounts of ammonia are formed by intestinal bacteria and absorbed into the blood. If the ammonia is not converted to urea by the liver, plasma ammonia concentrations rise to toxic levels and cause hepatic coma and death.

- **Production of body heat** by continuous cellular metabolism. The liver is the body organ with the highest rate of chemical activity during basal conditions, and it produces about 20% of total body heat.

SECRETIONS OF THE DIGESTIVE SYSTEM

Mucus

Mucus is secreted by mucous glands in every part of the gastrointestinal (GI) tract. The functions of mucus are to protect the lining of the tract from digestive juices, lubricate the food bolus for easier passage, promote adherence of the fecal mass, and neutralize acids and bases. Prostaglandins aid in protecting the gastrointestinal mucosa from injury.

Saliva

Saliva consists of mucus, ptyalin, and salivary amylase. It is produced by the salivary glands and totals about 1000 milliliters daily. Saliva has a slightly acidic to neutral pH (6–7); it lubricates the food bolus and begins starch digestion.

Gastric Juice

Gastric juice consists of mucus, digestive enzymes, hydrochloric acid, and electrolytes. The gastric glands secrete about 2000 milliliters of highly acidic (pH of 1–3) gastric juice daily. Secretion varies according to time of day, the time and type of food intake, psychological states, and other metabolic activities of the body. It is highest in the evening and lowest in the early morning. Secretion is stimulated by the parasympathetic nervous system (by the vagus nerve); the hormone gastrin; the presence of food in the mouth; and seeing, smelling, or thinking about food.

The major digestive enzyme in gastric juice is pepsin, a proteolytic enzyme (named before the "ase" system of naming enzymes) that functions best at a pH of 2 to 3. Hydrochloric acid provides the acid medium to promote pepsin activity. The major function of gastric juice is to begin digestion of proteins. There is also a weak action on fats by gastric lipase and on carbohydrates by gastric amylase. A large amount of mucus is secreted in the stomach to protect the stomach wall from the proteolytic action of pepsin. When mucus is not secreted, gastric ulceration occurs within hours.

Pancreatic Juices

Pancreatic juices are alkaline (pH of 8 or above) secretions that contain amylase for carbohydrate digestion, lipase for fat digestion, and trypsin and chymotrypsin for protein digestion. They also contain large amounts of sodium bicarbonate, a base (alkali) that neutralizes the acid chyme from the stomach by reacting with hydrochloric acid. This protects the mucosa of the small intestine from the digestive properties of gastric juice. The daily amount of pancreatic secretion is about 1200 milliliters. The hormone cholecystokinin stimulates secretion of pancreatic juices.

Bile

Bile is an alkaline (pH of about 8) secretion that is formed continuously in the liver, carried to the gallbladder by the bile ducts, and stored there. The hormone cholecystokinin causes the gallbladder to contract and release bile into the small intestine when fats are present in intestinal contents. The liver secretes about 600 milliliters of bile daily. This amount is concentrated to the 50- to 60-milliliter capacity of the gallbladder. Bile contains bile salts, cholesterol, bilirubin, fatty acids, and electrolytes. Bile salts are required for digestion and absorption of fats, including fat-soluble vitamins. Most of the bile salts are reabsorbed and reused by the liver (enterohepatic recirculation); some are excreted in feces.

EFFECTS OF DRUGS ON THE DIGESTIVE SYSTEM

The digestive system and drug therapy have a reciprocal relationship. Many common symptoms (ie, nausea, vomiting, constipation, diarrhea, abdominal pain) relate to GI dysfunction. These symptoms may result from a disorder in the digestive system, disorders in other body systems, or drug therapy. Many GI symptoms and disorders alter the ingestion, dissolution, absorption, and metabolism of drugs. Drugs may be administered to relieve these symptoms and disorders, but drugs administered for conditions unrelated to the digestive system may cause such symptoms and disorders. GI conditions may alter responses to drug therapy.

Drugs used in digestive disorders primarily alter GI secretion, absorption, or motility. They may act systemically or locally in the GI tract. The drug groups included in this section are laxatives, antidiarrheals, antiemetics, and drugs used for acid-peptic disorders. Other drug groups used in GI disorders include cholinergics (see Chap. 19), anticholinergics (see Chap. 20), corticosteroids (see Chap. 23), and anti-infective drugs (see Section 5).

Review and Application Exercises

Short Answer Exercises

1. What is the main function of the GI system?

2. What is the role of the parasympathetic nervous system in GI function?

3. List factors affecting GI motility and secretions.

4. Describe important GI secretions and their functions.

5. What factors stimulate or inhibit GI secretions?

6. How does the GI tract affect oral medications?

7. How do oral medications affect the GI tract?

Selected References

Goldman, L., & Ausiello, D. (2004). Approach to the patient with gastrointestinal disease. In L. Goldman & D. Ausiello (Eds.), *Cecil textbook of medicine* (22nd ed., pp. 782–785). Philadelphia: W. B. Saunders.

Porth, C. M. (2005). Control of gastrointestinal function. In C. M. Porth, *Pathophysiology: Concepts of altered health states* (7th ed., pp. 871–884). Philadelphia: Lippincott Williams & Wilkins.

Nutritional Support Products, Vitamins, and Mineral–Electrolytes

OBJECTIVES

After studying this chapter, you will be able to:

1. Assess clients for risk factors and manifestations of protein-calorie undernutrition.
2. Identify clients at risk for development of vitamin and/or mineral–electrolyte deficiency or excess.
3. Describe adverse effects associated with overdoses of vitamins.
4. Discuss the rationale for administering vitamin K to newborns.
5. Describe signs, symptoms, and treatment of sodium, potassium, magnesium, and chloride imbalances.
6. Describe signs, symptoms, and treatment of iron deficiency anemia.
7. Discuss the chelating agents used to remove excessive copper, iron, and lead from body tissues.
8. Apply nursing process skills to prevent, recognize, or treat nutritional imbalances.
9. Monitor laboratory reports that indicate nutritional status.

APPLYING YOUR KNOWLEDGE

Jane Farber is a 91-year-old female who suffers from heart failure, osteoarthritis, and Parkinson's disease. Upon evaluation, you find that Mrs. Farber is undernourished and slightly dehydrated.

INTRODUCTION

Water, carbohydrates, proteins, fats, vitamins, and minerals are required to promote or maintain health, to prevent illness, and to promote recovery from illness or injury. Water is required for cellular metabolism and excretion of metabolic waste products; 2000 to 3000 milliliters are needed daily. Proteins are structural and functional components of all body cells and tissues; the recommended amount for adults is 50 to 60 grams daily. Carbohydrates and fats mainly provide energy for cellular metabolism. Energy is measured in kilocalories (kcal) per gram of food oxidized in the body. Carbohydrates and proteins supply 4 kcal per gram; fats supply 9 kcal per gram.

Vitamins are required for normal body metabolism, growth, and development. They are components of enzyme systems that release energy from proteins, fats, and carbohydrates. They also are required for formation of red blood cells, nerve cells, hormones, genetic material, and bone and other tissues. Minerals and electrolytes are essential constituents of bone, teeth, cell membranes, connective tissue, and many essential enzymes. They function to maintain fluid, electrolyte, and acid–base balance; maintain osmotic pressure; maintain nerve and muscle function; assist in transfer of compounds across cell membranes; and influence the growth process.

For all of these nutrients, clients' requirements vary widely, depending on age, sex, size, health or illness status, and other factors. This chapter discusses products to improve nutritional status in clients with deficiency states and excess states of selected vitamins and mineral–electrolytes.

NUTRITIONAL DEFICIENCY STATES

Nurses encounter many clients who are unable to ingest, digest, absorb, or use sufficient nutrients to improve or maintain health. Debilitating illnesses such as cancer; acquired immunodeficiency syndrome; and chronic lung, kidney, or cardiovascular disorders often interfere with appetite and gastrointestinal (GI) function. Therapeutic drugs often cause anorexia, nausea, vomiting, diarrhea, or constipation. Nutritional deficiencies may impair the function of essentially every body organ. Signs and symptoms include unintended weight loss; increased susceptibility to infection; weakness and fatigability; impaired wound healing; impaired growth and development in children; edema; and decreased hemoglobin.

NUTRITIONAL PRODUCTS

Various products are available to supplement or substitute for dietary intake. These may consist of liquid enteral formulas, intravenous (IV) fluids, pancreatic enzymes, vitamins, and minerals.

Liquid Enteral Products

Numerous liquid enteral formulas are available over-the-counter or in health care settings for oral or tube feedings. Many are nutritionally complete, except for water, when given in sufficient amounts (eg, Ensure, Isocal, Sustacal, Resource). Additional water must be given to meet fluid needs. Most oral products are available in a variety of flavors and contain 1 kcal per milliliter. Additional products are formulated for clients with special conditions (eg, renal or hepatic failure, malabsorption syndromes) or needs (eg, high protein, increased calories).

Intravenous Fluids

IV fluids are used when oral or tube feedings are contraindicated. Most are nutritionally incomplete and used short term to supply fluids and electrolytes. Dextrose or dextrose and sodium chloride solutions are often used. When nutrients must be provided parenterally for more than a few days, a special parenteral nutritional formula can be designed to meet all nutritional needs or to supplement other feeding methods.

Pancreatic Enzymes

Pancreatic enzymes (amylase, protease, lipase) are required for absorption of carbohydrates, protein, and fat. Pancreatin and pancrelipase are commercial preparations used as replacement therapy in deficiency states, including cystic fibrosis, chronic pancreatitis, pancreatectomy, and pancreatic obstruction. Dosage is 1 to 3 capsules or tablets with each meal or snack.

Vitamins

Vitamins are obtained from foods or supplements. Although foods are considered the best source, studies indicate that most adults and children do not consume enough fruits, veg-

etables, cereal grains, dairy products, and other foods to consistently meet their vitamin requirements. In addition, some conditions increase requirements above the usual recommended amounts (eg, pregnancy, lactation, various illnesses).

Historically, the major concern about vitamins was sufficient intake to promote health and prevent deficiency diseases. To this end, the Food and Nutrition Board of the National Academy of Sciences established recommendations for daily vitamin intake (Dietary Reference Intakes [DRIs]; see Box 57-1).

Currently, concern extends to excessive vitamin intake, which may also cause disordered body metabolism and may be detrimental to health. Vitamin supplements are widely promoted to increase health and prevent or treat illness. However, the supplements can be harmful if overused. As a result, the DRIs include the maximum Tolerable Upper Intake Levels (ULs) of some vitamins. **These amounts should not be exceeded.**

Vitamins are classified as fat soluble (A, D, E, K) and water soluble (B complex, C). Fat-soluble vitamins are absorbed from the intestine with dietary fat and absorption requires the presence of bile salts and pancreatic lipase. Vitamin D is discussed mainly in Chapter 25 because of its major role in bone metabolism. Vitamin deficiencies occur with inadequate intake or disease processes that interfere with absorption or use of vitamins. Excess states occur with excessive intake of fat-soluble vitamins because these vitamins accumulate in the body. Excess states do not occur with dietary intake of water-soluble vitamins but may occur with vitamin supplements that exceed recommended amounts. Vitamins are described further in Table 57-1, and recommended dosages of vitamin preparations are listed in Table 57-2.

Vitamin Supplements

Vitamin supplements may be prescribed by health care providers, but most are self-prescribed. Because vitamins are essential nutrients, some people believe that large amounts (megadoses) promote health and provide other beneficial effects. However, excessive intake may cause harmful effects and "megavitamins" should never be self-prescribed. Additional characteristics include the following:

- Vitamins from supplements exert the same physiologic effects as those obtained from foods.
- Vitamin supplements do not require a prescription.
- Vitamin products vary widely in number, type, and amount of specific ingredients.
- Preparations should not contain more than recommended amounts of vitamin D, folic acid, and vitamin A.
- Synthetic vitamins have the same structure and function as natural vitamins derived from plant and animal sources and are less expensive.
- Multivitamin preparations often contain minerals as well. **Large doses of all minerals are toxic.**
- Vitamins are often marketed in combination products with each other (eg, antioxidant vitamins) and with herbal prod-

Box 57-1 Dietary Reference Intakes (DRIs)

Dietary Reference Intakes are the recommended amounts of vitamins (see Table 57-1) and some minerals (see Table 57-3). The current DRIs were established in 1997, 1998, and 2000 by the Food and Nutrition Board of the National Academy of Sciences and are intended to replace the Recommended Dietary Allowances (RDAs) used since 1989. DRIs consist of four subtypes of nutrient recommendations, as follows:

1. **Estimated Average Requirement** (EAR) is the amount estimated to provide adequate intake in 50% of healthy persons in a specific group.
2. **Recommended Dietary Allowance** (RDA) is the amount estimated to meet the needs of approximately 98% of healthy children and adults in a specific age and gender group. The RDA is used to advise various groups about nutrient intake. It should be noted, however, that RDAs were established to prevent deficiencies and that they were extrapolated from studies of healthy adults. Thus, they may not be appropriate for all groups, such as young children and older adults.
3. **Adequate Intake** (AI) is the amount thought to be sufficient when there is not enough reliable, scientific information to estimate an average requirement. The AI is derived from data that show an average intake that appears to maintain health.

4. **Tolerable Upper Intake Level (UL)** is the maximum intake considered unlikely to pose a health risk in almost all healthy persons in a specified group; it is not intended to be a recommended level of intake.

With **vitamins,** the ULs for adults (19–70 years and older) are D, 50 mg; E, 1000 mg; C, 2000 mg; folate, 1000 mcg; niacin, 35 mg; and pyridoxine, 100 mg. With vitamins C and D and pyridoxine, the UL refers to the total intake from food, fortified food, and supplements. With niacin and folate, the UL applies to synthetic forms obtained from supplements, fortified foods, or a combination of the two. With vitamin E, the UL applies to any form of supplemental alpha-tocopherol. These ULs should not be exceeded.

There are inadequate data for establishing ULs for biotin, cyanocobalamin (B_{12}), pantothenic acid, riboflavin, and thiamine. As a result, consuming more than the recommended amounts of these vitamins should generally be avoided.

With **minerals,** ULs have been established for calcium (2.5 g), phosphorus (3–4 g), magnesium (350 mg), fluoride (10 mg), and selenium (400 mcg). The UL should not be exceeded for any mineral–electrolyte because all minerals are toxic in overdose. Except for magnesium, which is set for supplements only and excludes food and water sources, the stated UL amounts include those from both foods and supplements.

ucts (eg, B-complex vitamins with ginseng, for "energy"). There is no reliable evidence to support the use of such products.

Mineral–Electrolytes

There are 22 minerals considered necessary for human nutrition. Some (calcium, phosphorus, sodium, potassium, magnesium, chlorine, sulfur) are required in relatively large amounts. Calcium and phosphorus are discussed mainly in Chapter 25 because of their major roles in bone metabolism. Sulfur is a component of cellular proteins, several amino acids, B vitamins, insulin, and other essential body substances. No recommended intake has been established; it is obtained from protein foods.

Other minerals are required in small amounts and are often called *trace elements*. Eight trace elements (chromium, cobalt, copper, fluoride, iodine, iron, selenium, and zinc) have relatively well-defined roles in human nutrition. Others (manganese, molybdenum, nickel, silicon, tin, and vanadium) are present in many body tissues and may be necessary for normal growth, structure, and function of connective tissue. However, requirements are unknown and states of deficiency or excess have not been identified in humans.

Minerals occur in the body and foods mainly in ionic form. Ions are electrically charged particles. Metals (eg, sodium, potassium, calcium, magnesium) form positive ions or cations; nonmetals (eg, chlorine, phosphorus, sulfur) form negative ions or anions. These cations and anions combine to form compounds that are physiologically inactive and electrically neutral. When placed in solution, such as a body fluid, the components separate into electrically charged particles called *electrolytes*. At any given time, the body must maintain an equal number of positive and negative charges. Therefore, the ions are constantly combining and separating to maintain electrical neutrality or electrolyte balance.

These electrolytes also maintain the acid–base balance of body fluids. When foods are digested, they produce mineral residues that react chemically as acids or bases. Acids are usually anions (eg, chloride, bicarbonate, sulfate, phosphate). Bases are usually cations (eg, sodium, potassium, calcium, magnesium). If approximately equal amounts of cations and anions are present in the mineral residue, the residue is essentially neutral, and the pH of body fluids does not require adjustment. If there is an excess of cations (base), the body must draw on its anions (acid) to combine with the cations, render them physiologically inactive, and restore the normal pH of the blood. Excess cations combine with anions (eg, phosphate) and are excreted in the urine; excess anions combine with hydrogen ions or other cations and are excreted in the urine.

Mineral–electrolytes are obtained from foods or supplements. Although most minerals are supplied by a well-balanced

(text continues on page 923)

TABLE 57-1   Vitamins

VITAMIN/FUNCTION	RECOMMENDED DAILY INTAKE	FOOD SOURCES	SIGNS & SYMPTOMS OF DEFICIENCY	SIGNS & SYMPTOMS OF EXCESS
Fat-Soluble Vitamins **Vitamin A** (retinol) Required for normal vision, growth, bone development, skin, and mucous membranes	DRIs* *Females:* 14 y and older, 700 mcg; in pregnancy, 750–770 mcg; lactation, 1200–1300 mcg *Males:* 14 y and older, 900 mcg *Children:* 1–3 y, 300 mcg; 4–8 y, 400 mcg; 9–13 y, 600 mcg *Infants (AIs):* 0–6 mo, 400 mcg; 6–12 mo, 500 mcg	Preformed vitamin A: meat, butter and fortified margarine, egg yolk, whole milk, cheese made from whole milk Carotenoids: turnip and collard greens, carrots, sweet potatoes, squash, apricots, peaches, cantaloupe	Night blindness; xerophthalmia, which may progress to corneal ulceration and blindness; changes in skin and mucous membranes that lead to skin lesions and infections, respiratory tract infections, and urinary calculi	Anorexia, vomiting, irritability, skin changes (itching, desquamation, dermatitis); pain in muscles, bones, and joints; gingivitis; enlargement of spleen and liver; increased intracranial pressure; other neurologic signs. Congenital abnormalities in newborns whose mothers took excessive vitamin A during pregnancy. Acute toxicity, with increased intracranial pressure, bulging fontanels, and vomiting, may occur in infants who are given vitamin A.
Vitamin E Antioxidant in preventing destruction of certain fats, including the lipid portion of cell membranes; may increase absorption, hepatic storage, and use of vitamin A	RDAs† *Females:* 14 y and older, 15 mg; in pregnancy, 15 mg (22.5 IU); lactation, 19 mg (28.5 IU) *Males:* 14 y and older, 15 mg *Children:* 1–3 y, 6 mg; 4–8 y, 7 mg; 9–13 y, 11 mg *Infants (AIs):* 0–6 mo, 4 mg; 7–12 mo, 6 mg	Cereals, green leafy vegetables, egg yolk, milk fat, butter, meat, vegetable oils	Deficiency is rare.	Fatigue; nausea; headache; blurred vision; diarrhea
Vitamin K Essential for normal blood clotting. Activates precursor proteins, found in the liver, into clotting factors II, VII, IX, and X	1 mcg/kg	Green leafy vegetables (spinach, kale, cabbage, lettuce), cauliflower, tomatoes, wheat bran, cheese, egg yolk, liver	Abnormal bleeding (melena, hematemesis, hematuria, epistaxis, petechiae, ecchymoses, hypovolemic shock)	Clinical manifestations rarely occur. However, when vitamin K is given to someone who is receiving warfarin (Coumadin), the client can be made "warfarin-resistant" for 2–3 wk.
Vitamin D (see Chap. 25)				
Water-Soluble Vitamins **B-Complex Biotin** Essential in fat and carbohydrate metabolism	AIs *Females:* 14–18 y, 25 mcg; 19 y and older, 30 mcg; in pregnancy, 30 mcg; lactation, 35 mcg	Meat, egg yolk, nuts, cereals, most vegetables	Anorexia, nausea, depression, muscle pain, dermatitis	Not established

TABLE 57-1 Vitamins (continued)

VITAMIN/FUNCTION	RECOMMENDED DAILY INTAKE	FOOD SOURCES	SIGNS & SYMPTOMS OF DEFICIENCY	SIGNS & SYMPTOMS OF EXCESS
	Males: 4–18 y, 25 mcg; 19 y and older, 30 mcg *Children:* 1–3 y, 8 mcg; 4–8 y, 12 mcg; 9–13 y, 20 mcg *Infants:* 0–6 mo, 5 mcg; 7–12 mo, 6 mcg			
Cyanocobalamin (B$_{12}$) Essential for normal metabolism of all body cells; normal red blood cells; normal nerve cells; growth; and metabolism of carbohydrate, protein, and fat	RDAs *Females:* 14 y and older, 2.4 mcg; in pregnancy, 2.6 mcg; lactation, 2.8 mcg *Males:* 14 y and older, 2.4 mcg *Children:* 1–3 y, 0.9 mcg; 4–8 y, 1.2 mcg; 9–13 y, 1.8 mcg *Infants (AIs):* 0–6 mo, 0.4 mcg; 7–12 mo, 0.5 mcg	Meat, eggs, fish, cheese	Pernicious anemia: decreased numbers of RBCs; large, immature RBCs; fatigue; dyspnea Severe deficiency: leukopenia, infection, thrombocytopenia, cardiac dysrhythmias, heart failure Neurologic signs and symptoms: paresthesias in hands and feet, unsteady gait, depressed deep-tendon reflexes Severe deficiency: loss of memory; confusion; delusions; hallucinations; and psychosis may occur. Nerve damage may be irreversible.	Not established
Folic acid (folate) Essential for normal metabolism of all body cells; normal red blood cells; and growth	RDAs *Females:* 14 y and older, 400 mcg; in pregnancy, 600 mcg; lactation, 500 mcg *Males:* 14 y and older, 400 mcg *Children:* 1–3 y, 150 mcg; 4–8 y, 200 mcg; 9–13 y, 300 mcg *Infants (AIs):* 0–6 mo, 65 mcg; 7–12 mo, 80 mcg	Liver, kidney beans, fresh green vegetables (spinach, broccoli, asparagus), fortified grain products (eg, breads, cereals, rice)	Megaloblastic anemia that cannot be distinguished from the anemia produced by B$_{12}$ deficiency; impaired growth in children; glossitis; GI problems	Not established
Niacin (B$_3$) Essential for glycolysis, fat synthesis, and tissue respiration. It functions as	DRIs *Females:* 14 y and older, 14 mg; in pregnancy, 18 mg; lactation, 17 mg	Meat, poultry, fish, peanuts	Pellagra: erythematous skin lesions, GI problems (stomatitis, glossitis, enteritis, diarrhea), central	Flushing; pruritus; hyperglycemia; hyperuricemia; increased liver enzymes

(continued)

TABLE 57-1 **Vitamins** (continued)

VITAMIN/FUNCTION	RECOMMENDED DAILY INTAKE	FOOD SOURCES	SIGNS & SYMPTOMS OF DEFICIENCY	SIGNS & SYMPTOMS OF EXCESS
a coenzyme in many metabolic processes (after conversion to nicotinamide, the physiologically active form).	*Males:* 14 y and older, 16 mg *Children:* 1–3 y, 6 mg; 4–8 y, 8 mg; 9–13 y, 12 mg *Infants (AIs):* 0–6 mo, 2 mg; 7–12 mo, 4 mg		nervous system problems (headache, dizziness, insomnia, depression, memory loss) Severe deficiency: delusions, hallucinations, impairment of peripheral motor and sensory nerves	
Pantothenic acid (B₅) Essential for metabolism of carbohydrate, fat, and protein (eg, release of energy from carbohydrate; fatty acid metabolism; synthesis of cholesterol, steroid hormones, and phospholipids)	AIs *Females:* 14 y and older, 5 mg; in pregnancy, 6 mg; lactation, 7 mg *Males:* 14 y and older, 5 mg *Children:* 1–3 y, 2 mg; 4–8 y, 3 mg; 9–13 y, 4 mg *Infants:* 0–6 mo, 1.7 mg; 7–12 mo, 1.8 mg	Eggs, liver, salmon, yeast, cauliflower, broccoli, lean beef, potatoes, tomatoes	No deficiency state established	Not established
Pyridoxine (B₆) A coenzyme in metabolism of carbohydrate, protein, and fat; required for formation of tryptophan and conversion of tryptophan to niacin; helps release glycogen from the liver and muscle tissue; functions in metabolism of the central nervous system; helps maintain cellular immunity	DRIs *Females:* 14–18 y, 1.2 mg; 19–50 y, 1.3 mg; 51–70 and older, 1.5 mg; in pregnancy, 1.9 mg; lactation, 2.0 mg *Males:* 14–50 y, 1.3 mg; 51–70 y and older, 1.7 mg *Children:* 1–3 y, 0.5 mg; 4–8 y, 0.6 mg; 9–13 y, 1.0 mg *Infants (AIs):* 0–6 mo, 0.1 mg; 7–12 mo, 0.3 mg	Yeast, wheat germ, liver and other glandular meats, whole grain cereals, potatoes, legumes	Skin and mucous membrane lesions (seborrheic dermatitis, intertrigo, glossitis, stomatitis), neurologic problems (convulsions, peripheral neuritis, mental depression)	Not established
Riboflavin (B₂) A coenzyme in metabolism; necessary for growth; may function in production of corticosteroids and red blood cells and gluconeogenesis	DRIs *Females:* 14–18 y, 1.0 mg; 19 y and older, 1.1 mg; in pregnancy, 1.4 mg; lactation, 1.6 mg *Males:* 14 y and older, 1.3 mg *Children:* 1–3 y, 0.5 mg; 4–8 y, 0.6 mg; 9–13 y, 0.9 mg *Infants (AIs):* 0–6 mo, 0.3 mg; 7–12 mo, 0.4 mg	Milk, cheddar and cottage cheeses, meat, eggs, green leafy vegetables	Glossitis, stomatitis, seborrheic dermatitis, eye disorders (burning, itching, lacrimation, photophobia, vascularization of the cornea)	Not established

TABLE 57-1 Vitamins (continued)

VITAMIN/FUNCTION	RECOMMENDED DAILY INTAKE	FOOD SOURCES	SIGNS & SYMPTOMS OF DEFICIENCY	SIGNS & SYMPTOMS OF EXCESS
Thiamine (B₁) A coenzyme in carbohydrate metabolism; essential for energy production	DRIs *Females:* 14–18 y, 1.0 mg; 19 y and older, 1.1 mg; in pregnancy, 1.4 mg; lactation, 1.4 mg *Males:* 14 y and older, 1.2 mg *Children:* 1–3 y, 0.5 mg; 4–8 y, 0.6 mg; 9–13 y, 0.9 mg *Infants (AIs):* 0–6 mo, 0.2 mg; 7–12 mo, 0.3 mg	Meat, poultry, fish, egg yolk, dried beans, whole-grain cereal products, peanuts	Mild deficiency: fatigue, anorexia, retarded growth, mental depression, irritability, apathy, lethargy Severe deficiency (beriberi): peripheral neuritis; personality disturbances; heart failure; edema; Wernicke-Korsakoff syndrome in alcoholics	Not established
Vitamin C (ascorbic acid) Essential for formation of skin, ligaments, cartilage, bone, and teeth; required for wound healing and tissue repair, metabolism of iron and folic acid, synthesis of fats and proteins, preservation of blood vessel integrity, and resistance to infection	DRIs *Females:* 14–18 y, 65 mg; 19 y and older, 75 mg; in pregnancy, 80–85 mg; lactation, 115–120 mg *Males:* 14–18 y, 75 mg; 19 y and older, 90 mg *Children:* 1–3 y, 15 mg; 4–8 y, 25 mg; 9–13 y, 45 mg *Infants (AIs):* 0–6 mo, 40 mg; 7–12 mo, 50 mg	Fruits and vegetables, especially citrus fruits and juices	Mild deficiency: irritability, malaise, arthralgia, increased tendency to bleed Severe deficiency: scurvy and adverse effects on most body tissues (gingivitis; bleeding of gums, skin, joints, and other areas; disturbances of bone growth; anemia; and loosening of teeth). If not treated, coma and death may occur.	Renal calculi

*DRIs for vitamin A are expressed in retinol activity equivalents (RAEs), which include both preformed vitamin A and carotenoids. 1 RAE = 1 mcg retinol or 12 mcg beta carotene.
†Vitamin E activity is expressed in milligrams of alpha-tocopherol equivalents (alpha TE).
AIs, Adequate Intake; DRIs, Dietary Reference Intakes; GI, gastrointestinal; RBCs, red blood cells; RDAs, Recommended Dietary Allowances.

diet, studies indicate that most adults and children do not ingest sufficient dietary calcium and that iron deficiency anemia is common in some populations. In addition, some conditions increase requirements (eg, pregnancy, lactation, various illnesses) and some drug–drug interactions decrease absorption or use of minerals.

As with vitamins, goals for daily mineral intake have been established as DRIs. Thus far, DRIs and ULs have been established for calcium, phosphorus, magnesium, iron, fluoride, and selenium. **The UL should not be exceeded for any mineral–electrolyte.** Except for magnesium, which is set for supplements only and excludes food and water sources, the stated amounts include those from both foods and supplements. Mineral–electrolytes are described further in Table 57-3.

Mineral Supplements

Many people take mineral preparations as dietary supplements, usually in a multivitamin–mineral combination. Health care providers and clients should consider the following factors in relation to mineral supplements.

● Nutritionists usually recommend dietary intake of nutrients rather than pharmaceutical supplements and emphasize that supplements do not compensate for an inadequate diet.
● In general, recommended daily doses should not be exceeded because all minerals are toxic at high doses.
● Multivitamin–mineral combinations recommended for age and gender groups contain different amounts of some minerals (eg, postmenopausal women need less

Table 57-2 Drugs at a Glance: Vitamin Drug Preparations

	ROUTES AND DOSAGE RANGES		
GENERIC/TRADE NAME	Adults	Children	COMMENTS
Fat-Soluble Vitamins			
Vitamin A (also called retinol)	*Deficiency,* PO, IM 100,000 IU daily for 3 d, then 50,000 IU daily for 2 wk, then 10,000–20,000 IU daily for another 2 mo	*Kwashiorkor,* Retinol 30 mg IM followed by intermittent oral therapy *Xerophthalmia (>1 y old),* retinyl palmitate 110 mg PO or 55 mg IM plus another 110 mg PO at 1 and 3 or 4 d later	IM administration indicated when oral not feasible, as in anorexia, nausea, vomiting, preoperative and postoperative conditions, or malabsorption syndromes With xerophthalmia, vitamin E 40 IU should be coadministered to increase effectiveness of the retinol.
Vitamin E	PO 100–400 IU daily	PO 15–30 IU daily	Should not be given IV because IV use has been associated with 38 infant deaths
Vitamin K Phytonadione (Mephyton)	Anticoagulant-induced prothrombin deficiency, PO, Sub-Q, IM 2.5–10 mg initially, repeat after 6–8 h (injected dose) or 12–48 h (oral dose) if needed (ie, if prothrombin time still prolonged) Hypoprothrombinemia due to other causes, PO, Sub-Q, IM 2.5–25 mg	*Older children,* same as adults *Newborns,* prevention of hemorrhagic disease, IM 0.5–1 mg within 1 h after birth; may be repeated after 2–3 wk if mother received anticoagulant, anticonvulsant, antitubercular, or recent antibiotic drug therapy during pregnancy Treatment of hemorrhagic disease, Sub-Q, IM 1 mg	Do not give IV; serious, anaphylaxis-like reactions have occurred.
Water-Soluble Vitamins **B-COMPLEX VITAMINS**			
Calcium pantothenate (B₅)	Total parenteral nutrition, IV 15 mg daily	Total parenteral nutrition, >11 y, IV 15 mg daily; 1–11 y, IV 5 mg daily	Deficiency states seen only with severe, multiple B-complex deficiency states
Cyanocobalamin (B₁₂)	PO 100–250 mcg daily IM 30 mcg daily for 5–10 d, then 100–200 mcg monthly	PO, IM, Sub-Q 10–100 mcg daily for 5–15 d, then 100–200 mcg monthly	Oral drug, alone or in multivitamin preparations, is given for nutritional deficiencies.
Nascobal	Intranasal gel, 1 spray (500 mcg) in one nostril, once per wk		Parenteral B₁₂ should be given for pernicious anemia. Intranasal drug should not be used if rhinitis, nasal congestion, or upper respiratory infection is present.
Folic acid	Deficiency, megaloblastic anemia, PO, Sub-Q, IM, IV up to 1 mg daily until symptoms decrease and blood tests are normal, then maintenance dose of 0.4 mg daily	PO, Sub-Q, IM, IV up to 1 mg daily until symptoms decrease and blood tests are normal, then a daily maintenance dose as follows: infants, 0.1 mg; <4 y, up to 0.3 mg; >4 y, 0.4 mg	Oral administration preferred unless severe intestinal malabsorption is present
Niacin (nicotinic acid) Niacinamide (nicotinamide)	Deficiency, PO 50–100 mg daily Pellagra, PO Up to 500 mg daily Hyperlipidemia, PO 2–6 g daily (maximum dose, 6 g/d)	Safety and effectiveness not established for amounts exceeding the RDA	To reduce flushing with larger doses, start with smaller doses and gradually increase them.

Table 57-2 Drugs at a Glance: Vitamin Drug Preparations (continued)

	ROUTES AND DOSAGE RANGES		
GENERIC/TRADE NAME	**Adults**	**Children**	**COMMENTS**
Pyridoxine (B₆)	Deficiency, PO, IM, IV 2–5 mg daily Anemia, peripheral neuritis, 50–200 mg daily	Safety and effectiveness not established for amounts exceeding the RDA	Usually given with isoniazid, an antitubercular drug, to prevent peripheral neuropathy
Riboflavin	Deficiency, PO 5–10 mg daily In total parenteral nutrition, 3.6 mg/d	In total parenteral nutrition, IV >11 y, 3.6 mg/d; 1–11 y, 1.4 mg/d	Deficiency rarely occurs alone; more likely with other vitamin deficiency states
Thiamine (B₁)	Deficiency, PO 10–30 mg daily; IM 10–20 mg 3 times daily for 2 wk, supplemented with 5–10 mg orally; IV 50–100 mg/d until able to take orally	Safety and effectiveness not established for amounts exceeding the RDA	Deficiency is common in alcoholics.
VITAMIN C Vitamin C (ascorbic acid)	Deficiency, PO, IM, IV 100–500 mg daily Urinary acidification, 2 g daily in divided doses Prophylaxis, 50–100 mg daily	Infants receiving formula, 35–50 mg daily for first few weeks of life	Excessive doses (eg, 2000 mg or more daily) cause adverse effects and should be avoided.

IM, intramuscular; IV, intravenous; PO, oral; RDA, Recommended Dietary Allowance; Sub-Q, subcutaneous.

iron than younger women). This should be considered in choosing a product.

- Iron supplements other than those in multivitamin–mineral combinations are usually intended for temporary use in the presence of deficiency or a period of increased need (eg, pregnancy). They should not be taken otherwise because of the risk of accumulation and toxicity.

- Most adolescent and adult females probably benefit from a calcium supplement to achieve the recommended amount (1000–1300 mg daily). The amounts consumed in dairy products and other foods should be considered and the UL of 2500 milligrams daily should not be exceeded.

- Although selenium is promoted as an antioxidant that decreases cardiovascular disease and cancer, there is limited evidence of such benefits and a selenium supplement is not recommended.

- Although zinc is promoted for treatment of the common cold and to promote wound healing, there is insufficient evidence to support such uses. With colds, zinc reportedly helps some people and does not help others. With wounds, zinc is reportedly beneficial only if the client has a zinc deficiency. More studies are needed before supplemental zinc can be recommended for general use.

AGENTS USED IN MINERAL–ELECTROLYTE IMBALANCES

Mineral–electrolyte imbalances include both deficiency states and excess states. Most deficiency states occur with inadequate intake or excessive losses (eg, vomiting, gastric suction, diarrhea, overuse of laxatives). Most excess states occur with excessive intake or impaired renal excretion.

Several pharmacologic agents are used to prevent or treat mineral–electrolyte imbalances. Usually, neutral salts of minerals (eg, potassium chloride) are used in deficiency states, and nonmineral drug preparations are used in excess states. These agents are described below; routes and dosage ranges are listed in Table 57-4.

Cation Exchange Resin

Sodium polystyrene sulfonate (Kayexalate) is used to treat hyperkalemia. Given orally or rectally, the resin combines with potassium in the colon. Potassium is then eliminated from the body in the feces. Each gram of resin removes about 1 milliequivalent of potassium. Because the resin requires several hours to lower serum potassium levels, it may be used after other measures (eg, IV insulin and glucose infusions)

(text continues on page 929)

TABLE 57-3 Minerals and Electrolytes

MINERAL/FUNCTION	RECOMMENDED DAILY INTAKE	FOOD SOURCES	SIGNS & SYMPTOMS OF DEFICIENCY	SIGNS & SYMPTOMS OF EXCESS
Macro Minerals				
Sodium				
Assists in regulating osmotic pressure, water balance, conduction of electrical impulses in nerves and muscles, and electrolyte and acid–base balance Influences permeability of cell membranes and assists in movement of substances across cell membranes Participates in many intracellular chemical reactions	Approximately 2 g	In most foods. Proteins contain large amounts, vegetables and cereals contain moderate to small amounts, fruits contain little or no sodium. Major source in the diet is table salt added to food in cooking, processing, or seasoning. One teaspoon contains 2.3 g of sodium. Water in some areas may contain significant amounts of sodium.	Serum sodium <135 mEq/L; anorexia, nausea, and vomiting; ataxia; confusion; delirium; hypotension and tachycardia; muscle tremors; oliguria and increased BUN; seizures; weakness	Serum sodium >145 mEq/L; disorientation; dry skin and mucous membranes; fever; hyperactive reflexes; hypotension; muscle rigidity; tremors and spasms; irritability; cerebral hemorrhage; coma; oliguria, concentrated urine, increased BUN
Potassium				
Within cells, helps maintain osmotic pressure, fluid and electrolyte balance, and acid–base balance In extracellular fluid, is required for conduction of nerve impulses and contraction of skeletal and smooth muscle (especially important in myocardium) Helps transport glucose into cells and is required for glycogen formation and storage Required for synthesis of muscle proteins	Approximately 40 mEq	Present in most foods, including meat, whole-grain breads or cereals, bananas, citrus fruits, tomatoes, and broccoli	Serum potassium <3.5 mEq/L; dysrhythmias and electrocardiographic changes; cardiac arrest; confusion; delirium; hyperglycemia; postural hypotension; muscle weakness; abdominal distention, constipation, paralytic ileus; polyuria, polydipsia, nocturia. Prolonged deficiency may increase serum creatinine and BUN.	Serum potassium >5 mEq/L; muscle weakness; cardiotoxicity, with dysrhythmias or cardiac arrest Cardiac effects are not usually severe until serum levels are 7 mEq/L or above.
Magnesium				
Required for conduction of nerve impulses and contraction of muscle (especially important in functions of cardiac and skeletal muscles) Serves as a component of many enzymes Essential for metabolism of carbohydrate and protein	*Adults (DRIs):* Males 19–30 y, 400 mg; 31–70 y and older, 420 mg; females 19–30 y, 310 mg; 31–70 y and older, 320 mg; in pregnancy, 350–360 mg; lactation, 310–320 mg Upper Level (UL) or maximum intake from pharmaceutical preparations,	Present in many foods; diet that is adequate in other respects contains adequate magnesium. Good food sources include nuts, cereal grains, dark green vegetables, and seafoods.	Serum magnesium <1.5 mEq/L; ataxia; confusion; dizziness; irritability; muscle tremors, carpopedal spasm, nystagmus, generalized spasticity; seizures; tachycardia, hypotension, premature atrial and ventricular beats	Serum magnesium >2.5 mEq/L; skeletal muscle weakness; cardiac dysrhythmias, hypotension; respiratory insufficiency; coma

TABLE 57-3 Minerals and Electrolytes (continued)

MINERAL/FUNCTION	RECOMMENDED DAILY INTAKE	FOOD SOURCES	SIGNS & SYMPTOMS OF DEFICIENCY	SIGNS & SYMPTOMS OF EXCESS
	350 mg (does not include intake from food and water) *Children (RDAs):* 1–3 y, 80 mg; 4–8 y, 130 mg; 9–13 y, 240 mg; 14–18 y, 410 mg *Infants (AIs):* 0–6 mo, 30 mg; 7–12 mo, 75 mg			
Chloride Helps maintain osmotic pressure and electrolyte, acid–base, and water balance Forms hydrochloric acid (HCl) in gastric mucosal cells	80–110 mEq	Most dietary chloride is ingested as sodium chloride (NaCl), and foods high in sodium are also high in chloride.	Serum chloride <95 mEq/L; arterial blood pH >7.45; dehydration; hypotension; low, shallow respirations; paresthesias of face and extremities; muscle spasms and tetany, which cannot be distinguished from the tetany produced by hypocalcemia	Serum chloride >103 mEq/L; arterial blood pH <7.35; increased rate and depth of respiration; lethargy, stupor, disorientation, and coma if acidosis is not treated
Trace Elements				
Chromium Aids glucose use by increasing effectiveness of insulin and facilitating transport of glucose across cell membranes	Not established	Brewer's yeast and whole-wheat products.	Impaired glucose tolerance (hyperglycemia, glycosuria); impaired growth and reproduction; decreased life span	Not established
Cobalt A component of vitamin B$_{12}$ that is required for normal function of all body cells and for maturation of red blood cells	Approximately 1 mg in the form of vitamin B$_{12}$	Animal foods, including liver, muscle meats, and shellfish. Fruits, vegetables, and cereals contain no cobalt as vitamin B$_{12}$.	Deficiency of vitamin B$_{12}$ produces pernicious anemia.	Not established
Copper A component of many enzymes Essential for correct functioning of the central nervous, cardiovascular, and skeletal systems Important in formation of red blood cells, apparently by regulating storage and release of iron for hemoglobin	Approximately 2 mg	Many foods, including liver, shellfish, nuts, cereals, poultry, dried fruits	Decreased serum levels; decreased iron absorption; anemia from impaired erythropoiesis; leukopenia. Death can occur. In infants, anemia, chronic malnutrition and diarrhea, or Menke's syndrome (retarded growth and progressive mental deterioration) can occur.	Increased serum levels; Wilson's disease (a rare disorder characterized by accumulation of copper in brain, liver, and kidneys). Signs and symptoms vary according to affected organs.

(continued)

TABLE 57-3 Minerals and Electrolytes (continued)

MINERAL/FUNCTION	RECOMMENDED DAILY INTAKE	FOOD SOURCES	SIGNS & SYMPTOMS OF DEFICIENCY	SIGNS & SYMPTOMS OF EXCESS
Fluoride A component of tooth enamel Strengthens bones Adequate intake before ages 50–60 years may decrease osteoporosis and fractures during later years.	*Adults (AIs):* males 19–70 y and older, 4 mg; females 19–70 y and older, 3 mg; in pregnancy and lactation, 5 mg *Children (AIs):* 1–3 y, 0.7 mg; 4–8 y, 1 mg; 9–13 y, 2 mg; 14–18 y, 3 mg *Infants (AIs):* 0–6 mo, 0.01 mg; 7–12 mo, 0.5 mg	Beef, canned salmon, eggs. Very little in milk, cereal grains, fruits, and vegetables. Fluoride content of foods depends on fluoride content of soil where they are grown.	Dental caries and possibly a greater incidence of osteoporosis	Mottling of teeth and osteosclerosis.
Iodine Essential component of thyroid hormones	*Adults (RDAs):* males and females 19–51 y and older, 150 mcg; in pregnancy, 175 mcg; lactation, 200 mcg *Children:* 1–10 y, 10 mg; males 11–18 y, 12 mg; females 11–18 y, 15 mg *Infants:* 0–6 mo, 40 mcg; 6–12 mo, 50 mcg	Seafood is the best source. In vegetables, iodine content varies with the amount of iodine in soil where grown. In milk and eggs, content depends on the amount present in animal feed.	Thyroid gland enlargement; possible hypothyroidism	Iodism, with coryza, edema, fever, conjunctivitis, lymphadenopathy, stomatitis, vomiting
Iron Essential component of hemoglobin, myoglobin, and several enzymes: hemoglobin is required for transport and use of oxygen by body cells; myoglobin aids oxygen transport and use by muscle cells; enzymes are important for cellular metabolism.	*Adults (RDAs):* males 19–51 y and older, 10 mg; females 19–50, 15 mg; 51 y and older, 10 mg; in pregnancy, 30 mg; lactation, 15 mg *Children:* 1–10 y, 10 mg; males 11–18 y, 12 mg; females 11–18 y, 15 mg *Infants:* 0–6 mo, 6 mg; 6–12 mo, 10 mg	Liver and other organ meats, lean meat, shellfish, dried beans and vegetables, egg yolks, dried fruits, molasses, whole-grain and enriched breads. Milk and milk products contain essentially no iron.	Iron deficiency anemia: with gradual development of anemia, minimal symptoms occur; with rapid development or severe anemia, dyspnea, fatigue, tachycardia, malaise and drowsiness occur.	Acute iron intoxication: vomiting, diarrhea, melena, abdominal pain, shock, convulsions, and metabolic acidosis. Death may occur within 24 h if treatment is not prompt. Chronic iron overload (hemochromatosis): cardiac dysrhythmias, heart failure, diabetes mellitus, bronze pigmentation of skin, liver enlargement, arthropathy, and others
Selenium Important for function of myocardium and probably other muscles	*Adults (RDAs):* males and females 19–70 y and older, 55 mcg; in pregnancy, 60 mcg; lactation, 70 mcg *Children (RDAs):* 1–3 y, 20 mcg; 4–8 y,	Fish, meat, breads, and cereals.	Deficiency most likely with long-term IV therapy. Signs and symptoms include myocardial abnormalities and other muscle discomfort and weakness.	Highly toxic in excessive amounts. Signs and symptoms include fatigue, peripheral neuropathy, nausea, diarrhea, and alopecia.

TABLE 57-3 Minerals and Electrolytes (continued)

MINERAL/FUNCTION	RECOMMENDED DAILY INTAKE	FOOD SOURCES	SIGNS & SYMPTOMS OF DEFICIENCY	SIGNS & SYMPTOMS OF EXCESS
	30 mcg; 9–13 y, 40 mcg; 14–18 y, 55 mcg *Infants (AIs):* 0–6 mo, 15 mcg; 7–12 mo, 20 mcg			
Zinc A component of many enzymes that are essential for normal metabolism (eg, carbonic anhydrase, lactic dehydrogenase, alkaline phosphatase) Necessary for normal cell growth, synthesis of nucleic acids (RNA and DNA), and synthesis of carbohydrates and proteins May be essential for use of vitamin A	*Adults (RDAs):* males 19–51 y and older, 15 mg; females, 19–51 y and older, 12 mg; in pregnancy, 15 mg; lactation, 16–19 mg *Children:* 1–10 y, 10 mg; males 11–18 y, 12 mg; females 11–18 y, 15 mg *Infants:* 0–6 mo, 40 mcg; 6–12 mo, 50 mcg	Animal proteins, such as meat, liver, eggs, and seafood. Wheat germ is also a good source.	Most evident in growing children and include impaired growth, hypogonadism in boys, anorexia, and sensory impairment (loss of taste and smell). Also, if the client has had surgery, wound healing may be delayed.	Unlikely with dietary intake but may develop with excessive ingestion or inhalation of zinc. Ingestion may cause nausea, vomiting, and diarrhea; inhalation may cause vomiting, headache, and fever.

AIs, Adequate Intake; BUN, blood urea nitrogen; DRIs, Dietary Reference Intakes; RDAs, Recommended Dietary Allowances.

have lowered serum levels. Insulin and glucose lower serum potassium levels by driving potassium into the cells; they do not remove potassium from the body.

Chelating Agents (Metal Antagonists)

Deferoxamine (Desferal) is used to remove excess iron from the body. When given orally within a few hours after oral ingestion of iron preparations, deferoxamine combines with the iron in the bowel lumen and prevents its absorption. When given parenterally, it removes iron from storage sites (eg, ferritin, hemosiderin) and combines with the iron to produce a water-soluble compound that can be excreted by the kidneys. The drug can remove 10 to 50 milligrams of iron per day. The urine becomes reddish brown from the iron content.

The major indication for use of deferoxamine is acute iron intoxication. The drug may also be used in chronic conditions characterized by accumulation of iron in tissues (eg, hemochromatosis with blood transfusions, hemosiderosis due to certain hemolytic anemias).

Penicillamine (Cuprimine) chelates copper, zinc, mercury, and lead to form soluble complexes that are excreted in the urine. It is used mainly to remove excess copper in clients with Wilson's disease, a rare condition characterized by accumulation of copper in vital organs. It also can be used pro-

phylactically, before clinical manifestations occur, in clients in whom this hereditary condition is likely to develop. Penicillamine may be used to treat cystinuria, a hereditary metabolic disorder characterized by large amounts of cystine in the urine and renal calculi. It may be used in lead poisoning and in severe rheumatoid arthritis that does not respond to conventional treatment measures.

Succimer (Chemet) chelates lead to form water-soluble complexes that are excreted in the urine. It is used to treat lead poisoning in children with blood levels above 45 micrograms per 100 milliliters. After oral administration, peak blood levels are reached in 1 to 2 hours. The drug is metabolized in the liver and excreted in urine and feces, with a half-life of 2 days. The most common adverse effects are anorexia, nausea, vomiting, and diarrhea.

Iron Preparations

Iron preparations are used to prevent or treat iron deficiency anemia. For prevention, they are often given during periods of increased need (eg, childhood, pregnancy). Oral ferrous salts (sulfate, gluconate, fumarate) are preferred, because they are well absorbed. Action starts in about 4 days, peaks in 7 to 10 days, and lasts 2 to 4 months. The drugs are not metabo-

(text continues on page 932)

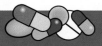

Table 57-4 Drugs at a Glance: Individual Agents Used in Mineral-Electrolyte and Acid-Base Imbalances

DRUG	INDICATIONS FOR USE	ROUTES AND DOSAGE RANGES	
		Adults	**Children**
Cation Exchange Resin			
Sodium polystyrene sulfonate (Kayexalate)	Treatment of hyperkalemia	PO 15 g in 100–200 mL of water and 70% sorbitol, 1–4 times daily Rectally (retention enema) 30–50 g in 100–200 mL of water and 70% sorbitol q6h	
Chelating Agents (Metal Antagonists)			
Deferoxamine (Desferal)	Acute iron intoxication Hemochromatosis due to blood transfusions Hemosiderosis due to hemolytic anemia	PO 4–8 g, within a few hours of oral ingestion of iron preparations IM 1 g initially, then 500 mg q4h for 2 doses, then 500 mg q4–12h if needed; maximum dose, 6 g/24h IV infusion (for patients in shock) 1 g slowly (not to exceed 15 mg/kg/h), then 500 mg q4h for 2 doses, then 500 mg q4–12h if necessary; maximum dose, 6 g/24 h	Same as adults
Penicillamine (Cuprimine)	Wilson's disease Rheumatoid arthritis Cystinuria	Wilson's disease, PO 250 mg 4 times daily, increased gradually if necessary, up to 2 g daily Rheumatoid arthritis, PO 125–250 mg/d for 4 wk, increased by 125–250 mg/d at 1- to 3-mo intervals, if necessary usual maintenance dose, 500–750 mg/d; maximum dose, 1000–1500 mg/d	*Older children:* same as adults *Infants >6 mo and young children:* Wilson's disease, PO 250 mg daily, dissolved in fruit juice
Succimer (Chemet)	Lead poisoning		PO 10 mg/kg or 350 mg/m² q8h for 5 days, then q12h for 14 days (total of 19 days of drug administration) For young children who cannot swallow capsules, the capsule contents can be sprinkled on soft food or given with a spoon.
Iron Preparations			
Ferrous gluconate (Fergon)	Iron deficiency anemia	PO 320–640 mg (40–80 mg elemental iron) 3 times daily	PO 100–300 mg (12.5–37.5 mg elemental iron) 3 times daily *Infants:* PO 100 mg or 30 drops of elixir initially, gradually increased to 300 mg or 5 mL (15–37.5 mg elemental iron) of elixir daily, in divided doses

Table 57-4 Drugs at a Glance: Individual Agents Used in Mineral-Electrolyte and Acid-Base Imbalances (continued)

| DRUG | INDICATIONS FOR USE | ROUTES AND DOSAGE RANGES | |
		Adults	Children
Ferrous sulfate (Feosol)	Iron deficiency anemia	PO 325 mg–1.2 g (60–240 mg elemental iron) daily in 3 or 4 divided doses	*6–12 y:* PO 120–600 mg (24–120 mg elemental iron) daily, in divided doses *<6 y:* 300 mg (60 mg elemental iron) daily, in divided doses
Iron dextran injection (InFeD)	Iron deficiency anemia	Dosage is calculated for individual clients according to hemoglobin and weight (see manufacturer's literature). A small test dose is required before therapeutic doses are given.	Dosage is calculated for individual clients according to hemoglobin and weight (see manufacturer's literature). A small test dose is required before therapeutic doses are given.
Magnesium Preparations **Magnesium oxide** **Magnesium hydroxide** **Magnesium sulfate**	Prevent or treat hypomagnesemia Treat hypertension or convulsions associated with toxemia of pregnancy or acute nephritis in children	Hypomagnesemia, PO magnesium oxide 250–500 mg 3–4 times daily, milk of magnesia 5 mL 4 times daily, or a magnesium-containing antacid 15 mL 3 times daily; IM (magnesium sulfate) 1–2 g (2–4 mL of 50% solution) 1–2 times daily based on serum magnesium levels Eclampsia, IM 1–2 g (2–4 mL of 50% solution) initially, then 1 g every 30 min until seizures stop Convulsive seizures, IM 1 g (2 mL of 50% solution) repeated PRN IV, do not exceed 150 mg/min (1.5 mL/min of a 10% solution, 3 mL/min of a 5% solution)	Convulsions, IM 20–40 mg/kg in a 20% solution; repeat as necessary
Potassium Preparation **Potassium chloride** (KCl)	Prevent or treat hypokalemia	PO 15–20 mEq 2–4 times daily IV 40–100 mEq/24 h, depending on serum potassium levels KCl **must** be diluted in dextrose or NaCl IV solution for IV use. **Maximum** *for serum K+ >2.5 mEq:* diluted 40 mEq/L, infused	IV infusion up to 3 mEq/kg or 40 mEq/m² daily Adjust amount of fluids to body size.

(continued)

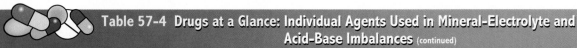

Table 57-4 Drugs at a Glance: Individual Agents Used in Mineral-Electrolyte and Acid-Base Imbalances (continued)

		ROUTES AND DOSAGE RANGES	
DRUG	**INDICATIONS FOR USE**	**Adults**	**Children**
		10 mEq/h to maximum dose of 200 mEq in 24 h **Maximum** *for serum K+* *<2.5 mEq:* diluted 80 mEq/L, infused 40 mEq/h to maximum dose of 400 mEq in 24 h	
Sodium Preparation **Sodium chloride** **(NaCl) injection**	Hyponatremia	IV 1500–3000 mL of 0.22% or 0.45% solution/24 h depending on the client's fluid needs; approximately 50 mL/h to keep IV lines open	
Zinc Preparation **Zinc sulfate**	Prevent or treat zinc deficiency	PO 25–50 mg elemental zinc (eg, zinc sulfate 110–220 mg) daily	
Multiple Mineral–Electrolyte Preparations Oral solutions (eg, Pedialyte) IV solutions (eg, Normosol, Plasma-Lyte 148, Ringer's solution)	Prevent or treat fluid and electrolyte deficiencies	IV 2000–3000 mL/24 h, depending on individual fluid and electrolyte needs	IV, PO, amount individualized according to fluid and electrolyte needs (ie, estimated fluid loss), age and weight (see manufacturer's literature)

IM, intramuscular; IV, intravenous; PO, oral; PRN, as needed.

---

lized; a portion of a dose is lost daily in feces. Otherwise, the iron content is recycled and its half-life is unknown. Sustained release or enteric-coated formulations are not as well absorbed as other preparations. Available ferrous salts differ in the amount of elemental iron they contain.

Adverse effects include nausea and other symptoms of GI irritation. Oral preparations also discolor feces, producing a black-green color that may be mistaken for blood in the stool. Iron preparations are contraindicated in clients with peptic ulcer disease, inflammatory intestinal disorders, anemias other than iron deficiency anemia, multiple blood transfusions, hemochromatosis, and hemosiderosis.

Ferrous sulfate (Feosol), which contains 20% elemental iron (ie, 65 mg per 325 mg tablet), is the prototype and often the preparation of choice. **Ferrous gluconate** (Fergon) may be less irritating to GI mucosa and therefore better tolerated than ferrous sulfate. It contains 12% elemental iron (ie, 36 mg per 325 mg tablet). **Ferrous fumarate** (Feostat) contains 33% elemental iron (ie, 33 mg per 100 mg tablet). As with dietary iron, only a portion is absorbed from pharmaceutical preparations and relatively large doses are needed to supply the 10 to

15 milligrams needed daily by most adults and children. Small amounts of iron are lost daily (about 0.5–1 mg) in urine, sweat, and sloughing of intestinal mucosal cells. Somewhat larger amounts (1–2 mg daily) are lost during menstruation. Thus, women of childbearing potential need larger amounts of iron than children, men, and postmenopausal women. Women who are pregnant have the greatest requirement and usually need an iron supplement. Although most iron products are available over-the-counter, their use should be discussed with a health care provider because of the toxicity that may occur with iron accumulation in body tissues.

Iron dextran injection (InFeD) is a parenteral form of iron useful in treating iron deficiency anemia when oral supplements cannot be used. One milliliter contains 50 milligrams of elemental iron. Indications for use include peptic ulcer or inflammatory bowel disease that is likely to be aggravated by oral iron preparations; the client's inability or unwillingness to take oral preparations; and a shortage of time for correcting the iron deficiency (eg, late pregnancy or preoperative status). Contraindications include anemias not associated with iron deficiency and clients with hypersensitivity to the drug (fatal anaphylactoid reactions have occurred).

The drug is usually given IV. Drug action has a slow onset and peaks in 1 to 2 weeks. Dosage is calculated according to hemoglobin level and weight. A small IV test dose should be given prior to a therapeutic dose.

Magnesium Preparations

Magnesium oxide or **hydroxide** may be given orally for mild hypomagnesemia in asymptomatic clients. **Magnesium sulfate** is given parenterally for moderate to severe hypomagnesemia; convulsions associated with pregnancy; and prevention of hypomagnesemia in total parenteral nutrition. Therapeutic effects in these conditions are attributed to the drug's depressant effects on the central nervous system and smooth, skeletal, and cardiac muscle. Oral magnesium salts may cause diarrhea; their uses as antacids and cathartics are discussed in Chapters 59 and 60, respectively.

Magnesium preparations are contraindicated in clients who have impaired renal function or who are comatose. Oral preparations of magnesium oxide or hydroxide act in 3 to 6 hours, are minimally absorbed systemically, and are excreted in urine. With parenteral magnesium sulfate, intramuscular (IM) injections act in 1 hour and last 3 to 4 hours; IV administration produces immediate action that lasts about 30 minutes. The products are excreted in urine.

Potassium Preparation

Potassium chloride (KCl) is usually the drug of choice for preventing or treating hypokalemia because deficiencies of potassium and chloride often occur together. It may be prescribed for clients who are receiving potassium-losing diuretics (eg, hydrochlorothiazide, furosemide); those who are receiving digoxin (hypokalemia increases risks of digoxin toxicity); and those who are receiving only IV fluids because of surgical procedures, GI disease, or other conditions. KCl also may be used to replace chloride in hypochloremic metabolic alkalosis. It is contraindicated in clients with renal failure and in those receiving potassium-saving diuretics, such as triamterene, spironolactone, or amiloride.

KCl can be given orally or IV. Oral preparations are available in flavored powders, liquids, effervescent tablets, and controlled- or extended-release tablets. Most clients prefer tablets to liquids. These preparations act slowly and peak in 1 to 2 hours. IV preparations act rapidly; IV KCl **must** be well diluted before administration to prevent hyperkalemia, cardiotoxicity, and severe pain at the injection site. Dosage must be individualized according to serum potassium levels; the usual range is 20 to 60 milliequivalents in 24 hours.

Zinc Preparations

Zinc sulfate and **zinc gluconate** are available over-the-counter in various forms and strengths (eg, tablets with 110 mg and capsules with 220 mg of zinc sulfate, equivalent to 25 or 50 mg

of elemental zinc). Zinc is also an ingredient in several vitamin–mineral combination products. Zinc preparations are given orally as a dietary supplement to prevent or treat zinc deficiency. They have a slow onset of action and a delayed peak. They are metabolized in the liver and excreted in feces.

Multiple Mineral–Electrolyte Preparations

There are numerous electrolyte solutions for IV use to maintain or replace electrolytes when the client is unable to eat and drink.

Oral electrolyte solutions (eg, Pedialyte) contain several electrolytes and a small amount of dextrose. They are used to supply maintenance amounts of fluids and electrolytes when oral intake is restricted. They are especially useful in children for treatment of diarrhea and may prevent severe fluid and electrolyte depletion. The amount given must be carefully calculated, prescribed, and administered to avoid excessive intake. Oral solutions should not be used in severe circumstances in which IV fluid and electrolyte therapy is indicated and they should not be mixed with other electrolyte-containing fluids, such as milk or fruit juices. In addition, they must be cautiously used in impaired renal function.

NURSING PROCESS

Assessment

Assess each client for current or potential nutritional deficiencies. Some specific assessment factors include the following:

● What are usual eating patterns?
● Does the client appear underweight? If so, assess for contributing factors (eg, appetite; ability to obtain, cook, or chew food). Calculate or estimate the body mass index (BMI); a BMI under $18.5 \ kg/m^2$ indicates undernutrition.
● Does the client have symptoms, disease processes, treatments, medications, or diagnostic tests that are likely to interfere with nutrition? For example, many illnesses and oral medications cause anorexia, nausea, vomiting, and diarrhea.

With vitamins, assessment factors include the following:

● Deficiency states are more common than excess states and people with other nutritional deficiencies are likely to have vitamin deficiencies as well.
● Deficiencies of water-soluble vitamins (B complex and C) are more common than those of fat-soluble vitamins.
● Vitamin deficiencies are usually multiple and signs and symptoms often overlap, especially with B-complex deficiencies.
● Vitamin requirements are increased during infancy, pregnancy, lactation, fever, hyperthyroidism, and many

illnesses. Thus, a vitamin intake that is normally adequate may be inadequate in certain circumstances.

- Vitamin deficiencies are likely to occur in people who are poor, elderly, chronically or severely ill, or alcoholic.
- Vitamin excess states are rarely caused by excessive dietary intake but may occur with use of vitamin drug preparations, especially if megadoses are taken.

With mineral–electrolytes, assessment factors include the following:

- Deficiency states are more common than excess states unless a mineral–electrolyte supplement is being taken. However, deficiencies and excesses may be equally harmful, and both must be assessed.
- Clients with other nutritional deficiencies are likely to have mineral–electrolyte deficiencies as well. Moreover, deficiencies are likely to be multiple, with overlapping signs and symptoms.
- Many drugs influence gains and losses of minerals and electrolytes, including diuretics and laxatives.
- Minerals and electrolytes are lost with gastric suction, polyuria, diarrhea, excessive perspiration, and other conditions.

Assess laboratory reports when available:

- Check the complete blood count for decreased red blood cells, hemoglobin, and hematocrit. Reduced values may indicate iron deficiency anemia, and further assessment is needed.
- Check serum electrolyte reports for abnormal values. All major minerals can be measured in clinical laboratories. The ones usually measured are sodium, chloride, and potassium; carbon dioxide content, a measure of bicarbonate, is also assessed.

Nursing Diagnoses

- Imbalanced Nutrition: Less Than Body Requirements related to inadequate intake or impaired ability to digest nutrients
- Imbalanced Nutrition: More Than Body Requirements related to excessive intake of pharmaceutical preparations of vitamins and minerals
- Risk for Injury related to complications of tube or IV feedings
- Risk for Injury related to nutrient deficiency or overdose
- Deficient Knowledge: Nutritional needs and sources of nutrients

Planning/Goals

The client will

- Improve nutritional status in relation to body needs
- Maintain fluid and electrolyte balance

- Ingest appropriate amounts of vitamins and mineral–electrolytes
- Avoid complications of enteral nutrition, including aspiration, diarrhea, and infection
- Avoid complications of parenteral nutrition
- Avoid overdoses and adverse effects of vitamins and minerals
- Avoid mineral–electrolyte supplements unless recommended by a health care provider
- Take mineral–electrolyte drugs as prescribed and have appropriate laboratory tests to monitor response

Interventions

- Promote a well-balanced diet for all clients. Five daily servings of fruits and vegetables provide adequate vitamins unless the client has increased requirements or conditions that interfere with absorption or use of vitamins. An oral multivitamin may benefit most people, but it is not a substitute for an adequate diet. A diet that is adequate in protein and calories usually provides adequate minerals and electrolytes. Exceptions are calcium and iron, which are often needed as a dietary supplement in women and children.
- Treat symptoms or disorders that are likely to interfere with nutrition, such as pain, nausea, vomiting, or diarrhea.
- For clients who need increased protein-calorie intake, provide palatable supplements at appropriate times and encourage clients to take them.
- Promote exercise and activity. For undernourished clients, this may increase appetite, improve digestion, and aid bowel elimination.
- Minimize the use of sedative-type drugs when appropriate. Although no one should be denied pain relief, strong analgesics and other sedatives may cause drowsiness and decreased desire or ability to eat and drink as well as constipation and a feeling of fullness.
- Weigh clients at regular intervals. Calculate or estimate BMI when indicated.
- For clients receiving parenteral nutrition, monitor weight, fluid intake, urine output, vital signs, blood glucose, serum electrolytes, and complete blood count daily or weekly, according to the client's status and whether he or she is hospitalized or at home.
- Mineral supplements are recommended only for current or potential deficiencies because all are toxic in excessive amounts.
- For clients who have nasogastric tubes to suction, irrigate the tubes with isotonic sodium chloride solution. The use of tap water is contraindicated because it is hypotonic and would pull electrolytes into the stomach. Electrolytes are then lost in the aspirated and discarded stomach contents. For the same reason, only small amounts of ice chips or water are allowed per hour. Clients often request

ice chips or water in larger amounts than desirable; the nurse must explain the reason for the restrictions.

● Provide appropriate client teaching regarding nutritional support products, vitamins, and minerals (see accompanying display).

Evaluation

● Observe undernourished clients for quantity and quality of nutrient intake, weight gain, and improvement in laboratory tests of nutritional status (eg, serum proteins, blood sugar, electrolytes).

● Observe children for quantity and quality of food intake and appropriate increases in height and weight.

● Interview and observe for signs and symptoms of complications of enteral and parenteral nutrition.

PRINCIPLES OF THERAPY

Managing Nutritional Deficiencies

When possible, oral administration of liquid formulas, vitamins, and minerals is preferred. With vitamin and mineral supplements, larger doses are needed to treat deficiencies than are needed to prevent them. Treatment of deficiency states should be cautious, to avoid excess states.

Enteral Nutrition: Oral and Tube Feedings

When the GI tract is functional but the client cannot ingest enough food and fluid, high-protein, high-calorie foods (eg, milkshakes) or nutritionally complete supplements (eg, Ensure) can be given with meals, between meals, and at bedtime. When oral feeding is contraindicated, tube feeding

---

CLIENT TEACHING GUIDELINES
Nutritional Support Products, Vitamins, and Minerals

General Considerations

☑ Nutrition is extremely important in promoting health and recovery from illness. For people who are unable to take in enough nutrients because of poor appetite or illness, nutritional supplements can be very beneficial in improving nutritional status. For example, supplemental feedings can slow or stop weight loss; increase energy and feelings of well-being; and increase resistance to infection.

☑ With oral or tube-feeding supplements, choose one or more that the client is able and willing to take when possible.

☑ With vitamins, supplements are often recommended because studies indicate that many adults and children do not ingest sufficient dietary vitamins. Supplements are also usually needed by pregnant women and by people who smoke, ingest large amounts of alcohol, have impaired immune systems, or are elderly. When choosing a vitamin supplement, the following factors should be considered:

☑ Avoid large doses of vitamins. They will not promote health, strength, or youth. In addition, excessive amounts of B vitamins and vitamin C are eliminated in urine and some can cause adverse effects (eg, large doses of vitamin C can cause kidney stones; niacin [B_3] can cause stomach upset, flushing, skin rashes, itching, and aggravation of asthma and gout; pyridoxine [B_6] may cause numbness in limbs and difficulty in walking). Excessive amounts of vitamins A, D, E, and K are stored in the body and often lead to toxic effects. For example, high doses of vitamin A can result in headaches; diarrhea; nausea; loss of appetite; dry, itching skin; and elevated blood calcium. Excessive doses during pregnancy may cause birth defects.

☑ Although natural vitamins are advertised as being better than synthetic vitamins, there is no evidence to support this claim. The two types are chemically identical and used in the same way by the human body. Natural vitamins are more expensive.

☑ Sexually active women of childbearing potential need an adequate intake of folic acid to prevent severe birth defects in infants. To help prevent birth defects from folic acid deficiency, the Food and Drug Administration requires that folic acid be added to breads and cereal-grain products. This is estimated to add about 100 mcg of folic acid to the daily diet of most people. However, the recommended daily intake for adults is 400 mcg.

☑ Vitamins from supplements exert the same physiologic effects as those obtained from foods.

☑ Multivitamin preparations often contain minerals as well, usually in smaller amounts than those recommended for daily intake. Large doses of minerals are toxic.

☑ With minerals, a well-balanced diet contains all the minerals needed for health in most people. Exceptions are calcium and iron, which are often needed as a dietary supplement in women and children. Note that herbal preparations of chamomile, feverfew, and St. John's wort may inhibit iron absorption. The safest action is to take mineral supplements only on a health care provider's advice, in the amounts and for the length of time prescribed. All minerals are toxic when taken in excess. Additional considerations include:

☑ Keep all mineral–electrolyte substances out of reach of children to prevent accidental overdose. Acute iron intoxication is a common problem among young children and can be fatal. Also, supervise children in using fluoride supplements (eg, remind them to spit out oral rinses and gels rather than swallow them).

☑ Keep appointments with health care providers for periodic blood tests and other follow-up procedures when mineral–electrolyte supplements are prescribed (eg, potassium chloride). This helps prevent ingestion of excessive amounts.

(continued)

✔ Minerals are often contained in multivitamin preparations, with percentages of the recommended dietary allowances supplied. These amounts differ in various preparations and should be included in estimations of daily intake.

Self- or Caregiver Administration

✔ For oral supplemental feedings, take or give at the preferred time and temperature, when possible.

✔ For tube feedings:

  ✔ Use or give with the client in a sitting position, if possible, to decrease risks of strangling and pulling formula into the lungs.

  ✔ Be sure the tube is placed correctly before each feeding. Ask a health care provider how to check placement with your type of tube.

  ✔ Be sure the solution is room temperature. Cold formulas may cause abdominal cramping.

  ✔ Do not take or give more than 1 pint (500 mL) per feeding, including 2 to 3 oz of water for rinsing the tube. This helps to avoid overfilling the stomach and possible vomiting.

  ✔ Take or give slowly, over approximately 30 to 60 minutes. Rapid administration may cause nausea and vomiting.

  ✔ With continuous feedings, change containers and tubing daily. With intermittent feedings, rinse all equipment after each use, and change at least every 24 hours. Most tube-feeding formulas are milk based and infection may occur if formulas become contaminated or equipment is not kept clean.

  ✔ Ask a health care provider about the amount of water to take or give. Most people receiving 1.5 to 2 quarts (1500–2000 mL) of tube feeding daily need approximately 1 quart (1000 mL) or more of water daily. However, clients' needs vary. Water can be mixed with the tube feeding formula, given after the tube feeding, or given between feedings. Be sure to include the amount of water used for rinsing the tube in the total daily amount.

✔ For giving medications by tube:

  ✔ Give liquid preparations when available. When not available, some tablets may be crushed and some capsules may be emptied and mixed with 1 to 2 tablespoons of water. Ask a health care provider which medications can safely be crushed or altered, because some (eg, long-acting or enteric-coated) can be harmful if crushed.

  ✔ Do not mix medications with the tube-feeding formula because some medications may not be absorbed.

  ✔ Do not mix medications; give each one separately.

  ✔ Rinse the tube with water before and after each medication to get the medication through the tube and to keep the tube open.

✔ With supplementary vitamins, preparations differ widely in amounts and types of vitamin content. The product should not contain more than recommended amounts of vitamin D and vitamin A because of possible adverse effects.

✔ When choosing a vitamin supplement, compare ingredients and costs. Store brands are usually effective and less expensive than name brands.

✔ Vitamin C supplements are available in tablet and powder forms of various dosages, often in multivitamin and other preparations sold as antioxidants. In 2000, the recommended dietary allowance was increased from 60 mg daily to 75 mg for adult women and 90 mg for adult men. Large doses (eg, 1000 mg or more daily) may cause adverse effects and should be avoided. An adequate amount of vitamin C can also be obtained by eating at least five servings of fruit and vegetables daily.

✔ Take oral niacin preparations, except for timed-release forms, with or after meals or at bedtime to decrease stomach irritation. In addition, sit or lie down for approximately 30 minutes after taking a dose. Niacin causes blood vessels to dilate and may cause facial flushing, dizziness, and falls. Facial flushing can be decreased by taking 325 mg of aspirin 30 to 60 minutes before a dose of niacin. Itching, tingling, and headache may also occur. These effects usually subside with continued use of niacin.

✔ Swallow extended-release products whole; do not break, crush, or chew them. Breaking the product delivers the entire dose at once and may cause adverse effects.

✔ Take prescribed vitamins as directed and for the appropriate time. In pernicious anemia, vitamin B_{12} injections must be taken for the remainder of life. In pregnancy and lactation, vitamin supplements are usually taken only during this period of increased need.

✔ Swallow vitamin E capsules whole; do not crush or chew.

✔ Take iron preparations with or after meals, with approximately 8 oz of fluid, to prevent stomach upset. Do not take iron with coffee or other caffeine-containing beverages, because caffeine decreases absorption (take iron and caffeine preparations at least 2 hours apart). Do not crush or chew slow-release tablets or capsules. With liquid preparations, dilute with water, drink through a straw, and rinse the mouth afterward to avoid staining the teeth. Expect that stools will be dark green or black.

✔ With potassium preparations, mix oral solutions or effervescent tablets with at least 4 oz of water or juice to improve the taste, dilute the drug, and decrease gastric irritation. Do not crush or chew slow-release preparations. Take after meals initially to decrease gastric irritation. If no nausea, vomiting, or other problems occur, the drug can be tried before meals because it is better absorbed from an empty stomach. Do *not* stop taking the medication without notifying the physician who prescribed it, especially if also taking digoxin or diuretics. Excessive amounts should also be avoided. Do not use salt substitutes unless they are recommended by a health care provider; they contain potassium chloride and may result in excessive intake. Serious problems may develop from either high or low levels of potassium in the blood.

helps to maintain GI tract and immune system functioning. Guidelines for tube feedings include the following:

- Several tubes and placement sites are available. For short-term use (about 4 weeks), a nasogastric tube may be used. For long-term feedings, a gastrostomy tube may be placed percutaneously or surgically. Naso-intestinal tubes are recommended for clients at risk of aspiration from gastric feedings or with gastric disorders. Except for gastrostomy tubes, the tubes should be soft and small bore to decrease trauma.
- When tube feedings are the client's only source of nutrients, they should be nutritionally complete and given in amounts calculated to provide adequate water, protein, calories, vitamins, and minerals.
- For feedings that enter the stomach, intermittent administration is often used. For feedings that enter the duodenum or jejunum, a continuous drip method is required because the small bowel cannot tolerate the larger volumes of intermittent feedings. Continuous feedings require an infusion pump for accurate control of the flow rate. Water can be given with, after, or between regular feedings and with medications, according to the client's fluid needs.
- A potential complication of tube feeding is aspiration of the formula into the lungs. This is more likely to occur with unconscious clients. It can be prevented by correctly positioning clients, verifying tube placement, and giving feedings slowly.

Parenteral Nutrition: IV Feedings

Parenteral feedings are indicated when the GI tract is nonfunctional, when nutritional needs cannot be met by enteral feedings, or when enteral feedings would aggravate conditions such as inflammatory bowel diseases or pancreatitis.

Short-Term IV Nutrition

For short-term use (eg, 3–5 days), the goal is to provide adequate amounts of fluids and electrolytes and enough carbohydrate to minimize oxidation of body protein and fat for energy. The choice of specific solution depends on individual needs, but it should contain at least 5% dextrose. A frequently used solution is 5% dextrose in 0.22% sodium chloride, 2000 to 3000 milliliters in 24 hours (provides approximately 170 kcal/L, water, sodium, and chloride). KCl is often added, and vitamins may be added. These solutions are nutritionally inadequate.

Long-Term IV Nutrition

For long-term use (weeks to months), the goal is to provide all nutrients required for normal body functioning, including tissue growth and repair. Basic solutions provide water, carbohydrate, protein, vitamins, and minerals; fat emulsions (eg, Intralipid) are usually given separately to provide additional calories and essential fatty acids (500 mL of 10% emulsion provides 550 kcal). Guidelines include the following:

- Parenteral nutritional solutions can be administered through central or peripheral IV lines. Some solutions are hypertonic (from high concentrations of glucose) and must be given in a central vein so they can be diluted rapidly. Solutions that contain 5% or 10% dextrose are less hypertonic and can be given in a peripheral vein. However, they are nutritionally incomplete and used for a limited time (about 5–7 days).
- Fat emulsions are isotonic and may be given centrally or peripherally. When given peripherally, they are coinfused with dextrose–protein solution, to help protect the vein from phlebitis.
- Dextrose–protein solutions are given through an in-line filter. Fat emulsions should not be filtered; they are "piggybacked" into the IV line beyond the filter.
- Solutions should be administered with an infusion pump to maintain a steady and accurate flow rate.
- Sterile technique should be used in all aspects of preparation, administration, and site care. Most agencies have specific protocols for changing solution containers, administration sets, and dressings at the venipuncture site.

Managing Vitamin Disorders

Early recognition and treatment of vitamin disorders can prevent a mild deficiency or excess from becoming severe. For deficiency states, oral vitamin preparations are preferred when possible. Multiple deficiencies are common and a multivitamin preparation used to treat them usually contains more than the recommended daily amount. These products should be used for limited periods. When fat-soluble vitamins are given to correct a deficiency, there is a risk of producing excess states. When water-soluble vitamins are given, excesses are less likely but may occur with large doses. For excess states, the usual treatment is to stop administration of the vitamin preparation. There are no specific antidotes or antagonists.

Vitamin A Disorders

With vitamin A deficiency, assist clients to increase intake of foods containing preformed vitamin A (eg, meat, egg yolk, whole milk) or beta carotene (eg, yellow fruits and vegetables such as cantaloupe, peaches, carrots, sweet potatoes) when feasible. If a supplement is required, vitamin A alone may be preferred over a multivitamin unless multiple deficiencies are present. Daily doses should not exceed 25,000 IU (approximately 7500 mcg RE; 1 mcg RE = 3.3 IU) daily unless a severe deficiency is present. Vitamin A may be given IM if GI absorption is severely impaired or ocular symptoms are severe. With vitamin A excess, immediately stop known sources of the vitamin.

Vitamin K Disorders

With vitamin K deficiency, bleeding may occur spontaneously or in response to trauma. Thus, administration of vitamin K and measures to prevent bleeding are indicated. If the deficiency is not severe, oral vitamin K may be given for a few days until serum prothrombin activity returns to a normal range. In obstructive jaundice, bile salts must be given at the same time as oral vitamin K, or vitamin K must be given parenterally. In malabsorption syndromes or diarrhea, parenteral administration is probably necessary. A single dose of vitamin K may be sufficient.

With severe bleeding, vitamin K may be given IV but must be given very slowly to decrease risks of hypotension and shock. Even with IV vitamin K, however, therapeutic effects do not occur for at least 4 hours. For more rapid control of bleeding, transfusions of plasma or whole blood are needed.

B-Complex Disorders

With B-complex vitamins, most deficiencies are multiple rather than single and treatment consists of increasing intake of foods containing B-complex vitamins (many foods, including meat, vegetables, and cereal grains) or giving multivitamin preparations. If a single deficiency seems predominant, that vitamin may be given alone or in addition to a multivitamin preparation. For example, *folic acid* deficiency may occur with inadequate dietary intake and intestinal disorders that inhibit absorption. In addition, folic acid is depleted by alcohol and several medications, including antibiotics containing trimethoprim (eg, Bactrim), phenytoin, methotrexate, and oral contraceptives. *Thiamine* deficiency is common in alcoholics because of inadequate dietary intake and the use of large amounts of thiamine to metabolize ethanol.

Anemias Associated With B-Complex Vitamin Deficiencies
One type of anemia occurs with pyridoxine deficiency and is relieved by administration of pyridoxine. Another type, called *megaloblastic anemias* (because they are characterized by abnormally large, immature red blood cells), occurs with deficiency of folic acid or vitamin B_{12}. If megaloblastic anemia is severe, treatment is usually instituted with both folic acid and vitamin B_{12}.

In pernicious anemia, vitamin B_{12} must be given by injection because oral forms are not absorbed from the GI tract. The injections must be continued for life. Vitamin B_{12} is also given to prevent pernicious anemia in clients who are strict vegetarians, who have had gastrectomy, or who have chronic small bowel disease. Although folic acid relieves hematologic disorders of pernicious anemia, giving folic acid alone allows continued neurologic deterioration. Thus, an accurate diagnosis is required.

In other megaloblastic anemias, vitamin B_{12} or folic acid is indicated. Although both of these are included in many multivitamin preparations, they usually must be given separately for therapeutic purposes. With vitamin B_{12}, doses in excess of 100 micrograms are rapidly excreted in urine. With folic acid, doses in excess of 1 milligram are excreted in the urine.

Vitamin C Disorders

Treatment of vitamin C deficiency involves increased intake of vitamin C from dietary (eg, fruits and vegetables) or pharmaceutical sources. Vitamin C is available alone for oral, IM, or IV administration. It is also an ingredient in most multivitamin preparations for oral or parenteral use.

In 2000, the DRI for vitamin C was increased from 60 milligrams daily to 75 milligrams for most adult women and 90 milligrams for most adult men. Some nutritionists recommend 120 milligrams per day; others recommend approximately 200 milligrams per day from five servings of fruits and vegetables or 100 milligrams per day of a vitamin C supplement. An additional recommendation is to avoid large doses (ie, more than 1 g/day). With excessive intake of vitamin C supplements, the main concern is formation of calcium oxalate kidney stones and potential obstruction or other renal damage. There is no known benefit of such large amounts, and their use should be discouraged.

Use of Vitamins in Preventing Cancer and Cardiovascular Disease

Vitamins with antioxidant effects (eg, C; E; beta carotene, a precursor of vitamin A) are thought to help prevent heart disease, cancer, and other illnesses. Antioxidants inactivate oxygen free radicals, potentially toxic substances formed during normal cell metabolism, and prevent or inhibit them from damaging body cells. In general, however, research studies are inconclusive and vitamin supplementation to prevent cancer and cardiovascular disease is not currently recommended. Clinical trials continue in this area.

Cancer

Vitamin A and beta carotene may reduce cancers of the lung, breast, oral mucosa, esophagus, and bladder. Vitamin A supplements are not recommended, but people are urged to increase dietary intake of fruits and vegetables that contain vitamin A and beta carotene. It is unknown whether anticancer effects stem from beta carotene or other components of fruits and vegetables.

Vitamin C, in diets with five or more daily servings of fruits and vegetables, is associated with reduced risk of cancers of the GI tract (eg, oral cavity, esophagus, stomach, colon) and lung. However, in some studies, vitamin C supplements did not decrease the occurrence of stomach or colorectal cancer. Thus, the cancer-preventing effects of fruits and vegetables may be associated with factors other than vitamin C. Vitamin E has also been promoted for cancer prevention, but supplementation to prevent cancer is not recommended (see accompanying Research Brief).

RESEARCH BRIEF

Effects of Vitamin E Supplementation

SOURCE:

Lonn, E., Bosch, J., Yusuf, S., et al. (2005). Effects of long-term vitamin E supplementation on cardiovascular events and cancer: A randomized controlled trial. *Journal of the American Medical Association, 293*(11), 1338–1347.

SUMMARY:

This report is from the Heart Outcomes Prevention Evaluation (HOPE) clinical trial, conducted between December 1993 and April 1999; and its extension (HOPE-The Ongoing Outcomes or HOPE-TOO), continued from April 1999 until May 2003. HOPE involved more than 9000 clients and HOPE-TOO involved more than 7000 clients 55 years of age or older who had vascular disease or diabetes mellitus. The purpose of the study was to evaluate whether long-term vitamin E supplementation would decrease risks of cancer, cancer death, or major cardiovascular events (ie, myocardial infarction, stroke, or cardiovascular death). The clients took a daily vitamin E supplement of 400 international units (IU) or placebo for a median duration of 7 years. Results indicated no differences between the vitamin E group and the placebo group in cancer incidence, cancer deaths, or major cardiovascular events. In addition, the vitamin E group had higher rates of heart failure and hospitalizations for heart failure than the placebo group. The researchers concluded that long-term vitamin E supplementation does not prevent cancer or major cardiovascular events in clients with vascular disease or diabetes mellitus, may increase the risk for heart failure, and should not be used in this population.

NURSING IMPLICATIONS:

The main implication for the nurse may be to correct a common misconception that high-dose, long-term vitamin supplementation, including vitamin E, is beneficial to health, and that even if it does not benefit the recipient, it "can't hurt." For people 11 years of age and older, the Recommended Dietary Allowance (RDA) for vitamin E is 15 IU for males and 12 IU for females. Single vitamin E supplements may contain 100 to 1000 IU per tablet or capsule; multivitamin preparations may contain various amounts but usually contain more than the RDA.

Cardiovascular Disease

Folic acid and vitamin C are thought to have cardioprotective effects. Folic acid is important in the metabolism of homocysteine, a toxic amino acid and a major risk factor for heart dis-

ease. Homocysteine is normally produced during metabolism of methionine, another amino acid. Several B vitamins, including folic acid, are required for the metabolism of homocysteine to a nontoxic substance, and an increased blood level of homocysteine occurs with folic acid deficiency. Excessive homocysteine damages the endothelial lining of arteries and leads to plaque formation, atherosclerosis, and thrombosis. Folic acid supplements can prevent or delay these effects by lowering blood levels of homocysteine. Although the Food and Drug Administration (FDA) requirement that folic acid be added to cereal-grain foods may be helpful, the folic acid intake that helps prevent cardiovascular disease is thought to be higher.

Vitamin C is thought to help prevent cardiovascular disease by antioxidant effects. The atherogenic effects of blood lipids, especially low-density lipoprotein (LDL) cholesterol (see Chap. 55), are attributed to their chemical breakdown or oxidation. Vitamin C may help prevent oxidation of LDL cholesterol. Overall, however, the effects of vitamin C on prevention of coronary artery disease (CAD) are unclear. Some studies indicate an increased risk for CAD only with a severe vitamin C deficiency and that vitamin C has little effect on ischemic heart disease and stroke after adjustment for other risk factors. More research is needed before vitamin C supplements are recommended for cardioprotective effects, but increased intake of fruits and vegetables may be beneficial.

Vitamin E has also been promoted for prevention of cardiovascular disease. Although some observational studies report beneficial effects of vitamin E supplements, randomized clinical trials do not.

Managing Mineral–Electrolyte Disorders

When a mineral is given to correct a deficiency state, there is a risk of producing an excess state. Because both deficiencies and excesses may be harmful, the amount of mineral supplement should be titrated closely to the amount needed by the body. Larger doses are needed to treat deficiency states than are needed to prevent deficiencies from developing. When mineral–electrolyte drug preparations are needed, oral products are preferred when possible. They are safer, less likely to produce toxicity, more convenient to administer, and less expensive than parenteral preparations.

Potassium Disorders

Hypokalemia

- Assess for conditions contributing to hypokalemia, and attempt to eliminate them or reduce their impact.
- Assess severity by checking serum potassium levels and clinical manifestations. Serum potassium levels alone are inadequate because they may not accurately reflect depletion of body potassium or shifts of potassium into cells.
- In general, potassium supplements are indicated when serum potassium is below 3 mEq/L; when symptoms

or electrocardiographic (ECG) changes indicate hypokalemia; and when clients are receiving digoxin, if necessary to maintain serum potassium above 3.5 mEq/L.

- KCl is the drug of choice in most instances. Controlled-release tablets or capsules with KCl in a wax matrix or microencapsulated form are preferred over liquids by most clients.
- IV KCl is indicated when a client cannot take an oral preparation or has severe hypokalemia. The serum potassium level should be measured and adequate urine output established before IV potassium therapy is started.
  - IV KCl must be well diluted to prevent sudden hyperkalemia, cardiotoxic effects, and phlebitis at the venipuncture site. The usual dilution is KCl 20 to 40 mEq per 1000 mL of IV fluid.
  - Dosage must be individualized. Clients receiving IV fluids only are usually given 40 to 60 mEq of KCl daily (eg, 20 mEq KCl per L of fluids at a flow rate of 100 to 125 mL/hour). An infusion pump should be used to control flow rate accurately. Also, serum potassium levels must be checked frequently and dosage adjusted if indicated.

Hyperkalemia

- Eliminate any exogenous sources of potassium, such as potassium supplements, penicillin G potassium, salt substitutes, and blood transfusion with old blood.
- Treat acidosis, if present, because potassium leaves cells and enters the serum with acidosis.
- Use measures that antagonize the effects of potassium, that cause potassium to leave the serum and re-enter cells, and that remove potassium from the body. Appropriate measures are determined mainly by serum potassium levels and ECG changes. Continuous cardiac monitoring is required. If the following measures fail to reduce hyperkalemia, peritoneal dialysis or hemodialysis may be used.

With severe hyperkalemia (serum potassium above 7 mEq/L and ECG changes indicating hyperkalemia), urgent treatment is required. IV **sodium bicarbonate** 45 milliequivalents, over a 5-minute period, causes rapid movement of potassium into cells. This can be repeated in a few minutes if ECG changes persist. **Calcium gluconate** 10%, 5 to 10 milliliters IV, is also given early in treatment to decrease the cardiotoxic effects of hyperkalemia. It is contraindicated if the client is receiving digoxin, and it cannot be added to fluids containing sodium bicarbonate because insoluble precipitates are formed. IV **glucose and insulin** may also be infused. This causes potassium to move into cells, though not as quickly as administration of sodium bicarbonate.

With less severe hyperkalemia (or when serum potassium levels have been reduced by other measures), sodium polystyrene sulfonate, a cation exchange resin, can be given orally or rectally to remove potassium from the body. Each gram of the resin combines with 1 milliequivalent of potassium, and both are excreted in feces. The resin is usually mixed with water and sorbitol, a poorly absorbed, osmotically active alcohol that has a laxative effect. The sorbitol offsets the constipating effect of the resin and aids in its expulsion. Oral administration is preferred, and several doses daily may be given until serum potassium is normal. When given as an enema, the solution must be retained from 1 to several hours, or repeated enemas must be given for therapeutic effect.

Magnesium Disorders

Hypomagnesemia

For mild hypomagnesemia, oral magnesium preparations may be given. For moderate to severe and symptomatic hypomagnesemia, parenteral (IV or IM) magnesium sulfate may be given daily as long as hypomagnesemia persists or continuing losses occur. Initial dosage may be larger, but the usual maintenance dose is approximately 8 milliequivalents daily. A 10% solution is available in 10-milliliter vials that contain 8 milliequivalents of magnesium sulfate for adding to IV solutions. A 50% solution is available in 2-milliliter vials (8 mEq) for IM administration. Serum magnesium levels should be measured daily during treatment with a magnesium preparation.

Hypermagnesemia

- Stop any source of exogenous magnesium, such as magnesium sulfate or magnesium-containing antacids and cathartics.
- Have calcium gluconate available for IV administration. It is an antidote for the sedative effects of magnesium excess.
- Increase urine output by increasing fluid intake, if feasible. This increases removal of magnesium from the body in urine.
- Clients with chronic renal failure are the most likely to become hypermagnesemic. They may require peritoneal dialysis or hemodialysis to lower serum magnesium levels.

Iron Deficiency and Excess

Iron Deficiency Anemia

- Anemia is a symptom, not a disease. Therefore, the underlying cause must be identified and eliminated, if possible.
- Encourage increased dietary intake of foods with high iron content.
- Ferrous sulfate is usually the drug of choice for oral iron therapy. Slow-release or enteric-coated products decrease absorption of iron, but may cause less gastric irritation.
- Dosage is calculated in terms of elemental iron. Iron preparations vary greatly in the amount of elemental iron they contain. Ferrous sulfate, for example, con-

tains 20% iron; thus, each 325-mg tablet furnishes about 65 mg of elemental iron. With the usual regimen of one tablet three times daily, a daily dose of 195 mg of elemental iron is given. For most clients, probably half that amount would correct the deficiency. However, tablets are not manufactured in sizes to allow this regimen, and liquid preparations are not popular with clients. Thus, relatively large doses are usually given, but smaller doses may be effective, especially if GI symptoms become a problem with higher dosages. Whatever the dose, only about 10% to 15% of the iron is absorbed. Most of the remainder is excreted in feces, which turn dark green or black.

- Oral iron preparations are better absorbed if taken on an empty stomach. However, because gastric irritation is a common adverse reaction, they are more often given with or immediately after meals.
- Although normal hemoglobin levels return after approximately 2 months of oral iron therapy, an additional 6-month period of drug therapy is recommended to replenish the body's iron stores.
- Reasons for failure to respond to iron therapy include continued blood loss, failure to take the drug as prescribed, or defective iron absorption. These factors must be re-evaluated if no therapeutic response is evident within 3 to 4 weeks after drug therapy is begun.
- Parenteral iron is indicated when oral preparations may further irritate a diseased GI tract, when the client is unable or unwilling to take the oral drugs, or when the anemia must be corrected rapidly.
- For severe iron deficiency anemia, blood transfusions may be most effective.

Iron Excess

- Acute iron overdosage requires treatment as soon as possible, even if overdosage is only suspected and the amount taken is unknown. It is unnecessary to wait until the serum iron level is measured.

  If treatment is begun shortly after oral ingestion of iron, aspiration of stomach contents by nasogastric tube or whole bowel irrigation with a polyethylene glycol solution (eg, CoLyte) may be performed. Gastric lavage can be followed by instillation of 1% sodium bicarbonate solution to form insoluble iron carbonate compounds, or 5 to 8 g of deferoxamine (Desferal) dissolved in 50 mL of distilled water to bind the iron remaining in the GI tract and prevent its absorption. Deferoxamine may also be given IM or IV to bind with iron in tissues and allow its excretion in the urine. Throughout the treatment period, supportive measures may be needed for GI hemorrhage, acidosis, and shock.
- For chronic iron overload or hemochromatosis, the first step in treatment is to stop the source of iron, if possible. Phlebotomy is the treatment of choice for most clients because withdrawal of 500 mL of blood removes about 250 mg of iron. Phlebotomy may be needed as often as weekly and for as long as 2 to 3 years. For clients resistant to or intolerant of phlebotomy, deferoxamine can be given. Ten to 50 mg of iron are excreted daily in the urine with deferoxamine administration.

Effects of Vitamins and Minerals on Other Drugs

Folic acid decreases effects of phenytoin, probably by accelerating phenytoin metabolism, and may decrease absorption and effects of zinc. *Niacin* may increase the risk of rhabdomyolysis (a life-threatening breakdown of skeletal muscle) with statin cholesterol-lowering drugs. *Vitamin A* in large doses, and possibly vitamin E, may increase the anticoagulant effect of warfarin. *Vitamin C,* 1 gram daily or more, may decrease metabolism and increase the effects of estrogens and oral contraceptives. It is recommended that the daily dose of vitamin C not exceed 100 milligrams, to prevent this interaction.

Iron salts may decrease absorption of levodopa, levothyroxine, methyldopa, penicillamine, fluoroquinolones, and tetracyclines. *Magnesium salts* may decrease absorption and therapeutic effects of digoxin, fluoroquinolones, nitrofurantoin, penicillamine, and tetracyclines. *Zinc salts* may decrease absorption of fluoroquinolones and most tetracyclines (doxycycline is apparently not affected).

Use in Special Populations

Nutritional Support in Children

Children usually need sufficient water, protein, carbohydrate, and fat in proportion to their size to support growth and increased physical activity. However, reports of childhood obesity and inadequate exercise are steadily increasing. Therefore, the goal of nutritional support is to meet needs without promoting obesity.

For children with special needs in relation to nutrients, various enteral formulations are available for use. Some examples include Lofenalac for children with phenylketonuria (a disorder in which the amino acid phenylalanine cannot be metabolized normally); Nursoy, Prosobee, and Soyalac, which contain soy protein, for children who are allergic to cow's milk; and Nutramigen and Pregestimil, which contain easily-digested nutrients for children with malabsorption or other GI problems.

With tube feedings, to prevent nausea and regurgitation, the recommended rate of administration is no more than 5 milliliters every 5 to 10 minutes for premature and small infants and 10 milliliters per minute for older infants and children. Preparation of formulas, positioning of children, and administration are the same as for adults to prevent aspiration and infection.

Parenteral nutrition may be indicated in infants and children who cannot eat or be fed enterally (eg, during medical illnesses or in perioperative conditions) to improve or maintain nutritional status. Overall, benefits include weight gain, increased height, increased liver synthesis of plasma proteins, and improved healing and recovery.

With **vitamins,** children need sufficient amounts to support growth and normal body functioning. If supplements are given, considerations include the following:

- Dosages should not exceed recommended amounts. There is a risk of overdosage by children and their parents. Because of manufacturers' marketing strategies, many supplements are available in flavors and shapes (eg, cartoon characters, animals) designed to appeal to children. Because younger children may think of these supplements as candy and take more than recommended, they should be stored out of reach and dispensed by an adult. Because parents' desires to promote health may lead them to give unneeded supplements or to give more than recommended amounts, parents may need information about the potential hazards of vitamin overdoses.
- The content of supplements for infants and children younger than 4 years of age is regulated by the FDA; the content of preparations for older children is not regulated.
- Supplements given to children and adolescents should provide recommended amounts of vitamins. Except for single supplements of vitamin K and vitamin E in infants, multivitamin products are commonly used. For infants, liquid formulations usually include vitamins A, D, C, and B complex. Folic acid is not included because it is unstable in liquid form. For older children, chewable tablets usually contain vitamins A, D, C, and B complex, including folic acid.
- A single IM dose of vitamin K is given to newborn infants to prevent hemorrhagic disease of newborns.
- Preterm infants need proportionately more vitamins than term infants because their growth rate is faster and their absorption of vitamins from the intestine is less complete. A multivitamin product containing the equivalent of DRIs for term infants is recommended.
- ULs have been established for some vitamins and these maximum daily amounts should not be exceeded. For

infants (birth to 12 months), the only UL is for vitamin D (25 mcg). For other children, ULs vary according to age, as listed in Table 57-5.

With **mineral–electrolytes,** children need sufficient amounts to support growth and normal body functioning. However, iron deficiency is common in young children and teenage girls, and an iron supplement is often needed. Guidelines include the following:

- A combined vitamin–mineral supplement every other day may be reasonable, especially for children who eat poorly.
- If supplements are given, dosages should be discussed with a health care provider and usually should not exceed recommended amounts for particular age groups. ULs for children have been established for some minerals and **these maximum daily amounts should not be exceeded.** They are listed in Table 57-6. The ULs for magnesium indicate maximum intake from pharmaceutical preparations; they do not include intake from food and water.
- All minerals and electrolytes are toxic in overdose and may cause life-threatening adverse effects. All such drugs should be kept out of reach of young children and should never be referred to as "candy."
- In areas where water is not fluoridated, a vitamin–mineral supplement containing fluoride may be indicated for infants and children. Fluoride must be prescribed by a physician, dentist, or nurse practitioner. Children must be guarded against excessive fluoride ingestion and possible toxicity. Fluoride supplements are used more often than formerly and numerous preparations are available for oral (tablets, chewable tablets, solutions) or topical (liquid rinse solutions or gels) uses. Supplements used by children or adults should be kept out of the reach of children; supplements prescribed for children should be used only with adult supervision; and children using topical preparations should be reminded to spit them out and not to swallow them.
- If KCl and other electrolyte preparations are used to treat deficiency states in children, serum electrolyte

TABLE 57-5 Vitamins: Tolerable Upper Intake Levels for Children

VITAMIN	1–3 YEARS	4–8 YEARS	9–13 YEARS	14–18 YEARS
D	50 mg	50 mg	50 mg	50 mg
E	200 mg	300 mg	600 mg	800 mg
C	400 mg	650 mg	1200 mg	1800 mg
Folate	300 mcg	400 mcg	600 mcg	800 mcg
Niacin	10 mg	15 mg	20 mg	30 mg
Pyridoxine	30 mg	40 mg	60 mg	80 mg

TABLE 57-6 Minerals: Tolerable Upper Intake Levels for Children

MINERAL	BIRTH–6 MONTHS	7–12 MONTHS	1–3 YEARS	4–8 YEARS	9–13 YEARS	14–18 YEARS
Calcium	No data	No data	2.5 g	2.5 g	2.5 g	2.5 g
Phosphorus	No data	No data	3 g	3 g	4 g	4 g
Fluoride	0.7 mg	0.9 mg	1.3 mg	2.2 mg	10 mg	10 mg
Magnesium	No data	No data	65 mg	110 mg	350 mg	350 mg
Selenium	45 mcg	60 mcg	90 mcg	150 mcg	280 mcg	400 mcg

levels must be monitored. In addition, doses must be carefully measured and given no more often than prescribed to avoid toxicity.

● Accidental ingestion of iron-containing medications and dietary supplements is a common cause of poisoning death in children younger than 6 years of age. To help combat accidental poisoning, products containing iron must be labeled with a warning and products with 30 mg or more of iron (eg, prenatal products) must be packaged as individual doses. All iron-containing preparations should be stored in places that are inaccessible to young children.

Nutritional Support in Older Adults

Older adults are at risk of undernutrition with all nutrients. Inadequate intake may result from the inability to obtain and prepare food; disease processes that interfere with the ability to digest and use nutrients; and the use of drugs that decrease absorption of nutrients. When alternative feeding methods (tube feedings, IV fluids) are used, careful assessment of nutritional status is required to avoid deficits or excesses. With the high incidence of atherosclerosis, cardiovascular disease, and diabetes mellitus in older adults, it is especially important that intake of animal fats and high-calorie sweets be reduced.

Vitamin requirements are the same as for younger adults, but deficiencies are common, especially of vitamins A and D, cyanocobalamin (B_{12}), folic acid, riboflavin, and thiamine. With vitamin B_{12}, for example, it is estimated that older adults only absorb 10% to 30% of the amount found in food. Every older adult should be assessed regarding vitamin intake (from foods and supplements) and use of drugs that interact with dietary nutrients. For most older adults, a daily multivitamin is probably desirable, even for those who seem healthy and able to eat a well-balanced diet. In addition, requirements may be increased during illnesses, especially those affecting GI function. Overdoses, especially of the fat-soluble vitamins A and D, may cause toxicity and should be avoided. ULs for older adults have been established for some vitamins (D, 50 mg; E, 1000 mg; C, 2000 mg; folate, 1000 mcg; niacin, 35 mg; pyridoxine, 100 mg) and **these amounts should not be exceeded.**

APPLYING YOUR KNOWLEDGE 57-1

You recognize that along with being undernourished, Mrs. Farber is also most likely deficient in vitamins. You confer with the physician. What will be the likely recommendation for Mrs. Farber?

Mineral–electrolyte requirements are also the same as for younger adults, but deficiencies of calcium and iron are common. Excess states also may occur in older adults. For example, decreased renal function promotes retention of magnesium and potassium. Hyperkalemia also may occur with the use of potassium supplements or salt substitutes. All minerals and electrolytes are toxic in overdose. ULs for older adults (>65 years of age) have been established for calcium (2.5 g), phosphorus (3–4 g), fluoride (10 mg), magnesium (350 mg), and selenium (400 mcg) and **these maximum daily amounts should not be exceeded.** In general, serum levels of minerals and electrolytes should be monitored carefully during illness, and measures taken to prevent either deficiency or excess states.

APPLYING YOUR KNOWLEDGE 57-2

It is important to assess clients for individual risk factors related to gender, health status, and age. For Mrs. Farber, what particular mineral–electrolyte deficiencies would you consider/explore?

Nutritional Support in Clients With Renal Impairment

Clients with impaired renal function usually have multiple metabolic disorders such as hyperglycemia, accumulation of urea nitrogen (the end product of protein metabolism), and increased serum triglyceride levels from disordered fat metabolism. With enteral nutrition, Amin-Aid may be given to provide amino acids, carbohydrates, and a few electrolytes for clients with acute or chronic renal failure. With parenteral nutrition, several amino acid solutions are formulated for clients with renal failure (eg, Aminosyn-RF). In addition, clients with acute renal failure (ARF) often have hyperkalemia, hyperphosphatemia, and hypermagnesemia, so that potassium, phosphorus, and magnesium should be omitted until serum levels return to normal. IV fat emulsions should not be given to clients with ARF if serum triglyceride levels exceed 300 milligrams per deciliter. With chronic renal failure

(CRF), high-calorie, low-electrolyte enteral formulations are usually indicated. Nepro is a formulation for clients receiving dialysis; Suplena, which is lower in protein and some electrolytes than Nepro, may be used in clients who are not receiving dialysis. Serum triglyceride levels should be measured before IV fat emulsions are given. Many clients with CRF have hypertriglyceridemia, which is worsened by fat emulsions and may cause pancreatitis.

With vitamins, clients with ARF who are unable to eat an adequate diet need a vitamin supplement to meet DRIs. Large doses of vitamin C should be avoided because urinary excretion is impaired. In addition, oxalate (a product of vitamin C catabolism) may precipitate in renal tubules or form calcium oxalate stones, obstruct urine flow, and worsen renal function. Clients with CRF often have deficiencies of water-soluble vitamins because many foods that contain these vitamins are restricted due to their potassium content. In addition, vitamin C is reabsorbed from renal tubules by a specific transport protein. When the transport protein becomes saturated, remaining vitamin C is excreted in urine. Vitamin C is removed by dialysis and clients receiving dialysis require vitamin C replacement. The optimal replacement dose is unknown but probably should not exceed 200 milligrams per day (to avoid increased oxalate and possible stones). Overall, a multivitamin with essential vitamins, including vitamin C 70 to 100 milligrams, pyridoxine 5 to 10 milligrams, and folic acid 1 milligram, is recommended for daily use.

With mineral–electrolyte products, several are contraindicated in clients with renal impairment, including magnesium and KCl, because of potential accumulation and toxicity. Frequent measurements of serum electrolyte levels may be indicated. In clients with CRF who are on hemodialysis and receiving supplemental erythropoietin therapy, two iron preparations have been developed to treat iron deficiency anemia. Sodium ferric gluconate complex (Ferrlecit) and iron sucrose (Venfor) may be given IV during dialysis.

Nutritional Support in Clients With Hepatic Impairment

The liver is extremely important in digestion and metabolism of carbohydrate, protein, and fat as well as storage of nutrients. Thus, clients with impaired hepatic function are often undernourished, with impaired metabolism of foodstuffs, vitamin deficiencies, and fluid and electrolyte imbalances. Depending on the disease process and the extent of liver impairment, these clients have special needs in relation to nutritional support.

- Clients with alcoholic hepatitis or cirrhosis have a high rate of metabolism and therefore need foods to supply extra energy. However, metabolic disorders interfere with the liver's ability to process and use foodstuffs. Clients with cirrhosis often have hyperglycemia. Clients with severe hepatitis often have hypoglycemia because of impaired hepatic production of glucose and possibly impaired hepatic metabolism of insulin.

- Protein restriction is usually needed in clients with cirrhosis to prevent or treat hepatic encephalopathy, which is caused by excessive protein or excessive production of ammonia (from protein breakdown in the GI tract). For clients able to tolerate enteral feedings (usually by GI tube), Hepatic Aid II is formulated for clients with liver failure. When parenteral nutrition is necessary for clients with hepatic failure and hepatic encephalopathy, HepatAmine, a special formulation of amino acids, may be used. Other amino acid preparations are contraindicated in clients with hepatic encephalopathy and coma.

- Enteral and parenteral fat preparations must be used very cautiously. Medium-chain triglycerides (eg, MCT oil), which are used to provide calories in other malnourished clients, may lead to coma in clients with advanced cirrhosis. Clients who require parenteral nutrition may develop high serum triglyceride levels and pancreatitis if given usual amounts of IV fat emulsions.

- Sodium and fluid restrictions are often needed to decrease edema.

- Vitamin deficiencies commonly occur in clients with chronic liver disease because of poor intake and malabsorption. With hepatic failure, hepatic stores of vitamin A, pyridoxine, folic acid, riboflavin, pantothenic acid, vitamin B_{12}, and thiamine are depleted. Folic acid deficiency may lead to megaloblastic anemia. Thiamine deficiency may lead to Wernicke's encephalopathy. Therapeutic doses of vitamins should be given for documented deficiency states.

  Niacin is contraindicated in liver disease because it may increase liver enzymes (alanine and aspartate aminotransferase, alkaline phosphatase) and bilirubin and cause further liver damage. Long-acting dosage forms may be more hepatotoxic than the fast-acting forms.

- Iron dextran must be used with extreme caution in clients with impaired hepatic function. Also, overdoses of chromium and copper are hepatotoxic and should be avoided.

Nutritional Support in Clients With Critical Illness

Critically ill clients often have organ failures that alter their ability to ingest and use essential nutrients. Thus, they may be undernourished in relation to protein-calorie, vitamin, and mineral–electrolyte needs. Some considerations include the following:

- With enteral nutrition, adequate calories and DRI-equivalent amounts of all vitamins are usually needed. Clients with respiratory impairment may need a formula that contains less carbohydrate and more fat than other products and produces less carbon dioxide (eg, Pulmocare, Nutrivent). Clients with cardiac or renal impairment who require fluid restriction may benefit from a more concentrated formula (eg, 1.5 kcal/mL).

● With parenteral nutrition, adequate types and amounts of nutrients are needed. When IV fat emulsions are given, they should be infused slowly, over 24 hours. With vitamins, the Nutrition Advisory Group of the American Medical Association (NAG-AMA) has established guidelines for daily intake, and parenteral multivitamin formulations are available for adults and children. Those for adults do not contain vitamin K, which is usually injected weekly. The usual dose is 2 to 4 mg, but some clinicians give 5 to 10 mg. Vitamin K is included in pediatric parenteral nutrition solutions.

● Electrolyte and acid–base imbalances often occur in critically ill clients and are usually treated as in other clients, with very close monitoring of serum electrolyte levels and avoiding excessive amounts of replacement products.

Nutritional Support in Home Care

The home care nurse is involved with nutritional matters in almost any home care setting. Because nutrition is so important to health, the home care nurse should take advantage of any opportunity for health promotion in this area. Health promotion may involve assessing the nutritional status of all members of the household, especially children, older adults, and those with obvious deficiencies, and providing assistance to improve nutritional status.

For clients receiving tube feedings at home, the home care nurse may teach about the goals of treatment, administration, preparation or storage of solutions, equipment (eg, obtaining, cleaning), and monitoring responses (eg, weight, urine output).

For clients receiving parenteral nutrition at home, solutions, infusion pumps, and other equipment are obtained from a pharmacy, home health agency, or independent company. The home care nurse may not be involved in the initial setup but is likely to participate in ongoing client care, monitoring of client responses, and supporting caregivers. In addition, the home care nurse may need to coordinate activities among physicians, IV therapy personnel, and other health care providers.

With vitamins, the home care nurse needs to assess for indications of vitamin deficiencies or use of supplements, especially megadoses. If difficulties are found, the nurse may need to counsel household members about dietary sources of vitamins and adverse effects of excessive vitamin intake.

With mineral–electrolytes, the home care nurse needs to assess for indications of mineral–electrolyte deficiency or excess. Depending on assessment data, teaching may be needed about dietary sources of these nutrients; when mineral supplements are indicated or should be avoided; and safety factors related to iron supplements or exposure to lead in homes with small children.

APPLYING YOUR KNOWLEDGE 57-3:
HOW CAN YOU AVOID THIS MEDICATION ERROR?
Mrs. Farber is taking an iron supplement. You tell the family to give her the iron supplement with her morning coffee.

N U R S I N G   A C T I O N S

Nutritional Products, Vitamins, and Mineral–Electrolytes

NURSING ACTIONS	RATIONALE/EXPLANATION
1. Administer accurately	
a. For **oral supplemental feedings,** chill liquids or pour over ice and give through a straw, from a closed container, between meals.	Chilling (or freezing) may improve formula taste and decrease formula odor. A straw directs the formula toward the back of the throat and decreases its contact with taste buds. A closed container also decreases odor. Giving between meals may have less effect on appetite at mealtimes.
b. For **tube feedings:**	
(1) Have the client sitting, if possible.	To decrease risks of aspirating formula into lungs
(2) Check tube placement before each feeding.	To prevent aspiration or accidental instillation of feedings into lungs
(3) Give the solution at room temperature.	Cold formulas may cause abdominal cramping.
(4) If giving by intermittent instillation, do not give more than 500 mL per feeding, including water for rinsing the tube.	To avoid gastric distention, possible vomiting, and aspiration into lungs
(5) Give by gravity flow (over 30–60 minutes) or infusion pump.	Rapid administration may cause nausea, vomiting, and other symptoms.
(6) With continuous feedings, change containers and tubing daily. With intermittent bolus feedings, rinse all equipment after each use, and change at least every 24 hours.	Most tube-feeding formulas are milk based and provide a good culture medium for bacterial growth. Clean technique, not sterile technique, is required.

(continued)

NURSING ACTIONS	RATIONALE/EXPLANATION
(7) Give additional water with, after, or between feedings.	To avoid dehydration and promote fluid balance. Most clients receiving 1500 to 2000 mL of tube-feeding formula daily will need 1000 mL or more of water daily.
(8) Rinse nasogastric tubes with at least 50–100 mL water after each bolus feeding or administration of medications through the tube.	To keep the tube patent and functioning. This water is included in calculation of fluid intake.
(9) When medications are ordered by tube, liquid preparations are preferred over crushed tablets or powders emptied from capsules.	Tablets or powders may stick in the tube lumen. This may mean the full dose of the medication does not reach the stomach. Also, the tube is likely to become obstructed.
c. With **pancreatic enzymes,** give before or with meals or food.	To be effective, these agents must be in the small intestine when food is present.
d. With **fat-soluble vitamins:**	
(1) Do not give oral preparations at the same time as mineral oil.	Mineral oil absorbs the vitamins and thus prevents their systemic absorption.
(2) For subcutaneous (Sub-Q) or intramuscular (IM) administration of vitamin K, aspirate carefully to avoid intravenous (IV) injection, apply gentle pressure to the injection site, and inspect the site frequently. For IV injection, vitamin K may be given by direct injection or diluted in IV fluids (eg, 5% dextrose in water or saline).	Vitamin K is given to clients with hypoprothrombinemia, which causes bleeding tendencies. Thus, any injection may cause trauma and bleeding at the injection site.
(3) Administer IV vitamin K slowly, at a rate not to exceed 1 mg/min, whether diluted or undiluted.	IV phytonadione may cause hypotension and shock from an anaphylactic type of reaction.
e. With **B-complex vitamins:**	
(1) Give parenteral cyanocobalamin (vitamin B_{12}) IM or deep Sub-Q.	
(2) Give oral niacin, except for timed-release forms, with or after meals or at bedtime. Have the client sit or lie down for about 30 minutes after administration.	To decrease anorexia, nausea, vomiting, diarrhea, and flatulence. Niacin causes vasodilation, which may result in dizziness, hypotension, and injury from falls. Vasodilation occurs within a few minutes and may last 1 hour.
(3) Give IM thiamine deeply into a large muscle mass. Avoid the IV route.	To decrease pain at the injection site. Hypotension and anaphylactic shock have occurred with rapid IV administration and large doses.
f. With **mineral–electrolyte preparations,** give oral drugs with food or immediately after meals; give IV preparations slowly, do not mix with any other drug in a syringe, and dilute as directed with compatible IV solutions.	Giving oral drugs with or after food decreases gastric irritation. Rapid IV administration may cause cardiac dysrhythmias or other serious problems. Mixing the drugs may cause drug inactivation or precipitation.
g. For **potassium supplements:**	
(1) For oral preparations, give with or after meals; do **not** crush controlled- or extended-release tablets; mix oral liquids, powders, and effervescent tablets in at least 4 oz of juice, water, or carbonated beverage.	Giving with food decreases gastric irritation; crushing extended-release tablets causes the drug to be absorbed immediately rather than over several hours, as intended; mixing dilutes, disguises the taste, and decreases gastric irritation.
(2) For IV potassium chloride (KCl), **never** give undiluted drug IV; dilute 20–60 mEq in 1000 ml of IV solution, such as dextrose in water; be sure that KCl is mixed well with the IV solution; as a general rule, give potassium-containing IV solutions at a rate that administers approximately 10 mEq/h or less; for life-threatening dysrhythmias caused by	Concentrated drug and transient hyperkalemia may cause life-threatening cardiotoxicity, severe pain, and vein sclerosis; adequate dilution decreases risks of hyperkalemia and cardiotoxicity and prevents or decreases pain at the infusion site; 10 mEq or less per hour is the safest amount and rate of potassium administration and it is usually effective; risks of hyperkalemia and life-threatening cardiotoxicity are

NURSING ACTIONS	RATIONALE/EXPLANATION
hypokalemia, potassium can be replaced with 20–40 mEq/h with constant electrocardiogram (ECG) monitoring. Use an infusion pump and do **not** give potassium-containing IV solutions into a central venous catheter.	greatly increased with high concentrations or rapid flow rates. Constant ECG monitoring can detect hyperkalemia. Infusion pumps can regulate the flow rate accurately. Administration through a central IV line can cause hyperkalemia and cardiac dysrhythmias or arrest.
h. For parenteral **magnesium sulfate** ($MgSO_4$):	
(1) Read the drug label carefully to be sure you have the correct preparation for the intended use.	$MgSO_4$ is available in concentrations of 10%, 25%, and 50% and in sizes of 2-, 10-, and 20-mL ampules, as well as a 30-mL multidose vial.
(2) For IM use, small amounts of 50% solution are usually given (1 g $MgSO_4$ = 2 mL of 50% solution).	
(3) For IV use, a 5% or 10% solution is used for direct injection, intermittent infusion, or continuous infusion. Whatever concentration is used, administer no more than 150 mg/min (1.5 mL/min of 10% solution; 3 mL/min of 5% solution).	
i. For **iron preparations:**	
(1) Give tablets or capsules before meals, with 8 oz of water or juice, if tolerated. If gastric upset occurs, give with or after meals. Instruct patients not to crush or chew sustained-release preparations.	Iron preparations are absorbed better if taken on an empty stomach. If taken with meals, note that bran, eggs, tea, coffee, and dairy products decrease iron absorption. Crushing or chewing releases all the medication at once, rather than over several hours, as intended.
(2) Dilute liquid iron preparations, give with a straw, and have the client rinse the mouth afterward.	To prevent temporary staining of teeth
(3) To give iron dextran IM, use a 2- to 3-inch needle and Z-track technique to inject the drug into the upper outer quadrant of the buttock.	To prevent discomfort and staining of Sub-Q tissue and skin
(4) To give iron dextran IV (either directly or diluted in sodium chloride solution and given over several hours), do not use the multidose vial.	The multidose vial contains phenol as a preservative and is not suitable for IV use. Ampules of 2 mL or 5 mL are available without preservative.
j. Refer to the individual drugs or package literature for instructions regarding administration of deferoxamine, penicillamine, IV sodium bicarbonate, and multiple electrolyte solutions.	
2. Observe for therapeutic effects	
a. With nutritional formulas given orally or by tube feeding, observe for weight gain and increased serum albumin. For infants and children receiving milk substitutes, observe for decreased diarrhea and weight gain.	Therapeutic effects depend on the reason for use (ie, prevention or treatment of undernutrition).
b. With pancreatic enzymes, observe for decreased diarrhea and steatorrhea.	The pancreatic enzymes function the same way as endogenous enzymes to aid digestion of carbohydrate, protein, and fat.
c. With vitamins, observe for decreased signs and symptoms of deficiency:	
(1) With vitamin A, observe for improved vision, especially in dim light or at night, less dryness in eyes and conjunctiva (xerophthalmia), and improvement in skin lesions.	Night blindness is usually relieved within a few days. Skin lesions may not disappear for several weeks.
(2) With vitamin K, observe for decreased bleeding and more nearly normal blood coagulation tests (eg, prothrombin time).	Blood coagulation tests usually improve within 4–12 hours.

(continued)

NURSING ACTIONS	RATIONALE/EXPLANATION
(3) With B-complex vitamins, observe for decreased or absent stomatitis, glossitis, seborrheic dermatitis, neurologic problems (neuritis, convulsions, mental deterioration, psychotic symptoms), cardiovascular problems (edema, heart failure), and eye problems (itching, burning, photophobia).	Deficiencies of B-complex vitamins commonly occur together and produce many similar manifestations.
(4) With vitamin B_{12} and folic acid, observe for increased appetite, strength and feeling of well-being, increased reticulocyte counts, and increased numbers of normal red blood cells, hemoglobin, and hematocrit.	Therapeutic effects may be rapid and dramatic. The client usually feels better within 24–48 hours, and normal red blood cells begin to appear. Anemia is decreased within approximately 2 weeks, but 4–8 weeks may be needed for complete blood count to return to normal.
(5) With vitamin C, observe for decreased or absent malaise, irritability, and bleeding tendencies (easy bruising of skin, bleeding gums, nosebleeds, and so forth).	
d. With mineral–electrolyte preparations, observe for decreased signs of deficiency.	
(1) With KCl or other potassium preparations, observe for decreased signs of hypokalemia and increased serum potassium levels.	
(2) With $MgSO_4$, observe for decreased signs of hypomagnesemia, increased serum magnesium levels, or control of convulsions.	
(3) With zinc sulfate ($ZnSO_4$), observe for improved wound healing.	
(4) With iron preparations, observe for increased vigor and feeling of well-being, improved appetite, less fatigue, and increased red blood cells, hemoglobin, and hematocrit. With parenteral iron, observe for an average increase in hemoglobin of 1 g/wk.	Therapeutic effects are usually evident within a month unless other problems are also present (eg, vitamin deficiency, achlorhydria, infection, malabsorption).
3. Observe for adverse effects	
a. With commercial nutritional formulas (except Osmolite and Isocal), observe for hypotension, tachycardia, increased urine output, dehydration, nausea, vomiting, or diarrhea.	These adverse reactions are usually attributed to the hypertonicity of the preparations. They can be prevented or minimized by starting with small amounts of formula, given slowly.
b. With vitamin A, observe for signs of hypervitaminosis A (anorexia; vomiting; irritability; headache; skin disorders; pain in muscles, bones, and joints; other clinical manifestations; and serum levels of vitamin A above 1200 U/dL).	Severity of manifestations depends largely on dose and duration of excess vitamin A intake. Very severe states produce additional clinical signs, including enlargement of liver and spleen, altered liver function, increased intracranial pressure, and other neurologic manifestations.
c. With vitamin K, observe for hypotension and signs of anaphylactic shock with intravenous phytonadione.	Vitamin K rarely produces adverse reactions. Giving IV phytonadione slowly may prevent adverse reactions.
d. With B-complex vitamins, observe for hypotension and anaphylactic shock with parenteral niacin, thiamine, cyanocobalamin, and folic acid; anorexia, nausea, vomiting and diarrhea, and postural hypotension with oral niacin.	Adverse reactions are generally rare. They are unlikely with B-complex multivitamin preparations. They are most likely to occur with large IV doses and rapid administration.
e. With vitamin C megadoses, observe for diarrhea and rebound deficiency if stopped abruptly.	Adverse reactions are rare with usual doses and methods of administration.
f. With mineral–electrolytes, observe for excess states.	These are likely to occur with excessive dosages of supplements. They can usually be prevented by using relatively low doses in non-emergency situations and by frequent monitoring of serum levels of electrolytes and iron.

NURSING ACTIONS	RATIONALE/EXPLANATION
g. With potassium preparations, observe for hyperkalemia.	This is most likely to occur with rapid IV administration, high dosages or concentrations, or in the presence of renal insufficiency and decreased urine output.
h. With magnesium preparations, observe for hypermagnesemia.	See potassium preparations, above.
i. Gastrointestinal (GI) symptoms—anorexia, nausea, vomiting, diarrhea, and abdominal discomfort from gastric irritation	Most oral preparations of minerals and electrolytes are likely to cause gastric irritation. Taking the drugs with food or 8 oz of fluid may decrease symptoms.
j. Cardiovascular symptoms—cardiac dysrhythmias, hypotension, tachycardia, other symptoms of shock	Potentially fatal dysrhythmias may occur with hyperkalemia or hypermagnesemia; shock may occur with deferoxamine and iron dextran injections.
k. With Kayexalate, observe for hypokalemia, hypocalcemia, hypomagnesemia, and edema.	Although this drug is used to treat hyperkalemia, it removes calcium and magnesium ions as well as potassium ions. Because it acts by trading sodium for potassium, the sodium retention may lead to edema.

4. Observe for drug interactions

a. With fat-soluble vitamins:	
(1) Bile salts *increase* effects.	Increase intestinal absorption
(2) Laxatives, especially mineral oil, *decrease* effects.	Mineral oil combines with fat-soluble vitamins and prevents their absorption if both are taken at the same time. Excessive or chronic laxative use decreases intestinal absorption.
(3) Antibiotics may *decrease* effects.	With vitamin K, antibiotics decrease production by decreasing intestinal bacteria. With others, antibiotics may cause diarrhea and subsequent malabsorption.
b. With B-complex vitamins:	
(1) Cycloserine (antituberculosis drug) *decreases* effects.	By increasing urinary excretion of vitamin B-complex
(2) Isoniazid (INH) *decreases* effect.	INH has an antipyridoxine effect. When INH is given for prevention or treatment of tuberculosis, pyridoxine is usually given also.
(3) With folic acid: alcohol, cholestyramine, methotrexate, oral contraceptives, phenytoin, sulfasalazine, and triamterene *decrease* effects.	Alcohol alters liver function and leads to poor hepatic storage of folic acid. Methotrexate and phenytoin act as antagonists to folic acid and may cause folic acid deficiency. Cholestyramine, oral contraceptives, and sulfasalazine decrease absorption of folic acid.
(4) With vitamin B_{12}, omeprazole (Prilosec) decreases effects.	Decreases absorption of B_{12} from foods
c. Drugs that *increase* effects of minerals and electrolytes and related drugs:	
(1) Cation exchange resin (Kayexalate): diuretics increase potassium loss; other sources of sodium increase the likelihood of edema.	Additive effects
(2) With iron salts:	
(a) Allopurinol (Zyloprim)	This drug may increase the concentration of iron in the liver. It should not be given concurrently with any iron preparation.
(b) Ascorbic acid (vitamin C)	Increases absorption of iron by acidifying secretions
(3) With potassium salts:	
(a) Angiotensin-converting enzyme (ACE) inhibitors (eg, captopril)	May increase risks of hyperkalemia

(continued)

NURSING ACTIONS	RATIONALE/EXPLANATION
(b) Diuretics, potassium-saving (spironolactone, triamterene, amiloride)	These drugs should *not* be given with a potassium supplement because of additive risks of producing life-threatening hyperkalemia.
(c) Salt substitutes	These contain potassium rather than sodium and may cause hyperkalemia if given with potassium supplements.
(d) Penicillin G potassium	This potassium salt of penicillin contains 1.7 mEq of potassium per 1 million units and increases risks of hyperkalemia.
d. Drugs that *decrease* effects of minerals and electrolytes and related drugs:	
(1) With oral iron salts:	
(a) Antacids	Decrease absorption. Iron is best absorbed in an acidic environment and antacids increase alkalinity.
(b) Caffeine	Decreases absorption. An iron preparation and a caffeine-containing substance (eg, coffee) should be separated by at least 2 hours.
(c) Cimetidine (Tagamet)	Decreases absorption
(d) Pancreatic extracts	Decrease absorption
(2) With potassium salts:	
(a) Calcium gluconate	Decreases cardiotoxic effects of hyperkalemia and is therefore useful in the treatment of hyperkalemia
(b) Sodium polystyrene sulfonate (Kayexalate)	Used in treatment of hyperkalemia because it removes potassium from the body

APPLYING YOUR KNOWLEDGE: ANSWERS

57-1 Include the administration of a multivitamin with her daily nourishment. The undernourished frequently have deficiencies in vitamins A, D, B$_{12}$, folic acid, riboflavin, and thiamine.

57-2 In the elderly, the most common mineral–electrolyte deficiencies are of calcium and iron. Excess states are also possible. Serum levels of minerals and electrolytes should be monitored carefully and measures taken to prevent both deficiency and excess.

57-3 Iron preparations are to be administered before meals for best absorption. When given with coffee, tea, or dairy products, absorption is decreased.

Review and Application Exercises

Short Answer Exercises

1. For clients who are unable to ingest food, which nutrients can be provided with enteral or IV nutritional formulas?

2. What is the role of lipid emulsions in parenteral nutrition?

3. What roles do vitamins play in normal body functioning?

4. Identify client populations who are at risk for vitamin deficiencies and excesses.

5. Are fat-soluble or water-soluble vitamins more toxic in overdoses? Why?

6. For a client who asks your advice about taking a multivitamin supplement daily, how would you reply? Justify your answer.

7. How do the vitamin requirements of children, older adults, and critically ill clients differ from those of healthy young and middle-aged adults?

8. What are the major roles of minerals and electrolytes in normal body functioning?

9. When a client is given potassium supplements for hypokalemia, how do you monitor for therapeutic and adverse drug effects?

10. List the main steps in treatment of hyperkalemia. Identify client populations at risk for development of hyperkalemia.

11. What are advantages and disadvantages of iron supplements?

12. List measures an adult can take to prevent accidental iron poisoning in small children.

NCLEX-Style Questions

13. Mr. H. develops respiratory distress while receiving continuous tube feeding. After stopping the feeding, the nurse should first
   a. Assess bowel sounds to determine if he has a paralytic ileus.
   b. Assess breath sounds to determine if he has aspirated tube-feeding formula.
   c. Perform nasal or tracheal suctioning.
   d. Aspirate stomach contents.

14. Which of the following statements by Mr. H.'s daughter, who will care for him at home, leads you to believe that she has understood your teaching regarding tube feedings? "I will . . .
   a. . . . store unopened cans of formula in the refrigerator."
   b. . . . stop the feedings if he has more than 2 stools per day."
   c. . . . place him in a sitting position for his feedings."
   d. . . . give no more than 50 mL per hour."

15. Which of the following is a fat-soluble vitamin that is toxic in overdose?
   a. vitamin A
   b. vitamin B_1
   c. vitamin C
   d. folic acid

16. Teaching for a client who is being started on an iron supplement should include information that the preparation
   a. may cause diarrhea
   b. may cause stools to be dark green or black
   c. should be taken with an antacid
   d. should not be taken with fruit juice

17. Which of the following IV electrolytes should be well diluted and never given as a bolus injection because it can cause fatal cardiac dysrhythmias?

   a. sodium bicarbonate
   b. magnesium sulfate
   c. sodium chloride
   d. potassium chloride

Selected References

Brophy, D. F., & Gehr, T. W. B. (2002). Disorders of potassium and magnesium homeostasis. In J. T. DiPiro, R. L. Talbert, G. C. Yee, G. R. Matzke, B. G. Wells, & L. M. Posey (Eds.), *Pharmacotherapy: A pathophysiologic approach* (5th ed., pp. 981–993). New York: McGraw-Hill.

DeHart, R. M., & Worthington, M. A. (2002). Nutritional considerations in major organ failure. J. T. DiPiro, R. L. Talbert, G. C. Yee, G. R. Matzke, B. G. Wells, & L. M. Posey (Eds.), *Pharmacotherapy: A pathophysiologic approach* (5th ed., pp. 2519–2542). New York: McGraw-Hill.

Drug facts and comparisons. (Updated monthly). St. Louis: Facts and Comparisons.

Giles, H., & Vijayan, A. (2004). Fluid and electrolyte management. In G. B. Green, I. S. Harris, G. A. Lin, et al. (Eds.), *The Washington manual of medical therapeutics* (31st ed., pp. 39–71). Philadelphia: Lippincott Williams & Wilkins.

Kim, R. B. (Ed.). (2001). *Handbook of adverse drug interactions.* New Rochelle, NY: Medical Letter.

Klein, S. (2004). Nutrition support. In G. B. Green, I. S. Harris, G. A. Lin, et al. (Eds.), *The Washington manual of medical therapeutics* (31st ed., pp. 23–38). Philadelphia: Lippincott Williams & Wilkins.

Mahan, L. K., & Escott-Stump, S. (Eds.). (2004). *Krause's food, nutrition, and diet therapy* (11th ed.). Philadelphia: W. B. Saunders.

Mason, J. B. (2004). Consequences of altered micronutrient status. In L. Goldman & D. Ausiello (Eds.), *Cecil textbook of medicine* (22nd ed., pp. 1326–1336). Philadelphia: W. B. Saunders.

Massey, P. B. (2002). Dietary supplements. *Medical Clinics of North America, 86*(1), 127–147.

McMahon, M. M. (2004). Parenteral nutrition. In L. Goldman & D. Ausiello (Eds.), *Cecil textbook of medicine* (22nd ed., pp. 1322–1326). Philadelphia: W. B. Saunders.

Pleuss, J. (2004). Alterations in nutritional status. In C. M. Porth, *Pathophysiology: Concepts of altered health states* (7th ed., pp. 217–238). Philadelphia: Lippincott Williams & Wilkins.

Pronsky, Z. M., & Crowe, J. P. (2005). In L. K. Mahan & S. Escott-Stump (Eds.), *Krause's food, nutrition, and diet therapy* (11th ed., pp. 455–474). Philadelphia: W. B. Saunders.

Reiter, P. D., & Sacks, G. S. (2002). Prevalence and significance of malnutrition. In J. T. DiPiro, R. L. Talbert, G. C. Yee, G. R. Matzke, B. G. Wells, & L. M. Posey (Eds.), *Pharmacotherapy: A pathophysiologic approach* (5th ed., pp. 2465–2474). New York: McGraw-Hill.

Rock, C. L. (2004). Nutrition in the prevention and treatment of disease. In L. Goldman & D. Ausiello (Eds.), *Cecil textbook of medicine* (22nd ed., pp. 1308–1311). Philadelphia: W. B. Saunders.

Rombeau, J. L. (2004). Enteral nutrition. L. Goldman & D. Ausiello (Eds.), *Cecil textbook of medicine* (22nd ed., pp. 1319–1322). Philadelphia: W. B. Saunders.

Smeltzer, S. C., & Bare, B. G. (2004). *Brunner & Suddarth's textbook of medical-surgical nursing* (10th ed.). Philadelphia: Lippincott Williams & Wilkins.

Drugs to Aid Weight Management

OBJECTIVES

After studying this chapter, you will be able to:

1. Promote healthful lifestyle measures to maintain body weight within a desirable range and avoid obesity.
2. Assess clients for risk factors and manifestations of obesity.
3. Calculate body mass index (BMI).
4. Counsel clients about the health consequences of obesity.
5. Assist overweight clients to develop and maintain a safe and realistic weight-loss program.
6. Identify reliable sources for information about nutrition, weight loss, and weight maintenance.
7. Assist clients with effective use of approved weight-loss drugs, when indicated.

APPLYING YOUR KNOWLEDGE

Pauline McKay, age 51, has had a weight problem all her life. She has been on countless diets, but always with the same result: she loses weight, then regains it plus additional weight. She is 5 feet 5 inches tall and weighs 265 pounds. Her physician starts her on orlistat.

INTRODUCTION

Carbohydrates, proteins, and fats are required for human nutrition. Either deficiencies or excesses impair health, cause illness, and impair recovery from illness or injury. Proteins are basic anatomic and physiologic components of all body cells and tissues; carbohydrates and fats serve primarily as sources of energy for cellular metabolism. Energy is measured in kilocalories (kcal, commonly called *calories*) per gram of food oxidized in the body. Carbohydrates and proteins supply 4 kcal per gram; fats supply 9 kcal per gram. Excessive amounts of any of these nutrients are converted to fat and stored in the body, resulting in overweight and obesity. This chapter discusses obesity and treatment strategies, including drugs to aid weight loss and weight maintenance.

Overweight and Obese Adults

Being overweight and obesity are widespread problems and are increasing in the United States, in both children and adults. They are considered major public health problems because of their association with high rates of morbidity and mortality. *Overweight* is defined as a body mass index (BMI) of 25 to 29.9 kilograms per square meter; *obese* is defined as a BMI of 30 or more kilograms per square meter. The BMI reflects weight in relation to height and is a better indicator than weight alone. The desirable range for BMI is 18.5 to 24.9 kilograms per square meter, with any values below 18.5 indicating underweight and any values of 25 or above indicating excessive weight (Box 58-1). A large waist circumference (>35 inches for women, >40 inches for men) is another risk factor for overweight and obesity. Obesity is further divided into three classes, depending on BMI (I=BMI 30–34.9; II=35–39.9; III=40 and above). These classes are used by medical insurance companies to determine eligibility for treatment benefits. Medicare recently approved policies that would allow payment for some obesity treatments.

Obesity may occur in anyone but is more likely to occur in women, minority groups, and poor people. It results from consistent ingestion of more calories than are used for energy and it substantially increases risks for development of numerous health problems (Box 58-2). Most obesity-related disor-

Box 58-1 Calculation of Body Mass Index (BMI) and Height and Weight Indicators for Overweight and Obese

BMI

Body mass index can be calculated as weight in kilograms divided by height in meters, squared; or as weight in pounds divided by height in inches, squared, multiplied by a conversion factor of 704.5 (listed as 703 in some sources), as follows:

$$\text{BMI} = \frac{\text{Weight (pounds)}}{\text{Height (inches)}^2} \times 704.5$$

Example: A person who weighs 150 lb and is 5'5" (65 in) tall

$$\text{BMI} = \frac{150 \text{ lb}}{65 \text{ in} \times 65 \text{ in}} \times 704.5 = \frac{105,675}{422.5} = 25$$

Weight Compared With Height as an Indicator for Being Overweight or Obese

Height (ft/in)	Weight (lb) Indicating Overweight (BMI 25)	Weight (lb) Indicating Obesity (BMI 30)
5'2" (62 inches)	135	165
5'3"	140	170
5'4"	145	175
5'5"	150	180
5'6"	155	185
5'7"	160	190
5'8"	165	195
5'9"	170	200
5'10"	175	205
5'11"	180	210
6'0"	185	220
6'1"	190	225
6'2" (74 inches)	195	230

ders are attributed mainly to the multiple metabolic abnormalities associated with obesity. Abdominal fat out of proportion to total body fat (also called *central* or *visceral obesity*), which often occurs in men and postmenopausal women, is considered a greater risk factor for disease and death than lower body obesity. In addition to the many health problems associated with obesity, obesity is increasingly being considered a chronic disease in its own right. Although it has been the focus of much research in recent years, no current theory adequately explains the disorder and its resistance to treatment.

Prevalence

The prevalence of overweight people and obesity has dramatically increased over the past 20 years. Some authorities estimate that 60% of American adults are overweight or obese.

There are differences in prevalence by gender, ethnicity, and socioeconomic status. In general, more women than men are obese, whereas more men than women are overweight; African-American women and Mexican Americans of both sexes have the highest rates of overweight and obesity in the United States; and women in lower socioeconomic classes are more likely to be obese than those in higher socioeconomic classes.

Etiology

The etiology of excessive weight is thought to involve complex and often overlapping interactions among physiologic, genetic, environmental, psychosocial, and other factors.

Physiologic Factors

In general, increased weight is related to an energy imbalance in which energy intake (food/calorie consumption) exceeds energy expenditure. Total energy expenditure represents the energy expended at rest (ie, the basal or resting metabolic rate), during physical activity, and during food consumption. When a person ingests food, about 10% of the energy content of that food is expended in the digestion, absorption, and metabolism of nutrients. Foods that contain carbohydrates and proteins stimulate energy expenditure; high-fat foods have little stimulatory effect. The energy required to metabolize and to use food reaches a maximum level about 1 hour after the food is ingested. In addition, men tend to expend more energy than women because they have proportionally more muscle mass. Energy expenditure usually decreases in older men and women of all ages because these groups have less muscle tissue and more adipose tissue. Muscle is more metabolically active (ie, has higher energy needs and burns more calories) than adipose tissue.

Excessive weight can result from eating more calories, exercising less, or a combination of the two factors. Consuming an extra 500 calories each day for a week results in 3500 excess calories or 1 pound of fat. Excess calories are converted to triglycerides and stored in fat cells (adipocytes). With continued intake of excessive calories, fat cells increase in both size and number.

Genetic Factors

Various studies indicate that a significant portion of weight variation within a given environment is genetic in origin. For example, identical twins raised in separate environments often have similar body types. Most cases of human obesity are attributed mainly to the combination of genetic susceptibility and environmental conditions.

Environmental Factors

Environmental factors contributing to the greater number of overweight and obese individuals include increased food consumption and decreased physical activity. The ready availability and relatively low cost of a wide variety of foods, in addition to large portion sizes and high-calorie foods, promote overeating. In addition, many social gatherings are associated with eating or overeating.

Box 58-2 Health Risks of Obesity

Obesity is associated with serious health risks. Several disease states and chronic health problems are more prevalent in obese clients, as well as increased mortality. Studies indicate that a high body mass index (BMI) is associated with an increased risk of death from all causes, among both men and women, and in all age groups. In addition, a higher death rate occurs in people who gain weight of 10 kg or more after 18 years of age. Some of the major health risks include the disorders listed below. In general, these conditions tend to worsen as the degree of obesity increases and improve with weight loss.

Cancer

Obesity is associated with a higher prevalence of breast, colon, and endometrial cancers. With breast cancer, risks increase in postmenopausal women with increasing body weight. Women who gain more than 20 lb from age 18 to midlife have double the risk of breast cancer compared with women who maintain a stable weight during this period of their life. In addition, central obesity apparently increases the risk of breast cancer independent of overall obesity. In women with central obesity, this additional risk factor may be related to an excess of estrogen (from conversion of androstenedione to estradiol in peripheral fatty tissue) and a deficiency of sex hormone–binding globulin to combine with the estrogen.

Colon cancer seems to be more common in obese men and women. In addition, a high BMI may be a risk factor for a higher mortality rate with colon cancer. Endometrial cancer is clearly more common in obese women, with adult weight gain again increasing risk.

Cardiovascular Disorders

Obesity is a major risk factor for cardiovascular disorders and increased mortality from cardiovascular disease. Studies have confirmed the relationship between obesity and increased risk of coronary heart disease (CHD) and stroke in both men and women. In addition, obesity during adolescence is associated with higher rates and greater severity of cardiovascular disease as adults.

Obesity increases risks by aggravating other risk factors such as hypertension, insulin resistance, low HDL cholesterol, and hypertriglyceridemia. In addition, obesity seems to be an independent risk factor for cardiovascular disorders, and central obesity may be more important than BMI as a risk factor for death from cardiovascular disease. The increased mortality rate is seen even with modest excess body weight.

Hypertension, dyslipidemia, insulin resistance, and glucose intolerance are known cardiac risk factors that tend to cluster in obese individuals. Hypertension often occurs in obese persons and is thought to play a major role in the increased incidence of cardiovascular disease and stroke observed in clients with obesity. Metabolic abnormalities that occur with obesity and type 2 diabetes mellitus (eg, insulin resistance and the resultant hyerinsulinemia) aggravate hypertension and increase cardiovascular risks. The combination of obesity and hypertension is associated with cardiac changes (eg, thickening of the ventricular wall, ischemia, and increased heart volume) that lead to heart failure more

rapidly. Weight loss of as little as 4.5 kg (10 lb) can decrease blood pressure and cardiovascular risk in many people with obesity and hypertension.

Diabetes Mellitus

Obesity is strongly associated with impaired glucose tolerance, insulin resistance, and diabetes mellitus. In addition, obesity during adolescence is associated with higher rates of diabetes as adults as well as more severe complications of diabetes at younger ages.

The cellular effects by which obesity causes insulin resistance are unknown. Proposed mechanisms include down-regulation of insulin receptors, abnormal postreceptor signals, and others. Whatever the mechanism, the impaired insulin response stimulates the pancreatic beta cells to increase insulin secretion, resulting in a relative excess of insulin called *hyperinsulinemia,* and causes impaired lipid metabolism (increased low-density lipoprotein [LDL] cholesterol and triglycerides and decreased high-density lipoprotein [HDL]). These metabolic changes increase hypertension and other risk factors for cardiovascular disease. As with cardiovascular disease and diabetes in general, central obesity seems to increase the likelihood of serious disease. The abdominal fat of central obesity seems to be more insulin resistant than peripheral fat deposited over the buttocks and legs. Intentional weight loss significantly reduces mortality in obese individuals with diabetes.

Dyslipidemias

Obesity strongly contributes to abnormal and undesirable changes in lipid metabolism (eg, increased triglycerides and LDL cholesterol; decreased HDL cholesterol) that increase risks of cardiovascular disease and other health problems.

Gallstones

Obesity apparently increases the risk for developing gallstones by altering production and metabolism of cholesterol and bile. The risk is higher in women, especially those who have had multiple pregnancies or who are taking oral contraceptives. However, rapid weight loss with very–low-calorie diets is also associated with gallstones.

Metabolic Syndrome

Metabolic syndrome is a group of risk factors and chronic conditions that occur together and greatly increase the risks of diabetes mellitus, serious cardiovascular disease, and death. The syndrome is thought to be highly prevalent in the United States. Major characteristics include many of the health problems associated with obesity (eg, dyslipidemias, hypertension, impaired glucose tolerance, insulin resistance, central obesity). More specifically, metabolic syndrome includes three or more of the following abnormalities:

- Central obesity (waist circumference >40 inches for men and >35 inches for women)
- Serum triglycerides of 150 mg/dL or more
- HDL cholesterol <40 mg/dL in men and <50 mg/dL in women
- Blood pressure of 135/85 mm Hg or higher
- Serum glucose of 110 mg/dL or higher

Box 58-2 Health Risks of Obesity (continued)

Osteoarthritis

Obesity is associated with osteoarthritis (OA) of both weight-bearing joints, such as the hip and knee, and non–weight-bearing joints. Extra weight can stress affected bones and joints, contract muscles that normally stabilize joints, and may alter the metabolism of cartilage, collagen, and bone. In general, obese people develop OA of the knees at an earlier age and are more likely than nonobese people to require knee replacement surgery.

The important role of obesity in OA is supported by the observation that weight loss delays onset and reduces symptoms and disability. Weight reduction may also decrease infection, wound complications, and blood loss if surgery is required. Despite the benefits of weight loss, however, persons with OA have difficulty losing weight because painful joints limit exercise and activity.

Sleep Apnea

Sleep apnea commonly occurs in obese persons. A possible explanation is enlargement of soft tissue in the upper airways that leads to collapse of the upper airways with inspiration during sleep. The obstructed breathing leads to apnea with hypox-

emia, hypercarbia, and a stress response. Sleep apnea is associated with increased risks of hypertension, possible right heart failure, and sudden death. Weight loss leads to improvement in sleep apnea.

Miscellaneous Effects

Obesity is associated with numerous difficulties in addition to those described above. These may include:

- Nonalcoholic fatty liver disease, which is being increasingly recognized and which may lead to liver failure
- Poor wound healing
- Poor antibody response to hepatitis B vaccine
- A negative perception of people who are obese that affects their education, socioeconomic, and employment status
- High costs associated with treatment of the medical conditions caused or aggravated by obesity as well as the costs associated with weight-loss efforts
- In women, obesity is associated with menstrual irregularities and increased complications of pregnancy (eg, gestational diabetes, higher rates of labor induction and cesarean section, and increased risk of neural tube and other congenital defects in offspring of obese women).

In relation to physical activity, usual activities of daily living for many people, including work-related activities, require relatively little energy expenditure. In addition, few Americans are thought to exercise in the optimal frequency, intensity, or duration to maintain health and prevent excessive weight gain. For both adults and children, increased time watching television, playing video or computer games, and working on computers contributes to less physical activity and is thought to promote weight gain and obesity. In general, though, it is still unknown whether less physical activity leads to obesity, or the physical effects of obesity lead to minimal physical activity.

Psychosocial Factors

Psychosocial disorders may be either a cause or an effect of obesity. Although much is still unknown about the psychological aspects of obesity development, depression and/or abuse may play a role. Obese people often report symptoms of depression and some people overeat and gain weight during depressive episodes. It may be that obesity and depression commonly occur together and reinforce each other. A depressed person is less likely to take the active measures in diet and exercise that are required to lose weight, even if obesity is a prominent factor in the development of depression. In women, sexual, physical, and emotional abuse can result in obesity. Abuse during childhood and adolescence tends to produce more severe effects.

Other Factors

Diseases are rarely a major cause of obesity development. However, numerous disease processes may limit a person's

ability to engage in calorie-burning physical activity. In addition, numerous prescription medications reportedly cause weight gain in some or most of the clients who take them (Box 58-3).

Overweight and Obese Children

Being overweight and obesity are common and increasing among children and adolescents, to the point of being called an "epidemic." Some studies estimate that 15% of children in the United States are overweight and that another 15% are at risk for becoming overweight, especially those with overweight parents. Overweight is defined as a BMI above the 85th percentile for the age group, and obesity as a BMI above the 95th percentile.

Childhood obesity is a major public health concern because these children have or are at risk of developing hypertension, dyslipidemias, type 2 diabetes, and other disorders that may lead to major disability and death at younger adult ages than nonobese children. Obesity, type 2 diabetes, and other health problems are mainly attributed to poor eating habits and too little exercise. In addition, the child who is obese after 6 years of age is highly likely to be obese as an adult, especially if a parent is obese. Obesity in adults that began in childhood tends to be more severe.

In addition to major health problems; reduced energy; and less physical agility, obese children are often ridiculed or bullied by other children and may be discriminated against by adults in schools and workplaces.

Box 58-3 Effects of Selected Medications on Weight

Antidepressants

Selective serotonin reuptake inhibitors (SSRIs), such as fluoxetine (Prozac, Sarafem) and related drugs, apparently promote weight loss with short-term use. However, with long-term use, they reportedly may cause as much weight gain as tricyclic antidepressants (TCAs) such as amitriptyline (Elavil). TCAs have long been associated with excessive appetite and weight gain. Mirtazapine (Remeron) and phenelzine (Nardil) are also associated with weight gain. The effects of bupropion (Wellbutrin, Zyban) on weight are unclear from clinical trials. Gain was reported when bupropion was used as a smoking deterrent but both gain and loss occurred when used as an antidepressant. However, anorexia and weight loss occurred at a higher percentage rate than increased appetite and weight gain.

Antidiabetic Drugs

Although little attention is paid to the topic in most literature about diabetic drugs, weight gain apparently occurs with insulin, sulfonylureas, and the glitazones (but not with metformin, acarbose, or miglitol). Almost all clients with type 2 diabetes eventually require insulin; those who are failing on oral agents generally gain a large amount of body fat when switched to insulin therapy. Although the mechanism of weight gain is unknown, it may be related to the chronic hyperinsulinism induced by long-acting insulins and the sulfonylureas (which increase insulin secretion). Less weight is gained when oral drugs are given during the day and an intermediate- or long-acting insulin is injected at bedtime. This strategy is thought to cause less daytime hyperinsulinemia than the more traditional insulin strategies.

For near–normal-weight diabetic clients who require drug therapy, a sulfonylurea may be given. However, for obese clients, metformin is usually the initial drug of choice because it does not promote weight gain. Metformin may also be used to treat obese diabetic children, aged 10 to 16 years, who require drug therapy.

Antiepileptic Drugs

Weight gain commonly occurs with the use of antiepileptic drugs (AEDs). This has been observed for many years with older drugs (eg, phenytoin, valproic acid, carbamazepine) and more recently with newer AEDs (eg, gabapentin, lamotrigine, tiagabine). Mechanisms by which the drugs promote weight gain are unclear, but may involve stimulation of appetite and/or a slowed metabolic rate. Consequences of weight gain may include increased risks of diabetes mellitus, hypertension, and other physical health problems as well as psychological distress over appearance, especially in children and adolescents.

Antihistamines

Histamine$_1$ (H$_1$) antagonists (eg, diphenhydramine, loratadine) reportedly increase appetite and cause weight gain.

Antihypertensives

The main antihypertensive drugs reported to cause weight gain are the widely-used beta blockers. The drugs can cause fatigue and decrease exercise tolerance and metabolic rate, all of which may contribute to weight gain. Other mechanisms may also be involved. As a result, some clinicians question the use of beta blockers in overweight or obese clients with uncomplicated hypertension. Alpha blockers may also cause weight gain, but apparently at a low incidence of 0.5% to 1%. Angiotensin-converting enzyme (ACE) inhibitors and calcium channel blockers are not reported to promote weight gain.

Antipsychotics

Weight gain is often reported and extensively documented with the use of atypical drugs, the most commonly used antipsychotic drugs. Although the exact mechanism is unknown, weight gain has been associated with antihistaminic effects, anticholinergic effects, and blockade of serotonin receptors. In addition, dietary factors and activity levels may also play significant roles.

Clozapine and olanzapine reportedly cause significant weight gain in 40% or more of clients. Compared with clozapine and olanzapine, risperidone causes less weight gain, and quetiapine and ziprasidone cause the least weight gain. Weight gain may lead to noncompliance with drug therapy. In addition to weight gain, clozapine and olanzapine adversely affect glucose regulation and can aggravate pre-exising diabetes or cause new-onset diabetes. The extent to which these effects are related to weight gain is unknown. For clients who are obese, diabetic, or at risk of developing diabetes, an antipsychotic drug that causes less weight gain would seem the better choice.

Cholesterol-Lowering Agents

Weight gain has been reported with the statin group of drugs; mechanisms and extent are unknown.

Corticosteroids

Systemic corticosteroids may cause increased appetite; weight gain; central obesity; and retention of sodium and fluid. Inhaled and intranasal corticosteroids have little effect on weight.

Gastrointestinal Drugs

Increased appetite and weight gain have been reported with the proton pump inhibitors (PPIs) such as omeprazole and others. The mechanisms and extent are unknown.

Hormonal Contraceptives

The weight gain associated with using hormonal contraceptives may be related more to retention of fluid and sodium than to increased body fat.

Mood Stabilizing Agent

Weight gain has been reported with long-term use of lithium, with approximately 20% of clients gaining 10 kg (22 lb) or more. This increased weight is attributed to fluid retention; consumption of high-calorie beverages as a result of increased thirst; or a decreased metabolic rate. Weight gain is a common reason for noncompliance with lithium therapy and weight gain may be more common in women with lithium-induced hypothyroidism and in those who are already overweight.

GENERAL CHARACTERISTICS OF DRUGS FOR OBESITY

The National Heart, Lung, and Blood Institute (NHLBI) of the National Institutes of Health and most other organizations generally recommend reserving drug therapy for those with a BMI of 30 kilograms per square meter or greater and health problems (eg, hypertension, dyslipidemia, coronary heart disease, type 2 diabetes, sleep apnea) that are likely to improve with weight loss. These organizations emphasize that drug therapy for obesity should be used as part of a weight-management program that also includes a sensible diet, physical activity, and behavioral modification. Guidelines also emphasize that drug therapy should be used to decrease medical risk and improve health rather than promote cosmetic weight loss.

Drug therapy for obesity has a problematic history, mainly because of serious adverse effects and rapid weight regain when the drugs were stopped. Some drugs (fenfluramine, dexfenfluramine, phenylpropanolamine) and a component of many over-the-counter and herbal weight-loss products (ephedra, ma huang) have been taken off the market because of their adverse effects.

Older drugs include amphetamines and similar drugs. Amphetamines (see Chap. 15) are not recommended because they are controlled substances (Schedule II) with a high potential for abuse and dependence. Benzphetamine, diethylpropion, phendimetrazine, and phentermine are adrenergic drugs (see Chap. 17) that stimulate the release of norepinephrine and dopamine in the brain. This action in nerve terminals of the hypothalamic feeding center suppresses appetite. These drugs are central nervous system (CNS) and cardiovascular stimulants and are contraindicated in cardiovascular disease, hyperthyroidism, glaucoma, and agitated states.

Of the adrenergic anorexiant drugs, only phentermine is commonly used. Two newer drugs, sibutramine and orlistat, are also commonly used and are the only weight-loss drugs approved for long-term use. According to some clinicians, sibutramine and orlistat may be continued as long as they are

effective and adverse effects are tolerable. The drugs are described below; dosage ranges are listed in Table 58-1.

INDIVIDUAL DRUGS

Phentermine

Phentermine hydrochloride (Adipex-P, Ionamin, Pro-Fast) is the most frequently prescribed adrenergic anorexiant. It is a Schedule IV drug and recommended only for short-term use (3 months or less). Its use is contraindicated in clients with hypertension or other cardiovascular disease and in those with a history of drug abuse. Because it increases blood pressure, phentermine should be used with caution even in clients with mild hypertension. The drug should also be used cautiously in clients with anxiety or agitation because of CNS stimulant effects. The most commonly reported adverse effects are nervousness, dry mouth, constipation, and hypertension.

Sibutramine

Sibutramine (Meridia) is a Schedule IV and the most commonly prescribed anti-obesity drug. It inhibits the reuptake of serotonin and norepinephrine in the brain, thereby increasing the amounts of these neurotransmitters. Clinical effects include increased satiety, decreased food intake, and a faster metabolism rate. Sibutramine is approved by the Food and Drug Administration (FDA) for long-term use, but effects are mostly unknown beyond 1 to 2 years. The drug increases blood pressure and heart rate and is contraindicated in clients with cardiovascular disorders (eg, coronary heart disease, dysrhythmias, heart failure, hypertension). It should be used cautiously in clients who take other medications that increase blood pressure and pulse rate. It should also be used cautiously in clients with impaired hepatic function, narrow-angle glaucoma (may cause mydriasis), or a history of substance abuse or dependency. Sibutramine has not been studied in children under 16 years of age and is not recommended for women who are pregnant or lactating. The drug

Table 58-1 Drugs at a Glance: Drugs for Obesity

GENERIC/TRADE NAME	ROUTE AND DOSAGE RANGES
Appetite Suppressants	
Phentermine hydrochloride (Adipex-P, Ionamin, Pro-Fast)	PO 8 mg 3 times daily, 30 min before meals, or 15–37.5 mg daily in the morning
Sibutramine (Meridia)	PO 10–15 mg once daily, in the morning, with or without food
Fat Blocker	
Orlistat (Xenical)	PO 120 mg with each main meal, up to 3 capsules daily
PO, oral.	

is contraindicated in people with severe renal or hepatic dysfunction.

Oral sibutramine is rapidly absorbed from the intestine and undergoes first-pass metabolism, during which time active metabolites are formed. Peak plasma levels of the active metabolites occur within 3 to 4 hours and drug half-life is 14 to 16 hours. The long half-lives of the active metabolites allow for once-daily dosing. The drug is highly bound to plasma proteins and rapidly distributed to most body tissues, with the highest concentrations in the liver and kidneys. It is metabolized in the liver, mainly by the cytochrome P450 3A4 enzymes. The active metabolites produced by first-pass metabolism are further metabolized to inactive metabolites, which are then excreted in urine and feces.

Common adverse effects of sibutramine include dry mouth, headache, insomnia, nervousness, and constipation; cardiovascular effects include hypertension, tachycardia, and palpitations. Potentially serious drug interactions may occur if sibutramine is taken with other cardiovascular stimulants (increased risk of hypertension and dysrhythmias), CNS stimulants (increased anxiety and insomnia), and serotonergic drugs (serotonin syndrome). Other drugs that increase serotonin include the selective serotonin reuptake inhibitors (eg, fluoxetine [Prozac] and related drugs); the triptan antimigraine drugs (eg, sumatriptan [Imitrex]); dextromethorphan (a common ingredient in cough syrups); and lithium. The combination of sibutramine with any of these drugs may cause serotonin syndrome, a condition characterized by agitation, confusion, hypomania, impaired coordination, loss of consciousness, nausea, tachycardia, and other symptoms.

In clinical trials, people lost the most weight during the first 6 months of sibutramine therapy. However, continued drug therapy helped to maintain weight loss for 12 to 24 months. Most of the clinical trials included diet and behavioral modification techniques in addition to sibutramine therapy. As with other weight-loss drugs, studies indicate that sibutramine therapy is more effective when it is combined with lifestyle modification and diet than when used alone.

Orlistat

Orlistat (Xenical) differs from phentermine and sibutramine because it decreases absorption of dietary fat from the intestine (by binding to gastric and pancreatic lipases in the gastrointestinal [GI] tract lumen and making them unavailable to break down dietary fats into absorbable free fatty acids and monoglycerides). The drug blocks absorption of approximately 30% of the fat ingested in a meal; increasing dosage does not increase this percentage. Decreased fat absorption leads to decreased caloric intake, resulting in weight loss and improved serum cholesterol values (eg, decreased total and low-density lipoprotein [LDL] cholesterol levels). The improvement in cholesterol levels is thought to be independent of weight-loss effects. The use of orlistat has not been studied in pregnant or lactating women.

Orlistat is not absorbed systemically and its action occurs in the GI tract. Consequently, it does not cause systemic adverse effects or drug interactions as phentermine and sibutramine do. Its main disadvantages are frequent administration (3 times daily) and GI symptoms (abdominal pain, oily spotting, fecal urgency, flatulence with discharge, fatty stools, fecal incontinence, and increased defecation). Adverse GI effects occur in almost all orlistat users but usually subside after a few weeks of continued drug usage. The drug also prevents absorption of the fat-soluble vitamins, A, D, E, and K. As a result, people taking orlistat should also take a multivitamin containing these vitamins daily. The multivitamin should be taken 2 hours before or after the orlistat dose. If taken at the same time, the orlistat prevents absorption of the fat-soluble vitamins.

Orlistat is intended for people who are clinically obese, not those wanting to lose a few pounds. In addition, high-fat foods still need to be decreased because total caloric intake is a major determinant of weight, and adverse effects (eg, diarrhea; fatty, malodorous stools) worsen with high fat consumption. Long-term effects of orlistat are unknown, although one study reported safe and effective use for 2 years. In addition to weight loss and reduced cholesterol levels, clinical trials found reduced severity and improved management of other health problems associated with obesity, such as diabetes and hypertension. In general, the addition of orlistat therapy to diet and other lifestyle changes produced greater weight loss than addition of a placebo. In some clients with impaired glucose tolerance, weight loss with orlistat and lifestyle changes prevented or delayed the occurrence of diabetes mellitus. After the medication was stopped, most clients regained weight.

APPLYING YOUR KNOWLEDGE 58-1

Pauline asks how orlistat will help her when nothing else in the past has been successful. How would you respond?

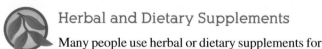

Herbal and Dietary Supplements

Many people use herbal or dietary supplements for weight loss, even though reliable evidence of safety and effectiveness are lacking. Some herbal products claim to decrease appetite and increase the rate at which the body burns calories. However, in most cases, there is no scientific evidence that they work at all. Some supplements for weight loss contain cardiovascular and CNS stimulants that may cause serious, even life-threatening, adverse effects.

In general, many consumers do not seem to appreciate the benefits of proven weight-management techniques (eg, appropriate diet and exercise) or the potential risks of taking unproven weight-loss products. Selected products are described below.

Ephedra (ma huang) is an herb that has long been a component of many weight-loss products (eg, Metabolife, Herbalife). It is not recommended for use by anyone, because it is a strong cardiovascular and CNS stimulant that increases risks of heart attack, seizure, stroke, and sudden death. Many ephedra-containing products also contained caffeine, which can further increase cardiovascular and CNS stimulation. In 2004, the FDA banned the sale of products containing ephedra.

Glucomannan expands on contact with body fluids. It is included in weight-loss regimens because of its supposed ability to produce feelings of stomach fullness, thereby causing a person to eat less. It also has a laxative effect. There is little evidence to support its use as a weight-loss aid. Products containing glucomannan should not be used by people with diabetes; glucomannan may cause hypoglycemia alone and increases hypoglycemic effects of antidiabetic medications.

Guarana, a major source of commercial caffeine, is found in weight-loss products as well as caffeine-containing soft drinks, bodybuilding supplements, smoking-cessation products, vitamin supplements, candies, and chewing gums. Caffeine is the active ingredient; the amount varies among products, and caffeine content of any particular product cannot be accurately predicted. Guarana is promoted to decrease appetite and increase energy and mental alertness. It is contraindicated in clients with dysrhythmias and may aggravate gastroesophageal reflux disease (GERD) and peptic ulcer disease.

Adverse effects include diuresis; cardiovascular symptoms (premature ventricular contractions, tachycardia); CNS symptoms (agitation, anxiety, insomnia, seizures, tremors); and GI symptoms (nausea, vomiting, diarrhea). Such effects are more likely to occur with higher doses or concomitant use of guarana and other sources of caffeine. Adverse drug–drug interactions include additive CNS and cardiovascular stimulation with beta-adrenergic agonists (eg, epinephrine, albuterol and related drugs, pseudoephedrine) and theophylline. In addition, concurrent use of cimetidine, fluoroquinolones, or oral contraceptives may increase or prolong serum caffeine levels and subsequent adverse effects.

Guar gum is a dietary fiber included in weight-loss products because it is bulk-forming and produces feelings of fullness. Several small studies indicated it is no more effective than placebo for weight loss. It may cause esophageal or intestinal obstruction if not taken with an adequate amount of water and may interfere with the absorption of other drugs if taken at the same time. Adverse effects include nausea, diarrhea, flatulence, and abdominal discomfort.

Hydroxycitric acid (in Citrimax and other supplements) apparently suppresses appetite in animals, but there are no reliable studies that indicate its effectiveness in humans. One 12-week study did not show weight loss.

Laxative and diuretic herbs (eg, aloe, rhubarb root, buckthorn, cascara, senna, parsley, juniper, dandelion leaves) are found in several products such as Super Dieter's Tea, Trim-Maxx Tea, and Water Pill. These products cause a significant loss of body fluids and electrolytes, not fat. Adverse effects may include low serum potassium levels, with subsequent cardiac dysrhythmias and other heart problems. In addition, long-term use of laxatives may lead to loss of normal bowel function and the necessity for continued use (ie, laxative dependency).

LipoKinetix, a combination dietary supplement, was associated with severe hepatotoxicity in seven young (ages 20–32 years), previously healthy people who developed acute hepatitis (four women and three men). Five Japanese clients were diagnosed within 1 month after beginning the drug; two Caucasian bodybuilders were diagnosed within 3 months. Three people were taking only LipoKinetix; four were also taking other supplements, which they resumed later without recurrence of hepatitis. All reported taking LipoKinetix according to the manufacturer's instructions; all recovered after the product was discontinued.

LipoKinetix contains norephedrine, caffeine, sodium usniate, 3,5-diiodothyronine, and yohimbe. The ingredient(s) responsible for the hepatotoxicity were unknown. The reactions were considered idiosyncratic and no other cause of hepatitis was found.

With the observation that the five Japanese clients developed hepatotoxicity more rapidly than the two Caucasians, there is a possibility that Asians are less able to metabolize and excrete this product. As discussed in the early chapters of this text, smaller doses of several prescription drugs are needed in this population because of genetic or ethnic differences in metabolism. This principle may also apply to some herbal and dietary supplements and should be considered in teaching clients of Asian descent.

NURSING PROCESS

Assessment

Assess each overweight or obese client for factors contributing to overweight and health risks related to excess weight, regardless of the reason for the contact. Some specific assessment factors include the following:

- Assess usual drinking and eating patterns, including healthful (eg, whole-grain breads and cereals, fruits, vegetables, low-fat dairy products) and unhealthful (eg, sugar-containing beverages and desserts, fried foods, saturated fat, fast foods, high-calorie snack foods) intake. The best way is to ask the client to keep a food diary for 2 or 3 days. If food intake is not written down, people tend to underestimate the amount and caloric content. (If available, consult a nutritionist to assess a client's diet and work with the client to improve health and weight status.)
- Assess any obviously overweight person for health problems caused or aggravated by excessive weight (eg, elevated blood pressure, other cardiovascular problems, diabetes mellitus, sleep apnea).
- Calculate or estimate the body mass index (see Box 58-1) and measure waist circumference.

- Check available reports of laboratory tests. Overweight clients may have abnormally high values for total and LDL cholesterol, triglycerides, and blood sugar, and low values for high-density lipoprotein (HDL) cholesterol. If no laboratory reports are available, ask clients if a health care provider has ever told them they have high cholesterol or blood sugar.
- List all prescription and nonprescription medications being taken and ask about vitamins, herbals, and other dietary supplements. Review the list for drugs used to treat health problems associated with obesity, drugs that may promote weight gain, and any products that may be used to promote weight loss.
- Assess usual patterns of physical activity and exercise, including work and recreational activities.
- Assess motivation to develop and adhere to a weight-management plan. Ask if there are concerns about weight; if there is interest in a weight-management program to improve health; and what methods, over-the-counter products, or herbal or dietary supplements have been previously used to reduce weight, if any. The nurse must be very tactful in eliciting information and assessing whether a client would like assistance with weight management. If the nurse–client contact stems from a health problem caused or aggravated by excessive weight, the nurse may use this information to help motivate the client to lose weight and improve health.

Nursing Diagnoses

- Imbalanced Nutrition: More Than Body Requirements related to excessive caloric intake
- Disturbed Body Image related to excessive weight gain
- Deficient Knowledge: Weight management

Planning/Goals

The client will
- Reduce the impact of excessive weight on chronic health problems
- Modify lifestyle behaviors toward weight loss and weight maintenance at a more healthful level
- Avoid overuse of anorexiant drugs
- Avoid unproven weight-loss dietary supplements

Interventions

- Support programs/efforts to help promote a healthful lifestyle and prevent obesity (eg, in families and schools).
- Serve as a role model by maintaining a healthful lifestyle and weight.
- Serve as a reliable source of information about weight loss and weight-loss products and programs (see accompanying Client Teaching Guidelines).

- For an obese client who reports interest and motivation in losing weight, assist to formulate realistic goals. Clients often expect to rapidly lose large amounts of weight with little or no effort. Most treatment programs result in a weight loss of 10% of body weight or less.
- Discuss health risks of obesity and anticipated benefits of achieving and maintaining a healthier weight. Emphasize that losing 5% to 10% of body weight is a reasonable goal and can significantly reduce the medical problems associated with being overweight.
- Assist clients to identify factors that support weight-loss efforts (eg, family and friend encouragement) and factors that sabotage weight-loss efforts (eg, having high-calorie snack foods readily available, frequently eating at fast-food restaurants).
- Promote exercise and activity. For overweight and obese clients, exercise may decrease appetite and distract from eating behaviors as well as increase calorie expenditure. For very sedentary, physically unfit clients, emphasize that any exercise can be beneficial and to start slowly, increasing the amount and intensity as physical condition improves.
- Encourage any efforts toward improving diet and increasing exercise to improve health.
- Weigh clients at regular intervals and measure waist circumference periodically.
- Refer clients to a nutritionist when indicated.
- Be alert for the psychological consequences of obesity and refer clients for counseling if indicated.
- Refer overweight and obese children to pediatric obesity specialists when possible.

Evaluation

- Observe overweight or obese clients for food intake, weight loss, decreased waist circumference, and appropriate use of exercise and anorexiant drugs.

APPLYING YOUR KNOWLEDGE 58-2

In addition to proper administration of her medication, what strategies should you review with Ms. McKay to assist her in being successful with weight loss?

PRINCIPLES OF THERAPY

Strategies to Prevent Becoming Overweight and Obese

Preventing excessive weight gain is a major struggle for many Americans as they fight the "battle of the bulge" daily. Many people want to lose weight, often more for appearance than for health. However, many are also unwilling or unable

General Considerations

☑ Because of the extensive health problems associated with over-weight and obesity, individuals whose weight is within a normal range should try to prevent excessive weight gain by practicing a healthful lifestyle in terms of diet and exercise. Following are selected recommendations from the *Dietary Guidelines for Americans 2005,* published by the United States Department of Health and Human Services and the Department of Agriculture in January 2005 (updated every 5 years; available online at www.healthierus. gov/dietaryguidelines).

1. Eat a variety of foods daily (eg, six to eleven servings of whole-grain bread and cereals, 2 cups of fruit, 2 ½ cups of vegetables, three or more servings of low-fat milk or other dairy products). Also limit intake of saturated fat (eg, in meats), *trans* fats (eg, hydrogenated oils in many commercial baked goods and other products), cholesterol, added sugars, salt, and alcohol. The amount of *trans* fat in commercial prod-ucts must soon be added to the Nutrition Facts label and many manufacturers are reformulating their products without *trans* fats. Canola oil and olive oil are healthy fats, but they have a high calorie content (120 calories per tablespoon), which must be considered in weight control efforts.

2. To maintain body weight in a healthy range, balance diet (ie, calories gained) with exercise (ie, calories used). To pre-vent gradual weight gain over time, make small decreases in food and beverage calories and increase physical activity. Engage in regular physical activity and reduce sedentary activities to promote health, psychological well-being, and a healthy body weight. To reduce the risk of chronic disease, engage in at least 30 to 60 minutes of moderate-intensity physical activity, above usual activity, at work or home on most days of the week. For most people, greater health ben-efits can be obtained by engaging in physical activity of more vigorous intensity or longer duration.

3. Physical fitness can be developed or improved by including cardiovascular conditioning, stretching exercises for flexibil-ity, and resistance exercises or calisthenics for muscle strength and endurance.

☑ Individuals who are already overweight or obese should try to lose weight and maintain a lower weight because the likelihood of seri-ous health problems and early death increases as weight increases. However, try to emphasize goals for improvement in health status rather than losing a large amount of weight. Remem-ber that even a modest weight loss of 10 to 30 lbs can benefit your health. Most people are unlikely to achieve their "ideal" weight, and having unrealistic expectations sets one up for failure in any weight-loss program.

☑ Obesity is considered a chronic disease that requires long-term treatment, much like the treatment of diabetes and hypertension. Weight loss can be induced by severe calorie restriction, but with-out lifestyle changes (eg, in eating and activity behavior), body fat is invariably regained. The safest and most effective way to lose weight and keep it off is permanent lifestyle changes that involve eating less and exercising more. Reducing caloric intake by 500 to 1000 calories per day allows the loss of 1 to 2 lb of fat per week, respectively. Higher levels of physical activity can help with weight loss and prevent weight regain. Additional health benefits include lower rates of cardiovascular disease and death.

☑ Use available resources. For example, if unable to implement needed changes alone, consult a nutritionist, qualified obesity expert, or behavioral therapist. Such clinicians can help modify the eating, activity, and thinking habits that predispose to obesity.

☑ In addition to feeling better, health benefits of weight loss may include reduced blood pressure, reduced blood fats, less likeli-hood of having a heart attack or stroke, and less risk for develop-ment of diabetes mellitus.

☑ Any weight loss program should include a nutritionally adequate diet with decreased calories and increased exercise.

☑ Regular physical examinations and follow-up care are needed during weight loss programs.

☑ Although many weight-loss supplements are available and heavily advertised in newspapers, magazines, and television, none are considered safe and effective and none are recommended for use. If you do choose to use any of these products, notify your primary health care provider. Depending on your condition (ie, whether you have chronic health problems such as diabetes mellitus, hypertension, or others), the medications you take, and so forth, some weight-loss supplements can be harmful to your health.

☑ Diet and exercise are recommended for people who want to lose a few pounds. Medications to aid weight loss are usually recom-mended only for people whose health is endangered (ie, those who are overweight and have other risk factors for heart disease, and those who are obese).

☑ Read package inserts and other available information about the drug being taken, who should not take the drug, instructions and precautions for safe usage, and so forth. Keep the material for later reference if questions arise. If unclear about any aspect of the information, consult a health care provider before taking the drug.

☑ Appetite-suppressant drugs must be used correctly to avoid potentially serious adverse effects. Because most of these drugs stimulate the heart and the brain, adverse effects may include increased blood pressure, fast heartbeat, irregular heartbeat, heart attack, stroke, dizziness, nervousness, insomnia (if taken late in the day), and mental confusion. In addition, prolonged use of prescription drugs may lead to psychological dependence.

☑ Avoid over-the-counter decongestants and allergy, asthma, and cold remedies, and weight-loss herbal or dietary supplements when taking a prescription appetite suppressant. The combination can cause serious adverse effects from excessive heart and brain stimulation.

☑ Inform health care providers when taking an appetite suppressant, mainly to avoid other drugs with similar effects.

☑ Orlistat (Xenical) is not an appetite suppressant and does not cause heart or brain stimulation. It works in the intestines to keep fats in foods from being absorbed. It should be taken with a low-fat diet. Adverse effects include fatty stools and bloating.

(continued)

C L I E N T   T E A C H I N G   G U I D E L I N E S

Weight Management and Drugs That Aid Weight Loss (Continued)

Self-Administration

✔ Take appetite suppressants in the morning to decrease appetite during the day and avoid interference with sleep at night.

✔ Do not crush or chew sustained-release products.

✔ With sibutramine (Meridia):

  ✔ Take once daily, with or without food.

  ✔ Have blood pressure and heart rate checked at regular intervals (the drug increases them).

  ✔ Notify a health care provider if a skin rash, hives, or other allergic reaction occurs.

✔ With orlistat (Xenical):

  ✔ Take one capsule with each main meal or up to 1 hour after a meal, up to three capsules daily. If you miss a meal or eat a meal with no fat, you may omit a dose of orlistat.

  ✔ Take a multivitamin containing fat-soluble vitamins (A, D, E, and K) daily, at least 2 hours before or after taking orlistat. Orlistat prevents absorption of fat-soluble vitamins from food or multivitamin preparations if taken at the same time.

---

to adapt their lifestyles toward more healthful eating, exercising, and weight-controlling habits. As a result, millions of dollars are spent annually on weight-loss diets, products, and programs in an effort to find an easy way to lose weight. Health care providers need to promote efforts to prevent overweight and obesity when possible. When prevention is not possible, efforts should be aimed toward early recognition and treatment, before obesity and major health problems develop. Some strategies include the following:

● Personally practice a healthful lifestyle, primarily for one's own health and well-being, but also to serve as a role model and proponent for healthful practices in daily life.

● Provide or assist others to obtain reliable information about healthful lifestyle habits. For example, the United States Department of Health and Human Services and the Department of Agriculture publish *Dietary Guidelines for Americans* every 5 years. The most recent update was published in January 2005 and is available online at www.healthierus.gov/dietaryguidelines. Selected recommendations include the following:

  ● Eat a variety of foods daily (eg, several servings of whole-grain bread and cereals; 2 cups of fruit and 2½ cups of vegetables; three or more servings of low-fat milk or other dairy products). Also limit intake of saturated fat (eg, in meats, cheeses), *trans* fats (eg, hydrogenated oils in many baked goods), cholesterol, added sugars, salt, and alcohol. (The amount of *trans* fat in commercial products must soon be added to the label and many manufacturers are reformulating their products without *trans* fats. Canola oil and olive oil are healthy fats, but they have 120 calories per tablespoon, which must be considered in weight-control efforts).

  ● To maintain body weight in a healthy range, balance diet (ie, calories gained) with exercise (ie, calories used). To prevent gradual weight gain over time,

make small decreases in food and beverage calories and increase physical activity. Engage in regular physical activity and reduce sedentary activities to promote health, psychological well-being, and a healthy body weight. To reduce the risk of chronic disease, engage in at least 30 to 60 minutes of moderate-intensity physical activity, above usual activity, at work or home on most days of the week. For most people, greater health benefits can be obtained by engaging in physical activity of more vigorous intensity or longer duration.

In addition to these recommendations, many books, magazine and newspaper articles, and Internet sites (Box 58-4) contain useful information. However, all of these resources are not equally reliable; they must be carefully evaluated.

Management of Overweight and Obese Clients

Treatment options for obesity include diet, exercise, behavioral modification, drug therapy, and, if these options fail, possibly referring a client for bariatric (weight-loss) surgery. The safest and most effective treatment for most people usually includes a combination of diet, exercise, and behavioral modification. Drug therapy and bariatric surgery are recommended only for seriously overweight people with major medical problems that can be improved by weight loss. In addition, neither of these treatments is a substitute for the necessary changes in eating and physical activity patterns.

In 1998, the NHLBI issued a report entitled "Clinical Guidelines on the Identification, Evaluation and Treatment of Overweight and Obesity in Adults." This report (available at www.nhlbi.nih.gov/guidelines/obesity/ob_gdlns.htm) provides definitions and recommendations for treatment. Recommendations include the following:

● Weight loss to reduce health problems of individuals: decrease blood pressure if hypertensive; lower elevated levels of total cholesterol, LDL cholesterol, and triglycerides, and raise low levels of HDL cholesterol if dyslipidemic; lower elevated blood glucose levels in persons with type 2 diabetes.

● Use the BMI to assess overweight and obesity and estimate disease risks. Measure waist circumference initially and periodically to assess abdominal fat content. Weigh regularly to monitor body weight for gain, loss, or maintenance—whether or not the person is involved in a weight-loss program.

● The initial goal of weight-loss therapy should be to reduce body weight by about 10 percent from baseline, at a rate of 1 to 2 pounds per week for a period of 6 months. Steady weight loss over a longer period reduces fat stores in the body, limits the loss of vital protein tissues, and avoids the sharp decline in metabolic rate that accompanies rapid weight loss. After weight loss, weight maintenance should be the priority goal, because weight regain is a problem with all weight-loss programs. In some cases, after a period of weight maintenance, additional losses may be desirable.

● Dietary recommendations include low-calorie diets for weight loss, mainly reducing caloric intake by 500 to 1000 calories daily. Reducing dietary fat can reduce calories. However, reducing dietary fat without reducing total caloric intake does not produce weight loss. Vitamin and mineral supplements that meet age-related requirements are usually recommended with weight-loss programs that provide less than 1200 kcal for women or 1800 kcal for men.

● Physical activity recommendations should be part of any weight-management program because physical activity contributes to weight loss; may decrease abdominal fat; increases cardiorespiratory fitness; and helps with weight maintenance. Initially, physical activity for 30 to 45 minutes, 3 to 5 days a week, is encouraged. Long-term, adults should try to accumulate at least 30 minutes or more of moderate-intensity physical activity on most days of the week.

● In general, weight-loss and weight-maintenance programs should combine reduced-calorie diets, increased physical activity, and behavior therapy. After weight loss, weight-loss maintenance with dietary therapy, physical activity, and behavior therapy should be continued indefinitely. Drug therapy can also be used. However, drug safety and efficacy beyond 1 to 2 years of total treatment have not been established.

● Behavioral modification can be helpful in a weight-loss program. The goals are to help clients modify their eating, activity, and thinking habits that predispose to obesity. Techniques include identifying triggers that promote overeating and barriers that keep one from adopting a more healthful lifestyle. One strategy is keeping an accurate record of food/calorie intake and physical activity (most people tend to underestimate food intake and overestimate activity). In addition, stress management, stimulus control, and social support are helpful. Clients who eat more when stressed can learn to manage stress more healthfully. Counseling by a behavioral therapist may be needed. Stimulus control has to do with avoiding or minimizing circumstances that promote overeating (eg, cooking calorie-dense foods; having high-calorie snacks and "junk food" readily available; eating high-fat, high-calorie foods at fast-food restaurants). Social support involves family, friends, co-workers, and fellow dieters who encourage weight-loss efforts rather than sabotage them by urging one to eat high-calorie foods. In general, weight-loss regimens that use several of these strategies seem to be most effective.

In addition to the NHLBI guidelines, additional recommendations and comments include the following:

● Emphasize health benefits of weight reduction. There is strong evidence that weight loss reduces risk factors for cardiovascular disease, including blood pressure, serum triglycerides, and total and LDL cholesterol. It also increases HDL cholesterol. In addition, in overweight and obese people without diabetes, weight loss reduces blood glucose levels and the risk for development of type 2 diabetes.

● For people who already have type 2 diabetes, weight loss reduces blood levels of glucose and glycosylated (A_{1c}) hemoglobin. These effects make the diabetes easier to manage, reduce complications of diabetes, and may allow smaller doses of antidiabetic medications. For people who already have hypertension, losing excess weight reduces blood pressure and may reduce the number or amount of antihypertensive drugs. For people who already have dyslipidemias, blood lipid profiles improve with weight loss.

● Weight-loss diets wax and wane in popularity with the American public (Box 58-5). Although all of them can lead to weight loss if adhered to long enough, some are healthier than others and most are discarded before significant weight loss is achieved. Actually, any diet that reduces caloric intake in relation to caloric expenditure can lead to weight loss, and adherence is probably more important than the particular diet. Regardless of what

---

Box 58-5 Characteristics of Selected Diets

Various diets all work if total caloric intake is less than energy expenditure. Many diets are quite restrictive, however, and most people soon drop out and rapidly regain the weight they lost. As a result, the best "diet" is nutritionally adequate except for calories and can be followed long term.

Low calorie. These diets provide about 1200 to 1600 kcal per day. The usual recommendation is to reduce caloric intake by 500 to 1000 calories daily, to allow weight loss of 1 to 2 lb weekly. This rate of loss is likely to be more successful in terms of weight loss, and continuing a reduced-calorie diet promotes weight maintenance rather than weight regain. Note that losing weight through diet alone, without increased physical activity, is unlikely to improve cardiovascular health.

Very-low calorie. These diets usually consist of 800 calories or fewer per day. Numerous commercial products that promise "magical" results have been marketed. These diets result in rapid initial weight losses due mainly to diuresis and loss of sodium and water. Multiple health risks accompany such diets, including abnormalities in electrolytes, trace elements, and vitamins; gout; gallstones; cold intolerance; fatigue; lightheadedness; anemia; menstrual irregularities; and other problems.

The National Institutes of Health (NIH) recommends against using diets that provide fewer than 800 calories daily. If used at all, very–low-calorie diets should be used intermittently, for short periods, with a diet that maintains weight and is more nutritionally adequate.

Low fat. These diets do not cause significant weight loss unless caloric intake is reduced. Because fats are energy dense (9 cal/g), reducing fat is a practical way to reduce caloric intake. For both health and weight loss, current recommendations emphasize reducing intake of "bad" fats (eg, saturated and *trans* fat) but including healthy mono- and polyunsaturated fats (eg, olive and canola oil) within the caloric allotment.

Low carbohydrate. Several diets emphasizing carbohydrate restriction have recently been popular with the American public and many manufacturers are marketing "low-carb" products. Many people do not seem to realize that these products may contain as many or more calories than the "regular" version. In addition, the FDA has not defined "low carbohydrate" and statements on food labels such as "reduced carbohydrate" or "low carb" are not based on any standard.

The weight loss that occurs with these diets is attributed to caloric reduction or water loss, rather than the carbohydrate restriction. There have been no studies evaluating the long-term safety of low-carbohydrate diets.

The Atkins diet is a high-fat, low-carbohydrate diet consisting of unlimited amounts of meat, fish, eggs, and some cheeses. Sweets, starchy snacks, many fruits, some starchy vegetables, and some grains are prohibited. The high-protein foods cause a feeling of satiety with less food, so fewer calories are consumed. Also, during the first 10 days of this diet, ketosis is induced (by burning fat for energy when carbohydrates are not available). Ketosis increases water loss, which can cause rapid weight loss initially. Then, weight loss occurs more slowly. The main premise of this diet is that carbohydrates increase insulin levels and induce metabolic changes that cause weight gain. Although the Atkins diet seems to cause more short-term weight loss than traditional low-fat diets, weight loss is similar with the two diets after a year.

The South Beach diet is an adaptation of the Atkins diet. This diet emphasizes "good" versus "bad" carbohydrates and the "glycemic index." The glycemic index indicates the effect of foods on blood glucose levels. Some carbohydrates with a high glycemic index (eg, potatoes, pasta, white rice, white bread) can increase blood glucose as much or more than similar amounts of sucrose. The elevated blood sugar level stimulates increased insulin secretion and leads to excessive insulin in the blood. In general, high glycemic index foods are thought to promote fat accumulation and obesity. Low glycemic index foods are digested and absorbed more slowly, do not produce surges in blood glucose and blood insulin levels, and therefore are thought to promote weight control.

Adverse effects of low-carbohydrate diets may include constipation, dehydration, electrolyte imbalance, headache, aggravation of renal impairment (increased breakdown of body protein and fat increases the workload of the kidneys), and hyperuricemia leading to gout. In addition, some people experience a worsening of blood lipid levels and one study of adolescents on a very–low-calorie, low-carbohydrate diet showed increased calcium excretion and decreased bone mineral content. This could lead to later development of osteoporosis.

some diet gurus and others say, total caloric intake must be considered because it is a major determinant of weight loss, gain, or maintenance.

- Various formula diets or meal-replacement programs are available. The good ones contain high-quality protein, sugar as fructose, and a moderate amount of mono-unsaturated fat. The usual recommendation is to replace two meals daily for weight loss and one meal for weight maintenance. They can also be used as single meal replacements.

- Although both calorie-reduced diets and sufficient exercise can lead to weight loss and maintenance, the NHLBI guidelines are based on studies indicating that a combination of the two strategies is more effective than either alone. However, many overweight and obese people may be physically unfit and unable or unwilling to increase activity. Thus, activity should be started slowly and gradually increased, with the goal of exercise becoming part of the daily routine. Aerobic exercise increases the metabolic rate during and for approximately 1 hour after activity. Consistent adherence to a reduced-calorie diet and exercise routine is a major factor in achieving weight control and health benefits.

- For any clients following a weight-loss regimen, provide psychological support and positive reinforcement for efforts toward weight management. Programs or support groups involving supervision or regular participation within a social group appear to be more successful over time. Weight Watchers seems more successful than most other commercial programs; Overeaters Anonymous and Take off Pounds Sensibly (TOPS) are large self-help support groups. For more information on commercial programs, see the accompanying Research Brief.

- There seems to be increasing support for the long-term use of weight-loss medications in treatment of obesity. When drug therapy is indicated, a single drug in the lowest effective dose is recommended. As with most other drugs, low doses decrease risks of adverse drug effects. In addition, the National Institutes of Health do not recommend combining weight-loss medications except in the context of clinical trials. Thus far, studies indicate that combining sibutramine and orlistat has no additional benefit over using one of the drugs alone.

APPLYING YOUR KNOWLEDGE 58-3

Ms. McKay says she needs to lose 140 pounds and would like to accomplish this by her next birthday. How should you respond?

Management of Obesity in Special Populations

Managing Obesity in Children

Children in general need increased amounts of protein, carbohydrate, and fat in proportion to their size to support

---

RESEARCH BRIEF

Commercial Weight-Loss Programs

SOURCE:

Tsai, A. G., & Wadden, T. A. (2005). Systematic review: An evaluation of major commercial weight loss programs in the United States. *Annals of Internal Medicine, 142*(1), 56–66.

SUMMARY:

The authors evaluated published studies of medically based weight loss programs (Health Management Resources and OPTIFAST), nonmedical programs (Weight Watchers, Jenny Craig, and L. A. Weight Loss), very–low-calorie diets, commercial Internet-based programs (eDiets.com), and two nonprofit self-help programs (Overeaters Anonymous and Take Off Pounds Sensibly). The studies included adults in the United States, had more than 10 participants, and lasted more than 12 weeks.

Few high-quality studies were found; many presented the best-case scenario because they did not account for people who dropped out of the program. Of the programs evaluated, Weight Watchers had the strongest studies to support it. No high-quality studies of Jenny Craig or L. A. Weight Loss were found. The studies of the medically based very–low-calorie diets were of limited quality. Clients who stayed on the program lost substantial weight over 6 months, but regained about half of the lost weight in 1 to 2 years; many dropped out. The few studies of Internet-based and self-help programs were of limited quality and found that these approaches produced minimal weight loss.

NURSING IMPLICATIONS:

This information can be used to counsel clients who are considering a commercial weight-loss program. Except for Weight Watchers, the programs demonstrate little evidence of effectiveness. Costs vary but may be extensive.

---

growth and increased physical activity. However, reports of childhood obesity have greatly increased over recent years and childhood obesity has become a major public health concern. Therefore, the goal of nutrition is to meet needs without promoting obesity. When possible, specialists in childhood obesity should design and supervise treatment programs.

Efforts are needed toward both prevention and treatment of childhood obesity. Prevention should focus on identifying at-risk and overweight children and adolescents at an early stage; educating families about the health consequences of being overweight; and encouraging weight-control measures (eg, a more active lifestyle, a low-fat diet, regular meals, avoidance of snacking, drinking water instead of calorie-containing beverages, decreasing the time spent watching television and playing computer games). These measures are implemented successfully mainly within a family unit and family support is needed to assist the child in weight control and a more healthful lifestyle. In addition, schools should teach children the basic principles of good nutrition and why eating a balanced diet is important to health.

Pediatric clinicians recommend treatment for children and adolescents who are overweight and have complications of obesity, and for all children who are obese. Treatment of childhood obesity should focus on healthy eating and increasing physical activity. In general, children should not be put on "diets." For a child who is overweight, the recommended goal is to maintain weight or slow the rate of weight gain so that weight and BMI gradually decline as the child grows in height. If the child has already reached his or her anticipated adult weight, maintenance of that weight and prevention of additional gain should be the long-term treatment goal. If the child already exceeds the optimal adult weight, the goal of treatment should be a slow weight loss of 10 to 12 pounds per year until the optimal adult weight is reached. As with adults, increased activity is required for successful weight loss or management in children.

Family involvement and support are vital to children's weight management. Actually, the goal beyond weight control for a child is to develop healthier eating and exercise habits for long-term health benefits for the entire family. Studies indicate that children who eat adequate amounts of fruits, vegetables, and dairy products tend to continue these healthy eating habits. In general, young children who learn to eat a healthy diet are likely to reap the benefits throughout their lives. Improved diets and increased activity are unlikely to occur without active participation of parents and other caregivers.

Although drug therapy has not been generally recommended for treatment of childhood obesity, orlistat is approved for use in children aged 12 to 16 years. Sibutramine has not been studied in children under 16 years of age.

Managing Obesity in Older Adults

Overweight and obesity are common among older adults. Although caloric needs are usually decreased, primarily because of slowed metabolism and decreased physical activity, most people continue usual eating patterns. With the high incidence of atherosclerosis and cardiovascular disease in older adults, it is especially important that fat intake be reduced. Anorexiant drugs should be used very cautiously, if at all, because older adults often have cardiovascular, renal, or hepatic impairments that increase risks of adverse drug effects. The use of orlistat in older

adults has not been studied. However, the manufacturer recommends conservative use and dosage because older adults often have decreased renal, cardiac, and hepatic function.

Managing Obesity in Clients With Renal Impairment

In relation to drugs for obesity, little information is available about their use in clients with renal impairment. With sibutramine, dosage reductions are not recommended with mild to moderate impairment because the drug and its active metabolites are eliminated by the liver. However, some inactive metabolites are also formed and these are excreted renally. The drug is contraindicated in clients with severe renal impairment.

Managing Obesity in Clients With Hepatic Impairment

In relation to drugs for obesity, little information is available about their use in clients with hepatic impairment. Because sibutramine is metabolized in the liver, it is contraindicated in clients with severe hepatic impairment.

Managing Obesity in Home Care

The home care nurse may be involved with weight-management issues in almost any home care setting. Because nutrition, exercise, and weight control are so important to health, the home care nurse should take advantage of any opportunity for health promotion in this area. Health promotion may involve assessing the nutritional and fitness status of all members of the household and providing counseling or other assistance to improve health status. Those who are obviously overweight or who have obesity-related health problems must be approached with diplomacy and tact; they have probably tried repeatedly to lose weight and been told by previous health care providers that they need to lose weight. The home care nurse should be able to provide accurate information about realistic and successful techniques for losing weight and keeping it off; health benefits of even modest weight loss; and reasons to avoid "fad" diets, weight-loss herbal and dietary supplements, and programs that promise rapid and easy weight loss with little effort.

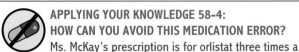

APPLYING YOUR KNOWLEDGE 58-4:
HOW CAN YOU AVOID THIS MEDICATION ERROR?
Ms. McKay's prescription is for orlistat three times a day. She takes the dose with breakfast, lunch, and dinner. She has a meeting today that runs through lunch and so she skips lunch but takes her pill on time.

NURSING ACTIONS

Drugs for Weight Loss and Maintenance

NURSING ACTIONS	RATIONALE/EXPLANATION
1. Administer accurately	
a. With phentermine:	
(1) Give single-dose drugs in the early morning.	For maximum appetite-suppressant effects during the day
(2) Give multiple-dose preparations 30 minutes before meals and the last dose of the day about 6 hours before bedtime.	For maximum appetite-suppressant effects at mealtime and to avoid interference with sleep from the drug's stimulating effects on the central nervous system (CNS)
b. With sibutramine, give once daily, in the morning.	
c. With orlistat, give one capsule with each main meal or up to 1 hour after a meal, up to three capsules daily. If a meal is missed or contains no fat, the dose can be omitted.	The drug needs to be in the gastrointestinal tract when fat-containing foods are eaten, to prevent fat absorption.
2. Observe for therapeutic effects	
a. With phentermine and sibutramine, observe for decreased caloric intake and weight loss.	The recommended rate of weight loss is 1–2 lb weekly.
b. With orlistat, observe for weight loss and improvements in health status (eg, reduced LDL cholesterol, elevated HDL cholesterol, improved glycemic control, and reduced blood pressure).	Most weight loss occurs in the first 6 months of therapy, but the reduced weight can be maintained as long as orlistat is continued. The metabolic improvements are very beneficial for people with obesity-related health problems such as diabetes, dyslipidemia, hypertension, and metabolic syndrome.
3. Observe for adverse effects	
a. With phentermine and sibutramine, observe for:	
(1) Nervousness, insomnia, hyperactivity	These effects result from excessive stimulation of the CNS. They are more likely to occur with large doses or too-frequent administration.
(2) Hypertension	Anorexiant drugs stimulate the sympathetic nervous system and may cause or aggravate hypertension.
(3) Development of tolerance to appetite-suppressant effects	This usually occurs within 4–6 weeks and is an indication for discontinuing drug administration. Continued administration and/or large doses do not maintain appetite-suppressant effects. Instead, they increase the incidence of adverse effects.
b. With orlistat, observe for abdominal cramping, gas pains, diarrhea, and fatty stools.	These effects commonly occur. They usually improve within a few weeks of continued drug use, but worsen with a high intake of dietary fat, which should be avoided.
4. Observe for drug interactions	
a. Drugs that *increase* effects of phentermine and sibutramine:	
(1) Antidepressants, tricyclic	May increase hypertensive effects
(2) Other CNS stimulants	Additive stimulant effects
(3) Other sympathomimetic drugs (eg, epinephrine)	Additive hypertensive and other cardiovascular effects
b. Drugs that *decrease* effects of phentermine and sibutramine:	
(1) Antihypertensive drugs	Decrease blood pressure–raising effects of anorexiants
(2) CNS depressants (eg, alcohol)	Antagonize or decrease effects
c. Drugs that *increase* effects of sibutramine:	
(1) Adrenergics (eg, epinephrine, pseudoephedrine)	Additive increases in blood pressure

(continued)

NURSING ACTIONS	RATIONALE/EXPLANATION
(2) Antidepressants (tricyclic antidepressants [TCAs; eg, amitriptyline], selective serotonin reuptake inhibitors [SSRIs; eg, fluoxetine])	TCAs and sibutramine increase levels of norepinephrine and serotonin in the brain; SSRIs increase serotonin levels. Concurrent use of these drugs may cause excessive CNS stimulation, hypertension, and serotonin syndrome and should be avoided.
(3) Antifungals (eg, itraconazole and related azoles)	Decrease metabolism and may increase adverse effects and toxicity of sibutramine
(4) Antimigraine triptans (eg, sumatriptan)	Additive serotonin effects
(5) Lithium	Additive serotonin effect

APPLYING YOUR KNOWLEDGE: ANSWERS

58-1 Orlistat works by blocking the fat absorbed from the intestine. This drug will block approximately 30% of the fat ingested in a meal. It is important to teach that increasing the dose will not increase the percentage of fat blocked. This drug also blocks the absorption of fat-soluble vitamins, so you should advise Ms. McKay to take a multivitamin at a different time than the orlistat.

58-2 Strategies should include the practice of a healthy lifestyle by eating a variety of foods daily and by eating a diet rich in whole grains, vegetables, and low-fat dairy products. Limit the intake of saturated fat, *trans* fat, cholesterol, added sugars, salt, and alcohol. Ms. McKay must also include some regular physical activity.

58-3 The initial goal of weight-loss therapy should be to reduce body weight by about 10 percent from baseline and to lose weight at a rate of 1 to 2 pounds per week for the first 6 months. Assist Ms. McKay to set a realistic and healthy goal.

58-4 The dose of orlistat should not be taken if the client misses a meal. Teach Ms. McKay to omit the dose if a meal is omitted.

Review and Application Exercises

Short Answer Exercises

1. Calculate the BMI for yourself, one or more members of your family, or a client.

2. Assess eating and physical activity habits of yourself, one or more members of your family, or a client. In general, do these habits promote health or obesity?

3. If you, the family member, or the client has health problems related to overweight and obesity, list at least three things that can be done to improve health.

4. Debate whether or not it is important that health care providers demonstrate healthful practices in diet, exercise, and weight control to the general public.

5. With an overweight or obese client who wants to lose weight, what are some nursing interventions to assist and support the client?

6. List advantages and disadvantages of drug therapy for weight loss or maintenance.

NCLEX-Style Questions

7. Which of the following is a characteristic of low-calorie or reduced-calorie diets?
   a. They provide about 500–1000 kcal per day.
   b. They reduce daily intake by about 1600 kcal per day.
   c. They are required for weight loss.
   d. They focus on high-fat, high-carbohydrate foods.

8. Drug therapy for weight management may be prescribed for clients with which of the following?
   a. a BMI of 22 and a desire to lose 10 pounds
   b. a BMI of 24.5 and physically fit
   c. a BMI of 27 or more with weight-related health problems
   d. a BMI of 25 to 29 and healthy

9. Sibutramine (Meridia) may be contraindicated for clients with which of the following disorders?
    a. cardiovascular disease
    b. diabetes mellitus
    c. chronic fatigue syndrome
    d. gastroesophageal reflux disease

10. Orlistat (Xenical) aids weight loss by
    a. decreasing appetite
    b. increasing satiety and feelings of fullness
    c. increasing metabolism
    d. decreasing absorption of dietary fat

11. To decrease diarrhea with orlistat (Xenical), a client should be instructed to
    a. Avoid large amounts of fatty foods.
    b. Drink eight glasses of water daily.
    c. Avoid caffeine-containing beverages.
    d. Increase physical activity.

Selected References

Campbell, M. L., & Mathys, M. L. (2001). Pharmacologic options for the treatment of obesity. *American Journal of Health-System Pharmacy, 58*(14), 1301–1308.

Dennis, K. E. (2004). Weight management in women. *Nursing Clinics of North America, 39,* 231–241.

Drug facts and comparisons. (Updated monthly). St. Louis: Facts and Comparisons.

Expert Panel. (1998). Clinical guidelines on the identification, evaluation, and treatment of overweight and obesity in adults: Executive summary. *American Journal of Clinical Nutrition, 68,* 899–917.

Favreau, J. T., Ryu, M. L., Braunstein, G., et al. (2002). Severe hepatotoxicity associated with the dietary supplement LipoKinetix. *Annals of Internal Medicine, 136*(8), 590–595.

Jensen, M. D. (2004). Obesity. In L. Goldman & D. Ausiello (Eds.), *Cecil textbook of medicine* (22nd ed., pp. 1339–1346). Philadelphia: W. B. Saunders.

LaQuatra, I. M. (2004). Nutrition for weight management. In L. K. Mahan & S. Escott-Stump (Eds.), *Krause's food, nutrition and diet therapy* (11th ed., pp. 558–593). Philadelphia: W. B. Saunders.

Mahan, L. K., & Escott-Stump, S. (Eds.) (2004). *Krause's food, nutrition and diet therapy* (11th ed.). Philadelphia: W. B. Saunders.

Miller, S. J. (2002). Energy balance and weight control. In I. Wolinsky & L. Williams (Eds.), *Nutrition in pharmacy practice* (pp. 307–340). Washington, DC: American Pharmaceutical Association.

National Institutes of Health. (2004, August). *Strategic plan for NIH obesity research: A report of the NIH obesity research task force* (NIH Publication No. 04-5493). Washington, DC: U.S. Department of Health and Human Services.

Pereira, M., Kartashov, A. I., Ebbeling, C. B., et al. (2005). Fast-food habits, weight gain, and insulin resistance (the CARDIA study): 15-Year prospective analysis. *Lancet, 365*(9453), 36–42.

Pleuss, J. (2005). Alterations in nutritional status. In C. M. Porth, *Pathophysiology: Concepts of altered health states* (7th ed., pp. 217–238). Philadelphia: Lippincott Williams & Wilkins.

Pronsky, Z. M., & Crowe, J. P. (2004). Food-drug interactions. In L. K. Mahan & S. Escott-Stump (Eds.), *Krause's food, nutrition and diet therapy* (11th ed., pp. 455–474). Philadelphia: W. B. Saunders.

St. Peter, J. V., & Khan, M. A. (2002). Obesity. In J. T. DiPiro, R. L. Talbert, G. C. Yee, G. R. Matzke, B. G. Wells, & L. M. Posey (Eds.), *Pharmacotherapy: A pathophysiologic approach* (5th ed., pp. 2543–2563). New York: McGraw-Hill.

Saper, R. B., Eisenberg, D. M., & Phillips, R. S. (2004). Common dietary supplements for weight loss. *American Family Physician, 70*(9), 1731–1738.

Smeltzer, S. C., & Bare, B. G. (2004). *Brunner & Suddarth's textbook of medical-surgical nursing* (10th ed.). Philadelphia: Lippincott Williams & Wilkins.

Waitman, J. A., & Aronne, L. J. (2004). Pharmacological treatment. In G. D. Foster & C. A. Nonas (Eds.), *Managing obesity: A clinical guide* (pp. 151–157). Chicago: American Dietetic Association.

Yancy, W. S., Jr., Olsen, M. K., Guyton, J. R., et al. (2004). A low-carbohydrate, ketogenic diet versus a low-fat diet to treat obesity and hyperlipidemia: A randomized, controlled trial. *Annals of Internal Medicine, 140*(10), 769–777.

Yanovski, S. Z., & Yanovski, J. A. (2002). Obesity. *New England Journal of Medicine, 346*(8), 591–601.

Drugs Used for Peptic Ulcer and Acid Reflux Disorders

OBJECTIVES

After studying this chapter, you will be able to:

1. Describe the main elements of peptic ulcer disease and gastroesophageal reflux disease (GERD).
2. Differentiate the types of drugs used to treat peptic ulcers and acid reflux disorders.
3. Discuss the advantages and disadvantages of proton pump inhibitors.
4. Differentiate between prescription and over-the-counter uses of histamine$_2$ receptor blocking agents.
5. Discuss significant drug–drug interactions with cimetidine.
6. Describe characteristics, uses, and effects of selected antacids.
7. Discuss the rationale for using combination antacid products.
8. Teach clients nonpharmacologic measures to manage peptic ulcers and GERD.

APPLYING YOUR KNOWLEDGE

Kathleen Daniels is a 54-year-old woman who has chronic GERD. She is prescribed rabeprazole 20 mg PO daily. She also takes OTC famotidine 10 mg twice a day as needed to control her heartburn. When needed, she takes Mylanta 5 mL also.

INTRODUCTION

Drugs to prevent or treat peptic ulcer and acid reflux disorders consist of several groups of drugs, most of which alter gastric acid and its effects on the mucosa of the upper gastrointestinal (UGI) tract. To aid understanding of drug effects, peptic ulcer disease and gastroesophageal reflux disease (GERD) are described below; related UGI disorders are described in Box 59-1.

Peptic Ulcer Disease

Peptic ulcer disease is characterized by ulcer formation in the esophagus, stomach, or duodenum, areas of the gastrointestinal (GI) mucosa that are exposed to gastric acid and pepsin. Gastric and duodenal ulcers are more common then esophageal ulcers.

Peptic ulcers are attributed to an imbalance between cell-destructive and cell-protective effects (ie, presence of increased destructive mechanisms or presence of decreased protective mechanisms). *Cell-destructive* effects include those of gastric acid (hydrochloric acid); pepsin; *Helicobacter pylori* (*H. pylori*) infection; and ingestion of nonsteroidal anti-inflammatory drugs (NSAIDs). Gastric acid, a strong acid that can digest the stomach wall, is secreted by parietal cells in the mucosa of the stomach antrum, near the pylorus. The parietal cells contain receptors for acetylcholine, gastrin, and histamine, substances that stimulate gastric acid production. Acetylcholine is released by vagus nerve endings in response to stimuli, such as thinking about or ingesting food. Gastrin is a hormone released by cells in the stomach and duodenum in response to food ingestion and stretching of the stomach wall. It is secreted into the bloodstream and eventually circulated to the parietal cells. Histamine is released from cells in the gastric mucosa and diffuses into nearby parietal cells. An enzyme system (hydrogen–potassium adenosine triphosphatase, or H$^+$, K$^+$-ATPase) catalyzes the production of gastric acid and acts as a gastric acid (proton) pump to move gastric acid from parietal cells in the mucosal lining of the stomach into the stomach lumen.

Pepsin is a proteolytic enzyme that helps digest protein foods and also can digest the stomach wall. Pepsin is derived

Box 59-1 Selected Upper Gastrointestinal Disorders

Gastritis

Gastritis, a common disorder, is an acute or chronic inflammatory reaction of gastric mucosa. Patients with gastric or duodenal ulcers usually also have gastritis. *Acute gastritis* (also called *gastropathy*) usually results from irritation of the gastric mucosa by such substances as alcohol, aspirin or other nonsteroidal anti-inflammatory drugs (NSAIDs), and others. *Chronic gastritis* is usually caused by *H. Helicobacter pylori* infection and it persists unless the infection is treated effectively. *H. pylori* organisms may cause gastritis and ulceration by producing enzymes (eg, urease, others) that break down mucosa; they also alter secretion of gastric acid.

Nonsteroidal Anti-Inflammatory Drug Gastropathy

NSAID gastropathy indicates damage to gastroduodenal mucosa by aspirin and other NSAIDs. The damage may range from minor superficial erosions to ulceration and bleeding. NSAID gastropathy is one of the most common causes of gastric ulcers, and it may cause duodenal ulcers as well. Many people take NSAIDs daily for pain, arthritis, and other conditions. Chronic ingestion of NSAIDs causes local irritation of gastroduodenal mucosa; inhibits the synthesis of prostaglandins (which normally protect gastric mucosa by inhibiting acid secretion, stimulating secretion of bicarbonate and mucus, and maintaining mucosal blood flow); and increases the synthesis of leukotrienes and possibly other inflammatory substances that may contribute to mucosal injury.

Stress Ulcers

Stress ulcers indicate gastric mucosal lesions that develop in patients who are critically ill from trauma, shock, hemorrhage, sepsis, burns, acute respiratory distress syndrome, major surgical procedures, or other severe illnesses. The lesions may be single or multiple ulcers or erosions. Stress ulcers are usually manifested by painless upper gastrointestinal (GI) bleeding. The frequency of occurrence has decreased, possibly because of prophylactic use of antacids and antisecretory drugs and improved management of sepsis, hypovolemia, and other disorders associated with critical illness.

Although the exact mechanisms of stress ulcer formation are unknown, several factors are thought to play a role, including mucosal ischemia, reflux of bile salts into the stomach, reduced GI-tract motility, and systemic acidosis. Acidosis increases severity of lesions, and correction of acidosis decreases their formation. In addition, lesions do not form if the pH of gastric fluids is kept at about 3.5 or above and lesions apparently form only when mucosal blood flow is diminished.

Zollinger-Ellison Syndrome

Zollinger-Ellison syndrome is a rare condition characterized by excessive secretion of gastric acid and a high incidence of ulcers. It is caused by gastrin-secreting tumors in the pancreas, stomach, or duodenum. Approximately two thirds of the gastrinomas are malignant. Symptoms are those of peptic ulcer disease, and diagnosis is based on high levels of serum gastrin and gastric acid. Treatment may involve long-term use of a proton pump inhibitor to diminish gastric acid, or surgical excision.

---

from a precursor called *pepsinogen,* which is secreted by chief cells in the gastric mucosa. Pepsinogen is converted to pepsin only in a highly acidic environment (ie, when the pH of gastric juices is 3 or less).

H. pylori is a gram-negative bacterium found in the gastric mucosa of most clients with chronic gastritis, about 75% of clients with gastric ulcers, and more than 90% of clients with duodenal ulcers. It is spread mainly by the fecal–oral route. However, iatrogenic spread by contaminated endoscopes, biopsy forceps, and nasogastric tubes has also occurred. After it moves into the body, the organism colonizes the mucus-secreting epithelial cells of the stomach mucosa and is thought to produce gastritis and ulceration by impairing mucosal function. Eradication of the organism accelerates ulcer healing and significantly decreases the rate of ulcer recurrence.

Cell-protective effects (eg, secretion of mucus and bicarbonate; dilution of gastric acid by food and secretions; prevention of diffusion of hydrochloric acid from the stomach lumen back into the gastric mucosal lining; the presence of prostaglandin E; alkalinization of gastric secretions by pancreatic juices and bile; perhaps other mechanisms) normally prevent autodigestion of stomach and duodenal tissues and ulcer formation.

A gastric or duodenal ulcer may penetrate only the mucosal surface or it may extend into the smooth muscle layers. When superficial lesions heal, no defects remain. When smooth muscle heals, however, scar tissue remains and the mucosa that regenerates to cover the scarred muscle tissue may be defective. These defects contribute to repeated episodes of ulceration.

Although there is considerable overlap in etiology, clinical manifestations, and treatment of gastric and duodenal ulcers, there are differences as well. **Gastric ulcers** (which may be preceded by less severe mucosal defects such as erosions or gastritis) are often associated with stress (eg, major trauma, severe medical illness), NSAID ingestion, or *H. pylori* infection of the stomach. They are often manifested by painless bleeding and take longer to heal than duodenal ulcers. Gastric ulcers associated with stress may occur in any age group and are usually acute in nature; those associated with *H. pylori* infection or NSAID ingestion are more likely to occur in older adults, especially in the sixth and seventh decades, and to be chronic in nature. **Duodenal ulcers** are strongly associated with *H. pylori* infection and NSAID ingestion, may occur at any age; occur about equally in men and women; are often manifested by abdominal pain; and are usually chronic in nature. They are also associated with cigarette smoking. Compared with nonsmokers, smokers are more likely to develop duodenal ulcers; their ulcers heal more slowly with treatment; and the ulcers recur more rapidly.

Gastroesophageal Reflux Disease (GERD)

GERD, the most common disorder of the esophagus, is characterized by regurgitation of gastric contents into the esophagus and exposure of esophageal mucosa to gastric acid and pepsin. The same amount of acid–pepsin exposure may lead to different amounts of mucosal damage, possibly related to individual variations in esophageal mucosal resistance.

Acid reflux often occurs after the evening meal and decreases during sleep. The main symptom is heartburn (pyrosis), which increases with a recumbent position or bending over. Effortless regurgitation of acidic fluid into the mouth, especially after a meal and at night, is often indicative of GERD. Depending on the frequency and extent of acid–pepsin reflux, GERD may result in mild to severe esophagitis or esophageal ulceration. Pain on swallowing usually means erosive or ulcerative esophagitis.

The main cause of GERD is thought to be an incompetent lower esophageal sphincter (LES). Normally, the LES is contracted or closed and prevents the reflux of gastric contents. It opens or relaxes on swallowing, to allow passage of food or fluid, then contracts again. Several circumstances contribute to impaired contraction of the LES and the resulting reflux, including foods (eg, fats, chocolate), fluids (eg, alcohol, caffeinated beverages), medications (eg, beta adrenergics, calcium channel blockers, nitrates), gastric distention, cigarette smoking, and recumbent posture.

GERD occurs in men, women, and children, but is especially common during pregnancy and after 40 years of age.

CLASSIFICATIONS AND INDIVIDUAL DRUGS

Drugs used in the treatment of acid-peptic disorders promote healing of lesions and prevent recurrence of lesions by decreasing cell-destructive effects or increasing cell-protective effects. Several types of drugs are used, alone and in various combinations. Antacids neutralize gastric acid and decrease pepsin production; antimicrobials and bismuth can eliminate *H. pylori* infection; histamine$_2$ receptor antagonists (H$_2$RAs) and proton pump inhibitors (PPIs) decrease gastric acid secretion; sucralfate provides a barrier between mucosal erosions or ulcers and gastric secretions; and misoprostol restores prostaglandin activity. Types of drugs and individual agents are

described in the following sections; dosages are listed in the Drugs at a Glance tables.

Antacids

Antacids are alkaline substances that neutralize acids. They react with hydrochloric acid in the stomach to produce neutral, less acidic, or poorly absorbed salts and to raise the pH (alkalinity) of gastric secretions. Raising the pH to approximately 3.5 neutralizes more than 90% of gastric acid and inhibits conversion of pepsinogen to pepsin. Commonly used antacids are aluminum, magnesium, and calcium compounds. Table 59-1 provides information for representative antacid products.

Antacids differ in the amounts needed to neutralize gastric acid (50–80 mEq of acid is produced hourly), in onset of action, and in adverse effects. *Aluminum compounds* have a low neutralizing capacity (ie, relatively large doses are required) and a slow onset of action. They can cause constipation. In people who ingest large amounts of aluminum-based antacids over a long period, hypophosphatemia and osteomalacia may develop because aluminum combines with phosphates in the GI tract and prevents phosphate absorption. Aluminum compounds are rarely used alone for acid-peptic disorders. *Magnesium-based antacids* have a high neutralizing capacity and a rapid onset of action. They may cause diarrhea and hypermagnesemia. *Calcium compounds* have a rapid onset of action but may cause hypercalcemia and hypersecretion of gastric acid ("acid rebound") due to stimulation of gastrin release, if large doses are used. Consequently, calcium compounds are rarely used in peptic ulcer disease.

Commonly used antacids are mixtures of aluminum hydroxide and magnesium hydroxide (eg, Gelusil, Mylanta, Maalox). Some antacid mixtures contain other ingredients, such as simethicone (contained in Mylanta) or alginic acid. Simethicone is an antiflatulent drug available alone as Mylicon. When added to antacids, simethicone does not affect gastric acidity. It reportedly decreases gas bubbles, thereby reducing GI distention and abdominal discomfort. Alginic acid (eg, in Gaviscon) produces a foamy, viscous layer on top of gastric acid and thereby decreases backflow of gastric acid onto esophageal mucosa while the person is in an upright position.

Antacids act primarily in the stomach and are used to prevent or treat peptic ulcer disease, GERD, esophagitis, heartburn, gastritis, GI bleeding, and stress ulcers. Aluminum-based antacids also are given to clients with chronic renal failure and hyperphosphatemia to decrease absorption of phosphates in food.

Magnesium-based antacids are contraindicated in clients with renal failure.

Helicobacter pylori Agents

Multiple drugs are required to eradicate *H. pylori* organisms and heal related ulcers. Effective combinations include two

Table 59-1 Drugs at a Glance: Representative Antacid Products

	COMPONENTS				
TRADE NAME	Magnesium Oxide or Hydroxide	Aluminum Hydroxide	Calcium Carbonate	Other	ROUTE AND DOSAGE RANGES (ADULTS)
Aludrox	103 mg/5 mL	307 mg/5 mL			PO 10 mL q4h, or as needed
Amphojel		300 or 600 mg/tab			PO 600 mg 5 or 6 times daily
Gelusil	200 mg/tab	200 mg/tab		Simethicone 25 mg/tab	PO 10 or more mL or 2 or more tablets after meals and at bedtime or as directed by physician to a maximum of 12 tablets or tsp/24 h
Maalox suspension	200 mg/5 mL	225 mg/5 mL			PO 30 mL 4 times daily, after meals and at bedtime or as directed by physician; maximal dose, 16 tsp/24 h
Mylanta	200 mg/tab, 200 mg/ 5 mL	200 mg/tab, 200 mg/5 mL		Simethicone 25 mg/tab, 20 mg/ 5 mL	PO 5–10 mL or 1–2 tablets q2–4h, between meals and at bedtime or as directed by physician
Mylanta Double strength	400 mg/tab, 400 mg/ 5 mL	400 mg/tab, 400 mg/5 mL		Simethicone 30 mg/tab, 30 mg/ 5 mL	Same as Mylanta
Titralac			420 mg/tab, 1 g/5 mL	Glycine 180 mg/ tab, 300 mg/ 5 mL	PO 1 tsp or 2 tablets, after meals or as directed by physician, to maximal dose of 19 tablets or 8 tsp/24 h

PO, oral.

antimicrobials and a PPI or an H₂RA. For the antimicrobial component, two of the following drugs—**amoxicillin, clarithromycin, metronidazole,** or **tetracycline**—are used. A single antimicrobial agent is not used because of concern about emergence of drug-resistant *H. pylori* organisms. For clients with an active ulcer, adding an antisecretory drug (eg, H₂RA or PPI) to an antimicrobial regimen accelerates symptom relief and ulcer healing. In addition, antimicrobial–antisecretory combinations are associated with low ulcer-recurrence rates.

A bismuth preparation is added to some regimens. Bismuth exerts antibacterial effects against *H. pylori* by disrupting bacterial cell walls, preventing the organism from adhering to gastric epithelium, and inhibiting bacterial enzymatic and proteolytic activity. It also increases secretion of mucus and bicarbonate, inhibits pepsin activity, and accumulates in ulcer craters.

Although several regimens are effective in *H. pylori* infection, three-drug regimens with a PPI and two antibacterial drugs may be preferred. The regimen using metronidazole, a bismuth compound, tetracycline, and an antisecretory drug is very effective in healing ulcers. However, this regimen is not well tolerated, partly because of the multiple daily doses required. Because client compliance is a difficulty with all the *H. pylori* eradication regimens, some drug combinations are packaged as individual doses to increase convenience. For example, Helidac contains bismuth, metronidazole, and tetracycline (taken with an H₂RA); Prevpac contains amoxicillin, clarithromycin, and lansoprazole. Table 59-2 provides further information.

Histamine₂ Receptor Antagonists (H₂RAs)

Histamine is a substance found in almost every body tissue and released in response to certain stimuli (eg, allergic reactions, tissue injury). After it is released, histamine causes contraction of smooth muscle in the bronchi, GI tract, and uterus; dilation and increased permeability of capillaries; dilation of cerebral blood vessels; and stimulation of sensory nerve endings to produce pain and itching.

(text continues on page 976)

Table 59-2 Drugs at a Glance: Drugs for Acid–Peptic Disorders

GENERIC/TRADE NAME	INDICATIONS FOR USE	ROUTES AND DOSAGE RANGES (ADULTS)
Histamine₂ Receptor Antagonists	Treatment of peptic ulcers and GERD to promote healing, then maintenance to prevent recurrence Prevention of stress ulcers, GI bleeding, and aspiration pneumonitis Treatment of Zollinger-Ellison syndrome Treatment of heartburn	
Cimetidine (Tagamet)		*Duodenal or gastric ulcer,* PO 800 mg once daily at bedtime or 300 mg 4 times daily or 400 mg twice daily *Maintenance,* PO 400 mg at bedtime *IV injection,* 300 mg diluted in 20 mL of 0.9% NaCl solution q6–8h *IV intermittent infusion,* 300 mg diluted in 50 mL of dextrose or saline solution q6h *IM* 300 mg q6–8h *GERD,* PO 800 mg twice daily or 400 mg 4 times daily *Prevention of upper GI bleeding,* IV continuous infusion, 50 mg/h *Heartburn,* PO 200 mg once or twice daily as needed *Impaired renal function,* PO, IV 300 mg q8–12h
Famotidine (Pepcid, Pepcid RPD) **Famotidine 10 mg, calcium carbonate 800 mg, & magnesium hydroxide 165 mg** (Pepcid Complete)		*Duodenal or gastric ulcer,* PO 40 mg once daily at bedtime or 20 mg twice daily for 4–8 wk; maintenance, PO 20 mg once daily at bedtime *Zollinger-Ellison syndrome,* PO 20 mg q6h, increased if necessary *IV injection,* 20 mg q12h, diluted to 5 or 10 mL with 5% dextrose or 0.9% sodium chloride *IV infusion,* 20 mg q12h, diluted with 100 mL of 5% dextrose or 0.9% sodium chloride *Impaired renal function (creatinine clearance <50 mL/min),* PO, IV 20 mg q24–48h *GERD,* PO 20 mg twice daily for 6–12 wk *Heartburn,* (Pepcid Complete) PO 1–2 tablets, chewed, daily as needed
Nizatidine (Axid)		*Duodenal or gastric ulcer,* PO 300 mg once daily at bedtime or 150 mg twice daily; maintenance, PO 150 mg once daily at bedtime *GERD,* PO 150 mg twice daily *Heartburn,* PO 75–150 mg twice daily as needed *Impaired renal function (creatinine clearance [CrCl] 20–50 mL/min),* PO 150 mg daily; CrCl <20 mL/min, PO 150 mg q48h
Ranitidine (Zantac)		*Duodenal ulcer,* PO 300 mg once daily at bedtime or 150 mg twice daily *IM* 50 mg q6–8h *IV injection,* 50 mg diluted in 20 mL of 5% dextrose or 0.9% sodium chloride solution q6–8h *IV intermittent infusion,* 50 mg diluted in 100 mL of 5% dextrose or 0.9% sodium chloride solution *Gastric ulcer or GERD,* PO 150 mg twice daily *Impaired renal function (CrCl <50 mL/min),* PO 150 mg q24h; IV, IM 50 mg q18–24h

Table 59-2 Drugs at a Glance: Drugs for Acid–Peptic Disorders (continued)

GENERIC/TRADE NAME	INDICATIONS FOR USE	ROUTES AND DOSAGE RANGES (ADULTS)
Proton Pump Inhibitors	Treatment of gastric and duodenal ulcers, for 4–8 wk Treatment of GERD with erosive esophagitis for 4–8 wk to promote healing, then maintenance to prevent recurrence Treatment of Zollinger-Ellison syndrome	
Esomeprazole (Nexium, Nexium IV, Nexium delayed-release capsules)		*GERD with erosive esophagitis,* PO 20–40 mg once daily for 4–8 wk; maintenance, 20 mg once daily, IV 20–40 mg daily up to 10 d
Lansoprazole (Prevacid, Prevacid IV)		*Duodenal ulcer,* PO 15 mg daily for healing and maintenance *Gastric ulcer,* PO 30 mg once daily, up to 8 wk *Erosive esophagitis,* PO 30 mg daily up to 8 wk; maintenance, 15 mg daily, IV 30 mg daily up to 7 d *H. pylori infection,* PO 30 mg (with amoxicillin and clarithromycin) twice daily for 14 d *Hypersecretory conditions,* PO 60–90 mg daily
Omeprazole (Prilosec)		*Gastric ulcer,* PO 40 mg once daily for 4–8 wk *Duodenal ulcer,* PO 20 mg once daily for 4–8 wk *GERD,* PO 20 mg once daily *Zollinger-Ellison syndrome,* PO 60 mg once daily
Pantoprazole (Protonix, Protonix IV)		*GERD with erosive esophagitis,* PO, IV 40 mg once daily *Zollinger-Ellison syndrome,* PO, IV 40–80 mg q12h
Rabeprazole (Aciphex)		*Duodenal ulcer,* PO 20 mg once daily up to 4 wk *GERD,* PO 20 mg once daily for healing and maintenance *Zollinger-Ellison syndrome,* PO 60 mg once or twice daily
Miscellaneous Agents		
Misoprostol (Cytotec)	Prevention of aspirin and NSAID-induced gastric ulcers in selected clients	PO 100–200 mg 4 times daily with meals and at bedtime
Sucralfate (Carafate)	Treatment of active duodenal ulcer to promote healing, then maintenance to prevent recurrence	*Treatment of active ulcer,* PO 1 g 4 times daily before meals and at bedtime *Maintenance therapy,* PO 1 g 2 times daily
Helicobacter pylori Agents ANTIMICROBIALS **Amoxicillin**	*H. pylori* infection causing gastric or duodenal ulcers	PO 500 mg 4 times daily
Clarithromycin		PO 500 mg 2–3 times daily
Metronidazole		PO 250 mg 4 times daily
Tetracycline		PO 500 mg 4 times daily
BISMUTH SUBSALICYLATE	*H. pylori* eradication and GI upset (abdominal cramping, indigestion, nausea, diarrhea)	*Adults:* PO 525 mg (2 tabs or 30 mL) 4 times daily *Children:* 9–12 y, PO 1 tab or 15 mL; 6–9 y, PO ⅔ tab or 10 mL; 3–6 y, PO ⅓ tab or 5 mL; <3 y, consult physician. Dosage may be repeated every 30–60 min, if needed, up to 8 doses in 24 h.

(continued)

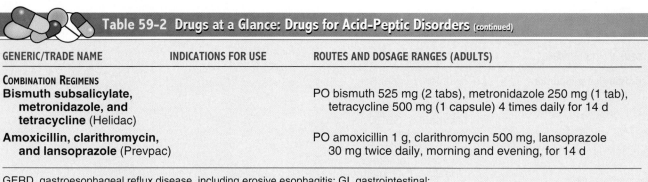

Table 59-2 Drugs at a Glance: Drugs for Acid-Peptic Disorders (continued)

GENERIC/TRADE NAME	INDICATIONS FOR USE	ROUTES AND DOSAGE RANGES (ADULTS)
COMBINATION REGIMENS		
Bismuth subsalicylate, metronidazole, and tetracycline (Helidac)		PO bismuth 525 mg (2 tabs), metronidazole 250 mg (1 tab), tetracycline 500 mg (1 capsule) 4 times daily for 14 d
Amoxicillin, clarithromycin, and lansoprazole (Prevpac)		PO amoxicillin 1 g, clarithromycin 500 mg, lansoprazole 30 mg twice daily, morning and evening, for 14 d

GERD, gastroesophageal reflux disease, including erosive esophagitis; GI, gastrointestinal; IM, intramuscular; IV, intravenous; NSAID, nonsteroidal anti-inflammatory drug; PO, oral.

Histamine also causes strong stimulation of gastric acid secretion. Vagal stimulation causes release of histamine from cells in the gastric mucosa. The histamine then acts on receptors located on the parietal cells to increase production of hydrochloric acid. These receptors are called the *H_2 receptors.*

Traditional antihistamines or H_1 receptor antagonists prevent or reduce other effects of histamine but do not block histamine effects on gastric acid production. The H_2RAs inhibit both basal secretion of gastric acid and the secretion stimulated by histamine, acetylcholine, and gastrin. They decrease the amount, acidity, and pepsin content of gastric juices. A single dose of an H_2RA can inhibit acid secretion for 6 to 12 hours and a continuous intravenous (IV) infusion can inhibit secretion for prolonged periods.

Clinical indications for use include prevention and treatment of peptic ulcer disease, GERD, esophagitis, GI bleeding due to acute stress ulcers, and Zollinger-Ellison syndrome. With gastric or duodenal ulcers, healing occurs within 6 to 8 weeks; with esophagitis, healing occurs in about 12 weeks. Over-the-counter (OTC) oral preparations, at lower dosage strengths, are approved for the treatment of heartburn.

There are no known contraindications, but the drugs should be used with caution in children, pregnant women, older adults, and clients with impaired renal or hepatic function. Dosage should be reduced in the presence of impaired renal function.

Adverse effects occur infrequently with usual doses and duration of treatment. They are more likely to occur with prolonged use of high doses and in older adults or those with impaired renal or hepatic function.

Cimetidine, ranitidine, famotidine, and nizatidine are the four available H_2RAs (see Table 59-2). **Cimetidine** was the first, and it is still widely used. It is well absorbed after oral administration. After a single dose, peak blood level is reached in 1 to 1.5 hours, and an effective concentration is maintained about 6 hours. The drug is distributed in almost all body tissues. Cimetidine should be used with caution during pregnancy because it crosses the placenta, and it should not be taken during lactation because it is excreted in breast milk. Most of an oral dose is excreted unchanged in the urine within 24 hours; some is excreted in bile and eliminated in feces. For acutely ill clients, cimetidine is given IV. A major disadvantage of cimetidine is that it inhibits the hepatic metabolism of numerous other drugs, thereby increasing blood levels and risks of toxicity with the inhibited drug.

Ranitidine is more potent than cimetidine on a weight basis, and smaller doses can be given less frequently. In addition, ranitidine causes fewer drug interactions than cimetidine. Oral ranitidine reaches peak blood levels 1 to 3 hours after administration, and is metabolized in the liver; approximately 30% is excreted unchanged in the urine. Parenteral ranitidine reaches peak blood levels in about 15 minutes; 65% to 80% is excreted unchanged in the urine. **Famotidine** and **nizatidine** are similar to cimetidine and ranitidine.

Compared with cimetidine, the other drugs cause similar effects except they are less likely to cause mental confusion and gynecomastia (antiandrogenic effects). In addition, they do not affect the cytochrome P450 drug-metabolizing system in the liver and therefore do not interfere with the metabolism of other drugs.

Proton Pump Inhibitors (PPIs)

PPIs are strong inhibitors of gastric acid secretion. These drugs bind irreversibly to the gastric proton pump (eg, the enzyme H^+, K^+-ATPase) to prevent the "pumping" or release of gastric acid from parietal cells into the stomach lumen, thereby blocking the final step of acid production. Inhibition of the proton pump suppresses gastric acid secretion in response to all primary stimuli, histamine, gastrin, and acetylcholine. Thus, the drugs inhibit both daytime (including meal-stimulated) and nocturnal (unstimulated) acid secretion.

Indications for use include treatment of peptic ulcer disease, erosive gastritis, GERD, and Zollinger-Ellison syndrome. PPIs are usually the drugs of choice for treatment of duodenal and gastric ulcers, GERD with erosive esophagitis, and Zollinger-Ellison syndrome. Compared with H_2RAs, PPIs suppress gastric acid more strongly and for a longer time. This effect provides faster symptom relief and faster healing in acid-related diseases. For example, healing of duodenal and gastric ulcers after 2 weeks is similar to the healing after 4 weeks of H$_2$RA therapy. The PPIs and H$_2$RAs are similarly effective in maintenance therapy of peptic ulcer disorders, with similar rates of ulcer recurrence. In clients with GERD, PPIs usually abolish symptoms within 1 to 2 weeks and heal esophagitis within 8 weeks. The drugs are also effective in maintenance therapy to prevent recurrence of esophagitis. In clients with *H. pylori*–associated ulcers, eradication of the organism with antimicrobial drugs is preferable to long-term maintenance therapy with antisecretory drugs.

The drugs usually are well tolerated; adverse effects are minimal with both short- and long-term use. Nausea, diarrhea, and headache are the most frequently reported adverse effects. However, long-term consequences of profound gastric acid suppression are unknown.

Omeprazole, esomeprazole, lansoprazole, pantoprazole, and **rabeprazole** are the available PPIs (see Table 59-2). Omeprazole was the first and is still widely used. It is well absorbed after oral administration, highly bound to plasma proteins (about 95%), metabolized in the liver, and excreted in the urine (about 75%) and bile or feces. Acid-inhibiting effects occur within 2 hours and last 72 hours or longer. When the drug is discontinued, effects persist for 48 to 72 hours or longer, until the gastric parietal cells can synthesize additional H$^+$, K$^+$-ATPase. The other drugs are very similar to omeprazole. Omeprazole (Prilosec) is expected to be approved for OTC sales for treating heartburn. If heartburn is not improved within 14 days of treatment, clients should be evaluated by their health care provider. Prescription omeprazole has been very expensive; with nonprescription use, the cost should be much lower.

Prostaglandin

Naturally occurring prostaglandin E, which is produced in mucosal cells of the stomach and duodenum, inhibits gastric acid secretion and increases mucus and bicarbonate secretion, mucosal blood flow, and perhaps mucosal repair. It also inhibits the mucosal damage produced by gastric acid, aspirin, and NSAIDs. When synthesis of prostaglandin E is inhibited, erosion and ulceration of gastric mucosa may occur. This is the mechanism by which aspirin and other NSAIDs are thought to cause gastric and duodenal ulcers (see Chap. 7).

Misoprostol (see Table 59-2) is a synthetic form of prostaglandin E approved for concurrent use with NSAIDs to protect gastric mucosa from NSAID-induced erosion and ulceration. It is indicated for clients at high risk of GI ulceration and bleeding, such as those taking high doses of NSAIDs for arthritis and older adults. It is contraindicated in women of childbearing potential, unless effective contraceptive methods are being used; and during pregnancy, because it may induce abortion. The most common adverse effects are diarrhea (occurs in 10%–40% of recipients) and abdominal cramping. Older adults may be unable to tolerate misoprostol-induced diarrhea and abdominal discomfort.

Sucralfate

Sucralfate is a preparation of sulfated sucrose and aluminum hydroxide that binds to normal and ulcerated mucosa. It is used to prevent and treat peptic ulcer disease. It is effective even though it does not inhibit secretion of gastric acid or pepsin and it has little neutralizing effect on gastric acid. Its mechanism of action is unclear, but it is thought to act locally on the gastric and duodenal mucosa. Possible mechanisms include binding to the ulcer and forming a protective barrier between the mucosa and gastric acid, pepsin, and bile salts; neutralizing pepsin; stimulating prostaglandin synthesis in the mucosa; and exerting healing effects through the aluminum component. Sucralfate is effective in healing duodenal ulcers and in maintenance therapy to prevent ulcer recurrence. In general, the rates of ulcer healing with sucralfate are similar to the rates with H$_2$RAs.

Adverse effects are low in incidence and severity because sucralfate is not absorbed systemically. Constipation and dry mouth are most often reported. The main disadvantages of using sucralfate are that the tablet is large; it must be given at least twice daily; it requires an acid pH for activation and should not be given with an antacid, H$_2$RA, or PPI; and it may bind to other drugs and prevent their absorption. In general, sucralfate should be given 2 hours before or after other drugs.

Herbal and Dietary Supplements

Several herbal supplements are promoted as aiding heartburn, gastritis, and peptic ulcer disease. Most have not been studied in humans and there is little, if any, evidence that they are either safe or effective for the proposed uses. Given the known safety and effectiveness of available drugs and the possible consequences of delaying effective treatment, the use of herbal supplements for any acid-peptic disorder should be discouraged.

NURSING PROCESS

Assessment

Assess the client's status in relation to peptic ulcer disease, GERD, and other conditions in which antiulcer drugs are used.
● Identify risk factors for peptic ulcer disease.
  ● Cigarette smoking. Effects are thought to include stimulation of gastric acid secretion and decreased

blood supply to gastric mucosa. (Nicotine constricts blood vessels.) Moreover, clients with peptic ulcers who continue to smoke heal more slowly and have more recurrent ulcers, despite usually adequate treatment, than those who stop smoking.
- Stress, including physiologic stress (eg, shock, sepsis, burns, surgery, head injury, severe trauma, medical illness) and psychological stress. One mechanism may be that stress activates the sympathetic nervous system, which then causes vasoconstriction in organs not needed for "fight or flight." Thus, stress may lead to ischemia in gastric mucosa, with ulceration if ischemia is severe or prolonged.
- Drug therapy with aspirin and other NSAIDs, corticosteroids, and antineoplastics.
● Signs and symptoms depend on the type and location of the ulcer.
- Periodic epigastric pain, which occurs 1 to 4 hours after eating or during the night and is often described as "burning" or "gnawing," is a symptom of a chronic duodenal ulcer.
- GI bleeding occurs with acute or chronic ulcers when the ulcer erodes into a blood vessel. Clinical manifestations may range from mild (eg, occult blood in feces, eventual anemia) to severe (eg, hematemesis, melena, hypotension, shock).
- GERD produces heartburn (a substernal burning sensation).

Nursing Diagnoses

- Pain related to effects of gastric acid on peptic ulcers or inflamed esophageal tissues
- Imbalanced Nutrition: Less Than Body Requirements related to anorexia and abdominal discomfort
- Constipation related to aluminum- or calcium-containing antacids and sucralfate
- Diarrhea related to magnesium-containing antacids and misoprostol
- Deficient Knowledge related to drug therapy and non-pharmacologic management of GERD and peptic ulcer disease

Planning/Goals

The client will
- Take or receive antiulcer, anti-heartburn drugs accurately
- Experience relief of symptoms
- Avoid situations that cause or exacerbate symptoms, when possible
- Be observed for GI bleeding and other complications of peptic ulcer disease and GERD
- Maintain normal patterns of bowel function
- Avoid preventable adverse effects of drug therapy

Interventions

Use measures to prevent or minimize peptic ulcer disease and gastric acid–induced esophageal disorders.
● With peptic ulcer disease, helpful interventions may include the following:
- General health measures such as a well-balanced diet, adequate rest, and regular exercise
- Avoiding cigarette smoking and gastric irritants (eg, alcohol, aspirin and NSAIDs, caffeine)
- Reducing psychological stress (eg, by changing environments) or learning healthful strategies of stress management (eg, relaxation techniques, physical exercise). There is no practical way to avoid psychological stress because it is part of everyday life.
- Long-term drug therapy with small doses of H$_2$RAs, antacids, or sucralfate. With "active" peptic ulcer disease, helping the client follow the prescribed therapeutic regimen helps to promote healing and prevent complications (see accompanying Client Teaching Guidelines).
- Diet therapy is of minor importance in prevention or treatment of peptic ulcer disease. Some physicians prescribe no dietary restrictions, whereas others suggest avoiding or minimizing highly spiced foods, gas-forming foods, and caffeine-containing beverages.
- With heartburn and esophagitis, helpful measures are those that prevent or decrease gastroesophageal reflux of gastric contents (eg, avoiding irritant, highly spiced, or fatty foods; eating small meals; not lying down for 1 to 2 hours after eating; elevating the head of the bed; avoiding obesity, constipation, or other conditions that increase intra-abdominal pressure).

Evaluation

- Observe and interview regarding drug use.
- Observe and interview regarding relief of symptoms.
- Observe for signs and symptoms of complications.
- Observe and interview regarding adverse drug effects.

APPLYING YOUR KNOWLEDGE 59-1
In addition to taking her medication properly, you should instruct Ms. Daniels to take measures to avoid gastric irritation. What content would be included in this teaching plan?

APPLYING YOUR KNOWLEDGE 59-2
Ms. Daniels suffers from acid reflux. She should be taught measures that can help reduce the pain associated with heartburn. What should you teach her with regard to minimizing the symptoms of acid reflux?

General Considerations

✓ These drugs are commonly used to prevent and treat peptic ulcers and heartburn. Peptic ulcers usually form in the stomach or first part of the small bowel (duodenum), where tissues are exposed to stomach acid. Two common causes of peptic ulcer disease are stomach infection with a bacterium called *Helicobacter pylori* and taking nonsteroidal anti-inflammatory drugs (NSAIDs) such as ibuprofen and many others. Heartburn (also called gastro-esophageal reflux disease) is caused by stomach acid splashing back onto the esophagus.

　Peptic ulcer disease and heartburn are chronic conditions that are usually managed on an outpatient basis. Complications such as bleeding require hospitalization. Overall, these conditions can range from mild to serious, and it is important to seek information about the disease process, ways to prevent or minimize symptoms, and drug therapy.

✓ With heartburn, try to minimize acid reflux by elevating the head of the bed; avoiding stomach distention by eating small meals; not lying down for 1 to 2 hours after eating; minimizing intake of fats, chocolate, citric juices, coffee, and alcohol; avoiding smoking (stimulates gastric acid production); and avoiding obesity, constipation, or other conditions that increase intra-abdominal pressure. In addition, take tablets and capsules with 8 oz of water and do not take medications at bedtime unless instructed to do so. Some medications (eg, tetracycline, potassium chloride tablets, iron supplements, nonsteroidal anti-inflammatory drugs [NSAIDS]) may cause "pill-induced" irritation of the esophagus (esophagitis) if not taken with enough liquid.

✓ Most medications for peptic ulcer disease and heartburn decrease stomach acid. An exception is the antibiotics used to treat ulcers caused by *H. pylori* infection. The strongest acid reducers are omeprazole (Prilosec), esomeprazole (Nexium), lansoprazole (Prevacid), pantoprazole (Protonix), and rabeprazole (Aciphex). These are prescription drugs, except for omeprazole, which is approved for nonprescription use. Histamine-blocking drugs such as cimetidine (Tagamet), famotidine (Pepcid), and others are available as both prescription and over-the-counter (OTC) preparations. OTC products are indicated for heartburn, and smaller doses are taken than for peptic ulcer disease. These drugs usually should not be taken longer than 2 weeks without the advice of a health care provider. The concern is that OTC drugs may delay diagnosis and treatment of potentially serious illness. In addition, cimetidine can increase toxic effects of numerous drugs and should be avoided if you are taking other medications.

　Misoprostol (Cytotec) is given to prevent ulcers from NSAIDs, which are commonly used to relieve pain and inflammation with arthritis and other conditions. This drug should be taken only while taking a traditional NSAID such as ibuprofen. A related drug, celecoxib (Celebrex) is less likely to cause peptic ulcer disease.

Do not take misoprostol if pregnant and do not become pregnant while taking the drug. If pregnancy occurs during misoprostol therapy, stop the drug and notify your health care provider immediately. Misoprostol can cause abdominal cramps and miscarriage.

　Numerous antacid preparations are available, but they are not equally safe in all people and should be selected carefully. For example, products that contain magnesium have a laxative effect and may cause diarrhea; those that contain aluminum or calcium may cause constipation. Some commonly used antacids (eg, Maalox, Mylanta) are a mixture of magnesium and aluminum preparations, an attempt to avoid both constipation and diarrhea. People with kidney disease should not take products that contain magnesium because magnesium can accumulate in the body and cause serious adverse effects. Thus, it is important to read product labels and, if you have a chronic illness or take other medications, ask your physician or pharmacist to help you select an antacid and an appropriate dose.

Self- or Caregiver Administration

✓ Take antiulcer drugs as directed. Underuse decreases therapeutic effectiveness; overuse increases adverse effects. For acute peptic ulcer disease or esophagitis, drugs are given in relatively high doses for 4 to 8 weeks to promote healing. For long-term maintenance therapy, dosage is reduced.

✓ With Prilosec, Aciphex, Nexium, and Protonix, swallow the capsule whole; do not open, chew, or crush. With Prevacid, the capsule can be opened and the granules sprinkled on applesauce for patients who are unable to swallow capsules. Also, the granules are available in a packet for preparing a liquid suspension. Follow instructions for mixing the granules exactly. The granules should not be crushed or chewed.

✓ Take cimetidine with meals or at bedtime. Take famotidine, nizatidine, and ranitidine with or without food. Do not take an antacid for 1 hour before or after taking one of these drugs.

✓ Take sucralfate on an empty stomach at least 1 hour before meals and at bedtime. Also, do not take an antacid for 1 hour before or after taking sucralfate.

✓ Take misoprostol with food.

✓ For treatment of peptic ulcer disease, take antacids 1 and 3 hours after meals and at bedtime (4 to 7 doses daily), 1 to 2 hours before or after other medications. Antacids decrease absorption of many medications if taken at the same time. Also, chew chewable tablets thoroughly before swallowing, then drink a glass of water; allow effervescent tablets to dissolve completely and almost stop bubbling before drinking; and shake liquids well before measuring the dose.

✓ Take Pepcid RPD orally disintegrating tablets by placing on tongue and allowing to dissolve with saliva. Taking with liquids not necessary.

PRINCIPLES OF THERAPY

Drug Selection

All of the drugs used for acid-peptic disorders are effective for indicated uses; the choice of drugs may depend on etiology, acuity, severity of symptoms, cost, and convenience. General guidelines include the following:

- *PPIs* are the drugs of first choice in most situations. They heal gastric and duodenal ulcers more rapidly and may be more effective in treating erosive esophagitis, erosive gastritis, and Zollinger-Ellison syndrome than H$_2$RAs. They are also effective in eradicating *H. pylori* infection when combined with two antibacterial drugs. Omeprazole and rabeprazole are given only orally; esomeprazole, lansoprazole, and pantoprazole may be given orally or IV. PPIs are more expensive than H$_2$RAs.

- *H. pylori* infection should be considered in most cases of peptic ulcer disease. If infection is confirmed by appropriate diagnostic tests, agents to eradicate the organisms should be drugs of first choice. The most-recommended drug regimen is a combination of a PPI and two antibacterial drugs.

- *H$_2$RAs* have been replaced as first-choice drugs by the PPIs for most indications, but are still widely used. Cimetidine may be less expensive but it may cause confusion and antiandrogenic effects. It also increases the risks of toxicity with several commonly used drugs. Compared with cimetidine, other H$_2$RAs are more potent on a weight basis and have a longer duration of action, so they can be given in smaller, less frequent doses. In addition, they do not alter the hepatic metabolism of other drugs. OTC H$_2$RAs are indicated for the treatment of heartburn. In some cases, clients may depend on self-medication with OTC drugs and delay seeking treatment for peptic ulcer disease or GERD. For prescription or nonprescription uses, cimetidine is preferably taken by clients who are taking no other medications.

- *Antacids* are often used as needed to relieve heartburn and abdominal discomfort. If used to treat acid-peptic disorders, they are more often used with other agents than alone and require a regular dosing schedule. The choice of antacid should be individualized to find a preparation that is acceptable to the client in terms of taste, dosage, and convenience of administration. Some guidelines include the following:
  - Most commonly used antacids combine aluminum hydroxide and magnesium hydroxide. The combination decreases the adverse effects of diarrhea (with magnesium products) and constipation (with aluminum products). Calcium carbonate is effective in relieving heartburn, but it is infrequently used to treat peptic ulcers or GERD.
  - Antacids may be used more often now that low doses (eg, two antacid tablets four times a day) have

been shown to be effective in healing gastric and duodenal ulcers. All of the low-dose regimens contained aluminum, and the aluminum rather than acid neutralization may be the important therapeutic factor. Compared with other drugs for acid-peptic disorders, low-dose antacids are inexpensive and cause few adverse effects. In addition, tablets are as effective as liquids and usually more convenient to use.

- Antacids with magnesium are contraindicated in renal disease because hypermagnesemia may result; those with high sugar content are contraindicated in diabetes mellitus.

- Additional ingredients may be helpful to some clients. Simethicone has no effect on intragastric pH but may be useful in relieving flatulence or gastroesophageal reflux. Alginic acid may be useful in clients with daytime acid reflux and heartburn.

- *Sucralfate* must be taken before meals, and this is inconvenient for some clients.

 APPLYING YOUR KNOWLEDGE 59-3:
HOW CAN YOU AVOID THIS MEDICATION ERROR?
Ms. Daniels finds that Maalox is less expensive than Mylanta so she switches her antacid brand. She complains that her heartburn is getting worse.

Guidelines for Therapy With Proton Pump Inhibitors

- Recommended doses of PPIs heal most gastric and duodenal ulcers in about 4 weeks. Large gastric ulcers may require 8 weeks.
- The drugs may be used to maintain healing of gastric and duodenal ulcers and decrease risks of ulcer recurrence.
- A PPI and two antimicrobial drugs is the most effective regimen for eradication of *H. pylori* organisms.
- With GERD, higher doses or longer therapy may be needed for severe disease and esophagitis. Lower doses can maintain symptom relief and esophageal healing.

Guidelines for Therapy With Histamine$_2$ Receptor Antagonists

- For an acute ulcer, full dosage may be given up to 8 weeks. When the ulcer heals, dosage may be reduced by 50% for maintenance therapy to prevent recurrence.
- For duodenal ulcers, a single evening or bedtime dose produces the same healing effects as multiple doses. Commonly used nocturnal doses are cimetidine 800 mg, ranitidine 300 mg, nizatidine 300 mg, or famotidine 40 mg.
- For gastric ulcers, the optimal H$_2$RA dosage schedule has not been established. Gastric ulcers heal more slowly than duodenal ulcers and most authorities prescribe 6 to 8 weeks of drug therapy.

- To maintain ulcer healing and prevent recurrence, long-term H$_2$RA therapy is often used. The drug is usually given as a single bedtime dose, but the amount is reduced by 50% (ie, cimetidine 400 mg, ranitidine 150 mg, nizatidine 150 mg, or famotidine 20 mg).
- For Zollinger-Ellison syndrome, high doses as often as every 4 hours may be required.
- For severe reflux esophagitis, multiple daily doses may be required for adequate symptom control.
- Dosage of all these drugs should be reduced in the presence of impaired renal function.
- Antacids are often given concurrently with H$_2$RAs to relieve pain. They should not be given at the same time (except for Pepcid Complete) because the antacid reduces absorption of the other drug. H$_2$RAs usually relieve pain after 1 week of administration.
- These drugs are available in a wide array of products. Precautions must be taken to ensure the correct formulation, dosage strength, and method of administration for the intended use. For example, cimetidine is available in tablets of 200, 300, 400, and 800 mg; an oral liquid with 300 mg/5 mL; and injectable solutions. Ranitidine is available in tablets of 75 mg; capsules (Zantac GEL-dose) of 150 and 300 mg; liquid syrup with 15 mg/mL; effervescent granules of 150 mg; and injectable solutions of 1 mg/mL and 25 mg/mL. Nizatidine is available in tablets of 75 mg and capsules of 150 and 300 mg; and famotidine in tablets of 10, 20, and 40 mg; chewable tablets of 10 mg; orally disintegrating tablets (Pepcid RPD) of 20 and 40 mg; a powder for oral suspension that contains 40 mg/5 mL when reconstituted; and injection solutions of 10 mg/mL and 20 mg/50 mL.
- All of the drugs are available by prescription and OTC. When prescriptions are given, clients should be advised to avoid concomitant use of OTC versions of the same or similar drugs.

Guidelines for Therapy With Sucralfate

- When sucralfate is used to treat an ulcer, it should be administered for 4 to 8 weeks unless healing is confirmed by radiologic or endoscopic examination.
- When used long term to prevent ulcer recurrence, dosage should be reduced.

Guidelines for Therapy With Antacids

- To prevent stress ulcers in critically ill clients and to treat acute GI bleeding, nearly continuous neutralization of gastric acid is desirable. Dose and frequency of administration must be sufficient to neutralize approximately 50 to 80 mEq of gastric acid each hour. This can be accomplished by a continuous intragastric drip through a nasogastric tube or by hourly administration.
- When a client has a nasogastric tube in place, antacid dosage may be titrated by aspirating stomach contents, determining pH, and then basing the dose on the pH. (Most gastric acid is neutralized and most pepsin activity is eliminated at a pH above 3.5.)
- When prescribing antacids to treat active ulcers, it has long been recommended to take them 1 hour and 3 hours after meals and at bedtime for greater acid neutralization. This schedule is effective but inconvenient for many clients. More recently, lower doses taken less often have been found effective in healing duodenal or gastric ulcers even though less acid neutralization occurs.
- It was formerly thought that liquid antacid preparations were more effective. Now, tablets are considered as effective as liquids.
- When antacids are used to relieve pain, they usually may be taken as needed. However, they should not be taken in high doses or for prolonged periods because of potential adverse effects.

Effects of Acid-Suppressant Drugs on Other Drugs

Antacids may prevent absorption of most drugs taken at the same time, including benzodiazepine antianxiety drugs, corticosteroids, digoxin, H$_2$RAs (eg, cimetidine), iron supplements, phenothiazine antipsychotic drugs, phenytoin, fluoroquinolone antibacterials, and tetracyclines. Antacids increase absorption of a few drugs, including levodopa, quinidine, and valproic acid. These interactions can be avoided or minimized by separating administration times by 1 to 2 hours.

H$_2$RAs may alter the effects of several drugs. Most significant effects occur with cimetidine, which interferes with the metabolism of many commonly used drugs. Consequently, the affected drugs are eliminated more slowly, their serum levels are increased, and they are more likely to cause adverse effects and toxicity unless dosage is reduced.

Interacting drugs include antidysrhythmics (lidocaine, propafenone, quinidine); the anticoagulant warfarin; anticonvulsants (carbamazepine, phenytoin); benzodiazepine antianxiety or hypnotic agents (alprazolam, diazepam, flurazepam, triazolam); beta-adrenergic blocking agents (labetalol, metoprolol, propranolol); the bronchodilator theophylline; calcium channel blocking agents (eg, verapamil); tricyclic antidepressants (eg, amitriptyline); and sulfonylurea antidiabetic drugs. In addition, cimetidine may increase serum levels (eg, fluorouracil, procainamide and its active metabolite) and pharmacologic effects of other drugs (eg, respiratory depression with opioid analgesics) by unidentified mechanisms. Cimetidine also may decrease effects of several drugs, including drugs that require an acidic environment for absorption (eg, iron salts, indomethacin, fluconazole, tetracyclines) and miscellaneous drugs (eg, digoxin, tocainide) by unknown mechanisms.

Ranitidine, famotidine, and nizatidine do not inhibit the cytochrome P450 metabolizing enzymes. Ranitidine decreases absorption of diazepam if given at the same time and increases hypoglycemic effects of glipizide. Nizatidine increases serum salicylate levels in people taking high doses of aspirin.

PPIs have relatively few effects on other drugs. Omeprazole increases blood levels of some benzodiazepines (diazepam, flurazepam, triazolam), phenytoin, and warfarin, probably by inhibiting hepatic metabolism. These interactions have not been reported with the other PPIs.

Sucralfate decreases absorption of ciprofloxacin and other fluoroquinolones, digoxin, phenytoin, and warfarin. Sucralfate binds to these drugs when both are present in the GI tract. This interaction can be avoided or minimized by giving the interacting drug 2 hours before sucralfate.

Effects of Acid-Suppressant Drugs on Nutrients

Dietary folate, iron, and vitamin B_{12} are better absorbed from an acidic environment. When gastric fluids are made less acidic by antacids, H_2RAs, or PPIs, deficiencies of these nutrients may occur. In addition, sucralfate interferes with absorption of fat-soluble vitamins, and magnesium-containing antacids interfere with absorption of vitamin A.

Use in Special Populations

Use in Children

Antacids may be given to ambulatory children in doses of 5 to 15 milliliters every 3 to 6 hours or after meals and at bedtime, as for adults with acid-peptic disorders. For prevention of GI bleeding in critically ill children, 2 to 5 milliliters may be given to infants and 5 to 15 milliliters to children every 1 to 2 hours. Safety and effectiveness of other antiulcer drugs have not been established for children.

Although PPIs are not approved by the Food and Drug Administration for use in children and are not available in pediatric dosage formulations, they are widely used in the treatment of peptic ulcer and gastroesophageal disease. They are also used to eradicate *H. pylori* organisms. Most published reports involve adult doses for children older than 3 years of age. Some clinicians titrate dosage by a child's weight, such as an initial dose of 0.7 milligrams per kilogram of body weight per day.

Use in Older Adults

All of the antiulcer, anti-heartburn drugs may be used in older adults. With antacids, smaller doses may be effective because older adults usually secrete less gastric acid than younger adults. Also, with decreased renal function, older adults are more likely to have adverse effects, such as neuromuscular effects with magnesium-containing antacids. Many physicians recommend calcium carbonate antacids (eg, Tums) as a calcium supplement to prevent or treat osteoporosis in older women.

With H_2RAs, older adults are more likely to experience adverse effects, especially confusion, agitation, and disorien-

tation with cimetidine. In addition, older adults often have decreased renal function, and doses need to be reduced.

Older adults often take large doses of NSAIDs for arthritis and therefore are at risk for development of acute gastric ulcers and GI bleeding. Thus, they may be candidates for treatment with misoprostol. Dosage of misoprostol may need to be reduced to prevent severe diarrhea and abdominal cramping.

PPIs and sucralfate are well tolerated by older adults. A PPI is probably the drug of choice for treating symptomatic GERD because evidence suggests that clients 60 years of age and older require stronger antisecretory effects than younger adults. No dosage reduction is recommended for older adults.

Use in Clients With Renal Impairment

A major concern with antacids is the use of magnesium-containing preparations (eg, Mylanta, Maalox). These are contraindicated in clients with impaired renal function (creatinine clearance <30 mL/minute) because 5% to 10% of the magnesium may be absorbed and accumulate to cause hypermagnesemia. In addition, antacids with calcium carbonate can cause alkalosis and raise urine pH; chronic use may cause renal stones, hypercalcemia, and renal failure.

Antacids containing aluminum hydroxide (eg, Amphogel, Rolaids) are the antacids of choice in clients with chronic renal failure. Aluminum tends not to accumulate and it binds with phosphate in the GI tract to prevent phosphate absorption and hyperphosphatemia.

With **PPIs,** no special precautions or dosage reductions are required in clients with renal impairment.

All of the available **H_2RAs** are eliminated through the kidneys, and dosage needs to be substantially reduced in clients with renal impairment to avoid adverse effects. Cimetidine may cause mental confusion in clients with renal impairment. It also blocks secretion of creatinine in renal tubules, thereby decreasing creatinine clearance and increasing serum creatinine level. With moderate to severe renal impairment, recommended dosages include cimetidine 300 milligrams every 12 hours, ranitidine 150 milligrams orally once daily or IV every 18 to 24 hours, and famotidine 20 milligrams at bedtime or every 36 to 48 hours if indicated. Dosage may be cautiously increased if necessary and if renal function is closely monitored. For clients on hemodialysis, an H_2RA should be given at the end of dialysis.

Use in Clients With Hepatic Impairment

PPIs are metabolized in the liver and may cause transient elevations in liver function tests. With omeprazole, bioavailability is increased because of decreased first-pass metabolism, and plasma half-life is increased. However, dosage adjustments are not recommended. Lansoprazole and rabeprazole should be used cautiously and dosage should be reduced in clients with severe liver impairment.

H₂RAs are partly metabolized in the liver and may be eliminated more slowly in clients with impaired liver function. A major concern with cimetidine is that it can inhibit hepatic metabolism of many other drugs.

Use in Clients With Critical Illness

Gastric acid–suppressant drugs (eg, PPIs, H₂RAs) and **sucralfate** are commonly used in critically ill clients. The **PPIs** are the strongest gastric acid suppressants and are usually well tolerated. For clients who cannot take drugs orally, a PPI can be given IV. The **H₂RAs** are used to prevent stress-induced gastric ulceration in adults and children. Except for clients with renal impairment, in whom dosage must be reduced, information about the pharmacokinetics of these drugs in critically ill clients is limited and only cimetidine and ranitidine have been studied. Compared with healthy people, critically ill clients had a longer half-life and lower clearance rate for

H₂RAs. The drugs are usually given by intermittent IV infusion. Ranitidine or famotidine is preferred because critically ill clients often require numerous other drugs with which cimetidine may interact and alter effects. Nizatidine is not available in a parenteral formulation.

Use in Home Care

All of the antiulcer, anti-heartburn drugs are commonly taken in the home setting, usually by self-administration. The home care nurse can assist clients by providing information about taking the drugs correctly and monitoring responses. If cimetidine is being taken, the home care nurse needs to assess for potential drug–drug interactions. With OTC H₂RAs, clients should be instructed to avoid daily use of maximum doses for longer than 2 weeks. If use of antacids or OTC H₂RAs seems to be excessive or prolonged, the client should be assessed for peptic ulcer disease or GERD.

N   U   R   S   I   N   G   A   C   T   I   O   N   S

Antiulcer Drugs

NURSING ACTIONS	RATIONALE/EXPLANATION
1. Administer accurately	
a. With proton pump inhibitors:	
(1) Give most of the drugs before food intake; give oral pantoprazole with or without food.	Manufacturer's recommendations
(2) Ask clients to swallow the tablets or capsules whole, without crushing or chewing.	Drug formulations are delayed-release and long-acting. Opening, crushing, or chewing destroys these effects.
(3) For clients who are unable to swallow capsules, the lansoprazole capsule can be opened and the granules mixed with 60 mL of orange or tomato juice or sprinkled on 1 tablespoon of applesauce, Ensure pudding, cottage cheese, or yogurt, and swallowed immediately, without chewing. Esomeprazole capsules can be mixed with applesauce and swallowed without chewing.	Manufacturer's recommendations. Enteric-coated, delayed-release granules are in oral capsules or separate packets. Chewing or crushing destroys the coating; mixing the granules with applesauce or other acidic substances preserves the coating of the granules, allowing them to remain intact until they reach the small intestine.
(4) To give lansoprazole granules as a liquid suspension, mix 1 packet with 30 mL of water (use no other liquids), stir well, and ask the client to swallow immediately, without chewing the granules. Esomeprazole capsules can be opened, mixed with 50 mL of water, and swallowed or administered via nasogastric tube. Flush tube with water after administration.	
(5) Give intravenous (IV) pantoprazole over 15 minutes, injected into a dedicated line or the Y-site of an IV infusion. Use the in-line filter provided; if injecting in a Y-site, the filter should be placed below the Y-site closest to the patient. Flush the IV line with 5% dextrose, 0.9% NaCl, or lactated Ringer's solution before and after pantoprazole administration. Ivesomeprazole can be injected over no less than 3 minutes or infused over 10–30 minutes into a dedicated IV line. Flush the IV line with 5% dextrose or lactated Ringer's solution before and after esomeprazole administration.	

(continued)

NURSING ACTIONS	RATIONALE/EXPLANATION
b. With histamine (H_2) blockers:	
(1) Give single oral doses at bedtime; give multiple oral doses of cimetidine with meals and at bedtime and other drugs without regard to food intake.	The drugs are effective and convenient in a single oral dose at bedtime.
(2) To give oral disintegrating tablets (Pepcid RPD), open blister package with dry hands immediately before use, place on tongue, and allow to dissolve with saliva to swallow. Administration with liquids not necessary.	
(3) To give cimetidine or ranitidine IV, dilute in 20 mL of 5% dextrose or normal saline solution, and inject over at least 2 minutes. For intermittent infusion, dilute in at least 50 mL of 5% dextrose or 0.9% sodium chloride solution, and infuse over 15–20 minutes.	
(4) To give famotidine IV, dilute with 5–10 mL of 0.9% sodium chloride injection, and inject over at least 2 minutes. For intermittent infusion, dilute in 100 mL of 5% dextrose or 0.9% sodium chloride, and infuse over 15–30 minutes.	
c. With antacids:	
(1) Do not give doses within approximately 1 hour of oral H_2 antagonists or sucralfate.	Antacids decrease absorption and therapeutic effectiveness of the other drugs.
(2) Shake liquids well before measuring the dose.	These preparations are suspensions and must be mixed thoroughly to give the correct dose.
(3) Instruct clients to chew antacid tablets thoroughly and follow with a glass of water.	To increase the surface area of drug available to neutralize gastric acid
d. Give sucralfate 1 hour before meals and at bedtime.	To allow the drug to form its protective coating over the ulcer before high levels of gastric acidity. Sucralfate requires an acidic environment. After it has adhered to the ulcer, antacids and food do not affect drug action.
e. Give misoprostol with food.	
f. Follow package instructions for administering combination drug regimens for *Helicobacter pylori* infection (eg, Prevpac, Helidac) and instruct client to avoid alcohol during and 72 hours after therapy.	Metronidazole may precipitate a disulfiram-like reaction if alcohol ingestion occurs with use.
2. Observe for therapeutic effects	Therapeutic effects depend on the reason for use.
a. Decreased epigastric pain with gastric and duodenal ulcers; decreased heartburn with *gastroesophageal reflux disorders*	Antacids should relieve pain within a few minutes. Proton pump inhibitors and H_2 antagonists relieve pain in 7–10 days by healing effects on peptic ulcers or esophagitis.
b. Decreased gastrointestinal (GI) bleeding (eg, absence of visible or occult blood in vomitus, gastric secretions, or feces)	
c. Higher pH of gastric contents	The minimum acceptable pH with antacid therapy is 3.5.
d. Radiologic or endoscopic reports of ulcer healing	Healing usually occurs within 4 to 8 weeks.
3. Observe for adverse effects	
a. With proton pump inhibitors, observe for headache, diarrhea, abdominal pain, nausea, and vomiting.	These effects occur infrequently and are usually well tolerated.
b. With H_2 antagonists, observe for diarrhea or constipation, headache, dizziness, muscle aches, fatigue, skin rashes, mental confusion, delirium, coma, depression, fever.	Adverse effects are uncommon and usually mild with recommended doses. Central nervous system effects have been associated with high doses in elderly clients or those with impaired renal function. With long-term administration of cimetidine, other adverse effects have been observed. These include decreased sperm count and gynecomastia in men, and galactorrhea in women.
c. With antacids containing magnesium, observe for diarrhea and hypermagnesemia.	Diarrhea may be prevented by combining these antacids with other antacids containing aluminum or calcium. Hypermagnesemia may occur in clients with impaired renal function. These antacids should not be given to clients with renal failure.

NURSING ACTIONS	RATIONALE/EXPLANATION
d. With antacids containing aluminum or calcium, observe for constipation.	Constipation may be prevented by combining these antacids with other antacids containing magnesium. A high-fiber diet, adequate fluid intake (2000–3000 mL daily), and exercise also help prevent constipation.
e. With sucralfate, observe for constipation.	The drug is not absorbed systemically and constipation is the most commonly reported adverse effect.
f. With misoprostol, observe for diarrhea, abdominal pain, nausea and vomiting, headache, uterine cramping, vaginal bleeding.	Diarrhea commonly occurs and may be severe enough to lead to dosage reduction or stopping the drug.
g. With bismuth, observe for black stools.	This is a harmless discoloration of feces; it does not indicate GI bleeding.
4. Observe for drug interactions	Most significant drug interactions alter the effect of the other drug rather than that of the antiulcer or anti–gastroesophageal reflux disease (GERD) drug.
a. Drugs that alter effects of proton pump inhibitors:	
(1) Clarithromycin *increases* effects of omeprazole.	May increase blood levels
(2) Sucralfate *decreases* effects of lansoprazole.	Decreases absorption of lansoprazole, which should be given about 30 minutes before sucralfate if both are used.
b. Drugs that *decrease* effects of H_2 antagonists:	
(1) Antacids	Antacids decrease absorption of cimetidine and probably ranitidine. The drugs should not be given at the same time.
c. Drugs that alter effects of antacids:	
(1) Anticholinergic drugs (eg, atropine) *increase* effects.	May increase effects by delaying gastric emptying and by decreasing acid secretion themselves
(2) Cholinergic drugs (eg, dexpanthenol [Ilopan]) *decrease* effects.	May decrease effects by increasing GI motility and rate of gastric emptying
d. Drugs that *decrease* effects of sucralfate:	
(1) Antacids	Antacids should not be given within 30 minutes before or after administration of sucralfate.

APPLYING YOUR KNOWLEDGE: ANSWERS

59-1 Teach Ms. Daniels to avoid cigarette smoking, alcohol, caffeine, aspirin, and NSAIDs.

59-2 Acid reflux can be reduced by avoiding stomach distention. Eating small meals will reduce gastric distention. Teach Ms. Daniels not to lie down for at least 1 to 2 hours after eating. Foods and drinks that can increase acid reflux include fats, chocolate, citric juices, coffee, and alcohol. Take medication with 8 oz of water. Control obesity, constipation, or other causes of increased intra-abdominal pressure. It may also be helpful to elevate the head of the bed to reduce acid reflux.

59-3 When providing client teaching about drug therapy, include the reasons why each medication has been selected. Make sure to encourage the client to ask questions. Teach Ms. Daniels that the reason she is to take Mylanta is because it contains simethicone; Maalox does not. Although simethicone will not reduce gastric acid, it does relieve gas and reflux.

Review and Application Exercises

Short Answer Exercises

1. What are risk factors for peptic ulcer disease?

2. What roles do gastric acid, pepsin, *H. pylori* organisms, prostaglandins, and mucus play in peptic ulcer occurrence?

3. How do the various drug groups heal ulcers or prevent their recurrence?

4. Compare H_2RAs and PPIs in indications for use and effectiveness.

5. What is the rationale for taking H_2 blockers at bedtime, sucralfate before meals, and antacids after meals?

6. Why are aluminum and magnesium salts often combined in antacid preparations?

7. For a client who smokes cigarettes and is newly diagnosed with peptic ulcer disease, how would you explain that smoking cessation aids ulcer healing?

8. Compare and contrast peptic ulcer disease and GERD in terms of risk factors, drug therapy, and client teaching needs.

NCLEX-Style Questions

9. When taking a client's history, the nurse notes that the client is taking warfarin and cimetidine concurrently. The nurse should anticipate that the
   a. warfarin effects would be increased
   b. cimetidine effects would be increased
   c. warfarin effects would be decreased
   d. cimetidine effects would be decreased

10. The nurse explains to the client being discharged who is taking sucralfate that the medication should be administered
    a. at the same time as an antacid
    b. after meals
    c. with meals
    d. 2 hours before other drugs

11. A client with *H. pylori* develops a related ulcer. He is placed on ranitidine and Helidac, a drug combination that contains bismuth, metronidazole, and tetracycline. The client had been instructed not to consume alcohol, ignored the teaching, and drank a six-pack of beer. The client presents to the emergency department with tachycardia, headache, diaphoresis, and nausea and vomiting. This disulfiram-like reaction likely occurred because of the interaction between the alcohol and which drug in the combination?
    a. ranitidine
    b. bismuth
    c. metronidazole
    d. tetracycline

12. A client asks the nurse how sucralfate (Carafate) works. The nurse replies that sucralfate
    a. inhibits gastric acid secretion
    b. increases mucus and bicarbonate secretion

    c. binds to normal and ulcerated mucosa, creating a protective barrier
    d. enhances prostaglandin synthesis

13. One of the most common adverse effects of misoprostol that makes the drug difficult to tolerate in older adults is
    a. headache
    b. constipation
    c. hyperphosphatemia
    d. diarrhea

Selected References

Chicella, M. F., Batres, L. A., Heesters, M. S., & Dice, J. E. (2005). Prokinetic drug therapy in children: A review of current options. *Annals of Pharmacotherapy, 39*(4), 706–711.

Drug facts and comparisons. (Updated monthly). St. Louis: Facts and Comparisons.

Go, M. F. (2005). Diagnosis and treatment of *Helicobacter pylori. Current Treatment Options in Gastroenterology, 8*(2), 163–174.

Guyton, A. C., & Hall, J. E. (2000). *Textbook of medical physiology* (10th ed.). Philadelphia: W. B. Saunders.

Hale-Pradhan, P. B., Landry, H. K., & Sypula, W. T. (2002). Esomeprazole for acid peptic disorders. *Annals of Pharmacotherapy, 36*(4), 655–663.

Hassall, E. (2005). Decisions in diagnosing and managing chronic gastroesophageal reflux in children. *Journal of Pediatrics, 146*(Suppl. 3), S3–S12.

Henderson, R. P., & Lander, R. D. (2000). Peptic ulcer disease. In E. T. Herfindal & D. R. Gourley (Eds.), *Textbook of therapeutics: Drug and disease management* (7th ed., pp. 515–531). Philadelphia: Lippincott Williams & Wilkins.

Lacy, C. F., Armstrong, L. L., Goldman, M. P., et al. (2004). *Lexi-Comp's drug information handbook* (12th ed.). Hudson, OH: Lexi-Comp.

Metz, D. C., & Walsh, J. H. (2000). Gastroduodenal ulcer disease and gastritis. In H. D. Humes (Ed.), *Kelley's Textbook of internal medicine* (4th ed., pp. 824–844). Philadelphia: Lippincott Williams & Wilkins.

Meurer, L. N., & Bower, D. J. (2002). Management of *Helicobacter pylori* infection. *American Family Physician, 65*(7), 1327–1336.

Porth, C. M. (2005). *Pathophysiology: Concepts of altered health states* (7th ed.). Philadelphia: Lippincott Williams & Wilkins.

Richter, J. E. (2000). Diseases of the esophagus. In H. D. Humes (Ed.), *Kelley's Textbook of internal medicine* (4th ed., pp. 813–824). Philadelphia: Lippincott Williams & Wilkins.

Vanderhoff, B. T., & Tahboub, R. M. (2002). Proton pump inhibitors: An update. *American Family Physician, 66*(2), 273–280.

Laxatives and Cathartics

CHAPTER

OBJECTIVES

After studying this chapter, you will be able to:

1. Differentiate the major types of laxatives according to effects on the gastrointestinal tract.
2. Differentiate the consequences of occasional use from those of chronic use.
3. Discuss rational choices of laxatives for selected client populations or purposes.
4. Discuss bulk-forming laxatives as the most physiologic agents.
5. Discuss possible reasons for and hazards of overuse and abuse of laxatives.

APPLYING YOUR KNOWLEDGE

Clay Lester is an 84-year-old man. His past health history includes heart disease (coronary artery disease). He is complaining about being constipated. You are his home care nurse.

INTRODUCTION

Laxatives and cathartics are drugs used to promote bowel elimination (defecation). The term *laxative* implies mild effects and elimination of soft, formed stool. The term *cathartic* implies strong effects and elimination of liquid or semiliquid stool. Because the different effects depend more on the dose than on the particular drug used, the terms often are used interchangeably.

Defecation

Defecation is normally stimulated by movements and reflexes in the gastrointestinal (GI) tract. When the stomach and duodenum are distended with food or fluids, gastrocolic and duodenocolic reflexes cause propulsive movements in the colon, which move feces into the rectum and arouse the urge to defecate. When sensory nerve fibers in the rectum are stimulated by the fecal mass, the defecation reflex causes strong peristalsis, deep breathing, closure of the glottis, contraction of abdominal muscles, contraction of the rectum, relaxation of anal sphincters, and expulsion of the fecal mass.

The cerebral cortex normally controls the defecation reflex so that defecation can occur at acceptable times and places. Voluntary control inhibits the external anal sphincter to allow defecation, or contracts the sphincter to prevent defecation. When the external sphincter remains contracted, the defecation reflex dissipates, and the urge to defecate usually does not recur until additional feces enter the rectum or several hours later.

In people who often inhibit the defecation reflex or fail to respond to the urge to defecate, constipation develops as the reflex weakens. *Constipation* is the infrequent and painful expulsion of hard, dry stools. Although there is no "normal" number of stools because of variations in diet and other factors, most people report more than three bowel movements per week. Normal bowel elimination should produce a soft, formed stool without pain.

GENERAL CHARACTERISTICS OF LAXATIVES AND CATHARTICS

Indications for Use

There are several rational indications for use:

- To relieve constipation in pregnant women; elderly clients whose abdominal and perineal muscles have become weak and atrophied; children with megacolon; and clients receiving drugs that decrease intestinal motility (eg, opioid analgesics, drugs with anticholinergic effects)
- To prevent straining at stool in clients with coronary artery disease (eg, post–myocardial infarction), hypertension, cerebrovascular disease, and hemorrhoids and other rectal conditions
- To empty the bowel in preparation for bowel surgery or diagnostic procedures (eg, colonoscopy, barium enema)
- To accelerate elimination of potentially toxic substances from the GI tract (eg, orally ingested drugs or toxic compounds)
- To prevent absorption of intestinal ammonia in clients with hepatic encephalopathy
- To obtain a stool specimen for parasitologic examination
- To accelerate excretion of parasites after anthelmintic drugs have been administered
- To reduce serum cholesterol levels (psyllium products)

Contraindications to Use

Laxatives and cathartics should not be used in the presence of undiagnosed abdominal pain. The danger is that the drugs may cause an inflamed organ (eg, the appendix) to rupture and spill GI contents into the abdominal cavity with subsequent peritonitis, a life-threatening condition. Oral drugs also are contraindicated with intestinal obstruction and fecal impaction.

CLASSIFICATIONS AND INDIVIDUAL DRUGS

Laxatives and cathartics are somewhat arbitrarily classified as bulk-forming laxatives; surfactant laxatives or stool softeners; saline cathartics; stimulant cathartics; lubricant or emollient laxatives; and miscellaneous. Individual drugs are listed in Table 60-1.

Bulk-Forming Laxatives

Bulk-forming laxatives (eg, polycarbophil, psyllium seed) are substances that are largely unabsorbed from the intestine. When water is added, these substances swell and become gel-like. The added bulk or size of the fecal mass stimulates peristalsis and defecation. The substances also may act by pulling water into the intestinal lumen. Bulk-forming laxatives are

the most physiologic laxatives because their effect is similar to that of increased intake of dietary fiber. They usually act within 12 to 24 hours, but may take as long as 2 to 3 days to exert their full effects.

Surfactant Laxatives (Stool Softeners)

Surfactant laxatives (eg, docusate calcium, potassium, or sodium) decrease the surface tension of the fecal mass to allow water to penetrate into the stool. They also act as a detergent to facilitate admixing of fat and water in the stool. As a result, stools are softer and easier to expel. These agents have little if any laxative effect. Their main value is to prevent straining while expelling stool. They usually act within 1 to 3 days and should be taken daily.

Saline Laxatives

Saline laxatives (eg, magnesium citrate, milk of magnesia) are not well absorbed from the intestine. Consequently, they increase osmotic pressure in the intestinal lumen and cause water to be retained. Distention of the bowel leads to increased peristalsis and decreased intestinal transit time for the fecal mass. The resultant stool is semifluid. These laxatives are used when rapid bowel evacuation is needed. With oral magnesium preparations, effects occur within 0.5 to 6 hours; with sodium phosphate–containing rectal enemas, effects occur within 15 minutes.

Saline laxatives are generally useful and safe for short-term treatment of constipation; cleansing the bowel prior to endoscopic examinations; and treating fecal impaction. However, they are not safe for frequent or prolonged usage or for certain clients because they may produce fluid and electrolyte imbalances. For example, clients with impaired renal function are at risk of developing hypermagnesemia with magnesium-containing laxatives because some of the magnesium is absorbed systemically. Clients with congestive heart failure are at risk of fluid retention and edema with sodium-containing laxatives.

Polyethylene glycol–electrolyte solution (eg, NuLytely) is a nonabsorbable oral solution that induces diarrhea within 30 to 60 minutes and rapidly evacuates the bowel, usually within 4 hours. It is a prescription drug used for bowel cleansing before GI examination (eg, colonoscopy) and is contraindicated in clients with GI obstruction, gastric retention, colitis, or bowel perforation. Combination products such as HalfLytely combine polyethylene glycol with a stimulant cathartic, bisacodyl, to evacuate the colon in preparation for a colonoscopy. Polyethylene glycol solution (MiraLax) is an oral laxative that may be used to treat occasional constipation. Effects may require 2 to 4 days. It is a prescription drug and should not be taken longer than 2 weeks.

Stimulant Cathartics

The stimulant cathartics are the strongest and most abused laxative products. These drugs act by irritating the GI mucosa

Table 60-1 Drugs at a Glance: Laxatives and Cathartics

	ROUTES AND DOSAGE RANGES	
GENERIC/TRADE NAME	**Adults**	**Children**
Bulk-Forming Laxatives		
Methylcellulose (Citrucel)	PO 1 heaping tbsp 1–3 times daily with water (8 oz or more)	PO 1 level tbsp 1–3 times daily in 4 oz of water
Polycarbophil (FiberCon, Mitrolan)	PO 1 g 4 times daily or PRN with 8 oz of fluid; maximum dose, 6 g/24 h	*6–12 y:* PO 500 mg 1–3 times daily or PRN; maximum dose, 3 g/24 h *2–6 y:* PO 500 mg 1 or 2 times daily or PRN; maximum dose, 1.5 g/24 h
Psyllium preparations (Metamucil, Effersyllium, Serutan, Perdiem Plain)	PO 4–10 g (1–2 tsp) 1–3 times daily, stirred in at least 8 oz of water or other liquid	
Surfactant Laxatives (Stool Softeners)		
Docusate sodium (Colace)	PO 50–200 mg daily	*>12 y:* same dosage as adults *3–12 y:* 20–120 mg daily *<3 y:* 10–40 mg daily
Docusate calcium (Surfak)	PO 50–240 mg daily	*>12 y:* same dosage as adults *2–12 y:* 50–150 mg daily *<2 y:* 25 mg daily
Saline Cathartics		
Magnesium citrate solution	PO 200 mL at bedtime	
Magnesium hydroxide (milk of magnesia, magnesia magma)	Regular liquid, PO 15–60 mL at bedtime. Concentrated liquid, PO 10–20 mL at bedtime	Regular liquid, PO 2.5–5 mL
Polyethylene glycol–electrolyte solution (PEG 3350, sodium sulfate, sodium bicarbonate, sodium chloride, potassium chloride) (CoLyte, GoLytely)	For bowel cleansing before gastrointestinal examination: PO 240 mL (8 oz) every 10 min until 4 L is consumed	No recommended children's dose
Sodium phosphate and sodium biphosphate (Fleet Phosphosoda, Fleet Enema)	PO 20–40 mL in 8 oz of water Rectal enema, 60–120 mL	*≥10 y:* PO 10–20 mL in 8 oz of water *5–10 y:* PO 5–10 mL in 8 oz of water Rectal enema, 60 mL
Stimulant Cathartics		
Bisacodyl (Dulcolax)	PO 10–15 mg Rectal suppository, 10 mg	*≥6 y:* PO 5–10 mg *<2 y:* rectal suppository 5 mg
Cascara sagrada	PO, tablets, 325 mg; fluid extract, 0.5–1.5 mL; aromatic fluid extract, 5 mL	*≥12 y:* same as adults
Castor oil (Neoloid)	PO 15–60 mL	*5–15 y:* PO 5–30 mL depending on strength of emulsion *<2 y:* PO 1.25–7.5 mL depending on strength of emulsion
Glycerin	Rectal suppository, 3 g	*<6 y:* rectal suppository 1–1.5 g

(continued)

Table 60-1 Drugs at a Glance: Laxatives and Cathartics (continued)

GENERIC/TRADE NAME	ROUTES AND DOSAGE RANGES	
	Adults	Children
Senna preparations (Senokot, Black Draught)	Granules, PO 1 level tsp once or twice daily; geriatric, obstetric, gynecologic clients, PO ½ level tsp once or twice daily Syrup, PO 2–3 tsp once or twice daily; geriatric, obstetric, gynecologic clients, 1–1½ tsp once or twice daily Tablets, PO 2 tablets once or twice daily; geriatric, obstetric, gynecologic clients, 1 tablet once or twice daily Suppositories, 1 suppository at bedtime	*Weight >27 kg:* granules, syrup, tablets, suppositories—½ adult dose
COMBINATION PRODUCT **Halflytely & Bisacodyl tablets Bowel Prep kit**	For bowel cleansing before colonoscopy: PO 4 bisacodyl tablets (5 mg each) with water. After bowel movement occurs, drink (8 oz) of Halflytely solution every 10 minutes (8 doses) until all 2 L of solution is consumed.	Pediatric dosage not established.
Lubricant Laxative **Mineral oil** (Agoral Plain, Milkinol, Fleet Mineral Oil Enema)	PO 15–30 mL at bedtime Rectal enema, 30–60 mL	*>6 y:* PO 5–15 mL at bedtime Rectal enema, 30–60 mL
Miscellaneous Laxatives **Lactulose** (Chronulac, Cephulac)	PO 15–30 mL daily; maximum dose, 60 mL daily Portal systemic encephalopathy, PO 30–45 mL 3 or 4 times daily, adjusted to produce two or three soft stools daily Rectally as retention enema, 300 mL with 700 mL water or normal saline, retained 30–60 min, q4–6h	*Infants:* PO 2.5–10 mL daily in divided doses *Older children:* PO 40–90 mL daily in divided doses
Sorbitol	PO 30–50 g daily	

PO, oral; PRN, as needed.

and pulling water into the bowel lumen. As a result, feces are moved through the bowel too rapidly to allow colonic absorption of fecal water, so a watery stool is eliminated. These drugs should not be used frequently or for longer than 1 week because they may produce serum electrolyte and acid–base imbalances (eg, hypocalcemia; hypokalemia; metabolic acidosis or alkalosis).

Oral stimulant cathartics include bisacodyl, cascara sagrada, castor oil, and senna products. These products produce laxative effects in 6 to 12 hours. As a result, a single bedtime dose usually produces a morning bowel movement. Rectal suppository products include bisacodyl, which produces effects within 15 minutes to 2 hours, and glycerin. In addition to irritant, stimulant effects, glycerin exerts hyperosmotic effects in the colon. It usually acts within 30 minutes. Glycerin is not given orally for laxative effects.

Lubricant Laxative

Mineral oil is the only lubricant laxative used clinically. It lubricates the fecal mass and slows colonic absorption of water from the fecal mass, but the exact mechanism of action is unknown. Effects usually occur in 6 to 8 hours. Oral mineral oil may cause several adverse effects and is not recommended for long-term use. Mineral oil enemas are sometimes used to soften fecal impactions and aid their removal.

Miscellaneous Laxatives

Lactulose is a disaccharide that is not absorbed from the GI tract. It exerts laxative effects by pulling water into the intestinal lumen. It is used to treat constipation and hepatic encephalopathy. The latter condition usually results from alcoholic liver disease in which ammonia accumulates and causes stupor or coma. Ammonia is produced by metabolism of dietary protein and intestinal bacteria. Lactulose decreases production of ammonia in the intestine. The goal of treatment is usually to maintain two to three soft stools daily; effects usually occur within 24 to 48 hours. The drug should be used cautiously because it may produce electrolyte imbalances and dehydration.

Sorbitol is a monosaccharide that pulls water into the intestinal lumen and has laxative effects. It is often given with sodium polystyrene sulfonate (Kayexalate), a potassium-removing resin used to treat hyperkalemia, to prevent constipation and aid expulsion of the potassium–resin complex.

Herbal and Dietary Supplements

Many of the commonly used laxatives are plant-based (eg, cascara, psyllium, senna, castor oil). These have long been used and are safe and effective when used as directed.

Aloe is used most often as a topical remedy for burns and possibly other minor wounds. When used for this purpose, a gel-like liquid can be squeezed directly from a plant leaf onto the burned area. Oral aloe is sometimes used as a laxative. However, it is not recommended for this use because it is a strong stimulant laxative. With oral ingestion, aloe can cause severe cramping and other potentially serious adverse effects including hypokalemia and cardiac dysrhythmias.

APPLYING YOUR KNOWLEDGE 60-1
Based on Mr. Lester's past health history, what will be the most likely drug of choice?

NURSING PROCESS

Assessment

Assess clients for current or potential constipation.
- Identify risk factors.
  - Diet with minimal fiber (eg, small amounts of fruits, vegetables, and whole-grain products)
  - Low fluid intake (eg, <2000 mL daily)
  - Immobility or limited activity
  - Drugs that reduce intestinal function and motility (eg, opioid analgesics, antacids containing aluminum or calcium, anticholinergics, calcium channel blockers, clozapine, diuretics, iron, phenothiazines, cholestyramine, colestipol, sucralfate, tricyclic antidepressants, vincristine). Overuse of antidiarrheal agents also may cause constipation.
  - Conditions that may reduce intestinal function and motility (eg, depression, eating disorders such as anorexia nervosa, hypothyroidism, hypercalcemia, multiple sclerosis, Parkinson's disease, spinal lesions)
  - Hemorrhoids, anal fissures, or other conditions characterized by painful bowel elimination
  - Elderly or debilitated clients

- Signs and symptoms include the following:
  - Decreased number and frequency of stools
  - Passage of dry, hard stools
  - Abdominal distention and discomfort
  - Flatulence

Nursing Diagnoses

- Constipation related to decreased activity; inadequate dietary fiber; inadequate fluid intake; drugs; or disease processes
- Pain (abdominal cramping and distention) related to constipation or use of laxatives
- Noncompliance with recommendations for nondrug measures to prevent or treat constipation
- Risk for Deficient Fluid Volume related to diarrhea from frequent or large doses of laxatives
- Deficient Knowledge: Nondrug measures to prevent constipation and appropriate use of laxatives

Planning/Goals

The client will
- Take laxative drugs appropriately
- Use nondrug measures to promote normal bowel function and prevent constipation
- Regain normal patterns of bowel elimination
- Avoid excessive losses of fluids and electrolytes from laxative use
- Be protected from excessive fluid loss, hypotension, and other adverse drug effects, when possible
- Be assisted to avoid constipation when at risk (eg, has illness or injury that prevents activity and food and fluid intake; takes medications that decrease GI function)

Interventions

- Assist clients with constipation and caregivers to
  - Understand the importance of diet, exercise, and fluid intake in promoting normal bowel function and preventing constipation
  - Increase activity and exercise
  - Increase intake of dietary fiber (eg, vegetables, fruits, cereal grains)
  - Drink at least 2000 mL of fluid daily
  - Establish and maintain a routine for bowel elimination (eg, going to the bathroom immediately after breakfast)
  - Understand and comply with drug therapy (see accompanying Client Teaching Guidelines)
- Monitor client responses.
  - Record number, amount, and type of bowel movements.
  - Record vital signs. Hypotension and weak pulse may indicate deficient fluid volume.

Evaluation

- Observe and interview for improved patterns of bowel elimination.
- Observe for use of nondrug measures to promote bowel function.
- Observe for appropriate use of laxatives.
- Observe and interview regarding adverse effects of laxatives.

APPLYING YOUR KNOWLEDGE 60-2

Given Mr. Lester's complaint of constipation, what would you assess with regard to his bowel pattern and risk for constipation?

PRINCIPLES OF THERAPY

Laxative Abuse

Laxatives and cathartics are widely available on a nonprescription basis and are among the most frequently abused drugs. One reason for overuse is the common misconception that a daily bowel movement is necessary for health and well-being, even with little intake of food or fluids. This notion may lead to a vicious cycle of events in which a person fails to have a bowel movement, takes a strong laxative, again fails to have a bowel movement, and takes another laxative before the fecal column has had time to become re-established (2–3 days with normal food intake). Thus, a pattern of laxative dependence and abuse is established.

Laxatives are also abused for weight control, probably most often by people with eating disorders and those who must meet strict weight requirements (eg, some athletes). This is a very dangerous practice because it may lead to life-threatening fluid and electrolyte imbalances.

Drug Selection

In 2005, a review of published studies of efficacy and safety of medications for chronic constipation was completed to provide evidence-based recommendations for treatment. This review concluded that there was good evidence for the use of polyethylene glycol, lactulose, and psyllium to treat chronic

---

CLIENT TEACHING GUIDELINES

Laxatives

General Considerations

- Diet, exercise, and fluid intake are important in maintaining normal bowel function and preventing or treating constipation.
- Eat foods high in dietary fiber daily. Fiber is the portion of plant food that is not digested. It is contained in fruits, vegetables, and whole-grain cereals and breads. Bran, the outer coating of cereal grains such as wheat or oats, is an excellent source of dietary fiber and is available in numerous cereal products.
- Drink at least 6 to 10 glasses (8 oz each) of fluid daily if not contraindicated.
- Exercise regularly. Walking and other activities aid movement of feces through the bowel.
- Establish a regular time and place for bowel elimination. The defecation urge is usually strongest after eating and the defecation reflex is weakened or lost if repeatedly ignored.
- Laxative use should be temporary and not regular, as a general rule. Regular use may prevent normal bowel function, cause adverse drug reactions, and delay treatment for conditions that cause constipation.
- *Never* take laxatives when acute abdominal pain, nausea, or vomiting is present. Doing so may cause a ruptured appendix or other serious complication.
- After taking a strong laxative, it takes 2 to 3 days of normal eating to produce enough feces in the bowel for a bowel movement. Frequent use of a strong laxative promotes loss of normal bowel function, loss of fluids and electrolytes that your body needs, and laxative dependence.
- If you have chronic constipation and are unable or unwilling to eat enough fiber-containing foods in your diet, the next-best action is

regular use of a bulk-forming laxative (eg, Metamucil) as a dietary supplement. These laxatives act the same way as increasing fiber in the diet and are usually best for long-term use. When taken daily, they can prevent constipation. However, they may take 2 to 3 days to work and are not effective in relieving acute constipation.
- Your urine may be discolored if you take a laxative containing senna (eg, Senokot) or cascara sagrada. The color change is not harmful.
- Some people use strong laxatives for weight control. This is an inappropriate use and a dangerous practice because it can lead to life-threatening fluid and electrolyte imbalances, including dehydration and cardiovascular problems.

Self- or Caregiver Administration

- Take all laxatives as directed and do not exceed recommended doses to avoid adverse effects.
- With bulk-forming laxatives, mix in 8 oz of fluid immediately before taking and follow with additional fluid, if able. *Never* take the drug dry. Adequate fluid intake is essential with these drugs.
- With bisacodyl tablets, swallow whole (do not crush or chew), and do not take within 1 hour of an antacid or milk. This helps prevent stomach irritation, abdominal cramping, and possible vomiting.
- Take magnesium citrate or milk of magnesia on an empty stomach with 8 oz of fluid to increase effectiveness.
- Refrigerate magnesium citrate before taking to improve taste and retain effectiveness.
- Mix lactulose with fruit juice, water, or milk, if desired, to improve taste.

constipation. There was minimal evidence in the published literature for many commonly used agents, including magnesium hydroxide, senna, bisacodyl, and stool softeners.

Clinically the choice of a laxative or cathartic often depends on the reason for use and the client's condition.

- For long-term use of laxatives or cathartics in clients who are older, unable or unwilling to eat an adequate diet, or debilitated, bulk-forming laxatives (eg, Metamucil) usually are preferred. However, because obstruction may occur, these agents should not be given to clients with difficulty in swallowing or adhesions or strictures in the GI tract, or to those who are unable or unwilling to drink adequate fluids.

- For clients in whom straining is potentially harmful or painful, stool softeners (eg, docusate sodium) are the agents of choice.

- For occasional use to cleanse the bowel for endoscopic or radiologic examinations, saline or stimulant cathartics are acceptable (eg, magnesium citrate, polyethylene glycol–electrolyte solution, bisacodyl). These drugs should not be used more than once per week. Frequent use is likely to produce laxative abuse.

- Oral use of mineral oil may cause potentially serious adverse effects (decreased absorption of fat-soluble vitamins and some drugs; lipid pneumonia if aspirated into the lungs). Thus, mineral oil is not an oral laxative of choice in any condition, although occasional use in the alert client is unlikely to be harmful. It should not be used regularly. Mineral oil is probably most useful as a retention enema to soften hard, dry feces and aid in their expulsion.

- In fecal impaction, a rectal suppository (eg, bisacodyl) or an enema (eg, oil retention or Fleet enema) is preferred. Oral laxatives are contraindicated when fecal impaction is present but may be given after the rectal mass is removed. After the impaction is relieved, measures should be taken to prevent recurrence. If dietary and other nonpharmacologic measures are ineffective or contraindicated, use of a bulk-forming agent daily or another laxative once or twice weekly may be necessary.

- Saline cathartics containing magnesium, phosphate, or potassium salts are contraindicated in clients with renal failure because hypermagnesemia, hyperphosphatemia, or hyperkalemia may occur.

- Saline cathartics containing sodium salts are contraindicated in clients with edema or congestive heart failure because enough sodium may be absorbed to cause further fluid retention and edema. They also should not be used in clients with impaired renal function or those following a sodium-restricted diet for hypertension.

- Polyethylene glycol–electrolyte solution is formulated for rapid and effective bowel cleansing without significant changes in water or electrolyte balance.

Use in Special Populations

Use in Children

Constipation is responsible for 3% of visits to pediatric clinics and up to 30% of visits to pediatric gasteroenterologists. As in adults, increasing fluids, high-fiber foods, and exercise is preferred when possible. For acute constipation, glycerin suppositories are often effective in infants and small children. Stool softeners may be given to older children. Children usually should not use strong, stimulant laxatives. Magnesium hydroxide is frequently prescribed for children with persistent constipation; however, saline laxatives are not recommended for children younger than 2 years old. Parents should be advised not to give children any laxative more than once a week without consulting a health care provider. Polyethylene glycol–electrolyte solution is effective in treating acute iron overdose in children, although it is not approved by the Food and Drug Administration for this indication.

Use in Older Adults

As many as 15% to 20% of community-dwelling older adults and up to 50% of nursing home residents experience constipation. Laxatives are often used or overused. Nondrug measures to prevent constipation (eg, increasing fluids and high-fiber foods; exercise) are much preferred to laxatives. If a laxative is required on a regular basis, a bulk-forming psyllium compound (eg, Metamucil) is best because it is most physiologic in its action. If taken, it should be accompanied by a full glass of fluid. There have been reports of obstruction in the GI tract when a psyllium compound was taken with insufficient fluid. Strong stimulant laxatives should be avoided.

APPLYING YOUR KNOWLEDGE 60-3:
HOW CAN YOU AVOID THIS MEDICATION ERROR?
Mr. Lester is concerned about not having a bowel movement. He takes a psyllium preparation at 8 A.M. He does not have a result by noon, so he takes milk of magnesia. He has not had a stool by supper, so he takes a glycerin suppository.

Use in Clients With Cancer

Many clients with cancer require moderate to large amounts of opioid analgesics for pain control. The analgesics slow GI motility and cause constipation. These clients need a bowel-management program that includes routine laxative administration. Stimulant laxatives (eg, a senna preparation, bisacodyl) increase intestinal motility, which is the action that opiates suppress. These drugs may cause abdominal cramping, which may be lessened by giving small doses three or four times daily.

Use in Clients With Spinal Cord Injury

Spinal cord injury (SCI) impairs the ability of an individual to sense that a bowel movement is imminent, and the ability to control the timing and place of bowel evacuation. Common problems that the individual with SCI must cope with include incontinence and fecal impaction, which if left untreated may result in perforation of the bowel.

SCIs above the twelfth thoracic vertebrae (T12) are referred to as *upper motor neuron injuries.* Individuals with this type of SCI are unable to sense when the bowel is full. The anal sphincter remains closed until the bowel becomes distended with stool, resulting in uncontrolled reflex emptying. Individuals with upper motor neuron injuries usually follow a bowel program that includes taking a daily stool softener such as docusate sodium, and stimulating bowel movements at the desired time using digital stimulation and rectal suppositories such as bisacodyl or glycerin.

SCIs below T12 are referred to as *lower motor neuron injuries.* With this type of SCI, the muscles of the colon and anus remain relaxed or flaccid, resulting in constipation and incontinence. The bowel-control program for individuals with lower motor neuron injuries involves digital stimulation and manual removal of the stool. Initially digital disempaction should be done every other day. It may be necessary to increase the frequency of digital disempaction to every day to avoid unplanned bowel movements, or constipation and impaction.

With both types of SCIs the goal of the bowel program is to have regular bowel movements at a predictable time and place and to minimize "accidents." It is recommended to implement the bowel program at the same time each day, preferably after a meal. Factors that will influence bowel activity must be considered in the bowel program. These factors include eating at regular intervals; including high-fiber foods in the diet; adequate intake of fluids in the diet; avoidance of medications and foods that may cause diarrhea or constipation; and an awareness of cues that a bowel movement may be imminent, such as sweating, restlessness, sensations of fullness in the lower abdomen, and piloerection or "goosebumps."

Use in Clients With Renal Impairment

Saline cathartics containing phosphate, sodium, magnesium, or potassium salts are usually contraindicated or must be used cautiously in the presence of impaired renal function. Ten percent or more of the magnesium in magnesium salts may be absorbed and cause hypermagnesemia; sodium phosphate and sodium biphosphate may cause hyperphosphatemia, hypernatremia, acidosis, and hypocalcemia; potassium salts may cause hyperkalemia.

Use in Clients With Hepatic Impairment

Because most laxatives are not absorbed or metabolized extensively, they can usually be used without difficulty in clients with hepatic impairment. In fact, they are used therapeutically in clients with hepatic encephalopathy to decrease absorption of ammonia from dietary protein in the GI tract. Lactulose is usually given in dosages to produce two to three soft stools daily.

Use in Home Care

Laxatives are commonly self-prescribed and self-administered in the home setting. The home care nurse may become involved when visiting a client for other purposes. The role of the home care nurse may include assessing usual patterns of bowel elimination; identifying clients at risk of developing constipation; promoting lifestyle interventions to prevent constipation; obtaining laxatives when indicated; and counseling about rational use of laxatives.

N U R S I N G   A C T I O N S

Laxatives and Cathartics

NURSING ACTIONS	RATIONALE/EXPLANATION
1. Administer accurately	
a. Give bulk-forming laxatives with at least 8 oz of water or other fluid. Mix with fluid immediately before administration.	To prevent thickening and expansion in the gastrointestinal (GI) tract with possible obstruction. These substances absorb water rapidly and solidify into a gelatinous mass.
b. With bisacodyl tablets, instruct the client to swallow the tablets without chewing and not to take them within an hour after ingesting milk or gastric antacids or while receiving cimetidine therapy.	The tablets have an enteric coating to delay dissolution until they reach the alkaline environment of the small intestine. Chewing or giving the tablets close to antacid substances or to cimetidine-treated clients causes premature dissolution and gastric irritation and results in abdominal cramping and vomiting.
c. Give saline cathartics on an empty stomach with 240 mL of fluid.	To increase effectiveness

NURSING ACTIONS	RATIONALE/EXPLANATION
d. Refrigerate magnesium citrate and polyethylene glycol–electrolyte solution before giving.	To increase palatability and retain potency
e. Castor oil may be chilled and followed by fruit juice or other beverage.	To increase palatability
f. Insert rectal suppositories to the length of the index finger, next to rectal mucosa.	These drugs are not effective unless they are in contact with intestinal mucosa.
2. Observe for therapeutic effects	
a. Soft to semiliquid stool	Therapeutic effects occur in approximately 1–3 days with bulk-forming laxatives and stool softeners; 6–8 hours with bisacodyl tablets, cascara sagrada, and senna products; 15–60 minutes with bisacodyl and glycerin suppositories.
b. Liquid to semiliquid stool	Effects occur in approximately 1–3 hours with saline cathartics and castor oil.
c. Decreased abdominal pain when used in clients with irritable bowel syndrome or diverticulosis	
d. Decreased rectal pain when used in clients with hemorrhoids or anal fissures	Pain results from straining to expel hard, dry feces.
3. Observe for adverse effects	
a. Diarrhea—several liquid stools, abdominal cramping. Severe, prolonged diarrhea may cause hyponatremia, hypokalemia, dehydration, and other problems.	Diarrhea is most likely to result from strong, stimulant cathartics (eg, castor oil, bisacodyl, senna preparations) or large doses of saline cathartics (eg, milk of magnesia).
b. With bulk-forming agents, impaction or obstruction	Impaction or obstruction of the GI tract can be prevented by giving ample fluids with these agents and not giving the drugs to clients with known dysphagia or strictures anywhere in the alimentary canal.
c. With saline cathartics, hypermagnesemia, hyperkalemia, fluid retention, and edema	Hypermagnesemia and hyperkalemia are more likely to occur in clients with renal insufficiency because of impaired ability to excrete magnesium and potassium. Fluid retention and edema are more likely to occur in clients with congestive heart failure or other conditions characterized by edema. Polyethylene glycol–electrolyte solution produces the least change in water and electrolyte balance.
d. With mineral oil, lipid pneumonia and decreased absorption of vitamins A, D, E, and K	Lipid pneumonia can be prevented by not giving mineral oil to clients with dysphagia or impaired consciousness. Decreased absorption of fat-soluble vitamins can be prevented by not giving mineral oil with or shortly after meals or for longer than 2 weeks.
4. Observe for drug interactions	
a. Drugs that *increase* effects of laxatives and cathartics:	
(1) GI stimulants (eg, metoclopramide)	Additive stimulation of intestinal motility
b. Drugs that *decrease* effects of laxatives and cathartics:	
(1) Anticholinergic drugs (eg, atropine) and other drugs with anticholinergic properties (eg, phenothiazine antipsychotic drugs, tricyclic antidepressants, some antihistamines, and antiparkinson drugs)	These drugs slow intestinal motility. Clients receiving these agents are at risk for development of constipation and requiring laxatives, perhaps on a long-term basis.
(2) Central nervous system depressants (eg, opioid analgesics)	Opioid analgesics commonly cause constipation.

APPLYING YOUR KNOWLEDGE: ANSWERS

60-1 Mr. Lester has heart disease and should not strain when having a bowel movement. Docusate sodium is most likely the drug of choice. This drug has little laxative effect. Docusate sodium will work by decreasing the surface tension of the fecal mass, thereby allowing water to enter the stool. It will also act as a detergent to facilitate the addition of fat and water to the stool, thereby making it easier to expel.

60-2 Assess for the number of stools, the appearance of the fecal mass, any abdominal distention or discomfort, or flatulence. Evaluate the drugs Mr. Lester is taking because they may reduce intestinal function. Also, assess risk factors such as decreased activity and a diet with minimal fiber intake and low fluid intake.

60-3 Mr. Lester has taken much more medication than needed. The psyllium preparation will usually act in 12 to 24 hours but may take as long as 2 to 3 days to exert the full effect. Milk of magnesia is a saline cathartic that will usually have an effect in 0.5 to 6 hours. Mr. Lester did not allow either of these medications enough time to work. He also administered a stimulant cathartic that should not be used in older clients. Teach Mr. Lester about drug actions, including how long before each drug takes effect. Also, provide guidance on appropriate drug selection.

Review and Application Exercises

Short Answer Exercises

1. What are risk factors for development of constipation?

2. Describe nonpharmacologic strategies to prevent constipation.

3. Which type of laxative is, in general, the most desirable for long-term use? Which is the least desirable?

4. What are the most significant adverse effects of strong laxatives?

5. If an adult client asked you to recommend an over-the-counter laxative, what information about the client's condition would you need, and what would you recommend? Why?

NCLEX-Style Questions

6. Important points to include when teaching measures to promote healthy bowel function include all of the following except
   a. Increase activity.
   b. Eat a low-residue diet.
   c. Increase fluid intake.
   d. Establish regular bowel habits.

7. Which of the following is safe to use in a 60-year-old constipated client with dysphagia?
   a. methylcellulose (Citrucel)
   b. psyllium (Metamucil)
   c. mineral oil (Agoral Plain)
   d. docusate sodium (Colace)

8. For which of the following clients is a laxative contraindicated?
   a. a client with cancer taking daily narcotics for pain control
   b. a client complaining of abdominal pain and distention
   c. a client scheduled for a colonoscopy
   d. a client with limited mobility due to Parkinson's disease

Selected References

Barnett, J. L. (2000). Approach to the patient with constipation, fecal incontinence, and gas. In H. D. Humes (Ed.), *Kelley's Textbook of internal medicine* (4th ed., pp. 755–763). Philadelphia: Lippincott Williams & Wilkins.

Borowitz, S. M., Cox, D. J., Kovatchev, B., Ritterband, L. M., Sheen, J., & Sutphen, J. (2005). Treatment of childhood constipation by primary care physicians: Efficacy and predictors of outcome. *Pediatrics, 115*(4), 873–877.

Bosshard, W., Dreher, R., Schnegg, J. F., & Bula, C. J. (2004). The treatment of chronic constipation in elderly people: An update. *Drugs Aging, 21*(14), 911–930.

Drug facts and comparisons. (Updated monthly). St. Louis: Facts and Comparisons.

Hogue, V. W. (2000). Constipation and diarrhea. In E. T. Herfindal & D. R. Gourley (Eds.), *Textbook of therapeutics: Drug and disease management* (7th ed., pp. 571–588). Philadelphia: Lippincott Williams & Wilkins.

Loening-Bauche, V. (2005). Prevalence, symptoms and outcome of constipation in infants and toddlers. *Journal of Pediatrics, 146*(3), 359–363.

Porth, C. M. (2005). Disorders of gastrointestinal function. In C. M. Porth, *Pathophysiology: Concepts of altered health states* (7th ed., pp. 885–916). Philadelphia: Lippincott Williams & Wilkins.

Ramkumar, D., & Rao, S. (2005). Efficacy and safety of traditional medical therapies for chronic constipation: Systematic review. *American Journal of Gastroenterology, 100*(4), 936–971.

Spruill, W. J., & Wade, W. E. (2002). Diarrhea, constipation, and irritable bowel syndrome. In J. T. DiPiro, R. L. Talbert, G. C. Yee, G. R. Matzke, B. G. Wells, & L. M. Posey (Eds.), *Pharmacotherapy: A pathophysiologic approach* (5th ed., pp. 655–669). New York: McGraw-Hill.

Antidiarrheals

OBJECTIVES

After studying this chapter, you will be able to:

1. Identify clients at risk for development of diarrhea.
2. Discuss guidelines for assessing diarrhea.
3. Describe types of diarrhea in which antidiarrheal drug therapy may be indicated.
4. Differentiate the major types of antidiarrheal drugs.
5. Discuss characteristics, effects, and nursing process implications of commonly used antidiarrheal agents.

APPLYING YOUR KNOWLEDGE

Max McGrath is a 47-year-old salesman who travels extensively as part of his job. He recently returned from a trip to Mexico. He has been having diarrhea for the past 10 days and seeks advice on how to manage his symptoms.

INTRODUCTION

Antidiarrheal drugs are used to treat diarrhea, defined as the frequent expulsion of liquid or semiliquid stools. Diarrhea is a symptom of numerous conditions that increase bowel motility; cause secretion or retention of fluids in the intestinal lumen; and cause inflammation or irritation of the gastrointestinal (GI) tract. As a result, bowel contents are rapidly propelled toward the rectum, and absorption of fluids and electrolytes is limited. Some causes of diarrhea include the following:

- Excessive use or abuse of laxatives. Laxative abuse may accompany eating disorders such as anorexia nervosa or bulimia.
- Intestinal infections with viruses, bacteria, or protozoa. A common source of infection is ingested food or fluid contaminated by a variety of organisms.
  - *Escherichia coli* O157:H7–related hemorrhagic colitis most commonly occurs with the ingestion of under-cooked ground beef. A serious complication of *E. coli*

O157:H7 colitis is hemolytic uremic syndrome (HUS), characterized by thrombocytopenia, microangiopathic hemolytic anemia, and renal failure. Children are especially susceptible to HUS, which is the leading cause of dialysis in pediatric clients. So-called *travelers' diarrhea* is usually caused by an enterotoxigenic strain of *E. coli* (ETEC). Fecal contamination of food or water is the most common source of ETEC-induced diarrhea.

- Consumption of improperly prepared poultry may result in diarrhea due to infection with *Campylobacter jejuni.* In the United States, this is the most common bacterial organism identified in infectious diarrhea. In addition to diarrhea, vomiting, fever, and abdominal discomfort, *Campylobacter* bacteria produce neurotoxins, which may result in paralysis.
- *Salmonella* infections may occur when contaminated poultry and other meats, eggs, and dairy products are ingested. Elderly clients are especially susceptible to *Salmonella*-associated colitis.

- Several strains of *Shigella* may produce diarrhea. Infection most often results from direct person-to-person contact, but may also occur via food or water contamination. Handwashing is especially important in preventing the spread of *Shigella* from person to person.
- Other diarrhea-producing organisms associated with contamination of specific foods include *Vibrio vulnificus* and *Vibrio parahaemolyticus* contamination of raw shellfish and oysters (particularly in the Gulf Coast States), *Clostridium perfringens* contamination of inadequately heated or reheated meats, *Staphylococcus aureus* contamination of processed meats and custard-filled pastries, *Bacillus cerus* contamination of rice and bean sprouts, and *Listeria monocytogenes* contamination of hot dogs and luncheon meats. Newborns, pregnant women, and older and immunocompromised individuals are especially susceptible to *L. monocytogenes* infection.
- Two of the most common viral organisms responsible for gastroenteritis and diarrhea are rotavirus or Norwalk-like virus (calicivirus). Vomiting is usually a prominent symptom accompanying virus-induced diarrhea.
- Undigested, coarse, or highly spiced food in the GI tract. The food acts as an irritant and attracts fluids in a defensive attempt to dilute the irritating agent. This may result from inadequate chewing of food or lack of digestive enzymes.
- Lack of digestive enzymes. Deficiency of pancreatic enzymes inhibits digestion and absorption of carbohydrates, proteins, and fats. Deficiency of lactase, which breaks down lactose to simple sugars (ie, glucose and galactose) that can be absorbed by GI mucosa, inhibits digestion of milk and milk products. Lactase deficiency commonly occurs among people of African and Asian descent.
- Inflammatory bowel disorders, such as gastroenteritis, diverticulitis, ulcerative colitis, and Crohn's disease. In these disorders, the inflamed mucous membrane secretes large amounts of fluids into the intestinal lumen, along with mucus, proteins, and blood, and absorption of water and electrolytes is impaired. In addition, when the ileum is diseased or a portion is surgically excised, large amounts of bile salts reach the colon, where they act as cathartics and cause diarrhea. Bile salts are normally reabsorbed from the ileum.
- Drug therapy. Many oral drugs irritate the GI tract and may cause diarrhea, including acarbose, antacids that contain magnesium, antibacterials, antineoplastic agents, colchicine, laxatives, metformin, metoclopramide, misoprostol, selective serotonin reuptake inhibitors, tacrine, and tacrolimus. Antibacterial drugs are commonly used offenders that also may cause diarrhea by altering the normal bacterial flora in the intestine.

Antibiotic-associated colitis (also called *pseudomembranous colitis*) is a serious condition that results from oral or parenteral antibiotic therapy. By suppressing normal flora in the colon, antibiotics allow proliferation of other bacteria, especially gram-positive, anaerobic *Clostridium difficile* organisms. These organisms produce a toxin that causes fever, abdominal pain, inflammatory lesions of the colon, and severe diarrhea with stools containing mucus, pus, and sometimes blood. Symptoms may develop within a few days or several weeks after the causative antibiotic is discontinued. Other enteric pathogens that may overgrow in the presence of antibiotic therapy and result in colitis include *Salmonella, Clostridium perfringens type A, S. aureus* and *Candida albicans*. Antibiotic-associated colitis is more often associated with ampicillin, cephalosporins, and clindamycin, but may occur with any antibiotic or combination of antibiotics that alters intestinal microbial flora.

- Intestinal neoplasms. Tumors may increase intestinal motility by occupying space and stretching the intestinal wall. Diarrhea sometimes alternates with constipation in colon cancer.
- Functional disorders. Diarrhea may be a symptom of stress or anxiety in some clients. No organic disease process can be found in such circumstances.
- Hyperthyroidism. This condition increases bowel motility.
- Surgical excision of portions of the intestine, especially the small intestine. Such procedures decrease the absorptive area and increase fluidity of stools.
- Human immunodeficiency virus (HIV) infection/acquired immunodeficiency syndrome (AIDS). Diarrhea occurs in most clients with HIV infection, often as a chronic condition that contributes to malnutrition and weight loss. It may be caused by drug therapy, infection with a variety of microorganisms, or other factors.

Diarrhea may be acute or chronic and mild or severe. Most episodes of acute diarrhea are defensive mechanisms by which the body tries to rid itself of irritants, toxins, and infectious agents. These episodes are usually self-limiting and subside within 24 to 48 hours without serious consequences. If it is severe or prolonged, acute diarrhea may lead to serious fluid and electrolyte depletion, especially in young children and older adults. Chronic diarrhea may cause malnutrition and anemia, and is often characterized by remissions and exacerbations.

CHARACTERISTICS, CLASSIFICATIONS, AND INDIVIDUAL ANTIDIARRHEAL DRUGS

Antidiarrheal drugs include a variety of agents, most of which are discussed in other chapters. When used for treatment of

(text continues on page 1002)

Table 61-1 Drugs at a Glance: Antidiarrheal Drugs

GENERIC/TRADE NAME	CHARACTERISTICS	CLINICAL INDICATIONS	ROUTES AND DOSAGE RANGES	
			Adults	Children
Opiate-Related Drugs **Paregoric**	Morphine is the active ingredient. Paregoric contains 0.4 mg/mL of morphine. A Schedule III drug alone and a Schedule V in the small amounts combined with other drugs. Recommended doses and short-term use do not produce euphoria, analgesia, or dependence.	Symptomatic treatment of acute diarrhea	PO 5–10 mL 1–4 times daily (maximum of 4 doses) until diarrhea is controlled	PO 0.25–0.5 mL/kg 1–4 times daily (maximum of 4 doses) until diarrhea is controlled
Difenoxin with atropine sulfate (Motofen)	An active metabolite of diphenoxylate Overdose may cause respiratory depression and coma. Each tablet contains 1 mg of difenoxin and 0.025 mg of atropine. The atropine is added to discourage overdose and abuse for opioid effects. Contraindicated in children <2 y of age and clients who are allergic to the ingredients or have hepatic impairment. A Schedule IV drug	Symptomatic treatment of acute or chronic diarrhea	PO 2 mg initially, then 1 mg after each loose stool or 1 mg q3–4h as needed; maximum dose, 8 mg (8 tablets)/ 24 h	Safety and effectiveness not established for children <12 y of age
Diphenoxylate with atropine sulfate (Lomotil)	A derivative of meperidine (Demerol) Commonly prescribed; decreases intestinal motility In recommended doses, does not produce euphoria, analgesia, or dependence. In high doses, produces morphine-like effects, including	Symptomatic treatment of acute or chronic diarrhea	PO 5 mg (2 tablets or 10 mL of liquid) 3 or 4 times daily; maximal daily dose, 20 mg	Liquid preparation (2.5 mg diphenoxylate and 0.025 mg atropine per 5 mL), PO 4 times daily, as follows: *9–12 y, 23–55 kg:* 3.5–5 mL *6–8 y, 17–32 kg:* 2.5–5 mL *5 y, 16–23 kg:* 2.5–4.5 mL *4 y, 14–20 kg:* 2–4 mL

(continued)

Table 61-1 Drugs at a Glance: Antidiarrheal Drugs (continued)

GENERIC/TRADE NAME	CHARACTERISTICS	CLINICAL INDICATIONS	ROUTES AND DOSAGE RANGES	
			Adults	Children
	euphoria, dependence, and respiratory depression Naloxone (Narcan) is the antidote for overdose. Each tablet or 5 mL of liquid contains 2.5 mg of diphenoxylate and 0.025 mg of atropine. The atropine is added to discourage drug abuse. Contraindicated in clients with severe liver disease or glaucoma A Schedule V drug			*3 y, 12–16 kg:* 2–3 mL *2 y, 11–14 kg:* 1.5–3 mL Contraindicated in children <2 y of age
Loperamide (Imodium)	A derivative of meperidine; decreases intestinal motility As effective as diphenoxylate, with fewer adverse effects in recommended doses. High doses may produce morphine-like effects. Naloxone (Narcan) is the antidote for overdose.	Symptomatic treatment of acute or chronic diarrhea	PO 4 mg initially, then 2 mg after each loose stool to a maximal daily dose of 16 mg. For chronic diarrhea, dosage should be reduced to the lowest effective amount (average 4–8 mg daily).	*8–12 y, >30 kg:* PO 2 mg 3 times daily *6–8 y, 20–30 kg:* PO 2 mg twice daily *2–5 y, 13–20 kg:* PO 1 mg 3 times daily Safety not established for children <2 y of age.
Antibacterial Agents **Azithromycin**	A macrolide (see Chap. 33)	Traveler's diarrhea acquired in SE Asia. Regardless of destination, may be preferred antibiotic for children and those unable to take quinolones.	PO 500 mg daily for 3 days.	PO 10 mg/kg on day 1, up to 500 mg; and 5 mg/kg on days 2 and 3, up to 250 mg.
Ciprofloxacin (Cipro)	A fluoroquinolone (See Chap. 31)	Diarrhea caused by susceptible strains of *Escherichia coli*, *Campylobacter jejuni*, and *Shigella* species	PO 500 mg q12h for 5–7 d	Not recommended for use
Erythromycin (E-Mycin)	A macrolide (see Chap. 33)	Intestinal amebiasis caused by *Entamoeba histolytica*	PO 250 mg 4 times daily for 10–14 d	PO 30–50 mg/kg/d, in divided doses, for 10–14 d
Metronidazole (Flagyl)	See Chap. 33	Diarrhea and colitis caused by *Clostridium difficile* organisms	*C. difficile* infection, PO 500 mg 3 times daily or 250 mg 4 times daily	Dosage not established for *C. difficile* infection

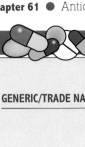

Table 61-1 Drugs at a Glance: Antidiarrheal Drugs (continued)

GENERIC/TRADE NAME	CHARACTERISTICS	CLINICAL INDICATIONS	ROUTES AND DOSAGE RANGES	
			Adults	Children
		Intestinal amebiasis	Intestinal amebiasis, PO 750 mg 3 times daily for 5–10 d	Intestinal amebiasis, PO 35–50 mg/kg/24 h (maximum 750 mg/dose), in 3 divided doses for 10 d
Nitazoxanide (Alinia)	Antiprotozoal agent	Diarrhea caused by *Giardia lamblia* or *Cryptosporidium parvum*	For *G. lamblia:* PO 500 mg tablet every 12 h with food or 25 mL (500 mg) oral suspension every 12 h with food for 3 d. For *C. parvum:* adult dose not established	For *G. lamblia* and *C. parvum:* >12 y, same as adults 4–11 y, 10 mL (200 mg) oral suspension every 12 h with food for 3 d 1–3 y, 5 mL (100 mg) oral suspension every 12 h with food for 3 d
Rifaximin (Xifaxan)	Structural analog of rifampin; a broad-spectrum, non-specific antibiotic that remains in the gut where it exerts its effects	Traveler's diarrhea caused by *E. coli*	PO 200 mg 3 times a day for 3 d	Dosage not established for children <12 y of age
Trimethoprim-sulfamethoxazole (TMP-SMX) (Bactrim, Septra)	See Chap. 32	Diarrhea caused by susceptible strains of *E. coli* or *Shigella* organisms Traveler's diarrhea	PO 160 mg of TMP and 800 mg of SMX q12h for 5 d or longer	PO 8 mg/kg of TMP and 40 mg/kg of SMX daily, in 2 divided doses, q12h, for 5 d or longer
Vancomycin	Cell wall synthesis inhibitor (see Chap. 33)	Diarrhea and colitis caused by *C. difficile* organism	PO 500 mg to 2 g per day in 3–4 divided doses for 7–10 d *or* PO 125 mg 3 or 4 times daily	PO 400 mg/kg/d in 4 divided doses for 7–10 d. Do not exceed 2 g/d.
Miscellaneous Drugs Bismuth subsalicylate (Pepto-Bismol)	Has antimicrobial, antisecretory, and possibly anti-inflammatory effects	Control of diarrhea, including traveler's diarrhea, and relief of abdominal cramping	PO 2 tablets or 30 mL every 30–60 min, if needed, up to 8 doses in 24 h	9–12 y, PO 1 tablet or 15 mL 6–9 y, PO ⅔ tablet or 10 mL 3–6 y, PO ⅓ tablet or 5 mL <3 y, consult pediatrician
Cholestyramine (Questran)	Binds and inactivates bile salts in the intestine	Diarrhea due to bile salts reaching the colon and causing a cathartic effect. "Bile salt diarrhea" is associated with Crohn's disease or surgical excision of the ileum.	PO 16–32 g/d in 120–180 mL of water, in 2–4 divided doses before or during meals and at bedtime	

(continued)

Table 61-1 Drugs at a Glance: Antidiarrheal Drugs (continued)

GENERIC/TRADE NAME	CHARACTERISTICS	CLINICAL INDICATIONS	ROUTES AND DOSAGE RANGES	
			Adults	Children
Colestipol (Colestid)	Same as cholestyramine, above	Same as cholestyramine	PO 15–30 g/d in 120–180 mL of water, in 2–4 divided doses before or during meals and at bedtime	
Octreotide (Sandostatin)	In GI tract, decreases secretions and motility	Diarrhea associated with carcinoid tumors, HIV/AIDS, cancer chemotherapy or radiation, or diarrhea unresponsive to other drugs	Sub-Q, IV 50 mcg 2–3 times daily initially, then adjusted according to response	Dosage not established
Pancreatin or pancrelipase (Viokase, Pancrease, Cotazym)	Pancreatic enzymes used only for replacement	Diarrhea and malabsorption due to deficiency of pancreatic enzymes	PO 1–3 tablets or capsules or 1–2 packets of powder with meals and snacks	PO 1–3 tablets or capsules or 1–2 packets of powder with each meal
Psyllium preparations (Metamucil)	Absorbs water and decreases fluidity of stools	Possibly effective for symptomatic treatment of diarrhea	PO 1–2 tsp, 2 or 3 times daily, in 8 oz of fluid	

AIDS, acquired immunodeficiency syndrome; GI, gastrointestinal; HIV, human immunodeficiency virus; IV, intravenous; PO, oral; Sub-Q, subcutaneous.

diarrhea, the drugs may be given to relieve the symptom (nonspecific therapy) or the underlying cause of the symptom (specific therapy). Individual drugs are listed in Table 61-1.

Nonspecific Therapy

A major element of nonspecific therapy is adequate fluid and electrolyte replacement. When drug therapy is required, nonprescription antidiarrheal drugs (eg, loperamide) may be effective.

Loperamide (Imodium) is a synthetic derivative of meperidine that decreases GI motility by its effect on intestinal muscles. Because loperamide does not penetrate the central nervous system (CNS) well, it does not cause the CNS effects associated with opioid use and lacks potential for abuse. Although adverse effects are generally few and mild, loperamide can cause abdominal pain, constipation, drowsiness, fatigue, nausea, and vomiting. For nonprescription use, dosages for adults should not exceed 8 milligrams per day; with supervision by a health care provider, maximum daily dosage is 16 milligrams per day. In general, loperamide should be discontinued after 48 hours if clinical improvement has not occurred.

Overall, opiates and opiate derivatives (see Chap. 6) are the most effective agents for symptomatic treatment of diarrhea. These drugs decrease diarrhea by slowing propulsive movements in the small and large intestines. Morphine, codeine,

and related drugs are effective in relieving diarrhea but are rarely used for this purpose because of their adverse effects. Opiates have largely been replaced by the synthetic drugs diphenoxylate, loperamide, and difenoxin, which are used only for treatment of diarrhea and do not cause morphine-like adverse effects in recommended doses. Diphenoxylate and difenoxin require a prescription.

Bismuth salts have antibacterial and antiviral activity; **bismuth subsalicylate** (Pepto-Bismol, a commonly used over-the-counter [OTC] drug) also has antisecretory and possibly anti-inflammatory effects because of its salicylate component.

Octreotide acetate is a synthetic form of somatostatin, a hormone produced in the anterior pituitary gland and in the pancreas. The drug may be effective in diarrhea because it decreases GI secretion and motility. It is used for diarrhea associated with carcinoid syndrome, intestinal tumors, HIV/AIDS, and diarrhea that does not respond to other antidiarrheal drugs.

Other nonspecific agents sometimes used in diarrhea are anticholinergics (see Chap. 20) and polycarbophil and psyllium preparations (see Chap. 60). Anticholinergic drugs, of which atropine is the prototype, are infrequently used because doses large enough to decrease intestinal motility and secretions cause intolerable adverse effects. The drugs are occasionally used to decrease abdominal cramping and pain (antispasmodic effects) associated with acute nonspecific diarrhea and chronic diarrhea associated with inflammatory bowel disease.

Polycarbophil (eg, FiberCon) and psyllium preparations (eg, Metamucil) are most often used as bulk-forming laxatives. They are occasionally used in diarrhea to decrease fluidity of stools. The preparations absorb large amounts of water and produce stools of gelatin-like consistency. They may cause abdominal discomfort and bloating.

Specific Therapy

Specific drug therapy for diarrhea depends on the cause of the symptom and may include the use of antibacterial, enzymatic, and bile salt–binding drugs. Antibacterial drugs are recommended for bacterial enteritis when diarrhea lasts longer than 48 hours; when the client passes six or more loose stools in 24 hours; when diarrhea is associated with fever; or when blood or pus is seen in the stools. Although effective in preventing travelers' diarrhea, antibiotics usually are not recommended because their use may promote the emergence of drug-resistant microorganisms. Although effective in reducing diarrhea due to *Salmonella* and *E. coli* intestinal infections, antibiotics may induce a prolonged carrier state during which the infection can be transmitted to other people.

Rifaximin (Xifaxan) is a structural analog of the antimycobacterial drug, rifampin. It is a *nonsystemic* antibiotic that remains in the gut and is not absorbed into the bloodstream. It was specifically developed to treat travelers' diarrhea due to noninvasive strains of *E. coli* in clients older than 12 years of age. It should not be used for diarrhea in the presence of fever or bloody stools or for diarrhea due to pathogens other than *E. coli*. As with the use of other broad-spectrum antibiotics, superinfections may occur with rifaximin therapy, requiring termination of the medication and treatment.

Nitazoxanide (Alinia) is an antiprotozoal agent used specifically for treating diarrhea resulting from infection with *Giardia lamblia* or *Cryptosporidium parvum*. Caution should be used when administering Alinia concurrently with highly plasma-protein–bound medications such as warfarin, because the active metabolite of nitazoxanide is highly plasma-protein bound and such concurrent use may result in competitive drug interactions.

Indications for Use

Despite the limitations of drug therapy in the prevention and treatment of diarrhea, antidiarrheal drugs are indicated in the following circumstances.

- Severe or prolonged diarrhea (>2–3 days), to prevent severe fluid and electrolyte loss
- Relatively severe diarrhea in young children and older adults. These groups are less able to adapt to fluid and electrolyte losses.
- In chronic inflammatory diseases of the bowel (ulcerative colitis and Crohn's disease), to allow a more nearly normal lifestyle
- In ileostomies or surgical excision of portions of the ileum, to decrease fluidity and volume of stool

- HIV/AIDS–associated diarrhea
- When specific causes of diarrhea have been determined

Contraindications to Use

Contraindications to the use of antidiarrheal drugs include diarrhea caused by toxic materials; microorganisms that penetrate intestinal mucosa (eg, pathogenic *E. coli*, *Salmonella*, *Shigella*); or antibiotic-associated colitis. In these circumstances, antidiarrheal agents that slow peristalsis may aggravate and prolong diarrhea. Opiates (morphine, codeine) usually are contraindicated in chronic diarrhea because of possible opiate dependence. Difenoxin, diphenoxylate, and loperamide are contraindicated in children younger than 2 years of age.

Herbal and Dietary Supplements

Several herbal remedies are promoted for treatment of diarrhea. Most include tannins, substances with astringent properties that reduce intestinal inflammation and secretions. The leaves of edible berry plants (ie, blackberry, blueberry, raspberry) are sometimes used in a "tea" made by pouring boiling water over 1 to 2 teaspoons of leaves, drunk up to six times daily. There is little objective evidence of effectiveness or toxicity.

NURSING PROCESS

Assessment

Assess for acute or chronic diarrhea.

- Try to determine the duration of diarrhea; number of stools per day; amount, consistency, color, odor, and presence of abnormal components (eg, undigested food, blood, pus, mucus) in each stool; precipitating factors; accompanying signs and symptoms (ie, nausea, vomiting, fever, abdominal pain or cramping); and measures used to relieve diarrhea. When possible, look at stool specimens for possible clues to causation. Blood may indicate inflammation, infection, or neoplastic disease; pus or mucus may indicate inflammation or infection. Infections caused by *Shigella* organisms produce blood-tinged mucus. Infections caused by *Salmonella* or *E. coli* usually produce green, liquid or semiliquid stools. Inflammatory bowel disorders often produce nonbloody mucus.
- Try to determine the cause of the diarrhea. This includes questioning about such causes as chronic inflammatory diseases of the bowel, food intake, possible exposure to contaminated food, living or traveling in areas of poor sanitation, and use of laxatives or other drugs that may cause diarrhea. When available, check laboratory reports on stool specimens (eg, culture reports).
- With severe or prolonged diarrhea, especially in young children and older adults, assess for dehydration, hypokalemia, and other fluid and electrolyte disorders.

Nursing Diagnoses

- Diarrhea related to GI infection or inflammatory disorders, other disease processes, dietary irritants, or overuse of laxatives
- Anxiety related to availability of bathroom facilities
- Deficient Fluid Volume related to excessive losses in liquid stools
- Pain (abdominal cramping) related to intestinal hypermotility and spasm
- Deficient Knowledge: Factors that cause or aggravate diarrhea and appropriate use of antidiarrheal drugs

Planning/Goals

The client will
- Take antidiarrheal drugs appropriately
- Obtain relief from acute diarrhea (reduced number of liquid stools, reduced abdominal discomfort)
- Maintain fluid and electrolyte balance
- Maintain adequate nutritional intake
- Avoid adverse effects of antidiarrheal medications
- Re-establish normal bowel patterns after an episode of acute diarrhea
- Have fewer liquid stools with chronic diarrhea

Interventions

Use measures to prevent diarrhea.
- Prepare and store food properly and avoid improperly stored foods and those prepared under unsanitary conditions. Dairy products, cream pies, and other foods may cause diarrhea ("food poisoning") if not refrigerated.
- Wash hands before handling any foods, after handling raw poultry or meat, and always before eating.
- Chew food well.
- Do not overuse laxatives (ie, amount per dose or frequency of use). Many OTC products contain senna or other strong stimulant laxatives.

Provide education about drug therapy (see accompanying Client Teaching Guidelines).

Regardless of whether antidiarrheal drugs are used, supportive therapy is required for the treatment of diarrhea. Elements of supportive care include the following:

- Replacement of fluids and electrolytes (2–3 quarts daily). Fluids such as weak tea; water; bouillon; clear soup; non-carbonated, caffeine-free beverages; and gelatin are usually tolerated and helpful. If the client cannot tolerate adequate amounts of oral liquids or if diarrhea is severe or prolonged, intravenous fluids may be needed (ie, solutions containing dextrose, sodium chloride, and potassium chloride).
- Avoid foods and fluids that may further irritate GI mucosa (eg, highly spiced foods; "laxative" foods, such as raw fruits and vegetables).

- Increase frequency and length of rest periods, and decrease activity. Exercise and activity stimulate peristalsis.
- If perianal irritation occurs because of frequent liquid stools, cleanse the area with mild soap and water after each bowel movement, then apply an emollient, such as white petrolatum (Vaseline).

Evaluation

- Observe and interview for decreased number of liquid or loose stools.
- Observe for signs of adequate food and fluid intake (eg, good skin turgor and urine output, stable weight).
- Observe for appropriate use of antidiarrheal drugs.
- Observe and interview for return of pre-diarrheal patterns of bowel elimination.
- Interview regarding knowledge and use of measures to prevent or minimize diarrhea.

APPLYING YOUR KNOWLEDGE 61-1
What factors would you include in your assessment of Mr. McGrath?

PRINCIPLES OF THERAPY

In most cases of acute, nonspecific diarrhea in adults, fluid losses are not severe and clients need only simple replacement of fluids and electrolytes lost in the stool. Acceptable replacement fluids during the first 24 hours include 2 to 3 liters of clear liquids (eg, flat ginger ale, decaffeinated cola drinks or tea, broth, gelatin). Also, the diet should consist of bland foods (eg, rice, soup, bread, salted crackers, cooked cereals, baked potatoes, eggs, applesauce). A regular diet may be resumed after 2 to 3 days.

Drug Selection

The choice of antidiarrheal agent depends largely on the cause, severity, and duration of diarrhea.

- For symptomatic treatment of diarrhea, difenoxin with atropine (Motofen), diphenoxylate with atropine (Lomotil), or loperamide (Imodium) is probably the drug of choice for most people.
- In bacterial gastroenteritis or diarrhea, the choice of antibacterial drug depends on the causative microorganism and susceptibility tests.
- In ulcerative colitis, sulfonamides, adrenal corticosteroids, and other anti-inflammatory agents such as balsalazide (Colazal), mesalamine (Pentasa), and olsalazine (Dipentum) are the drugs of choice. The latter drugs are related to aspirin and nonsteroidal anti-inflammatory

C L I E N T   T E A C H I N G   G U I D E L I N E S

Antidiarrheals

General Considerations

☑ Taking a medication to stop diarrhea is not always needed or desirable because diarrhea may mean the body is trying to rid itself of irritants or bacteria. Treatment is indicated if diarrhea is severe, prolonged, or occurs in young children or older adults, who are highly susceptible to excessive losses of body fluids and electrolytes.

☑ Try to drink 2 to 3 quarts of fluid daily. This helps prevent dehydration from fluid loss in stools. Water, clear broths, and noncarbonated, caffeine-free beverages are recommended because they are unlikely to cause further diarrhea.

☑ Avoid highly spiced or "laxative" foods, such as fresh fruits and vegetables, until diarrhea is controlled.

☑ Frequent and thorough handwashing and careful food storage and preparation can help prevent diarrhea.

☑ Consult a health care provider if diarrhea is accompanied by severe abdominal pain or fever, lasts longer than 3 days, or if stools contain blood or mucus. These signs and symptoms may indicate more serious disorders for which other treatment measures are needed.

☑ Stop antidiarrheal drugs when diarrhea is controlled to avoid adverse effects such as constipation.

☑ Bismuth subsalicylate (Pepto-Bismol) and loperamide (Imodium A-D) are available over the counter; difenoxin (Motofen) and diphenoxylate (Lomotil) are prescription drugs.

☑ Difenoxin, diphenoxylate, and loperamide may cause dizziness or drowsiness and should be used with caution if driving or performing other tasks requiring alertness, coordination, or physical dexterity. In addition, alcohol and other drugs that cause drowsiness should be avoided.

☑ Pepto-Bismol may temporarily discolor bowel movements a grayish-black.

☑ Keep antidiarrheal drugs out of reach of children. Accidental overdose of Motofen may cause fatal respiratory depression.

Self- or Caregiver Administration

☑ Take or give antidiarrheal drugs only as prescribed or directed on nonprescription drug labels.

☑ Do not exceed maximal daily doses of diphenoxylate (Lomotil), loperamide, difenoxin, or paregoric.

☑ With liquid diphenoxylate, use only the calibrated dropper furnished by the manufacturer for accurate measurement of dosages.

☑ With Pepto-Bismol liquid, shake the bottle well before measuring the dose; with tablets, chew them well or allow them to dissolve in the mouth.

☑ Add at least 30 mL of water to each dose of paregoric to help the drug dose reach the stomach. The mixture appears milky.

☑ Take cholestyramine or colestipol with at least 4 oz of water. These drugs should never be taken without fluids because they may block the gastrointestinal tract. Also, do not take within 4 hours of other drugs because they may combine with and inactivate other drugs.

☑ Take rifaximin with or without food for 3 days. Notify health care provider if your condition worsens or does not improve after 1 to 2 days.

☑ Use caution driving or operating machinery if experiencing dizziness while using rifaximin.

☑ Diabetic clients should be aware that Alinia oral suspension contains 1.48 g of sucrose per 5 mL.

---

drugs (see Chap. 7 and Appendix A) and are contraindicated in clients with hypersensitivity to salicylates or any other product component. They are given orally or rectally and are thought to exert topical anti-inflammatory effects in ulcerative colitis.

● In antibiotic-associated colitis, stopping the causative drug is the initial treatment. If symptoms do not improve within 3 or 4 days, oral metronidazole or vancomycin is given for 7 to 10 days. Both are effective against *C. difficile,* but metronidazole is the drug of first choice and is much less expensive. Vancomycin may be given for severe disease or when metronidazole is ineffective. For approximately 6 weeks after recovery, relapse often occurs and requires re-treatment. Because relapse is not due to emergence of drug-resistant strains, the same drug used for the initial bout may be used to treat the relapse.

● In diarrhea caused by enzyme deficiency, pancreatic enzymes are given rather than antidiarrheal drugs.

● In bile-salt diarrhea, cholestyramine or colestipol may be effective.

● Although morphine and codeine are contraindicated in chronic diarrhea, they may occasionally be used in the treatment of acute, severe diarrhea. Dosages required for antidiarrheal effects are smaller than those required for analgesia. The following oral drugs and dosages are approximately equivalent in antidiarrheal effectiveness: 4 mg morphine, 30 mg codeine, 10 mL paregoric, 5 mg diphenoxylate, and 2 mg loperamide. A common and potentially fatal drug error is confusing paregoric (camphorated tincture of opium) with the much more potent drug Opium Tincture. Paragoric contains only 0.4 mg/mL of morphine, while Opium Tincture is much more concentrated, containing 10 mg/mL of morphine. Labels should be in place on Opium Tincture packaging identifying it as a poison, identifying the strength of morphine per mL as 10 mg/mL, and containing the statement, "Warning! DO NOT use Opium Tincture in place of paregoric."

APPLYING YOUR KNOWLEDGE 61-2

What is the most likely drug of choice for Mr. McGrath?

Use in Special Populations

Use in Children

Antidiarrheal drugs, including antibiotics, are often used in children to prevent excessive losses of fluids and electrolytes. In small children, serious fluid volume deficit may rapidly develop with diarrhea. Worldwide, from 2000 to 2003, the World Health Organization estimated that diarrhea accounted for 18% of deaths in children under 5 years of age during the first 28 days of life. Drug therapy should be accompanied by appropriate fluid replacement and efforts to decrease further stimuli. Oral rehydration solutions (eg, **Pedialyte** solution and freezer popsicles) are commercially available in ready-to-use formulations in the United States. Packets of powder (containing glucose, sodium, potassium, chloride, and citrate), to be mixed with 1 liter of boiled or treated water, are available in developing countries and are usually provided by the World Health Organization.

    Difenoxin and **diphenoxylate** contain atropine, and signs of atropine overdose may occur with usual doses. Difenoxin and diphenoxylate are contraindicated in children younger than 2 years of age; **loperamide** should not be used in children younger than 6 years, except with a pediatrician's supervision, and should generally not be used for longer than 2 days in older children. Loperamide is a nonprescription drug.

Use in Older Adults

Diarrhea is less common than constipation in older adults, but it may occur from laxative abuse and bowel-cleansing procedures before GI surgery or diagnostic tests. Fluid volume deficits may rapidly develop in older adults with diarrhea. General principles of fluid and electrolyte replacement; measures to decrease GI irritants; and drug therapy apply as for younger adults. Most antidiarrheal drugs may be given to older adults, but cautious use is indicated to avoid inducing constipation.

Use in Clients With Renal Impairment

Difenoxin and **diphenoxylate** should be used with extreme caution in clients with severe hepatorenal disease because hepatic coma may be precipitated.

Use in Clients With Hepatic Impairment

Difenoxin and **diphenoxylate** should be used with extreme caution in clients with abnormal liver-function test results or severe hepatorenal disease because hepatic coma may be precipitated. With **loperamide,** monitor clients with hepatic impairment for signs of CNS toxicity. Loperamide normally undergoes extensive first-pass metabolism, which may be lessened by liver disease. As a result, a larger portion of a dose reaches the systemic circulation and may cause adverse effects. Dosage may need to be reduced.

Use in Immunocompromised Clients

Diarrhea often occurs in immunocompromised clients (eg, those with AIDS, organ transplant, or anticancer chemotherapy) and may be difficult to treat with the usual antidiarrheal drugs. **Octreotide** may be effective, but it should be used only after other medications have failed because it is given by injection and is expensive.

Use in Home Care

Prescription and OTC antidiarrheal aids are often taken in the home setting. The role of the home care nurse may include advising clients and caregivers about appropriate use of the drugs; trying to identify the cause and severity of the diarrhea (ie, risk of fluid and electrolyte deficit); and teaching strategies to manage the current episode and prevent future episodes. If octreotide is taken at home, the home care nurse may need to teach the client or a caregiver how to administer subcutaneous injections.

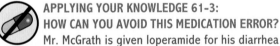 **APPLYING YOUR KNOWLEDGE 61-3:**
HOW CAN YOU AVOID THIS MEDICATION ERROR?
Mr. McGrath is given loperamide for his diarrhea and sent home. He has a stool specimen examined for microorganisms. His report shows the presence of salmonella organisms. He continues to have diarrhea so you increase the dose of **loperamide.**

N U R S I N G   A C T I O N S

Antidiarrheals

NURSING ACTIONS	RATIONALE/EXPLANATION
1. Administer accurately	
a. With liquid diphenoxylate, use only the calibrated dropper furnished by the manufacturer for measuring dosage.	For accurate measurement

NURSING ACTIONS	RATIONALE/EXPLANATION
b. Add at least 30 mL of water to each dose of paregoric. The mixture appears milky.	To add sufficient volume for the drug to reach the stomach
c. Do not exceed maximal daily doses of diphenoxylate, loperamide, difenoxin, and paregoric. Also, stop the drugs when diarrhea is controlled.	To decrease risks of adverse reactions, including drug dependence
d. Give cholestyramine and colestipol with at least 120 mL of water. Also, do not give within approximately 4 hours of other drugs.	The drugs may cause obstruction of the gastrointestinal (GI) tract if swallowed in a dry state. They may combine with and inactivate other drugs.
2. Observe for therapeutic effects **a.** Decreased number, frequency, and fluidity of stools	Therapeutic effects are usually evident within 24–48 hours.
b. Decreased or absent abdominal cramping pains	
c. Signs of normal fluid and electrolyte balance (adequate hydration, urine output, and skin turgor)	
d. Resumption of usual activities of daily living	
3. Observe for adverse effects **a.** Constipation	Constipation is the most common adverse effect. It can be prevented by using antidiarrheal drugs only as prescribed and stopping the drugs when diarrhea is controlled.
b. Drug dependence	Dependence is unlikely with recommended doses but may occur with long-term use of large doses of paregoric, diphenoxylate, and difenoxin.
c. With diphenoxylate, anorexia, nausea, vomiting, dizziness, abdominal discomfort, paralytic ileus, toxic megacolon, hypersensitivity (pruritus, urticaria, angioneurotic edema), headache, and tachycardia	Although numerous adverse reactions have been reported, their incidence and severity are low when diphenoxylate is used appropriately.
With overdoses of a diphenoxylate–atropine or difenoxin–atropine combination, respiratory depression and coma may result from diphenoxylate or difenoxin content and anticholinergic effects (eg, dry mouth, blurred vision, urinary retention) from atropine content.	Deliberate overdose and abuse are unlikely because of unpleasant anticholinergic effects. Overdose can be prevented by using the drug in recommended doses and only when required. Overdose can be treated with naloxone (Narcan) and supportive therapy.
d. With loperamide, abdominal cramps, dry mouth, dizziness, nausea, and vomiting	Abdominal cramps are the most common adverse effect. No serious adverse effects have been reported with recommended doses of loperamide. Overdose may be treated with naloxone, gastric lavage, and administration of activated charcoal.
e. With cholestyramine and colestipol, constipation, nausea, and abdominal distention	Adverse effects are usually minor and transient because these drugs are not absorbed from the GI tract.
f. With octreotide, diarrhea, headache, cardiac dysrhythmias, and injection-site pain	These are commonly reported adverse effects.
g. With rifaximin, flatulence, headache, stomach pain, urgent bowel movements, nausea, constipation, fever, vomiting, dizziness	These are commonly reported adverse effects.
4. Observe for drug interactions	Few clinically significant drug interactions have been reported with commonly used antidiarrheal agents.
a. Drugs that *increase* effects of antidiarrheal agents: (1) Central nervous system (CNS) depressants (alcohol, sedative-hypnotics, opioid analgesics, antianxiety agents, antipsychotic agents)	Additive CNS depression with opiate and related antidiarrheals. Opioid analgesics have additive constipating effects.

(continued)

NURSING ACTIONS	RATIONALE/EXPLANATION
(2) Anticholinergic agents (atropine and synthetic anticholinergic antispasmodics; antihistamines and antidepressants with anticholinergic effects)	Additive anticholinergic adverse effects (dry mouth, blurred vision, urinary retention) with diphenoxylate–atropine (Lomotil) and difenoxin–atropine (Motofen)
b. Nitazoxanide may increase the effect of highly protein-bound, narrow therapeutic-index drugs, such as warfarin, resulting in toxicity.	The active metabolite of nitazoxanide is 99.9% protein bound and may compete with other protein-bound medications at plasma protein binding sites.

APPLYING YOUR KNOWLEDGE: ANSWERS

61-1 Determine the number of stools each day and the amount, consistency, color, odor, and presence of abnormal components in each stool. Ask Mr. McGrath what measures he has initiated to relieve the diarrhea and if he has any other symptoms, such as nausea and vomiting or fever. The most obvious cause of Mr. McGrath's diarrhea is his recent trip to Mexico; however, also consider chronic inflammatory diseases of the bowel, use of laxative or other drugs, and food intake.

61-2 The drug of choice to treat diarrhea is loperamide. Mr. McGrath should be instructed to take no more than 8 mg per day: 4 mg initially then 2 mg after each loose stool. If his symptoms persist for more than 48 hours, Mr. McGrath should consult his physician.

61-3 Mr. McGrath should discontinue the use of loperamide. Antidiarrheal agents are contraindicated in diarrhea caused by microorganisms. In these circumstances, antidiarrheal agents that slow peristalsis may aggravate and prolong diarrhea.

Review and Application Exercises

Short Answer Exercises

1. What are some common causes of diarrhea?

2. In which populations is diarrhea most likely to cause serious problems?

3. Which types of diarrhea do not require antidiarrheal drug therapy, and why?

4. How do antidiarrheal drugs decrease frequency or fluidity of stools?

5. What are adverse effects of commonly used antidiarrheal drugs?

6. If a client asked you to recommend an OTC antidiarrheal agent, which would you recommend, and why?

7. Would your recommendation differ if the proposed recipient were a child? Why or why not?

NCLEX-Style Questions

8. An appropriate nursing measure when treating a young child with diarrhea would be to
   a. Encourage a regular diet.
   b. Encourage intake of clear liquids.
   c. Encourage intake of milk products.
   d. Encourage use of herbal tea.

9. A client on antibiotic therapy begins to experience fever, abdominal pain, and diarrhea containing mucus, pus, and blood. The best nursing action in this situation is
   a. Continue the antibiotic because the client has signs of a GI infection.
   b. Monitor the client's vital signs and notify the physician if there is further deterioration.
   c. Withhold the antibiotic and notify the physician of the client's condition.
   d. Encourage fluid intake because fever is a sign of dehydration.

10. A client with diarrhea begins to complain of eye pain after administration of diphenoxylate with atropine (Lomotil). The nurse should
    a. Offer an OTC analgesic such as acetaminophen.
    b. Discontinue the diphenoxylate with atropine and notify the physician.
    c. Tell the client this is a common side effect and will soon pass.
    d. Apply a cool compress to the eyes for relief of the discomfort.

Selected References

Brye, J., Boschi-Pinto, C., Shibuya, K., Black, R. E., WHO Child Health Epidemiology Reference Group. (2005). WHO estimates of the causes of death in children. *Lancet, 365*(9465), 1147–1152.

Drug facts and comparisons. (Updated monthly). St. Louis: Facts and Comparisons.

Guerrant, R., Gilder, T., Steiner, T., Thielman, N., Slutsker, L., Tauxe, R., et al. (2001). Practice guidelines for the management of infectious diarrhea. *Clinical Infectious Diseases, 32,* 331–351.

Hogue, V. W. (2000). Constipation and diarrhea. In E. T. Herfindal & D. R. Gourley (Eds.), *Textbook of therapeutics: Drug and disease management* (7th ed., pp. 571–588). Philadelphia: Lippincott Williams & Wilkins.

Institute for Safe Medication Practices. (2002, February 20). *Hazard alert! Recurring confusion between tincture of opium and paregoric.* Retrieved August 22, 2005, from http://ismp.org/MSAarticles/recruitingPring/htm

Jabbar, A., & Wright, R. (2003). Gastroenteritis and antibiotic-associated diarrhea. *Primary Care Clinical Office Practice, 30,* 63–80.

Juckett, G. (2005). Travel medicine. *West Virginia Medical Journal, 100*(6), 222–225.

McCray, W., Jr., & Krevsky, B. (1999). Diarrhea in adults: When is intervention necessary? *Hospital Medicine, 35*(1), 39–46.

Musher, D. M., & Musher, B. L. (2004). Contagious acute gastrointestinal infections. *The New England Journal of Medicine, 351*(23), 2417–2427.

Porth, C. M. (2005). Disorders of gastrointestinal function. In C. M. Porth, *Pathophysiology: Concepts of altered health states* (7th ed., pp. 885–916). Philadelphia: Lippincott Williams & Wilkins.

Scheidler, M. D., & Giannella, R. A. (2001, July 15). Practical management of acute diarrhea. *Hospital Practice, 36*(7), 49–56.

Scheindlin, S. (2002, February). Advising patients on OTC antidiarrheals. *Pharmacy Times, 68*(2), 58–61.

Schroeder, M. S. (2005). Clostridium difficile–associated diarrhea. *American Family Physician, 71*(5), 921–928.

Semrad, C. E., & Powell, D. W. (2004). Approach to the patient with diarrhea and malabsorption. L. Goldman & D. Ausiello (Eds.), *Cecil textbook of medicine* (22nd ed., pp. 842–847). Philadelphia: W. B. Saunders.

Spruill, W. J., & Wade, W. E. (2002). Diarrhea, constipation, and irritable bowel syndrome. In J. T. DiPiro, R. L. Talbert, G. C. Yee, G. R. Matzke, B. G. Wells, & L. M. Posey (Eds.), *Pharmacotherapy: A pathophysiologic approach* (5th ed., pp. 655–669). New York: McGraw-Hill.

Antiemetics

OBJECTIVES

After studying this chapter, you will be able to:

1. Identify clients at risk of developing nausea and vomiting.
2. Discuss guidelines for preventing, minimizing, or treating nausea and vomiting.
3. Differentiate the major types of antiemetic drugs.
4. Discuss characteristics, effects, and nursing process implications of selected antiemetic drugs.

APPLYING YOUR KNOWLEDGE

Nellie Snyder is a 38-year-old woman who has breast cancer. She is receiving radiation and chemotherapy. Ms. Snyder is experiencing significant nausea and vomiting. Her physician orders ondansetron 32 mg IV to be administered 30 minutes prior to her chemotherapy, and 8 to 16 mg PO every 8 hours as needed. She also receives metoclopramide 10 mg PO four times a day: 30 minutes before meals, and at bedtime.

INTRODUCTION

Antiemetic drugs are used to prevent or treat nausea and vomiting. *Nausea* is an unpleasant sensation of abdominal discomfort accompanied by a desire to vomit. *Vomiting* is the expulsion of stomach contents through the mouth. Nausea may occur without vomiting, and vomiting may occur without prior nausea, but the two symptoms often occur together.

Nausea and vomiting are common symptoms experienced by virtually everyone. These symptoms may accompany almost any illness or stress situation. Causes of nausea and vomiting include the following:

- Gastrointestinal (GI) disorders, including infection or inflammation in the GI tract, liver, gallbladder, or pancreas; impaired GI motility and muscle tone (eg, gastroparesis); and overeating or ingestion of foods or fluids that irritate the GI mucosa
- Cardiovascular, infectious, neurologic, or metabolic disorders
- Drug therapy. Nausea and vomiting are the most common adverse effects of drug therapy. Although the symptoms may occur with most drugs, they are especially associated with alcohol, aspirin, digoxin, anticancer drugs, antimicrobials, estrogen preparations, and opioid analgesics.
- Pain and other noxious stimuli, such as unpleasant sights and odors
- Emotional disturbances; physical or mental stress
- Radiation therapy
- Motion sickness
- Postoperative status, which may include pain, impaired GI motility, and receiving various medications

Vomiting occurs when the vomiting center (a nucleus of cells in the medulla oblongata) is stimulated. Stimuli are relayed to the vomiting center from peripheral sites (eg, gastric mucosa, peritoneum, intestines, joints) and central sites (eg, cerebral cortex; vestibular apparatus of the ear; neurons in the fourth ventricle, called the *chemoreceptor trigger zone* [CTZ]). The vomiting center, CTZ, and GI tract contain benzodiazepine, cholinergic, dopamine, histamine, opiate, and serotonin receptors, which are stimulated by emetogenic drugs and toxins circulating in blood and cerebrospinal fluid.

For example, in cancer chemotherapy, emetogenic drugs are thought to stimulate the release of serotonin from the enterochromaffin cells of the small intestine; this released serotonin then activates 5-HT$_3$ receptors located on vagal afferent nerves in the CTZ to initiate the vomiting reflex. In motion sickness, rapid changes in body motion stimulate receptors in the inner ear (vestibular branch of the auditory nerve, which is concerned with equilibrium), and nerve impulses are transmitted to the CTZ and the vomiting center.

When stimulated, the vomiting center initiates efferent impulses that cause closure of the glottis; contraction of abdominal muscles and the diaphragm; relaxation of the gastroesophageal sphincter; and reverse peristalsis, which moves stomach contents toward the mouth for ejection.

GENERAL CHARACTERISTICS OF ANTIEMETIC DRUGS

Indications for Use

Antiemetic drugs are indicated to prevent and treat nausea and vomiting associated with surgery, pain, motion sickness, cancer chemotherapy, radiation therapy, and other causes.

Contraindications to Use

Antiemetic drugs are usually contraindicated when their use may prevent or delay diagnosis, when signs and symptoms of drug toxicity may be masked, and for routine use to prevent postoperative vomiting.

CLASSIFICATIONS AND INDIVIDUAL DRUGS

Drugs used to prevent or treat nausea and vomiting belong to several different therapeutic classifications, and most have anticholinergic, antidopaminergic, antihistaminic, or antiserotonergic effects. In general, the drugs are more effective in prophylaxis than treatment. Most antiemetics prevent or relieve nausea and vomiting by acting on the vomiting center, CTZ, cerebral cortex, vestibular apparatus, or a combination of these. Major drugs are described in the following sections and in Table 62-1.

Phenothiazines

Phenothiazines, of which chlorpromazine (Thorazine) is the prototype, are central nervous system depressants used in the treatment of psychosis and psychotic symptoms in other disorders (see Chap. 9). These drugs have widespread effects on the body. Their therapeutic effects in nausea and vomiting (as in psychosis) are attributed to their ability to block dopamine from receptor sites in the brain and CTZ (antidopaminergic effects). When used as antiemetics, phenothiazines act on the

CTZ and the vomiting center. Not all phenothiazines are effective antiemetics.

Phenothiazines are usually effective in preventing or treating nausea and vomiting induced by drugs, radiation therapy, surgery, and most other stimuli, but are usually ineffective in motion sickness. These drugs cause sedation; **prochlorperazine** (Compazine) and **promethazine** (Phenergan) are commonly used. Because of their adverse effects (eg, sedation, cognitive impairment), phenothiazines are mainly indicated when other antiemetic drugs are ineffective or only a few doses are needed.

Antihistamines

Antihistamines are used primarily to prevent histamine from exerting its widespread effects on body tissues (see Chap. 45). Antihistamines used as antiemetic agents are the "classic" antihistamines or H$_1$ receptor blocking agents (as differentiated from cimetidine and related drugs, which are H$_2$ receptor blocking agents). The drugs are thought to relieve nausea and vomiting by blocking the action of acetylcholine in the brain (anticholinergic effects). Antihistamines may be effective in preventing and treating motion sickness. Not all antihistamines are effective as antiemetic agents.

Corticosteroids

Although corticosteroids are used mainly as antiallergic, antiinflammatory, and antistress agents (see Chap. 23), they have antiemetic effects as well. The mechanism by which the drugs exert antiemetic effects is unknown; they may block prostaglandin activity in the cerebral cortex. Dexamethasone and methylprednisolone are commonly used in the management of chemotherapy-induced emesis, usually in combination with one or more other antiemetic agents. Regimens vary from a single dose before chemotherapy to doses every 4 to 6 hours for 24 to 48 hours. With this short-term use, adverse effects are mild (eg, euphoria, insomnia, mild fluid retention).

Benzodiazepine Antianxiety Drugs

These drugs (see Chap. 8) are not antiemetics, but they are often used in multidrug regimens to prevent nausea and vomiting associated with cancer chemotherapy. The drugs produce relaxation and inhibit cerebral cortex input to the vomiting center. They are often prescribed for clients who experience anticipatory nausea and vomiting before administration of anticancer drugs. Lorazepam (Ativan) is commonly used.

Prokinetic Agents

Metoclopramide (Reglan) is a prokinetic agent that increases GI motility and the rate of gastric emptying by increasing the release of acetylcholine from nerve endings in the GI tract (peripheral cholinergic effects). As a result, it can decrease nausea and vomiting associated with gastroparesis and other nonobstructive disorders characterized by gastric

Table 62-1 Drugs at a Glance: Antiemetic Drugs

	ROUTES AND DOSAGE RANGES	
GENERIC/TRADE NAME	Adults	Children
Phenothiazines		
Prochlorperazine (Compazine)	PO 5–10 mg 3 or 4 times daily (sustained-release capsule, 10 mg twice daily) IM 5–10 mg q3–4h to a maximum of 40 mg daily Rectal suppository 25 mg twice daily	>10 kg, PO 0.4 mg/kg/d, in 3 or 4 divided doses IM 0.2 mg/kg as a single dose Rectal suppository 0.4 mg/kg/d, in 3 or 4 divided doses
Promethazine (Phenergan)	PO, IM, rectal suppository 12.5–25 mg q4–6h	>3 mo, PO, IM, rectal suppository 0.25–0.5 mg/kg q4–6h
Antihistamines		
Cyclizine (Marezine)	Motion sickness, PO 50 mg 30 min before departure, then q4–6h as needed, to a maximal daily dose of 200 mg IM 50 mg q4–6h as needed	6–12 y, Motion sickness, PO 25 mg up to three times daily (maximal daily dose 75 mg)
Dimenhydrinate (Dramamine)	PO 50–100 mg q4–6h as needed (maximal dose, 400 mg in 24 h) IM 50 mg as needed IV 50 mg in 10 mL of sodium chloride injection, over 2 min	6–12 y, PO 25–50 mg q6–8h (maximal dose, 150 mg in 24 h) IM 1.25 mg/kg 4 times daily (maximal dose, 300 mg in 24 h)
Hydroxyzine (Vistaril)	IM 25–100 mg q4–6h as needed	IM 0.5 mg/lb q4–6h as needed
Meclizine (Antivert, Bonine)	Motion sickness, PO 25–50 mg 1 h before travel Vertigo, PO 25–100 mg daily in divided doses	Dosage not established
Prokinetic Agent		
Metoclopramide (Reglan)	PO 10 mg 30 min before meals and at bedtime for 2–8 wk IV 2 mg/kg 30 min before injection of cisplatin and 2 h after injection of cisplatin, then 1–2 mg/kg q2–3h if needed, up to 4 doses	Dosage not established
5-HT₃ (Serotonin) Receptor Antagonists		
Dolasetron (Anzemet)	Prevention of PONV, PO 100 mg 2 h before surgery Prevention or treatment of PONV, IV 12.5 mg as a single dose, 15 min before cessation of anesthesia or as soon as nausea or vomiting develops Prevention of chemotherapy-induced nausea and vomiting, PO 100 mg within 1 h before chemotherapy; IV 1.8 mg/kg as a single dose approximately 30 min before chemotherapy	2–16 y, prevention of PONV, PO 1.2 mg/kg within 2 h before surgery. Maximum dose, 100 mg Prevention or treatment of PONV, IV 0.35 mg/kg as a single dose, 15 min before cessation of anesthesia or as soon as nausea or vomiting develops. Maximum dose, 12.5 mg Prevention of chemotherapy-induced nausea and vomiting, PO 1.8 mg/kg within 1 h before chemotherapy, maximum dose 100 mg; IV 1.8 mg/kg as a single dose approximately 30 min before chemotherapy, maximum dose 100 mg
Granisetron (Kytril)	Cancer chemotherapy, PO 1 mg twice daily, first dose approximately 1 h before emetogenic drug, second dose 12 h later, only on days receiving chemotherapy; IV 10 mcg/kg infused over 5 min, 30 min before emetogenic drug, only on days receiving chemotherapy	2–16 y, IV 10 mcg/kg
Ondansetron (Zofran)	*Nausea and vomiting associated with highly emetogenic cancer chemotherapy:*	

Table 62-1 Drugs at a Glance: Antiemetic Drugs (continued)

GENERIC/TRADE NAME	ROUTES AND DOSAGE RANGES	
	Adults	Children
	PO 24 mg 30 min before start of single day chemotherapy	Pediatric dosage not established
	IV 0.15 mg/kg for 3 doses given 30 minutes before chemotherapy, repeat in 4 and 8 h; IV 32 mg as a single dose. Infuse over 15 min	*6–18 mos,* IV 0.15 mg/kg for 3 doses given 30 minutes before chemotherapy, repeat in 4 and 8 h. Infuse over 15 min.
	Nausea and vomiting associated with moderately emetogenic cancer chemotherapy: PO 8 mg for 2 doses given 30 min before chemotherapy, repeat in 8 h.	≥12 y, PO dosage same as adult 4–11 y, PO 4 mg given for 3 doses given 30 min before chemotherapy, repeat in 8 and 16 h.
	Post operative nausea and vomiting: PO 16 mg 1h before anesthesia	PO dosage not established
	IV 4 mg given over 2–5 min. IM 4 mg	*1 mo–12 y,* ≤40kg: IV 0.1 mg/kg; ≥40 kg: IV 4 mg. Given over 2–5 min.
Palonosetron (Aloxi)	Cancer chemotherapy, IV 0.25 mg 30 min before emetogenic drug. Repeat dosing within a 7-day interval is not recommended.	Dosage not established
Miscellaneous Agents **Dronabinol** (Marinol)	PO 5 mg/m² (square meter of body surface area) 1–3 h before chemotherapy, then q2–4h for a total of 4–6 doses daily. Dosage can be increased by 2.5 mg/m² increments to a maximal dose of 15 mg/m² if necessary.	Same as adults for treatment of chemotherapy-induced nausea and vomiting
Phosphorated carbohydrate solution (Emetrol)	PO 15–30 mL repeated at 15-min intervals until vomiting ceases	PO 5–10 mL repeated at 15-min intervals until vomiting ceases
Scopolamine (Transderm Scop)	Motion sickness, PO, Sub-Q, 0.6–1 mg/kg as a single dose Transdermal disc (1.5 mg scopolamine) placed behind the ear every 3 d if needed	Motion sickness, PO, Sub-Q 0.006 mg as a single dose

IM, intramuscular; IV, intravenous; PO, oral; PONV, postoperative nausea and vomiting; Sub-Q, subcutaneous.

retention of food and fluids. Metoclopramide also has central antiemetic effects; it antagonizes the action of dopamine, a catecholamine neurotransmitter. Metoclopramide is given orally in diabetic gastroparesis and esophageal reflux. Large doses of the drug are given IV during chemotherapy with cisplatin (Platinol) and other emetogenic antineoplastic drugs.

With oral administration, action begins in 30 to 60 minutes and peaks in 60 to 90 minutes. With intramuscular (IM) use, action onset occurs in 10 to 15 minutes and peaks in 60 to 90 minutes. With IV use, action onset occurs in 1 to 3 minutes and peaks in 60 to 90 minutes. Adverse effects include sedation, restlessness, and extrapyramidal reactions (eg, akathisia, dystonia, symptoms of Parkinson's disease).

Metoclopramide may increase the effects of alcohol and cyclosporine (by increasing their absorption) and decrease the effects of cimetidine and digoxin (by accelerating passage through the GI tract and decreasing time for absorption).

Metoclopramide is relatively contraindicated in Parkinson's disease because it further depletes dopamine and reduces the effectiveness of levodopa, a major antiparkinson drug.

5-Hydroxytryptamine₃ (5-HT₃ or Serotonin) Receptor Antagonists

Ondansetron (Zofran), **granisetron** (Kytril), **dolasetron** (Anzemet), and **palonosetron** (Aloxi) are used to prevent or treat moderate to severe nausea and vomiting associated with cancer chemotherapy, radiation therapy, and postoperative status. These drugs antagonize serotonin receptors, preventing their activation by the effects of emetogenic drugs and toxins.

Odansetron, granisetron, and dolasetron may be given intravenously (IV) or orally. Palonosetron is only given IV. All four of these drugs are metabolized in the liver. Adverse effects are usually mild to moderate, and common ones include diarrhea, headache, dizziness, constipation, muscle aches, and transient elevation of liver enzymes.

Ondansetron was the first drug of this group. Its half-life is 3 to 5.5 hours in most clients and 9 to 20 hours in clients with moderate or severe liver impairment. With oral drug, action begins in 30 to 60 minutes and peaks in about 2 hours. With IV drug, onset and peak of drug action are immediate.

Granisetron has a half-life of 6 hours with oral drug and 5 to 9 hours with IV drug; its half-life in clients with liver impairment is unknown. Action begins rapidly with IV injection and peaks in 30 to 45 minutes; action begins more slowly with oral drug and peaks in 60 to 90 minutes.

Dolasetron has a half-life of about 7 hours with both IV and oral drug, which is extended to 11 hours in clients with severe liver impairment. Action onset and peak occur rapidly with IV administration; with oral drug, onset is rapid and peak occurs in 1 to 2 hours.

The newest serotonin receptor antagonist, palonosetron, is 62% plasma-protein bound and has a half-life of 40 hours. This prolonged half-life makes palonosetron effective for prevention of delayed emesis after chemotherapy. It is administered over 30 seconds and is given 30 minutes before chemotherapy via the same IV access. Drug action begins rapidly after IV administration.

APPLYING YOUR KNOWLEDGE 62-1
What adverse effects would you assess Ms. Snyder for, in relation to ondansetron?

Miscellaneous Antiemetics

Dronabinol is a cannabinoid (derivative of marijuana) used in the management of nausea and vomiting associated with anticancer drugs and unrelieved by other drugs. Dronabinol causes the same adverse effects as marijuana, including psychiatric symptoms, has a high potential for abuse, and may cause a withdrawal syndrome when abruptly discontinued. As a result, it is a Schedule III drug under federal narcotic laws.

Withdrawal symptoms (eg, insomnia, irritability, restlessness) may occur if dronabinol is abruptly stopped. Onset occurs within 12 hours, with peak intensity within 24 hours and dissipation within 96 hours. These symptoms are most likely to occur with high doses or prolonged use. Sleep disturbances may persist for several weeks.

Phosphorated carbohydrate solution (Emetrol) is a hyperosmolar solution with phosphoric acid. It is thought to reduce smooth muscle contraction in the GI tract and is available over the counter.

Scopolamine, an anticholinergic drug (see Chap. 20), is effective in relieving nausea and vomiting associated with motion sickness and radiation therapy for cancer. A transdermal patch is often used to prevent seasickness.

Herbal and Dietary Supplements

Ginger, commonly used in cooking, is promoted for use in preventing nausea and vomiting associated with motion sickness, pregnancy, postoperative status, and other conditions. A few studies have investigated its antiemetic activity in humans. In one randomized, double-blind study (Fetrow & Avila, 2001), 60 women undergoing gynecologic surgery were given either 1000 milligrams of powdered ginger root orally, 10 milligrams of metoclopramide (Reglan) IV, or a placebo, 1.5 hours before surgery. Results indicated that ginger was comparable to metoclopramide and that both treatments were more effective than placebo in preventing postoperative nausea and vomiting. Similar results were obtained in another study with 120 clients having gynecologic surgery; in this study, metoclopramide was given orally. Although these studies support the use of ginger, other studies do not. The general consensus seems to be that it is premature to recommend ginger for any therapeutic use until long-term, controlled studies are done.

NURSING PROCESS

Assessment

Assess for nausea and vomiting.
- Identify risk factors (eg, digestive or other disorders in which nausea and vomiting are symptoms; drugs associated with nausea and vomiting).
- Interview regarding frequency, duration, and precipitating causes of nausea and vomiting. Also, question the client about accompanying signs and symptoms, characteristics of vomitus (amount; color; odor; presence of abnormal components, such as blood), and any measures that relieve nausea and vomiting. When possible, observe and measure the vomitus.

Nursing Diagnoses

- Deficient Fluid Volume related to uncontrolled vomiting
- Imbalanced Nutrition: Less Than Body Requirements related to impaired ability to ingest and digest food
- Altered Tissue Perfusion: Hypotension related to fluid volume depletion or antiemetic drug effect
- Risk for Injury related to adverse drug effects
- Deficient Knowledge related to nondrug measures to reduce nausea and vomiting and appropriate use of antiemetic drugs

Planning/Goals

The client will
- Receive antiemetic drugs at appropriate times, by indicated routes
- Take antiemetic drugs as prescribed for outpatient use
- Obtain relief of nausea and vomiting
- Eat and retain food and fluids
- Have increased comfort
- Maintain body weight
- Maintain normal bowel elimination patterns

● Have fewer vomiting episodes and less discomfort with cancer chemotherapy or surgical procedures

Interventions

Use measures to prevent or minimize nausea and vomiting.

● Assist clients to identify situations that cause or aggravate nausea and vomiting.
● Avoid exposure to stimuli when feasible (eg, unpleasant sights and odors; excessive ingestion of food, alcohol, or nonsteroidal anti-inflammatory drugs).
● Because pain may cause nausea and vomiting, administration of analgesics before painful diagnostic tests and dressing changes or other therapeutic measures may be helpful.
● Administer antiemetic drugs 30 to 60 minutes before a nausea-producing event (eg, radiation therapy, cancer chemotherapy, travel), when possible.
● Many oral drugs cause less gastric irritation, nausea, and vomiting if taken with or just after food. For any drug likely to cause nausea and vomiting, check reference sources to determine whether it can be given with food without altering beneficial effects.
● When nausea and vomiting occur, assess the client's condition and report to the physician. In some instances, a drug (eg, digoxin, an antibiotic) may need to be discontinued or reduced in dosage. In other instances (eg, paralytic ileus, GI obstruction), preferred treatment is restriction of oral intake and nasogastric intubation.
● Eating dry crackers before rising in the morning may help prevent nausea and vomiting associated with pregnancy.
● Avoid oral intake of food, fluids, and drugs during acute episodes of nausea and vomiting. Oral intake may increase vomiting and risks of fluid and electrolyte imbalances.
● Minimize activity during acute episodes of nausea and vomiting. Lying down and resting quietly are often helpful.

Give supportive care during vomiting episodes.

● Give replacement fluids and electrolytes. Offer small amounts of food and fluids orally when tolerated and according to client preference.
● Record vital signs, intake and output, and body weight at regular intervals if nausea or vomiting occurs frequently.
● Decrease environmental stimuli when possible (eg, noise, odors). Allow the client to lie quietly in bed when nauseated. Decreasing motion may decrease stimulation of the vomiting center in the brain.
● Help the client rinse his or her mouth after vomiting. Rinsing decreases the bad taste and corrosion of tooth enamel caused by gastric acid.
● Provide requested home remedies when possible (eg, a cool, wet washcloth to the face and neck).

Provide appropriate education for any drug therapy (see accompanying Client Teaching Guidelines).

Evaluation

● Observe and interview for decreased nausea and vomiting.
● Observe and interview regarding ability to maintain adequate intake of food and fluids.
● Compare current weight with baseline weight.
● Observe and interview regarding appropriate use of antiemetic drugs.

APPLYING YOUR KNOWLEDGE 62-2
What nursing measures, in addition to the administration of medication, should you implement to reduce Ms. Snyder's nausea and vomiting?

PRINCIPLES OF THERAPY

Drug Selection

Choice of an antiemetic drug depends largely on the cause of nausea and vomiting and the client's condition.

● The 5-HT$_3$ receptor antagonists (ondansetron, granisetron, dolasetron, and palonosetron) are usually the drugs of first choice for clients with chemotherapy-induced or postoperative nausea and vomiting. In chemotherapy, studies indicate greater effectiveness when combined with a corticosteroid (eg, dexamethasone).
● Drugs with anticholinergic and antihistaminic properties are preferred for motion sickness. Antihistamines such as meclizine and dimenhydrate are also useful for vomiting caused by labyrinthitis, uremia, or postoperative status.
● For ambulatory clients, drugs causing minimal sedation are preferred. However, most antiemetic drugs cause some sedation in usual therapeutic doses.
● Promethazine (Phenergan), a phenothiazine, is often used clinically for its antihistaminic, antiemetic, and sedative effects.
● Although phenothiazines are effective antiemetic agents, they may cause serious adverse effects (eg, hypotension, sedation, anticholinergic effects, extrapyramidal reactions that simulate signs and symptoms of Parkinson's disease). Consequently, phenothiazines other than promethazine usually should not be used, especially for pregnant, young, older, and postoperative clients, unless vomiting is severe and cannot be controlled by other measures.
● Metoclopramide (Reglan) may be preferred when nausea and vomiting are associated with nonobstructive gastric retention.

General Considerations

✔ Try to identify the circumstances that cause or aggravate nausea and vomiting and avoid them when possible.

✔ Drugs are more effective in preventing nausea and vomiting than in stopping them. Thus, they should be taken before the causative event when possible.

✔ Do not eat, drink, or take oral medications during acute vomiting episodes, to avoid aggravating the stomach upset.

✔ Lying down may help nausea and vomiting to subside; activity tends to increase stomach upset.

✔ After your stomach has settled down, try to take enough fluids to prevent dehydration and potentially serious problems. Tea, broth, and gelatins are usually tolerated.

✔ Do not drive an automobile or operate dangerous machinery if drowsy from antiemetic drugs, to avoid injury.

✔ If taking antiemetic drugs regularly, do not drink alcohol or take other drugs without consulting a health care provider. Several drugs interact with antiemetic agents, to increase adverse effects.

✔ Dronabinol, which is derived from marijuana and recommended only for nausea and vomiting associated with cancer chemo-

therapy, can cause dizziness, drowsiness, mood changes, and other mind-altering effects. You should avoid alcohol and other drugs that cause drowsiness. Also, do not drive or perform hazardous tasks requiring alertness, coordination, or physical dexterity, to decrease risks of injury.

Self- or Caregiver Administration

✔ Take the drugs as prescribed: Do not increase dosage, take more often, or take when drowsy, dizzy, or unsteady on your feet. Several of the drugs cause sedation and other adverse effects, which are more severe if too much is taken.

✔ To prevent motion sickness, take medication 30 minutes before travel and then every 4 to 6 hours, if necessary, to avoid or minimize adverse effects.

✔ Take or give antiemetic drugs 30 to 60 minutes before a nausea-producing event, when possible. This includes cancer chemotherapy, radiation therapy, painful dressings, or other treatments.

✔ Take dronabinol only when you can be supervised by a responsible adult because of its sedative and mind-altering effects.

Drug Dosage and Administration

Dosage and route of administration depend primarily on the reason for use.

- Doses of phenothiazines are much smaller for antiemetic effects than for antipsychotic effects.
- Most antiemetic agents are available in oral, parenteral, and rectal dosage forms. As a general rule, oral dosage forms are preferred for prophylactic use and rectal or parenteral forms are preferred for therapeutic use.
- Antiemetic drugs are often ordered PRN (as needed). As for any PRN drug, the client's condition should be assessed before drug administration.
- The use of antiemetic drugs is usually short term, from a single dose to a few days.
- When nausea and vomiting are likely to occur because of travel, administration of emetogenic anticancer drugs, diagnostic tests, or therapeutic procedures, an antiemetic drug should be given before the emetogenic event. Pretreatment usually increases client comfort and allows use of lower drug doses. It also may prevent aspiration and other potentially serious complications of vomiting.

Use in Special Populations

Use in Clients Undergoing Chemotherapy

Several anticancer drugs may cause severe nausea and vomiting and much discomfort for clients. Cisplatin is one of the

most emetogenic drugs. For this reason, new antiemetics are usually compared with older drugs in the treatment of cisplatin-induced nausea and vomiting. Some general management guidelines include the following:

- Chemotherapy may be given during sleeping hours.
- Some clients may experience less nausea and vomiting if they avoid or decrease food intake for a few hours before scheduled chemotherapy.
- Antiemetic drugs should be given before the emetogenic drug to prevent nausea and vomiting when possible. Most often, they are given IV for rapid effects and continued for 2 to 3 days. Continuous IV infusion may be more effective than intermittent bolus injections.
- The 5-HT$_3$ receptor antagonists (eg, ondansetron) are usually considered the most effective antiemetics. They may be given in a single daily dose.
- Metoclopramide, given IV in high doses, may be used alone or in combination with various other drugs. Diphenhydramine (Benadryl) may be given at the same time or PRN because high doses of metoclopramide often cause extrapyramidal effects (see Chap. 9).
- Various combinations of antiemetic and sedative-type drugs are used, and research continues in this area. A commonly used regimen for prophylaxis is a corticosteroid (eg, dexamethasone 8–10 mg) and a 5-HT$_3$ receptor antagonist (eg, dolasetron 1.8 mg/kg, granisetron 10 mcg/kg, ondansetron 16–32 mg, or palonosetron 0.25 mg).

Use in Children

Few studies of antiemetics have been done in children and their usage is not clearly defined. Thus, antiemetic drug therapy should be cautious and limited to prolonged vomiting of known etiology.

- With the 5-HT$_3$ receptor antagonists, safety and efficacy of granisetron and dolasetron have not been established for children younger than 2 years of age, and there is little information available about the use of ondansetron in children 3 years of age and younger. Safety and efficacy of palonosetron has not been established in clients below the age of 18 years.
- Phenothiazines are more likely to cause dystonias and other neuromuscular reactions in children than in adults. Promethazine is preferred because its action is more like that of the antihistamines than the phenothiazines. However, promethazine should not be used in children with hepatic disease, Reye's syndrome, a history of sleep apnea, or a family history of sudden infant death syndrome. Excessive doses may cause hallucinations, convulsions, and sudden death.
- Several antiemetics (eg, cyclizine, scopolamine) are not recommended for use in children younger than 12 years of age.
- Metoclopramide often causes extrapyramidal reactions (eg, dystonia) in children, even in small doses.
- Dronabinol may be used to prevent or treat chemotherapy-induced nausea and vomiting in children who do not respond to other antiemetic drugs. However, the drug should be used cautiously in children because of its psychoactive effects.

Use in Older Adults

Most antiemetic drugs cause drowsiness, especially in older adults, and therefore should be used cautiously. Efforts should be made to prevent nausea and vomiting when possible. Older adults are at risk of fluid volume depletion and electrolyte imbalances with vomiting.

Dronabinol should be used cautiously because older adults are usually more sensitive to the drug's psychoactive effects than young or middle-aged adults.

Use in Clients With Renal Impairment

Several drugs are commonly used for clients with renal impairment who have nausea and vomiting.

- Metoclopramide dosage should be reduced in clients with severe renal impairment to decrease drowsiness and extrapyramidal effects.

- Phenothiazines are metabolized primarily in the liver, and dosage reductions are not usually needed for clients with renal impairment. However, these drugs have anticholinergic effects and can cause urinary retention and orthostatic hypotension. They also can cause extrapyramidal symptoms and sedation in clients with end-stage renal disease (ESRD).

Use in Clients With Hepatic Impairment

Most antiemetic drugs are metabolized in the liver and should be used cautiously in clients with impaired hepatic function.

- With oral ondansetron, do not exceed an 8-mg dose; with IV use, a single, maximal daily dose of 8 mg is recommended.
- Phenothiazines are metabolized in the liver and eliminated in urine. In the presence of liver disease (eg, cirrhosis, hepatitis), metabolism may be slowed and drug elimination half-lives prolonged, with resultant accumulation and increased risk of adverse effects. Thus, the drugs should be used cautiously in clients with hepatic impairment. Cholestatic jaundice has been reported with promethazine.
- Dronabinol normally undergoes extensive first-pass hepatic metabolism to active and inactive metabolites. Resultant plasma levels consist of approximately equal portions of the parent drug and the main active metabolite. In addition, the drug is eliminated mainly by biliary excretion, over several weeks. Thus, long-term use at recommended doses may lead to accumulation of toxic amounts of the drug and its metabolite, even in clients with normal liver function.

    In clients with hepatic impairment, more of the parent drug and less of the active metabolite are likely to reach the bloodstream. Thus, therapeutic and adverse effects are less predictable. Also, impaired liver function can decrease metabolism and excretion in bile so that accumulation is likely and adverse effects may be increased and prolonged. The drug should be used very cautiously, if at all, in clients with moderate to severe hepatic impairment.

Use in Home Care

Antiemetics are usually given orally or by rectal suppository in the home setting. The home care nurse may need to assess clients for possible causes of nausea and vomiting and assist clients and caregivers with appropriate use of the drugs and other interventions to prevent fluid and electrolyte depletion. Teaching safety precautions with sedating drugs may also be needed.

N U R S I N G   A C T I O N S

Antiemetics

NURSING ACTIONS	RATIONALE/EXPLANATION
1. Administer accurately	
a. For prevention of motion sickness, give antiemetics 30 minutes before travel and q4–6h, if necessary.	To allow time for drug dissolution and absorption
b. For prevention of vomiting with cancer chemotherapy and radiation therapy, give antiemetic drugs 30–60 minutes before treatment.	Drugs are more effective in preventing than in stopping nausea and vomiting.
c. Inject intramuscular antiemetics deeply into a large muscle mass (eg, gluteal area).	To decrease tissue irritation
d. In general, do not mix parenteral antiemetics in a syringe with other drugs.	To avoid physical incompatibilities
e. Omit antiemetic agents and report to the physician if the client appears excessively drowsy or is hypotensive.	To avoid potentiating adverse effects and central nervous system (CNS) depression
f. Mix intravenous (IV) ondansetron in 50 mL of 5% dextrose or 0.9% sodium chloride injection and infuse over 15 minutes.	
g. Mix granisetron in 20–50 mL of 5% dextrose or 0.9% sodium chloride injection and infuse over 5 minutes.	
h. With dolasetron:	
(1) Give oral drug 1–2 hours before chemotherapy; give IV drug about 30 minutes before chemotherapy.	For oral administration to clients who cannot swallow tablets, dolasetron injection can be mixed in apple or apple–grape juice. Specific instructions should be obtained from a pharmacy. When kept at room temperature, the diluted oral solution should be used within 2 hours.
(2) Give IV drug (up to 100-mg dose) by direct injection over 30 seconds or longer or dilute up to 50 mL with 0.9% sodium chloride, 5% dextrose, or 5% dextrose and 0.45% sodium chloride and infuse over 15 minutes.	
i. Infuse palonosetron IV over 30 seconds. Do not mix with other drugs. Flush the IV line with normal saline before and after administration of palonosetron.	Manufacturer's instructions
2. Observe for therapeutic effects	
a. Verbal reports of decreased nausea	
b. Decreased frequency or absence of vomiting	
3. Observe for adverse effects	
a. Excessive sedation and drowsiness	Excessive sedation may occur with usual doses of antiemetics and is more likely to occur with high doses. This may be minimized by avoiding high doses and assessing the client's level of consciousness before each dose.
b. Anticholinergic effects—dry mouth, urinary retention	These effects are common to many antiemetic agents and are more likely to occur with large doses.
c. Hypotension, including orthostatic hypotension	Most likely to occur with phenothiazines; may also occur with 5-HT$_3$ antagonists
d. Extrapyramidal reactions—dyskinesia, dystonia, akathisia, parkinsonism	These disorders may occur with phenothiazines and metoclopramide.
e. With ondansetron and related drugs, observe for headache, diarrhea or constipation, dizziness, fatigue, and muscle aches. Bradycardia and hypotension may also occur.	These drugs are usually well tolerated, with mild to moderate adverse effects.

NURSING ACTIONS	RATIONALE/EXPLANATION
f. With dronabinol, observe for alterations in mood, cognition, and perception of reality; dysphoria; drowsiness; dizziness; anxiety; tachycardia; and conjunctivitis.	Tachycardia may be prevented with a beta-adrenergic blocking drug, such as propranolol (Inderal).
4. Observe for drug interactions	
a. Drugs that *increase* effects of antiemetic agents:	
(1) CNS depressants (alcohol, sedative-hypnotics, anti-anxiety agents, other antihistamines or antipsychotic agents)	Additive CNS depression
(2) Anticholinergics (eg, atropine)	Additive anticholinergic effects. Some phenothiazines and antiemetic antihistamines have strong anticholinergic properties.
(3) Antihypertensive agents	Additive hypotension
b. Drugs that alter effects of 5-HT$_3$ receptor antagonists:	
(1) Atenolol and cimetidine *increase* effects of dolasetron.	The drugs decrease dolasetron metabolism and clearance.
(2) Rifampin (and presumably other enzyme inducers) *decreases* effects of dolasetron and granisetron.	Enzyme inducers accelerate metabolism of affected drugs.

APPLYING YOUR KNOWLEDGE: ANSWERS

62-1 Assess for headache, diarrhea or constipation, dizziness, fatigue, and muscle aches.

62-2 Encourage Ms. Snyder to minimize activity during acute nausea and vomiting. Avoid oral intake of food, fluids, and drugs, because this may increase vomiting. Encourage Ms. Snyder to take antiemetics 30 to 60 minutes before meals or a nausea-producing event such as radiation or chemotherapy. Avoid exposure to stimuli as much as possible; this includes unpleasant sights and odors, alcohol, and excessive ingestion of food or drugs that irritate the gastric mucosa.

62-3 Diphenhydramine is given with metoclopramide to decrease metoclopramide's extrapyramidal effects.

62-4 You should follow the client's wishes whenever possible; however, Ms. Snyder needs to understand that the antiemetic medication will work much better when given to *prevent* nausea and vomiting rather than to *treat* it. Convey to her that the pretreatment approach will increase her comfort and allow the use of lower doses of the drugs.

Review and Application Exercises

Short Answer Exercises

1. List common causes of nausea and vomiting or circumstances in which nausea and vomiting often occur.

2. How do antiemetic drugs prevent or relieve nausea and vomiting?

3. What are adverse effects of commonly used antiemetics?

4. Are antiemetics more effective if given before, during, or after nausea and vomiting?

5. Which antiemetics are usually given to control the nausea and vomiting that occur with certain antineoplastic drugs?

NCLEX-Style Questions

6. Antiemetics are most effective when administered
   a. before an emetogenic event occurs
   b. during an episode of nausea, but before vomiting has occurred

c. after the client has experienced nausea and vomiting

d. timing of administration has no impact on drug effectiveness

7. The nurse would question an order for which of the following antiemetics for treatment of motion sickness–induced nausea?

a. prochlorperazine (Compazine)

b. dimenhydrinate (Dramamine)

c. meclizine (Antivert)

d. scopolamine (Transderm Scop)

8. When administering 5-HT$_3$ receptor antagonists prior to cancer chemotherapy, the nurse should also be prepared to administer which of the following adjunctive medications?

a. promethazine

b. dexamethasone

c. dronabinol

d. hydroxyzine

Selected References

Bender, C. M., McDaniel, R. W., Murphy-Ende, K., et al. (2002). Chemotherapy-induced nausea and vomiting. *Oncology Nursing, 6,* 94–102.

Drug facts and comparisons. (Updated monthly). St. Louis: Facts and Comparisons.

Fetrow, C. W., & Avila, J. R. (2001). *Professional's handbook of complementary & alternative medicines* (2nd ed.). Springhouse, PA: Springhouse.

Hasler, W. L. (2000). Approach to the patient with nausea and vomiting. In H. D. Humes (Ed.), *Kelley's Textbook of internal medicine* (4th ed., pp. 729–738). Philadelphia: Lippincott Williams & Wilkins.

Porth, C. M. (2005). Disorders of gastrointestinal function. In C. M. Porth, *Pathophysiology: Concepts of altered health states* (7th ed., pp. 885–916). Philadelphia: Lippincott Williams & Wilkins.

Powell, D. W. (2004). Approach to the patient with gastrointestinal disease. L. Goldman & D. Ausiello (Eds.), *Cecil textbook of medicine* (22nd ed., pp. 782–785). Philadelphia: W. B. Saunders.

Rosen, R. H. (2002). Management of chemotherapy-induced nausea and vomiting. *Journal of Pharmacy Practice, 15*(1), 32–41.

Taylor, A. T. (2002). Nausea and vomiting. In J. T. DiPiro, R. L. Talbert, G. C. Yee, G. R. Matzke, B. G. Wells, & L. M. Posey (Eds.), *Pharmacotherapy: A pathophysiologic approach* (5th ed., pp. 641–653). New York: McGraw-Hill.

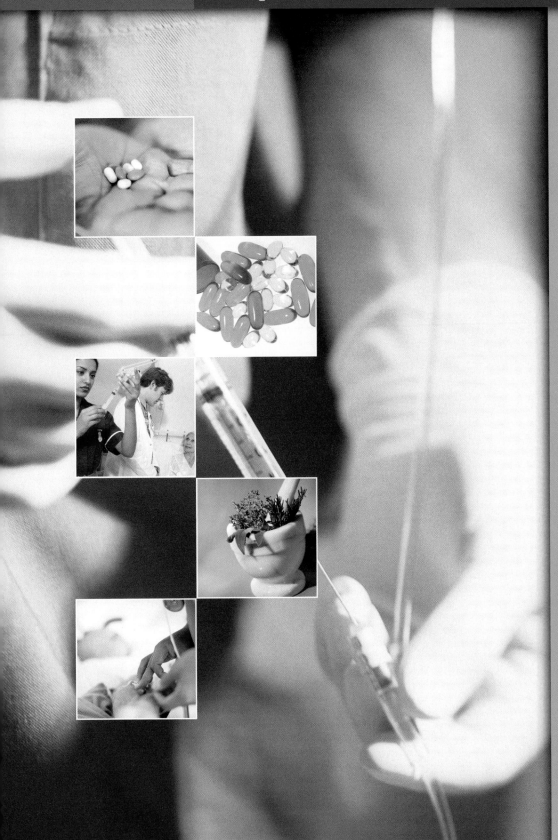

CHAPTER OUTLINE

63 Drugs Used in
Ophthalmic Conditions

64 Drugs Used in
Dermatologic
Conditions

65 Drug Use During
Pregnancy and
Lactation

Drugs Used in Ophthalmic Conditions

OBJECTIVES

After studying this chapter, you will be able to:

1. Review characteristics of ocular structures that influence drug therapy for eye disorders.
2. Discuss selected drugs in relation to their use in ocular disorders.
3. Use correct techniques to administer ophthalmic medications.
4. Assess for ocular effects of systemic drugs and systemic effects of ophthalmic drugs.
5. Teach clients, family members, or caregivers correct administration of eye medications.
6. For a client with an eye disorder, teach about the importance of taking medications as prescribed to protect and preserve eyesight.

APPLYING YOUR KNOWLEDGE

Irene Molnar is a 75-year-old woman who has glaucoma. You are a home care nurse visiting Mrs. Molnar. Her physician has prescribed the following:

Acetazolamide (Diamox), 250 mg PO, every 6 hours

Timolol (Timoptic), one drop in each eye, twice daily

Pilocarpine (Isopto-Carpine) one drop of 2% solution in each eye, three times daily

INTRODUCTION

Basic Structure and Function of the Eye

The eye is the major sensory organ through which a person receives information about the external environment. Extensive discussion of vision and ocular anatomy is beyond the scope of this chapter, but some characteristics and functions are described to facilitate understanding of ocular drug therapy. These include the following:

- The eyelids and lacrimal system function to protect the eye. The *eyelid* is a barrier to the entry of foreign bodies, strong light, dust, and other potential irritants. The *conjunctiva* is the mucous membrane lining of the eyelids. The *canthi* (singular, *canthus*) are the angles where the upper and lower eyelids meet. The *lacrimal system* produces a fluid that constantly moistens and cleanses the anterior surface of the eyeball. The fluid drains through two small openings in the inner canthus and flows through the nasolacrimal duct into the nasal cavity. When the conjunctiva is irritated or certain emotions are experienced (eg, sadness), the lacrimal gland produces more fluid than the drainage system can accommodate. The excess fluid overflows the eyelids and becomes *tears*.

- The eyeball is a spherical structure composed of the sclera, cornea, choroid, and retina, plus special refractive tissues. The *sclera* is a white, opaque, fibrous tissue that covers the posterior five sixths of the eyeball. The *cornea* is a transparent, special connective tissue that covers the anterior sixth of the eyeball. The cornea contains no blood vessels. The *choroid,* composed of blood vessels and connective tissue, continues forward to form the iris. The *iris* is composed of pigmented cells, the opening called the *pupil,* and muscles that control the size of the pupil by contracting or dilating in response to stimuli. The *retina* is the innermost layer of the eyeball.

- For vision to occur, light rays must enter the eye through the cornea; travel through the pupil, lens, and vitreous body (discussed later in chapter); and be focused on the retina. Light rays do not travel directly to the retina. Instead, they are deflected in various directions according to the density of the ocular structures through which they pass. This process, called *refraction,* is controlled by the aqueous humor, lens, and vitreous body. The *optic disk* is the area of the retina where ophthalmic blood vessels and the optic nerve enter the eyeball.

- The structure and function of the eyeball are further influenced by the lens, aqueous humor, and vitreous body. The *lens* is an elastic, transparent structure; its function is to focus light rays to form images on the retina. It is located behind the iris and is held in place by suspensory ligaments attached to the ciliary body. The *aqueous humor* is a clear fluid produced by capillaries in the ciliary body. Most of the fluid flows through the pupil into the anterior chamber (between the cornea and the lens and anterior to the iris). A small amount flows into a passage called *Schlemm's canal,* from which it enters the venous circulation. Normally, production and drainage of aqueous humor are approximately equal, and normal intraocular pressure (IOP) is maintained. Impaired drainage of aqueous humor causes increased IOP. The *vitreous body* is a transparent, jelly-like mass located in the posterior portion of the eyeball. It functions to refract light rays and maintain the normal shape of the eyeball.

Disorders of the Eye

The eye is subject to the development of many disorders that threaten its structure, function, or both. Some disorders in which ophthalmic drugs play a prominent role are discussed in the following sections.

Refractive Errors

Refractive errors include myopia (nearsightedness), hyperopia (farsightedness), presbyopia, and astigmatism. These conditions impair vision by interfering with the eye's ability to focus light rays on the retina. Ophthalmic drugs are used only in the diagnosis of the conditions; treatment involves prescription of eyeglasses or contact lenses.

Glaucoma

Glaucoma, a common preventable cause of blindness, is a group of diseases characterized by optic nerve damage and changes in visual fields. It is often characterized by increased IOP (>22 mm Hg), but may also occur with normal IOP (<21 mm Hg; average 15–16 mm Hg). Diagnostic tests for glaucoma include ophthalmoscopic examination of the optic disk, measurement of IOP (tonometry), and testing of visual fields.

The most common type of glaucoma is called primary open-angle glaucoma. Its etiology is unknown, but contributing factors include advanced age, a family history of glaucoma and elevated IOP, diabetes mellitus, hypertension, myopia, long-term use of corticosteroid drugs, and previous eye injury, inflammation, or infection. In addition, the incidence of glaucoma in African Americans is about three times higher than in non–African Americans. Closed-angle glaucoma is usually an acute situation requiring emergency surgery. It may occur when pupils are dilated and the outflow of aqueous humor is blocked. Darkness and drugs with anticholinergic effects (eg, atropine, antihistamines, tricyclic antidepressants) may dilate the pupil, reduce outflow of aqueous humor, and precipitate acute glaucoma.

Inflammatory or Infectious Conditions

Inflammation may be caused by bacteria, viruses, allergic reactions, or irritating chemicals. Infections may result from foreign bodies, contaminated hands, contaminated eye medications, or infections in contiguous structures (eg, nose, face, sinuses). Common inflammatory and infectious disorders include the following:

- **Conjunctivitis** is a common eye disorder that may be caused by allergens (eg, airborne pollens), bacterial or viral infections, or physical or chemical irritants. Symptoms include redness, tearing, itching, edema, and burning or gritty sensations. Bacterial conjunctivitis is often caused by *Staphylococcus aureus, Streptococcus pneumoniae,* or *Haemophilus influenzae* and produces mucopurulent drainage. Conjunctivitis with a purulent discharge is most often caused by the gonococcus; corneal ulcers and scarring may result.
- **Blepharitis** is a chronic infection of glands and lash follicles on the margins of the eyelids characterized by burning, redness, and itching. A hordeolum (commonly called a "stye") is often associated with blepharitis. The most common causes are seborrhea and staphylococcal infections.
- **Keratitis** (inflammation of the cornea) may be caused by microorganisms, trauma, allergy, ischemia, and drying of the cornea (eg, from inadequate lacrimation). The major symptom is pain, which ranges from mild to severe. Vision may not be affected initially. However, if not treated effectively, corneal ulceration, scarring, and impaired vision may result.
- **Bacterial corneal ulcers** are most often caused by pneumococci and staphylococci. Pseudomonal ulcers are less common but may rapidly progress to perforation. Fungal ulcers may follow topical corticosteroid therapy or injury with plant matter, such as a tree branch. Viral ulcers are usually caused by the herpesvirus.
- **Fungal infections** commonly occur and may often be attributed to frequent use of ophthalmic antibiotics and corticosteroids.

OPHTHALMIC DRUG THERAPY

Drug therapy of ophthalmic conditions is unique because of the location, structure, and function of the eye. Many systemic drugs are unable to cross the blood–eye barrier and achieve therapeutic concentrations in ocular structures. In general, penetration is greater if the drug achieves a high concentration in the blood, is fat soluble, and is poorly bound to serum proteins, and if inflammation is present.

Because of the difficulties associated with systemic therapy, various methods of administering drugs locally have been developed. The most common and preferred method is topical application of ophthalmic solutions or suspensions (eye drops) to the conjunctiva. Drugs are distributed through the tear film covering the eye and may be used for superficial disorders (eg, conjunctivitis) or for relatively deep ocular disorders (eg, glaucoma). Topical ophthalmic ointments may also be used. In addition, ophthalmologists may inject medications (eg, antibiotics, corticosteroids, local anesthetics) into or around various eye structures.

Classifications of Ophthalmic Drugs

Drugs used to diagnose or treat ophthalmic disorders represent numerous therapeutic classifications, most of which are discussed in other chapters. Major classes used in ophthalmology are described below.

Anesthetics (Local)

Topical ophthalmic anesthetics are used for various diagnostic and therapeutic procedures (eg, tonometry, removal of foreign bodies or sutures, minor surgery on the cornea and conjunctivae). Proparacaine is a commonly used agent; after administration of 1 drop, anesthesia begins within 20 seconds and lasts 10 to 15 minutes. Injectable local anesthetics are administered by ophthalmologists, usually for eye surgery. Lidocaine is commonly used; it has a rapid onset and lasts 1 to 2 hours.

Antihistamines and Mast Cell Stabilizers

Antihistamines (H_1 receptor antagonists) and mast cell stabilizers (eg, cromolyn) are used to decrease redness and itching associated with allergic conjunctivitis. Cromolyn acts by inhibiting the release of histamine and slow reacting substance of anaphylaxis (SRS-A) from mast cells. It is not useful in treatment of acute symptoms, and several days to weeks of use may be needed to elicit a therapeutic response.

Antimicrobials

Antimicrobials are used to treat bacterial, viral, and fungal infections of the external portion of the eye. Bacterial infections include conjunctivitis, keratitis, blepharitis, and corneal ulcers. The drugs are usually applied topically but may be given orally or intravenously. Sulfonamides (eg, sulfacetamide) are commonly used to treat bacterial conjunctivitis. They have activity against both gram-positive and gram-negative organisms. Bacitracin, neomycin, polymyxin, erythromycin, tetracycline, gentamicin, tobramycin, and several fluoroquinolones

(eg, ciprofloxacin, ofloxacin) are also commonly used topical antibacterial drugs. Natamycin is usually the drug of choice for fungal infections; trifluridine is used for viral infections.

Autonomic Nervous System Drugs

These drugs are used for diagnostic and therapeutic purposes (see Chaps. 16 through 20). Phenylephrine is often used to dilate the pupil before ophthalmologic examinations or surgical procedures. Dosage is usually 1 drop initially and a second drop in 5 to 10 minutes. Dilation occurs within 30 minutes and lasts 2 to 3 hours. Numerous drugs are used to decrease IOP in glaucoma; they act by decreasing formation or increasing outflow of aqueous humor. Ophthalmic beta-adrenergic blocking agents (eg, timolol) are most commonly used. Adrenergic vasoconstricting drugs are commonly used to decrease redness associated with allergic conjunctivitis.

Autonomic drugs indicated in one disorder may be contraindicated in another (eg, anticholinergic drugs may be contraindicated in glaucoma). In addition, adrenergic mydriatics (eg, phenylephrine) should be used cautiously in clients with hypertension, cardiac dysrhythmias, arteriosclerotic heart disease, and hyperthyroidism. Ophthalmic beta blockers usually have the same contraindications and precautions as oral or injected drugs (eg, bradycardia, heart block, bronchospastic disorders).

Corticosteroids

Corticosteroids (see Chap. 23) are often used to treat inflammatory conditions of the eye (eg, conjunctivitis, uveitis, keratitis), to reduce scarring and prevent loss of vision. The duration of treatment varies with the type of lesion and may range from a few days to several months. Corticosteroids are generally more effective in acute than chronic inflammatory conditions. Because these drugs are potentially toxic, they should not be used to treat minor disorders or disorders that can be effectively treated with safer drugs. When used, corticosteroids should be administered in the lowest effective dose and for the shortest effective time. Long-term use should be avoided when possible, because it may result in glaucoma, increased IOP, optic nerve damage, defects in visual acuity and fields of vision, cataracts, or secondary ocular infections.

Ophthalmologic corticosteroids may be administered topically, systemically, or both. They are contraindicated in eye infections caused by the herpesvirus because the drugs increase the severity of the infection. Ophthalmic preparations of corticosteroids combined with antimicrobial drugs are also available and commonly used for conditions in which both types of drugs are needed (eg, keratoconjunctivitis, postoperatively).

Nonsteroidal Anti-inflammatory Drugs (NSAIDs)

NSAIDs, in ophthalmic formulations for topical use, may be used in eye disorders (see Table 63-3 and Chap. 7). As in other conditions, the drugs are thought to act by blocking the synthesis of inflammatory prostaglandins. Some clinicians use combinations of topical NSAIDs and corticosteroids to manage inflammatory disorders.

Prostaglandin Analogs

These are antiglaucoma drugs that apparently reduce IOP by increasing the outflow of aqueous humor. The drugs may be used when a client's IOP is not lowered adequately with a beta blocker or when a beta blocker is contraindicated for a client. When compared with twice-daily ophthalmic timolol, the drugs were considered as effective as timolol. The drugs may be used in conjunction with other antiglaucoma medications (eg, a beta blocker or carbonic anhydrase inhibitor [CAI]) if multiple drugs are required.

In clinical trials, the incidence of systemic adverse effects was about the same as with placebo. The most common adverse effects were ocular burning, stinging, and itching. However, the drugs may cause a permanent darkening of eye color, especially in light-colored eyes, and alter eyelashes.

Nurses who are pregnant should be careful in handling prostaglandin analogs because these drugs may be absorbed through the skin. If accidental contact occurs, the exposed area should be washed immediately with soap and water.

Carbonic Anhydrase Inhibitors (CAIs) and Osmotic Agents

CAIs and osmotic agents are given to decrease IOP in glaucoma and before certain surgical procedures. CAIs lower IOP by decreasing production of aqueous humor. Oral CAIs are rarely used since the development of topical CAIs, beta blockers, and other newer glaucoma medications. Topical CAIs may be used alone but are most often used in combination with other glaucoma medications. With glycerin, a commonly used osmotic agent, maximum lowering of IOP occurs in 1 hour and lasts 4 to 5 hours.

Fluorescein

Fluorescein is a dye used in diagnosing lesions or foreign bodies in the cornea, fitting contact lenses, and studying the lacrimal system and flow of aqueous humor.

Individual Drugs

Individual drugs are described in Tables 63-1, 63-2, and 63-3.

(text continues on page 1031)

Table 63-1 Drugs at a Glance: Drugs Used in Ocular Disorders*

CLASSES OF DRUGS/ OCULAR EFFECTS	CLINICAL INDICATIONS	GENERIC/TRADE NAME	DOSAGE RANGES
Autonomic Nervous System Drugs			
ADRENERGICS			
Decreased production of aqueous humor	Glaucoma	**Dipivefrin (0.1% solution)** (Propine)	1 drop in affected eye(s) q12h
Mydriasis	Ophthalmoscopic examination	**Phenylephrine (2.5% and 10% solutions)**	Before ophthalmoscopy or refraction, 1 drop of
Decreased IOP	Reduction of adhesion	(Neo-Synephrine)	2.5% or 10% solution
Vasoconstriction	formation with uveitis		Preoperatively, 1 drop of
Photophobia	Preoperative and post-		2.5% or 10% solution
	operative mydriasis		30–60 min before
	Local hemostasis		surgery
			Postoperatively, 1 drop of 10% solution once or twice daily
			Children: Refraction, 1 drop of 2.5% solution
ALPHA₂ ADRENERGIC AGONISTS			
Decreased IOP	Glaucoma	**Apraclonidine** (Iopidine)	1 or 2 drops in affected eye(s) 3 times daily
	Prevention of increased IOP after ocular surgery	**Brimonidine** (Alphagan P)	1 drop in affected eye(s) 3 times daily, q8h
BETA BLOCKERS			
Decreased production of aqueous humor	Glaucoma	**Betaxolol** (Betoptic)	1 or 2 drops in affected eye(s) twice daily
Reduced IOP		**Carteolol**	1 drop in affected eye(s) twice daily

Table 63-1 Drugs at a Glance: Drugs Used in Ocular Disorders* (continued)

CLASSES OF DRUGS/ OCULAR EFFECTS	CLINICAL INDICATIONS	GENERIC/TRADE NAME	DOSAGE RANGES
		Levobunolol (Betagan)	1 or 2 drops in affected eye(s) once or twice daily
		Metipranolol (OptiPranolol)	1 drop in affected eye(s) twice daily
		Timolol maleate (Timoptic, Timoptic-XE)	1 drop in affected eye(s) twice daily; gel, 1 drop once daily
CHOLINERGICS Increased outflow of aqueous humor Miosis	Glaucoma	**Pilocarpine (0.25%–10% solutions)** (Isopto Carpine, Pilocar)	Glaucoma, 1 drop of 1% or 2% solution in each eye 3 or 4 times daily
		Pilocarpine ocular system (Ocusert Pilo-20 or -40)	One system in conjunctival sac per wk
		Carbachol (Carboptic)	2 drops of 0.75%–3% solution into eye(s) up to 3 times daily
ANTICHOLINERGICS Mydriasis Cycloplegia Photophobia	Mydriasis for refraction and other diagnostic purposes Before and after intraocular surgery Treatment of uveitis	**Atropine sulfate (0.5%– 3% solutions)**	Before intraocular surgery, 1 drop After intraocular surgery, 1 drop once daily
		Cyclopentolate hydrochloride (Cyclogyl)	For refraction, 1 drop of 0.5% or 2% solution Before ophthalmoscopy, 1 drop of 0.5% solution *Children:* For refraction, 1 drop of 0.5%, 1%, or 2% solution, repeated in 10 min
		Homatropine hydrobromide (2% and 5% solutions)	Refraction, 1 drop of 5% solution every 5 min for 2 or 3 doses or 1 or 2 drops of 2% solution every 10–15 min for 5 doses Uveitis, 1 drop of 2% or 5% solution 2 or 3 times daily
		Tropicamide (0.5% and 1% solutions) (Mydriacyl)	Before refraction or ophthalmoscopy, 1 drop, repeated in 5 min, then every 20–30 min as needed to maintain mydriasis
Diuretics **CARBONIC ANHYDRASE INHIBITORS** Decreased production of aqueous humor Decreased IOP	Glaucoma Preoperatively in intraocular surgery	**Acetazolamide** (Diamox)	PO 250 mg q6h; sustained-release capsules, PO 500 mg q12h IV, IM 5–10 mg/kg/d in divided doses, q6h *Children:* PO 10–15 mg/kg/d in divided doses, q6–8h IV, IM 5–10 mg/kg q6h

(continued)

Table 63-1 Drugs at a Glance: Drugs Used in Ocular Disorders* (continued)

CLASSES OF DRUGS/ OCULAR EFFECTS	CLINICAL INDICATORS	GENERIC/TRADE NAME	DOSAGE RANGES
		Brinzolamide (Azopt)	1 drop 3 times daily
		Dorzolamide (Trusopt)	1 drop 3 times daily
OSMOTIC AGENTS Reduced volume of vitreous humor Decreased IOP	Before intraocular surgery Treatment of acute glaucoma	**Glycerin** (Osmoglyn)	PO 1–1.5 g/kg, usually as a 50% or 75% solution 1–1½ h before surgery *Children:* Same as adults
		Isosorbide (Ismotic)	Emergency reduction of IOP, PO 1.5 g/kg up to 4 times daily
		Mannitol (Osmitrol)	IV 1.5–2 g/kg as a 20% solution over 30–60 min *Children:* Same as adults
Prostaglandin Analogs Decreased IOP	Glaucoma	**Bimatoprost** (Lumigan)	1 drop once daily in the evening
		Latanoprost (Xalatan)	1 drop once daily in the evening
		Travoprost (Travatan)	1 drop once daily in the evening
		Unoprostone (Rescula)	1 drop twice daily
Miscellaneous Agents **ANESTHETICS, LOCAL** Surface anesthesia of conjunctiva and cornea	Tonometry Removal of foreign bodies Removal of sutures	**Proparacaine** (Alcaine, Ophthaine)	Minor procedures, 1 or 2 drops of 0.5% solution
		Tetracaine (Pontocaine)	Minor procedures, 1 or 2 drops of 0.5% solution
LUBRICANTS Serve as "artificial tears"	Protect the cornea during keratitis or diagnostic procedures Moisten contact lenses	**Methylcellulose** (Methulose)	1 or 2 drops as needed
		Polyvinyl alcohol (Liquifilm)	1 or 2 drops as needed

*Antimicrobial agents are listed in Table 63-2; anti-allergic and anti-inflammatory agents are listed in Table 63-3.

IM, intramuscular; IOP, intraocular pressure; IV, intravenous; PO, oral.

Table 63-2 Drugs at a Glance: Ophthalmic Antimicrobial Agents

GENERIC/TRADE NAME	DOSAGE RANGES	
	Adults	Children
Antibacterial Agents **Ciprofloxacin 3.5 mg/mL solution** (Ciloxan)	Corneal ulcer: Day 1, 2 drops q 15min for 6 h, then q30min for rest of day; day 2, 2 drops q1h; days 3–14, 2 drops q4h Conjunctivitis: 1 or 2 drops q2h while awake for 2 d, then 1 or 2 drops q4h while awake for 5 d	Safety and efficacy not established in infants <1 y
Erythromycin 5% ointment (Ilotycin)		Prevention of neonatal gonococcal or chlamydial conjunctivitis, 0.5–1 cm in each eye

Table 63-2 Drugs at a Glance: Ophthalmic Antimicrobial Agents (continued)

| GENERIC/TRADE NAME | DOSAGE RANGES | |
	Adults	Children
Gatifloxacin (Zymar)	1 drop in affected eye(s) every 2 h while awake, up to 8 times daily, for 2 d, then 1 drop up to 4 times daily while awake, for 5 d	Dosage not established
Gentamicin 3 mg/mL solution or 3 mg/g ointment (Garamycin)	1 drop q1–4h; ointment, apply 2 or 3 times daily	Same as adults
Levofloxacin 5 mg/mL solution (Quixin)	1 or 2 drops q2h up to 8 doses/d for 1 or 2 d, then q4h up to 4 doses/d for 5 d	Dosage not established
Moxifloxacin (Vigamox)	1 drop in affected eye(s) 3 times daily for 7 d	Same as adults for children 1 y and older
Norfloxacin 3mg/mL (Chibroxacin)	1–2 drops, 4 times daily up to 7 d	Same as adults for children 1 y and older
Ofloxacin 3 mg/mL solution (Ocuflox)	Conjunctivitis: 1 or 2 drops q2–4h while awake for 2 d, then 4 times daily for 3–5 d	Same as adults for children 1 y and older
	Corneal ulcer: 1 or 2 drops q30min while awake, q4–6h during sleep, for 1–2 d, then q1h while awake for 4–6 d, then q4h while awake until healed	Dosage not established
Sulfacetamide 10% solution or ointment (Bleph-10), **15% solution** (Isopto Cetamide), **10% and 30% solution, 10% ointment** (Sodium Sulamyd)	Conjunctivitis, corneal ulcers, or other superficial infections caused by susceptible organisms: 1 or 2 drops q4h or 0.5 inch ointment 3 or 4 times daily, for 7–10 days	Safety and efficacy not established. Contraindicated in infants <2 mo of age
Sulfisoxazole 4% solution (Gantrisin)	1 or 2 drops 3 or more times daily	Safety and efficacy not established. Contraindicated in infants <2 mo of age
Tobramycin (0.3% solution and 3 mg/g ointment) (Tobrex)	1 or 2 drops 2–6 times daily or ointment 2 or 3 times daily	See manufacturer's instructions
Antiviral Agent **Trifluridine 1% solution** (Viroptic)	Keratoconjunctivitis or corneal ulcers caused by herpes simplex virus: 1 drop q2h while awake (maximum, 9 drops/d) until corneal ulcer heals, then 1 drop q4h (minimum, 5 drops/d), for 7 d	>6 y: Same as adults
Antifungal Agent **Natamycin 5% suspension** (Natacyn)	1 drop q1–2h for 3–4 d, then q3–4h for 14–21 d	Safety and efficacy not established

Table 63-3 Drugs at a Glance: Topical Ophthalmic Antiallergic and Anti-Inflammatory Agents

GENERIC/TRADE NAME	INDICATIONS FOR USE	ROUTES AND DOSAGE RANGES
Antiallergic Agents **Azelastine** (Optivar)	Allergic conjunctivitis	1 drop in affected eye(s) twice daily
Cromolyn (Crolom, Opticrom)	Treatment of seasonal allergic conjunctivitis, keratitis, and keratoconjunctivitis	1 or 2 drops in each eye 4–6 times daily at regular intervals

(continued)

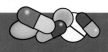

Table 63-3 Drugs at a Glance: Topical Ophthalmic Antiallergic and Anti-Inflammatory Agents (continued)

GENERIC/TRADE NAME	INDICATIONS FOR USE	DOSAGE RANGES
Emedastine (Emadine)	Allergic conjunctivitis	1 or 2 drops twice daily
Epinastine (Elestat)	Allergic conjunctivitis	1 drop in each eye twice daily
Ketotifen (Zaditor)	Allergic conjunctivitis	1 drop in affected eye(s) q8–12h
Levocabastine (Livostin)	Treatment of seasonal allergic conjunctivitis	1 drop in affected eyes 4 times daily, for up to 2 wk
Lodoxamide (Alomide)	Conjunctivitis Keratitis	1 or 2 drops in affected eye(s) 4 times daily, for up to 3 mo
Olopatadine (Patanol)	Allergic conjunctivitis	1 or 2 drops twice daily
Corticosteroids		
Dexamethasone (Decadron, Maxidex)	Inflammatory disorders of the conjunctiva, cornea, eyelid, and anterior eyeball (eg, conjunctivitis, keratitis) Corneal injury from chemical, radiation, or thermal burns, or penetration of foreign bodies Prevention of graft rejection after corneal transplant	Solution or suspension 1 or 2 drops q1h daytime, q2h nighttime until response; then 1 drop q4h Postoperative inflammation, 1 or 2 drops 4 times daily, starting 24 h after surgery, for 2 wk Ointment thin strip 3 or 4 times daily until response, then once or twice daily
Fluorometholone (FML)	Inflammatory disorders	Solution 1 drop q1–2h until response, then less often Ointment thin strip 3 or 4 times daily until response, then once or twice daily
Loteprednol (Lotemax, Alrex)	Allergic conjunctivitis Keratitis Treatment of inflammation after ocular surgery	Allergic conjunctivitis, 0.2%, 1 drop in affected eye(s) 4 times daily Keratitis, 0.5%, 1 or 2 drops in affected eye(s) 4 times daily Postoperative inflammation, 0.5%, 1 or 2 drops in affected eye(s) 4 times daily starting 24 h after surgery and continuing for 2 wk
Medrysone (HMS)	Inflammatory disorders	1 drop q1–2h until response obtained, then less frequently
Prednisolone (Econopred, others)	Inflammatory disorders	Solution or suspension 1 or 2 drops q1–2h until response, then 1 drop q4h, then less frequently Ointment thin strip 3 or 4 times daily until response, then once or twice daily
Rimexolone (Vexol)	Treatment of anterior uveitis Treatment of inflammation after ocular surgery	Uveitis, 1 or 2 drops in affected eye q1h during waking hours for 1 wk, then 1 drop q2h for 1 wk, then taper until uveitis resolved Postoperative inflammation, 1 or 2 drops in affected eye(s) 4 times daily starting 24 h after surgery and continuing for 2 wk
Nonsteroidal Anti-Inflammatory Drugs		
Diclofenac (Voltaren)	Treatment of inflammation after cataract surgery	1 drop to affected eye 4 times daily, starting 24 h after surgery, for 2 wk
Flurbiprofen (Ocufen)	Inhibition of pupil constriction during eye surgery	1 drop q30min for 4 doses, starting 2 h before surgery
Ketorolac (Acular)	Treatment of ocular itching due to seasonal allergic conjunctivitis	1 drop 4 times daily for approximately 1 wk
Suprofen (Profenal)	Inhibition of pupil constriction during eye surgery	2 drops at 3, 2, and 1 h before surgery or q4h while awake the day before surgery

NURSING PROCESS

Assessment

Assess the client's condition in relation to ophthalmic disorders.

● Determine whether the client has impaired vision and, if so, the extent or severity of the impairment. Minimal assessment includes the vision-impaired client's ability to participate in activities of daily living, including safe ambulation. Maximal assessment depends on the nurse's ability and working situation. Some nurses do vision testing and ophthalmoscopic examinations.
● Identify risk factors for eye disorders. These include trauma, allergies, infection in one eye (a risk factor for infection in the other eye), use of contact lenses, infections of facial structures or skin, and occupational exposure to chemical irritants or foreign bodies.
● Signs and symptoms vary with particular disorders:
  ● Pain is usually associated with corneal abrasions or inflammation. Sudden, severe pain may indicate acute glaucoma, which requires immediate treatment to lower IOP and minimize damage to the optic nerve.
  ● Signs of inflammation (redness, edema, heat, tenderness) are especially evident with infection or inflammation of external ocular structures, such as the eyelids and conjunctiva. A watery or mucoid discharge also often occurs.
  ● Pruritus is most often associated with allergic conjunctivitis.
  ● Photosensitivity commonly occurs with keratitis.

Nursing Diagnoses

● Disturbed Sensory Perception: Visual, related to eye disorders
● Risk for Injury: Blindness related to inadequately treated glaucoma or ophthalmic infections
● Deficient Knowledge related to prevention and treatment of ocular disorders

Planning/Goals

The client will
● Take ophthalmic medications as prescribed
● Follow safety precautions to protect eyes from trauma and disease
● Experience improvement in signs and symptoms (eg, decreased drainage with infections, decreased eye pain with glaucoma)
● Avoid injury from impaired vision (eg, falls)
● Avoid systemic effects of ophthalmic drugs
● Have regular eye examinations to monitor effects of antiglaucoma drugs

Interventions

Use measures to minimize ocular disorders.

● Promote regular eye examinations. This is especially important among middle-aged and older adults, who are more likely to have several types of ocular disorders. These clients are also more likely to experience ocular disorders as adverse effects of drugs taken for non-ocular disorders.
● Assist clients at risk of eye damage from IOP (eg, those with glaucoma; those who have had intraocular surgery, such as cataract removal) to avoid straining at stool (use laxatives or stool softeners if needed), heavy lifting, bending over, coughing, and vomiting when possible.
● Promote handwashing and keeping hands away from eyes to prevent eye infections.
● Cleanse contact lenses or assist clients in lens care, when needed.
● Treat eye injuries appropriately:
  ● For chemical burns, irrigate the eyes with copious amounts of water as soon as possible (ie, near the area where the injury occurred). Do not wait for transport to a first-aid station, hospital, or other health care facility. Damage continues as long as the chemical is in contact with the eye.
  ● For thermal burns, apply cold compresses to the area.
  ● Superficial foreign bodies may be removed by irrigation with water. Foreign bodies embedded in ocular structures must be removed by a physician.
  ● Warm, wet compresses are often useful in ophthalmic inflammation or infections. They relieve pain and promote healing by increasing the blood supply to the affected area.

Provide appropriate teaching for any drug therapy (see accompanying Client Teaching Guidelines).

Evaluation

● Observe and interview for compliance with instructions regarding drug therapy and follow-up care.
● Observe and interview for relief of symptoms.
● Observe for systemic adverse effects of ophthalmic drugs (eg, tachycardia and dysrhythmias with adrenergics; bradycardia or bronchoconstriction with beta blockers).

APPLYING YOUR KNOWLEDGE 63-1
When you arrive at Mrs. Molnar's house, she is in the middle of brushing her hair. She drops her hair brush and bends over to pick it up. This provides an opportunity to provide what client teaching?

General Considerations

✔ Prevent eye disorders, when possible. For example, try to avoid long periods of reading and computer work; minimize exposure to dust, smog, cigarette smoke, and other eye irritants; wash hands often and avoid touching the eyes to decrease risks of infection. Use protective eyewear when indicated.

✔ Do not use nonprescription eye drops (eg, Murine, Visine) on a regular basis for longer than 48 to 72 hours. Persistent eye irritation and redness should be reported to a health care provider.

✔ Have regular eye examinations and testing for glaucoma after 40 years of age.

✔ Eye-drop preparations often contain sulfites, which can cause allergic reactions in some people.

✔ If you have glaucoma, do not take any drugs without the ophthalmologist's knowledge and consent. Many drugs given for purposes other than eye disorders may cause or aggravate glaucoma. Also, wear a medical alert bracelet or carry identification that states you have glaucoma. This helps to avoid administration of drugs that aggravate glaucoma or to maintain treatment of glaucoma, in emergencies.

✔ If you have an eye infection, wash hands before and after contact with the infected eye to avoid spreading the infection to the unaffected eye or to other people. Also, avoid touching the unaffected eye.

✔ If you wear contact lenses, wash your hands before inserting them and follow instructions for care (eg, cleaning, inserting or removing, and duration of wear). Improper or infrequent cleaning may lead to infection. Overwearing is a common cause of corneal abrasion and may cause corneal ulceration. The lens wearer should consult an ophthalmologist when eye pain occurs. Antibiotics are often prescribed for corneal abrasions to prevent development of ulcers.

✔ If you wear soft contact lenses, do not use any eye medication without consulting a specialist in eye care. Some eye drops contain benzalkonium hydrochloride, a preservative, which is absorbed by soft contacts. The medication should not be applied while wearing soft contacts and should be instilled 15 minutes or longer before inserting soft contacts.

✔ Never use eye medications used by someone else and never allow your eye medications to be used by anyone else. These preparations should be used by one person only and they are dispensed

in small amounts for this purpose. Single-person use minimizes cross-contamination and risks of infection.

✔ Many eye drops and ointments cause temporary blurring of vision. Do not use such medications just before driving or operating potentially hazardous machinery.

✔ Avoid straining at stool (use laxatives or stool softeners if necessary), heavy lifting, bending over, coughing, and vomiting when possible. These activities increase intraocular pressure, which may cause eye damage in glaucoma and after eye surgery.

Self-Administration

✔ If using more than one eye medication, be sure to administer the correct one at the correct time. Benefits depend on accurate administration.

✔ Check expiration dates; do not use any eye medication after the expiration date and do not use any liquid medications that have changed color or contain particles.

✔ Shake the container if instructed to do so on the label. Solutions do not need to be shaken; suspensions should be shaken well to ensure the drug is evenly dispersed in the liquid and not settled in the bottom of the container.

✔ Wash hands thoroughly.

✔ Tilt head back or lie down and look up.

✔ Pull the lower eyelid down to expose the conjunctiva (mucous membrane).

✔ Place the dropper directly over the eye. Avoid contact of the dropper with the eye, finger, or any other surface. Such contact contaminates the solution and may cause eye infections and serious damage to the eye, with possible loss of vision.

✔ Look up just before applying a drop; look down for several seconds after applying a drop.

✔ Release the eyelid, close the eyes, and press on the inside corner of the eye with a finger for 3 to 5 minutes. Closing the eyes and blocking the tear duct helps the medication be more effective by slowing its drainage out of the eye.

✔ Do not rub the eye; do not rinse the dropper.

✔ If more than one eye drop is ordered, wait 5–10 minutes before instilling the second medication.

✔ Use the same basic procedure to insert eye ointments.

PRINCIPLES OF THERAPY

General Guidelines for Ophthalmic Drug Therapy

● Topical application is the most common route of administration for ophthalmic drugs, and correct administration is essential for optimal therapeutic effects.

● Systemic absorption of eye drops can be decreased by closing the eye and applying pressure over the tear

duct (nasolacrimal occlusion) for 3 to 5 minutes after instillation.

● When multiple eye drops are required, there should be an interval of 5 to 10 minutes between drops because of limited eye capacity and rapid drainage into tear ducts.

● Absorption of eye medications is increased in eye disorders associated with hyperemia and inflammation.

● Many ophthalmic drugs are available as eye drops (solutions or suspensions) and ointments. Ointments are administered less frequently than drops and often produce higher concentrations of drug in target tissues. However, they also cause blurred vision, which limits their daytime use, at least for ambulatory clients. In some situations, drops may be used during waking hours and ointments at bedtime.

- Topical ophthalmic medications should not be used after the expiration date; cloudy, discolored solutions should be discarded.
- Topical eye medications contain a number of inactive ingredients, such as preservatives, buffers, tonicity agents, antioxidants, and so forth. Some contain sulfites, to which some people may have allergic reactions.
- Some eye drops contain benzalkonium hydrochloride, a preservative, which is absorbed by soft contact lenses. The medications should not be applied while wearing soft contacts and should be instilled 15 minutes or longer before inserting soft contacts.
- To increase safety and accuracy of ophthalmic drug therapy, the labels and caps of eye medications are color coded.

APPLYING YOUR KNOWLEDGE 63-2

You are teaching Mrs. Molnar how to administer her medication. What do you teach her about administering eye drops?

Ocular Infections

Guidelines for drug therapy of ocular infections include the following:

- Drug therapy is usually initiated as soon as culture material (eye secretions) has been obtained, often with a broad-spectrum antibacterial agent or a combination of two or more antibiotics.
- Topical administration is used most often, and recommended drugs include bacitracin, polymyxin B, and sulfacetamide. These agents are rarely given systemically. They do not cause sensitization to commonly used systemic antibiotics and do not promote growth of drug-resistant microorganisms. Other antibacterial drugs available in ophthalmic formulations include erythromycin, gentamicin, tobramycin, several fluoroquinolones (ciprofloxacin, gatifloxacin, moxifloxacin, norfloxacin, ofloxacin), and combination products.
- In severe infections, antibacterial drugs may be given both topically and systemically. Because systemic antibiotics penetrate the eye poorly, large doses are required to attain therapeutic drug concentrations in ocular structures. Drugs that reach therapeutic levels in the eye when given in proper dosage include ampicillin and dicloxacillin. Gentamicin and other antibiotics penetrate the eye when inflammation is present.
- Combination products containing two or more antibacterials are available for topical treatment of external ocular infections. These products are most useful when

therapy must be initiated before the infecting microorganism is identified. Mixtures (eg, polymyxin B and bacitracin) provide a broader spectrum of antibacterial activity than a single drug.

- Fixed-dose combinations of an antibacterial agent and a corticosteroid are available for topical use in selected conditions (eg, staphylococcal keratitis, blepharoconjunctivitis, bacterial conjunctivitis, some postoperative inflammatory reactions). Neomycin and corticosteroid mixtures include NeoDecadron. Neomycin, polymyxin B, and corticosteroid mixtures include Poly-Pred and Maxitrol. Neomycin, polymyxin B, bacitracin, and corticosteroid mixtures include Cortisporin. Sulfacetamide and corticosteroid mixtures include Blephamide, Metimyd, and Vasocidin.
- Trifluridine (Viroptic) is the drug of choice in eye infections caused by the herpes simplex virus. Ganciclovir and fomiversin are available for treatment of cytomegalovirus (CMV) retinitis in clients with acquired immunodeficiency syndrome (AIDS). These intravitreal preparations are administered by an ophthalmologist.
- Natamycin (Natacyn) is the drug of choice in fungal eye infections. It has a broad spectrum of antifungal activity and is nonirritating and nontoxic.

Corneal Abrasions

Injuries to the cornea cause pain, tearing, photophobia, and a foreign-body sensation or gritty feeling in the eye. These symptoms can be worsened by exposure to light, blinking, and rubbing the injured surface against the inside of the eyelid. Initial management involves removal of foreign bodies, and analgesia with topical NSAIDs or oral analgesics. Topical antibiotics also may be used. Most corneal abrasions heal in 24 to 72 hours.

Clients who wear contact lenses are at higher risk of developing abrasions that become infected and ulcerate. For these clients, an antipseudomonal antibiotic (eg, gentamicin or a fluoroquinolone) should be used. In addition, the client should avoid wearing contact lenses until the abrasion is healed and antibiotic therapy completed.

Glaucoma

For chronic glaucoma, the goal of drug therapy is to slow disease progression by reducing IOP. Topical beta blockers are first-line drugs and commonly used. They may be used alone or in combination with other antiglaucoma drugs. Several are available for ophthalmic use. Most adverse effects of systemic beta blockers may also occur with ophthalmic preparations and their use may be restricted in clients with respiratory or cardiac disease.

Other first-line drugs, which may be used with or instead of beta blockers, include brimonidine, prostaglandin analogs, and topical CAIs. Apraclonidine, dipivefrin, epinephrine, and pilocarpine are second-line drugs, mainly because of more adverse effects than first-line agents.

Use in Special Populations

Use in Children

Topical ophthalmic drug therapy in children differs little from that in adults. Few studies of ophthalmic drug therapy in children have been reported, and many conditions for which adults need therapy (eg, cataract, glaucoma) rarely occur in children. A major use of topical ophthalmic drugs in children is to dilate the pupil and paralyze accommodation for ophthalmoscopic examination. As a general rule, the short-acting mydriatics and cycloplegics (eg, cyclopentolate, tropicamide) are preferred because they cause fewer systemic adverse effects than atropine and scopolamine. In addition, lower drug concentrations are usually given empirically because of the smaller size of children and the potential risk of systemic adverse effects.

Use in Older Adults

Older adults are at risk for development of ocular disorders, especially glaucoma and cataracts. General principles of ophthalmic drug therapy are the same as for younger adults. In addition, older adults are likely to have cardiovascular disorders that may be aggravated by systemic absorption of topical eye medication. Thus, accurate dosage and occlusion of the nasolacrimal duct in the inner canthus of the eye are needed to prevent adverse drug effects (eg, hypertension, tachycardia, or dysrhythmias with adrenergic drugs; bradycardia, heart block, or bronchoconstriction with beta blockers).

Use in Home Care

The home care nurse may be involved in the care of clients with acute or chronic eye disorders. As with other drug therapy, the nurse may need to teach clients and caregivers reasons for use, accurate administration, and assessment of therapeutic and adverse responses to eye medications. The nurse may also need to encourage periodic eye examinations and measurements of IOP to promote optimal vision and prevent blindness.

N U R S I N G   A C T I O N S

Ophthalmic Drugs

NURSING ACTIONS	RATIONALE/EXPLANATION
1. Administer accurately	
a. Read labels of ophthalmic medications carefully.	To avoid error, because many drugs are available in several concentrations
b. Read medication orders carefully and accurately.	To avoid error. Avoid abbreviations (eg, OS, OD, OU) when possible.
c. For hospitalized clients, keep eye medications at the bedside.	Eye medications should be used by one person only. They are dispensed in small amounts for this purpose. This minimizes cross-contamination and risk of infection.
d. Wash hands before approaching the client for instillation of eye medications.	To reduce risks of infection
e. To administer eye drops, have the client lie down or tilt the head backward and look upward. Then, pull down the lower lid to expose the conjunctival sac, and drop the medication into the sac. After instillation, have the client close the eyes gently, and apply pressure to the inner canthus.	Drug absorption and concentration in ocular tissues depend partly on the length of time the medication is in contact with ocular tissues. Contact time is increased by closing the eyes (delays outflow into the nasolacrimal duct) and by placing pressure on the inner canthus (delays outflow and decreases side effects resulting from systemic absorption).
f. When instilling ophthalmic ointments, position the client as above, and apply a ¼-inch to ½-inch strip of ointment to the conjunctiva.	
g. Do not touch the dropper tip or ointment top to the eye or anything else.	To avoid contamination of the medication and infection
h. When crusts or secretions are present, cleanse the eye before administering medication.	If the eye is not cleansed, the drug may not be absorbed.

NURSING ACTIONS	RATIONALE/EXPLANATION
i. When two or more eye drops are scheduled for the same time, they should be instilled at least 5 minutes, but preferably 10 minutes apart.	To avoid drug loss by dilution and outflow into the nasolacrimal duct
2. Observe for therapeutic effects	Therapeutic effects depend on the reason for use.
a. With beta-blocking agents, observe for decreased intraocular pressure (IOP).	Lowering of IOP usually occurs within a month; periodic measurements should be done.
b. With mydriatics, observe for dilation of the pupil.	Mydriasis begins within 5–15 minutes after instillation.
c. With miotics, observe for constriction of the pupil.	
d. With antimicrobial drugs, observe for decreased redness, edema, and drainage.	
e. With osmotic agents, observe for decreased IOP.	With oral glycerin, maximal decrease in IOP occurs approximately 1 hour after administration, and effects persist for about 5 hours. With intravenous (IV) mannitol, maximal decreased IOP occurs within 30–60 minutes and lasts 6–8 hours.
3. Observe for adverse effects	
a. Local effects:	
(1) Irritation, burning, stinging, blurred vision, discomfort, redness, itching, tearing, conjunctivitis, keratitis, allergic reactions	These effects may occur with any topical ophthalmic agent. Burning and stinging occur with instillation and are usually transient. Allergic reactions may occur with the active ingredient, preservatives, or other components.
(2) With prostaglandin analogs—permanent darkening of eye color may occur, especially in light-colored eyes. Changes in the length and thickness of eyelashes may also occur.	Changes in eye color and eyelashes may not be noticeable for months to years after starting drug use. These effects are most problematic in clients receiving treatment in one eye.
(3) With antibacterial agents—superinfection or sensitization	Superinfection caused by drug-resistant organisms may occur. Sensitization means that topical application induces antibody formation. Therefore, if the same or a related drug is subsequently administered systemically, an allergic reaction may occur. Sensitization can be prevented or minimized by avoiding topical administration of antibacterial agents that are commonly given systemically.
(4) With anticholinergics, adrenergics, corticosteroids—glaucoma or increased IOP	Mydriatic drugs (anticholinergics and adrenergics) may cause an acute attack of angle closure in clients with closed-angle glaucoma by blocking outflow of aqueous humor. Topical corticosteroids raise IOP in some clients. The "glaucomatous" response occurs most often in clients with chronic, primary open-angle glaucoma and their relatives. It also may occur in clients with myopia or diabetes mellitus. The magnitude of increased IOP depends on the concentration, frequency of administration, duration of therapy, and anti-inflammatory potency of the corticosteroid. This effect can be minimized by checking IOP every 2 months in clients receiving long-term therapy with topical corticosteroids.
(5) With miotic drugs—decreased vision in dim light	These agents prevent pupil dilation, which normally occurs in dim light or darkness.

(continued)

NURSING ACTIONS	RATIONALE/EXPLANATION
b. Systemic effects:	Systemic absorption and adverse effects of eye drops can be prevented or minimized by closing the eyes or applying pressure to the inner canthus (nasolacrimal occlusion) after instillation of the medications. Pressure may be applied by the nurse or the client.
(1) With beta-blocking agents—bradycardia, bronchospasm, and others (see Chap. 18)	These agents may be absorbed systematically and cause all the adverse effects associated with oral or injected drugs.
(2) With miotics—sweating, nausea, vomiting, diarrhea, abdominal pain, bradycardia, hypotension, bronchoconstriction. Toxic doses produce ataxia, confusion, convulsions, coma, respiratory failure, and death.	These cholinergic or parasympathomimetic effects occur rarely with pilocarpine or carbachol. Acute toxicity may be reversed by an anticholinergic agent, atropine, given IV.
(3) With anticholinergic mydriatics—dryness of the mouth and skin, fever, rash, tachycardia, confusion, hallucinations, delirium	These effects are most likely to occur with atropine and in children and older adults. Tropicamide (Mydriacyl) rarely causes systemic reactions.
(4) With adrenergic mydriatics—tachycardia, hypertension, premature ventricular contractions, tremors, headache	Systemic effects are uncommon. They are more likely to occur with repeated instillations of high drug concentrations (eg, epinephrine 2%, phenylephrine [Neo-Synephrine] 10%).
(5) With carbonic anhydrase inhibitors—anorexia, nausea, vomiting, diarrhea, paresthesias, weakness, lethargy	Nausea, malaise, and paresthesias (numbness and tingling of extremities) commonly occur with oral drugs, which are given only when topical drugs are not effective.
(6) With osmotic diuretics—dehydration, nausea, vomiting, headache, hyperglycemia and glycosuria with glycerin (Osmoglyn)	These agents may produce profound diuresis and dehydration. Oral agents (eg, glycerin) are less likely to cause severe systemic effects than IV agents (eg, mannitol). These agents are usually given in a single dose, which decreases the risks of serious adverse reactions unless large doses are given.
(7) With corticosteroids, see Chapter 23.	Serious adverse effects may occur with long-term use of corticosteroids.
(8) With antibacterial agents, see Chapter 29 and the chapter on the individual drug group.	Adverse effects may occur with all antibacterial agents.
(9) With apraclonidine—bradycardia, orthostatic hypotension, headache, insomnia	This drug is related to clonidine, an alpha-adrenergic agonist antihypertensive agent (see Chaps. 18 and 52).
(10) With ophthalmic nonsteroidal anti-inflammatory drugs—potential for increased bleeding	Systemic absorption may interfere with platelet function and increase risks of bleeding with surgery or anticoagulant therapy.
(11) With prostaglandin analogs—headache, cold/flu/upper respiratory infection, bronchitis, sinusitis, muscle and joint pain, chest pain	These were the most commonly reported systemic adverse effects in clinical trials, similar in incidence to placebo.
4. Observe for drug interactions	
a. Drugs that *increase* effects of antiglaucoma drugs:	
(1) Other antiglaucoma drugs	Antiglaucoma drugs may be used in various combinations for additive effects when a single drug does not decrease IOP sufficiently.
b. Drugs that *increase* effects of adrenergic (sympathomimetic) ophthalmic drugs:	
(1) Anticholinergic ophthalmic drugs	The combination (eg, atropine and phenylephrine) produces additive mydriasis.
(2) Systemic adrenergic drugs	Additive risks of adverse effects (eg, tachycardia, cardiac dysrhythmias, hypertension)

NURSING ACTIONS	RATIONALE/EXPLANATION
c. Drugs that *decrease* effects of adrenergic ophthalmic preparations:	
(1) Cholinergic ophthalmic drugs	Antagonize mydriatic effects of adrenergic drugs
d. Drugs that *increase* effects of antiadrenergic ophthalmic preparations:	
(1) Systemic antiadrenergics (eg, propranolol, atenolol, metoprolol, nadolol, timolol)	When the client is receiving a topical beta blocker in ocular disorders, administration of systemic beta-blocking agents in cardiovascular disorders may cause additive systemic toxicity.
e. Drugs that *increase* effects of anticholinergic ophthalmic drugs:	
(1) Adrenergic ophthalmic agents	Additive mydriasis
(2) Systemic anticholinergic drugs (eg, atropine) and other drugs with anticholinergic effects (eg, some antihistamines, antipsychotic agents, and tricyclic antidepressants)	Additive anticholinergic effects (mydriasis, blurred vision, tachycardia). These drugs are hazardous in narrow-angle glaucoma.
f. Drugs that *decrease* effects of cholinergic ophthalmic drugs:	
(1) Anticholinergics and drugs with anticholinergic effects (eg, atropine, antipsychotic agents, tricyclic antidepressants, some antihistamines)	Antagonize antiglaucoma (miotic) effects of cholinergic drugs
(2) Corticosteroids	Long-term use of corticosteroids, topically or systemically, raises IOP and may cause glaucoma. Therefore, corticosteroids decrease effects of all drugs used for glaucoma.
(3) Sympathomimetic drugs	Antagonize miotic (antiglaucoma) effect

APPLYING YOUR KNOWLEDGE: ANSWERS

63-1 Instruct Mrs. Molnar to avoid activities that increase IOP. She should avoid straining at stool, heavy lifting, bending over, coughing, and vomiting when possible.

63-2 Wash hands before applying the medication. To decrease the systemic absorption of eye drops, instruct Mrs. Molnar to close the eye and apply pressure to the tear duct for 3 to 5 minutes after instillation. When multiple eye drops are prescribed, there should be an interval of 5 to 10 minutes between the medications.

Review and Application Exercises

Short Answer Exercises

1. List common disorders of the eye for which drug therapy is indicated.

2. Do ophthalmic medications need to be sterile? Why or why not?

3. What are important principles and techniques related to the nurse's administration of ophthalmic drugs?

4. For a client with newly prescribed eye drops, how would you teach self-administration principles and techniques?

NCLEX-Style Questions

5. What is a major purpose of occluding tear ducts after administering eye drops?
   a. to prevent eye infections
   b. to prevent systemic absorption of the drug
   c. to make self-administration easier
   d. to use a smaller drug dosage

6. When a client has two eye drops ordered at the same time, how should the nurse administer them?
   a. The drops should be given one immediately after the other.
   b. Wait 5 to 10 minutes between drops.
   c. Wait 30 seconds between drops.
   d. Reschedule the medications to be given 1 hour apart.

7. For a client receiving an ophthalmic beta blocker and a systemic beta blocker, which of the following effects is likely to occur?
   a. increased bradycardia
   b. increased nausea
   c. increased antiglaucoma effect
   d. increased blood pressure

8. People who wear contact lenses are at high risk of developing which of the following eye disorders?
   a. cataract
   b. glaucoma
   c. corneal abrasion
   d. allergic conjunctivitis

9. Corticosteroid eye drops are used to
   a. dilate pupils prior to surgery
   b. constrict pupils in glaucoma
   c. prevent cataract development
   d. prevent scarring and loss of vision

Selected References

Alexander, C. L., Miller, S. J., & Abel, S. R. (2002). Prostaglandin analog treatment of glaucoma and ocular hypertension. *The Annals of Pharmacotherapy, 36*(3), 504–511.

Alm, A., Schoenfelder, J., & McDermott, J. (2004). A 5-year, multicenter, open-label, safety study of adjunctive latanoprost therapy for glaucoma. *Archives of Ophthalmology, 122*(7), 957–965.

Carroll, E. W., Porth, C. M., & Curtis, R. L. (2005). Alterations in vision. In C. M. Porth, *Pathophysiology: Concepts of altered health states* (7th ed., pp. 1291–1327). Philadelphia: Lippincott Williams & Wilkins.

Drug facts and comparisons. (Updated monthly). St. Louis: Facts and Comparisons.

Fay, A., & Jakobiec, F. A. (2004). Diseases of the visual system. In L. Goldman & D. Ausiello (Eds.), *Cecil textbook of medicine* (22nd ed., pp. 2406–2420). Philadelphia: W. B. Saunders.

Flach, A. J., & Fraunfelder, F. W. (2004). Ophthalmic therapeutics. In P. Riordan-Eva & J. P. Whicher (Eds.), *Vaughan & Asbury's general ophthalmology* (16th ed., pp. 62–79). New York: McGraw-Hill.

Lesar, T. S. (2002). Glaucoma. In J. T. DiPiro, R. L. Talbert, G. C. Yee, G. R. Matzke, B. G. Wells, & L. M. Posey (Eds.), *Pharmacotherapy: A pathophysiologic approach* (5th ed., pp. 1665–1678). New York: McGraw-Hill.

Sackett, C. (2004). Assessment and management of patients with eye and vision disorders. In S. C. Smeltzer & B. G. Bare (Eds.), *Brunner & Suddarth's textbook of medical-surgical nursing* (10th ed., pp. 1746–1788). Philadelphia: Lippincott Williams & Wilkins.

Wilson, S. A., & Last, A. (2004). Management of corneal abrasions. *American Family Physician, 70*(1), 123–128.

Drugs Used in Dermatologic Conditions

OBJECTIVES

After studying this chapter, you will be able to:

1. Review characteristics of skin structures that influence drug therapy of dermatologic disorders.
2. Discuss antimicrobial, anti-inflammatory, and selected miscellaneous drugs in relation to their use in dermatologic disorders.
3. Use correct techniques to administer dermatologic medications.
4. Teach clients, family members, or caregivers correct administration of dermatologic medications.
5. For clients with "open lesion" skin disorders, teach about the importance and techniques of preventing infection.
6. Practice and teach measures to protect the skin from the damaging effects of sun exposure.

APPLYING YOUR KNOWLEDGE

Ginger Hertzfeld is a 15-year-old female student at the high school where you are the school nurse. She tells you that she has a red and itchy rash. Ginger is very modest and shy and will not show you the rash, but wants advice on an over-the-counter preparation she can use to treat it.

INTRODUCTION

Basic Structure and Function of the Skin

The skin is the largest body organ and acts as the interface between the internal and external environments. It is composed of the epidermis and dermis. Epidermal or epithelial cells begin in the basal layer of the epidermis and migrate outward, undergoing degenerative changes in each layer. The outer layer, called the *stratum corneum,* is composed of dead cells and keratin. The dead cells are constantly being shed (desquamated) and replaced by newer cells. Normally, approximately 1 month is required for cell formation, migration, and desquamation. When dead cells are discarded, keratin remains on the skin. Keratin is a tough protein substance that is insoluble in water, weak acids, and weak bases. Hair and nails, which are composed of keratin, are referred to as *appendages* of the skin.

Melanocytes are pigment-producing cells located at the junction of the epidermis and the dermis. These cells produce yellow, brown, or black skin coloring in response to genetic influences, melanocyte-stimulating hormone released from the anterior pituitary gland, and exposure to ultraviolet (UV) light (eg, sunlight).

The dermis is composed of elastic and fibrous connective tissue. Dermal structures include blood vessels, lymphatic channels, nerves and nerve endings, sweat glands, sebaceous glands, and hair follicles. The dermis is supported underneath by subcutaneous tissue, which is composed primarily of fat cells.

The skin has numerous functions, most of which are protective, including the following:

- Serves as a physical barrier against loss of fluids and electrolytes and against entry of microorganisms, foreign bodies, and other potentially harmful substances
- Detects sensations of pain, pressure, touch, and temperature through sensory nerve endings
- Assists in regulating body temperature through production and elimination of sweat
- Serves as a source of vitamin D when exposed to sunlight or other sources of UV light. Skin contains a precursor for vitamin D.
- Excretes water, sodium, chloride, lactate, and urea in sweat

● Inhibits growth of many microorganisms by its acidic pH (4.5–6.5)

Mucous membranes are composed of a surface layer of epithelial cells, a basement membrane, and a layer of connective tissue. They line body cavities that communicate with the external environment (eg, mouth, vagina, anus). Mucous membranes receive an abundant blood supply because capillaries lie just beneath the epithelial cells.

Disorders of the Skin

Dermatologic disorders may be primary (ie, originate in the skin or mucous membranes) or secondary (ie, result from a systemic condition, such as measles or adverse drug reactions). This chapter emphasizes selected primary skin disorders and the medications used to prevent or treat them.

Inflammatory Disorders

Dermatitis

Dermatitis is a general term denoting an inflammatory response of the skin to injuries from irritants, allergens, or trauma. *Eczema* is often used as a synonym for dermatitis. Whatever the cause, dermatitis is usually characterized by erythema (redness), pruritus (itching), and skin lesions. It may be acute or chronic.

● **Atopic dermatitis** is a common disorder characterized mainly by pruritus and lesions that vary according to the extent of inflammation, stages of healing, and scratching. Scratching damages the skin and increases the risks of secondary infection. Acute lesions are reddened skin areas containing papules and vesicles; chronic lesions are often thick, fibrotic, and nodular.

   The cause is uncertain but may involve allergic, hereditary, or psychological elements. Approximately 50% to 80% of clients have asthma or allergic rhinitis; some have a family history of these disorders. Thus, exposure to possible causes or exacerbating factors such as allergens, irritating chemicals, foods, and emotional stress should be considered. The condition may occur in all age groups but is more common in children.

● **Contact dermatitis** results from direct contact with irritants (eg, soaps, detergents) or allergens (eg, clothing materials or dyes; jewelry; cosmetics) that stimulate inflammation. Irritants cause tissue damage and dermatitis in anyone with sufficient contact or exposure. Allergens cause dermatitis only in sensitized or hypersensitive people. The location of the dermatitis may indicate the cause (eg, facial dermatitis may indicate an allergy to cosmetics).

● **Seborrheic dermatitis** is a disease of the sebaceous glands characterized by excessive production of sebum. It may occur on the scalp, face, or trunk. A simple form involving the scalp is dandruff, which is characterized by flaking and itching of the skin. More severe forms are characterized by greasy, yellow scales or crusts with variable amounts of erythema and itching.

● **Urticaria** ("hives") is an inflammatory response characterized by a skin lesion called a *wheal,* a raised edematous area with a pale center and red border, which itches intensely. Histamine is the most common mediator of urticaria and it causes vasodilation, increased vascular permeability, and pruritus.

   Histamine is released from mast cells and basophils by both allergic (eg, insect bites, foods, drugs) and nonallergic (eg, radiocontrast media, opiates, heat, cold, pressure, UV light, some antibiotics) stimuli. An important difference between allergic and nonallergic reactions is that many allergic reactions require prior exposure to the stimulus, whereas nonallergic reactions can occur with the first exposure.

● **Drug-induced skin reactions** can occur with virtually any drug and can resemble the signs and symptoms of virtually any skin disorder. Topical drugs usually cause a localized, contact-dermatitis type of reaction and systemic drugs cause generalized skin lesions. Skin manifestations of serious drug reactions include erythema, facial edema, pain, blisters, necrosis, and urticaria. Systemic manifestations may include fever, enlarged lymph nodes, joint pain or inflammation, shortness of breath, hypotension, and leukocytosis. Drug-related reactions usually occur within the first or second week of drug administration and subside when the drug is discontinued.

Psoriasis

Psoriasis is a chronic, inflammatory skin disorder attributed to activated T lymphocytes, which produce cytokines that stimulate abnormal growth of affected skin cells and blood vessels. The abnormal growth results in excessively rapid turnover of epidermal cells. Instead of 30 days from formation to elimination of normal epidermal cells, epidermal cells involved in psoriasis are abnormal in structure and have a lifespan of about 4 days. Skin lesions of psoriasis are erythematous, dry, and scaling. The lesions may occur anywhere on the body but commonly involve the skin covering bony prominences, such as the elbows and knees. Skin lesions may be tender, but they do not usually cause severe pain or itching. However, the lesions are unsightly and usually cause embarrassment and mental distress.

The disease is characterized by remissions and exacerbations. Exacerbating factors include infections, winter weather, some drugs (eg, beta blockers, lithium), and possibly stress, obesity, and alcoholism.

Rosacea

Rosacea is characterized by erythema, flushing, telangiectases (fine, red, superficial blood vessels) and acne-like lesions of facial skin. Hyperplasia of the nose (rhinophyma) eventually develops. Rosacea is a chronic disease of unknown etiology that usually occurs in middle-aged and older people, more often in men than women.

Dermatologic Infections

Bacterial Infections

Bacterial infections of the skin are common; they are most often caused by streptococci or staphylococci.

- **Cellulitis** is characterized by erythema, tenderness, and edema, which may spread to subcutaneous tissue. Generalized malaise, chills, and fever may occur.
- **Folliculitis** is an infection of the hair follicles that most often occurs on the scalp or bearded areas of the face.
- **Furuncles** and **carbuncles** are infections usually caused by staphylococci. Furuncles (boils) may result from folliculitis. They usually occur in the neck, face, axillae, buttocks, thighs, and perineum. Furuncles tend to recur. Carbuncles involve many hair follicles and include multiple pustules. Carbuncles may cause fever, malaise, leukocytosis, and bacteremia. Healing of carbuncles often produces scar tissue.
- **Impetigo** is a superficial skin infection caused by streptococci or staphylococci. An especially contagious form is caused by group A beta-hemolytic streptococci. This form occurs most often in children.

Fungal Infections

Fungal infections of the skin and mucous membranes are most often caused by *Candida albicans*.

- **Oral candidiasis** (thrush) involves mucous membranes of the mouth. It often occurs as a superinfection after the use of broad-spectrum systemic antibiotics.
- **Candidiasis of the vagina and vulva** occurs with systemic antibiotic therapy and in women with diabetes mellitus.
- **Intertrigo** involves skin folds or areas where two skin surfaces are in contact (eg, groin, pendulous breasts).
- **Tinea** infections (ringworm) are caused by fungi (dermatophytes). These infections may involve the scalp (tinea capitis), the body (tinea corporis), the foot (tinea pedis), and other areas of the body. Tinea pedis, commonly called *athlete's foot,* is the most common type of ringworm infection.

Viral Infections

Viral infections of the skin include verrucal (warts) and herpes infections. There are two types of herpes simplex infections: type 1 usually involves the face or neck (eg, fever blisters or cold sores on the lips), and type 2 involves the genitalia. Other herpes infections include varicella (chickenpox) and herpes zoster (shingles).

Trauma

Trauma refers to a physical injury that disrupts the skin. When the skin is broken, it may not be able to function properly. The major problem associated with skin wounds is infection. Common wounds include lacerations (cuts or tears); abrasions (shearing or scraping of the skin); puncture wounds; surgical incisions; and burn wounds.

Ulcerations

Cutaneous ulcerations are usually caused by trauma and impaired circulation. They may become inflamed or infected.

- **Pressure ulcers** (also called *decubitus ulcers*) may occur anywhere on the body when external pressure decreases blood flow. They are most likely to develop in clients who are immobilized, incontinent, malnourished, and debilitated. Common sites include the sacrum, trochanters, ankles, and heels. In addition, abraded skin is susceptible to infection and ulcer formation.
- **Venous stasis ulcers,** which usually occur on the legs, result from impaired venous circulation. Other signs of venous insufficiency include edema, varicose veins, stasis dermatitis, and brown skin pigmentation. Bacterial infection may occur in the ulcer.

Acne

Acne is a common disorder characterized by excessive production of sebum and obstruction of hair follicles, which normally carry sebum to the skin surface. As a result, hair follicles expand and form comedones (blackheads and whiteheads). Acne lesions vary from small comedones to acne vulgaris, the most severe form, in which follicles become infected and irritating secretions leak into surrounding tissues to form inflammatory pustules, cysts, and abscesses. Most clients have a variety of lesion types at one time. At least four pathologic events take place within acne-infected hair follicles: (1) androgen-mediated stimulation of sebaceous gland activity, (2) abnormal keratinization leading to follicular plugging (comedone formation), (3) proliferation of the bacterium *Propionibacterium acnes* within the follicle, and (4) inflammation.

Acne occurs most often on the face, upper back, and chest because large numbers of sebaceous glands are located in these areas. One etiologic factor is increased secretion of male hormones (androgens), which occurs at puberty in both sexes. This leads to increased production of sebum and proliferation of *P. acnes* bacteria, which depend on sebum for survival. The *P. acnes* organisms contain lipase enzymes that break down free fatty acids and produce inflammation in acne lesions. Other causative factors may include medications (eg, phenytoin, corticosteroids) and stress (ie, the stress mechanism may involve stimulation of androgen secretion). There is no evidence that certain foods (eg, chocolate) or lack of cleanliness cause acne.

External Otitis

External otitis is an infection of the external ear characterized by pain, itching, and drainage. The external ear is lined with epidermal tissue, which is susceptible to the same skin disorders that affect other parts of the body. External otitis is most often caused by *Pseudomonas aeruginosa* and *Staphylococcus aureus* organisms and may be treated with antimicrobial ear drops for approximately 7 to 10 days.

Anorectal Disorders

Hemorrhoids and anal fissures are common anorectal disorders characterized by pruritus, bleeding, and pain. Inflammation and infection may occur.

DERMATOLOGIC DRUG THERAPY

Many dermatologic medications are applied topically to skin and mucous membranes. The drugs may improve barrier function; soften and remove scaly lesions; alter inflammation in the skin; alter blood flow; exert antimicrobial effects; or affect proliferating cells. Components of topical medications include an active drug and additives that facilitate application of the preparation to skin and mucous membranes. Numerous dosage forms have been developed for topical application of drugs to various parts of the body and for various therapeutic purposes (see Box 64-1). Many topical drug preparations are available in several dosage forms.

Topical medications are used primarily for local effects and systemic absorption is undesirable. Major factors that increase systemic absorption of topical agents include damaged or inflamed skin; high concentrations of drug; and application of drug to the face or mucous membranes, to large areas of the body, or for prolonged periods.

Types of Dermatologic Drugs

Many different drugs are used to prevent or treat dermatologic disorders; most fit into one or more of the following categories.

Antimicrobials

Antimicrobials are used to treat infections caused by bacteria, fungi, and viruses (see Chaps. 29 through 36). When used in dermatologic infections, antimicrobials may be administered locally (topically) or systemically (orally or parenterally). Topical antibacterials (eg, erythromycin, clindamycin, metronidazole, tetracycline [Table 64-1]) are used to treat superficial skin disorders such as acne, folliculitis, and skin wounds or ulcers. Systemic antibacterials (eg, penicillins, cephalosporins) are used for soft-tissue infections such as impetigo, furuncles, carbuncles, cellulitis, and postoperative wound infections. Tetracycline, doxycycline, and minocycline are used for acne and rosacea; fluoroquinolones (eg, ciprofloxacin) are often used to treat soft-tissue infections caused by gram-negative organisms.

Antiseptics

These drugs kill or inhibit the growth of bacteria, viruses, or fungi. They are used primarily to prevent infection. They are

---

Box 64-1   Dosage Forms of Topical Medications

Medications for application to skin and mucous membranes mix an active drug with preservatives, emulsifying agents, and an appropriate base or vehicle. Numerous dosage forms are available for various conditions and therapeutic uses, as follows.

- **Creams** are emulsions of oil in water that may be greasy or nongreasy. They leave a thin coating of oil on the skin as the water evaporates. Creams retain moisture in the skin and are cosmetically acceptable for use on the face and other visible areas of the body. They also may be used in hairy, moist, intertriginous areas. Creams are especially useful in subacute dermatologic disorders.
- **Gels** are transparent colloids, which are solid at room temperature but melt on contact with the skin. They dry and leave a film over the area that helps retain moisture in the skin. They are especially useful in subacute dermatologic disorders.
- **Lotions** are suspensions of insoluble substances in water. They cool, dry, and protect the skin. They are most useful in subacute dermatologic disorders.
- **Ointments** are oil-based substances that usually contain a medication in an emollient vehicle, such as petrolatum or lanolin. Ointments occlude the skin and promote retention of moisture. Thus, they are especially useful in chronic skin dis-

orders characterized by dry lesions. Ointments should usually be avoided in hairy, moist, and intertriginous areas of the body because of potential maceration, irritation, and secondary infection.
- **Pastes** are a mixture of powder and ointment.
- **Powders** have absorbent, cooling, and protective effects. Powders usually should not be applied in acute exudative disorders or on denuded areas because they tend to cake, occlude the lesions, and retard healing. Also, some powders (eg, cornstarch) may lead to secondary infections by promoting growth of bacteria and fungi.
- **Solutions** include water, alcohol, and propylene glycol, but not oil.
- **Sprays** and **aerosols** are similar to lotions.
- **Topical otic medications** are usually liquids. However, creams or ointments may be used for dry, crusted lesions, and powders may be used for drying effects.
- **Topical vaginal medications** may be applied as douche solutions, vaginal tablets, or vaginal creams used with an applicator.
- **Anorectal medications** may be applied as ointments, creams, foams, and rectal suppositories.

Table 64-1 Drugs at a Glance: Topical Antimicrobial Agents

GENERIC/TRADE NAME	INDICATIONS FOR USE	APPLICATION
Antibacterial Agents		
Azelaic acid (Azelex, Finacea)	Acne	To lesions, twice daily
Bacitracin	Bacterial skin infections	To affected area, after cleansing, 1–3 times daily, small amount Cover with a sterile dressing, if desired. Do not use longer than 1 wk.
Benzoyl peroxide	Acne	To affected areas, after cleansing, 1–3 times daily
Clindamycin (Cleocin T)	Acne vulgaris	To affected areas, twice daily
Erythromycin (Aknemycin)	Acne vulgaris	To affected areas, after cleansing, twice daily, morning and evening
Gentamicin (Garamycin)	Skin infections caused by susceptible strains of streptococci, staphylococci, and gram-negative organisms	To infected areas, 3 or 4 times daily. Cover with dressing if desired.
Mafenide (Sulfamylon)	Treatment of burn wounds	To affected area, after cleansing, once or twice daily, using sterile technique
Metronidazole (MetroLotion)	Rosacea	To affected areas, after cleansing, twice daily, morning and evening
Mupirocin (Bactroban)	Impetigo caused by *Staphylococcus aureus*, beta-hemolytic streptococci, or *Streptococcus pyogenes* Eradication of nasal colonization with methicillin-resistant *S. aureus*	Impetigo: Ointment, to affected areas, 3 times daily. Cover with dressing, if desired. Other skin lesions: Cream, 3 times daily for 10 d. Cover with dressing, if desired. Eradication of nasal colonization: Ointment from single-use tube, one half in each nostril, morning and evening for 5 d
Silver sulfadiazine (Silvadene)	Prevent or treat infection in burn wounds caused by *Pseudomonas* and many other organisms	To affected area, after cleansing, once or twice daily, using sterile technique
Combination Products		
Bacitracin and polymyxin B (Polysporin)	Bacterial skin infections	To lesions, 2 or 3 times daily
Erythromycin/benzoyl peroxide (Benzamycin)	Acne	To affected areas, after cleansing, twice daily, morning and evening
Neomycin, polymyxin B, and bacitracin (Neosporin)	Bacterial skin infections	To lesions, 2 or 3 times daily
Antifungal Agents		
Butenafine (Mentax)	Tinea pedis	To affected area, once daily for 4 wk
Ciclopirox (Loprox)	Tinea infections Cutaneous candidiasis	To affected area, twice daily for 2–4 wk
Clotrimazole (Lotrimin)	Tinea infections Cutaneous candidiasis	To affected areas, twice daily, morning and evening
Econazole (Spectazole)	Tinea infections Cutaneous candidiasis	Tinea infections: To affected areas, once daily Cutaneous candidiasis: To affected areas, twice daily
Haloprogin (Halotex)	Tinea infections	To affected area, twice daily for 2–4 wk

(continued)

Table 64-1 Drugs at a Glance: Topical Antimicrobial Agents (continued)

GENERIC/TRADE NAME	INDICATIONS FOR USE	APPLICATION
Ketoconazole (Nizoral)	Tinea infections Cutaneous candidiasis Seborrheic dermatitis	Tinea infections and cutaneous candidiasis: To affected areas, once daily for 2–4 wk Seborrheic dermatitis: To affected areas twice daily for 4 wk or until clinical clearing
Miconazole (Micatin)	Tinea infections Cutaneous candidiasis	To affected areas, twice daily for 2–4 wk
Naftifine (Naftin)	Tinea infections	To affected areas, once daily with cream, twice daily with gel
Nystatin (Mycostatin)	Candidiasis of skin and mucous membranes	To affected areas, after cleansing, 2 or 3 times daily until healing is complete
Oxiconazole (Oxistat)	Tinea infections	To affected areas, once or twice daily for 2–4 wk
Sertaconazole (Ertaczo)	Tinea infections	To affected areas, twice daily for 4 wk
Sulconazole (Exelderm)	Tinea infections	To affected areas, once or twice daily
Terbinafine (Lamisil)	Tinea infections	To affected areas, twice daily for 1–4 wk
Tolnaftate (Tinactin)	Tinea infections	To affected areas, twice daily for 2–4 wk
Antiviral Agents **Acyclovir** (Zovirax)	Herpes genitalis Herpes labialis in immunosuppressed clients	To lesions, q3h 6 times daily for 7 d
Penciclovir (Denavir)	Herpes labialis	To lesions, q2h while awake for 4 d

occasionally used to treat dermatologic infections. Skin surfaces should be clean before application of antiseptics.

Corticosteroids

Corticosteroids are used to treat the inflammation present in many dermatologic conditions. They are most often applied topically (Table 64-2), but also may be given orally or parenterally. Chapter 23 provides additional information about corticocosteroids.

Emollients

Emollients or lubricants (eg, mineral oil, lanolin) are used to relieve pruritus and dryness of the skin.

Enzymes

Enzymes (Table 64-3) are used to débride burn wounds, decubitus ulcers, and venous stasis ulcers. They promote healing by removing necrotic tissue.

Immunomodulators

Immunomodulators are drugs with immunosuppressant and anti-inflammatory effects. They are not steroids, do not cause

the adverse effects associated with corticosteroids, and may be used as corticosteroid substitutes. They are used to treat moderate to severe atopic dermatitis.

Tacrolimus (Protopic) ointment and pimecrolimus (Elidel) cream are considered safe and effective in adults and children as young as 2 years of age. They may cause increased burning and itching during the first week of use, but they are not associated with significant systemic absorption or increased risk of infections.

Keratolytic Agents

These agents are used to treat keratin-containing skin conditions. Alpha hydroxy acids (eg, glycolic acid and others) are often used to treat wrinkles and sun-damaged skin. These acids are a component of many "anti-aging" cosmetics and other products. Salicylic acid is used to remove warts, corns, and calluses.

Retinoids

Retinoids are vitamin-A derivatives that are active in proliferation and differentiation of skin cells. These agents are commonly used to treat acne; psoriasis; aging and wrinkling of skin from sunlight exposure; and skin cancers. Retinoids (eg, isotretinoin) are contraindicated in women

Table 64–2 Drugs at a Glance: Topical Corticosteroids

GENERIC/TRADE NAME	DOSAGE FORMS	POTENCY
Alclometasone (Aclovate)	Cream, ointment	Low
Amcinonide (Cyclocort)	Cream, lotion, ointment	High
Augmented betamethasone dipropionate (Diprolene)	Cream, gel, lotion, ointment	Ointment, very high; cream, high
Betamethasone dipropionate (Alphatrex, others)	Aerosol, cream, lotion, ointment	Cream and ointment, high; lotion, medium
Betamethasone valerate (Valisone, others)	Cream, foam, lotion, ointment	Ointment, high; cream, medium
Clobetasol (Temovate)	Cream, gel, ointment, scalp application	Very high
Clocortolone (Cloderm)	Cream	Medium
Desonide (Tridesilon)	Cream, lotion, ointment	Low
Desoximetasone (Topicort)	Cream, gel, ointment	Medium
Dexamethasone (Decadron)	Aerosol, cream	Low
Diflorasone (Florone, Maxiflor)	Cream, ointment	Ointment, very high; cream, high
Fluocinolone (Synalar, others)	Cream, oil, ointment, shampoo, solution	High
Fluocinonide (Lidex)	Cream, gel, ointment, solution	High
Flurandrenolide (Cordran)	Cream, lotion, ointment, tape	Medium
Fluticasone (Cutivate)	Cream, ointment	Medium
Halcinonide (Halog)	Cream, ointment, solution	High
Halobetasol (Ultravate)	Cream, ointment	Very high
Hydrocortisone (Cortaid, others)	Cream, lotion, ointment, solution, spray, roll-on stick	Medium or low
Mometasone (Elocon)	Cream, lotion, ointment	Medium
Triamcinolone acetonide (Aristocort, Kenalog, others)	Aerosol, cream, lotion, ointment	0.5% cream and ointment, high; lower concentrations, medium

of childbearing potential unless the women have negative pregnancy tests; agree to use effective contraception before, during, and after drug therapy; and agree to take the drugs as prescribed. These drugs have been associated with severe fetal abnormalities. In 2004, the FDA tightened control of prescription isotretinoin (Accutane) to require manufacturers to maintain records of doctors who prescribe the drug, pharmacies that distribute it, and clients who take it. Physicians and pharmacies must inform clients about the risks of taking the drug, have them sign informed-consent documents, and obtain proof of negative pregnancy tests. Previous requirements, which were mainly voluntary, included two negative pregnancy tests before starting isotretinoin and a monthly pregnancy test during therapy.

Sunscreens

Sunscreens are used to protect the skin from the damaging effects of UV radiation, thereby decreasing skin cancer and signs of aging, including wrinkles. Dermatologists recommend sunscreen preparations that block both UVA and UVB

and have a "sun protection factor" (SPF) value of 30 or higher. The SPF is determined by the ratio of sunlight exposure needed to cause erythema in users of a sunscreen versus the exposure needed to cause erythema in nonusers. These highly protective sunscreens are especially needed by people who are fair skinned, allergic to sunlight, or using medications that increase skin sensitivity to sunlight (eg, estrogens, tetracycline).

Individual Drugs

Individual Drugs are described in Tables 64-1, 64-2, and 64-3.

APPLYING YOUR KNOWLEDGE 64-1

You ask Ginger to describe her rash. She says that it is red and very itchy. Upon further questioning, she tells you that she has had it before but cannot remember what it is called. She also has a history of seasonal allergies. Ginger agrees to let you look at the rash. Her history and the appearance of the rash suggest dermatitis. What can Ginger use to help relieve the itching and inflammation?

Table 64-3 Drugs at a Glance: Miscellaneous Dermatologic Agents

GENERIC/TRADE NAME	DERMATOLOGIC EFFECTS	CLINICAL INDICATIONS	METHOD OF ADMINISTRATION
Enzymes			
Collagenase (Santyl)	Débriding effects	Enzymatic débridement of infected wounds (eg, burn wounds, decubitus ulcers)	Topically once daily until the wound is cleansed of necrotic material
Papain (Panafil)	Débriding effects	Débridement of surface lesions	Topically 1 or 2 times daily
Trypsin (Granulex)	Débriding effects	Débridement of infected wounds (eg, decubitus and varicose ulcers)	Topically by spray twice daily
Immunomodulators			
Pimecrolimus (Elidel)	Anti-inflammatory	Atopic dermatitis	Topically to affected skin, twice daily
Tacrolimus (Protopic)	Anti-inflammatory	Atopic dermatitis	Topically to affected skin, twice daily
Retinoids			
Acitretin (Soriatane)	Related to vitamin A	Severe psoriasis	PO 25–50 mg/d
Adapalene (Differin)	Reportedly causes less burning, itching, redness, and dryness than tretinoin	Acne vulgaris	Topically to skin lesions once daily
Isotretinoin (Accutane)	Inhibits sebum production and keratinization	Severe cystic acne Disorders characterized by excessive keratinization (eg, pityriasis, ichthyosis) *Mycosis fungoides*	PO 1–2 mg/kg/d, in 2 divided doses, for 15–20 wk
Tazarotene (Tazorac)	A prodrug; mechanism of action is unknown	Acne Psoriasis	Topically to skin, after cleansing, once daily in the evening
Tretinoin (Retin-A)	Irritant	Acne vulgaris	Topically to skin lesions once daily
Other Agents			
Anthralin (Anthra-Derm, others)	Slows the rate of skin-cell growth and replication	Psoriasis	Topically to skin lesions once daily or as directed
Becaplermin (Regranex)	A recombinant human platelet-derived growth factor	Diabetic skin ulcers	Topically to ulcer; amount calculated according to size of the ulcer
Calcipotriene (Dovonex)	Synthetic analog of vitamin D that helps to regulate skin-cell production and development	Psoriasis	Topically to skin lesions twice daily
Capsaicin (Zostrix)	Depletes substance P (which transmits pain impulses) in sensory nerves of the skin	Relief of pain associated with rheumatoid arthritis, osteoarthritis, and neuralgias	Topically to affected area, up to 3 or 4 times daily
Coal tar (Balnetar, Zetar, others)	Irritant	Psoriasis Dermatitis	Topically to skin, in various concentrations and preparations (eg, creams, lotions, shampoos, bath emulsion). Also available in combination with hydrocortisone and other substances

Table 64-3 Drugs at a Glance: Miscellaneous Dermatologic Agents (continued)

GENERIC/TRADE NAME	DERMATOLOGIC EFFECTS	CLINICAL INDICATIONS	METHOD OF ADMINISTRATION
Colloidal oatmeal (Aveeno)	Antipruritic	Pruritus	Topically as a bath solution (1 cup in bathtub of water)
Dextranomer (Debrisan)	Absorbs exudates from wound surfaces	Cleansing of ulcers (eg, venous stasis, decubitus) and wounds (eg, burn, surgical, traumatic)	Apply to a clean, moist wound surface q12h initially, then less often as exudate decreases
Fluorouracil (Efudex)	Antineoplastic	Actinic keratoses Superficial basal cell carcinomas	Topically to skin lesions twice daily for 2–6 wk
Masoprocol (Actinex)	Inhibits proliferation of keratin-containing cells	Actinic keratoses	Topically to skin lesions morning and evening for 28 d
Salicylic acid	Keratolytic, antifungal	Removal of warts, corns, calluses Superficial fungal infections Seborrheic dermatitis Acne Psoriasis	Topically to skin lesions
Selenium sulfide (Selsun)	Antifungal, antidandruff	Dandruff Tinea versicolor	Topically to scalp as shampoo once or twice weekly

Herbal Remedies/Preparations

Many supplements are promoted for use in skin conditions. Most have not been tested adequately to ensure effectiveness. At the same time, however, topical use rarely causes serious adverse effects or drug interactions. Two topical agents for which there is some support of safety and effectiveness are aloe and oat preparations.

Aloe is often used as a topical remedy for minor burns and wounds (eg, sunburn, cuts, abrasions) to decrease pain, itching, and inflammation and to promote healing. Its active ingredients are unknown. Wound healing is attributed to moisturizing effects and increased blood flow to the area. Reduced inflammation and pain may result from inhibition of arachidonic acid metabolism and formation of inflammatory prostaglandins. Reduced itching may result from inhibition of histamine production.

Commercial products are available for topical use, but fresh gel from the plant may be preferred. When used for this purpose, a clear, thin, gel-like liquid can be squeezed directly from a plant leaf onto the burned or injured area several times daily if needed.

Aside from oral use as a cereal, a good source of dietary fiber, and a well-documented cholesterol-lowering product, **oat** preparations have long been used topically to treat minor skin irritation and pruritus associated with common skin disorders. Oats contain gluten, which forms a sticky mass that holds moisture in the skin when it is mixed with a liquid and has emollient effects. For topical use, oats are contained in bath products, cleansing bars, and lotions (eg, Aveeno products) that can be used once or twice daily. They should not be used near the eyes or on inflamed skin. After use, bath products should be washed off with water.

NURSING PROCESS

Assessment

Assess the client's skin for characteristics or lesions that may indicate current or potential dermatologic disorders.

- When a skin rash is present, interview the client and inspect the area to determine the following:
  - **Appearance of individual lesions.** Lesions should be described as specifically as possible so that changes can be identified. Terms commonly used in dermatology include *macule* (flat spot), *papule* (raised spot), *nodule* (small, solid swelling), *vesicle* (blister), *pustule* (pus-containing lesion), *petechia* (flat, round, purplish-red spot the size of a pinpoint, caused by intradermal or submucosal bleeding), and *erythema* (redness). Lesions also may be described as *weeping, dry and scaly,* or *crusty.*
  - **Location or distribution.** Some skin rashes occur exclusively or primarily on certain parts of the body (eg, face, extremities, trunk), and this distribution may indicate the cause.

- **Accompanying symptoms.** Pruritus occurs with most dermatologic conditions. Fever, malaise, and other symptoms may occur as well.
- **Historic development.** Appropriate questions include
  - When and where did the skin rash appear?
  - How long has it been present?
  - Has it changed in appearance or location?
  - Has it occurred previously?
- **Etiologic factors.** In many instances, appropriate treatment is determined by the cause. Some etiologic factors include the following:
  - **Drug therapy.** Many commonly used drugs may cause skin lesions, including antibiotics (eg, penicillins, sulfonamides, tetracyclines), narcotic analgesics, and thiazide diuretics. Skin rashes due to drug therapy are usually generalized and appear abruptly.
  - **Irritants or allergens** may cause contact dermatitis. For example, dermatitis involving the hands may be caused by soaps, detergents, or various other cleansing agents. Dermatitis involving the trunk may result from allergic reactions to clothing.
  - **Communicable diseases** (eg, measles, chickenpox) cause characteristic skin rashes and systemic signs and symptoms.
- When skin lesions other than rashes are present, assess appearance; size or extent; amount and character of any drainage; and whether the lesion appears infected or contains necrotic material. Bleeding into the skin is usually described as *petechiae* (pinpoint hemorrhages) or *ecchymoses* (bruises). Burn wounds are usually described in terms of depth (partial or full thickness of skin) and percentage of body surface area. Burn wounds with extensive skin damage are rapidly colonized with potentially pathogenic microorganisms. Venous stasis, pressure, and other cutaneous ulcers are usually described in terms of diameter and depth.
- When assessing the skin, consider the age of the client. Infants are likely to have "diaper" dermatitis, miliaria (heat rash), and tinea capitis (ringworm infection of the scalp). School-aged children have a relatively high incidence of measles, chickenpox, and tinea infections. Adolescents often have acne. Older adults are more likely to have dry skin, actinic keratoses (premalignant lesions that occur on sun-exposed skin), and skin neoplasms.
- Assess for skin neoplasms. *Basal cell carcinoma* is the most common type of skin cancer. It may initially appear as a pale nodule, most often on the head and neck. *Squamous cell carcinomas* may appear as ulcerated areas. These lesions may occur anywhere on the body but are more common on sun-exposed parts, such as the face and hands. *Malignant melanoma* is the most serious skin cancer. It involves melanocytes, the pigment-producing cells of the skin. Malignant melanoma may occur in pigmented nevi (moles) or previously normal skin. In nevi, malignant melanoma may be manifested by enlargement and ulceration. In previously normal skin, lesions appear as irregularly shaped pigmented areas. Although it can occur in almost any area, malignant melanoma is most likely to be located on the back in caucasian people and in toe webs and on soles of the feet in African-American or Asian people.

- Color changes and skin rashes are more difficult to detect when assessing dark-skinned clients. Some guidelines include the following:
  - Adequate lighting is required; nonglare daylight is best. The illumination provided by overbed lights or flashlights is inadequate for most purposes.
  - Some skin rashes may be visible on oral mucous membranes.
  - Petechiae are not visible on dark-brown or black skin, but they may be visible on oral mucous membranes or the conjunctiva.
- When skin disorders are present, assess the client's psychological response to the condition. Many clients, especially those with chronic disorders, feel self-conscious and depressed.

Nursing Diagnoses

- Disturbed Body Image related to visible skin lesions
- Anxiety related to potential for permanent scarring or disfigurement
- Pain related to skin lesions and pruritus
- Risk for Injury: Infection related to entry of microbes through damaged skin

Planning/Goals

The client will
- Apply topical drugs correctly
- Experience relief of symptoms
- Use techniques to prevent or minimize skin damage and disorders
- Avoid scarring and disfigurement when possible
- Be encouraged to express concerns about acute and chronic body-image changes

Interventions

Use measures to prevent or minimize skin disorders.
- Use general measures to promote health and increase resistance to disease (ie, maintain nutrition, rest, and exercise).
- Practice good personal hygiene, with at least once-daily cleansing of skin areas with high bacterial counts, such as underarms and perineum.
- Practice safety measures to avoid injury to the skin. Any injury, especially one that disrupts the integrity of the

skin (eg, lacerations, puncture wounds, scratching of skin lesions) increases the likelihood of skin infections.

- Avoid known irritants or allergens. Have the client substitute nonirritating soaps or cleaning supplies for irritating ones; use hypoallergenic jewelry and cosmetics if indicated; wear cotton clothing if indicated.
- Use measures to relieve dry skin and pruritus. Dry skin causes itching, and itching promotes scratching. Scratching relieves itching only if it is strong enough to damage the skin and serve as a counterirritant. Skin damaged or disrupted by scratching is susceptible to invasion by pathogenic microorganisms. Thus, dry skin may lead to serious skin disorders. Older adults are especially likely to have dry, flaky skin. Measures to decrease skin dryness include the following:
  - Alternating complete and partial baths. For example, the client may alternate a shower or tub bath with a sponge bath (of face, hands, underarms, and perineal areas). Warm water, mild soaps, and patting dry are recommended because hot water, harsh soaps, and rubbing with a towel have drying effects on the skin.
  - Liberal use of lubricating creams, lotions, and oils. Bath oils, which usually contain mineral oil or lanolin oil and a perfume, are widely available. If bath oils are used, precautions against falls are necessary because the oils make bathtubs and shower floors slippery. Creams and lotions may be applied several times daily.
- Prevent pressure ulcers by avoiding trauma to the skin and prolonged pressure on any part of the body. In clients at high risk for development of pressure ulcers, major preventive measures include frequent changes of position and correct lifting techniques. Various pressure-relieving devices (eg, special beds and mattresses) also are useful. Daily inspection of the skin is needed for early detection and treatment of beginning pressure ulcers.
- Avoid excessive exposure to sunlight and other sources of UV light. Although controlled amounts of UV light are beneficial in some dermatologic disorders (eg, acne, psoriasis), excessive amounts cause wrinkling, dryness, and malignancies. If prolonged exposure is necessary, protective clothing and sunscreen lotions decrease skin damage.
- When skin rashes are present, cool, wet compresses or baths are often effective in relieving pruritus. Water or normal saline may be used alone or with additives, such as colloidal oatmeal (Aveeno) or baking soda. A cool environment also tends to decrease pruritus. The client's fingernails should be cut short and kept clean to avoid skin damage and infection from scratching.
- For severe itching, a systemic antihistamine may be needed.

Provide appropriate teaching for any drug therapy (see accompanying Client Teaching Guidelines).

Evaluation

- Observe and interview regarding use of dermatologic drugs.
- Observe for improvement in skin lesions and symptoms.
- Interview regarding use of measures to promote healthy skin and prevent skin disorders.

APPLYING YOUR KNOWLEDGE 64-2
What nonpharmacologic measures would you recommend for Ginger?

APPLYING YOUR KNOWLEDGE 64-3
Ginger requires teaching about applying the hydrocortisone. What points should you cover?

PRINCIPLES OF THERAPY

Goals of Therapy

General treatment goals for many skin disorders are to relieve symptoms (eg, dryness, pruritus, inflammation, infection), eradicate or improve lesions, promote healing and repair, restore skin integrity, and prevent recurrence. Specific goals often depend on the condition being treated. With acne, for example, goals are to reduce inflammatory, noninflammatory, and total lesion counts.

General Guidelines for Dermatologic Drug Therapy

- Pharmacologic therapy may include a single drug or multiple agents used concurrently or sequentially.
- For severe skin conditions, a dermatologist is best qualified to prescribe medications and other treatments. Because many skin conditions are so visible, early and aggressive treatment may be needed to prevent additional tissue damage, repeated infections, scarring, and mental anguish.
- Topical medications are preferred, when effective, and many preparations are available. Astringents and lotions are usually used as drying agents for "wet," oozing lesions, and ointments and creams are used as "wetting" agents for dry, scaling lesions.
- To relieve pruritus, a common symptom of inflammatory skin disorders, skin lubricants, systemic antihistamines, and topical corticosteroids are important elements.
- Topical corticosteroids are used for both acute and chronic inflammatory and pruritic lesions. However, when acute lesions involve extensive areas, or chronic lesions are resistant to topical drugs, systemic corticosteroid therapy may be needed. Prednisone 0.5 to 1 mg/kg/day is often used for 1 to 3 weeks.

C L I E N T   T E A C H I N G   G U I D E L I N E S

Topical Medications for Skin Disorders

General Considerations

☑ Severe dermatologic disorders should be treated by a dermatologist. Promote healthy skin by a balanced diet, personal hygiene measures, avoiding excessive exposure to sunlight, avoiding skin injuries, and lubricating dry skin. Healthy skin is less susceptible to inflammation, infections, and other disorders. It also heals more rapidly when disorders or injuries occur.

☑ Common symptoms of skin disorders are inflammation, infection, and itching and the goal of most drug therapy is to relieve these symptoms and promote healing. Systemic medications (eg, oral antihistamines, antibiotics and corticosteroids) may be used for severe disorders, at least initially, but most medications are applied directly to the skin. There is a wide array of topical products, both prescription and over-the-counter.

☑ It is extremely important to use the correct topical medication and the correct amount for the condition being treated. Topical corticosteroids, for example, come in many vehicles (eg, creams, lotions, ointments). These products cannot be used interchangeably. In addition, they should not be combined (ie, using a prescription and a nonprescription product) and should not be covered with occlusive dressings unless specifically instructed to do so. Correct use increases beneficial effects, decreases risks of worsening the condition being treated, and decreases risks of adverse effects.

☑ Adverse effects of topical medications may involve the skin (eg, irritation, excessive drying, infection) where the drug is applied or the entire body, when the drug is absorbed into the bloodstream. Systemic absorption is increased when the drug is strong; applied to inflamed skin, over a large surface area, or frequently; or covered with an occlusive dressing (eg, plastic wrap). Systemic absorption is of most concern with corticosteroid preparations.

☑ Some ways to prevent or decrease skin disorders include:
  ☑ Identifying and avoiding, when possible, substances that cause skin irritation and inflammation (eg, harsh cleaning products, latex gloves, cosmetics, wool fabrics, pet dander)
  ☑ Bathing in warm water with a mild cleanser (eg, Dove, Basis, Cetaphil), patting skin dry, and applying lotions or oils (eg, Aquaphor, Eucerin, mineral oil, or baby oil) to lubricate skin and decrease dryness
  ☑ Avoiding scratching, squeezing, or rubbing skin lesions. These behaviors cause additional skin damage and increase risks of infection. Fingernails should be cut short; cotton gloves can be worn at night.
  ☑ Maintaining a cool environment; preventing sweating
  ☑ Applying cold compresses to inflamed, itchy skin
  ☑ Using baking soda or colloidal oatmeal (Aveeno) in bath water to relieve itching

☑ If you are taking an oral antihistamine to relieve itching, it should be taken on a regular schedule, around the clock, for greater effectiveness.

☑ Misinformation about acne is common. Acne is not caused by dirt; washing does not improve acne; and vigorous scrubbing and squeezing may worsen acne lesions. There is also no evidence that acne is caused by eating chocolate or other foods. Recommendations for managing acne include using non–acne-producing cosmetics, moisturizers, and sunscreens; washing and bathing with a gentle, nonirritating cleanser (eg, Dove or Purpose bar); and avoiding sun exposure if taking a tetracycline or retinoid antiacne medication. (The drugs increase risks of sunburn.) After treatment is started, significant improvement in acne lesions may take as long as 6 to 12 weeks. It is very important to not give up or stop treatment prematurely.

☑ People with psoriasis can obtain information and support from:
  National Psoriasis Foundation (NPF)
  6600 SW 92nd Avenue, Suite 300
  Portland, OR 97223
  Telephone: 1-800-723-9166
  E-mail: getinfo@npfusa.org
  Web site: http//www.psoriasis.org

☑ Unavoidable skin lesions or scars can often be hidden or rendered less noticeable with makeup or clothing.

☑ Women can wear cosmetics over most topical medications. If unclear, ask a health care provider whether makeup is permissible. With acne, use noncomedogenic make-up, moisturizers, and sunscreens.

☑ If taking an oral retinoid (eg, Accutane), avoid vitamin supplements containing vitamin A and excessive exposure to sunlight, to decrease risks of excessive vitamin A intake and photosensitivity.

☑ Because adult household contacts of children with ringworm of the scalp may be asymptomatic carriers, they should use a shampoo containing ketoconazole daily until the infected child is clear of signs and symptoms.

Self-Administration

☑ Use topical medications only as prescribed or according to the manufacturer's instructions (for over-the-counter products). Use the correct preparation for the intended area of application (ie, skin, ear, vagina).

☑ For topical application to skin lesions, cleanse the skin and remove previously applied medication to promote drug contact with the affected area of the skin.
  ☑ Wash the skin and pat it dry.
  ☑ Apply a small amount of the drug preparation and rub it in well. A thin layer of medication is effective and decreases the incidence and severity of adverse effects. With acne and rosacea, preventing skin lesions is easier than eliminating lesions that are already present. As a result, topical medications should be applied to the general area of involvement rather than individual lesions.

☑ For burn wounds, broken skin, or open lesions, apply the drug with sterile gloves or sterile cotton-tipped applicators to prevent infection.

☑ Wash hands before and after application. Wash before to avoid infection; wash afterward to avoid transferring the drug to the face or eyes and causing adverse reactions.

☑ For minor wounds and abrasions, cleansing with soap and water is usually adequate. If an antiseptic is used, an iodine preparation (eg, aqueous iodine solution 1%) is preferred. Alcohol should not be applied to open wounds. Hydrogen peroxide may help with cleansing but it is a weak antiseptic.

☑ With azelaic acid (Azelex) for acne, use for the full prescribed period; do not use occlusive dressings or wrappings; and keep away from mouth, eyes, and other mucous membranes (if it gets into eyes, wash eyes with a large amount of water).

☑ With benzoyl peroxide for acne:

   ☑ With cleansing solutions, wash affected areas once or twice daily. Wet skin areas to be treated before applying the

cleanser. Rinse thoroughly and pat dry. Reduce use if excessive drying or peeling occurs.

☑ With other dosage forms, apply once daily initially and gradually increase to two or three times daily if needed. Cleanse skin, let dry completely, and apply a small amount over the affected area. Reduce dosage if excessive drying, redness, or discomfort occurs. If excessive stinging or burning occurs after any single application, remove with mild soap and water and resume use the next day. Keep away from eyes, mouth, and inside of nose. Rinse with water if contact occurs with these areas. Avoid other sources of skin irritation (eg, sunlight, sunlamps, other topical acne medications).

Use of Topical Corticosteroids

Because of the extensive use of topical corticosteroids and the risks of potentially serious adverse effects, numerous precautions, guidelines, and recommendations have evolved to increase safety and effectiveness of these drugs.

Drug Selection

Choice of drug depends mainly on the acuity, severity, location, and extent of the condition being treated. For acute lesions, a more potent corticosteroid may be needed, at least initially; for chronic lesions, the least-potent preparation that is effective is indicated (see Table 64-2).

- Low-potency drugs (eg, hydrocortisone) are preferred when likely to be effective. They are especially recommended for use in children, on large areas, and on body sites especially prone to corticosteroid damage (eg, face, scrotum, axillae, flexures, skin folds).
- Mid-potency drugs (eg, flurandrenolide) are usually effective in nonintertriginous areas in children and adults.
- High-potency drugs (eg, amcinonide) are used for acute or severe disorders and areas resistant to lower-potency agents. Short-term or intermittent use (eg, every other day, 3 or 4 consecutive days per week, once per week) may be more effective and cause fewer adverse effects than continuous use of lower-potency products. These drugs may also be alternated with lower-potency agents.
- Very–high-potency drugs (eg, clobetasol, halobetasol) usually are used for less absorptive areas such as soles of feet, palms of hands, and thick skin plaques. Usage should not exceed 2 consecutive weeks and total dosage should not exceed 50 g/week because of the potential for these drugs to suppress the hypothalamic–pituitary–adrenal (HPA) axis. Clobetasol suppresses the

HPA axis at doses as low as 2 g/day. *These drugs should not be used with occlusive dressings or for children younger than 12 years of age.*

- Drug potency and clinical use vary with the dosage form, and many topical corticosteroids are available in creams, ointments, and other preparations. Creams are usually the most acceptable to clients; ointments penetrate the epidermis better and are often used for chronic dry or scaly lesions; lotions are recommended for intertriginous areas and the scalp. Some preparations are available in aerosol sprays, gels, and other dosage forms.

Drug Dosage

Dosage depends on the drug concentration, the area of application, and the method of application.

- The skin covering the face, scalp, scrotum, and axillae is more permeable to corticosteroids than other skin surfaces, and these areas can usually be treated with less potent formulations, smaller amounts, or less frequent applications.
- Drug absorption and risks of systemic toxicity are significantly increased when the drug is applied to inflamed skin or covered by an occlusive dressing. Application should be less frequent and limited to isolated, resistant areas when occlusive dressings are used.
- The drug should be applied sparingly. Some clinicians recommend twice-daily applications until a clinical response is obtained, then decreasing to the least-frequent schedule needed to control the condition.
- With continuous use, one or two applications daily may be as effective as three or four applications, because the drugs have a repository effect.
- If an occlusive dressing is applied, leave it on overnight or for at least 6 hours. However, do not leave it in place for more than 12 hours in a 24-hour period.

- After long-term use or after using a potent drug, taper dosage by switching to a less potent agent or applying the drug less frequently. Discontinuing the drug abruptly can cause a rebound effect, in which the skin condition worsens.

Drug Therapy in Selected Skin Conditions

The choice of topical dermatologic agents depends primarily on the reason for use and client response.

Acne

Numerous prescription and nonprescription anti-acne products are available.

- **Antimicrobial drugs** include both topical and systemic agents. Topical drugs usually are indicated for mild to moderate acne, often in combination with a topical retinoid to maximize reduction in severity and number of lesions. *Azelaic acid* (Azelex, Finacea) has antibacterial activity against *P. acnes* and is reportedly as effective in mild to moderate acne as benzoyl peroxide or topical erythromycin. *Benzoyl peroxide* is an effective topical bactericidal agent that is available in numerous preparations (eg, gel, lotion, cream, wash) and concentrations (eg, 2.5%–10%). Lotion and cream preparations are the least irritating. *Clindamycin* and *erythromycin* are also available in topical dosage forms. These drugs reduce *P. acnes* bacteria and are approximately equally effective. Combination products of topical clindamycin or erythromycin and benzoyl peroxide are more effective than antibiotics alone. Best results require 8 to 12 weeks of therapy, and maintenance therapy is usually required. Adverse effects of topical antibiotics include erythema, peeling, dryness, and burning. An additional difficulty is the development of resistant strains of *P. acnes.* Recommendations for reducing drug resistance include using topical retinoids or benzoyl peroxide or both when using topical antibiotics and avoiding long-term use of topical or oral antibiotics when feasible. Benzoyl peroxide can also cause an irritant dermatitis and bleach hair, clothes, and bed linens.

    Oral antimicrobials are first-line treatment for clients with moderate to severe inflammatory acne. These drugs have both antimicrobial and anti-inflammatory effects. They reduce *P. acnes* organisms and thereby inhibit production of *P. acnes*–induced inflammatory cytokines. Commonly used oral antibiotics include tetracycline, doxocycline, minocycline, and erythromycin. Tetracycline and erythromycin suppress leukocyte chemotaxis and bacterial lipase activity; minocycline and doxycycline inhibit cytokines and proteinase enzymes that contribute to inflammation and tissue breakdown. Resistance to the tetracyclines is less common than to erythromycin and is least with minocycline. All oral antibiotics require at least 6 to 8 weeks of use. Although there are no established guidelines for duration of use, some clinicians encourage using the drugs for shorter periods and avoiding long-term use as maintenance therapy, to decrease the development of resistant *P. acnes* organisms.

- **Retinoids**, in both systemic and topical forms, may be used for moderate to severe acne. All topical retinoids (tretinoin, adalapene, tazarotene) reduce acne lesions, usually within 12 weeks. Tretinoin is often used with other products because it may require several months to decrease acne lesions significantly if used alone. Adapalene gel causes less skin irritation and is better tolerated than tretinoin and tazarotene, but tazarotene may be more effective. Topical retinoids should be applied to the entire area of involvement, starting with about 30 seconds' duration and building up to an hour or more. Maintenance therapy is usually required.

    Oral isotretinoin (Accutane) may be used for clients with severe acne who do not respond to safer drugs. Its anti-acne effects include suppression of sebum production, inhibition of comedone formation, and inhibition of inflammation. Approximately 70% to 80% of clients treated appropriately (usually 1 mg/kg/day for 5 months) have a long-term remission. Major drawbacks are teratogenic and other adverse effects. This drug must never be given to a woman of childbearing age unless she agrees to baseline and monthly pregnancy tests and to practice adequate contraceptive measures during and for 6 months after the drug is discontinued. In addition, baseline and 1-month measurements of cholesterol, fasting triglycerides, and liver function are recommended because the drug may increase these values.

Anorectal Disorders

In anorectal disorders, most preparations contain a local anesthetic, emollients, and perhaps a corticosteroid. These preparations relieve pruritus and pain but do not cure the underlying condition. Some preparations contain ingredients of questionable value, such as vasoconstrictors, astringents, and weak antiseptics. No particular mixture is clearly superior.

Dermatitis

Both systemic and topical agents are usually needed. Sedating, systemic antihistamines such as diphenhydramine or hydroxyzine are often used to relieve itching and promote rest and sleep. An oral antibiotic such as clindamycin, dicloxacillin, a cephalosporin, or a macrolide may be given for a week to treat secondary infections. An oral corticosteroid such as prednisone may be needed initially for severe inflammation, but topical corticosteroids are most often used.

Coal-tar preparations have anti-inflammatory and antipruritic actions and can be used alone or with topical corticosteroids. However, these agents have an unpleasant odor and they stain clothing. They are usually applied at bedtime.

Additional preparations include moisturizers and lubricants (eg, Aquaphor) for dry skin and itching; mild skin cleansers (eg, Basis, Cetaphil) to avoid further skin irritation; and baking soda or colloidal oatmeal (eg, Aveeno) in baths or soaks for pruritus.

External Otitis

Otic preparations of various dermatologic medications are used. Hydrocortisone is the corticosteroid most often included in topical otic preparations. It relieves pruritus and inflammation in chronic external otitis. Systemic analgesics are usually required.

Pressure Ulcers

In pressure ulcers, the only clear-cut guideline for treatment is avoiding further pressure on the affected area. Many topical agents are used, most often with specific procedures for dressing changes, skin cleansing, and so on. No one agent or procedure is clearly superior. Consistent implementation of a protocol (eg, position changes; inspection of current or potential pressure areas; dressing changes; use of alternating, pressure-relieving mattresses) may be more effective than drug therapy.

Psoriasis

Localized lesions are usually treated by a combination of topical agents, such as a corticosteroid during daytime hours and a coal-tar ointment at night. Coal-tar preparations work slowly but produce longer remissions. Newer antipsoriasis drugs such as calcipotriene (Dovonex) or tazarotene (Tazorac) may also be used. Calcipotriene is reportedly as effective as topical fluocinonide. However, its onset of action is slower than that of a topical corticosteroid. A combination of calcipotriene and a topical corticosteroid may be used initially for rapid improvement, after which the calcipotriene can be continued as monotherapy. Tazarotene is a topical retinoid that may cause cutaneous irritation.

Generalized psoriasis, which requires systemic treatment or body phototherapy, should be managed by dermatologists. Systemic therapy may involve oral retinoids, methotrexate, or monoclonal antibodies. Acitretin is the oral retinoid of choice for treatment of severe psoriasis. Like other oral retinoids, acitretin is teratogenic. Thus, women of childbearing potential who take acitretin should be instructed to avoid ingesting alcohol and to use adequate contraception while taking the drug and for at least 3 years thereafter. Methotrexate is an antineoplastic drug that has long been used to treat psoriasis because it suppresses inflammation and proliferation of T lymphocytes. It may cause significant adverse effects. The monoclonal antibodies (see Chap. 41) are newer biologic agents that reduce the activity of T lymphocytes and the

inflammation of skin lesions. Alefacept (Amevive) and efalizumab (Raptiva) are used to treat moderate to severe psoriasis. Alefacept is given IM or IV once weekly for 12 weeks. Its adverse effects include lymphopenia and injection-site reactions (eg edema, inflammation, pain). Efalizumab is given subcutaneously once weekly for 12 weeks. Its adverse effects include infection, lymphocytosis, and a first-dose reaction characterized by chills, fever, muscle aches, and nausea.

Phototherapy can involve natural sunlight, which is highly effective. Most clients with psoriasis notice some remission during summer months. Office phototherapy treatments are usually performed three to five times weekly.

Rosacea

Mild skin cleansers (eg, Cetaphil), oral tetracycline, and topical metronidazole are commonly used; oral isotretinoin and topical metronidazole are also effective. These medications prevent or treat acneiform lesions; they have little to no effect on other aspects (eg, erythema; telangiectasia; hyperplasia of connective tissue and sebaceous glands).

Urticaria

Systemic drug therapy with antihistamines (H_1 receptor antagonists) is the major element of drug therapy. In addition, an epinephrine injection may be used initially, and topical medications may be applied to relieve itching. With chronic urticaria, the goal of treatment is symptom relief. Antihistamines are most effective when given before histamine-induced urticaria occurs and should be given around the clock, not just when lesions appear.

Use in Special Populations

Use in Children

Children may develop a wide range of dermatologic disorders, including dermatitis and skin rashes in younger children and acne in adolescents. Few guidelines have been developed for drug therapy of these disorders. Infants, and perhaps older children, have more permeable skin and are more likely to absorb topical drugs than adults. In addition, absorption is increased in the presence of broken or damaged skin. Therefore, cautious use of topical agents is advised.

With topical corticosteroids, suppression of the HPA axis (see Chap. 23), Cushing's disease, and intracranial hypertension have been reported in children. Signs of impaired adrenal function may include delayed growth and low plasma cortisol levels. Signs of intracranial hypertension may include headaches and swelling of the optic nerve (papilledema) on ophthalmoscopic examination. The latter may lead to blindness if pressure on the optic nerve is not relieved.

Because children are at high risk for development of systemic adverse effects with topical corticosteroids, these drugs should be used only if clearly indicated, in the smallest effective dose, for the shortest effective time, and usually without occlusive dressings. In addition, a low-potency agent should be used initially in infants and in intertriginous areas of older children. If a more potent drug is required for severe dermatitis, the child should be examined often and the strength of the drug reduced as skin lesions improve.

Use in Older Adults

Older adults often have thin, dry skin and are at risk of pressure ulcers if mobility, nutrition, or elimination is impaired. Principles of topical drug therapy are generally the same as for younger adults. In addition, topical corticosteroids should be used with caution on thinned or atrophic skin.

Use in Home Care

Skin disorders are commonly treated at home by clients or caregivers. When a home care nurse is involved, responsibilities may include assessing clients, other members of the household, and the home environment for risks of skin disorders; teaching preventive or treatment measures; assisting with treatment; and assessing response to treatment.

APPLYING YOUR KNOWLEDGE 64-4

Ginger's rash has spread to her face. As a teenager, she thinks it looks horrible. What would be an appropriate nursing diagnosis?

NURSING ACTIONS

Dermatologic Drugs

NURSING ACTIONS	RATIONALE/EXPLANATION
1. Administer accurately	
a. Use the correct preparation for the intended use (ie, dermatologic, otic, vaginal, anorectal)	Preparations may differ in drug contents and concentrations.
b. For topical application to skin lesions:	
(1) Wash the skin, and pat it dry.	To cleanse the skin and remove previously applied medication. This facilitates drug contact with the affected area of the skin.
(2) Apply a small amount of the drug preparation, and rub it in well.	A thin layer of medication is effective and decreases the incidence and severity of adverse effects.
(3) For burn wounds, broken skin, or open lesions, apply the drug with sterile gloves or sterile cotton-tipped applicators.	To prevent infection
(4) Use the drug only for the individual client.	To avoid bacterial cross-contamination between clients
(5) Wash hands before and after application.	Wash hands before to avoid exposing the client to infection; wash hands afterward to avoid transferring the drug to your own face or eyes and causing adverse reactions.
2. Observe for therapeutic effects	Therapeutic effects depend on the medication being used and the disorder being treated.
a. With dermatologic conditions, observe for healing of skin lesions.	With acne and rosacea, improvement may require 6–12 weeks of therapy.
b. With external otitis, observe for decreased pain and pruritus.	
c. With vaginal disorders, observe for decreased vaginal discharge and pruritus.	
d. With anorectal disorders, observe for decreased pain and pruritus.	
3. Observe for adverse effects	Incidence of adverse effects is low with topical agents. Local effects may occur with most topical agents but may be more likely with antiseptics, local anesthetics, and antimicrobials.
a. Local irritation or inflammation—burning on application, erythema, skin rash, pruritus	

NURSING ACTIONS	RATIONALE/EXPLANATION
b. With topical corticosteroids, observe for local and systemic effects.	
(1) Local effects include skin atrophy, striae, telangiectasia, hypopigmentation, rosacea, dermatitis, acne, and allergic and irritant reactions.	These effects commonly occur with prolonged use, frequent application, and higher-potency drugs. Atrophy or thinning of skin is more likely in the face, groin, and axillae.
	Allergic and irritant reactions to preservatives, fragrances, and other ingredients may prevent healing or worsen dermatitis.
(2) Systemic effects include suppression of adrenal function, hypertension, hyperglycemia, muscle weakness, osteoporosis, cataracts, glaucoma, and growth retardation in children.	Systemic effects are more likely with more potent agents (eg, clobetasol can cause suppression of the hypothalamic–pituitary–adrenal axis with as little as 2 g daily); application over large areas of skin; prolonged use; and the use of occlusive dressings. In addition, children are at higher risk because they may absorb proportionally larger amounts and be more sensitive to systemic toxicity.
	Little adrenal suppression is likely to occur with doses less than 50 grams weekly for an adult and 15 grams weekly for a small child, unless occlusive dressings are used.
c. With topical antibiotics, superinfection and sensitization may occur.	Superinfection with drug-resistant organisms may occur with any antibacterial agent; diarrhea and pseudomembranous colitis may occur with topical clindamycin. Sensitization may cause serious allergic reactions if the same drug is given systemically at a later time.
d. With oral retinoids, observe for hypervitaminosis A (nausea, vomiting, headache, blurred vision, eye irritation, conjunctivitis, skin disorders, abnormal liver function, musculoskeletal pain, increased plasma triglycerides, depression, and suicidal ideation).	Adverse effects commonly occur with usual doses but are more severe with higher doses.
4. Observe for drug interactions	Clinically significant drug interactions rarely occur with topical agents.

APPLYING YOUR KNOWLEDGE: ANSWERS

64-1 The drug of choice for Ginger is most likely a low-potency, topical hydrocortisone.

64-2 Teach Ginger that dry skin and pruritus are aggravated by hot water and harsh soap, so she should take warm baths and use a gentle cleanser. Patting the skin dry with a towel and using a lotion will reduce the irritation. She may also take a colloidal-oatmeal bath to help relieve the pruritus.

64-3 Apply hydrocortisone sparingly, in a thin layer. Ginger may apply it twice daily until the itch and redness are resolved. If she experiences relief with less frequent application, she should use the drug less often.

64-4 The most appropriate nursing diagnosis based on this data is Disturbed Body Image related to visible skin lesions.

Review and Application Exercises

Short Answer Exercises

1. What are the main functions of the skin?

2. Describe interventions to promote skin health and integrity.

3. During initial assessment of a client, what signs and symptoms may indicate common skin disorders?

4. Which client groups are at risk for development of common skin disorders (eg, skin infections, pressure ulcers)?

5. Compare topical and systemic corticosteroids in terms of adverse effects.

6. If an adolescent client with acne asks your advice about over-the-counter topical drugs, which would you recommend, and why?

7. List general principles of using topical agents for common skin disorders.

NCLEX-Style Questions

8. Topical medications are usually applied for what kinds of effects?
   a. rapid
   b. slow
   c. local
   d. systemic

9. Systemic absorption of topical medications is greatest in
   a. damaged skin
   b. intact skin
   c. soles of the feet
   d. skin of the elbows and knees

10. With a teenage boy taking tretinoin (Retin-A), which of the following statements indicates that he understands the teaching you have done?
   a. "I will apply the medication three times daily for 6 weeks."
   b. "My skin may become red and irritated from the medication."
   c. "I will soak my face in cold water before each application."
   d. "This medication will increase my tolerance to sunlight."

11. Over-the-counter benzoyl peroxide is an effective treatment for many cases of
   a. acne
   b. psoriasis
   c. tinea infections
   d. dermatitis

12. In general, a dermatologist should prescribe the use of all topical
   a. antifungal drugs
   b. anti-acne drugs
   c. antibacterial drugs
   d. high-potency corticosteroids

Selected References

Goldman, R. D. (2004). ELA-max: A new topical lidocaine formulation. *Annals of Pharmacotherapy, 38,* 892–894.

Haider, A., & Shaw, J. C. (2004). Treatment of acne vulgaris. *Journal of the American Medical Association, 292*(6), 726–735.

Is Accutane really dangerous? (2002, September 16). *The Medical Letter on Drugs and Therapeutics, 44*(1139).

Joseph, M. G. (2002). *Dermatology for clinicians: A practical guide to common skin conditions.* New York: Parthenon Publishing.

Patel, N. M., Elias, S. S., & Cheigh, N. H. (2002). Acne and psoriasis. In J. T. DiPiro, R. L. Talbert, G. C. Yee, G. R. Matzke, B. G. Wells, & L. M. Posey (Eds.), *Pharmacotherapy: A pathophysiologic approach* (5th ed., pp. 1689–1704). New York: McGraw-Hill.

Simandl, G. (2005). Alterations in skin function and integrity. In C. M. Porth, *Pathophysiology: Concepts of altered health states* (7th ed., pp. 1449–1493). Philadelphia: Lippincott Williams & Wilkins.

Werth, V. P. (2004). Principles of therapy. In L. Goldman & D. Ausiello (Eds.), *Cecil textbook of medicine* (22nd ed., pp. 2455–2466). Philadelphia: W. B. Saunders.

Drug Use During Pregnancy and Lactation

OBJECTIVES

After studying this chapter, you will be able to:

1. Discuss reasons for avoiding or minimizing drug therapy during pregnancy and lactation.
2. Describe selected teratogenic drugs.
3. Discuss guidelines for drug therapy of pregnancy-associated signs and symptoms.
4. Discuss guidelines for drug therapy of selected chronic disorders during pregnancy and lactation.
5. Discuss the safety of immunizations given during pregnancy.
6. Teach adolescent and young-adult women to avoid prescribed and over-the-counter drugs when possible and to inform physicians and dentists if there is a possibility of pregnancy.
7. Discuss the role of the home care nurse working with the pregnant woman.
8. Discuss drugs used during pregnancy complications (eg, preterm labor, preeclampsia, selected infections) and normal labor and delivery in terms of their effects on the mother and newborn infant.
9. Describe abortifacients in terms of characteristics and nursing process implications.

APPLYING YOUR KNOWLEDGE

Annie Blevins is a 30-year-old woman who comes to the primary care facility where you work to receive her annual checkup. She was recently married and both she and her husband want to start trying to get pregnant. Before her marriage, Mrs. Blevins took Ortho Tri-Cyclen to prevent pregnancy. She has since discontinued taking the oral contraceptive.

INTRODUCTION

Drug use before and during pregnancy and during lactation requires special consideration and, in general, should be avoided or minimized when possible. In sexually active women of reproductive age and ability who may become pregnant (ie, are not consistently using effective contraception), the concern is that the woman may ingest drugs that are potentially harmful to the fetus before she knows she is pregnant. Fetal organs are formed during the first 2 to 8 weeks after conception. During pregnancy, any drugs ingested by the mother may affect the fetus. Drug effects on the fetus are often unknown, especially with newer drugs, and few drugs are considered safe. During lactation, many drugs are excreted in breast milk and reach the nursing infant in varying amounts. Some drugs should be avoided during lactation; some can be continued with precautions to decrease infant exposure.

Despite these very real concerns, however, many prepregnant, pregnant, and lactating women take drugs for var-

ious reasons, including acute disorders that may or may not be associated with pregnancy; chronic disorders that require continued treatment during pregnancy or lactation; and habitual use of nontherapeutic drugs (eg, alcohol, tobacco, others). Most of the drugs in this chapter are described elsewhere; they are discussed here in relation to pregnancy and lactation. Other drugs covered in this chapter are used mainly to influence some aspect of pregnancy. These drugs are discussed in greater detail and include those used to terminate pregnancy (abortifacients); drugs used to stop preterm labor (tocolytics); and drugs used during labor and delivery.

PREGNANCY

During pregnancy, mother and fetus undergo physiologic changes that influence drug effects. In the pregnant woman, physiologic changes alter drug pharmacokinetics (Table 65-1), and drug effects are less predictable than in the nonpregnant state.

TABLE 65-1 Pregnancy: Physiologic and Pharmacokinetic Changes

PHYSIOLOGIC CHANGE	PHARMACOKINETIC CHANGE
Increased plasma volume and body water, approximately 50% in a normal pregnancy	After it is absorbed into the bloodstream, a drug (especially if water soluble) is distributed and "diluted" more than in the nonpregnant state. Drug dosage requirements may increase. However, this effect may be offset by other pharmacokinetic changes of pregnancy.
Increased weight (average 25 lb) and body fat	Drugs (especially fat-soluble ones) are distributed more widely. Drugs that are distributed to fatty tissues tend to linger in the body because they are slowly released from storage sites into the bloodstream.
Decreased serum albumin. The rate of albumin production is increased. However, serum levels fall because of plasma volume expansion. Also, many plasma-protein binding sites are occupied by hormones and other endogenous substances that increase during pregnancy.	The decreased capacity for drug binding leaves more free or unbound drug available for therapeutic or adverse effects on the mother and for placental transfer to the fetus. Thus, a given dose of a drug is likely to produce greater effects than it would in the nonpregnant state. Some commonly used drugs with higher unbound amounts during pregnancy include dexamethasone (Decadron), diazepam (Valium), lidocaine (Xylocaine), meperidine (Demerol), phenobarbital, phenytoin (Dilantin), and propranolol (Inderal).
Increased renal blood flow and glomerular filtration rate secondary to increased cardiac output	Increased excretion of drugs by the kidneys, especially those excreted primarily unchanged in the urine. These include penicillins, digoxin (Lanoxin), and lithium. In late pregnancy, the increased size and weight of the uterus may decrease renal blood flow when the woman assumes a supine position. This may result in decreased excretion and prolonged effects of renally excreted drugs.

Maternal–Placental–Fetal Circulation

Drugs ingested by the pregnant woman reach the fetus through the maternal–placental–fetal circulation, which is completed about the third week after conception. On the maternal side, arterial blood pressure carries blood and drugs to the placenta. In the placenta, maternal and fetal blood are separated by a few thin layers of tissue over a large surface area. Drugs readily cross the placenta, mainly by passive diffusion. Placental transfer begins approximately the fifth week after conception. When drugs are given on a regular schedule, serum levels reach equilibrium, with fetal blood usually containing 50% to 100% of the amount in maternal blood.

After drugs enter the fetal circulation, relatively large amounts are pharmacologically active because the fetus has low levels of serum albumin and thus low levels of drug binding. Drug molecules are distributed in two ways. Most are transported to the liver, where they are metabolized. Metabolism occurs slowly because the fetal liver is immature in quantity and quality of drug-metabolizing enzymes. Drugs metabolized by the fetal liver are excreted by fetal kidneys into amniotic fluid. Excretion also is slow and inefficient due to immature development of fetal kidneys. In addition, the fetus swallows some amniotic fluid, and some drug molecules are recirculated.

Other drug molecules are transported directly to the heart, which then distributes them to the brain and coronary arteries. Drugs enter the brain easily because the blood–brain barrier is poorly developed in the fetus. Approximately half of the drug-containing blood is then transported through the umbilical arteries to the placenta, where it re-enters the maternal circulation. Thus, the mother can metabolize and excrete some drug molecules for the fetus.

Drug Effects on the Fetus

The fetus, which is exposed to any drugs circulating in maternal blood, is very sensitive to drug effects because it is small, has few plasma proteins that can bind drug molecules, and has a weak capacity for metabolizing and excreting drugs. After drug molecules reach the fetus, they may cause teratogenicity (anatomic malformations) or other adverse effects. The teratogenicity of many drugs is unknown. However, since 1984, the Food and Drug Administration (FDA) has required that new drugs be assigned a risk category (Box 65-1).

Drug teratogenicity is most likely to occur when drugs are taken during the first trimester of pregnancy, when fetal organs are formed (Fig. 65-1). For drugs taken during the second and third trimesters, adverse effects are usually manifested in the neonate (birth to 1 month) or infant (1 month to 1 year) as growth retardation, respiratory problems, infection, or bleeding. It should be emphasized, however, that drugs taken at any time during pregnancy can affect the baby's brain because brain development continues throughout pregnancy and after birth. Overall, effects are determined mainly by the type and amount of drugs, the duration of exposure, and the level of fetal growth and development when exposed to the drugs. Both therapeutic and nontherapeutic drugs may affect the fetus. Fetal effects of commonly used *therapeutic* drugs are listed in Box 65-2; effects of *nontherapeutic* drugs are listed in Box 65-3.

Box 65-1 U.S. Food and Drug Administration Drug Risk Categories Regarding Pregnancy

A. Adequate studies in pregnant women demonstrate no risk to the fetus.

B. Animal studies indicate no risk to the fetus, but there are no adequate studies in pregnant women; or animal studies show adverse effects, but adequate studies in pregnant women have not demonstrated a risk.

C. A potential risk, usually because animal studies have either not been performed or have indicated adverse effects, and there are no data from human studies. These drugs may be used when potential benefits outweigh the potential risks.

D. There is evidence of human fetal risk, but the potential benefits to the mother may be acceptable despite the potential risk.

X. Studies in animals or humans or adverse reaction reports or both have demonstrated fetal abnormalities; the risk of use in a pregnant woman clearly outweighs any possible benefit.

FETAL THERAPEUTICS

Although the major concern about drugs ingested during pregnancy is adverse effects on the fetus, a few drugs are given to the mother for therapeutic effects on the fetus. These include digoxin for fetal tachycardia or heart failure, levothyroxine for hypothyroidism, penicillin for exposure to maternal syphilis, and prenatal corticosteroids to promote surfactant production to improve lung function and decrease respiratory distress syndrome in preterm infants.

MATERNAL THERAPEUTICS

Thus far, the main emphasis on drug use during pregnancy has related to actual or potential adverse effects on the fetus. Despite the general principle that drug use should be avoided when possible, pregnant women may require drug therapy for various illnesses, increased nutritional needs, pregnancy-associated problems, chronic disease processes, treatment of preterm labor, induction of labor, and pain management during labor.

Herbal and Dietary Supplements

Pregnancy increases nutritional needs, and vitamin and mineral supplements are commonly used. **Folic acid** supplementation is especially important, to prevent neural-tube birth defects (eg, spina bifida). Such defects occur early in pregnancy, often before the woman realizes she is pregnant. For this reason, it is recommended that all women of childbearing potential ingest 400 or 600 micrograms of folic acid daily from food and/or a supplement. In addition, pregnancy increases folic acid requirements five- to

(text continues on page 1064)

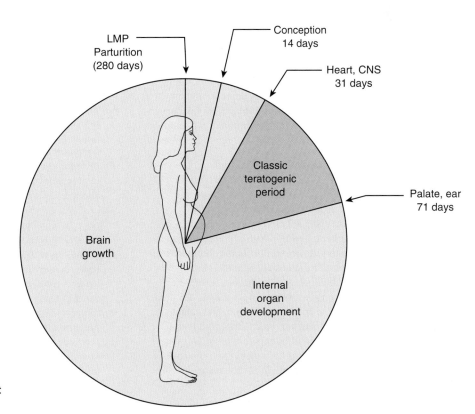

FIGURE 65-1 The gestational clock showing the classic teratogenic risk assessment. (Adapted from Niebyl, J. [1999]. Drugs and related areas in pregnancy. In J. Sciarra [Ed.], *Obstetrics and gynecology*. Philadelphia: Lippincott Williams & Wilkins.)

Box 65-2 Effects of Therapeutic Drugs During Pregnancy

Some drugs (eg, Food and Drug Administration [FDA] risk category X) are contraindicated and should not be used at all during pregnancy. All systemically absorbed drugs are relatively contraindicated because any drug in the pregnant woman's bloodstream reaches the fetus. The majority of commonly used drugs are classified as FDA risk category C, meaning that adequate studies have not been done in pregnant women and effects on the fetus are unknown. These drugs should be used only if potential benefit to the mother justifies potential harm to the fetus.

Adrenergics
Adrenergics are cardiac stimulants that increase rate and force of cardiac contractions and may increase blood pressure. Most are risk category C. Some were teratogenic and embryocidal in animal studies, but there is no evidence of such effects in humans. These drugs are common ingredients in over-the-counter decongestants, cold remedies, and appetite suppressants.

Oral and parenteral adrenergics may inhibit uterine contractions during labor; cause hypokalemia, hypoglycemia, and pulmonary edema in the mother; and cause hypoglycemia in the neonate. These effects are unlikely with inhaled adrenergics (eg, albuterol), which are commonly used to control asthma during pregnancy. Oral *albuterol* and oral or intravenous (IV) *terbutaline* relax uterine muscles and inhibit preterm labor.

Analgesics, Opioid
Opioids rapidly cross the placenta and reach the fetus. Maternal addiction and neonatal withdrawal symptoms result from regular use. Use of *codeine* during the first trimester has been associated with congenital defects.

When given to women in labor, opioids may decrease uterine contractility and slow progress toward delivery. They may also cause respiratory depression in the neonate. *Meperidine* reportedly causes less neonatal respiratory depression than other opioids. *Butorphanol* is also used. If respiratory depression occurs, it can be reversed by administration of *naloxone* (Narcan), an opioid antagonist.

Angiotensin-Converting Enzyme (ACE) Inhibitors
These drugs (risk category C during first trimester; category D during the second and third trimesters) can cause fetal and neonatal morbidity and death; several dozen cases have been reported worldwide. Adverse fetal effects apparently do not occur during first-trimester exposure. With exposure during the second and third trimesters, however, effects may include fetal and neonatal injury such as hypotension, neonatal skull hypoplasia, anuria, renal failure, and death. As a result, the drugs should be discontinued as soon as pregnancy is detected.

Prematurity, intrauterine growth retardation, and patent ductus arteriosus also have been reported, although it is not clear that these effects resulted from exposure to ACE inhibitors. Neonates with histories of in utero exposure to ACE inhibitors should be observed closely for hypotension, oliguria, and hyperkalemia.

Angiotensin II Receptor Blockers (ARBs)
See "ACE Inhibitors," above. The ARBs are also risk category C during the first trimester and category D during the second and third trimesters, and also affect the renin–angiotensin system. They should be discontinued when pregnancy is detected because drugs that act directly on the renin–angiotensin system can cause fetal and neonatal morbidity and death.

Antianginal Agents (Nitrates)
These drugs lower blood pressure and may decrease blood supply to the fetus. Thus, they should be used only if necessary.

Antianxiety and Sedative-Hypnotic Agents (Benzodiazepines)
These drugs should generally be avoided. They and their metabolites cross the placenta freely and accumulate in fetal blood. If taken during the first trimester, they may cause physical malformations. If taken during labor, they may cause sedation, respiratory depression, hypotonia, lethargy, tremors, irritability, and sucking difficulties in the neonate.

Antibacterials
Beta lactams. Penicillins cross the placenta but apparently produce no adverse effects on the fetus. They are considered safer than other antibiotics. *Cephalosporins* cross the placenta and seem to be safe, although they have not been studied extensively in pregnancy. They have shorter half-lives, lower serum concentrations, and a faster rate of elimination in pregnancy. *Carbapenems* vary in risk category, with ertapenem and meropenem being category B and imipenem-cilastatin being category C. *Aztreonam* is risk category B.

Aminoglycosides (risk category D) cross the placenta; fetal serum levels may reach 15% to 50% of maternal levels. Ototoxicity may occur with gentamicin. Serious adverse effects on the fetus or neonate have not been reported with other aminoglycosides, but there is potential harm because the drugs are nephrotoxic and ototoxic.

Clindamycin (risk category B) should be used mainly when infection with *Bacteroides fragilis* is suspected. In addition, it may be used in penicillin-allergic women to treat group B streptococcal infection.

Fluoroquinolones are risk category C but are contraindicated in pregnancy (because of joint damage in animals) if safer alternatives are likely to be effective.

Macrolides. Erythromycin (risk category B) crosses the placenta to reach fetal serum levels up to 20% of maternal levels, but no fetal abnormalities have been reported. In animal studies, adverse fetal effects were reported with *clarithromycin* and *dirithromycin* (risk category C) but not with *azithromycin* (category B). Clarithromycin is contraindicated if a safer alternative is available.

Nitrofurantoin (risk category B) should not be used during late pregnancy because of possible hemolytic anemia in the neonate.

Sulfonamides are category C and should not be used during the third trimester because they may cause kernicterus in the neonate.

Box 65-2 Effects of Therapeutic Drugs During Pregnancy (continued)

Tetracyclines are risk category D and are contraindicated. They cross the placenta and interfere with development of teeth and bone in the fetus. Animal studies indicate embryotoxicity.

Trimethoprim, often given in combination with sulfamethoxazole (Bactrim), is risk category C but contraindicated during the first trimester. It crosses the placenta to reach levels in fetal serum that are similar to those in maternal serum. It is a folate antagonist and may interfere with folic acid metabolism in the fetus. In addition, cardiovascular and neural-tube defects have been reported in infants whose mothers took a *trimethoprim–sulfonamide* combination in early pregnancy. Alternative antibacterials are recommended to treat UTIs during early pregnancy.

Vancomycin, risk category C, is not recommended because fetal effects are unknown.

Anticholinergics

Atropine (category C) crosses the placenta rapidly with IV injection; effects on the fetus depend on the maturity of its parasympathetic nervous system. *Scopolamine* (category C) may cause respiratory depression in the neonate and may contribute to neonatal hemorrhage by reducing vitamin K–dependent clotting factors in the neonate.

Anticoagulants

Heparin (risk category C) does not cross the placenta and has not been associated with congenital defects. It is the anticoagulant of choice during pregnancy. However, its use has been associated with 13% to 22% unfavorable outcomes, including stillbirths and prematurity. *Warfarin* (risk category D) crosses the placenta and fetal hemorrhage, spontaneous abortion, prematurity, stillbirth, and congenital anomalies may occur. Approximately 31% of fetuses exposed to warfarin may experience a problem related to the anticoagulant. If a woman becomes pregnant during warfarin therapy, inform her of the potential risks to the fetus, and discuss the possibility of terminating the pregnancy.

Antidepressants

Selective serotonin reuptake inhibitors (SSRIs; eg, fluoxetine and others) are risk category C, but considered relatively safe during pregnancy when compared with the risks of untreated depression. Few studies have been done; most of the available data are related to fluoxetine. In one study of 228 women who took *fluoxetine* during the first trimester, 5.5% of the infants had major birth defects. In addition, late exposure to fluoxetine resulted in more preterm births than early exposure (14.3% vs. 4.1%). Some neonates exposed to SSRIs late in the third trimester have developed complications requiring extended hospitalization, respiratory support, and tube feeding. Such complications can occur immediately after birth. Additional signs and symptoms among these neonates have included apnea, constant crying, cyanosis, feeding difficulty, hyperactive muscle tone and reflexes, hypoglycemia, irritability, respiratory distress, seizures, and vomiting. It is unknown whether these effects are due to drug toxicity, a drug withdrawal syndrome, or serotonin syndrome. Other SSRIs (*sertraline, paroxetine, fluvoxamine, citalopram*) are not thought to increase risks of major birth defects.

Newer, non-SSRI antidepressants are also risk category C and relatively little is known about their effects during pregnancy. Most information has been derived from their use by women who became pregnant while taking the drugs. In one study of 150 women who had taken *venlafaxine* in the first trimester (35 of these women took the drug throughout pregnancy), researchers compared them with two control groups. In the venlafaxine group, there were 125 live births, 18 spontaneous abortions, seven therapeutic abortions, and two major malformations. There were no statistically significant differences between the venlafaxine group and the control groups. There is little information available about the effects of *bupropion* and *mirtazepine,* but they are not thought to cause major birth defects or other adverse effects. For women who require an antidepressant drug, but who do not respond to or who experience adverse effects with SSRIs, available information suggests the newer antidepressants are safe.

Tricyclic antidepressants (*amitriptyline, imipramine,* and *nortriptyline* are risk category D; others are category C) have been associated with teratogenicity and embryotoxicity when given in large doses, and there have been reports of congenital malformations and neonatal withdrawal syndrome. Monoamine oxidase inhibitors (eg, *phenelzine*) are risk category C; large doses were associated with fewer viable offspring and growth retardation in animal studies.

Antidiabetic Drugs

Insulin (most are risk category B; insulin aspart and glargine are category C) is the only antidiabetic drug recommended for use during pregnancy. *Sulfonylureas* (risk category C), except *glyburide,* are teratogenic in animals and there has been concern about their causing hypoglycemia and hyperinsulinemia in fetuses. Fetal effects of other oral agents are largely unknown. *Acarbose, metformin,* and *miglitol* are FDA category B; *nateglinide, pioglitazone, repaglinide,* and *rosiglitazone* are category C.

Antiemetics

None of the available antiemetic drugs has been proven safe for use and nondrug measures are preferred for controlling nausea and vomiting when possible. If drug therapy is necessary, the antihistamines *cyclizine* and *dimenhydrinate* are risk category B and considered safer for the fetus than other drugs.

Antiepileptic Drugs (AEDs)

More than 90% of women receiving antiseizure drugs deliver normal infants. After years of questioning whether teratogenesis resulted from epilepsy or AEDs, a study confirmed that use of the drugs by pregnant women causes physical abnormalities in their offspring. Moreover, infants exposed to one drug had a higher rate of abnormalities than infants not exposed (20.6% vs. 8.5%), and infants exposed to two or more drugs had a still

(continued)

Box 65-2 Effects of Therapeutic Drugs During Pregnancy (continued)

higher rate (28%). Infants whose nonepileptic mothers took the drugs for bipolar disorder also had higher rates of birth defects.

Older drugs such as *carbamazepine, phenytoin,* and *valproate* are known teratogens and FDA risk category D. Valproate can produce neural-tube defects such as spina bifida. The Centers for Disease Control and Prevention (CDC) estimate the risk of valproate-exposed women having children with spina bifida to be approximately 1% to 2%. Newer drugs (eg, *gabapentin, lamotrigine, oxcarbazepine, tiagabine, topiramate, zonisamide*) are FDA risk category C, and their effects on human fetuses are largely unknown. They were all fetotoxic and/or teratogenic in animal studies. In addition, oxcarbazepine is closely related structurally to carbamazepine and is likely to be teratogenic in humans. Zonisamide use during the first trimester is considered significantly teratogenic and women of childbearing potential who take the drug should be advised to use effective contraception.

Antifungals

Systemic antifungals vary in their risk categories and expected effects during pregnancy. *Amphotericin B,* including lipid formulations, is risk category B. It has been used successfully in serious fungal infections without adverse fetal effects, but only a small number of cases have been reported. *Caspofungin, fluconazole, itraconazole,* and *ketoconazole* are risk category C. They were teratogenic in animal studies. With fluconazole, risk is considered minimal when used as a single oral dose of 150 milligram or less, but chronic use may be teratogenic. *Voriconazole* is risk category D and is teratogenic in animals; if the drug is prescribed for women of childbearing potential, the client should be advised to use effective contraception.

Antihistamines

Histamine₁ receptor blocking agents vary in risk category. *Azatadine, cetirizine, chlorpheniramine, clemastine, cyproheptadine, dexchlorpheniramine, diphenhydramine,* and *loratadine* are category B. *Brompheniramine, carbinoxamine, desloratadine, fexofenadine, hydroxyzine, pheniramine, phenyltoloxamine, promethazine, pyrilamine,* and *triprolidine* are category C. The drugs have been associated with teratogenic effects, but the extent is unknown. The drugs should generally not be used during the third trimester because of possible adverse effects in the neonate. Of the histamine₂ receptor blocking agents, *cimetidine* and *ranitidine* are risk category B and considered acceptable for treatment of gastroesophageal reflux disease that does not respond to dietary and other lifestyle changes.

Antihypertensives

Methyldopa (oral, risk category B; IV, risk category C) crosses the placenta and reaches fetal concentrations similar to those in maternal serum. However, no teratogenic or other adverse fetal effects have been reported despite widespread use during pregnancy. Neonates of mothers receiving methyldopa may have decreased blood pressure for about 48 hours. *Hydralazine* (risk category C) has also been widely used during pregnancy and is considered safe.

Clonidine and *guanabenz* are risk category C; *guanfacine* is category B. Clonidine crosses the placenta and plasma levels in neonates are about half the maternal levels. The effects of guanabenz and guanfacine are unknown.

ACE inhibitors (eg, *captopril* and others) and ARBs (eg, *losartan* and others) are contraindicated during pregnancy (see above). See "Beta-Adrenergic Blocking Agents" and "Calcium Channel Blocking Agents," below, for additional information about these antihypertensive drugs.

Antimanic Agent

Lithium (risk category D) crosses the placenta and fetal concentrations are similar to those in the mother. Cardiac and other birth defects may occur. In the neonate, lithium is eliminated slowly and may cause bradycardia, cyanosis, diabetes insipidus, hypotonia, hypothyroidism, and electrocardiographic (ECG) abnormalities. Most of these effects resolve within 1 to 2 weeks.

Antipsychotics

Phenothiazines (eg, *chlorpromazine*) are risk category C and readily cross the placenta. Studies indicate that the drugs are not teratogenic, but animal studies indicate potential embryotoxicity, increased neonatal mortality, and decreased performance. The possibility of permanent neurologic damage cannot be excluded. Use near term may cause abnormal movements, abnormal reflexes, and jaundice in the neonate, and hypotension in the mother.

Clozapine is risk category B. Animal studies and clinical experiences have not indicated teratogenic effects with clozapine, molindone, or thiothixene. The newer drugs *olanzapine, quetiapine, risperidone,* and *ziprasidone* are risk category C. Fetal effects of newer drugs are largely unknown. However, fetotoxic effects occurred in animal studies.

Antitubercular Drugs

These drugs are recommended for treatment of active tuberculosis in pregnant women; use for prophylaxis should be delayed until after delivery. *Isoniazid, pyrazinamide,* and *rifampin* are risk category C. Isoniazid crosses the placenta and had embryocidal effects in animals but was not teratogenic. It is recommended that neonates of isoniazid-treated mothers be observed for adverse drug effects. Rifampin crosses the placenta and was teratogenic in animal studies. If taken during the last few weeks of pregnancy, rifampin can cause postnatal hemorrhage in the mother and infant. Vitamin K may be indicated. The effects of pyrazinamide are unknown. *Ethambutol* is risk category B and has no detectable effects on the fetus. Overall, these drugs are always given in combination to treat active tuberculosis and the effects of the combinations on the fetus are unknown.

Antivirals

These drugs vary in risk category. *Acyclovir, atazanivir, didanosine, emtricitabine, enfuvirtide, famciclovir, nelfinavir, ritonavir, saquinavir, tenofovir,* and *valacyclovir* are category B. *Abacavir, adefovir, amantadine, cidofovir, delavirdine,*

Box 65-2 Effects of Therapeutic Drugs During Pregnancy (continued)

foscarnet, efavirenz, ganciclovir, indinavir, lamivudine, nevirapine, oseltamivir, rimantidine, stavudine, valganciclovir, zalcitabine, zanamivir, and *zidovudine* are category C. *Ribavirin* is category X and contraindicated; significant teratogenic effects occurred in all animals studied. Zidovudine is widely used to prevent transmission of HIV infection to the fetus and well-controlled studies support such usage.

Aspirin
Aspirin is risk category D and contraindicated because of potential adverse effects on the mother and fetus. Maternal effects include prolonged gestation, prolonged labor, and antepartum and postpartum hemorrhage. Fetal effects include constriction of the ductus arteriosus, low birth weight, and increased incidence of stillbirth and neonatal death.

Beta-Adrenergic Blocking Agents
Beta blockers vary in risk categories, and the safety of their use has not been established. Teratogenicity has not been reported in humans, but problems may occur during delivery. These include maternal bradycardia and neonatal bradycardia, hypoglycemia, apnea, low Apgar scores, and low birth weight. Neonatal effects may last up to 72 hours.

Acebutolol, pindolol, and *sotalol* are risk category B. Acebutolol and its major metabolite cross the placenta. Neonates of mothers who received acebutolol during pregnancy have decreased birth weight, blood pressure, and heart rate. Subnormal birth weight has occurred with sotalol also. *Betaxolol, bisoprolol, carteolol, esmolol, metoprolol, nadolol, penbutolol, propranolol,* and *timolol* are risk category C. These drugs had embryotoxic effects in animals at doses higher than the maximum recommended doses in humans. *Atenolol* is category D; it crosses the placenta and can cause fetal harm.

Calcium Channel Blocking Agents
These drugs are risk category C. Teratogenic and embryotoxic effects occurred in small animals given large doses. *Amlodipine* and *bepridil* decreased litter size and increased intrauterine deaths. *Diltiazem* caused fetal death, skeletal abnormalities, and increased incidence of stillbirths. *Felodipine* caused fetal anomalies and prolongation of parturition, with difficult labor and increased frequency of fetal and early postnatal deaths. *Isradipine* decreased fetal and postnatal survival. *Nicardipine* reduced birth weights and neonatal survival. *Nifedipine* was associated with a variety of embryotoxic, placentotoxic, and fetotoxic effects. *Nisoldipine* was fetotoxic but not teratogenic. *Verapamil* was embryocidal and retarded fetal growth.

Because these drugs decrease maternal blood pressure, there is a potential risk of inadequate blood flow to the placenta and the fetus.

Corticosteroids
Systemic corticosteroids are risk category C. They cross the placenta (prednisone apparently less than others), and animal studies indicate that large doses early in pregnancy may produce cleft palate, stillbirth, and decreased fetal size. Chronic maternal ingestion during the first trimester has shown a 1%

incidence of cleft palate in humans. Infants of mothers who received substantial amounts of corticosteroids during pregnancy should be closely observed for signs of adrenal insufficiency. In cases of preterm labor, *betamethasone* is used to promote fetal production of surfactant to increase lung maturity. Inhaled corticosteroids (eg, those used to treat allergic rhinitis or asthma) are less likely to cause adverse effects in the fetus because of less systemic absorption. Inhaled *budesonide* is risk category B and studies of more than 2000 infants born to mothers who used the drug for asthma indicate that it does not cause congenital malformations.

Digoxin
Digoxin is risk category C, but is considered safe for use during pregnancy. It crosses the placenta to reach fetal serum levels that are 50% to 80% those of maternal serum. Fetal toxicity and neonatal death have occurred with maternal overdose. Dosage requirements may be less predictable during pregnancy, and serum drug levels and other assessment parameters must be closely monitored. Digoxin also has been administered to the mother for treatment of fetal tachycardia and heart failure.

Diuretics
Thiazides and related drugs vary in risk category. *Chlorothiazide, chlorthalidone, hydrochlorothiazide, indapamide, and metolazone* are category B. *Bendroflumethiazide, hydroflumethiazide, methyclothiazide,* and *trichlormethiazide* are category C. These drugs cross the placenta. They are not associated with teratogenesis, but they may cause other adverse effects. The drugs decrease plasma volume and may decrease blood flow to the uterus and placenta, with resultant impairment of fetal nutrition and growth. Other adverse effects may include fetal or neonatal jaundice, thrombocytopenia, hyperbilirubinemia, hemolytic jaundice, fluid and electrolyte imbalances, and impaired carbohydrate metabolism. These drugs are not indicated for treatment of dependent edema caused by uterine enlargement and restriction of venous blood flow. They also are not effective in prevention or treatment of pregnancy-induced hypertension (preeclampsia). They may be used for treatment of pathologic edema.

Loop diuretics also vary in risk category. *Ethacrynic acid* and *torsemide* are category B; *bumetanide* and *furosemide* are category C. The drugs are not considered teratogenic, but animal studies indicated fetal toxicity and death. Like the thiazides, loop diuretics may decrease plasma volume and blood flow to the placenta and fetus.

The potassium-conserving diuretics *amiloride* and *triamterene* are risk category B. The drugs cross the placenta in animal studies, but effects on the human fetus are unknown.

Dyslipidemics
Colesevelam is risk category B; *cholestyramine* and *colestipol* are risk category C. These drugs are considered safe for use during pregnancy because they are not absorbed systemically. HMG-CoA reductase inhibitors or "statins" (eg, *lovastatin*) are risk category X and contraindicated during

(continued)

Box 65-2 Effects of Therapeutic Drugs During Pregnancy (continued)

pregnancy. They should be given to women of childbearing age only if they are highly unlikely to become pregnant and are informed of potential hazards. If a woman becomes pregnant while taking one of these drugs, the drug should be stopped and the client informed of possible adverse drug effects on the fetus.

Nonsteroidal Anti-Inflammatory Drugs (NSAIDs)
NSAIDs vary in risk category. *Diclofenac, fenoprofen, flurbiprofen, ibuprofen, indomethacin, ketoprofen, naproxen,* and *sulindac* are risk category B. *Etodolac, ketorolac, meloxicam, nabumetone, oxaprozin, piroxicam, tolmetin* and the COX-2 inhibitor *celecoxib* is category C. **All of the drugs are category D in the third trimester or near delivery.** Thus, use of NSAIDs should generally be avoided, especially during the third trimester. If these drugs are taken in the third trimester, effects on human fetuses include constriction of the ductus arteriosus prenatally; nonclosure of the ductus arteriosus postnatally; impaired function of the tricuspid valve in the heart; pulmonary hypertension; degenerative changes in the myocardium; impaired platelet function with resultant bleeding; intracranial bleeding; renal impairment or failure; oligohydramnios; gastrointestinal bleeding or perforation; and increased risk of necrotizing enterocolitis, a life-threatening disorder. If NSAIDs are taken near delivery, maternal effects

include delayed onset of labor and delivery and increased risk of excessive bleeding.

Retinoids
Oral retinoids are derivatives of vitamin A that are used for severe skin disorders. *Acitretin* (Soriatane), used for severe psoriasis, and *isotretinoin* (Accutane), used for severe acne, are risk category X and are known teratogens. With isotretinoin, teratogenic effects can occur with any dose and with short duration of use. These drugs are contraindicated during pregnancy and precautions should be taken to ensure that women are not pregnant when they start one of the drugs (eg, have a negative pregnancy test) and that they do not become pregnant while taking one of the drugs (ie, use effective contraception). Topical retinoids are risk category C and are not thought to be teratogens.

Excessive oral doses of *vitamin A* (those above the Recommended Dietary Allowance) are also risk category X and should be avoided by women of childbearing potential.

Thyroid Hormone
Levothyroxine is risk category A. It does not readily cross the placenta and it seems safe in appropriate dosages. However, it may cause tachycardia in the fetus. When given as replacement therapy in hypothyroid women, the drug should be continued through pregnancy.

---

tenfold and deficiencies are common. A supplement is usually needed to supply adequate amounts. For deficiency states, 1 milligram or more daily may be needed.

Herbal supplements are not recommended during pregnancy. **Ginger** has been used to relieve nausea and vomiting during pregnancy, with a few studies supporting its use. Overall, it has not been proven effective, but is probably safe for use.

APPLYING YOUR KNOWLEDGE 65-1
What nutritional advice should you give to Mrs. Blevins?

Pregnancy-Associated Symptoms and Their Management

Anemias

Three types of anemia are common during pregnancy. One is physiologic anemia, which results from expanded blood volume. A second is iron-deficiency anemia, which is often related to long-term nutritional deficiencies. Iron supplements are usually given for prophylaxis (eg, ferrous sulfate 300 milligrams or ferrous gluconate 600 milligrams three times daily). Iron preparations should be taken with food to decrease gastric irritation. Citrus juices enhance absorption. A third type is megaloblastic anemia, caused by folic acid deficiency. A folic acid supplement is often prescribed for prophylaxis.

Constipation

Constipation often occurs during pregnancy, probably from decreased peristalsis. Preferred treatment, if effective, is to increase exercise and intake of fluids and high-fiber foods. If a laxative is required, a bulk-producing agent (eg, Metamucil) is the most physiologic for the mother and safest for the fetus because it is not absorbed systemically. A stool softener (eg, docusate) or an occasional saline laxative (eg, milk of magnesia) may also be used. Mineral oil should be avoided because it interferes with absorption of fat-soluble vitamins. Reduced absorption of vitamin K can lead to bleeding in newborns. Castor oil, all strong laxatives, and excessive amounts of any laxative should be avoided because they can cause uterine contractions and initiate labor.

Gastroesophageal Reflux Disease

Gastroesophageal reflux disease (GERD), of which heartburn (pyrosis) is the main symptom, occurs in one third or more of pregnant women. Hormonal changes relax the lower esophageal sphincter, and the growing fetus increases abdominal pressure. These developments allow gastric acid to splash into the esophagus and cause irritation, discomfort, and esophagitis. In addition, GERD may trigger asthma attacks in pregnant women with asthma.

Nonpharmacologic interventions include eating small meals; not eating for 2 to 3 hours before bedtime; avoiding

Box 65-3 Effects of Nontherapeutic Drugs During Pregnancy

Alcohol is a known teratogen that is contraindicated during pregnancy. Alcohol crosses the placenta easily and reaches fetal concentrations as high as maternal concentrations. In addition, harmful effects on the fetus extend throughout pregnancy. The harmful effects can vary in severity according to the timing of alcohol ingestion in relation to fetal development, the amount of alcohol ingested, and other hereditary and environmental factors.

No amount of alcohol is considered safe and even small amounts ingested during critical periods of fetal development (eg, during the first 2–8 weeks of pregnancy, when the woman may not even know she is pregnant) may be teratogenic. Alcohol ingestion during organ formation may result in a variety of skeletal and organ defects. Alcohol ingestion later in gestation, when the fetal brain is undergoing rapid development, may result in behavioral and cognitive disorders without obvious physical abnormalities. Some evidence indicates that binge drinking, when large amounts of alcohol are ingested during short periods of time, may be especially significant, with resulting abnormalities determined by the period of exposure. Chronic or heavy alcohol ingestion throughout pregnancy may cause intrauterine growth retardation and fetal alcohol syndrome, a condition characterized by multiple congenital defects and mental retardation.

Caffeine is the most commonly ingested nontherapeutic drug during pregnancy. It is present in coffee, tea, cola drinks, over-the-counter analgesics, antisleep preparations, and chocolate. Although ingestion of moderate amounts has not been associated with birth defects, spontaneous abortions, preterm births, and low birth weights have occurred. In addition, high doses may cause cardiac dysrhythmias in the fetus.

Cigarette smoking (nicotine and carbon monoxide ingestion) is one of the few preventable causes of perinatal morbidity and mortality and is contraindicated. Effects include increased fetal, neonatal, and infant mortality (estimated at approximately 4600 infant deaths annually in the United States); decreased birth weight and length; shortened gestation; and increased complications of pregnancy (eg, abruptio placentae; spontaneous abortion; preterm delivery).

These effects are attributed to decreased flow of blood and oxygen to the placenta and uterus. Nicotine causes vasoconstriction and decreases blood flow to the fetus; carbon monoxide decreases the oxygen available to the fetus. Chronic fetal hypoxia from heavy smoking has been associated with mental retardation and other long-term effects on physical and intellectual development. Overall, effects of smoking are dose related, with light smoking (<1 pack/day) estimated to increase fetal deaths by 20% and heavy smoking (1 or more packs/day) increasing deaths by 35%.

Nicotine replacement therapy for smoking cessation is also considered harmful to the fetus. Nicotine gum is risk category C, and other forms of nicotine replacement (inhaler, spray, transdermal patch) are category D. The specific effects on fetal development are unknown. Spontaneous abortion during nicotine replacement treatment has been reported and use of nicotine replacement products in the third trimester has been associated with decreased fetal breathing. Pregnant smokers should be encouraged to quit by using educational and behavioral techniques rather than nicotine replacement products.

Cocaine, marijuana, methamphetamine, and **heroin** are illegal drugs of abuse, and their use during pregnancy is particularly serious. **Cocaine** may cause maternal vasoconstriction, tachycardia, hypertension, cardiac dysrhythmias, and seizures. These effects may impair fetal growth and neurologic development; increase the risk of spontaneous abortion during the first and second trimesters; and cause fetal cerebrovascular accidents and multiple congenital defects. During the third trimester, cocaine causes increased uterine contractility; vasoconstriction and decreased blood flow in the placenta; fetal tachycardia; and increased risk of fetal distress. Maternal complications include premature delivery, spontaneous abortion, abruptio placentae, and death. These life-threatening effects on mother and fetus are even more likely to occur with "crack" cocaine, a highly purified and potent form. Maternal malnutrition, use of other drugs and teratogens, lack of prenatal care, and other factors may also contribute to fetal disorders.

Marijuana impairs formation of DNA and RNA, the basic genetic material of body cells. It also may decrease the oxygen supply of mother and fetus. Maternal use of marijuana may be associated with fetal growth retardation, but other factors such as multiple drug use, lifestyles, diseases, socioeconomic status, and nutrition may also play important roles. **Methamphetamine** is a potent form of amphetamine. It produces central nervous system- and cardiovascular-stimulating effects similar to those produced by cocaine. It is highly addictive and its effects last longer than those of cocaine. Methamphetamine had teratogenic and embryocidal effects in animals given large doses. Infants born to mothers dependent on amphetamines have an increased risk of premature delivery, low birth weight, and symptoms of withdrawal (eg, agitation). **Heroin** ingestion increases the risks of pregnancy-induced hypertension, third-trimester bleeding, complications of labor and delivery, and postpartum morbidity.

---

caffeine, gas-producing foods, and constipation; and sitting in an upright position. For clients who do not obtain adequate relief with these measures, drug therapy may be needed. Antacids may be used if necessary. Because little systemic absorption occurs, the drugs are unlikely to harm the fetus if used in recommended doses. Histamine$_2$ (H$_2$) receptor antagonists (other than nizatidine) may be used safely during pregnancy and ranitidine (Zantac) is preferred. Proton pump inhibitors such as esomeprazole (Nexium) are thought to be safe. However, experience with their use during pregnancy is limited and some clinicians reserve them for clients for whom H$_2$ blockers are ineffective.

Gestational Diabetes

Some women first show signs of glucose intolerance during pregnancy. This is called *gestational diabetes.* Women with risk factors (eg, obesity; age older than 35 years; family history of diabetes; being Hispanic, Native American, Asian, or African American; previous pregnancy with stillbirth, spontaneous abortion, fetal anomalies, or large baby) should be screened at the first prenatal visit. Most women without risk factors, or whose initial test was normal, should be tested between 24 and 28 weeks of gestation. The criterion for a diagnosis of diabetes is a fasting plasma glucose level of more than 126 milligrams per deciliter or a nonfasting glucose level of more than 200 milligrams per deciliter. Women with gestational diabetes are at higher risk for complications of pregnancy, including fetal abnormalities such as a large body size (eg, 9 lb or more), hypoglycemia, hypocalcemia, polycythemia, and bilirubinemia.

Management includes close observation and frequent self-monitoring of fasting and postprandial blood glucose levels because even mild hyperglycemia is detrimental to the fetus. Nutrition is the major treatment strategy. For women who are obese, mild calorie restriction may be indicated (highly calorie-restricted weight-loss diets should be avoided because severe calorie restriction can lead to ketosis and harm the developing fetus). Moderate exercise may also be helpful. If these interventions are ineffective, recombinant human insulin is needed to keep blood glucose levels as nearly normal as possible. Oral antidiabetic drugs are generally contraindicated, although acarbose, metformin, and miglitol seem to cause minimal fetal risk.

When the pregnancy ends, blood glucose levels usually return to a normal range within a few weeks. However, two thirds of these women will have gestational diabetes in subsequent pregnancies and up to half will develop overt diabetes within 15 years.

Nausea and Vomiting

Nausea and vomiting often occur, especially during early pregnancy. Dietary management (eg, eating a few crackers when awakening, waiting a few minutes before arising) and maintaining fluid and electrolyte balance are recommended. Antiemetic drugs should be given only if nausea and vomiting are severe enough to threaten the mother's nutritional or metabolic status. Meclizine, 25 to 50 milligrams daily, and dimenhydrinate, 50 milligrams every 3 to 4 hours, are thought to have low teratogenic risks. Pyridoxine (vitamin B_6) also may be helpful. If used, recommended dosage is 10 to 25 milligrams daily.

Pregnancy-Induced Hypertension

Pregnancy-induced hypertension includes preeclampsia and eclampsia, conditions that endanger the lives of mother and fetus. Preeclampsia is most likely to occur during the third trimester of pregnancy, before, during, or after delivery. It is manifested by hypertension and proteinuria (blood pressure with systolic >140 mm Hg or diastolic >90 mm Hg and proteinuria above 300 mg in 24 hours).

Preeclampsia may occur in women with chronic hypertension, diabetes mellitus, or multiple fetuses, but it most often occurs suddenly, during a first pregnancy. Some women can be observed on an outpatient basis, with frequent monitoring of mother and fetus. Women who are noncompliant with follow-up care or who have severe preeclampsia should be hospitalized. Drug therapy for severe or progressive preeclampsia includes intravenous (IV) hydralazine or labetalol (see Chap. 52) for blood pressure control, and magnesium sulfate (see Chap. 57 and "Tocolytics," below) for prevention or treatment of seizures. Drug therapy reduces perinatal deaths and severe maternal hypertension. If not effectively treated, preeclampsia may progress to eclampsia, which is characterized by potentially fatal seizures. The only cure for preeclampsia is delivery of the baby. Indications for delivery include fetal distress or severe growth restriction and maternal gestation of 38 weeks or longer; low platelet counts; progressive deterioration of hepatic or renal function; development of severe headache, epigastric pain, nausea, or vomiting; or eclampsia. Vaginal delivery is preferred, but cesarean section may be needed in some cases.

For women at risk of developing preeclampsia, aspirin 60 milligrams daily, from 24 to 28 weeks of gestation until onset of labor, may be used for prophylaxis.

Selected Infections

Group B streptococcal infections may affect the pregnant woman and the neonate. Women colonized with group B streptococci (estimated at 10%–30% of pregnant women) have increased risks of premature delivery and transmitting the bacteria to the infant during delivery. During late pregnancy, urinary tract infections (UTIs) or amnionitis may occur. After cesarean delivery, endometritis, bacteremia, or wound infection may occur. In the infant, bacteremia, meningitis, or pneumonia may occur.

Because of the potentially serious consequences of infection with group B streptococci, pregnant women should have a vaginal culture performed at 35 to 37 weeks of gestation. A positive culture indicates infection that should be treated. However, antibiotics given at this time may not provide coverage during labor and delivery. An IV antibiotic should also be started at the onset of labor or with rupture of membranes and continued until delivery. Penicillin G (5 million units followed by 2.5 million units q4h) or ampicillin (2 g followed by 1 g q4h) are recommended. For clients who are allergic to penicillin, clindamycin (900 mg q8h) or erythromycin (500 mg q6h) may be used.

Human immunodeficiency virus (HIV) infection and **acquired immunodeficiency syndrome (AIDS)** in pregnant women require antiretroviral drug therapy for the mother and to prevent transmission to the infant. For pregnant women, two reverse transcriptase inhibitors (eg, zidovudine, lamivudine, didanosine, nevirapine) and a protease inhibitor (eg, indinavir, saquinavir, others) are usually given, as for non-pregnant women, unless there are contraindications. The goal of treatment is to achieve an HIV plasma RNA load of less than 400 copies per milliliter. When possible, zidovudine (AZT) should be one of the reverse transcriptase inhibitors because of its safety for mother and infant and its demonstrated ability to decrease transmission to the infant.

For young children, almost all HIV infections are transmitted perinatally, either in utero, during labor and delivery, or in breast milk. Antiretroviral drug therapy for the pregnant woman reduces perinatal transmission by about two thirds. In addition to the above regimen, monotherapy with oral AZT may be used after 14 weeks of gestation. During labor, IV AZT is given until delivery. After delivery, the infant should be given AZT for 6 weeks, with or without other antiretroviral drugs. The long-term impact of antiretroviral agents on infants is unknown.

Children with HIV infection have failure to thrive, central nervous system abnormalities, and developmental delays as major manifestations. *Pneumocystis jiroveci* pneumonia (formerly called *Pneumocystis carinii* pneumonia or PCP) is an opportunistic infection that may occur in infants, most often between 3 and 6 months of age, and is a major cause of early mortality in HIV-infected children. Trimethoprim-sulfamethoxazole (TMP-SMZ; eg, Bactrim) is recommended for prophylaxis and should be started by 4 to 6 weeks of age for all infants born to HIV-infected mothers.

Because of the potentially serious consequences for infants born to HIV-infected mothers, it is recommended that all pregnant women undergo testing for HIV infection; that women with HIV infection or AIDS should be strongly urged to avoid pregnancy; and that, if pregnancy does occur, the mother should not breast-feed her infant.

Urinary tract infections (UTIs) commonly occur during pregnancy and may include asymptomatic bacteriuria, cystitis, and pyelonephritis. Although treatment of asymptomatic bacteriuria is controversial in some populations, the condition should be treated in pregnant women because of its association with cystitis and pyelonephritis. If untreated, symptomatic cystitis occurs in approximately 30% of pregnant women. Asymptomatic bacteriuria and UTIs are also associated with increased preterm deliveries and low birth weights. Amoxicillin, cephalexin, and nitrofurantoin are commonly used drugs. Hospitalization and IV cephalosporin may be needed for management of pyelonephritis.

APPLYING YOUR KNOWLEDGE 65-2
Mrs. Blevins becomes pregnant. She calls the office complaining of constipation. What do you recommend?

Management of Chronic Diseases During Pregnancy

Asthma

Asthma is one of the most common, potentially serious medical conditions to complicate pregnancy. It is associated with increased risk of infant death, preeclampsia, premature birth, low birth weight, and congenital malformations. These risks are higher with severe asthma and lower with well-controlled asthma. Asthma attacks, which are usually accompanied by hypoxia, hypocapnia, and alkalemia, should be treated promptly and effectively, with hospitalization if indicated. Respiratory infections are common triggers for acute asthma exacerbations.

Because asthma is unpredictable during pregnancy (ie, symptomatology may improve, worsen, or stay about the same), all women with asthma should be monitored closely when pregnant and treated when indicated. Some women with asthma do not require drug therapy during pregnancy. For those who need drug therapy, treatment is considered safer for the fetus than poor asthma control. In general, drug therapy during pregnancy is similar to that in nonpregnant individuals. Commonly used drugs include orally inhaled beta$_2$ agonists (eg, albuterol), inhaled cromolyn, and inhaled and systemic corticosteroids (eg, budesonide, beclomethasone, prednisone). The regular use of inhaled corticosteroids decreases the number of asthma exacerbations during pregnancy and systemic corticosteroids are used for severe exacerbations. Women taking an oral corticosteroid near term require "stress doses" at the time of delivery. Oral theophylline may also be used. Serum theophylline levels should be monitored, and values of 5 to 12 micrograms per milliliter are recommended during pregnancy.

In 2004, the National Asthma Education and Prevention Program (NAEPP) issued recommendations for drug therapy and other aspects of managing asthma during pregnancy. These recommendations are summarized in Box 65-4.

Antiasthma drug therapy is continued during lactation for mothers breast-feeding their baby. The amount of medication reaching the infant through breast milk is less than the amount received in utero through the placenta.

Diabetes Mellitus

Diabetes increases the risks of pregnancy for both mother and fetus, and the hormonal changes of pregnancy have diabetogenic effects that may cause or aggravate diabetes. Maternal risks include retinopathy, preeclampsia, and pyelonephritis; fetal risks include congenital malformations and perinatal death. Despite careful management, congenital malformations occur in 6% to 10% of pregnancies in women with diabetes. Because diabetic retinopathy progresses in many pregnant women, clients should be examined by an ophthalmologist each trimester.

Some women first show signs of diabetes during pregnancy (gestational diabetes). Others, who were previously able to control diabetes with diet alone, may become insulin dependent during pregnancy. Still others, already insulin dependent, are likely to need larger doses as pregnancy advances. Overall, pregnancy makes diabetes more difficult to control. In addition, insulin requirements fluctuate during

---

Box 65-4 **National Asthma Education and Prevention Program (NAEPP) Expert Panel Report: Managing Asthma During Pregnancy: Recommendations for Pharmacologic Treatment—2004 Update**

General Recommendations

- Controlling asthma during pregnancy is important because poorly controlled asthma can lead to serious medical problems for pregnant women and their fetus(es).
- Because asthma severity changes during pregnancy for most women, pregnant clients with persistent asthma should have their asthma checked at least monthly by a health care provider (eg, clinicians providing obstetric care should monitor asthma severity during each prenatal visit).
- Assist clients to identify and avoid or limit exposure to triggers that precipitate or worsen acute asthma symptoms (eg, tobacco smoke; allergens such as dust mites).
- Women with other conditions that can worsen asthma (eg, allergic rhinitis, sinusitis, gastroesophageal reflux) should have those conditions treated as well. Such conditions often become more troublesome during pregnancy.

Drug Therapy Recommendations

- Evidence indicates that it is safer to take medications than to have asthma exacerbations.
- A stepwise approach to asthma care similar to that used in the NAEPP general asthma treatment guidelines for children and nonpregnant adults is recommended (see Chap. 44). Under this approach, medication is stepped up in intensity if needed, and stepped down when possible, depending on asthma severity.
- For quick relief of acute asthma symptoms, albuterol, a short-acting, inhaled beta$_2$ agonist, should be used, and preg-

nant women with asthma should have this medication available at all times.

- For treatment of persistent asthma (eg, women who have symptoms at least 2 days a week or 2 nights a month), asthma medication is needed daily to prevent exacerbations. Inhaled corticosteroids are preferred to control the underlying inflammation. Budesonide (Pulmicort) is often used because there are more data on its safety during pregnancy than for other inhaled corticosteroids. However, there are no data indicating that other inhaled corticosteroids are unsafe during pregnancy, and other inhaled corticosteroids may be continued if they effectively control a client's asthma. Alternative daily medications are leukotriene receptor antagonists such as montelukast (Singulair) or zafirlukast (Accolate); cromolyn (Intal); or theophylline.
- For clients whose persistent asthma is not well controlled on low doses of inhaled corticosteroids alone, the guidelines recommend either increasing the dose of inhaled corticosteroid or adding another medication (eg, a long-acting beta agonist such as salmeterol [Serevent]).
- Oral corticosteroids may be required for the treatment of severe asthma. The guidelines note that there are conflicting data regarding the safety of oral corticosteroids during pregnancy. However, severe, uncontrolled asthma poses a definite risk to the mother and fetus and use of oral corticosteroids may be warranted.

---

pregnancy. Recommendations for management include the following:

- For a planned pregnancy, women with diabetes can have a better outcome if they can maintain normal or near-normal blood glucose levels and normal glycosylated hemoglobin (A_{1C}) levels for at least 2 months prior to conception. In addition, women taking oral hypoglycemic agents should be switched to insulin prior to pregnancy, because these drugs cross the placenta, may be teratogenic, and can cause prolonged fetal hyperinsulinemia. If the drugs are not discontinued prior to pregnancy, they should be discontinued as soon as pregnancy is suspected. This recommendation may change because acarbose (Precose), miglitol (Glyset), and metformin (Glucophage) are thought to have little risk for the fetus.
- Tight blood glucose control is needed throughout pregnancy. It is especially important early in the first trimester, when fetal organs are being formed, because poor glycemic control increases the risks of birth defects. The usual goals for tight glucose control are fasting and preprandial capillary blood glucose levels

of approximately 65 mg/dL (equivalent to a plasma concentration of 75 mg/dL), and 1-hour postprandial levels of less than 120 mg/dL (plasma value less than 140 mg/dL). During this time, it is recommended that women monitor their blood glucose levels at least four times daily (eg, fasting, following breakfast, late afternoon, and evening).

- Insulin is the antidiabetic drug of choice during pregnancy. Human insulin should be used because it is least likely to cause an allergic response. Because insulin requirements vary according to the stage of pregnancy, the diabetic client's blood glucose levels must be monitored closely and insulin therapy individualized. It is especially important that sufficient insulin is given to prevent maternal acidosis. Uncontrolled acidosis is likely to interfere with neurologic development of the fetus. Careful dietary control and other treatment measures are also necessary throughout pregnancy.
- Insulin requirements usually decrease during the first trimester and increase during the second and third trimesters. During the ninth month, insulin needs are approximately 50% greater than at preconception and

the increase is greater among women with type 2 diabetes. Obese women with type 2 diabetes may need much higher insulin doses because of the additional insulin resistance of pregnancy.

● During labor and delivery, short-acting insulin and frequent blood glucose tests are used to control diabetes, as during other acute situations.

● During the postpartum period, insulin requirements fluctuate because stress, trauma, infection, surgery, or other factors associated with delivery tend to increase blood glucose levels and insulin requirements. At the same time, termination of the pregnancy reverses the diabetogenic hormonal changes and decreases insulin requirements. Short-acting insulin is given, and dosage is based on frequent measurements of blood glucose. After the insulin requirement is stabilized, the client may be able to return to the prepregnancy treatment program.

Hypertension

Chronic hypertension is defined as blood pressure above 140/90 mm Hg that begins before conception or in the first 20 weeks of pregnancy and persists after delivery. Hypertension that is initially diagnosed during pregnancy and does not resolve after pregnancy also is classified as chronic. Whenever it occurs, chronic hypertension is associated with increased maternal and fetal risks (eg, preeclampsia, abruptio placentae, intrauterine growth restriction, preterm delivery, perinatal death). In women with chronic hypertension, blood pressure often decreases during the first and second trimesters and increases during the third trimester. The early decrease in blood pressure may allow antihypertensive medications to be stopped temporarily.

Management of chronic hypertension during pregnancy consists of nonpharmacologic and pharmacologic therapies. Nonpharmacologic interventions (eg, avoiding excessive weight gain, sodium restriction, increased rest) should be emphasized. If drug therapy is required, methyldopa is the drug of first choice because it has not been associated with adverse effects on the fetus or neonate. Alternatives include labetalol and other beta blockers, clonidine, hydralazine, isradipine, nifedipine, and prazosin. With beta blockers, fetal and neonatal bradycardia, hypotension, hypoglycemia, and respiratory depression have been reported. As a result, some authorities recommend avoiding the drugs during the first trimester and stopping them 2 to 3 days before delivery. Angiotensin-converting enzyme (ACE) inhibitors and angiotensin II receptor blockers (ARBs) should be avoided during pregnancy because of potential renal damage in the fetus.

Although diuretics are commonly used in the treatment of hypertension, they should not be given during pregnancy. They decrease blood volume, cardiac output, and blood pressure and may cause fluid and electrolyte imbalances, all of which may have adverse effects on the fetus.

Seizure Disorders

Although antiepileptic drugs (AEDs) are known teratogens, they must often be taken during pregnancy because seizures may also be harmful to mother and fetus. Fortunately, most pregnancies (>90%) result in normal infants. Despite the usually good outcomes, women with epilepsy have higher risks of complications of pregnancy, including intrapartum bleeding, preeclampsia, abruptio placentae, premature labor, and stillborn births. In addition, the incidence of birth defects is 2 to 3 times higher in fetuses exposed to AEDs than in those not exposed. If an AED is required, monotherapy with the lowest dose that controls seizures should be used because the rate of major birth defects (eg, cardiac defects, cleft lip or palate, neural-tube defects including spina bifida) in infants exposed to one AED is significantly higher than those not exposed and even higher in infants exposed to two or more AEDs. Infants whose mothers took AEDs for bipolar disorder rather than for epilepsy also have higher rates of birth defects. The effects of newer AEDs during pregnancy are largely unknown.

Plasma drug levels should be checked monthly during pregnancy. Approximately one third of women with epilepsy have an increased number of seizures during pregnancy. This is attributed to physiologic changes of pregnancy (eg, increased blood volume) that lower plasma levels of AEDs.

Women with epilepsy should take a folic acid supplement (at least 400 mcg daily) all the time and 800 mcg or more during pregnancy, to prevent or reduce neural-tube defects. Supplemental vitamin K (eg, 10 mg/day) is also recommended during the last month of pregnancy, to prevent bleeding in neonates. AEDs are associated with a neonatal bleeding disorder characterized by decreased levels of vitamin K–dependent clotting factors. The prenatal vitamin K supplement is in addition to the injection of vitamin K usually given to all neonates immediately after birth.

DRUGS THAT ALTER UTERINE MOTILITY

Abortifacients

Abortion is the termination of pregnancy before 20 weeks. It may occur spontaneously or be intentionally induced. Medical abortion may be induced by prostaglandins and an antiprogestin (Table 65-2). Prostaglandins may be used to terminate pregnancy during the second trimester. In the female reproductive system, prostaglandins E and F are found in the ovaries, myometrium, and menstrual fluid. They stimulate uterine contraction and probably help initiate and maintain the normal birth process. Drug preparations of prostaglandins are capable of inducing labor at any time during pregnancy. Misoprostol (Cytotec), a prostaglandin developed to prevent gastric ulcers associated with nonsteroidal anti-inflammatory drugs (NSAIDs) (see Chap. 59), is being

Table 65-2 Drugs at a Glance: Abortifacients, Prostaglandins, Tocolytics, and Oxytocics

GENERIC/TRADE NAME	ROUTES AND DOSAGE RANGES
Progesterone Antagonist **Mifepristone** (Mifeprex)	PO 600 mg as a single dose or smaller amounts for 4–7 d
Prostaglandins **Carboprost** tromethamine (Hemabate)	IM 250 mcg q1.5–3.5h, depending on uterine response, increased to 500 mcg per dose if uterine contractility is inadequate after several 250-mcg doses
Dinoprostone (Prostin E₂ vaginal suppository)	Intravaginally 20 mg, repeated q3–5h until abortion occurs
Misoprostol (Cytotec)	PO or intravaginally 200–400 mcg q12h for second-trimester termination. Termination usually complete within 48 h
Tocolytics **Ritodrine** (Yutopar)	IV infusion 0.1 mg/min initially, increased by 50 mcg/min every 10 min to a maximal dose of 350 mcg/min if necessary to stop labor. The infusion should be continued for 12 h after uterine contractions cease.
Terbutaline (Brethine)	IV infusion 10 mcg/min, titrated up to a maximum dose of 80 mcg/min until contractions cease PO 2.5 mg q4–6h as maintenance therapy until term
Magnesium sulfate	IV infusion, loading dose 3–4 g mixed in 5% dextrose injection and administered over 15–20 min Maintenance dose 1–2 g/h, according to serum magnesium levels and deep-tendon reflexes PO 250–450 mg q3h, to maintain a serum level of 2.0–2.5 mEq/L
Nifedipine (Procardia)	PO 10 mg every 20 min for 3 or 4 doses; maximum dose 40 mg in 1 h; then 10–20 mg q4–6h
Oxytocics **Oxytocin** (Pitocin)	During labor and delivery, IV 2 milliunits/min, gradually increased to 10 milliunits/min, if necessary, to produce three or four contractions within 10-min periods. Prepare solution by adding 10 units (1 mL) of oxytocin to 1000 mL of 0.9% sodium chloride or 5% dextrose in 0.45% sodium chloride. To control postpartum hemorrhage, IV 10–40 units added to 1000 mL of 0.9% sodium chloride, infused at a rate to control bleeding To prevent postpartum bleeding, IM 3–10 units (0.3–1 mL) as a single dose
Methylergonovine maleate (Methergine)	After delivery of the placenta, IM, IV 0.2 mg; repeat in 2–4 h if bleeding is severe. To prevent excessive postpartum bleeding, PO 0.2 mg 2–4 times daily for 2–7 d, if necessary

IM, intramuscular; IV, intravenous; PO, oral.

given orally or intravaginally for first- or second-trimester termination. It is not FDA approved for this use.

Mifepristone (Mifeprex) is a progesterone antagonist used to terminate pregnancy during the first trimester. A prostaglandin (eg, **misoprostol**) is given approximately 48 hours after the mifepristone to augment uterine contractions and ensure expulsion of the conceptus.

Tocolytics

Drugs given to inhibit labor and maintain the pregnancy are called *tocolytics*. Uterine contractions with cervical changes between 20 and 37 weeks of gestation are considered *preterm labor*. Preterm labor may occur spontaneously or be precipitated by premature rupture of membranes or other factors. Nonpharmacologic treatment includes bed rest, hydration, and sedation. Drug therapy is most effective when the cervix is dilated less than 4 centimeters and membranes are intact. Tocolytic drugs do not reduce the number of preterm births, but they may prolong pregnancy from 2 to 7 days. The goal of tocolytic treatment is to postpone birth long enough to reduce problems associated with prematurity (eg, respiratory distress, bleeding in the brain, infant death). For example, the delay may allow antenatal administration of a corticosteroid (eg, betamethasone [Celestone]) to the mother to improve pulmonary maturity and function in the infant when it is born. In addition, the mother may need to be transported to a facility equipped to deal with high-risk deliveries. After uterine contractions are stopped, opinions differ regarding continuation of tocolytic drug therapy.

Magnesium sulfate, nifedipine, some NSAIDs, ritodrine, and terbutaline are used as tocolytics. Of these drugs, ritodrine is the only one approved by the FDA for tocolysis. The drugs are equivalent in effectiveness but cause different adverse effects. They are described below and in Table 65-2.

Magnesium sulfate, often given by continuous IV infusion, is used as a first-line agent. It inhibits uterine contraction by suppressing nerve impulses to the uterine smooth muscles. When possible, IV infusions should be administered in an obstetric labor and delivery unit with adequate staffing to provide constant observation of the client during the first hour of therapy and at least hourly monitoring during the remainder of the infusion. Other safety measures include a unit protocol that standardizes drug concentration, flow rate, type of infusion pump, and frequency and type of assessment data to be documented (eg, serum drug levels, respiratory status, reflexes, uterine activity, urine output). The antidote, calcium gluconate, should be readily available for use if hypermagnesemia occurs.

These safety measures are needed because hypotension, muscle paralysis, respiratory depression, and cardiac arrest can occur with overdoses of magnesium sulfate. Hypermagnesemia is more likely to occur when magnesium sulfate is used as a tocolytic than when it is used to prevent or treat seizures in eclampsia, because tocolytic serum levels (4–7 mEq/L or 4.8–8.4 mg/dL) are higher than antiseizure levels (2.5–5 mEq/L or 3–6 mg/dL). Close monitoring of serum levels and signs of hypermagnesemia is required. (*Note that hospital laboratories may report serum magnesium levels in mEq/L, mg/dL, or mmol/L. The same values must be used for accurate comparisons of serial measurements.*) In addition, infants born to mothers who recently received tocolytic doses of magnesium sulfate should be assessed for hypermagnesemia and respiratory depression. Endotracheal intubation and assisted ventilation may be needed, as well as IV calcium gluconate.

Nifedipine is a calcium channel blocking drug that decreases uterine contractions. Its use is associated with fewer adverse effects than magnesium sulfate or beta adrenergic drugs. However, a common adverse effect is maternal hypotension, which may reduce blood flow between the placenta and the uterus.

NSAIDs, such as indomethacin (Indocin), ketorolac (Toradol), and sulindac (Clinoril), inhibit uterine prostaglandins that help to initiate the uterine contractions of normal labor. Maternal adverse effects include nausea, heartburn, dizziness, and GI bleeding. In addition, a few instances of serious neonatal complications, including necrotizing enterocolitis, intravascular hemorrhage, and patent ductus arteriosus have been reported.

Ritodrine and **terbutaline** are beta-adrenergic agents that inhibit uterine contractions by reducing intracellular calcium levels. These drugs cause more maternal adverse effects than other tocolytics. Adverse effects may include hyperkalemia, hyperglycemia, cardiac dysrhythmias, hypotension, and pulmonary edema.

DRUGS USED DURING LABOR AND DELIVERY AT TERM

At the end of gestation, labor usually begins spontaneously and proceeds through delivery of the neonate. If labor does not occur spontaneously, it may be induced or stimulated by drugs that stimulate uterine contraction. Drugs often used during labor, delivery, and the immediate postpartum period include oxytocics, analgesics, and anesthetics.

Labor Induction

Prostaglandin preparations (eg, Prepidil or Cervidil formulations of dinoprostone) may be administered to promote cervical ripening (ie, the cervix becomes softer and thinner, to facilitate labor) or induce labor at or near full-term gestation. Prostaglandins F_{2alpha} and E_2 stimulate uterine contractions by increasing intracellular calcium concentrations and activating the actin–myosin contractile units of uterine muscle. About 13% of pregnancies end in labor induction. Reasons for induction include gestation longer than 42 weeks, suspected fetal growth retardation, maternal hypertension, and premature rupture of membranes with no active labor within 4 hours.

Oxytocics

Oxytocic drugs include **oxytocin** and **methylergonovine.** Oxytocin is a hormone produced in the hypothalamus and released by the posterior pituitary gland (see Chap. 22). Pitocin, a synthetic form of oxytocin, is the most commonly used agent for labor induction after cervical ripening. It can also be used to augment labor when uterine contractions are weak and ineffective. Physiologic doses produce a rhythmic uterine contraction–relaxation pattern that approximates the normal labor process. An IV solution of 10 milliunits per milliliter is used for infusion, and dosage (flow rate) is titrated according to frequency and strength of contractions. Oxytocin is contraindicated for antepartum use in the presence of fetal distress, cephalopelvic disproportion, preterm labor, placenta previa, previous uterine surgery, and severe preeclampsia. Maternal condition and fetal heart rate must be closely monitored during oxytocin administration. Maternal adverse effects include hypotension, excessive uterine stimulation, and uterine rupture.

After delivery, oxytocin is the drug of choice for prevention or control of postpartum uterine bleeding because it is less likely to cause hypertension than methylergonovine. The drug reduces uterine bleeding by contracting uterine muscle. It also plays a role in letdown of breast milk to the nipples during lactation.

Methylergonovine (Methergine) may be used for management of postpartum hemorrhage related to uterine atony.

Analgesics

During early labor, pain occurs with uterine contractions; during later stages, pain occurs with perineal stretching. Parenteral opioid analgesics (eg, IV or intramuscular meperidine, morphine, fentanyl) are commonly used to control discomfort and pain during labor and delivery. They may prolong labor and cause sedation and respiratory depression in the mother and neonate. Meperidine may cause less neonatal depression than other opioid analgesics. Butorphanol is also widely used. If neonatal respiratory depression occurs, it can be reversed by naloxone (Narcan).

Regional analgesia may also be used and may be more effective than IV analgesics. Epidural analgesia involves administration of an opioid (eg, fentanyl, preservative-free morphine) through a catheter placed in the epidural space for that purpose. Following a cesarean section, a long-acting form of morphine (eg, Duramorph) can be injected into the epidural catheter to provide analgesia up to 24 hours. Possible adverse effects include maternal urinary retention, but no significant effects on the fetus have been noted.

Anesthetics

Local anesthetics also are used to control discomfort and pain. They are injected by physicians for regional anesthesia in the pelvic area. Epidural blocks involve injection into the epidural space of the spinal cord. Bupivacaine is commonly used. With regional anesthesia, the mother is usually conscious and comfortable, and the neonate is rarely depressed. Fentanyl may be combined with a small amount of an anesthetic drug for both analgesia and anesthesia. No significant effects on the fetus occurred in clinical studies.

NEONATAL THERAPEUTICS

In the neonate, any drug must be used cautiously. Drugs are usually given less often because they are metabolized and excreted slowly. Immature liver and kidney function prolongs drug action and increases risks of toxicity. Also, drug therapy should be initiated with low doses, especially with drugs that are highly bound to plasma proteins. Neonates have few binding proteins, which leads to increased amounts of free, active drug and increased risk of toxicity. When a health care provider is assessing the neonate, drugs received by the mother during pregnancy, labor and delivery, and lactation must be considered.

At birth, some drugs are routinely administered to prevent hemorrhagic disease of the newborn and ophthalmia neonatorum. Hemorrhagic disease of the newborn occurs because the intestinal tract lacks the bacteria that normally synthesize vitamin K and there is little if any dietary intake of vitamin K. Vitamin K is required for liver production of several clotting factors, including prothrombin. Thus, the neonate is at increased risk of bleeding during the first week of life. One dose of phytonadione 0.5 to 1 milligram is injected at delivery or on admission to the nursery.

Ophthalmia neonatorum is a form of bacterial conjunctivitis that may cause ulceration and blindness. It may be caused by several bacteria, most commonly *Chlamydia trachomatis,* a sexually transmitted organism. Erythromycin ointment 0.5% is applied to each eye at delivery. It is effective against both chlamydial and gonococcal infections.

NURSING PROCESS

Assessment

Assess each female client of reproductive age for possible pregnancy. If the client is known to be pregnant, assess status in relation to pregnancy, as follows:
- Length of gestation
- Use of prescription, over-the-counter, herbal, nontherapeutic, and illegal drugs
- Acute and chronic health problems that may influence the pregnancy or require drug therapy
- With premature labor, assess length of gestation, the frequency and quality of uterine contractions, the amount of vaginal bleeding or discharge, and the length of labor. Also determine whether any tissue has been expelled from the vagina. When abortion is inevitable, an oxytocic drug may be given. When stopping labor is possible or desired, a tocolytic drug may be given.
- When spontaneous labor occurs in normal, full-term pregnancy, assess frequency and quality of uterine contractions, amount of cervical dilatation, fetal heart rate and quality, and maternal blood pressure.
- Assess antepartum women for intention to breast-feed.

Nursing Diagnoses

- Risk for Injury: Damage to mother, fetus, or neonate from maternal ingestion of drugs
- Noncompliance related to ingestion of nonessential drugs during pregnancy
- Risk for Injury related to possible damage to mother or infant during the birth process
- Deficient Knowledge: Drug effects during pregnancy and lactation

Planning/Goals

The client will

- Avoid unnecessary drug ingestion when pregnant or likely to become pregnant
- Use nonpharmacologic measures to relieve symptoms associated with pregnancy or other health problems when possible
- Obtain optimal care during pregnancy, labor and delivery, and the postpartum period
- Avoid behaviors that may lead to complications of pregnancy and labor and delivery
- Breast-feed safely and successfully if desired

Interventions

- Use nondrug measures to prevent or minimize the need for drug therapy during pregnancy.
- Promote or provide optimal prenatal care to promote a healthy pregnancy (eg, regular monitoring of blood pressure, weight, blood sugar, urine protein; counseling about nutrition and other healthful activities).
- Assist women with chronic health problems (eg, asthma, diabetes, hypertension) to manage the disorders effectively and decrease risks of harm to themselves and their babies.
- Help clients and families cope with complications of pregnancy, including therapeutic abortion.
- Counsel candidates for therapeutic abortion about methods and expected outcomes; counsel abortion clients about contraceptive techniques.
- Provide teaching about drug use during pregnancy and lactation (see accompanying display).

Evaluation

- Observe and interview regarding actions taken to promote reproductive and general health.
- Observe and interview regarding compliance with instructions for promoting and maintaining a healthy pregnancy.
- Interview regarding ingestion of therapeutic and nontherapeutic drugs during prepregnant, pregnant, and lactating states.
- Observe and interview regarding the health status of the mother and neonate.

PRINCIPLES OF THERAPY

General Guidelines: Pregnancy

- Give medications only when clearly indicated, weighing anticipated benefits to the mother against the risk of harm to the fetus.

- When drug therapy is required, the choice of drug should be based on the stage of pregnancy and available drug information (see Boxes 65-1 and 65-2). During the first trimester, for example, an older drug that has not been associated with teratogenic effects is usually preferred over a newer drug of unknown teratogenicity.
- Any drugs used during pregnancy should be given in the lowest effective doses and for the shortest effective time.
- Counsel pregnant women about the use of immunizations during pregnancy. Live-virus vaccines (eg, measles, mumps, polio, rubella, yellow fever) should be avoided because of possible harmful effects to the fetus.

  Inactive-virus vaccines, such as influenza, rabies, hepatitis B (if the mother is high risk and negative for hepatitis B antigen), and toxoids (eg, diphtheria, tetanus) are considered safe for use. In addition, hyperimmune globulins can be given to pregnant women who are exposed to hepatitis B, rabies, tetanus, or varicella (chicken pox).

APPLYING YOUR KNOWLEDGE 65-3

Mrs. Blevins asks you about over-the-counter and prescription drug use during her pregnancy. What do you tell her?

General Guidelines: Lactation

- Most systemic drugs taken by the mother reach the infant in breast milk. For some, the amount of drug is too small to cause significant effects; for others, effects on the nursing infant are unknown or potentially adverse. Drugs that are considered safe, those to be used with caution, and those that are contraindicated are listed in Box 65-5.
- Give medications only when clearly indicated, weighing potential benefit to the mother against possible harm to the nursing infant. For contraindicated drugs, it is usually recommended that the mother stop the drug or stop breast-feeding.
- Any drugs used during lactation should be given in the lowest effective dose for the shortest effective time.
- The American Academy of Pediatrics (AAP) supports breast-feeding as optimal nutrition for infants and does not recommend stopping maternal drug therapy unless necessary. In some instances, mothers may pump and discard breast milk while receiving therapeutic drugs, to maintain lactation.
- Women with HIV infection should not breast-feed. The virus can be transmitted to the nursing infant.

Home Care

Many obstetric clients with conditions such as preterm labor, hyperemesis, and elevated blood pressure are managed in the home. The home care nurse who assists in managing these

General Considerations

☑ Any systemic drug ingested by a pregnant woman reaches the fetus and may interfere with fetal growth and development. For most drugs, safety during pregnancy has not been established, and all drugs are relatively contraindicated. Therefore, any drug use must be cautious and minimal to avoid potential damage to the fetus.

☑ Avoid drugs when possible and use them very cautiously when necessary. **If women who are sexually active and not using effective contraception take any drugs, there is a high risk that potentially harmful agents may be ingested before pregnancy is suspected or confirmed.** It is estimated that 50% or more of pregnancies are unplanned.

☑ Lifestyle or nontherapeutic drugs associated with problems during pregnancy include alcohol, caffeine, and cigarette smoking. Women should completely avoid alcohol when trying to conceive and throughout pregnancy; no amount is considered safe. Caffeine intake should be limited to about three caffeinated beverages per day; excessive intake should be avoided. Women who smoke should quit if possible during pregnancy, to avoid the effects of nicotine, carbon monoxide, and other chemicals on the fetus. However, the use of nicotine replacement products during pregnancy is not recommended.

☑ Herbal supplements are not recommended; their effects during pregnancy are largely unknown.

☑ Measures to prevent the need for drug therapy include a healthful lifestyle (adequate nutrition, exercise, rest, and sleep; avoiding alcohol and cigarette smoking) and avoiding infection (personal hygiene, avoiding contact with people known to have infections, maintaining indicated immunizations).

☑ Nondrug measures to relieve common health problems include positioning, adequate food and fluid intake, and deep breathing.

☑ See a health care provider as soon as pregnancy is suspected.

☑ Inform any health care provider from whom treatment is sought if there is a possibility of pregnancy.

☑ Many drugs are excreted in breast milk to some extent and reach the nursing infant. The infant's health care provider should be informed about medications taken by the nursing mother and consulted about potential drug effects on the infant. Before taking over-the-counter medications, consult a health care provider. In regard to nontherapeutic drugs, recommendations include the following:

1. Alcohol should be used in moderation and nursing should be withheld temporarily after alcohol consumption (1–2 hours per drink). Alcohol reaches the baby through breast milk, with the highest concentration about 30 to 60 minutes after drinking (60–90 minutes if taken with food). The effects of alcohol on the baby are directly related to the amount of alcohol the mother consumes. Moderate to heavy drinking (2 or more drinks per day) can interfere with the ability to breast-feed, harm the baby's motor development, and slow the baby's weight gain. If you plan to drink (eg, wine with dinner), you can avoid breast-feeding for a few hours (until the alcohol has time to leave your system) or you can pump your milk before drinking alcohol and give it to the baby after you have had the alcohol. You can also pump and discard the milk that is most affected by the ingested alcohol.

2. Caffeine is considered compatible with breast-feeding. However, large amounts should be avoided because infants may be jittery and have difficulty sleeping.

3. Cigarette smoking is contraindicated. Nicotine and an active metabolite are concentrated in milk and the amounts reaching the infant are proportional to the number of cigarettes smoked by the mother. Ideally, the mother who smokes would stop. If unable or unwilling to stop, she should decrease the number of cigarettes as much as possible, avoid smoking before nursing, and avoid smoking (or allowing other people to smoke) in the same room with the infant. The risk for sudden infant death syndrome (SIDS) is greater when a mother smokes or when the baby is around secondhand (passive) smoke. Maternal smoking and passive smoke may also increase respiratory and ear infections in infants.

---

clients should be an obstetric specialist who is knowledgeable about normal pregnancy and potential complications. The nurse should be aware of the drugs being used to treat the complicated obstetric client as well as maternal use of any nonprescription and nontherapeutic drugs. A systematic assessment of maternal and fetal responses should be made on each visit.

Home care visits also allow for assessment of compliance with the proposed management plan. Understanding of previous teaching should be evaluated on each visit. It is especially important for the client to know the danger signs and symptoms that may necessitate notifying a health care provider.

The overall goal of home care is to maintain the pregnancy to the most advanced gestational age possible. Home care follow-up by a nurse has been demonstrated to positively affect the outcome of a high-risk pregnancy.

APPLYING YOUR KNOWLEDGE 65-4:
HOW CAN YOU AVOID THIS MEDICATION ERROR?
Mrs. Blevins delivers a healthy baby and is breast-feeding. At her 6-week checkup, she is told she can resume normal sexual relations. Mrs. Blevins does not want to have another child for a while, so she resumes taking the birth control pills that she took prior to becoming pregnant.

Box 65-5 Drug Effects During Lactation

Overview

The American Academy of Pediatrics (AAP) recommends breast-feeding for optimal nutrition during the first year of life and is considered the most authoritative source of information about drug effects in lactation. Most drugs have not been tested in nursing women and no one knows exactly how a given drug will affect a nursing infant. Even the clinical practice guidelines from the AAP emphasize that the reported effects of drug safety or nonsafety are often anecdotal and based on observations in a single infant or a few infants rather than on well-designed studies. In general, maternal drug use during lactation should be cautious and based on the following assumptions:

1. There is some degree of risk with any systemic medication ingested by the mother. Some of the drug reaches the nursing infant, with the amount usually proportional to the amount in the mother's bloodstream. However, in many instances, the infant may not receive sufficient drug to produce adverse effects.
2. The lowest dose and the shortest effective duration are recommended.
3. Potential drug effects on nursing infants should be considered and the infant's health care provider should be consulted when indicated.
4. Most over-the-counter and prescription drugs, taken in moderation and only when needed, are thought to be safe.

Drugs Generally Considered Safe During Lactation

Acetaminophen, antibacterials (penicillins and cephalosporins), anticoagulants (heparin or warfarin), antiepilepsy medications, antihistamines, antihypertensives (angiotensin-converting enzyme [ACE] inhibitors, calcium channel blockers), butorphanol, caffeine (in moderate amounts), corticosteroids (prednisolone or inhaled products), cromolyn, decongestants (oxymetolazine nose drops or spray), digoxin, famotidine, ibuprofen, insulin, levothyroxine, progestin-only birth control pills (the "mini-pill"), sucralfate

Drugs To Be Used With Caution During Lactation

Alcohol (within 2 hours of breast-feeding), aluminum-containing antacids, amantadine, antianxiety agents (benzodiazepines), antibacterials (chloramphenicol, metronidazole, nitrofurantoin, sulfonamides), antidepressants (bupropion, tricyclics, selective serotonin reuptake inhibitors), antihistamine (clemastine), antipsychotics (older agents), aspirin, beta blockers (acebutolol, atenolol), corticosteroids (systemic drugs may suppress growth, interfere with endogenous corticosteroid production, or cause other adverse effects in nursing infants), diuretics, dyslipidemics (cholestyramine [may cause severe constipation in the infant], statins), methadone, metoclopramide, theophylline

Drugs That Are Contraindicated During Lactation

If these drugs are required, breast-feeding should usually be stopped: amiodarone, antibacterials (fluoroquinolones, tetracyclines, trimethoprim [may interfere with folic acid metabolism in the infant]), antineoplastics (cyclophosphamide, doxorubicin, methotrexate, most others), bromocriptine (decreases milk production), caffeine (large amounts), cyclosporine, drugs of abuse (amphetamines, cocaine, heroin, marijuana, phencyclidine, nicotine), ergotamine, immunosuppressants, isotretinoin, lithium, phenytoin

N U R S I N G   A C T I O N S

Abortifacients, Prostaglandins, Tocolytics, and Oxytocics

NURSING ACTIONS	RATIONALE/EXPLANATION
1. Administer accurately	These drugs are given according to specific protocols and should be administered only by nurses experienced in their use and aftercare of clients.
a. With mifepristone (Mifeprex), prostaglandin abortifacients (eg, Hemabate, Prostin E₂) and prostaglandin cervical ripening agents (eg, Cervidil), consult manufacturers' instructions.	
b. Give intravenous (IV) magnesium sulfate via an infusion pump; read the drug label carefully to be sure of using the correct preparation for the intended use; when available, use premixed IV bags of 20 grams of magnesium sulfate in 500 milliliters of IV fluid; clearly label IV bags; use a separate 100-milliliter (4-gram) or 150-milliliter (6-gram) IV piggyback solution for the initial bolus dose; give the initial bolus over 20–30 minutes; titrate the maintenance dose (1–2 g/hour) according to uterine activity and serum magnesium levels;	Magnesium sulfate is a high-risk drug and should be given only by experienced labor and delivery nurses who are knowledgeable about safe administration and monitoring clients. The nurse should assess and document maternal status and fetal status before starting the drug infusion; remain at the bedside during bolus infusions; and monitor the client frequently throughout drug administration.
	Magnesium sulfate is available in different concentrations and sizes as well as a multidose vial.

(continued)

NURSING ACTIONS	RATIONALE/EXPLANATION
have a second nurse check all IV bags containing magnesium sulfate and all infusion pump settings; have IV calcium gluconate readily available.	Calcium gluconate is an antidote for an overdose of magnesium sulfate. One ampule of 1 gram (10 milliliters of a 10% solution) can be given IV over 3 minutes to relieve signs and symptoms of hypermagnesemia.
c. Give IV ritodrine via an infusion pump, with the client lying in the left lateral position.	To decrease risks of hypotension
d. Give terbutaline IV initially, via an infusion pump, then by mouth (PO) for maintenance.	Although not Food and Drug Administration–approved for tocolysis, there is extensive clinical experience with the drug.
e. For IV oxytocin, dilute the drug in an IV sodium chloride solution, and piggyback the solution into a primary IV line. Use an infusion pump to administer.	Oxytocin may cause water intoxication, which is less likely to occur if the drug is given in a saline solution. Piggybacking allows regulation of the oxytocin drip without interrupting the main IV line.
f. Give intramuscular (IM) oxytocin immediately after delivery of the placenta.	To prevent excessive postpartum bleeding
2. Observe for therapeutic effects	
a. When an abortifacient is given, observe for the onset of uterine bleeding and the expulsion of the fetus and placenta.	Abortion usually occurs within 24 hours after a prostaglandin is given and approximately 5 days after mifepristone administration.
b. When a tocolytic drug is given in threatened abortion or premature labor, observe for absent or decreased uterine contractions.	The goal of drug therapy is to stop the labor process. Uterine activity may be assessed by maternal self-report, palpation, or electronic fetal monitoring. Tocolytic blood levels of magnesium sulfate range from 4.8–9.6 mg/dL.
c. When magnesium sulfate is given in preeclampsia, observe for an absence or decrease of seizures.	Blood levels of 3–6 mg/dL are considered optimal for antiseizure effects.
d. When oxytocin is given to induce or augment labor, observe for firm uterine contractions at a rate of three to four per 10 minutes. Each contraction should be followed by a palpable relaxation period. Examine periodically for cervical dilatation and effacement.	Uterine contractions should become regular and increase in duration and intensity.
e. When oxytocin or methylergonovine is given to prevent or control postpartum bleeding, observe for a small, firm uterus and minimal vaginal bleeding.	These agents control bleeding by causing strong uterine contractions. The uterus can be palpated in the lower abdomen.
3. Observe for adverse effects	
a. With mifepristone, observe for excessive uterine bleeding and abdominal pain.	These effects are uncommon but may occur.
b. With prostaglandins, observe for:	
(1) Nausea, vomiting, diarrhea	These are the most common adverse effects; they result from stimulation of gastrointestinal smooth muscle.
(2) Fever, cardiac dysrhythmias, bronchospasm, convulsions, chest pain, muscle aches	These effects occur less often. Bronchospasm is more likely to occur in clients with asthma; seizures are more likely in clients with known epilepsy.
c. With magnesium sulfate, observe for:	
(1) Hypermagnesemia—respiratory depression and failure, depressed deep-tendon reflexes, muscle weakness, hypotension, cardiac dysrhythmias, cardiac arrest	Hypermagnesemia is most likely to occur with rapid IV administration; high dosages or concentrations; in the presence of renal insufficiency and decreased urine output; and when relatively high blood levels are required for tocolytic effects.
(2) Headache, vomiting, nausea, chest pain, lethargy, visual disturbances, weakness	
(3) Change in fetal heart rate	
d. With ritodrine, observe for:	
(1) Change in fetal heart rate	This is a common adverse effect and may be significant if changes are extreme or prolonged.

NURSING ACTIONS	RATIONALE/EXPLANATION
(2) Maternal effects (eg, palpitations, dysrhythmias, changes in blood pressure, nausea and vomiting, hyperglycemia, dyspnea, chest pain, anaphylactic shock)	
e. With oxytocin, observe for:	
(1) Excessive stimulation of uterine contractility (hypertonicity; tetany; rupture; cervical and perineal lacerations; fetal hypoxia; dysrhythmias; death or damage from rapid, forceful propulsion through the birth canal)	Most likely to occur when excessive doses are given to initiate or augment labor.
(2) Hypotension or hypertension	Usual obstetric doses do not cause significant change in blood pressure. Large doses may cause an initial drop in blood pressure, followed by a sustained elevation.
(3) Water intoxication (convulsions, coma)	
f. With ergot preparations, observe for:	
(1) Nausea, vomiting, diarrhea	These drugs stimulate the vomiting center of the brain and stimulate contraction of gastrointestinal smooth muscle.
(2) Symptoms of ergot poisoning—coolness, numbness, and tingling of extremities; headache; vomiting; dizziness; thirst; convulsions; weak pulse; confusion; chest pain; muscle weakness and pain	The ergot alkaloids are highly toxic. Circulatory impairments may result from vasoconstriction and vascular insufficiency. Large doses also damage capillary endothelium and may cause thrombosis and occlusion.
(3) Hypertension	Hypertension may result from generalized vasoconstriction.
4. Observe for drug interactions	
a. Drugs that *alter* effects of prostaglandins:	
(1) Aspirin and other nonsteroidal anti-inflammatory agents, such as ibuprofen	These drugs inhibit effects of prostaglandins. When given concurrently with abortifacient prostaglandins, the abortive process is prolonged.
b. Drug that *alters* effects of magnesium sulfate:	
(1) Calcium gluconate	Calcium gluconate is an antidote for magnesium sulfate overdose.
c. Drugs that *alter* effects of ritodrine:	
(1) Beta-adrenergic blocking agents (eg, propranolol)	Decreased effectiveness of ritodrine, which is a beta-adrenergic stimulating (agonist) agent
(2) Corticosteroids	Increased risk of pulmonary edema
d. Drugs that *alter* effects of oxytocin:	
(1) Vasoconstrictors, such as epinephrine and other adrenergic drugs	Additive vasoconstriction with risks of severe, persistent hypertension and intracranial hemorrhage
e. Drugs that *alter* effects of ergot alkaloids:	
(1) Propranolol (Inderal)	Additive vasoconstriction
(2) Vasoconstrictors	See oxytocin at 4d above

APPLYING YOUR KNOWLEDGE: ANSWERS

65-1 Instruct Mrs. Blevins to begin to take 400 to 600 micrograms of folic acid daily. Folic acid supplementation can prevent neural-tube birth defects.

65-2 Tell Mrs. Blevins that constipation is a common occurrence during pregnancy. The best treatment is to increase amount of exercise and intake of fluids and high-fiber foods. If a laxative is needed, a bulk-producing agent is recommended because it is safest for both mother and fetus.

65-3 All systemically absorbed drugs in the mother's bloodstream will reach the fetus. Drugs are listed with an FDA pregnancy risk category based on the amount of risk to the fetus. Drugs categorized as risk category X should not be used at all during pregnancy. Most drugs are risk category C and should be discussed with the physician. These drugs should only be used when the potential benefit to the mother outweighs the risk to the fetus.

65-4 Mrs. Blevins needs a new prescription for birth control without estrogen. Ortho Tri-Cyclen contains estrogen; estrogen is contraindicated while she is breast-feeding.

Review and Application Exercises

Short Answer Exercises

1. Why should drugs be avoided during pregnancy and lactation when possible?

2. How does insulin therapy for diabetes mellitus differ during pregnancy?

3. What is the rationale for using methyldopa and hydralazine to treat hypertension during pregnancy?

4. How are asthma and seizure disorders managed during pregnancy?

5. In a client receiving a tocolytic drug to inhibit uterine contractions, how and when would you assess the client for adverse drug effects?

6. In a client receiving an oxytocin infusion to induce or augment labor, what interventions are needed to increase safety and decrease adverse drug effects?

7. Which immunizations are safe to be administered during pregnancy? Which are contraindicated?

8. A pregnant client asks you about using herbal supplements. What would you tell her? Why?

NCLEX-Style Questions

9. A daily vitamin-K supplement is recommended during the last month of pregnancy for women receiving long-term drug therapy for which of the following conditions?
   a. asthma
   b. diabetes mellitus
   c. hypertension
   d. seizure disorders

10. For a client receiving a continuous IV magnesium sulfate infusion for tocolysis, which of the following medications needs to be readily available at the client's bedside?
    a. diazepam (Valium)
    b. hydralazine (Apresoline)
    c. calcium gluconate
    d. phenytoin (Dilantin)

11. Betamethasone (Celestone) is ordered for a client experiencing preterm labor at 34 weeks' gestation. The nurse explains to the client that the drug is being given to
    a. enhance fetal lung maturity
    b. counteract the effects of tocolytic therapy
    c. treat intrauterine infection
    d. decrease need for a cesarean section

12. A drug of choice for treating group B streptococcal infection in a pregnant woman is a
    a. penicillin
    b. fluoroquinolone
    c. aminoglycoside
    d. tetracycline

13. Oxytocin is usually preferred over methylergonovine for prevention and control of postpartum uterine bleeding because it is less likely to cause
    a. hypotension
    b. hypertension
    c. bradycardia
    d. tachycardia

Selected References

Drug facts and comparisons. (Updated monthly). St. Louis: Facts and Comparisons.

Elliot, D. L. (2004). Pregnancy: Hypertension and other common medical problems. In L. Goldman & D. Ausiello (Eds.), *Cecil textbook of medicine* (22nd ed., pp. 1521–1528). Philadelphia: W. B. Saunders.

Gibbs, R. S., Schrag, S., & Schuchat, A. (2004). Perinatal infections due to Group B streptococci. *Obstetrics & Gynecology, 104*(5), 1062–1076.

Lacy, C. F., Armstrong, L. L., Goldman, M. P., Lance, L. L. (2004). *Lexi-Comp's drug information handbook* (12th ed.). Hudson, OH: Lexi-Comp.

McCarter-Spaulding, D. E. (2005). Medications in pregnancy and lactation. *MCN: The Journal of Maternal/Child Nursing, 30*(1), 12–17.

National Asthma Education and Prevention Program (NAEPP) Expert Panel. Managing asthma during pregnancy: Recommendations for pharmacologic treatment—2004 update. *Journal of Allergy & Clinical Immunology, 115*(1), 34–46.

Patka, J. H., Lodolce, A. E., & Johnston, A. K. (2005). High- versus low-dose oxytocin for augmentation or induction of labor. *The Annals of Pharmacotherapy, 39*(1), 95–101.

Pigarelli, D. L., & Kraus, C. K. (2002). Pregnancy and lactation: Therapeutic considerations. In J. T. DiPiro, R. L. Talbert, G. C. Yee, G. R. Matzke, B. G. Wells, & L. M. Posey (Eds.), *Pharmacotherapy: A pathophysiologic approach* (5th ed., pp. 1413–1429). New York: McGraw-Hill.

Porth, C. M. (2005). *Pathophysiology: Concepts of altered health states* (7th ed.). Philadelphia: Lippincott Williams & Wilkins.

Pschirrer, E. R. (2004). Seizure disorders in pregnancy. *Obstetric and Gynecology Clinics of North America, 31,* 373–384.

Ressel, G. (2002). Practice guidelines: AAP updates statement for transfer of drugs and other chemicals into breast milk. *American Family Physician, 65*(5), 979–980.

Schroeder, B. M. (2002). Practice guidelines: ACOG practice bulletin on diagnosing and managing preeclampsia and eclampsia. *American Family Physician, 66*(2), 330–331.

Simpson, K. R., & Knox, G. E. (2004). Obstetrical accidents involving intravenous magnesium sulfate: Recommendations to promote patient safety. *MCN: The Journal of Maternal/Child Nursing, 29*(3), 161–169.

Spector, S. A. (2004). HIV in pregnancy. In L. Goldman & D. Ausiello (Eds.), *Cecil textbook of medicine* (22nd ed., pp. 1528–1531). Philadelphia: W. B. Saunders.

Watts, D. H. (2002). Management of human immunodeficiency virus infection in pregnancy. *New England Journal of Medicine, 346*(24), 1879–1891.

Young, V. S. L. (2005). Teratogenicity and drugs in breast milk. In M. A. Koda-Kimble, L. Y. Young, W. A. Kradjan, et al., *Applied therapeutics: The clinical use of drugs* (8th ed., pp. 47-1–47-32). Philadelphia: Lippincott Williams & Wilkins.

Recently Approved and Miscellaneous Drugs

GENERIC/TRADE NAME	CLINICAL USE	CHARACTERISTICS	ROUTES AND DOSAGE RANGES
Alprostadil (Caverject, Muse)	Erectile dysfunction	A form of prostaglandin E Induces erection within 5–20 min	Caverject, injection into penis Muse, insertion into urethra Dosage, lowest effective dose
Antithrombin III, human (Thrombate III)	Antithrombin III deficiency in clients with thrombotic disorders	Replaces a substance normally found in plasma	Dosage individualized
Azacitidine (Vidaza)	Myelodysplastic syndrome	Antimetabolite antineo-plastic agent	Variable—see literature
Balsalazide (Colazal)	Ulcerative colitis	Anti-inflammatory effects	PO 2250 mg 3 times daily for 8–12 wk
Bromfenac (Xibrom)	Eye inflammation after cataract extraction	A nonsteroidal anti-inflammatory drug (NSAID)	1 drop to affected eye twice daily, starting 24 h after cataract surgery and con-tinuing for 2 wk
Clofarabine (Clolar)	Relapsed or refractory acute lymphoblastic leukemia in children (1–21 y)	Antimetabolite antineo-plastic agent	IV 52 mg/m^2 once daily for 5 consecutive d; repeat q2–6wk
Darifenacin (Enablex)	Overactive bladder	An anticholinergic drug that reduces incontinence, urgency, and frequency	PO 7.5 mg once daily ini-tially, increased to 15 mg once daily if necessary
Duloxetine (Cymbalta)	Neuropathic pain associated with diabetic peripheral neuropathy Major depressive disorder	Inhibits serotonin and norepinephrine reuptake Adverse effects include nau-sea, dizziness, insomnia, drowsiness.	Neuropathic pain, PO 60 mg once daily Depression, PO 40 mg (20 mg twice daily) or 60 mg (30 mg twice daily or 60 mg once daily)
Entecavir (Baraclude)	Chronic hepatitis B	Antiviral agent Adverse effects include dizziness, fatigue, headache, nausea, lactic acidosis, hepatomegaly.	PO 0.5 mg once daily for clients beginning treat-ment; 1 mg daily for those who have developed resis-tance to lamivirdine
Eszopidone (Lunesta)	Insomnia	Nonbenzodiazepine hypnotic A Schedule IV drug	PO 2–3 mg immediately before bedtime
Exenatide (Byetta)	Adjunctive treatment of type 2 diabetes mellitus with metformin, a sulfonylurea, or a metformin-sulfonylurea combination in clients who have not achieved ade-quate glycemic control	An incretin mimetic agent. Incretin has antihyper-glycemic activity. Adverse effects include hypoglycemia, dizziness, diarrhea, nausea, vomiting.	Sub-Q 5 mcg twice daily, within 60 min before morn-ing and evening meals
Insulin detemir (Levemir)	Type 1 and type 2 diabetes mellitus	A long-acting form of insulin Effects last up to 24 h Can be used alone, with oral antidiabetic agents, or with a rapid-acting insulin	Sub-Q, dosage variable, once or twice daily
Lanthanum (Fosrenol)	Reduce serum phosphate levels in patients with end-stage renal disease	Binds to dietary phosphate and inhibits its absorption	PO 750–1500 mg daily, in divided doses with meals. To be chewed before swallowing

(continued)

GENERIC/TRADE NAME	CLINICAL USE	CHARACTERISTICS	ROUTES AND DOSAGE RANGES
Mesalamine (Pentasa, Rowasa)	Ulcerative colitis Proctitis	Anti-inflammatory effects	Tablets, PO 800 mg 3 times daily for 6 wk Capsules, PO 1 g 4 times daily for up to 8 wk Rectally, 1 suppository (500 mg) twice daily or enema (60 mL) once daily
Micafungin (Mycamine)	Prevent *Candida* infections in clients undergoing hematopoietic stem cell transplantation (HSCT) and treatment of esophageal candidiasis	Similar to caspofungin Adverse effects include liver and renal function changes and a possible histamine-related reaction with rash, itching, facial swelling, and vasodilation.	IV infusion, 50 mg daily for HSCT recipients; 150 mg daily for esophageal candidiasis, infused over 1 h
Mitodrine (ProAmatine)	Orthostatic hypotension	For severe symptoms only	PO 10 mg 3 times daily
Osalazine (Dipentum)	Ulcerative colitis	Anti-inflammatory effects	PO 500 mg twice daily
Palifermin (Kepivance)	Oral mucositis associated with hematologic malignancies	Drug decreases incidence and severity of mucositis.	IV 60 mcg/kg/d for 3 d before and after myelotoxic drug therapy (6 doses)
Pentosan polysulfate sodium (Elmiron)	Bladder pain associated with interstitial cystitis	May prevent mucosal irritation	PO 100 mg 3 times daily
Pramlintide (Symlin)	Used with insulin to treat type 1 and type 2 diabetes mellitus	A synthetic analog of amylin, an endogenous hormone produced in pancreatic beta cells that works with insulin and glucagons to maintain normal glucose levels Insulin dosage must be reduced when pramlintide therapy is initiated.	See drug literature; dosage varies with type of diabetes
Pregabalin (Lyrica)	Neuropathic pain associated with diabetic peripheral neuropathy and postherpetic neuralgia	May cause dizziness, drowsiness, ankle edema, blurred vision, weight gain	PO 50–100 mg 3 times daily
Rasburicase (Elitek)	Prevent elevated serum uric acid levels in children with malignancies	May cause anaphylaxis	IV infusion 0.15–0.2 mg/kg once daily for 5 d, 4–24 h before chemotherapy
Riluzole (Rilutek)	Amyotrophic lateral sclerosis (ALS)	May cause nausea and increased liver enzymes	PO 50 mg q12h
Sevelamer (Renagel)	Hyperphosphatemia in clients with end-stage renal disease	Reduces serum phosphorus levels	PO 800–1600 mg with each meal, depending on serum phosphorus level
Sildenafil (Viagra)	Erectile dysfunction	Associated with myocardial infarction	PO 50 mg 1 h before sexual activity
Solifenacin (Vesicare)	Overactive bladder	An anticholinergic drug that reduces incontinence, urgency, and frequency	PO 5–10 mg once daily
Sulfasalazine (Azulfidine)	Ulcerative colitis Rheumatoid arthritis	Anti-inflammatory effects	PO 2–4 g daily in divided doses
Tadalafil (Cialis)	Erectile dysfunction	Adverse effects include hypertension and myocardial infarction.	PO 10 mg before anticipated sexual activity
Tegaserod (Zelnorm)	Constipation-dominant irritable bowel syndrome (IBS)	May cause diarrhea and abdominal pain	PO 6 mg twice daily for 4–6 wk

GENERIC/TRADE NAME	CLINICAL USE	CHARACTERISTICS	ROUTES AND DOSAGE RANGES
Tigecycline (Tygacil)	Complicated skin, skin structures, and intra-abdominal infections caused by susceptible organisms	The first of a new class of antibiotics called *glycylcyclines,* which are derivatives of tetracyclines Has a broad spectrum of antimicrobial activity, including against methicillin-resistant *Staphylococcus aureus* (MRSA)	IV infusion, 100 mg initially, then 50 mg q12h over 30–60 min for 5–14 d
Tipranavir	Human immunodeficiency virus/acquired immuno-deficiency syndrome (HIV/AIDS) infection	A protease inhibitor (see Chap. 35)	
Vardenafil (Levitra)	Erectile dysfunction	Adverse effects include flushing, headache, dizziness.	PO 10 mg 60 min before sexual activity
Ziconotide (Prialt)	Analgesic for severe chronic pain in clients who require intrathecal therapy	May cause psychosis and neurologic impairment	See literature

IV, intravenous; PO, oral; Sub-Q, subcutaneous.

The International System of Units

The International System of Units (Système International d'Unites or SI units), which is based on the metric system, has been adopted by many countries in an attempt to standardize reports of clinical laboratory data among nations and disciplines. A major reason for using SI units is that biologic substances react in the human body on a molar basis.

The International System, like the conventional or traditional system, uses the kilogram for measurement of mass or weight and the meter for measurement of length. The major difference is that the International System uses the mole for measurement of amounts per volume of a substance. A mole is the amount of a chemical compound of which its weight in grams equals its molecular weight. Thus, the concentrations of solutions are expressed in moles, millimoles, or micromoles per liter (mol/L, mmol/L, micromol/L) rather than the conventional measurement of mass per volume, such as grams or milligrams per 100 mL or dL. A few laboratory values are the same in conventional and SI units, but many differ dramatically. Moreover, "normal values" in both systems often vary, depending on laboratory methodologies and reference sources. Thus, *laboratory data should be interpreted in light of the client's clinical status and with knowledge of the "normal values" of the laboratory performing the test.*

Serum Drug Concentrations

Measuring the amount of a drug in blood plasma or serum is often useful in the clinical management of various disorders. For example, serum drug levels may be used to guide drug dosage (eg, with aminoglycoside antibiotics such as gentamicin); to evaluate an inadequate therapeutic response; and to diagnose or manage drug toxicity. Listed below are generally accepted therapeutic serum drug concentrations, in conventional and SI units, for some commonly used drugs. In addition, toxic concentrations are listed for acetaminophen and salicylate. Note that SI units have not been established for some drugs.

DRUG	CONVENTIONAL UNITS	SI UNITS
Acetaminophen	0.2–0.6 mg/dL	13–40 µmol/L
	Toxic >5 mg/dL	>300 µmol/L
Amikacin	(Peak) 16–32 mcg/mL	20–30 mg/L
	(Trough) ≤8 mcg/mL	
Amitriptyline	110–250 ng/mL	375–900 nmol/L
Carbamazepine	4–12 mcg/mL	17–50 µmol/L
Desipramine	125–300 ng/mL	470–825 nmol/L
Digoxin	0.5–2.2 ng/mL	1–2.6 nmol/L
Disopyramide	2–8 mcg/mL	6–18 µmol/L
Ethosuximide	40–110 mcg/mL	280–780 µmol/L
Gentamicin	(Peak) 4–8 mcg/mL	5–10 mg/L
	(Trough) ≤2 mcg/mL	
Imipramine	200–350 ng/mL	530–950 nmol/L
Lidocaine	1.5–6 mcg/mL	6–21 µmol/L
Lithium	0.5–1.5 mEq/L	0.5–1.5 mmol/L
Maprotiline	50–200 ng/mL	180–270 nmol/L
Nortriptyline	50–150 ng/mL	190–570 nmol/L
Phenobarbital	15–50 mcg/mL	65–170 µmol/L
Phenytoin	10–20 mcg/mL	40–80 µmol/L
Primidone	5–12 mcg/mL	25–45 µmol/L
Procainamide	4–8 mcg/mL	17–40 µmol/L
Propranolol	50–200 ng/mL	190–770 nmol/L
Protriptyline	100–300 ng/mL	380–1140 nmol/L
Quinidine	2–6 mcg/mL	4.6–9.2 µmol/L
Salicylate	100–200 mg/L	724–1448 µmol/L
	Toxic >200 mg/L	>1450 µmol/L
Theophylline	10–20 mcg/mL	55–110 µmol/L
Tobramycin	(Peak) 4–8 mcg/mL	5–10 mg/L
	(Trough) ≤2 mcg/mL	
Valproic acid	50–100 mcg/mL	350–700 µmol/L
Vancomycin	(Peak) 30–40 mg/mL	(Peak) 20–40 mg/L
	(Trough) 5–10 mg/mL	(Trough) 5–10 mg/L

dL, deciliter; mcg, microgram; mEq, milliequivalent; mmol, micromole; ng, nanogram; nmol, nanomole; µmol, micromole.

Canadian Drug Laws and Standards

OVERVIEW

Canadian drug laws are federal and provincial. The two main federal laws are the Food and Drugs Act, initially passed in 1953, and the Controlled Drugs and Substances Act, passed in 1997 to replace and update the former Narcotic Control Act. These national laws, with their amendments, regulate drug-related standards and practices. Health Canada is the national authority that evaluates and regulates the safety and effectiveness of drugs and medical devices available to Canadians. The Health Products and Food Branch (HPFB) of Health Canada regulates the use of therapeutic substances such as pharmaceutical products; narcotic, controlled, and restricted drugs; and biologic drug products. Health Canada is similar to the Food and Drug Administration in the United States and has a similar drug review process.

THE FOOD AND DRUGS ACT

The Food and Drugs Act applies to all food, drugs, cosmetics, and medical devices sold in Canada. In relation to drugs, the Act controls the manufacture, distribution, sale, advertising, labeling, and use of all drugs except controlled substances. In addition, the Act specifies that drugs cannot be marketed without a notice of compliance and a drug identification number from Health Canada. Amended guidelines date back to 1953, stating that the use of foods, drugs, cosmetics, and therapeutic devices must follow established guidelines. Any drug that does not comply with standards established by recognized pharmacopeiae and formularies in the United States, Europe, Britain, or France cannot be labeled, packaged, sold, or advertised in Canada.

Specific provisions:

- Empower the government to control the marketing of drugs according to proof of safety and effectiveness
- Require that drugs comply with the standards under which the drugs are approved for sale or the standards listed in "specific pharmacopeiae"
- Direct the government to supervise the manufacturing processes of some drugs
- Classify drugs that require a prescription and specify that refills must be designated on the original prescription and obtained within 6 months (Schedule F)
- Specify symbols to be placed on containers of the different classifications of drugs (eg, **Pr** for "Prescription required" drugs)

- Require proof of appropriate drug release from oral dosage formulations
- Prohibit advertising of prescription and controlled drugs to the public
- Prohibit the sale of contaminated, adulterated, or unsafe drugs
- Establish requirements for labeling
- Prohibit false, misleading, or deceptive labeling of drug products

Drug regulations stemming from the Act separate drugs sold in Canada into several categories referred to as *schedules,* which are described below.

Schedule F lists drugs such as antihypertensives, psychotropics, and other medications that are available to the general public only with a prescription from a medical practitioner. Prescriptions for Schedule F drugs may be written or oral (eg, telephone order to the pharmacist), and can be refilled as often as indicated by the licensed prescriber. Several hundred drugs are listed in Schedule F and new drugs are often added to the list. The symbol **Pr** must appear on all manufacturing labels. A few drugs (eg, digoxin) are classified federally as nonprescription, but the provinces may require a prescription.

Schedule G lists certain controlled drugs. These drugs have a moderate potential for abuse and require greater control than **Schedule F** drugs (which have essentially no potential for abuse). Schedule G contains about 14 drugs, including some non-narcotic potent analgesics (eg, nalbuphine, butorphanol), amphetamines and derivatives, anabolic steroids, and barbiturates. These drugs can be obtained by a written or oral prescription but refills are only allowed with a written order. The symbol **C** must appear on labels of these drugs and a health care provider may only dispense these drugs to clients suffering from specific diseases or illnesses. Schedule G is similar to Schedule III of the Controlled Substances Act in the United States.

Schedule H lists potentially dangerous hallucinogens that have no recognized medical use, such as lysergic acid diethylamide (LSD), MDMA (ecstasy), mescaline, and peyote. This category is similar to Schedule I of the Controlled Substances Act in the United States.

THE CONTROLLED DRUGS AND SUBSTANCES ACT

The Controlled Drugs and Substances Act and its amendments regulate the manufacture, distribution, sale, possession, and use of substances classified as narcotics or controlled substances (eg, opiates, cocaine, marijuana, methadone, and benzodiazepine antianxiety and hypnotic agents).

Additional provisions:

- Restrict possession of the drugs to authorized people
- Require people possessing the drugs to keep them in a secure place, maintain strict dispensing records, and promptly report any thefts or other losses

- Require prescriptions for dispensing narcotics. An exception is low-dose codeine preparations (eg, 8-mg tablets and 20 mg/30 mL solutions) that contain at least two additional medicinal ingredients. These preparations can be purchased without a prescription but they can be sold only by a pharmacist.
- Require that containers with prescribed narcotics be labeled with the symbol **N** and containers with other controlled substances be labeled with the symbol **C.**
- Specify eight levels or schedules of controlled drugs. Drugs representing each schedule are listed below.

  Schedule I. Opium derivatives (eg, codeine, morphine, heroin, hydrocodone, hydromorphone, oxycodone, oxymorphone), buprenorphine, cocaine, dextropropoxyphene, diphenoxylate, difenoxin, fentanyl and related drugs, levomethorphan, levorphanol, methadone, pentazocine, phencyclidine, pethidine

  Schedule II. Cannabis, cannabinol, nabilone, tetrahydrocannabinol

  Schedule III. Amphetamines, methamphetamine, 3,4-methylenedioxyamphetamine (MDMA or ecstasy), methylphenidate, lysergic acid diethylamide (LSD), mescaline, psilocin, flunitrazepam (Rohypnol, a "date rape" drug), 4-hydroxybutanoic acid (GHB, a "date rape" drug)

  Schedule IV. Barbiturates (eg, pentobarbital, secobarbital), benzodiazepines (alprazolam, chlordiazepoxide, clonazepam, clorazepate, diazepam, estazolam, flurazepam, lorazepam, midazolam, oxazepam, quazepam, temazepam, triazolam), anabolic steroids (androstenediol, fluoxymesterone, nandrolone, oxandrolone, stanozolol, testosterone), butorphanol, chlorphentermine, diethylpropion, mazindol, nalbuphine, phendimetrazine, phentermine, zolpidem

  Schedule V. Ephedrine, ergotamine

  Schedule VI. Drugs alone or in preparations or mixtures that contain precursor drugs used to manufacture controlled drugs (ephedrine, ergotamine, lysergic acid, norephedrine [phenylpropanolamine], pseudoephedrine)

  Schedule VII. 3 kilograms of cannabis (marijuana) or cannabis resin

  Schedule VIII. 30 grams of cannabis or 1 gram of cannabis resin

PROVINCIAL REGULATIONS

Provincial regulations of prescription drugs promote substitution of cheaper drugs (eg, generic rather than brand-name products) over expensive drugs and focus on cost-effectiveness to determine if a new drug should be included in the provincial formulary. These regulations direct prescribers to prescribe generic drugs and the pharmacists to dispense the cheapest generic drug available for all prescriptions.

NURSING IMPLICATIONS

In drug therapy, nurses in Canada are governed by federal and provincial laws as well as professional standards. With prescribed drugs, for example, nurses must safely and accurately administer the drugs to the clients for whom they are prescribed. In addition, nurses need a strong knowledge base about the drugs they administer and about the clients who receive the drugs in order to assess for therapeutic and adverse effects, drug–drug and drug–food interactions, and client and family teaching needs. Nursing interventions include actions to maximize therapeutic effects, minimize adverse effects, educate clients, and evaluate the effectiveness of drug therapy.

With controlled drugs, legal possession by a nurse is restricted to the following circumstances:

- When administering to a client according to an order from a health care provider legally licensed to give such an order
- When performing custodial care of controlled substances as an agent of a health care facility
- When receiving a prescribed controlled substance for personal medical treatment

Additional regulations include storing the drugs in a locked container, allowing only authorized persons access to the drugs, and maintaining accurate counts and special records for each drug and each dose administered.

Canadian Drug Names

The purpose of this appendix is to assist the Canadian reader to identify the drugs discussed in this book. Many drugs are distributed by international pharmaceutical companies, and many names (generic and brand) are the same in the United States and Canada. The following drug names are those listed in the 2005 edition of the *Compendium of Pharmaceuticals and Specialties* (CPS), published by the Canadian Pharmacists Association. Drugs are listed alphabetically by generic name, followed by the number of the chapter in which the drug is discussed in the text and Canadian brand names. Drugs listed without a brand name are usually available only by generic names. Numerous brand names have been discontinued by their manufacturers in recent years and this seems to be a continuing trend.

Canadian trade names that begin with Apo, Gen, Novo, Nu, ratio, or Rhoxal are drugs manufactured by Apotex, Genpharm, Novopharm, Nu-Pharm, ratiopharm, and Rhoxalpharma companies, respectively. Many brand names consist of a company prefix and a generic name (eg, Apo-Cimetidine, Gen-Alprazolam, Novo-Acebutolol, Nu-Clonidine, ratio-Atenolol, Rhoxal-Ciprofloxacin). Because these names are easy to identify, they are not included in the accompanying list. However, some trade names consisting of a company prefix and a shortened version of the generic name (eg, Apo-Alpraz for alprazolam) are included.

GENERIC/CANADIAN BRAND NAMES	GENERIC/CANADIAN BRAND NAMES
Abacavir (35)	Fosamax
Ziagen	**Alfuzosin (18)**
Abciximab (54)	Xatral
ReoPro	**Allopurinol (7)**
Acarbose (26)	Novo-Purol, Zyloprim
Prandase	**Almotriptan (7)**
Acebutolol (18)	Axert
Monitan, Rhotral, Sectral	**Alprazolam (8)**
Acetaminophen (7), Paracetamol*	Apo-Alpraz, Novo-Alprazol, Nu-Alpraz, Xanax
Abenol, Atasol, Novo-Gesic, Pediatrix, Tempra, Tylenol	**Alteplase (54)**
Acetazolamide (63)	Activase rt-PA, Cathflo
Diamox	**Aluminum hydroxide (59)**
Acetylcysteine (46)	Amphojel
Mucomyst, Parvolex	**Aluminum hydroxide gel/magnesium hydroxide (59)**
Acitretin (64)	Diovol, Gelusil, Mylanta
Soriatane	**Amantadine (12, 35)**
Acyclovir (35, 64)	Endantadine, Symmetrel
Zovirax	**Amcinonide (64)**
Adalapene (64)	Cyclocort
Differin	**Amikacin (31)**
Adalimumab (40)	Amikin
Humira	**Amiloride (53)**
Adenosine (49)	Apo-Amiloride
Adenocard	**Aminocaproic acid (54)**
Albuterol (17, 44), Salbutamol*	Amicar
Airomir, Apo-Salvent, Ventolin	**Aminophylline (44)**
Alendronate (25)	Phyllocontin

(continued)

GENERIC/CANADIAN BRAND NAMES	GENERIC/CANADIAN BRAND NAMES
Amiodarone (49) Cordarone	**Bitolterol (44)** Tornalate
Amitriptyline (10) Novo-Triptyn	**Bleomycin (42)** Blenoxane
Amlodipine (50) Norvasc	**Brimonidine (63)** Alphagan
Amoxicillin (30) Apo-Amoxi, Lin-Amox, Novamoxin, Nu-Amoxi	**Budesonide (47)** Entocort, Pulmicort, Rhinocort
Amoxicillin/clavulanate (30) Apo-Amoxi Clav, Clavulin	**Bumetanide (53)** Burinex
Amphotericin B (36) Abelcet, Amphotec, Fungizone	**Bupropion (10, 14)** Wellbutrin, Zyban
Ampicillin (30) Apo-Ampi, Nu-Ampi	**Buspirone (8)** Buspar
Anagrelide (54) Agrylin	**Calcitonin-salmon (25)** Calcimar, Caltine, Miacalcin NS
Anakinra (40) Kineret	**Calcitriol (25)** Calcijex, Rocaltrol
Asparaginase (42) Kidrolase	**Calcium carbonate (25)** Apo-Cal, Caltrate, Os-Cal, Tums
Aspirin (7) Asaphen, Novasen	**Candesartan (52)** Atacand
Atenolol (18, 50, 52) Apo-Atenol, Novo-Atenol, Nu-Atenol, Tenormin	**Capecitabine (42)** Xeloda
Atomoxetine (15) Strattera	**Captopril (52)** Apo-Capto, Capoten, Novo-Captoril, Nu-Capto
Atorvastatin (55) Lipitor	**Carbachol (63)** Isopto Carbachol, Miostat
Atropine sulfate (20, 63) Isopto Atropine	**Carbamazepine (11)** Novo-Carbamaz, Tegretol
Azatadine (45) Optimine	**Carboplatin (42)** Paraplatin-AQ
Azathioprine (41) Imuran	**Carmustine (42)** BiCNU
Azelastine (45) Astelin	**Caspofungin (36)** Cancidas
Azithromycin (33) Zithromax	**Cefaclor (30)** Ceclor
Bacitracin (63, 64) Baciguent	**Cefadroxil (30)** Duricef
Baclofen (13) Lioresal, Nu-Baclo	**Cefazolin (30)**
Becaplermin (64) Regranex	**Cefepime (30)** Maxipime
Beclomethasone (23, 44) Gen-Beclo AQ, Propaderm, Qvar, Rivanase AQ, Vanceril	**Cefixime (30)** Suprax
Benzoyl peroxide (64) Acetoxyl, Benoxyl, Benzac, Benzagel, Desquam-X, Oxyderm, Panoxyl, Solugel	**Cefotaxime (30)** Claforan
Benztropine (12, 20)	**Cefotetan (30)** Cefotan
Betamethasone (23, 64) Betaderm, Betaject, Betnesol, Celestone, Tara-Sone, Valisone	**Cefoxitin (30)**
Betaxolol (18, 63) Betoptic S	**Cefprozil (30)** Cefzil
Bethanechol (19) Duvoid	**Ceftazidime (30)** Ceptaz, Fortaz
Biperiden (12, 20) Akineton	**Ceftizoxime (30)** Cefizox
Bisacodyl (60) Dulcolax, Gentlax	**Ceftriaxone (30)** Rocephin
	Cefuroxime (30) Ceftin, Zinacef
	Celecoxib (7) Celebrex

GENERIC/CANADIAN BRAND NAMES	GENERIC/CANADIAN BRAND NAMES
Cephalexin (30) Apo-Cephalex, Novo-Lexin, Nu-Cephalex	**Dacarbazine (42)** DTIC
Cetirizine (45) Reactin	**Dactinomycin (42)** Cosmegen
Chlorambucil (42) Leukeran	**Dalteparin (54)** Fragmin
Chloramphenicol (33, 63) Chloromycetin, Pentamycetin	**Danazol (28)** Cyclomen
Chloroquine (37) Aralen	**Dantrolene (13)** Dantrium
Chlorpheniramine (45) Novo-Pheniram	**Daunorubicin (daunomycin) (42)** Cerubidine
Chlorpromazine (9, 62) Largactil	**Deferoxamine (57)** Desferal
Chlorthalidone (53)	**Demeclocycline (32)** Declomycin
Cholestyramine (55) Questran	**Desipramine (10)** Norpramin
Ciclopirox (64) Loprox, Penlax, Stieprox	**Desloratadine (45)** Aerius
Cilazapril (52) Inhibace	**Desonide (64)** Desocort
Cimetidine (59) Novo-Cimetine, Nu-Cimet	**Desoximetasone (64)** Topicort
Ciprofloxacin (31, 63) Apo-Ciproflox, Ciloxan, Cipro	**Dexamethasone (23, 63, 64)** Dexasone, Maxidex
Cisplatin, *cis*-platinum (42)	**Dextroamphetamine (15)** Dexedrine
Citalopram (10) Celexa	**Dextromethorphan (46)** Balminil DM, Benylin DM, Koffex DM
Clarithromycin (33) Biaxin	**Diazepam (8)** Diastat, Diazemuls, Novo-Dipam, Valium
Clindamycin (33) Clindets, Dalacin C	**Diclofenac (7)** Apo-Diclo, Novo-Difenac, Nu-Diclo, Voltaren
Clomipramine (8) Anafranil	**Dicyclomine (20)** Bentylol
Clonazepam (8) Clonapam, Rivotril	**Didanosine (35)** Videx
Clonidine (52) Catapres, Dixarit	**Diflunisal (7)**
Clopidogrel (54) Plavix	**Digoxin (48)** Lanoxin
Clorazepate (8) Novo-Clopate	**Digoxin immune fab (48)** Digibind
Clotrimazole (36) Canesten, Clotrimaderm	**Diltiazem (49, 50, 52)** Apo-Diltiaz, Cardizem, Novo-Diltazem, Nu-Diltiaz, Tiazac
Cloxacillin (30) Apo-Cloxi, Novo-Cloxin, Nu-Cloxi	**Dimenhydrinate (45, 62)** Gravol, Novo-Dimenate
Clozapine (9) Clozaril	**Dinoprostone (prostaglandin E$_2$) (65)** Cervidil, Prepidil, Prostin E$_2$
Colestipol (55) Colestid	**Diphenhydramine (12, 45)** Allerdryl, Allernix, Benadryl, Nytol, Unisom
Cromolyn (44), Sodium cromoglycate* Intal, Nalcrom, Opticrom	**Diphenoxylate (61)** Lomotil
Cyclobenzaprine (13) Flexeril, Novo-Cycloprine	**Dipivefrin (63)** Propine
Cyclopentolate (63) Cyclogyl	**Dipyridamole (54)** Persantine
Cyclophosphamide (42) Cytoxan, Procytox	**Disopyramide (49)** Rythmodan
Cyclosporine (41) Neoral, Sandimmune	**Dobutamine (17, 51)** Dobutrex
Cytarabine (42) Cytosar	

(continued)

GENERIC/CANADIAN BRAND NAMES	GENERIC/CANADIAN BRAND NAMES
Docetaxel (42) Taxotere	**Ethosuximide (11)** Zarontin
Docusate (60) Colace, Selax, Soflax	**Etidronate (25)** Didronel
Donepezil (19) Aricept	**Etodolac (7)**
Dopamine (17, 51)	**Etoposide (42)** Vepesid
Doxazosin (18, 52) Cardura	**Famciclovir (35)** Famvir
Doxepin (10) Sinequan	**Famotidine (59)** Pepcid
Doxorubicin (42) Adriamycin, Caelyx, Myocet	**Felodipine (50)** Plendil, Renedil
Doxycycline (32) Apo-Doxy, Doxycin, Doxytec, Novo-Doxylin, Vibra-Tabs	**Fenofibrate (55)** Apo-Feno-Micro, Lipidil
Econazole (36) Ecostatin	**Fentanyl (6)** Duragesic
Edrophonium (19) Enlon	**Ferrous sulfate (57)** Fer-In-Sol, Ferodan
Efavirenz (35) Sustiva	**Fexofenadine (45)** Allegra
Eletriptan (7) Relpax	**Filgrastim (40)** Neupogen
Enalapril (52) Vasotec	**Flavoxate (20)**
Enfuvirtide (35) Fuzeon	**Flecainide (49)** Tambocor
Enoxaparin (54) Lovenox	**Fluconazole (36)** Diflucan
Epinephrine (17, 44, 51) Adrenalin, EpiPen, Vaponefrin	**Fludarabine (42)** Fludara
Epoetin alfa (40) Eprex	**Fludrocortisone (23)** Florinef
Eprosartan (52) Teveten	**Flumazenil (8)** Anexate
Ergocalciferol (25) Drisdol, Ostoforte	**Flunisolide (23, 44)** Rhinalar
Ertapenem (30) Invanz	**Fluocinolone (64)** Liderm, Tiamol
Erythromycin (33, 63) Apo-Erythro, Erybid, Eryc	**Fluorometholone (63)** Flarex, FML
Esmolol (49) Brevibloc	**Fluorouracil, 5-FU (42)** Efudex
Estradiol (27) Climara, Estraderm, Estradot, Estrace, Estring	**Fluoxetine (10)** Prozac
Estrogens, conjugated (27) C.E.S, Premarin	**Fluphenazine (9)** Modicate
Estropipate (27), Piperazine estrone sulfate* Ogen	**Flurazepam (8)**
Etanercept (41) Enbrel	**Flurbiprofen (7, 63)** Ansaid, Froben, Ocufen
Ethambutol (34) Etibi	**Flutamide (42)** Euflex
Ethinyl estradiol/ethynodiol (27) Demulen	**Fluticasone (23)** Flonase, Flovent
Ethinyl estradiol/levonorgestrel (27) Alesse, Min-Ovral, Triphasil, Triquilar	**Fluvastatin (55)** Lescol
Ethinyl estradiol/norethindrone (27) Brevicon, Ortho, Synphasic	**Fluvoxamine (10)** Luvox
Ethinyl estradiol/norgestrel (27) Ovral	**Fosfomycin (32)** Monurol
	Fosinopril (52) Monopril

GENERIC/CANADIAN BRAND NAMES	GENERIC/CANADIAN BRAND NAMES
Fosphenytoin (11) Cerebyx	**Insulins (26)** Humalog, Humulin, Iletin, Novolinge, NovoRapid
Furosemide (25, 53) Lasix	**Interferons (40)** Alfa-2a (Pegasys, Roferon A); alfa-2b (Intron A); beta-1a (Avonex, Rebif); beta-1b (Betaseron)
Gabapentin (11) Neurontin	**Ipratropium (44)** Apo-Ipravent, Atrovent, Novo-Ipramide
Ganciclovir (35) Cytovene	**Irbesartan (52)** Avapro
Gatifloxacin (31) Tequin	**Irinotecan (42)** Camptosar
Gefitinib (42) Iressa	**Isoproterenol (17, 44)**
Gemcitabine (42) Gemzar	**Isosorbide dinitrate (50)** Apo-ISDN, Novo-Sorbide
Gemfibrozil (55) Lopid	**Isosorbide mononitrate (50)** Imdur
Gentamicin (31, 63) Alcomicin, Garamycin	**Isotretinoin, (64)** Accutane
Glimepiride (26) Amaryl	**Ketoconazole (40)** Ketodrem, Nizoral
Glyburide (26), Glibenclamide* DiaBeta, Gen-Glybe	**Ketoprofen (7)** Apo-Keto, Novo-Keto, Rhodis, Rhovail
Goserelin (42) Zoladex	**Ketorolac (7)** Acular, Toradol
Granisetron (62) Kytril	**Labetalol (18, 52)** Trandate
Guaifenesin (46), Glyceryl guaiacolate* Balminil Expectorant, Benylin-E, Robitussin	**Lamivudine (35)** Heptovir
Halcinonide (64) Halog	**Lamotrigine (11)** Lamictal
Haloperidol (9) Novo-Peridol	**Lansoprazole (59)** Prevacid
Hydralazine (52) Apresoline, Novo-Hylazin, Nu-Hydral	**Leuprolide (42)** Eligard, Lupron
Hydrochlorothiazide (53) Apo-Hydro, Novo-Hydrazide	**Levetiracetam (11)** Keppra
Hydrocodone (6, 46) Hycodan	**Levobunolol (18, 63)** Betagan
Hydrocortisone (23, 44, 64) Cortef, Emo-Cort, Hycort	**Levofloxacin (31)** Levaquin
Hydromorphone (6, 46) Dilaudid, Hydromorph Contin	**Levothyroxine (24)** Eltroxin, Synthroid
Hydroxyurea (42) Hydrea	**Lidocaine (49), Lignocaine*** Xylocaine, Xylocard
Hydroxyzine (8, 45, 62)	**Linezolid (33)** Zyvoxam
Ibandronate (25) Bondronat	**Lisinopril (52)** Prinivil, Zestril
Ibuprofen (7) Advil, Motrin, Novo-Profen	**Lithium (10)** Carbolith, Duralith, Lithane
Idarubicin (42) Idamycin	**Loperamide (61)** Imodium
Ifosfamide (42) Ifex	**Loratadine (45)** Claritin
Imatinib (42) Gleevec	**Lorazepam (8)** Ativan, Novo-Lorazem, Nu-Loraz
Imipenem/cilastatin (30) Primaxin	**Losartan (52)** Cozaar
Imipramine (10) Novo-Pramine, Tofranil	**Lovastatin (55)** Mevacor
Indomethacin (7) Indocid, Novo-Methacin, Nu-Indo, Rhodacine	**Mannitol (53)** Osmitrol

(continued)

GENERIC/CANADIAN BRAND NAMES	GENERIC/CANADIAN BRAND NAMES

Mebendazole (37)
Vermox
Meclizine (45, 62)
Bonamine
Medroxyprogesterone (27)
Apo-Medroxy, Depo-Provera, Gen-Medroxy,
  Novo-Medrone, Provera
Megestrol (27)
Megace
Meloxicam (7)
Mobicox
Melphalan (42)
Alkeran
Meperidine (6), Pethidine*
Demerol
Mercaptopurine (42)
Purinethol
Meropenem (30)
Merrem
Mestranol/norethindrone (27)
Ortho-Novum
Metaproterenol (17, 44), Orciprenaline*
Metformin (26)
Glucophage
Methenamine (32)
Dehydral, Hip-Rex, Mandelamine
Methimazole (24)
Tapazole
Methocarbamol (13)
Robaxin
Methotrexate (41, 42)
Methyldopa (52)
Nu-Medopa
Methylphenidate (15)
Concerta, Ritalin
Methylprednisolone (23, 44, 64)
Depo-Medrol, Medrol, Solu-Medrol
Metoclopramide (62)
Apo-Metoclop
Metolazone (53)
Zaroxolyn
Metoprolol (18, 52)
Betaloc, Novo-Metoprol, Nu-Metop
Metronidazole (33, 37, 64)
Flagyl, Florazole, MetroCream, Metrogel, NidaGel,
  Noritate, Rosasol
Miconazole (36, 64)
Micatin, Micozole, Monistat
Midazolam (8)
Milrinone (48)
Primacor
Minocycline (32)
Minocin
Minoxidil (52)
Apo-Gain, Loniten, Minox, Rogaine
Misoprostol (7, 59)
Mometasone (45)
Elocom, Nasonex
Montelukast (44)
Singulair
Morphine (6)
Kadian, M-Eslon, M.O.S., MS Contin

Moxifloxacin (31)
Avelox, Vigamox
Muromonab-CD3 (41)
Orthoclone OKT 3
Mycophenolate (41)
CellCept
Nabumetone (7)
Relafen
Nadolol (18, 50, 52)
Apo-Nadol, Corgard
Naloxone (6)
Naphazoline (17, 46)
Naphcon, Vasocon
Naproxen (7)
Anaprox, Naprosyn, Novo-Naprox, Nu-Naprox
Naratriptan (7)
Amerge
Nateglinide (26)
Starlix
Nedocromil (44)
Alocril
Nelfinavir (35)
Viracept
Neostigmine (19)
Prostigmin
Nevirapine (35)
Viramune
Nifedipine (50)
Adalat XL, Apo-Nifed, Nu-Nifed
Nilutamide (42)
Anandron
Nitrofurantoin (32)
MacroBID, Novo-Furantoin
Nitroglycerin (50)
Gen-Nitro, Minitran, Nitro-Dur, Nitrol, Nitrostat,
  Transderm-Nitro
Nitroprusside (52)
Nitropride
Nizatidine (59)
Norepinephrine (17, 51), Noradrenaline*
Levophed
Norethindrone (27)
Micronor
Norfloxacin (31, 63)
Apo-Norflox
Nortriptyline (10)
Aventyl
Nystatin (36, 64)
Candistatin, Mycostatin, Nyaderm
Ofloxacin (31, 63)
Apo-Oflox, Floxin, Ocuflox
Olanzapine (9)
Zyprexa
Omeprazole (59)
Losec
Ondansetron (62)
Zofran
Orlistat (58)
Xenical
Orphenadrine (12, 13)
Norflex

GENERIC/CANADIAN BRAND NAMES	GENERIC/CANADIAN BRAND NAMES
Oseltamivir (35) Tamiflu	**Propantheline (20)** Pro-Banthine
Oxaprozin (7) Daypro	**Propranolol (18, 49, 50, 52)** Inderal, Novo-Pranol
Oxazepam (8)	**Propylthiouracil (24)** Propyl-Thyracil
Oxcarbazepine (11) Trileptal	**Pseudoephedrine (46)** Eltor, Sudafed
Oxycodone (6) OxyContin, Supeudol	**Pyridostigmine (19)** Mestinon
Paclitaxel (42) Taxol	**Quetiapine (9)** Seroquel
Pamidronate (25) Aredia	**Quinapril (52)** Accupril
Pantoprazole (59) Panto IV, Pantoloc	**Quinidine (49)** Biquin
Paroxetine (10) Paxil	**Rabeprazole (59)** Pariet
Peginterferon alfa-2a (40) Pegasys	**Raloxifene (25)** Evista
Pemetrexed (42) Alimta	**Ramipril (52)** Altace
Penicillin V (30) Apo-Pen VK, Novo-Pen-VK, Nu-Pen-VK	**Ranitidine (59)** Novo-Ranidine, Nu-Ranit, Zantac
Pentamidine (37)	**Repaglinide (26)** GlucoNorm
Perphenazine (9) Trilafon	**Ribavirin (35)** Virazole
Phenelzine (10) Nardil	**Rifampin (34)** Rifadin, Rofact
Phenobarbital (8, 11), Phenobarbitone*	**Risedronate (25)** Actonel
Phenylephrine (17, 46) Mydfrin, Neo-Synephrine	**Risperidone (9)** Risperdal
Phenytoin (11) Dilantin	**Ritonavir (35)** Norvir
Pindolol (18, 52) Apo-Pindol, Novo-Pindol, Nu-Pindol, Visken	**Rituximab (42)** Rituxan
Pioglitazone (26) Actos	**Rizatriptan (7)** Maxalt
Piperacillin (30)	**Ropinirole (12)** ReQuip
Piperacillin/tazobactam (30) Tazocin	**Rosiglitazone (26)** Avandia
Piroxicam (7) Novo-Pirocam, Nu-Pirox	**Rosiglitazone/metformin (26)** Avandamet
Potassium chloride (32) Apo-K, K-Dur, K-Lor, Micro-K, Slow-K	**Salmeterol (44)** Serevent
Pramipexole (12) Mirapex	**Saquinavir (35)** Fortovase, Invirase
Pravastatin (55) Pravachol	**Scopolamine (20, 62)** Transderm-V
Prazosin (52) Apo-Prazo, Novo-Prazin, Nu-Prazo	**Selegiline (12)**
Prednisolone (23), Deltahydrocortisone* Pediapred, Pred Forte	**Sertraline (10)** Zoloft
Prednisone (23) Winpred	**Simvastatin (55)** Zocor
Procainamide (49) Procan-SR, Pronestyl	**Sodium polystyrene sulfonate (57)** Kayexalate
Prochlorperazine (9) Stemetil	**Sotalol (18, 49)** Sotacor
Procyclidine (12)	
Promethazine (9, 45, 62)	
Propafenone (49) Rythmol	

(continued)

GENERIC/CANADIAN BRAND NAMES	GENERIC/CANADIAN BRAND NAMES
Spironolactone (53) Aldactone, Novo-Spiroton	**Trandolapril (52)** Mavik
Stavudine (35) Zerit	**Tranexamic acid (54)** Cyklokapron
Streptokinase (54) Streptase	**Trastuzumab (42)** Herceptin
Sucralfate (59) Sulcrate	**Tretinoin (retinoic acid) (64)** Rejuva-A, Renova, Retin-A
Sulfacetamide (63) Cetamide	**Triamcinolone (23, 44, 64)** Aristocort, Kenalog, Nasacort, Triaderm
Sulfamethoxazole/trimethoprim (32) Apo-Sulfatrim, Novo-Trimel, Nu-Cotrimox, Septra	**Triazolam (8)** Apo-Triazo, Halcion
Sulindac (7) Apo-Sulin, Novo-Sundac	**Trifluridine (35, 63)** Viroptic
Sumatriptan (7) Imitrex	**Trihexyphenidyl (12)** Apo-Trihex
Tamoxifen (42) Apo-Tamox, Nolvadex, Tamofen	**Trimipramine (10)** Apo-Trimip, Rhotrimine, Surmontil
Telmesartan (52) Micardis	**Tropicamide (63)** Mydriacyl
Temazepam (8) Restoril	**Valacyclovir (35)** Valtrex
Teniposide (42) Vumon	**Valdecoxib (7)** Bextra
Tenofovir (35) Viread	**Valganciclovir (35)** Valcyte
Terazosin (18, 52) Hytrin	**Valproic acid (11)** Depakene, Epiject
Terbinafine (36) Lamisil	**Valsartan (52)** Diovan
Terbutaline (17, 44) Bricanyl	**Vancomycin (33)** Vancocin
Terconazole (36) Terazol	**Venlafaxine (10)** Effexor XR
Testosterone (28) Androderm, Delatestryl	**Verapamil (49, 50, 52)** Apo-Verap, Chronovera, Isoptin, Novo-Veramil, Nu-Verap
Tetracycline (32, 63) Apo-Tetra, Nu-Tetra	**Vinblastine (42)**
Theophylline (16, 47) Apo-Theo LA, Novo-Theophyl, Theolair	**Vincristine (42)**
Thiothixene (9) Navane	**Voriconazole (36)** Vfend
Ticarcillin/clavulanate (30) Timentin	**Warfarin (54)** Coumadin
Timolol (18, 52, 63) Apo-Timol, Apo-Timop, Novo-Timol, Timoptic	**Xylometazoline (17, 46)** Balminil Nasal Decongestant
Tiotropium (20) Spiriva	**Zafirlukast (44)** Accolate
Tirofiban (54) Aggrastat	**Zalcitabine (35)** Hivid
Tobramycin (31, 63) Tobrex	**Zaleplon (8)** Starnoc
Tolcapone (12) Tasmar	**Zanimivir (35)** Relenza
Tolnaftate (36, 64) ZeaSorb AF	**Zidovudine (35)** Retrovir
Topiramate (11) Topamax	**Zoledronic acid (25)** Zometa
Topotecan (42) Hycamtin	**Zolmitriptan (7)** Zomig

Repchinsky, C. (Ed.). (2005). *Compendium of pharmaceuticals and specialities*. Ottawa, Ontario: Canadian Pharmacists Association.

Anesthetics, Adjunctive Drugs, and Nursing Considerations

Anesthetics interrupt the conduction of painful nerve impulses from a site of injury to the brain. They are given to prevent pain and promote relaxation during surgery, childbirth, and some diagnostic tests and treatments.

GENERAL ANESTHETICS

General anesthetics produce profound central nervous system (CNS) depression, during which there is complete loss of sensation, consciousness, pain perception, and memory. The drugs include inhalation and intravenous (IV) agents and can be used for almost any surgical, diagnostic, or therapeutic procedure. General anesthesia is often started with a fast-acting IV drug (eg, propofol, thiopental) then maintained with a mixture of an anesthetic gas and oxygen given by inhalation. The IV agent produces rapid loss of consciousness and provides a pleasant induction and recovery. An anesthetic barbiturate or propofol may be used alone for anesthesia during brief diagnostic tests or surgical procedures. Selected agents and their characteristics and uses are listed in Table F-1.

General Anesthetic Adjunctive Drugs

Several drugs are used along with general anesthetics. *Antianxiety agents* and *sedative-hypnotics* are given to decrease anxiety, promote rest, allow easier induction of anesthesia, and allow smaller doses of anesthetics. These drugs may be given the night before to aid sleep and 1 or 2 hours before the scheduled procedure. In addition, midazolam (Versed) is often used in ambulatory surgical or invasive diagnostic procedures and for regional anesthesia. It has a rapid onset and short duration of action, causes amnesia, produces minimal cardiovascular adverse effects, and reduces the dose of opioid analgesics required during surgery. *Anticholinergic drugs* are given to prevent vagal effects (eg, bradycardia, hypotension) associated with general anesthesia and surgery. Vagal stimulation occurs with some inhalation anesthetics and with surgical procedures in which there is manipulation of the pharynx, trachea, peritoneum, stomach, intestine, or other viscera, and procedures in which pressure is exerted on the eyeball.

Neuromuscular blocking agents (see Table F-1) cause muscle relaxation, an important component of general anesthesia, and allow the use of smaller amounts of anesthetic agents. They are also used to facilitate mechanical ventilation, control increased intracranial pressure, and treat status epilepticus. Artificial ventilation is necessary because these drugs paralyze muscles of respiration as well as other skeletal muscles. The drugs do not cause sedation; therefore, unless recipients are unconscious, they can see and hear environmental activities and conversations. These commonly used drugs prevent acetylcholine from acting at neuromuscular

TABLE F-1   General Anesthetics and Neuromuscular Blocking Agents

GENERIC/TRADE NAME	CHARACTERISTICS
General Inhalation Anesthetics	
Desflurane (Suprane), **enflurane** (Ethrane), **isoflurane** (Forane), **sevoflurane** (Ultane)	These drugs are similar volatile liquids used for induction and maintenance of general anesthesia. They are given by anesthesiologists or nurse anesthetists.
Nitrous oxide	One of the oldest and safest anesthetics; given with oxygen to prevent hypoxia; has rapid induction and recovery; used for anesthesia with IV barbiturates, neuromuscular blocking agents, opioid analgesics, and stronger inhalation anesthetics; used alone for analgesia in dentistry, obstetrics, and brief surgical procedures
General Intravenous Anesthetics	
Alfentanil (Alfenta), **remifentanil** (Ultiva), **sufentanil** (Sufenta)	These drugs are rapid-acting opioid-analgesic anesthetics used as a primary anesthetic or as an analgesic adjunct with other general anesthetics.
Etomidate (Amidate)	A nonanalgesic hypnotic used for induction and maintenance of general anesthesia; may be used with nitrous oxide for short operative procedures
Methohexital (Brevital), **thiopental** (Pentothal)	Ultra–short-acting barbiturates used to induce general anesthesia. For major surgery, the drugs are used with inhalation anesthetics and muscle relaxants.
Midazolam (Versed)	A short-acting benzodiazepine. Given IV or IM for preoperative sedation. Given IV for conscious sedation during short endoscopic or other diagnostic procedures; induction of general anesthesia; and maintenance of general anesthesia with nitrous oxide and oxygen for short surgical procedures. Adverse effects of IV drug include respiratory depression, apnea, and death.
Propofol (Diprivan)	A rapid-acting hypnotic used for induction or maintenance of general anesthesia, with other agents. Also used alone for sedation in critical care units. Recovery occurs a few minutes after the drug is stopped. Adverse effects include hypotension, apnea, and other signs of central nervous system depression.
Neuromuscular Blocking Agents	
Atracurium (Tracium), **Cisatracurium** (Nimbex), **Rocuronium** (Zemuron), **Vecuronium** (Norcuron)	These are intermediate-acting, nondepolarizing skeletal muscle relaxants used with general anesthesia for surgical procedures and to facilitate endotracheal intubation and mechanical ventilation. They may cause hypotension and their effects can be reversed by neostigmine (Prostigmin).
Mivacurium (Mivacron)	Similar to the above agents except it is short acting.
Pancuronium	An older, long-acting drug used during surgery after general anesthesia has been induced or to aid endotracheal intubation or mechanical ventilation. It may cause hypotension and effects can be reversed by neostigmine (Prostigmin).
Succinylcholine	A depolarizing, short-acting drug that may be used during surgery and brief procedures, such as endoscopy and endotracheal intubation. It is used less often than the nondepolarizing agents described above. Adverse effects include malignant hyperthermia, a life-threatening condition.

IM, intramuscular; IV, intravenous.

junctions. As a result, the nerve cell membrane is not depolarized, the muscle fibers are not stimulated, and skeletal muscle contraction does not occur. The drugs should be used very cautiously in clients with renal or hepatic impairment because the drug or its metabolites may accumulate and cause prolonged paralysis.

Nursing Considerations With General Anesthetics and Neuromuscular Blocking Agents

- General anesthetics should be administered *only* by anesthesiologists or nurse anesthetists and *only* in locations where staff, equipment, and drugs are available for emergency use or cardiopulmonary resuscitation. Most nurses care for clients before and after administration of general anesthetics.
- If a medical disorder of a vital organ system (cardiovascular, respiratory, renal) is present, it should be corrected before anesthesia is given, when possible. Such disorders increase the risks of complications with anesthesia and surgery. Additional risk factors include cigarette smoking, obesity, and limited exercise or activity.
- Compared with adults, children are at greater risk of complications (eg, laryngospasm, bronchospasm, aspi-

ration, postoperative nausea and vomiting) and death from general anesthetics and adjunctive drugs.

- Compared with younger adults, older adults often have physiologic changes and pathologic conditions that make them more susceptible to adverse effects of anesthetics, neuromuscular blocking agents, and adjunctive medications. Thus, lower doses of these agents are usually needed.

- During preanesthetic nursing assessments, clients should be asked about drug allergies and the use of prescription drugs, nonprescription drugs, and herbal or dietary supplements. With herbal products, the American Society of Anesthesiologists recommends that all herbals be stopped 2 or 3 weeks before any surgical procedure because some (eg, feverfew, garlic, ginkgo biloba, ginseng) can increase risks of bleeding and some (eg, kava, valerian) can increase effects of sedatives.

- Effects of anesthetics wear off gradually and the nurse must observe and safeguard clients during this recovery period. With general anesthetics and neuromuscular blocking agents, frequent (eg, every 5–15 minutes) assessment of cardiovascular and respiratory function is needed until the client wakes up and is breathing well. This is usually done in a postanesthesia recovery (PAR) area. Observe for adverse effects, including excessive sedation (eg, delayed awakening, failure to respond to verbal or tactile stimuli); respiratory problems (eg, laryngospasm, hypoxia, hypercarbia); cardiovascular problems (eg, hypotension, tachycardia and other cardiac dysrhythmias, fluid and electrolyte imbalances); and other problems (eg, restlessness, nausea, vomiting).

- Propofol and neuromuscular blocking agents are commonly used in critical care units, usually for clients who are intubated and mechanically ventilated. These drugs should be administered and monitored only by health care personnel who are skilled in the management of critically ill clients, including cardiopulmonary resuscitation and airway management. Critical care nurses must often care for clients receiving IV infusions of the drugs and titrate dosage and flow rate to achieve desired effects and minimize adverse effects. Consult drug literature regarding accurate administration and monitoring of these drugs.

LOCAL ANESTHETICS

Local anesthetics, given to produce loss of sensation and motor activity, are applied to or injected into localized areas of the body. The drugs decrease the permeability of nerve cell membranes to ions, especially sodium. This action reduces excitability of cell membranes; when excitability falls low enough, nerve impulses cannot be initiated or conducted by the anesthetized nerves. As a result, the drugs prevent the cells from responding to pain impulses and other sensory stimuli.

Anesthetic effects dwindle as drug molecules diffuse out of neurons into the bloodstream. The drugs are then transported to the liver for metabolism, mainly to inactive metabolites. The metabolites are excreted in the urine, along with a small amount of unchanged drug. Commonly used local anesthetics are listed in Table F-2.

Selected Types of Local Anesthesia

- *Spinal* anesthesia involves injecting the anesthetic agent into the cerebrospinal fluid, usually in the lumbar spine. The anesthetic blocks sensory impulses at the root of peripheral nerves as they enter the spinal cord. Spinal anesthesia is especially useful for surgery involving the lower abdomen and legs.

- *Epidural* anesthesia, which involves injecting the anesthetic into the epidural space, is used most often in obstetrics during labor and delivery. This route is also used to provide analgesia (often with a combination of a local anesthetic and an opioid) for clients with postoperative or other pain. When the combination is used, the dosage of both drugs must be reduced to avoid respiratory depression and other adverse effects.

- *Topical* anesthesia involves application of a local anesthetic to skin and mucous membranes. The anesthetic is usually an ingredient in ointments, solutions, or lotions designed for use at particular sites. For example, preparations are available for use on eyes, ears, nose, oral mucosa, perineum, hemorrhoids, and skin. These preparations are used to relieve pain and itching of dermatoses, sunburn, minor skin wounds, hemorrhoids, sore throat, and other conditions. The main adverse effect is allergic reactions.

Nursing Considerations With Local Anesthetics

- Some local anesthetic is absorbed into the bloodstream and circulated through the body, especially when injected or applied to mucous membrane. *Systemic absorption accounts for most of the potentially serious adverse effects of local anesthetics.* These adverse effects include CNS stimulation (eg, hyperactivity, excitement, seizure activity) followed by CNS depression; cardiovascular depression (eg, hypotension, dysrhythmias); and allergic reactions (eg, hives and other skin lesions; itching; edema; possible anaphylactoid symptoms, including severe hypotension). Serious adverse effects are more likely to occur with large doses, high concentrations, injections into highly vascular areas, or accidental injection into a blood vessel.

- Except with IV lidocaine for cardiac dysrhythmias, local anesthetic solutions must not be injected into blood vessels because of the high risk of serious adverse reactions involving the cardiovascular system and CNS.

TABLE F-2 Local Anesthetics

GENERIC/TRADE NAME	CHARACTERISTICS
Injectable Drugs	
Articaine (Septodont)	Used for local infiltration (injection) and nerve block for dental and periodontal procedures or oral surgery. Effects occur in 1–6 min and last 1 h.
Bupivacaine (Marcaine)	Used for infiltration, nerve block, and epidural anesthesia during childbirth. With injection, effects occur in 5 min and last 2–4 h. With epidural administration, effects occur in 10–20 min and last 3–5 h. May cause systemic toxicity (eg, decreased cardiac output, dysrhythmias, CNS stimulation possibly proceeding to seizures).
Chloroprocaine (Nesacaine)	Used for infiltration, nerve block, and epidural anesthesia. Effects occur in 6–12 min and last 30 min. Rapidly metabolized and less likely to cause systemic toxicity than other local anesthetics
Levobupivacaine (Chirocaine)	Given by local infiltration and epidurally for surgery and obstetrics and for postoperative pain management. When given epidurally, effects occur within 10 min and last about 8 h.
Lidocaine (Xylocaine)	Used for local infiltration, nerve block, and spinal and epidural anesthesia. With injection, effects occur in less than 2 min and last 30–60 min. With epidural use, effects occur in 5–15 min and last 1–3 h. Lidocaine is also given IV to prevent or treat cardiac dysrhythmias. (**Warning:** Do not use preparations containing epinephrine for dysrhythmias.)
Mepivacaine (Carbocaine)	Used for infiltration, nerve block, and epidural anesthesia. With injection, effects occur in 3–5 min and last 0.75–1.5 h. With epidural use, effects occur in 5–15 min and last 1–3 h.
Prilocaine (Citanest)	Used for infiltration, nerve block, and epidural anesthesia. With injection, effects occur in less than 2 min and last 60 min. With epidural use, effects occur in 5–15 min and last 1–3 h.
Ropivacaine (Naropin)	Used for local or regional surgical anesthesia and obstetric or postoperative analgesia. Given by injection or epidural infusion. With epidural use, effects occur in 10–30 min and last up to 6 h.
Topical Drugs	
Benzocaine (Americaine, Lanacane, Solarcaine, others)	Used on skin and mucous membranes to relieve pain and itching of sunburn, other minor burns and wounds, skin abrasions, earache, hemorrhoids, sore throat, and other conditions. Available over-the-counter in aerosol sprays, throat lozenges, rectal suppositories, lotions, and ointments. May cause allergic reactions.
Butamben (Butesin)	Used on skin only, mainly for minor burns and skin irritations
Dibucaine (Nupercainal)	Used on skin and mucous membranes. Anesthetic effects occur in less than 15 min and last 3–4 h. May cause local allergic reactions
Dyclonine (Dyclone)	Used to relieve pain of mouth or anogenital lesions and to anesthetize mucous membranes of throat and gastrointestinal tract for endoscopic procedures. Effects occur in less than 10 min and last less than 60 min.
Lidocaine (Xylocaine, Dentipatch, others)	One of the most commonly used local anesthetics. Available in several preparations, including lidocaine viscous, which is used orally for numbing of the mouth and throat, and topical patches for relief of painful conditions such as postherpetic neuralgia and to provide oral anesthesia for superficial dental procedures. With topical use, effects occur in 2–5 min and last 15–45 min.
Pramoxine (Tronothane)	Used for skin wounds, dermatoses, hemorrhoids, endotracheal intubation, and sigmoidoscopy
Proparacaine (Alcaine)	Used to anesthetize the eye for tonometry and for removal of sutures, foreign bodies, and cataracts
Tetracaine (Pontocaine)	Used for topical anesthesia

- Local anesthetics given during labor cross the placenta and may depress muscle strength, muscle tone, and rooting behavior in newborns. In addition, if a local anesthetic (eg, bupivacaine) is infused epidurally with an opioid analgesic (eg, fentanyl), dosage of both agents must be reduced to decrease risks of respiratory arrest.

- Epinephrine, a vasoconstrictor, is often added to a local anesthetic to slow systemic absorption, prolong anesthetic effects, and control bleeding. This combination should *not* be given IV or in excessive dosage because the drugs can cause serious systemic toxicity, including cardiac dysrhythmias. In addition, the combination should *not* be used for nerve blocks in areas supplied by end arteries (fingers, ears, nose, toes, penis) because it may produce ischemia and gangrene.

- For topical anesthesia, use the local anesthetic only on the body part and condition for which it was prescribed. Most preparations are specifically made to apply on certain areas, and they cannot be used effectively and safely on other body parts. Also, teach clients to cleanse the site before application, if needed, so that the drug has direct contact with the affected area; and to avoid using the product longer or applying more often than directed because skin irritation, rash, and hives can develop.

- When used to anesthetize nasal, oral, pharyngeal, laryngeal, tracheal, bronchial, or urethral mucosa, local anesthetics should be given in low concentrations and at the lowest effective dosages. The drugs are well absorbed through mucous membranes and may cause systemic adverse reactions.

- A mixture of lidocaine and prilocaine (Eutectic Mixture of Local Anesthetics [EMLA]) was formulated to penetrate intact skin, provide local anesthesia, and decrease pain of vaccinations and venipuncture, especially in children. The cream is applied at the injection site with an occlusive dressing at least 60 minutes before vaccination or venipuncture. It should not be used on abraded skin or mucous membranes.

Index

Note: Page numbers followed by f, t, or b indicate figures, tables, and boxed material.

A

abacavir (Ziagen), 566t, 574–575
abarelix (Plenaxis), 342
Abbokinase (urokinase), 883t, 885
abbreviations, 34t
abciximab (ReoPro), 882t, 884
Abelcet (amphotericin B lipid complex), 587b, 596–597, 600
Abilify (aripiprazole), 156t, 159t, 161, 168, 171–172
abortifacients, 1069–1070, 1070t, 1075–1077
absence seizure, 194
absolute refractory period, 795
absorption
    hepatic disorders' effect on, 22t
    inflammatory bowel disorders' effect on, 22t
    principles of, 12, 14
    renal impairments' effect on, 23t
acamprosate (Campral), 238t, 240
acarbose (Precose), 414t, 433
accelerin, 877t
Accolate (zafirlukast), 736t, 740, 745
AccuNeb (albuterol), 732, 732t–733t
Accupril (quinapril), 843t
Accutane (isotretinoin), 1046t, 1052
acebutolol (Sectral), 293t, 801t, 804, 844t
Aceon (perindopril), 843t
acetaminophen (Tylenol)
    antidote for, 28t, 123
    in children, 125
    client teaching about, 120–121
    dosage of, 110t, 123
    in hepatic-impaired patients, 126
    in home care, 126
    indications for, 106b, 107, 123
    in older adults, 125
    opioid/acetaminophen products, 94t
    pharmacokinetics of, 115
    in renal-impaired patients, 125
    serum levels of, 1083
    toxicity, 123
acetazolamide (Diamox), 1027t
acetic acid derivatives, 109
acetylcholine
    cholinergic receptor stimulation by, 307
    description of, 77, 266
    dopamine and, 214
    functions of, 307
acetylcysteine (Mucomyst)
    antidote uses of, 28t
    description of, 123
    mucolytic uses of, 764t
acetyltransferase, 21
Achromycin (tetracycline)
    administration of, 524–525
    adverse effects of, 525–526
    antiprotozoal uses of, 606
    characteristics of, 516t
    in children, 479, 523
    client teaching about, 522
    contraindications, 520
    in critical illness, 524
    dairy products interaction with, 19
    definition of, 515
    drug interactions, 526
    in hepatic-impaired clients, 524
    indications for, 519
    mechanism of action, 516
    nursing actions for, 524–526
    nursing process for, 520, 522
    in older adults, 524
    in renal-impaired clients, 524
    self-administration of, 522
    therapeutic effects of, 525
    therapeutic principles for, 522–523
acid-base balance, 919
acidosis, 423
acitretin (Soriatane), 1046t
Aclovate (alclometasone), 1045t
acne, 1041, 1052
acquired immunodeficiency syndrome
    description of, 368
    human immunodeficiency virus progression to, 561b
ACTH (corticotropin), 341–342, 343t
Acthar Gel (corticotropin), 341–342, 343t
ActHIB (Haemophilus influenzae b conjugate vaccine), 635t
Actifed Cold & Allergy, 764t
Actimmune (interferon gamma-1b), 654t
Actinex (masoprocol), 1047t
Actinomycin D (dactinomycin), 696t
Activase (alteplase), 882t, 885
activated charcoal, 27b, 259
activated partial thromboplastin time, 888
active immunity, 625, 634
active transport, 13b
active tuberculosis, 543
Activelle, 444t
Actonel (risedronate), 390, 393t, 401
Actos (pioglitazone), 414t, 430–431, 433
Acular (ketorolac), 1030t
acute ingestion, 237
acute pain
    description of, 84b, 95
    opioid analgesics for, 95, 99
acute renal failure, 66, 943–944
acyclovir (Zovirax), 563, 564t, 575, 577–578, 1044t
Adalat (nifedipine), 819t, 845t
adalizumab (Humira), 669t, 674–675
adapalene (Differin), 1046t
adaptive immunity, 625
Addison's disease, 353, 357
additive effects, 19
adefovir (Hepsera), 564t
A-delta fibers, 83
Adenocard (adenosine), 802t, 805
adenosine (Adenocard), 802t, 805
adenosine diphosphate receptor antagonists, 884
adequate intake, 919b
Adipex-P (phentermine hydrochloride), 957, 957t, 967
adjuvant chemotherapy, 710
administration of drugs
    abbreviations commonly used in, 34t
    in critical-illness patients, 69
    dosages. See drug dosages
    drug preparations for, 70
    ear medications, 36t, 48
    eye solutions, 36t, 48
    gastrointestinal, 39t
    intramuscular injections
        advantages and disadvantages of, 39t
        antipsychotic drugs, 164, 168
        in children, 63
        drug actions after, 19
        nursing action for, 47
        sites for, 40, 43f
    intravenous injections
        absorption of, 14
        administration technique, 42b
        advantages and disadvantages of, 39t
        in children, 32b
        continuous infusion, 41b
        in critical-illness patients, 69
        drug preparation for, 42b
        equipment for, 41b
        of illicit drugs, 236–237
        intermittent infusion, 41b
        nursing action for, 47–48
        of opioid analgesics, 94
        principles of, 41b–42b
        sites for, 40, 41b–42b, 43f–44f
    legal responsibilities, 32
    medication errors, 32b, 32–33
    medication systems, 33
    nasogastric tube, 46
    needleless systems, 40
    nose drops, 48
    nursing actions for, 44–48, 70–71
    in older adults, 66
    opioid analgesics, 94–96
    oral, 38, 39t, 45–46
    parenteral
        ampules used in, 38
        definition of, 38
        equipment for, 38, 41
        injection sites, 40, 43f
    pharmacokinetics affected by, 18–19
    principles of, 31–32
    psychological considerations, 25
    rectal suppositories, 36t, 48
    rights of, 31, 70
    self-administration, 55–56
    to skin, 48
    subcutaneous injections
        absorption after, 14
        advantages and disadvantages of, 39t
        insulin, 423
        nursing action for, 46–47
        sites for, 40, 43f
    topical, 40t
    using IV line already established, 47–48
    vaginal suppositories, 36t, 48
adolescents. See also Children; Infants
    antipsychotic drugs in, 165b, 165–166
    diabetes mellitus in, 426–427
    growth hormone levels in, 341
    immunizations in, 646
    latent tuberculosis infection in, 546b

adrenal cortex
  disorders of, 353
  sex hormones of, 353
adrenal insufficiency
  description of, 368
  hypothyroidism and, 381
Adrenalin (epinephrine)
  administration of, 284–285
  adrenergic drugs in, 283
  anaphylactic shock treated with, 280
  cardiopulmonary resuscitation using, 281
  characteristics of, 273t, 275, 276t
  concentrations of, 278t
  in critical illness, 835
  shock treated with, 831t, 832
  therapeutic effects of, 285
  vasopressin vs., 281–282
adrenergic drugs. *See also specific drug*
  administration of, 279, 284–285
  adverse effects of, 285
  allergic disorders treated with, 274–275
  asthma treated with, 732, 732t–733t, 734
  cardiopulmonary resuscitation using, 281
  in children, 283
  client teaching about, 280
  contraindications, 275
  in critical illness, 283–284
  description of, 272
  drug interactions, 286
  heart failure treated with, 780b
  in hepatic-impaired clients, 283
  in home care, 284
  hypotension treated with, 282
  indications for, 274–275
  indirect action of, 274f
  mechanism of action, 272–274
  monoamine oxidase inhibitor contraindications, 286
  nasal congestion treated with, 282
  nursing actions for, 284–286
  nursing process for, 278–279
  in older adults, 283
  ophthalmic preparations of, 283
  during pregnancy, 1060b
  in renal-impaired clients, 283
  selection of, 279
  self-administration of, 280
  shock treated with, 282
  therapeutic effects of, 285
  therapeutic principles for, 279–284
  toxicity of, 282–283
adrenergic fibers, 266
adrenergic receptors, 269–270
adrenocortical hyperfunction, 353
adrenocortical insufficiency
  corticosteroids for prevention of, 367
  description of, 353, 357
  signs and symptoms of, 369
adrenocorticotropic hormone, 175
Adriamycin (doxorubicin), 696t, 714
Adrucil (fluorouracil), 695t–696t
adult respiratory distress syndrome, 368
Advair (fluticasone/salmeterol), 734t
adventitia, 774
adverse effects
  of adrenergic drugs, 285
  of alpha-adrenergic agonists, 303
  of alpha-adrenergic blockers, 303
  of aminoglycosides, 512–513
  of anabolic steroids, 461–462
  of analgesic–antipyretic–anti-inflammatory drugs, 127–128
  of androgens, 461–462

  of antianginal drugs, 827
  of antianxiety drugs, 150–151
  of antiasthmatic drugs, 745
  of anticholinergic drugs, 222, 330
  of anticoagulants, 893–894
  of antidepressants, 189
  of antidiabetic drugs, 430–431
  of antidiarrheal drugs, 1007
  of antidysrhythmic drugs, 810–811
  of antiemetic drugs, 1018–1019
  of antiepileptic drugs, 205, 210
  of antifungal drugs, 599–600
  of antihistamines, 758
  of antihypertensive drugs, 858–859
  of antimicrobial drugs, 482–483
  of antineoplastic drugs, 694, 717–718
  of antiparasitic drugs, 615–616
  of antiparkinson drugs, 223–224
  of antiplatelet drugs, 893–894
  of antipsychotic drugs, 166b, 169–171
  of antiseizure drugs, 205, 210
  of antishock drugs, 836
  of antitubercular drugs, 557
  of antitussives, 768–769
  of antiviral drugs, 577–578
  of beta blockers, 303, 827
  of beta-lactam antibacterials, 500–501
  of calcium channel blockers, 827
  of central nervous system stimulants, 260–261
  of cholinergic drugs, 316
  of corticosteroids, 369
  definition of, 25
  of dermatologic drugs, 1054–1055
  of diuretics, 873–874
  of dyslipidemic drugs, 908
  of estrogens, 451–452
  of fluoroquinolones, 513
  of growth hormone, 348
  of hematopoietic drugs, 663
  of hypothalamic hormones, 349
  of immunizations, 647–648
  of immunostimulant drugs, 663
  of immunosuppressants, 685–687
  of insulin, 430
  of ketolides, 538
  of laxatives, 995
  of macrolides, 538
  of monoamine oxidase inhibitors, 189
  of nasal decongestants, 768
  of nonsteroidal anti-inflammatory drugs, 108
  nursing actions for, 71
  of nutritional support, 948–949
  in older adults, 64
  of ophthalmic drugs, 1035–1036
  of opioid analgesics, 85, 100
  of pituitary hormones, 349
  of progestins, 452
  of sedative-hypnotics, 150
  of selective serotonin reuptake inhibitors, 177
  of skeletal muscle relaxants, 233
  of sulfonamides, 525–526
  of tetracyclines, 525–526
  of thyroid drugs, 384
  of tricyclic antidepressants, 189
  types of, 25–26
  of urinary antiseptics, 525–526
  of vasopressin, 349
  of vitamins, 948–947
Advil Cold and Sinus Tablets, 764t
Advil (ibuprofen), 109, 111t
AeroBid (flunisolide), 358t, 731b, 736t
African Americans
  antidepressants in, 186

  antihypertensive drug actions in, 21
  antipsychotic drugs in, 167
Afrin (oxymetazoline), 763t
Afrin (oxymetazoline hydrochloride), 273t
age
  drug actions affected by, 20
  immune system based on, 629–630
Agenerase (amprenavir), 568t, 570
Aggrastat (tirofiban), 882t, 884, 887, 891
Aggrenox (dipyridamole and aspirin), 882t
Agilect (rasagiline), 221
agonists
  alpha-adrenergic. *See* alpha-adrenergic agonists
  definition of, 18
  dopamine, 220
  opioid, 85–89, 86t–87t
  partial, 161
agonists/antagonists, 87t, 89
Agoral Pain (mineral oil), 990t, 993
Agrylin (anagrelide), 882t, 885, 891
akathisia, 169
akinetic seizure, 194
Akineton (biperiden), 323t, 325
Aknemycin (erythromycin), 1043t
alanine aminotransferase, 315
albumin, 22t–23t
albuterol (Proventil, Ventolin, AccuNeb, Repetab), 273t, 732, 732t–733t
Alcaine (proparacaine), 1028t, 1098t
alclometasone (Aclovate), 1045t
alcohol (ethanol) abuse
  absorption, 237
  acute intoxication, 240
  assessment of, 248
  dependence on, 239–241
  drug interactions, 237, 239
  metabolism of, 237
  pharmacokinetics of, 237
  during pregnancy, 1065b
  prevention of, 250
  seizures caused by, 240
  systemic effects of, 239b
  withdrawal symptoms, 240
alcoholic hepatitis, 944
Alcoholics Anonymous, 251
Aldactazide, 867t
Aldactone (spironolactone), 865t, 866, 871
aldesleukin (Proleukin), 653t, 656, 658, 663–664
Aldoril, 847t
aldosterone
  antagonist of, 781
  endogenous, 862
  renal functions of, 862
alefacept (Amevive), 669t, 673
alemtuzumab (Campath), 699, 700t
alendronate (Fosamax), 390, 393t, 398, 401
Alesse, 445t
Aleve (naproxen sodium), 113t
Alfenta (alfentanil), 87, 1096t
alfentanil (Alfenta), 87, 1096t
alfuzosin (UroXatral), 292t, 295
alimentary canal, 913, 914f
Alimta (pemetrexed), 696t, 698
Alinia (nitazoxanide), 609t, 611, 1001t, 1003
Alkeran (melphalan), 695t, 713
alkylating drugs, 695t, 698
Allegra (fexofenadine), 752, 754, 756, 758
allergens, 625, 748
allergic asthma, 678
allergic conjunctivitis, 752
allergic contact dermatitis, 749

allergic disorders
  adrenergic drugs for, 274
  assessment of, 278–279
allergic drug reactions, 749–750
allergic reaction, 25
allergic rhinitis, 365, 748–750, 751t, 754t
allergies, 631
allopurinol (Zyloprim), 115, 116t, 121, 129
almotriptan (Axert), 116, 117t, 121, 128
aloe, 991, 1047
alopecia, 706b
Aloxi (palonosetron), 1013t, 1013–1014
alpha₂ agonists, 844t
alpha₁ receptors, 269, 269t
alpha₂ receptors, 269, 269t
alpha₁–acid glycoprotein, 23t–24t
alpha-adrenergic agonists. *See also specific drug*
  administration of, 302
  adverse effects of, 303
  characteristics of, 291–295, 292t
  in children, 299–300
  client teaching about, 298
  contraindications, 291
  in critical illness, 301
  drug interactions, 303–304
  in ethnic groups, 300
  in home care, 301
  mechanism of action, 290
  nursing actions for, 302–304
  nursing process for, 297–298
  in older adults, 300
  selection of, 298
  therapeutic effects of, 302
alpha-adrenergic blockers. *See also specific drug*
  adverse effects of, 303
  antihypertensive uses of, 844t
  characteristics of, 292t–293t
  in children, 299–300
  client teaching about, 298
  contraindications, 291
  in critical illness, 301
  drug interactions, 303–304
  in ethnic groups, 300
  in hepatic-impaired clients, 301
  in home care, 301
  indications for, 290–291
  mechanism of action, 290
  nonselective, 293t
  nursing actions for, 302–304
  nursing process for, 297–298
  in older adults, 300
  in renal-impaired clients, 301
  selection of, 298
  selective, 292t
  therapeutic effects of, 302
alpha-adrenergic receptors, 77
alpha₁–adrenergic receptors, 272–273
alpha₂–adrenergic receptors, 175
alpha–beta-adrenergic blockers, 845t
alpha–beta-blockers, 293t
alpha-fetoprotein, 707–708
Alphagan P (brimonidine), 1026t
alpha-glucosidase inhibitors, 413, 414t, 424–425, 427–428
Alphatrex (betamethasone dipropionate), 1045t
alprazolam (Xanax, Xanax XR), 136t, 138, 143–144, 149
alprostadil (Caverject, Muse), 1079
Alrex (loteprednol), 1030t
Altace (ramipril), 843t
alteplase (Activase), 882t, 885
alternate-day therapy, 365

Altocor (lovastatin), 901, 902t, 905–906
Alupent (metaproterenol), 273t, 732, 733t, 734
alveoli, 726
Alzheimer's disease
  description of, 307
  indirect-acting cholinergics for, 310t, 311–314
Amanita muscaria, 314
amantadine (Symmetrel)
  adverse effects of, 578
  in children, 574
  influenza A virus treated with, 565t, 570
  Parkinson's disease treated with, 215, 217t, 218, 222, 224
  in renal-impaired clients, 575
Amaryl (glimepiride), 414t
ambenonium (Mytelase), 309, 310t
Ambien (zolpidem), 139t, 140, 143, 148
amcinonide (Cyclocort), 1045t
amebiasis, 603–604, 612
amebic dysentery, 603
amebicides, 606, 607t
Amerge (naratriptan), 116, 117t, 128
Americaine (benzocaine), 1098t
American drug laws, 4–6, 5t
American Hospital Formulary Service, 8
American Society of Anesthesiologists, 61
Amevive (alefacept), 669t, 673
Amicar (aminocaproic acid), 29t, 885, 886t
Amidate (etomidate), 1096t
amifostine (Ethyol), 705, 708t
amikacin (Amikin), 505t, 550, 1083
Amikin (amikacin), 505t, 550, 1083
amiloride (Midamor), 865t, 866
amines, 76
amino acid decarboxylase, 216
amino acids, 76, 78
aminocaproic acid (Amicar), 29t, 885, 886t
aminoglycosides. *See also specific drug*
  administration of, 512
  adverse effects of, 512–513
  in children, 479, 510
  contraindications, 507
  in critical illness, 511
  definition of, 504
  description of, 504
  dosage of, 509–510
  drug interactions, 513
  in hepatic-impaired clients, 511
  in home care, 511
  indications for, 506–507
  infections treated with, 506
  mechanism of action, 506
  nursing actions for, 512–513
  nursing process for, 507–509
  in older adults, 479, 511
  penicillins and, 497
  pharmacokinetics of, 504, 506
  during pregnancy, 1060b
  in renal-impaired clients, 511
  therapeutic principles for, 509–510
  toxicity of, 510
  tuberculosis treated with, 506–507
aminopenicillins, 487
Aminophylline (short-acting theophylline), 733t, 1083
amiodarone (Cordarone), 801t, 804, 808, 811t
amitriptyline (Elavil), 178t, 1083
amlodipine (Norvasc), 819t, 845t
amoxapine (Asendin), 178t
amoxicillin (Amoxil, Trimox, Wymox)
  description of, 486t, 487, 488t
  trade names of, 4

amoxicillin clavulanate (Augmentin), 488t, 489
Amoxil (amoxicillin), 486t, 487, 488t
amphetamines
  abuse of, 242–243
  characteristics of, 254, 255t
  drug interactions, 261
  indications for, 254, 255t
Amphotec (amphotericin B cholesteryl), 587b, 596–597, 600
amphotericin B cholesteryl (Amphotec), 587b, 596–597, 600
amphotericin B deoxycholate (Fungizone), 583, 586, 587t, 596–597, 600
amphotericin B lipid complex (Abelcet), 587b, 596–597, 600
ampicillin (Marcillin, Omnipen), 487, 488t
ampicillin-sulbactam (Unasyn), 488t, 489
amprenavir (Agenerase), 568t, 570
ampules, 38
anabolic steroids
  abuse of, 456–457
  administration of, 461
  adverse effects of, 461–462
  characteristics of, 457–458
  contraindications, 458
  description of, 455–456
  in hepatic-impaired clients, 460
  indications for, 457–458
  mechanism of action, 457
  nursing actions for, 461–462
  nursing process for, 459
  therapeutic effects of, 461
  therapeutic principles for, 460–461
Anafranil (clomipramine), 138, 139t, 150, 178t, 187
anagrelide (Agrylin), 882t, 885, 891
anakinra (Kineret), 669t, 674
analeptics, 254–256, 255t
analgesia
  endogenous, 83
  patient-controlled, 95
analgesic–antipyretic–anti-inflammatory drugs
  adverse effects of, 127–128
  drug interactions, 128–129
  mechanism of action, 104, 106–107
  nursing actions for, 126–129
  nursing process for, 119
  overview of, 103–104
  therapeutic effects of, 127
  therapeutic principles for, 119–130
analgesics
  nonopioid, 93
  opioid. *See* opioid analgesics
anaphylactic reactions, 750
anaphylactic shock
  characteristics of, 830t
  definition of, 829
  description of, 25, 275
  epinephrine for, 279–280
  management of, 834
anaphylactoid reactions, 750
anaphylatoxins, 105
anaphylaxis
  antihistamines for, 752
  description of, 748
  epinephrine for, 280
Anaprox (naproxen sodium), 113t
Anaspaz (hyoscyamine), 321, 322t
anastrozole (Arimidex), 704, 705t
Ancef (cefazolin), 486t, 492t, 496
Ancobon (flucytosine), 587b, 588b, 592, 597
Androderm, 457
Androgel (testosterone gel), 458t

androgens
  abuse of, 456–457
  administration of, 457, 461
  adverse effects of, 461–462
  characteristics of, 457–458
  in children, 460
  client teaching about, 460
  contraindications, 458
  definition of, 455
  description of, 353
  drug interactions, 460, 462
  in hepatic-impaired clients, 460
  indications for, 457–458
  mechanism of action, 457
  nursing actions for, 461–462
  nursing process for, 459
  in older adults, 460
  self-administration of, 460
  therapeutic effects of, 461
  therapeutic principles for, 460–461
Android (methyltestosterone), 458t
androstendione, 458
anemia
  iron deficiency, 940–941, 1064
  megaloblastic, 938
  pernicious, 938
  during pregnancy, 1064
anesthesia
  epidural, 1097
  spinal, 1097
anesthetics
  general
    adjunctive drugs, 1095–1096
    neuromuscular blocking agents and,
      1095–1097
    physiologic effects of, 1095
  during labor, 1072
  local, 1097–1099, 1098t
angina pectoris
  Canadian Cardiovascular Society classification
    of, 815b
  definition of, 814, 824
  description of, 291
  nonpharmacologic management of, 816–817
  nursing process for, 821–823
  pharmacologic management of, 817. See also
    antianginal drugs
  stable, 815b
  types of, 814, 815b
  unstable, 815b, 816
  variant, 815b
anginal pain, 814, 815b
Angiomax (bivalirudin), 881t, 883
angiotensin II, 337
angiotensin II receptor blockers, 780b, 842, 843t,
    846, 852, 854, 856, 1060b
angiotensin-converting enzyme, 840b
angiotensin-converting enzyme inhibitors. See
    also specific drug
  in African Americans, 21
  antihypertensive uses of, 842, 851–852
  characteristics of, 842
  in children, 854
  in diabetes mellitus patients, 419
  heart failure treated with, 780b
  in hepatic-impaired clients, 854
  mechanism of action, 842
  nonsteroidal anti-inflammatory drugs effect on,
    122
  pharmacokinetics of, 842
  during pregnancy, 1060b
  in renal-impaired clients, 855–856
  types of, 843t

anorectal medications, 1042b
anorexia, 706b
Ansaid (flurbiprofen), 109, 112t
Anspor (cephradine), 490t
Antabuse (disulfiram), 238t, 239–241
antacids, 18
antagonism, 19
antagonists
  definition of, 18
  opioid, 89–90, 90t
anterior pituitary gland, 336, 339, 456
anterior pituitary hormones, 336, 340–342,
    343t–344t, 345
Anthra-Derm (anthralin), 1046t
anthralin (Anthra-Derm), 1046t
anthrax, 515
antiadrenergic drugs
  administration of, 302
  alpha-adrenergic agonists. See alpha-
    adrenergic agonists
  alpha-adrenergic blockers. See alpha-
    adrenergic blockers
  beta-adrenergic blockers. See beta blockers
  definition of, 289
  mechanisms of action, 289–290
  nursing actions for, 302–304
antiandrogens, 704, 705t
antianginal drugs. See also specific drug
  adjunctive, 821
  administration of, 826
  adverse effects of, 827
  beta blockers, 818t, 819–820
  calcium channel blockers, 819t, 820–821
  in children, 823
  client teaching about, 824–825
  in critical illness, 825–826
  dosage of, 823
  drug interactions, 827
  in hepatic-impaired clients, 825
  in home care, 826
  nursing actions for, 826–827
  nursing process for, 821–823
  in older adults, 823
  organic nitrates, 817–819, 823–824
  in renal-impaired clients, 823, 825
  selection of, 823
  self-administration of, 824
  therapeutic effects of, 826–827
  therapeutic principles for, 823–826
antianxiety drugs. See also specific drug
  administration of, 144
  adverse effects of, 150–151
  antidepressants as, 146
  benzodiazepines. See also specific drug
    administration of, 144
    antidote for, 28t
    contraindications, 138
    in critical illness clients, 148
    cytochrome P450 metabolism of, 135, 146
    description of, 132
    duration of activity, 144
    frequency of use, 144
    in hypoalbuminemia, 147
    indications for, 135, 138, 145
    mechanism of action, 135
    nursing actions for, 149–150
    in older adults, 144
    pharmacokinetics of, 135, 136t
    in renal-impaired clients, 147
    self-administration of, 143
    toxicity of, 145
    variations among, 135
    withdrawal from, 144–145

  in children, 146–147
  client teaching about, 143
  in critical-illness clients, 148
  dosage of, 142, 144
  drug interactions, 151
  duration of activity, 144
  frequency of use, 144
  in hepatic-impaired clients, 147–148
  in home care, 148
  in hypoalbuminemia, 147
  nonbenzodiazepine, 138–140
  nursing actions for, 149–151
  nursing process for, 141–142
  in older adults, 147
  in renal-impaired clients, 147
  self-administration of, 143
  therapeutic effects of, 150
antiasthmatic drugs. See also specific drug
  administration of, 739, 741, 744
  adrenergics, 732, 732t–733t, 734
  adverse effects of, 745
  anticholinergics, 734
  anti-inflammatory, 735–738
  bronchodilators
    adrenergics, 732, 732t–733t, 734
    description of, 730, 732
    drug interactions, 745
    overdose of, 742
  in children, 742–743
  client teaching about, 740–741
  in critical illness, 744
  dosage of, 741–742
  drug interactions, 745
  in hepatic-impaired clients, 743
  in home care, 744
  immunosuppressant monoclonal antibody, 738
  leukotriene modifiers, 736t, 737
  mast cell stabilizers, 736t, 738, 754t
  nursing actions for, 744–745
  nursing process for, 738–739
  in older adults, 743
  in renal-impaired clients, 743
  selection of, 739, 741
  self-administration of, 740
  therapeutic effects of, 744–745
  therapeutic principles for, 739–744
  toxicity of, 742
  xanthines, 734–735
antibiotic(s)
  definition of, 474
  intravenous, 481
  mechanism of action, 474
  microorganisms resistant to, 471, 472b–473b,
    473, 478
antibiotic-associated colitis, 536, 998, 1005
antibiotic-resistant microorganisms, 471,
    472b–473b
antibodies, 625, 633, 673
anticholinergic drugs. See also specific drug
  administration of, 329
  adverse effects of, 222, 330
  antidote for, 28t
  antispasmodic, 320, 324
  asthma treated with, 734
  belladonna alkaloids and derivatives, 321,
    322t–323t, 324
  biliary colic treated with, 326
  centrally acting, 324–325
  in children, 327–328
  client teaching about, 326
  contraindications, 216, 321
  in critical illness, 328
  description of, 319

drug interactions, 224, 317, 330
extrapyramidal reactions, 327
in glaucoma patients, 327
in hepatic-impaired clients, 328
in home care, 328
indications for, 216, 321, 326–327
mechanism of action, 216, 319–320, 320f
muscarinic agonist poisoning, 327
nursing actions for, 329–330
nursing process for, 325–326
in older adults, 222, 328
ophthalmic, 328
opioid analgesic interactions with, 101
overactive urinary bladder treated with, 327
during pregnancy, 1061b
preoperative use of, 321
renal colic treated with, 326
in renal-impaired clients, 328
selection of, 220
self-administration of, 326
systemic effects of, 320
therapeutic effects of, 329
toxicity of, 327
types of, 217t
anticholinesterase drugs
mechanism of action, 308
myasthenia gravis treated with, 312–313
toxicity of, 314
anticoagulants. See also specific drug
administration of, 892–893
adverse effects of, 893–894
in children, 890
client teaching about, 889
description of, 879–880
drug interactions, 894
heparin
administration of, 892–893
antidote for, 28t
characteristics of, 880, 881t, 883, 888, 890
drug interactions, 894
low-molecular-weight, 880, 881t, 883,
890–891, 893
during pregnancy, 1061b
therapeutic effects of, 893
in hepatic-impaired clients, 891
herbal and dietary supplements, 891–892
in home care, 891
nonsteroidal anti-inflammatory drugs effect on,
122
nursing actions for, 892–895
nursing process for, 886–888
in older adults, 890
during pregnancy, 1061b
in renal-impaired clients, 890–891
selection of, 888
self-administration of, 889
therapeutic effects of, 893
therapeutic principles for, 888–891
warfarin
antidote for, 29t
characteristics of, 881t, 883, 888–891
drug interactions, 894–895
during pregnancy, 1061b
vitamin K interactions with, 19
anticonvulsants. See also specific drug
bipolar disorder treated with, 181
definition of, 193
antidepressants. See also specific drug
administration of, 184, 188–189
adverse effects of, 189
in African Americans, 186
anxiety treated with, 146
characteristics of, 176

in children, 187
client teaching about, 183
contraindications, 177
in critical illness, 188
dosage of, 184
duration of use, 184
in ethnic groups, 186–187
herbal and dietary supplements, 181
in home care, 188
indications for, 177
mechanism of action, 176–177
monoamine oxidase inhibitors. See monoamine
oxidase inhibitors
nursing actions for, 188–191
nursing process for, 181–182
in older adults, 187–188
perioperative use of, 186
during pregnancy, 1061b
in renal-impaired clients, 188
selection of, 182, 184
selective serotonin reuptake inhibitors. See
selective serotonin reuptake inhibitors
suicidality and, 185
therapeutic effects of, 189
toxicity of, 185–186
tricyclic. See tricyclic antidepressants
weight gain caused by, 956b
withdrawal from, 186
antidiabetic drugs. See also specific drug
adverse effects of, 430–431
hypoglycemic drugs. See hypoglycemia, drugs
for
insulin. See insulin
nursing actions for, 428–433
during pregnancy, 1061b
therapeutic effects of, 430
weight gain secondary to, 956b
antidiarrheal drugs. See also specific drug
administration of, 1006–1007
adverse effects of, 1007
antibacterial, 1000t–1001t
characteristics of, 998–1003
in children, 1006
client teaching about, 1005
contraindications, 1003
drug interactions, 1007–1008
in hepatic-impaired clients, 1006
in home care, 1006
in immunocompromised clients, 1006
indications for, 1003
nonspecific, 1002–1003
nursing actions for, 1006–1008
nursing process for, 1003–1004
opiate-related, 999t–1000t
overview of, 997–998
selection of, 1004–1005
self-administration of, 1005
therapeutic effects of, 1007
therapeutic principles for, 1004–1006
antidiuretic hormone, 79, 341, 840b
antidote
definition of, 19
half-life of, 27b
antidysrhythmic drugs. See also specific drug
administration of, 810
adverse effects of, 810–811
beta blockers, 801t, 803–804
calcium channel blockers, 802t, 805
characteristics of, 796
in children, 808–809
client teaching about, 807
in critical illness, 809
drug interactions, 811–812

in hepatic-impaired clients, 809
in home care, 809
indications for, 796
mechanism of action, 796
nursing actions for, 810–811
nursing process for, 805–806
in older adults, 809
potassium channel blockers, 801t–802t,
804–805
in renal-impaired clients, 809
self-administration of, 807
sodium channel blockers
class IA, 796, 800t, 802
class IB, 800t
class IC, 800t
therapeutic effects of, 810
therapeutic range for, 811t
antiemetic drugs. See also specific drug
administration of, 1018
adverse effects of, 1018–1019
antihistamines, 1011, 1012t
benzodiazepines, 1011
characteristics of, 1011
in chemotherapy patients, 1015
in children, 1017
client teaching about, 1015
contraindications, 1011
corticosteroids, 1011, 1012t
dosage of, 1015
drug interactions, 1019
in hepatic-impaired clients, 1017
in home care, 1017
indications for, 1011
nursing actions for, 1018–1019
nursing process for, 1014–1015
in older adults, 1017
overview of, 1010–1011
phenothiazines, 1011, 1012t, 1015, 1017
during pregnancy, 1061b
prokinetic agents, 1011–1013, 1012t
in renal-impaired clients, 1017
self-administration of, 1015
serotonin receptor antagonists, 1012t–1013t,
1013–1014, 1019
therapeutic principles for, 1015–1017
antiepileptic drugs. See also specific drug
administration of, 209
adverse effects of, 205, 210
characteristics of, 194–195
in children, 207
client teaching about, 204
combination therapy using, 205
contraindications, 195
costs of, 205
in critical illness, 208
definition of, 193
dosage of, 205–206
drug interactions, 210–212
duration of use, 206
forms of, 205
goals of, 203–204
in home care, 208
indications for, 194–195
mechanism of action, 194
monitoring of, 206
nonantiepileptic drugs affected by, 206–207
nursing actions for, 209–212
nursing process for, 202–203
in older adults, 207–208
pharmacokinetics of, 195
during pregnancy, 1061b–1062b, 1069
pregnancy risks, 205
in renal-impaired clients, 208

antiepileptic drugs (*continued*)
    selection of, 204–205
    therapeutic effects of, 210
    therapeutic principles for, 203–208
    toxicity of, 206
    weight gain caused by, 956b
antiestrogens, 391, 394, 704
antifungal drugs. *See also specific drug*
    administration of, 598–599
    adverse effects of, 599–600
    azoles, 583, 588t–590t, 591–592, 596–597
    in cancer patients, 597
    in children, 597
    client teaching about, 594
    in critical illness, 597
    description of, 583
    dosage of, 595
    drug interactions, 596–597, 600–601
    duration of use, 595
    in hepatic-impaired clients, 598
    in home care, 597
    indications for, 595–596
    nursing actions for, 598–601
    nursing process for, 593–594
    in older adults, 597
    polyenes, 583, 586, 587t
    during pregnancy, 1062b
    in renal-impaired clients, 597
    selection of, 595
    self-administration of, 594
    therapeutic effects of, 599
    therapeutic principles for, 595–598
antigen, 468, 625, 748
antigen–antibody interactions, 625
antigen-presenting cells, 626
antigen–T lymphocyte interactions, 625
antigout drugs, 115, 121
antihelmintics, 605, 609t–610t, 615
antihemophilic factor, 877t
antihistamines. *See also specific drug*
    administration of, 758
    adverse effects of, 758
    antiemetic uses of, 1011, 1012t
    characteristics of, 750–753
    in children, 756
    client teaching about, 756
    contraindications, 753t
    in critical illness, 757
    definition of, 747
    drug interactions, 758
    first-generation histamine₁ receptor antago-
        nists, 753
    in hepatic-impaired clients, 757
    in home care, 757
    indications for, 750, 752–753
    mechanism of action, 750, 753f
    nursing actions for, 758, 768
    nursing process for, 754–755
    in older adults, 756
    ophthalmic uses of, 1025
    during pregnancy, 1062b
    in renal-impaired clients, 757
    second-generation histamine₁ receptor antago-
        nists, 754
    selection of, 755–756
    therapeutic effects of, 758
    therapeutic principles for, 755–757, 767
    weight gain caused by, 956b
antihypertensive drugs. *See also specific drug*
    administration of, 858
    adverse effects of, 858–859
    in African Americans, 21
    alpha₂ agonists, 844t

alpha-adrenergic blockers, 844t, 846, 849
alpha–beta-adrenergic blockers, 845t
angina pectoris treated with, 821
angiotensin II receptor blockers, 780b, 842,
    843t, 846, 852, 854, 856, 1060b
angiotensin-converting enzyme inhibitors. *See*
    angiotensin-converting enzyme inhibitors
antiadrenergics, 846, 849, 852–853
    beta blockers, 844t, 853
    calcium channel blockers, 845t, 849, 853
    in children, 854–855
    classification of, 842–849
    client teaching about, 852
    combination products, 847t–848t, 853
    in critical illness, 857
    description of, 838
    diuretics, 849, 853
    dosage of, 853
    drug interactions, 859
    ethnicity and, 853–854
    in home care, 857
    nursing actions for, 858–859
    nursing process for, 850–851
    in older adults, 855
    opioid analgesic interactions with, 101
    postganglionic-active drugs, 844t
    during pregnancy, 1062b
    in renal-impaired clients, 855–856
    selection of, 851–853
    self-administration of, 852
    in surgery patients, 857
    therapeutic effects of, 858
    therapeutic principles for, 851–858
    types of, 843t–849t
    vasodilators, 781, 839, 846t, 849, 853
    weight gain caused by, 956b
antilipemics, 821
Antilirium (physostigmine salicylate), 309–311,
    310t, 327
antimalarial drugs, 604, 606, 608t–609t, 611
antimetabolites, 695t–696t, 698–699
antimicrobial drugs. *See also specific drug*
    administration of, 478, 481
    adverse effects of, 482–483
    characteristics of, 474–475
    in children, 479
    client teaching about, 477
    combination therapy, 478
    in critical illness, 480
    dosage of, 478
    duration of use, 479
    in hepatic-impaired clients, 480
    in home care, 480–481
    indications for, 474–475
    mechanism of action, 474
    nursing actions for, 481–483
    nursing process for, 475–476
    in older adults, 479
    ophthalmic, 1028t–1029t
    perioperative use of, 479
    purpose of, 467
    rational use of, 476–477
    in renal-impaired clients, 480
    selection of, 477–478
    self-administration of, 477
    terminology associated with, 474
    therapeutic effects of, 481–482
    therapeutic principles for, 476–481
antimuscarinic drugs, 319
antineoplastic drugs. *See also specific drug*
    administration of, 711, 715–716
    adverse effects of, 694, 717–718
    alkylating drugs, 695t, 698

antiandrogens, 704, 705t
antiestrogens, 704
antimetabolites, 695t–696t, 698–699
antitumor antibiotics, 696t, 699
aromatase inhibitors, 704, 705t
biologic targeted, 699–702, 719
characteristics of, 694, 698
in children, 712
classification of, 698–699
cytoprotectant drugs, 705, 707
description of, 691
dosage of, 710–711
drug interactions, 718–719
growth factors, 701–702
in hepatic-impaired clients, 714–715
in home care, 715
hormone inhibitor drugs, 702–705, 711, 719
indications for, 698
luteinizing hormone releasing hormone
    analogs, 704–705, 705t
monoclonal antibodies, 699–701, 700t,
    716–718
nitrosoureas, 695t, 698
nursing actions for, 715–719
nursing process for, 707–709
in older adults, 712
overview of, 694
plant alkaloids, 697t, 699
platinum compounds, 695t, 698
podophyllotoxins, 697t, 699
proteasome inhibitors, 700t, 702
in renal-impaired clients, 713–714
safety precautions with, 712
selection of, 710
taxanes, 697t, 699
therapeutic effects of, 716
therapeutic principles for, 709–715
tyrosine kinase inhibitors, 700t, 701–702
vinca alkaloids, 697t, 699, 719
antiparasitic drugs. *See also specific drug*
    administration of, 615
    adverse effects of, 615–616
    antihelmintics, 605, 609t–610t, 615
    antimalarials, 606, 608t–609t, 611
    antiprotozoals. *See antiprotozoal drugs*
    in children, 614
    client teaching about, 614
    drug interactions, 616
    in home care, 614–615
    nursing actions for, 615–616
    nursing process for, 612–614
    in older adults, 614
    pediculicides, 610t, 612
    scabicides, 610t, 612
    self-administration of, 614
    therapeutic effects of, 615
antiparkinson drugs. *See also specific drug*
    administration of, 222–223
    adverse effects of, 223–224
    anticholinergic drugs. *See anticholinergic*
        drugs
    in children, 221–222
    client teaching about, 220
    dopaminergic drugs, 215, 217t, 225
    dosage of, 221
    drug interactions, 224–225
    goals of, 220
    in hepatic-impaired clients, 222
    in home care, 222
    nursing actions for, 222–225
    in older adults, 222
    overview of, 214–215
    in renal-impaired clients, 222

selection of, 220–221
self-administration of, 220
therapeutic effects of, 223
therapeutic principles for, 220–222
antiplatelet drugs. *See also specific drug*
adenosine diphosphate receptor antagonists, 884
administration of, 892–893
adverse effects of, 893–894
characteristics of, 882t
client teaching about, 889
glycoprotein IIb/IIIa receptor antagonists, 884–885
nursing actions for, 892–895
nursing process for, 886–888
phosphodiesterase inhibitor, 885
in renal-impaired clients, 890–891
self-administration of, 889
therapeutic effects of, 893
therapeutic principles for, 888–891
thrombolytic agents, 882t, 885
thromboxane A$_2$ inhibitors, 884
antiprostaglandin drugs, 103
antiprotozoal drugs, 606, 607t
antipsychotic drugs. *See also specific drug*
administration of, 168–169
adverse effects of, 166b, 169–171
in African Americans, 167
antidote for, 29t
in Asians, 167
atypical, 154, 159t–160t, 160–161
bipolar disorder treated with, 181
in children, 165b, 165–166
client teaching about, 163
contraindications, 155
in critical illness patients, 167–168
D2 dopamine receptor binding of, 154
description of, 154
dosage of, 164, 166b
drug interactions, 171–172
duration of use, 164
in ethnic groups, 167
extrapyramidal reactions, 164, 169–170
first-generation, 154–156, 158t–159t
goals of, 163
in hepatic-impaired patients, 167
in Hispanics, 167
in home care, 168
hypersensitivity reactions to, 170
indications for, 155
intramuscular administration of, 164, 168
mechanism of action, 154–155
nonphenothiazines, 155–156, 158t–160t, 160–161
nursing actions for, 168–172
nursing process for, 161–162
in older adults, 166, 166b
perioperative use of, 165
pharmacokinetics of, 156t
phenothiazines, 155
during pregnancy, 1062b
principles of, 163–168
in renal-impaired patients, 167
second-generation, 154, 159t–160t, 160–161
selection of, 163–164
therapeutic effects of, 169
typical, 154–156, 158t–159t, 164
weight gain caused by, 164, 956b
withdrawal from, 164
antirejection agents, 672–673
antiretroviral drugs. *See also specific drug*
client teaching about, 573
combination, 570, 573–574

description of, 563
drug interactions, 574
fusion inhibitor, 569t, 570
monitoring of, 574
non-nucleoside reverse transcriptase inhibitors, 563, 566t–567t, 569–570
nucleoside reverse transcriptase inhibitors, 563, 566t–567t
nucleotide reverse transcriptase inhibitor, 563, 567t
protease inhibitors, 565, 568t, 569
self-administration of, 573
therapeutic principles for, 572–574
antiseizure drugs. *See also antiepileptic drugs*
administration of, 209
adverse effects of, 205, 210
characteristics of, 194–195
in children, 207
client teaching about, 204
combination therapy using, 205
contraindications, 195
costs of, 205
in critical illness, 208
definition of, 193
dosage forms for, 205
dosage of, 205–206
drug interactions, 210–212
duration of use, 206
goals of, 203–204
in hepatic-impaired clients, 208
in home care, 208
indications for, 194–195
mechanism of action, 194
nursing actions for, 209–212
nursing process for, 202–203
in older adults, 207–208
pharmacokinetics of, 195
selection of, 204–205
therapeutic effects of, 210
therapeutic principles for, 203–208
toxicity of, 206
antishock drugs. *See also specific drug*
administration of, 835
adverse effects of, 836
characteristics of, 830
in children, 834
drug interactions, 836
nursing actions for, 835–836
nursing process for, 832–833
selection of, 833
therapeutic effects of, 835–836
types of, 831t
antispasmodics
anticholinergics, 320, 324
urinary, 325
antithrombin III (Thrombate III), 1079
antithyroid drugs, 376–378, 377t, 381–385
antitrichomonal drugs, 604
antitubercular drugs. *See also specific drug*
adherence to, 553–554
administration of, 556
adverse effects of, 557
in children, 555
drug interactions, 557–558
drugs affected by, 554
in hepatic-impaired clients, 555–556
in home care, 556
monitoring of, 554
nursing actions for, 556–558
during pregnancy, 1062b
primary, 544, 547–550
combination, 549–550
in renal-impaired clients, 555

secondary, 550
therapeutic effects of, 556–557
antitumor antibiotics, 696t, 699
antitussives. *See also specific drug*
adverse effects of, 768–769
characteristics of, 762
client teaching about, 766
narcotic, 763t
non-narcotic, 763t
nursing actions for, 768
therapeutic effects of, 768
therapeutic principles for, 766–767
Antivert (meclizine), 1012t
antiviral drugs. *See also antiretroviral drugs; specific drug*
administration of, 576–577
adverse effects of, 577–578
in children, 574–575
description of, 562
drug interactions, 578–580
in hepatic-impaired clients, 576
herpesvirus treated with, 563, 564t–565t
in home care, 576
human immunodeficiency virus treated with. *See antiretroviral drugs*
influenza A treated with, 565t, 570
nursing actions for, 576–580
in older adults, 575
during pregnancy, 1062b–1063b
in renal-impaired clients, 575–576
respiratory syncytial virus infection treated with, 565t, 570
therapeutic effects of, 577
Anturane (sulfinpyrazone), 115, 116t, 129
anxiety
antidepressants for, 146
assessment of, 141
benzodiazepines for. *See Benzodiazepines*
in children, 146–147
cognitive behavioral therapy for, 146
description of, 132–133
drug therapy for, 145–146. *See also antianxiety drugs*
herbal and dietary supplements for, 140
nursing process for, 141–142
situational, 133
anxiety disorders
definition of, 133
generalized, 134b, 145–146
obsessive-compulsive disorder, 134b
panic disorder, 134b
pathophysiology of, 133
post-traumatic stress disorder, 134b
social phobia, 134b
Anzemet (dolasetron), 1012t, 1013, 1018
aortic valve, 774
Apidra (insulin glulisine), 408, 410t
apothecary system, 37, 37t
apraclonidine (Lopidine), 1026t
Apresoline (hydralazine), 21, 846t, 855
Apri, 445t
aprotinin (Trasylol), 886, 886t
Aqua-Ban, 257t
Aquachloral (chloral hydrate), 138, 139t
aqueous humor, 1024
arachidonic acid metabolism
corticosteroid effects on, 355
description of, 103, 105b
Aralen (chloroquine), 606, 607t, 616
Aramine (metaraminol), 273t, 831t, 832
Aranesp (darbepoetin alfa), 652t, 655, 658, 663
Arava (leflunomide), 124, 670t, 675, 681–683, 682, 686, 688

Aredia (pamidronate), 390, 393t, 401
argatroban, 881t, 883
Aricept (donepezil), 310t, 311, 314
Arimidex (anastrozole), 704, 705t
aripiprazole (Abilify), 156t, 159t, 161, 168, 171–172
Aristocort Forte (triamcinolone diacetate), 359t, 731b
Aristocort (triamcinolone), 359t, 731b, 1045t
Arixtra (fondaparinux), 881t, 883
Aromasin (exemestane), 704, 705t
aromatase inhibitors, 704, 705t
arteries, 774
arthritis
    osteoarthritis, 106b, 118, 124, 955b
    psoriatic, 678–679
    rheumatoid, 124, 679
Arthropan (choline salicylate), 109, 111t
articaine (Septodont), 1098t
Ascaris lumbricoides, 605b
Asendin (amoxapine), 178t
Asians
    antidepressants in, 186–187
    antipsychotic drugs in, 167
Asmanex Twisthaler (mometasone), 359t, 736t
aspartate, 78
aspergillosis, 584b, 595
Aspergillosis fumigatus, 584b
Aspergillus, 582
aspirin (acetylsalicylic acid)
    angina pectoris treated with, 821
    antiplatelet effects of, 106, 882t
    characteristics of, 109
    in children, 108
    client teaching about, 120
    contraindications, 108–109
    description of, 103
    dosage of, 110t
    indications for, 106b, 107, 110t, 119, 122
    mechanism of action, 104
    pain management using, 122
    perioperative use of, 124
    pharmacokinetics of, 109
    during pregnancy, 1063b
    in renal-impaired patients, 125
    rheumatoid arthritis treated with, 124
    self-administration of, 120
assessment
    of alcohol abuse, 248
    of allergic disorders, 278–279
    of anxiety, 141
    of asthma, 279
    of chronic obstructive pulmonary disorders, 279
    description of, 51–52
    of diabetes mellitus, 417–418
    of heart failure, 784–785
    of hypersensitivity reactions, 755
    of hypertension, 850
    of hypocalcemia, 395
    of myasthenia gravis, 311
    of pain, 91–92
    of Parkinson's disease, 219
    of psychosis, 161–162
    of substance abuse, 248
    of urinary tract infections, 520
Astelin (azelastine), 752, 754
asthma
    antiasthmatic drugs for. See antiasthmatic drugs
    assessment of, 738–739
    corticosteroids for, 365–366, 731b
    description of, 279, 729

exacerbations, 731b
    herbal and dietary supplements for, 738
    National Asthma Education and Prevention Program, 730, 731b, 1068b
    nursing process for, 738–739
    pathophysiology of, 730
    during pregnancy, 1067
    symptoms of, 729–730
Atacand (candesartan), 843t
atazanavir (Reyataz), 568t
atenolol (Tenormin), 293t, 818t, 844t
Atgam (lymphocyte immune globulin, antithymocyte globulin), 670t, 673, 686
atheromas, 898
atherosclerosis, 815–816, 876–877, 898
Ativan (lorazepam)
    antianxiety uses of, 136t–137t, 138, 148–149
    antiseizure uses of, 198t, 200
    substance abuse disorders treated with, 238t
Atkins diet, 964b
atomoxetine (Strattera), 256, 256t, 259
atopic dermatitis, 1040
atorvastatin (Lipitor), 901, 902t, 905–906
atovaquone (Mepron), 609t, 611
atovaquone/proguanil (Malarone), 608t
atracurium (Tracium), 1096t
atria, 773
atrial fibrillation, 797b, 808
atrial flutter, 797b–798b
atropine sulfate
    anticholinergic properties of, 321, 322t, 327
    antidote uses of, 28t, 327
    characteristics of, 322t
    cholinergic drugs reversed using, 314
    in critical illness, 328
    description of, 216
    ophthalmic, 322t, 1027t
    sinus bradycardia treated with, 320
    toxicity of, 327
Atrovent (ipratropium bromide), 321, 322t, 324, 732t–733t, 734, 767
attention deficit-hyperactivity disorder
    central nervous system stimulants for, 259–260
    cholinergic drugs for, 314
    definition of, 253
    methylphenidate for, 242, 248, 254, 255t, 258–260
Attenuvax (measles vaccine), 637t
augmented betamethasone dipropionate (Diprolene), 1045t
Augmentin (amoxicillin clavulanate), 488t, 489
autoantigens, 665–666
autoimmune disorders
    description of, 631, 665–667
    immunosuppressants for, 678–679
autonomic drugs, 271
autonomic nervous system
    divisions of, 266–271
    functions of, 265
    neurotransmitters of, 266
    parasympathetic nervous system, 270–271
    structure of, 265–266
    sympathetic nervous system, 267–270
Avalide, 847t
Avandamet (rosiglitazone/metformin), 415t
Avandia (rosiglitazone), 414t, 430–431
Avapro (irbesartan), 843t
Avastin (bevacizumab), 699, 700t
Aveeno (colloidal oatmeal), 1047t
Avelox (moxifloxacin), 508t, 1029t
Aventyl (nortriptyline), 178t, 1083
Aviane, 445t
Avlosulfon (dapsone), 609t, 611

Avonex (interferon beta-1a), 654t
Axert (almotriptan), 116, 117t, 121, 128
axon, 75
Aygestin (norethindrone acetate), 443t
azacitidine (Vidaza), 1079
Azactam (aztreonam), 486t, 494, 500
azathioprine (Imuran), 669t, 671, 679–682, 685
azelaic acid (Azelex, Finacea), 1043t, 1052
azelastine (Astelin, Optivar), 752, 754, 1029t
Azelex (azelaic acid), 1043t, 1052
azithromycin (Zithromax), 528, 529t, 530, 539, 551, 1000t
Azmacort, 359t
azoles, 583, 588t–590t, 591–592, 596–597
Azopt (brinzolamide), 1028t
AZT (zidovudine), 563, 566t, 574, 576, 578–580
aztreonam (Azactam), 486t, 494, 500
Azulfidine (sulfasalazine), 517t, 1080

B

B cells, 625, 628–629
Bacillus anthracis, 515
Bacillus Calmette-Guérin vaccine, 651, 654t, 656, 662
bacitracin, 1043t
bacitracin and polymyxin B (Polysporin), 1043t
baclofen (Lioresal), 228–230, 229t
bacteria
    classification of, 468
    gram-negative, 470b–471b
    gram-positive, 469b–470b
    host defense mechanisms against, 473–474
    normal flora, 468
    normal types of, 468
    types of, 469b–471b
bacterial endocarditis, 474
bactericidal, 474
bacteriostatic, 474
Bacteroides fragilis, 470b, 530
Bactocill (oxacillin), 487, 488t
Bactrim (trimethoprim-sulfamethoxazole)
    antidiarrheal uses of, 1001t
    characteristics of, 517t–518t
    description of, 479
    during pregnancy, 1061b
    urinary tract infections treated with, 515
Bactroban (mupirocin), 1043t
Balnetar (coal tar), 1046t
balsalazide (Colazal), 1079
bar coding, 33
Baraclude (entecavir), 1079
barbiturates abuse, 241–242
basal cell carcinoma, 1048
basal ganglia, 80, 214
basil, 416
basiliximab (Simulect), 669t, 674, 679
bay leaf, 416
BayGam (immune globulin), 641t
BayHep B (hepatitis B immune globulin, human), 641t
BayRab (rabies immune globulin), 642t
BayTet (tetanus immune globulin), 642t
B-complex biotin
    administration of, 946
    deficiency of, 920t
    disorders of, 938
    food sources of, 920t
    function of, 920t
    recommended daily intake of, 920t–921t
becaplermin (Regranex), 1046t
beclomethasone (Beconase AQ), 736t, 754t
beclomethasone (QVAR), 736t

beclomethasone (QVAR, Vancenase), 358t, 363, 731b, 732t, 735
Beconase AQ (beclomethasone), 736t, 754t
bee pollen, 416
belladonna alkaloids and derivatives, 321, 322t–323t, 324
belladonna tincture, 321
Benadryl (diphenhydramine), 29t, 217t, 751t, 753, 756
benazepril (Lotensin), 843t
bendroflumethiazide (Naturetin), 864t
Benemid (probenecid), 115, 116t, 129, 497
Benicar (olmesartan), 843t
benign prostatic hyperplasia, 290, 459, 834
Bentyl (dicyclomine hydrochloride), 323t
Benylin DM (dextromethorphan), 763t, 769
Benzamycin (erythromycin/benzoyl peroxide), 1043t
Benzedrex (propylhexedrine), 273t
benzocaine (Americaine, Lanacane, Solarcaine), 1098t
benzodiazepines. See also specific drug
    abuse of, 241–242
    administration of, 144
    alcohol abuse treated with, 240
    antidote for, 28t
    contraindications, 138
    in critical illness clients, 148
    cytochrome P450 metabolism of, 135, 146
    description of, 132
    duration of activity, 144
    frequency of use, 144
    in hypoalbuminemia, 147
    indications for, 135, 138, 145
    mechanism of action, 135
    nursing actions for, 149–150
    in older adults, 144
    pharmacokinetics of, 135, 136t
    during pregnancy, 1060b
    in renal-impaired clients, 147
    self-administration of, 143
    toxicity of, 145
    variations among, 135
    withdrawal from, 144–145
benzoyl peroxide, 1043t
benztropine (Cogentin), 217t, 323t, 325
benzylpenicilloyl polylysine (Pre-Pen), 497
beta blockers. See also specific drug
    administration of, 297, 299
    adverse effects of, 303, 827
    angina pectoris treated with, 818t, 819–820
    antidote for, 28t
    antihypertensive uses of, 844t, 853
    characteristics of, 819–820
    in children, 300, 854
    class II, 801, 803–804
    client teaching about, 299
    contraindications, 291
    in critical illness, 301
    discontinuation of, 299
    drug interactions, 304
    duration of action, 297
    dysrhythmias treated with, 801t
    elimination of, 297
    in ethnic groups, 300
    heart failure treated with, 780b
    in hepatic-impaired clients, 301, 856
    in home care, 301
    indications for, 291, 295
    intrinsic sympathomimetic activity of, 296
    lipid solubility of, 296–297
    mechanism of action, 290, 290f

membrane-stabilizing activity of, 296
nonselective, 296
nonsteroidal anti-inflammatory drugs effect on, 122
nursing actions for, 302–304
nursing process for, 297–298
in older adults, 300
ophthalmic uses of, 1026t–1027t
potassium channel blockade, 296
during pregnancy, 1063b
receptor selectivity of, 296
in renal-impaired clients, 301, 856
selection of, 298–299
selective, 296
self-administration of, 299
therapeutic effects of, 302
weight gain caused by, 956b
beta₁ receptors, 269, 269t, 274
beta₂ receptors, 269, 269t, 274
beta₃ receptors, 274
beta-adrenergic receptors, 77
Betagan (levobunolol), 293t, 1026t
beta-lactam antibacterials
    administration of, 496, 499–500
    adverse effects of, 500–501
    carbapenems, 491, 494, 494t, 498, 500–501, 1060b
    cephalosporins. See cephalosporins
    in children, 497
    in critical illness, 498–499
    description of, 485
    dosage of, 496
    drug interactions, 501
    in hepatic-impaired clients, 498
    in home care, 499
    mechanism of action, 485
    monobactam, 494, 498
    nursing actions for, 499–501
    nursing process for, 494–495
    in older adults, 497–498
    penicillin–beta-lactamase inhibitor combinations, 487–489, 488t
    penicillins. See penicillin(s)
    during pregnancy, 1060b
    in renal-impaired clients, 498
    therapeutic effects of, 500
    types of, 485
betamethasone acetate and sodium phosphate (Celestone Soluspan), 358t
betamethasone (Celestone), 358t
betamethasone dipropionate (Alphatrex), 1045t
betamethasone valerate (Valisone), 1045t
Betapace (sotalol), 293t, 802t, 804–805
Betaseron (interferon beta-1b), 654t
betaxolol (Betoptic, Kerlone), 293t, 844t, 1026t
bethanechol (Urecholine), 308, 310t, 314–315
Betoptic (betaxolol), 293t, 1026t
bevacizumab (Avastin), 699, 700t
Bexxar (tositumomab and iodine 131–itositu-momab), 700t, 701
Biavax II (rubella and mumps vaccine), 639t
bicalutamide (Casodex), 704, 705t, 715
Bicillin (penicillin G benzathine), 488t
BiCNU (carmustine), 695t, 713–714
biguanides, 413, 414t, 425
bile, 916
bile acid sequestrants, 901–903, 902t
biliary colic, 326
bimatoprost (Lumigan), 1028t

biologic response modifiers, 632, 651, 668
biologic targeted antineoplastic drugs, 699–702, 719
biperiden (Akineton), 323t, 325
bipolar disorder
    anticonvulsants for, 181
    antipsychotic drugs for, 181
    definition of, 175b
    etiology of, 176
bisacodyl (Dulcolax), 989t
bismuth subsalicylate (Pepto-Bismol), 1001t, 1002
bisoprolol (Zebeta), 293t, 844t
bisphosphonates, 390, 393t, 396, 399–402
bitolterol (Tornalate), 273t
bivalirudin (Angiomax), 881t, 883
black cohosh, 58t, 443–444
Black Draught (senna preparations), 990t
blastomycosis, 583, 584b, 593, 595
Blenoxane (bleomycin), 696t, 714
bleomycin (Blenoxane), 696t, 714
blepharitis, 1024
Blocadren (timolol), 293t, 845t
blood
    components of, 775–776
    functions of, 775
blood dyscrasias, 170
blood flow, 838–839
blood pressure
    classification of, 839
    elevated. See hypertension
    hormonal regulation of, 840b
    measurement of, 851
    neural regulation of, 840b
    regulation of, 838–839, 840b–841b
    vascular regulation of, 840b–841b
blood vessels, 774–775
body mass index, 952, 953b
body surface area, 62, 64f
body weight
    drug action affected by, 20
    loss of. See weight loss
    obesity. See obesity
bone disorders
    bisphosphonates for, 390, 393t, 396, 399–402
    description of, 391b
    nursing process for, 395–396
    osteoporosis, 391b, 394, 396, 398, 450
bone marrow transplantation, 660, 667–668, 681
bone metabolism, 390
bone remodeling, 390
Bonine (meclizine), 1012t
bortezomib (Velcade), 700t, 702, 715, 718
bosentan (Tracleer), 782t, 784
bradykinin, 82, 105b, 839
brain, 80
brand name, 4
Bravelle (Urofollitropin), 344t, 345
Brethine (terbutaline), 273t
bretylium (Bretylol), 801t, 804, 811t
Bretylol (bretylium), 801t, 804, 811t
Brevibloc (esmolol), 293t, 801t, 804, 809
Brevicon, 445t
Brevital (methohexital), 1096t
brimonidine (Alphagan P), 1026t
brinzolamide (Azopt), 1028t
bromfenac (Xibrom), 1079
bromocriptine (Parlodel), 217t, 218, 224
brompheniramine (LoHist), 751t, 753
bronchi, 726
bronchioles, 726
bronchodilation, 320

bronchodilators
    adrenergics, 732, 732t–733t, 734
    description of, 730, 732
    drug interactions, 745
    overdose of, 742
bronchospasm, 730
b-type natriuretic peptide, 782t, 783–784
budesonide (Pulmicort Terbuhaler, Pulmicort Respules, Rhinocort, Entocort EC), 358t, 363, 731b, 732t, 736t, 754t
bulk-forming laxatives, 988, 989t
bumetanide (Bumex), 864t, 871
Bumex (bumetanide), 864t, 871
bupivacaine (Marcaine), 1098t
Buprenex (buprenorphine), 87t, 89
buprenorphine (Buprenex), 87t, 89
bupropion (Wellbutrin, Wellbutrin SR, Wellbutrin XL, Zyban)
    antidepressant uses of, 179t, 180, 182–184, 186
    smoking cessation uses of, 238t, 244
burns, 97
bursitis, 106b
BuSpar (buspirone), 138, 139t, 143, 145–148, 151
buspirone (BuSpar), 138, 139t, 143, 145–148, 151
butamben (Butesin), 1098t
butenafine (Mentax), 588b, 1043t
Butesin (butamben), 1098t
butoconazole (Femstat, Gynazole), 588b
butorphanol (Stadol), 87t, 89, 101
Byetta (exenatide), 1079
BZ1, 135
BZ2, 135

C
C fibers, 83
Cafergot (ergotamine tartrate and caffeine), 116, 117t, 257t
Caffedrine, 257t, 1065b
caffeine, 254, 256, 257t, 259, 261
Calan (verapamil), 802t, 805, 811t, 819t, 845t
Calciferol (ergocalciferol), 392t
calciferol (vitamin D), 387–388
Calcijex (calcitriol), 392t
Calcimar (salmon calcitonin), 390, 393t
calcipotriene (Dovonex), 1046t
calcitonin, 373, 388
calcitriol (Rocaltrol, Calcijex), 388, 392t
calcium
    in children, 943t
    daily requirements, 389b
    description of, 337
    disorders involving, 391b
    functions of, 389b
    metabolism of
        hormones involved in, 387–388, 388f
        parathyroid hormone in, 336, 387, 393t
        therapeutic principles for, 396–399
    in osteoporotic patients, 398
    phosphorus and, 388, 389b
    serum levels of, 395
    sources of, 389b
calcium acetate (PhosLo), 392t
calcium carbonate, 390
calcium carbonate precipitated (Os-Cal, Tums), 392t
calcium channel blockers. See also specific drug
    adverse effects of, 827
    angina pectoris treated with, 819t, 820–821
    antidote for, 28t
    antidysrhythmic uses of, 802t, 805

antihypertensive uses of, 845t, 849, 853
    in children, 854
    in hepatic-impaired clients, 856–857
    mechanism of action, 821f
    in older adults, 823
    during pregnancy, 1063b
    in renal-impaired clients, 856
calcium chloride, 392t
calcium citrate (Citracal), 392t
calcium gluconate
    antidote uses of, 28t
    characteristics of, 390, 392t
calcium lactate, 392t
calcium pantothenate, 924t
calcium preparations, 390, 400
calmodulin, 337
calories, 952
Campath (alemtuzumab), 699, 700t
Campral (acamprosate), 238t, 240
Camptosar (irinotecan), 697t, 713
camptothecins, 697t, 699
Campylobacter jejuni, 997
Canada
    Controlled Drugs and Substances Act, 1085
    drug names, 1087–1094
    Food and Drugs Act, 1084–1085
    provincial regulations in, 1085–1086
cancer
    carcinogens associated with, 693b
    classification of, 692–694
    colony-stimulating factors in patients with, 659
    corticosteroids for, 366
    description of, 691
    development of, 692
    immunizations in patients with, 646
    immunosuppression-related, 678
    interferons in patients with, 660
    interleukins in patients with, 659–660
    laxatives for patients with, 993
    malignant cells, 691–692
    obesity and, 954b
    treatment of, 709–710
    vitamins for prevention of, 938–939
cancer pain
    acetaminophen for, 124–125
    description of, 84b
    opioid analgesics for, 96–97, 99
Cancidas (caspofungin), 588b, 592, 597–598, 600
candesartan (Atacand), 843t
Candida albicans, 468, 582–583
candidiasis, 583, 584b–585b, 593, 595, 1041
cannabinoids, 245, 1013t, 1014
canthi, 1023
Capastat (capreomycin), 550
capecitabine (Xeloda), 695t, 714
capillaries, 774–775
capillary hydrostatic pressure, 863
Capoten (captopril), 842, 843t, 857
Capozide, 847t
capreomycin (Capastat), 550
capsaicin (Zostrix), 58t, 91, 1046t
capsules, 34, 35t
captopril (Capoten), 842, 843t, 857
carbachol (Carboptic), 1027t
carbamazepine (Tegretol), 194–195, 196t, 200, 207, 211, 1083
carbapenems, 491, 494, 494t, 498, 500–501, 1060b
carbenicillin (Geocillin), 487, 488t
carbidopa (Lodosyn), 215–216, 217t, 218
Carbocaine (mepivacaine), 1098t
carbon dioxide, 726
carbonic anhydrase inhibitors, 1026, 1027t–1028t

carboplatin (Paraplatin), 695t
carboprost tromethamine (Hemabate), 1070t
Carboptic (carbachol), 1027t
carboxyhemoglobin, 817
carbuncles, 1041
carcinoembryonic antigen, 708
carcinogenicity, 26
carcinogens, 693b
carcinomas, 693
Cardene IV (nicardipine), 845t
Cardene (nicardipine), 819t, 845t
Cardene SR (nicardipine), 845t
cardiac glycosides, 778–784
cardiac orifice, 914
cardiac output, 838
cardiac remodeling, 778
cardiac transplantation, 680
cardiogenic shock, 829, 830t
cardiopulmonary resuscitation
    epinephrine for, 281
    vasopressin for, 281
cardiovascular disease, 939
cardiovascular disorders, 22t
cardiovascular system
    alcohol abuse effects on, 239b
    anabolic steroids' effect on, 456
    androgens' effect on, 456
    blood vessels, 774–775
    cocaine effects on, 244b
    in diabetes mellitus patients, 418
    disorders of, 776
    glucocorticoids' effect on, 354
    heart, 773–774
    physiology of, 773–776
Cardizem (diltiazem), 802t, 805, 819t, 845t
Cardura (doxazosin), 292t, 294, 844t
care maps, 56
caregiver teaching, 54b
carisoprodol (Soma), 229t, 230
carmustine (BiCNU, Gliadel), 695t, 713–714
carrier proteins, 13b
carteolol (Cartrol), 293t, 844t, 1026t
Cartrol (carteolol), 293t, 844t, 1026t
carvedilol (Coreg), 293t, 295, 298, 845t
cascara sagrada, 989t
Casodex (bicalutamide), 704, 705t, 715
caspofungin (Cancidas), 588b, 592, 597–598, 600
castor oil (Neoloid), 989t
Cataflam (diclofenac potassium), 111t
Catapres (clonidine)
    agonist effects of, 289
    antihypertensive uses of, 844t, 857
    characteristics of, 291, 292t
    indications, 290–291
    opioid withdrawal uses of, 96
    substance abuse disorders treated with, 238t, 240
Catechol-O-methyltransferase, 268, 834
Catechol-O-methyltransferase inhibitors, 214, 216, 218
cathartics
    contraindications, 988
    definition of, 987
    drug interactions, 995
    indications for, 988
    long-term use of, 993
    in renal-impaired clients, 994
    saline, 993
    stimulant, 988–990, 989t
catheters
    description of, 41b
    peripherally inserted central, 41b
cation exchange resin, 925, 929, 930t

Caverject (alprostadil), 1079
CCNU (lomustine), 695t, 713
CD4⁺ cells, 628
CD8⁺ cells, 628
Ceclor (cefaclor), 486t, 490t
Cedax (ceftibuten), 491t
cefaclor (Ceclor), 486t, 490t
cefadroxil (Duricef, Ultracef), 490t
cefazolin (Kefzol, Ancef), 486t, 492t, 496
cefdinir (Omnicef), 490t
cefditoren pivoxil (Spectracef), 490t
cefepime (Maxipime), 486t, 493t
cefixime (Suprax), 486t, 490t
Cefizox (ceftizoxime), 493t
Cefobid (cefoperazone), 486t, 492t, 498
cefoperazone (Cefobid), 486t, 492t, 498
Cefotan (cefotetan), 486t, 492t
cefotaxime (Claforan), 492t
cefotetan (Cefotan), 486t, 492t
cefoxitin (Mefoxin), 492t
cefpodoxime (Vantin), 490t
cefprozil (Cefzil), 490t
ceftazidime (Fortaz), 486t, 493t
ceftibuten (Cedax), 491t
ceftizoxime (Cefizox), 493t
ceftriaxone (Rocephin), 486t, 493t
cefuroxime (Ceftin, Kefurox, Zinacef), 486t,
    490t, 492t
Cefzil (cefprozil), 490t
Celebrex (celecoxib), 107–108, 111t, 115,
    128–129
celecoxib (Celebrex), 107–108, 111t, 115,
    128–129
Celestone (betamethasone), 358t
Celestone Soluspan (betamethasone acetate and
    sodium phosphate), 358t
Celexa (citalopram), 177, 178t
cell(s)
    functions of, 11b
    physiology of, 10, 12
    structures of, 11b
cell cycle, 691–692, 692f
cell membrane
    corticosteroid effects on, 355
    drug transport through, 12
    structure of, 11b
CellCept (mycophenolate mofetil), 670t, 671,
    680–683, 687–688
cellulitis, 1041
Cenestin (conjugated estrogens), 440, 441t
central nervous system
    adverse effects on, 25
    anabolic steroids' effect on, 457
    androgens' effect on, 457
    anticholinergic drugs' effect on, 320
    basal ganglia, 80
    blood pressure regulation by, 840b
    brain, 80
    cerebellum, 79
    cerebral cortex, 78
    cocaine effects on, 244b
    components of, 78–80
    definition of, 75
    depressants of, 80
    description of, 265
    disorders of, 22t
    drug distribution into, 14
    drugs that affect, 80
    extrapyramidal system, 80
    hypothalamus, 79
    limbic system, 79
    lymphomas of, 366
    medulla oblongata, 79

neurons of, 75
opioids effect on, 83, 85
pyramidal system, 80
reticular activating system, 79
spinal cord, 80
stimulants of, 80
thalamus, 78–79
central nervous system stimulants. *See also spe-
    cific drug*
    administration of, 260
    adverse effects of, 260–261
    amphetamines
        abuse of, 242–243
        characteristics of, 254, 255t
        drug interactions, 261
        indications for, 254, 255t
    analeptics, 254–256, 255t
    caffeine, 254, 256, 257t, 259, 261
    characteristics of, 254
    in children, 259–260
    client teaching about, 258
    cocaine, 243, 244b
    dosage of, 259
    drug interactions, 261
    drugs affected by, 259
    goals of, 258–259
    herbal and dietary supplements, 257
    nursing actions for, 260–261
    nursing process for, 257–258
    in older adults, 260
    therapeutic effects of, 260
    therapeutic principles for, 258–260
    toxicity of, 259
    xanthines, 254, 256, 257t
central obesity, 953
centrally acting anticholinergic drugs, 324–325
cephalexin, 486t
cephalexin (Keflex), 490t
cephalosporins. *See also specific drug*
    administration of, 499
    in children, 479, 497
    classification of, 489–491, 490t–491t
    client teaching about, 496
    contraindications, 489
    description of, 489
    drug interactions, 501
    first-generation, 489, 492t, 496
    fourth-generation, 491, 493t, 496
    indications for, 489
    nursing actions for, 499–501
    nursing process for, 496
    in older adults, 479
    oral, 490t–491t
    parenteral, 492t–493t
    perioperative use of, 497
    pharmacokinetics of, 486t, 489
    during pregnancy, 1060b
    in renal-impaired clients, 497
    second-generation, 489, 491, 492t, 496
    third-generation, 491, 492t–493t, 496
cephradine (Anspor, Velosef), 486t, 490t
Cephulac (lactulose), 990, 990t
cerebellum, 79
cerebral cortex, 78
Cerebyx (fosphenytoin), 195, 196t–197t, 200,
    206, 209
certified nurse assistant, 32
cetirizine (Zyrtec), 752, 754, 756
cetuximab (Erbitux), 699–701, 700t
chamomile, 58t
charcoal, activated, 27b, 259
chelating agents, 929
Chemet (succimer), 29t, 929, 930t

chemical gating, 13b
chemical synapse, 76
chemoreceptor trigger zone, 1010–1011
chemoreceptors, 840b
chemotaxis, 624, 625
chemotherapy
    adjuvant, 710, 713
    antiemetic drugs, 1016
    client teaching about, 710
    complications of, 706b–707b
    definition of, 694
    description of, 709–710
    emesis induced by, 366, 706b, 1016
    neoadjuvant, 710
    palliative, 710
Cheracol D Cough Liquid, 764t
children. *See also* adolescents; infants; neonates
    acetaminophen in, 125
    adrenergic drugs in, 283
    alpha-adrenergic agonists in, 299–300
    alpha-adrenergic blockers in, 299–300
    aminoglycosides in, 479, 510
    androgens in, 460
    angiotensin II receptor blockers in, 854
    angiotensin-converting enzyme inhibitors in,
        854
    antianginal drugs in, 823
    antianxiety drugs in, 146–147
    antiasthmatic drugs in, 742–743
    anticholinergic drugs in, 327–328
    anticoagulants in, 890
    antidepressants in, 187
    antidiarrheal drugs in, 1006
    antidysrhythmic drugs in, 808–809
    antiemetic drugs in, 1017
    antiepileptic drugs in, 207
    antifungal drugs in, 597
    antihistamines in, 756
    antihypertensive drugs in, 854–855
    antimicrobial drugs in, 479
    antineoplastic drugs in, 712
    antiparasitic drugs in, 614
    antiparkinson drugs in, 221–222
    antipsychotic drugs in, 165b, 165–166
    antitubercular drugs in, 555
    antiviral drugs in, 574–575
    anxiety in, 146–147
    aspirin contraindication in, 108
    beta blockers in, 300, 854
    calcium channel blockers in, 854
    central nervous system stimulants in, 259–260
    cephalosporins in, 497
    cholinergic drugs in, 314
    corticosteroids in, 367, 743
    dermatologic drugs in, 1053–1054
    diabetes mellitus in, 426–427
    diarrhea in, 1006
    digoxin in, 788
    diuretics in, 870–871
    drug administration in, 63
    drug therapy in, 62–63
    dyslipidemic drugs in, 906
    erythromycin in, 535
    estrogens in, 450
    fluoroquinolones in, 479, 510
    growth hormone in, 346
    heparin in, 890
    hypercalcemia in, 399
    hypertension in, 854
    hypocalcemia in, 399
    hypotension in, 834
    ibuprofen in, 125
    immunizations in, 645–646

children (*continued*)
  immunostimulant drugs in, 660
  immunosuppressants in, 681–682
  intramuscular injections in, 63
  latent tuberculosis infection in, 546b, 555
  laxatives in, 993
  leukotriene modifiers in, 743
  lithium in, 187
  medication errors in, 32b
  mineral–electrolytes for, 942–943
  nonsteroidal anti-inflammatory drugs in, 125
  nutritional support in, 941–943
  obesity in, 955, 965–966
  ophthalmic drugs in, 1034
  opioid analgesics in, 97–98
  penicillins in, 479, 497
  pharmacodynamics in, 165
  pharmacokinetics in, 20, 63t, 165
  physiologic characteristics of, 63t
  respiratory disorders in, 767
  shock in, 834
  skeletal muscle relaxants in, 232
  sulfonamides in, 523–524
  tetracyclines in, 479, 523
  thiazide diuretics in, 854
  thyroid drugs in, 382
  tricyclic antidepressants in, 187
  tuberculosis in, 555
  urinary tract infections in, 523
  vitamins for, 942, 942t
Chirocaine (levobupivacaine), 1098t
Chlamydia trachomatis, 515, 530
chloral hydrate (Aquachloral, Noctec), 138, 139t
chlorambucil (Leukeran), 695t
chloramphenicol (Chloromycetin), 530, 531t,
    534, 537–539
chlordiazepoxide (Librium), 136t, 238t, 240
chloride, 927t
Chloromycetin (chloramphenicol), 530, 531t,
    534, 537–539
chloroprocaine (Nesacaine), 1098t
chloroquine (Aralen), 606, 607t, 616
chloroquine with primaquine, 606, 608t
chlorothiazide (Diuril), 864t
chlorpheniramine (Chlor-Trimeton), 751t, 753
chlorpromazine (Thorazine), 156t–157t
chlorthalidone (Hygroton), 864t
Chlor-Trimeton (chlorpheniramine), 751t, 753
cholecalciferol (Delta-D), 392t
cholestatic hepatitis, 170
cholesterol, 897, 898b
cholesterol absorption inhibitors, 902t, 903,
    906–907
cholestyramine (Questran), 901, 902t, 905, 1001t
cholic acid, 897
choline salicylate (Arthropan), 109, 111t
cholinergic crisis, 312–313
cholinergic drugs. *See also specific drug*
  administration of, 315–316
  adverse effects of, 316
  Alzheimer's disease treated with, 310t,
      311–314
  antidote for, 28t
  atropine reversal of, 314
  in children, 314
  client teaching about, 313
  contraindications, 308–309
  description of, 307
  direct-acting, 308–309, 317
  drug interactions, 317
  in hepatic-impaired clients, 315
  in home care, 315

indications for, 308
  indirect-acting, 308–309, 309f, 310t, 311
  mechanism of action, 308, 308f
  myasthenia gravis treated with, 312–313
  nursing process for, 311–312
  in older adults, 315
  in renal-impaired clients, 315
  therapeutic effects of, 316
  toxicity of, 314
cholinergic fibers, 266
cholinergic receptors, 270–271
cholinergic system, 77
chondroitin sulfate
  description of, 58t, 117–118
  with glucosamine, 118–119
Chorex (human chorionic gonadotropin), 342,
    344t, 349
choriogonadotropin alfa (Ovidrel), 344t
choroid, 1023
Choron (human chorionic gonadotropin), 342,
    344t, 349
Christmas factor, 877t
chromium, 416, 927t
chronic bronchitis, 279, 730
chronic ingestion, 237
chronic obstructive pulmonary disease
  acute respiratory failure in, 368
  corticosteroids for, 366
  description of, 735
chronic obstructive pulmonary disorders, 279
chronic pain
  description of, 84b
  opioid analgesics for, 95, 99
chronic renal failure, 943–944
Chronulac (lactulose), 990, 990t
Chvostek's sign, 395
chylomicrons, 898b
ciclopirox (Loprox), 588b, 1043t
cidofovir (Vistide), 563, 564t, 574–575
cilia, 726
cilostazol (Pletal), 882t, 885, 891
cimetidine (Tagamet)
  cytochrome P450 inhibition by, 19
  opioid analgesic interactions with, 101
Cipro (ciprofloxacin), 507, 508t, 1000t, 1028t
ciprofloxacin (Cipro), 507, 508t, 1000t, 1028t
cirrhosis, 944
cisatracurium (Nimbex), 1096t
cisplatin (Platinol), 695t, 713–714
citalopram (Celexa), 177, 178t
Citanest (prilocaine), 1098t
Citracal (calcium citrate), 392t
Citrucel (methylcellulose), 989t
cladribine (Leustatin), 695t
Claforan (cefotaxime), 492t
Clarinex (desloratadine), 752, 754, 756
clarithromycin (Biaxin, Biaxin XL), 528, 529t,
    539, 551, 1060b
Claritin (loratadine), 752, 754t, 756, 758
clemastine (Tavist), 751t
Cleocin (clindamycin hydrochloride), 479, 530,
    531t, 534–538, 1043t
Cleocin phosphate (clindamycin phosphate),
    531t, 534–538, 1043t
clindamycin hydrochloride (Cleocin), 479, 530,
    531t, 534–538, 1043t
clindamycin phosphate (Cleocin phosphate),
    531t, 534–538
clinical pathways, 56
clinical trials, 6–7
Clinoril (sulindac), 109, 114t
clobetasol (Temovate), 1045t

clocortolone (Cloderm), 1045t
Cloderm (clocortolone), 1045t
clofarabine (Clolar), 1079
Clolar (clofarabine), 1079
clomipramine (Anafranil), 138, 139t, 150, 178t,
    187
clonazepam (Klonopin)
  antianxiety uses of, 136t, 138, 143, 149
  antiseizure uses of, 196t, 200
clonidine (Catapres)
  agonist effects of, 289
  antihypertensive uses of, 844t, 857
  characteristics of, 291, 292t
  indications, 290–291
  opioid withdrawal uses of, 96
  substance abuse disorders treated with, 238t,
      240
cloning, 6
clopidogrel (Plavix), 882t, 884, 891
clorazepate (Tranxene)
  antianxiety uses of, 136t–137t
  antiseizure uses of, 196t, 200
Clostridium difficile, 998, 1005
clot lysis, 877
clotrimazole (Lotrimin, Mycelex, Gyne-
    Lotrimin), 588b, 1043t
cloxacillin (Cloxapen), 487
Cloxapen (cloxacillin), 487
clozapine (Clozaril), 156t, 159t, 160, 171, 956b
Clozaril (clozapine), 156t, 159t, 160, 171, 956b
"club" drugs, 246–248
clusters of differentiation, 674
coagulation, 879b
coagulation factors, 877t
coal tar (Balnetar, Zetar), 1046t
cobalt, 927t
cocaine, 1065b
coccidioidomycosis, 583, 585b, 593, 595
codeine, 86t, 87, 763t, 769, 1060b
Cogentin (benztropine), 217t, 323t, 325
Cognex (tacrine), 310t, 311, 315
cognitive behavioral therapy, 146
Colace (docusate sodium), 989t
Colazal (balsalazide), 1079
colchicine, 115, 116t, 121, 124, 127
cold remedies
  characteristics of, 762
  client teaching about, 766
  selection of, 766–767
  therapeutic effects of, 768
  therapeutic principles for, 766–767
colesevelam (Welchol), 902t
Colestid (colestipol), 902t, 1002t
colestipol (Colestid), 902t, 1002t
collagenase (Santyl), 1046t
collateral circulation, 774, 904
colloidal oatmeal (Avenno), 1047t
colony-forming unit, 621
colony-stimulating factors
  in cancer patients, 659
  characteristics of, 622t, 623, 652t–653t,
      655–656
CoLyte (polyethylene glycol–electrolyte solu-
    tion), 988, 989t
Combi-Patch, 444t
Combivent (ipratropium/albuterol), 734t
Combivir (zidovudine and lamivudine), 567t, 570
common cold
  description of, 760
  remedies for. *See* cold remedies
community-acquired infection, 468, 471
Compazine (prochlorperazine), 1011, 1012t
complement, 105

compliance, 726
Comprehensive Drug Abuse Prevention and Control Act, 4, 5t
computerized ordering of medications, 33
Comtan (entacapone), 217t, 218, 220
Comtrex Cold & Sinus Tablets, 764t
Comvax (*Haemophilus influenzae* b conjugate vaccine with hepatitis B vaccine), 635t
concentration-dependent bactericidal effects, 510
confusion, 153
congenital adrenal hyperplasia, 353
conjugated estrogens (Cenestin, Premarin), 440, 441t
conjunctiva, 1023
conjunctivitis, 1024
constipation, 100, 987, 1064
Contact Day & Night Cold & Flu Tablets, 764t
contact dermatitis, 749, 1040
continuous infusion, 41b
continuous renal replacement therapy, 480
contraception, 449
Controlled Drugs and Substances Act (Canada), 1085
Controlled Substances, 6b
Controlled Substances Act, 4
convoluted tubules, 861, 862f
convulsion, 193
coping, 141–142
copper, 927t
Cordarone (amiodarone), 801t, 804, 808, 811t
Cordran (flurandrenolide), 1045t
Coreg (carvedilol), 293t, 295, 298, 845t
Corgard (nadolol), 293t, 818t, 844t
Coricidin D Cold, Flu, & Sinus Tablets, 764t
Corlopam (fenoldopam), 846t, 857
cornea, 1023
corneal abrasions, 1033
corneal ulcers, 1024
coronary artery disease, 814
coronary atherosclerosis, 815–816, 876–877, 898
Cortef (hydrocortisone), 357, 358t
Cortenema (hydrocortisone retention enema), 359t
corticospinal tract, 80
corticosteroids. *See also specific drug*
  administration of, 364–365, 368
  adrenal insufficiency and, 743
  adrenocortical insufficiency prevented by, 367
  adverse effects of, 369
  allergic rhinitis treated with, 365
  alternate-day therapy for, 365
  antiemetic uses of, 1011, 1012t
  anti-inflammatory actions of, 356f
  arthritis treated with, 365
  asthma treated with, 365–366, 731b, 735–737
  cancer treated with, 366
  chemotherapy-induced emesis treated with, 366
  in children, 367, 743
  chronic obstructive pulmonary disease treated with, 366
  client teaching about, 362–363
  in critical illness, 368
  Crohn's disease treated with, 366
  definition of, 352
  dermatologic uses of, 1044
  description of, 336
  dosage of, 364
  drug interactions, 369–370
  endogenous, 352–353
  goals of, 363
  in hepatic-impaired clients, 368
  in home care, 368

  hypercalcemia treated with, 394
  immunosuppressive use of, 668, 680
  indications for, 355–357
  inflammatory bowel disease treated with, 366
  long-term use of, 364
  mechanism of action, 355
  nursing actions for, 368–371
  nursing process for, 360–361
  in older adults, 367, 743
  ophthalmic uses of, 1025, 1030t
  during pregnancy, 1063b
  in renal-impaired clients, 367–368
  selection of, 363–364
  self-administration of, 363
  spinal cord injury treated with, 366–367
  therapeutic effects of, 368–369
  therapeutic principles for, 363–368
  topical, 1044, 1051–1052, 1055
  types of, 357–360, 358t–359t
  ulcerative colitis treated with, 366
corticotropin (ACTH, Acthar Gel), 341–342, 343t, 348
corticotropin-releasing factor
  in depression, 175
  description of, 133, 339
  hypothalamic, 175
Cortifoam (hydrocortisone acetate intrarectal foam), 359t
cortisol, 353
cortisone (Cortone), 358t
Cortone (cortisone), 358t
Cortrosyn (cosyntropin), 342, 343t
Corzide, 847t
Cosmegen (dactinomycin), 696t
cosyntropin (Cortrosyn), 342, 343t
cough, 761
Coumadin (warfarin)
  antidote for, 29t
  characteristics of, 881t, 883, 888–889
  during pregnancy, 1061b
  vitamin K interactions with, 19
COX-1, 104, 106
COX-2, 104, 106
COX-2 inhibitors
  contraindications, 108
  description of, 106, 114–115
Cozaar (losartan), 843t
"crack," 243
C-reactive protein, 901
creams, 1042b
creatine, 58t
creatinine clearance, 66, 480
Crestor (rosuvastatin), 901, 902t
cretinism, 374
critical illness. *See also specific drug, in critical illness*
  adrenergic drugs in, 283–284
  alpha-adrenergic agonists in, 301
  alpha-adrenergic blockers in, 301
  aminoglycosides in, 511
  antianginal drugs in, 825–826
  antianxiety drugs in, 148
  antiasthmatic drugs in, 744
  anticholinergic drugs in, 328
  antidepressants in, 188
  antidysrhythmic drugs in, 809
  antiepileptic drugs in, 208
  antifungal drugs in, 597
  antihistamines in, 757
  antihypertensive drugs in, 857
  antimicrobial drugs in, 480
  antipsychotic drugs in, 167–168
  antiseizure drugs in, 208

  atropine in, 328
  beta-lactam antibacterials in, 498–499
  cholinergic drugs in, 315
  clindamycin in, 536
  corticosteroids in, 368
  definition of, 68
  diabetic clients with, 425–426, 428
  diuretics in, 871
  drug administration considerations, 69
  drug dosage in, 68–69
  drug therapy considerations for, 68–69
  epinephrine in, 835
  erythromycin in, 536
  fluoroquinolones in, 511
  nutritional support in, 944–945
  opioid analgesics in, 98–99
  sulfonamides in, 524
  tetracyclines in, 524
critical paths, 56
Crixivan (indinavir), 568t, 569–570, 575, 578–579
Crohn's disease, 366, 678
Crolom (cromolyn), 1029t
cromolyn (Intal, Crolom, Opticrom), 736t, 738, 743, 754t, 1029t
cross-tolerance, 25
cryptococcosis, 585b, 593, 595
Cryptococcus neoformans, 582
Cubicin (daptomycin), 479, 530–532, 531t, 535, 537–539
Cultivate (fluticasone), 1045t
culture, 468, 477–478
Cuprimine (penicillamine), 929, 930t
Cushing's disease, 353, 370
cyanocobalamin
  deficiency of, 921t
  food sources of, 921t
  function of, 921t
  recommended daily intake of, 921t
cyclic adenosine monophosphate, 17, 76, 337
cyclic guanosine monophosphate, 730
cyclizine (Marezine), 1012t
cyclobenzaprine (Flexeril), 229t, 230
Cyclocort (amcinonide), 1045t
Cyclogyl (cyclopentolate hydrochloride), 1027t
cyclopentolate hydrochloride (Cyclogyl), 1027t
cyclophosphamide (Cytoxan), 695t, 713, 718
cycloplegia, 320
cycloserine (Seromycin), 550
cyclosporine (Sandimmune, Neoral), 122–123, 669t, 672, 677, 680–683, 685–687
cyclothymia, 175b
Cyklokapron (tranexamic acid), 885–886, 886t
Cymbalta (duloxetine), 1079
CYP3A inhibitors, 534
cyproheptadine, 751t
cytarabine (Cytosar-U), 695t, 714
cytochrome P450
  benzodiazepine metabolism by, 135, 146
  definition of, 15
  selective serotonin reuptake inhibitor effects on, 184–185
CytoGam (cytomegalovirus immune globulin, intravenous, human), 641t
cytokine(s)
  definition of, 621
  description of, 105
  hematopoietic, 621–622
  immune system, 629, 630f
  inhibitors of, 674–675
  mechanism of action, 621–622
cytokine receptors, 621, 623
cytomegalovirus, 561b

cytomegalovirus immune globulin, intravenous, human (CytoGam), 641t
Cytomel (liothyronine), 376, 377t
cytoplasm, 11b
cytoprotectant drugs, 705, 707
Cytosar-U (cytarabine), 695t, 714
Cytotec (misoprostol), 1070t
cytotoxic antiproliferative agents, 668, 671
cytotoxic T cells, 628, 667
Cytovene (ganciclovir), 563, 564t, 575, 578–579
Cytoxan (cyclophosphamide), 695t, 713, 718

D

daclizumab (Zenapax), 669t, 674, 679
dactinomycin (Actinomycin D, Cosmegen), 696t
Dalmane (flurazepam), 136t–137t
dalteparin (Fragmin), 881t
danazol (Danocrine), 457–458
Danocrine (danazol), 457–458, 458t
Dantrium (dantrolene), 229t, 230, 233
dantrolene (Dantrium), 229t, 230, 233
dapsone (Avlosulfon), 609t, 611
daptomycin (Cubicin), 479, 530–532, 531t, 535, 537–539
Daraprim (pyrimethamine), 609t, 611
darbepoetin alfa (Aranesp), 652t, 655, 658, 663
darifenacin (Enablex), 1079
Darvon (propoxyphene), 86t, 88–89
"date-rape" drugs, 246–248
daunorubicin liposomal (DaunoXome), 696t, 714
DaunoXome (daunorubicin liposomal), 696t, 714
Daypro (oxaprozin), 109, 114t
DDAVP (desmopressin), 344t, 345
ddI (didanosine), 566t, 576–577
Debrisan (dextranomer), 1047t
Decadron (dexamethasone), 358t, 363–364, 1030t, 1045t
Declomycin (demeclocycline), 516t, 519
decubitus ulcers, 1041
deep vein thrombosis, 880, 886–887, 891
defecation, 987
deferoxamine (Desferal), 28t, 929, 930t
Delatestryl (testosterone enanthate), 458t
delavirdine (Rescriptor), 555, 567t, 573, 577
delayed hypersensitivity, 748
Delestrogen (estradiol valerate), 441t
delirium, 153
Delta-Cortef (prednisolone), 359t
Delta-D (cholecalciferol), 392t
Deltasone (prednisone), 359t, 363
delta-9–tetrahydrocannabinol, 245
delusions, 153
Demadex (torsemide), 865t, 868
demeclocycline (Declomycin), 516t, 519
Demerol (meperidine), 86t, 88, 1060b
Demulen, 445t
demyelination, 227
Denavir (penciclovir), 1044t
dendrite, 75
dendritic cells, 626
Depacon injection (sodium valproate), 199t
Depakene capsules (valproic acid), 199t, 202, 204, 208, 1083
Depakene syrup (sodium valproate), 199t
Depakote enteric-coated tablets (divalproex sodium), 199t
dependence
    alcohol, 239–241
    amphetamine, 243
    barbiturates, 241
    benzodiazepines, 241
    cocaine, 243

drug, 26, 235–237
    hallucinogen, 246
    nicotine, 244–245
    opioid, 242
dependent edema, 863
Depo-Estradiol (estradiol cypionate), 441t
Depo-Provera (medroxyprogesterone acetate), 442t, 446t, 715
Depo-Testosterone (testosterone cypionate), 458t
depression
    antidepressants for. See antidepressants
    definition of, 175b
    environmental factors for, 176
    etiology of, 174–176
    monoamine neurotransmitter dysfunction theory of, 174–175
    neuroendocrine factors associated with, 175–176
    nursing process for, 181–182
dermatitis, 1040, 1052–1053
dermatologic drugs. See also specific drug
    administration of, 1054
    adverse effects of, 1054–1055
    antimicrobials, 1042
    antiseptics, 1042, 1044
    in children, 1053–1054
    client teaching about, 1050–1051
    corticosteroids, 1044
    emollients, 1044
    enzymes, 1044, 1046t
    guidelines for, 1049, 1051
    immunomodulators, 1044, 1046t
    keratolytic agents, 1044
    nursing actions for, 1054–1055
    nursing process for, 1047–1049
    in older adults, 1054
    overview of, 1042
    retinoids, 1044–1045, 1046t, 1052, 1064b
    self-administration of, 1050–1051
    sunscreens, 1045
    therapeutic effects of, 1054
    therapeutic principles for, 1049, 1051–1054
dermatophytes, 582
dermis, 1039
Desenex (zinc undecylenate), 590t
Desferal (deferoxamine), 28t, 929, 930t
desflurane (Suprane), 1096t
desloratadine (Clarinex), 752, 754, 756
desmopressin (DDAVP, Stimate), 344t, 345
Desogen, 445t
desogestrel, 440
desonide (Tridesilon), 1045t
desoximetasone (Topicort), 1045t
Desoxyn (methamphetamine), 254, 255t
Desyrel (trazodone), 179t, 180
Detrol LA (tolterodine), 324t, 325
Detrol (tolterodine), 324t, 325
dexamethasone acetate, 358t, 363–364
dexamethasone (Decadron, Maxidex), 358t, 363–364, 1030t, 1045t
dexamethasone sodium phosphate, 358t, 363–364
dexchlorpheniramine, 751t, 753
Dexedrine (dextroamphetamine), 254, 255t
dexmedetomidine and propofol (Diprivan), 148, 1096
dexmedetomidine (Precedex), 138, 139t
dexmethylphenidate (Focalin), 254, 255t, 258–259
dexrazoxane (Zinecard), 707, 708t
dextranomer (Debrisan), 1047t
dextroamphetamine (Dexedrine), 254, 255t
dextromethorphan (Benylin DM), 763t, 769

DHE 45 (dihydroergotamine mesylate), 116–117, 117t
DiaBeta (glyburide), 414t
diabetes mellitus
    angiotensin-converting enzyme inhibitors in, 419
    assessment of, 417–418
    in children, 426–427
    client teaching about, 420–421
    complications of, 407, 408b
    in critically ill patients, 428
    definition of, 406
    fluoroquinolones in, 511
    gestational, 1065–1069
    herbal and dietary supplements for, 415–416
    in home care, 428
    illness with, 425–426
    insulin for. See insulin
    nursing process for, 417–419
    obesity and, 954b, 955
    in older adults, 427
    signs and symptoms of, 407
    type 1, 406, 426–427
    type 2, 406–407, 427
    unconscious patient with, 423
diabetic ketoacidosis, 407, 408b, 423
diacylglycerol, 338
Diamox (acetazolamide), 1027t
Diamox Sequels (acetazolamide), 1027t
diarrhea
    antidiarrheal drugs for. See antidiarrheal drugs
    in children, 1006
    description of, 997–998
    herbal and dietary supplements, 1003
    nursing process for, 1003–1004
    therapeutic principles for, 1004–1006
diastole, 774
diazepam (Valium)
    antianxiety uses of, 135, 136t–137t, 138, 147–149
    antiseizure uses of, 196t, 200
    muscle relaxant uses of, 229t
dibucaine (Dyclone), 1098t
diclofenac potassium (Cataflam), 111t
diclofenac sodium (Voltaren, Voltaren XR), 111t, 114–115, 1030t
dicloxacillin (Dycill, Dynapen, Pathocil), 486t, 487, 488t
dicyclomine hydrochloride (Bentyl), 323t, 324
didanosine (ddI, Videx, Videx EC), 566t, 576–577
Didronel (etidronate), 390, 393t
dienestrol, 441t
Dietary Guidelines for Americans, 962
dietary reference intakes, 919b
Dietary Supplement Health and Education Act, 56
dietary supplements
    anticoagulation using, 891–892
    asthma, 738
    central nervous system stimulants, 257
    client teaching about, 61
    definition of, 56
    for diabetes mellitus, 415–416
    dyslipidemia managed using, 900, 907
    heart failure treated with, 789
    nurse's role in, 57
    obesity treated with, 958–959
    during pregnancy, 1059, 1064
    regulation of, 56–57
    respiratory disorders treated with, 762, 765
diet–drug interactions, 19
diets, 964b

difenoxin with atropine sulfate (Motofen), 999t, 1006
Differin (adapalene), 1046t
diffusion, 13b
diflorasone (Florone, Maxiflor), 1045t
Diflucan (fluconazole), 587b, 588b, 591, 596–597, 600
diflunisal (Dolobid), 109, 111t
digestive system
  description of, 913, 914f
  esophagus, 913–914
  gallbladder, 914
  large intestine, 914
  liver, 914–915
  oral cavity, 913
  pancreas, 914
  secretions of, 915–916
  small intestine, 914
  stomach, 914
Digibind (digoxin immune Fab), 28t, 788
digitalizing dose, 781
digoxin immune Fab (Digibind), 28t, 788
digoxin (Lanoxin)
  administration of, 781–782, 789–790
  adverse effects of, 791–792
  antidote for, 28t
  characteristics of, 778–779
  in children, 788
  contraindications, 781
  digitalization of, 781–782
  diuretics and, 869–870
  dosage of, 782t, 787–788
  drug interactions, 792
  electrolyte balance while using, 787–788
  in hepatic-impaired clients, 789
  in home care, 789
  indications for, 781
  mechanism of action, 779, 781
  nonsteroidal anti-inflammatory drugs effect on, 123
  in older adults, 788
  pharmacokinetics of, 779
  during pregnancy, 1063b
  in renal-impaired clients, 788–789
  serum levels of, 1083
  toxicity of, 783, 788
dihydroergotamine mesylate (DHE 45), 116–117, 117t
dihydrotachysterol (Hytakerol), 392t
dihydrotestosterone, 455, 458–459, 704
Dilantin (phenytoin)
  adverse effects of, 195
  characteristics of, 198t
  dysrhythmias treated with, 800t, 803, 811t
  nonantiepileptic drugs affected by, 207
  nonsteroidal anti-inflammatory drugs effect on, 123
  osteoporosis risks, 398
  pharmacokinetics of, 195
  serum levels of, 1083
Dilaudid (hydromorphone), 86t, 87–88
diltiazem (Cardizem), 802t, 805, 819t, 845t
dimenhydrinate (Dramamine), 1012t
Dimetapp Cold and Allergy Elixir, 764t
Dimetapp (pseudoephedrine), 763t
dinoprostone (Prostin E2), 1070t
Diovan HCT, 847t
Diovan (valsartan), 843t
Dipentum (olsalazine), 1080
diphenhydramine (Benadryl), 29t, 217t, 751t, 753, 756
diphenoxylate with atropine sulfate (Lomotil), 999t–1000t, 1006

diphtheria and tetanus toxoids, absorbed, 640t, 645, 648
diphtheria and tetanus toxoids and acellular pertussis and *Haemophilus influenza* type B conjugate vaccines (TriHIBit), 640t, 645, 648
diphtheria and tetanus toxoids and acellular pertussis vaccine (Tripedia, Infanrix), 640t, 645, 648
dipivefrin (Propine), 1026t
Diprivan (dexmedetomidine and propofol), 148, 1096
Diprolene (augmented betamethasone dipropionate), 1045t
dipyridamole and aspirin (Aggrenox), 882t
dipyridamole (Persantine), 882t, 885
Disalcid (salsalate), 109, 114t
disease-modifying antirheumatic drugs, 679
disease-modifying effects, 124
disopyramide (Norpace), 800t, 803, 811t, 1083
displacement, 19
disseminated intravascular coagulation, 880
distribution, 14, 23t
distributive shock, 829, 830t, 833
disulfiram (Antabuse), 238t, 239–241
Ditropan (oxybutynin), 324t, 325
Ditropan XL (oxybutynin), 324t, 325
diuretics. *See also specific drug*
  administration of, 872
  adverse effects of, 873–874
  antihypertensive uses of, 849, 853
  characteristics of, 863
  in children, 870–871
  client teaching about, 869
  combination products, 866, 867t
  in critical illness, 871
  definition of, 861
  digoxin and, 869–870
  dosage of, 868–869
  drug interactions, 874
  edema treated with, 869
  heart failure treated with, 780b–781b
  in hepatic-impaired clients, 871
  in home care, 871
  loop, 864t–865t, 866, 868, 871
  nonsteroidal anti-inflammatory drugs effect on, 122
  nursing actions for, 872–874
  nursing process for, 867–868
  in older adults, 871
  osmotic, 18, 866
  potassium imbalances secondary to, 869–870
  potassium-losing, 868
  potassium-sparing, 780b–781b, 865t, 866, 868, 871
  during pregnancy, 1063b
  renal sites of action for, 863f
  in renal-impaired clients, 855, 871
  selection of, 868
  self-administration of, 869
  therapeutic effects of, 872
  therapeutic principles for, 868–871
  thiazide
    characteristics of, 864t, 865–866
    in children, 854
    description of, 849
    indications for, 868
    in older adults, 871
    in renal-impaired clients, 871
  types of, 864t
Diuril (chlorothiazide), 864t
divalproex sodium (Depakote enteric-coated tablets), 199t

DNA viruses, 560
dobutamine (Dobutrex), 273t, 831t, 832
Dobutrex (dobutamine), 273t, 831t, 832
docetaxel (Taxotere), 697t, 711
docusate calcium (Surfak), 989t
docusate sodium (Colace), 989t
dofetilide (Tikosyn), 801t, 804–805
dolasetron (Anzemet), 1012t, 1013, 1018
Dolobid (diflunisal), 109, 111t
Dolophine (methadone), 86t, 88, 238t, 242
donepezil (Aricept), 310t, 311, 314
dopamine
  acetylcholine and, 214
  characteristics of, 273t
  neurotransmitter uses of, 77
  shock treated with, 830, 831t
dopamine agonists, 220
dopamine receptors, 77, 154
dopaminergic drugs, 215, 217t, 225
dopaminergic receptors, 269–270, 830
dopaminergic system
  description of, 77
  in schizophrenia pathogenesis, 154
Dopar (levodopa), 215–216, 217t, 223–225
Dopram (doxapram), 254, 255t
Doral (quazepam), 136t–137t
dorzolamide (Trusopt), 1028t
dosages. *See* drug dosages
Dovonex (calcipotriene), 1046t
down-regulation, 18
down-regulation, 337
doxapram (Dopram), 254, 255t
doxazosin (Cardura), 292t, 294, 844t
doxepin (Sinequan), 178t
Doxercalciferol (Hectorol), 392t
Doxil (doxorubicin liposomal), 696t, 714
doxorubicin (Adriamycin), 696t, 714
doxorubicin liposomal (Doxil), 696t, 714
doxycycline (Vibramycin), 516t, 519, 606, 607t
Dramamine (dimenhydrinate), 1012t
Drisdol (ergocalciferol), 392t
Dristan Cold Formula, 764t
dronabinol (Marinol), 245, 1013t, 1014, 1017
drop factor, 42b
drotrecogin alfa (Xigris), 882t, 885
drug(s). *See also specific drug*
  adverse effects of, 25–26
  American laws regarding, 4–6, 5t
  biotechnology of, 6
  classification of, 4
  clinical trials of, 6–7
  cross-tolerance, 25
  definition of, 10
  development of, 6–8
  Drug Enforcement Administration regulation of, 4–5
  Food and Drug Administration approval of, 7
  information sources about, 8
  marketing of, 7–8
  names of, 4
  overdose of, 26, 28t–29t
  over-the-counter, 7
  pharmacodynamics of, 17–18
  pharmacokinetics of. *See* pharmacokinetics
  prototype, 4
  serum concentrations, 1083
  sources of, 6
  testing of, 6–7
  variables that affect, 18–25
drug action
  age effects on, 20
  body weight effects on, 20
  client-related variables that affect, 20–25

drug action (*continued*)
  ethnicity effects on, 21
  gender effects on, 21
  genetics effect on, 20–21
  pathologic conditions that affect, 21, 22t–24t
drug administration
  abbreviations commonly used in, 34t
  in critical-illness patients, 69
  dosages. *See* drug dosages
  drug preparations for, 70
  ear medications, 36t, 48
  eye solutions, 36t, 48
  gastrointestinal, 39t
  intramuscular injections
    advantages and disadvantages of, 39t
    antipsychotic drugs, 164, 168
    in children, 63
    drug actions after, 19
    nursing action for, 47
    sites for, 40, 43f
  intravenous injections
    absorption of, 14
    administration technique, 42b
    advantages and disadvantages of, 39t
    in children, 32b
    continuous infusion, 41b
    in critical-illness patients, 69
    drug preparation for, 42b
    equipment for, 41b
    of illicit drugs, 236–237
    intermittent infusion, 41b
    nursing action for, 47–48
    of opioid analgesics, 94
    principles of, 41b–42b
    sites for, 40, 41b–42b, 43f–44f
  legal responsibilities, 32
  medication errors, 32b, 32–33
  medication systems, 33
  nasogastric tube, 46
  needleless systems, 40
  nose drops, 48
  nursing actions for, 44–48, 70–71
  in older adults, 66
  opioid analgesics, 94–96
  oral, 38, 39t, 45–46
  parenteral
    ampules used in, 38
    definition of, 38
    equipment for, 38, 41
    injection sites, 40, 43f
  pharmacokinetics affected by, 18–19
  principles of, 31–32
  psychological considerations, 25
  rectal suppositories, 36t, 48
  rights of, 31, 70
  self-administration, 55–56
  to skin, 48
  subcutaneous injections
    absorption after, 14
    advantages and disadvantages of, 39t
    insulin, 423
    nursing action for, 46–47
    sites for, 40, 43f
  topical, 40t
  using IV line already established, 47–48
  vaginal suppositories, 36t, 48
drug allergies, 752
drug delivery systems, 34
drug dependence, 26, 235–237
drug dosages. *See also specific drug, dosage of*
  abbreviations commonly used in, 34t
  calculation of, 36–38
  for children, 62–63

controlled-release forms, 34
for critical illness patients, 68–69
definition of, 18
fixed, 62
forms of, 34, 35t–36t
in hepatic-impaired patients, 67–68
for infants, 62–63
initial loading dose, 509
maintenance dose, 509
measurement systems for, 37, 37t
for neonates, 62–63
for older adults, 65–66
in renal-impaired patients, 67
selection of, 62
transdermal, 34
Drug Enforcement Administration, 4–5
Drug Facts and Comparisons, 8
drug fever, 26
drug interactions. *See also specific drug, drug*
        interactions
  with drugs, 19–20
  effects of, 19–20
  with foods, 19
  nursing actions for, 71
drug reactions
  allergic, 749–750
  pseudoallergic, 750
drug receptors, 17–18
Drug Regulation Reform Act, 5t
drug therapy
  in children, 62–63
  critical paths, 56
  in critical-illness patients, 68–69
  goals of, 62
  in hepatic-impaired patients, 67–68
  in home care, 69–70
  nursing actions for, 70–71
  nursing process in
    assessment, 51–52
    definition of, 51
    evaluation, 53–54
    interventions, 53
    nursing diagnoses, 52–53
    planning/goals, 53
  in older adults, 63–66
  overview of, 50–51
  principles of, 62–70
  in renal-impaired patients, 66–67
drug tolerance, 25
drug toxicity
  acetaminophen, 123
  adrenergic drugs, 282–283
  aminoglycosides, 510
  antiasthmatic drugs, 742
  anticholinergic drugs, 327
  anticholinesterase drugs, 314
  antidepressants, 185–186
  antiepileptic drugs, 206
  antiseizure drugs, 206
  atropine sulfate, 327
  benzodiazepine, 145
  benzodiazepines, 145
  causes of, 26
  central nervous system stimulants, 259
  cholinergic drugs, 314
  management of, 26, 27b
  monoamine oxidase inhibitors, 185
  opioid, 96
  opioid analgesics, 96
  selective serotonin reuptake inhibitors, 185
  tricyclic antidepressants, 185
drug transport
  description of, 12

mechanisms of, 13b
pathways of, 13b
schematic diagram of, 13f
drug-resistant tuberculosis, 543–544
Dulcolax (bisacodyl), 989t
duloxetine (Cymbalta), 1079
DuoNeb (ipratropium/albuterol), 734t
duration of action, 16
Durham-Humphrey Amendment, 4, 5t
Duricef (cefadroxil), 490t
Dyazide, 867t
Dycill (dicloxacillin), 487, 488t
Dyclone (dibucaine, dyclonine), 1098t
dyclonine (Dyclone), 1098t
DynaCirc (isradipine), 819t, 845t
Dynapen (dicloxacillin), 487, 488t
Dyrenium (triamterene), 865t, 866
dyskinesia, 223
dyskinesias, 169
dyslipidemia
  description of, 898–900
  herbal and dietary supplements for, 907
  obesity and, 954b
dyslipidemic drugs
  administration of, 907–908
  adverse effects of, 908
  bile acid sequestrants, 901–903, 902t
  characteristics of, 900–901
  in children, 906
  cholesterol absorption inhibitors, 902t, 903,
        906–907
  client teaching about, 905
  definition of, 897
  drug interactions, 908–909
  ethnicity and, 906
  fibrates, 902t, 903, 906–907
  in hepatic-impaired clients, 907
  HMG-CoA reductase inhibitors, 901, 902t
  in home care, 907
  niacin, 902t, 903, 907
  nursing actions for, 907–909
  nursing process for, 903–905
  in older adults, 906
  during pregnancy, 1063b–1064b
  in renal-impaired clients, 906–907
  selection of, 905–906
  self-administration of, 905
  therapeutic effects of, 908
  therapeutic principles for, 905–907
dysmenorrhea, 106b
dysrhythmias
  characteristics of, 795
  definition of, 792, 795
  nonpharmacologic management of, 796, 807
  nursing process for, 805–806
  pharmacologic management of, 807–808
  types of, 797b–800b
dysthymia, 175b
dystonias, 169

E
ear solutions, 36t
ecchymoses, 1048
echinacea, 58t, 417, 762, 765
echinocandins, 583
econazole (Spectazole), 588b, 1043t
Econopred (prednisolone), 1030t
ectasy, 246–247
Edecrin (ethacrynic acid), 864t
edema, 863, 869
edrophonium (Tensilon), 309, 310t, 313
E.E.S. (erythromycin ethylsuccinate), 529t

efalizumab (Raptiva), 670t, 673
efavirenz (Sustiva), 567t
Effersyllium (psyllium), 988, 989t
Effexor (venlafaxine), 138, 139t, 179t, 180, 182, 186, 1061b
Effexor XR (venlafaxine), 179t, 180, 186, 1061b
Efudex (fluorouracil), 695t–696t, 1047t
Elavil (amitriptyline), 178t, 1083
electrolytes. *See also specific electrolyte*
 definition of, 919
 drug interactions, 949–950
 functions of, 919
electronic infusion devices, 41b
Elestat (epinastine), 1030t
eletriptan (Relpax), 116, 117t, 128–129
Elidel (pimecrolimus), 1046t
Eligard (leuprolide), 704, 705t
elimination half-life, 16
Elimite (permethrin), 610t, 612, 616
Elitek (rasburicase), 1080
Ellence (epirubicin), 696t
Elmiron (pentosan polysulfate sodium), 1080
Elocon (mometasone), 1045t
Eloxatin (oxaliplatin), 695t
Elspar (L-asparaginase), 697t, 699, 714
Emadine (emedastine), 1030t
embolus, 876
emedastine (Emadine), 1030t
emergency contraception, 449
Emetrol (phosphorated carbohydrate solution), 1013t, 1014
EMLA, 63, 1099
emphysema, 279, 730
emtricitabine (Emtriva), 566t, 575
Emtriva (emtricitabine), 566t, 575
E-mycin (erythromycin base), 529t, 1000t
Enablex (darifenacin), 1079
enalapril (Vasotec), 843t
Enbrel (etanercept), 124, 670t, 675, 682
endocardium, 773
endocrine disorders, 22t
endocrine system
 alcohol abuse effects on, 239b
 elements of, 335
 functions of, 335
 nervous system interactions with, 336
endoplasmic reticulum, 11b
endothelial cells, 774, 878b
endothelium, 727
endothelium-derived relaxing factors, 816
endotracheal intubation, 27b
end-stage renal disease, 66
Enduron (methyclothiazide), 864t
enemas, 36t
enflurane (Ethrane), 1096t
enfuvirtide (Fuzeon), 569t, 570
Engerix-B (hepatitis B vaccine), 636t
enkephalins, 83
enoxaparin (Lovenox), 881t
entacapone (Comtan), 217t, 218, 220
Entamoeba histolytica, 603
entecavir (Baraclude), 1079
enteral nutrition, 918, 935, 937, 945–946
enteric-coated tablets, 35t
Enterobius vermicularis, 605b
enterococci
 description of, 470b
 vancomycin-resistant, 472b–473b, 532–533
Enterococcus faecalis, 470b, 532
Enterococcus faecium, 470b
enterohepatic recirculation, 15
Entocort EC (budesonide), 358t

enzyme inducers, 20
enzyme induction, 15
enzyme inhibition, 15
eosinophils, 626
ephedra, 278, 958–959
ephedrine, 273t, 275, 277t, 278, 763t
epicardium, 773
Epidermal growth factor receptor, 701
epidermis, 1039
epidural anesthesia, 1097
epilepsy
 characteristics of, 193
 in infancy, 193
epinastine (Elestat), 1030t
epinephrine (Adrenalin)
 administration of, 284–285
 adrenergic drugs in, 283
 anaphylactic shock treated with, 280
 asthma treated with, 732t
 cardiopulmonary resuscitation using, 281
 characteristics of, 273t, 275, 276t
 concentrations of, 278t
 in critical illness, 835
 local anesthetics and, 1099
 shock treated with, 831t, 832
 therapeutic effects of, 285
 vasopressin vs., 281–282
epinephrine (endogenous), 268–269
epirubicin (Ellence), 696t
epitopes, 624
Epivir (lamivudine), 566t, 575
epoetin alfa (Epogen, Procrit), 652t, 655, 658, 663
Epogen (epoetin alfa), 652t, 655, 658, 663
Epogen (erythropoietin), 707, 708t
eprosartan (Teveten), 843t
eptifibatide (Integrilin), 882t, 884, 887, 891
Erbitux (cetuximab), 699–701, 700t
Ergamisol (levamisole), 697t
ergocalciferol (Calciferol, Drisdol), 392t
Ergomar (ergotamine tartrate), 116, 117t
ergotamine tartrate and caffeine (Cafergot), 116, 117t, 257t
ergotamine tartrate (Ergomar), 116, 117t, 121
ergotism, 128
erlotinib (Tarceva), 700t, 701
Ertaczo (sertaconazole), 1044t
ertapenem (Invanz), 494, 494t
Erythrocin stearate (erythromycin stearate), 529t
erythrocytes, 775
erythromycin
 in children, 535
 in critical illness, 536
 CYP3A inhibitors and, 534
 description of, 528–529
 drug interactions, 533–534, 539
 in hepatic-impaired clients, 535
 indications for, 530
 in older adults, 535
 ophthalmic uses of, 1028t
erythromycin (Aknemycin), 1043t
erythromycin base (E-mycin), 529t, 1000t
erythromycin estolate (Ilosone), 529t
erythromycin ethylsuccinate (E.E.S.), 529t
erythromycin lactobionate, 529t
erythromycin stearate (Erythrocin stearate), 529t
erythromycin/benzoyl peroxide (Benzamycin), 1043t
erythropoietin, 622t
erythropoietin (Epogen, Procrit), 707, 708t
Escherichia coli, 470b
Escherichia coli O157:H7, 997
escitalopram (Lexapro), 178t, 183

Esidrix (hydrochlorothiazide), 864t, 868, 870
esmolol (Brevibloc), 293t, 801t, 804, 809
esophageal candidiasis, 595
esophagus, 913–914
essential hypertension, 839
estazolam (ProSom), 136t–137t
esterified estrogens (Estratab), 441t
estimated average requirement, 919b
Estinyl (ethinyl estradiol), 440, 442t
Estrace (estradiol), 437, 440
Estraderm (estradiol transdermal system), 441t
estradiol cypionate (Depo-Estradiol), 441t
estradiol (Estrace), 437, 440
estradiol hemihydrate (Vagifem), 441t
estradiol transdermal gel (Estragel), 441t
estradiol transdermal system (Estraderm), 441t
estradiol valerate (Delestrogen), 441t
Estragel (estradiol transdermal gel), 441t
Estratab (esterified estrogens), 441t
estriol, 437
estrogen(s)
 administration of, 449
 adverse effects of, 451–452
 characteristics of, 440, 441t–442t
 in children, 450
 conjugated, 440, 441t
 description of, 336, 391, 394, 436
 dosage of, 449
 drug interactions, 449, 452–453
 endogenous, 437, 437b
 esterified, 441t
 exogenous, 440, 441t–442t
 in hepatic-impaired clients, 450
 in home care, 450
 indications for, 438
 mechanism of action, 438
 nursing actions for, 451–453
 nursing process for, 444, 446–447
 in older adults, 450
 selection of, 448
 synthesis of, 436
 therapeutic effects of, 451
estrogen replacement therapy, 391, 394, 438, 450
estrogen–progestin combinations, 439b, 444t, 452
estrone, 437, 442t
estropipate (Ogen), 442t
Estrostep 21, 445t
Estrostep Fe, 445t
eszopidone (Lunesta), 1079
etanercept (Enbrel), 124, 670t, 675, 682
ethacrynic acid (Edecrin), 864t
ethambutol (Myambutol), 548t, 549
ethinyl estradiol (Estinyl), 440, 442t
ethionamide (Trecator SC), 550
Ethmozine (moricizine), 801t, 803, 808
ethnicity
 antihypertensive drugs and, 853–854
 drug action affected by, 21
 dyslipidemic drugs and, 906
ethosuximide (Zarontin), 196t, 200, 1083
Ethrane (enflurane), 1096t
ethynodiol, 440
Ethyol (amifostine), 705, 708t
etidronate (Didronel), 390, 393t
etodolac (Lodine), 109, 111t, 114
etomidate (Amidate), 1096t
etoposide (VePesid), 697t
Eulexin (flutamide), 704, 705t, 715
evaluation, 53–54
Evista (raloxifene), 398
excretion, 15
Exelderm (sulconazole), 590t, 1044t
Exelon (rivastigmine), 310t, 311

exemestane (Aromasin), 704, 705t
exenatide (Byetta), 1079
expectorants, 762, 763t
expiration, 727
extended-release capsules, 35t
extended-release tablets, 35t
extended-spectrum penicillins, 487
external otitis, 1041–1042, 1053
extrapyramidal symptoms, 164, 169–170
extrapyramidal system, 80
extravasation, 707b
extrinsic pathway, 879b
eye
    anatomy of, 1023–1024
    disorders of, 1024
    structure of, 1023–1024
eye ointments, 36t
eye solutions, 36t, 48
eyeball, 1023
eyelid, 1023
ezetimibe (Zetia), 902t, 903

F
facilitated diffusion, 13b
Factive (gemifloxacin), 508t
Factrel (gonadorelin), 342, 343t, 349
famciclovir (Famvir), 563, 564t, 575
Famvir (famciclovir), 563, 564t, 575
Fareston (toremifene), 704, 705t, 715
Faslodex (fulvestrant), 704, 705t
fast channels, 795
fast metabolizers, 167
fat-soluble vitamins, 918, 920t, 946, 949
FDA Modernization Act, 5t
febrile seizure, 194
Feldene (piroxicam), 114, 114t
felodipine (Plendil), 819t, 845t
Femara (letrozole), 704, 705t
Femhrt, 444t
Femstat (butoconazole), 588b
fenofibrate (Tricor), 902t, 903, 905
fenoldopam (Corlopam), 846t, 857
fenoprofen (Nalfon), 109, 112t, 129
fentanyl (Sublimaze), 86t, 87, 95, 99–100
Feosol (ferrous sulfate), 931t
Feostat (ferrous fumarate), 932
Fergon (ferrous gluconate), 930t
ferrous fumarate (Feostat), 932
ferrous gluconate (Fergon), 930t, 932
ferrous sulfate (Feosol), 931t, 932, 1064
fertility drugs, 347
fetus
    development of, 456b
    drug effects on, 1058
    immune system of, 629
    maternal–placental–fetal circulation, 1058
    teratogenicity, 1058
    therapeutics, 1059
fever
    aspirin for, 122
    definition of, 103
    drug, 26
    drug reactions and, 750
    physiology of, 103–104
feverfew, 59t, 118
fexofenadine (Allegra), 752, 754, 756, 758
FiberCon (polycarbophil), 988, 989t
fibrates, 902t, 903, 906–907
fibrinogen, 877t
fibrinolysin, 885
fibrin-stabilizing factor, 877t
fight-or-flight reaction, 267

filgrastim (Neupogen), 652t, 659–661, 707, 708t
Finacea (azelaic acid), 1043t, 1052
Fiorinal, 257t
first messenger, 266
first-degree heart block, 798b
first-pass effect, 15
fixed doses, 62
Flagyl (metronidazole)
    antidiarrheal uses of, 1000t–1001t
    description of, 531t, 532, 535–536, 539, 604
    drug interactions, 616
    protozoal infections treated with, 606
flavoxate (Urispas), 324t, 325
flecainide (Tambocor), 800t, 803, 811t
Fleet Enema (sodium phosphate and sodium
    biphosphate), 989t
Fleet Mineral Oil Enema (mineral oil), 990t
Fleet Phosphosoda (sodium phosphate and
    sodium biphosphate), 989t
Flexeril (cyclobenzaprine), 229t, 230
Flomax (tamsulosin hydrochloride), 292t,
    294–295
Flonase (fluticasone), 358t, 736t, 754t
Florinef (fludrocortisone), 359t
Florone (diflorasone), 1045t
Flovent (fluticasone aerosol), 736t
Flovent Rotadisk (fluticasone powder), 736t
Floxin (ofloxacin), 508t
fluconazole (Diflucan), 587b, 588b, 591,
    596–597, 600
flucytosine (Ancobon), 587b, 588b, 592, 597
Fludara (fludarabine), 695t
fludarabine (Fludara), 695t
fludrocortisone (Florinef), 359t
Flumadine (rimantadine), 565t, 570, 578
flumazenil (Romazicon)
    antidote uses of, 28t, 145, 241
    substance abuse disorders treated with, 238t
FluMist (influenza vaccine), 636t
flunisolide (AeroBid, Nasalide, Nasarel), 358t,
    731b, 736t, 754t
flunitrazepam (Rohypnol), 247
fluocinolone (Synalar), 1045t
fluocinonide (Lidex), 1045t
fluorescein, 1026
fluoride, 928t, 943t
fluorometholone, 1030t
Fluoroplex (fluorouracil), 695t–696t
fluoroquinolones. See also specific drug
    administration of, 512
    adverse effects of, 513
    in children, 479, 510
    client teaching about, 509
    contraindications, 507
    in critical illness, 511
    definition of, 507
    description of, 504
    in diabetes mellitus patients, 511
    dosage of, 510
    drug interactions, 513
    in hepatic-impaired clients, 480
    indications for, 507
    mechanism of action, 507
    nursing actions for, 512–513
    nursing process for, 507–509
    in older adults, 511
    during pregnancy, 1060b
    in renal-impaired clients, 511
fluorouracil (Adrucil, Efudex, Fluoroplex), 695t,
    1047t
fluoxetine (Prozac, Sarafem)
    characteristics of, 178t
    description of, 177

half-life of, 186
    in hepatic-impaired patients, 188
    marketing of, 8
fluoxymesterone (Halotestin), 458t
fluphenazine decanoate (Prolixin Decanoate),
    156t–157t, 168
fluphenazine enanthate (Prolixin Enanthate),
    156t–157t, 168
flurandrenolide (Cordran), 1045t
flurazepam (Dalmane), 136t–137t
flurbiprofen (Ansaid, Ocufen), 109, 112t, 1030t
flutamide (Eulexin), 704, 705t, 715
fluticasone aerosol (Flovent), 736t
fluticasone (Flonase, Cultivate), 358t, 736t, 754t,
    1045t
fluticasone powder (Flovent Rotadisk), 736t
fluticasone/salmeterol (Advair), 734t
fluvastatin (Lescol, Lescol XL), 901, 902t, 905–906
Fluvirin (influenza vaccine), 636t
fluvoxamine (Luvox), 179t, 185
Fluzone (influenza vaccine), 636t
Focalin (dexmethylphenidate), 254, 255t,
    258–259
folate (folic acid)
    in children, 942t
    deficiency of, 921t
    food sources of, 921t
    function of, 921t
    preparations, 924t
    recommended daily intake of, 921t
folic acid (folate)
    in children, 942t
    deficiency of, 921t, 938
    food sources of, 921t
    function of, 921t
    preparations, 924t
    recommended daily intake of, 921t
follicle-stimulating hormone, 341
folliculitis, 1041
Follistim (follitropin beta), 344t, 345
follitropin alfa (Gonal-F), 344t, 345
follitropin beta (Follistim), 344t, 345
fondaparinux (Arixtra), 881t, 883
Food, Drug, and Cosmetic Act of 1938, 4, 5t
Food and Drug Administration
    drug approval by, 7
    responsibilities of, 6
Food and Drugs Act, 1084–1085
food–drug interactions, 19
Foradil (formoterol), 732, 732t, 740
Forane (isoflurane), 1096t
formoterol (Foradil), 732, 732t, 740
Fortaz (ceftazidime), 493t
Forteo (teriparatide), 393t, 394
Fortovase (saquinavir), 568t, 569, 578–579
Fosamax (alendronate), 390, 393t, 398, 401
fosamprenavir (Lexiva), 568t
foscarnet (Foscavir), 563, 564t, 575, 578
Foscavir (foscarnet), 563, 564t, 575, 578
fosfomycin (Monurol), 521t
fosinopril (Monopril), 843t
fosphenytoin (Cerebyx), 195, 196t–197t, 200,
    206, 209, 211
Fosrenol (lanthanum), 1079
Fragmin (dalteparin), 881t
Frova (frovatriptan), 116, 117t, 128
frovatriptan (Frova), 116, 117t, 128
fulvestrant (Faslodex), 704, 705t
fungal infections
    antifungal drugs for. See antifungal drugs
    description of, 583
    skin, 1041
    types of, 584b–586b

fungi, 468, 582
Fungizone (amphotericin B deoxycholate), 583, 586, 587t, 596–597, 600
Fungoid (triacetin), 590t
Furadantin (nitrofurantoin), 521t, 526, 1060b
furosemide (Lasix), 393t, 394, 864t–865t, 866, 868, 870
furuncles, 1041
Fuzeon (enfuvirtide), 569t, 570

G

GABA
    benzodiazepine receptor binding to, 135
    definition of, 133
GABA receptors, 77, 133
GABA-ergic system, 77
gabapentin (Neurontin), 197t, 200, 211
Gabitril (tiagabine), 199t, 201, 208
galantamine (Razadyne), 310t, 311, 314
gallbladder, 914
gallstones, 954b
Gamimune N (immune globulin intravenous), 642t
gamma benzene hexachloride (Lindane), 610t, 612
Gammagard (immune globulin intravenous), 642t
gamma-hydroxybutyrate (GHB), 247
ganciclovir (Cytovene), 563, 564t, 575, 578–579
ganglia, 265
Gantrisin (sulfisoxazole), 517t, 1029t
Garamycin (gentamicin), 505t, 507, 1029t, 1043t, 1083
garlic, 59t, 417, 907
gastric juice, 915
gastroesophageal reflux disease, 730, 1064–1065
gastrointestinal candidiasis, 584b, 595
gastrointestinal system
    adverse effects on, 25
    alcohol abuse effects on, 239b
    cocaine effects on, 244b
    disorders of, 22t, 321
    glucocorticoids' effect on, 354
gatifloxacin (Tequin), 508t, 511, 1029t
gauge, 38, 40
gefitinib (Iressa), 700t, 701, 715
gels, 1042b
gemcitabine (Gemzar), 696t, 714
gemfibrozil (Lopid), 902t, 903, 905
gemifloxacin (Factive), 508t
gemtuzumab ozogamicin (Mylotarg), 700t, 701
Gemzar (gemcitabine), 696t, 714
gender, 21
general anesthetics
    adjunctive drugs, 1095–1096
    neuromuscular blocking agents and, 1095–1097
    physiologic effects of, 1095
general interventions, 53
generalized anxiety disorder, 134b, 145–146
generalized seizures, 194
genetics, 20–21
genitourinary system
    cocaine effects on, 244b
    in diabetes mellitus patients, 418
    disorders of, 321
Genotropin (somatropin), 344t
gentamicin (Garamycin), 505t, 507, 1029t, 1043t, 1083
Geocillin (carbenicillin), 487
Geodon (ziprasidone), 156t, 160t, 161, 169, 171
gestational diabetes, 1065–1069

GHB (gamma-hydroxybutyrate), 247
giardiasis, 604
ginger, 59t, 1014
ginkgo biloba, 59t, 416
ginseng, 59t, 417
glaucoma, 1024, 1033–1034
Gleevec (imatinib), 700t, 701
glia, 75
Gliadel (carmustine), 695t, 713–714
glimepiride (Amaryl), 414t
glipizide (Glucotrol, Glucotrol XL), 414t, 429
glitazones, 413–415, 414t, 425, 428
glomerular filtration, 861–862
glucagon, 28t
glucagon-like peptide-1, 405
glucocorticoids
    anti-inflammatory effects of, 357, 360
    characteristics of, 336, 353, 354b
glucomannan, 417, 959
Glucophage (metformin), 413, 414t, 427–428, 430–431
Glucophage XR (metformin), 413, 414t, 427–428, 430–431
glucosamine
    with chondroitin sulfate, 118–119
    description of, 60t, 118
    glucose levels affected by, 416
glucose
    blood testing, 420
    herbal and dietary supplements that affect, 416–417
    insulin secretion and, 405
    metabolism of, 404, 405f
glucose-dependent insulinotropic peptide, 405
glucose-6–phosphate dehydrogenase deficiency, 21
Glucotrol (glipizide), 414t, 429
Glucotrol XL (glipizide), 414t, 429
Glucovance (glyburide/metformin), 415, 415t
glutamate, 78, 83
glutamate receptors, 154
glyburide (DiaBeta, Micronase, Glynase Pres Tab), 414t
glyburide/metformin (Glucovance), 415, 415t
glycated hemoglobin, 418
glycemic index, 964b
glycerin (Osmoglyn), 865t, 1028t
glycerin (suppository), 989t
glycine, 78
glycoprotein IIb/IIIa complexes, 879b
glycoprotein IIb/IIIa receptor antagonists, 884–885
glycoproteins, 11
glycopyrrolate (Robinul), 323t
glycosylated hemoglobin, 964
Glynase Pres Tab (glyburide), 414t
Glyset (miglitol), 414t, 429, 433
goals, in nursing process, 53
Golgi complex, 11b
GoLytely (polyethylene glycol–electrolyte solution), 988t, 989t
gonadorelin (Factrel), 342, 343t, 349
gonadotropin-releasing hormone, 340
Gonal-F (follitropin alfa), 344t, 345
goserelin (Zoladex), 342, 343t, 704, 705t
gout, 106b, 115, 124
graft-versus-host disease, 667–668
gram-negative bacteria, 470b–471b
gram-positive bacteria, 469b–470b
Gram's stain, 468
granisetron (Kytril), 1012t, 1013–1014, 1018
Granulex (trypsin), 1046t
granulocyte-colony stimulating factor, 622t, 623

granulocyte-macrophage colony stimulating factor, 622t, 623
griseofulvin, 588b, 592–593, 597–598, 601
group B streptococcal infections, 1066
growth factors, 701–702
growth hormone
    abuse of, 348
    adverse effects of, 348
    characteristics of, 341–342, 344t
    client teaching about, 347
    in older adults, 348
growth hormone release–inhibiting hormone, 339–340
growth hormone–releasing hormone, 339
guaifenesin (Robitussin), 763t
guanabenz (Wytensin), 291, 292t, 294, 844t
guanadrel (Hylorel), 844t
guanfacine (Tenex), 292t, 294, 844t
guar gum, 417, 959
guarana, 257, 959
Gynazole (butoconazole), 588b
Gyne-Lotrimin (clotrimazole), 588b

H

Habitrol (nicotine), 238t
Haemophilus influenzae, 519
Haemophilus influenzae b conjugate vaccine (ActHIB, HibTITER, PedvaxHIB), 635t, 645, 648
Haemophilus influenzae b conjugate vaccine with hepatitis B vaccine (Comvax), 635t, 645, 648
Hageman factor, 877t
halcinonide (Halog), 1045t
Halcion (triazolam), 136t–137t
Haldol (haloperidol)
    antipsychotic uses of, 156, 156t, 158t, 167, 243
    substance abuse disorders treated with, 238t
half-life
    of antidotes, 27b
    definition of, 16
halflytely & bisacodyl tablets, 990t
hallucinations, 153
hallucinogens, 246
halobetasol (Ultravate), 1045t
Halog (halcinonide), 1045t
haloperidol decanoate, 156t, 158t, 167
haloperidol (Haldol)
    antipsychotic uses of, 156t, 158t, 167, 243
    substance abuse disorders treated with, 238t
haloprogin (Halotex), 588b, 1043t
Halotestin (fluoxymesterone), 458t
Halotex (haloprogin), 588b, 1043t
haptens, 625
Harrison Narcotic Act, 5t
Hashimoto's thyroiditis, 374
Havrix (hepatitis A vaccine), 635t
hay fever, 748
heart
    anatomy of, 773–774
    automaticity of, 794–795
    conductivity of, 795
    electrophysiology of, 794–795
heart block, 798b
heart failure
    acute, 784, 787
    assessment of, 784–785
    causes of, 777
    chronic, 787
    compensatory mechanisms for, 777–778
    definition of, 777
    description of, 298–299

heart failure (*continued*)
drug therapy for
adverse effects of, 791–792
b-type natriuretic peptide, 782t, 783–784
cardiac glycosides, 778–784
in children, 788
digoxin. *See* digoxin (Lanoxin)
drug interactions, 792
endothelial receptor antagonists, 782t, 784
in home care, 789
inotropes, 778–784
nursing actions for, 789–792
in older adults, 788–789
overview of, 777
phosphodiesterase inhibitors, 782t, 783
therapeutic effects of, 791
herbal and dietary supplements for, 789
mild, 784
moderate, 784
New York Heart Association classification of, 778, 779t
nonpharmacologic management of, 785–786
nursing process for, 784–785
severe, 784
signs and symptoms of, 777, 779t
therapeutic principles for, 785–790
heart valves, 774
Hectorol (Doxercalciferol), 392t
Helicobacter pylori, 106
helminthiasis, 605, 613
helper T cells, 628
Hemabate (carboprost tromethamine), 1070t
hematologic system, 25, 239b
hematopoiesis
drugs that affect, 632
schematic diagram of, 627f
hematopoietic drugs. *See also specific drug*
administration of, 658, 661–662
adverse effects of, 663
characteristics of, 651, 655
in children, 660
client teaching about, 658
description of, 655
dosage of, 658–659
drug interactions, 663–664
in hepatic-impaired clients, 661
in home care, 661
laboratory monitoring of, 659
nursing actions for, 661–664
nursing process for, 656–658
in older adults, 660
in renal-impaired clients, 661
therapeutic effects of, 662–663
types of, 652t
hemochromatosis, 941
hemodialysis, 27b, 206
hemolytic-uremic syndrome, 714
hemostasis
definition of, 877
drugs for, 885–886
heparin
administration of, 892–893
antidote for, 28t
characteristics of, 880, 881t, 883, 888, 890
drug interactions, 894
low-molecular-weight, 880, 881t, 883, 890–891, 893
during pregnancy, 1061b
therapeutic effects of, 893
heparin-induced thrombocytopenia, 880
hepatic impairment
acetaminophen in, 126
adrenergic drugs in, 283

alpha-adrenergic blockers in, 301
aminoglycosides in, 511
anabolic steroids in, 460
androgens in, 460
angiotensin II receptor blockers in, 856
angiotensin-converting enzyme inhibitors in, 854
antianginal drugs in, 825
antianxiety drugs in, 147–148
antiasthmatic drugs in, 743
anticholinergic drugs in, 328
anticoagulants in, 891
antidepressants in, 188
antidysrhythmic drugs in, 809
antiemetic drugs in, 1017
antiepileptic drugs in, 208
antifungal drugs in, 598
antihistamines in, 757
antimicrobial drugs in, 480
antineoplastic drugs in, 714–715
antiplatelet agents in, 891
antipsychotic drugs in, 167
antiseizure drugs in, 208
antitubercular drugs in, 555–556
antiviral drugs in, 576
beta blockers in, 301, 856
beta-lactam antibacterials in, 498
calcium channel blockers in, 856–857
cholinergic drugs in, 315
corticosteroids in, 368
digoxin in, 789
diuretics in, 871
drug therapy considerations in, 67–68
dyslipidemic drugs in, 907
erythromycin in, 535
estrogens in, 450
fluoroquinolones in, 480, 511
hematopoietic drugs in, 661
immunostimulants in, 661
immunosuppressants in, 682–683
insulin in, 427–428
macrolides in, 535
nitrates in, 825
nutritional support in, 944
opioid analgesics in, 98
penicillins in, 480
sedative-hypnotics in, 147–148
skeletal muscle relaxants in, 232
sulfonamides in, 524
tetracyclines in, 524
hepatitis A, inactivated, and hepatitis B, recombinant (Twinrix), 636t
hepatitis A vaccine (Havrix, Vaqta), 635t
hepatitis B immune globulin, human (BayHep B, Nabi-HB), 641t
hepatitis B vaccine (Recombivax HB, Engerix-B), 636t, 645
hepatitis B virus, 633
herbal supplements. *See also specific herb*
anticoagulation using, 891–892
anxiety treated with, 140
asthma, 738
central nervous system stimulants, 257
client teaching about, 61
definition of, 56
for diabetes mellitus, 415–416
dyslipidemia, 907
heart failure treated with, 789
list of, 58t–61t
migraines treated with, 118
nurse's role in, 57
obesity treated with, 958–959
pain management using, 91, 117–118
during pregnancy, 1059, 1064

regulation of, 56–57
respiratory disorders treated with, 762, 765
for weight control, 278
Herceptin (trastuzumab), 700t, 701
heroin, 242
herpes simplex virus
antiviral drugs for, 563, 564t–565t
description of, 561b
herpes zoster, 561b
HibTITER (*Haemophilus influenzae* b conjugate vaccine), 635t
high-density lipoprotein, 897, 898b
Hiprex (methenamine-hippurate), 521t
Hispanics
antidepressants in, 187
antipsychotic drugs in, 167
histamine, 105, 747–748, 838–839
histamine₁ receptor antagonists
first-generation, 753
second-generation, 754
histamine receptors, 747–748
histoplasmosis, 583, 585b–586b, 593, 595–596
histrelin (Suprelin), 342
Hivid (zalcitabine), 567t, 575, 579
HMG-CoA reductase inhibitors, 901, 902t
HMS (medrysone), 1030t
Hodgkin's lymphoma, 646
Homans' sign, 887
homatropine hydrobromide, 1027t
homatropine hydrobromide (Isopto-Homatropine), 321, 322t
home care
acetaminophen use in, 126
adrenergic drugs in, 284
antianginal drugs in, 826
antianxiety drugs in, 148
antiasthmatic drugs in, 744
anticholinergic drugs in, 328
anticoagulants in, 891
antidepressants in, 188
antidysrhythmic drugs in, 809
antiemetic drugs in, 1017
antiepileptic drugs in, 208
antihistamines in, 757
antihypertensive drugs in, 857
antimicrobial drugs in, 480–481
antineoplastic drugs in, 715
antiparasitic drugs in, 614–615
antipsychotic drugs in, 168
antiseizure drugs in, 208
antiviral drugs in, 576
beta blockers in, 301
cholinergic drugs in, 315
corticosteroids in, 368
diabetes mellitus in, 428
digoxin use in, 789
diuretics in, 871
drug therapy in, 69–70
estrogens in, 450
hematopoietic drugs in, 661
heparin in, 891
hormonal contraceptives in, 450
immunostimulant drugs in, 661
immunosuppressants in, 683
intravenous antibiotics in, 481
macrolides in, 536
nutritional support in, 945
ophthalmic drugs in, 1034
opioid analgesics in, 99
progestins in, 450
respiratory disorders in, 767, 769
sedative-hypnotics in, 148
theophylline in, 744

hookworm infections, 605b
hormonal contraceptives
  characteristics of, 443
  client teaching about, 448
  contraindications, 440
  drug interactions, 449, 452–453
  in home care, 450
  indications for, 439–440, 449
  mechanism of action, 438
  nursing actions for, 451–453
  nursing process for, 444, 446–447
  selection of, 448
  types of, 445t–446t
hormonal drugs, 338
hormone(s)
  anterior pituitary, 336, 340–342, 343t–344t, 345
  calcium metabolism regulated by, 387–388, 388f
  cellular actions of, 337
  characteristics of, 336–338
  cyclic secretion of, 336–337
  definition of, 335
  disorders of, 338
  elimination of, 337
  function of, 336
  hyperfunction caused by, 338
  hypothalamic, 336, 339–340, 342
  neoplasms that produce, 335
  pharmacokinetics of, 337
  pharmacologic use of, 338
  physiologic use of, 338
  posterior pituitary, 336, 341, 344t–345t, 345–346
  protein-derived, 337
  thyroid, 336
hormone inhibitor drugs, 702–705, 711, 719
hormone replacement therapy
  client teaching about, 447
  description of, 438, 439b
household system, 37, 37t
human chorionic gonadotropin (Chorex, Choron, Pregnyl), 342, 344t, 349, 456b
human immunodeficiency virus
  description of, 561b–562b, 631
  drugs for. See antiretroviral drugs
  immunizations in, 646
  during pregnancy, 1066–1067
  progression to AIDS, 561b
  tuberculosis infection in patients with, 547b, 554–555
Humatin (paromomycin), 505t–506t
Humatrope (somatropin), 342, 344t
Humira (adalizumab), 669t, 674–675
Humulin (insulin lispro), 408, 410t
Humulin L (insulin zinc suspension), 409t
Humulin N (isophane insulin suspension), 409t, 422
Humulin R (insulin injection), 409t
Humulin U (insulin zinc suspension), 409t
Hycamtin (topotecan), 697t
Hycodan (hydrocodone bitartrate), 763t
Hydeltrasol (prednisolone sodium phosphate), 359t
hydralazine (Apresoline), 21, 846t, 855
Hydrea (hydroxyurea), 697t
Hydrocet (hydrocodone), 94t
hydrochloric acid, 916
hydrochlorothiazide (HydroDIURIL, Esidrix, Oretic), 864t, 865, 868, 870
hydrocodone, 87
hydrocodone bitartrate (Hycodan), 763t
hydrocodone/acetaminophen products, 94t

hydrocortisone acetate intrarectal foam (Cortifoam), 359t
hydrocortisone (Hydrocortone, Cortef), 357, 358t
hydrocortisone retention enema (Cortenema), 359t
hydrocortisone sodium phosphate, 358t
hydrocortisone sodium phosphate and sodium succinate, 736t
hydrocortisone sodium succinate, 358t
Hydrocortone (hydrocortisone), 357, 358t
HydroDIURIL (hydrochlorothiazide), 864t, 868, 870
hydroflumethiazide (Saluron), 864t
hydromorphone (Dilaudid), 86t, 87–88
hydroxychloroquine (Plaquenil), 606, 608t
hydroxycitric acid, 959
hydroxyprogesterone caproate (Hylutin), 442t
hydroxyurea (Hydrea), 697t
hydroxyzine (Vistaril), 138, 139t, 150, 751t, 1012t
Hygroton (chlorthalidone), 864t
Hylorel (guanadrel), 844t
Hylutin (hydroxyprogesterone caproate), 442t
hyoscyamine (Anaspaz), 321, 322t
hyperaldosteronism, 353
hypercalcemia
  acute, 397
  in children, 399
  description of, 388, 391b
  drugs used for, 390–395, 397–398
  in older adults, 399
  in renal-impaired clients, 399
hyperglycemia, 416, 873
hyperinsulinemia, 954b
hyperkalemia, 869–870, 940
hyperlipidemia, 898–900
hypermagnesemia, 940
hyperosmolar hyperglycemic nonketotic coma, 407, 408b, 423–424
hyperparathyroidism, 387
hypersensitivity reactions
  allergic drug reactions, 749–750
  allergic rhinitis, 748–750, 751t, 754t
  antimicrobial drugs and, 482
  antipsychotic drugs and, 170
  assessment of, 755
  definition of, 25
  to penicillins, 497
  type I, 748
  type II, 748
  type III, 748
  type IV, 748
hypertension
  antihypertensive drugs for. See antihypertensive drugs
  assessment of, 850
  in children, 854
  definition of, 839
  description of, 295
  essential, 839
  herbal and dietary supplements for, 857–858
  isolated systolic, 839
  JNC 7 guidelines for, 851
  nursing process for, 850–851
  obesity and, 954b
  in older adults, 855
  physiologic effects of, 839, 841
  pregnancy-induced, 1066, 1069
  prevention of, 850–851
  primary, 854
  secondary, 854
  signs and symptoms of, 850
  sodium restriction for, 853

  systemic response to, 839
  systolic, 855
  systolic–diastolic, 855
  target organs for, 841
  World Health Organization guidelines for, 851
hypertensive emergencies, 841–842, 857
hypertensive urgencies, 842, 857
hyperthyroidism
  in children, 382
  description of, 374, 375t
  drugs for, 376–378, 377t
  in older adults, 382
  symptoms of, 378–379
hyperuricemia, 124, 127, 707b, 873
hypoalbuminemia, 147
hypocalcemia
  assessment of, 395
  in children, 399
  description of, 391b
  drugs for, 397
  nursing process for, 396–397
  in older adults, 399
  treatment of, 787–788
hypoglycemia
  in children, 426
  description of, 411b
  drugs for
    alpha-glucosidase inhibitors, 413, 414t, 424–425, 427–428
    biguanides, 413, 414t, 425
    client teaching about, 420–421
    glitazones, 413–415, 414t, 425
    insulin. See insulin
    meglitinides, 415, 415t, 425, 427–428, 430
    in older adults, 427
    oral, 412–415, 413f, 421, 424–425
    in renal-impaired clients, 427
    sulfonylureas, 412–413, 414t, 424–425, 429–432, 460
    therapeutic principles for, 419–428
  signs and symptoms of, 420
hypoglycemic reaction, 420
hypogonadism, 458
hypokalemia, 869–870, 939–940
hypomagnesemia, 940
hypomania, 175b, 176
hypoparathyroidism, 387
hypotension
  in children, 834
  description of, 282
  management guidelines for, 834
  from opioid analgesics, 100
  systemic response to, 839
hypothalamic hormones
  adverse effects of, 349
  characteristics of, 336, 339–340, 342, 343t
  drug interactions, 349–350
  nursing actions for, 348–350
  nursing process for, 346
  therapeutic effects of, 348–349
hypothalamic-pituitary-adrenal axis, 175
hypothalamic–pituitary–adrenocortical axis, 336, 357
hypothalamus, 79, 336, 339
hypothyroidism
  adrenal insufficiency and, 381
  in children, 382
  description of, 374, 375t
  drugs for, 376
  in older adults, 382
  symptoms of, 378–379
hypovolemic shock, 829, 830t, 834
hypoxemia, 27b

Hytakerol (dihydrotachysterol), 392t
Hyzaar, 847t

I

ibritumomab tiuxetan (Zevalin), 700t, 701
ibuprofen (Motrin, Advil), 109, 111t, 125
ibutilide, 805
Idamycin (idarubicin), 696t, 714
idarubicin (Idamycin), 696t, 714
idiosyncrasy, 26
Ifex (ifosfamide), 695t, 713
ifosfamide (Ifex), 695t, 713
Ilosone (erythromycin estolate), 529t
imatinib (Gleevec), 700t, 701
Imdur (isosorbide mononitrate), 817, 818t
imipenem-cilastatin (Primaxin), 486t, 491, 494,
    494t
imipramine (Tofranil), 178t, 1083
Imitrex (sumatriptan), 116, 117t, 121, 128
immediate hypersensitivity, 748
immune globulin (BayGam), 641t
immune globulin intravenous (Gamimune N,
    Gammagard, Iveegam, Polygam S/D,
    Panglobulin, Sandoglobulin,
    Venoglobulin-S), 642t, 649
immune responses
    altered, 665
    description of, 354, 624, 665
    drugs that alter, 632
immune serums, 634, 641t–643t
immune system
    age-related changes, 629–630
    cytokines of, 629, 630f
    description of, 624
    disorders of, 631–632
    fetal, 629
    neonatal, 629–630
    nutritional status and, 631
    in older adults, 630–631
    secretory, 625
    stress effects on, 631
immunity
    active, 625, 634
    adaptive, 625
    antigens, 625
    definition of, 624
    description of, 624
    innate, 625
    passive, 625, 634
immunizations. See also vaccines
    administration of, 647
    in adolescents, 646
    adverse effects of, 647–648
    in cancer clients, 646
    CDC recommendations, 644–645
    in children, 645–646
    client teaching about, 644
    contraindications, 634
    definition of, 634
    drug interactions, 649
    in immunosuppressed clients, 646
    indications for, 634
    nursing actions for, 647–649
    nursing process for, 643–644
    in older adults, 646
    recommendations for, 633–634, 644–645
    toxoids, 640t–641t
    types of, 635t–640t
immunodeficiency disorders, 631–632
immunoglobulin(s), 625, 629
immunoglobulin A, 629
immunoglobulin D, 629

immunoglobulin E, 629, 674
immunoglobulin G, 629
immunoglobulin M, 629
immunomodulators, 632, 651, 668, 1044
immunorestoratives, 651
immunostimulant drugs
    administration of, 661–662
    adverse effects of, 663
    characteristics of, 651, 655
    in children, 660
    drug interactions, 663–664
    in hepatic-impaired clients, 661
    in home care, 661
    nursing actions for, 661–664
    in older adults, 660
    therapeutic effects of, 662–663
immunosuppressants
    administration of, 684–685
    adverse effects of, 685–687
    antibody preparations, 673
    antirejection agents, 672–673
    in children, 681–682
    client teaching about, 677
    corticosteroids, 668, 680
    cytokine inhibitors, 674–675
    cytotoxic antiproliferative agents, 668, 671
    definition of, 665
    dosage of, 680
    drug interactions, 687–689
    in hepatic-impaired clients, 682–683
    in home care, 683
    monoclonal antibody, 738
    nursing actions for, 684–689
    nursing process for, 675–676
    in older adults, 681–682
    in renal-impaired clients, 682
    risk–benefit factors, 676, 678
    risks associated with, 676, 678
    self-administration of, 677
    sites of action for, 666f
    therapeutic effects of, 685
    therapeutic principles for, 676, 678
immunosuppression
    cancer secondary to, 678
    description of, 646
    history of, 668
    for organ transplantation, 667
    risks associated with, 676, 678
    in transplantation patients, 679–681
Imodium (loperamide), 1000t, 1002, 1006
Imogam (rabies immune globulin), 642t
Imovax (rabies vaccine), 638t
impetigo, 1041
Imuran (azathioprine), 669t, 671, 679–682, 685
inactivated poliomyelitis vaccine, 633, 638t, 645,
    648
inamrinone, 782t, 783, 790, 792
incretin hormones, 405
indapamide (Lozol), 864t
Inderal (propranolol)
    angina pectoris treated with, 818t, 820
    antidysrhythmic uses of, 801t, 804, 808–809
    antihypertensive uses of, 845t
    characteristics of, 293t, 295, 300, 377t, 378
    serum levels of, 1083
Inderide, 847t
indinavir (Crixivan), 568t, 569–570, 575,
    578–579
Indocin (indomethacin), 109, 112t, 129
indomethacin (Indocin), 109, 112t, 129
Infanrix (diphtheria and tetanus toxoids and acel-
    lular pertussis vaccine), 640t
infants. See also children; neonates

    antiepileptic drugs in, 207
    drug administration in, 63
    drug therapy in, 62–63
    epilepsy in, 193
    pharmacokinetics in, 20, 63t
    physiologic characteristics of, 63t
infections
    aminoglycosides for, 506
    chemotherapy-related, 706b–707b
    community-acquired, 468, 471
    nosocomial, 468, 471
    ocular, 1033
    opportunistic, 468
    protozoal. See protozoal infections
    viral. See viral infections
infectious diseases, 468
InFeD (iron dextran injection), 931t, 932–933
Infergen (interferon alfacon-1), 654t, 656
inflammation
    aspirin for, 122
    chemical mediators of, 105b
    definition of, 104
    glucocorticoids' effect on, 354
inflammatory bowel disease, 366
infliximab (Remicade), 124, 670t, 675, 686
influenza virus
    description of, 565t, 570
    vaccine against, 636t, 648
INH (isoniazid)
    administration of, 556
    adverse effects of, 544, 547
    antidote for, 28t–29t
    characteristics of, 548t
    client teaching about, 552
    drug interactions, 554, 557–558
    genetic variations that affect, 21
    in hepatic-impaired clients, 555–556
    pharmacokinetics of, 544
    tuberculosis treated with, 544, 546b, 547
inhalant abuse, 248
injections. See specific injection
innate immunity, 625
Innohep (tinzaparin), 881t
inositol triphosphate, 337–338
insomnia
    definition of, 133
    drug therapy for, 146
    sedative-hypnotics for, 147
inspiration, 727
insulin
    administration of, 421, 423, 428–429
    adverse effects of, 430
    analogs, 408, 410t
    combination therapies, 425
    description of, 407
    dosage of, 422
    drug interactions, 431–432
    elimination of, 405
    endogenous, 404–405
    glucose effects on, 405
    guidelines for, 422–423
    in hepatic-impaired clients, 427–428
    human, 407
    indications for, 407
    injection of, 423, 429
    intermediate-acting, 408, 409t, 412
    long-acting, 408, 409t, 412
    metabolism affected by, 406b
    mixtures, 410t
    pancreatic production of, 404
    perioperative, 424
    pork, 407
    during pregnancy, 1068

preparation of, 422
rapid-acting, 408
in renal-impaired clients, 427
self-administration of, 421
serum levels of, 404
short-acting, 408, 424, 429
storage of, 420
subcutaneous infusion pump of, 412f, 422
syringes for, 40
insulin aspart (Novolog), 408, 410t, 422
insulin detemir (Levemir), 1079
insulin glargine (Lantus), 408, 410t, 422
insulin glulisine (Apidra), 408, 410t, 422
insulin injection (Regular Iletin II, Humulin R,
  Novolin R), 409t
insulin lispro (Humulin), 408, 410t
insulin lispro protamine, 410t
insulin pumps, 412f, 422
insulin resistance, 406, 413
insulin sensitizers, 413
insulin zinc suspension (Lente Iletin II, Lente L,
  Humulin L), 409t
Intal (cromolyn), 736t, 738, 743, 754t
integral proteins, 11
Integrilin (eptifibatide), 882t, 884, 887, 891
intensive care unit, 68
interference, 19
interferon alfa, 622t
interferon alfa-2a (Roferon-A), 653t, 656
interferon alfa-2b and ribavirin (Rebetron), 654t
interferon alfa-2b (Intron A), 653t–654t, 656
interferon alfacon-1 (Infergen), 654t, 656
interferon alfa-n1, 656
interferon beta, 622t, 656
interferon beta-1a (Avonex, Rebif), 654t
interferon beta-1b (Betaseron), 654t
interferon gamma, 622t, 656
interferon gamma-1b (Actimmune), 654t
interferons, 105, 660, 662
interleukin(s)
  blockers of, 674
  description of, 105, 653t, 656, 659–660
interleukin-1, 622t, 841b
interleukin-2, 622t
interleukin-3, 622t
interleukin-4, 622t
interleukin-5, 622t
interleukin-6, 622t
interleukin-7, 622t
interleukin-8, 622t, 841b
interleukin-9, 622t
interleukin-10, 622t
interleukin-11, 623t
interleukin-12, 623t
interleukin-13, 623t
interleukin-14, 623t
interleukin-15, 623t
interleukin-16, 623t
interleukin-17, 623t
interleukin-18, 623t
intermediate-acting insulins, 408, 409t, 412
intermittent infusion, 41b
International System of Units, 1082
interstitial cell-stimulating hormone. See luteinizing hormone
intertrigo, 1041
interventions, 53
intestinal amebiasis, 603, 612
intima, 774
intramuscular injections
  advantages and disadvantages of, 39t
  antipsychotic drugs, 164, 168
  in children, 63

drug actions after, 19
nursing action for, 47
sites for, 40, 43f
intraocular pressure, 1024
intravenous injections
  absorption of, 14
  administration technique, 42b
  advantages and disadvantages of, 39t
  in children, 32b
  continuous infusion, 41b
  in critical-illness patients, 69
  drug preparation for, 42b
  equipment for, 41b
  of illicit drugs, 236–237
  intermittent infusion, 41b
  nursing action for, 47–48
  of opioid analgesics, 94
  principles of, 41b–42b
  sites for, 40, 41b–42b, 43f–44f
intrinsic pathway, 879b
Intron A (interferon alfa-2b), 653t–654t, 656
Invanz (ertapenem), 494, 494t
iodine, 928t
iodine, radioactive, 381–382
iodoquinol (Yodoxin), 603–604, 606
Iodotope (sodium iodide 131), 377t, 378
Ionamin (phentermine hydrochloride), 957, 957t,
  967
ipecac, 27b
IPOL (poliomyelitis vaccine, inactivated), 638t
ipratropium bromide (Atrovent), 321, 322t, 324,
  732t–733t, 734, 754t, 767
ipratropium/albuterol (Combivent, DuoNeb),
  734t
irbesartan (Avapro), 843t
Iressa (gefitinib), 700t, 701, 715
irinotecan (Camptosar), 697t, 713
iris, 1023
iron, 28t, 928t, 941
iron deficiency anemia, 239b, 940–941, 1064
iron dextran injection (InFeD), 931t, 932–933
iron preparations, 929, 930t–931t, 932–933, 947
Ismo (isosorbide mononitrate), 817, 818t, 819
Ismotic (isosorbide), 1028t
isocarboxazid (Marplan), 179t
isoflurane (Forane), 1096t
isolated systolic hypertension, 839
isoniazid (INH)
  administration of, 556
  adverse effects of, 544, 547
  antidote for, 28t–29t
  characteristics of, 548t
  client teaching about, 552
  drug interactions, 554, 557–558
  genetic variations that affect, 21
  in hepatic-impaired clients, 555–556
  pharmacokinetics of, 544
  tuberculosis treated with, 544, 546b, 547
isophane insulin suspension (NPH, NPH Iletin II,
  Humulin N, Novolin N), 409t, 422, 429
isoproterenol (Isuprel), 273t, 277t, 278, 285, 831t,
  832
Isoptin (verapamil), 802t, 805, 811t, 819t, 845t
Isopto Carpine (pilocarpine), 1027t
Isopto-Homatropine (homatropine hydrobromide), 321, 322t
Isordil (isosorbide dinitrate), 817–819, 818t
isosorbide dinitrate (Isordil), 817–819, 818t
isosorbide (Ismotic), 1028t
isosorbide mononitrate (Ismo, Imdur), 817, 818t,
  819
isotretinoin (Accutane), 1046t, 1052
isradipine (DynaCirc), 819t, 845t

Isuprel (isoproterenol), 273t, 277t, 278, 285, 831t,
  832
itraconazole (Sporanox), 587b, 589t, 591–592,
  597, 600
IV push, 41b–42b. See also intravenous injection
Iveegam (immune globulin intravenous), 642t
ivermectin (Stromectol), 610t, 611

J
jaundice, 167
Jenest-28, 445t
JNC 7, 851
juvenile rheumatoid arthritis, 106b

K
Kaletra (lopinavir and ritonavir), 568t, 570
kanamycin (Kantrex), 505t, 550
Kantrex (kanamycin), 505t, 550
kava
  anxiety treated with, 140
  characteristics of, 60t
Kayexalate (sodium polystyrene sulfonate), 925,
  929, 930t
Kefauver-Harris Amendment, 5t
Keflex (cephalexin), 490t
Kefurox (cefuroxime), 492t
Kefzol (cefazolin), 486t, 492t, 496
Kemadrin (procyclidine), 323t, 325
Kenacort (triamcinolone), 359t, 731b
Kenalog-40 (triamcinolone acetonide), 359t,
  1045t
Kepivance (palifermin), 1080
Keppra (levetiracetam), 198t, 200–201, 207
keratitis, 1024
keratolytic agents, 1044
Kerlone (betaxolol), 293t, 844t
ketamine, 247–248
Ketek (telithromycin), 529t, 529–530, 539
ketoconazole (Nizoral), 587b, 589t, 591, 600, 1044t
ketolides
  administration of, 536–537
  adverse effects of, 538
  client teaching about, 534
  description of, 529
  mechanism of action, 529
  nursing actions for, 536–539
  nursing process for, 533
  self-administration of, 534
  therapeutic effects of, 537
  therapeutic principles for, 533–536
ketones, 419
ketoprofen (Oruvail), 109, 112t
ketorolac (Toradol, Acular), 108–109, 113t, 114,
  1030t
ketotifen (Zaditor), 1030t
kidneys
  adverse effects on, 25
  diuretic sites of action in, 863f
  function alterations in, 862–863
  glomerular filtration by, 861–862
  nephron of, 861–862, 862f
  pharmacokinetics affected by, 23t–24t
  physiology of, 861–862
  tubular reabsorption, 862
Kineret (anakinra), 669t, 674
Klebsiella pneumoniae, 470b
Klonopin (clonazepam)
  antianxiety uses of, 136t, 138, 143, 149
  antiseizure uses of, 196t, 200
Kupffer's cells, 626, 915
Kytril (granisetron), 1012t, 1013–1014, 1018

L

labetalol (Trandate, Normodyne), 293t, 845t
labor
  analgesics during, 1072
  anesthetics during, 1072
  induction of, 1071–1072
  opioid analgesics during, 97
lacrimal system, 1023
lactation, 1073, 1075b
lactulose (Chronulac, Cephulac), 990, 990t
Lamictal (lamotrigine), 197t, 200, 211
Lamisil (terbinafine), 583, 587b, 590t, 593, 597–598, 601, 1044t
lamivudine (Epivir), 566t, 575
lamotrigine (Lamictal), 197t, 200, 211
Lanacane (benzocaine), 1098t
Lanoxin (digoxin)
  administration of, 781–782
  adverse effects of, 791–792
  antidote for, 28t
  characteristics of, 778–779
  client teaching about, 786
  contraindications, 781
  digitalization of, 781–782
  diuretics and, 869–870
  dosage of, 782t, 787–788
  drug interactions, 792
  electrolyte balance while using, 787–788
  indications for, 781
  mechanism of action, 779, 781
  nonsteroidal anti-inflammatory drugs effect on, 123
  pharmacokinetics of, 779
  during pregnancy, 1063b
  self-administration of, 786
  serum levels of, 1083
  toxicity of, 783, 788
lanthanum (Fosrenol), 1079
Lantus (insulin glargine), 408, 410t
large intestine, 914
Lariam (mefloquine), 608t, 611
Larodopa (levodopa), 215–216, 217t, 223–225
larynx, 726
Lasix (furosemide), 393t, 394, 864t–865t, 866, 868, 870
L-asparaginase (Elspar), 697t, 699, 714
latanoprost (Xalatan), 1028t
latent tuberculosis infection
  in adolescents, 546b
  in children, 546b
  definition of, 543
  in HIV-infected persons, 547b
  isoniazid for, 546b
  nursing process for, 551–552
  during pregnancy, 546b
  prevention of, 544
  targeted tuberculin testing for, 545b
  treatment of, 546b–547b
laxatives. *See also specific drug*
  abuse of, 992
  administration of, 994–995
  adverse effects of, 995
  bulk-forming, 988, 989t
  in cancer patients, 993
  in children, 993
  client teaching about, 992
  contraindications, 988
  definition of, 987
  drug interactions, 995
  in hepatic-impaired clients, 994
  herbal supplements, 991
  in home care, 994
  indications for, 988

long-term use of, 993
lubricant, 990, 990t
  nursing actions for, 994–995
  nursing process for, 991–992
  in older adults, 993
  in renal-impaired clients, 994
  saline, 988
  selection of, 992–993
  self-administration of, 992
  in spinal cord injury patients, 993–994
  surfactant, 988, 989t
  therapeutic effects of, 995
L-dopa (levodopa), 215, 223–224
lead, 29t
leflunomide (Arava), 124, 670t, 675, 681–683, 686, 688
lens, 1024
Lente Iletin II (insulin zinc suspension), 409t
Lente L (insulin zinc suspension), 409t
lepirudin (Refludan), 881t, 883, 891
Lescol (fluvastatin), 901, 902t, 905–906
Lescol XL (fluvastatin), 901, 902t, 905–906
lethal doses, 18
letrozole (Femara), 704, 705t
leucovorin (Wellcovorin), 707, 708t
leukemias, 692
Leukeran (chlorambucil), 695t
Leukine (sargramostim), 652t–653t, 659–660, 662, 707, 708t
leukocytes, 775–776
leukotriene modifiers
  in children, 743
  description of, 736t, 737
leukotrienes, 105
leuprolide (Eligard, Lupron, Viadur), 704, 705t
leuprolide (Lupron), 342, 343t
Leustatin (cladribine), 695t
levalbuterol (Xopenex), 732, 732t–733t
levamisole (Ergamisol), 697t
Levaquin (levofloxacin), 508t, 1029t
Levatol (penbutolol), 293t, 844t
Levemir (insulin detemir), 1079
levetiracetam (Keppra), 198t, 200–201, 207
Levitra (vardenafil), 1081
Levlen, 445t
Levlite, 445t
levobunolol (Betagan), 293t, 1026t
levobupivacaine (Chirocaine), 1098t
levocabastine (Livostin), 1030t
levodopa (L-dopa, Larodopa, Dopar), 215–216, 217t, 223–225
levodopa/carbidopa (Sinemet), 216, 217t, 220–221
levodopa/carbidopa/entacapone (Stalevo), 217t
Levo-Dromoran (levorphanol), 86t, 88
levofloxacin (Levaquin), 508t, 1029t
Levophed (norepinephrine), 273t, 831t, 832, 835
levorphanol (Levo-Dromoran), 86t, 88
Levothroid (levothyroxine), 374, 376, 377t, 379, 382–383
levothyroxine (Synthroid, Levothroid), 374, 376, 377t, 379, 382–383
Lexapro (escitalopram), 178t
Lexiva (fosamprenavir), 568t
Lexxel, 847t
Librium (chlordiazepoxide), 136t, 238t, 240
Lidex (fluocinonide), 1045t
lidocaine
  anesthetic uses of, 1098t
  digoxin toxicity treated with, 788
  dysrhythmias treated with, 803, 809, 811t
  in hepatic-impaired patients, 68

ligand gating, 13b
ligands, 266
limbic system, 79
Lindane (gamma benzene hexachloride), 610t, 612
linezolid (Zyvox), 531t, 532, 535, 537–538
Lioresal (baclofen), 228–230, 229t
liothyronine (Cytomel, Triostat), 376, 377t
liotrix (Thyrolar), 376, 377t
lipids, 897, 898b
lipid-soluble drugs, 13b
Lipitor (atorvastatin), 901, 902t, 905–906
LipoKinetix, 959
lipoproteins, 897, 898b
liposomal amphotericin B (AmBisome), 587b, 596–597, 600
Liquifilm (polyvinyl alcohol), 1028t
lisinopril (Prinivil, Zestril), 843t
Listeria monocytogenes, 998
lithium carbonate (Lithotab, Lithobid)
  adverse effects of, 189
  characteristics of, 179t, 180–181
  in children, 187
  drug interactions, 191
  mechanism of action, 176–177
  nonsteroidal anti-inflammatory drugs effect on, 123
  perioperative considerations for, 186
  precautions for, 183
  in renal-impaired clients, 188
  serum levels of, 1083
  therapeutic levels of, 184
  weight gain caused by, 956b
Lithobid (lithium carbonate)
  adverse effects of, 189
  characteristics of, 179t, 180–181
  in children, 187
  drug interactions, 191
  mechanism of action, 176–177
  nonsteroidal anti-inflammatory drugs effect on, 123
  perioperative considerations for, 186
  precautions for, 183
  in renal-impaired clients, 188
  serum levels of, 1083
  therapeutic levels of, 184
  weight gain caused by, 956b
Lithotab (lithium carbonate)
  adverse effects of, 189
  characteristics of, 179t, 180–181
  in children, 187
  drug interactions, 191
  mechanism of action, 176–177
  nonsteroidal anti-inflammatory drugs effect on, 123
  perioperative considerations for, 186
  precautions for, 183
  in renal-impaired clients, 188
  serum levels of, 1083
  therapeutic levels of, 184
  weight gain caused by, 956b
liver
  adverse effects on, 25
  alcohol abuse effects on, 239b
  anabolic steroids' effect on, 456
  anatomy of, 914–915
  androgens' effect on, 456
liver impairment
  acetaminophen in, 126
  adrenergic drugs in, 283
  alpha-adrenergic blockers in, 301
  aminoglycosides in, 511
  anabolic steroids in, 460

androgens in, 460
angiotensin II receptor blockers in, 856
angiotensin-converting enzyme inhibitors in, 854
antianginal drugs in, 825
antianxiety drugs in, 147–148
antiasthmatic drugs in, 743
anticholinergic drugs in, 328
anticoagulants in, 891
antidepressants in, 188
antidysrhythmic drugs in, 809
antiemetic drugs in, 1017
antiepileptic drugs in, 208
antifungal drugs in, 598
antihistamines in, 757
antimicrobial drugs in, 480
antineoplastic drugs in, 714–715
antiplatelet agents in, 891
antipsychotic drugs in, 167
antiseizure drugs in, 208
antitubercular drugs in, 555–556
antiviral drugs in, 576
beta blockers in, 301, 856
beta-lactam antibacterials in, 498
calcium channel blockers in, 856–857
cholinergic drugs in, 315
corticosteroids in, 368
digoxin in, 789
diuretics in, 871
drug therapy considerations in, 67–68
dyslipidemic drugs in, 907
erythromycin in, 535
estrogens in, 450
fluoroquinolones in, 480, 511
hematopoietic drugs in, 661
immunostimulants in, 661
immunosuppressants in, 682–683
insulin in, 427–428
macrolides in, 535
nitrates in, 825
nutritional support in, 944
opioid analgesics in, 98
penicillins in, 480
sedative-hypnotics in, 147–148
skeletal muscle relaxants in, 232
sulfonamides in, 524
tetracyclines in, 524
liver transplantation, 681
Livostin (levocabastine), 1030t
local anesthetics, 1097–1099, 1098t
locus ceruleus, 133
Lodine (etodolac), 109, 111t, 114
Lodosyn (carbidopa), 215–216, 217t, 218
Loestrin, 445t
Loestrin Fe, 445t
LoHist (brompheniramine), 751t, 753
Lomotil (diphenoxylate with atropine sulfate), 999t–1000t, 1006
lomustine (CCNU), 695t, 713
long-acting insulins, 408, 409t, 412
Loniten (minoxidil), 846t
loop diuretics, 864t–865t, 866, 868, 871
Lo/Ovral, 445t
loperamide (Imodium), 1000t, 1002, 1006
Lopid (gemfibrozil), 902t, 903, 905
Lopidine (apraclonidine), 1026t
lopinavir and ritonavir (Kaletra), 568t, 570
Lopressor HCT, 847t
Lopressor (metoprolol), 293t, 818t, 844t
Loprox (ciclopirox), 588b, 1043t
Lorabid (loracarbef), 490t
loracarbef (Lorabid), 490t
loratadine (Claritin), 752, 754, 756, 758

lorazepam (Ativan)
    antianxiety uses of, 136t–137t, 138, 148–149
    antiseizure uses of, 198t, 200
    substance abuse disorders treated with, 238t
Lorcet (hydrocodone), 94t
Lortab (hydrocodone), 94t
losartan (Cozaar), 843t
Lotemax (loteprednol), 1030t
Lotensin (benazepril), 843t
Lotensin HCT, 848t
loteprednol (Lotemax, Alrex), 1030t
lotions, 1042b
Lotrel, 848t
Lotrimin (clotrimazole), 588b, 1043t
lovastatin (Mevacor, Altocor), 901, 902t, 905–906
Lovenox (enoxaparin), 881t
low-calorie diet, 964b
low-carbohydrate diet, 964b
low-density lipoprotein, 897, 898b, 901
low-fat diet, 964b
low-molecular-weight heparins, 880, 881t, 883, 890–891, 893
Low-Orgestrel, 445t
loxapine (Loxitane), 156, 156t, 159t
Loxitane (loxapine), 156, 156t, 159t
Lozol (indapamide), 864t
LSD, 246
lubricant laxatives, 990, 990t
Lugol's solution (strong iodine solution), 376, 377t
Lumigan (bimatoprost), 1028t
Lunesta (eszopidone), 1079
lung circulation, 726–727
lungs, 726
Lupron (leuprolide), 342, 343t, 704, 705t
luteinizing hormone, 341, 703f
luteinizing hormone releasing hormone analogs, 704–705, 705t
Luvox (fluvoxamine), 179t
lymphatic system, 775
lymphocyte(s)
    B, 625, 628–629
    definition of, 626
    natural killer cells, 626
    T, 626, 628
lymphocyte immune globulin, antithymocyte globulin (Atgam), 670t, 673, 679, 686
lymphomas, 366, 692–693
lymphotoxin, 629
Lyrica (pregabalin), 1080
lysosomes, 11b, 355

M
ma huang, 278, 958–959
Macrodantin (nitrofurantoin), 521t, 526, 1060b
macrolides
    administration of, 536–537
    adverse effects of, 538
    client teaching about, 534
    definition of, 528
    in hepatic-impaired clients, 535
    in home care, 536
    indications for, 530
    mechanism of action, 529
    nursing actions for, 536–539
    nursing process for, 533
    during pregnancy, 1060b
    in renal-impaired clients, 535
    self-administration of, 534

therapeutic effects of, 537
therapeutic principles for, 533–536
macrophages, 630f
mafenide (Sulfamylon), 518t, 1043t
magnesium
    in children, 943t
    description of, 926t–927t
    disorders involving, 940
magnesium citrate, 988, 989t
magnesium hydroxide, 931t, 933, 988, 989t, 993
magnesium oxide, 931t, 933
magnesium preparations, 931t, 933
magnesium sulfate, 802t, 805, 931t, 933, 947, 1071, 1076
major depression, 175b
major histocompatibility complex, 624
malaria
    antimalarial drugs, 606, 608t–609t, 611
    description of, 604, 612–613
Malarone (atovaquone/proguanil), 606, 608t, 611
malathion (Ovide), 610t, 612
malignant melanoma, 1048
malnutrition, 21
Mandelamine (methenamine mandelate), 521t, 523
mania, 175b, 176
mannitol (Osmitrol), 865t, 866, 1028t
maprotiline, 179t, 180, 1083
Marcaine (bupivacaine), 1098t
Marcillin (ampicillin), 487, 488t
Marezine (cyclizine), 1012t
marijuana, 245–246
Marinol (dronabinol), 245, 1013t, 1014, 1017
marketing, 7–8
Marplan (isocarboxazid), 179t
masoprocol (Actinex), 1047t
mast cell stabilizers, 736t, 738, 754t, 1025
Matulane (procarbazine), 697t, 715
Mavik (trandolapril), 843t
Maxair (pirbuterol), 273t, 732, 732t–733t
Maxalt (rizatriptan), 116, 117t, 121, 128
Maxidex (dexamethasone), 1030t
Maxiflor (diflorasone), 1045t
Maxipime (cefepime), 493t
Maxzide, 867t
MDMA. See 3,4–methylenedioxy-methamphetamine
measles, mumps, and rubella vaccine (M-M-R II), 637t, 647–648
measles and rubella vaccine (M-R-Vax II), 637t
measles vaccine (Attenuvax), 637t
mebendazole (Vermox), 609t, 611–612
mechanical ventilation, 27b
meclizine (Antivert, Bonine), 1012t
media, 774
medication(s). See also drug(s); specific drug
    bar coding of, 33
    computerized ordering of, 33
    definition of, 31
    reasons for giving, 3–4
medication administration record, 33, 44
medication errors, 32b, 32–33
medication history, 52b
medication orders, 33–34, 34b
medication systems, 33
Mediterranean diet, 900
Medrol (methylprednisolone), 359t
medroxyprogesterone acetate (Depo-Provera, Provera), 442t, 715
medrysone (HMS), 1030t
medulla oblongata, 79
mefenamic acid (Ponstel), 113t, 114
mefloquine (Lariam), 608t, 611

Mefoxin (cefoxitin), 492t
Megace (megestrol acetate), 443t
megakaryocytes, 776, 878b
megaloblastic anemia, 239b, 938
megestrol acetate (Megace), 443t
meglitinides, 415, 415t, 425, 427–428, 430
melanocytes, 1039
melanocyte-stimulating hormone, 341
melatonin
    anxiety treated with, 140
    characteristics of, 60t
    sleep–wake cycles affected by, 140
Mellaril (thioridazine), 164
meloxicam (Mobic), 113t, 114
melphalan (Alkeran), 695t, 713
memantine (Namenda), 314
meningitis vaccine (Menomune-A/C/Y/W-135),
        637t
Menomune-A/C/Y/W-135 (meningitis vaccine),
        637t
menopause, 438, 443, 450
menotropins (Pergonal), 342, 344t, 349
menstrual cycle, 437
Mentax (butenafine), 588b, 1043t
mepenzolate, 323t
meperidine (Demerol), 86t, 88, 98, 1060b
Mephyton (vitamin K)
    deficiency of, 920t
    food sources of, 920t
    function of, 920t
    preparations, 924t
    recommended daily intake of, 920t
    warfarin interactions with, 19, 886t, 886t
mepivacaine (Carbocaine), 1098t
Mepron (atovaquone), 609t, 611
mercaptopurine (Purinethol), 696t, 713–714,
        719
Meridia (sibutramine), 957t, 957–958, 967
meropenem (Merrem), 494, 494t
Merrem (meropenem), 494, 494t
Meruvax II (rubella vaccine), 638t–639t
mesalamine (Pentasa, Rowasa), 1080
mescaline, 246
mesna (Mesnex), 707, 708t
Mesnex (mesna), 707, 708t
Mestinon (pyridostigmine), 310t, 311, 314
metabolic syndrome, 954b
metabolism
    carbohydrate, 406b
    drug
        age effects on, 20
        definition of, 15
        drug–drug interaction effects on, 19
        endocrine disorders' effect on, 22t
        hepatic disorders' effect on, 22t
        malnutrition effects on, 21
        respiratory impairment effects on, 24t
    estrogen effects on, 437b
    fat, 406b
    insulin effects on, 406b
    protein, 406b
Metaglip (metformin/glipizide), 415t
Metamucil (psyllium), 988, 989t, 1002t
metaproterenol (Alupent), 273t, 732, 733t, 734
metaraminol (Aramine), 273t, 831t, 832
metaxalone (Skelaxin), 229t, 230, 232
metered dose inhalers, 36t, 732
metformin (Glucophage, Glucophage XR), 413,
        414t, 427–428, 431
metformin/glipizide (Metaglip), 415t
methadone (Dolophine), 86t, 88, 238t, 242
methamphetamine, 243
methamphetamine (Desoxyn), 254, 255t

methenamine mandelate (Mandelamine), 521t,
        523
methenamine-hippurate (Hiprex), 521t
Methergine (methylergonovine maleate), 1070t
methicillin-resistant *Staphylococcus aureus*, 468,
        471, 472b, 487, 532
methimazole (Tapazole), 376, 377t, 380
methocarbamol (Robaxin), 229t, 230
methohexital (Brevital), 1096t
methotrexate (Rheumatrex)
    adverse effects of, 686
    antineoplastic uses of, 696t
    drug interactions, 688, 719
    in hepatic-impaired clients, 683
    immunosuppressive uses of, 670t, 671
    nonsteroidal anti-inflammatory drugs effect on,
        123
    in renal-impaired clients, 682, 713–714
    rheumatoid arthritis treated with, 124
Methulose (methylcellulose), 1028t
methyclothiazide (Enduron), 864t
methylcellulose (Citrucel, Methulose), 989t
3,4–methylenedioxy-methamphetamine, 246–247
methylergonovine maleate (Methergine), 1070t
methylphenidate (Ritalin), 242, 248, 254, 255t,
        258–260
methylprednisolone (Medrol), 359t
methylprednisolone sodium succinate (Solu-
        Medrol), 359t, 736t
methyltestosterone (Android, Testred), 458t
metipranolol (OptiPranolol), 293t, 1027t
metoclopramide (Reglan), 1011–1013, 1012t,
        1016
metolazone (Zaroxolyn, Mykrox), 864t, 870
metoprolol (Lopressor), 293t, 818t, 844t
metric system, 37, 37t
MetroLotion (metronidazole), 1043t
metronidazole (Flagyl)
    antidiarrheal uses of, 1000t–1001t
    description of, 531t, 532, 535–536, 539, 604
    drug interactions, 616
    protozoal infections treated with, 606
metronidazole (MetroLotion), 1043t
Mevacor (lovastatin), 901, 902t, 905–906
mexiletine (Mexitil), 800t, 803, 811t
Mexitil (mexiletine), 800t, 803, 811t
Miacalcin (salmon calcitonin), 390, 393t
micafungin (Mycamine), 1080
Micardis (telmisartan), 843t
miconazole (Monistat), 589t, 1044t
microdrip, 42b
Microgestin Fe, 445t
Micronase (glyburide), 414t
Micronor, 446t
microorganisms
    antibiotic-resistant, 471, 472b–473b, 473, 478
    classification of, 468
    description of, 467
    host defense mechanisms against, 473–474
    normal, 468
Midamor (amiloride), 865t, 866
midazolam (Versed), 136t–137t, 149, 1096t
Mifeprex (mifepristone), 1070, 1070t, 1076
mifepristone (Mifeprex), 1070, 1070t, 1076
miglitol (Glyset), 414t, 429, 433
migraine
    acetaminophen for, 124
    characteristics of, 106b
    client teaching about, 121
    drugs for, 115–117, 117t
    herbal medicines for, 118
    nursing process for, 119
milk of magnesia, 988

Milkinol (mineral oil), 990t, 993
milliequivalents, 37
milrinone (Primacor), 782t, 783, 790, 831t, 832
mineral(s)
    chloride, 927t
    client teaching about, 935–936
    description of, 919
    drug interactions, 949–50
    magnesium, 926t–927t
    nursing actions for, 945–950
    nursing process for, 933–935
    potassium, 926t
    self-administration of, 936
    sodium, 785, 926t, 932t
    supplements, 923, 925
    tolerable upper intake levels for, 919b
mineral oil (Agoral Pain, Milkinol, Fleet Mineral
        Oil Enema), 990t, 993
mineral–electrolyte imbalances
    cation exchange resin for, 925, 929, 930t
    chelating agents for, 929, 930t
    description of, 925
    iron preparations, 929, 930t–931t, 932–933,
        947
    magnesium preparations, 931t, 933
    nursing process for, 933–935
    potassium preparations, 931t, 933
    sodium preparations, 932t
mineralocorticoids, 336, 353, 355b
minimum effective concentration, 15–16
minimum inhibitory concentration, 478, 536
Minipress (Prazosin), 292t, 294, 844t
Minizide, 848t
Minocin (minocycline), 516t
minocycline (Minocin), 516t
minoxidil (Loniten), 846t
Mintezol (thiabendazole), 610t, 612
Mirapex (pramipexole), 217t, 218, 221
Mircette, 445t
mirtazapine (Remeron), 146, 179t, 180, 182,
        189–190
misoprostol (Cytotec), 1070t
mitochondria, 11b
mitodrine (ProAmatine), 1080
mitomycin (Mutamycin), 696t
mitoxantrone (Novantrone), 696t
mitral valve, 774
Mitrolan (polycarbophil), 988, 989t
Mivacron (mivacurium), 1096t
mivacurium (Mivacron), 1096t
mixed seizure, 194
mixed-acting drugs, 273
M-M-R II (measles, mumps, and rubella vaccine),
        637t
Moban (molindone), 156, 156t, 159t
Mobic (meloxicam), 113t, 114
Mobitz type I heart block, 798b
modafinil (Provigil), 254–256, 255t, 259, 261
Modicon, 445t
Moduretic, 867t
moexipril (Univasc), 843t
molds, 582
molindone (Moban), 156, 156t, 159t
mometasone (Asmanex Twisthaler, Nasonex,
        Elocon), 359t, 736t, 754t, 1045t
Monistat (miconazole), 589t, 1044t
monoamine oxidase, 834
monoamine oxidase inhibitors. *See also specific
        drug*
    adrenergic drug contraindications, 286
    adverse effects of, 189
    description of, 180
    drug interactions, 191

food interactions with, 19
indications for, 182
levodopa contraindications, 215
mechanism of action, 176
in older adults, 188
opioid analgesic interactions with, 101
selective serotonin reuptake inhibitors and, 177
toxicity of, 185
triptan drugs affected by, 129
types of, 179t–180t
tyramine-containing foods and, 19
monoamine oxidase-A, 218–219
monoamine oxidase-B, 218–219
monobactam, 494, 498
monoclonal antibodies, 673–674, 699–701, 700t, 716–718, 738
monocyte-colony stimulating factor, 622t, 623
monocytes, 626
Monopril (fosinopril), 843t
montelukast (Singulair), 736t, 737–738
Monurol (fosfomycin), 521t
mood disorders
bipolar disorder. See bipolar disorder
definition of, 174
depression. See depression
mood stabilizers, 180–181, 956b
Moraxella catarrhalis, 519
moricizine (Ethmozine), 801t, 803, 808
morphine (MSIR, MS Contin)
cancer-related pain treated with, 96
characteristics of, 85–87, 86t
classification of, 4
codeine metabolism to, 87
metabolites of, 98
pain management using, 85–87, 86t, 93
Motofen (difenoxin with atropine sulfate), 999t, 1006
motor areas, 78
Motrin (ibuprofen), 109, 111t
Motrin Sinus Tablets, 764t
moxifloxacin (Avelox, Vigamox), 508t, 1029t
M-R-Vax II (measles and rubella vaccine), 637t
MS Contin (morphine)
cancer-related pain treated with, 96
characteristics of, 85–87, 86t
classification of, 4
codeine metabolism to, 87
metabolites of, 98
pain management using, 85–87, 86t, 93
MSIR (morphine)
cancer-related pain treated with, 96
characteristics of, 85–87, 86t
chronic diarrhea contraindications, 1005
classification of, 4
codeine metabolism to, 87
metabolites of, 98
pain management using, 85–87, 86t, 93
mucolytics, 762
Mucomyst (acetylcysteine)
antidote uses of, 28t
description of, 123
mucolytic uses of, 764t
mucositis, 706b
mucus, 915
multidrug-resistant *Streptococcus pneumoniae,* 469b
multidrug-resistant tuberculosis, 506–507, 544, 550, 553, 555
multiple myeloma, 693
multiple sclerosis, 227–228
mumps vaccine (Mumpsvax), 637t
Mumpsvax (mumps vaccine), 637t
mupirocin (Bactroban), 1043t

muromonab-CD3 (Orthoclone OKT3), 670t, 674, 680–683, 686–687
muscarinic agonist poisoning, 327
muscarinic receptors, 270–271
muscle relaxants. *See also specific drug*
adverse effects of, 233
in children, 232
client teaching about, 231–233
contraindications, 228
drug interactions, 233
goals of, 231
in hepatic-impaired clients, 232
in home care, 232
indications for, 228
mechanism of action, 228
nursing actions for, 232–233
nursing process for, 230–231
in older adults, 232
in renal-impaired clients, 232
selection of, 232
self-administration of, 231
therapeutic effects of, 233
muscle spasm, 227, 230
musculoskeletal system
alcohol abuse effects on, 239b
glucocorticoids' effect on, 354
Muse (alprostadil), 1079
Mutamycin (mitomycin), 696t
Myambutol (ethambutol), 548t, 549
myasthenia gravis
anticholinesterase drugs for, 312–313, 316
assessment of, 311
description of, 307–308
myasthenic crisis, 312–313
Mycamine (micafungin), 1080
Mycelex (clotrimazole), 588b
Mycobacterium avium complex
clarithromycin for, 530
definition of, 528
description of, 550–551
prevention of, 551
Mycobacterium tuberculosis, 542
mycophenolate mofetil (CellCept, Myfortic), 670t, 671, 680–683, 687–688
Mycoplasma pneumoniae, 515
mycoses, 583
Mycostatin (nystatin), 589t, 591, 1044t
Mydriacyl (tropicamide), 1027t
mydriasis, 320
myelin, 75
myelosuppression, 532
Myfortic (mycophenolate mofetil), 670t
Mykrox (metolazone), 864t, 870
Mylotarg (gemtuzumab ozogamicin), 700t, 701
myocardial infarction, 291, 299, 776, 814
myocardial ischemia, 816
myocardium, 773
myoclonic seizure, 194
Mytelase (ambenonium), 309, 310t
myxedema coma, 374

N

Nabi-HB (hepatitis B immune globulin, human), 641t
nabumetone (Relafen), 109, 113t, 114
nadolol (Corgard), 293t, 818t, 844t
nafarelin (Synarel), 342, 343t
nafcillin (Unipen), 486t, 487, 488t
naftifine (Naftin), 589t, 1044t
Naftin (naftifine), 589t, 1044t
Na,K-adenosine triphosphatase, 779
nalbuphine (Nubain), 87t, 89, 101

Nalfon (fenoprofen), 109, 112t, 129
nalidixic acid (NegGram), 521t
nalmefene (Revex), 89–90, 90t
naloxone (Narcan)
antidote uses of, 19, 27b, 29t
characteristics of, 89, 90t
substance abuse disorders treated with, 238t
toxicity indications for, 27b
withdrawal uses of, 96
naltrexone (ReVia), 90, 90t, 238t, 240–241, 242
Namenda (memantine), 314
naphazoline hydrochloride (Privine), 273t, 763t
Naprelan (naproxen sodium), 113t
Naprosyn (naproxen), 109, 113t
naproxen (Naprosyn), 109, 113t, 126
naproxen sodium (Aleve, Anaprox, Naprelan), 113t
Naqua (trichlormethiazide), 864t
naratriptan (Amerge), 116, 117t, 128
Narcan (naloxone)
antidote uses of, 19, 27b, 29t
characteristics of, 89, 90t
substance abuse disorders treated with, 238t
toxicity indications for, 27b
narcolepsy, 253
narcotic antitussives, 763t
Narcotics Anonymous, 251
Nardil (phenelzine), 179t
Naropin (ropivacaine), 1098t
Nasacort (triamcinolone acetonide), 359t, 731b, 754t
nasal congestion, 761
nasal decongestants
adverse effects of, 768
characteristics of, 761–762
client teaching about, 766
contraindications, 761–762
drug interactions, 769
nursing actions for, 768
therapeutic effects of, 768
therapeutic principles for, 766–767
types of, 763t
Nasalide (flunisolide), 358t, 731b, 736t, 754t
Nasarel (flunisolide), 754t
Nascobal, 924t
nasogastric tubes, 46, 934
Nasonex (mometasone), 359t, 736t, 754t
Natacyn (natamycin), 589t, 1029t
natamycin (Natacyn), 589t, 1029t
nateglinide (Starlix), 415, 415t, 430, 433
National Asthma Education and Prevention Program, 730, 731b, 1068b
Natrecor (nesiritide), 782t, 783–784, 790
natural killer cells, 626
Naturetin (bendroflumethiazide), 864t
nausea and vomiting
causes of, 1010
herbal and dietary supplements, 1014
nursing process for, 1014–1015
from opioid analgesics, 100
physiology of, 1010–1011
during pregnancy, 1066
therapeutic principles for, 1015–1017
Navane (thiothixene), 156, 156t, 159t
Navelbine (vinorelbine), 697t
N-desmethyldiazepam, 135
Nebcin (tobramycin), 506t, 1083
NebuPent (pentamidine), 609t, 611, 614–616
Necator americanus, 605b
Necon, 445t
nedocromil (Tilade), 736t, 738
needleless systems, 40, 41b
needles, 38, 40

negative feedback system, 336, 352
NegGram (nalidixic acid), 521t
Neisseria gonorrhoeae, 489, 507
nelfinavir (Viracept), 568t, 573
Nembutal (pentobarbital), 241
neoadjuvant chemotherapy, 710
Neoloid (castor oil), 989t
neomycin, 505t
neomycin, polymyxin B, and bacitracin
　　(Neosporin), 1043t
neonates. *See also* children; infants
　　digoxin in, 788
　　drug therapy in, 62–63
　　immune system of, 629–630
　　pharmacokinetics in, 63t
　　physiologic characteristics of, 63t
　　therapeutics for, 1072
neoplasms, 692–694
neoplastic disorders, 632
Neoral (cyclosporine), 669t, 677
Neosporin (neomycin, polymyxin B, and baci-
　　tracin), 1043t
neostigmine (Prostigmin), 309, 310t, 314, 316
Neo-Synephrine (phenylephrine), 273t, 277t, 278,
　　283, 763t, 831t, 832, 1026t
nephron, 861–862, 862f
nephrotoxicity, 25
nerve fiber, 75
nervous system
　　autonomic. *See* autonomic nervous system
　　central. *See* central nervous system
　　divisions of, 265, 266f
　　endocrine system interactions with, 336
　　glucocorticoids' effect on, 354
　　peripheral. *See* peripheral nervous system
Nesacaine (chloroprocaine), 1098t
nesiritide (Natrecor), 782t, 783–784, 790
Neulasta (pegfilgrastim), 652t, 662
Neumega (oprelvekin), 653t, 656, 660, 663, 707,
　　708t
Neupogen (filgrastim), 652t, 659–661, 707, 708t
neurogenic shock, 829, 830t
neuroleptic malignant syndrome, 170
neuromodulators, 195
neuromuscular blocking agents
　　anticholinesterase drugs' effect on, 308
　　general anesthetics and, 1095–1097
neurons, 75
Neurontin (gabapentin), 197t, 200, 211
neuropathic pain, 84b
neurotransmission
　　in central nervous system disorders, 78
　　description of, 75
　　neurotransmitters, 75–76
　　receptors involved in, 76
　　synapses, 76
　　systems for, 77–78
neurotransmitters, 75–76
Neutra-Phos (phosphate salts), 393t, 394, 402
Neutrexin (trimetrexate), 609t, 611, 616
neutrophils, 626
nevirapine (Viramune), 567t, 576
niacin, 902t, 903, 907, 921t–922t, 924t
niacinamide (nicotinamide), 924t
nicardipine (Cardene), 819t, 845t
Nicoderm CQ (nicotine), 238t
Nicorette (nicotine), 238t
nicotinamide (niacinamide), 924t
nicotine (Habitrol, Nicoderm CQ, Nicorette,
　　Nicotrol, Nicotrol Inhaler, Nicotrol NS),
　　238t, 243–245, 244b
nicotinic receptors, 270–271
Nicotrol Inhaler (nicotine), 238t

Nicotrol (nicotine), 238t
Nicotrol NS (nicotine), 238t
nifedipine (Adalat, Procardia), 819t, 845t
nifedipine (Procardia), 1070t, 1071
Nilandron (nilutamide), 704, 705t, 715
nilutamide (Nilandron), 704, 705t, 715
Nimbex (cisatracurium), 1096t
nimodipine (Nimotop), 819t
nimodipine (Nimotop), 819t
Nimotop (nimodipine), 819t
Nipent (pentostatin), 696t
Nipress (sodium nitroprusside), 846t, 857
Nisoldipine (Sular), 819t, 845t
nitazoxanide (Alinia), 609t, 611, 1001t, 1003
nitrates, 817–819, 823–824
nitric oxide, 816, 840b–841b
Nitro-Bid (nitroglycerin), 817–818, 818t, 824,
　　826, 857
nitrofurantoin (Furadantin, Macrodantin), 521t,
　　526, 1060b
nitrogen mustard derivatives, 695t, 698
nitroglycerin (Nitro-Bid), 817–818, 818t, 824,
　　826, 857
nitrosoureas, 695t, 698
nitrous oxide, 1096t
Nix (permethrin), 610t, 612, 616
Nizoral (ketoconazole), 587b, 589t, 591, 600,
　　1044t
N-methyl D-aspartate, 78
nociceptors, 82–83
Noctec (chloral hydrate), 138, 139t
NoDoz, 257t
Nolahist (phenindamine), 752
Nolvadex (tamoxifen), 704, 705t, 715
nomogram, 62, 64f
non-narcotic antitussives, 763t
non-nucleoside reverse transcriptase inhibitors,
　　563, 566t–567t, 569–570
nonopioid analgesics, 93
nonphenothiazines, 155–156, 158t–160t, 160–161
nonsteroidal anti-inflammatory drugs
　　adverse effects of, 108
　　Alzheimer's disease and, 314
　　antiplatelet activity of, 884
　　in children, 125
　　client teaching about, 120
　　contraindications, 108–109
　　drugs affected by, 122–123
　　in home care, 126
　　indications for, 106b, 107, 122
　　labeling of, 108
　　mechanism of action, 104
　　in older adults, 125
　　ophthalmic uses of, 1025–1026, 1030t
　　during pregnancy, 1064b
　　in renal-impaired patients, 125
　　rheumatoid arthritis treated with, 124
　　self-administration of, 120
　　types of, 109, 114–115
noradrenergic neurons, 236
noradrenergic system
　　in anxiety disorders, 133
　　description of, 77, 236
Norcuron (vecuronium), 1096t
Nordette, 445t
Norditropin (somatropin), 344t
norepinephrine (endogenous)
　　depression and, 174
　　functions of, 268
　　in sympathetic nervous system, 267–268
　　synthesis of, 266–267
norepinephrine (Levophed), 273t, 831t, 832, 835
norethindrone acetate (Aygestin), 440, 443t
Norflex (orphenadrine citrate), 229t, 230

norfloxacin (Noroxin), 508t
norgestimate, 440
norgestrel, 440
Norinyl, 445t
Normodyne (labetalol), 293t, 845t
Noroxin (norfloxacin), 508t
Norpace (disopyramide), 800t, 803, 811t, 1083
Norplant, 446t
Nor-QD, 446t
Nortrel, 445t
nortriptyline (Aventyl, Pamelor), 178t, 1083
Norvasc (amlodipine), 819t, 845t
Norvir (ritonavir), 568t, 569, 578–579
nose drops, 48
nosocomial infections, 468, 471
Novantrone (mitoxantrone), 696t
Novolin N (isophane insulin suspension), 409t,
　　422
Novolin R (insulin injection), 409t
Novolog (insulin aspart), 408, 410t
NPH Iletin II (isophane insulin suspension), 409t,
　　422, 429
NPH (isophane insulin suspension), 409t, 429
Nubain (nalbuphine), 87t, 89, 101
nucleoside reverse transcriptase inhibitors, 563,
　　566t–567t
nucleotide reverse transcriptase inhibitor, 563,
　　567t
nucleus, 11b
Numorphan (oxymorphone), 86t, 88
nurse, 32
nursing diagnoses
　　description of, 52–53
　　for pain, 92
nursing process
　　assessment, 51–52
　　definition of, 51
　　evaluation, 53–54
　　interventions, 53
　　nursing diagnoses, 52–53
　　for pain, 91–92
　　planning/goals, 53
nutrition
　　enteral, 918, 935, 937, 945–946
　　parenteral, 937
nutritional deficiencies
　　description of, 917–918
　　management of, 935, 937
　　nursing process for, 933–935
nutritional products, 918–919
nutritional status, 631
nutritional support
　　adverse effects of, 948–949
　　in children, 941–943
　　in critical illness, 944–945
　　enteral, 918, 935, 937, 945–946
　　in hepatic-impaired clients, 944
　　in home care, 945
　　nursing actions for, 945–950
　　in older adults, 943
　　parenteral, 937
　　in renal-impaired clients, 943–944
Nutropin (somatropin), 344t
nystatin (Mycostatin), 589t, 591, 1044t

O

obesity
　　behavioral modification for, 963
　　cancer and, 954b
　　cardiovascular disorders and, 954b
　　central, 953
　　in children, 955, 965–966

client teaching about, 961–962
description of, 952–953
diabetes mellitus and, 954b, 955
drugs for, 957–959
dyslipidemias and, 954b
etiology of, 953, 955
factors associated with, 953, 955
gallstones and, 954b
health risks of, 954b–955b
in hepatic-impaired clients, 966
herbal and dietary supplements for, 958–959
in home care, 966
management of, 962–964
medications associated with, 956b
metabolic syndrome and, 954b
nursing process for, 959–960
in older adults, 966
orlistat for, 957t, 958, 962, 967
osteoarthritis and, 955b
phentermine hydrochloride for, 957, 957t, 967
prevalence of, 953
prevention of, 960, 962
psychosocial factors of, 955
in renal-impaired clients, 966
sibutramine for, 957t, 957–958, 962, 967
visceral, 953
obsessive-compulsive disorder, 134b
octreotide (Sandostatin), 342, 343t, 349, 1002, 1002t
Ocufen (flurbiprofen), 1030t
Ocuflox (ofloxacin), 508t, 1029t
ocular infections, 1033
ofloxacin (Floxin, Ocuflox), 508t, 1029t
Ogen (estropipate), 442t
Ogestrel, 445t
ointments, 1042b
olanzapine (Zyprexa), 156t, 159t, 160, 168, 171, 956b
older adults
    acetaminophen in, 125
    adrenergic drugs in, 283
    adverse effects in, 64
    alpha-adrenergic agonists in, 300
    alpha-adrenergic blockers in, 300
    aminoglycosides in, 479, 511
    androgens in, 460
    antianginal drugs in, 823
    antiasthmatic drugs in, 743
    anticholinergic drugs in, 328
    anticoagulants in, 890
    antidepressants in, 187–188
    antidysrhythmic drugs in, 809
    antiemetic drugs in, 1017
    antiepileptic drugs in, 207–208
    antifungal drugs in, 597
    antihistamines in, 756
    antihypertensive drugs in, 855
    antimicrobial drugs in, 479
    antineoplastic drugs in, 712
    antiparasitic drugs in, 614
    antiparkinson drugs in, 222
    antipsychotic drugs in, 166, 166b
    antitubercular drugs in, 555
    antiviral drugs in, 575
    benzodiazepine use in, 144
    beta blockers in, 300
    beta-lactam antibacterials in, 497–498
    calcium channel blockers in, 823
    central nervous system stimulants in, 260
    cephalosporins in, 479
    cholinergic drugs in, 315
    corticosteroids in, 367, 743
    dermatologic drugs in, 1054

diabetes mellitus in, 427
digoxin in, 788
diuretics in, 871
drug administration in, 66
drug dosage for, 65–66
drug selection for, 65–66
drug therapy in, 63–66
dyslipidemic drugs in, 906
erythromycin in, 535
estrogens in, 450
fluoroquinolones in, 511
growth hormone in, 348
heparin in, 890
hypercalcemia in, 399
hypertension in, 855
hypocalcemia in, 399
hypoglycemic drugs in, 427
immune system in, 630–631
immunizations in, 646
immunosuppressants in, 681–682
laxatives in, 993
mineral–electrolytes for, 943
monoamine oxidase inhibitors in, 188
nonsteroidal anti-inflammatory drugs in, 125
nutritional support in, 943
obesity in, 966
ophthalmic drugs in, 1034
opioid analgesics in, 98
penicillins in, 479, 497–498
pharmacokinetics in, 20, 65t
physiologic considerations in, 65t
progestins in, 450
respiratory disorders in, 767
selective serotonin reuptake inhibitors in, 187
shock in, 834
skeletal muscle relaxants in, 232
sulfonamides in, 524
tetracyclines in, 524
theophylline in, 743
thiazide diuretics in, 871
thyroid drugs in, 382
tricyclic antidepressants in, 187–188
tuberculosis in, 555
vitamins for, 943
warfarin in, 890
olmesartan (Benicar), 843t
olopatadine (Patanol), 1030t
omalizumab (Xolair), 670t, 674, 738
Omnicef (cefdinir), 490t
Omnipen (ampicillin), 487, 488t
Oncaspar (pegaspargase), 699
oncogenes, 692
oncology, 691
Oncovin (vincristine), 697t, 715
ondansetron (Zofran), 1012t–1013t, 1013–1014
Opthaine (proparacaine), 1028t
ophthalmic drugs. *See also specific drug*
    adverse effects of, 1035–1036
    anesthetics, 1025
    antihistamines, 1025
    antimicrobials, 1025
    autonomic nervous system drugs, 1025
    carbonic anhydrase inhibitors, 1026, 1027t–1028t
    in children, 1034
    classification of, 1025–1026
    client teaching about, 1032
    corticosteroids, 1025, 1030t
    drug interactions, 1036–1037
    fluorescein, 1026
    in home care, 1034
    mast cell stabilizers, 1025
    nonsteroidal anti-inflammatory drugs, 1025–1026, 1030t

nursing actions for, 1034–1037
nursing process for, 1031
in older adults, 1034
overview of, 1024–1025
prostaglandin analogs, 1026
therapeutic effects of, 1035
therapeutic principles for, 1032–1034
ophthalmic neonatorum, 1072
opiate receptors, 83
opioid analgesics
    abuse of, 242
    administration of
        in children, 97
        description of, 83
        frequency of, 95–96
        guidelines for, 99–100
        routes of, 94–96
    adverse effects of, 85, 100
    agonists, 85–89, 86t–87t
    agonists/antagonists, 87t, 89
    antagonists, 89–90, 90t
    antidote for, 29t
    in burn patients, 97
    central nervous system effects, 83, 85
    characteristics of, 83, 85
    in children, 97–98
    client teaching guidelines for, 93
    colic treated with, 97
    contraindications, 85
    in critical illness clients, 98–99
    definition of, 83
    dependence on, 242
    dosage of, 94
    equianalgesic doses of, 85
    in hepatic-impaired clients, 98
    in home care, 99
    indications for, 85, 96–97
    interactions, 100–101
    mechanism of action, 85
    nursing actions for, 99–101
    in older adults, 98
    in opiate-tolerant clients, 97
    pharmacokinetics of, 83
    postoperative use of, 97
    during pregnancy, 1060b
    PRN dosing of, 95
    in renal-impaired clients, 98
    self-administration of, 93
    storage of, 33
    therapeutic effects of, 100
    toxicity, 96
    withdrawal from, 96, 242
opioid receptors, 85
opportunistic infections, 468
oprelvekin (Neumega), 653t, 656, 660, 663, 707, 708t
optic disk, 1024
Opticrom (cromolyn), 1029t
OptiPranolol (metipranolol), 293t, 1027t
Optivar (azelastine), 1029t
oral administration
    description of, 38, 39t
    nursing action for, 45–46
oral cavity, 913
oral contraceptives, 448. *See also* hormonal contraceptives
oral solutions, 35t
Orap (pimozide), 156
Oretic (hydrochlorothiazide), 864t, 868, 870
organ transplantation
    immunosuppression for, 667
    rejection reactions, 667
organic nitrates, 817–819, 823–824

organophosphate insecticides, 314
orlistat (Xenical), 957t, 958, 962, 967
Orphan Drug Act, 5t
orphenadrine citrate (Norflex), 229t, 230
Ortho Evra, 446t
Ortho Tri-Cyclen, 446t
Ortho-Cept, 445t
Orthoclone OKT3 (muromonab-CD3), 670t, 674, 680–683, 686–687
Ortho-Cyclen, 445t
Ortho-Novum, 445t
orthostatic hypotension, 223
Orth-Prefest, 444t
Oruvail (ketoprofen), 109, 112t
olsalazine (Dipentum), 1080
Os-Cal (calcium carbonate precipitated), 392t
oseltamivir (Tamiflu), 565t, 570
Osmitrol (mannitol), 865t, 866, 1028t
Osmoglyn (glycerin), 865t, 1028t
osmotic diuretics, 18, 866
osteoarthritis, 106b, 118, 124, 955b
osteoporosis, 391b, 394, 396, 398, 450
Otrivin (xylometazoline hydrochloride), 273t, 763t
ovarian hormones, 336
Ovcon, 445t
overdosage, 18
overdose, 26, 28t–29t
over-the-counter medications
    client teaching about, 57
    Food and Drug Administration approval of, 7
overweight
    definition of, 952
    management of, 962–964
    prevention strategies, 960, 962
Ovide (malathion), 610t, 612
Ovidrel (choriogonadotropin alfa), 344t
Ovrette, 446t
oxacillin (Bactocill), 487, 488t
oxaliplatin (Eloxatin), 695t
oxaprozin (Daypro), 109, 114t
oxazepam (Serax), 136t–137t
oxcarbazepine (Trileptal), 198t, 201, 204, 207, 209, 211
oxiconazole (Oxistat), 590t, 1044t
Oxistat (oxiconazole), 590t, 1044t
oxybutynin (Ditropan, Ditropan XL), 324t, 325
oxycodone (OxyContin; Roxicodone), 86t, 88
OxyContin (oxycodone), 86t, 88
oxymetazoline hydrochloride (Afrin), 273t, 763t
oxymorphone (Numorphan), 86t, 88
oxytocics, 1075–1077
oxytocin (Pitocin), 79, 341, 345t, 345–346, 349–350, 1070t, 1071–1072, 1077

P
p53, 692
paclitaxel (Taxol), 697t, 711, 714
Paget's disease, 390, 391b
pain
    acute, 84b, 95, 99
    assessment of, 91–92
    cancer-related
        acetaminophen for, 124–125
        description of, 84b
        opioid analgesics for, 96–97, 99
    chronic, 84b, 95, 99
    classification of, 83, 84b
    definition of, 103
    description of, 82
    endogenous analgesia system for, 83
    herbal medicines for, 117–118
    intensity of, 91
    location of, 91
    muscle spasm-related, 230
    neuropathic, 84b
    nociceptors' role in, 82–83
    nursing process for, 91–92
    perception of, 91
    physiology of, 82–83
    referred, 91
    somatic, 84b
    treatment of
        drug dosages, 94
        drug selection, 93
        goals, 92
        nonopioid analgesics, 93
        opioids. See opioid analgesics
    visceral, 84b
palifermin (Kepivance), 1080
palliative chemotherapy, 710
palonosetron (Aloxi), 1013t, 1013–1014
Pamelor (nortriptyline), 178t, 1083
pamidronate (Aredia), 390, 393t, 401
Panafil (papain), 1046t
pancreas, 914
Pancreas (pancreatin), 1002t
pancreatic juices, 915
pancreatin (Viokase, Pancrease), 1002t
pancuronium, 1096t
Panglobulin (immune globulin intravenous), 642t
panic disorder, 134b
panthothenic acid
    deficiency of, 922t
    food sources of, 922t
    function of, 922t
    recommended daily intake of, 922t
papain (Panafil), 1046t
para-aminobenzoic acid, 516
para-aminosalicylic acid, 550
paranoia, 153
Paraplatin (carboplatin), 695t
parasite, 603
parasympathetic nervous system, 270–271, 319
parathyroid hormone, 336, 387, 393t
paregoric, 999t
parenteral nutrition, 937
parenteral solutions, 35t
paricalcitol (Zemplar), 392t
parietal pleura, 726
parkinsonism, 169, 214, 220
Parkinson's disease
    anticholinergic drugs for, 321
    assessment of, 219
    definition of, 214
    description of, 77
    nursing process for, 219
Parlodel (bromocriptine), 217t, 218, 224
Parnate (tranylcypromine), 179t
paromomycin (Humatin), 505t–506t
paroxetine (Paxil), 177, 179t, 186
partial agonists, 161
partial dopamine agonists, 161
partial seizures, 193, 204–205
passive diffusion, 13b
passive immunity, 625, 634
pastes, 1042b
Patanol (olopatadine), 1030t
Pathocil (dicloxacillin), 487, 488t
patient-controlled analgesia, 95
Paxil (paroxetine), 177, 179t, 186
peak expiratory flow rate, 739
PediaCare (ibuprofen), 111t
pediculicides, 610t, 612
pediculosis, 605–606, 613
PedvaxHIB (*Haemophilus influenzae* b conjugate vaccine), 635t
pegaspargase (Oncaspar), 699
Pegasys (peginterferon alfa-2a), 653t
pegfilgrastim (Neulasta), 652t, 662
peginterferon alfa-2a (Pegasys), 653t
peginterferon alfa-2b (PEG-Intron), 653t
PEG-Intron (peginterferon alfa-2b), 653t
pegvisomant (Somavert), 342
pemetrexed (Alimta), 696t, 698
penbutolol (Levatol), 293t, 844t
penciclovir (Denavir), 1044t
penicillamine (Cuprimine), 929, 930t
penicillin(s)
    absorption of, 486
    administration of, 499
    aminoglycosides and, 497
    aminopenicillins, 487
    in children, 479, 497
    client teaching about, 495
    contraindications, 487
    in critical illness, 499
    description of, 485–486
    drug interactions, 501
    extended-spectrum, 487
    in hepatic-impaired clients, 480
    hypersensitivity to, 497
    indications for, 486–487
    nursing actions for, 499–501
    in older adults, 479
    penicillinase-resistant, 487, 488t
    during pregnancy, 1060b
    probenecid and, 497
    in renal-impaired clients, 497
    self-administration of, 495
    streptococcal infections treated with, 497
    therapeutic principles for, 495–499
penicillin G benzathine (Bicillin), 488t
penicillin G (Pfizerpen, Wycillin), 486t, 487
penicillin G potassium and sodium (Pfizerpen), 488t
penicillin G procaine (Wycillin), 488t
penicillin V (Beepen VK, Pen-Vee-K, Veetids), 486t, 487, 488t
penicillinase-resistant penicillins, 487, 488t
penicillin–beta-lactamase inhibitors, 487–489, 488t
penicillin-binding proteins, 473, 485
penicillin-resistant *Streptococcus pneumoniae*, 472b
Pentam 300 (pentamidine), 609t, 611, 614–616
pentamidine (Pentam 300, NebuPent), 609t, 611, 614–616
Pentasa (mesalamine), 1080
pentobarbital (Nembutal), 241
pentosan polysulfate sodium (Elmiron), 1080
pentostatin (Nipent), 696t
Pentothal (thiopental), 1096t
Pen-Vee-K (penicillin V), 486t, 487
peptides, 76
Pepto-Bismol (bismuth subsalicylate), 1001t, 1002
Percocet (oxycodone), 94t
Perdiem Plain (psyllium), 988, 989t
pergolide (Permax), 217t, 218, 224
Pergonal (menotropins), 342, 344t, 349
pericardium, 773
perindopril (Aceon), 843t
peripheral arterial insufficiency, 903–904
peripheral nervous system, 265
peripheral proteins, 11
peripherally inserted central catheters, 41b
Permax (pergolide), 217t, 218, 224

permethrin (Nix, Elimite), 610t, 612, 616
pernicious anemia, 938
perphenazine (Trilafon), 156t–157t
Persantine (dipyridamole), 882t, 885
petechiae, 1048
Pfizerpen (penicillin G), 486t, 487
Pfizerpen (penicillin G potassium and sodium), 488t
phagocytosis, 355
pharmacodynamics, 17–18
pharmacoeconomics, 8
pharmacokinetics
    absorption, 12, 14
    in children, 20, 63t
    client-related variables that affect, 20–25
    definition of, 12
    distribution, 14
    in elderly, 20
    excretion, 15
    in infants, 20, 63t
    metabolism, 15
    in neonates, 63t
    in older adults, 65t
    of opioid analgesics, 83
    pathologic conditions that affect, 21, 22t–24t
    pregnancy-related changes, 1058b
    renal impairments' effect on, 23t
pharmacology, 3, 8
pharmacotherapy, 3
pharynx, 726
phenazopyridine (Pyridium), 521t
phencyclidine, 246
phenelzine (Nardil), 179t
Phenergan (promethazine), 155, 752, 756, 1011, 1012t
phenindamine (Nolahist), 752
phenobarbital, 198t, 201, 208, 212, 1083
phenothiazines, 29t, 155, 1011, 1012t, 1015, 1017
phentermine hydrochloride (Adipex-P, Ionamin, Pro-Fast), 957, 957t, 967
phenylephrine (Neo-Synephrine), 273t, 277t, 278, 283, 763t, 831t, 832, 1026t
phenytoin (Dilantin)
    administration of, 209
    adverse effects of, 195
    characteristics of, 198t
    client teaching about, 204
    drug interactions, 211
    dysrhythmias treated with, 800t, 803, 811t
    nonantiepileptic drugs affected by, 207
    nonsteroidal anti-inflammatory drugs effect on, 123
    osteoporosis risks, 398
    pharmacokinetics of, 195
    in renal-impaired clients, 208
    serum levels of, 1083
pheochromocytoma, 291
PhosLo (calcium acetate), 392t
phosphate metabolism, 387
phosphate salts (Neutra-Phos), 393t, 394, 402
phosphodiesterase inhibitors, 782t, 783
phospholipids, 337
phosphorated carbohydrate solution (Emetrol), 1013t, 1014
phosphorus
    calcium and, 388, 389b
    in children, 943t
    daily requirements, 389b
    functions of, 389b
    sources of, 389b
physical dependence, 236
Physicians' Desk Reference, 8

physostigmine salicylate (Antilirium), 28t, 309–311, 310t, 327
piggyback method, 48
Pilocar (pilocarpine), 1027t
pilocarpine (Isopto Carpine, Pilocar), 1027t
pimecrolimus (Elidel), 1046t
pimozide (Orap), 156
pindolol (Visken), 293t, 844t
Pin-Rid (pyrantel), 610t, 612
pinworm infections, 605b
pioglitazone (Actos), 414t, 430–431, 433
piperacillin (Pipracil), 486t, 487
piperacillin-tazobactam (Zosyn), 488t, 489
Pipracil (piperacillin), 487
pirbuterol (Maxair), 273t, 732, 732t–733t
piroxicam (Feldene), 114, 114t
Pitocin (oxytocin), 79, 341, 345t, 345–346, 349–350, 1070t, 1071–1072
pituitary gland
    anterior, 336, 339, 456
    disorders of, 347
    posterior, 339, 341
pituitary hormones
    adverse effects of, 349
    anterior, 336, 340–342, 343t–344t, 345
    drug interactions, 349–350
    nursing actions for, 348–350
    nursing process for, 346
    posterior, 336, 341, 344t–345t, 345–346
    therapeutic effects of, 348–349
    therapeutic principles for, 346–348
placebo, 25
placebo response, 25
placental hormones, 336
planning, 53
plant alkaloids, 697t, 699
Plaquenil (hydroxychloroquine), 606, 608t
plasma thromboplastin antecedent, 877t
Plasmodium spp., 604, 606
platelet(s)
    activation of, 878b
    adhesion of, 878b–879b
    aggregation of, 879b
    description of, 776
    procoagulant activity of, 878b–879b
platelet-activating factor, 105b
Platinol (cisplatin), 695t, 713–714
platinum compounds, 695t, 698
Plavix (clopidogrel), 882t, 884, 891
Plenaxis (abarelix), 342
Plendil (felodipine), 819t, 845t
Pletal (cilostazol), 882t, 885, 891
pleura, 726
pleural cavity, 726
pneumococcal meningitis, 469b
pneumococcal sinusitis, 469b
pneumococcal vaccine, polyvalent (Pneumovax 23, Pnu-Imune 23), 637t–638t, 648
pneumococcal 7–valent conjugate vaccine (Prevnar), 638t, 645, 648
Pneumocystis jiroveci
    description of, 604
    drugs for, 609t, 611
    during pregnancy, 1067
pneumocystosis, 604–605
Pneumovax 23 (pneumococcal vaccine, polyvalent), 637t–638t
Pnu-Imune 23 (pneumococcal vaccine, polyvalent), 637t–638t
podophyllotoxins, 697t, 699
poliomyelitis vaccine, inactivated (IPOL), 638t, 645, 648
polycarbophil (FiberCon, Mitrolan), 988, 989t

polyclonal antibodies, 673
polyenes, 583, 586
polyethylene glycol–electrolyte solution (CoLyte, GoLytely), 988, 989t
Polygam S/D (immune globulin intravenous), 642t
Polysporin (bacitracin and polymyxin B), 1043t
polyvinyl alcohol (Liquifilm), 1028t
Ponstel (mefenamic acid), 113t, 114
Pontocaine (tetracaine), 1028t, 1098t
postantibiotic effects, 510
posterior pituitary hormones, 336, 341, 344t–345t, 345–346
postganglionic fibers, 266
postganglionic-active drugs, 844t
postherpetic neuralgia, 195
postmenopausal women, 439b
postsynaptic adrenergic receptors, 273
post-traumatic stress disorder, 134b
Posture (tricalcium phosphate), 392t
potassium
    administration of, 946–947
    description of, 926t
    disorders involving, 939–940. See also hyper-kalemia; hypokalemia
potassium channel blockers, 801t–802t, 804–805
potassium chloride, 788, 931t–932t, 933
potassium preparations, 931t–932t, 933
potassium-losing diuretics, 868
potassium-sparing diuretics, 780b–781b, 865t, 866, 868, 871
potentiation, 19
powders, 1042b
pralidoxime (Protopam), 314
pramipexole (Mirapex), 217t, 218, 221
pramlintide (Symlin), 1080
pramoxine (Tronothane), 1098t
Prandin (repaglinide), 415, 415t, 430, 433
Pravachol (pravastatin), 901, 902t, 905
pravastatin (Pravachol), 901, 902t, 905
Prazosin (Minipress), 292t, 294, 844t
Precedex (dexmedetomidine), 138, 139t
Precose (acarbose), 414t, 433
prednisolone acetate, 359t
prednisolone (Delta-Cortef, Econopred), 359t, 1030t
prednisone (Deltasone), 359t, 363, 393t
preeclampsia, 1066
pregabalin (Lyrica), 1080
preganglionic fibers, 266
pregnancy
    acquired immunodeficiency syndrome during, 1066–1067
    adrenergics during, 1060b
    alcohol use during, 1065b
    anemia during, 1064
    angiotensin II receptor blockers during, 1060b
    angiotensin-converting enzyme inhibitors, 1060b
    antibacterials during, 1060b–1061b
    anticholinergics during, 1061b
    anticoagulants during, 1061b
    antidepressants during, 1061b
    antidiabetics during, 1061b
    antiemetics during, 1061b
    antiepileptic drugs during, 1061b–1062b, 1069
    antifungal drugs during, 1062b
    antihistamines during, 1062b
    antihypertensives during, 1062b
    antipsychotics during, 1062b
    antitubercular drugs during, 1062b

pregnancy (*continued*)
  antiviral drugs during, 1062b–1063b
  aspirin during, 1063b
  asthma during, 1067
  benzodiazepines during, 1060b
  beta blockers during, 1063b
  caffeine use during, 1065b
  calcium channel blockers during, 1063b
  cholinergic drug contraindications during, 308–309
  cigarette smoking during, 1065b
  client teaching about, 1074
  cocaine use during, 1065b
  constipation during, 1064
  corticosteroids during, 1063b
  description of, 1057
  diabetes mellitus during, 1065–1069
  digoxin during, 1063b
  diuretics during, 1063b
  drug distribution during, 14, 20
  dyslipidemics during, 1063b–1064b
  Food and Drug Administration drug risk cate-
    gories, 1058, 1059b
  gastroesophageal reflux disease during,
    1064–1065
  herbal and dietary supplements during, 1059,
    1064
  home care, 1073–1074
  human immunodeficiency virus during,
    1066–1067
  hypertension during, 1066, 1069
  infections during, 1066–1067
  latent tuberculosis infection during, 546b
  marijuana use during, 1065b
  maternal–placental–fetal circulation, 1058
  methamphetamine use during, 1065b
  nausea and vomiting during, 1066
  nonsteroidal anti-inflammatory drugs, 1064b
  nursing process for, 1072–1073
  opioid analgesics during, 1060b
  pharmacokinetics changes, 1058b
  physiologic changes, 1058b
  retinoids during, 1064b
  seizure disorders during, 1069
  therapeutic principles for, 1073
  urinary tract infections during, 1067
Pregnyl (human chorionic gonadotropin), 342,
    344t, 349
Premarin (conjugated estrogens), 440, 441t
premature ventricular contracts, 798b–799b
Premphase, 444t
Prempro, 444t
Pre-Pen (benzylpenicilloyl polylysine), 497
Prescription Drug User Fee Act, 5t
prescription medicine
  client teaching about, 55–56
  self-administration of, 55–56
pressor effect, 274
pressure ulcers, 1041, 1053
presystemic metabolism, 15
Preven, 446t, 449
Prevnar (pneumococcal 7–valent conjugate vac-
    cine), 638t
Prialt (ziconotide), 1081
Priftin (rifapentine), 548t, 549
prilocaine (Citanest), 1098t
Primacor (milrinone), 782t, 783, 790, 831t, 832
primaquine, 608t, 611
primary open-angle glaucoma, 1024
Primaxin (imipenem-cilastatin), 486t, 491, 494,
    494t
Prinivil (lisinopril), 843t
Prinzide, 848t

Privine (naphazoline hydrochloride), 273t, 763t
ProAmatine (mitodrine), 1080
Pro-Banthine (propantheline bromide), 323t
probenecid (Benemid), 115, 116t, 129, 497
procainamide (Pronestyl, Procanbid), 21, 800t,
    803, 811t, 1083
Procanbid (procainamide), 800t, 803, 811t, 1083
procarbazine (Matulane), 697t, 715
Procardia (nifedipine), 819t, 845t, 1070t, 1071
Procardia XL (nifedipine), 845t
prochlorperazine (Compazine), 1011, 1012t
proconvertin, 877t
Procrit (epoetin alfa, erythropoietin), 652t, 655,
    658, 663, 707, 708t
procyclidine (Kemadrin), 323t, 325
prodrugs, 15
Pro-Fast (phentermine hydrochloride), 957, 957t,
    967
Profenal (suprofen), 1030t
Progestasert intrauterine, 446t
progesterone, 336, 437–438, 443t
progestin(s)
  adverse effects of, 452
  characteristics of, 440, 441t–442t
  description of, 436
  drug interactions, 452–453
  formulations, 440, 442t–443t, 443
  in home care, 450
  indications for, 438–439
  nursing actions for, 451–453
  nursing process for, 444, 446–447
  in older adults, 450
  selection of, 448
  synthesis of, 436
  therapeutic effects of, 451
progestin–estrogen combinations, 439b, 444t, 452
proglotids, 605b
Prograf (tacrolimus), 671t, 672–673, 677,
    680–683, 687–689
prokinetic agents, 1011–1013, 1012t
prolactin, 341
prolactin-inhibitory factor, 79, 340
prolactin-releasing factor, 340
Proleukin (aldesleukin), 653t, 656, 658, 663–664
Prolixin Decanoate (fluphenazine decanoate),
    156t–157t, 168
Prolixin Enanthate (fluphenazine enanthate),
    156t–157t, 168
Proloprim (trimethoprim), 522t
promethazine (Phenergan), 155, 752, 756, 1011,
    1012t
Pronestyl (procainamide), 800t, 803, 811t, 1083
propafenone (Rythmol), 800t, 803, 811t
propantheline bromide (Pro-Banthine), 323t
proparacaine (Alcaine, Opthaine), 1028t, 1098t
Propine (dipivefrin), 1026t
Propionibacterium acnes, 1041, 1052
propionic acid derivatives, 109
propoxyphene (Darvon), 86t, 88–89
propranolol (Inderal)
  angina pectoris treated with, 818t, 820
  antidysrhythmic uses of, 801t, 804, 808–809
  antihypertensive uses of, 845t
  characteristics of, 293t, 295, 300, 377t, 378
  serum levels of, 1083
propylhexedrine (Benzedrex), 273t
propylthiouracil, 376, 377t, 380, 384
ProSom (estazolam), 136t–137t
prostacyclin, 104t, 841b
prostaglandins
  COX-1 production of, 104, 106
  D2, 104t
  definition of, 103, 839

description of, 82–83
  E₂, 104t
  F₂, 104t
  I₂, 104t, 108
  pathologic, 107f
  physiologic, 107f
  types of, 104t
Prostigmin (neostigmine), 309, 310t, 314, 316
Prostin E₂ (dinoprostone), 1070t
protamine sulfate, 28t, 886, 886t
protease inhibitors, 101, 565, 568t, 569
proteasome inhibitors, 700t, 702
protein binding, 14, 14f, 19
protein channels, 13b
protein-derived hormones, 337
Proteus spp., 470b, 519–520
prothrombin, 877t
prothrombin time, 888
proto-oncogenes, 692
Protopam (pralidoxime), 314
Protopic (tacrolimus), 1046t
protoplasm, 11b
prototype drugs, 4
protozoal infections
  amebiasis, 603–604, 612
  giardiasis, 604
  helminthiasis, 605
  malaria, 604, 612–613
  pediculosis, 605–606
  pneumocystosis, 604–605
  scabies, 605–606, 613
  toxoplasmosis, 604
  trichomoniasis, 604, 613
protriptyline (Vivactil), 178t
Proventil (albuterol), 273t, 732, 732t–733t
Provera (medroxyprogesterone acetate), 442t,
    715
Provigil (modafinil), 254–256, 255t, 259, 261
Prozac (fluoxetine)
  characteristics of, 178t
  description of, 177
  half-life of, 186
  marketing of, 8
pseudoallergic drug reactions, 750
pseudoallergies, 752
pseudoephedrine (Sudafed, Dimetapp), 273t,
    277t, 278, 763t
Pseudomonas aeruginosa, 470b–471b
psoriasis, 678–679, 1040, 1053
psoriatic arthritis, 678–679
psychological dependence, 235–236
psychosis
  acute, 153
  chronic, 153
  definition of, 153
psyllium preparations (Metamucil, Effersyllium,
    Serutan, Perdiem Plain), 988, 989t, 1002t
Pulmicort Respules (budesonide), 358t, 363,
    731b, 732t
Pulmicort Terbuhaler (budesonide), 358t, 363,
    731b, 732t, 736t
pulmonic valve, 774
pupil, 1023
Pure Food and Drug Act, 5t
Purinethol (mercaptopurine), 696t, 713–714, 719
pyrantel (Pin-Rid), 610t, 612
pyrazinamide, 548t, 552
Pyridium (phenazopyridine), 521t
pyridostigmine (Mestinon), 310t, 311, 314
pyridoxine
  antidote uses of, 28t–29t
  in children, 942t
  deficiency of, 922t

food sources of, 922t
function of, 922t
preparations, 925t
recommended daily intake of, 922t
pyrimethamine (Daraprim), 609t, 611

Q

quaternary amines, 319, 320t
quazepam (Doral), 136t–137t
Questran (cholestyramine), 901, 902t, 905, 1001t
quetiapine (Seroquel), 156t, 159t, 161, 168, 171–172
quinapril (Accupril), 843t
quinidine, 800t, 802, 811t
quinidine salts, 802–803
quinine (Quinamm), 609t, 611
quinupristin-dalfopristin (Synercid), 479, 531t, 532, 537–538
QVAR (beclomethasone), 358t, 363, 731b, 732t, 735, 736t

R

R on T phenomenon, 799b
rabies immune globulin (BayRab, Imogam), 642t
rabies vaccine (human diploid cell rabies vaccine [HDCV]) (Imovax), 638t
radioactive iodine, 381–382
raloxifene (Evista), 398
ramipril (Altace), 843t
Ramsay scale, 148
Rapamune (Sirolimus), 670t, 672, 677, 680–683, 687–688
rapid-acting insulins, 408
Raptiva (efalizumab), 670t, 673
rasagiline (Agilect), 221
rasburicase (Elitek), 1080
Razadyne (galantamine), 310t, 311, 314
Rebetron (interferon alfa-2b and ribavirin), 654t
Rebif (interferon beta-1a), 654t
receptor(s)
alpha₁, 269, 269t
alpha₂, 269, 269t
beta₁, 269, 269t
beta₂, 269, 269t
central nervous system, 76
cholinergic, 270–271
desensitization of, 270
dopamine, 77
dopaminergic, 269–270
hormone, 337
muscarinic, 270–271
nicotinic, 270–271
opioid, 85
serotonin, 77, 133
receptor desensitization, 18
receptor protein, 17
Recombivax HB (hepatitis B vaccine), 636t
recommended dietary allowance, 919b
rectal suppositories
description of, 36t, 48
fecal impaction treated with, 993
opioid, 98
reentry excitation, 795
referred pain, 91
Refludan (lepirudin), 881t, 883, 891
refraction, 1024
refractive errors, 1024
Reglan (metoclopramide), 1011–1013, 1012t, 1016
Regranex (becaplermin), 1046t
Regular Iletin II (insulin injection), 409t

rejection reactions
antirejection agents, 672–673
description of, 667
Relafen (nabumetone), 109, 113t, 114
relative refractory period, 795
Relenza (zanamivir), 565t, 570
Relpax (eletriptan), 116, 117t, 128–129
REM sleep, 133
Remeron (mirtazapine), 146, 179t, 180, 182, 189–190
Remicade (infliximab), 124, 670t, 675
remifentanil (Ultiva), 87, 1096t
remodeling, 390
Remodulin (treprostinil), 882t
Renagel (sevelamer), 1080
renal colic, 326
renal impairment
acetaminophen in, 125
adrenergic drugs in, 283
alpha-adrenergic agonists in, 301
alpha-adrenergic blockers in, 301
aminoglycosides in, 511
angiotensin II receptor blockers in, 856
angiotensin-converting enzyme inhibitors in, 855–856
antianginal drugs in, 823, 825
antianxiety drugs in, 147
antiasthmatic drugs in, 743
anticholinergic drugs in, 328
anticoagulants in, 890–891
antidepressants in, 188
antidysrhythmic drugs in, 809
antiemetic drugs in, 1017
antiepileptic drugs in, 208
antihistamines in, 757
antihyperitensive drugs in, 855–856
antimicrobial drugs in, 480
antineoplastic drugs in, 713–714
antiplatelet agents in, 890–891
antipsychotic drugs in, 167
antiseizure drugs in, 208
antiviral drugs in, 575–576
aspirin in, 125
beta blockers in, 301, 856
beta-lactam antibacterials in, 498
calcium channel blockers in, 856
cholinergic drugs in, 315
corticosteroids in, 367–368
digoxin use in, 788–789
diuretics in, 855, 871
drug therapy considerations in, 66–67
dyslipidemic drugs in, 906–907
fluoroquinolones in, 511
hematopoietic drugs in, 661
hypercalcemia in, 399
hypoglycemic drugs in, 427
immunostimulants in, 661
immunosuppressants in, 682
insulin in, 427
macrolides in, 535
nonsteroidal anti-inflammatory drugs in, 125
nutritional support in, 943–944
opioid analgesics in, 98
penicillins in, 498
sedative-hypnotics in, 147
skeletal muscle relaxants in, 232
sulfonamides in, 524
tetracyclines in, 524
thiazide diuretics in, 871
renal transplantation, 680–681
renin–angiotensin–aldosterone system, 778, 840b, 856
ReoPro (abciximab), 882t, 884

repaglinide (Prandin), 415, 415t, 433
Repetab (albuterol), 732, 732t–733t
Requip (ropinirole), 217t, 218, 221–222
Rescriptor (delavirdine), 555, 567t, 573, 577
Rescula (unoprostone), 1028t
resistant organisms, 478
RespiGam (respiratory syncytial virus immune globulin intravenous), 642t
respiration, 725
respiratory depression, 100
respiratory disorders
in children, 767
common cold, 760
description of, 727
herbal and dietary supplements for, 762, 765
in home care, 767, 769
nasal congestion associated with, 761
nursing process for, 765
in older adults, 767
signs and symptoms of, 761
sinusitis, 761
respiratory syncytial virus immune globulin intravenous (RespiGam), 642t
respiratory syncytial virus infection
description of, 562b
drugs for, 565t, 570
respiratory system
cocaine effects on, 244b
glucocorticoids' effect on, 354
overview of, 725–727
respiratory tract, 725–726
Restoril (temazepam), 136t–137t
Retavase (reteplase), 883t, 885
reteplase (Retavase), 883t, 885
reticular activating system, 79
retina, 1023
Retin-A (tretinoin), 1046t, 1052
retinitis, 561b
retinoids, 1044–1045, 1046t, 1052, 1064b
retinol (vitamin A)
deficiency of, 920t
food sources of, 920t
function of, 920t
preparations, 924t
recommended daily intake of, 920t
Retrovir (zidovudine), 563, 566t, 574, 576, 578–580
reverse transcriptase, 562
Revex (nalmefene), 89–90, 90t
ReVia (naltrexone), 90, 90t, 238t, 240–242
Reyataz (atazanavir), 568t
Reye's syndrome, 108, 649
rheumatoid arthritis, 106b, 124, 679
Rheumatrex (methotrexate)
adverse effects of, 686
antineoplastic uses of, 696t
drug interactions, 688, 719
in hepatic-impaired clients, 683
immunosuppressive uses of, 670t, 671
nonsteroidal anti-inflammatory drugs effect on, 123
in renal-impaired clients, 682, 713–714
rheumatoid arthritis treated with, 124
Rhinocort (budesonide), 358t, 363, 731b, 754t
rhinorrhea, 761
Rho(D) immune globulin (RhoGAM), 642t
RhoGAM (Rho(D) immune globulin), 642t
ribavirin (Virazole), 565t, 570, 578
riboflavin
deficiency of, 922t
food sources of, 922t
function of, 922t
preparations, 925t
recommended daily intake of, 922t

rifabutin (Mycobutin), 548t, 548–549, 554
Rifadin (rifampin), 547–548, 548t, 552, 554, 556, 558
Rifamate, 549–550
rifampin and pyrazinamide (RIF-PZA), 546b
rifampin (Rifadin), 547–548, 548t, 552, 554, 556, 558
rifapentine (Priftin), 548t, 549, 554
Rifater, 549–550
rifaximin (Xifaxan), 531t, 532, 538, 1001t, 1003
Rilutek (riluzole), 1080
riluzole (Rilutek), 1080
rimantadine (Flumadine), 565t, 570, 578
rimexolone (Vexol), 1030t
risedronate (Actonel), 390, 393t, 401
Risperdal Consta (risperidone), 156t, 160t, 169, 171
Risperdal (risperidone), 156t, 160t, 161, 168, 171
risperidone (Risperdal; Risperdal Consta), 156t, 160t, 161, 168, 171
Ritalin (methylphenidate), 242, 248, 254, 255t, 258–260
ritodrine (Yutopar), 1070t, 1071, 1076
ritonavir (Norvir), 568t, 569, 578–579
Rituxan (rituximab), 699, 700t
rituximab (Rituxan), 699, 700t
rivastigmine (Exelon), 310t, 311
rizatriptan (Maxalt), 116, 117t, 121, 128
RNA viruses, 560, 562
Robaxin (methocarbamol), 229t, 230
Robinul (glycopyrrolate), 323t
Robitussin Cold and Flu Tablets, 764t
Robitussin (guaifenesin), 763t
Rocaltrol (calcitriol), 392t
Rocephin (ceftriaxone), 493t
rocuronium (Zemuron), 1096t
Roferon-A (interferon alfa-2a), 653t, 656
Rohypnol (flunitrazepam), 247
Romazicon (flumazenil), 28t, 145
ropinirole (Requip), 217t, 218, 221–222
ropivacaine (Naropin), 1098t
rosacea, 1040, 1053
rosiglitazone (Avandia), 414t, 430–431
rosiglitazone/metformin (Avandamet), 415t
rosuvastatin (Crestor), 901, 902t
roundworm infections, 605b
Rowasa (mesalamine), 1080
Roxicet (oxycodone), 94t
Roxicodone (oxycodone), 86t, 88
rubella and mumps vaccine (Biavax II), 639t
rubella vaccine (Meruvax II), 638t–639t
Rythmol (propafenone), 800t, 803, 811t

S

salicylate
    intoxication, 122
    serum levels of, 1083
salicylic acid, 1047t
saline cathartics, 993
saline laxatives, 988
saliva, 915
salmeterol (Serevent), 273t, 732, 732t–733t, 740
salmon calcitonin (Calcimar, Miacalcin), 390, 393t
Salmonella, 471b, 997
salsalate (Disalcid), 109, 114t
Saluron (hydroflumethiazide), 864t
Sanctura (trospium chloride), 323t, 325
Sandimmune (cyclosporine), 669t, 672, 677, 680–683, 685–686
Sandoglobulin (immune globulin intravenous), 642t

Sandostatin (octreotide), 342, 343t, 349, 1002, 1002t
Santyl (collagenase), 1046t
saquinavir (Fortovase), 568t, 569, 578–579
Sarafem (fluoxetine), 177, 178t
sarcomas, 693
Sarcoptes scabiei, 605
sargramostim (Leukine), 652t–653t, 659–660, 662, 707, 708t
saturated solution of potassium iodide (SSKI), 376–378, 377t
saw palmetto, 60t
scabicides, 610t, 612
scabies, 605–606, 613
schizophrenia
    behavioral manifestations of, 154
    dopaminergic system in, 154
    etiology of, 154
    glutamatergic system in, 154
    hallucinations associated with, 153
    risk factors for, 153
    serotonergic system in, 154
    symptoms of, 154
Schlemm's canal, 1024
sclera, 1023
scopolamine (Transderm Scop), 216, 322t–323t, 324, 1013t, 1014
seborrheic dermatitis, 1040
secobarbital (Seconal), 241
Seconal (secobarbital), 241
second messenger, 266
second-degree heart block, 798b
second-messenger systems, 337–338
secretory immune system, 625
Sectral (acebutolol), 293t, 801t, 804, 844t
sedative-hypnotics. *See also specific drug*
    adverse effects of, 150
    in children, 146–147
    client teaching about, 143
    in critical-illness clients, 148
    dosage of, 142, 144
    drug interactions, 151
    in hepatic-impaired clients, 147–148
    in home care, 148
    insomnia treated with, 147
    nursing actions for, 149–151
    nursing process for, 141–142
    in older adults, 147
    oral, 149
    in renal-impaired clients, 147
    self-administration of, 143
    therapeutic effects of, 150
    types of, 138, 139t
seizure
    absence, 194
    akinetic, 194
    alcohol-related, 240
    definition of, 193
    febrile, 194
    generalized, 194
    mixed, 194
    myoclonic, 194
    partial, 193, 204–205
    tonic-clonic, 194
seizure threshold, 194
selective serotonin 5–HT1 receptor agonists, 116, 117t
selective serotonin reuptake inhibitors. *See also specific drug*
    adverse effects of, 177
    characteristics of, 178t–179t
    cytochrome P450 inhibition by, 184–185
    drug interactions, 190

mechanism of action, 176–177
monoamine oxidase inhibitors and, 177
pharmacokinetics of, 177
during pregnancy, 1061b
self-administration of, 183
suicidality risks, 185
toxicity of, 185
selegiline (Eldepryl), 215, 217t, 218–220, 224
selenium, 928t–929t, 943t
selenium sulfide (Selsun), 1047t
self-antigens, 665
Selsun (selenium sulfide), 1047t
senna preparations (Senokot, Black Draught), 990t
Senokot (senna preparations), 990t
sensory areas, 78
sepsis, 24t, 368
Septa (trimethoprim-sulfamethoxazole)
    antidiarrheal uses of, 1001t
    characteristics of, 517t–518t
    description of, 479
    during pregnancy, 1061b
    urinary tract infections treated with, 515
septic shock, 829, 830t, 834
Septodont (articaine), 1098t
Serax (oxazepam), 136t–137t
Serevent (salmeterol), 273t, 732, 732t–733t, 740
serology, 468
Seroquel (quetiapine), 156t, 159t, 161, 168, 171–172
Serostim (somatropin), 344t
serotonergic system
    description of, 77
    in schizophrenia, 154
serotonin
    in anxiety disorders, 133
    depression and, 174
    description of, 77, 839
serotonin receptor antagonists, 1012t–1013t, 1013–1014, 1019
serotonin receptors, 133
serotonin syndrome, 532
Serratia marcescens, 471b
sertaconazole (Ertaczo), 1044t
sertraline (Zoloft), 138, 139t, 179t, 188
serum drug level, 15–16, 16f
serum half-life, 16
serum sickness, 748, 750
Serutan (psyllium), 988, 989t
sevelamer (Renagel), 1080
sevoflurane (Ultane), 1096t
sex hormone-binding globulin, 455
sex hormones, 702–703
Sherley Amendment, 5t
Shigella, 471b, 998
shock
    anaphylactic
        characteristics of, 830t
        definition of, 829
        description of, 25, 275
        epinephrine for, 279–280
        management of, 834
    cardiogenic, 829, 830t
    corticosteroids for, 357
    in critical illness, 834
    definition of, 829
    description of, 282
    distributive, 829, 830t, 833
    in hepatic-impaired clients, 834
    hypovolemic, 829, 830t, 834
    management guidelines for, 834
    neurogenic, 829, 830t
    nursing process for, 832–833
    in older adults, 834

pharmacokinetics affected by, 24t
in renal-impaired clients, 834
septic, 829, 830t, 834
signs and symptoms of, 829
therapeutic principles for, 833–835
vasogenic, 829
short-acting insulins, 408, 424, 429
sibutramine (Meridia), 957t, 957–958, 962, 967
sideroblastic anemia, 239b
signal transduction, 266, 268f
Silvadene (silver sulfadiazine), 519t, 1043t
silver sulfadiazine (Silvadene), 519t, 1043t
Simulect (basiliximab), 669t, 674, 679
Sinemet (levodopa/carbidopa), 216, 217t, 220
Sinequan (doxepin), 178t
Singulair (montelukast), 736t, 737–738
sinoatrial node, 774, 794
sinus bradycardia, 320, 797b
sinus tachycardia, 797b
sinusitis, 761
Sinutab Sinus Allergy Maximum Strength
  Tablets, 764t
sirolimus (Rapamune), 670t, 672, 677, 680–683,
  687–688
situational anxiety, 133
Skelaxin (metaxalone), 229t, 230, 232
skeletal muscle relaxants. *See also specific drug*
  adverse effects of, 233
  in children, 232
  client teaching about, 231–233
  contraindications, 228
  drug interactions, 233
  goals of, 231
  in hepatic-impaired clients, 232
  in home care, 232
  indications for, 228
  mechanism of action, 228
  nursing actions for, 232–233
  nursing process for, 230–231
  in older adults, 232
  in renal-impaired clients, 232
  selection of, 232
  self-administration of, 231
  therapeutic effects of, 233
Skelid (tiludronate), 390, 393t, 402
skin
  anatomy of, 1039
  drug administration to, 48
  functions of, 1039–1040
skin cancer, 1048
skin disorders
  acne, 1041, 1052
  bacterial infections, 1041
  client teaching about, 1050–1051
  dermatitis, 1040
  external otitis, 1041–1042, 1053
  fungal infections, 1041
  pressure ulcers, 1041, 1053
  prevention of, 1050–1051
  psoriasis, 678–679, 1040, 1053
  rosacea, 1040, 1053
  trauma, 1041
  ulcerations, 1041
  urticaria, 748, 1040, 1053
skin flora, 468
sleep
  description of, 133
  melatonin effects on, 140
sleep apnea, 955b
slow channels, 795
slow metabolizers, 167
slow releasing substances of anaphylaxis, 737
small intestine, 914

smoking
  cessation of, 238t, 244, 249
  during pregnancy, 1065b
social phobia, 134b
sodium, 785, 926t, 932t
sodium bicarbonate, 29t
sodium chloride injection, 393t, 394
sodium iodide 131I (Iodotope), 377t, 378
sodium nitroprusside (Nipress), 846t, 857
sodium phosphate and sodium biphosphate (Fleet
    Phosphosoda, Fleet Enema), 989t
sodium polystyrene sulfonate (Kayexalate), 925,
    929, 930t
sodium valproate (Depakene syrup, Depacon
    injection), 199t
Solarcaine (benzocaine), 1098t
solifenacin (Vesicare), 1080
Solu-Medrol (methylprednisolone sodium succi-
    nate), 359t
solutions, 1042b
Soma (carisoprodol), 229t, 230
somatic pain, 84b
somatomedin, 348
somatostatin, 339–340
somatotropin, 341
somatropin (Humatrope), 342, 344t
Somavert (pegvisomant), 342
Sonata (zaleplon), 138–140, 139t, 148
sorbitol, 990t, 991
Soriatane (acitretin), 1046t
sotalol (Betapace), 293t, 802t, 804–805
South Beach diet, 964b
spasticity, 227–228
Spectazole (econazole), 588b, 1043t
spectinomycin (Trobicin), 531t, 532
Spectracef (cefditoren pivoxil), 490t
spinal anesthesia, 1097
spinal cord
  description of, 80
  dorsal horn of, 83
spinal cord injury
  corticosteroids for, 367
  laxatives for patients with, 993–994
  lower motor neuron, 994
  upper motor neuron, 994
Spiriva (tiotropium bromide), 323t, 733t
spironolactone (Aldactone), 865t, 866, 871
Sporanox (itraconazole), 587b, 589t, 591–592,
    597, 600
sporotrichosis, 586b, 593, 596
squamous cell carcinoma, 1048
SSKI (saturated solution of potassium iodide),
    376–378, 377t
St. John's wort, 60t, 181
stable angina, 815b
Stadol (butorphanol), 87t, 89, 101
Stalevo (levodopa/carbidopa/entacapone), 217t
staphylococci, 469b
Staphylococcus aureus
  description of, 469b
  methicillin-resistant, 468, 471, 472b, 487,
    532
Staphylococcus epidermidis, 469b
Starlix (nateglinide), 415, 415t, 430, 433
statins, 901, 902t
status asthmaticus, 744
status epilepticus, 194, 207
stavudine (Zerit), 566t, 575
steady-state concentration, 16
Stelazine (trifluoperazine), 156t, 158t
stem cell transplantation, 660
stem cells, 621
Stevens-Johnson syndrome, 210

Stimate (desmopressin), 344t, 345
stimulant cathartics, 988–990, 989t
stimulants. *See* central nervous system stimulants
Stokes-Adams syndrome, 274
stomach, 914
stomatitis, 706b
stool softeners, 988
Strattera (atomoxetine), 256, 256t, 259
stratum corneum, 1039
Streptase (streptokinase), 883t, 885
streptococci, 469b
Streptococcus pneumoniae
  description of, 469b
  penicillin-resistant, 471b
Streptococcus pyogenes, 470b
streptokinase (Streptase), 883t, 885
streptomycin, 506t, 548t
stress response, 352
Stromectol (ivermectin), 610t, 611
strong iodine solution (Lugol's solution), 376,
    377t
Strongyloides stercoralis, 605b
Stuart factor, 877t
subcutaneous injections
  absorption after, 14
  advantages and disadvantages of, 39t
  insulin, 423
  nursing action for, 46–47
  sites for, 40, 43f
Sublimaze (fentanyl), 86t, 87, 95, 99–100
substance abuse
  alcohol. *See* alcohol
  amphetamines, 242–243
  assessment of, 248
  barbiturates, 241–242
  benzodiazepines, 241–242
  characteristics of, 236–237
  "club" drugs, 246–248
  cocaine, 243, 244b
  "date-rape" drugs, 246–248
  definition of, 235
  drugs used to treat, 238t
  gamma-hydroxybutyrate (GHB), 247
  hallucinogens, 246
  inhalants, 248
  intravenous abuse, 236–237
  ketamine, 247–248
  LSD, 246
  marijuana, 245–246
  mescaline, 246
  nicotine, 243–245, 244b
  nursing process for, 248–249
  opioids, 242
  phencyclidine, 246
  prevention of, 250
  treatment of, 250–251
  volatile solvents, 248
substance P, 83, 84b
subtotal thyroidectomy, 381
succimer (Chemet), 29t, 929, 930t
succinylcholine, 1096t
Sudafed (pseudoephedrine), 273t, 277t, 278, 763t
sudden cardiac death, 799b
Sufenta (sufentanil), 87, 1096t
sufentanil (Sufenta), 87, 1096t
suicidality, 185
Sular (Nisoldipine), 819t, 845t
sulconazole (Exelderm), 590t, 1044t
sulfacetamide, 1029t
sulfadiazine, 517t
Sulfamylon (mafenide), 518t, 1043t
sulfasalazine (Azulfidine), 517t, 1080
sulfinpyrazone (Anturane), 115, 116t, 129

sulfisoxazole (Gantrisin), 517t, 1029t
sulfonamides. *See also specific drug*
    administration of, 525
    adverse effects of, 525–526
    characteristics of, 517t–519t
    in children, 523–524
    client teaching about, 523
    contraindications, 520
    in critical illness, 524
    definition of, 515
    drug interactions, 526
    in hepatic-impaired clients, 524
    indications for, 519–520
    mechanism of action, 516, 519
    nursing actions for, 524–526
    in older adults, 524
    during pregnancy, 1060b
    in renal-impaired clients, 524
    self-administration of, 523
    therapeutic effects of, 525
    topical, 518t–519t
    types of, 517t–519t
sulfonylureas, 412–413, 414t, 424–425, 429–432,
    460
sulindac (Clinoril), 109, 114t, 126
sumatriptan (Imitrex), 116, 117t, 121, 128
Sumycin (tetracycline), 607t
sunscreens, 1045
suppositories
    rectal, 36t, 48, 993
    vaginal, 36t, 48
Suprane (desflurane), 1096t
supraventricular tachydysrhythmias, 808
suprofen (Profenal), 1030t
surfactant laxatives, 988, 989t
Surfak (docusate calcium), 989t
Surmontil (trimipramine maleate), 178t
susceptible organisms, 478
suspensions, 36t
Sustiva (efavirenz), 567t
Symlin (pramlintide), 1080
Symmetrel (amantadine)
    adverse effects of, 578
    in children, 574
    influenza A virus treated with, 565t, 570
    Parkinson's disease treated with, 215, 217t,
        218, 222, 224
    in renal-impaired clients, 575
sympathetic nervous system
    adrenergic receptors of, 269–270
    blood pressure regulation by, 839, 840b
    description of, 352–353, 839
    stimulation of, 267
Synalar (fluocinolone), 1045t
synapses, 76
synaptic cleft, 76
synaptic vesicles, 76
Synarel (nafarelin), 342, 343t
Synercid (quinupristin-dalfopristin), 479, 531t,
    532, 537–538
synergism, 19
Synthroid (levothyroxine), 374, 376, 377t, 379,
    382–383
syringes, 40
systemic candidiasis, 595
systemic lupus erythematosus, 750

T

T cells, 625–626, 628, 667
tablets, 34, 35t
tachydysrhythmias, 808

tacrolimus (Prograf, Protopic), 671t, 672–673,
    677, 680–683, 687–689, 1046t
tadalafil (Cialis), 1080
Tagamet (cimetidine), 19
Tambocor (flecainide), 800t, 803, 811t
Tamiflu (oseltamivir), 565t, 570
tamoxifen (Nolvadex), 704, 705t, 715
tamsulosin hydrochloride (Flomax), 292t, 294–295
Tapazole (methimazole), 376, 377t, 380
tapeworms, 605b
Tarceva (erlotinib), 700t, 701
tardive dyskinesia, 170
Tarka, 848t
Tasmar (tolcapone), 215, 217t, 218
Tavist (clemastine), 751t
taxanes, 697t, 699
Taxol (paclitaxel), 697t, 711, 714
Taxotere (docetaxel), 697t, 711
tazarotene (Tazorac), 1046t
Tazorac (tazarotene), 1046t
tears, 1023
Teczem, 848t
tegaserod (Zelnorm), 1080
Tegretol (carbamazepine), 194–195, 196t, 200,
    207, 211, 1083
telithromycin (Ketek), 529t, 529–530, 539
telmisartan (Micardis), 843t
temazepam (Restoril), 136t–137t
Temodar (temozolomide), 697t
Temovate (clobetasol), 1045t
temozolomide (Temodar), 697t
tenecteplase (TNKase), 883t, 885
Tenex (guanfacine), 292t, 294, 844t
teniposide (Vumon), 697t
tenofovir (Viread), 563, 567t
Tenoretic, 848t
Tenormin (atenolol), 293t, 818t, 844t
Tensilon (edrophonium), 309, 310t, 313
Tequin (gatifloxacin), 508t, 511, 1029t
teratogenicity, 26, 1058
Terazol (terconazole), 590t
terbinafine (Lamisil), 583, 587b, 590t, 593,
    597–598, 601, 1044t
terbutaline (Brethine), 273t
terconazole (Terazol), 590t
teriparatide (Forteo), 393t, 394
tertiary amines, 319, 320t
testicular hormone, 336
testolactone (Teslac), 458t
testosterone
    body tissue effects of, 456b
    endogenous, 455
    transdermal formulations of, 457
testosterone cypionate (Depo-Testosterone), 458t
testosterone enanthate (Delatestryl), 458t
testosterone gel (Androgel), 458t
testosterone transdermal systems (Androderm),
    458t
Testred (methyltestosterone), 458t
tetanus and diphtheria toxoids, adsorbed, 641t
tetanus immune globulin (BayTet), 642t
tetanus toxoid, absorbed, 641t
tetracaine (Pontocaine), 1028t, 1098t
tetracyclines (Achromycin)
    administration of, 524–525
    adverse effects of, 525–526
    characteristics of, 516t
    in children, 479, 523
    client teaching about, 522
    contraindications, 520
    in critical illness, 524
    dairy products interaction with, 19
    definition of, 515

drug interactions, 526
    in hepatic-impaired clients, 524
    indications for, 519
    mechanism of action, 516
    nursing actions for, 524–526
    nursing process for, 520, 522
    in older adults, 524
    during pregnancy, 1061b
    in renal-impaired clients, 524
    self-administration of, 522
    skin disorders treated with, 1043t
    therapeutic effects of, 525
    therapeutic principles for, 522–523
tetrahydrozoline hydrochloride (Tyzine, Visine),
    273t, 763t
tetraiodothyronine, 336
Teveten (eprosartan), 843t
thalamus
    description of, 78–79
    pain perception role of, 83
Theochron (long-acting theophylline), 734t
theophylline
    in children, 742–743
    client teaching about, 740
    dosage of, 742
    long-acting (Theochron), 734t
    in older adults, 743
    overdose of, 742
    serum levels of, 1083
    short-acting (Aminophylline), 733t
TheraFlu Flu, Cold, and Cough Powder, 764t
therapeutic effects, 25, 71. *See also specific drug,*
    therapeutic effects of
thiabendazole (Mintezol), 610t, 612
thiamine
    deficiency of, 923t, 938
    description of, 80
    food sources of, 923t
    function of, 923t
    preparations, 925t
    recommended daily intake of, 923t
thiazide diuretics
    characteristics of, 864t, 865–866
    in children, 854
    description of, 849
    indications for, 868
    in older adults, 871
    in renal-impaired clients, 871
thiazolidinediones, 413
thioamide drugs, 381
thiopental (Pentothal), 1096t
thioridazine (Mellaril), 164
thiothixene (Navane), 156, 156t, 159t
third-degree heart block, 798b
Thorazine (chlorpromazine), 156t–157t
threadworm infections, 605b
throat lozenges, 36t
Thrombate III (antithrombin III), 1079
thrombolytic therapy, 29t, 882t, 885, 890
thrombophlebitis, 886–887
thromboplastin, 877t
thrombopoietin, 622t
thrombosis, 877–879, 878b–879b
thromboxane A_2
    description of, 104t, 106, 108
    inhibitors of, 884
thrombus, 877
thrush, 584b
thymosin, 628
Thyrogen (thyrotropin alfa), 344t, 345
thyroid disorders
    description of, 374, 375t
    nursing process for, 378–379

thyroid drugs
administration of, 383
adverse effects of, 384
in children, 382
contraindications, 376
dosage of, 380
drug interactions, 380–381, 384–385
goals of, 379–380
for hypothyroidism, 376
indications for, 376
mechanism of action, 374, 376
nursing actions for, 383–385
in older adults, 382
selection of, 380
therapeutic effects of, 383
therapeutic principles for, 379–382
thyroid gland, 373
thyroid hormones
description of, 336
functions of, 373–374
thyroid storm, 374
thyroid-stimulating hormone, 373, 380
Thyrolar (liotrix), 376, 377t
thyrotoxic crisis, 374
thyrotropin, 341
thyrotropin alfa (Thyrogen), 344t, 345
thyrotropin-releasing hormone, 340, 374
thyroxine, 373
tiagabine (Gabitril), 199t, 201, 208
Ticar (ticarcillin), 487, 488t
ticarcillin (Ticar), 486t, 487, 488t
ticarcillin-clavulanate (Timentin), 488t, 489
TICE BCG (tuberculosis vaccine [bacillus
Calmette-Guérin]), 639t
Ticlid (ticlopidine), 882t, 884, 891
ticlopidine (Ticlid), 882t, 884, 891
tigecycline (Tygacil), 1081
Tikosyn (dofetilide), 801t, 804–805
Tilade (nedocromil), 736t, 738
tiludronate (Skelid), 390, 393t, 402
Timentin (ticarcillin-clavulanate), 488t, 489
Timolide, 848t
timolol (Blocadren, Timoptic), 293t, 845t, 1027t
Timoptic (timolol), 293t, 1027t
Tinactin (tolnaftate), 590t, 1044t
Tindamax (tinidazole), 606, 607t
tinea infections, 1030t
tinidazole (Tindamax), 606, 607t
tinzaparin (Innohep), 881t
tioconazole (Vagistat), 590t
tiotropium bromide (Spiriva), 323t, 324, 733t
tipranavir, 1081
tirofiban (Aggrastat), 882t, 884, 887, 891
tizanidine (Zanaflex), 228–230, 229t, 232
TNKase (tenecteplase), 883t, 885
tobramycin (Nebcin, Tobrex), 506t, 1029t
Tobrex (tobramycin), 1029t
tocainide, 811t
tocolytics, 1070t, 1070–1071, 1075–1077
Tofranil (imipramine), 178t, 1083
tolcapone (Tasmar), 215, 217t, 218
Tolectin (tolmetin), 109, 114t
tolerable upper intake level, 919b
tolerance, 25
tolmetin (Tolectin), 109, 114t
tolnaftate (Tinactin), 590t, 1044t
tolterodine (Detrol, Detrol LA), 324t, 325
tonic-clonic seizure, 194
Topamax (topiramate), 199t, 201–202, 207–208
topotecan (Hycamtin), 697t
topical medications, 1042b
topical otic medications, 1042b
topical vaginal medications, 1042b

Topicort (desoximetasone), 1045t
topiramate (Topamax), 199t, 201–202, 207–208
topotecan, 715
Toradol (ketorolac), 108–109, 113t, 114
toremifene (Fareston), 704, 705t, 715
Tornalate (bitolterol), 273t
torsades de pointes, 799b
torsemide (Demadex), 865t, 868
tositumomab and iodine 131–itositumomab
(Bexxar), 700t, 701
toxic concentration, 15
toxic doses, 18
toxicity
acetaminophen, 123
adrenergic drugs, 282–283
aminoglycosides, 510
antiasthmatic drugs, 742
anticholinergic drugs, 327
anticholinesterase drugs, 314
antidepressants, 185–186
antiepileptic drugs, 206
antiseizure drugs, 206
atropine sulfate, 327
benzodiazepine, 145
benzodiazepines, 145
causes of, 26
central nervous system stimulants, 259
cholinergic drugs, 314
management of, 26, 27b
monoamine oxidase inhibitors, 185
opioid, 96
opioid analgesics, 96
selective serotonin reuptake inhibitors, 185
tricyclic antidepressants, 185
toxoids
definition of, 634
indications for, 634
types of, 640t–641t
Toxoplasma gondii, 604
toxoplasmosis, 604
trace elements, 919, 927t–929t
trachea, 726
Tracium (atracurium), 1096t
Tracleer (bosentan), 782t, 784
trade name, 4
tramadol (Ultram), 86t–87t, 89
Trandate (labetalol), 293t, 845t
trandolapril (Mavik), 843t
tranexamic acid (Cyklokapron), 885–886, 886t
Transderm Scop (scopolamine), 1013t, 1014
transdermal formulations, 34
transient ischemic attacks, 884
transplantation
antirejection agents, 672–673
bone marrow, 660, 667–668, 681
cardiac, 680
immunosuppressants use in, 679–681
liver, 681
malignancies after, 678
organ, 667
renal, 680–681
Tranxene (clorazepate)
antianxiety uses of, 136t–137t
antiseizure uses of, 196t, 200
tranylcypromine (Parnate), 179t
trastuzumab (Herceptin), 700t, 701
Trasylol (aprotinin), 886, 886t
Travatan (travoprost), 1028t
travelers' diarrhea, 997
travoprost (Travatan), 1028t
trazodone (Desyrel), 179t, 180
Trelstar (triptorelin), 342, 704, 705t
treprostinil (Remodulin), 882t

tretinoin (Retin-A), 1046t, 1052
triacetin (Fungoid), 590t
triamcinolone acetonide (Kenalog-40, Azmacort,
Nasacort), 359t, 731b, 754t, 1045t
triamcinolone (Aristocort, Kenacort), 359t, 731b
triamcinolone diacetate (Aristocort Forte), 359t,
731b
triamterene (Dyrenium), 865t, 866
triazolam (Halcion), 136t–137t
tricalcium phosphate (Posture), 392t
Trichinella spiralis, 605b
trichinosis, 605b
trichlormethiazide (Naqua), 864t
Trichomonas vaginalis, 604
trichomoniasis, 604, 613
Trichuris trichiura, 605b
Tricor (fenofibrate), 902t, 903, 905
tricuspid valve, 774
tricyclic antidepressants. *See also specific drug*
adverse effects of, 189
antidote for, 29t
cancer-related pain treated with, 96–97
in children, 187
dosage of, 178t, 184
drug interactions, 190
indications for, 178t
mechanism of action, 176–177
metabolism of, 185
in older adults, 187–188
pharmacokinetics of, 177
during pregnancy, 1061b
selection of, 182
self-administration of, 183
toxicity of, 185
Tridesilon (desonide), 1045t
trifluoperazine (Stelazine), 156t, 158t
trifluridine (Viroptic), 563, 564t, 1029t
Trihexy (trihexyphenidyl), 324t, 324–325
trihexyphenidyl (Trihexy), 217t, 324t, 324–325
TriHIBit (diphtheria and tetanus toxoids and acellular pertussis and *Haemophilus influenza*
type B conjugate vaccines), 640t
triiodothyronine, 336, 373
Trilafon (perphenazine), 156t–157t
Trileptal (oxcarbazepine), 198t, 201, 204, 207,
209, 211
Tri-Levlen, 446t
trimethoprim (Proloprim, Trimpex), 522t
trimethoprim-sulfamethoxazole (Bactrim, Septra)
antidiarrheal uses of, 1001t
characteristics of, 517t–518t
description of, 479
in older adults, 524
Pneumocystis jiroveci treated with, 609t, 611
during pregnancy, 1061b
urinary tract infections treated with, 515
trimetrexate (Neutrexin), 609t, 611, 616
trimipramine maleate (Surmontil), 178t
Trimox (amoxicillin), 487
Trimpex (trimethoprim), 522t
Tri-Norinyl, 446t
Triostat (liothyronine), 376, 377t
Tripedia (diphtheria and tetanus toxoids and acellular pertussis vaccine), 640t
Triphasil, 446t
triprolidine (Zymine), 752
triptorelin (Trelstar), 342, 704, 705t
Trivora-28, 446t
Trizivir (zidovudine, lamivudine, and abacavir),
567t, 570
Trobicin (spectinomycin), 531t, 532
Tronothane (pramoxine), 1098t
tropicamide (Mydriacyl), 1027t

trospium chloride (Sanctura), 323t, 325
Trousseau's sign, 395
Trusopt (dorzolamide), 1028t
trypsin (Granulex), 1046t
tryptophan, 77
Tuamine (tuaminoheptane), 273t
tuaminoheptane (Tuamine), 273t
tuberculin, 40
tuberculosis
    active, 543, 550
    aminoglycosides for, 506–507
    in children, 555
    definition of, 542
    drug-resistant, 543–544
    drug-susceptible, 553
    in HIV-infected persons, 547b, 554–555
    latent
        in adolescents, 546b
        in children, 546b, 555
        definition of, 543
        in HIV-infected persons, 547b
        isoniazid for, 546b
        nursing process for, 551–552
        during pregnancy, 546b
        prevention of, 544
        targeted tuberculin testing for, 545b
        treatment of, 546b–547b
    multidrug-resistant, 506–507, 544, 550, 553, 555
    natural history of, 542–543
    nurse's role in preventing, 544
    nursing process for, 551–552
    in older adults, 555
    phases of, 542–543, 543f
    prevention of, 544, 552
    therapeutic principles for, 552–556
tuberculosis vaccine (bacillus Calmette-Guérin), 639t
tubular reabsorption, 862
tumor lysis syndrome, 694
tumor necrosis factor-alpha
    blocking agents, 674–675
    description of, 623t, 629, 666
tumor necrosis factor-beta, 623t, 629
tumor-infiltrating lymphocytes, 659
tumor-suppressor genes, 692
Tums (calcium carbonate precipitated), 392t
Twinrix (hepatitis A, inactivated, and hepatitis B, recombinant), 636t
Tygacil (tigecycline), 1081
Tylenol (acetaminophen)
    antidote for, 28t, 123
    in children, 125
    client teaching about, 120–121
    dosage of, 110t, 123
    in hepatic-impaired patients, 126
    in home care, 126
    indications for, 106b, 107, 123
    in older adults, 125
    opioid/acetaminophen products, 94t
    pharmacokinetics of, 115
    in renal-impaired patients, 125
    serum levels of, 1083
    toxicity, 123
Tylenol with codeine, 94t
Tylox (oxycodone), 94t
type 1 diabetes mellitus, 406, 426–427
type 2 diabetes mellitus, 406–407, 427
Typhim Vi (typhoid vaccine), 639t
typhoid vaccine (Vivotif Berna, Typhim Vi), 639t
tyrosine kinase inhibitors, 700t, 701–702
Tyzine (tetrahydrozoline hydrochloride), 273t, 763t

U

ulcerations, 1041
ulcerative colitis, 366, 1004
Ultane (sevoflurane), 1096t
Ultiva (remifentanil), 87, 1096t
Ultracef (cefadroxil), 490t
Ultracet (tramadol), 94t
Ultralente (insulin zinc suspension), 409t
Ultram (tramadol), 86t–87t, 89
Ultravate (halobetasol), 1045t
Unasyn (ampicillin-sulbactam), 488t, 489
Unipen (nafcillin), 487, 488t
units, 37
Univasc (moexipril), 843t
unoprostone (Rescula), 1028t
unstable angina, 815b, 816
up-regulation, 337
Urecholine (bethanechol), 308, 310t, 314–315
urinary antiseptics
    adverse effects of, 525–526
    description of, 515–516
    nursing actions for, 524–526
    therapeutic effects of, 525
    therapeutic principles for, 523
    types of, 521t–522t
urinary antispasmodics, 325
urinary catheterization, 520
urinary tract infections
    aminoglycosides for, 510
    assessment of, 520
    in children, 523
    description of, 487
    during pregnancy, 1067
    trimethoprim-sulfamethoxazole for, 515
urine, 862
Urispas (flavoxate), 324t, 325
Urofollitropin (Bravelle), 344t, 345
urokinase (Abbokinase), 883t, 885
UroXatral (alfuzosin), 292t, 295
urticaria, 748, 1040, 1053

V

vaccines. *See also* immunizations
    definition of, 634
    shortages of, 645
    storage of, 645
    types of, 635t–640t
    viral, 571–572
Vagifem (estradiol hemihydrate), 441t
vaginal candidiasis, 584b, 595, 1041
vaginal creams, 36t
vaginal suppositories, 36t, 48
Vagistat (tioconazole), 590t
valacyclovir (Valtrex), 563, 565t
valerian
    characteristics of, 61t
    sedative-hypnotic properties of, 140–141
valganciclovir, 563
Valisone (betamethasone valerate), 1045t
Valium (diazepam)
    antianxiety uses of, 135, 136t–137t, 138, 147–149
    antiseizure uses of, 196t, 200
valproate, 194, 212
valproic acid (Depakene capsules), 199t, 202, 204, 208, 1083
valrubicin (Valstar), 696t
valsartan (Diovan), 843t
Valstar (valrubicin), 696t
Valtrex (valacyclovir), 563, 565t
Vancenase (beclomethasone), 358t, 363, 731b, 732t, 735
Vanceril (beclomethasone), 358t, 363, 731b, 732t, 735
Vancocin (vancomycin), 531t, 532–533, 535, 538–539, 1001t, 1083
vancomycin (Vancocin), 531t, 532–533, 535, 538–539, 1001t, 1083
vancomycin-intermediate *Staphylococcus aureus*, 472b
vancomycin-resistant enterococci, 472b–473b, 532–533
Vantas (histrelin), 342
Vantin (cefpodoxime), 490t
Vaqta (hepatitis A vaccine), 635t
vardenafil (Levitra), 1081
variant angina, 815b
varicella virus vaccine (Varivax), 639t–640t, 648
varicella-zoster immune globulin, 643t
Varivax (varicella virus vaccine), 639t–640t, 648
vascular remodeling, 841b
Vaseretic, 848t
vasoconstrictors, 840b
vasodilators, 781, 839, 840b, 846t, 849
vasogenic shock, 829
vasomotor center, 79
vasopressin, 840b
    adverse effects of, 349
    cardiopulmonary resuscitation using, 281
    characteristics of, 341, 344t
    drug interactions, 349–350
    epinephrine vs., 281–282
Vasotec (enalapril), 843t
vecuronium (Norcuron), 1096t
Veetids (penicillin V), 486t, 487, 488t
veins, 774
Velban (vinblastine), 697t, 715
Velcade (bortezomib), 700t, 702, 715, 718
Velosef (cephradine), 490t
venipuncture, 47
venlafaxine (Effexor, Effexor XR), 138, 139t, 179t, 180, 182, 186, 1061b
Venoglobulin-S (immune globulin intravenous), 642t
venous stasis ulcers, 1041
Ventolin (albuterol), 732, 732t–733t
ventricles, 773
ventricular fibrillation, 799b
ventricular remodeling, 778
ventricular tachycardia, 799b
VePesid (etoposide), 697t
verapamil (Calan, Isoptin), 802t, 805, 811t, 819t, 845t
Vermox (mebendazole), 609t, 611–612
Versed (midazolam), 136t–137t, 149, 1096t
very-low calorie diet, 964b
very-low-density lipoprotein, 897, 898b
vesicants, 707b
Vesicare (solifenacin), 1080
vesicles, 75
Veterans Health Administration, 33
Vexol (rimexolone), 1030t
Vfend (voriconazole), 587b, 590t, 592, 597
Viadur (leuprolide), 704, 705t
vials, 38
Vibramycin (doxycycline), 516t, 519, 606, 607t
Vibrio parahaemolyticus, 998
Vibrio vulnificus, 998
Vicks NyQuil Cold & Flu Capsules, 764t
Vicodin (hydrocodone), 94t
vidarabine (Vira-A), 563, 565t
Vidaza (azacitidine), 1079
Videx (didanosine), 566t, 576–577
Videx EC (didanosine), 566t, 576–577
Vigamox (moxifloxacin), 1029t
vinblastine (Velban), 697t, 715
vinca alkaloids, 697t, 699, 719

vincristine (Oncovin), 697t, 715
vinorelbine (Navelbine), 697t
Viokase (pancreatin), 1002t
Vira-A (vidarabine), 563, 565t
Viracept (nelfinavir), 568t, 573
viral infections
  antibacterial drugs used in, 572
  course of, 562
  description of, 561b–562b
  nursing process for, 571
  prevention of, 571
  therapeutic principles for, 571–576
  vaccines for, 571–572
Viramune (nevirapine), 567t, 576
Virazole (ribavirin), 565t, 570, 578
Viread (tenofovir), 563, 567t
Viroptic (trifluridine), 563, 564t, 1029t
viruses. See also specific viruses
  antibodies induced by, 562
  course of, 562
  description of, 468, 560
  DNA, 560
  nursing process for, 571
  protein coat of, 562
  replication of, 560, 562
  RNA, 560, 562
  structure of, 560, 562
  therapeutic principles for, 571–576
  vaccines for, 571–572
visceral obesity, 953
visceral pain, 84b
Visine (tetrahydrozoline hydrochloride), 273t
Visken (pindolol), 293t, 844t
Vistaril (hydroxyzine), 138, 139t, 150, 751t, 1012t
Vistide (cidofovir), 563, 564t, 574–575
vitamin(s)
  adverse effects of, 948–949
  cancer prevention using, 938–939
  for children, 942, 942t
  classification of, 918
  client teaching about, 935–936
  drug interactions, 947
  fat-soluble, 918, 920t, 946, 949
  functions of, 917
  nursing actions for, 945–950
  nursing process for, 933–935
  self-administration of, 936
  supplements, 918–919
  therapeutic effects of, 947–948
  tolerable upper intake levels for, 919b
  water-soluble, 918, 920t–923t
vitamin A (retinol)
  deficiency of, 920t, 937
  food sources of, 920t
  function of, 920t
  preparations, 924t
  recommended daily intake of, 920t
vitamin B₁
  deficiency of, 923t
  food sources of, 923t
  function of, 923t
  preparations, 925t
  recommended daily intake of, 923t
vitamin B₂
  deficiency of, 922t
  food sources of, 922t
  function of, 922t
  recommended daily intake of, 922t
vitamin B₅
  deficiency of, 922t
  food sources of, 922t
  function of, 922t
  preparations, 924t
  recommended daily intake of, 922t

vitamin B₆
  deficiency of, 922t
  food sources of, 922t
  function of, 922t
  preparations, 925t
  recommended daily intake of, 922t
vitamin B₁₂
  deficiency of, 921t
  food sources of, 921t
  function of, 921t
  preparations, 924t
  recommended daily intake of, 921t
vitamin C
  antioxidant effects of, 939
  cancer risks and, 938
  in children, 942t
  deficiency of, 923t, 938
  description of, 765
  food sources of, 923t
  function of, 923t
  preparations, 925t
  recommended daily intake of, 923t, 938
vitamin D (calciferol)
  calcium salts and, 397
  in children, 942t
  deficiency of, 388
  description of, 388
  drug interactions, 401–402
  home care assessments, 399
  parathyroid hormone effects on, 387
  preparations, 390, 392t
vitamin E
  in children, 942t
  deficiency of, 920t
  food sources of, 920t
  function of, 920t
  preparations, 924t
  recommended daily intake of, 920t
vitamin K₁, 29t
vitamin K (Mephyton)
  deficiency of, 920t
  disorders of, 937–938
  food sources of, 920t
  function of, 920t
  preparations, 924t
  recommended daily intake of, 920t
  warfarin interactions with, 19, 886, 886t
vitreous body, 1024
Vivactil (protriptyline), 178t
Vivarin, 257t
Vivotif Berna (typhoid vaccine), 639t
volatile solvents, 248
voltage gating, 13b
Voltaren (diclofenac sodium), 111t, 1030t
Voltaren XR (diclofenac sodium), 111t, 1030t
vomiting
  antiemetic drugs. See antiemetic drugs
  causes of, 1010
  herbal and dietary supplements, 1014
  nursing process for, 1014–1015
  from opioid analgesics, 100
  physiology of, 1010–1011
  during pregnancy, 1066
  therapeutic principles for, 1015–1017
von Willebrand factor, 878b–879b
voriconazole (Vfend), 587b, 590t, 592, 597
Vumon (teniposide), 697t

W

warfarin (Coumadin)
  antidote for, 29t
  characteristics of, 881t, 883, 888–891

drug interactions, 894–895
  during pregnancy, 1061b
  vitamin K interactions with, 19
water, 917
water-soluble vitamins, 918, 920t–923t
weight loss
  behavioral modification for, 963
  client teaching about, 961–962
  nursing actions for, 967–968
  orlistat for, 957t, 958, 962, 967
  phentermine hydrochloride for, 957, 957t
  sibutramine for, 957t, 957–958, 962, 967
  web sites for, 963b
Welchol (colesevelam), 902t
Wellbutrin (bupropion), 179t, 180, 182–184, 186
Wellbutrin SR (bupropion), 179t, 180, 182–184, 186
Wellbutrin XL (bupropion), 179t, 180, 182–184, 186
Wellcovorin (leucovorin), 707, 708t
whipworm infections, 605b
white blood cells
  basophils, 626
  dendritic cells, 626
  description of, 624, 626
  eosinophils, 626
  monocytes, 626
  neutrophils, 626
whole bowel irrigation, 27b
withdrawal
  from alcohol, 240
  from antidepressants, 186
  from antipsychotic drugs, 164
  from benzodiazepines, 144–145
  from opioid analgesics, 96, 242
Wycillin (penicillin G), 486t, 487
Wycillin (penicillin G procaine), 488t
Wymox (amoxicillin), 487
Wytensin (guanabenz), 291, 292t, 294, 844t

X

Xalatan (latanoprost), 1028t
Xanax (alprazolam), 136t, 138, 143–144, 149
Xanax XR (alprazolam), 136t, 138, 143–144, 149
xanthine oxidase, 115
xanthines, 254, 256, 257t
Xeloda (capecitabine), 695t, 714
Xenical (orlistat), 957t, 958, 967
Xibrom (bromfenac), 1079
Xifaxan (rifaximin), 531t, 532, 538, 1001t, 1003
Xigris (drotrecogin alfa), 882t, 885
Xolair (omalizumab), 670t, 674, 738
Xopenex (levalbuterol), 732, 732t–733t
Xylocaine (lidocaine), 1098t
xylometazoline hydrochloride (Otrivin), 273t, 763t

Y

Yasmin, 445t
yeasts, 582
yellow-fever vaccine (YF-Vax), 640t
YF-Vax (yellow-fever vaccine), 640t
Yodoxin (iodoquinol), 603–604, 606
Yutopar (ritodrine), 1070t, 1071, 1076

Z

Zaditor (ketotifen), 1030t
zafirlukast (Accolate), 736t, 740, 745
zalcitabine (Hivid), 567t, 575, 579
zaleplon (Sonata), 138–140, 139t, 148

Zanaflex (tizanidine), 228–230, 229t, 232
zanamivir (Relenza), 565t, 570
Zarontin (ethosuximide), 196t, 200, 1083
Zaroxolyn (metolazone), 864t, 870
Zebeta (bisoprolol), 293t, 844t
Zelnorm (tegaserod), 1080
Zemplar (paricalcitol), 392t
Zemuron (rocuronium), 1096t
Zenapax (daclizumab), 669t, 674, 679
Zerit (stavudine), 566t, 575
Zestoretic, 848t
Zestril (lisinopril), 843t
Zetar (coal tar), 1046t
Zetia (ezetimibe), 902t, 903
Zevalin (ibritumomab tiuxetan), 700t, 701
Ziac, 848t
Ziagen (abacavir), 566t, 574–575
ziconotide (Prialt), 1081
zidovudine, lamivudine, and abacavir (Trizivir), 567t, 570

zidovudine and lamivudine (Combivir), 567t, 570
zidovudine (AZT, ZVD, Retrovir), 563, 566t, 574, 578–580
zileuton (Zyflo), 736t, 737–738, 740, 743
Zinacef (cefuroxime), 492t
zinc, 631, 929t
zinc gluconate, 765, 933
zinc sulfate, 932t, 933
zinc undecylenate (Desenex), 590t
Zinecard (dexrazoxane), 707, 708t
ziprasidone (Geodon), 156t, 160t, 161, 169, 171
Zithromax (azithromycin), 528, 529t, 530, 539, 551, 1000t
Zofran (ondansetron), 1012t–1013t, 1013–1014
Zoladex (goserelin), 342, 343t, 704, 705t
zoledronate (Zometa), 390, 393t
zolmitriptan (Zomig), 116, 117t, 121, 128
Zoloft (sertraline), 138, 139t, 179t, 188
zolpidem (Ambien), 139t, 140, 143, 148

Zometa (zoledronate), 390, 393t
Zomig (zolmitriptan), 116, 117t, 121, 128
Zonegran (zonisamide), 199t, 202, 207, 212
zonisamide (Zonegran), 199t, 202, 207, 212
Zostrix (capsaicin), 58t, 91, 1046t
Zosyn (piperacillin-tazobactam), 488t, 489
Zovia, 445t
Zovirax (acyclovir), 563, 564t, 575, 577–578, 1044t
ZVD (zidovudine), 563, 566t, 574, 576, 578–580
Zyban (bupropion), 179t, 183, 238t
Zyflo (zileuton), 736t, 737–738, 740, 743
Zyloprim (allopurinol), 115, 116t, 121, 129
Zymine (triprolidine), 752
Zyprexa (olanzapine), 156t, 159t, 160, 168, 171, 956b
Zyrtec (cetirizine), 752, 754, 756
Zyvox (linezolid), 531t, 532, 535, 537–538